I. **NCLEX® Examination Review Questions:** Chapter-specific practice questions help evaluate knowledge of important topics.

II. **Final Exam Preparation Questions:** Quick examination questions to reveal which chapters you need to review in more detail.

III. **Pharmacology Animations:** Improve your grasp of complex pharmacology concepts with these easy-to-understand animations.

- Nursing, Medical, and Pharmacology Domains
- Patient Nonadherence
- Agonists/Antagonists
- Receptor Interaction
- Passive Diffusion
- Impact of Surface Area
- Overview of Pharmacokinetics: Oral Administration
- Distribution: Fat vs. Water-Soluble Drugs
- Cytochrome P450 Drug Metabolism
- Half-Life of Intravenously Administered Ampicillin
- Drug Movement Through the Body
- Normal Electrophysiology
- Renin-Angiotensin in Control of Blood Pressure
- Time to Steady State
- Time to Steady State: Starting and Stopping Drug
- Pharmacokinetic Profiles: Normal, Renal Failure, and Hemodialysis
- Zero Order Elimination
- Dose-Dependent Elimination
- Effect of Repeated Dosing on Levels
- Load Plus Repeated Maintenance Dose

IV. **Printable Chapter Summaries:** Print these summaries of each chapter in *Mosby's Pharmacology in Nursing* for studying on the go.

V. **Electronic Calculators:** To help you do quick and accurate calculations of everything from absolute neutrophil count to the six-item cognitive impairment test.

- Absolute Neutrophil Count (ANC)
- Body Mass Index (BMI)
- Body Surface Area - Pediatric
- Body Surface Area (BSA)
- Corrected Phenytoin
- Corrected QT
- Corrected Serum Calcium
- Corrected Serum Sodium
- Creatinine Clearance - Estimated (Cockroft-Gault)
- Creatinine Clearance - Measured
- Fluid Deficit
- Heart Rate
- Ideal Body Weight (IBW) - Females
- Ideal Body Weight (IBW) - Males
- IV Infusion Rate
- LDL
- Metric Units Conversion
- Predicted Peak Flow (PPF)- Females
- Predicted Peak Flow (PPF)- Males
- Risk Assessment Tool for Falls
- Six-Item Cognitive Impairment Test

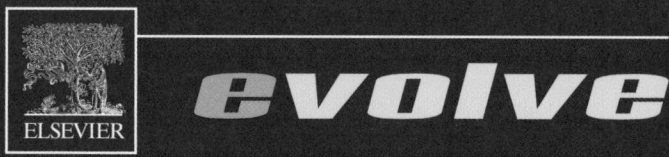

To access your Student Resources, visit:

http://evolve.elsevier.com/mckenry

Evolve® Student Resources for *McKenry: Mosby's Pharmacology in Nursing*, 22nd edition, offer the following features:

- **Case Studies**
  In-depth, interactive cases prepare you for nursing practice.

- **Concept Maps**
  This resource promotes critical thinking related to the nursing process.

- **Critical Thinking Answer Guidelines**
  Guidelines to answering the critical thinking questions found in the textbook chapters.

- **Content Updates/New Drugs List**
  The latest content updates and list of new drugs from the authors of the textbook to keep you current with recent developments in this area of study.

- **WebLinks**
  Allows you to link to hundreds of websites carefully chosen to supplement the content of the textbook. The WebLinks are regularly updated, with new ones added as they develop.

- **Mosby/Saunders ePharmacology Update Newsletter**
  An online newsletter covering the newest information in pharmacology released twice each semester.

- **Mosby's Drug Consult Internet Edition**
  Basic-level access to this comprehensive database of the most current, unbiased, accurate, and reliable drug information available. Includes drug updates, free information on the top 200 drugs by prescription, and online extras, including new drug approvals, safety notices, new drug indications, and links to pharmaceutical manufacturers for more information.

- **Supplemental Resources**
  Additional appendixes and links to information from the textbook.

The following is a list of disorders and conditions common in medical-surgical, maternity and women's health, pediatric, and psychiatric patients, as well as selected drugs administered for these disorders. Tear out this card and take it with you for reference during your clinical rotations. Also listed are page numbers in *Mosby's Pharmacology in Nursing* where you can find more information on these drugs.

Disorder/ Condition	Drug(s) Commonly Administered	Page No.
MEDICAL-SURGICAL		
Alzheimer's disease	donepezil (Aricept)	485
	galantamine (Razadyne)	484
	memantine (Namenda)	485
	rivastigmine (Exelon)	484
Asthma/Chronic obstructive pulmonary disease (COPD)	albuterol (Proventil)	702
	cromolyn (Intal)	713
	ipratropium (Atrovent)	704
	prednisone	852
	theophylline (Bronkodyl)	704
Burns	mafenide (Sulfamylon)	1188
	silver sulfadiazine (Silvadene)	1188
Cancer	doxorubicin (Adriamycin)	973
	interferon alfa-2a (Roferon-A)	988
	methotrexate (MTX, Folex PFS)	973
	topotecan (Hycamtin)	977
	vincristine (Oncovin)	975
Cirrhosis	furosemide (Lasix)	658
	spironolactone (Aldactone)	665
Coronary heart disease (CHD)/ Hyperlipidemia	atorvastatin (Lipitor)	638
	cholestyramine (Questran)	642
	gemfibrozil (Lopid)	644
	lovastatin (Mevacor)	638
	niacin	641
Crohn's disease	infliximab (Remicade)	769
	mesalamine (Asacol)	768
Cushing's syndrome	aminoglutethimide (Cytadren)	860
Diabetes mellitus	acarbose (Precose)	880
	glyburide (DiaBeta)	877
	insulin	866
	metformin (Glucophage)	879
	repaglinide (Prandin)	880
	rosiglitazone (Avandia)	881
Disseminated intravascular coagulation (DIC)	heparin (Liquiprin)	606
Deep vein thrombosis (DVT)	enoxaparin (Lovenox)	606
	heparin (Liquiprin)	606
	warfarin (Coumadin)	607

Disorder/ Condition	Drug(s) Commonly Administered	Page No.
Dysrhythmia	amiodarone (Cordarone)	534
	diltiazem (Cardizem)	538
	lidocaine (Xylocaine)	531
	procainamide (Procan)	527
	sotalol (Betapace)	536
Epilepsy	carbamazepine (Tegretol)	340
	phenytoin (Dilantin)	350
	valproate	353
End-stage renal disease (ESRD)	calcitriol (Calcijex, Rocaltrol)	1216
	calcium acetate (PhosLo)	686
	epoetin (Epogen)	687
	sevelamer (Renalgel)	686
Gastroesophageal reflux disease (GERD)	cimetidine (Tagamet)	750
	metoclopramide (Reglan)	760
	omeprazole (Prilosec)	748
Genital herpes	acyclovir (Zovirax)	1067
	famciclovir (Famvir)	1068
	valacyclovir (Valtrex)	1068
Glaucoma	betaxolol (Betoptic)	795
	carbachol (Carbastat)	797
	dipivefrin (Propine)	796
	echothiophate iodide (Phospholine Iodide)	797
	latanoprost (Xalatan)	795
	timolol (Istalol)	795
Gout	allopurinol (Zyloprim)	675
	colchicine	672
Heart failure	captopril (Capoten)	556
	digoxin (Lanoxin)	510
	furosemide (Lasix)	658
	losartan (Cozaar)	557
	spironolactone (Aldactone)	665
Hepatitis	adefovir (Hepsera)	1071
	immune globulin	1158, 1159
	ribavirin (Virazole)	1072
Human immunodeficiency virus	enfuvirtide (Fuzeon)	1089
	indinavir (Crixivan)	1088
	nevirapine (Viramune)	1087
	saquinavir (Fortovase)	1088
	zidovudine (AZT)	1081
Hyperparathyroidism	cinacalcet (Sensipar)	836

Disorder/ Condition	Drug(s) Commonly Administered	Page No.
Hypertension	amlodipine (Norvasc)	560
	atenolol (Tenormin)	554
	captopril (Capoten)	556
	clonidine (Catapres)	563
	hydralazine (Apresoline)	569
	hydrochlorothiazide (HydroDiuril)	551
	lisinopril (Zestril)	556
	losartan potassium (Cozaar)	557
	propranolol (Inderal)	462
Hyperthyroidism	propylthiouracil	846
	sodium iodide (^{131}I, Iodotope)	844
Hypoglycemia	dextrose 50% (25 g/50 mL)	884
	glucagon	884
	glucose (Glutose)	876
Hypothyroidism	levothyroxine (Levothroid)	840
Impotence	sildenafil (Viagra)	943
	tadalafil (Cialis)	943
	vardenafil (Levitra)	944
Malignant hyperthermia	abciximab (ReoPro)	601
	alteplase (Activase)	617
	aspirin (ASA)	268
	dantrolene (Dantrium)	488
Myocardial infarction/ Acute coronary syndrome	atenolol (Tenormin)	554
	clopidogrel (Plavix)	598
	enoxaparin (Lovenox)	606
	nitroglycerin	580
Osteoarthritis	acetaminophen (Tylenol)	274
	celecoxib (Celebrex)	269
Osteoporosis	alendronate (Fosamax)	836
	calcitonin (Miacalcin)	834
	raloxifene (Evista)	837
	teriparatide (Forteo)	838
Pain	acetaminophen (Tylenol)	274
	aspirin (ASA)	268
	ibuprofen (Motrin)	269
	morphine (Astramorph)	253
Parkinson's disease	benztropine (Cogentin)	470
	carbidopa/levodopa (Sinemet)	474
	selegiline (Eldepryl)	476
Peptic ulcer disease	clarithromycin (Biaxin)	1030
	omeprazole (Prilosec)	748
Rheumatoid arthritis	adalimumab (Humira)	1191
	celecoxib (Celebrex)	269
	etanercept (Enbrel)	1191
	ibuprofen (Motrin)	269
	methotrexate (Rheumatrex)	973
Tuberculosis	isoniazid (Nydrazid)	1102
	pyrazinamide (Tebrazid)	1103
	rifampin (Rifadin)	1102
Ulcerative colitis	mesalamine (Asacol)	768
	olsalazine (Dipentum)	768
	sulfasalazine (Azulfidine)	769
Urinary incontinence	oxybutynin (Ditropan)	440
	tolterodine (Detrol, Detrol LA)	440

Disorder/ Condition	Drug(s) Commonly Administered	Page No.
Wounds	collagenase (Santyl)	1203
	flexible hydroactive dressings and granules (DuoDerm)	1204

MATERNITY AND WOMEN'S HEALTH

Disorder/ Condition	Drug(s) Commonly Administered	Page No.
Breast cancer	anastrozole (Arimidex)	987
	tamoxifen (Nolvadex)	986
Infertility	chorionic gonadotropin (APL)	898
	clomiphene citrate (Clomid)	915
	menotropins (Pergonal)	898
Menopause	estrogen	900
Ovarian cancer	paclitaxel (Taxol)	975
Preeclampsia/ Eclampsia	magnesium sulfate	539
Vaginitis	estrogen	900

PEDIATRIC

Disorder/ Condition	Drug(s) Commonly Administered	Page No.
Attention deficit–hyperactivity disorder (ADHD)	atomoxetine (Strattera)	368
	dextroamphetamine and amphetamine (Adderall)	366
	methylphenidate (Concerta)	367
Cystic fibrosis	dornase alfa (Pulmozyme)	718
	pancrelipase (Creon)	757
Diabetes mellitus, type 1	insulin	866
Otitis media	amoxicillin/potassium clavulanate (Augmentin)	1017
	azithromycin (Zithromax)	1030
	sulfamethoxazole-trimethoprim (SMZ-TMP)	1047

PSYCHIATRIC

Disorder/ Condition	Drug(s) Commonly Administered	Page No.
Alcohol abuse	disulfiram (Antabuse)	167
	naltrexone (ReVia)	168
Anxiety disorders	alprazolam (Xanax)	319
	buspirone (BuSpar)	322
	diazepam (Valium)	320
	lorazepam (Ativan)	319
Bipolar disorder	lithium (Eskalith)	409
	valproic acid (Depakene)	409
Depression	bupropion (Wellbutrin)	401
	fluoxetine (Prozac)	406
	imipramine (Tofranil)	397
Drug abuse	buprenorphine/naloxone (Suboxone)	161
	clonidine (Catapres)	159
	methadone	160
Obsessive-compulsive disorder	clomipramine (Anafranil)	397
	fluoxetine (Prozac)	406
Schizophrenia	haloperidol (Haldol)	383
	olanzapine (Zyprexa)	389
	quetiapine (Seroquel)	390

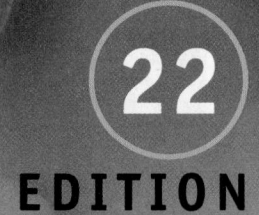

22
EDITION

MOSBY'S PHARMACOLOGY IN NURSING

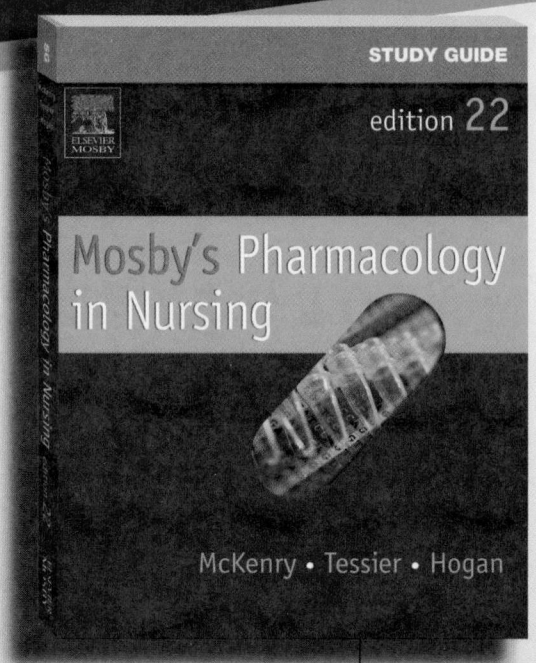
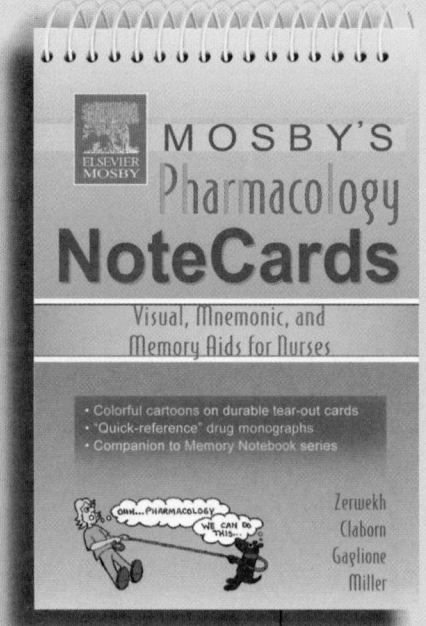
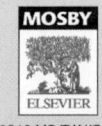

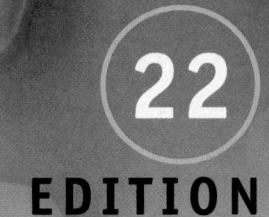

22 EDITION

MOSBY'S PHARMACOLOGY IN NURSING

LEDA MCKENRY, PhD, C-APN, FAAN
Professor Emeritus
School of Nursing, University of Massachusetts—Amherst
Amherst, Massachusetts

ED TESSIER, PharmD, MPH, BCPS
Lecturer, University of Massachusetts
School of Nursing, University of Massachusetts—Amherst
Amherst, Massachusetts

MARYANN HOGAN, RN, MSN
Clinical Assistant Professor
School of Nursing, University of Massachusetts—Amherst
Amherst, Massachusetts

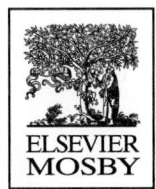

ELSEVIER
MOSBY

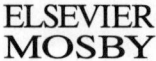

**ELSEVIER
MOSBY**

11830 Westline Industrial Drive
St. Louis, Missouri 63146

ISBN-13: 978-0-323-03008-3
ISBN-10: 0-323-03008-4

MOSBY'S PHARMACOLOGY IN NURSING

Notice

Previous editions copyrighted 2003, 2001, 1998, 1995, 1992, 1989, 1986, 1982, 1979, 1976, 1973, 1969, 1966, 1963, 1960, 1955, 1951, 1948, 1945, 1942, 1940, 1936

ISBN-13: 978-0-323-03008-3
ISBN-10: 0-323-03008-4

Acquisitions Editor: Kristin Geen
Associate Developmental Editor: Jamie Horn
Editorial Assistant: Rebecca Williams
Publishing Services Manager: Debbie Vogel
Senior Project Manager: Jodi Willard
Senior Book Designer: Amy Buxton

Printed in the United States of America

Last digit is the print number: 9   8   7   6   5   4   3   2

Barbara Allerton, RN, MSN
Assistant Professor
Boise State University
Boise, Idaho

Shelly Anderson, MSN, MBA, RN,
  ARNP-BC, CNA
Acting Dean of Nursing—Graduate
  Programs
School of Nursing
Graceland University
Lamoni, Iowa/Independence, Missouri

Susan Gail Auten, RN, BSN, MA
Nursing Instructor
Southeastern Community College
Whiteville, North Carolina

Diane S. Benson, RN, EdD
Associate Professor
Humboldt State University
Arcata, California

Teresa S. Burckhalter, MSN, RN, C
Nursing Faculty
Technical College of the Lowcountry
Beaufort, South Carolina

Sue Burnell-Jones, RN
Clinical Coordinator and Nurse Educator
Carlingview Manor
Ottawa, Ontario, Canada

Darlene A. Clark, RN, MS
Nursing Instructor
Pennsylvania State University
University Park, Pennsylvania

Maureen M. Covelli, PhD, RN
Assistant Professor
University of Central Florida
Orlando, Florida

Marina Davydov, RN
Beth Israel Medical Center
New York, New York

Mary M. Fabick, BSN, MEd, MSN, CEN
Associate Professor
Milligan College
Milligan, Tennessee

Brenda Rushing French
Assistant Professor of Nursing
Columbus State University
Columbus, Georgia

Lisa Hawthorne, RN, MSN
Maric College
San Diego, California

Elizabeth A. Henneman, PhD, RN, CCNS
Assistant Professor
University of Massachusetts
Amherst, Massachusetts

Anne Cowley Herzog, MSN, RN
Professor of Nursing
Cypress College
Cypress, California

Janice J. Hoffman, RN, MSN
SPRING Program Director
The Johns Hopkins Hospital
Baltimore, Maryland

Ilko Iliev, PhD
Professor and Chairman
Southern University at Shreveport
Shreveport, Louisiana

Judith Ann Kilpatrick, DNSc, BSN,
  MSN, RN
Assistant Professor
Widener University
Chester, Pennsylvania

Jack R. Kless, RN, CRNA, BS, MA, MSN
Instructor and Program Director
Frances Payne Bolton School of
  Nursing/Case Western Reserve
  University
Cleveland, Ohio

Wilma LaCava, BSN, MSN, ANCC
Associate Professor, Nursing
Riverside Community College
Riverside, California

Carolyn Lee, PharmD, CSPI
Louisiana Poison Control Center
Monroe, Louisiana

Natasha Leskovsek, RN, BSN, MBA,
  MPM, JD
Nurse Attorney
Heller Ehrman
Washington, D.C.

Anthony McGuire, RN, CCRN, MSN,
  ACNP
Advanced Practice Nurse
St. Joseph Hospital
Orange, California

Lora McGuire, RN, MS
Professor of Nursing
Joliet Junior College
Joliet, Illinois

Sherry Neely, MSN, RN, CRNP
Assistant Professor
Butler County Community College
Butler, Pennsylvania

Joan Reale, PhD, RN
Associate Professor
Carlow University
Pittsburgh, Pennsylvania

Gwen Scarborough, RN, MSN
Assistant Professor
University of Tennessee at Martin
Martin, Tennessee

Linda J. Scheetz, EdD, APRN, BC, CEN
Assistant Professor, College of Nursing
Rutgers, The State University of New
  Jersey
Newark, New Jersey

Stephen M. Setter, PharmD, CDE, CGP,
  DVM
Associate Professor of Pharmacotherapy
Washington State University
Spokane, Washington

Brenda Shelton, MS, RN, CCRN, AOCN
Clinical Nurse Specialist
The Sidney Kimmel Comprehensive
  Cancer Center at Johns Hopkins
Baltimore, Maryland

Mary M. Sullivan-Whalen, RN, MSN,
  FNP
The Rockefeller University
Laboratory for Investigative Dermatology
New York, New York

Robi Thomas, MS, RN, AOCN, CHPN
Assistant Professor of Nursing and Chair,
  Grand Rapids Campus
McAuley School of Nursing
University of Detroit Mercy
Grand Rapids, Michigan

Angela S. Wilson, PhD, RN, BC
Associate Professor and Department Chair
The University of Virginia's College at
  Wise
Wise, Virginia

Kathleen M. Wolz, RN, MSN, CCRN
Assistant Professor
Joliet Junior College
Joliet, Illinois

Mosby's Pharmacology in Nursing—now in its twenty-second edition—is a classic text with a long and distinguished tradition of providing nurses with a sound basis for the clinical application of pharmacology. It remains one of the most comprehensive and current pharmacology texts available for nurses. Through twenty-two editions, it has enjoyed tremendous success as a textbook for students who, when confronted with the rigorous content of their pharmacology course work, find our organization and presentation both accessible and conducive to learning.

The focus of *Mosby's Pharmacology in Nursing* is on a sound understanding of the pharmacologic properties of major drug classes and individual drugs, with special emphasis on the clinical application of drug therapy through the nursing process.

Nursing students undertaking the study of pharmacology today face a growing challenge: how to master a body of knowledge that is growing at the speed of the digital age while also studying in an increasingly compressed time frame. *Mosby's Pharmacology in Nursing* equips students to meet that challenge by covering each major drug and drug class in concise, easy-to-locate passages of text, which we call **drug monographs.** It also provides **specific applications of the nursing process** to each major drug and drug class. The use of a question-and-answer format supplemented with clinical cases helps make this twenty-second edition more relevant to the student nurse. As an additional tool to help students grasp the action of drug classes, *Mosby's Pharmacology in Nursing* identifies **key drugs** throughout; these are noted with a special key icon. Mastering the content of the key drugs helps students better grasp the pharmacologic properties of all drugs in the same class.

Mosby's Pharmacology in Nursing has additional appeal as a **pharmacology reference** because of its thorough coverage of the very latest drug classes and individual drugs and its emphasis on clinical nursing management. This makes the book useful both as a primary textbook and as a clinical reference for nursing practice.

Organization

Macrostructure

The book is divided into two major parts. Part One, Basic Concepts, includes three units: Unit 1, Principles of Pharmacology and Nursing; Unit 2, Biopsychosocial Aspects of Pharmacology; and Unit 3, Current Issues in Pharmacology. Part Two: Clinical Concepts consists of broad pharmacologic units and makes up the largest portion of this text. In general, the 16 units in Part Two begin with a chapter that reviews the body system and then proceed with chapters on the major drug categories used for that system.

Chapter Organization

Each chapter of *Mosby's Pharmacology in Nursing* begins with a **Chapter Focus,** followed by **Learning Objectives** and lists of **Key Terms** (boldfaced in the text) and **Key Drugs** to help students focus on important material in the chapter. A reader-friendly and **case-based chapter format** features a case study at the beginning of each pharmacology discussion, followed by a series of questions with answers that focus on application of the content to nursing practice. Case studies can be located easily; they are identified by an orange icon. Green icons are used to identify headings that start new discussions. Summary tables and boxes are included throughout to supplement and reinforce the material and to help the student make comparisons among similar drugs.

The drug chapters that make up the bulk of *Mosby's Pharmacology* in Nursing begin with a discussion of a drug group or classification. Individual drugs are then discussed by generic name, followed by a **pronunciation guide** and **U.S. and Canadian trade** names. (Canadian trade names are highlighted with a maple leaf icon ✹.) If the generic name is a key drug, it is highlighted with a icon and receives special, in-depth coverage. The drug monograph continues in a step-by-step, clinically oriented format that includes mechanism of action, indications, pharmacokinetics/dosing, adverse effects, and significant drug interactions (when appropriate). It concludes with a Nursing Management section.

The Nursing Management section uses the following nursing process format:
- Assessment
- Nursing diagnosis
- Planning
- Implementation (with subheads for Monitoring, Intervention, and Education, when appropriate)
- Evaluation

The text of each chapter concludes with a **summary** that provides students with a succinct review of the chapter. Following the summary, **Critical Thinking Questions** present "real-life" scenarios to help apply the chapter material. (Answer guidelines for these questions are now available on the book's **Evolve website.**)

New to This Edition

In the twenty-second edition, a new and innovative **case-based chapter format** features case studies followed by a series of questions with answers that pertain to pharmacology in nursing practice. An attractive **full-color design** makes the book more engaging, and approximately **200 photos and illustrations** clearly depict key pharmacologic principles and show how drugs work in the body. Content throughout the book has been streamlined and includes more **readable, relevant explanations** and an increased use of summary tables and boxes to highlight key information.

New boxed material includes **Evidence-Based Practice** boxes, which cover the latest research topics in pharmacology; **Pharmacologic Issues in an Age of Terrorism** boxes, which cover timely topics such as the role of vaccination in terrorism response and toxicology management in terrorism; and **Special Considerations for Pharmacogenetics** boxes, which highlight the relevance of genetics to selected drug categories. At the end of each chapter, **e-Learning Supplement** boxes remind students of related content and exercises on the student CD-ROM and Evolve website.

A new chapter on **Medication Errors** discusses factors that contribute to medication errors and practical methods that nurses can use to reduce these errors. Separate **Medication Safety Alert** boxes apply these ideas to real-life nursing practice and can be found throughout the textbook.

A perforated **Clinical Rotation Disorders Guide** in the front of the book is subdivided into four clinical sections (medical-surgical, maternity and women's health, pediatric, and psychiatric) and alphabetically lists disorders for which drugs are commonly administered—perfect for programs that integrate pharmacology into the curriculum.

A **companion CD-ROM** contains 600 NCLEX questions (including a special Final Exam preparation section that can be used to test a student's knowledge of specific chapters to see which areas they need to review more closely), drug mechanism animations, printable chapter summaries highlighting the key points in each chapter for studying on the go, and multiple electronic calculators.

Additional Features

This book is **organized by body system**, which facilitates access and enhances learning. This twenty-second edition retains many special feature boxes, including **Special Considerations for Children** and **Special Considerations for Older Adults** boxes, which highlight important life span implications of drug therapy; **Management of Drug Overdose** boxes, which alert the nurse to important information and guidelines regarding overdoses for specific drugs; **Cultural Considerations** boxes, which teach students key cultural and ethnic considerations in drug therapy; **Pregnancy Safety** boxes, which list FDA Pregnancy Categories for drugs covered in each chapter; **Nursing Care Plans**, which illustrate the application of relevant nursing diagnoses, corresponding outcome criteria, and nursing interventions for selected drug groups; **TechnologyLink** boxes, which list website resources that can serve as a springboard to individual student research; **Complementary and Alternative Therapies** boxes, which profile the most commonly used herbs in clinical practice; and **Community and Home Health Considerations** boxes, which underscore today's trend toward nursing in the community. **Drug reference** tables summarize key pharmacologic information (e.g.,

mechanism of action, pharmacokinetics, dosages) and enhance the text's utility as a reference.

A comprehensive index includes **entries for every trade name, followed by the generic name in parentheses.** Page numbers for drug monographs are highlighted in bold type. A separate **Disorders Index** alphabetically references disorders in the text to aid in integrating the text with medical-surgical nursing course content.

Ancillaries

Mosby's Pharmacology in Nursing, twenty-second edition, is not just a textbook but also the core of a state-of-the art learning system.

For students, we have created a printed **Study Guide.** This guide has been extensively revamped and expanded by text co-author MaryAnn Hogan to include NCLEX® review questions and a variety of creative and engaging learning activities such as "Staying on Top of Terminology," "Focusing on the Facts," and "Connecting with Clients."

The **Evolve student resources** (http://evolve.elsevier.com/mckenry) features interactive case studies, concept maps, answers to the critical thinking questions in the textbook, WebLinks, access to *Mosby's Drug Consult Internet Edition,* and other supplemental information. By accessing the Evolve website, students can also subscribe to the Mosby/Saunders ePharmacology Update newsletter, which is e-mailed twice every semester and keeps students and instructors up-to-date on the latest drug news, warnings and precautions, questions and answers, and much more. Be sure to check the website often for content updates and information on new drugs.

For instructors, we offer a comprehensive **Instructor's Electronic Resource.** This single CD-ROM includes four main components: (1) an **Instructor's Resource Manual** with chapter focus, key terms, key drugs, learning objectives, chapter outlines, teaching/learning strategies, case studies, and collaborative learning activities; (2) an **ExamView Test Bank** with more than 1500 questions in an NCLEX® examination-style format with rationales, page number references, cognitive level, nursing process, and NCLEX® category listed for each question; (3) an **Image Collection** with over 200 full-color illustrations and boxes from the text; and (4) over 1000 **PowerPoint Lecture Slides** with images integrated where appropriate.

The **Evolve instructor resources** include all of the student resources listed above and downloads of the content on the *Instructor's Electronic Resource,* plus course communication tools to enhance the classroom experience.

Acknowledgments

We would like to thank the many people who have contributed to the development of the twenty-second edition of *Mosby's Pharmacology in Nursing.* Our students, academic and clinical colleagues, and mentors have influenced our practice and our revised approach to this text. Reviewers have been instrumental in providing suggestions, constructive comments, and additional clinical perspective during development.

In addition, the editorial staff was outstanding in their professional support of this project. We are grateful to Robin Carter, Executive Publisher, and Kristin Geen, Acquisitions Editor, for their creative ideas and essential support throughout the project; and to Jodi Willard, Senior Project Manager, for her exceptional work in the production phase. We are particularly grateful to Jamie Horn, Associate Developmental Editor, who was tireless in following up on endless details throughout the preproduction phase and without whom this text in its current form would not have been possible.

Finally, we would like to thank our families and friends for their unfailing patience and encouragement. Without your support, this edition would not have been possible.

Publisher's Historical Perspective

Mosby's Pharmacology in Nursing has a tradition of providing the nursing student, educator, and practicing nurse with thorough and up-to-date coverage of pharmacology and nursing management.

Through twenty-one editions, this book has sold well over 2,000,000 copies, making it the most widely used and successful nursing pharmacology textbook ever published.

Currently in its twenty-second edition, *Mosby's Pharmacology in Nursing* has its roots in *A Textbook of Materia Medica for Nurses* by A. L. Muirhead, which was published in 1919. In 1936, Hugh Alister McGuigan became the primary author, at which time the book was renamed *Materia Medica and Pharmacology.* In 1940, Elsie E. Krug joined McGuigan as coauthor—a role she was to hold until 1948, when she became the primary author. After 10 successful editions, the book was renamed *Pharmacology in Nursing* in 1955.

SPECIAL FEATURES

Special features such as new *Special Considerations for Pharmacogenetics* **boxes**, *Complementary and Alternative Considerations* **boxes,** and new *Evidence-Based Practice* **boxes** highlight important information students need to know.

Cultural Considerations **boxes** prepare students to work with a diverse patient population.

Students learn real-world application of pharmacology through new *integrated case studies* in each chapter, followed by a series of questions with answers that focus on nursing practice.

Nursing Care Plans illustrate the application of relevant nursing diagnoses, corresponding outcome criteria, and nursing interventions.

***Medication Safety Alert* boxes** highlight key information students need for safe medication administration.

Drug monographs cover each major drug and drug class in concise, easy-to-locate passages of text.

262 CHAPTER 14 Analgesics

Medication Safety Alert

Analgesics

The Institute for Safe Medication Practices (ISMP) has identified a number of issues related to safety with the use of analgesics, including the following:

- Acetaminophen dosing with combination products (e.g., orders for acetaminophen plus orders for combination products with acetaminophen such as oxycodone/acetaminophen, hydrocodone/acetaminophen) leading to client acetaminophen intake greater than 4 g daily and hepatotoxicity
- Assessing pain without assessing level of sedation and respiratory status
- Dangerous abbreviations:
  - DPT: Demerol, promethazine, Thorazine vs. diphtheria, pertussis, tetanus vaccine
  - MSO_4: $MgSO_4$ vs. morphine sulfate vs. magnesium sulfate
- Dosing and labeling confusion with liquid and rapidly dissolving acetaminophen formulations
- Interchange of tincture of opium (10 mg/mL morphine) for paregoric (2 mg/5 mL and 45% ethanol)
- Patient-controlled analgesia (PCA): errors risking client safety include:
  - Inappropriate client selection
  - Inadequate client education
  - Inadequate lockout periods
  - Inadequate staff training
  - Inadequate monitoring
  - Drug product mix-ups
  - Inappropriate programming of pump
  - Flaws in pump design
  - Dose calculation errors
- Polypharmacy orders given in rapid sequence (e.g., moderate dose of opioid if moderate pain, high dose for severe pain, where inadequate time to evaluate response to the first order occurs)
- Sound-alike names:
  - Toradol vs. Foradil
  - Hydroxyzine vs. hydralazine

For more information, see the ISMP website: http://www.ismp.org

sidered as a last resort. A discussion of safety is presented in the Medication Safety Alert box above. The management of drug overdose of opioids is presented in Chapter 9.

Opioid Antagonists

Opioid antagonists bind to opioid receptors and competitively displace the opioid analgesics from their receptor sites. As such, these agents reverse the effects of opioid agonists such as morphine and heroin. Naloxone is the prototype opioid antagonist. Naltrexone and nalmefene are also opioid antagonists. Nalmefene is a chemical analogue of naltrexone and at full dosages has a longer duration of action than naloxone. Nalmefene and naloxone are administered parenterally, whereas naltrexone is available as an oral drug.

Antagonists block opioid effects and can precipitate withdrawal symptoms in individuals who are physically dependent on opioids. These products are used to reverse the adverse or overdose effects of opioids (codeine, diphenoxylate, fentanyl, heroin, hydromorphone, levorphanol, meperidine, methadone, morphine, oxymorphone, opium derivatives, and propoxyphene) and most partial agonists (agonist-antagonist drugs such as butorphanol, nalbuphine, and pentazocine).

Respiratory depression induced by nonopioids (e.g., barbiturates), CNS depression, or disease progression does not usually respond to opioid antagonist drug therapy. It has also been reported that larger drug dosages are necessary to antagonize the effects of buprenorphine, butorphanol, nalbuphine, and pentazocine. However, a buprenorphine overdose may not respond to the opioid antagonists or, at best, may only partially respond (*USP DI*, 2005).

In an opioid analgesic overdose, naloxone and naltrexone reverse respiratory depression, sedation, miosis (constriction of pupils), and euphoric effects; they may also reverse the psychotomimetic effects of the agonist-antagonist analgesics (pentazocine and others). The drugs are believed to work at all three receptor sites, but their greatest activity is at the mu receptors (see Figure 14-9).

naloxone hydrochloride [nal **ox** one]
(Narcan)
Naloxone is inactivated orally but is very effective parenterally.

Indications
Naloxone is used for partial or complete reversal of CNS and respiratory depression associated with opioid agonists and partial agonists as discussed above.

Pharmacokinetics/Dosing
Naloxone has an onset of action is 1 to 2 minutes (IV) and 2 to 5 minutes (IM or subcutaneous). The half-life is between 60 and 100 minutes. Duration of action depends on the dose administered and the route of administration. Usually the IM dose results in a prolonged effect. Naloxone is widely distributed throughout the body and also crosses the placenta. It is metabolized in the liver and excreted via the kidneys.

The adult dose of naloxone is 0.4 to 2 mg as single dose or 0.1 to 0.2 mg for postoperative opioid depression. Naloxone may be diluted with sterile water for injection if a larger volume is needed (*USP DI*, 2005). For continuous infusion, 2 mg of naloxone may be diluted in 500 mL of normal saline or 5% dextrose injection. Because naloxone is shorter acting than most opioids, repeat naloxone injections or continuous infusion is necessary to prevent the recurrence of respiratory depression.

Adverse Effects
Adverse effects include nausea, vomiting, dizziness, hypertension, tachycardia, sweating, nervousness, abdominal cramps or pain, headache, weakness, joint and muscle pain, insomnia, hallucinations, confusion, mood alterations, tinnitus, and fever.

naltrexone [nal **trex** one]
(ReVia)

Indications
Naltrexone is indicated for adjuvant treatment in detoxified, opioid-dependent clients. It is also used in the management of ethanol dependence.

432 CHAPTER 21 Drugs Affecting the Parasympathetic Nervous System and the Neurotransmitter Acetylcholine

Pharmacologic Issues in an Age of Terrorism

Chemical Warfare

Chemical weapons are the most common type of unconventional warfare, which also includes biologic and nuclear weapons. It is estimated that as much as a third of the world's arsenal consists of chemical weapons. Concerns about the use of these agents for terrorist attacks have escalated since the events of September 11, 2001. Among these agents are the organophosphates, VX, and the G agents (sarin, tabun, and soman). Immediate care, including decontamination, could save many lives.

Nerve Agents

Nerve agents affect both the autonomic and central nervous systems. The extent of the signs and symptoms may be localized or systemic, depending on the exposure. It is critical that health care providers recognize the symptoms of chemical agents in order to begin decontamination and treatment, and for their own protection. Many of these agents saturate the clothing as well as the skin, and can contaminate those persons who are treating the victims.

Name/Symbol	Means of Exposure	Lethal Dosage	Rate of Action	Effects	Antidotes/Methods of Treatment
Tabun (GA)	Skin contact and/or inhalation	Via inhalation: 400 LCt_{50} mg/min/m^3 Via skin exposure: 1000 LD_{50}	Very rapid Incapacitating effects occur within 1-10 min; lethal effects occur within 10-15 min	Effects seen in eyes (contraction of pupils, pain, dim or blurred vision), nose (runny nose), and airways (chest tightness) Nausea and vomiting also possible Twitching/seizures result when skeletal muscle reached Fluctuations in heart rate Loss of consciousness and seizure activity can occur within 1 min of exposure in cases of exposure to high concentration of agent Eventual paralysis, death	4 steps to management of exposure to nerve agents: decontamination; ventilation; antidotes; supportive therapy Therapeutic drug options: Atropine and pralidoxime chloride (autoinjectors packaged together in kits provided to military personnel) Diazepam, lorazepam (for seizures)
Sarin (GB)	Skin contact and/or inhalation	Via inhalation: 100 LCt_{50} mg/min/m^3 Via skin exposure: 1700 LD_{50}	Very rapid Incapacitating effects occur within 1-10 min; lethal effects occur within 2-15 min		
Soman (GD)	Skin contact and/or inhalation	Via inhalation: 70 LCt_{50} mg/min/m^3 Via skin exposure: 50 LD_{50}	Very rapid Incapacitating effects occur within 1-10 min; lethal effects occur within 1-15 min		
VX	Skin contact and/or inhalation	Via inhalation: 50 LCt_{50} mg/min/m^3 Via skin exposure: 10 LD_{50}	Rapid Incapacitating effects occur within 1-10 min; lethal effects occur within 4-42 hr		
Novichok agents		Novichok 5 estimated to exceed the toxicity effectiveness of VX by 5 to 8 times Novichok 7 estimated to exceed the toxicity effectiveness of soman by 10 times	Very rapid	Assumed to be similar to the effects of other nerve agents listed above	Assumed to be similar to treatment methods for other nerve agents listed above

Modified from http://faculty.ncwc.edu/toconnor/429/429lect18.htm
LCt_{50}, Lethal mass exposure dose; *LD_{50}*, median lethal dose.

***Pharmacologic Issues in an Age of Terrorism* boxes** cover timely topics, such as the role of vaccination and toxicology management in terrorism response.

Special Considerations for Children and ***Special Considerations for Older Adults* boxes** help students understand important life span implications of drug therapy.

CHAPTER 21 Drugs Affecting the Parasympathetic Nervous System and the Neurotransmitter Acetylcholine 439

obstruction), urinary retention (aggravates symptoms), prostatic hypertrophy (aggravates symptoms), or myasthenia gravis (aggravates condition by inhibition of acetylcholine). Do not use in clients with open-angle glaucoma (mydriatic effect increases intraocular pressure), ulcerative colitis, or renal or hepatic disease (increases effects of drug). Administer systemic forms carefully to clients with chronic pulmonary disease because bronchial secretions may be sufficiently decreased to result in bronchial plugs. Use with caution in infants and young children and in children with blonde hair and blue eyes, Down's syndrome, spastic paralysis, or brain damage; these individuals tend to be more sensitive to the effects of the drug (*USP DI*, 2005). Review the client's current medication regimen for the risk of significant drug interactions, such as other drugs with anticholinergic properties that would have an additive effect.

Obtain a baseline assessment of the client's vital signs and urinary and bowel status. For older adults and debilitated clients, a mental status assessment is helpful in determining if the client is experiencing any drug-related drowsiness or CNS stimulation. A baseline ECG is required if the drug is used as an antidysrhythmic. A baseline intraocular pressure determination is indicated for clients undergoing long-term therapy.

Nursing Diagnosis The client receiving atropine therapy is at risk for the following nursing diagnoses/collaborative problems: hyperthermia related to the suppression of sweat gland activity; risk for injury related to blurred vision, dizziness, or light-headedness; impaired tissue integrity (irritation at injection site); disturbed thought processes (confusion, agitation); impaired comfort related to dry mouth or increased sensitivity of the eyes to light; urinary retention related to the antimuscarinic effects of the drug; constipation related to decreased motility of the GI tract; and the potential complications of allergic reaction and decreased cardiac output related to the ineffectiveness of the drug.

Planning During atropine therapy, the client will:

- Experience relief from symptoms for which the drug was prescribed.
- Effectively manage the therapeutic drug regimen, including knowledge of the medication, its adverse effects, and which adverse effects are reportable, and compliance with medication schedule.
- Be free of injury related to drug action or adverse effects.

Special Considerations for Older Adults | ANTICHOLINERGIC AGENTS

- Older adults are highly susceptible to anticholinergic adverse effects, especially constipation, dry mouth, and urinary retention (usually in men).
- Avoid using anticholinergic agents in clients with narrow-angle glaucoma or a history of urinary retention.
- Memory impairment has been reported with continuous administration of these agents, especially in older clients.
- When usual adult dosages are administered, some older adults may experience a paradoxical reaction: hyperexcitability, agitation, confusion, and sedation.
- Chronic use decreases or inhibits the flow of saliva, which may contribute to oral discomfort, periodontal disease, and candidiasis.
- Overheating resulting in heat stroke has been reported in persons receiving anticholinergic drugs during vigorous exercise or in periods of hot weather.
- Blurred vision and/or increased sensitivity to light may occur.
- Anticholinergic dosing in older adults should begin with the lowest dosage, with gradual increases until maximum improvement is noted or intolerable adverse effects occur.

Special Considerations for Children | ANTICHOLINERGIC AGENTS

- Infants and young children are very susceptible to anticholinergic adverse effects.
- Closely monitor children with spastic paralysis or brain damage because they usually have an increased reaction to anticholinergic agents and thus require a dosage reduction.
- Anticholinergics, especially in high doses, may cause a paradoxical-type reaction of increased nervousness, confusion, and hyperexcitability.
- Anticholinergic drugs suppress sweat gland activity. Therefore children receiving these agents in environments where hot weather prevails or temperatures are high have an increased risk of developing a rapid body temperature increase.
- Dosage adjustments are often necessary for infants and young children and in children with blonde hair, blue eyes, Down's syndrome, spastic paralysis, or brain damage because they usually have an increased response to this drug category. Flushing, increased temperature, irritability, increased pulse, and increased respiratory rate may occur (*USP DI*, 2005).
- Start with low dosages and increase gradually as needed and as tolerated.

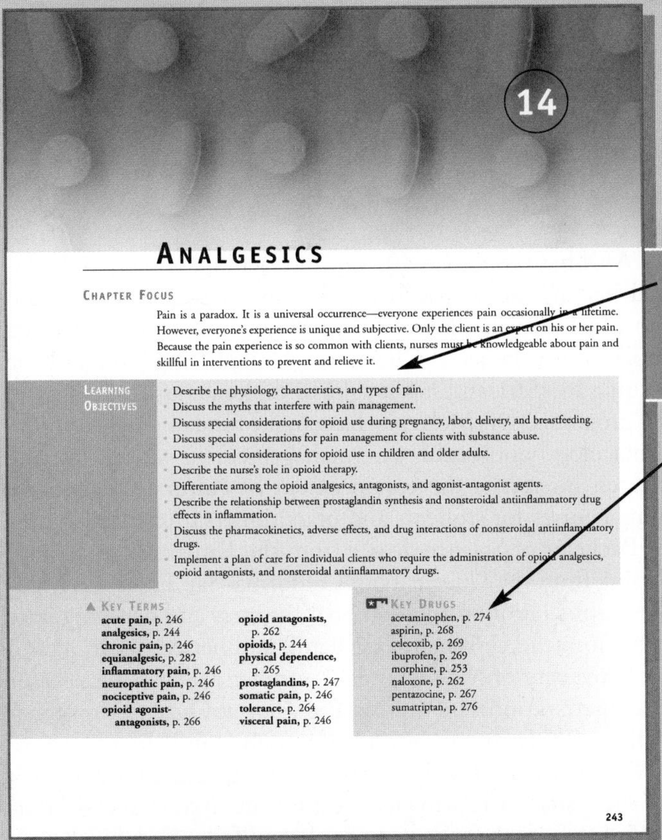

14

ANALGESICS

CHAPTER FOCUS

Pain is a paradox. It is a universal occurrence—everyone experiences pain occasionally in a lifetime. However, everyone's experience is unique and subjective. Only the client is an expert on his or her pain. Because the pain experience is so common with clients, nurses must be knowledgeable about pain and skillful in interventions to prevent and relieve it.

LEARNING OBJECTIVES

- Describe the physiology, characteristics, and types of pain.
- Discuss the myths that interfere with pain management.
- Discuss special considerations for opioid use during pregnancy, labor, delivery, and breastfeeding.
- Discuss special considerations for pain management for clients with substance abuse.
- Discuss special considerations for opioid use in children and older adults.
- Describe the nurse's role in opioid therapy.
- Differentiate among the opioid analgesics, antagonists, and agonist-antagonist agents.
- Describe the relationship between prostaglandin synthesis and nonsteroidal antiinflammatory drug effects in inflammation.
- Discuss the pharmacokinetics, adverse effects, and drug interactions of nonsteroidal antiinflammatory drugs.
- Implement a plan of care for individual clients who require the administration of opioid analgesics, opioid antagonists, and nonsteroidal antiinflammatory drugs.

KEY TERMS

acute pain, p. 246
analgesics, p. 244
chronic pain, p. 246
equianalgesic, p. 282
inflammatory pain, p. 246
neuropathic pain, p. 246
nociceptive pain, p. 246
opioid agonist-antagonists, p. 266
opioid antagonists, p. 262
opioids, p. 244
physical dependence, p. 265
prostaglandins, p. 247
somatic pain, p. 246
tolerance, p. 264
visceral pain, p. 246

KEY DRUGS

acetaminophen, p. 274
aspirin, p. 268
celecoxib, p. 269
ibuprofen, p. 269
morphine, p. 253
naloxone, p. 262
pentazocine, p. 267
sumatriptan, p. 276

243

Chapter Focus, Learning Objectives, and lists of ***Key Terms*** and ***Key Drugs*** help students focus on important material in the chapter.

Management of Drug Overdose **boxes** provide important information on overdoses for specific drugs.

Pregnancy Safety **boxes** list the FDA Pregnancy Categories for the drugs covered in each chapter.

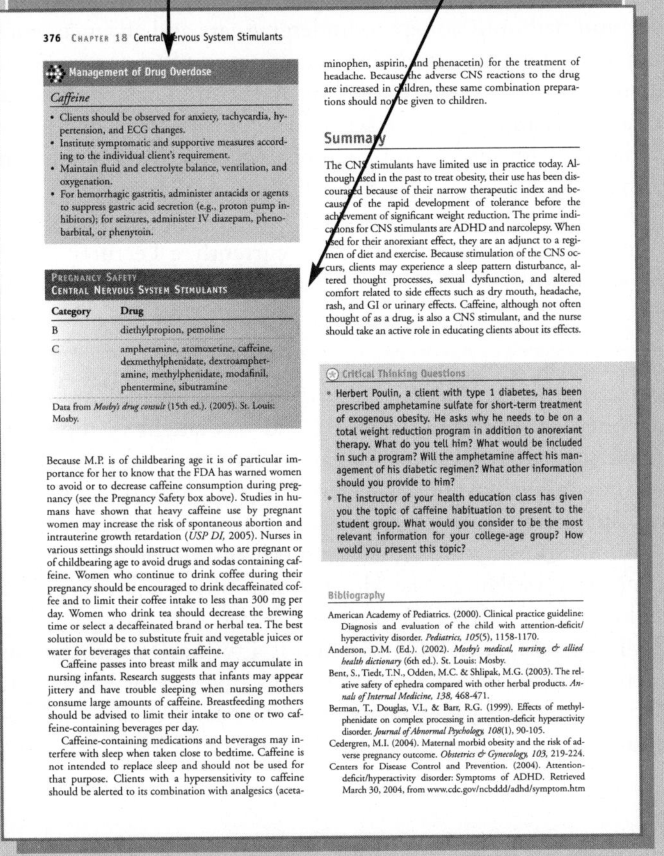

376 CHAPTER 18 Central Nervous System Stimulants

Management of Drug Overdose

Caffeine

- Clients should be observed for anxiety, tachycardia, hypertension, and ECG changes.
- Institute symptomatic and supportive measures according to the individual client's requirement.
- Maintain fluid and electrolyte balance, ventilation, and oxygenation.
- For hemorrhagic gastritis, administer antacids or agents to suppress gastric acid secretion (e.g., proton pump inhibitors); for seizures, administer IV diazepam, phenobarbital, or phenytoin.

PREGNANCY SAFETY
CENTRAL NERVOUS SYSTEM STIMULANTS

Category	Drug
B	diethylpropion, pemoline
C	amphetamine, atomoxetine, caffeine, dexmethylphenidate, dextroamphetamine, methylphenidate, modafinil, phentermine, sibutramine

Data from *Mosby's drug consult* (15th ed.). (2005). St. Louis: Mosby.

Because M.P. is of childbearing age it is of particular importance for her to know that the FDA has warned women to avoid or to decrease caffeine consumption during pregnancy (see the Pregnancy Safety box above). Studies in humans have shown that heavy caffeine use by pregnant women may increase the risk of spontaneous abortion and intrauterine growth retardation (*USP DI,* 2005). Nurses in various settings should instruct women who are pregnant or of childbearing age to avoid drugs and sodas containing caffeine. Women who continue to drink coffee during their pregnancy should be encouraged to drink decaffeinated coffee and to limit their coffee intake to less than 300 mg per day. Women who drink tea should decrease the brewing time or select a decaffeinated brand or herbal tea. The best solution would be to substitute fruit and vegetable juices or water for beverages that contain caffeine.

Caffeine passes into breast milk and may accumulate in nursing infants. Research suggests that infants may appear jittery and have trouble sleeping when nursing mothers consume large amounts of caffeine. Breastfeeding mothers should be advised to limit their intake to one or two caffeine-containing beverages per day.

Caffeine-containing medications and beverages may interfere with sleep when taken close to bedtime. Caffeine is not intended to replace sleep and should not be used for that purpose. Clients with a hypersensitivity to caffeine should be alerted to its combination with analgesics (acetaminophen, aspirin, and phenacetin) for the treatment of headache. Because the adverse CNS reactions to the drug are increased in children, these same combination preparations should not be given to children.

Summary

The CNS stimulants have limited use in practice today. Although used in the past to treat obesity, their use has been discouraged because of their narrow therapeutic index and because of the rapid development of tolerance before the achievement of significant weight reduction. The prime indications for CNS stimulants are ADHD and narcolepsy. When used for their anorexiant effect, they are an adjunct to a regimen of diet and exercise. Because stimulation of the CNS occurs, clients may experience a sleep pattern disturbance, altered thought processes, sexual dysfunction, and altered comfort related to side effects such as dry mouth, headache, rash, and GI or urinary effects. Caffeine, although not often thought of as a drug, is also a CNS stimulant, and the nurse should take an active role in educating clients about its effects.

Critical Thinking Questions

- Herbert Poulin, a client with type 1 diabetes, has been prescribed amphetamine sulfate for short-term treatment of exogenous obesity. He asks why he needs to be on a total weight reduction program in addition to anorexiant therapy. What do you tell him? What would be included in such a program? Will the amphetamine affect his management of his diabetic regimen? What other information should you provide to him?
- The instructor of your health education class has given you the topic of caffeine habituation to present to the student group. What would you consider to be the most relevant information for your college-age group? How would you present this topic?

Bibliography

American Academy of Pediatrics. (2000). Clinical practice guideline: Diagnosis and evaluation of the child with attention-deficit/hyperactivity disorder. *Pediatrics, 105*(5), 1158-1170.
Anderson, D.M. (Ed.). (2002). *Mosby's medical, nursing, & allied health dictionary* (6th ed.). St. Louis: Mosby.
Bent, S., Tiedt, T.N., Odden, M.C. & Shlipak, M.G. (2003). The relative safety of ephedra compared with other herbal products. *Annals of Internal Medicine, 138,* 468-471.
Berman, T., Douglas, V.I., & Barr, R.G. (1999). Effects of methylphenidate on complex processing in attention-deficit hyperactivity disorder. *Journal of Abnormal Psychology, 108*(1), 90-105.
Cedergren, M.I. (2004). Maternal morbid obesity and the risk of adverse pregnancy outcome. *Obstetrics & Gynecology, 103,* 219-224.
Centers for Disease Control and Prevention. (2004). Attention-deficit/hyperactivity disorder: Symptoms of ADHD. Retrieved March 30, 2004, from www.cdc.gov/ncbddd/adhd/symptom.htm

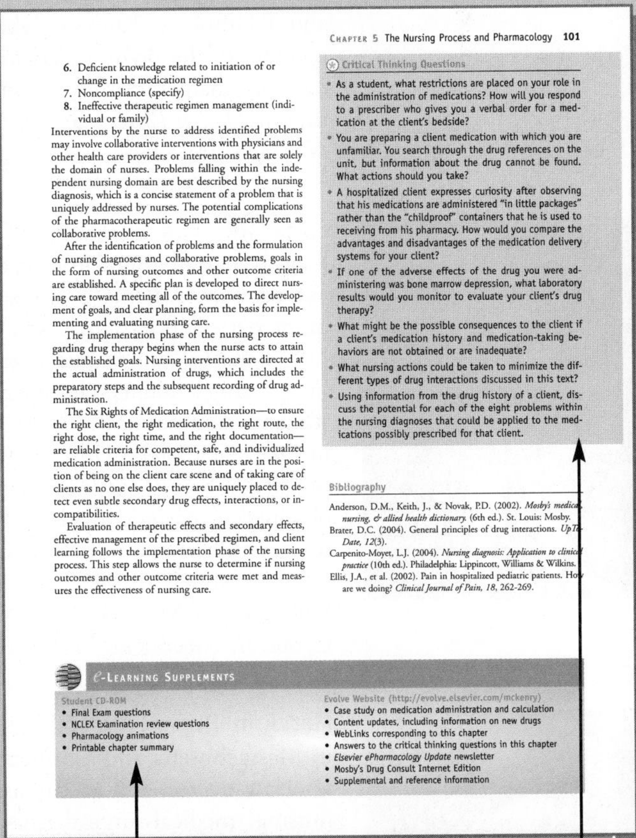

CHAPTER 5 The Nursing Process and Pharmacology 101

6. Deficient knowledge related to initiation of or change in the medication regimen
7. Noncompliance (specify)
8. Ineffective therapeutic regimen management (individual or family)

Interventions by the nurse to address identified problems may involve collaborative interventions with physicians and other health care providers or interventions that are solely the domain of nurses. Problems falling within the independent nursing domain are best described by the nursing diagnosis, which is a concise statement of a problem that is uniquely addressed by nurses. The potential complications of the pharmacotherapeutic regimen are generally seen as collaborative problems.

After the identification of problems and the formulation of nursing diagnoses and collaborative problems, goals in the form of nursing outcomes and other outcome criteria are established. A specific plan is developed to direct nursing care toward meeting all of the outcomes. The development of goals, and clear planning, form the basis for implementing and evaluating nursing care.

The implementation phase of the nursing process regarding drug therapy begins when the nurse acts to attain the established goals. Nursing interventions are directed at the actual administration of drugs, which includes the preparatory steps and the subsequent recording of drug administration.

The Six Rights of Medication Administration—to ensure the right client, the right medication, the right route, the right dose, the right time, and the right documentation—are reliable criteria for competent, safe, and individualized medication administration. Because nurses are in the position of being on the client care scene and of taking care of clients as no one else does, they are uniquely placed to detect even subtle secondary drug effects, interactions, or incompatibilities.

Evaluation of therapeutic effects and secondary effects, effective management of the prescribed regimen, and client learning follows the implementation phase of the nursing process. This step allows the nurse to determine if nursing outcomes and other outcome criteria were met and measures the effectiveness of nursing care.

Critical Thinking Questions

- As a student, what restrictions are placed on your role in the administration of medications? How will you respond to a prescriber who gives you a verbal order for a medication at the client's bedside?
- You are preparing a client medication with which you are unfamiliar. You search through the drug references on the unit, but information about the drug cannot be found. What actions should you take?
- A hospitalized client expresses curiosity after observing that his medications are administered "in little packages" rather than the "childproof" containers that he is used to receiving from his pharmacy. How would you compare the advantages and disadvantages of the medication delivery systems for your client?
- If one of the adverse effects of the drug you were administering was bone marrow depression, what laboratory results would you monitor to evaluate your client's drug therapy?
- What might be the possible consequences to the client if a client's medication history and medication-taking behaviors are not obtained or are inadequate?
- What nursing actions could be taken to minimize the different types of drug interactions discussed in this text?
- Using information from the drug history of a client, discuss the potential for each of the eight problems within the nursing diagnoses that could be applied to the medications possibly prescribed for that client.

Bibliography

Anderson, D.M., Keith, J., & Novak, P.D. (2002). *Mosby's medical, nursing, & allied health dictionary.* (6th ed.). St. Louis: Mosby.
Brater, D.C. (2004). General principles of drug interactions. *UpToDate, 12*(3).
Carpenito-Moyet, L.J. (2004). *Nursing diagnosis: Application to clinical practice* (10th ed.). Philadelphia: Lippincott, Williams & Wilkins.
Ellis, J.A., et al. (2002). Pain in hospitalized pediatric patients. How are we doing? *Clinical Journal of Pain, 18,* 262-269.

e-LEARNING SUPPLEMENTS

Student CD-ROM
- Final Exam questions
- NCLEX Examination review questions
- Pharmacology animations
- Printable chapter summary

Evolve Website (http://evolve.elsevier.com/mckenry)
- Case study on medication administration and calculation
- Content updates, including information on new drugs
- WebLinks corresponding to this chapter
- Answers to the critical thinking questions in this chapter
- *Elsevier ePharmacology Update* newsletter
- Mosby's Drug Consult Internet Edition
- Supplemental and reference information

At the end of each chapter, ***e-Learning Supplements*** **boxes** remind students of related content and exercises on the new companion CD-ROM and Evolve website, and ***Critical Thinking Questions*** help reinforce key concepts.

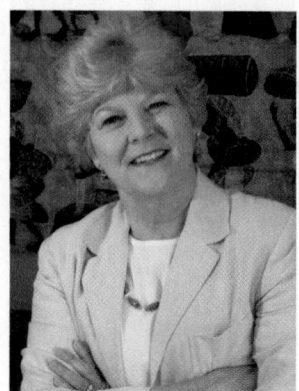

Leda M. McKenry, PhD, APN-BC, FAAN has more than 40 years of teaching, service, and consultation experience in nursing and health care management that includes community and acute care settings in Florida, California, Louisiana, Nevada, and Massachusetts in the United States and in the Bahamas, Colombia, Spain, Jamaica, Ghana, the United Kingdom, and the Republic of Ireland. She began teaching in 1961 and has taught in diploma, associate-degree, baccalaureate, and graduate nursing programs. Dr. McKenry has taught fundamentals of nursing, medical-surgical nursing, pharmacology, and health care management in various nursing programs. Her current area of research interest is the enhancement of cultural competence through cross-cultural service learning courses for students and practitioners in the health professions. Dr. McKenry received her Bachelor of Science degree from the University of Miami, her Master of Science degree in Nursing from the University of California–San Francisco Medical Center, her Master of Business Administration in International Business and her Doctorate in International Health Development from the University of Miami, and her certification as a Family Nurse Practitioner from the University of Massachusetts—Amherst. She is a Professor Emeritus at the University of Massachusetts–Amherst; Visiting Professor at Queen's University in Belfast, Northern Ireland; and Adjunct Professor at Nwame Nkrumah University of Science and Technology, Kumasi, Ghana, West Africa—and she is still teaching. Dr. McKenry is a member of the Board of Trustees of the Sisters of Providence Health Care System and is President of Ghana Health Mission. Her interest in pharmacology has been life-long; she is the author of *Mosby's Patient Guides to Medications* and has been co-author of *Mosby's Pharmacology in Nursing* since 1986.

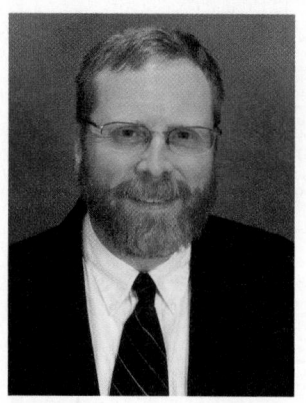

Ed Tessier, PharmD, MPH, BCPS has practiced as a clinical pharmacist and consultant in acute, long-term, and ambulatory care settings since 1980. His practice interests include gerontology and general medicine, and his practice is focused on assisting clients and clinicians at all levels in the better understanding of pharmacotherapy to improve the safe and effective use of drugs. Dr. Tessier has taught pharmacology and pathophysiology to undergraduate and advance practice nursing students, pharmacy students, emergency medicine practitioners, physician assistant students, and physical therapy students since 1995. He received his Bachelor of Science Degree in Pharmacy at the University of Rhode Island; completed a residency in hospital pharmacy practice at Saint Mary's Hospital affiliated with the Mayo Clinic in Rochester, Minnesota; and obtained a Masters of Public Health at the University of Massachusetts–Amherst and a Doctorate of Pharmacy at Idaho State University. Dr. Tessier is Board Certified as a Pharmacotherapy Specialist with the Board of Pharmaceutical Specialties. He is currently a Lecturer at the University of Massachusetts–Amherst and works as a clinical pharmacist at Franklin Medical Center in Greenfield, Massachusetts.

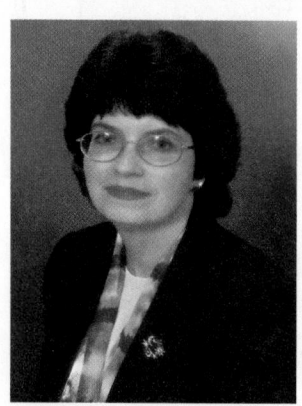

MaryAnn Hogan, RN, MSN has practiced nursing in critical care and adult acute care units in Massachusetts and Connecticut. She began teaching in 1981 and has taught in diploma, associate-degree, and baccalaureate nursing programs. Ms. Hogan has taught fundamentals of nursing, medical-surgical nursing, and leadership and management in various nursing programs. Her interest in pharmacology stems from the tremendous importance this therapy plays in health maintenance and restoration for so many individuals and the knowledge that this aspect of therapy is complex and constantly evolving. Ms. Hogan's area of research interest is health-related behavior changes in older adults. She has an ongoing interest in assisting nursing students to prepare for the NCLEX-RN licensing examination and is a former NCLEX® item writer. Ms. Hogan received her Bachelor of Science degree from the University of Massachusetts–Amherst and her Master of Science degree in Nursing from Anna Maria College in Paxton, Massachusetts. She is a Clinical Assistant Professor at the University of Massachusetts–Amherst.

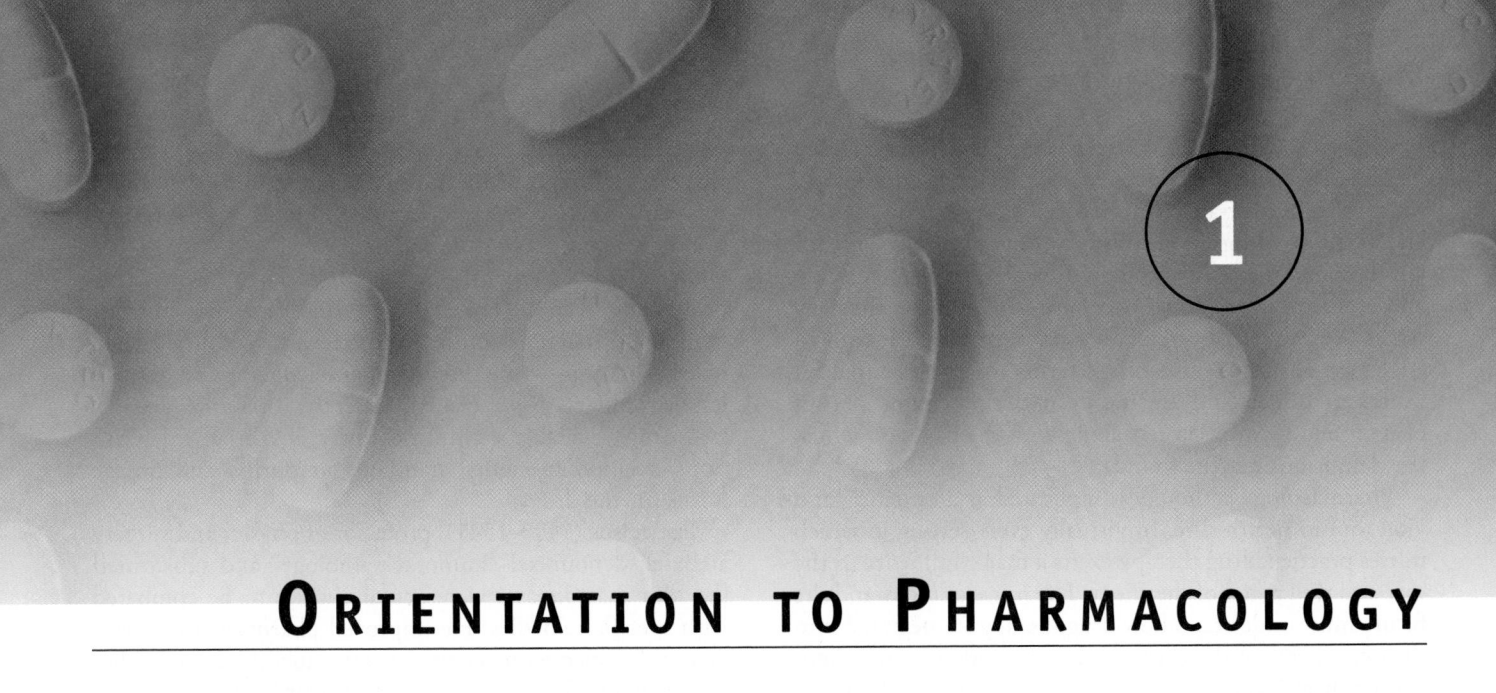

ORIENTATION TO PHARMACOLOGY

CHAPTER FOCUS

To administer medications safely and teach clients and caregivers how to manage a therapeutic drug regimen effectively, nurses need to understand and apply the principles of pharmacology. This chapter will focus on the historical development of pharmacology as a science for the improvement of health, the terminology associated with it, and the scope of nursing practice related to it.

LEARNING OBJECTIVES

- Define key terms used in pharmacology.
- Cite significant historical events in the development of pharmacology.
- Describe the difference between chemical, generic, and trade names of drug products.
- Identify authoritative sources for drug information.
- Identify the scope of nursing responsibilities related to pharmacology.
- Correlate the steps of the nursing process with the study of pharmacology.
- Plan effective ways to study pharmacology.

▲ KEY TERMS

adverse effects, p. 9
allopathic medicine, p. 2
chemical name, p. 4
collaborative problems, p. 10
complementary/alternative drugs, p. 2
dosage, p. 9
drug, p. 4
drug interactions, p. 9
generic (nonproprietary) name, p. 4

indications, p. 9
mechanism of action, p. 9
nonprescription or over-the-counter (OTC) drug, p. 4
pharmacokinetics, p. 9
pharmacopeia, p. 2
pregnancy safety, p. 9
prescription drug or legend drug, p. 4
trade, brand, or proprietary name, p. 4

✱ **What is pharmacology and why is the study of pharmacology essential for nurses?**

Pharmacology is a science that studies the effects of drugs within a living system. It deals with all legal and illegal drugs used in society today, including street, prescription, nonprescription or over-the-counter (OTC), and complementary/ alternative medications. The pharmacologic agents available today have controlled, prevented, cured and, in a few instances, eradicated disease. The result has been an improved quality of life and, perhaps, an extension of the life span. In

the practice of nursing, pharmacology applies knowledge from many different disciplines, including anatomy and physiology, pathology, microbiology, organic chemistry and biochemistry, mathematics, anthropology, psychology, and sociology. Thus clinical drug therapy can be considered an applied science for nursing.

Although medications are beneficial, they can also potentially harm the client, which is reflected by the fact that the term *pharmaceutical* is actually derived from the Greek word for poison (Siler, 1982). Therefore the nurse should have a thorough understanding of any medication *before* giving it to a client. The nurse must know the usual dosage, route of administration, indication(s), significant adverse effects, major drug interactions, contraindications, and the appropriate nursing assessment, planning, implementation, and evaluation techniques necessary to administer the drug safely. A number of terms are fundamental to the knowledge base of nurses. Lists of key terms that are essential for nurses to understand are found at the beginning of this chapter and future chapters along with the pages on which the definitions may be found.

Pharmacology, although complicated, is an exciting and vital tool in health care. In virtually every setting in which nurses practice, drug therapy exerts a major influence in the care and well being of the client. The nurse of today and the future must understand how drug therapy is integrated into the overall care of the client, and must work with the client and the health care team to assure that pharmacotherapy is safe, effective and optimal. As you approach an understanding of pharmacology, most learners find it helpful to relate theoretical concepts to actual practice. This text will assist your application of theoretical knowledge through the use of a "question and answer" format and the use of case studies integrated in the presentation of content.

Historical Trends

Since the beginning of time people have searched for substances to treat illness and cure disease. The oldest known prescriptions were found on a clay tablet written by a Sumerian physician in approximately 3000 BC.

Primitive people through the Egyptian period (3500 BC to 300 AD) believed that evil spirits living in the body caused disease. Asclepius, who lived between 600 and 700 BC, was considered the principal Greek god of healing. He combined religion and healing in a temple setting, and his large family represented health or medical ideology. For example, his wife Epeione soothed pain; daughter Hygieia, the goddess of health, represented the prevention of disease; and Panaceia, another daughter, represented treatment. His temple settings were used to treat both the rich and poor to cure their illnesses.

In the fifth century BC, Hippocrates advanced the idea that disease resulted from natural causes and could be understood only through a study of natural laws. He believed the body to have recuperative powers and saw the role of the health care provider as assisting the recuperative process. Called the Father of Medicine, Hippocrates influenced the principles that control the practice of medicine today.

The fall of the Roman Empire marked the beginning of the medieval period (400 to 1580 AD). Germanic barbarians overran Western Europe, which reverted to a medicine of folklore and tradition similar to that of the Greeks before Hippocrates. At the same time, Christian religious orders built monasteries that became sites for all learning, including pharmacy and medicine. They aided the sick and needy with food, rest, and medicinals from their monastery gardens. The Arabs' interest in medicine, pharmacy, and chemistry was reflected in the hospitals and schools they built, the many new drugs they contributed, and their formulation of the first set of drug standards.

In 1240 AD, Emperor Frederick II declared pharmacy to be separate from medicine, but pharmacy was not truly established separately until the sixteenth century, when Valerius Cordus wrote the first pharmacopeia as an authoritative standard. A **pharmacopeia** is the total of all authorized drugs available within a country; it contains descriptions, recipes, strengths, standards of purity, and dosage forms for the drugs.

Paracelsus (1493-1541), professor of physics and surgery at Basel, denounced "humoral pathology" and substituted the idea that diseases were actual entities to be combated with specific remedies. He improved pharmacy and therapeutics for succeeding centuries, introducing new remedies and reducing the overdosing so prevalent in that period.

Great progress was made in pharmacy and chemistry during the seventeenth and eighteenth centuries. The first London pharmacopeia appeared in 1618, and many preparations introduced then are still in use today, including opium tincture, coca, and ipecac. The first important national pharmacopeia was the French *Codex* (1818); this was followed by the *United States Pharmacopeia* in 1820, Great Britain in 1864, and Germany in 1872. Table 1-1 summarizes a number of the major drug discoveries.

The study of accurate dosages in the nineteenth century led to the establishment of large-scale manufacturing plants for the production of drugs. Drug dosages and knowledge of their expected action became more precise. **Allopathic medicine,** or evidenced-based practice of medicine, had begun to replace empiricism. In the twenty-first century, change will continue to reform the health care systems in the United States and Canada. The emphasis on providing quality health care in a more cost-effective manner is leading to a redefinition of professional roles and decision-making responsibilities among health care professionals. More clients and health care providers are using **complementary/alternative therapies** for health promotion and the treatment of illness and injury. Complementary/alternative therapies are techniques different from allopathic medicine, such as herbal preparations, acupuncture, aromatherapy, and therapeutic touch. An integrated health care delivery team is evolving; this team centers on client-focused care that at a minimum includes assessment, planning, monitoring, client counseling, accountability for therapeutic outcomes, and client advocacy. A health promotion focus and managed care approaches are changing the content of professional education. Drug therapy is the mainstay in the application of restorative and rehabilitative care and a component of preventive medicine, and therefore the nurse needs to have a solid foundation in pharmacology.

As a result of the current and projected trends, the health care consumer will be asking for more information; one of the persons most often questioned is the nurse (Oermann, Harris, & Dammeyer, 2001). Nurses in all

TABLE 1-1 EXAMPLES OF MAJOR DRUG DISCOVERIES

Drug	Time Period	Comments
opium tincture, coca (cocaine), and ipecac	17th century	Important drugs; still used today
digitalis	1785	Cardiac medication; source of digoxin
smallpox vaccine	1796	Important vaccine in its time; smallpox considered eradicated worldwide in 1980 by the World Health Organization; potential bioterrorism risk today
morphine	1815	Most important analgesic derived from opium; used to treat severe pain
quinine, atropine, and codeine	19th century	Still available for use today
ether and chloroform	1840s	First general anesthetics; rare or obsolete today
insulin	1922	Most important discovery for treatment of diabetes mellitus
heparin	1942	Anticoagulant that decreased postpartum and postsurgical deaths related to immobility
penicillin	Mid-1940s	Revolutionized treatment of microbial infections; precursor of many other antibiotics
cortisone	1949	Important hormone from adrenal gland cortex; also synthetically prepared
phenothiazines	Mid-1950s	First psychotherapeutic agents; revolutionized the care for the mentally ill
polio vaccines	1955, 1961	Discovery of inactivated and live oral poliovirus vaccines very significant in eliminating polio epidemics
oral contraceptives	Late 1950s	Chemicals similar to natural estrogen or progesterone hormones; used by millions of women worldwide
benzodiazepines	Early 1960s	Sedatives and antianxiety medication used by millions
antivirals	Mid-1970s	Useful for the prophylaxis and treatment of viral diseases
H_2 blockers	Mid-1970s	Antiulcer drugs that decrease need for gastric surgery
AZT	1987	First antiretroviral agent for HIV
SSRIs	Late 1980s	Revolutionized the treatment of depression
HMG-CoA reductase inhibitors	Late 1980s	Drugs to treat dyslipidemias
HIV protease inhibitors	1996	Potent class of antiretroviral agents; dramatically reduce HIV-related mortality when used in combination with other drugs
proton pump inhibitors	2001	Suppress gastric acid secretions; major advance in the treatment of gastroesophageal reflux disease (GERD) and other gastric disorders

AZT, Zidovudine; *HIV*, human immunodeficiency virus; *HMG-CoA*, hepatic 3-methylglutaryl coenzyme A; *SSRIs*, selective serotonin reuptake inhibitors.

practice roles and settings need to understand the therapeutic uses of and potential for injury with prescription, OTC, complementary/alternative, and illicit drugs. Nursing roles—which include administering medications in health care agencies, community, and home care settings; teaching clients safe and effective self-administration of medications; and detecting drug-related problems—require thorough preparation with comprehensive and current knowledge. Nurses will assume greater responsibility for professional judgment in the administration and supervision of drug therapy and, in advanced roles, prescriptive authority (Byrne, Richardson, Brunsdon, & Patel, 2000). Therefore nurses must recognize a variety of factors, including social, cultural, and environmental factors and the individual client's lifestyle to more effectively use drug information to better care for their clients. Acquiring knowledge about drugs is a lifelong component of the nursing role for safe and effective practice.

✳ What is a drug?

A **drug** is any substance used in the diagnosis, cure, treatment, or prevention of a disease or condition. A drug collects three different types of names as it passes through the investigational stages before being approved and marketed. The first is the chemical name, the second is the generic or nonproprietary name, and the third is the trade, brand, or proprietary name.

✳ Studying pharmacology seems complex enough; why is it that each drug has at least three names?

The **chemical name** is a precise description of the chemical composition and molecular structure of the drug. This name is particularly meaningful to the chemist. For example, the chemical name of a popular analgesic is *N*-(4-hydroxyphenyl) acetamide. Its generic name is acetaminophen, and it is also sold under a number of brand or trade names—Tylenol, Tempra, and Panadol, among others.

The manufacturer, with the approval of the United States Adopted Name (USAN) Council, often assigns the **generic** or **nonproprietary name.** The USAN Council helps to select simple, informative, and unique nonproprietary names for drugs by establishing logical nomenclature classifications based on pharmacologic and/or chemical relationships. Because the generic name is simpler than the chemical name, it is the official name listed in official compendiums, such as the *United States Pharmacopeia (USP)*.

When drug companies market a particular drug product, they often select and copyright a **trade, brand,** or **proprietary name** for their drug. This copyright restricts the use of the name to only the individual drug company. Because numerous brand names may exist for the same ingredient, such as for acetaminophen, prescribers are encouraged to use the generic name. The use of generic names is also widely advocated to avoid confusion between similar-sounding trade names (see the Medication Safety Alert box below). On occasion, the manufacturer may reformulate a drug product using a new generic drug yet retain the older, recognized, brand name. This is an additional source of confusion for clients and health care professionals alike.

In the hospital setting, it is more common to see generic names used, but in the community, in which pharmaceutical companies market directly to prescribers with representatives visiting health providers' practices or to consumers by television ads, it is more common to see trade names. The brand, trade, or proprietary name of drugs discussed in this text will be enclosed in parentheses following the generic name.

Extensive advertising is often used to encourage health care provider prescribing and to promote sales of the trade name drug. Pharmaceutical manufacturers are now extensively advertising prescription drugs directly to consumers, with the expense of this advertising borne mainly by the consumer. However, much of the research in new drugs is performed in laboratories of reputable drug firms. To realize a legitimate return for the cost of research, drug companies need to patent their products and have exclusive rights to their manufacture and sale for a specified time period.

With some exceptions, the majority of generic drug products sold are considered therapeutically equivalent to the trade name product. Most states in the United States and provinces in Canada allow pharmacists to substitute generic drugs when filling a prescription unless the prescriber has indicated that the trade name form of the drug is essential. Generic products are often much less expensive than trade name drugs.

A drug may be considered a **prescription drug** or a **legend drug,** which means it requires a legal prescription to be dispensed; or it may be a **nonprescription** or **over-the-counter (OTC) drug,** a drug that may be purchased without a prescription. Some prescription drugs may be purchased in lower doses that are considered relatively safe for sale OTC. Such a drug is ibuprofen, which is sold as an OTC drug in its 200-mg strength (Advil or Motrin IB) but requires a prescription for the 400-, 600-, or 800-mg tablet.

✳ Where do drugs come from?

Drugs and biologic products are identified or derived from four main sources: (1) plants, from which drugs such as digoxin, vincristine, and colchicine are obtained (Figure 1-1); (2) animals and humans, from which drugs such as epinephrine, insulin, and adrenocorticotropic hormone are obtained; (3) minerals or mineral products, such as iron, iodine, and zinc; and (4) synthetic or chemical substances made in the laboratory. The drugs made of chemical substances are pure drugs, and some of them are simple sub-

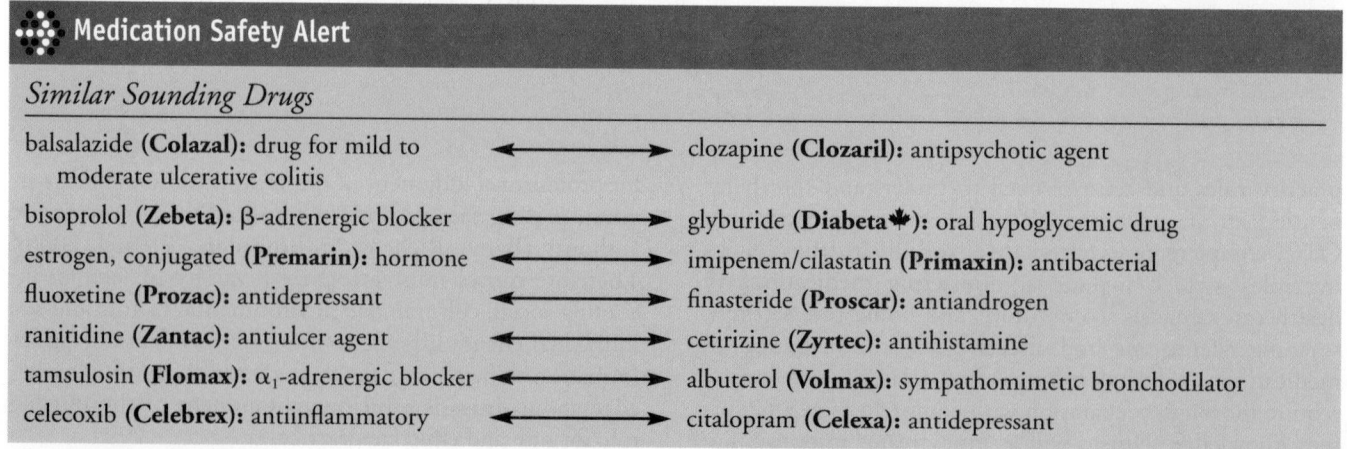

⁛ Medication Safety Alert

Similar Sounding Drugs

balsalazide (**Colazal**): drug for mild to moderate ulcerative colitis	⟷	clozapine (**Clozaril**): antipsychotic agent
bisoprolol (**Zebeta**): β-adrenergic blocker	⟷	glyburide (**Diabeta**✿): oral hypoglycemic drug
estrogen, conjugated (**Premarin**): hormone	⟷	imipenem/cilastatin (**Primaxin**): antibacterial
fluoxetine (**Prozac**): antidepressant	⟷	finasteride (**Proscar**): antiandrogen
ranitidine (**Zantac**): antiulcer agent	⟷	cetirizine (**Zyrtec**): antihistamine
tamsulosin (**Flomax**): α₁-adrenergic blocker	⟷	albuterol (**Volmax**): sympathomimetic bronchodilator
celecoxib (**Celebrex**): antiinflammatory	⟷	citalopram (**Celexa**): antidepressant

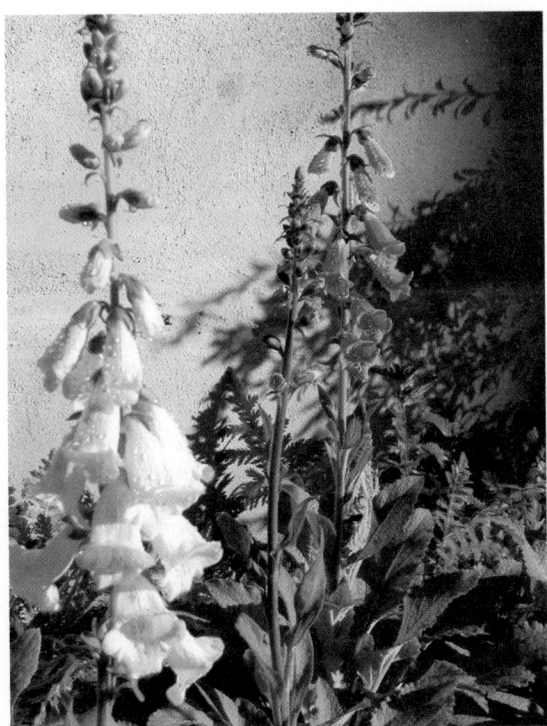

FIGURE 1-1 Foxglove—source of digitoxin and digoxin.

stances, such as sodium bicarbonate and magnesium hydroxide. Others are products of complex synthesis, such as the sulfonamides and the adrenocorticosteroids.

The leaves, roots, seeds, and other parts of plants may be dried or otherwise processed for use as a medicine and, as such, are known as crude drugs. The chemical substances they contain produce their therapeutic effect; however, because of differences in growing conditions, the amount of active ingredient in the product varies. When the pharmacologically active constituents are separated from the crude preparation, the resulting substances are more potent and usually produce effects more reliably than does the crude drug. Today, most drugs in common use are synthetic preparations.

✳ Why is a system of drug classification important?
The thousands of drugs available would present a formidable study if they had to be approached as individual agents. Fortunately, drugs can be systematically classified into a reasonable number of drug groups on the basis of chemical, pharmacologic, or therapeutic relatedness.

Drug classification may be approached from a number of perspectives: clinical indication, mechanism of action, or body system. This book uses these approaches when appropriate. Two examples of drugs classified by clinical indication are Chapter 37: "Bronchodilator, Antiasthmatic, and Mucolytic Drugs" and Chapter 59: "Antifungal and Antiviral Drugs." An example of drugs classified by body system is Unit Four: "Drugs Affecting the Central Nervous System."

These drug groupings can assist you to understand and learn about the individual agents available for drug therapy. Understanding the characteristic effects of a particular class of drugs at the cellular, tissue, organ, and functional system levels permits you to extrapolate information to a wide variety of drugs. A typical representative drug can be selected and studied and its specific characteristics compared with those of others in the same class. In this way, the individual gradually builds a knowledge base.

Pharmacology becomes easier when you understand the common characteristics of each drug classification and when a *key* or *prototype* drug within each group is studied thoroughly. When a new drug becomes available, you will be able to associate it with its drug classification and make inferences about many of its basic qualities before reading about its specific properties. Learning which of the qualities of a new drug are different from those of the prototype drug and its dosage is extremely helpful.

The basic information to be learned about each major drug includes its generic name and original trade name, the category to which it belongs, its clinical uses, mechanism of action, adverse effects, contraindications, precautions, significant drug interactions, and nurse's role in managing the care of a client who is receiving that drug. Nursing management of a client's drug regimen includes initial assessment of the client, making nursing diagnoses for which the client may be at risk during the drug regimen, monitoring the drug therapy, appropriate administration of the drug, client education, and evaluation of the drug's effectiveness for this client. "Looking it up" should become second nature to both nursing students and practicing nurses. *Nurses are professionally, morally, legally,* and *personally* responsible for every dose of medication they administer.

The release of new drugs and new information on old drugs are ongoing events. Much remains to be learned about the actual mode of action of many commonly prescribed drugs and the effects from prolonged use. Furthermore, there is increasing concern about drug-induced disease. Fortunately, drug therapy is temporary for most conditions or for illness prevention. However, some diseases require lifelong use of drugs to sustain life (such as insulin for type 1 diabetes mellitus) or prolonged use to maintain relatively normal physiologic or psychological functioning (such as phenytoin [Dilantin] for seizure disorders).

Lists of drugs, dosages, and their indications should not be regarded as dogma. Laboratory research and new scientific methods of evaluation are constantly generating new information. Sometimes there are reports that a drug, even an old and trusted one, is suspected of causing mutations, birth defects, cancer, cardiac dysrhythmias, or less serious secondary effects. Not only nursing students but also practicing nurses are challenged by the proliferation of drugs; most of the drugs on the market today were developed recently. Change is the only constant in pharmacology.

✳ How does a nurse keep pharmacology knowledge current?
News releases and numerous articles, journals, and books are written in an attempt to keep up with the new discoveries about new and old drugs. This text provides you with a basic foundation of drug knowledge. However, it is unrealistic to believe that a nurse can know everything there is to know

about all medications on the market. Therefore the practitioner must know how and where to obtain general and detailed drug information. Many excellent drug references are available, each with a specific focus and/or emphasis. Because no single reference is a complete source of drug data to meet the varied and specialized needs of clinical practice today, be familiar with the primary drug reference sources available. Table 1-2 lists major drug information resources.

TABLE 1-2 MAJOR DRUG INFORMATION RESOURCES*	
Reference	**Comments**
BOOKS	
American Hospital Formulary Service (AHFS) Drug Information (Bethesda, MD: American Society of Hospital Pharmacists, Inc.)	Objective overview in monograph form Comprehensive source of comparative, unbiased drug information on nearly every available drug in United States Issues supplements; updated annually Widely used drug information source for all health care professionals
Compendium of Pharmaceuticals and Specialties (CPS) (Ottawa, Ontario, Canada: Canadian Pharmaceutical Association)	Widely used reference source in Canada for all health care professionals Published annually Contains manufacturers' addresses and phone numbers
Drug Facts and Comparisons (St. Louis: Facts and Comparisons)	Comprehensive drug information arranged to facilitate comparisons and evaluations Contains package sizes and strengths plus cost index information Contains manufacturers' addresses and phone numbers Contains section for orphan drugs, diagnostic aids, radiopaque agents, antidotes, and drugs in development Widely used reference source, especially for pharmacists
Handbook of Nonprescription Drugs (Washington, DC: American Pharmaceutical Association)	Comprehensive OTC drug information Reviews physiology, the primary minor illnesses, and the drugs used in treatment Has tables with specific OTC drug information
Lexicomp's Drug Information Handbook (Hudson, OH: Lexi-Comp)	Widely used by pharmacists and prescribers Contains drug monographs Modest nursing implications Revised annually
Mosby's Drug Consult (St. Louis: Mosby)	Comprehensive drug information Contains drug product identification charts Includes product ratings (equivalent/not equivalent classifications) from FDA Has drug cost comparisons Lists foreign brand availability Published annually
Physicians' Desk Reference (PDR) (Oradell, NJ: Medical Economics)	Widely used source for health care professionals Pharmaceutical industry finances the book Drug information same as drug package insert Lacks comparative information on safety and efficacy Lacks nursing information Contains drug product identification section and manufacturers' addresses and phone numbers
USP DI: Drug Information for the Health Care Professional (Greenwood Village, CO:MICROMEDEX Thomson Healthcare)	Available in several volumes; volume I is for health care professionals, and volume II offers advice for clients in lay language Consists of extensive drug monographs with practical information Highlights clinically significant information to reduce drug risks Issues monthly updates; updated annually Highly recommended drug reference for all health care professionals

*All of these references are available in an electronic format.

Any nursing process is only as effective as the knowledge base and the analytic thought that goes into it. Logic and judgment improve as the nurse's information base is perfected, partly as experience is tested against knowledge. Nowhere is ongoing self-learning more essential than in nursing pharmacotherapeutics. The "need to know" escalates, for example, when a nurse who is responsible for administering medications is confronted with an order for an unfamiliar drug or with an unexpected client symptom not usually associated with the diagnosis.

❋ **Is drug information available in the clinical setting?**
Health care agencies commonly furnish sources of drug information. The area or unit in which a nurse works often has a nursing library shelf and/or electronic resources within the clinical setting that contains pharmacology information and other material of interest. Any nurse can initiate the development of such material and request funds or supplies. The agency's nursing staff development department is responsible for promoting ongoing and updated learning and can facilitate audiovisual aids, references, or a seminar program. A call to the agency's pharmacist will always provide the needed information.

With the proliferation of medical sites on the Internet, many search engines and directories are available to provide both general and specialized drug information for health care professionals and clients. Many professional journals (nursing, pharmacy, medical) also provide current drug information, and a number of them are also available on the Internet. Select the Internet site carefully when seeking drug information, because erroneous information may also be posted. Because there is no screening tool for Internet information, the best approach is to be knowledgeable about the reputation of the provider of the information, for example: drug information from drug information centers; pharmacy, medical, or nursing school posted information; professional journals; and the American Cancer Society, the Food and Drug Administration (FDA), the National Institutes of Health (NIH), and numerous other organizations.

Building a personal library and keeping it current are also important professional activities. No one text is a complete source of all the pharmacology information necessary for nursing practice. Nurses must gather reliable information from various sources to meet clinical needs.

❋ **What is the scope of nursing responsibility for drug therapy?**
Drugs can either help or harm. Nurses, physicians, nurse practitioners, physician assistants, and clinical pharmacists are held legally responsible for safe and therapeutically effective drug administration. Specifically, nurses are liable for their actions and omissions and for the duties they delegate to others, including medication technicians, pharmacy technicians, practical nurses, and even physicians. They are personally responsible—legally, morally, and ethically—for every drug they administer or have administered, no matter

TABLE 1-2 DRUG INFORMATION RESOURCES*—cont'd	
Reference	**Comments**
NEWSLETTERS	
The Medical Letter (New Rochelle, NY: The Medical Letter)	Biweekly newsletter with evaluation of the efficacy, safety, rationale, and price comparison of current medications Objective summaries Valuable newsletter, highly recommended
Prescriber's Letter: The Most Practical Alerts and Advice, for Prescribers, on Developments in Drug Therapy (Stockton, CA: Prescriber's Letter)	Monthly newsletter provided concise information Subscribers can obtain detailed information about any item Provides unbiased and evidence-based approach to medications
OTHER RESOURCES	
Epocrates Rx Online (San Mateo, CA)	Drug and formulary reference available for both Palm and Pocket PC OS users
Various drug handbooks for nurses	Give brief overviews of drugs in outline format Helpful as quick refreshers on the unit to remind nurse of important points once nurse has had a course in pharmacology Drug information is formatted according to the nursing process; gives nursing considerations
Computerized pharmacology databases	Available in most health agencies Allow drug information to be printed so clients have it for personal use Some systems allow individualization of information for clients Many databases are adapted for handheld systems

who actually prescribed it. Indeed, all members of a health care team may be held liable for a single injury to a client. The increase in litigation against nurses and physicians indicates that society tolerates only a minimal margin of error in relation to human injury and life. Claims have been brought against health care professionals for drug errors that caused loss of life and permanent injury. When these claims are supported with evidence that the conduct of one or more health care professionals helped to bring about the loss or injury, those parties may be held liable. The law, a legal and social norm, requires health care professionals to be safe and competent practitioners and permits compensation to those harmed or injured.

However, the law is also a protective force for the knowledgeable, competent, and responsible nurse. Nurses who are determined to safeguard clients from drug-induced harm will, for example:

- Keep their knowledge base current
- Refer to authoritative sources in professional literature and to prescribers and pharmacists
- Use correct techniques and precautions
- Observe and chart drug effects explicitly
- Question a drug order that is unclear or that appears to contain an error
- Refuse to administer or refuse to allow others to order or administer a drug if there is reason to believe it will be harmful
- Use sound nursing judgment

The law, in turn, protects such nurses from unfair litigation. Chapter 2 discusses in greater detail the legal role of the nurse related to drug therapy.

Nurses are entrusted with potent and habit-forming drugs, and they must not abuse or misuse this trust. Drugs are comforting and lifesaving when used respectfully and intelligently, but they can lead to tragedy when used unwisely or with undue dependence. The nurse who combines diligent and intelligent observation with moral integrity and factual knowledge is a safe and competent practitioner and a credit to the nursing profession.

In addition, the nurse must establish with the client a "therapeutic alliance," a respectful and trusting relationship to facilitate the highest attainable level of self-care. The client is the most important participant in the team effort for safe and effective drug administration. Clients are not expected to be submissive, acquiescent, and unquestioning followers of the health team's instructions; they must be motivated to assume responsibility for their own care. Nurses must recognize that the willingness to participate is ultimately the client's. All the nurse's knowledge, skill, and ability are brought to bear on the establishment of a therapeutic alliance to facilitate the most appropriate level of self-care related to medications.

Paying close attention to all drugs the nurse administers helps the nurse to learn to identify them, tailor their application, and spot errors before they occur. Expertise is built in just this fashion. Learning the names of drugs, their formulations, and their pharmacologic actions is best accomplished in small increments and in a systematic way by making associations with information about a known drug

in a classification, its close analogues, and clients for whom the nurse has provided care. The learning value of the analysis and synthesis of data in actual practice far outweighs that of memorizing long lists of unrelated drugs and their properties.

Nurses in emergency departments (EDs) and in community health practices are often challenged to identify medications from a client's personal unlabeled pillboxes or containers. Often many varieties of drugs and pieces of tablets are mixed together. Clients are often unable to assist in identifying their drugs, having never been properly educated by health care providers. The *Physician's Desk Reference (PDR)*, the *USP DI: Drug Information for the Health Care Professional (USP DI)*, and *Mosby's Drug Consult* provide actual photographs of drugs to assist the health care professional in identifying an unknown tablet or capsule. In addition, manufacturers often place an identification code consisting of letters or numbers on their solid oral dosage forms. Although these markings may not be meaningful to the practicing nurse, pharmacists and local drug information centers can use them as aids in identifying generic and trade products. Difficult identification problems can be referred to the FDA Drug Listing Branch or the FDA Division of Poison Control, both of which are located in Rockville, Maryland.

Pharmacology books must be kept up-to-date in the nurse's library. In addition, official current literature on drugs must be followed carefully, because new drugs only slowly make their way into more permanent literature. For the nurse working in a hospital or home health service, physicians, instructors, in-service educators, and pharmacists are on hand to help. In a more isolated practice, greater personal effort is required to maintain currency. In all cases, nurses must pay close attention to the drug therapy of their clients.

Learning is an active process. Clinical experience with drugs is invaluable, because it enables you to do the following:

- Note which drugs are most commonly used to treat certain diseases or specific signs and symptoms
- Note the dosage of and the frequency with which drugs are administered
- Observe which drugs are most effective in relieving particular signs and symptoms
- Witness individual differences in clients' reactions to a specific drug
- Relate knowledge obtained from authoritative sources to real-life situations
- Apply the nursing process to drug therapy

Regardless of what is to be learned, reasoning and the ability to analyze and synthesize information are prerequisites to understanding. These cognitive skills, along with perceptual skills, permit you to see meaningful relationships, make comparisons, and determine significance, all of which are essential for sound decision making in nursing.

How does pharmacology relate to the nursing process?

The nursing process is a systematic method for identifying actual or potential health care problems or impediments to the activities of daily living. It points the way to rational nursing actions and the objective evaluation of care, which care, in the case of pharmacology, is related to the client's drug regimen.

The direction of the nursing process is fairly universal in the field, although its structure may vary from the widely used pattern of four phases or steps: (1) assessment of data (which may culminate in a nursing diagnosis), (2) planning, (3) implementation, and (4) evaluation.

To apply the nursing process to drug therapy, nurses *assess* the medication needs of their clients partly in terms of how these needs are matched by the prescriber's orders; to do this they consider the indications of the drug, the client's preexisting health conditions, and any medications the client is currently taking. The result of this assessment is the *nursing diagnosis*. These may be expressed as actual nursing diagnoses, or ones for which the client is at risk with this drug regimen. Collaborative problems, certain physiologic complications that nurses monitor to detect onset or changes in status, should also be considered. Nurses make *plans* that include goals directly related to the client's nursing diagnoses and specific outcome criteria. This sets the stage for *implementation* of the goals using specific, evidenced-based nursing actions. Implementation may include *monitoring* the client for therapeutic and nontherapeutic effects of the drug and ability to manage the therapeutic regimen; *intervention* related to preparing and administering a medication as ordered, or to withholding a dose and obtaining a change in the medication order; and *client education* for the safe and accurate self-administration of the drug by the client or caregiver. The final step is the *evaluation* of the nursing care provided based on the level of achievement of the outcome criteria for which the client and nurse have planned. Each time nursing care is evaluated, the knowledge base of a nurse increases and becomes more valuable. The nursing process is discussed in more detail in Chapter 5.

How will this textbook help me to gain knowledge in pharmacology?

This text orients the reader to nursing pharmacology and therapeutics by presenting a firm theoretic foundation and a practical approach to drug therapy that is applicable in many settings—the home, the clinic, the extended care facility, the office, the classroom, and the hospital.

Part I provides general principles, theories, and facts about drugs and their administration. Practical information about the integration of the nursing process with pharmacology is presented, and general principles of action are given to facilitate your learning in both academic and clinical environments. The rest of the book presents specific drug information about clinical applications and nursing management of the care of clients receiving specific medications. Thus this book can be used both as a text and as a reference.

To find information about a particular drug in this book, do the following:

- Look it up in the index.
- When you find the information about the drug, refer back to the beginning of the chapter or unit and read the material that precedes the specific discussion.

Reading only the pages listed in the index will illuminate only the specifics of the drug, which will be out of context and without the necessary fundamental information about that class of drugs. Reading the background information offers an overall perspective and places the drug information into an understandable framework.

What is an effective way to learn pharmacology?

One of the more effective ways to study pharmacology is to understand the pharmacologic characteristics of a classification of drugs: its major uses; mechanisms of action; absorption, distribution, metabolism, and excretion; onset and duration of action; and adverse effects. Identify the key drug in each classification. Throughout the book, key drugs are highlighted with the symbol ■. These drugs can be studied as representatives of the drug classification under discussion. Other drugs within the classification can then be identified by the manner in which they differ from the prototype. This approach will enhance learning rather than the rote memorization of a multiplicity of facts about each and every drug.

The specific drug information in the text summarizes what is needed to administer drugs safely and competently. Each discussion is titled with some of the common names by which the particular drug is known. The trade names of drugs that are available in Canada but not in the United States are followed by a maple leaf symbol (❖).

In the sections that present specific drug information, the **mechanism of action** explaining how the drug acts at the biochemical or cellular level to produce its therapeutic effects is initially presented. The officially approved therapeutic purposes of the drug or the conditions for which it is used are detailed as **indications**. The **pharmacokinetics** section specifies how the drug is absorbed, distributed, associated with tissue, biotransformed or metabolized, and excreted. This section is often combined with the **dosage** section, which presents the currently approved regimen governing the amount, frequency, and number of doses of a therapeutic agent. The section titled **adverse effects** details most of the common nontherapeutic effects that may be experienced when the drug is administered. When applicable, **drug interactions** are also listed. It must be noted that not all drugs have been tested for safety and efficacy in administration to adults older than 65 years of age, pregnant women, women who are breastfeeding, or children. The routes and special techniques for drug preparation are also listed. **Pregnancy Safety** boxes list the FDA pregnancy safety category associated with various drugs, which indicates the documented problems with the use of a drug during pregnancy.

The nursing management sections describe distinctive nursing measures:

Assessment involves gathering data about an individual's experience with medications and allergies, identifying preexisting health status and medical conditions that might influence the choice of dosage of drug and/or concurrent drugs that might cause significant interactions, determining the potential outcome and suggested management of such interactions, and performing baseline observations that are essential for measuring changes in the client's health status during the medication regimen or for determining whether administration of the drug is appropriate.

Nursing diagnosis involves identifying selected nursing diagnoses that nurses, by virtue of their education and experience, are able and licensed to treat, and **collaborative problems,** which are physiologic complications that nurses monitor to detect their onset or changes in status (Carpenito-Moyet, 2004).

Planning is an important step in the nursing process; these are expressed as goals for the drug regimen. However, to prevent redundancies within the discussion of each drug, modifications to administration of the drug are found in the intervention section, and outcome criteria are discussed in the evaluation section.

Implementation incorporates the nursing activities of monitoring, intervention, and client education, which need to be planned to administer a specific drug safely and accurately: *Monitoring:* significant observations relative to the client's health status, including diagnostic and laboratory tests that ensure a safe and effective drug regimen; *Intervention:* special handling, timing of doses, and other significant aspects of the actual administration of a drug; and *Education:* client teaching to enable the client and/or caregiver to effectively manage the therapeutic medication regimen at home.

Evaluation provides the planned outcome criteria or nursing outcomes for reviewing care of the client in regard to safe and effective drug therapy.

Safe, therapeutically effective drug administration is a major responsibility of nurses. It depends on sound, current knowledge of medications and careful monitoring of their effects on clients. With increasingly shorter lengths of stay by clients in acute and subacute care settings, nurses have an increasing responsibility to ensure that clients and caregivers can effectively manage the medication regimen at home. Ongoing laboratory and clinical research modifies and enlarges available drug information, necessitating a continual effort to keep one's knowledge up-to-date. The modes of action of many commonly prescribed drugs, the effects of their prolonged use, and the possibility of drug-induced disease are yet to be completely understood. There are many sources of current drug information, but even the most diligent student of these sources requires clinical experience to develop competence in drug administration. Few areas of nursing demand more intellectual curiosity, integrity, factual knowledge, and motivation to use reference sources than pharmacology.

Summary

Pharmacology, the study of drug effects within a living system, has always been linked to our concept of health and illness and therefore has held importance for humanity through the ages.

Each drug is identified by three names: the chemical name; the generic (nonproprietary) name, which is generally a simplification of the chemical name; and the trade, brand, or proprietary name under which the pharmaceutical company markets the drug. Because generic drugs are less expensive than trade name drugs, most states allow pharmacists to substitute them for trade name drugs within limitations.

Drugs are classified either by clinical indication, mechanism of action, or by body system. Drug classifications facilitate the nurse's understanding of pharmacology by allowing the conceptualization of the common characteristics of each grouping and the key or prototype drug, and the association of new drugs with a particular classification.

Pharmacology is a field of ever-increasing importance for nursing. Because nurses are held by law to be responsible for the drugs they administer, they should maintain a current knowledge base and be competent in the assessment, planning, implementation, and evaluation of the client's nursing care. This text will assist the learner in achieving that knowledge and competence within pharmacology.

✸ Critical Thinking Questions

- Why is the study of pharmacology important for nurses? Think of three clinical examples that would indicate its importance to the care of clients.

- Review the structure of one of the later chapters that discusses a classification of drugs. Consider how you might go about studying for an examination on that chapter.

- A nurse in the process of administering medications is confronted with a prescriber's order for a drug with which the nurse is unfamiliar. What sources of drug information could the nurse use?

---

 e-**LEARNING SUPPLEMENTS**

Student CD-ROM
- Final Exam questions
- NCLEX® Examination review questions
- Pharmacology animations
- Printable chapter summary

Evolve Website (http://evolve.elsevier.com/mckenry)
- Content updates, including information on new drugs
- WebLinks corresponding to this chapter
- Answers to the critical thinking questions in this chapter
- *Elsevier ePharmacology Update* newsletter
- *Mosby's Drug Consult* Internet Edition
- Supplemental and reference information

Bibliography

American Medical Association. (2003). United States Adopted Names. Retrieved September 27, 2003, from http://www.ama-assn.org/ama/pub/category/2956.htmlAnderson, D.M. (2002). *Mosby's medical, nursing, and allied health dictionary* (6th ed.). St. Louis: Mosby.

Byrne, G., Richardson, M., Brunsdon, J., & Patel, A. (2000). Patient satisfaction with emergency nurse practitioners in A&E. *Journal of Clinical Nursing 9*(1), 83-93.

Carpenito-Moyet, L.J. (2004). *Nursing diagnosis: Applications to clinical practice* (10th ed.). Philadelphia: Lippincott, Williams & Wilkins.

Drug facts and comparisons (58th ed.). (2005). St. Louis: Facts and Comparisons.

Gebbie, K., Rosenstock, L., & Hernandez, L.M. (Eds.). (2002). *Who will keep the public healthy: Educating public health professionals for the 21st century.* Washington, DC: Institute of Medicine.

Leake, C.D. (1975). *An historical account of pharmacology to the twentieth century.* Springfield, IL: Charles C. Thomas.

Lyons, A.S., & Petrucelli, R.J. II. (1978). *Medicine: An illustrated history.* New York: Harry N. Abrams.

Mosby's drug consult (15th ed.). (2005). St. Louis: Mosby.

Oermann, M.H., Harris, C.H., & Dammeyer, J.A. (2001). Teaching by the nurse: How important is it to patients? *Applied Nursing Research 14*(1), 11-17.

Roger, F.B. (1972). *A syllabus of medical history.* Boston: Little, Brown.

Ross, M., Mutnick, B., & Murhammer, J. (2003). Look-alike, sound-alike drug name confusion, virtual hospital. Retrieved September 27, 2003, from http://www.vh.org/adult/provider/pharmacyservices/RXUpdate/2001/08RXU.html

Siler, W.A. (1982). *Death by prescription* (Revised 2nd ed.). Tallahassee, FL: Health Care Projects.

USP DI: Drug information for the health care professional (25th ed.). (2005). Greenwood Village, CO: MICROMEDEX Thomson Healthcare.

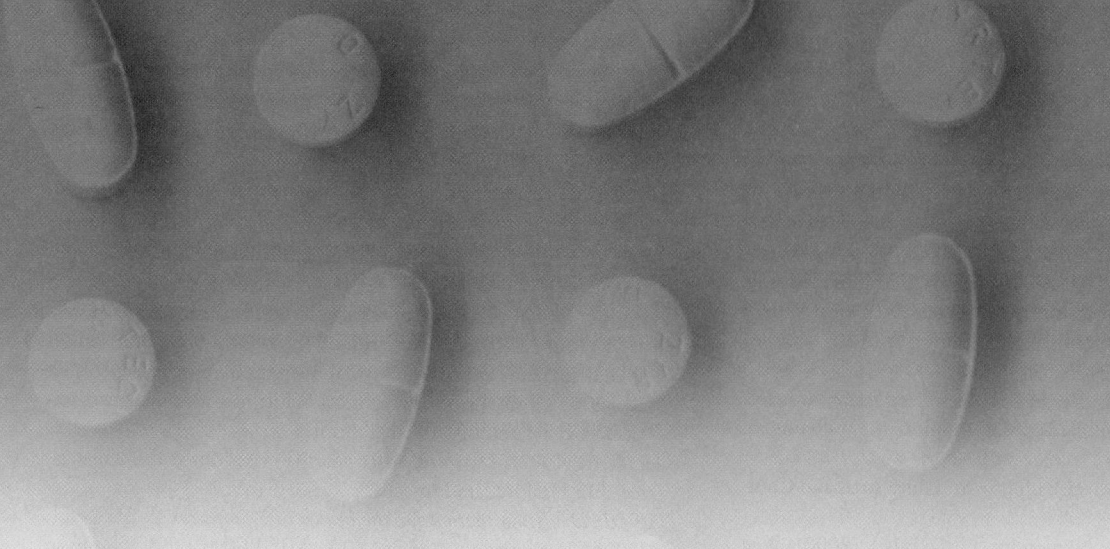

LEGAL AND ETHICAL ASPECTS OF MEDICATION ADMINISTRATION

CHAPTER FOCUS

As the professional role changes to keep pace with technologic advances, the role of nursing becomes more complex and nurses have gained autonomy over their practice. With this autonomy has come greater legal accountability, and nurses must consider this responsibility as they practice. However, even the law and the technologic advances in health care are not sufficient to cope with many of the ethical dilemmas faced by nurses. This chapter discusses the legal foundations for and ethical considerations of the nursing management of pharmacotherapeutics.

LEARNING OBJECTIVES

- Describe the historical development of governmental regulation to protect the public from harmful drugs.
- Differentiate between over-the-counter and prescription drugs.
- Identify the process used in the development and evaluation of a new drug before marketing.
- Describe the government's regulatory procedure for evaluating over-the-counter drugs and prescription drugs for safety and effectiveness.
- Identify legislative or authoritative source(s) for drug standards.
- Explain the difference between permissive and mandatory drug substitution in the United States.
- Describe the U.S. Food and Drug Administration's pregnancy categories for drugs.
- Describe the nurse's role in drug research.
- Explore the ethical issues involved in the administration of medications.

▲ KEY TERMS

Many remedies of the past lacked the information taken for granted today, such as the strength of the substance in a preparation or even the ingredients themselves. This type of medical practice, although not always ineffective, extended well into the nineteenth century. Not until the twentieth century were standards for drug identification, drug preparation, and proof of drug effectiveness and safety required.

✱ How have U.S. legislation and drug standardization come about to protect the public?

Before 1906, patent medicines and remedies were sold by medicine men in traveling wagon shows, in drugstores, by mail order, and by doctors, real or self-titled. Such products were not required to have a list of ingredients on the label,

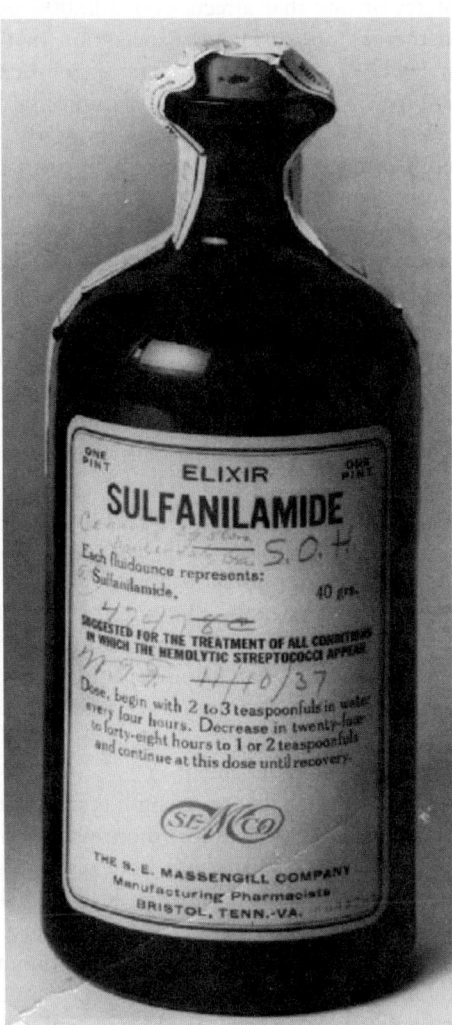

FIGURE 2-1 Continuing problems with dangerous drugs that fell outside the parameters of the Pure Food and Drugs Act finally received national attention with the Elixir Sulfanilamide disaster in 1937. Massengill distributed this preparation without testing for safety (which was not required by law). Because it contained diethylene glycol as a vehicle, a chemical analogue of antifreeze, over 100 people died, many of whom were children.

From Center for Drug Evaluation and Research. *A brief history of the Center for Drug Evaluation and Research.* Rockville, MD: Department of Health and Human Services, Public Health Service, Food and Drug Administration.

so many contained potent and dangerous drugs such as opium, morphine, heroin, chloral hydrate, and alcohol. Many persons, especially infants and children, were reportedly injured, became addicted, or died as a result of ingesting the ingredients contained in these preparations

In 1906, the first U.S. law, the federal Pure Food and Drug Act, was passed to protect the public from adulterated or mislabeled drugs. The law required a drug company to declare on the package label the presence of any of 11 drugs identified as being dangerous and perhaps addictive (some of which were in the list just mentioned). However, this first law had loopholes and required subsequent legislative change.

The Pure Food and Drug Act of 1906 designated the *United States Pharmacopeia* and the *National Formulary* as official drug standards and empowered the federal government to enforce them. Drugs had to meet the standards of strength and purity professed for them, and labels had to indicate the type and amount of morphine or other narcotic ingredients present. In 1912, Congress passed the Sherley Amendment, prohibiting the use of fraudulent therapeutic claims.

The next drug legislation occurred in 1938 with the passage of the Federal Food, Drug, and Cosmetic Act. This Act was important because it prevented new drugs from being marketed before being properly tested for safety. Although introduced in 1933, it was not passed until more than 100 deaths had occurred from ingestion of a diethylene glycol solution of sulfanilamide that had been marketed as an "elixir" without investigation of its toxicity (Figure 2-1).

The Durham-Humphrey Amendment of 1952 further changed the 1938 drug act by specifying how prescription, or legend, drugs and refills could be ordered and dispensed (Box 2-1). This amendment also recognized a second class of drugs, over-the-counter (OTC) drugs, for which prescriptions are not required.

In 1958, the U.S. Senate began investigating the drug industry, which reported huge profits and used false or misleading promotions of some drugs. This investigation received little support until the thalidomide tragedy in Europe. Thalidomide, a sedative marketed in Europe, was found to be responsible for severe deformities in thousands of infants

---

BOX 2-1 PRESCRIPTION (LEGEND) DRUGS

Legend drugs must bear the legend "Caution: Federal law prohibits dispensing without prescription." These include most drugs given by injection and the following:

- Hypnotic, narcotic, or habit-forming drugs or derivatives thereof as specified in the law
- Drugs that because of their toxicity or method of use are not safe unless administered under the supervision of a licensed practitioner (physician, dentist, nurse practitioner, or physician assistant)
- New drugs that are limited to investigational use or new drugs that are not considered safe for indiscriminate use by the public.

whose mothers had taken the drug during early pregnancy. These events led to passage of the Kefauver-Harris Amendment in 1962. (Thalidomide is currently available in the United States for the treatment and maintenance therapy of erythema nodosum leprosum [leprosy]. It is also available as an **orphan drug**—a drug developed under the Orphan Drug Act [see later]—for use in bone marrow transplantation, acquired immunodeficiency syndrome [AIDS], and several other conditions.) Thalidomide—as do other high-risk drugs—carries a **"black box" warning,** which is the most serious type of warning in prescription drug labeling by the U.S. Food and Drug Administration (FDA).

The Kefauver-Harris Amendment required proof of both the safety and efficacy of a new drug before it could be approved for use. It also required that informed consent be obtained from research study subjects. To uphold the new safety and efficacy standard, the FDA signed a contract in 1966 with the National Academy of Sciences and the National Research Council (NAS/NRC) to study all supporting data for therapeutic claims for drugs introduced since 1938. This program of study was called the Drug Efficacy Study Implementation (DESI).

Under DESI review, thousands of drugs and therapeutic claims have been evaluated and many ineffective drugs have been withdrawn from the market. For example, guaifenesin

---

BOX 2-2 IMPORTANT DRUG LEGISLATION (UNITED STATES)

Food, Drug, and Cosmetic Act of 1938: Mandated that drug manufacturers must test all drugs for harmful effects and that drug labels must be accurate and complete

Durham-Humphrey Amendment of 1952: Distinguished more clearly between drugs that can be sold with or without a prescription and those that cannot be refilled

Drug Amendment of 1962 (Kefauver-Harris Act): Tightened controls over drug safety and statements about adverse effects and contraindications, drug testing methods, and drug effectiveness criteria

Controlled Substances Act of 1970 (Comprehensive Drug Abuse Prevention and Control Act of 1970): Categorized controlled substances on the basis of their relative potential for abuse

Drug Regulation Reform Act of 1978: Shortened the drug investigation process to release drugs sooner to the public

Orphan Drug Act of 1983: Allowed drug companies to take tax deductions for about three-quarters of the cost of clinical studies for drugs that may offer little or no profit, but may benefit people with rare diseases

Drug Price Competition and Patent Term Restoration Act of 1984: Expanded the number of drugs suitable for an ANDA and allowed restoration of the time needed for drug approval to be added a pharmaceutical company's patent time.

(Robitussin) is the only expectorant classified as effective; others, such as terpin hydrate and ammonium chloride, are not approved for sale as expectorants. Drugs rated as "possibly effective" or "probably effective" are withdrawn or reformulated; however, a drug may remain on the market while claims are being modified and scientific data collected to substantiate its claims. An approved drug can be prescribed for a disorder for which the drug has not been FDA approved; this is called "off-label" use of the drug. Informed consent for this nonresearch application is generally not required.

In 1983, the Orphan Drug Act authorized the FDA to provide pharmaceutical manufacturers with grants and tax incentives to encourage drug research for the treatment of rare diseases or conditions. A rare disease is defined in the law as one that affects less than 200,000 people in the United States or one that affects over 200,000 people but for which there is no reasonable expectation that development costs will be recovered from U.S. sales of the drug. Because this type of research is typically unprofitable, it was limited before the passage of this act. Among the disorders that benefit from this research are cystic fibrosis, von Willebrand disease, leprosy (Hansen disease), Huntington disease, and rare cancers. Over 500 orphan drugs have been discovered and 200 have been marketed since passage of this Act (U.S. Food and Drug Administration, 2003c).

The Drug Price Competition and Patent Term Restoration Act of 1984 expanded the number of drugs suitable for an abbreviated new drug application (ANDA). ANDAs make it less costly and time-consuming for generics of already approved drugs, which are usually sold at lower prices than trade name drugs, to reach the market. Twenty years of legal protection are given to a pharmaceutical firm for each drug patent. Some of that time allowance is used while the drug goes through the approval process, so within this law, the "Patent Term Restoration" allows restoration of up to 5 years of lost patent time to the pharmaceutical manufacturer (U.S. Food and Drug Administration, 2003a). Box 2-2 provides a summary of important legislation.

✱ How are drugs standardized?

Drugs may vary considerably in strength and activity. Drugs obtained from plants (e.g., opium [morphine] and digitalis [digoxin]) may fluctuate in strength from plant to plant depending on where the plants are grown, the age at which they are harvested, and how they are preserved. Because accurate dosage and reliability of a drug's effect depend on uniformity of strength and purity, standardization is necessary.

The chemical or biologic technique by which the strength and purity of a drug are measured is known as **assay.** Chemical assay is a chemical analysis to determine the types and amounts of ingredients present. For example, opium is known to contain certain alkaloids, and these may vary greatly in different preparations. The U.S. official standard demands that opium contain not less than 9.5% and not more than 10.5% of anhydrous morphine. Opium of a higher morphine content may be reduced to the official standard by admixture with opium of a lower percentage or with certain other pharmacologically inactive diluents such as sucrose, lactose, glycyrrhiza, or magnesium carbonate.

With some drugs, either the active ingredients are not known or there are no available methods of analyzing and standardizing them. These drugs may be standardized by biologic methods in a process called bioassay. **Bioassay** is performed by determining the amount of a preparation required to produce a defined effect on a suitable laboratory animal under certain standard conditions. For example, the potency of a certain sample of insulin is measured by its ability to lower the blood sugar of rabbits.

❊ Who establishes the drug standards in the United States?

Since 1980, the only official book of drug standards in the United States has been the *United States Pharmacopeia (USP)*. Any drug included in this book has met high standards of quality, purity, and strength. Drugs meeting these criteria can be identified by the letters "USP" following the official name. The *USP DI: Drug Information for the Health Care Professional* is a distillation of the *USP* authoritative information for use by pharmacists, physicians, nurses, other health care professionals, and consumers and serves as a valuable resource in a clinical setting. Other valuable references more frequently available in the clinical setting are the *Physician's Desk Reference (PDR)*, which contains full text product labels, and the *American Hospital Formulary Service (AHFS) Drug Information*. Other drug information resources are reviewed in Chapter 1.

❊ Are OTC preparations regulated differently?

Of the estimated 400,000 drug products marketed in the United States and Canada, more than 300,000 are OTC drugs. These 300,000 individual drug products contain approximately 700 to 1000 active ingredients. In 1972, the FDA assembled an advisory review panel to perform an ingredient review, asking primarily the following questions: Are the ingredients safe and effective for consumers to self-medicate? and Are the labeling, indications, dosage instructions, and warnings sufficient? If they were found lacking, appropriate recommendations had to be developed.

This study, completed in 1983, found that approximately one-third of the ingredients reviewed were safe and effective for the labeled indications. Ingredients found particularly or potentially dangerous were either transferred to prescription status only (e.g., hexachlorophene, an antibacterial topical with a potential for inducing neurologic toxicities) or removed entirely from the market (e.g., camphorated oil or camphor liniment). (See Chapter 11 for a discussion of OTC medications.)

❊ Can a drug be changed from prescription status to OTC?

In the United States, the OTC review panels are primarily responsible for switching a number of prescription drugs to nonprescription or OTC status. These drug products are considered to be safe for self-treatment by consumers without professional guidance. Cimetidine (Tagamet HB), famotidine (Pepcid AC), diphenhydramine (Benadryl), and topical hydrocortisone are examples of products switched from prescription to OTC status. There may be differences in the OTC status of other drugs from country to country.

❊ Can a trade name drug be substituted for a generic drug on a prescription?

Although the prescriber retains the prerogative to require the dispensing of a particular brand of drug, nearly every state has a drug substitution law that either permits or mandates generic substitution by the pharmacist. In permissive states the prescriber must give express permission for substitution by either signing a special section on the prescription form or by checking the correct phrase on the prescription. If substitution is not wanted, the prescriber may note this by indicating "dispense as written," "brand necessary," or "medically necessary."

In states with a mandatory law, the pharmacist is required to dispense approved, less expensive, generic drugs to the client. Several exceptions apply in such situations; for example, the client's consent may be required before substitution, or the prescriber may mark the individual prescription with a term that prohibits substitution, such as "medically necessary."

❊ Are controlled substances regulated differently than other drugs?

The Harrison Narcotic Act (1914) was the first federal law aimed at curbing drug addiction or dependence. This law not only established the word "narcotic" as a legal term but also regulated the importation, manufacture, sale, and use of opium, cocaine, and all of their compounds and derivatives. Marijuana and its derivatives were also included in this act, as were many synthetic analgesic drugs that could produce or sustain either physical or psychological dependence. It made criminals of the estimated 200,000 users of narcotics in the United States at that time. Physicians were unable to write a narcotic prescription for an individual with an addition, even when it was part of a "cure" program. Although this was reversed in 1925, physicians were loathe to prescribe narcotics to addicts and an illegal drug distribution chain had become well-established.

This Act and other substance abuse amendments now have only historical import; they have been superseded by the Comprehensive Drug Abuse Prevention and Control Act of 1970, also known as the **Controlled Substances Act (CSA)**, which took effect May 1, 1971. This law was designed to prevent and provide increased research into substance abuse and dependence and to provide for treatment and rehabilitation of those who abuse drugs and those who are dependent on drugs. It also improved the administration and regulation of the manufacturing, distribution, and dispensing of **controlled substances** (drugs covered by this Act, which are classified according to their use and abuse potential) by legitimate handlers of these drugs to help reduce their widespread dispersion into illicit markets.

The CSA classifies controlled substances solely according to their potential for use and abuse. Drugs are classified into numbered levels, or schedules, from Schedule I to Schedule V (Table 2-1). Drugs with the highest abuse potential are placed in Schedule I; those with the lowest potential for abuse are in Schedule V. These classifications are flexible because drugs may occasionally be added or changed from one

TABLE 2-1 SCHEDULE OF CONTROLLED SUBSTANCES

Schedule	Characteristics	Dispensing Restrictions	Examples
I	High abuse potential No accepted medical use—for research, analysis, or instruction only May lead to severe dependence	Approved protocol necessary	Some opiates, opium derivatives (e.g., heroin), hallucinogenic substances (e.g., LSD), and others
II	High abuse potential Accepted medical uses May lead to severe physical and/or psychological dependence	Written prescription necessary (signed by the practitioner) Emergency verbal prescriptions must be confirmed in writing within 72 hours No prescription refills allowed Container must have warning label*	Opiates (e.g., fentanyl, methadone), methamphetamine, and others Codeine in combination with acetaminophen Stimulants (e.g., amphetamine, methylphenidate)
III	Less abuse potential than Schedules I and II Accepted medical uses May lead to moderate/low physical dependence or high psychological dependence	Written or oral prescription required Container must have warning label*	Depressants (e.g., some barbiturates), some opiates (e.g., codeine, morphine), anabolic steroids, and others
IV	Lower abuse potential than Schedule III Accepted medical uses May lead to limited physical or psychological dependence	Written or oral prescription required Prescription expires in 6 months with no more than five prescription refills allowed Container must have warning label	Some sedatives, antianxiety drugs, some nonopioid analgesiscs, and others
V	Lower abuse potential than Schedule IV Accepted medical uses May lead to limited physical or psychological dependence	May require written prescription or may be sold without a prescription but may not be dispensed for other than a medical reason (check state law)	Medications (generally for relief of coughs or diarrhea) that contain limited quantities of codeine and others

Data from U.S. Food and Drug Administration. (2005). Food and drugs, Chapter 13, Drug abuse prevention and control, subchapter 1, control and enforcement. Accessed July 10, 2005, from http://www.fda.gov/opacom/laws/cntrlsub/ctlsbtoc.htm.
*The warning label states the following: "Caution: Federal law prohibits the transfer of this drug to any person other than the client for whom it was prescribed."

schedule to another without new legislation. For example, dronabinol (Marinol), a derivative of marijuana used to treat cancer chemotherapy-induced nausea, was changed from Schedule II to Schedule III in 1999. Certain drugs with a potential for dependence, such as ethanol and certain analgesics, are not listed as controlled substances. Anyone handling controlled substances must follow the more inclusive or stringent requirements of federal and state laws (U.S. Food and Drug Administration, 2003b).

In July 1973, the Drug Enforcement Administration (DEA), in the Department of Justice, became the sole legal drug enforcement agency in the United States.

How are controlled substances managed in nursing practice?

It is unlawful for any person to possess a controlled substance unless it has been obtained by a valid prescription or order or unless its possession is pursuant to actions in the course of professional practice. It is a federal offense to transfer a drug listed in Schedule II, III, or IV to any person other than the one for whom the drug was ordered.

Drug suppliers and hospitals—as well as physicians, pharmacists, and nurses—are individually and collectively responsible for accounting for the inventory and management of the flow and distribution of controlled substances. Institutional control of the flow of controlled substances is maintained by carefully recorded checks of the balance on hand, supplies added, and doses administered. All doses of controlled substances should be kept in double-locked cabinets or other secure areas, with the keys in the custody of a designated nurse. The nurse who carries the keys to the "narcotics box" is responsible for stock supplies of controlled substances. This person is required to perform actual counts of the doses of each controlled substance in the unit's stock at the beginning and end of each shift or workday. Many health care agencies use computerized systems for the dispensing of controlled substances; these systems tabulate the counts, thus minimizing the physical counting of these substances at the beginning and end of the shift. Complete documentation and high accountability are demanded of the nurses who count or otherwise handle controlled substances during the work period. Each dose is accounted for as it is administered, discarded, wasted, or withheld. Although these protocols may seem to entail a needless waste of time, they are necessary to safeguard the control of drug flow.

Additional Regulatory Bodies or Services

Food and Drug Administration

The FDA is charged with enforcement of the federal Food, Drug, and Cosmetic Act. The FDA enforces the Act by seizure of offending (improperly manufactured or packaged) goods and criminal prosecution of responsible persons or firms in federal courts. At regular intervals, pharmaceutical firms must report to the FDA all adverse effects associated with their new drugs.

Public Health Service

The Public Health Service (PHS) is part of the Department of Health and Human Services. One of this agency's many functions is the regulation of biologic products, "biologics" (viral preparations, serums, antitoxins, or analogous products used to prevent, treat, or cure diseases). The PHS Act provides the FDA with statutory authority to regulate biologics.

Do nurses need to be concerned with product liability?

In a majority of the states the rule of strict manufacturer's liability has been adopted. This doctrine holds manufacturers liable for injuries caused by defects in their products, drugs, or devices. Product liability exists if (1) a product is defective or not fit for its reasonably foreseeable uses, (2) the defect arose before the product left the control of the manufacturer, and (3) the defect caused some person harm. If these three criteria are met, the manufacturer must pay monetary damages for harm unless the liability can be shifted to some other party. Anyone harmed by a defective product has the right to sue the manufacturer for compensation.

Manufacturers are legally responsible for knowing the effects of their products. If an unknown risk could have been discovered through a reasonable amount of research, the manufacturer is held liable for any resulting harm. Because nurses are accountable, they need to stay alert to defects in the drugs they administer. Despite manufacturers' quality assurance programs, drug products are susceptible to errors in the manufacturing, packaging, and delivery processes. Although the detection of chemical defects is usually outside the nurse's province, the detection of observable physical defects is not. Nurses should learn to be keenly aware of the physical characteristics of the drugs they administer and make comparisons before administering them. For exam-

ple, unusual discolorations, precipitates, other inconsistencies, or foreign bodies in parenteral fluids should be considered suspect. Such observations warrant withholding the drug and contacting the pharmacy department or other authoritative source. Recall of defective drugs is necessary to prevent client harm.

Occasionally, human error causes the wrong medication to be dispensed from the pharmacy. Again, the nurse is responsible for every medication administered. In this case, both the nurse who administered the wrong drug and the pharmacist who labeled it may be held liable for any resulting client harm. This liability has been sustained in the courts on several occasions. Helpful color photographs of many drug formulations can be found in the *PDR, Mosby's Drug Consult,* and the *USP DI.* The pharmacist can be contacted for assistance in the verification of any questionable medication.

How is the use of drugs legislated in Canada?

In Canada, the Health Protection Branch (HPB) of Health Canada, formerly the Department of National Health and Welfare is responsible for the administration and enforcement of the Food and Drugs Act, as well as the Controlled Drugs and Substances Act. These acts are designed to protect the consumer from health hazards and fraud or deception in the sale and use of foods, drugs, cosmetics, and medical devices. Canadian drug legislation began in 1875 when the Parliament of Canada passed an act to prevent the sale of adulterated food, drink, and drugs. Since that time foods and drugs have been controlled on a national basis.

Canadian Food and Drugs Act

In 1953, the present Canadian Food and Drugs Act was passed by the Senate and House of Commons of Canada, and since that time the law has been amended often. The act stipulates that no food, drug, cosmetic, or device is to be advertised or sold to the general public as a treatment, preventive, or cure for certain diseases listed in Schedule A of the act. Among the diseases included in the list are alcoholism, arteriosclerosis, cancer, epilepsy, and other diseases. When it is necessary to provide adequate directions for the safe use of a drug to treat or prevent diseases mentioned in Schedule A, that disease or disorder may be mentioned on the labels and inserts accompanying the drug. In addition, the act prohibits the sale of drugs that are contaminated, adulterated, or unsafe for use and those whose labels are false, misleading, or deceptive. According to the act, drugs must comply with prescribed standards as stated in the recognized pharmacopoeias and formularies listed in Schedule B of the act, or with the professed standards under which the drug is sold. Recognized pharmacopoeias and formularies include the following:

- *European Pharmacopoeia*
- *Pharmacopée Française*
- *Pharmacopoeia Internationalis*
- *The British Pharmacopeia*
- *The Canadian Formulary*

- *The Pharmaceutical Codex*
- *United States Pharmacopeia*

The legend "Canadian standard drug" or the abbreviation CSD must appear on the inner and outer labels of a drug to signify that it meets the standards prescribed for it.

The sale of certain drugs is prohibited unless the premises in which they were manufactured and the process and conditions of manufacture have been approved by the Minister of Health. These drugs are listed in Schedules C and D, and some of these drugs include insulin, anterior pituitary extracts, radioactive isotopes, blood and blood derivatives, and immunizing agents. The distribution of samples of drugs is also prohibited, with the exception of distribution to duly licensed individuals such as physicians, dentists, or pharmacists. Schedule F of the act contains a list of drugs that can be sold and refilled only on prescription. Refills may be permitted at specified intervals but cannot exceed 6 months. The drugs listed in Schedule F include antibiotics, hormones, and tranquilizers. They must always be properly and clearly labeled and include directions for use. Labels on containers of Schedule F drugs must be marked with the symbol **Pr**. These drugs cannot be advertised to the general public other than giving the name, price, and quantity of the drug. Box 2-3 contains a summary of Canadian prescription drugs.

Controlled drugs for Canada are those listed in Part G of the act and include amphetamines, barbituric acid and its derivatives (barbiturates), and phenmetrazine. Controlled drugs must be marked with the symbol ⟨C⟩ in a clear and conspicuous color and size on the upper left quarter of the label. The proper name of the drug must appear on the label either before or after the proprietary or trade name. Controlled drugs can be dispensed only by prescription.

When a controlled drug is dispensed by prescription, the labels must carry the following:

- Name and address of the pharmacy or pharmacist
- Date and number of the prescription
- Name of the person for whom the controlled drug is dispensed

- Name of the practitioner
- Directions for use
- Any other information that the prescription requires be shown on the label

Prescriptions for controlled drugs cannot be refilled unless the practitioner so directed in writing at the time the prescription was issued and also specified the number of refills and the dates for or intervals between refilling. All information on the labels must be clearly and prominently displayed and readily discernible. Controlled drugs cannot be advertised to the general public.

Restricted drugs are those listed in Schedule H of the act and include the hallucinogenic drugs lysergic acid diethylamide (LSD), diethyltryptamine (DET), dimethyltryptamine (DMT), mescaline, and dimethoxyamphetamine (STP, DOM). The sale of these drugs is prohibited. These drugs may be obtained for research by a qualified investigator if authorized by the Minister of Health. Precautions must be taken to ensure against the loss or theft of a restricted drug.

The following list includes some of the additional requirements found in the Canadian Food and Drugs Act:

1. Labels of drugs must show the following:
   a. Proper name of the drug immediately preceding or following the proprietary or brand name.
   b. Name and address of the manufacturer or distributor.
   c. Lot number of the drug.
   d. Adequate directions for use.
   e. Quantitative list of medicinal ingredients and their proper or common names.
   f. Net amount of drug.
   g. Common or proper name and proportion of any preservatives used in parenteral drugs.
   h. Expiration date if the drug does not maintain its potency, purity, and physical characteristics for at least 3 years from the date of manufacture.
   i. Recommended single and daily adult dose; if the drug is for children, the label must state "Children: As directed by physician" or:

AGE (IN YEARS)	PROPORTION OF ADULT DOSE
10-14	One-half
5-9	One-fourth
2-4	One-sixth
Under 2	As directed by physician

   j. A warning that the drug be kept out of the reach of children and any precautions to be taken (e.g., "Caution: May be injurious if taken in large doses for a long time. Do not exceed the recommended dose without consulting a physician"). This warning is to be preceded by a symbol—octagonal in shape, red in color, and on a white background.
   k. Contraindications and side effects of nonprescription drugs.
   l. On and after July 1, 1974, the drug identification number assigned to the drug, preceded by the

---

BOX 2-3 CANADIAN PRESCRIPTION AND RESTRICTED DRUGS

PRESCRIPTION DRUGS

Schedule F

- May be used only after professional consultation
- Includes more than 200 drugs
- Identified by **Pr** on the label

CONTROLLED DRUGS

- Affect the central nervous system (stimulants, sedatives)
- Identified by ⟨C⟩ on the label in a clear manner and a conspicuous color and size

RESTRICTED DRUGS

- Available only to institutions for research
- Identified by the wording "Restricted Drug" on the label

words "Drug Identification Number" or the abbreviation "D.I.N." is to be shown on the main labels of a drug sold in dosage form (one ready for use by the consumer).

2. Other specific regulations are the following:

   a. Manufacturers must be able to demonstrate that a drug in oral dosage form represented as releasing the drug at certain time intervals actually is released and available as represented.

   b. Oral tablets must disintegrate within 45 minutes. Enteric-coated tablets must not disintegrate for 60 minutes when exposed to gastric juice but must disintegrate within an additional 60 minutes when exposed to intestinal juices.

   c. Drugs containing boric acid or sodium borate as a medicinal ingredient must carry a statement that the drug should not be administered to infants or children younger than 3 years of age.

   d. Acetylsalicylic acid (aspirin) for internal use shall carry a cautionary statement to the effect that it should not be administered to a child under 2 years of age except on the advice of a physician and that it not be administered to or used by children or adolescents who have chickenpox or who manifest flu symptoms because of the risk of Reye's syndrome (a rare and serious illness).

   e. The inner label of chloramphenicol must carry a warning that bone marrow depression has been associated with its use.

   f. Safety factors such as sterility and the absence of pyrogens must be ensured in parenteral drugs.

These regulations allow the government to withdraw from the market any drugs found to be unduly toxic. New drugs introduced to the market must have demonstrated effectiveness and safety in human clinical studies to the satisfaction of the manufacturer and the government. For more specific information, see Departmental Consolidation of the Food and Drugs Act and of the Food and Drug Regulations with Amendments to December 31, 2004 (http://www.hc-sc.gc.ca/food-aliment/friia-raaii/food_drugs-aliments_drogues/act-loi/pdf/e_index.html).

Canadian Controlled Drugs and Substances Act

The regulations of the Canadian Controlled Drugs and Substances Act govern the possession, sale, manufacture, production, and distribution of narcotics. The Canadian Narcotic Control Act was passed in 1961 and revoked the Canadian Opium and Narcotic Act of 1952. The 1961 act has been amended a number of times and finally revoked, culminating in the Canadian Controlled Drugs and Substances Act of 1996.

Only authorized persons can be in possession of a controlled drug or substance. Authorized persons include a licensed dealer, pharmacist, practitioner, person in charge of a hospital, or a person acting as an agent for a practitioner. A licensed dealer is one who has been given permission to manufacture, produce, import, export, or distribute a controlled substance. Practitioners include persons registered under the laws of a province to practice the profession of medicine, dentistry, or veterinary medicine or any person or class of persons prescribed as a practitioner. However, persons other than these may be licensed by the Minister of Health to produce (either by cultivation, manufacturing, or synthesizing) or to purchase and possess for scientific purposes any substance included in Schedules I to IV. Peace officers and members of technical or scientific departments of the government of Canada or of a province or university may possess controlled substances in connection with their employment. A person who is undergoing treatment by a medical practitioner may be prescribed a controlled substance. This person may possess the prescribed controlled substance but may not knowingly obtain a controlled substance from any other medical practitioner without notifying that practitioner that he or she is already undergoing treatment and obtaining a controlled drug on prescription. Penalties for unauthorized possession or trafficking are determined by the Schedule number of the controlled substance.

All persons authorized to be in possession of controlled drugs must keep a record of the name and quantity of all such substances received, from whom they were obtained, and to whom the drugs were supplied (including quantity, form, and dates of all transactions). In addition, they must ensure the safekeeping of all controlled drugs and substances, keep full and complete records on all such drugs for at least 2 years, and report any loss or theft within 10 days of discovery.

The schedule of the Canadian Controlled Drugs and Substances Act lists those drugs—and their preparations, derivatives, alkaloids, and salts—that are subject to the act. Although the act describes eight categories of drugs, only Schedules I to V are considered controlled substances (Table 2-2).

Before a pharmacist may legally dispense a drug included in Schedules I to IV or a medication containing such a drug, he or she must receive a prescription from a designated practitioner. A signed and dated prescription issued by such a duly authorized practitioner is essential in the case of any controlled substance prescribed as such or any preparation containing a substance in a form intended for parenteral administration. Prescriptions of any controlled substance may not be refilled.

There is one exception to the prescription requirement. Certain compounds with a small codeine content may be sold to the public by a pharmacist without a prescription. In such instances the narcotic content cannot exceed 8 mg per tablet or 20 mg/28 mL. In products of this type, codeine must be in combination with two or more nonnarcotic substances and in recognized therapeutic doses. In addition, the labels for items of this nature are required to show the true formula of the medicinal ingredients and contain a caution to the following effect: "This preparation contains codeine and should not be administered to children except on the advice of a physician." These preparations cannot be advertised or displayed in a pharmacy. It is also unlawful to publish any narcotic advertisement for the general public.

TABLE 2-2 CANADIAN SCHEDULE OF CONTROLLED SUBSTANCES

Schedule	Examples
I	Opium poppy, its preparations, derivatives, alkaloids, and salts, including opium, codeine, morphine, and thebaine; coca, phenylpiperidines, phenazepines, amidones, methadols, phenalkoxams, thiambutenes, moramides, most morphinans, some benzazocines, ampromides, benzimidazoles, phenocyclidine, piritramide, fentanyls and their derivatives, and tilidine
II	Cannabis, its preparations, derivatives, and similar synthetic preparations
III	Amphetamines, methylphenidate, methaqualone, LSD, mescaline, and similar drugs and their derivatives
IV	Barbiturates, meprobamate, most benzodiazepines, anabolic steroids, zolpidem, and similar drugs and their derivatives
V	Propylhexedrine and any salt thereof
VI	Part 1, Class A precursors: ephedrine, ergotamine, lysergic acid, pseudoephedrine, and other similar drugs Part 2, Class B precursors: acetone, ethyl ether, hydrochloric acid, methyl ethyl ketone, sulphuric acid, toluene Part 3: Any preparation or mixture that contains a precursor set out in Part 1 or Part 2
VII	Cannabis resin (3 kg); cannabis (marijuana) (3 kg)
VIII	Cannabis resin (1 g); cannabis (marijuana) (30 g)

Data from http://laws.justice.gc.ca/en/C-38.8/37534.html. Updated to August 31, 2004. Accessed April 19, 2005.

Labels of containers of narcotics must legibly and conspicuously bear the proprietary and proper or common names of the narcotic, the names of the manufacturer and distributor, the symbol "N" in the upper left quarter, and the net contents of the container and of each tablet, capsule, or ampule.

Application to Nursing A nurse may be in violation of the Canadian Controlled Drugs and Substances Act if in illegal possession of controlled substances. Ignorance of the content of a drug in the nurse's possession is not considered a justifiable excuse. Proof of possession without a prescription is sufficient to constitute an offense. Legal possession of narcotics by a nurse is limited to times when a drug is administered to a client on the order of a physician, when the nurse is acting as the official custodian of narcotics in a department of a hospital or clinic, and when the nurse is a client for whom a physician has prescribed a controlled substance. A nurse engaged in illegal distribution or transportation of controlled substances may be held liable, and heavy penalties are imposed for violation of the Canadian Controlled Drugs and Substances Act.

Apart from the general rules for prescription drugs, certain rules for controlled drugs apply in most health agencies:

- A PRN order (an "as required for pain" order) for controlled drugs must be rewritten every 7 days in Canada.
- A standing order (i.e., drug dose administered by the nurse for the physician without obtaining a signed order) is not permitted for such drugs.
- In an emergency situation a verbal order is permitted if the nurse documents the nature of the emergency in the chart and validates the order within 24 hours.

- When a controlled drug is administered to a client, the nurse must record the date, time of administration, client's name, and physician's name, and he or she must sign the entry.
- When a client refuses a dose of a controlled drug, it should be placed in the sewage system in the presence of a witness. If a dose of the drug is contaminated or wasted, the nurse should make an entry in the records book explaining how the dose was disposed of, and a witness should sign the entry.
- All controlled substances stored on nursing units must be kept in locked cabinets so that only authorized personnel have access to them.

Drug Standards in the United Kingdom and Canada The *British Pharmacopoeia (BP)* is similar to the *USP* in scope and purpose. See pp. 14 and 15 for a general statement about the standardization of drugs in general by assay and bioassay. Drugs listed in the *BP* are considered official and are subject to legal control in the United Kingdom and in those parts of the British Commonwealth in which the *BP* has statutory force. The *USP* is used a great deal in Canada, and some preparations used in Canada conform to the *USP* instead of the *BP* because many of the drugs used in Canada are manufactured in the United States.

The *Canadian National Formulary* contains formulas for preparations used extensively in Canada. It also contains standards for new drugs prescribed in Canada but not included in the *BP*. The publication has been given official status by the Canadian Food and Drugs Act.

The *Physician's Formulary* contains formulas for preparations that are representative of the needs of medical practice in Canada. It is published by the Canadian Medical Association.

✱ **Countries such as the United States and Canada have drug control, but is there international cooperation for the control of drugs?**

International control of drugs legally began in 1912 when the first "Opium Conference" was held in The Hague, Netherlands. International treaties were drawn up legally obligating governments to (1) limit to medical and scientific needs the manufacturing of and trade in medicinal opium, (2) control the production and distribution of raw opium, and (3) establish a system of governmental licensing to control the manufacture of and trade in drugs covered by the convention.

In 1961, government representatives formulated the "Single Convention on Narcotic Drugs," which became effective in 1964. This act consolidated all existing treaties into one document for the control of all narcotic substances. An International Narcotics Control Board made up of government representatives was established to enforce this law. Enforcement is an immense task, and it is impossible to prevent illicit trafficking in drugs. For example, during a 1-year period it was estimated that 1200 tons of opium were circulated in the illicit market when only 800 tons were considered sufficient to meet world medical needs. Its activities also include psychotropic substances. In 2002, the Board, in cooperation with the government of China, prevented an export of 5 tons of diazepam to Afghanistan, a quantity that is far in excess of the annual medical requirements of that substance. It was believed that diazepam diverted to Afghanistan was used to adulterate heroin.

Laws need to be frequently updated and strictly enforced, but the unfortunate fact is that financial support for regulation and enforcement is sometimes not equal to the task.

✱ **What is the process by which drugs come to the market?**

The multibillion-dollar pharmaceutical industry is constantly screening substances that have the potential to be marketed as new drugs. It may take years and huge amounts of capital for a prospective drug to progress through the following FDA-required testing sequence:

A. Animal studies, to ascertain the following:
   1. Toxicity
      a. Acute toxicity as represented by the LD_{50} (the median lethal dose—the dose that is lethal to 50% of the laboratory animals tested)
      b. Subacute toxicity
      c. Chronic toxicity
   2. Therapeutic index—a quantitative measure of the relative safety of a drug; the ratio of the LD_{50} to the median effective dose (the dose that has a therapeutic effect in 50% of the animals tested)
   3. Modes of absorption, distribution, metabolism (biotransformation), and excretion
B. Human studies
   1. Phase I—initial pharmacologic evaluation
   2. Phase II—limited controlled evaluation
   3. Phase III—extended clinical evaluation

A noteworthy lack of correlation exists between levels of toxicity in animals and adverse effects in humans. In addition, many symptoms of adverse effects in humans simply cannot be determined in animals. A partial list of common human symptoms that are not measurably distinguishable in animals includes dizziness, nausea, drowsiness, nervousness, indigestion, headache, and weakness.

FDA Approval Process

The FDA approval process and specifications are as follows:

• **Investigational New Drug (IND).** An IND application must be submitted to the FDA if a pharmaceutical company or clinician wants to investigate either a new drug or an old drug for a new indication or at a different, unapproved dosage in humans. The IND will include evidence of drug safety by providing animal or clinical information, proof of the investigator's qualifications to perform this research, and evidence of the drug product's proven quality and strength. The investigation covered under the IND is divided into three phases:

Phase I: initial pharmacologic evaluation. A small number of normal individuals (usually volunteers) take the drug so that the investigators can determine the pharmacokinetics of the agent (absorption, distribution, metabolism, routes of elimination or excretion). Blood tests, urine analysis, vital signs, and specific monitoring tests are performed during this phase.

Phase II: limited controlled evaluation. The drug is now administered at gradually increasing dosages to selected individuals with the targeted disease. For example, if the product is believed to have antihypertensive properties, individuals with documented hypertension are chosen for this phase. During this phase the individual is closely monitored for drug effectiveness and side effects. If no serious side or adverse effects occur, the study progresses to phase III.

Phase III: extended clinical evaluation. The drug is now ready for testing in various centers in the United States in larger numbers of individuals. Standards (protocols) have been developed and must be followed at all investigative sites. The three objectives for this phase are to (1) determine clinical effectiveness, (2) determine drug safety, and (3) establish tolerated dosage or dosage range.

Several other factors are involved with this program. First, the investigator reports to the FDA after completion of each phase and needs its approval before progressing to the following phases. Second, a double-blind study may be instituted, usually in phase II or phase III. A double-blind study involves the administration of the research drug or a placebo (such as lactose) and/or a marketed drug with the same pharmacologic effects as the drug being studied. All of the products are formulated to look the same and are then packaged, usually by code numbers. In general, no one involved with the study knows if the client is taking the study drug (the active drug) or the placebo. This eliminates bias and allows the evaluation to be performed accurately—on the basis of therapeutic response.

• **New Drug Application (NDA).** After completing phase III of the IND, and assuming the data collected indicate that the new drug is very promising, investigators submit all data to the FDA. After careful review of the information, the FDA may approve or reject the NDA. If the NDA is approved, the drug product can be marketed for the selected indication in the dosing schedules as studied. If the NDA is rejected, the FDA may require additional studies or information before reconsideration.

- *Abbreviated New Drug Application (ANDA) (for generic drug approval).* Generic formulations of currently marketed medications are not usually required to repeat all of the previous steps before marketing. A company is required to prove that its product can produce the same therapeutic effects as the already marketed drug. Although nearly all generic drugs require an ANDA, the FDA may require different methods to prove generic equivalency, depending on the drug. For example, chlordiazepoxide (Librium) and amitriptyline (Elavil) require *in vivo* studies; the generic drug must be given to humans, and data from blood and urine studies should be equivalent to data obtained when the name brand product is given, according to statistical analysis. Other drug products, such as chlorpheniramine (Chlor-Trimeton) and dexamethasone (Decadron) need only prove that the manufacturing process is in compliance with Good Manufacturing Practice (GMP) guidelines and that their quality control standards are equivalent. Thus the FDA establishes criteria according to the drug product, the possibility of bioequivalence problems, or the lack of such problems. Drugs marketed before 1938, such as chloral hydrate and phenobarbital, do not require an approved ANDA before marketing.

Nurses should be aware of several limitations in the testing and marketing process. The number of persons studied and the time allotted for the study are limited. Most drugs will not have been tested in pregnant women, persons with multiple disease states, or persons on multiple medications. In addition, certain types of individuals may be excluded from the study, such as children and older adults. However, the Pediatric Research Equity Act of 2003 indicates that all applications for new ingredients, new indications, new dosage forms, new dosing regimens, and new routes of administration must contain a pediatric assessment unless the sponsor has obtained either a waiver or a deferral of pediatric studies. A drug is marketed if it is considered safe and effective during the time of study, subject to the previously mentioned limitations.

✳ **Are there ways in which new drugs may need to be classified?**

New drugs are also classified according to pregnancy safety category. Before any drug is used during pregnancy, the expected benefits should be considered against the possible risks to the fetus. The FDA has established a scale to indicate drugs that may have documented problems in animals and/or humans during pregnancy, but for many drugs this information is unknown. The prescriber, nurse, and client should carefully review any precautionary information before using the drug product. The categories are as follows (*USP DI*, 2005):

- **Category A:** Adequate and well-controlled studies indicate no risk to the fetus in the first trimester of pregnancy, and there is no evidence of risk in later trimesters.
- **Category B:** Animal reproduction studies have not demonstrated a risk to the fetus, but there are no adequate and well-controlled studies in pregnant women.
- **Category C:** Animal reproduction studies have reported an adverse effect on the fetus, but there are no adequate and well-controlled studies in humans; the benefits of the drugs in pregnant women may be acceptable despite its potential risks.
- **Category D:** There is evidence of human fetal risk, but the potential benefits from the use of the drug in pregnant women may be acceptable despite its potential risks—if the situation is life-threatening or if safer drugs either are not available or are ineffective.
- **Category X:** Studies in animals or humans demonstrate fetal abnormalities, or adverse effect reports indicate evidence of fetal risk. The risk of use in a pregnant woman clearly outweighs any possible benefit. These drugs should not be used in pregnant women.

✳ **Once a drug is marketed, is it considered safe?**

Once marketed, a drug is used by greater numbers of clients and probably for longer periods; thus it is inevitable that it will be reported to produce additional effects (possibly therapeutic but often adverse) that were not noted during the trial studies. Therefore a phase IV, or postmarketing, surveillance period has been advocated to monitor and tabulate information about new drugs and disseminate it to health care professionals and consumers. This is a more difficult phase to supervise because it depends on the voluntary reports of persons in the medical field. The importance of this phase should not be underestimated—it affects many more people than the previous three phases combined.

This voluntary adverse-reaction reporting program called MedWatch was initiated by the FDA in 1993. The program's purpose is to detect drug reactions that have not been revealed by previous clinical or pharmaceutical studies. Adverse events may occur once a product is on the open market and widely used—often by clients who have multiple health problems and are taking many other drugs. All health care professionals, including nurses, are encouraged to report an unusual occurrence or an unusually high number of occurrences associated with a drug, its formulation, its packaging, and so forth (Figure 2-2). The nurse need not verify the cause of an adverse effect but does need to inform the FDA of medication- or medical device-related events that are suspected to have resulted in death or the risk of death, hospitalization, persistent or permanent disability, birth defects, or the need for medical intervention to prevent permanent impairment. The FDA requests that nurses and other health care professionals provide information about products even if clients are not involved (e.g., contaminated products or product labeling that might be confusing). Nurse and client confidentiality are maintained in the reporting. The paperwork is a one-

U.S. Department of Health and Human Services

Form Approved: OMB No. 0910-0291, Expires: 03/31/05
See OMB statement on reverse.

MEDWATCH

The FDA Safety Information and
Adverse Event Reporting Program

For VOLUNTARY reporting of
adverse events and product problems

Page ____ of ____

FDA USE ONLY

Triage unit
sequence #

A. PATIENT INFORMATION

1. Patient Identifier	2. Age at Time of Event:	3. Sex	4. Weight
In confidence	or ____ Date of Birth:	☐ Female ☐ Male	____ lbs or ____ kgs

B. ADVERSE EVENT OR PRODUCT PROBLEM

1. ☐ Adverse Event and/or ☐ Product Problem (e.g., defects/malfunctions)

2. Outcomes Attributed to Adverse Event
(Check all that apply)
☐ Death: ____ (mo/day/yr)
☐ Life-threatening
☐ Hospitalization - initial or prolonged
☐ Disability
☐ Congenital Anomaly
☐ Required Intervention to Prevent Permanent Impairment/Damage
☐ Other: ____

3. Date of Event (mo/day/year)

4. Date of This Report (mo/day/year)

5. Describe Event or Problem

6. Relevant Tests/Laboratory Data, Including Dates

7. Other Relevant History, Including Preexisting Medical Conditions (e.g., allergies, race, pregnancy, smoking and alcohol use, hepatic/renal dysfunction, etc.)

PLEASE TYPE OR USE BLACK INK

C. SUSPECT MEDICATION(S)

1. **Name** (Give labeled strength & mfr/labeler, if known)

#1 ____

#2 ____

2. **Dose, Frequency & Route Used**
#1 ____
#2 ____

3. **Therapy Dates** (If unknown, give duration) from/to (or best estimate)
#1 ____
#2 ____

4. **Diagnosis for Use** (Indication)
#1 ____
#2 ____

5. **Event Abated After Use Stopped or Dose Reduced?**
#1 ☐ Yes ☐ No ☐ Doesn't Apply
#2 ☐ Yes ☐ No ☐ Doesn't Apply

6. **Lot #** (if known)
#1 ____
#2 ____

7. **Exp. Date** (if known)
#1 ____
#2 ____

8. **Event Reappeared After Reintroduction?**
#1 ☐ Yes ☐ No ☐ Doesn't Apply
#2 ☐ Yes ☐ No ☐ Doesn't Apply

9. **NDC#** (For product problems only)
____ - ____ - ____

10. **Concomitant Medical Products and Therapy Dates** (Exclude treatment of event)

D. SUSPECT MEDICAL DEVICE

1. **Brand Name**

2. **Type of Device**

3. **Manufacturer Name, City and State**

4. **Model #**	**Lot #**	5. **Operator of Device**
Catalog #	**Expiration Date** (mo/day/yr)	☐ Health Professional ☐ Lay User/Patient
Serial #	**Other #**	☐ Other: ____

6. **If Implanted, Give Date** (mo/day/yr)

7. **If Explanted, Give Date** (mo/day/yr)

8. **Is this a Single-use Device that was Reprocessed and Reused on a Patient?**
☐ Yes ☐ No

9. **If Yes to Item No. 8, Enter Name and Address of Reprocessor**

10. **Device Available for Evaluation?** (Do not send to FDA)
☐ Yes ☐ No ☐ Returned to Manufacturer on: ____ (mo/day/yr)

11. **Concomitant Medical Products and Therapy Dates** (Exclude treatment of event)

E. REPORTER (See confidentiality section on back)

1. **Name and Address**

Phone #

2. **Health Professional?**
☐ Yes ☐ No

3. **Occupation**

4. **Also Reported to:**
☐ Manufacturer
☐ User Facility
☐ Distributor/Importer

5. **If you do NOT want your identity disclosed to the manufacturer, place an "X" in this box:** ☐

FDA

Mail to: **MEDWATCH**
5600 Fishers Lane
Rockville, MD 20852-9787
-or-
FAX to:
1-800-FDA-0178

FORM FDA 3500 (12/03) Submission of a report does not constitute an admission that medical personnel or the product caused or contributed to the event.

FIGURE 2-2 MedWatch form and advice about voluntary reporting.

From MedWatch: The FDA Medical Products Reporting Program. Rockville, MD: U.S. Department of Health and Human Services, Public Health Service, Food and Drug Administration.

Continued

ADVICE ABOUT VOLUNTARY REPORTING

Report adverse experiences with:
- Medications *(drugs or biologics)*
- Medical devices *(including in-vitro diagnostics)*
- Special nutritional products *(dietary supplements, medical foods, infant formulas)*
- Cosmetics
- Medication errors

Report product problems - quality, performance or safety concerns such as:
- Suspected counterfeit product
- Suspected contamination
- Questionable stability
- Defective components
- Poor packaging or labeling
- Therapeutic failures

Report SERIOUS adverse events. An event is serious when the patient outcome is:
- Death
- Life-threatening *(real risk of dying)*
- Hospitalization *(initial or prolonged)*
- Disability *(significant, persistent or permanent)*
- Congenital anomaly
- Required intervention to prevent permanent impairment or damage

Report even if:
- You're not certain the product caused the event
- You don't have all the details

How to report:
- Just fill in the sections that apply to your report
- Use section C for all products except medical devices
- Attach additional blank pages if needed
- Use a separate form for each patient
- Report either to FDA or the manufacturer *(or both)*

Confidentiality: The patient's identity is held in strict confidence by FDA and protected to the fullest extent of the law. FDA will not disclose the reporter's identity in response to a request from the public, pursuant to the Freedom of Information Act. The reporter's identity, including the identity of a self-reporter, may be shared with the manufacturer unless requested otherwise.

If your report involves a serious adverse event with a device and it occurred in a facility outside a doctor's office, that facility may be legally required to report to FDA and/or the manufacturer. Please notify the person in that facility who would handle such reporting.

Important numbers:
- 1-800-FDA-0178 -- To FAX report
- 1-800-FDA-1088 -- To report by phone or for more information
- 1-800-822-7967 -- For a VAERS form for vaccines

To Report via the Internet:
http://www.fda.gov/medwatch/report.htm

FIGURE 2-2 **Cont'd.**—MedWatch form and advice about voluntary reporting.

From *MedWatch: The FDA Medical Products Reporting Program*. Rockville, MD: U.S. Department of Health and Human Services, Public Health Service, Food and Drug Administration.

page form that can be obtained from the hospital's risk manager or copied from any of the drug reference books previously discussed (see Figure 2-2). It can also be downloaded from http://www.fda.gov/medwatch/SAFETY/3500.pdf with an addressed and stamped envelope. The American Nurses Association was involved in the development of MedWatch and supports the program for providing another way in which nurses can advocate for client safety. Nurses have emerged as very active reporters to the MedWatch system, submitting approximately 25% of the 5000 voluntary reports received by the FDA each year (Worthington, 2002).

The FDA has come under closer scrutiny over the past few years regarding its role in monitoring adverse drug events and providing warning statements or removing drugs from the market. Cholesterol-lowering drugs and cyclo-oxygenase 2 (COX-2) inhibitors have recently prompted medical experts to reexamine how the FDA uses adverse drug reaction information in ensuring safety for marketed drugs (Kimmel et al., 2005; Psaty, Furberg, Ray, & Weiss, 2004). Typically, the FDA requires manufacturers to notify prescribers of any serious adverse events or warnings. This is often done via a "Dear Doctor" or a "Dear Healthcare Provider" letter sent by the manufacturer, but it may not reach all health care providers. The FDA regularly reports new adverse events and warnings on its web page (http://www.fda.gov/medwatch/safety.htm), and health care providers should review this site regularly for adverse event reports and recommendations.

Nurses and Drug Research

Pharmaceutical research is common in the clinical setting. In 2001, more than 400 anticancer drugs alone were tested in 722 clinical trials in the United States (Jameson, 2003). Nurses involved in research projects involving human subjects must be knowledgeable about informed consent and must protect clients by being ever alert to the possibility of subtle errors in protocol or oversights in adherence to ethical tenets. The most important elements of a nurse's responsibility relate to a client's right to informed consent and to participation that is fully voluntary and without coercion.

✺ When clients are involved in drug studies, how are nurses involved in informed consent?

All participants in experimental drug studies should be true volunteers and not subjected to any coercion. **Informed consent** must be obtained from all participants. This is the written consent to an experimental procedure by an individual after he or she has been given a careful explanation of the nature, purpose, procedures, drugs, or devices involved; identification of any experimental procedures; potential benefits, risks, and discomforts to participant; alternative treatments; confidentiality of research records, compensation if injury occurs; persons to contact about rights, and what to do if research results in injury, and a statement that research is voluntary and that withdrawal does not incur penalty (Karigan, 2001). Although an informed consent must be obtained in writing, this particular consent is heir to the flaws of other client consents: the information conveyed may be incomplete, or not delivered in nonmedical language, or presented at a time when the client is sleepy or sedated and not fully cognizant of the ramifications of what is being signed. It is the nurse's obligation to ensure that this does not happen and that it is the researcher who gives a full explanation and answers pertinent questions.

The rights of human participants in medical research have come to be protected under the umbrella of the **Nuremberg Code.** This 1947 code was developed under the aegis of American physicians as a result of the post–World War II Nuremberg trials of Nazi physicians who had conducted experiments on political prisoners without their consent. In essence, the Nuremberg Code states the following:

- Truly voluntary consent of the human subject is critical.
- The experiment must be proved to be valid or made possible only through the use of human subjects.
- The study justifies the results and risks.
- Unnecessary suffering, death, or disability will be avoided.
- The experiment will be conducted in a careful and professional manner by scientifically qualified persons.
- Either the subject or the investigator can terminate the experiment at any point that the experiment is thought to be unendurable or impossible.

In 1964, the rules and regulations of clinical research were further refined by the Declaration of Helsinki, which emphasized written informed consent, patients' rights, the integrity of the investigator, and strict protocols for experimenting on humans. A research protocol is a written document describing in detail how a clinical trial is to be conducted, including background information, study design, treatment plan, objectives, eligible participants, study requirements, and evaluation. Nurses need to know the outline of the protocol and how to find specific information related to it, such as drug dosages, adverse effects, and nursing implications (Karigan, 2001).

The Declaration of Helsinki was followed by the National Research Act of 1974 after the details of the Tuskegee Syphilis Study were made public. The Tuskegee Syphilis Study allowed 600 men to unknowingly participate in a research study in which appropriate treatment was denied. The Act again emphasized protection of human subjects, informed consent, Institutional Review Board (IRB) guidelines, and overall good clinical practice in research. An IRB is a committee in the institution or agency sponsoring a site for the research; it is responsible for reviewing and approving studies to ensure that clinical research is ethical, safe, and scientifically sound. Such a committee is required by the federal government in any organization receiving federal funds for research.

In 1979, the *Belmont Report: Ethical Principles and Guidelines for the Protection of Human Subjects of Research* provided additional guidelines for more stringent protection of subjects and focused on respect, beneficence, and justice as a basis for interdisciplinary research.

New drug studies in children require special consideration; there are stipulations that require both children's and parents' consent for research that involves children for studies funded by the Department of Health and Human Services. In addition, researchers must follow more rigorous guidelines to protect a child's rights.

Expanding roles in nursing often include nurses on a team that is researching experimental drug development. Indeed, more nurses than ever before are conducting research of their own using human subjects; much of this research is clinical even if not directly related to investigational drugs. Because of a healthy professional commitment to client well-being, nurses may find themselves caught in an ethical dilemma. They appreciate a client's right to know and yet are aware that some information may unduly influence a person's behavior or condition in some way and thereby adversely influence the variable under study. Nurses involved in clinical drug studies should be fully informed about the study and the drug under investigation. All information available to the prescriber, researcher, or pharmacist should also be available to the nurse. Ethical and legal responsibilities mandate that a nurse's actions be based on adequate knowledge and skill and that clients are protected from foreseeable harm. Thus, the nurse needs to know the recommended dosage range and route of administration, desired therapeutic effect, and undesired and toxic effects of the drug being investigated. Throughout the entire investigation the nurse must strictly adhere to the protocols of the study. The nurse should also record all observations as precisely as possible because they will have a direct influence on the outcome of the study.

✸ What other regulations affect nursing management of pharmacotherapeutics?

Nursing practice is regulated not only by the previous drug standards and legislation but also by individual state nurse practice acts; joint policy statements among the state nursing associations, medical associations, and hospital associations; and institutional and agency policies. Institutions and agencies may set policies that interpret more specifically those actions allowable under state nursing practice acts, but they may not modify, expand, or restrict the intent of such acts. Personal and professional ethical standards further govern actual nursing decisions and judgments in practice.

The nurse practice acts of individual states define conditions under which nurses may be licensed to practice professionally. One function of these acts is to protect the public from unskilled, undereducated, or unlicensed nurses and to delineate clearly the scope of nursing as a health care profession. These statutes protect nurses by clearly defining their responsibilities and freedoms. Every state nurse practice act includes laws and regulations on reciprocity and suspension or revocation of nurse licenses.

✸ With expansion of nursing roles, how does regulation of practice remain current?

The traditional roles of the nurse have changed and expanded along with newer techniques and approaches to

BOX 2-4 PRESCRIPTIVE AUTHORITY FOR NURSE PRACTITIONERS WITHIN THE UNITED STATES

STATES WITH INDEPENDENT NURSE PRACTITIONER PRESCRIBING AUTHORITY*

Including Controlled Substances

Alaska	Maine	Utah†
Arizona	Montana	Washington
District of Columbia	New Hampshire	Wisconsin
Iowa	New Mexico	Wyoming
Idaho	Oregon	

STATES WITH DEPENDENT NURSE PRACTITIONER PRESCRIBING AUTHORITY

Including Controlled Substances

Arkansas	Maryland	Ohio
California	Massachusetts	Oklahoma
Colorado	Michigan	Pennsylvania
Connecticut	Minnesota	Rhode Island
Delaware	Mississippi	South Carolina†
Georgia‡	Nebraska	South Dakota
Hawaii	Nevada	Tennessee
Illinois	New Jersey	Texas
Indiana	New York	Vermont
Kansas	North Carolina	Virginia
Louisiana	North Dakota	West Virginia

Excluding Controlled Substances

Alabama	Kentucky
Florida	Missouri

Modified from Phillips, S.J. (2005). Annual legislative update: A comprehensive look at the legislative issues affecting advanced nursing practice. *Nurse Practitioner: The American Journal of Primary Healthcare, 30*(1), 14-47.

*Independent prescribing means that prescribing is defined by the State Board of Nursing of a state as an activity within the actual practice of a nurse practitioner. It is not statutorily defined as a delegated medical act and so does not require physician collaboration or supervision.

†Schedule IV and/or V controlled substances only.

‡Nurse practitioners do not have written prescribing or dispensing authority; the process falls under delegated medical authority.

drug therapy. Two such areas are prescription writing and certain modes of drug administration.

In the past, prescribing medications was a purely medical function as determined by state law, and medication administration was usually delegated to nurses and occasionally to licensed pharmacists and other trained personnel. In reality, astute nurses have been indirectly prescribing for many years, using diplomatic ploys with physicians to attend to changing client needs: "Will you write an order for Dulcolax for Mrs. Rommel? She hasn't had a bowel movement for 3 days." Today certain expanding roles in nursing, along with increased education and expertise (e.g., certification as a nurse practitioner by the American Nurses Credentialing Center and other organizations), have led states to legitimize the prescribing function of nurse practitioners.

Two reports helped to define this prescribing role—one from the American Medical Association in 1970, and the other from the Department of Health, Education, and Welfare in 1971. Both reports clearly state that the prescribing of medications may be the practice of medicine when carried out by a physician and the practice of nursing when carried out by the nurse. In response to this change, all states amended their nurse practice acts. These amendments have predominantly given authorization to the nurse practitioner to write prescriptions within established protocols, under physician supervision or collaboration, or independently according to the statutes of any given state. As of September 1998, nurse practitioners in all 50 states and the District of Columbia have legislative authority to prescribe (Pearson, 2000). However, within these states there is a wide disparity, with some states having almost no barriers to prescriptive rights by nurse practitioners and others having limitations that are still significant (Box 2-4).

Research has supported that the quality of basic care provided by nurse practitioners was not distinguishable from that given by physicians in terms of process, outcomes and client satisfaction (Boodhoo et al., 2004; Lambin, Adams, Fox, & Divine, 2004; Rosenfeld, Kobayashi, Barber, & Mezey, 2004; Crowther, 2003; Bryant & Graham, 2002; Mundinger, 1994; McGrath, 1990). Nurse practitioners prescribe fewer drugs than physicians and are less likely to opt for pharmacologic management of the client's condition (Pan, Straub, & Geller, 1997). The plethora of studies attesting to the nurse practitioner's functional effectiveness, safety, and acceptance by the client may offer one solution to the high costs, long waits, and depersonalization in health care today.

In general, changing roles and functions and the laws that govern them are not enacted simultaneously. Usually a time lag exists between the adoption of a new function and official approval. Thus nurses who fill drug reservoirs for epidural administration of analgesia and inject some medications intravenously are breaking new legal ground. Such procedures are potentially more risky than other medication procedures, and nurses who perform them are probably placing themselves in a tenuous legal position unless (1) they are qualified by virtue of adequate training, education, and experience, and (2) written sanction exists. Policies should be drawn up jointly by the administration of the health care agency and nursing representatives. These policy statements should carefully delineate the roles of nurses, nurse practitioners, physicians, and physician assistants, and should present guidelines for these procedures. These statements should also include a list of drugs and routes to be used only by physicians and a list of criteria for permitting nurses to give medications by an intravenous (IV) route or other system. Currently in most pharmacy departments, personnel draw up and prepare admixtures in large-volume IV solutions before delivering the medication to the nursing area. This procedure is performed under controlled conditions in agency pharmacies, with the goal of reducing IV solution contamination and medication errors.

✴ **What legal requirements need to be met before I may administer a drug?**

At the implementation stage, three conditions must be met before a medication can legally be administered by any route:

1. The medication order must be valid.
2. The physician/prescriber and the nurse must be licensed. The nonphysician prescriber must be prescribing within the regulations of the state.
3. The nurse must know the purpose, actions, effects, and major adverse effects of the drug, and the teaching required to enable the client or caregiver to self-administer the drug safely and accurately.

A valid order is one that leaves no room for doubt regarding the medication prescribed, its dosage and route, the dosing interval, and the prescriber's name/signature. Moreover, the drug must also be deemed appropriate for that specific client. Because nurses are legally, morally, and ethically responsible for their actions, *they must assess the medication order for its preciseness, accuracy, and appropriateness.* Orders signed by medical students, physician assistants, and, in some states, nurse practitioners are not legally accepted as having been signed by a duly licensed physician (this is the wording of many nursing practice acts) and should not be until a physician actually sign the orders (unless the law is changed). Nurses should be aware of the policy of their health agency and state regulation. The validity of orders written and signed by an unlicensed intern or resident may be equivocal depending on local law or policy.

The medication order must be written and worded in a way that is correct, complete, legible, and clearly understandable. If it is not, clarification must be sought from the prescriber. Creating a healthy, open, questioning atmosphere in the prescriber-nurse relationship avoids the very real hazard lurking behind "guessing," "assuming," and "not wanting to bother the doctor."

Although not every medication given in error results in actual client harm, the potential always exists. See Chapter 4, entitled "Medication Errors."

The order may be judged by the nurse to be incorrect or inappropriate for the client. An example of this would be a dose too high for a client of low body weight or impaired renal function as evidenced by low creatinine clearance or a medication that is noted to have secondary effects of tachycardia or dysrhythmias and is ordered for a client with a recent myocardial infarction. Such a situation may be quite intimidating to the nurse, who is now in the position of challenging the judgment of the prescriber at the risk of incurring embarrassment, a job threat, or both. Of course, such intimidation is not justifiable. It is the nurse's or nursing student's absolute right and responsibility to question any proposed action that is potentially harmful to a client. Medications are written by the prescriber at a given time in the treatment of the client. However, the condition of the client may change, requiring the nurse to exercise critical judgment regarding the appropriateness of each dose for that client before administering it.

Prescribers and some nurses (and many consumers) often are under the mistaken impression that nurses who merely act by following a prescriber's order are absolved from any untoward results of that act. Actually, *no one can relieve a nurse of responsibility for the nurse's actions*; for a

nurse to carry out an order that the nurse knows to be incorrect constitutes negligence. Changing an order by modifying any part of it without consultation with the prescriber is similarly illegal.

✳ What do I do if I believe a medication order is in error?

If an order is believed to be in error, some suggested actions are as follows:

- Validate the order by consulting with the pharmacist, an authoritative reference source, such as the *USP DI, AHFS Drug Information,* or the health care agency's computerized drug information system.
- If the order is apparently incorrect, objectively report the conflicting facts and discuss it with the prescriber in a factual, nonblaming manner.

If the prescriber still wants the medication given as ordered after the nurse's objections have been raised, can the nurse give the medication if the prescriber takes full responsibility? Again, *no one* can release nurses from full responsibility for every medication they give just because they are acting under a prescriber's order. To do so is to court a lawsuit for negligence. This fact must be made clear to the prescriber as the rationale for the nurse's refusal to medicate.

If the prescriber chooses to administer the medication personally after the nurse refuses to do so in the belief that it could be potentially harmful to the client, the nurse should see that the facts of the situation are made known to the nurse's immediate supervisors, and consultation should be sought if necessary. Every health care agency should have in place a mechanism for such reporting. If the drug is given, the medication record should reflect that it was the prescriber who gave it.

✳ What if the medication order contains a drug with which I am not familiar?

Orders for a medication that is unfamiliar to the administering nurse must stimulate a nearly reflex reaction to "look it up" or to "ask the pharmacist." It is also important to realize that many trade names for drugs look and sound alike, as discussed in Chapter 1, so added caution is needed. Administering an unfamiliar drug even though remaining in ignorance of its actions and its intended effects and adverse effects (at the very minimum) is considered nursing negligence if it results in harm to the client. In one instance a nurse was found liable when a 3-month-old infant died after being given an injectable form of digoxin instead of the pediatric elixir. In another instance hospital staff members were found negligent when prolonged infiltration of a dopamine infusion went unobserved, causing permanent injury (*Macon-Bibb Hosp. Authority v. Ross*, 335 SE2d 633, GA, 1986) (Box 2-5).

✳ Do nurses commit malpractice?

Astute nurses are alert to both the set limits of functioning and to the quality of functioning within those limits. Most lawsuits are brought by clients or families who believe they were subjected to a behavior or procedure that was not of the quality reasonably expected of someone with a nurse's professional education and experience under the particular circumstances. This is identified legally as **malpractice.** The nurse can take precautions against malpractice resulting from errors of medication administration by observing the **Six Rights of Medication Administration:**

- The *right medication* (the one that was prescribed and one that is not contraindicated)
- The *right client* (not someone else's medication by mistake, nor the medication of the person in the next bed)
- The *right dose* as prescribed and appropriate (this may involve simple mathematic computations)
- The *right route*, form of the drug, and administration technique as prescribed
- The *right time* for the dose (usually within 30 minutes of the time indicated and at beneficial intervals as ordered)
- The *right documentation*

Other examples of nursing actions that support and facilitate meeting nursing responsibilities for preventing medication errors are discussed in Chapter 4.

For the nurse's part, *accountability* is a term that has gained increasing importance, particularly as related to pharmacotherapeutics. Nurses are no longer considered to be merely "physicians' handmaidens" or to be accorded "umbrella protection from litigation" by the prescriber and the health care agency. Nurses are expected to take the responsibility for and be answerable for the service they provide or make available.

The basic guidelines to litigation-free, professional nursing practice and to medication administration in particular include the following:

- Knowing the limitations of nursing practice in the community by being aware of and abiding by agency policies, joint medical and nursing practice statements, nursing practice acts, and state and federal laws.
- Knowing the limitations of one's own skills, expertise, knowledge, and experience and never exceeding them.
- Informing involved personnel of and documenting thoroughly and carefully all happenings related to client care, especially those with potential legal implications.
- Maintaining a professional, caring, and collaborative relationship with clients and their families. Aside from this approach being proper, it can act to dissolve the potential dissatisfaction of clients with health care, the institution, or its policies.

✷ What are the ethical considerations of nursing management of drug therapy?

Value conflicts for nurses occur as a result of the changing legislation governing many of their activities in relation to medication administration, the increasing role of nurses in clinical research in pharmacotherapeutics, and day-to-day practice in which nurse, client, and prescriber may have differing opinions regarding what measures to take in a specific situation.

Probably the most powerful fundamental force at work in the actual implementation of right and proper nursing practice is the nurse's own concept of ethical and moral correctness and responsibility. The American Nurses Association (1985), the Canadian Nurses Association (1980), and the International Council of Nurses (1973) (Ellis & Hartley, 2003) have

---

BOX 2-5 LEGAL ASPECTS OF THE NURSING ROLE

How often do nurses encounter an infiltrating IV in the routine care of clients? The assessment and action taken by the nurse can be significant for the client, as in the case of *Macon-Bibb Hosp. Authority v. Ross,* 335 SE2d 633, GA, 1986.

Ms. Ross was brought to the emergency department (ED) with dyspnea, bradycardia, and a blood pressure of 250/150 mm Hg. She went into respiratory arrest at 2:55 PM; she was intubated with an endotracheal tube, and nitroprusside was administered intravenously to decrease her blood pressure. Because of the rapid drop in blood pressure, an IV administration of dopamine was started at 3:28 PM in her right wrist to increase her blood pressure. When her blood pressure stabilized, she was transferred to the cardiac care unit at 4:30 PM. At midnight, a nurse noted that the IV site had a "bruise bluish in color." The next notation was at 11:00 AM the following day, in which it was recorded that the client's right arm was swollen and painful with a large blistered area around the IV site. The same notation was made at 4:00 PM. It was not until 6:50 PM that a note indicated that a physician was informed of the infiltration. As a result of the extravasation of dopamine, the client's lower right arm was permanently scarred. On a jury verdict, the court entered judgment for the client.

The hospital appealed, but the court of appeals affirmed the judgment of the lower court. It was noted that although an in-

filtration may result from an improper technique, it may also be a result of the size of the needle, the status of the client's veins, or a particular intolerance to an IV. According to the expert nurse's testimony and supported by suitable references, dopamine should be infused into a "large vein," such as in the antecubital fossa, to minimize the risk of extravasation. In addition, dopamine should be monitored continuously for free flow. If extravasation of dopamine occurs, the recommended treatment of the site is infiltration with a saline solution of phentolamine (Regitine) within 12 hours.

The nurses were criticized for not being sufficiently knowledgeable regarding dopamine, which resulted in their failure to notify a physician of the client's impaired tissue integrity.

CRITICAL THINKING QUESTIONS

- How could the ED nurse caring for Ms. Ross have prevented this incident?
- What action should have been taken by Ms. Ross's admitting nurse in the intensive care unit to prevent this incident?
- What action should have been taken by the nurse who noted that the IV site had a "bruise bluish in color"?
- In what way could this hospital prevent a similar occurrence in the future?

adopted similar codes of ethics for nurses, which can serve as guides to standards of conduct, relationships, and practice. The nurse's responsibilities to clients as defined by these codes of ethics are to promote health, prevent illness, restore health, and alleviate suffering. The core of any such professional code is that its precepts spring from the reality that the client is a person with rights and dignity not to be subsumed under the needs or rights of any other person or the machinations of a health care agency or society at large. Thus nurses are obligated to respect the wishes of clients and to treat them with dignity. For example, a client has every right to know the necessary information about a drug he or she is receiving and to refuse to take a drug after having been given an explanation, no matter what the consequences. A client's right to respect from the nurse is independent of nationality, race, creed, color, age, gender, sexual orientation, politics, or physical or social status.

When ethical dilemmas occur, nurses may experience conflicting loyalties to their profession, colleagues, clients, agencies, spiritual/religious beliefs, and society. Nursing ethics, which provide guidance for nursing action, are based on the principles of **nonmalfeasance** (the duty to do no harm), **beneficence** (the duty to do good), autonomy (client empowerment), justice (fair and equal treatment for all), fidelity (faithfulness to one's obligations), and integrity (being true to one's word). These issues are essential to the bond of trust in the nurse-client relationship and demonstrate the caring perspective that is at the heart of nursing practice. The tenets of the codes of practice for nurses assure the client that the nurse will act in the client's best interest.

This obligation of the nurse to the client includes respecting the client's values, whether or not the nurse agrees with the client's decision in relation to his or her health care. For example, some clients might value remaining mentally alert and in control of their experiences rather than taking medications that would offer pain relief but could also alter their thought processes. The responsibility of the nurse is to assist the client in the decision-making process by ensuring that the client is informed of the risks and benefits of the therapy and can make a knowledgeable decision.

✳ How do these legal and ethical issues affect nursing practice?

Early in a nursing career, the study of legal issues related to the administration of medications can seem a somewhat less than fascinating exercise. However, as the nurse builds practical experience, this study proves its worth time and time again. Laws, acts, codes, and regulations shaping pharmacologic practice provide the boundaries for safe practice. Experience proves that knowing the accepted scope of nursing practice of one's nation, state, local, and institutional community provides security and support for the nurse who aspires to provide harm-free care. Legal statutes only guide; nurses must translate these guides into action. Often what provides the best guidance within legal constraints is the judgment of the individual nurse on the basis of his or her own code of ethics, professionalism, and sense of accountability. A fundamental precept is that what is best for the client usually turns out to be best for the nurse.

There are few hard and fast rules in nursing practice. Many specific questions about legalities in drug administration must be answered, and often the answer is "It depends. . . ." This should not immobilize nurses and prevent them from acting in healthy, assertive ways. If they function within the accepted boundaries of practice, continue to stretch for new knowledge, and act accountably for the benefit of their clients, little exists that can harm their clients, themselves, their professional reputations, or their jobs. The sureness that comes with experience flourishes as these skills are exercised. Exercising these skills often demands standing

---

⚙ TECHNOLOGY LINK

Legal and Ethical Aspects of Medication Administration

American Nurses Association (www.ana.org)

This site contains the ANA Code for Nursing, which includes guidelines for self-determination of clients, social and economic status of clients, and patient rights.

Food and Drug Administration (www.fda.gov)

This site is a comprehensive information source about the history of drug regulation, current processes for drug approval, and drug information.

Nursing Ethics Resources (www.nursingethics.ca)

This Canadian site is a good source of general nursing ethics resources, such as codes of ethics, nursing ethics in the news, books and articles on nursing ethics, and links to other biomedical and health care ethics websites.

Nursing Ethics Network (NEN) (www.nursingethicsnetwork.org)

The Nursing Ethics Network is an organization of professional nurses dedicated to advancing nursing ethics in clinical settings. It is supported by the Boston College of Nursing.

National Council of State Boards of Nursing (www.ncsbn.org)

This site contains a variety of nursing resources and documents about nurse regulation and licensure in each state. This organization is also the developer of the NCLEX examinations.

Public Responsibility in Medicine and Research (www.primr.org)

PRIM&R is committed to the advancement of strong research programs and to the consistent application of ethical precepts in both medicine and research. Through the website, PRIM&R addresses a broad range of issues in biomedical and behavioral research, clinical practice, ethics, and the law.

up for what is right in client care despite pressures generated by time constraints or by others who want them to "just get on with it." Being human, nurses will occasionally fail to use the best judgment or to be perfect. This is reasonable, but it is also reasonable for nurses to aspire to structure their practice in ways that make it difficult to fail.

The neophyte nurse may be somewhat shaken by the wealth of background information necessary to safe practice. The more experienced nurse will probably grapple with the temptation to become complacent and to make dangerous assumptions about the limits of the nurse's practice. Both have an equal need to continue to read and question in order to improve the quality of their decisions, whether the issues stem from legal, ethical, or moral considerations. See the Technology Link box on p. 29 for recommended sources of online information.

Although sophisticated and well-regulated in theory, the art of drug development, evaluation, and prescribing may sometimes be inadequate in practice. Because all chemical substances create adverse effects and interactions and because many have been identified as having questionable efficacy, it becomes increasingly compelling to avoid medicating when feasible and to substitute rational nursing measures. For example, if instituted effectively and early in the pain cycle, nursing interventions to promote comfort can often substantially reduce pain so that "as necessary" medications become less necessary.

Summary

Although substances to treat illness and cure disease have always existed, it was not until the twentieth century that the need to standardize and regulate such substances became apparent. In the United States, the Pure Food and Drug Act of 1906 was the first to limit false and misleading claims for drugs, but only those involved in interstate commerce. The *United States Pharmacopeia* was established as official standards for drugs. Further legislation in 1938 required the testing of drugs for safety, and in 1952 the requirements for distinction between legend drugs and OTCs were established. The Orphan Drug Act of 1983 has provided for the development of drugs for the treatment of rare diseases. To ease the movement of generic drugs to the marketplace the Drug Price Competition and Patent Restoration Act of 1984 was legislated. Since that time both generic, prescription, and OTC preparations have proliferated and there has been constant review to ensure their safety and efficacy.

The Harrison Narcotic Act of 1914 was the first law passed by any nation to regulate opium and other substances producing drug dependence. Currently such drugs are governed by the Controlled Substances Act which, in addition to other regulations, classifies controlled substances into their compared use and abuse potential. This law influences the daily routine of many nurses; a controlled substances count is performed at the beginning and end of every shift in settings in which supplies of these drugs are maintained. Other protection in effect for consumers includes the reporting of drug reactions by clinicians to the FDA, the reg-

ulation of biologic products by the Public Health Service, and the legislation of product liability by many states.

Similar legislation exists in Canada for the protection of its citizens. Although often amended, the Canadian Food and Drugs Act of 1953 stipulates the standards for drugs through a variety of pharmacopoeias and formularies, prohibits the sale of unsafe drugs and those with misleading labels, and in general regulates biologic, legend, controlled, and designated drugs. The Canadian Controlled Drugs and Substances Act of 1996 governs the possession, sale, manufacture, production, and distribution of narcotics. By this Act a nurse can be in legal possession of a narcotic only when administering a drug on the order of a physician, acting as the official custodian of narcotics in a hospital or clinic, or being a client for whom a physician has prescribed a drug.

Because drugs vary in strength and activity, standardization is necessary to ensure uniformity of strength and purity by either chemical or biologic assay. The only official book of drug standards in the United States is the *USP*, whereas Canada uses the *USP*, the *Canadian Formulary*, and the *British Pharmacopoeia*.

The progress of any drug from concept to acceptance in general practice is lengthy and costly. The FDA approval process ensures that each drug progresses sequentially after being classified as an IND, with an initial pharmacologic evaluation, a limited controlled evaluation, and an extended clinical evaluation. If the drug is promising, an NDA is submitted to the FDA for approval. If the NDA is approved, a postmarketing surveillance period follows. All participants in the experimental studies of this process should have given informed consent. Because nurses have increasing contact with clinical drug studies, they need to understand the precepts of the Nuremberg Code and other patient-protective measures and be alert to their implementation in the clinical setting to protect clients' rights.

Nurses in their practice are regulated not only by the legislation previously discussed but also by the nurse practice acts of the individual state in which they practice. These statutes define the scope of nursing practice as a health care profession within that state. As the roles of nurses change and expand in drug therapy, all states are allowing nurse practitioners to prescribe, albeit within limitations in some states. Even for nurses without a practitioner qualification, medication administration has become more of an interdependent function. Three conditions are essential for the administration of any drug by a nurse: (1) the medication order must be valid; (2) both the physician/prescriber and the nurse must be licensed; and (3) the nurse must be knowledgeable about the drug. In addition, nurses can safeguard themselves from errors of medication administration by observing the Six Rights of Medication Administration. With increasing accountability for their role in pharmacotherapeutics, nurses should be aware of guides to litigation-free, professional nursing practice.

Bibliography

American Nurses Association. (1985). *Code for nurses with interpretive statements.* Kansas City, MO: Author.

Anderson, D.M. (Ed.). (2002). *Mosby's medical, nursing, & allied health dictionary* (6th ed.). St. Louis: Mosby.

✳ Critical Thinking Questions

- A nurse is working with a client with advanced cancer for whom the physician orders chemotherapy. The client has reservations about starting the chemotherapy regimen and asks numerous questions about the benefits and risks associated with it. The nurse has been told that the client's condition is terminal and knows that the chemotherapy may alter the client's comfort with severe nausea and vomiting. Although realizing that the physician recommends the chemotherapy, the nurse feels a conflict between the need to follow orders and the nurse's role as client advocate. What action should the nurse take?

- When preparing to administer medications to a client in a home setting, the nurse notices that the container for one of the medications, instead of having a drug name, bears a number as an experimental drug with instructions to be given "one tablet three times a day." What action should the nurse take?

Blake J.B. (Ed.). (1968). *Safeguarding the public: Historical aspects of medicinal drug control.* Baltimore: The Johns Hopkins University Press.

Boodhoo, L. Bordoli, G., Mitcell, A.R., Lloyd, G., Sulka, N., & Patel, N. (2004). The safety and effectiveness of a nurse led cardioversion service under sedation, *Heart 90*(12), 1443-1446.

Bryant, R. & Graham, M.C. (2002). Advanced practice nurses: A study of client satisfaction. Journal of *American Academy of Nurse Practitioners, 14*(2), 88-92.

Canadian Nurses Association. (1980). *CNA code of ethics: An ethical basis for nursing in Canada.* Ottawa: Author.

Cowen, D.L. & Helfand, W.H. (1990). *Pharmacy: An illustrated history.* New York: Harry N. Abrams.

Crowther, M. (2003). Optimal management of outpatients with heart failure used advanced practice nurses in a hospital-based heart failure center. Journal of *American Academy of Nurse Practitioners, 15*(6), 260-265.

DiMasi, J.A., Hansen, R.W. & Grabowski, H.G. (2003). The price of innovation: New estimates of drug development costs. *Journal of Health Economics, 22*, 151-185.

Drug facts and comparisons (58th ed.). (2005). St. Louis: Facts and Comparisons.

Ellis, J.R. & Hartley, C.L. (2003). *Nursing in today's world: Challenges, issues, and trends* (8th ed.). Philadelphia: Lippincott, Williams & Wilkins.

International Narcotics Control Board. (2003). The role of the INCB. Retrieved October 17, 2003 from http://www.incb.org/e/index.htm

Jameson, S. (2003). Developing and maintaining a community research program. *Oncology Issues, 18*(4), 22-30.

Karigan, M. (2001). Ethics in clinical research: The nursing perspective. *American Journal of Nursing, 101*(9), 26-31.

Kimmel, S.E., Berlin, J.A., Reilly, M., Jaskowiak, J., Kishel, L., Chittams, J., et al. (2005). Patients exposed to rofecoxib and celecoxib have different odds of nonfatal myocardial infarction. *Annals of Internal Medicine, 142*(3), 157-164.

Lambing, A.Y., Adams, D.L., Fox, D.H., & Divine, G. (2004). Nurse practitioners' and physicians' care activities and clinical outcomes with an inpatient geriatric population, *Journal of the American Academy of Nursing Practitioners, 16*(8), 343-352.

McGrath, S. (1990). The cost-effectiveness of nurse practitioners. *Nurse Practitioner 15*, 40-42.

Mundinger, M.O. (1994). Advanced practice nursing: Good medicine for physicians? *New England Journal of Medicine, 330*, 211-214.

Pan, S., Straub, L.A., & Geller, J.M. (1997). Restrictive practice environment and nurse practitioners' prescriptive authority. *Journal of the American Academy of Nurse Practitioners, 9*(1), 9-15.

Pearson, L.J. (2000). Annual legislative update: How each state stands on legislative issues affecting advanced nursing practice. *Nurse Practitioner, 25*(1), 16-21.

Psaty, B.M., Furberg, C.D., Ray, W.A., & Weiss, N.S. (2004). Potential for conflict of interest in the evaluation of suspected adverse drug reactions: Use of cerivastatin and risk of rhabdomyolysis, *Journal of the American Medical Association, 292*(21), 2622-2631.

Public Citizen's Congress Watch. *America's other drug problem: A briefing book on the Rx drug debate.* Retrieved September 30, 2003 from http://www.citizen.org/documents/drugbriefingbk.pdf

Rosenfeld, P., Kobayashi, M., Barber, P., & Mezey, M. (2004). Utilization of nurse practitioners in long-term care: Findings and implications of a national survey. *Journal of American Medical Directors Association, 5*(1), 9-15.

Tabak, N. (1995). Decision making in consenting to experimental cancer therapy. *Cancer Nursing, 18*(2), 89-96.

Tschudini, V. (2003). *Ethics in nursing: The caring relationship* (Rev. 2nd ed.). Philadelphia: Elsevier.

U.S. Food & Drug Administration. (2003a). *Abbreviated new drug application (ANDA): Process for generic drugs.* Retrieved October 19, 2003, from http://www.fda.gov/cder/regulatory/applications/ANDA.htm

U.S. Food & Drug Administration. (2003b). Consulting the controlled substance staff on abuse liability, drug dependence, risk management and drug scheduling. *Manual of Policies and Procedures,* Center for Drug Evaluation and Research. Retrieved October 1, 2003, from http://www.fda.gov/cder/mapp/4200.3.pdf

U.S. Food & Drug Administration. (2003c). *The Orphan Drug Act (as amended).* Retrieved October 1, 2003, from http://www.fda.gov/orphan/oda.htm

USP DI: Drug information for the health care professional (25th ed.). (2005). Greenwood Village, CO: MICROMEDEX Thomson Healthcare.

Worthington, K.A. (2002). MedWatch: Promoting patient, worker safety by reporting medical device problems. *American Journal of Nursing, 102*(11), 112-115.

Young, J.H. (1961). *The toadstool millionaires: A social history of patent medicines in America before federal regulation.* Princeton, NJ: Princeton University Press.

*e-*LEARNING SUPPLEMENTS

Student CD-ROM
- Final Exam questions
- NCLEX Examination review questions
- Pharmacology animations
- Printable chapter summary

Evolve Website (http://evolve.elsevier.com/mckenry)
- Content updates, including information on new drugs
- WebLinks corresponding to this chapter
- Answers to the critical thinking questions in this chapter
- *Elsevier ePharmacology Update* newsletter
- *Mosby's Drug Consult* Internet Edition
- Supplemental and reference information

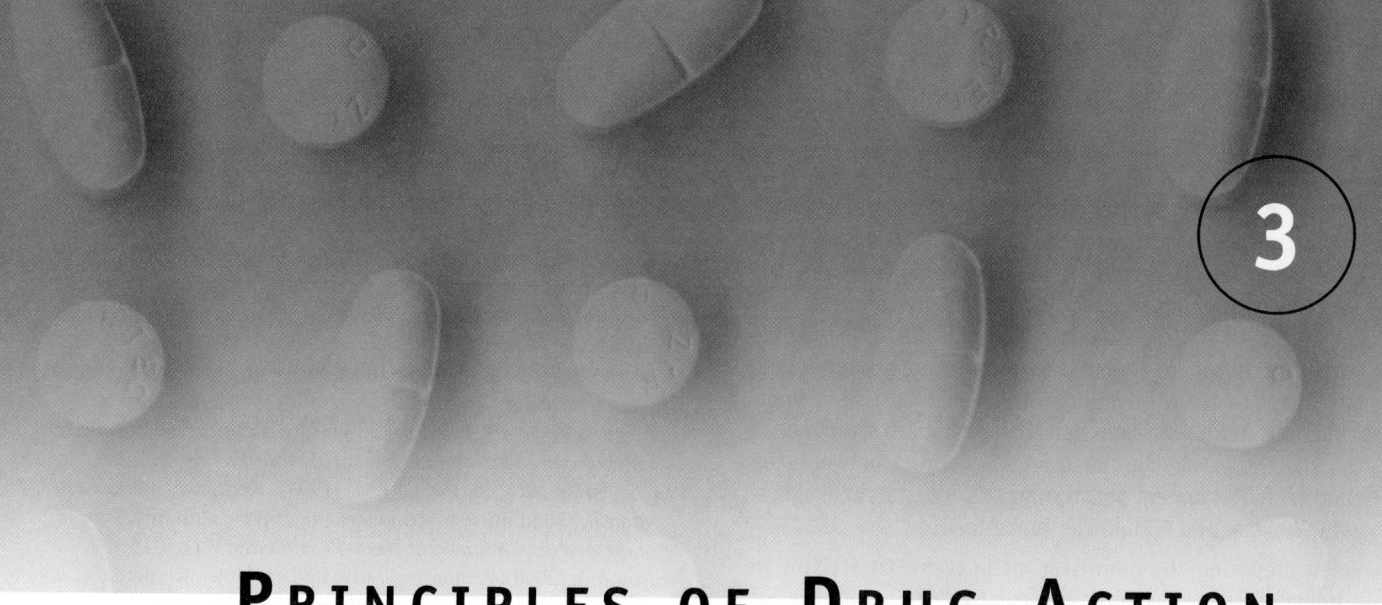

3

PRINCIPLES OF DRUG ACTION

CHAPTER FOCUS

The number of drugs used therapeutically is increasing tremendously, and because of this, the nurse's responsibilities concerning these agents have also expanded. To approach the level of knowledge needed to meet these increased responsibilities, all health care professionals must develop a fundamental theoretical framework within which to study and apply an understanding of drug therapy. This chapter presents theories of drug action, physiologic processes mediating drug action, variables affecting drug action, and unusual and adverse effects of drug therapy. The nurse can transfer this knowledge to the care of the unique problems of individual clients. Although these concepts may seem complex initially, an understanding of them is essential to the safe and effective management of a client's drug therapy. With continued study these concepts will become integral to your nursing knowledge and provide the reasoning for sound nursing judgment in relation to drug therapy for each of your clients.

LEARNING OBJECTIVES

- Identify the four general properties of drugs.
- Describe the three phases of drug activity: pharmaceutical, pharmacokinetic, and pharmacodynamic.
- Cite examples of drug properties that influence pharmacokinetics.
- Describe the physiochemical processes mediating drug action.
- Explain the client variables that influence the rate and extent of absorption, distribution, metabolism, and elimination.
- Explain current theories of drug action: drug-receptor interaction, drug-enzyme interaction, and nonspecific drug interaction.
- Discuss conditions that can alter the body's response to drugs.
- Use nursing assessments to identify unusual and adverse effects of drug therapy.
- Implement nursing management of drug therapy related to client variables that alter drug responses.

▲ KEY TERMS

Nurses have traditionally administered drugs to clients. In many health care delivery settings today, the nurse's responsibility has shifted to include educating clients for safe and effective self-management of drug therapy and the observing, interpreting, and documenting the client's response to and management of the drug regimen. The nurse may also be responsible for ensuring the safe administration of drugs by delegating that task to a variety of specially educated health workers. Because the moral, ethical, and legal responsibilities for drug therapy remain the nurse's, an understanding of the principles of drug action—pharmacokinetics and pharmacodynamics—is essential.

What are drugs?

A drug is a chemical that interacts with a living organism to produce a biologic response. Such a broad definition may be considered by some as controversial. For instance, is tobacco a drug? Under this definition it would be considered a drug because it contains a number of chemicals that interact with the human body to produce specific and measurable biologic effects. Similarly, many dietary supplements may be considered drugs because they contain chemicals that interact with the human body and produce quantifiable biologic effects. Yet in the United States and Canada, their legal recognition as drugs has been hotly debated and currently both tobacco and dietary supplements (herbs, vitamins, plant by-products—often referred to as "nutraceuticals") are not viewed by the U.S. Food and Drug Administration (FDA) (or, in Canada, by the Health Protection Branch [HPB] of Health Canada) in the same way as prescription and over-the-counter (OTC) medications. The ban on ephedra demonstrates that the role of the FDA and HPB is evolving to include oversight of nutraceuticals.

How do drugs work?

Drugs interact with the body to produce a specific response or set of responses. These effects are achieved through a biochemical and/or physiologic interaction between the drug and a functionally important tissue component (usually, but not always, a receptor) in the body. Drugs have four general properties:

- *Drugs only modify existing functions on a tissue or body organ; they do not create new functions.* Drugs do not "create" new sites of action in the body. The effects of drugs can be recognized only by alterations of a known physiologic function or process, such as replacing, interrupting, or potentiating a physiologic process in specialized tissues. For example, drugs used to treat anemia can replace iron to re-store the adequate production of red blood cells. Atropine reduces the rate of salivation in preoperative clients, which is an abnormal state, but that action decreases the surgical risk of aspiration. The administration of a cathartic can potentiate the rate of evacuation of the large intestine.

- *Drugs in general exert multiple actions rather than a single effect.* Receptors in which drugs work are located throughout the body and may be strikingly similar in their structure and their affinity for a drug. Different tissues may use similar or identical systems or processes (e.g., enzymes, electrolytes) and a drug that impacts such systems or processes affects multiple tissues. The beneficial effect observed in one set of tissues may be counterbalanced by undesirable effects observed in another set of tissues. As a rule, drugs that are more specific for their site of action are associated with fewer adverse effects. An example is atropine, a drug that has an affinity for heart, lung, gastrointestinal (GI), genitourinary (GU), and other tissues throughout the body. If atropine is administered to improve lung function in a client with chronic obstructive pulmonary disease (COPD), we observe the desired improved bronchodilation, but may also observe elevated heart rate, constipation, dry mouth and urinary retention. An alternative, ipratropium (Atrovent), works like atropine in the lung tissue, but when given by inhalation, is not absorbed in other tissue and as such does not produce the cardiac, GI, or GU tissue effects.

- *Drug action results from a physiochemical interaction between the drug and a functionally important molecule in the body.* Some drugs act by combining with a small molecule in the cellular environment (e.g., antacids neutralize gastric acid) or by altering membrane function (e.g., local anesthetics). However, the majority of drugs work by interacting with specific macromolecular components in tissues (typically receptors). The nature of this interaction is highly specific. The study of these interactions is referred to as **pharmacodynamics** and this phase of drug action is called the pharmacodynamic phase (Figure 3-1).

- *For a drug to achieve its function and interaction in the body, it must be present in adequate quantities at its specific site of action.* If a drug has an effect in heart tissue, an adequate quantity of that drug must reach cardiac tissue to exert its pharmacologic effect. To reach tissues, we must consider the dosage forms, or **pharmaceutics**, that are available and how those forms can be delivered to the body as individual molecules (the pharmaceutical phase of drug action). Once the dose form is in the body and is available as the individual molecule, it often needs to cross membranes to reach the site of action. The body will also attempt to alter and/or remove the drug from the body. The study of this process is known as **pharmacokinetics** (or the pharmacokinetic phase of drug action) (see Figure 3-1).

✳ How do drugs interact with the body at the tissue level?

Drugs typically work at the cellular or tissue level to modify existing physiologic properties. These pharmacodynamic interactions may involve altering enzyme function, hormone secretion, or metabolic functions either within the individual to whom the drug was administered, or on a pathogen (e.g., bacteria, virus) that is infecting the client. The process by which the drug exerts its effect is referred to as the drug's **mechanism of action**. The mechanism of drug action varies from drug to drug, but usually includes drug-receptor interactions, drug-enzyme interactions, or other nonspecific drug interactions (Ross & Kenakin, 2001).

Drug-Receptor Interactions

Many drugs work by binding to drug receptors in a very specific way to produce a quantifiable pharmacologic effect. A **receptor** is a location on a cell surface where certain mol-

ecules, such as drugs, enzymes, and neurotransmitters, attach to interact with cellular components. Most drug receptors possess a very specific three-dimensional configuration. Typically a portion of the drug molecule (considered the active site or sites) interacts with the specific molecular structure of the drug receptor to produce a tight fit. An analogy is a key (i.e., drug) fitting into a specific lock (i.e., drug receptor) in a three-dimensional configuration (Figure 3-2). The nature of drug "binding" to these receptor sites varies from drug to drug and receptor to receptor. It is characterized by the following principles:

- **Drug–receptor binding is reversible.** The interaction between drug and receptor is usually transient with drugs "hopping" on and off receptors frequently. The degree and duration of receptor binding are functions of how well the drug fits the receptor, the nature of the bond or attraction, and the concentration of the drug at the site of the receptor.
- **Drug-receptor binding is selective.** The interaction between drug and receptor is very specific. Each drug and receptor has a three-dimensional configuration that fits like a lock and key. Drugs that fit receptors very tightly or are strongly attracted to the receptor are considered to have a high **affinity** for the receptors.
- **Drug-receptor binding is graded.** Typically a "threshold" number of receptors must be filled with the drug before a pharmacologic response is observed. As more receptors are occupied, a greater pharmacologic response is observed. Once most or all of the receptors are occupied, a maximal pharmacological effect is observed and further increases in drug concentration at the receptor site will not produce added effect.
- **Drugs that bind to receptors may be agonistic, partial agonistic, or antagonistic.** Drugs that are **agonists** at the receptor display both a high affinity for the receptor and also produce a pharmacologic response (also referred to as intrinsic activity or **efficacy**) (Figure 3-3). Once a drug binds to a receptor, a series of events occur to transfer a signal from the occupied receptor site to an intracellular system to acti-

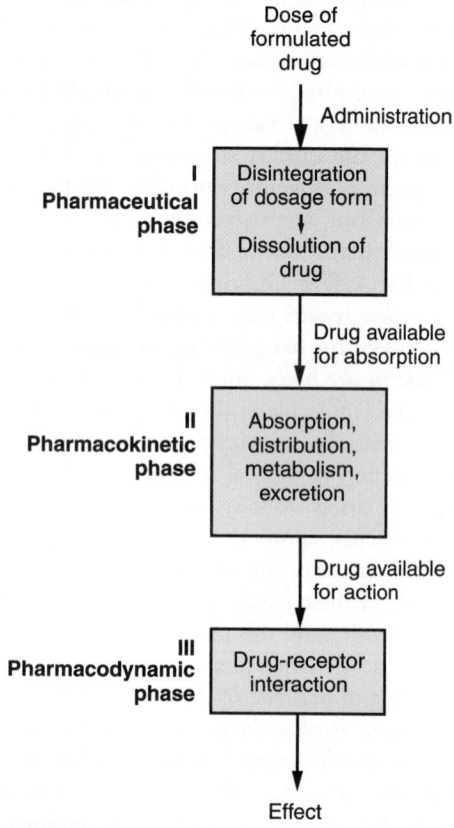

Dose of formulated drug

↓ Administration

I Pharmaceutical phase — Disintegration of dosage form → Dissolution of drug

↓ Drug available for absorption

II Pharmacokinetic phase — Absorption, distribution, metabolism, excretion

↓ Drug available for action

III Pharmacodynamic phase — Drug-receptor interaction

↓

Effect

FIGURE 3-1 Phases of drug activity.

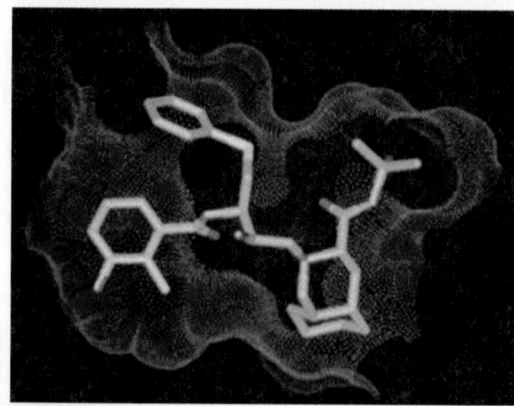

FIGURE 3-2 The anti-HIV drug nelfinavir (Viracept) is depicted binding to HIV-1 protease.

vate an event. The elements of this process include the drug binding to the receptor and a transducer effect involving an electrical or chemical signal to an intermediary (referred to as an effector) that facilitates an intracellular reaction producing a pharmacologic effect (Figure 3-4).

An **antagonist** is an agent that has an affinity for the receptor (or an area near the receptor) and counteracts the action of other drugs or substances at the receptor. Antagonists may be either competitive (e.g., compete with agonists to bind to the receptor) (Figure 3-5) or noncompetitive (e.g., bind to a site near the receptor and change the three-dimensional structure of the receptor in a way that renders the receptor inactive; typically these are less reversible or irreversible reactions) (Figure 3-6).

Drug-Enzyme Interaction

Enzymes are biologic catalysts that control all biochemical reactions of the cell. Drugs can inhibit the action of a specific enzyme and alter a physiologic process. For example, neostigmine (Prostigmin) is an agent used to manage the muscle weakness caused by myasthenia gravis, a degenerative neurologic disease. Neostigmine acts chemically by combining with the enzyme acetylcholinesterase to prevent it from inactivating the neurotransmitter acetylcholine at the neuromuscular junction. This prolongs the action of acetylcholine and helps to maintain muscle strength.

Drugs that combine with enzymes may do so because of their structural resemblance to an enzyme's substrate molecule (the substance acted on by an enzyme). A drug may resemble an enzyme's substrate so closely that the enzyme combines with the drug instead of with the normal substrate. Drugs resembling enzyme substrates are termed "antimetabolites" and can either block normal enzymatic action or result in the production of other substances with unique biochemical properties. The antimetabolites become the receptors for the enzyme. An example of an antimetabolite is the anticancer drug methotrexate, which inhibits the enzyme that allows the reduction of folic acid for deoxyribonucleic acid (DNA), ribonucleic acid (RNA), and protein synthesis.

Nonspecific Drug Interaction

Some drugs demonstrate no structural specificity and presumably act by producing more general effects on cell membranes and cellular processes. These drugs may penetrate into cells or accumulate in cellular membranes, by which they interfere, through physical or chemical means, with cell function or fundamental metabolic processes.

Cell membranes are complex lipoprotein structures that regulate the flow of ions and metabolites in a highly selective manner, to maintain an electrochemical gradient between the interior and exterior surfaces of the cell. Structurally

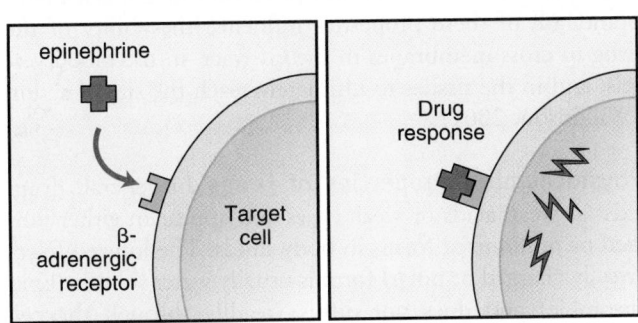

FIGURE 3-3 Agonist activity at the drug receptor.

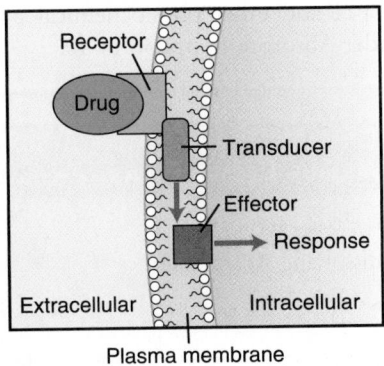

FIGURE 3-4 Cellular response to drug binding. This figure depicts actions that occur once a drug binds to a receptor, including drug binding at the receptor and transduction of a chemical or electrical signal via a transducer to an intermediary effector resulting in a pharmacologic response.

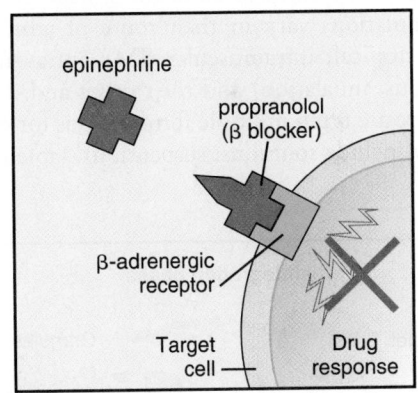

FIGURE 3-5 Competitive antagonistic activity at the receptor site.

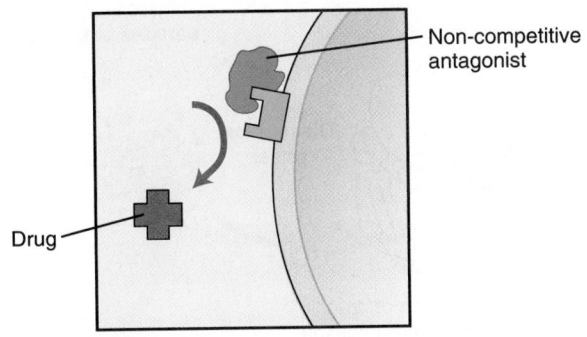

FIGURE 3-6 Noncompetitive antagonist activity at the receptor site.

nonspecific drugs include the general anesthetics, which are lipid-soluble compounds that have unrelated chemical structures but similar properties. It is believed that the general anesthetics alter the properties of lipids in the cell membranes of nerves rather than act on specific receptors.

Other structurally nonspecific drugs may act by biophysical means that do not affect cellular or enzymatic functions. Drugs acting as a result of their obvious physical properties include ointments and emollients. Hydrophilic (water-seeking) indigestible substances exert a laxative effect because of their physical action on the bowel. Examples of true chemical reactions that produce biologic effects include the interaction of a molecule such as lead with an antidotal drug and the neutralization of the hydrochloric acid in gastric juice by antacid drugs. Neither is considered a receptor interaction because no macromolecular tissue elements are involved. Detergents, isopropyl alcohol, hydrogen peroxide, and phenol derivatives such as phenylphenol (Lysol) are also structurally nonspecific and act by irreversibly destroying the functional integrity of the living cell.

✳ How do drugs get into the body?

The two phases of drug activity that are important for drugs to reach their site of action are the pharmaceutical phase and the pharmacokinetic phase.

Pharmaceutical Phase

Drugs administered in clinical practice are manufactured and packaged in a form to allow for storage and stability. Drug formulations vary in their route of administration (e.g., oral, topical, intramuscular (IM), intravenous (IV), subcutaneous, inhalation) and their onset and duration of effect. There are often multiple formulations for oral drugs, which may include solutions, suspensions, tablets, capsules

and sustained release formulations. For an oral drug to be absorbed, it must be available to cross the membranes of the GI tract in solution. The process by which a drug goes into solution and becomes available for absorption is known as **dissolution.** More rapid dissolution increases the rate at which the compound crosses the cell membrane. The dosage form of the drug influences the rate of dissolution. Oral drugs in liquid or in rapidly dissolving forms are more rapidly available for GI absorption than those in solid form (Figure 3-7 and Box 3-1).

Pharmacokinetic Phase

Pharmacokinetics is the study of drug concentrations during the processes of absorption, distribution, biotransformation, and excretion. The concentration of a drug at the site of its action is influenced by four primary factors: the rate and extent to which a drug is (1) absorbed into body fluids, (2) distributed to sites of action or storage areas, (3) biotransformed or metabolized to pharmacologically active or inactive metabolites, and (4) excreted from the body (Figure 3-8).

A number of variables influence the degree to which a drug is absorbed, distributed, metabolized, and excreted. These variables include the physiochemical properties of drugs, (e.g., molecular size of the drug, the degree of water or lipid solubility of the drug, and electrical charge of the drug) and the physiochemical properties of the cell membrane. All of these properties influence the ability of the drug to cross membranes in the GI tract, in the blood vessels, and in the tissues to ultimately reach the site of action (Wilkinson, 2001).

Physiochemical Properties of Drugs In general, drugs exist as weak acids or weak bases and appear in either ionized or nonionized forms in body fluids. The ionized (electrically charged or polar) form is usually water soluble (lipid insoluble) and does not diffuse readily through the cell membranes of the body. By contrast, the nonionized (electrically neutral or nonpolar) form is more lipid soluble (less water-soluble) and is more apt to cross cell membranes. The influence of pH and other physiochemical properties are discussed under Absorption, pp. 38 to 40.

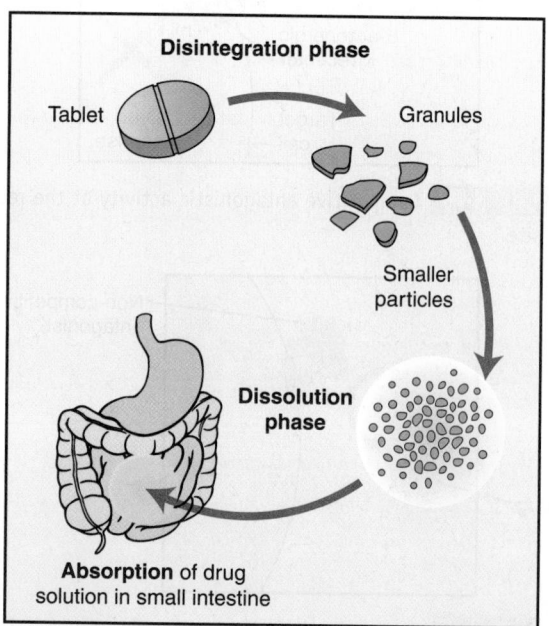

Disintegration phase

Tablet → Granules

Smaller particles

Dissolution phase

Absorption of drug solution in small intestine

FIGURE 3-7 Pharmaceutical phase.

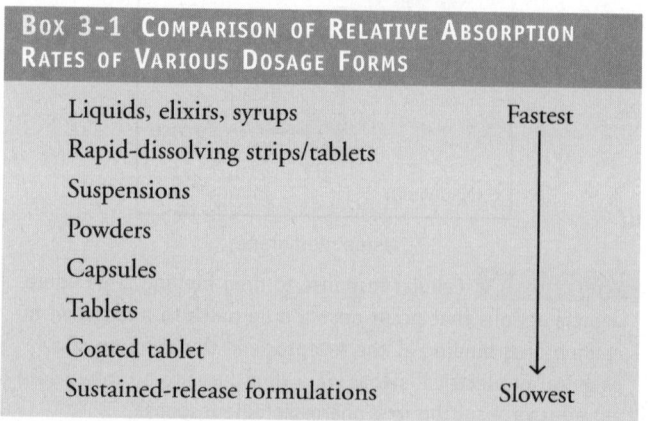

BOX 3-1 COMPARISON OF RELATIVE ABSORPTION RATES OF VARIOUS DOSAGE FORMS

Liquids, elixirs, syrups	Fastest
Rapid-dissolving strips/tablets	
Suspensions	
Powders	
Capsules	
Tablets	
Coated tablet	
Sustained-release formulations	Slowest

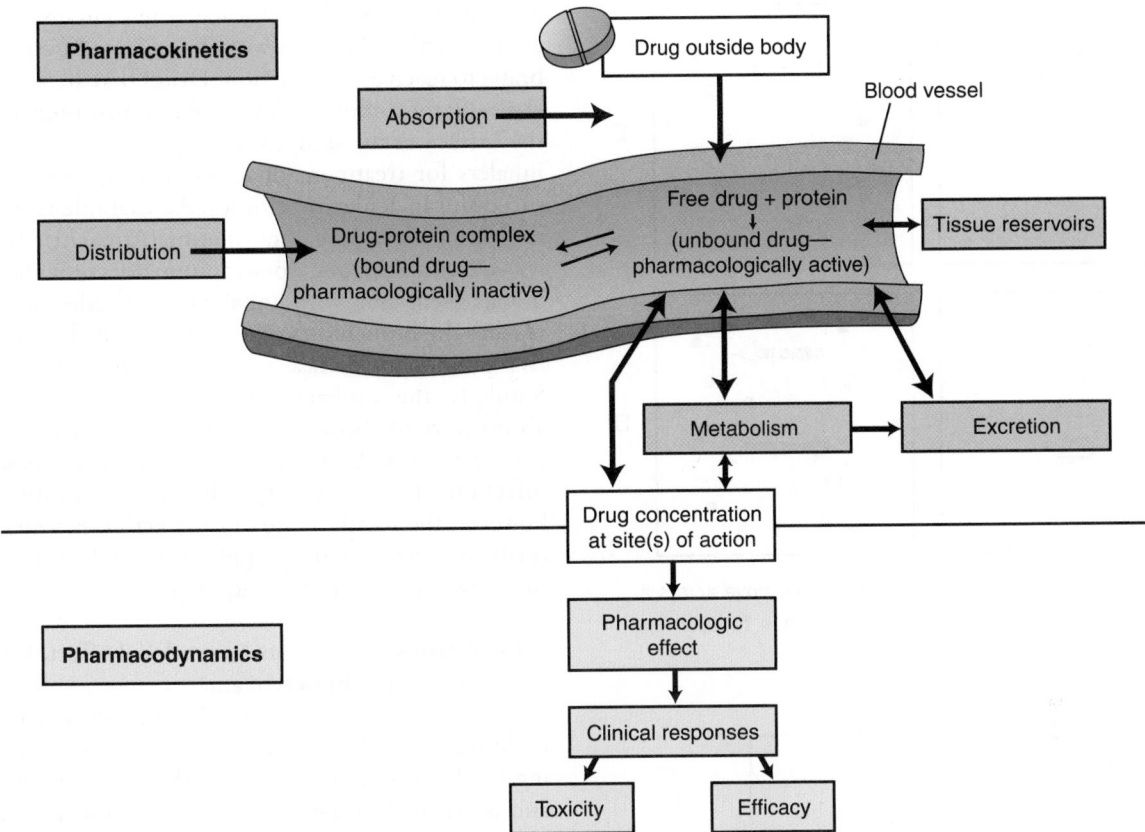

FIGURE 3-8 The interplay of pharmacokinetics and pharmacodynamics in drug action.

Physiochemical Properties of Cell Membranes The extent to which a drug attains pharmacokinetic activity (absorption, distribution, biotransformation, and excretion) depends on the rate at which it crosses cell membranes. The cell membrane consists of a bimolecular layer of lipids. Protein molecules are irregularly dispersed throughout this lipid bilayer and may act as carriers, enzymes, receptors, or antigenic sites (Figure 3-9). Drugs that are lipid (fat) solu-

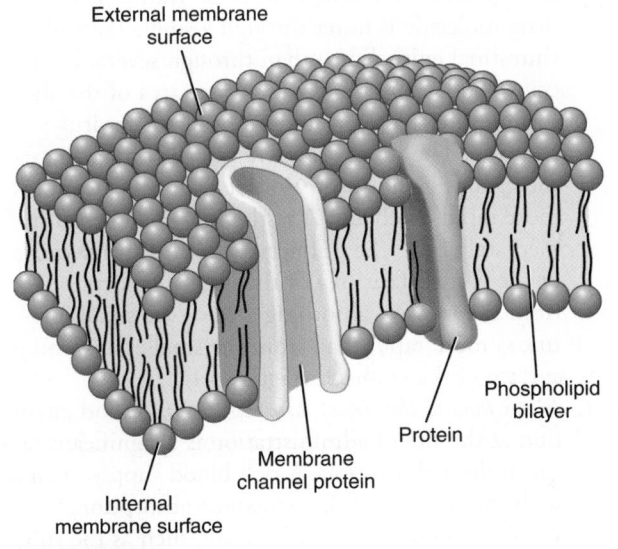

FIGURE 3-9 Cell membrane.

ble, or nonionized, pass easily through the lipid membrane, whereas ionized or water-soluble drugs have difficulty crossing cell membranes. The membrane has pores that permit the passage of small water-soluble substances such as urea, alcohol, electrolytes, and water.

Drug molecules, when free to move to sites of action, are transported from one body compartment to another by way of the plasma. However, free movement can be somewhat limited because these various sites are enclosed by membranes. Barriers to drug transport may consist of a single layer of cells (e.g., the villus in intestinal epithelium) or several layers of cells (e.g., the skin). A drug must penetrate these cell membranes to gain access to the interior of a cell or body compartment. All of the physiologic processes mediating drug action—absorption, distribution, metabolism, and excretion—rely on two physiochemical properties: passive transport and active transport across membranes.

Passive Transport Passive transport, or diffusion, of drugs occurs when the membrane is not required to generate energy to carry out the process. This mechanism involves the random movement of a substance from a region of higher concentration to a region of lower concentration (Figure 3-10, *A-C*) until equilibrium is established at the membrane (Figure 3-10, *D*). The higher the concentration gradient, the greater the amount of drug that will cross the membrane per unit of time. The vast majority of drugs are transported by this mechanism.

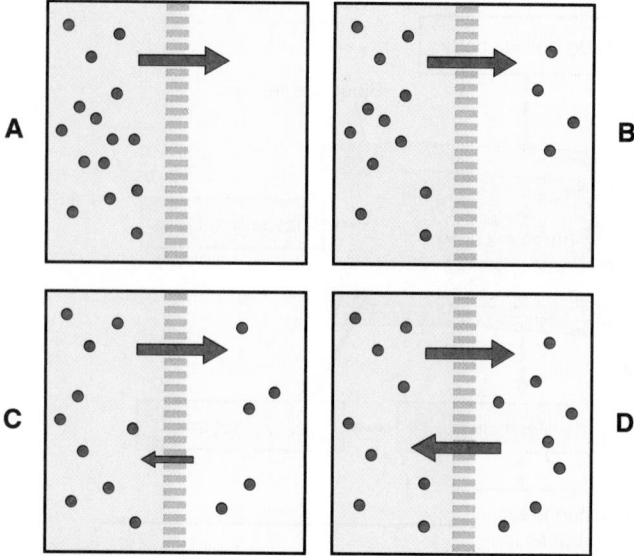

FIGURE 3-10 Passive transport. Molecules move across a membrane from a region of higher concentration to lower concentration.

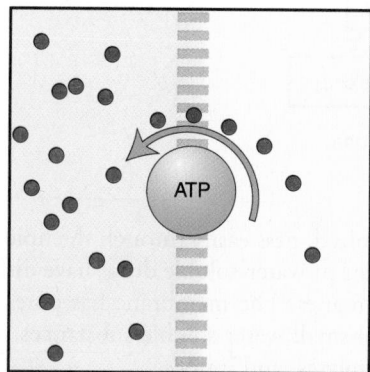

FIGURE 3-11 Active or carrier transport. In this example, adenosine triphosphate (ATP) moves a molecule across a membrane from an area of low concentration to high concentration.

Active or Carrier Transport Active or carrier transport is usually more rapid than passive diffusion. This mechanism involves the movement of drug molecules against a concentration gradient (from areas of low concentration to areas of high concentration) or, in the case of ions, against an electrochemical potential gradient (such as occurs with the "sodium pump"). An energy source is therefore required. Active or carrier transport is necessary for the transport of moderate-sized ions and water-soluble molecules such as amino acids, glucose and a few drugs (e.g., methyldopa [Aldomet] and levodopa [L-Dopa]). These drugs are transported by carriers that form complexes with drug molecules on the membrane surface, carry them through the membrane, and dissociate from them on the other side (Figure 3-11).

⊛ **Do drugs always have to cross a membrane to reach their site of action?**
For most drugs, the site of action is an internal tissue, and the drug must cross membranes and circulate in the

bloodstream to achieve efficacy. A few circumstances may exist in which the drug would not have to cross a membrane to reach a site of action. Drugs that are administered topically for a topical effect (e.g., dermal preparations for the surface of the skin, ear and eye drops for local effects, inhalers for treatment of respiratory conditions) may be successful in achieving efficacy. An example is the respiratory inhalation drug ipratropium (Atrovent). Because of its electrical charges, ipratropium does not cross membranes well, but with inhalation, an adequate amount reaches the bronchioles of the client with chronic obstructive pulmonary disease to have a beneficial local effect. Similarly, the antibacterial drug vancomycin is not well absorbed orally because of its large molecular weight, but can be used orally to treat localized *Clostridium difficile* infection of the colon. For the great majority of drugs, however, the receptor site of drug action is below the immediate surface of drug application and some degree of membrane penetration is required.

⊛ **For drugs that do not have a local effect, how do they get into the bloodstream?**
Absorption is a process involving the movement of drug molecules in the body from the site of entry to the circulating fluids. Absorption begins at the site of administration and is essential to the three subsequent processes of distribution, metabolism, and excretion. The rate of drug absorption is significant because it determines when a drug becomes pharmacologically available to exert its action. Both the duration and the intensity of drug action are greatly influenced by the rate of this process. The type of response depends on the selection of the *route* of administration, the *dose* of the drug, and the *dosage form* (tablet, capsule, or liquid) of the agent administered.

⊛ **What factors affect drug absorption?**
The rate at and extent to which a drug is absorbed are influenced by seven factors:
 1. *Nature of the absorbing surface (cell membrane) through which the drug must cross:* Transport of a drug molecule is faster through a single layer of cells (intestinal epithelium) than through several layers of cells (skin). The size of the surface area of the absorbing site is also an important factor in drug absorption. The more extensive the absorbing surface, the greater is the absorption of the drug and the more rapid its effects. Anesthetics are absorbed immediately from the pulmonary epithelium because of the vast surface area of the lungs. Absorption from the massive absorbing area of the small intestine is more rapid than from the smaller absorbing surface of the stomach (Figure 3-12).
 2. *Blood flow to the site of administration:* Blood circulation at the site of administration is a significant factor in drug absorption. A rich blood supply, such as with the sublingual site, enhances absorption, whereas a poorly vascularized site, such as the subcutaneous tissue, delays it. An individual in shock, for example, may not respond to drugs administered

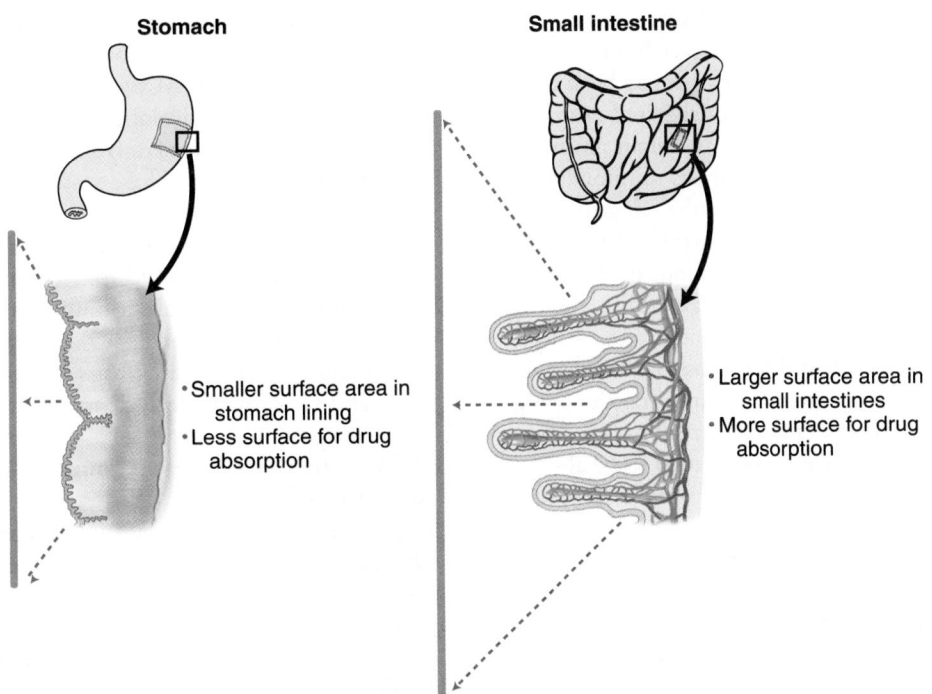

Stomach

- Smaller surface area in stomach lining
- Less surface for drug absorption

Small intestine

- Larger surface area in small intestines
- More surface for drug absorption

FIGURE 3-12 Surface area of the stomach vs. the small intestine.

IM or subcutaneously because of poor peripheral circulation. This has implications for the client in anaphylaxis secondary to bee stings, peanut allergy or some other allergic exposure. Subcutaneous administration of epinephrine (Epi-Pen) early in anaphylaxis can be successful in aborting anaphylactic vasodilation and bronchoconstriction. If anaphylaxis has progressed to a shocklike state with low blood pressure and poor tissue blood flow, epinephrine must be given IV. Similarly, the decreased peripheral blood flow in clients with heart failure (HF) may cause a significant reduction in the rate of transport of subcutaneously or IM administered drugs to target tissues, thereby considerably altering their efficacy. On the other hand, drugs injected IV are placed directly into the circulatory system and are totally available. IV administration is desirable when speedy drug effects are necessary, but this mode of administration carries the potential danger of temporarily toxic responses in vital organs such as the heart or brain. To prevent such adverse effects, most drugs must be injected slowly.

3. *Solubility of the drug:* To be absorbed, a drug must be in solution. The more soluble the drug, the more rapidly it is absorbed. Because cell membranes contain a fatty acid layer, lipid solubility is a valuable attribute of drugs to be absorbed from certain areas, such as the alimentary tract and the placental barrier. Chemicals and minerals that form insoluble precipitates in the GI tract (e.g., barium salts) or drugs that are not soluble in water or lipids cannot be absorbed.

4. *pH:* When in solution, drugs are a mixture of ionized and nonionized forms. The nonionized drug is lipid soluble and readily diffuses across the cell

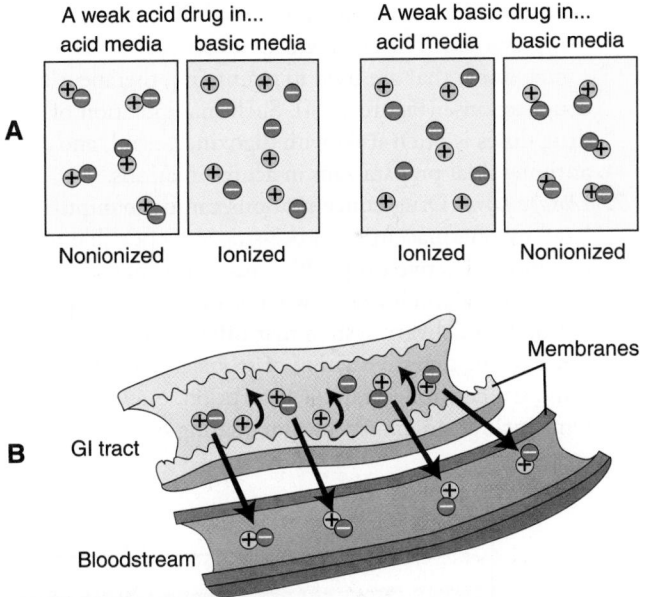

A weak acid drug in...
acid media   basic media

Nonionized   Ionized

A weak basic drug in...
acid media   basic media

Ionized   Nonionized

A

Membranes

B   GI tract

Bloodstream

FIGURE 3-13 Effect of pH on drug ionization and transport.

membrane. The ionized drug is lipid insoluble and nondiffusible (Figure 3-13, *B*). An acidic drug (e.g., aspirin) remains relatively undissociated in an acidic environment such as the stomach and therefore can readily diffuse across the membranes into the circulation. In contrast, an alkaline drug tends to ionize in an acidic environment and is not absorbed through the gastric membrane. Its absorption is enhanced in the less acidic or more alkaline sites, such as the small intestine. The reverse occurs when a drug is in an alkaline medium (Figure 3-13, *A*).

5. *Molecular weight:* Drugs that have a very large chemical structure and molecular weight are less likely to easily cross membranes and may have decreased oral absorption. A previously cited example was vancomycin, a large molecular weight antibacterial drug that, when given orally, is minimally absorbed into systemic circulation enhancing its effectiveness for treating *C. difficile* diarrhea. But for treating most other bacterial infections in the body, vancomycin must be given IV because of its molecular weight.

6. *Drug concentration:* Most drugs cross membranes by passive diffusion with the rate of drug transfer being a concentration-dependent phenomenon. Drugs administered in high concentrations tend to be absorbed more rapidly than drugs administered in low concentrations. In certain situations a drug may be initially administered in large doses that temporarily exceed the body's capacity for excretion of the drug. In this way, active drug levels are rapidly reached at the receptor site. Once an active drug level is established, smaller daily doses of the drug can be administered to replace only the amount of the drug excreted since the previous dose. The initial, temporary large doses of the drug are **loading,** or **priming doses** and are used to obtain a rapid therapeutic drug response. The smaller daily doses are **maintenance doses** that are used to maintain a therapeutic drug response (Figure 3-14). Such manipulation of drug doses is often used with digoxin, steroid, and antimicrobial preparations in acute situations.

7. *Dosage form:* Drug concentrations can be manipulated by pharmaceutical processing. It is possible to combine an active drug with a resin or other substance from which it is slowly released, or to prepare a drug in a delivery system that offers relative resistance to the digestive action of stomach contents, to achieve a controlled rate of absorption. Such systems include an enteric or film coating on the tablet that may only dissolve in the alkaline pH of the small intestines, drug bound to resins that slowly dissociate in the GI tract over hours, or liquid dose forms that are enveloped in a membrane type coating that allows for controlled release in the duodenum or jejunum. These systems may achieve drug delivery goals such as to (1) prevent decomposition of chemically sensitive drugs by gastric secretions (penicillin G and erythromycin are unstable in an acidic pH), (2) prevent dilution of the drug before it reaches the intestine, (3) prevent nausea and vomiting induced by the drug's effect in the stomach, and (4) provide delayed action of the drug.

❋ Why are there different routes of drug administration?

The mode of drug administration affects both the speed at which onset of action occurs and the magnitude of the therapeutic response that follows. The choice of route of administration is crucial in determining the suitability of a drug for an individual client. For example, a client who is vomiting will have little or no appreciable GI absorption of a drug when it is administered orally. In such a case, rectal or parenteral administration would be more beneficial in obtaining a therapeutic drug response.

A drug may enter the circulation either by being injected directly IV or by being absorbed from sites in which it has been placed. The routes of drug administration can be classified into the following categories: (1) enteral (administered along any portion of the GI tract); (2) parenteral (administered subcutaneously, IM, IV, or intrathecally); (3) pulmonary; and (4) topical.

❋ How is absorption of an orally administered drug achieved?

Enteral Route In general, oral, or enteral ingestion is the most commonly used method of drug administration. It is also the safest (because the drug might be retrieved), most convenient, least invasive, and most economical route of

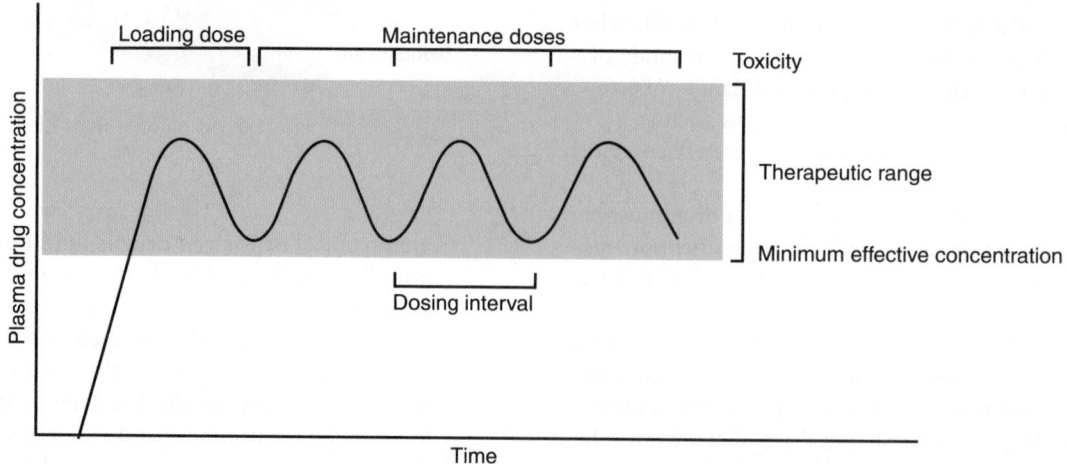

FIGURE 3-14 A loading dose is administered to reach a therapeutic response level rapidly. Maintenance doses are administered at prescribed intervals to maintain a therapeutic drug response.

administration. However, the frequent changes of the GI environment produced by food, emotion, physical activity, and concurrent diseases may make it the most unreliable and slowest of the commonly used routes. Drugs are absorbed from several sites along the GI tract.

Oral Absorption The oral cavity is lined with mucous membranes that consist of epithelial cells; these cells secrete saliva to begin food digestion. Although the oral cavity possesses a thin lining, a rich blood supply, and a slightly acidic pH, little absorption occurs in the mouth. Despite its small surface area, the oral mucosa is capable of absorbing certain drugs as long as they dissolve rapidly in the salivary secretions. The oral mucosa absorbs drugs given by the sublingual and buccal routes. In sublingual administration the drug is placed under the tongue to permit tablet dissolution in salivary secretions. Nitroglycerin is administered in this manner, and the client is advised to refrain as long as possible from swallowing the saliva containing the dissolved drug. Because nitroglycerin is nonionic with high lipid solubility, the drug readily diffuses through the lipid mucosal membranes. After absorption it enters the systemic circulation without preliminary passage through the portal circulation to the liver. Absorption is therefore rapid, and the effects of the drug may become apparent within 2 minutes. In buccal administration the drug is placed between the gum and the mucous membrane of the cheek. Testosterone and nitroglycerin may be administered by this route and are rapidly absorbed. Both the sublingual and the buccal routes avoid drug destruction by GI fluids by bypassing the stomach. They also avoid initial hepatic metabolism (known as the first-pass effect of the liver, see p. 46).

Gastric Absorption Although the stomach has a rich blood supply and a relatively large surface area, it is not usually an important absorption site. The length of time a substance remains in the stomach is a significant variable in determining the extent of gastric absorption.

In the stomach the pH is low (approximately 1.4), and drugs such as barbiturates, which are slightly acidic, tend to remain nonionized and are readily absorbed into the circulation. Morphine and quinine are slightly basic, ionize in the stomach, and are poorly absorbed there. Most drugs are weak bases and are absorbed on entering the small intestine because of the alkaline pH of that environment.

In general, slowing the gastric emptying rate delays drug absorption, whereas increasing the gastric emptying rate hastens drug absorption. Many drugs are administered on an empty stomach with sufficient water (8 ounces) to ensure dissolution, rapid passage into the small intestine, and drug absorption in the larger surface area. Drugs that cause gastric irritation are usually given with food. After the administration of a solid, the client should sit upright for at least 30 minutes to hasten gastric emptying time (time required for the drug to reach the small intestine) and to reduce the potential for tablets or capsules to lodge in the esophageal area. Gastroparesis or delayed gastric emptying time is often observed in individuals with diabetes and de-

layed onset of drugs given orally to these individuals is often observed. Prolonging gastric emptying time increases the risk of destruction of unstable drugs (e.g., acetaminophen [Tylenol]) by gastric juices.

Absorption in the Intestine The small intestine with its many villi has a larger absorption area than the stomach and is highly vascularized. Drugs that are poorly soluble in the stomach pass into this region and are absorbed primarily in the upper part of the small intestine. The pH of the intestinal fluid is alkaline (7 to 8), which strongly influences the rate of absorption of the nonionized basic drugs. Transport proteins like P-glycoprotein in the cells of the small intestine may also be involved in drug absorption. The amount and function of these proteins may vary based on genetic makeup (Evans & McLeod, 2003). Increased intestinal motility caused by diarrhea or laxatives may decrease exposure to the intestinal membrane and diminish absorption. Prolonged exposure to the intestinal surface, such as with constipation, allows more time for absorption.

The large intestine typically plays a smaller role in drug absorption due in part to a smaller overall surface area. Additionally, the drug concentration in the intestinal lumen is reduced once the medication reaches the colon.

Rectal Absorption Although the surface area of the rectum is not very large, drug absorption can occur because of its extensive vascularity. Drugs administered rectally are not immediately subjected to hepatic alteration because the blood that perfuses this region initially bypasses the portal circulation to the liver. Disadvantages to rectal drug administration include erratic absorption because of rectal contents, local drug irritation with some medications, and uncertainty of drug retention.

❊ **How does the absorption of injectable drugs differ from orally administered drugs?**
Parenteral Route The parenteral route refers to the administration of drugs by injection and commonly refers to the intradermal, subcutaneous, intramuscular, and intravenous routes.

Intradermal Route Intradermal (ID) or intracutaneous injections are made into the upper layers of the skin, almost parallel to the skin surface. Only a very small amount of drug or other substance may be administered by this route. It is used primarily used to determine the extent of allergies (e.g., extracts of grass), to test for infectious exposures (e.g., tuberculin), to test the nature of the immune system (e.g., *Candida* extracts), and to administer local anesthetics prior to a minor surgical procedure (e.g., lidocaine prior to suturing).

Subcutaneous Route A subcutaneous injection is given beneath the skin into the connective tissue or fat immediately underlying the dermis. This site is used only for drugs that are not irritating to the tissue; otherwise severe pain, necrosis, and sloughing of tissue may occur. The rate of absorption is relatively slow and may be irregular but can provide a sustained effect.

Intramuscular Route With IM administration, a drug is injected into skeletal muscle. Absorption occurs more rapidly than with subcutaneous injection because of greater tissue blood flow. As with subcutaneous administration, IM sites should only be used for drugs that are not irritating to tissues.

Intravenous Route The IV route produces an immediate pharmacologic response because the desired concentration of drug is injected directly into the bloodstream, thereby circumventing the absorption process. IV drugs should be administered slowly to prevent adverse reactions. Figure 3-15 compares onsets and duration of action of IV with that of other administration routes.

Intrathecal Route Many compounds cannot enter the cerebrospinal fluid (CSF) or are absorbed in this region very slowly because of the protective properties of the blood-brain barrier. With intrathecal administration, the drug is injected directly into the spinal subarachnoid space, thereby bypassing the blood-brain barrier. This route may be used when rapid effects are desired, such as in spinal anesthesia or in the treatment of acute infection of the central nervous system (CNS).

Epidural Route With epidural administration, a drug is injected via a small catheter into the epidural space of the spinal column—the space outside of the dura mater. This route is increasingly being used with opioids for pain management. Drugs administered by this route also have a rapid onset of action.

Other Parenteral Routes Drugs may be injected into other cavities of the body. Intraarticular administration delivers the medication into the synovial cavity of a joint, usually to relieve pain, reduce inflammation, and maintain joint mobility. Intraosseous administration delivers drugs or blood into the bone marrow when IV access is difficult. Intraperitoneal and intrapleural administration of antineoplastic or antimicrobial agents allows these drugs to be delivered directly to tumor or infection sites respectively.

✻ What about drug administration via the lungs?

Pulmonary Route To ensure that the normal gas exchange of oxygen and carbon dioxide is continuous in the lungs, drugs must be in the form of gases or fine mists (aerosols) when administered by inhalation. The lungs provide a large surface area for absorption, and the rich capillary network adjacent to the alveolar membrane tends to promote ready entry of medication into the bloodstream. Drugs such as bronchodilators, mucolytics, and antibiotics can be administered by various inhalation devices (oral inhalers, nebulizers), which propel the agents into the alveolar sacs and produce primarily local effects and, at times, unwanted systemic effects.

During a cardiac arrest, certain drugs (lidocaine, epinephrine, atropine, naloxone) can be administered via the endotracheal tube into the respiratory tract if IV access cannot be established. Certain anesthetic gases are also administered via this route during surgery.

✻ What about topically administered drugs?

Topical Route In general, drugs are applied topically to the skin and mucous membranes of various structures in the body to achieve local or systemic effects.

Skin Drugs applied to the skin produce a local or systemic effect through use of ointments, creams, or transdermal patches. Only lipid-soluble compounds are absorbed through the skin. To provide a consistent rate of absorption, only intact skin surfaces are used for topical applications. Adverse effects might occur from the systemic absorption of certain topical agents through broken or excoriated skin. Massaging the skin enhances drug absorption because capillaries become dilated and local blood flow is increased from the warmth created by the friction of rubbing.

Transdermal Transdermal drugs usually consist of a disk or patch that contains a 1-day to 1-week supply of medication. After being applied to the skin, the medication is absorbed at a steady rate. Examples of drugs applied transdermally are clonidine (Catapres-TTS), contraceptives (Ortho Evra), estrogen (Estraderm), fentanyl (Duragesic), nitroglycerin (Nitrodisc), and scopolamine (Transderm-Scop).

Eyes The administration of ophthalmic drugs produces a local effect on the conjunctiva or anterior chamber. Movement of the eyeball promotes distribution of the drug over the surface of the eye. Pressure applied to the inner canthus during drug administration and for a few minutes afterward will reduce systemic absorption. Examples of medications administered directly at this site include antiglaucoma and antimicrobial agents.

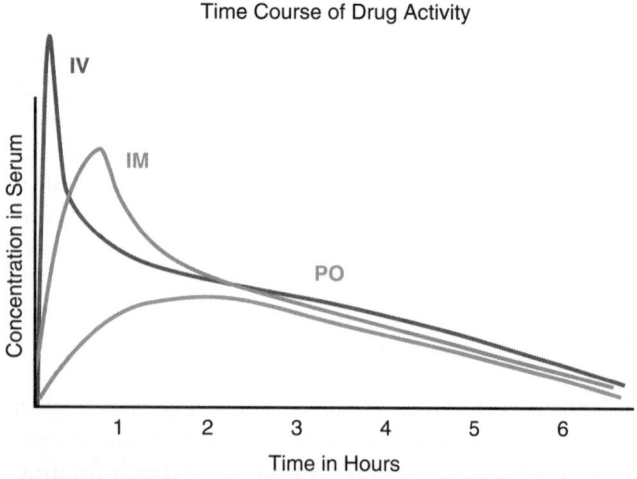

Time Course of Drug Activity

FIGURE 3-15 A comparison of drug onsets and duration of action by route of administration.

Ears The administration of drops into the auditory canal may be done to treat local infection, inflammatory conditions, or wax in the external ear. Otic drugs are primarily limited to treatments for otitis externa and drops to help remove ear wax.

Nasal Mucosa Drugs may be instilled in droplet or spray form or in a prepackaged specific-dose swab intended for direct intranasal application. This mode of administration can be used for systemic absorption or to facilitate shrinkage of the mucosa to enhance breathing or to enable insertion of a nasotracheal tube. Nasal administration of corticosteroid sprays has become quite popular as a localized treatment for allergic rhinitis.

✱ **What happens once drugs get into the circulation?**

Distribution

Once absorbed, a drug is immediately distributed throughout the body by blood circulation. **Distri-bution** is defined as the transport of a drug in body fluids from the bloodstream to various tissues of the body and ultimately to its site of action (see Figure 3-8). The rate at which a drug enters the different areas of the body depends on the permeability of capillaries to the molecules of the drug. Lipid-soluble drugs can readily cross capillary membranes to enter most tissues and fluid compartments, whereas water-soluble drugs require more time to arrive at their point of action. Cardiac function also affects the rate and extent of drug distribution. Cardiac output (the amount of blood pumped by the heart each minute) and regional blood flow (the amount of blood supplied to a specific organ or tissue) determine how much time is required for distribution. Most of the drug is first distributed to organs that have a rich blood supply, such as the heart, liver, kidney, and brain. Next, the drug enters organs with a less rich blood supply, such as muscles and fat.

Drug Reservoirs

Storage reservoirs allow a drug to accumulate by binding to specific tissues in the body. This binding sustains the pharmacologic effect of a drug at its point of action. The storage reservoirs in the body are the results of plasma protein binding and tissue binding.

Plasma Protein Binding On entry into the circulatory system, drugs may become attached to proteins, mainly albumin contained in the blood. As a free drug enters the plasma, it binds to the protein to form a drug-protein complex. This combination can also be reversed:

Free Drug + Protein ⇌ Drug-Protein complex

Equilibrium is established between the amount of free drug and the amount of drug that is bound to protein (drug-protein complex). Protein binding decreases the concentration of free drug in the circulation, thereby limiting the amount of drug that travels to the site of action. Because

the drug-albumin molecule is too large to diffuse through the membrane of the blood vessel, the bound molecule is trapped in the bloodstream and is pharmacologically inactive. It thus becomes a circulating drug reservoir or storage depot (see Figure 3-8).

The equilibrium process is dynamic. As free drug is eliminated from the body, the drug-protein complex begins to dissociate so that more free drug is released to replace what is lost. Temporary storage of drug molecules in the drug-protein complex allows the drug to be available for a longer period of time. For example, ceftriaxone (Rocephin), an antibiotic, is highly bound to protein; because free drug molecules are released slowly from the bound form, its antiinfective action is long lasting.

Degree of Drug Binding Plasma protein binding is expressed as a percentage, which represents the percent of total drug that is bound. One example of a *highly* protein-bound drug is warfarin (Coumadin), an anticoagulant. A ratio exists between free and bound warfarin, in which 99% is bound to plasma proteins at any given time; only 1% of free drug is available for therapeutic use, eventual biotransformation, and excretion. With few exceptions, this ratio remains consistent independent of dose (e.g., if 1 mg of warfarin is in the bloodstream, 0.99 mg is typically bound to plasma proteins; if 10 mg of warfarin is in the bloodstream, 9.9 mg is typically bound to plasma protein). Factors other than drug concentration may alter this ratio. These factors include a change in the amount of plasma protein (e.g., low albumin levels) or concurrently administered drugs that also bind to the same protein sites (see below). In such circumstances, a greater percentage of the drug could be unbound and toxicity may result. Drugs that are greater than 90% bound to plasma proteins are considered highly protein bound.

Competition for Binding Sites Because albumin and other plasma proteins provide a finite number of binding sites, two drugs can compete with one another for the same site and displace each other, creating more free drug of one or the other, or both. This competition may have unpredictable consequences if particular combinations of drugs are administered. This increase in free drug levels allows for more drug to be available to cross membranes and be pharmacologically active and also to be available for metabolism and/or excretion. The net effect may be an increased risk for toxicity, no net change, and/or increase elimination of the drug. This effect is of greatest concern when using two drugs that both have a high degree of plasma protein binding. The range of levels of one or both of those drugs must be carefully maintained to avoid toxicity or complications. An example is the frequently used combination of phenytoin (Dilantin) and valproic acid (Depakene) to prevent seizures. Because both drugs are highly bound to plasma proteins, increased unbound levels of phenytoin (and sometimes also valproic acid) can be observed and may be associated with either serious toxicity (because more drug is available at receptors) or subtherapeutic response (seizures because more drug is available for elimination).

Although increases in unbound drug concentrations as the result of plasma protein binding displacement could contribute to drug toxicity theoretically, the body will respond to increased unbound drug by increasing the rate of elimination of the unbound drug. If renal clearance is not impaired, the unbound drug concentration will return to its previous steady state value after four to five half-lives. When clinically significant drug interactions associated with competition for protein binding sites have been studied, it has been found that the displacing drug is also an inhibitor of clearance. This change in the clearance of unbound drug is the important mechanism in the drug interaction (Katzung, 2004).

Hypoalbuminemia Hypoalbuminemia is a state of low levels of albumin in the blood, which may be caused by malnutrition, hepatic damage (e.g., cirrhosis of the liver), certain kidney diseases (e.g., glomerulonephritis), or some type of body cavity drainage. When a client with low plasma protein is given the normal dosage of a plasma protein bound drug (plasma albumin for acidic drugs and α_1-acid glycoprotein for basic drugs), more of the free form of the drug enters the circulation, resulting in possible overdosage and toxicity.

❂ **Are drugs equally distributed in all tissues?**

Tissue Binding Most drugs that reach the plasma will diffuse into other body tissues. Various areas of the body differ in their affinity for different drugs. These different tissues are often referred to as compartments. Examples of compartments include the plasma, adipose (or fat) tissue, and bone. If an area is more highly separated from the rest of the body, it may be a hindrance to drug distribution. Such areas often involve specialized structures made up of biologic membranes, which serve as barriers to the passage of drugs. Such barriers include the blood-brain barrier and the placental barrier.

Fat Lipid-soluble drugs have a high affinity for adipose tissue, and this is where these drugs are stored. The relatively low blood flow in fat tissue makes it a stable reservoir for drugs. For example, a lipid-soluble drug such as thiopental (Pentothal) may stay in low concentrations in body fat for as long as 3 hours after administration. Administering this drug again before all of it has been excreted can produce a cumulative effect, because an additional amount of the agent will be stored in the fat tissue.

Bone Some drugs have an unusual affinity for bone; for example, tetracycline, an antibiotic, accumulates in bone after being absorbed onto the bone-crystal surface. Tetracycline can interfere with bone growth when it accumulates in the skeletal tissues of the fetus (by crossing the placenta from the mother) or young children. Tooth discoloration results when this drug is distributed to unerupted teeth in a fetus or young child. Brownish pigmentation of permanent teeth also may result if this drug is given during the prenatal period or early childhood.

Blood-Brain Barrier The blood-brain barrier is a special anatomic arrangement that allows the distribution of only lipid-soluble drugs (e.g., general anesthetics, barbiturates) into the brain and CSF. The blood-brain barrier consists of a row of capillary endothelial cells covered by a fatty sheath of glial cells joined by continuous tight intercellular junctions. Consequently, compounds that are strongly ionized and poorly soluble in fat cannot enter the brain. Antibiotics that are limited in their ability to cross the blood-brain barrier cannot be used to treat infections of the CNS. If the drug is instilled intrathecally, however, it bypasses the blood-brain barrier and directly treats the bacterial infection.

An additional set of factors that may affect distribution of drug in the brain is a number of transport proteins found in various membranes. One such transport protein is P-glycoprotein, which may serve as a pump to limit accumulation of drug in the brain. Drugs such as digoxin (Lanoxin), a cardiotonic used for HF and certain cardiac dysrhythmias, dexamethasone (Decadron), an antiinflammatory corticosteroid, and loperamide (Imodium), an antidiarrheal agent, have limited levels in the CNS in part secondary to this transport protein (Evans & McLeod, 2003).

Placental Barrier The membrane layers that separate the blood vessels of the mother and the fetus constitute the placental barrier. Tissue enzymes in the placenta can metabolize certain agents (e.g., catecholamines) by inactivating them as they travel from the maternal circulation to the embryo. This enzyme function may be genetically determined. Despite the thickness of the placenta, it does not afford complete protection to the fetus. Unlike the relative impermeability of the blood-brain barrier, many drugs cross the placenta to the fetus. Although lipid-soluble substances preferentially diffuse across the placenta, the barrier is also permeable to a great number of lipid-insoluble drugs. Among the drugs easily transported across the placenta are steroids, opioids, anesthetics, alcohol, and some antibiotics. Many agents intended to produce a therapeutic response in the mother may also cross the placental barrier and exert harmful effects on the developing embryo. Drugs that produce harmful effects on the developing fetus are referred to as *teratogens*. A full discussion of risks of drugs in pregnancy is presented in Chapter 7.

❂ **What is drug metabolism? Why is it important?**
Drug metabolism, or **biotransformation,** is the process of chemically inactivating a drug by converting it into a more water-soluble compound or metabolite that can then be excreted from the body (see Figure 3-8). The liver is the primary site of drug metabolism, but other tissues may be involved in the process, such as the plasma, kidneys, lungs, and intestinal mucosa.

Biotransformation

Drugs undergo one or both of two general types of chemical reactions in the liver. One type of transformation (referred to as Phase I metabolism) consists of the chemical reactions of oxidation, hydrolysis, or reduction to increase the water solubility of drug molecules. The second type of transformation (Phase II or conjugation) involves the union of the drug with a water-soluble substance in the body—glucuronide, glycine, methyl, or other alkyl groups. The conjugated molecule also becomes more ionized, or more water soluble, resulting is acceleration in renal excretion. In general, these responses convert an active drug to an inactive substance (a decrease or loss of pharmacologic activity) and to a substance that is more easily excreted in the urine.

The majority of drugs are metabolized in the liver by the hepatic microsomal enzyme system. A key element of the hepatic microsomal enzyme system is the cytochrome P450 system. The microsomal enzymes (and subvariants or isoenzymes) usually affect the biotransformation of lipid-soluble, nonionized drugs. Over the past 2 decades, there has been a greater awareness of these isoenzymes of the cytochrome P450 system and their clinical importance. These isoenzymes are categorized in family groups related to the similarity of amino acid structure. The most common isoenzyme families involved in drug metabolism are cytochrome P450 1A2, 2C9, 2C19, 2D6, and 3A4. Each family or isoenzyme group is specific for a substrate, a type of chemical or drug that it metabolizes. Although a drug may be metabolized by more than one isoenzyme, it is typical that one isoenzyme is predominant in metabolizing that drug (Table 3-1).

Many drugs can affect the hepatic enzymes by either increasing or decreasing the activity of the enzyme. The metabolism of some drugs can be enhanced by induction, or increasing hepatic enzymes, so that drug effectiveness is decreased. By inhibiting hepatic enzymes, such as the cytochrome P450 (CYP) system, drug metabolism is decreased and the potential for drug interactions and toxicity is possibly increased. The nature of this induction or inhibition is typically very specific for isoenzyme type. Some drugs that serve as inducers or inhibitors for one isoenzyme may actually be substrates of a different isoenzyme. An example is cimetidine (Tagamet), which is metabolized by CYP3A4 but inhibits the CYP2C9 isoenzyme, which then can diminish the metabolism of warfarin (Coumadin), phenytoin (Dilantin), and many other drugs and lead to toxic reactions.

Another example of hepatic metabolism is the chemical or enzymatic alterations needed to activate a prodrug. A prodrug is a pharmacologically inert compound that can be chemically converted to a pharmacologically active metabolite. Examples of prodrugs include the cardiovascular drugs losartan (Cozaar) and benazepril (Lotensin), and the anti-inflammatory agent sulindac (Clinoril).

Metabolism often involves the conversion of an active drug to other active metabolites with similar therapeutic effects. Examples include the partial conversion of codeine to morphine, which increases the analgesic effect of codeine. Another is the conversion of the antidepressant amitriptyline (Elavil) to the active metabolite nortriptyline, which was later marketed individually as Aventyl and Pamelor. Active metabolites often serve to extend the pharmacologic properties or duration of effect of the administered drug.

Occasionally, the metabolite may be toxic or contribute undesirable pharmacologic properties. An example is meperidine (Demerol), which is metabolized to normeperidine. Normeperidine can accumulate in clients with renal insufficiency and lead to seizures. Toxic metabolites may also be produced when one metabolic pathway is saturated (overwhelmed and working at capacity), and a minor metabolic pathway is utilized to a greater extent. This is observed with acetaminophen (Tylenol) overdosage and a metabolite injurious to the liver accumulates, leading to hepatic injury and potential hepatic failure and death.

In summary, drug metabolism may result in the following:
- Inactivation of the drug
- Alteration of the drug molecule to increase renal excretion of the drug
- Induction (increasing) or inhibition of the liver metabolizing enzyme (P450), which may affect the metabolism of other medications administered (e.g., decreasing drug effectiveness or increasing the potential for drug toxicity)
- Activation of a prodrug to an active substance
- Conversion of an active drug to active metabolite(s) with similar effects.

TABLE 3-1 ISOENZYMES OF THE CYTOCHROME P450 SYSTEM

Isoenzyme Family	Examples of Substrates (Drugs Metabolized by Specific Isoenzyme)
CYP1A2	acetaminophen (Tylenol), caffeine, diazepam (Valium), theophylline
CYP2C9	celecoxib (Celebrex), ibuprofen (Motrin), phenytoin (Dilantin), warfarin (Coumadin)
CYP2C19	phenobarbital, valproic acid (Depakene), omeprazole (Prilosec)
CYP2D6	codeine, captopril (Capoten), morphine, oxycodone (OxyContin)
CYP3A4	amiodarone (Cordarone), atorvastatin (Lipitor), cannabinoids (e.g., marijuana), cimetidine (Tagamet), erythromycin (E-Mycin), fluoxetine (Prozac), hormonal contraceptives, sildenafil (Viagra)

Modified from Lacy, C.F., Armstrong, L.L., Goldman, M.P., & Lance, L.L. (2004). *Drug information handbook* (12th ed.). Cleveland: Lexi-Comp.

The impact of drug metabolism on drug interactions is discussed throughout this text.

✱ Does everyone metabolize drugs the same way?

Individuals vary considerably in the rates at which they metabolize drugs. The microsomal enzyme system can be depressed by conditions that affect hepatic function, such as starvation and obstructive jaundice. Smokers metabolize a number of drugs more rapidly (e.g., theophylline, some antipsychotics) and typically require higher doses of these drugs to achieve the same therapeutic effect. Individuals with liver disease, severe cardiovascular dysfunction, or renal problems may be expected to have prolonged or decreased drug metabolism. Infants with immature metabolizing enzyme systems and older adults with degenerative enzyme function are the primary populations that experience depressed biotransformation.

Genetically determined differences also affect metabolism. Recognition of the significance of genetics on drug metabolism has contributed greatly to the new science of **pharmacogenetics.** Some drugs (e.g., procainamide [Pronestyl], hydralazine [Apresoline], and isoniazid [INH]) are metabolized by the acetyltransferase system. This system divides the population into "rapid acetylators" and "slow acetylators." The rapid acetylators metabolize a greater proportion of a drug dose than do the slow acetylators. The rapid (extensive) acetylators may develop reactions caused by the metabolic products of a drug, whereas the slow (poor) acetylators may appear more sensitive to a drug by experiencing severe toxic effects. For example, an individual who is a slow acetylator and is receiving hydralazine (Apresoline) is apt to develop a lupus-like syndrome—a serious adverse effect. An individual who is a rapid acetylator of the same drug might require higher doses of hydralazine to control hypertension. There is mounting evidence describing the genetic predisposition of individuals to express various cytochrome P450 isoenzymes. These genetic differences among individuals in part explain the broad range of response to drugs observed in the population. Genetic differences in pharmacodynamic action and drug toxicity have also been observed. Refer to Chapter 6 for a discussion of the principles of pharmacogenetics. Additionally, boxes throughout the text refer to pharmacogenetic trends in drug therapy.

If drug metabolism is delayed, cumulative drug effects may be expected and may be manifested as excessive or prolonged responses to ordinary doses of drugs. If drug metabolism is stimulated, a state of apparent drug tolerance is produced. A number of substances cause increased activity by hepatic microsomal enzymes, including CNS depressants, xanthines, pesticides, food preservatives, and dyes. Grapefruit and grapefruit juice contribute to decreased activity of cytochrome P450 3A4 typically resulting in elevated levels of drugs that are metabolized by this enzyme. Repeated administration of some drugs may stimulate the formation of new microsomal enzymes. This is the case with some antiepileptic drugs (e.g., phenobarbital, carbamazepine, phenytoin).

✱ Where in the body does drug metabolism occur?

Hepatic First-Pass Effect Orally administered drugs absorbed from the GI tract travel by the venous portal system to the liver before entering the general circulation. Some drugs are first taken up by the hepatic microsomal enzyme system, and a significant amount of the drug is metabolized before ever reaching the systemic circulation. This concept is referred to as the first-pass effect. Consequently, only a small fraction of the dose of these drugs is available for distribution to produce a pharmacologic effect. With such medications, the oral drug dose is calculated to compensate for this effect. For example, propranolol (Inderal) has a very significant hepatic first-pass effect; the oral dose may range from 10 mg to 80 mg, whereas the parenteral dose is usually 1 mg to 3 mg to achieve the same therapeutic effect. The hepatic first-pass effect helps to explain why an IV dose of some drugs is so much smaller than an oral dose.

Some drugs may have a hepatic first-pass effect that totally eliminates pharmacologic activity. These medications, such as lidocaine, require a different route of drug administration (e.g., parenteral) to enter the general circulation, thereby preventing the significant biotransformation as a result of first pass through the liver.

✱ How do drugs and their metabolites get out of the body?

Excretion

A drug continues to act in the body until it is biotransformed or excreted. Drug molecules (intact, changed, or inactivated) must ultimately be removed from their sites of action by physiologic channels involving mechanisms of excretion. **Excretion** is a process by which drugs and pharmacologically active or inactive metabolites are eliminated from the body, primarily through the kidneys (Figure 3-16).

Kidneys Drug excretion via the kidneys is the most important route for elimination. Some drugs are excreted unchanged in the urine, whereas other drugs are so extensively metabolized that only a small fraction of the original chemical substance is excreted intact.

Excretion is accomplished by passive glomerular filtration, active tubular secretion, and partial reabsorption (Figure 3-17). The availability of a drug for glomerular filtration depends on its concentration in unbound form in plasma. Free, unbound drugs and water-soluble metabolites are filtered by the glomeruli, whereas protein-bound substances do not pass into the tubular filtrate through the glomeruli. After filtration, lipid-soluble compounds are not excreted but instead are reabsorbed by the tubular nephron and reenter the systemic circulation. Water-soluble compounds fail to be reabsorbed and therefore are eliminated from the body.

Urinary pH varies between 4.6 and 8.2 and affects the degree of ionization (and therefore lipid or water solubility) of the drug. The amount of drug reabsorbed in the renal tubule by passive diffusion may then be altered. By chang-

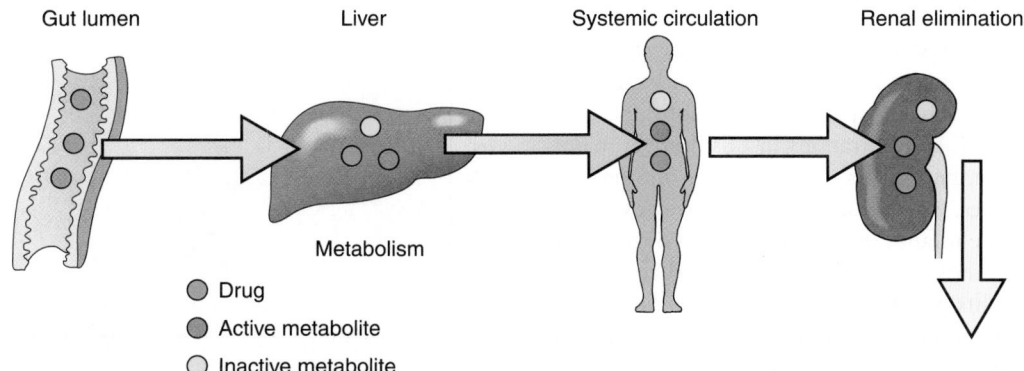

Gut lumen   **Liver**   **Systemic circulation**   **Renal elimination**

Metabolism

- Drug
- Active metabolite
- Inactive metabolite

FIGURE 3-16 Renal excretion of drugs as unchanged, active metabolite, and inactive metabolite.

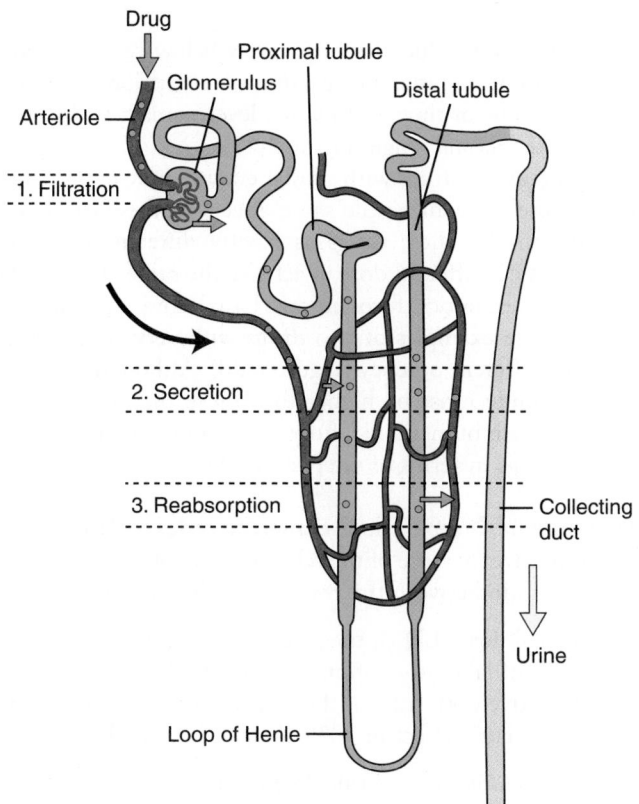

FIGURE 3-17 The drug excretion process.

ing the pH of urine, decreased reabsorption of the drug occurs resulting in increased elimination of certain drugs, thus preventing prolonged action or overdosage of a toxic compound. Weak acids are excreted more readily in alkaline urine and more slowly in acidic urine; the reverse is true for weak bases. Alkalinizing the urine can result in increased urinary drug excretion in cases of poisoning by weak organic acids such as aspirin or phenobarbital. Raising the pH of the urine causes weak acids to become ionized, and subsequently these agents are excreted, rather than reabsorbed. Urine may be alkalinized by administering sodium bicarbonate or tromethamine (Tham). In contrast, high doses of vitamin C or ammonium chloride acidify the urine and promote the excretion of alkaline drugs.

Another technique to alter the rate of excretion of a drug is to produce a competitively blocking effect. For example, probenecid may be used to block the renal tubular excretion of penicillin. This prolongs the effect of the antibiotic by maintaining a higher therapeutic plasma level.

✱ Are there ways other than the kidney that drugs can get out of the body?

Gastrointestinal Tract Some drugs may be excreted by biliary excretion. After metabolism by the liver, the metabolite is secreted into the bile, passed into the duodenum, and eliminated with feces.

Other drugs that are fat-soluble agents, such as estrogen, may be reabsorbed by the bloodstream from the intestine and returned to the liver. This is called the *enterohepatic cycle*. These compounds are later excreted by the kidney.

Lungs General anesthetics in gas and volatile liquid form are administered and excreted via the pulmonary route, generally in intact form. On inspiration, these agents enter the bloodstream and, after crossing the alveolar membrane, are distributed by the general circulation. The rate of gas loss depends on the rate of respiration. Therefore exercise or deep breathing, which causes a rise in cardiac output and a subsequent increase in pulmonary blood flow, promotes excretion. In contrast, decreased cardiac output, such as occurs in shock, prolongs the period of drug elimination. Other volatile substances, such as ethyl alcohol and paraldehyde, are highly soluble in blood and are excreted in limited amounts by the lungs. These substances are easily detected because the individual exhales the gases into the atmosphere.

Sweat and Salivary Glands Drug excretion through sweat and saliva is relatively unimportant because this process depends on the diffusion of lipid-soluble drugs through the epithelial cells of the glands. The elimination of drugs and metabolites in sweat may be responsible for adverse effects such as dermatitis and several other skin reactions. Drugs excreted in the saliva are usually swallowed and undergo the same fate as other orally administered agents. Certain compounds that are given IV may be excreted into saliva and cause the individual to complain of the "taste of the drug."

Mammary Glands Many drugs or their metabolites cross the epithelium of the mammary glands and are excreted in breast milk. Breast milk is acidic (pH 6.5), and therefore basic compounds, such as opioids (e.g., morphine and codeine) achieve high concentrations in this fluid. A major concern arises over the transfer of drugs from mothers to their breastfed babies, which can result in a cumulative drug effect because of the infant's undeveloped metabolizing system. The nursing mother should be instructed to discuss the risks and benefits of taking any medications (including OTC and complementary/alternative products) with her health care provider before breastfeeding.

✳ How does organ function affect drug excretion?

Renal function is an important consideration in dosing drugs that are either excreted unchanged in the urine or as pharmacologically active metabolites. Drugs may also be eliminated through the use of extracorporeal dialysis, which was originally designed to substitute for renal function in cases of severe but temporary renal shutdown. Overdosage of drugs may lead to just such a situation. By an artificial process resembling glomerular filtration, dialysis can rapidly reduce high plasma levels of a drug. As a general rule, substances that are completely or almost completely excreted by the normal kidney can be removed by hemodialysis. A more thorough discussion of drug dosing in renal failure is presented in Chapter 35.

Hepatic function is also an important aspect to evaluate in drug use. Although difficult to predict, enzyme systems and drug metabolism typically remains intact with mild to moderate hepatic insufficiency, but may be affected adversely in individuals with fulminant hepatic failure.

✳ How are drug doses determined?

A number of factors affect the dose of a drug, including the dose-response relationship, therapeutic index, plasma level profile, half-life, and bioavailability.

Drug-Response Relationship When a drug is first developed, it is studied in a range of individuals to establish how the drug behaves pharmacodynamically and pharmacokinetically. After administration, each drug has its own characteristic pharmacokinetic profile. In study subjects, serial plasma drug levels are evaluated after administration of a set amount of drug. At the same time, the subject is monitored for pharmacologic response. When similar data is assembled for larger numbers of subjects, a pattern emerges in the population studied that identifies a set range of doses associated with a set of pharmacologic properties. This is considered the dose-response curve (Figure 3-18). Typically, doses below the established dose range do not produce meaningful pharmacologic responses. Doses above this range often do not produce much additional pharmacologic change and/or may be associated with other unwanted effects. For many drugs, this dose range is associated with efficacy and minimal toxicity. Additionally, there is typically a range of plasma drug levels correlated with this dose range (referred to as the therapeutic plasma level range). Plasma levels above the upper limit of this range typically produce no further beneficial

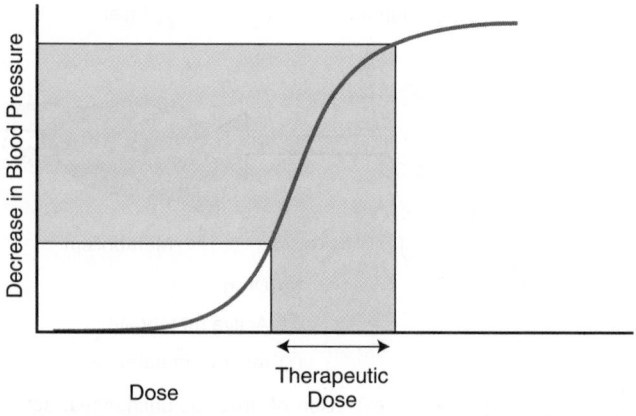

FIGURE 3-18 Dose-response curve for an antihypertensive.

effect or may produce toxicity; levels below the range are usually subtherapeutic. A drug's duration of action is defined as the window of time that plasma levels remain within the therapeutic plasma range (Figure 3-19).

On occasion, drugs with similar efficacy may require different doses to achieve the same effect. In these cases, we would consider these drugs as having different potency; they require a different dose to achieve the same range of effects. The diuretics furosemide (Lasix) and bumetanide (Bumex) are examples of two drugs with very similar efficacy but different potency (Figure 3-20). Although the dose of furosemide must be higher to achieve the same effects observed with bumetanide, furosemide and bumetanide are similar drugs in terms of safety and efficacy.

Therapeutic Index The therapeutic index (TI) provides a quantitative measure of the relative safety of a drug. It represents a ratio between the two factors that follow:

- Lethal dose (LD_{50}), the drug dose that is lethal in 50% of laboratory animals tested; and
- Effective dose (ED_{50}), the dose required to produce a therapeutic effect in 50% of a similar population.

The therapeutic index is calculated as follows:

$$TI = LD_{50}/ED_{50}$$

The closer the ratio is to 1, the greater the danger involved in administering that drug to human beings. In humans the dose that promotes a side effect or the first sign of a toxic response is obviously of greater importance than the therapeutic index of the drug, because the prescriber's major concern is avoiding even an isolated fatality caused by drug toxicity.

Plasma Level Profile of a Drug The plasma or serum level profile graphically demonstrates the relationship between the plasma drug concentration and the level of therapeutic effectiveness over time. After one dose is administered, the time course of the amount of drug in the body depends on its rates of absorption, distribution, metabolism, and elimination. For example, the drug in Figure 3-19 has an onset of action of approximately 2 hours, a peak level at 5 hours, and an 8-hour duration of action or effect. By monitoring the plasma level of a compound, the efficacy

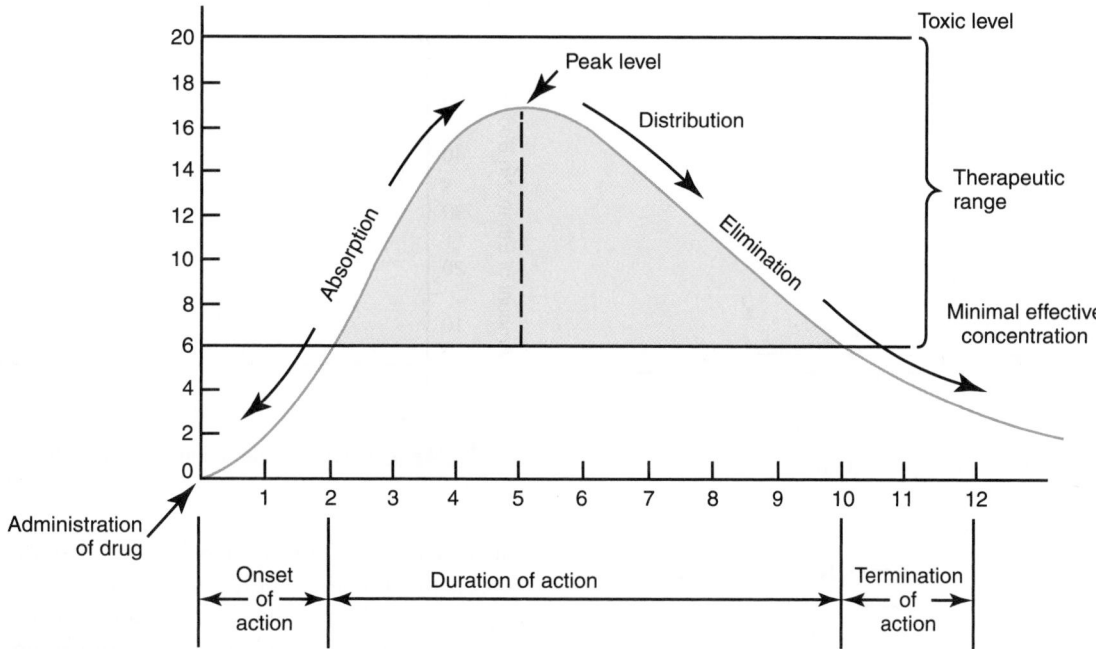

FIGURE 3-19 Plasma level profile of a drug.

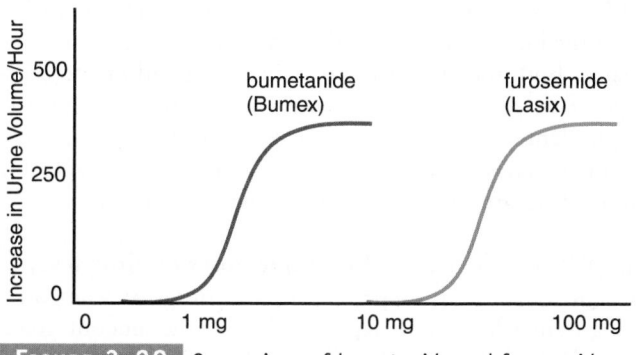

FIGURE 3-20 Comparison of bumetanide and furosemide, drugs with different potency but similar efficacy.

and safety of drug therapy can be more closely controlled. Box 3-2 lists important terms used in plasma level profiles and explains their interrelationships.

Once a drug is approved to be marketed and is in clinical use, serum levels of the drug may be used to fine-tune dosing. In many instances, nurses are required to monitor serum drug levels to help the prescriber determine the dose, scheduling, and route of administration for an individual client. These data provide information concerning the degree of therapeutic effectiveness and toxic levels or levels below the therapeutic range so that potential adverse effects can be predicted and serious clinical problems can be prevented.

Biologic Half-Life Drug elimination typically occurs in a concentration-dependent manner, with a greater quantity of drug eliminated per unit of time at higher concentrations. This process is referred to as first order or concentration-dependent elimination. The rate of biotransformation and excretion of a drug under first order elimination deter-

BOX 3-2 PLASMA LEVEL PROFILE TERMS

duration of action: the period from onset of drug action to the time when a response is no longer perceptible
half-life ($t_{1/2}$): the time required to reduce by one half the amount of unchanged drug in the body; used only for drugs that display concentration-dependent elimination
minimal effective concentration: the lowest plasma concentration that produces the desired drug effect
onset of action (latent period): the interval between the time a drug is administered and the first sign of its effect
peak plasma level: the highest plasma concentration attained from a dose
steady state: the point in time when the amount of drug going into the body equals the amount leaving the body and is reached in four to five half-lives for drugs that display concentration-dependent elimination
termination of action: the point at which a drug effect is no longer seen
therapeutic range: the range of plasma concentrations that produce the desired drug effect without toxicity (the range between minimal effective concentration and toxic level)
toxic level: the plasma concentration at which a drug produces serious adverse effects

mines its biologic **half-life** ($t_{1/2}$), the time required to reduce by one half the amount of unchanged drug in the body at the time equilibrium is established. The duration of the dosing interval is a function of the biologic half-life (see Figure 3-21). A drug with a short $t_{1/2}$, such as 2 or 3 hours, needs to be administered more often than one with a long $t_{1/2}$, such as 12 hours.

The half-life does not change with the size of the drug dose; it always takes the same amount of time to eliminate

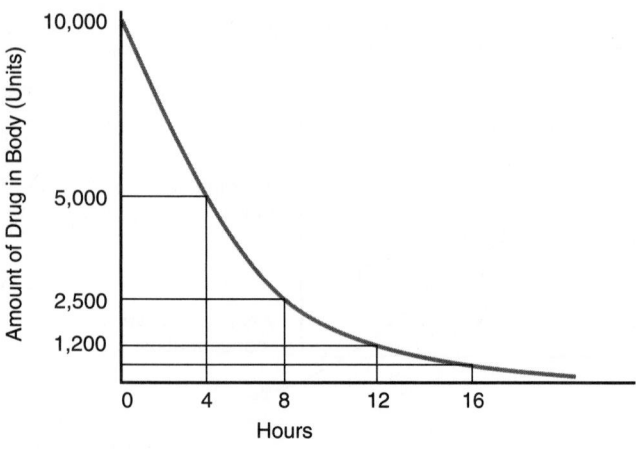

FIGURE 3-21 Biologic half-life ($t_{1/2}$).

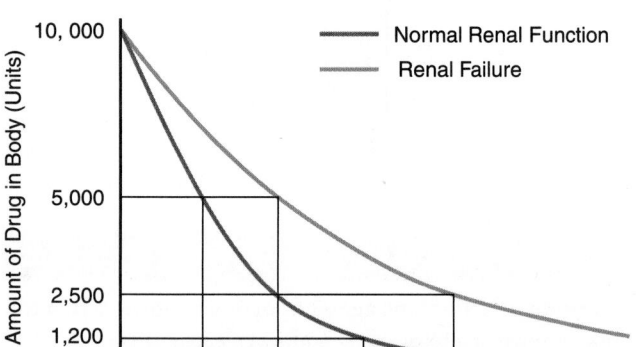

FIGURE 3-22 Biologic half-life ($t_{1/2}$) in renal failure.

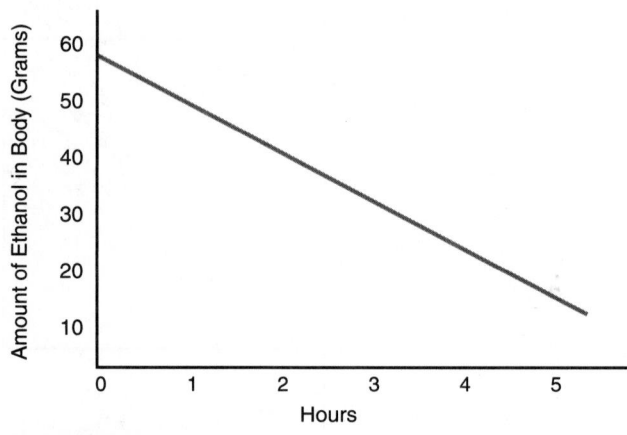

FIGURE 3-23 Zero order elimination of ethanol.

one half of the drug present in the body. If, for example, 10,000 units of a drug are administered IV and that drug has a half-life of 4 hours, then 5000 units of the drug will be excreted in 4 hours. In the next 4 hours, 2500 units will be excreted, with 1250 units more being excreted in the third 4-hour period (Figure 3-21). For clients with hepatic dysfunction or renal disorders, drug elimination may be prolonged and drug half-life lengthened, which usually necessitates reduction of the drug dose (Figure 3-22).

Under rare circumstances, drug elimination is not concentration-dependent (referred to as *zero order elimination*). This pattern is occasionally observed when normal pathways of elimination are saturated. Under such circumstances, the amount of drug eliminated per unit time is consistent (e.g., the same amount of drug eliminated each hour). This pattern is observed for ethanol, and for high-dose aspirin and high doses of the antiepileptic drug phenytoin (Dilantin) (Figure 3-23).

Drug Bioavailability Bioavailability refers to the percentage of active drug substances absorbed and available to reach the target tissues following drug administration. Drugs are considered to be biologically equivalent if they attain similar concentrations in blood and tissues at similar times; they are therapeutically equivalent if they provide equal therapeutic effectiveness in clinical trials. Of importance is the similarity of the absorption and therapeutic performances of drugs, which can be altered markedly by the ingredients and method of drug manufacture. Different brands of the same drug can vary, and even different lots from a single manufacturer may show different levels of effectiveness. Thus the U.S. Food and Drug Administration (FDA) pays close attention to drug preparation to ensure that the bioavailability of a drug conforms to uniform standards. Both the proportion of active drug and the percentage of its absorption are essential in attaining therapeutic equivalence among all chemically similar drugs. In the United States, ratings of bioavailability are available for most drugs on the FDA website (www.FDA.gov).

✷ What is the effect of multiple doses on drug levels?
Clients often receive repeated doses of drugs to maintain a long-term effect. With repeated dosing, the amount going into the body becomes equalized with the amount going out of the body. This concept is only valid with the great majority of drugs that exhibit first order (concentration-dependent) elimination. That point of equilibration is known as **steady state**. Steady state is essentially reached after four to five half-lives have passed while receiving a consistent dose, for example, continuous IV infusion or regular, repeated doses by any consistent route of administration (Figure 3-24).

Similarly, when stopping a drug, it takes about five half-lives before it is virtually eliminated out of the body (Figure 3-25). For some drugs with a very high affinity for binding to adipose or other tissue, a small amount of drug will continuously be leaving the adipose tissue beyond the five half-lives, but this is usually not clinically significant.

Repeated intermittent doses will also result in accumulation of drug over time until five half-lives have passed and steady state is achieved; occasionally a bit longer to reflect time for absorption and distribution. Once steady state is achieved, daily blood levels obtained each morning before the first dose will be consistent. For most drugs used clinically, blood levels are not routinely used for monitoring. However, blood levels may be monitored for drugs with a narrow therapeutic index in which there is a clear correlation between plasma level and efficacy and/or toxicity. Ex-

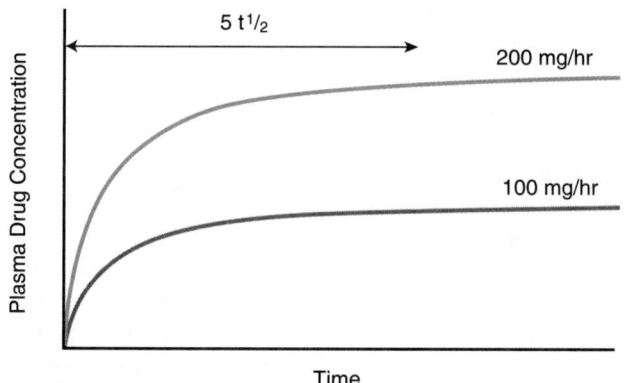

FIGURE 3-24 Time to steady-state drug concentration.

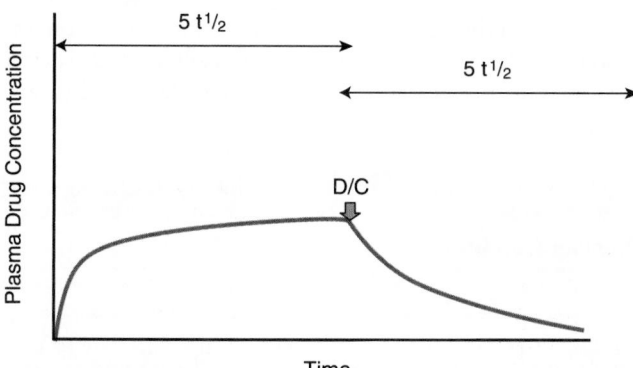

FIGURE 3-25 Half-life timing to steady-state drug concentration and elimination with discontinuation of the drug.

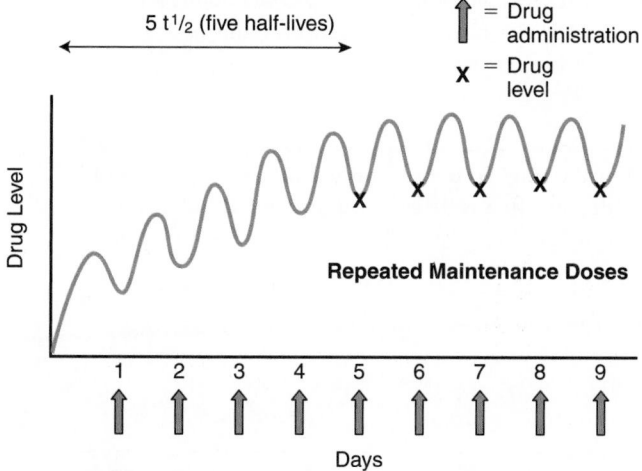

FIGURE 3-26 Morning serum drug concentrations for a drug with a morning dosing and a β elimination half-life of approximately 24 hours.

amples of such drugs are antiepileptic drugs, lithium, some antidepressants, digoxin, some drugs used for cardiac rhythm problems, and some antimicrobial agents. In most circumstances, a blood level before a dose (also known as a trough level) is used. Obtaining such a level before steady state is reached may be misleading (Figure 3-26).

✳ What about adverse effects?

In addition to producing therapeutic effects, drugs have the potential for causing undesirable responses, such as side effects or adverse reactions. **Side effects** are usually predictable and often unavoidable secondary effects produced by the drug at the usual therapeutic drug doses. For example, an opioid analgesic often causes the side effects of drowsiness and constipation. These effects occur at the usual prescribed dose, with drowsiness occurring soon after drug administration and constipation often being a delayed side effect that occurs later in therapy. The intensity of side effects is often dose-dependent.

The most commonly reported side effects are anorexia, nausea, vomiting, dizziness, drowsiness, dry mouth, abdominal gas or distress, constipation, and diarrhea. For some side effects, health care providers can provide nonpharmacologic advice, such as advising the individual to do the following:

- Use caution when getting up suddenly from a lying or sitting position to reduce the potential for dizziness or hypotension
- Use sugarless gum or candy or ice chips to relieve a dry mouth
- Avoid driving or using dangerous machinery until the individual's response to the medication can be assessed

Persistent or troublesome side effects may require pharmacological interventions, such as using laxatives, antiemetics, and antidiarrheals for constipation, vomiting, and diarrhea, respectively. In general, many side effects are manageable, and in some instances tolerance may develop to the side effect. Clients should be taught the most common side effects reported with a particular medication, how to avoid or self-manage it when possible, and when to report especially persistent effects to the prescriber.

Adverse reactions are unintended, undesirable, and often unpredictable drug effects. Every medication has a potential for causing harm. Sometimes adverse reactions are immediately apparent, whereas at other times they may take weeks or months to develop. Often new drugs are approved by the FDA or Health Canada after study in a small population (e.g., a few hundred to few thousand persons). With such relatively small sample sizes, not all potential adverse reactions may be detected before the drug is marketed. Adverse reactions can range from mild (e.g., rashes, phototoxic or photosensitivity reactions to light) to potentially fatal (anaphylaxis). With an increasing number of drugs being used, the incidence of adverse reactions has increased and is presently a significant problem in clinical practice (Nies, 2001). The nurse should be alert to any unusual individual responses to drugs, especially with newly released medications. Throughout this text, the term *adverse effects is used to identify the nontherapeutic effects of drugs and includes both side effects and adverse reactions.*

✳ How can adverse effects be predicted?

An **iatrogenic** condition is any adverse mental or physical condition induced in a client by a prescribed treatment or diagnostic procedure. Because these often involve prescribed medications, this term has also been used to define a disease caused by a prescriber (e.g., the use of phenothiazines in psychotic persons, which results in drug-induced Parkinson's disease). Other drug-induced diseases may include blood dyscrasias, hepatotoxicity, nephrotoxicity, and teratogenicity. With careful prescribing and monitoring, iatrogenic conditions are usually avoidable. With careful evaluation of a client's response to a drug, the nurse may be able to avoid or limit an iatrogenic disease.

Factors such as age, body mass, gender, environment, time of administration, pathologic state, genetics, and psychologic characteristics can alter an individual's response to drug therapy.

Adverse drug effects are often traced to the predictable influence of such variables. The nurse must be aware of characteristics that modify cell conditions and, therefore, the activity of a drug (Table 3-2).

Age Young children and older adults are usually highly responsive to medications. Infants often have immature hepatic and renal systems and, therefore, incomplete metabolic and excretory mechanisms. Older adults may demonstrate different responses to drug therapy because of a decline in hepatic and renal function, which is often accompanied by a concurrent disease process.

Body Mass The relationship between body mass and amount of drug administered influences the distribution and concentration of a drug. To maintain a desired drug concentration in individuals of various sizes, the drug dosage must be adjusted in proportion to body mass. The average adult drug dosage is calculated on the basis of the drug quantity that produces a particular effect in 50% of persons who are between the ages of 18 and 65 years and weigh approximately 150 pounds (70 kg). With children, drug dosage is commonly determined on the basis of amount of drug per kilogram of body weight or body surface area. For very lean and very obese individuals, drug dosage is often based on the amount of drug per kilogram of body weight or body surface area as well. Because water-soluble drugs do not distribute

TABLE 3-2 FACTORS THAT MODIFY CELL CONDITIONS AND DRUG ACTIVITY

Factor	Nursing Conditions
AGE	
Infants—immature body systems	Modify dosages.
Children—dosage adjustment usually necessary	Children have a different physiologic profile and body mass distribution. Thus the dose per kilogram is individualized and can be more or less than in an adult.
Older adults—depressed hepatic and renal systems	Older adults may also have concomitant physical conditions that alter drug effects; an altered distribution and excretion mechanism may also necessitate less drug or different scheduling of medication. Older adults are also at increased risk for drug interactions resulting from the use of multiple drugs.
BODY MASS	
The greater the volume of distribution of the drug in body mass, the lower the concentration of the drug in the body compartments. Calculation: average adult dose is based on a drug quantity that will produce a particular effect in 50% of the population between 18 and 65 years of age and approximately 150 pounds (70 kg) in weight	Adjust dosage in proportion to body mass. For children, the dosage often is determined on the basis of an amount of drug per kilogram of body weight or body surface area.
GENDER	
Women—smaller than men; definite differences during pregnancy and in relative proportions of fat and water; drugs vary by water or fat solubility	Allow for size differential and whether a drug is water or lipid soluble. Avoid drugs during pregnancy unless an absolute necessity exists.
ENVIRONMENTAL MILIEU	
Mood and behavior modified by (1) drug itself, (2) personality of the user, (3) environment of the user, and (4) interaction of these three factors. Other factors: sensory—deprivation or overload; physical environment—cold vs. heat; oxygen deprivation (altitude)	Be aware of the physical situation of the client with regard to heat and cold, interactions with other individuals, drug effects, and the way the client generally reacts to situations.

well into adipose tissue, such drugs (e.g., aminoglycoside antibiotics like tobramycin) are often dosed differently than are fat-soluble drugs in morbidly obese clients.

Gender Differences in drug effects related to gender result in part from the size differences between men and women. Women are usually smaller than men, which may lead to higher drug concentrations in women if the drug dosage is prescribed indifferently. Demonstrable differences also exist in relative proportions of fat and water in the bodies of men and women, and some drugs may be more soluble in one or the other. An increased drug response to zidovudine (AZT, Retrovir) and lamivudine (Epivir) in women with HIV compared to men appears related to elevated intracellular levels of active forms of these drugs in women (Anderson, 2003). Gender disparity in analgesic, cardiovascular, and antidepressant drug levels and/or response has also been reported (Hildebrandt et al., 2003; Pinn, 2003; Kornstein et al., 2000). Whether this variation is related to genetic pre-

disposition, hormonal fluctuation, differences in drug absorption or distribution is unclear.

Environmental Milieu Drugs affecting mood and behavior are particularly susceptible to the influence of environment. With such drugs one must consider the effects of (1) the drug itself, (2) the personality of the user, (3) the environment of the user, and (4) the interaction of these three components. Sensory deprivation and sensory overload may also affect responses to drugs. The physical environment can modify drug effects. For example, temperature affects drug activity, with heat relaxing the peripheral vessels and thus intensifying the actions of vasodilators; cold has the opposite effect. The relative oxygen deprivation at high altitudes may increase sensitivity to some drugs.

Time of Administration It is well known that drugs are absorbed more rapidly if the GI tract is free of food and that irritating drugs are more readily tolerated if there is food in

TABLE 3-2 FACTORS THAT MODIFY CELL CONDITIONS AND DRUG ACTIVITY—cont'd	
Factor	**Nursing Conditions**
TIME OF ADMINISTRATION	
Food—presence or absence Biologic rhythms—sleep-wake cycle, drug-metabolizing enzyme rhythms, corticosteroid secretion rhythm, blood pressure rhythms, circadian (24-hour) cycle in absorption and urinary excretion; also rhythm of drug receptor susceptibility Insufficient fluid intake with solid dosage forms	Give irritating drugs when food is in the client's stomach. The presence of food in the stomach may delay the absorption of oral drugs. Follow manufacturer's recommendations. Make every effort to understand the client's normal and abnormal rhythms, and seek possible relationships between the client's biologic rhythms and reactions to drug therapy. Administer drugs at the same time each day with a full glass of water. Altered body cycles (shift workers) may result in an altered response to a drug.
PATHOLOGIC STATE	
Presence and severity of pathologic state—pain intensifies the need for opioids; anxiety may produce resistance to large doses of tranquilizing drugs; the presence of circulatory, hepatic, and/or renal dysfunctions interferes with physiologic processes of drug action	Take into account any pain, disease, or altered metabolic state of the client and adjust dosage accordingly.
GENETIC FACTORS	
Genetically determined abnormal susceptibility to a chemical, or "idiosyncratic response"	Be aware that any client may show an idiosyncratic response. Always monitor closely for abnormal susceptibility, especially when beginning therapy. Be aware of common drug idiosyncrasies.
PSYCHOLOGICAL FACTORS	
Symbolic investment in drugs and faith in their efficacy Placebo effect Hostility toward or mistrust of medicine or health personnel	Be aware of the attitude and impression the nurse creates at the time of drug administration, and use them to enhance the effects of the drug.

the stomach. Research has indicated that the time of drug administration in relation to human biologic rhythms can significantly affect the response to certain medications. It seems quite plausible that in humans the sleep-wake rhythm, drug-metabolizing enzyme rhythms, and circadian (24-hour) variations contribute to the effective, ineffective, adverse, or toxic response to particular drugs. For example, cyclophosphamide (Cytoxan), an antineoplastic agent, should be administered in the morning to reduce the risk of hemorrhagic cystitis (blood in the urine) (*USP DI*, 2005). Body cortisol levels are at their highest in the morning; corticosteroids like prednisone, which mimic cortisol, are best dosed early in the day. Chronopharmacology (pharmacology concerned with the effects of drugs relative to body rhythms) and chronotoxicology (the study of poisons and their effects relative to body rhythms) are new areas that health care professionals are monitoring with great interest.

Pathologic State The presence of a pathologic condition and the severity of symptoms may call for careful consideration of the type of drug administered and for an adjustment in dosage. For example, the presence of severe pain tends to increase a client's requirement for an analgesic, and an extremely anxious individual can prove resis-tant to very large doses of tranquilizing and sedating drugs. Aspirin administered to a client with a fever will produce a decrease in temperature, whereas a client taking the drug for its analgesic effects will show no temperature change at all. Additionally, it bears repeating that the presence of circulatory, hepatic, or renal dysfunction will interfere with the physiologic processes of drug action.

Genetic Factors Genetic differences may affect an individual's response to a number of drugs (Evans & McLeod, 2003; Weinshilboum, 2003). Such differences may arise from genetic differences in drug metabolism or in receptor sensitivity. This pharmacogenetic variation often manifests as an "idiosyncrasy" and may be mistakenly diagnosed as a drug allergy. For example, some individuals may lack pseudocholinesterase activity in their plasma. If they receive an injection of succinylcholine (Anectine), which is normally hydrolyzed by plasma cholinesterase, they may become paralyzed and remain that way for a long time. Some individuals metabolize drugs by acetylation so significantly that they can be classified as slow acetylators or rapid acetylators, another example of a genetically based difference (Lin, Han, & Lin, 1993). The field of pharmacogenetics is of great interest because it may provide a rational explanation for many so-called drug idiosyncrasies (Johnson & Lima, 2003). See Chapter 6 for further discussion of this topic.

Psychological Factors A client's symbolic investment in drugs and faith in their effects strongly influence and usually potentiate drug effects. The placebo effect is an outstanding example of how strong motivation can influence the emergence of desired drug effects, whereas hostility and mistrust of medicine and health personnel can diminish drug effects. It is important for nurses to realize that their attitudes and the impressions created at the

time of drug administration may influence the therapeutic result.

✳ **What about unpredictable adverse effects?**

Allergic Drug Effects

The most frequently observed unpredictable adverse drug effect is drug allergy or hypersensitivity. A drug allergy is an altered state of reaction to a drug that results from previous sensitizing exposure and the development of an immunologic mechanism. Substances foreign to the body act as antigens and stimulate the production of antibodies or immunoglobulins (IgE, IgG, IgM). When a previously sensitized individual is again exposed to the foreign substance, the antigen reacts with the antibodies to release substances such as histamine, which then provoke allergic symptoms. The most widely used classification for allergic reactions is divided into Type I, Type II, Type III, and Type IV.

Type I (anaphylactic reaction) is an immediate reaction that occurs in a previously sensitized person within minutes of exposure to the chemical. This reaction is mediated by IgE antibodies located on the surface of mast cells and basophils. An immediate, severe reaction results and may be fatal if not recognized and treated quickly. The most dramatic form of anaphylaxis is sudden and severe bronchospasm, vasospasm, severe hypotension, and rapid death. Signs and symptoms are largely caused by the contraction of smooth muscles and may begin with irritability, extreme weakness, nausea, and vomiting and may proceed to dyspnea, cyanosis, seizures, and cardiac arrest. Less severe symptoms include hives and urticaria, which occur minutes after exposure. Drugs associated with this type of reaction include penicillins and cephalosporins. Antihistamines, epinephrine, and bronchodilators are indispensable in the treatment of anaphylactic shock.

Type II (cytotoxic reaction) involves a drug and IgG or IgM; it has sometimes been called an autoimmune response. This reaction manifests as hemolytic anemia (methyldopa [Aldomet]- or penicillin-induced), thrombocytopenia (quinidine gluconate [Quinaglute Dura-Tabs]-induced), or lupus erythematosus (procainamide [Pronestyl]-induced). Removal of the medication usually results in improvement, but it may take several months for the reaction to subside.

Type III (or Arthus reaction, an immune complex reaction) is sometimes called "serum sickness." With this reaction the drug forms a complex with IgG antibodies in the blood vessel, resulting in angioedema, arthralgia, fever, swollen lymph nodes (lymphadenopathy), and splenomegaly approximately 1 to 3 weeks after drug exposure. Penicillins, sulfonamides, and phenytoin (Dilantin) can cause this type of delayed reaction.

Type IV is a cell-mediated or delayed hypersensitivity reaction. For example, direct skin contact between the drug and sensitized cells results in an inflammatory reaction, such as contact dermatitis from poison ivy. This type of reaction occurs 24 to 48 hours after exposure and involves sensitized T lymphocytes and macrophages.

An individual who has had a mild allergic response to a particular drug should avoid reexposure to that drug and, optimally, should have skin tests performed to more definitively diagnose the response. Mild allergic reactions may be characterized by the development of a delayed rash, rhinitis, fever, and pruritus. Reinstitution of therapy with the same drug in a client who manifests an IgE-mediated allergic reaction (e.g., hives, urticaria) is always dangerous because an anaphylactic reaction may occur.

❋ How else can drug response be characterized?

A number of patterns in drug response emerge in different clients and with different drugs. These responses include tolerance, tachyphylaxis, cumulative effects, idiosyncratic effects, drug dependence, drug antagonism, summation, synergy, potentiation, and drug interactions.

Tolerance refers to a decreased physiologic response that occurs after repeated administration of a drug or a chemically related substance. This type of reaction necessitates an increase in dosage to maintain a given therapeutic effect. A cross tolerance to pharmacologically similar drugs may also develop, and drugs that act at the same receptor sites may also need their dosage increased to maintain an effect.

Although the actual mechanism of tolerance is unknown, multiple mechanisms have been proposed, such as an increase in hepatic drug metabolizing enzymes and pharmacodynamic tolerance. Pharmacodynamic tolerance refers to chronic or long-term drug use in an individual who requires larger drug doses to achieve the same effect as before. Drugs well known for their propensity to produce tolerance are tobacco, opium alkaloids, nitrates, and ethyl alcohol. The exact reason for this is unknown, but it is believed that receptor or cellular adaptation may occur (Nies, 2001).

Tachyphylaxis refers to a quickly developing tolerance that occurs after repeated administration of a drug. It is typically rapid in onset, and the client's initial response to the drug cannot be reproduced, even with larger doses of the drug. Many drugs may produce a tachyphylactic response in isolated individuals. Certain drugs may be more inclined to produce such a response, including some central nervous stimulants (e.g., amphetamines), and sedative-hypnotics (e.g., benzodiazepines).

A *cumulative effect* occurs when the body cannot metabolize one dose of a drug before another dose is administered. When drugs are excreted more slowly than they are absorbed, each new dose adds more to the total quantity in the blood and organs than is lost in the same amount of time by excretion. Unless drug administration is adjusted, high concentrations can be reached, producing toxic effects. Cumulative toxicity can occur rapidly, as dramatically illustrated in ethyl alcohol intoxication, or it can occur insidiously, as is the case in poisoning with heavy metals such as lead. Lead is stored in many body tissues and deposited in bones, thus having prolonged effects on the body while accumulation continues.

Idiosyncrasy is any abnormal or peculiar response to a drug, which may manifest itself by (1) overresponse or abnormal susceptibility to a drug; (2) underresponse, which demonstrates abnormal tolerance; (3) a qualitatively different effect from the one expected, such as excitation after the administration of a sedative; or (4) unpredictable and unexplainable symptoms. Idiosyncratic reactions are generally thought to result from genetic enzymatic deficiencies that lead to an abnormal mechanism of drug metabolism. This term has been used rather vaguely to describe drug reactions that are qualitatively different from the usual effects obtained in the majority of clients and that cannot be attributed to drug allergy.

Drug dependence is the term preferred over the previous terminology of "habituation" and "addiction." The World Health Organization has suggested the use of the term *dependence* in conjunction with the drug being described (e.g., barbiturate dependence or opioid dependence) (WHO, 2003). Dependence can be physical or psychological. Physical dependence refers to a state of physiologic drug adaptation that manifests itself by intense physical disturbance when the drug is withdrawn. Psychological dependence is a state of emotional reliance on a drug to maintain an effect. Its manifestations may range from a mild desire for a drug to craving to compulsive use of the drug. Drug dependence is explored in greater detail in Chapter 9.

Drug interaction occurs when the effects of one drug are modified by the prior or concurrent administration of another drug, thereby increasing or decreasing the pharmacologic action of each. Drug interactions may be either beneficial (e.g., probenecid [Benemid] prolongs the action of penicillins) or detrimental (e.g., sulfa antibacterials increase the action of oral anticoagulants, causing increased risk for hemorrhage). Drug interactions can be further characterized as pharmacodynamic (competitive or additive effects at the receptor) or pharmacokinetic (one agent affecting the absorption, distribution, metabolism, and/or excretion of a second agent). Common drug interactions and their mechanisms will be discussed throughout the text.

Drug antagonism occurs when the combination effect of two drugs is less than the sum of the drugs acting separately.

Summation (addition or additive effect) occurs when the combined effect of two drugs produces a result that equals the sum of the individual effects of each agent. The mathematical equivalent is $1 + 1 = 2$. For example, codeine and aspirin both act as analgesics and when given together they provide an additive or greater pain relief than when either one is used alone. This combination allows the administration of a lower dose of each drug, with a resultant decrease in adverse effects.

Synergism describes a drug interaction in which the combined effect of drugs is greater than the sum of each individual agent acting independently. Mathematically the response can be written as $1 + 1 = 3$ or more. Synergism can be exemplified by the use of a combination of drugs in treating hypertension. Each of the drugs lowers blood pressure but in a different way; the combined effect may produce a greater decrease in hypertension than the sum effect of each.

Potentiation refers to the concurrent administration of two drugs in which one drug increases the effect of the other drug.

❋ How do the principles of drug action relate to the nursing management of drug therapy?

Your responsibilities in drug administration extend beyond memorization of specific drugs, their actions, and their dosages. Effective implementation depends on a sound comprehension of the theories of drug action, constituting clinical judgment that can be applied to the individual client, each with a specific diagnosis and definable individual needs. Such a background necessitates that you understand theories of drug action, physiologic processes mediating drug action, variables affecting drug action, and unusual and adverse effects of drug therapy.

It is essential to use critical thinking in the nursing management of a client's therapeutic regimen. A prescriber writes an order for a specific medication for an individual client at a particular time when this pharmacologic intervention is deemed appropriate. However, circumstances change and a client may have a different response to a medication than was intended. Assess whether that dose is appropriate for the client each time it is to be administered. An analogy would be that the prescriber's order exists in time and space much like a pedestrian sign flashing "walk" or "don't walk" regardless of what is occurring in the environment. What is important is whether it is safe to cross the street at a given time—that the traffic has really stopped—regardless of what the sign indicates. In the same way, monitor for both therapeutic and nontherapeutic medication effects with each and every dose to ensure client safety in drug therapy.

On entry into the body, a drug initiates a series of physiologic events before it reaches its site of action. The extent of drug absorption depends on the form of the drug. Tablets or capsules must first disintegrate and then dissolve before absorption through the intestinal membrane can occur. Be sure to assess the client's ability to tolerate a particular form or route (e.g., testing the client's ability to swallow before an oral medication is administered). Also, do not crush or break open enteric-coated tablets because the coating protects the tablet from destruction by the acid pH of the stomach until the drug can reach the alkaline pH of the intestine, and thereby maintain its effectiveness. Drugs that irritate the gastric mucosa are also coated and should not be crushed or chewed.

The time of administration is another important concern. Drugs that require multiple daily doses and steady-state serum levels need to be evenly spaced throughout a 24-hour period. Drugs with more infrequent dosing need to be taken at the same time each day. To obtain the maximal pharmacokinetic benefit, give oral drugs with a glass of water (8 ounces) 30 to 60 minutes before meals. Remember that the presence of food, which delays stomach emptying, tends to delay the therapeutic effect of the drug. Occasionally, you will need to administer an agent with meals to prevent GI irritation. Always anticipate a rapid response when administering a drug by the IV route because the full dose is placed directly into the bloodstream, thus bypassing the need for absorption.

Individuals with hepatic dysfunction are susceptible to drug overdosage, especially if the drug is highly bound to plasma proteins. Additionally, clients with renal dysfunction may require adjustments in the amount and frequency of medication dosages. Because most agents are excreted by the kidneys, observe the client for a cumulative effect that may result from the continued administration of the drug. Usually drug dosage is adjusted in individuals with hepatic or renal disorders so that adverse effects are prevented.

In instances in which you are required to monitor serum drug levels, carefully observe the client's response to the drug and report this to the prescriber. This will assist the prescriber in determining the drug's dosage, frequency, and route of administration. These data are essential for promoting the optimal therapeutic benefit to the client while preventing potential adverse effects.

Finally, advise child-bearing women and sexually active women of child-bearing age who are not practicing contraception to check with their primary care provider before taking any drug because of the risk of teratogenic effects. If a medication is required, the lowest possible dose of the prescribed drug should be administered.

Chapter 5 explores the principles that will assist you to develop the nursing judgment necessary for safe and accurate medication administration.

Summary

Drugs are chemicals that interact with a living organism to produce biologic responses. They produce these responses according to certain theories of drug action, physiologic processes mediating drug action, variables affecting drug action, and unusual and adverse effects of drug therapy. Drugs modify only existing functions and exert multiple actions rather than a single effect. These actions result from a physiochemical interaction between the drug and a functionally important molecule in the body.

To produce the desired effect, a drug must have an appropriate concentration at its site of action. This concentration is influenced by a number of processes that can be divided into three phases: pharmaceutical, pharmacokinetic, and pharmacodynamic. The pharmaceutical phase focuses on the form of the drug, solid or liquid, and its dissolution to achieve absorption. The pharmacokinetic phase is concerned with the concentration of the drug during the processes of absorption, distribution, biotransformation, and excretion. Absorption involves the movement of drug molecules from the site of entry into the body to the circulating fluids. Several factors influence absorption: the nature of the absorbing surface through which the drug must pass, blood flow to the site of administration, solubility of the drug, pH, drug concentration, and dosage form. Drugs may be given for either local or systemic effect. The routes of drug administration are classified as enteral, parenteral, pulmonary, and topical. Distribution is the transport of a drug in body fluids to various tissues of the body and ultimately to the site of action. It is influenced by the body's storage reservoirs for drugs—plasma protein binding and tissue binding—and by barriers to drug distribution, such as the blood-brain barrier and the placental barrier. In biotransformation, the liver—the primary site for drug metabolism—inactivates the drug by converting it to a metabolite that can be excreted from the body. Excretion, the elimination of pharmacologically active or inactive metabolites from the body, occurs primarily through the kidneys, with some elimination through the intestine, lungs, mammary glands, and sweat and salivary glands.

The pharmacodynamic phase is concerned with the response of tissues to specific chemical agents at various sites in the body. The mechanism for action between the drug and a functionally important component of the living system may be a drug-receptor interaction, a drug-enzyme interaction, or a nonspecific drug interaction. Because each drug has its own characteristic pharmacokinetic activity, it may be necessary to monitor a client by obtaining a plasma level of a drug. The biologic half-life and the therapeutic index of a drug also provide information to assist the prescriber in determining the dose, scheduling, and route of administration for an individual client.

No drug is totally safe; it can sometimes react in the body to produce unpredictable and harmful effects. However, some identifiable factors do alter the response to drug therapy: age, body mass, gender, environmental milieu, time of administration, pathologic states, genetic factors, and psychological factors. The adverse effects caused unintentionally by treatment are known as iatrogenic disease. With drug therapy, iatrogenic diseases may be manifested in five major ways: blood dyscrasias, hepatic toxicity, renal damage, teratogenic effects, and dermatologic effects. Other, somewhat unpredictable adverse effects may be evidenced as drug allergy, tolerance, tachyphylaxis, cumulation, idiosyncrasy, drug dependence, drug interaction, drug antagonism, summation, synergism, potentiation, or immediate reactions such as anaphylaxis.

It is important to understand the principles involved in drug action and their influence on nursing practice to administer each medication with the greatest safety and efficacy.

✱ Critical Thinking Questions

- If you were administering a medication with a long half-life, what types of clients would be more at risk for cumulative effects?
- Both diazepam (Valium), an anxiolytic drug, and warfarin (Coumadin), an oral anticoagulant, are highly protein-bound medications. If you were administering both of these to the same client, what assessments of the client would be particularly important?
- How can a drug that has CNS activity but cannot cross the blood-brain barrier be administered for effectiveness?

Bibliography

Anderson, P.L., Kakuda, T.N., Kawle, S., & Fletcher, C.V. (2003). Antiviral dynamics and sex differences of zidovudine and lamivudine triphosphate concentrations in HIV-infected individuals. *AIDS, 17*(15), 2159-2168.

Bauer, L.A. (2002). Clinical pharmacokinetics and pharmacodynamics. In J.T. DiPiro, et al. (Eds.), *Pharmacotherapy: A pathophysiological approach* (5th ed.). Stamford, CT: Appleton & Lange.

Evans, W.E., & McLeod, H.L. (2003). Drug therapy: Pharmacogenomics—drug disposition, drug targets, and side effects. *New England Journal of Medicine, 348*(6), 538-549.

Hildebrandt, M.G., Steyerberg, E.W., Stage, K.B., Passchier, J., Kragh-Soerensen, P.; Danish University Antidepressant Group. (2003). Are gender differences important for the clinical effects of antidepressants? *American Journal of Psychiatry, 160*(9), 1643-1650.

Humma, L.M., & Lam, Y.W.F. (2002). Pharmacogenetics. In J.T. DiPiro, et al. (Eds.), *Pharmacotherapy: A pathophysiological approach* (5th ed.). Stamford, CT: Appleton & Lange.

Johnson, J.A., & Lima, J.J. (2003). Drug receptor/effector polymorphisms and pharmacogenetics: current status and challenges. *Pharmacogenetics 13*(9), 525-534.

Katzung, B.G. (2004). *Basic and clinical pharmacology* (9th ed.). Stamford, CT: Appleton & Lange.

Klaassen, C.D. (2001). Principles of toxicology and treatment of poisoning. In J.G. Hardman, & L.E. Limbird (Eds.), *Goodman & Gilman's the pharmacological basis of therapeutics* (10th ed.). New York: McGraw-Hill.

Koda-Kimble, M.A., Young, L.Y., Kradjan, W.A., Guglielmo, B.J., Alldredge, B.K., & Corelli, R.L. (Eds.). (2005). *Applied therapeutics: The clinical use of drugs* (8th ed.). Philadelphia: Lippincott, Williams & Wilkins.

Kornstein, S.G., Yonkers, K.A., McCullough, J.P., Keitner, G.I., Gelenbery, A.J., Davis, S.M., et al. (2000). Gender differences in treatment response to sertraline versus imipramine in chronic depression. *American Journal of Psychiatry, 157,* 1445-1452.

Lin, H.J., Han, C.Y., & Lin, B.K. (1993). Slow acetylator mutations in the human polymorphic *N*-acetyltransferase gene in 786 Asians, blacks, Hispanics, and whites: Application to metabolic epidemiology. *American Journal of Human Genetics, 52,* 827-834.

McCarver, D.G., Thomasson, H.R., & Martier, S.S. (1997). Alcohol dehydrogenase-2*3 allele protects against alcohol-related birth defects among African Americans. *Journal of Pharmacology and Experimental Therapeutics, 283*(3), 1095-1101.

Nies, A.S. (2001). Principles of therapeutics. In J.G. Hardman, & L.E. Limbird (Eds.), *Goodman & Gilman's the pharmacological basis of therapeutics* (10th ed.). New York: McGraw-Hill.

e-LEARNING SUPPLEMENTS

Student CD-ROM
- Final Exam questions
- NCLEX® Examination review questions
- Pharmacology animations
- Printable chapter summary

Evolve Website (http://evolve.elsevier.com/mckenry)
- Case study on principles of drug action
- Content updates, including information on new drugs
- WebLinks corresponding to this chapter
- Answers to the critical thinking questions in this chapter
- *Elsevier ePharmacology Update* newsletter
- *Mosby's Drug Consult* Internet Edition
- Supplemental and reference information

Phillips, K., Veenstra, D.L., Oren, E., Lee, J.K., & Sadee, W. (2001). Potential role of pharmacogenomics in reducing adverse drug reactions: A systematic review. *Journal of the American Medical Association, 286*(18), 2270-2279.

Pinn, V.W. (2003). Sex and gender factors in medical studies: Implications for health and clinical practice. *Journal of the American Medical Association, 289*(4), 397-400.

Polifka, J. E., & Friedman, J.M. (2002). Medical genetics: 1. Clinical teratology in the age of genomics. *CMAJ Canadian Medical Association Journal, 167*(3), 265-273.

Ross, E.M., & Kenakin, T.P. (2001). Pharmacodynamics: Mechanisms of drug action and the relationship between drug concentration and effect. In J.G. Hardman, & L.E. Limbird (Eds.), *Goodman & Gilman's the pharmacological basis of therapeutics* (10th ed.). New York: McGraw-Hill.

USP DI: Drug information for the health care professional (25th ed.). (2005). Greenwood Village, CO: MICROMEDEX Thomson Healthcare.

van Gelder, T., Hesselink, D.A., van Hest, R.M., Mathot, R.A.A., & van Schaik, R. (2004). Pharmacogenetics in immunosuppressive therapy: The best thing since TDM? *Therapeutic Drug Monitoring, 26*(4), 343-346.

Weinshilboum, R. (2003). Genomic medicine: Inheritance and drug response. *New England Journal of Medicine, 348*(6), 529-537.

Wilkinson, G.R. (2001). Pharmacokinetics: The dynamics of drug absorption, distribution, and elimination. In J.G. Hardman, & L.E. Limbird (Eds.), *Goodman & Gilman's the pharmacological basis of therapeutics* (10th ed.). New York: McGraw-Hill.

World Health Organization (2003). *WHO Expert Committee on Drug Dependence 33rd Report—WHO Technical Report Series 915.* Retrieved October 30, 2004, from http://www.who.int/medicines/library/qsm/915-en.pdf

MEDICATION ERRORS

4

CHAPTER FOCUS

Medication errors occur on a much larger scale in the United States than is acceptable. In recent years, much attention has been drawn to the frequency and severity of medication errors in health care agencies, primarily hospitals. Medication errors constitute one type of error that is part of a larger category of medical errors. This chapter provides an introduction to the scope of medication errors as a problem in our health care system, the factors that contribute to it, and what nurses can do to reduce them individually and as a member of the team working within a health care delivery system.

LEARNING OBJECTIVES

- Explore the nature and significance of medication errors in current clinical practice.
- Describe national initiatives to reduce the incidence of medication errors.
- Explain processes used by health care agencies to decrease the risk of medication errors.
- Identify the role of the nurse in preventing medication errors.

▲ KEY TERMS

adverse drug event, p. 60
medical error, p. 59
medication error, p. 60
medication reconciliation, p. 62

✱ Why are medical errors of such concern today?
Large-scale national attention was drawn to the topic of medical errors when the Institute of Medicine (IOM) released its landmark report, *To Err is Human: Building a Safer Health Care System* (1999). It defines **medical error** essentially as the failure to complete a planned aim in the manner intended or using the wrong plan to achieve an aim (IOM, 1999). The report identified client safety as a growing concern, incorporating data from the 1992 Harvard Medical Practice study and a 1984 study of hospitals in Utah and Colorado. These studies found that medical errors occur at an alarming rate (3.7% and 2.9%, respectively), and that more than half were preventable. Medication errors represent one subgroup of all medical errors. The

Harvard study found that medication-related errors resulted in adverse events in 19.4% of cases. Furthermore, if the proportions in these data were expanded to a national scale, the cost of these events in the United States was about $37.6 billion dollars ($17 billion preventable) and the approximate number of deaths in 1997 attributable to medication error was 7000.

Reaction to the report was immediate and widespread within the health care industry, and with public policy makers and private payers. Subsequent IOM reports, *Crossing the Quality Chasm* (2001) and *Priority Areas for National Attention: Transforming Health Care Quality* (2002), identified reduction of medication errors as a priority area of concern. Since the publication of those reports, several groups and agencies have responded, and this information is integrated in the remainder of the chapter.

✱ What is a medication error?

The current literature abounds with terms that may confuse the reader rather than provide clarity. A **medication error** is an error related to medication therapy and includes errors in prescribing, dispensing, administration, or monitoring. Medication errors may or may not constitute an **adverse drug event** for the client, which is a negative or untoward response to a medication. If a client experiences an adverse drug event as a result of a medication error, that event is considered preventable. However, not all adverse drug events are preventable; some clients exhibit negative or unanticipated responses to medications that were given in a proper manner or dose. Nurses and other health care providers are particularly committed to reducing the number of preventable adverse drug events, such as those caused by medication errors. There are many causes of medication errors, including human factors (performance or knowledge deficits, miscalculation of doses, and others), communication problems (written or oral miscommunications), name confusion (generic or trade name sound-alikes or look-alikes), and packaging and labeling issues. This means that efforts to significantly reduce medication error rates must include initiatives that consider each of these areas. Health care institutions today are working to develop both institutional and provider-specific remedies to reduce medication error rates. National initiatives are also underway to decrease medication error rates across the United States.

National Proposed Solutions

In a comprehensive review of current initiatives, Clancy (2004) recommended that public policy makers should focus efforts on developing error-prevention strategies and solutions that do the following:

- Incorporate appropriate design components (such as automated medication dispensing units)
- Have the greatest likelihood for reducing errors
- Have support based in research
- Address cost and implementation issues

To formulate successful strategies, it is crucial to keep in mind that the medication delivery system in any health care institution is a complex process consisting of many steps and linkages among departments and providers, such as physicians, pharmacists, nurses, and unit clerks (if they transcribe medication orders). With this in mind, any successful initiative toward error reduction must analyze each unique institutional system, and then select, design, and implement system changes that will best achieve the goals for that institution. Key organizations such as the IOM, the Agency for Healthcare Research and Quality (AHRQ) of the U.S. Department of Health and Human Services, the Institute for Safe Medication Practices (ISMP), and the Joint Commission on the Accreditation of Healthcare Organizations (JCAHO), among others, have also weighed in

with specific recommendations for decreasing the rate of medication errors.

The original IOM report (1999) concluded that the medical errors are generally not the result of careless providers. Rather, errors commonly result from system-related problems, processes, and conditions. This finding formed the basis of a recommendation to implement institution-specific safety systems to heighten safety practices at the point of care delivery. Other recommendations called for raised performance standards, creating a national focus of safety, and developing a nationwide public mandatory reporting system for errors. Much work at the national and local levels has occurred since that report was published, with varying degrees of outcome achievement.

The AHRQ developed an action plan in response to the IOM report, and was given $50 million dollars from Congress to support efforts at reducing medical errors. Its efforts are broad and comprehensive, and include the following:

- Developing and testing new technologies that support safety
- Conducting demonstration projects related to error prevention and error reporting
- Supporting ongoing research into medical errors
- Supporting projects that assess how the environment of care affects providers' ability to improve safety
- Funding research that enhances provider education about error reduction

The ISMP was the first organization to promote the use of *failure mode and effects analysis* (FMEA) to pinpoint areas in medication delivery systems that are most likely to fail. It also has a Medication Errors Reporting Program (MERP), which independently reviews reports submitted to the editorial staff of the *United States Pharmacopeia (USP)*. Any health care provider (physician, pharmacist, nurse, student) can report an error using this program via telephone, fax, or the Internet (www.usp.org/reporting/mer.htm). Information gained from these reports is also shared among the USP, ISMP, U.S. Food and Drug Administration (FDA), and the product manufacturer. The ISMP also participates as a partner in the MedWatch, the safety information and adverse event reporting program of the FDA (see Chapter 2). The ISMP is currently advocating for medication bar coding, electronic prescribing, and a national medical-error-reporting program.

JCAHO publishes annual patient safety goals that are part of the accreditation process for health care organizations seeking JCAHO accreditation. Goals are selected based on sentinel event reporting and provide both evidence-based and expert-based solutions to these problems. Annual patient safety goals become part of the criteria for accreditation. JCAHO has mandated that, effective January 1, 2004, accredited health care organizations must have a policy that prohibits use of dangerous abbreviations, acronyms, and symbols when prescribing drugs or otherwise documenting in the medical record. There is a core list of five abbreviations that all health care organizations must avoid. Additionally, each organization must choose three

TABLE 4-1 JCAHO LIST OF ABBREVIATIONS, ACRONYMS, AND SYMBOLS TO AVOID

Do Not Use	Potential Problem	Use Instead
OFFICIAL "DO NOT USE" LIST*		
U (unit)	Mistaken for "0" (zero), the number "4" (four) or "cc"	Write "unit"
IU (International Unit)	Mistaken for IV (intravenous) or the number 10 (ten)	Write "International Unit"
Q.D., QD, q.d., qd (daily) Q.O.D., QOD, q.o.d, qod (every other day)	Mistaken for each other Period after the Q mistaken for "I" and the "O" mistaken for "I"	Write "daily" Write "every other day"
Trailing zero (X.0 mg)† Lack of leading zero (.X mg)	Decimal point is missed	Write X mg Write 0.X mg
MS MSO4 and MgSO4	Can mean morphine sulfate or magnesium sulfate Confused for one another	Write "morphine sulfate" Write "magnesium sulfate"
ADDITIONAL ABBREVIATIONS, ACRONYMS AND SYMBOLS (FOR POSSIBLE FUTURE INCLUSION IN THE OFFICIAL "DO NOT USE" LIST)		
> (greater than) < (less than)	Misinterpreted as the number "7" (seven) or the letter "L"	Confused for one another Write "greater than" Write "less than"
Abbreviations for drug names	Misinterpreted due to similar abbreviations for multiple drugs	Write drug names in full
Apothecary units	Unfamiliar to many practitioners Confused with metric units	Use metric units
@	Mistaken for the number "2" (two)	Write "at"
cc	Mistaken for U (units) when poorly written	Write "ml" or "milliliters"
μg	Mistaken for mg (milligrams) resulting in one thousand–fold overdose	Write "mcg" or "micrograms"

© Joint Commission on Accreditation of Healthcare Organizations, 2005. Reprinted with permission.
*Applies to all orders and all medication-related documentation that is handwritten (including free-text computer entry) or on pre-printed forms.
†**Exception:** A "trailing zero" may be used only where required to demonstrate the level of precision of the value being reported, such as for laboratory results, imaging studies that report size of lesions, or catheter/tube sizes. It may not be used in medication orders or other medication-related documentation.

additional items to include in an agency-specific "Do Not Use" list (Table 4-1). This strategy will hopefully decrease the number of medication errors caused by transcription error and poor handwriting.

In summary, an enormous amount of time, energy, and resources is being directed to the study of medical errors as a broad focus and to medication errors as a subset of that focus. Efforts in this area are likely to continue for some time.

✱ **What efforts are being made in health care organizations to reduce medication errors?**

Although some of the conversation at the national level about reducing medication errors addresses national policy-

making strategies, a number of organization-specific initiatives have been proposed in the literature. A brief discussion of some of the key topics follows.

Systems Thinking: Eliminating a Culture of Blame

Typically in the past, when a medication occurred on a nursing unit, the event was written up on an incident report, "investigated" by a nurse manager, and resulted in a verbal or written reprimand of the nurse. In essence, this practice created a culture of "blaming" nurses for errors, while doing little or nothing to change the system that helped lead to the error in the first place. Current thought is that medication errors result from a multitude of factors, each of which must be discovered and addressed systematically. In this way, the root causes of errors can be identified and fixed, rather than target the nurse as the last link in the chain of medication delivery. Medication errors can occur at any of five points in the medication process: prescribing, documenting, dispensing, administering, and monitoring. The presence of distractions during any of these phases can be a major contributing factor for errors. Thus the entire system must be examined and repaired before significant progress can occur.

Medication Reconciliation

Medication reconciliation is a process that consists of identifying an accurate list of all client medications (name, dosage, frequency, and route), and using the list to ensure that the client receives the correct medications, regardless of where he or she is in the health care system. To complete a medication reconciliation, compare the client's current list of medications against the list of medications previously taken at home, and against the physician's admission, transfer, and/or discharge orders. Poor communication of medical information when transferring clients within the health care delivery system may account for up to 50% of all medication errors and up to 20% of adverse drug events for hospitalized clients. Whenever a client is transferred to another unit in the hospital, the nurse or other provider should compare previous medication orders to new orders, and reconcile any differences. Completing this process in a standardized manner may help to prevent medication errors that occur because of failure to administer medications that are needed by the client.

Computerized Physician Order Entry

Computerized physician order entry systems may dramatically reduce or eliminate medication errors by targeting the first step of the medication process, prescribing. Handwritten orders may be ineligible because of a variety of factors, such as the prescriber being rushed or having poor handwriting. A computerized order entry system provides menu-driven options for drug dosage and frequency, which can reduce prescribing errors (Teich et al., 2000). Furthermore, the computer can access individual client profile information, which could lead to decreased prescribing of drugs that could cause allergic reaction or adverse interactive drug effects. A final benefit is improved workflow on the nursing unit by reducing medication turnaround times, medication error rates, verbal orders, telephone calls/pages to clarify orders, and elimination of medication transcription errors (Lykowski & Mahoney, 2004).

Machine-Readable (Bar) Coding

The use of a machine-readable or "bar" code reader device is a potentially powerful tool to intercept medication errors in the administration stage of a medication. Because this is the "last stop" before a harmful medication reaches the client, this device is appealing to many clinicians. Nonetheless, the actual use of this technology lacks far behind the retail industry, another sector of the workplace requiring rapid filling of large orders and inventory control (ISMP, 2002). In 1999, only slightly more than 1% of hospitals in the United States used bar code technology. In 2002, approximately 35% of unit dose medications typically used in hospitals had bar codes applied by the manufacturer. This number needs to drastically increase to effectively implement this strategy for error prevention. The Veterans' Health Administration (VHA) began using bar code technology in the last few years, and there is likely to be keen interest in the outcome of their use. Although error reduction has been an early outcome, disadvantages include the high initial outlay for start-up costs and an increased amount of time needed to dispense medications by the nursing staff (Roark, 2004).

Pharmacist Presence on the Clinical Unit

Adopting the practice of having pharmacists and physicians collaborate in the clinical review of clients may be another successful strategy to reduce errors made in the prescribing phase of the medication process. Kucukarslan, Peters, Mlynarek, and Nafziger (2003) found that when pharmacists "rounded," or made clinical visits to the bedside, with physicians and made recommendations about drug therapy, there was a 78% drop in the rate of preventable adverse drug events. The most common types of interactions pertained to dosing-related changes and recommendations to add a medication to therapy. This error-reduction strategy could have a huge impact on the overall rate of medication errors if implemented on a large enough scale. However, a shortage of pharmacists may preclude this intervention for most institutions.

✳ What is the individual nurse's role in preventing medication errors?

Although many health care team members play a role in prescription, delivery, administration of drugs, and monitoring of clients to prevent medication errors, the nurse is the final point in the medication delivery system before the medication reaches the client. For this reason, the nurse must be especially vigilant in all aspects of medication administration. The nurse has key roles to play in both medication delivery and monitoring. Additionally, the nurse has a responsibility to report medication errors when they occur.

Proper Procedures and Techniques for Medication Administration

To ensure that the right client gets the right medication, it is essential to accurately and fully identify the client before administering each dose. Use the client's full name on all paperwork and in all references to help prevent mix-ups, and be alert to similarities in names. When clients on the same nursing unit have similar names, place them in rooms that are geographically distant as an extra precaution. Do not rely on memory to identify clients. In an institutional setting, medications should be administered only to clients wearing an identification wristband or tag. *Checking the client's name and date of birth on the identification wristband or bracelet against the name* on the accompanying medication sheet is the most reliable mode of identification. A common additional procedure is to ask the client to state his or her name and date of birth and compare it to the information on the medication Kardex, computer sheet, or medication administration record (MAR). However, just asking the client to state his or her name is not foolproof. For example, a client may give his name as "James" or "Santiago" (first name), and then be given medication intended for "Mr. James" or "Mr. Santiago" (last name). Avoid checking the client's name by calling it out and waiting for a corroborating answer, which is particularly risky (e.g., do *not* ask, "Are you James Santiago?"). Clients have been known to answer to almost any name when in a sleepy state. Do not rely on names on bed tags or labels. This practice is dangerous because clients are often away from their beds, and a client who is confused or in a groggy state after returning from a test or procedure could inadvertently occupy the wrong bed. Do not ask family members, either, because a distraught family member could answer inappropriately.

Each institution has a policy for replacing identification bands or tags that are inadvertently removed or lost, and this policy should be followed to replace the identification before administering any medications. An exception might be an emergency, in which a delay might be detrimental. However, even in an emergency the client's identity should be verified by some method before drug administration.

Before administering medications, make sure the drug order has not been changed in any way (e.g., discontinued or dosage changed) from what appears on the medication sheet or MAR. It is also important to check the MAR to see that the dose about to be given has not already been given by someone else caring for the client (such as another nurse or nursing student). Individual agency policies outline the checking procedure to be used, and these policies must be followed routinely to avoid error.

The following guidelines are recommended when distributing or administering drugs to clients:

1. When preparing or administering medications, concentrate your whole attention on what you are doing. Do not permit yourself to be distracted while working with medications.
2. Be certain you have a written order for every medication that you administer. (Verbal and telephone orders should be written out and signed by the prescriber as soon as possible. These types of orders should be used only in limited circumstances [e.g., emergencies]—not for the convenience of the prescriber).
3. Be certain that the data on the computer sheet or MAR corresponds exactly with the prescriber's written order and with the label on the client's medicine container. Do not decipher illegible orders or make assumptions.

Do not accept incomplete orders. Nonstandard abbreviations and symbols should not be used.

4. Make a habit of reading the medication container label and comparing it with the MAR at least three times: first, when removing the drug from the supply drawer or medication cart; second, when placing the medication in a soufflé cup, ounce cup, or syringe; and third, just before administering it to the client, before the container is discarded. Never give a medication from an unlabeled container or one that has an illegible label.
5. Look up information on all new or unfamiliar drugs before administering them. When administering a drug for the first time, read the package insert carefully for specific instructions.
6. If you must calculate the client's dose from the preparation on hand and you are uncertain of the calculation, verify your work on paper by having another responsible person (instructor, another nurse, or pharmacist) check it. In some hospitals, a second nurse routinely verifies certain drug doses (e.g., insulin). It is highly unusual for more than two units (e.g., tablets, vials) of a single drug to be administered in a single dose. Therefore, double check a calculation whenever the result calls for three or more units of a drug to make a dose.
7. Measure ordered quantities using proper equipment: graduated containers for milliliters or fluidounces and the manufacturers' droppers that are packaged with medications to be administered in drops. When measuring liquids, hold the container so that the line indicating the desired quantity is at eye level. Read the quantity when the lowest part of the concave surface of the fluid (meniscus) is on this line.
8. Handle dosage forms such as tablets, capsules, and pills so that the fingers do not come into contact with the medication. Use the cap of the container to place the medication into the container you will be taking to the client's bedside. Administer the medication with 8 ounces of water.
9. Avoid wasting medications; doing so tends to be expensive. In some instances, a single capsule may cost the client several dollars. Dropping medication on the floor is one way of being wasteful. When preparing medications, work over a clean and dry counter surface.
10. When pouring liquid medications, hold the bottle so the liquid does not run over the side and obscure the label. This is known as "palming the label." Wipe the rim of the bottle with a clean piece of paper tissue before replacing the stopper or cover.
11. Always prepare an intravenous (IV) admixture before labeling the container, and verify the dose on the emptied additive container when labeling the IV container.
12. When preparing an injection, always label the syringe immediately. Keep the vial with the syringe, and do not rely on memory to determine what solution is in which syringe.

13. *Never* administer a medication prepared by another person. In doing so, you accept the responsibility for accuracy, dose, correct medication, and so forth. If the person who prepared the medication made an error, you are accountable for any harm done to the client.

14. Positively identify the client by comparing the wristband and the name on the MAR, as well as any secondary information required by agency policy, such as date of birth.

15. If the client expresses doubt or concern about a medication or its dose, recheck to make certain there is no error; do this *before* administering the medication. You may need to recheck the order, the medication label, or the client's chart.

16. *Remain with the client until the medication has been taken.* Most clients are very cooperative about taking medications when the nurse brings them. However, some clients are more ill than they appear, and have been known to hoard medications until they have accumulated a lethal amount, which is then taken with fatal results. In some instances, clients have a prescriber's order allowing them to keep certain medications (e.g., nitroglycerin and antacids) at the bedside and take them as necessary.

17. If the client is receiving the first dose of an IV medication, especially an antibiotic, stay with the client for at least 5 minutes and monitor closely for adverse effects.

18. Do not leave a medication tray or cart unattended. If you are in a client's room and must leave, take the medications with you. Similarly, do not leave the medication cart unattended in the hall; either lock the cart in the hall or take it into the client's room with you.

19. Record the administration of each dose on the MAR as soon as possible. Never chart a medication as being given until it has been administered. Nursing students should check the MAR or computerized medication sheet before giving a medication. MARs should list all medications, including as required for pain (PRN), one-time-only, and special medications (e.g., heparin) in one place so the nurse can consider incompatibilities and/or duplication of similar drugs. Note the drug name, dosage, time, and route of administration on the medication record. Include the injection site when recording parenteral medications. Record the client's response to the medication, both adverse and intended, in the progress notes or nursing notes.

20. Develop a comprehensive approach to overseeing a client's medication therapy. Obtain a complete and accurate medication history from each client; reconcile the client's medication list, and monitor the client for anticipated and unanticipated responses to medications.

21. Within an institutional setting, return any unused medication to the pharmacy. Institutional policy and, in some states, the law requires the unused portion to be credited to the client's account. If the medication can be used for another client, the pharmacy will verify that it has been stored correctly and relabel it. Borrowing medications from one client's supply for another client is inappropriate and leads to dosing errors. Only medications issued by the pharmacy and labeled for a specific client should be used for that client, except in the case of a stock medication kept on the nursing unit. If the facility has a unit dose system, unpackaged or "loose" medications are never administered. Medications brought into the hospital by a client should be sent back home with a family member or, if they are to be used in the institutional setting, they should be sent to the hospital pharmacy to be verified and relabeled per agency policy.

Reporting Errors

Despite sincere efforts to administer medications safely, errors do happen. Box 4-1 outlines actual examples of errors related to medication administration. Note that these errors, when taken as a group, include prescriber errors, system-induced errors, and nurse errors.

Regardless of the originating point of the error, however, the nurse administering the medication is the last link in the chain to maintain client safety. What does one do when that link breaks, and an error is suspected? The first step in a suspected medication error is to take action to safeguard the client. Stop and backtrack, double-checking all actions or computations to see if an error occurred. If an error has occurred, it is critically important to be accountable for the error following a series of generally accepted steps. Notify the nursing instructor and/or supervising nurse for appropriate guidance and objective support. Assess the client for untoward effects of the drug at the time the error is discovered and notify the prescriber. Take any corrective action ordered and continue to monitor the client frequently until the client's health status is stable. Document the medication administered, the client's status, and the corrective actions taken factually in the progress notes section of the client's medical record. The client and family also should be informed. If intentional concealment occurs, the client could be awarded punitive damages, because intentional acts are not covered by malpractice insurance.

The final documentation of the error occurs when completing an agency-specific form called a patient safety report or incident report. The form used depends on agency policy and the nature of the report. A patient safety report is usually anonymous but needs to be thoroughly completed so that the "root cause" of a problem leading to an error can be identified. If an incident report is used, it is also important to fill out this form completely and factually, agency risk management personnel use it to develop procedures for preventing similar or identical incidents in the future. Do not write in the medical record that an incident report was completed and do not place a copy in the client record; the factual information already charted is sufficient. Incident

BOX 4-1 ERRORS RELATED TO MEDICATION ADMINISTRATION

- *Not knowing why a medication is to be administered.* This type of error caused one nurse to irrigate a client's bladder with a topical astringent-antiinflammatory agent (Burow solution) instead of with a genitourinary antibiotic irrigant distributed by a manufacturer of a similar name. In another instance, a nurse delayed giving a dose of medication essential to recuperation after cancer chemotherapy because she believed it to be "just a vitamin" instead of folinic acid.
- *Not identifying clients by their wristbands.* This type of error caused several nurses to give medication to the wrong individual in the right beds. One nurse even asked a client his name, which turned out to be similar to that of another client. One nurse called out her client's name, and the wrong person responded. The result was the same—all of the clients received the wrong medication.
- *Not checking with the prescriber.* This type of error caused one nurse to give her client 30 mL of milk of magnesia every hour rather than every night because she misinterpreted the "qn" (an unacceptable abbreviation) for "qh." Another nurse gave 2.5 mg of digoxin instead of 0.25 mg; the order was wrong, but the nurse did not recognize that it was excessive. As a result, the client received a toxic dose of medication.

- *Storing vials with a similar appearance in the same area.* Because of this type of error, the nurse gave a neuromuscular blocker instead of the flu vaccine. The nurse admitted to not reading the label (Cohen, 1996).
- *Poor handwriting.* Because of this type of error, a nurse administered Ritalin (methylphenidate) sent by the pharmacy instead of ritodrine (Yutopar). Neither the pharmacist nor the nurse questioned why the client would be receiving a central nervous system stimulant during her sixth month of pregnancy (Cohen, 1997b).
- *Not investigating a questionable dose.* A client's daughter questioned an insulin dose of 60 units, but the nurse did not investigate. The correct dose was 6 units; the client died from receiving the 60 units (Cohen, 1997a).
- *Knowledge and performance deficits.* Three Colorado nurses were indicted on charges of negligent homicide in a drug error that resulted in the death of a neonate. Knowledge deficits (not being familiar with the drug) and performance deficits (fatigue, use of a complex technique, and being interrupted while preparing medications) were considered to be the cause of the error (Smetzer, 1998).

reports are tools used by an agency to monitor for safety issues and agency practices that could result in legal exposure. Expect the incident to be investigated by the nurse manager and possibly others. It is important to cooperate fully in this process, even if it is uncomfortable, so that client safety and protection always remains first priority.

Summary

Medication error is one subgroup of the larger category of medical error. The number of medication errors that occur annually in the United States continues to be alarming. National groups such as the IOM, the ISMP, the JCAHO, and the AHRQ have recognized the scope of the problem and have provided recommendations to reduce the error rate in the United States. Many of the recommendations are aimed at the national and institutional levels. However, the nurse

is often the last link in the medication administration chain, so the role of the nurse in preventing medication errors cannot be underestimated.

⊛ Critical Thinking Questions

- Think about a recent experience in giving medications to an assigned client. What systems were in place that really worked well in preventing medication error? Were there any potential pitfalls in the system?
- How can physicians, nurses, and pharmacists work more effectively together in health care institutions to reduce the risk of medication error?
- How would you react if you made a medication error? What is the first thing you would do? What other priorities are important to address?

e-LEARNING SUPPLEMENTS

Student CD-ROM
- Final Exam questions
- NCLEX® Examination review questions
- Pharmacology animations
- Printable chapter summary

Evolve Website (http://evolve.elsevier.com/mckenry)
- Content updates, including information on new drugs
- WebLinks corresponding to this chapter
- Answers to the critical thinking questions in this chapter
- *Elsevier ePharmacology Update* newsletter
- *Mosby's Drug Consult* Internet Edition
- Supplemental and reference information

Bibliography

Berger, R., & Kichak, J. (2004). Computerized physician order entry: Helpful or harmful? *Journal of the American Medical Informatics Association, 11*(2), 100-103.

Beyea, S. (2004a). Best practices for abbreviation use. *AORN Journal, 79*(3), 641-642.

Beyea, S. (2004b). Creating a just safety culture. *AORN Journal, 79*(2), 412-414.

Caprioti, T. (2004). Basic concepts to prevent medication calculation errors. *Dermatology Nursing, 16(3),* 245-248.

Cavanaugh, M., & Vernarec, E. (2001). New regulations focus on medical errors. *RN, 64*(4), 71-72, 74.

Christianson, D. (2004). Medication management: Saving lives one order at a time. *Nursing Management, 35*(5), 16.

Clancy, T. (2004). Medication error prevention: Progress of initiatives. *JONA's Healthcare Law, Ethics Regulations, 6*(1), 3-12.

Cohen, M.R. (1996). Medication errors. *Nursing, 26*(2), 16.

Cohen, M.R. (1997a). Medication errors. *Nursing, 27*(4), 18.

Cohen, M.R. (1997b). Medication errors. *Nursing, 27*(9), 22.

Hall, L., Doran, D., & Pink, G. (2004). Nurse staffing models, nursing hours, and patient safety outcomes. *Journal of Nursing Administration, 34*(1), 41-45.

Henneman, E., & Gawlinski, A. (2004). A "near miss" model for describing the nurse's role in the recovery of medical errors. *Journal of Professional Nursing, 20*(3), 196-201.

Institute of Medicine. (2002). *Priority areas for national attention: Transforming health care quality.* Washington, DC: National Academy Press.

Institute of Medicine. (2001). *Crossing the quality chasm.* Washington, DC: National Academy Press.

Institute of Medicine. (1999). *To err is human: Building a safer health care system.* Washington, DC: National Academy Press.

Institute of Safe Medication Practices. (2002). White paper. *Bar coding of unit doses can reduce medication errors.* Huntington Valley, PA: Author.

Kucukarslan, S., et al. (2003). Pharmacists on rounding teams reduce preventable adverse drug events in hospital general medicine units. *Archives of Internal Medicine, 163*(17), 2014-2018.

Lykowski, G., & Mahoney, D. (2004). Computerized provider order entry improves workflow and outcomes. *Nursing Management, 35*(Suppl 2), 40G-40H.

Roark, D. (2004). Bar codes and drug administration: Can new technology reduce the number of medication errors? *American Journal of Nursing, 104*(1), 63-66.

Rudman, W., Brown, C., Hewitt, C., Carpenter, W., Campbell, B., Tubb, T., et al. (2002). The use of data mining tools in identifying medication error near misses and adverse drug events. *Topics in Healthcare Information Management, 23*(2), 94-103.

Smetzer, J.L. (1998). Lesson from Colorado: Beyond blaming individuals. *Nursing Management, 29*(6), 49-51.

Teich, J., Merchia, P., Schmiz, J., Kuperman, J., Spurr, C., & Bates, D. (2000). Effects of computerized physician order entry on prescribing practices. *Archives in Internal Medicine,* 160(8), 2741-2747.

THE NURSING PROCESS AND PHARMACOLOGY

CHAPTER FOCUS

Whether contact with clients occurs in the home, ambulatory care setting, extended care facility, or hospital, the nurse uses the nursing process to work with clients in relation to drug therapy. When its five components—assessment, nursing diagnosis, planning, implementation, and evaluation—are applied to drug therapy, the nurse develops a systematic and organized approach to handling the wealth of data about clients and their drugs. This chapter focuses on the nursing management of drug therapy utilizing the nursing process.

LEARNING OBJECTIVES

- Obtain an accurate and thorough drug history from a client.
- Articulate the components and types of drug orders essential for safe, effective drug administration.
- Assess contraindications to the administration of a drug and take appropriate action.
- Identify the variables influencing drug interactions, and common drug interactions and incompatibilities.
- Describe the clinical assessments needed by a client requiring drug therapy.
- Use the nursing process step of analysis to identify common nursing diagnoses for a client receiving drug therapy.
- Explain how to write appropriate outcome criteria for clients that relate to drug therapy.
- Identify common pharmaceutical preparations and dosage forms.
- Identify nursing activities related to proper drug storage and distribution.
- Describe the factors considered in establishing the dose, dosing intervals, and scheduling of medication.
- Differentiate between systemic effects and local effects of medications.
- Cite the advantages and disadvantages of the various routes of medication administration.
- Implement appropriate monitoring, nursing intervention, and client education about drug therapy.
- Evaluate the effectiveness of a client's drug therapy in progress toward outcomes and response to therapy.

▲ KEY TERMS

When applied to drug therapy, the **nursing process** provides the nurse with a systematic observational and problem-solving technique to collaborate with the client on appropriate medication-related interventions and to evaluate the effectiveness of these interventions. It provides direction for rational nursing actions to prevent and manage problems related to drug therapies. Its process and phases are analogous to scientific and problem-solving methods. Figure 5-1 diagrams these phases or steps. It should be kept in mind that the steps of the nursing process have an ongoing, cyclic nature—no step should be considered complete or static.

✸ **How will the nursing process be used in this text?**
- **Assessment,** which culminates in nursing diagnoses and collaborative problems includes:
  Client history for health practices and preexisting conditions
  Assessment of the prescription and concurrent drug therapy
  Baseline clinical assessment for monitoring future therapeutic and nontherapeutic drug responses
- **Planning,** which results in goals and outcome criteria for the client's drug therapy

- **Implementation** of nursing activities related to the drug regimen
  Ongoing monitoring of client response to drug therapy
  Specific interventions for safe and effective administration of drug therapy
  Client education for effective management of the therapeutic regimen
- **Evaluation,** which assesses the client's progress toward treatment goals and response to therapy

Assessment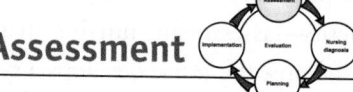

The assessment phase of the nursing process is both the first phase and a continuous processing of client-related data. During assessment of data, all the data relating to clients and their drug therapy are collected and organized so the nurse can begin to make inferences about the client's drug therapy. These data form the basis for developing nursing diagnoses and/or collaborative problems.

The client's status and the assessment data derived from a variety of sources will constantly change. As a result, the nursing diagnostic statements also will change. In collaboration with the prescriber, these changes may result in revision of the treatment plan, such as drug deletions, additions, or dosage changes.

Nurses must have a sound base of knowledge about a client's health issues and the drugs being administered, and the skill to use references to answer questions that arise. The ability to ask questions and seek answers about the data collected will form a solid foundation for the planning, implementation, and evaluation phases of the nursing process.

Assessment of the Client

Client data are collected through subjective and objective observations. In addition to observing clients and their environment, other sources of data are the interactions of clients with others and notes from the history and physical examination sections of the clinical record. At the initial interview the client's health care provider notes the past health history and performs a physical examination to assess the client's current health status. The resulting prioritized problem list helps to direct the therapeutic approach of the

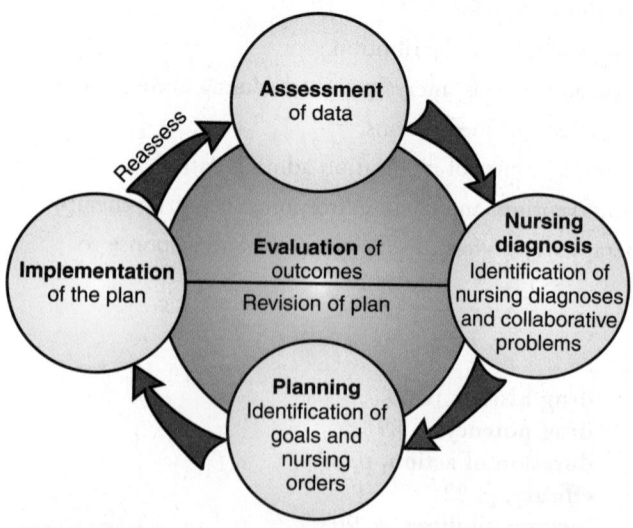

FIGURE 5-1 The nursing process.

health care team. The client's history and physical examination is reviewed by the nurse for relevant data in assessing the appropriateness of the planned drug therapy. Additionally, the nurse's clinical assessment, including reviewing laboratory data, develops a baseline for the future monitoring of the client for therapeutic and nontherapeutic responses to drug therapy. To develop a safe and effective drug regimen, a complete drug history should be obtained.

✳ Why is it important to obtain a thorough drug history from a client?

Obtaining a drug history, the process of gathering information that is relevant to the management of a client's medication regimen, is essential for planning nursing interventions and client education. Obtaining a comprehensive drug history requires a combination of nursing knowledge, interviewing skills, and a review of specific drug reference resources whenever necessary. A drug history should explore the client's general and specific health history, use of medications (e.g., prescription, over-the-counter [OTC] medications, self-treatment with complementary/alternative therapy) and specific behavioral factors (see Chapter 6) that influence individual drug therapies. A nurse should give particular attention to other substances the client may be taking, such as home remedies, OTC medications, and recreational drugs. Glover, Rybeck, and Tracy (2004) determined that 97% of their study participants took one OTC drug and that 59% took more than four. The client's readiness and ability to provide information is assessed. The purpose of a drug history is explained so the client understands why some questions may sound personal. Figure 5-2 shows a sample drug history form.

A thorough drug history can provide extremely useful information for the entire health care team. For example, it can do the following:

- Provide information crucial to prevent drug interactions, allergies, or adverse effects
- Identify the risk for drug-drug and drug-food interactions
- Provide clues about unreported chronic disorders
- Help interpret laboratory tests reliably
- Reveal learning needs or concerns regarding the client's effective management of a therapeutic regimen

When obtaining a drug history, it is important to communicate at the level of understanding appropriate for the client. Medical terms may be confusing to many people; therefore the nurse should be familiar with local observances and, when applicable, ethnic or cultural terms for specific diseases, illnesses, symptoms, and other information. The client's own words are used if appropriate. Rapport must be established if the transfer of relevant information is to be made freely.

Open-ended questioning is preferred to direct "yes" or "no" questions during the interview. For example, in obtaining information about a client's use of analgesics, a "yes" or "no" question would be "Do you take analgesics? If 'yes,' name them." If the person is unsure of the meaning of the term analgesic, a "no" answer might be the natural response.

The more descriptive information the nurse is seeking may be elicited if the question is reworded to ask "What do you take when you have pain, such as a headache, backache, muscle sprain, or other type of ache or pain?" Reminders must often accompany questions concerning OTC drugs; commonly used product names or currently advertised brands may be suggested to jog the memory of the client. For example, aspirin is an ingredient in hundreds of OTC preparations, therefore simply asking the client about aspirin consumption may limit the answer to only products labeled as aspirin. Suggesting trade name products, such as Anacin, Bufferin, or Alka-Seltzer, increases the possibility of obtaining a more thorough drug history.

If the interview is performed in the client's residence, the nurse may ask to see the medications. In an ambulatory care setting, clients may be asked to bring all of their medications into the office for review. Many individuals, especially older adults, forget to report all the medications they have on hand for self-medicating purposes. The storage place for medications should be noted; this information may be important if a potentially hazardous site is used. Areas of heat and moisture are not recommended as proper storage areas for most drugs, so storage in a bathroom cabinet or over a kitchen sink or stove may adversely affect many medications. Unless they are to be refrigerated, almost all medications are to be stored below 40° C (104° F), preferably between 15° C and 30° C (59° F and 86° F), and are to be protected from freezing.

Evaluating the client's knowledge about the proper disposal of drugs (see the Medication Safety Alert box on p. 71), the ability to read the print and the language and understand the terms and instructions on the medication labels, and the ability to locate expiration dates is part of assessing the individual's ability to store and consume medications safely. Studies have indicated that many persons (from one third to one half of various older adult populations) cannot read or do not understand drug package labels. This high incidence prompted the FDA to regulate labels for OTC drugs requiring larger print and clearer instructions in 1999. But the issue of "label literacy" clearly indicates an area of concern that requires nursing assessment. See Chapter 11 and Figure 11-1 for further discussion.

Information should also be obtained regarding the client's general lifestyle, dietary patterns, consumption of alcohol, use of caffeine-containing products, and smoking habits. All of these factors may affect or modify a typical drug response.

Preexisting Health Conditions In the assessment phase of the nursing process, it is essential to discover any health status issues that might influence the appropriateness of the medication or the dosage of the drug prescribed for the client such as gender, body size, age, childbearing, and breastfeeding status. Preexisting health conditions should be ascertained to assess for contraindications to the drug—conditions that would preclude the administration of a drug or any condition that would require special monitoring or care. Examples of contraindications include a drug with a Pregnancy Category X

DRUG HISTORY

Client's name _____ Date of interview _____

Mailing address: _____

DOB: _____ Height: _____ Weight: _____ BP: _____ HR: _____

Occupation _____ Physician(s) or other provider(s) _____

Gender: _____ Pregnancy Status: _____

Allergies (drug/food) _____ Reactions: _____
_____

Medical diagnosis and relevant past medical history:

Current prescribed medications; include name, strength, daily dosage, start date, purpose, and therapeutic/nontherapeutic responses: (Note client's knowledge about medications and the need for teaching.)

Prescription medications taken during the previous 3 months other than ones mentioned above:

Have you used a nonprescription (over-the-counter medication or complementary/alternative medication) for:

_____ headache	_____ eye/ear problems	_____ heartburn/GI upset/gas
_____ muscle/joint pain	_____ constipation	_____ rash/itching
_____ cough	_____ diarrhea	_____ vitamins
_____ colds/flu	_____ hemorrhoids	_____ herbal products
_____ sinus problems	_____ insomnia	_____ organic products
_____ allergy	_____ drowsiness	_____ other:

What nonprescription (other over-the-counter medications, herbal remedies, or health food products) do you take for the symptoms above? (Obtain complete listing and daily consumption.)

Do you use any salt substitutes? (Obtain brand name; Morton Lite Salt, CoSalt, etc.)

Do you use any food supplements? Name and quantity per day:

Close family members with drug allergies (relationship, drug, and reaction):

Lifestyle issues:
Caffeine Intake
_____ Never consumed
_____ Drinks per day
_____ Stopped _____ year(s) ago

Nicotine Use
_____ Never smoked
_____ Packs per day for _____ years
_____ Stopped _____ year(s) ago

Alcohol Consumption
_____ Never consumed
_____ Drinks per day
_____ Stopped _____ year(s) ago

Dietary Patterns:
_____ Meals a day
_____ Food restrictions: _____

Nurse _____

FIGURE 5-2 Sample drug history.

rating in a pregnant woman, use of penicillin in a client with a known history of anaphylaxis to penicillins, and use of a vasoconstrictive agent for migraine headache in a client with coronary artery disease. In each case, administering the drug would have a high potential for harm (e.g., birth defect, anaphylaxis, or myocardial infarction, respectively). Determine each medication's clinical indications and potential efficacy and any contraindications, especially any allergy or pathologic condition, such as renal, cardiac, or hepatic function impairment that would preclude its administration.

The client's allergy history, even if unrelated to the medication, must be explored to rule out and prevent any possible allergic reaction. Box 5-1 summarizes the medications often implicated in allergic reactions. The occurrence of drug allergy reactions is extremely individualized, unpredictable except for history, and not usually closely dose-related. The reaction may result in a very serious and life-threatening situation; consequently the drug must not be given. Reactions may vary from mild rash to severe exfoliative dermatitis and from asthma to anaphylactic shock.

Medication Safety Alert

How Do I Dispose of Unused Prescription and OTC Drugs?

Proper drug disposal is an emerging issue with the environment. Usually a household has the option of placing waste medicines in the trash or flushing them down the toilet. In the past, advice has been to flush the drugs down the toilet rather than risk the inadvertent access by children or pets if the drugs were placed in the trash. Once flushed, all medications have the potential to be transported into sewage systems. Even with septic systems, medicines can harm the beneficial bacteria that are responsible for breaking down waste. The major concerns to date have been the pathogen resistance to antibiotics and the disruption of endocrine systems of aquatic life and possibly humans, by hormones because many medications are not captured or are only partially captured by a wastewater treatment plant (WWTP). High risk agents (e.g., some cancer chemotherapy) may require special precautions in handling. In these cases, the pharmaceutical manufacturer may provide Material Safety Data Sheets (MSDS), which identify risk, handling precautions, and disposal information.

The options are to ask the pharmacy that sold the drug to dispose of it; but many pharmacies are unwilling do this. Second, ask if the community has a community household hazardous waste (HHW) collection program, the recommended option. Lacking this preferred option, placement in the garbage with transport to a landfill is a practical solution. In either case, keep the drugs in their original container because the label may contain safety information and the caps are typically watertight and childproof. Add a small amount of water or liquid glue to the solid drug and flour or kitty litter to liquid drugs before recapping to discourage any unintended use of the drug. Double enclose the contained drugs in a bag to prevent immediate identification of the drug container or to help prevent breakage of glass containers (Michigan Department of Environmental Quality, 2004).

BOX 5-1 MEDICATIONS COMMONLY IMPLICATED IN HYPERSENSITIVITY REACTIONS*

ANTIMICROBIALS

abacavir	**penicillins**
amphotericin B	protease inhibitors
cephalosporins	rifampin
erythromycin	**sulfa drugs**
fluoroquinolones	tetracyclines
neomycin	trimethoprim
nitrofurantoin	vancomycin

OTHER DRUGS

acetaminophen	gold salts
allopurinol	**histamine**
angiotensin converting enzyme inhibitors (ACE inhibitors)	**iron dextran**
	lamotrigine
angiotensin receptor blockers (ARBs)	local anesthetics
	nonsteroidal antiinflammatory drugs (NSAIDS)
aspirin (ASA)	phenytoin
atenolol	quinidine/quinine
carbamazepine	thiazide diuretics
clomipramine	

DIAGNOSTIC AGENTS

dehydrocholic acid	iodinated contrast dyes

BIOLOGICALS

adrenocorticotropic hormone (ACTH)	insulin
	monoclonal antibodies
antitoxins	**vaccines**
gamma globulin	

*Items marked in **bold** may be at higher risk. Serious hypersensitivity reactions can occur with most drugs. Lack of inclusion on this list does not necessarily indicate a low risk for hypersensitivity reactions.

They may include urticaria, angioneurotic edema, and drug fever (see Chapter 3).

It is essential to place alerting stickers or notations regarding the client's allergic history in the clinical record, computerized information system, Kardex, or other places according to agency policy. These locations need to be checked before any medications are given. Records may denote "no known drug allergies" (NKDA), but a correlation often exists between one allergic response and the development of another; therefore the client's description of any past allergic manifestations—to drugs, inhalants, foods (typically eggs, orange juice, chocolate, shellfish, or strawberries), or whatever—must be clarified and evaluated. Often the client erroneously defines an unexpected response as an allergic one. For example, the nausea that occurs following a meperidine (Demerol) injection may be labeled an allergic reaction by the client, when in actuality it is likely to be only a normal, if exaggerated, adverse effect. Correcting such misinformation with the client and in the records may be important because it makes that drug available for therapy when necessary. Before any questionable medications are administered, nurses should specifically inquire about previous experiences with these agents and, if necessary for a client who has many allergies, discuss with the prescriber the need for a test dose. Special methods for those who must take a medication to which they are allergic (e.g., aspirin, local anesthetics, or contrast media in diagnostic agents) include pretreatment medications in the form of antihistamines, prednisone, and ephedrine or cautiously increasing dosages of the allergy-provoking drug under super-

BOX 5-2 ALLERGIC REACTIONS TO FOOD ADDITIVES

Allergic reactions have been reported after the ingestion of food additives such as monosodium glutamate (MSG), tartrazine, and sulfites. Tartrazine and sulfites are also used as additives, preservatives, and antioxidants in various medications. The most serious adverse effect has occurred most often in clients who are asthmatic and has resulted in some reported deaths. Current lists of foods and drug products containing tartrazine and sulfites should be reviewed in assessing reported allergic reactions.

vision. Clients may also have allergies to the additives found in foods and drug products (Box 5-2).

Other contraindications to drug therapy must be assessed before administration. Clients may have medical problems that contraindicate a given drug or, if the drug is deemed necessary, that require careful consideration of the risk benefit ratio and careful monitoring of the client. Occasionally contraindications to drugs are differentiated into *absolute* contraindications (never use), or *relative* contraindications (use limited to circumstances in which benefit clearly outweighs risk and very careful monitoring is required). For example, opioid analgesics are *absolutely* contraindicated in clients with acute respiratory depression who do not have respiratory support, because the respiratory depressive effects of the drug would exacerbate the condition. Most drugs, including opioid analgesics, are *relatively* contraindicated for clients with hepatic or renal impairment. For such clients, they may be administered with caution and probably with dosage modifications that account for the degree of drug metabolism in the liver and/or excretion by the kidneys. As part of the assessment, note should be taken of the client's serum creatinine as an indicator of renal function and the serum bilirubin, alkaline phosphatase (ALP), alanine aminotransferase (ALT), aspartate aminotransferase (AST), lactate dehydrogenase (LDH) or a prothrombin time (PT) as indicators of hepatic function. If these values are not within the normal range, adjustments in the client's drug dosage might need to be made from the "normal" dosage, with either the dosage or the frequency of the doses decreased. It is essential to assess for and plan the pharmacologic therapeutic regimen to minimize the adverse effects and provide for client safety.

Assessment of the Drug (Prescription and Concurrent Drug Therapy)

The Prescription Drug data include information derived from a prescriber's orders or prescription and nursing knowledge about the pharmacokinetics and pharmacodynamics of the prescribed drug. The characteristics of the drugs administered and the manner in which the prescriber orders them to be administered have an impact on the client's nursing care.

"Medicating" a client begins when the medication is suggested and authorized by a legally sanctioned prescriber, usually a licensed physician or dentist. In many states nurse practitioners, pharmacists, or physician assistants are given this function legally within specified limitations. Practicing nurses should be aware of and follow the limitations outlined in the state nurse practice act for the state in which they practice.

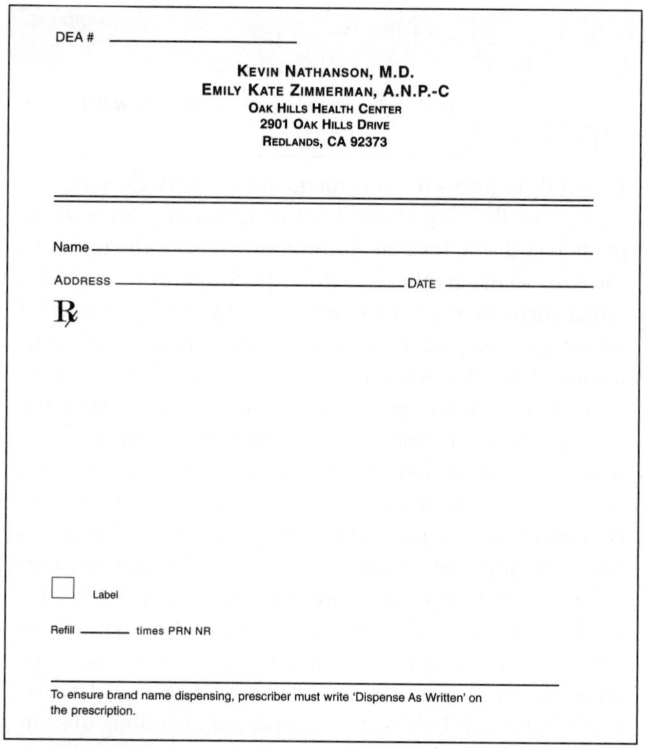
DEA # ______

KEVIN NATHANSON, M.D.
EMILY KATE ZIMMERMAN, A.N.P.-C
OAK HILLS HEALTH CENTER
2901 OAK HILLS DRIVE
REDLANDS, CA 92373

Name ______

ADDRESS ______ DATE ______

℞

☐ Label

Refill ______ times PRN NR

To ensure brand name dispensing, prescriber must write 'Dispense As Written' on the prescription.

FIGURE 5-3 Example of a prescription pad order form.

The prescriber's orders are meant for the individual who dispenses the medication. There are two different formats: the prescription blank and the order sheet. The prescription blank is given to clients in an ambulatory care setting or on discharge from the health care agency and is to be filled by a community pharmacist; it may look similar to the one shown in Figure 5-3. For clients in an institutional setting, the order is entered into a computerized clinical record or written on an order sheet found in the client's chart (Figure 5-4). It is filled by the pharmacy within the institution or contracted for by the institution and sent to the medication area on the client's unit for access by the nurse administering medications for the client. Many health care settings have computerized the process of ordering medications for clients, but the principles remain the same, with the computer printouts often resembling the former noncomputerized hospital stationery for medication administration.

The prescriber's order has seven elements that should be present and identifiable. These elements and the associated Six Rights of Medication Administration are in Table 5-1 and are also discussed in Chapter 2. All parts of the order should be legible and clearly expressed. If there is any question about the order or the prescription, *the prescriber who wrote the order or prescription must be contacted* to validate or clarify. Obviously, to administer a drug under questionable

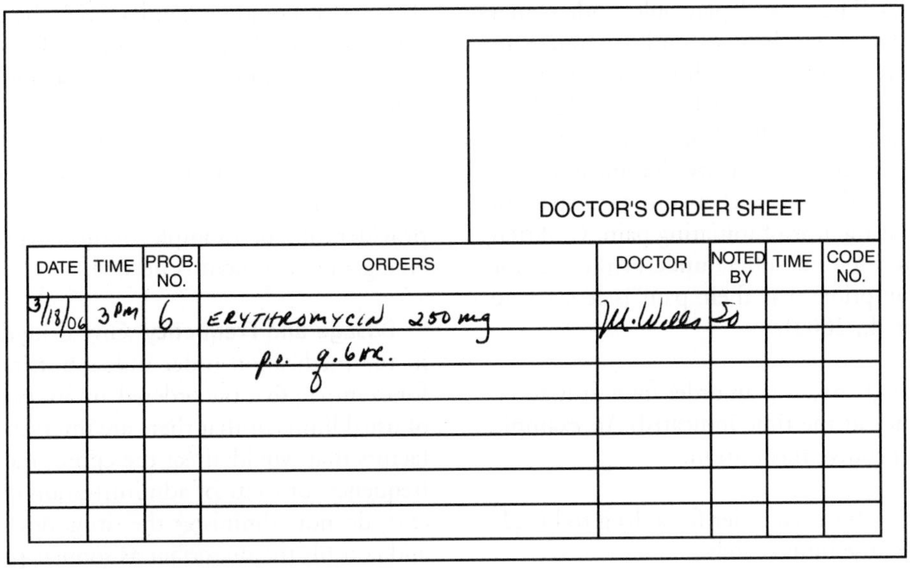

FIGURE 5-4 Example of an order sheet.

TABLE 5-1 ELEMENTS ESSENTIAL FOR MEDICATION ADMINISTRATION	
Six Rights of Medication Administration	Elements of Medication Order
Right client	Client's name Date order written
Right drug	Medication name
Right dose	Dosage
Right route	Route
Right time	Frequency
Right documentation	Prescriber signature

instructions is to risk harm to the client in an area with a high potential for error (see Chapter 4).

Safe nursing practice requires following approved procedures in the particular work environment and administering only drugs that are ordered in writing. Nursing students should be aware of special limitations imposed on their actions by the educational and/or clinical institution. In particular, they should be advised to follow only written orders. However, a verbal or telephoned order from a prescriber, often in response to the nurse's telephoned request, is sometimes unavoidable. When this occurs it is best for the nurse, not a student, to copy the order as it is being given, then verify it by repeating it back to the prescriber. Verbal or telephoned orders should be rare and involve circumstances of some urgency rather than convenience. Such orders must be clearly communicated and noted on the client's chart by the nurse. The prescriber must countersign the order, usually within 24 hours in most institutions, in order for it to be legal. Allowing the order to remain unsigned is careless and

negligent because it violates both the law and institutional policy. This allows a precarious period of nursing vulnerability to malpractice charges (see Chapter 2).

✱ What are the various types of drug orders?

Although clients in the community are free to medicate themselves with any accessible medication, usually neither the client nor the nurse may legally administer any medication without a written order once an individual is admitted to a clinical institution. The content of the prescriber's orders dictates the conditions under which the ordered drug may be administered. Several types of orders are described in the following sections.

Routine Order The most common type of order is the **routine order,** in which the drug is to be regularly administered as ordered until a formal discontinuation order is written or until a specified termination date is reached. Automatic termination or "automatic stops" may be explicit in agency policy. Automatic stop policies may be mandated for institutional accreditation or licensure requirements, or they may be applied variously by institutions. Such policies act as a stimulus to the prescriber to reevaluate the client's continued need for drugs that require especially close attention.

PRN Order An "as needed" order (**PRN order**) is an order for drugs to be administered according to client need. Within the other criteria specified by the order, the decision of when to medicate is left to the nurse's judgment. This type of order has implications for nursing autonomy similar to protocol orders.

Medications to reduce the perception of pain make up the bulk of PRN orders. Keen nursing assessments of pain are required to carry out these PRN orders appropriately. (See Chapter 14 for specifics for the evaluation of pain.) It is sufficient to note that pain is a very complex phenomenon that is influenced by factors of subjectivity, emotions, and age, among others. The most dependable guide is that the pain is what and when the client says it is; assumptions by the nurse are not as reliable. Research has demonstrated that clients are often undermedicated for pain (Glajchen, 2001; Winstein et al., 2000). A PRN order allows for the prophylactic use of pain medications by the nurse to prevent the onset of pain and to allow clients to participate in their therapies without the fear of initiating pain. Children in particular are often left to suffer, undermedicated for pain, under the assumption that their pain is less severe than it seems (Ellis et al., 2002).

Single Order A **single order** is an order for a drug to be administered only once at the time indicated. An example is an order for a preoperative medication.

Stat Order A **stat order** is an order for a drug to be administered as a single dose immediately.

Protocol A **protocol** is a set of criteria that serves as a directive under which medication may be given. Protocols may typically be one of two types: standing orders or flow-diagram protocols. Standing orders are officially accepted sets of orders (not only for medications) that are to be applied routinely by nurses in caring for clients with certain conditions or under certain circumstances (e.g., as part of admission orders in some critical care units). Flow-diagram protocols are criteria that give nurses guidelines for the administration of certain treatments and medications on the basis of client variables. Of all the types of orders, protocols provide the widest scope for the application of nursing judgment and decision making. Criteria and direction may be either very specific, for those with limited expertise or responsibility, or less specific and allow for greater latitude, self-reliance, and sophistication in decision making.

✳ **What components of the prescription need to be assessed?**

Client Every possible effort should be made to ensure that the client receives the intended medication in the manner planned by the prescriber. Toward this end, clients with similar names should be widely separated in the health care setting, and all their paperwork must be clearly distinguishable. Keep an identifying wristband on every client in an institutional setting and compare it with the identifying information that accompanies each dose of medication.

Date Check the date that a medication order was written against other information for accuracy or for confirmation of when the last dose is to be given.

Medication The name of the medication may be written in either generic or trade form. To prevent medical errors, many prescribers include both the generic and trade drug names, and may include the indication for use to assist the pharmacy in correctly interpreting and filling the prescription.

Clients should be familiar with the names of their medications. Tell clients the names of their drugs when the drugs are administered. Doing so begins the educational process so that clients may effectively manage their medication regimen at home. It is dangerous for clients not to know their medications. Exact names and dosages are crucial drug information for clients to provide to health care providers if, for example, multiple providers are used or emergency treatment is needed.

Dosage and Frequency Give drug dosages as prescribed in the medication order unless nursing judgment detects, for example, that the ordered amount falls outside the range of usual limits or that there are intervening individual client factors that would affect the appropriateness of the dosage, frequency, or route of administration of the drug. In such a case, do not administer the drug, document the omission, and consult the prescriber as soon as possible.

During the development of a drug, the manufacturer makes determinations regarding the optimal range of dosage, frequency, and effective route of administration for most people. These determinations are based on the known pharmacokinetics and pharmacodynamics of the drug. For example, a drug that routinely undergoes a slow biotransformation may remain in the body system longer and produce more prolonged effects than another drug. This type of drug may therefore be given effectively on a once-a-day basis; a drug that is excreted rapidly may need to be given every 4 hours around-the-clock if effective serum levels are to be maintained. Nursing judgments must be made to align an individual client's medication schedule with agency policy at appropriate intervals or to keep to a single schedule to meet a specific drug requirement (e.g., before or after meals) or a special need of the client. Reasons to individualize administration time include client convenience and the avoidance of disturbing the client's rest, sleep, meals, visiting hours, activities, or treatments. The rationale for other modifications in the therapeutic regimen should be discussed with the prescriber.

Route Every medication order should include a specified route for administration. Making assumptions in this area is negligent. The choice of the actual site of administration of injectables is a nursing or nurse-client decision. For example, subcutaneous, intramuscular (IM), and intravenous (IV) sites to avoid include any areas of obvious injury, disease, or lesions, even if minor; any areas that are noticeably erythematous (reddened), vesicular (blistered), open and weeping or pustular, ecchymotic (bruised), or scarred; and areas previously overused for injection. Such areas may have impaired circulation or may be adversely affected by the injection itself or by the material injected. Injection sites are rotated to avoid tissue damage from injections.

Assess the ordered route of administration routinely for efficacy, feasibility, or practicality. For example, the oral route would naturally be precluded for a client who is nauseated or vomiting. Obtain a change of drug order before administering a drug by a different route, because dosage or other factors may need to be readjusted if bioavailability is affected by such changes.

Concurrent Drug Therapy The complexity of modern pharmacotherapy is nowhere more obvious than in the ever-growing list of drugs that either interact nontherapeutically with one another, with foods, and with fluids or that distort laboratory test results. That these chemical substances interact with or potentiate one another is not surprising. Keep this fact in mind when medications appear either ineffective or harmful or when the accuracy of laboratory tests is crucial. Many prescribers, pharmacies, and agencies use automated systems to assist in the identification, interpretation of significance, and management of these interactions. The clinical pharmacist may be helpful in assisting the health care team in drug interaction management.

Drug-Drug and Drug-Food Interactions Some drugs commonly involved in clinically significant drug-drug interactions include antacids, warfarin (Coumadin), aspirin, tricyclic antidepressants (monoamine oxidase [MAO] inhibitors), aminoglycosides, amphetamines, corticosteroids, digoxin, diuretics, cimetidine (Tagamet), sulfonamides, alcohol, phenytoin (Dilantin), quinidine gluconate (Quinaglute Dura-Tabs), antihypertensives, β blockers, and theophylline (Elixophyllin). Interactions that are significant are ones that involve a drug with a narrow therapeutic index or if an interaction would constitute a change of at least 30% (Brater, 2004). Before giving any such medication, consult an appropriate source to assess the drug, its mechanism, and any other medications given concurrently to determine the probability of interactions. This text provides this information in the context of specific drug discussions.

Variables influencing drug interaction include pharmacokinetic mechanisms: absorption, distribution, metabolism, and excretion; pharmacodynamic mechanisms; and combined toxicity. With the following discussion of interactions, some of the classic drug interactions will be used as examples.

✳ **What pharmacokinetic mechanisms are involved in drug interactions?**

Absorption Gastrointestinal (GI) absorption of drugs may be affected by the concurrent use of other agents that (1) bind or chelate, (2) alter gastric pH, or (3) alter GI motility. A delay in the absorption rate of the drug is seldom clinically important, but a reduction in the extent of absorption will be clinically important if it results in subtherapeutic serum levels (Katzung, 2004).

Binding or Chelation Cholestyramine (Questran) and colestipol (Colestid), drugs indicated for hypercholesteremia, adsorb and combine with bile acids to form an insoluble complex that is excreted through the feces; this loss of bile acids lowers blood cholesterol levels. However, these drugs also adsorb other medications, as well as the fat-soluble vitamins A, D, E, and K; instead of being absorbed into the body, these substances are excreted from the body.

Many commonly used antimicrobials, including tetracyclines and fluoroquinolones, can form insoluble complexes in the GI tract if given at the same time as foods or drugs containing ions of calcium, aluminum, magnesium, or iron. Thus, avoid administering these medications with milk-based tube feedings, dairy products, antacids, minerals, or calcium supplements.

Milk, coffee, eggs, tea, whole-grain breads and cereals, dietary fiber, and foods containing bicarbonates, carbonates, phosphates, or oxalates may reduce iron absorption if given concurrently. Iron products should be ingested no sooner than 1 hour before or 2 hours after the mentioned food substances are given.

Drug interactions may also increase the extent of absorption. Approximately 10% of clients have bacteria in the gut that are able to metabolize digoxin, and thereby decrease the quantity available for absorption. If such a client is prescribed a broad spectrum antibiotic that eliminates many of these bacteria, then the bioavailability of digoxin increases and can lead to digoxin toxicity because of the drug's narrow therapeutic margin.

Alteration of Gastric pH The most common of these interactions, such as when a drug is taken with food or antacids, will delay the onset of drug action, not cause a decrease in total absorption or bioavailability (Brater, 2004).

Ascorbic acid from citrus fruits or juices enhances the absorption of iron. However, carbonated soft drinks or acid juices (fruit or vegetable) can cause drugs to dissolve more quickly in the stomach than in the intestine or can neutralize them, thereby changing the intended rate or completeness of absorption (Lowenthal & Parnetti, 1996).

Alteration of GI Motility Drugs that change gastric or intestinal motility can alter the digestion or absorption of other drugs and nutrients. Important drugs that affect these changes are GI prokinetic drugs, such as metoclopramide (Reglan) and stimulant cathartics, which increase bowel motility. At the other extreme are anticholinergics and opioids, which inhibit bowel motility. Some hormonal contraceptives impair the absorption of folic acid in undernourished clients.

Fatty foods and foods low in fiber delay stomach emptying by up to 2 hours, which may result in delayed and/or reduced drug absorption. Other medications, such as griseofulvin (Grisactin), exhibit enhanced bioavailability (absorption) following a high-fat meal.

Distribution Theoretically, competition for plasma protein binding sites may occur. For example, if a drug is avidly bound to serum proteins, a second drug might displace the first drug from these binding sites, leading sequentially to a dramatic elevation in the unbound and pharmacologically active drug concentration and an increased risk of adverse effects. However, it is now known that such interactions are usually of negligible clinical importance because of a concurrent rise in drug clearance as a result of the increased availability of the unbound drug (Brater, 2004). Clients with decreased renal function would be at higher risk for drug accumulation with any drug renally excreted.

Metabolism The MAO inhibitors prevent the biotransformation of tyramine, which is present in aged cheese, liver, overripe fruit, and preserved meat (e.g., sausage, bologna, pepperoni, salami) and may provoke a hypertensive crisis (a rapid and severe increase in blood pressure). Grapefruit juice inhibits the metabolism of carbamazepine (Tegretol), calcium channel blockers, "statins" for hyperlipidemias, and other drugs in the GI tract, which allows more of the drug to be absorbed. Higher carbamazepine levels can cause nausea, dizziness, tremor, and confusion. High levels of calcium channel blockers can lead to hypotension or cardiac dysrhythmias. High levels of the "statin" drugs can pose a risk for muscle injury, rhabdomyolysis, and renal failure. (*USP DI*, 2005).

Alteration of Enzymes Enzyme alterations, either induction or inhibition, may affect the metabolism of a food or drug and are the most frequently pharmacokinetic drug interactions observed in practice. An increased synthesis of cytochrome P450 isoenzymes by a drug is referred to as **induction**. The antiepileptic drug carbamazepine (Tegretol), for example, induces the biotransformation of other drugs by increasing the amount of isoenzymes that are specific for drug metabolism. In this process, carbamazepine is relatively unique in that it also induces its own metabolism. One of its metabolites is associated with increased central nervous system (CNS) toxicity. With certain other drugs, such as barbiturates, increased induction decreases the availability of the parent drug and other drugs as they are metabolized to inactive substances. In the example of barbiturates, this activity contributes to the development of drug tolerance.

Inhibition, in a sense the opposite of induction, is noted when one drug interferes with the normal metabolism of a second drug. This type of interaction is frequently noted for drugs that are metabolized by the same cytochrome P450 isoenzymes. Typically, two drugs compete for a unique enzyme system, and for one or both drugs, metabolism is reduced resulting in elevated levels. A common example includes administration of the azole antifungal fluconazole (Diflucan) to a client who is receiving the cholesterol-lowering drug atorvastatin (Lipitor). Fluconazole interferes with the P450 enzyme system that normally metabolizes atorvastatin, resulting in increased levels of atorvastatin. Such high levels of atorvastatin may result in muscle injury and rhabdomyolysis.

Alcohol Consumption It is important to elicit information about patterns of alcohol consumption when obtaining a history. Of the more than 100 most commonly prescribed drugs, more than half contain at least one ingredient known to interact adversely with imbibed alcohol. An interaction is probable if the drug is known to affect the CNS or is metabolized by the liver. The effects are dose-related, and the interactive effects are determined by how the alcohol is used—habitually, chronically, or only occasionally. Patterns of alcohol consumption are likely to affect the client's concurrence with drug treatment and follow through. Alcohol

consumption should be limited or completely avoided if a client is taking opioids, tranquilizers, sedatives, and other CNS depressant-type drugs, which may cause additive or synergistic respiratory and CNS depression.

The fact that many elixirs and tinctures are liquid formulations of drugs dissolved in alcohol is significant, especially in the assessment of pharmacotherapy for children, who are more at risk for the hypoglycemic effects of alcohol. Preparations with ethanol content must be reassessed and cannot be assumed to have the same rates and degrees of absorption as the same drugs in aqueous solution, because bioavailability may be altered.

Cigarette Smoking The main pharmacokinetic effect of heavy cigarette smoking is the lowering of drug plasma levels by the induction of microsomal enzyme systems responsible for increased drug metabolism or excretion. The rate of theophylline (Theo-24) breakdown is increased, necessitating an increase of 1.5 times to twice the average dose. The usual doses of other drugs have diminished effectiveness in the heavy cigarette smoker, such as with the antidepressant imipramine (Tofranil); analgesics such as pentazocine (Talwin) and propoxyphene (Darvon); vitamins C, B_{12}, and B_6; and the influenza vaccine. The absorption rate of insulin by the subcutaneous route is twice as slow as usual. Smoking also interacts with furosemide (Lasix) and propranolol (Inderal). Drowsiness and depression of the CNS are less common with diazepam (Valium), and drowsiness is reduced with chlorpromazine (Thorazine) with smoking. The risk of heart attack, stroke, and other circulatory disorders increases when smoking when combined with the use of estrogens.

Laboratory test results may also be somewhat outside the range of normal, depending on inhalation practices and the duration of smoking history. The white cell count is increased (in the absence of clinical infection); hemoglobin concentration, hematocrit, and red blood cell (RBC) size are increased; and clotting time is reduced. Some investigators of cigarette smoking have found an abnormal increase in cholesterol, and others have found carcinoembryonic antigen levels as high as those for persons with colon cancer, yet without other evidence of it. Therefore smokers sometimes can be expected to exhibit more numerous drug therapy "failures" or adverse effects, or they may even have fewer or different reactions to drugs than do nonsmoking clients. Certain laboratory test results must be interpreted in light of the client's history of smoking.

Caffeine Consumption Caffeinated beverages present a medical problem in that many people consume enough caffeine to produce substantial effects on a number of organ systems. Caffeine stimulates the CNS and cardiac muscle, and it acts on the kidney to produce diuresis. Individuals ingesting caffeine or caffeinated beverages usually experience less drowsiness and fatigue and more rapid and clearer flow of thought. As the dose is increased, however, signs of progressive CNS stimulation occur, including nervousness, anxiety, restlessness, insomnia, and tremors. Caffeine produces tachycardia and, in higher doses, dysrhythmias. Increases in blood pressure with caffeine ingestion are the result of an increase in systemic vascular resistance. Caffeine causes the secretion of both pepsin and gastric acid from the parietal cells of the stomach. The cardiac-stimulating effects of caffeine may inhibit the therapeutic effect of β-adrenergic blockers. Excessive CNS stimulation may occur with the concurrent use of caffeine and other CNS stimulants, progressing from nervousness to possibly seizures or cardiac dysrhythmias. Caffeine inhibits the absorption of calcium and promotes the excretion of lithium and other drugs. Caffeine may also produce severe hypertension when combined with MAO inhibitors. The normal metabolism of caffeine is significantly impaired with the use of the antimicrobial fluoroquinolones like ciprofloxacin (Cipro), necessitating caffeine restrictions while taking these agents.

Renal Excretion Because pH influences the ionization of weak acids and bases, changes in the pH of urine caused by drugs or food (making the urine overly acidic or alkaline) can have a significant effect on the excretion rates of some drugs. A drug in a nonionized state will diffuse more easily from the urine back into the blood, thereby prolonging drug action. For this reason, the action of acidic drugs is prolonged when urine is acidic. Although it is quite difficult to override the ability of the kidneys to regulate urine pH, an alkaline-ash or acid-ash diet, whether or not it is intentional, can drive urinary pH above 8 or below 5 and create a medium for potential drug reactions. The continued use of many antacid tablets each day in concert with quinidine administration has created quinidine intoxication by shifting urinary pH toward the alkaline levels and caused hearing loss or a dysrhythmia serious enough to require hospitalization. Probenecid (Benemid), an antigout medication, inhibits the renal clearance of penicillin because it inhibits the active renal tubular secretion of many weak organic acids, of which penicillin is one.

What pharmacodynamic mechanisms are involved in drug interactions?

Numerous examples exist of one drug intensifying or antagonizing the action of another drug at the receptor site. The nurse needs to consider drugs that have pharmacodynamic interactions. Pharmacodynamic interactions are caused by the concurrent administration of two drugs that have the opposite effect or similar effects. The interactions of drugs having similar effects (e.g., alcohol and sedatives, or drugs having hypotensive effects) may be easier to identify than the interactions of drugs having opposite effects. An example of such an interaction is a client with asthma who is being treated with a β-adrenergic drug such as albuterol (Proventil, Ventolin) for its bronchodilating effects while also being given a β-adrenergic blocking drug, which has bronchoconstricting properties, as an antihypertensive agent.

The natural extract of black licorice is chemically similar to that of aldosterone; therefore if taken in excess, licorice can cause hypokalemia, sodium, and water retention with resultant hypertension and alkalosis. The ingestion of large amounts of natural extract of black licorice is contraindicated for clients who are concurrently taking potassium-losing diuretics or for those who have cardiovascular disease.

Similarly, the consumption of large amounts of foods high in vitamin K (such as liver and green leafy vegetables) may reduce or antagonize the effectiveness of oral anticoagulants. Difficulty in maintaining the desired anticoagulant response with the appropriately prescribed dosages indicates the need for an assessment of food and drug consumption.

MAO inhibitors act by inhibiting the breakdown of norepinephrine, a vasopressor substance. The excess norepinephrine is stored in the neurons. Ingesting certain tyramine-containing foods (aged cheeses, beef and chicken liver, pickled herring, broad beans, canned figs, bananas, avocados, soy sauce, active yeast preparations, beer, sherry in large quantities, Chianti wine, chocolate, anchovies, caffeine, mushrooms, raisins, sausages, dried fish, tuna fish, cola drinks, and many fermented foods) may elevate the quantity of norepinephrine to toxic levels and precipitate a hypertensive crisis. OTC cold remedies containing ephedrine, phenylephrine, and phenylpropanolamine, and amphetamines in general can act similarly, releasing stored quantities of norepinephrine. The net effect may be a headache, a sudden climb in blood pressure to dangerous levels, cardiac dysrhythmias, or intracranial bleeding.

How does combination toxicity contribute to drug interactions?

The combined use of two or more drugs, each of which has toxic effects on the same organ, can greatly increase the likelihood of organ damage (Katzung, 2004). For example, concurrent administration of two hepatotoxic drugs can produce liver damage even though the dose of either drug alone may be insufficient to produce toxicity.

Not all drug interactions are dangerous; some are relatively insignificant or even beneficial. In the hospital setting, tables listing known harmful drug interactions are posted in the medication area as a reference for nurses. Most nurses practicing in the home setting carry drug handbooks that list significant drug interactions.

What baseline clinical assessment is required for drug therapy?

Baseline Assessment of the Condition for Which the Drug Has Been Prescribed Assessment of the client's condition for which the drug has been indicated allows the team to determine the drug's therapeutic effects. An example is a client presenting to the emergency department (ED) with an acute asthmatic attack who has a baseline assessment of cough, chest tightness, breathlessness, wheezing on auscultation, use of accessory muscles to breathe, pulse rate of 132 beats/min, respiratory rate of 38 breaths/min, peak expiratory flow rate (PEFR) of less than 25% of predicted and blood gases of Po_2 less than 60 mm Hg and Pco_2 greater than 40 mm Hg. If the β_2 agonist albuterol, a bronchodilator, is administered via nebulizer, and the drug is therapeutic, the client's cough will decrease in frequency and severity, the client's breathing effort will decrease (no evidence of the use of accessory muscles to breathe, client statement of decreased breathlessness and anxiety), respiratory rate of 24 breaths/min, pulse rate of 88 beats/min, and improved PEFR, and blood gases. The baseline assessment provides objective indicators by which to evaluate the drug's effectiveness.

Baseline Assessment of the Client's Health Status Relative to Potential Adverse Effects

The intent is to obtain an objective measure by which to evaluate whether the client is experiencing an adverse effect of a drug. For example, if an older client is prescribed an opioid analgesic, one of the most common adverse effects of the drug is constipation secondary to the drug's action of decreasing GI motility. As part of the client's baseline assessment, determine this client's normal bowel pattern to more effectively evaluate the opioid's adverse effect of constipation.

This baseline assessment should also include the results of various laboratory studies, if available. Renal and hepatic function impairment studies allow the nurse to anticipate if a client may experience issues with drug accumulation and toxicity. Also, if an adverse effect involves blood dyscrasias, a baseline complete blood count (CBC) will allow the nurse to determine hematologic adverse effects earlier. These assessments are as plentiful as drug adverse effects and unique to each client. With a sound background in drug knowledge, these assessments will become easier with experience.

✳ How is all of this assessment data processed?

When data from the nursing assessment have been collected, the next phase is analysis—the critical evaluation of information to determine its meaning and importance. It is the process of interpreting data based on sound pharmacologic and nursing principles. As with all phases of the nursing process, analysis is continuous.

The nurse may follow several steps to facilitate analysis. Initially, data are organized into categories. These data include the client's history of preexisting health conditions and present health status, concurrent medication regimen, understanding of the drug and the condition for which the drug is prescribed, and ability to manage a therapeutic regimen. Categorization of information is accomplished with a planned systematic assessment, and gaps in data are noted. Once identified, this missing information can be obtained to complete the assessment. Accepted standards and norms are then applied to determine discrepancies between what is and what should or could be, and conclusions are drawn regarding what actual problems may be present and those for which the client may be at high risk. The culmination of analysis is the diagnostic statement, which includes nursing diagnoses and collaborative problems toward which nursing care may be directed.

Nursing Diagnoses/ Collaborative Problems

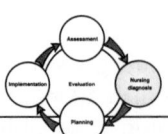

The North American Nursing Diagnosis Association (NANDA) defines a nursing diagnosis as "a clinical judgment about individual, family, or community responses to actual or potential health problems/life processes. A nursing

diagnosis provides the basis for the selection of nursing interventions to achieve outcomes for which the nurse is accountable" (North American Nursing Diagnosis Association, 2002). NANDA is the formal organization sanctioned by the American Nurses Association (ANA) to govern the development of a classification system for nursing diagnoses. Proposed nursing diagnoses are submitted to NANDA for official acceptance.

Additionally, because nurses routinely work to prevent problems, "high risk for" or "risk for" is the appropriate terminology for risk nursing diagnoses and is defined by NANDA (2002) to indicate "a clinical judgment that an individual, family, or community is more vulnerable to develop the problem than others in the same or similar situation." In the current health care climate the cost of health care may limit nurse-client interaction, and thus the use of "high risk for" nursing diagnoses assist nurses to identify the most vulnerable clients, families, and community populations.

Collaborative problems are "certain physiologic complications that nurses monitor to detect onset or changes of status. Nurses manage collaborative problems utilizing physician-prescribed and nursing-prescribed interventions to minimize the complications of the events" (Carpenito-Moyet, 2004). With nursing diagnoses, assessment involves detecting signs and symptoms of actual problems and risk factors for high-risk nursing diagnoses. In contrast, assessment for collaborative problems focuses on determining the status of the collaborative problem, that is, that certain conditions are present (which increase the client's vulnerability to the complication) or that the client has experienced the complication. The nurse's responsibilities are to monitor the client's physiologic status, perform specific activities to manage and minimize the severity of the situation, and consult with a health care provider to obtain orders for appropriate interventions. Collaborative problems can be written as "Potential complication (PC): (specify)." An example of a collaborative problem with the administration of a nonsteroidal antiinflammatory analgesic would be "PC: GI bleeding," or with methotrexate, an antineoplastic agent, "PC: hepatotoxicity."

The nurse makes independent decisions for both nursing diagnoses and collaborative problems. The difference is that in nursing diagnoses, nursing prescribes the definitive treatment, whereas with collaborative problems both nursing and medicine prescribe for the definitive treatment to achieve the desired outcomes for client care.

The nursing profession is working actively toward developing a classification system for nursing practice in a scientifically sound manner. Standardization of terminology facilitates communication among practitioners. Diagnostic statements used in this book are drawn from the list of NANDA-approved nursing diagnoses whenever possible. The NANDA list and other widely circulated lists are not considered complete; nurses are encouraged to test nursing diagnoses and develop new ones.

Several examples of nursing diagnoses follow. There are countless ways to convey the same thoughts, all equally correct; variations arise from differences among individuals constructing the diagnoses and from the wording chosen. Nursing diagnoses may be a one-part statement (e.g., wellness nursing diagnoses, syndrome nursing diagnoses), a two-part statement (e.g., risk nursing diagnoses, possible nursing diagnoses) or a three-part statement (actual nursing diagnoses). The two most common nursing diagnosis types related to pharmacology are risk nursing diagnoses that include two main components: a description of altered health status and an inferred reason for it (etiology or risk factors) and actual nursing diagnoses, which also include the symptoms by which the client demonstrates the problem, in addition to the nursing diagnosis title and its etiology. The following list presents some sample nursing diagnoses:

- Risk for impaired urinary elimination: urinary retention related to history of benign prostatic hyperplasia and concurrent anticholinergic therapy
- Risk for constipation related to decreased GI motility secondary to morphine administration
- Excess fluid volume: edema related to steroid therapy evidenced by 2+ pitting edema of ankles and weight gain of 4 pounds over 3 days
- Ineffective therapeutic regimen management: failure to refill prescriptions related to inadequate financial resources to buy drugs as evidenced by client's statement "I wish I could afford my heart pills"

Box 5-3 contains a current list of NANDA-approved nursing diagnoses that commonly result from drug therapy. However, the nurse should consider the full range of nursing diagnoses during assessment.

✳ What are the essential nursing diagnoses/potential complications for drug therapy?

For each medication there is a combination of nursing diagnoses and collaborative problems that should be anticipated or for which the client should be assessed. In addition to quite specific ones that may be particular to the individual client, assessment for the following eight specific nursing diagnoses/collaborative problems are basic to the management of every client's drug regimen:

1. *Risk nursing diagnoses/PC related to the client's preexisting health status.* These may be stated as " PC: (specify the physiologic complication related to the client's preexisting medical conditions, age, and childbearing status)," such as "PC: acute respiratory depression related to client's preexisting chronic obstructive pulmonary disease and the administration of morphine." On the other hand, a number of nursing diagnoses might also relate to the client's preexisting health status and the administration of morphine, such as "Risk for constipation related to the client's age (76 years), low fiber intake, and the administration of morphine" or "Risk for urinary retention related to client's history of benign prostatic hypertrophy and the administration of morphine."

2. *Risk nursing diagnoses/PC related to concurrent drug therapy.* An appropriate nursing diagnosis related to concurrent drug therapy might be "Risk for injury related to postural hypotension secondary to the concur-

BOX 5-3 NURSING DIAGNOSES COMMONLY SEEN WITH DRUG THERAPY*	
Activity intolerance	Infection, risk for
Activity intolerance, risk for	Injury, risk for
Anxiety	Injury, perioperative positioning, risk for
Aspiration, risk for	
Body image, disturbed	Knowledge, deficient
Body temperature, imbalanced, risk for	Knowledge of (Specify), readiness for enhanced
Breastfeeding, effective	Memory, impaired
Breathing pattern, ineffective	Nausea
Cardiac output, decreased	Nutrition: less than body requirements, imbalanced
Comfort, impaired	Oral mucous membrane, impaired
Confusion, acute	
Constipation	Poisoning, risk for
Coping, ineffective	Protection, ineffective
Denial, ineffective	Sensory perception, disturbed
Diarrhea	
Falls, risk for	Sexual dysfunction
Fatigue	Skin integrity, impaired
Fluid volume, excess	Skin integrity, impaired, risk for
Fluid volume, deficient, risk for	Sleep patterns, disturbed
	Suicide, risk for
Gas exchange, impaired	Swallowing, impaired
Growth and development, delayed	Therapeutic regimen management, ineffective
Health maintenance, ineffective	Therapeutic regimen management, readiness for enhanced
Health-seeking behaviors	
Home maintenance, impaired	Thought processes, disturbed
Incontinence, urinary, functional	Tissue perfusion, ineffective

Modified from North American Nursing Diagnosis Association (2005). *Nursing diagnoses: Definitions and classifications, 2005-2006.* Philadelphia: Author.
*For a complete listing of nursing diagnoses approved by the North American Nursing Diagnosis Association, visit http://evolve.elsevier.com/mckenry.

rent administration of propranolol (Inderal) and diuretic therapy." A PC might be "PC: (specify the physiologic complication related to concurrent drug therapy)," such as "PC: digoxin toxicity related to the concurrent administration of digoxin and furosemide therapy."

3. *Risk nursing diagnoses/PC related to the ineffectiveness of the drug.* A nursing diagnosis related to the ineffective-

ness of therapy might be "Chronic pain related to ineffective pain management program." A potential complication might be "PC: (specify the physiologic complication of the client's underlying condition related to the ineffectiveness of the drug)," such as "PC: sepsis related to the ineffectiveness of antibiotic therapy." The assessment of the effectiveness of the client's drug regimen is essential. If the outcome criteria for the client's drug therapy are not met, the drug is considered to be ineffective and the prescriber will need to alter the client's medications.

4. *Risk nursing diagnoses/PC related to the drug's adverse effects.* An appropriate nursing diagnosis related to drug adverse effects might be "Disturbed sleep pattern related to caffeine ingestion." "PC: (specify the physiologic complication related to the adverse effects of the administered drug)," such as "PC: thrombocytopenia related to heparin therapy" or "PC: GI bleeding related to aspirin therapy" might be applicable. Carpenito-Moyet (2004) has described "PC: medication therapy adverse effects" and specific potential complications for anticoagulant, antianxiety, adrenocorticosteroid, antineoplastic, antiepileptic, antidepressant, antidysrhythmic, antipsychotic, antihypertensive, β-adrenergic blocker, calcium channel blocker, and angiotensin-converting enzyme therapy.

5. *Risk for poisoning:* drug toxicity, which is the accentuated risk of accidental exposure to or ingestion of drugs or dangerous products in doses sufficient to cause poisoning. Older adults are particularly prone to this nursing diagnosis because of reduced vision, forgetfulness, polypharmacy, and the effects of drugs in the aging body.

6. *Deficient knowledge related to initiation of or change in the medication regimen.* Deficient knowledge, the state in which an individual or group experiences a deficiency in cognitive knowledge or psychomotor skills concerning the condition or treatment plan, is a common nursing diagnosis with clients receiving drug therapy. However, each client must be assessed for the level of knowledge related to his or her health condition and medication regimen. Client education is necessary if the client requests information or expresses inadequate knowledge of his or her health condition or medications to self-administer the prescribed drugs accurately and safely.

7. *Noncompliance,* the state in which an individual or group desires to comply but is prevented from doing so by factors that deter adherence to health-related advice given by health care professionals, is another nursing diagnosis that should be considered in the client's assessment. Indicators that noncompliance may be an issue are that the client does not participate in therapy, the client's symptoms persist, the disease progresses, or drug therapy outcome criteria are not met. "Noncompliance" is not a value judgment used when a client is not kowtowing to a higher authority, but it simply means that there are issues that need to be discovered by the team that are keeping the client from adhering to the prescribed drug regimen. Some authors will use the term "adherence" or "concordance" with therapy to indicate that the client is compliant; they may be considered synonymous. Also, the nursing diagnosis "noncompliance" is not used to describe a client who has made an informed autonomous decision not to comply.

8. *Ineffective therapeutic regimen management related to (specify)* is a pattern in which the individual experiences or is at high risk to experience difficulty integrating into daily living a program for the treatment of illness and its sequelae to meet specific health goals (NANDA, 2002). Factors that contribute to ineffective management may be a lack of trust in health care providers or insufficient confidence, knowledge, or resources.

In the interests of producing a text that is still manageable in size, these eight client issues will not be listed with every drug when client assessment is discussed. However, the reader should keep all of these issues in mind, because they are considered to be universal and are relevant to every medication.

Nursing diagnoses and collaborative problems form the basis for the design of subsequent phases of the nursing process—planning, implementation, and evaluation. The nursing diagnostic statement differentiates among wellness nursing diagnoses, syndrome nursing diagnoses, risk nursing diagnoses, possible nursing diagnoses, and actual nursing diagnoses.

By describing human responses, a nursing diagnosis distinguishes nursing from other health care disciplines. Nursing interventions may be categorized into three domains: dependent (or delegated), collaborative, and independent. Medicine both diagnoses and treats pathologic or cellular responses, whereas nursing both diagnoses and treats the human response. Activities that legally require a physician directive, or in some states, a nurse practitioner or physician assistant, are considered to be within the **dependent domain** of general nursing interventions; these activities constitute a significant portion of nursing practice related to pharmacology. A significant number of interventions within the **collaborative domain** involve interdependent activity between nurses and other health care providers. Client conditions require different ratios of medical (or other health care provider) input and nursing input (Figure 5-5). Neither nurses nor other health care providers possess exclusive responsibility for the diagnosis and treatment of collaborative problems. Each group maintains its own responsibility throughout its involvement with the client. The **independent domain** involves the diagnosis and treatment of problems that are primarily nursing in nature. The nurse identifies these problems and assumes primary responsibility for ordering the necessary interventions.

Nursing diagnoses are most useful in the independent domain. A nursing diagnosis is a clear, concise description of a problem that is uniquely addressed by nurses; the use of nursing diagnoses provides a focus for goals and interventions. Much of the nurse's role in pharmacotherapeutics

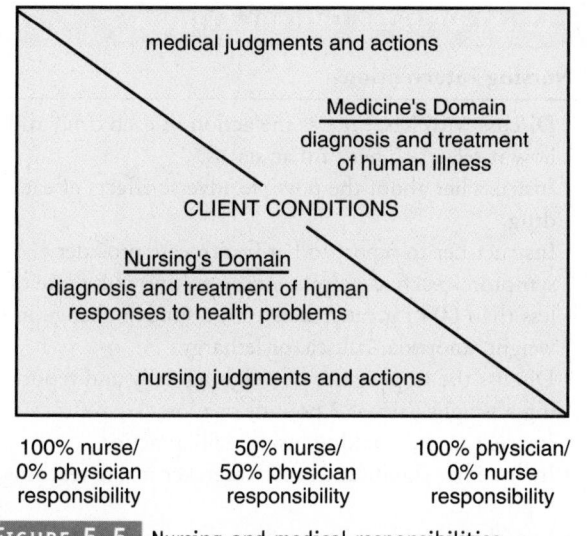

FIGURE 5-5 Nursing and medical responsibilities.

From McLane, A.M. (Ed.). (1987). *Classification of nursing diagnoses: Proceedings of the seventh conference.* St. Louis: Mosby.

encompasses the dependent and collaborative domains; these areas are not thoroughly addressed by nursing diagnoses but are more appropriately addressed by the identification of collaborative problems as potential complications. As the evolution of nursing diagnoses continues, their application to pharmacotherapeutics will become increasingly appropriate and useful.

Planning for Drug Therapy

The planning phase of the nursing process has two parts: setting goals and creating specific plans for interventions that will implement those goals. In this text, the goals are usually stated as the desired outcomes of the drug therapy, nursing outcomes (nursing-sensitive client outcomes to evaluate nursing interventions) or other outcome criteria (statements of observable or measurable results that should occur as the result of nursing and other health service activities). Goals for the effective management of the client's pharmacotherapeutic regimen include nursing outcomes and other outcome criteria because of the dependent, collaborative, and independent nature of the nursing activities involved. The planning to meet the pharmacotherapeutic nursing needs of clients should be characterized by an orientation to (1) the client, (2) resources in the environment, and (3) the future. The desired outcomes are to be established in collaboration with the client and others on the health care team, and in turn these outcomes should be characterized by a balance between the real and the ideal.

Outcome criteria associated with the medication needs of clients may be stated in many ways to encompass these three orientations. They must actually be stated (e.g., in the nursing care plan or protocol of care) to provide communication with the rest of the staff and to give clear direction for the subsequent implementation and evaluation phases of the nursing process. Without such statements, the implementa-

tion and evaluation of the client's care will be based on vague events and partially remembered and incomplete actions. When written as part of the goals for the resolution of nursing diagnoses or the prevention of collaborative problems (PCs)—stated as potential complications—in the nursing care plan, the outcome criteria are known as nursing outcomes. Nursing outcomes usually focus on enhancing the client's compliance behavior and resolving any deficient knowledge the client might have about his or her medication. Other outcome criteria are more the result of collaboration between the nurse and the prescriber. The nursing role focuses on monitoring for the "onset or any change in the client's status of physiologic complications and responding to any such changes with prescriber- and nurse-prescribed nursing interventions" (Carpenito-Moyet, 2004). Such therapeutic outcomes might relate to the normalization of the white blood cell (WBC) count, maintenance of adequate control of blood glucose, control of hypertension, or elimination of fever.

✳ How are goals and outcome criteria written?

Nursing outcomes or other outcome criteria are to be met sometime in the future. Therefore the use of the words "will be" in the outcome statement is appropriate. An approximation of time limits for accomplishing the outcome should be included in the statement to provide a way of measuring progress toward the outcome, whether short term, intermediate, or long term (e.g., "by date of discharge," "in 3 days," "3 weeks after surgery"). The time limit should be the best estimate, not an edict carved in stone. The outcome indicator or criterion is client oriented in that it *should describe what the client's condition or behavior will be* at the outcome of nursing care, not what the nurse intends to do for the client. For example, an outcome is best stated as "Client will demonstrate the safe and accurate self-administration of insulin in 3 days," rather than "To promote understanding of the drug regimen by the time of discharge from the hospital." If the goal describes only what nurses do, nurses could work diligently to promote a client's understanding of a drug regimen, with success being measured only in terms of what procedures were performed; however, the client may never have actually learned, which is the intent of the goal. The sample nursing care plan on p. 82 illustrates client-oriented outcome criteria. The nurse can prevent the blurring of the distinction between outcomes and interventions—two entirely different phases of the nursing process—by stating nursing or other outcome criteria in terms of behavioral objectives for the client. If criteria are stated in words that depict nursing interventions or actions, such as "prevent," "provide," "promote," or "maintain," the evaluation of care becomes more an appraisal of what the nurse did than of the client's response to therapy.

Finally, nursing outcomes and outcome criteria related to each nursing diagnosis or potential complication identified earlier may be ranked in priority to meet the client's needs.

The rest of the planning phase lays the groundwork for carrying out specific actions in the implementation phase.

NURSING CARE PLAN SELECTED NURSING DIAGNOSES RELATED TO CLIENT-ORIENTED OUTCOME CRITERIA		
Nursing Diagnosis	**Goals/Expected Outcomes**	**Nursing Interventions**
Deficient knowledge related to new drug regimen of digoxin, furosemide, and potassium chloride	Before discharge, Ms. Strauss will do the following: • State the action of each drug and how it relates to her cardiac status. • Identify at least three adverse effects that should be reported to her health care provider. • Weigh herself accurately and report results to nurse daily. • Demonstrated the ability to take her own pulse accurately.	• Discuss with Ms. Strauss the action of each drug and how it relates to her cardiac status. • Instruct her about the possible adverse effects of each drug. • Instruct her to report to her health care provider symptoms such as palpitations, a resting pulse rate of less than 60 or greater than 100, a sudden change in weight, anorexia, nausea, or lethargy. • Discuss the importance of weighing daily and reporting a weight gain of 2 pounds or more. • Instruct in pulse taking, using daily practice. • Include her significant other/caretaker in the teaching, if possible. • Provide her with written instructions concerning all of her care as a guide for her use at home.

Such plans for nursing actions should be supportable by research for best practice.

Development of a positive, accountable attitude by setting goals with expected outcomes and planning for each nursing action strengthens what nurses do for clients and why. The completed abbreviated nursing care plan, as a blueprint for action, can be entered in writing in the Kardex, in the computerized nursing information system, or on the client's chart and makes up the plan for nursing management of the client's nursing care. The nursing outcomes and other outcome criteria related to drug therapy may also be incorporated into interdisciplinary protocols for care, such as critical paths or protocols for client care. Outcome criteria and specific planning provide documentation for peers and preclude legal challenge, although guiding the selection of appropriate caring actions is first and foremost.

The last two components of the nursing process—implementation and evaluation—involve monitoring the client's health status, nurse- or health care provider-prescribed interventions and client education, and determining the effectiveness of the therapeutic regimen.

Implementation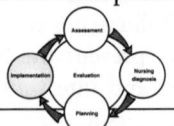

The implementation phase of the nursing process consists of putting goals into action. It is the actual giving of care as prescribed by the nursing care plan or nursing orders. The nurse is guided by the nursing care plan (formal or informal), with the goals (expected nursing and other outcomes) clearly in focus, and can initiate the proposed actions in an orderly way. The best chance for success lies in clear, frequent communication and collaboration with clients, because any action or outcome not viewed by clients as congruent with their own goals will decrease participation.

The implementation phase in drug therapy comprises all the steps of the act of administering medications. It includes collaborating with the prescriber and medicating clients according to the prescriber's orders using nursing judgment, preparing drugs (including performing any necessary mathematical calculations), using techniques and procedures with modifications for individual clients, being alert to errors, recording medications given, monitoring for therapeutic and adverse drug effects, and teaching clients about their drugs.

Drug Administration

The nursing function most closely identified with nursing by the public, and the one that carries the most legal vulnerability, is that of administering medications. This function requires much preparation, a solid knowledge base, skilled decision-making abilities, and close attention to the Six Rights of Medication Administration.

Pharmaceutical Preparations Pharmaceutical preparations are the formulations that make a drug suited to various methods of administration. They may be made up by the pharmacist but more often are prepared by the pharmaceutical company from which they are purchased. The nurse who is informed about various preparations can make more astute judgments about their individual applications and can make appropriate recommendations to the prescriber when necessary. Common preparations and their various applications are detailed in Box 5-4.

Drug Storage The appropriate storage of drugs on the nursing unit is a nursing responsibility and usually occurs with the guidance and supervision of pharmacy staff.

The **potency** (strength per milligram of drug) and **efficacy** (maximum ability of a drug to produce a result) of drugs are affected by the way in which they are handled and stored. Proper storage of a drug is necessary to maintain drug stability. Most drugs can be stored in the medication

BOX 5-4 COMMON DRUG PREPARATIONS AND THEIR APPLICATIONS

PREPARATIONS FOR ORAL USE

Liquids

Aqueous solutions—substances dissolved in water and syrups

Aqueous suspensions—solid particles suspended in liquid

Emulsions—fats or oils suspended in liquid with an emulsifier

Spirits—alcohol solution

Elixirs—aromatic, sweetened alcohol and water solution

Tinctures—alcohol extract of plant or vegetable substance

Fluidextracts—concentrated alcoholic liquid extract of plant or vegetables

Extracts—syrup or dried form of pharmacologically active drug, usually prepared by evaporating solution

Solids

Capsules—soluble case (usually gelatin) that contains liquid, dry, or beaded drug particles

Rapidly dissolving tablets/lozenges—formulations that dissolve quickly in the mouth (formulations of loratadine [Alavert] in tablet formulation, Dimetapp, Listerine Strip type formulations)

Tablets—compressed, powdered drug(s) in small disk

Troches/lozenges—medicated tablets that dissolve slowly in mouth

Powders/granules—loose or molded drug substance for drug administration, with or without liquids

PREPARATIONS FOR PARENTERAL USE

Ampules—sealed glass container for liquid injectable medication

Vials—glass container with rubber stopper for liquid or powdered medication

Cartridge/Tubex—single-dose unit of parenteral medication to be used with a specific injecting device

INTRAVENOUS INFUSIONS (SUSPENDED ON HANGER AT BEDSIDE)

Glass bottles, flexible collapsible plastic bags, and semi-rigid plastic containers in sizes from 150 to 1000 mL—used for continuous infusion of fluid replacement with or without medications

Intermittent IV infusions—usually a secondary IV setup of a small plastic or glass bottle (volume between 50 to 250 mL) to which medication is added; runs as a "piggyback" and is hung separately from the primary IV infusion via a secondary administration tubing set, usually for a period of 20 to 120 minutes; the primary IV solution is run during the time between medication doses

Heparin lock or angiocath—a port site for direct administration or intermittent IV medications without the need for a primary IV solution

PREPARATIONS FOR TOPICAL USE

Liniments—liquid suspensions for lubrication that are applied by rubbing

Lotions—liquid suspensions that can be protective, emollient, cooling, astringent, antipruritic, cleansing, etc.

Ointment—semisolid medicine in a base for local protective, soothing, astringent, or transdermal application for systemic effects (e.g., nitroglycerin, scopolamine, estrogen)

Paste—thick ointment primarily used for skin protection

Plasters—solid preparations that are adhesive, protective, or soothing

Creams—emulsions that contain an aqueous and an oily base

Aerosols—fine powders or solutions in volatile liquids that contain a propellant

Transdermal patches—patches containing medication that is absorbed continuously through the skin and acts systemically

PREPARATIONS FOR USE ON MUCOUS MEMBRANES

Drops—aqueous solutions with or without a gelling agent to increase retention time in the eye; used for eyes, ears, or nose

Instillations or an aqueous solution of medications—usually for topical action but occasionally used for systemic effects, including enemas, douches, mouthwashes, throat sprays, and gargles

Aerosol sprays, nebulizers, and inhalers—deliver aqueous solutions of medication in droplet form to the target membrane, such as the bronchial tree (e.g., bronchodilators)

Foams—powders or solutions of medication in volatile liquids with a propellant, such as vaginal foams for contraception

Suppositories—usually contain medicinal substances mixed in a firm but malleable base (cocoa butter) to facilitate insertion into a body cavity (e.g., rectal or vaginal)

MISCELLANEOUS DRUG DELIVERY SYSTEMS

Intradermal implants—pellets containing a small deposit of medication; are inserted in a dermal pocket; designed to allow medication to leach slowly into tissue; usually used to administer hormones such as testosterone or estradiol

Micropump system—a small, external pump that is attached by belt or implanted to delivery medication via a needle in a continuous, steady dose (e.g., insulin, anticancer chemotherapy, and opioids)

Membrane delivery systems—drug-laden membranes that are instilled in the eye to deliver a steady flow of medications (e.g., pilocarpine or corticosteroids)

cart, but some must be stored according to specific manufacturer's directions (on the label or package insert) to slow deterioration (e.g., live vaccines, most reconstituted drugs, and most suppositories). Many drugs change composition or potency when exposed to light, heat, moisture, or gases in the environment. The *USP DI: Drug Information for the Health Care Professional* (2005) has defined the nomenclature used in instructions for the prevention of changes from heat:

- Freeze: below $-20°$ C to $-10°$ C ($-4°$ F to $14°$ F)
- Store in a cold place: temperature no higher than $8°$ C ($46°$ F)
- Refrigerate: $2°$ C to $8°$ C ($36°$ F to $46°$ F)
- Warm: any temperature between $30°$ C to $40°$ C ($86°$ F to $104°$ F)
- Avoid excessive heat: temperature no higher than $40°$ C ($104°$ F)

Most drugs may be stored at room temperature, which is considered to be between $20°$ C and $25°$ C ($68°$ F and $77°$ F). Brief deviations from these temperatures are acceptable, such as $15°$ C and $30°$ C ($59°$ F and $86°$ F) (*Quality Review*, 1999).

Use medication refrigerators solely for the storage of drugs and related necessities and clean them out regularly, returning expired drugs or drugs belonging to discharged clients to the pharmacy. To ensure a more constant cool temperature, store medications within the refrigerator—not on the door shelves or within the freezer compartment. Keep at least one thermometer inside to monitor temperature maintenance.

The use of amber-colored containers protects some medications (e.g., furosemide [Lasix] and nitroglycerin) against deterioration by light. Point out this fact and its significance to clients who are self-medicating and who might otherwise transfer medications to a different container (to take to work, on vacation, etc.). Storage in a closed cabinet or other dark place should also be advised. If feasible, give clients information about how to tell if their medication has deteriorated. Also tell them that the medication needs to be replaced if storage requirements have not been maintained or if the appearance or effects of the medication have changed.

Certain drugs given intravenously are significantly sensitive to light: an antifungal, amphotericin B deoxycholate (Fungizone); B-complex vitamins; cancer chemotherapy drugs, cisplatin (Platinol), daunorubicin (Cerubidine), and doxorubicin (Adriamycin RDF); and the antihypertensive, nitroprusside (Nitropress). These medications should be checked for visible signs of deterioration, such as color change, precipitation, or gas formation. Deterioration may neutralize the drugs or make them toxic, and this can occur without any warning signs. Nitroprusside (Nitropress) and amphotericin B deoxycholate (Fungizone) solutions for infusions should be kept covered with foil or an amber plastic bag (not a brown paper bag, which is not light protective) while being administered by continuous IV infusion. Unless freshly prepared, all the other solutions should also be kept covered. Some drugs, such as the antidysrhythmic amiodarone, or the vasodilator nitroglycerin degrade in the presence of vinyl or plastics and may require preparation in

glass containers and/or use of special tubing to assure adequate drug integrity.

Tight lids can prevent the drug form or its active constituents from degrading or changing by preventing the exchange of moisture or gases within the container.

The expiration dates printed on drug labels mean simply that the drug contained is probably at its peak effectiveness until some point in time past that date. Because quality controls in drug production are subject to error rates similar to all other control programs, pharmaceutical companies tend to estimate these expiration dates somewhat conservatively. Thus the drug is not instantly rendered useless or harmful by that date, but the effectiveness of the therapy may be gradually diminished and the drug may produce inadequate or occasionally even toxic results some time after the printed date. Do not administer doses from an outdated lot of drug or container; obtain a fresh supply.

Certain precepts should guide the way in which clients' drugs are stored, distributed, and managed. Health care agencies have developed policies that, with some variations, support these precepts as rules for client protection and prevent nurses from making errors. Additionally, rational nursing judgments must enter into decision making; such judgments allow a departure from these rules as a wise and necessary choice, but these should never be undertaken lightly. It should also be a practice to consult other expert personnel or authorities.

The following are additional guidelines for handling medications and are not necessarily listed in order of importance:

- Keep all medicines in a special place, which may be a cart or room. This area should not be freely accessible to the public.
- Keep controlled substances and those dispensed under special legal regulations in a locked box or compartment (many states require double locks) and account for them at the end of each shift. Another nurse must attest to any dose that is wasted or discarded by initialing such a notation. Many automated dispensing systems help facilitate accountability.

✳ What guidelines are there for handling drugs?

- In most institutions, each client's medicines are kept in a designated drawer of the medication cart or computerized dispensing system. The nurse must be careful to keep the client's medicines in the right area and must make certain that the medicines are returned to the pharmacy when the client leaves the hospital.
- If stock supplies are maintained, they should be arranged in an orderly manner. Preparations for internal use should be kept separate from those for external use.
- Some preparations, such as serums, vaccines, certain suppositories, certain antibiotics, and insulin, may need to be refrigerated.
- The labels of all medicines should be clean and legible. If they are not, they should be sent to the pharmacist for relabeling. *Nurses should not label or relabel medicines.*
- Bottles of medicines should always be capped and protected from light, heat, and high humidity as necessary.

TABLE 5-2 STORAGE REQUIREMENTS AND EXPIRATION TIMES OF SELECTED INTRAVENOUS DRUGS

| Drug | Stability After Reconstitution | | |
	Room Temperature*	Refrigeration*	If Frozen*
cefamandole (Mandol)	24 hours	96 hours	6 months
cefazolin sodium (Ancef, Kefzol)	24 hours	10 days	—
cefoperazone (Cefobid) and parenteral solution used	24 hours	5 days	3 to 5 weeks, depending on concentration
sterile cefoxitin (Mefoxin)	6 to 18 hours	48 hours to 7 days	At least 30 weeks, depending on method of preparation
cefotetan for injection (Cefotan)	24 hours	96 hours	1 week

From *USP DI: Drug information for the health care professional* (25th ed.). (2005). Greenwood Village, CO: MICROMEDEX Thomson Healthcare.
*Recommended temperatures: room temperature, 20° C to 25° C (68° F to 77° F); refrigeration, 2° C to 8° C (36° F to 46° F); frozen, −20° C to −10° C (−4° F to 14° F).

Many IV drugs require a diluent to dissolve the medication, which then can be added to a larger volume of solution for administration. The storage times for such medications can vary, depending on the following:

- The expiration date on the fresh package of medication stored under the specific instructions of the manufacturer
- The expiration time period allotted for the dissolved medication
- The expiration time period allotted for the dissolved medication added to a larger volume of solution

To obtain accurate information for an individual drug, refer to the package insert or the *USP DI*. As an example, Table 5-2 illustrates the differing storage requirements and expiration times within the same drug classification (cephalosporin antibiotics).

Preparation of the Dose Technically, written medical orders are the only legal means for the administration of medications by nurses. Written orders constitute permanent legal records of the prescriber's plans and can be submitted as evidence in litigation. Because nurses are held legally accountable for every dose of medication they administer, they must routinely ensure that (1) each order is appropriate, accurate, and complete; and (2) the order is followed unerringly to completion, or the prescriber is consulted regarding why it was not completed. The free flow of communication between prescriber and nurse is crucial to fulfillment of this responsibility. Nurses must be ready to consult with the prescriber as necessary to clarify, understand, or suggest medication therapy as needed.

What is the process by which a prescriber's order is translated into the administration of a medication? The order is first transcribed by a unit secretary, nurse manager (or nursing care coordinator), or primary nurse from an order sheet onto the Kardex or medication administration record (MAR) (Figure 5-6); this entire process may also be com-

BOX 5-5 CHECKING TRANSCRIPTION

WHICH MEDICATION?

Is it quinine sulfate (a medication for leg cramps) or quinidine sulfate (a cardiac depressant)? Pentobarbital or phenobarbital? Ornade or Orinase? Decadron or Doriden?

WHICH DOSE?

Is it a loop of an f, g, or q, or is it another zero?

Vital signs q 4 h
Gentamycin 60 mg IV 6 h

ANYTHING MISSING?

Does Halcion i HS mean 0.125 mg or 0.25 mg?

puterized. In many health agencies the prescriber places the medication order into a computer that requisitions the drug from the pharmacy, and the order is automatically transcribed directly onto a computerized MAR from which the nurse prepares the medication. Such systems improve safety by avoiding the inaccuracy of hand transcription of the medication order to the MAR. If hand transcribed (e.g., a unit secretary has processed a handwritten order), it should be verified by a nurse, who can better relate the medication to the client and the diagnosis. To prevent error, the nurse must check the dosage of the medication and the age of the client, check for drug interaction possibilities and allergies, and ensure the completeness and clarity of the order (Box 5-5). Whatever the question concerning the prescriber's order, legally it can be clarified only with the prescriber who

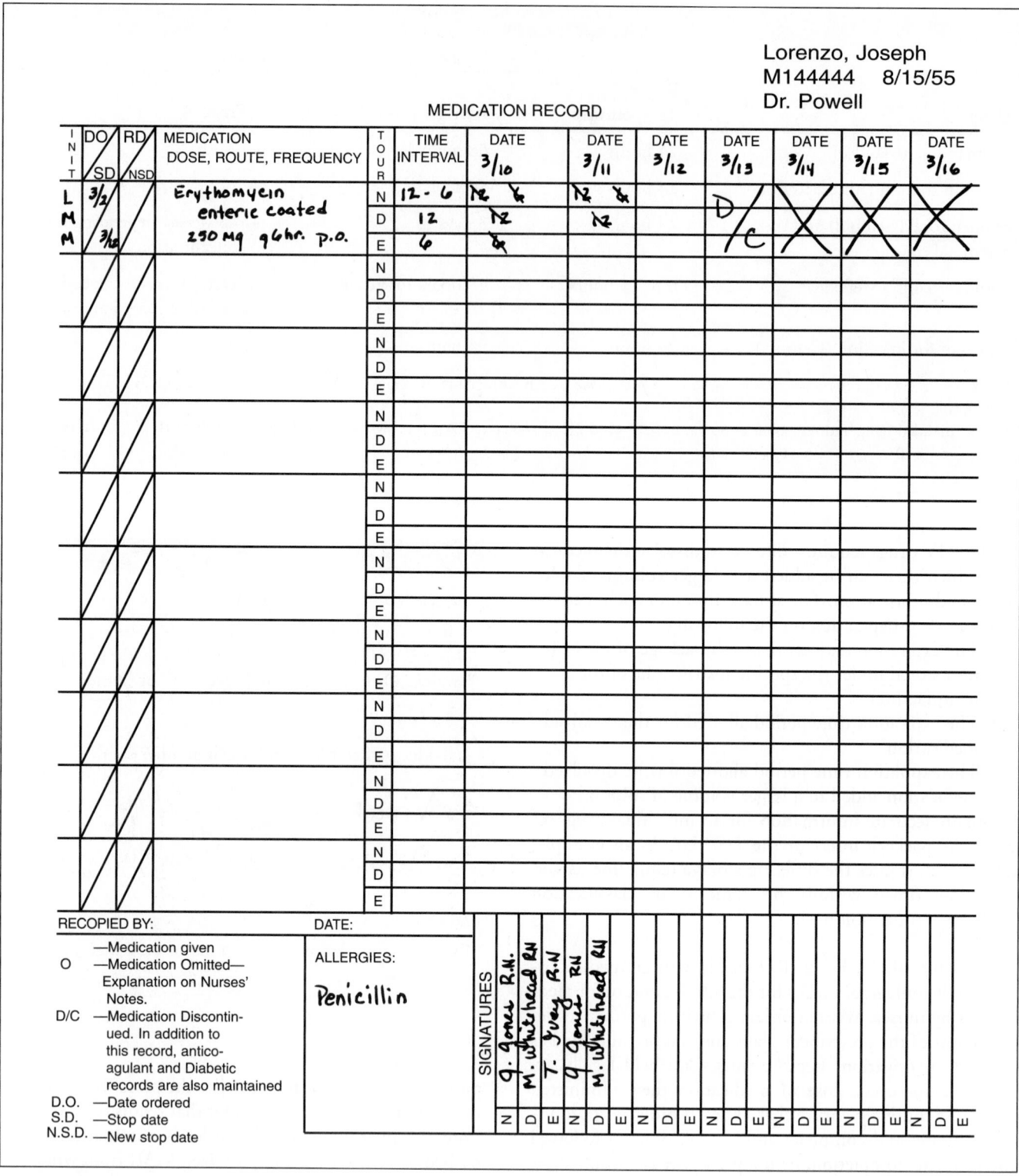

FIGURE 5-6 Sample medication administration record (MAR). In most health care agencies, this form has been computerized.

has written the order. Verifying an order with the physician or nursing colleague who happens to be present in the clinical or home setting does not suffice.

In the hospital or extended care facility, the institution's pharmacy department supplies the drug. When the supply arrives, it is appropriately stored in an individual client's own medication box, in the drawer of a medication cart, or in the computerized dispensing system. In the home, a local pharmacy or mail order pharmaceutical supplier may supply the drug to the client or client's family, with the nurse, client, or family member administering the medication as scheduled.

Because of space limitations, prescribers, pharmacists, and nurses rely on pharmacologic abbreviations or symbols for communication. These abbreviations are often from

TABLE 5-3 COMMON ABBREVIATIONS AND SYMBOLS RELATED TO MEDICATION ADMINISTRATION*

Abbreviation	Unabbreviated Form	Meaning	Abbreviation	Unabbreviated Form	Meaning
ac	ante cibum	before meals	p.m.	post meridiem	after noon
ad lib	ad libitum	freely	PO	per os	by mouth, orally
a.m.	ante meridiem	morning	PRN	pro re nata	according to necessity
bid	bis in die	twice each day	pt	patient	patient
caps	capsule	capsule	qh	quaque hora	every hour
elix	elixir	elixir	q4h, q4°	every 4 hours	every 4 hours around-the-clock
gtt	guttae	drops			
h, hr	hora	hour	qid	quater in die	4 times each day
IM	intramuscular	into a muscle	℞	recipe	take
IV	intravenous	into a vein	SL	sub lingua	under the tongue
IVPB	IV piggyback	secondary IV line	SOS	si opus sit	if it is necessary, one dose only
kg	kilogram	2.2 pounds			
KVO	keep vein open	very slow infusion rate	stat	statim	at once
			SubQ	subcutaneous	into subcutaneous tissue
L	liter	liter			
mcg	microgram	one millionth of a gram	tbsp	tablespoon	tablespoon (15 mL)
mg	milligram	one thousandth of a gram	tid	ter in die	three times a day
			TO	telephone order	order received over the telephone
mEq	milliequivalent	the number of grams of solute dissolved in one milliliter of a *normal* solution	tsp	teaspoon	teaspoon (4 or 5 mL)
			VO	verbal order	order received verbally
ml, mL	milliliter	one thousandth of a liter	×	times	as in two times a week
ng	nanogram	one billionth of a gram	=	equal to	equal to
			↑, ↗	increase or increasing	increase or increasing
OTC	over-the-counter	nonprescription drug	↓, ↙	decrease or decreasing	decrease or decreasing
pc	post cibum	after meals			

*It is recommended that certain abbreviations be abandoned if they are found to be confusing.

Latin and are universally used. Abbreviations are a key to communication in the busy health field and should be learned. Table 5-3 lists the most commonly used abbreviations and symbols common to clinical practice.

A number of prescribers also use abbreviations for ordering specific medications (Table 5-4). Because of the danger of misinterpretation, variant or nonstandard abbreviations should not be used. The nurse should review the approved abbreviation listing for the specific health agency.

When transcribed, the prescriber's order must contain all the elements for a complete prescription order described

earlier. It must contain the *full name* of the client (and bed location, such as "Room 212, Bed A"); the *date* the order was written; the *medication name*, dosage, *route of administration*, and *frequency of administration*; and, according to agency policy, the *name* or *initials* of the nurse responsible for the transcription or computer entry.

Types of Drug Delivery Systems There are several approaches to distributing and dispensing drugs to clients in an institutional setting: the floor stock system, unit-dose drug distribution, or a combination of these. In the floor

TABLE 5-4 ABBREVIATIONS FOR SPECIFIC MEDICATIONS

Abbreviation	Definition
ACTH	adrenocorticotropic hormone
ASA	acetylsalicylic acid (aspirin)
DES	diethylstilbestrol
DM	dextromethorphan
D_5W	5% dextrose in water
D_5NS	5% dextrose in normal saline
DSS or DOSS	dioctyl sodium sulfosuccinate
DW	distilled water
EC	enteric-coated
Fe	iron
5-FU	5-fluorouracil
FUDR	floxuridine
HC	hydrocortisone
INH	isoniazid
K	potassium
KCl	potassium chloride
LOC	laxative of choice
MOM	milk of magnesia
6-MP	6-mercaptopurine
Na	sodium
NS	normal saline
NSAID	nonsteroidal antiinflammatory drug
NTG	nitroglycerin
PAS	para-aminosalicylic acid
PB	phenobarbital
PCN	penicillin

stock system, all medications except those infrequently used are stored in bulk in the medication room of the nursing unit. The floor stock system is rarely used because of (1) the increased potential for medication errors caused by the large array of stock medications from which to choose, (2) the financial loss caused by misplaced or forgotten charges and expired drugs to be returned, (3) the need for frequent total drug inventories, and (4) the storage problems inherent in crowded medication rooms. Therefore this system is more costly and less safe for the client.

The national norm for institutions is unit-dose dispensing of most if not all prescribed medications. With this system, single-dose packages of drugs are dispensed. For example, each oral dose may be a tablet encased in a blister pack or in a paper tear-off strip of tablets. This packaging is said to be the safest and most economical method of drug distribution. However, in many instances drug wastage occurs in long-term care settings in which the drugs are issued in 30-day blister packages; these packages must be discarded when the drug is discontinued for the client—even if only a few of the total doses have been administered. The regulations governing this practice are being reviewed in many states.

The advantages of using the unit-dose system far outweigh the disadvantages. The most important advantages are increased medication safety and decreased errors, because drug computations are largely eliminated. The drug is already properly labeled and does not need to be prepared. All the nurse needs to do is deliver the package to the client; it is opened at the bedside and administered. This system may permit clients to check on their own drugs and be assured that they are receiving the proper medication and the proper dose. Unit-dose packaging also decreases the chances of deterioration and, in many instances clients can be given financial credit for drugs that are not used. In many circumstances, the use of bar code technology, including a handheld barcode reader, assists the pharmacist and nurse in assuring the correct drug and dose is dispensed, administered, and charted. Disadvantages include increased cost to set up the system and the need for additional pharmacy personnel to fill new orders and resupply the client's units every 24 hours. Because the drugs are not immediately available on the unit, the administration of new and stat medication orders may be delayed while the medication order is sent to the pharmacy, filled, and delivered back to the nurse. However, the safety features of the unit-dose system far outweigh any temporary inconvenience.

Strip packages make controlled substance counting more convenient for nurses, because all packages in the strip are numbered. Prefilled unit dose disposable syringes are also available.

Unit-dose dispensing systems in hospitals, rehabilitation centers, or extended care facilities may be centralized, decentralized, or a combination of both. In the centralized system, the pharmacist and pharmacy are located in a central area from which drugs are distributed to client care areas. In the decentralized system, clinical pharmacists and satellite pharmacies are located in client care areas, and drugs are prepared and distributed to clients from those particular areas. In the combined system, medications are prepared in a central area, and clinical pharmacists are assigned to various client care areas to oversee drug therapy, thus providing safer and more controlled drug ordering and drug distribution.

In the home setting the nurse is not usually administering drugs to multiple clients. In this case the individual drugs for the client are kept in a common container or may be in a blister pack.

✵ What is the role of the clinical pharmacist?

A present trend in drug delivery is toward more extensive use of clinical pharmacists stationed in nursing areas to work closely with prescribers, nurses, therapists, and dietitians. Because pharmacists are educated in the action, interaction, compounding, dispensing, and control of drugs, they can be an invaluable resource for assistance in solving pharmacologic problems in the institutional or community setting. Nurses often consult them about medication administration methods, dosages, drug identification, and secondary effects. Health care professionals from all disciplines consult with clinical pharmacists with questions relating to drug therapy. Today's health care system demands more of this type of interdisciplinary collaboration and shared expertise for the benefit of all, especially the client.

Many pharmacies can have special "clean rooms" and specially filtered air for compounding various parenteral solutions. A pharmacist or supervised designee may be responsible for putting all additives into IV solutions and checking all such solutions for compatibility reactions.

✳ What is the role of the nurse?

Regardless of any changes in ordering, distributing, or administering drugs, nurses share in the responsibility for their clients' medication safety. This is true whether they practice in a home, a primary health care setting, or an institution. Advanced technology and the availability of more potent drugs make it crucial for the nurse to be better informed about drugs and their actions. Nurses must observe clients and their response to drug therapy, determine whether PRN orders are to be given, and consult with prescribers about withholding, discontinuing, or changing drugs. They must continue to obtain histories, teach clients about medications and their effects, work collaboratively with pharmacists, and work with clients to plan the management of drug therapy in the home setting.

✳ How does one prepare to give drugs?

Doses, Dosing Intervals, and Scheduling Understanding the rationale for selecting a particular dose and frequency of administration requires a basic understanding of the drug in question. Within limits, increasing a dose or frequency of administration increases the pharmacologic effect, but it can also increase the risk of adverse effects. The various relationships involved can be represented as follows:

Optimal doses → Dose-response relationship
Optimal frequencies → Time-response relationship

The variables to deal with in *dose-response* relationships are defined as follows:

- **Drug potency:** absolute amount of drug required to produce a desired effect
- **Therapeutic index:** relative margin of safety; the ratio of lethal dose to effective dose
- **Maximum effect:** greatest response possible regardless of dose given

Time-response relationships deal with the following variables:

- **Latency:** time necessary for therapeutic effect
- **Time for maximum effect:** time after administration for the effect of the drug to peak
- **Duration of action:** length of time of a drug effect

These last variables are affected by the route of administration used, the pharmacokinetics involved, and the biorhythms of the individual client.

Doses are given at appropriate intervals to avoid wide fluctuations in the serum concentration of a drug and to avoid drug accumulation and toxicity. If the interval is too short, drug accumulation with the potential for toxicity will occur. If it is too long, serum concentration will drop because the drug continues to be excreted and not replaced. Drugs with very short half-lives do not accumulate and therefore need to be given frequently to achieve a steady state (see Chapter 3). Drugs with very long half-lives are often given once a day.

Dosing relationships are interpreted on the basis of a normal curve in drug studies. Doses and dosing intervals are derived for treating the ideal "average" person in a population. Although dosing intervals have been studied statistically, drug therapy regimens must be reassessed continually for individual needs. Some people will always fall outside the "average" range in responding to a drug. Additionally, dosing intervals may be modified in consideration of client convenience and their effect on the client's management of the therapeutic regimen.

The time for administering routine medications may be determined by agency policy. For example, drugs ordered four times a day may be given at 10 AM, 2 PM, 6 PM, and 10 PM, or at 9 AM, 1 PM, 5 PM, and 9 PM, and so forth. Special units, such as pediatrics, have other medication hours to coincide with the special needs of their clients. In the home the client may determine the times as long as the timing of the doses maintains therapeutic drug blood levels and client safety. Depending on the pharmacokinetics of the drug, client convenience, and the need to avoid mealtimes or other activities that might interfere with drug administration, nurses may choose autonomously to vary the administration times (but not the intervals)—if the decision is based on solid rationale (Box 5-6). For example, calcium supplements might be given at bedtime rather than at 9 AM on a daily schedule because calcium is better absorbed at night. Drugs administered once daily can usually be given according to a flexible schedule, perhaps just before or after a treatment that would interfere with a dosing time, such as a client's trip off the nursing unit to the physical therapy department or radiology department. At home, clients are encouraged to take their medications at the same time each day. This helps to establish a daily pattern and enhances adherence to the drug regimen.

Drugs should be administered as close to the time indicated as possible, but obviously a nurse practicing within an institutional setting cannot medicate each of a group of assigned clients at exactly the same time. Agency policies may vary but usually stipulate administration within a half hour before or after the indicated time. Exempt from this flexibility are stat or one-time-only drug orders, such as those given before diagnostic procedures or surgery, and those medications administered at more frequent intervals, such as every 2 hours or every 4 hours.

Drug effects are monitored by the prescriber and the nurse according to either direct assessment (subjective, by observation for clinical responses) or indirect assessment (objective, by serum concentrations of the drug or by relevant laboratory values). Because of their unique presence and expertise, nurses are most capable of assisting the prescriber in making keen assessments of clients' responses.

Drug Incompatibilities Interactions that occur when drugs are mixed before administration, as in a single syringe or in IV fluids, are termed drug **incompatibilities.** Drugs that are physically incompatible may produce unwanted changes through processes such as liquefaction, deliquescence, or precipitation. Chemical incompatibilities may result when ingredients interact to form new compounds or are neutralized. Separate administration routes should be sought if drug incompatibilities are anticipated.

Some drugs are highly incompatible in solution with many other drugs. Because solution incompatibilities are often time-dependent, fewer difficulties may be associated with mixing drugs in one syringe than with IV solutions; both drugs should be administered as soon after mixing as possible. Drugs that are noted for being incompatible with many other drugs in a syringe include chlordiazepoxide (Librium), diazepam (Valium), pentobarbital (Nembutal), phenobarbital (Luminal), phenytoin (Dilantin), and sodium bicarbonate; these drugs should be administered alone.

Many drugs have explicit manufacturer's instructions for preparation (dilution and method of adding to select parenteral solutions); these instructions should be followed closely. A check for drug compatibility is indicated before two or more drugs are added to the same IV solution. Standard IV parenteral drug charts and guides are available for reference use. Most hospital pharmacies provide an IV preparation service that screens for incompatibilities before preparation and delivery to the nursing area or the client's home.

With the increase in the number of potent drugs and the variety of combinations, use of the pharmacist's expertise in a controlled environment is a wise policy. If the nurse is required to prepare IV solutions on the nursing unit, adequate references, including a list of incompatibilities,

should be posted in the area in which this duty is performed. Open and regular communication with the pharmacy department is necessary for obtaining new or additional information and assistance whenever necessary.

Dosage Measurement If the drug is formulated in units that are multiples of the prescribed dose (tablet or liquid), the computation to determine the correct dosage is simple. However, dosage calculations are necessary if the drug does not come in units that are multiples of the prescribed dose or if the drug must be dissolved in water. For certain therapies, flow-rate calculations are necessary to set the proper amount for the desired dose effect. IV infusions necessitate careful calculations of flow rate. The calculation of dosages is a necessary skill to administer drugs safely. Many excellent nursing texts are available for developing and practicing the arithmetic skills necessary in the administration of medications (see the Bibliography at the end of this chapter).

Procedures and Techniques of Administration Accurate and full identification of the client before the administration of each dose of medication ensures that the right person gets the right medication as described in Chapter 4. Additionally, activities that reduce the risk of medication errors during administration are discussed.

The route of administration is determined by the physical and chemical properties of the drug, the condition or status of the client, the desired action of the drug, its speed of absorption, and the rapidity of response desired. As a rule, drugs are administered for either local or systemic effects (see Chapter 3). Some drugs given locally, such as epinephrine eyedrops, may produce both local and systemic effects if they are partly or entirely absorbed; some drugs (such as transdermal patches) are applied for local absorption yet are targeted solely for systemic effect, such as nitroglycerin (Transderm-Nitro), fentanyl (Duragesic), and scopolamine (Transderm-Scop). A drug may be injected into a joint cavity and have little or no effect beyond the tissues of that structure.

There is an increasing awareness that many more substances are absorbed through the skin than previously believed. Incidents of toxicity in infants exposed to topically applied dermal medications are increasing. These drugs include boric acid, iodides, hexachlorophene, corticosteroids, and rubbing alcohol. Care is advised in the use of any drug topically applied to an infant's skin.

✹ How are drugs administered for local effects?

Application to Skin Medications are applied to the skin primarily for the following effects:
- *Astringent:* to constrict or draw together; this substance may result in vasoconstriction, tissue contraction, and decreased secretions and sensitivity
- *Antiseptic* or *bacteriostatic:* to inhibit the growth and development of microorganisms

• *Emollient:* to soothe and soften to overcome dryness and hardness
• *Cleansing:* to remove dirt, debris, secretions, or crusts

These medications may be applied in the form of a lotion, tincture, ointment or cream, foam, wet dressing, bath, or soak. The effectiveness of medicinals applied to the skin for local effect is limited by the fact that, to protect the internal body environment, highly specialized layers of skin resist the penetration of many (but not all) foreign substances. Topical absorption is increased when the skin is thin or macerated, when drug concentration is increased, when contact of the drug with the skin is prolonged, or when the drug is combined with a solvent-penetrant such as dimethyl sulfoxide (DMSO). (See Chapter 65 for information on dermatologic drugs and Chapter 66 for information on debriding agents.)

Application to Mucous Membranes Drugs are well absorbed across mucosal surfaces, and therapeutic effects are easily obtained. However, mucous membranes are highly selective in their absorptive capacity and vary in sensitivity. To produce the same effect, a drug applied to the oral (buccal or sublingual) mucosa may be twice as concentrated as that applied to the nasal mucosa, and the concentration of the same drug may be reduced one fourth to one half for application to delicate membranes of the eye or urethra. Aqueous solutions are quickly absorbed from mucous membranes; oily liquids are not. Oily preparations should not be applied to nasal or respiratory mucosa by sprays or nebulae because the droplets of oil may be carried to terminal portions of the respiratory tract and be retained there, causing lipid pneumonia.

The respiratory mucosa may be medicated by means of inhalation or insufflation. The inhalation method uses sprays or nebulae whereby the drug is sprayed in the nose or throat by a nebulizer; aerosols are delivered by a flow of air or oxygen under pressure to disperse the drug throughout the lower respiratory tract. In the insufflation method a fine powder is blown or sprayed. Drugs administered by means of inhalation or insufflation tend to produce both a local respiratory and a systemic effect. The respiratory mucosa offers an enormous surface of absorbing epithelium. The drug is instantaneously absorbed (1) if the drug is volatile and can be absorbed chemically, and (2) if there is more in the inspired air than in the blood. This fact is of significance in emergencies. Amyl nitrite and oxygen are examples of volatile and gaseous agents given by inhalation.

Drugs in suppository form can be used for their local effects on the mucous membranes of the vagina, urethra, or rectum. Packs and tampons may be impregnated with a drug and placed in a body cavity; these are used particularly in the nose, ears, and vagina. Drugs may also be painted or swabbed on a mucosal surface, instilled (e.g., a vaginal douche), or administered via irrigation.

✿ **How are drugs administered for systemic effects?**
Drugs that produce a systemic effect must be absorbed into the bloodstream and carried to the cells or tissues capable of responding to them. The route of administration used depends on the nature and amount of drug to be given, the desired rapidity of effect, and the general condition of the client. Routes selected for systemic effect include the following: dermal, oral, sublingual, rectal, and parenteral (injection). Routes of parenteral administration include intradermal (or intracutaneous), subcutaneous, intramuscular, intravenous, intraspinal (or intrathecal), epidural, and sometimes intraarticular, intracardiac, intrapericardiac, intraosseous, and intraperitoneal.

Application to Skin Now that microquantitative assay capabilities make possible precise unit doses using transdermal modes, topical applications of some medications can be administered in patch form for systemic effect. Nitroglycerin (Nitrodisc, Nitro-Dur, Transderm-Nitro), which is used to treat anginal pain, is available in small unit-dose adhesive bandages that slowly release the medication over a 24-hour period. Some bandages use a semipermeable, rate-controlling membrane placed next to the skin; others disperse the nitroglycerin evenly throughout a gel matrix. See Box 28-2 for a diagram of some transdermal patches. Motion sickness is treated with scopolamine (Transderm-Scop); the duration of effect of one application behind the ear is approximately 3 days. Fentanyl (Duragesic), an analgesic, is also available in a transdermal system to provide continuous release of the potent opioid for 72 hours. Clonidine, estrogen, hormonal contraceptives for birth control, and nicotine are other medications available in patch form. The nurse should apply the patch over a clean, dry, and hair-free area; the application sites should be rotated.

Oral Administration Oral administration is the safest, most economical, and most convenient way of giving medicines. It is the preferred route unless some distinct advantage is to be gained by using another way. Most drugs are absorbed from the small intestine; only a few are absorbed from the stomach and colon. This explains the ineffectiveness of cathartics and enemas in removing most toxins and overdoses in cases of poisoning.

The effects of orally administered drugs are slower in onset and more prolonged but are less potent than those of parenterally administered drugs. Therefore when a steady state in pharmacokinetics is desired, it is often more closely approached with oral than with parenteral administration. The parenteral route may be used when rapid, high doses are needed as loading doses or in emergencies. If carefully tailored to individual needs, strategies for wise pain management can exploit the characteristics of the oral and parenteral routes for analgesics. For clients with low-level pain or chronic pain, the oral route for analgesics can be more successful than other routes in promoting a steady state (fewer oscillations) of pain relief. Acute pain may submit to an initial dose of analgesic by the parenteral route, followed by oral doses.

Altered effects from oral administration may result from (1) variation in absorption as a result of drug composition, gastric or intestinal pH and motility, food content, or a pathologic condition within the GI tract; or (2) alteration of the drug resulting from its retention, inactivation, or bio-transformation in the liver.

Disadvantages of the oral administration of certain drugs are that (1) they may have an objectionable odor or taste or be bulky to swallow; (2) they may irritate the gastric mucosa, causing nausea and vomiting; (3) they may be aspirated by a seriously ill or uncooperative client; (4) they may be destroyed by digestive enzymes; and (5) they may be inappropriate for some clients, such as those who must be given nothing by mouth.

Assist weak or impaired clients to take their medications, and do so as patiently and unhurriedly as possible. Taking a small sip of water before taking a tablet assists with swallowing solid forms of medications. With the exception of rapidly dissolving dose forms intended for dissolution in saliva, clients without a fluid restriction should be encouraged to take 8 ounces of water with their oral medications. This facilitates dissolution in the stomach and reduces gastric irritation. Esophageal erosion caused by an adherent tablet or pill has been reported when inadequate amounts of water were given. Having the client sit upright after taking oral medications also helps medication pass into the stomach. Some medications may be crushed (others may not) and mixed with a small amount of jam to make them easier to swallow and more palatable (Box 5-7).

Many liquid medicines may be diluted with water or another liquid. This practice is especially desirable if the medicine has a bad taste. Exceptions to this rule include cough medicines that are given for a local effect in the throat.

All medicine containers and trays should be scrupulously clean, and water supplied to the client with the medicine should be fresh. Carelessly prepared medicines and a lack of consideration in the way a medicine is handed to a client can convey a demeaning or insulting message, whether intended or not.

When administering medicine with an unpleasant taste, it is better to admit that it may be unpleasant than to make a client feel that his or her reaction is grossly exaggerated or silly. The nurse can attempt to improve the taste by diluting the medicine (if possible) or by offering chewing gum or hard candy immediately after administering the medicine.

Sublingual Administration Drugs given sublingually are placed under the tongue, where they should be retained until they are dissolved and absorbed. The thin epithelium and rich network of capillaries on the underside of the tongue permit both rapid absorption and rapid drug action. There is greater potency than with oral administration, because the drug gains access to the general circulation without initially entering the portal circulation of the liver or being affected by gastric and intestinal enzymes. Many of the same effects apply to buccal administration, whereby a tablet is held in the mouth in the pocket between the gums and the cheek for local dissolution and absorption.

The number of drugs that can be given sublingually is limited (e.g., nitroglycerin tablets). The drug must dissolve readily and the client must be able to cooperate. The client must understand that the drug is not to be swallowed and that taking a drink or falling asleep must be avoided until the drug has been absorbed. However, usually little harm is

---

BOX 5-7 MEDICATIONS THAT SHOULD NOT BE CRUSHED

The following is a partial listing of drugs that should not be crushed.* It is suggested that if a liquid dosage form of the medication is available, it should be used instead of a crushed tablet whenever possible. In general, coated tablets should not be crushed because the coating has been applied for a specific reason, such as (1) to prevent stomach irritation (e.g., Dulco-lax Tablet); (2) to prevent destruction by stomach acids (e.g., Ananase); (3) to produce a prolonged or extended effect (e.g., Dimetapp); or (4) to avoid an unwanted reaction (e.g., chloral

hydrated in capsule has a very bitter taste and Povan tablets will stain the mouth red; Kaon tablets may produce a burning effect on sensitive mucosa).

Do not crush drugs that have the following as part of their trade names: Sequel (sustained release), Spansule (sustained release), CR (controlled release), CRT (controlled-release tablet), LA (long acting), SR (sustained release), TR (time release), TD (time delay), SA (sustained action), XL (extended release), or XR (extended release).

Allegra-D	Depakene	Feosol tablet	Norpace CR
ASA Enseals	Depakote	Flomax	OxyContin
Azulfidine EN-tabs	Diamox Sequels	Isordil sublingual	Pentasa
Bisacodyl (various)	Donnatal Extentab	Kaon tablet	Prevacid
Cipro	Drixoral	Lithobid	Prilosec
Claritin D	Dulcolax tablet	Motrin tablet	Prozac
Colace	Ecotrin tablet	Nexium	Slow K tablet
Compazine Spansule	E-Mycin tablet	Nitroglycerin tablet	Sudafed 12-hour capsule

*Data from *Drug facts and comparisons*. (2005) (58th ed.). St. Louis: Facts and Comparisons.

done if a sublingual drug is inadvertently swallowed; the effects may be neutralized or delayed slightly.

Rectal Administration

Rectal administration of certain preparations can be used advantageously when the stomach is nonretentive or traumatized, when the medicine has an objectionable taste or odor, or when the medicine can be changed by digestive enzymes. It is also a reasonably convenient and safe method of giving drugs when the oral method is unsuitable, such as when the individual is either a small child (or infant) or is unconscious. Rectal administration is contraindicated if the anal area is irritated or if diarrhea, rectal bleeding, or hemorrhoids are present. It is also not typically used for drugs that require precise plasma levels since absorption via this site is more variable than oral administration.

Use of the rectal route avoids irritation of the upper GI tract and may promote higher bloodstream drug titers because venous blood from the lower part of the rectum does not initially traverse the liver before entering the general circulation. The suppository is often superior to the retention enema because with the suppository the drug is released at a slow but steady rate to ensure a protracted effect. One disadvantage of the retention enema is unpredictable retention of the drug; another is that some of the fluid may pass above the lower rectum and be absorbed into the portal circulation. Administering an evacuant enema before administering a rectal medication is usually advisable to ensure that there is no fecal bulk in the rectum to obstruct free flow of the medicated enema or the action of a suppository. The amount of solution that can be given rectally is usually small.

Refrigerated suppositories will soften and cannot be inserted if they are handled or carried in the pocket for even a brief period. Cold running water will restore rigidity to suppositories. To be retained for effective therapy, suppositories and enema tubing must be inserted beyond the internal anal sphincter (2 to 3 inches). The dose of a drug in suppository form cannot be divided by cutting the suppository in sections because the active drug constituent may not be evenly distributed throughout the suppository.

Parenteral Administration

Strictly speaking, parenteral administration means administration by any route other than oral and thus can technically be defined to include topical or inhalation administration. In practical usage, however, parenteral usually means administration by the use of a needle.

Parenteral administration of drugs includes all forms of drug injection into body tissues or fluids using a syringe and needle or catheter and container. Drugs given parenterally must be sterile, readily soluble and absorbable, and relatively nonirritating. Because the parenteral administration of drugs can be hazardous, several precautions are required: (1) aseptic technique must be used to avoid infection, and (2) accurate drug dose, proper rate of injection, and proper site of injection are essential to avoid harm such as lipodystrophy (atrophy or hypertrophy of subcutaneous fat tissue), abscesses, necrosis, skin slough, nerve injuries, prolonged pain, or periostitis. *An injected drug is irretrievable*, and an error in dose or method or site of injection is not easily corrected.

There are several differences between drugs given parenterally and drugs administered orally. The following is true of parenteral drugs: (1) the onset of drug action is more rapid (except as noted previously), (2) the dosage is often smaller because of the lack of a hepatic first-pass effect, and (3) the cost of drug therapy may be greater. Parenteral administration requires specialized knowledge, aseptic technique, and manual skill to ensure safety and therapeutic effectiveness. The nurse may perform most methods of parenteral administration, but some are usually performed only by a physician or other health care provider with advanced educational preparation. The nurse should know and adhere to agency policy. Clients and family members may also learn to administer injections.

If an injection is likely to sting or hurt, it is honest to tell the client beforehand. The client who is told is also more likely to deal with the pain more effectively than one who is not told. It is better to tell a child just before the injection rather than much beforehand so there is little time for the child to anticipate and grow anxious, thereby actually increasing the pain.

As the administration of the various parenteral injections is a nursing skill, the reader is referred to a text in fundamentals of nursing or a text on nursing skills for techniques for the psychomotor component of these techniques.

Intradermal Injection

An intradermal or intracutaneous injection is made into the upper layers of the skin, almost parallel to the skin surface. The amount of drug given is small, and absorption is slow. This method is advantageous in testing for allergic reactions and for giving small amounts of a local anesthetic. In a test for allergic reactions, minute amounts of the solution to be tested are injected just under the outer layers of the skin. The medial surface of the forearm and the skin of the back are commonly used sites. These injections are best made with a fine, short needle (26- or 27-gauge) and a small-barrel syringe (such as a tuberculin syringe).

Subcutaneous Injection

Small amounts of drug in solution are given subcutaneously into the fat pads of the abdomen, the outer surface of the upper arm, the anterior surface of the thigh or, occasionally, the lower abdominal surface for drugs such as heparin and insulin. In these locations there are fewer large blood vessels, and sensation is less keen than on the medial surfaces of the extremities. Massaging the part after injection tends to increase the rate of absorption but should be avoided after the injection of certain drugs (e.g., heparin) to minimize bruising as the drug spreads through the tissues. Subcutaneously injected medicines are limited to drugs that are highly soluble and nonirritating and to solutions of limited volume (ideally no more than 1 mL).

Irritating drugs given subcutaneously can result in the formation of sterile abscesses and necrotic tissue, especially if injections are made repeatedly in the same site. Care should be exercised to avoid contamination and to rotate sites. Subcutaneous injections are not effective in individuals with sluggish peripheral circulation (e.g., the client in shock).

Intramuscular Injection When a drug is too irritating to be given subcutaneously, deeper injections are made into muscular tissue, through the skin and subcutaneous tissue. However, irritation may occur with some drugs given intramuscularly. Larger doses can be given with IM injection, up to 5 mL. The deltoid can readily absorb up to 2 mL of drug. The gluteals and vastus lateralis are preferred for many IM injections because of fewer nerve endings and less discomfort at this site. The needle must be long enough to avoid depositing the drug into the subcutaneous or fatty tissue. The depth of insertion depends on the amount of subcutaneous tissue and varies with the weight of the client. IM absorption of drugs is delayed in circulatory collapse (e.g., shock states); in such cases the IV route should be chosen.

A drug may be given intramuscularly in an aqueous solution, an aqueous suspension, or a solution or suspension of oil. Suspensions form a depot of drug in the tissue, and slow, gradual absorption usually results; this allows the drug to act over a longer period of time. Few drugs are formulated in oil. Two disadvantages are sometimes encountered when preparations in oil are used: (1) the client may be sensitive to the oil, or (2) the oil may not be absorbed. In the latter case, incision and drainage of the oil may be necessary.

To prevent local postinjection complications (e.g., discomfort, scars, abscesses), no two injections should be made in the same spot during a course of treatment. Injection sites should be rotated, and the site for each IM injection should be recorded on the clinical record.

Intravenous Injection/Intravenous Infusion When an immediate effect is desired, when for any reason a drug cannot be injected into other tissues, or when absorption may be inhibited by poor circulation, the drug may be given directly into a vein as an intravenous **injection** (the act of forcing a liquid into the body by means of a syringe) or as an intravenous **infusion** (the introduction of a substance directly into a vein by means of gravity flow). The terms *injection* and *infusion* also refer to the substances so administered. These methods require skill and asepsis, and the drugs used in these methods must be highly soluble and capable of withstanding sterilization.

These methods are of great value in emergencies. Additionally, the dose and amount of absorption can be determined with accuracy. However, the rapidity of absorption and the fact that there is no recall once the drug has been given are dangers worthy of consideration. From this standpoint it is one of the least safe methods of administration. Precautions must be taken to prevent extravasation, or leakage, of the drug or fluids into surrounding tissue (**infiltration**).

With an IV injection ("IV push"), a comparatively small amount of solution (also referred to as a bolus) is given by means of a syringe into IV tubing, into a heparin lock, or

directly into a vein over a 1- to 7-minute period. Before injection, the drug is dissolved in a suitable amount of normal (physiologic) saline solution or some other isotonic solution. An IV bolus dose is the method of choice for rapidly administering drugs in an emergency because it is a reliable way to achieve optimal drug blood levels rapidly. It is also the way to administer certain IV medications that may be incompatible in solution: digoxin (Lanoxin), diazepam (Valium), furosemide (Lasix), diazoxide (Hyperstat), certain anticancer drugs, and diagnostic agents in dye form. Many drugs given intravenously must be given slowly to avoid cardiac, neurologic, otic, or respiratory changes. It is necessary for the nurse to know the appropriate IV dosage rate to avoid a potentially fatal problem.

With an IV infusion a larger amount of fluid is given (usually to adults), starting with 1 L. The solution flows by gravity from a graduated glass bottle or plastic bag through tubing, a connecting tip, and a needle or catheter into a vein, or it may be infused with an IV controller or pump.

There are many infusion pumps and controllers on the market, and manufacturers produce new models frequently. Infusion controllers are useful in 80% to 85% of cases calling for IV therapy. They work simply by using the force of gravity. Controllers are not capable of delivering rates with the accuracy of infusion pumps in special situations in which increases in back pressure are transmitted to the fluid in the tubing (e.g., arterial infusions, a restless child, a woman in labor). However, unlike infusion pumps, infusion controllers will not pump fluid into interstitial tissue if the infusion needle infiltrates.

There are at least two types of infusion pumps, both of which deliver infusion fluids under positive pressure: (1) nonvolumetric ("infusion pumps"), which measure fluid volume delivery by drop rate (not as accurate because drop volume may vary); and (2) volumetric ("volume pumps"), which can measure very precisely even smaller volumes of infusion solution by milliliter per hour. This latter pump is especially useful for small children, total parenteral nutrition, and the administration of potent drugs by continuous IV infusion (such as streptokinase, dopamine, or nitroglycerin). Alarm readout messages (e.g., "fix me") may be displayed on the front panel of the instrument.

IV infusions are most commonly given to relieve tissue dehydration, to restore depleted blood volumes, to dilute toxic substances in the blood and tissue fluids, to supply electrolytes or drugs, to provide an IV line if an emergency is anticipated, or to provide a fluid challenge to evaluate kidney function.

The fluid is usually given slowly to prevent a reaction or fluid overload, which may impair cardiac or pulmonary function, especially in older adults or in those with cardiac disease. Eight hours are usually required for every 1000 mL of fluid, depending on the condition of the client and the nature of and reason for the solution. This rate is slower in children, or may be more rapid in critical care clients and is determined by age, weight, and urinary output.

A number of commercial solutions are used in IV replacement therapy. Some solutions contain not only salts of sodium and potassium but also salts of calcium and magnesium. Vitamins are also added to IV fluids when necessary. (See Chapters 68 and 69 for a discussion of various IV infusion solutions including parenteral nutrition and, and Chapter 30 for a discussion of blood products.)

Some drugs, such as antibiotics, are administered by intermittent infusion (known as "IV piggyback" [IVPB] or "IV rider" in some parts of the United States). They are given via a setup that is secondary to the primary IV infusion and hung in tandem and connected to the primary setup. Most intermittent diluted drug infusions are meant to have a total infusion time of 20 or 30 minutes to 1 hour, depending on factors such as the amount of diluent required and the potential for vein wall irritation by the drug.

The presence of particulate matter (which can consist of tiny chunks of rubber stoppers or glass slivers from ampules) in IV infusion solutions is disturbingly common. Such matter can be introduced during manufacture, during changing of the solution bottle, or during administration of a medication. The resulting potential for phlebitis is high. Therefore it is recommended that in-line filtering devices be used for all IV therapy. Optimal filtration is provided by 0.22-micrometer filters; most organisms, except certain strains of *Pseudomonas* and the viruses, are filtered out by 0.45-micrometer in-line filters. To prevent the injection of larger particles, disposable needles with 5-micrometer filters can be used to draw medication up.

Central venous infusion is the administration of fluid through an IV catheter placed in a central vein. The catheter tip rests in the superior vena cava if the subclavian vein and internal and external jugular veins are cannulated; the catheter tip rests in the inferior vena cava if the femoral vein is cannulated. With peripheral central venous therapy, the central catheter is inserted in a peripheral vein, usually the basilic or cephalic vein, and the distal end of the catheter rests in the superior vena cava. Central venous infusion is used when poor venous access prohibits the use of peripheral veins or when irritating solutions must be infused directly into a large central vein to avoid phlebitis. Central IV devices are inserted by physicians for either short-term or long-term use. For short-term use, the central venous catheter has multiple lumens to allow simultaneous administration of more than one solution. Catheters for long-term use are more flexible and less thrombogenic but must be surgically implanted. These catheters are for long-term central access for the infusion of fluids, antibiotics, parenteral nutrition, chemotherapy, and home IV therapy.

Epidural Injection Epidural analgesia is being used increasingly for the management of acute and chronic pain. For this route of drug administration, the physician implants an epidural catheter beneath the client's skin with its tip in the epidural space, which lies just outside the subarachnoid space in which the CSF circulates. The drug bypasses the blood-brain barrier and diffuses into the CSF. This route of administration works well for opioid analgesics such as morphine, fentanyl (Sublimaze), and hydromorphone (Dilaudid), administered either by IV bolus dose or by continuous infusion because opioid receptors are found along the spinal cord, which allows the drugs to produce localized analgesia without loss of motor function. Once the epidural catheter is in place, the nurse is responsible for monitoring the infusion and the client's status relative to it.

Intrathecal Injection Intrathecal (into a sheath) injection is also known as intraspinal, subdural, subarachnoid, or lumbar injection. The technique is the same as that required for a lumbar puncture. Nurses do not usually directly administer drugs intraspinally, but they may be required to fill the drug reservoir of an implanted intraspinal delivery system. The nurse needs to be specially trained, and the manufacturer's instructions should be followed closely.

Additionally, drugs are occasionally administered by intracardiac, intrapericardiac, intraventricular, intraperitoneal, intraarticular, and intraosseous injections; however, state regulation and institutional policy may not allow nurses to administer drugs by these routes.

Alternative Drug Delivery Systems Innovative advances in scientific technology and computerization provide impetus for the development of increasingly sophisticated drug delivery systems, particularly in the treatment of diabetes mellitus and cancer. Examples of these technologies include implanted drug deposits and needle-syringe pump assemblies.

Small pumps weighing approximately half a pound are now available as portable infusion systems for continuous drug treatment of certain clients with type I diabetes or cancer. The systems currently approved and in use usually consist of a battery, a programmable electronic "brain," an electric motor and pump, and a syringe, all of which are detachable as a unit from the small needle kept in place either in subcutaneous abdominal or thigh tissue (for diabetes), or by Silastic catheter inserted into an artery supplying the malignant tumor. These programmable pumps allow for various flow rates and have an on and off feature. They appear to be quite efficient for clients with varying clinical needs. Some systems are designed to be worn externally over clothing, stored in a pocket, or suspended from a belt or a neck chain (Figure 5-7). The Quick-set cannula procedure is illustrated in Figure 5-8.

Monitoring

Although evaluation is considered to be the final step of the nursing process, this text presents a cluster of nursing actions to be included in monitoring the client for therapeutic effect and the occurrence of adverse drug reactions. These actions fall within the implementation activities of the nursing process related to drug therapy. The nurse constantly monitors the client to assess the progress toward the outcome criteria for the pharmacologic therapies and to assess the client's response to the pharmacologic interventions. Such monitoring is important, because approximately 30% of hospitalized clients experience an adverse drug effect, and as many as 1.5 million persons are hospitalized because of an adverse drug effect.

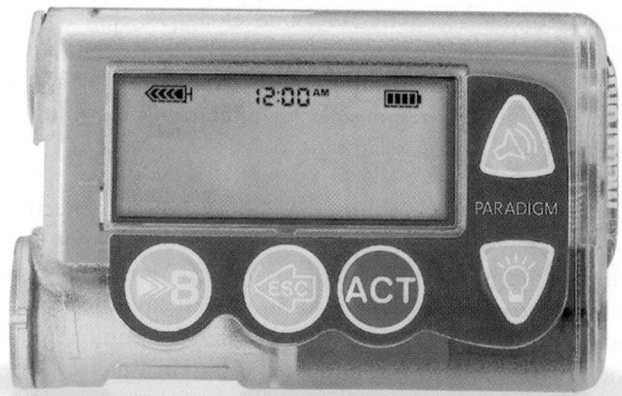

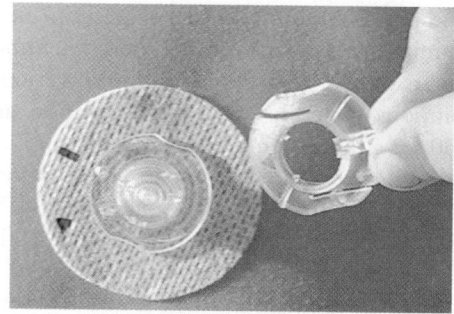

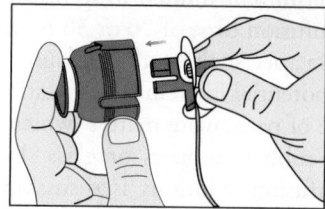

Step 1

FIGURE 5-7 An external insulin pump is the most advanced method for precise and adjustable insulin delivery. Medtronic's "smart" Paradigm insulin pumps simplify diabetes management by calculating precise insulin dosages for clients. The pump also keeps track of insulin used by the body to help clients avoid "insulin stacking," which can cause hypoglycemia. Pump users can deliver insulin at the touch of a few buttons, and insulin is delivered automatically around-the-clock, much like a healthy pancreas. Many clients experience improved quality of life with pump therapy, ridding themselves of multiple injections, strict meal schedules, and rigid sleep patterns. Insulin pump therapy is covered by private insurance, Medicare, and Medicaid. Medtronic Diabetes can be reached at (800) MINIMED.

Courtesy of Medtronic Diabetes, Northridge, CA.

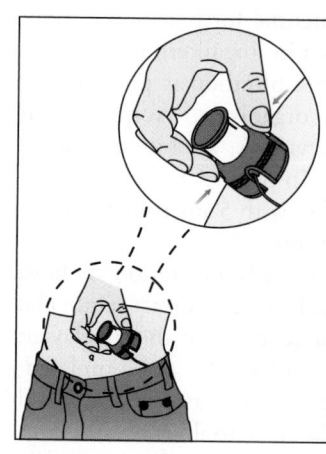

Step 2

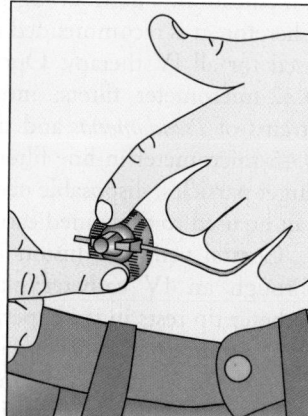

Step 3

Adverse drug effects might be related to an underlying condition of the client (medical condition, age, childbearing status), other drugs that the client might be taking, and adverse effects of the drug itself. These reactions fall into two broad categories. The first of these, type A, has predictability; if the properties of the drug are known, the nurse has a fair idea of the type of reaction that may occur. Most of these reactions relate to the mechanism of action of the drug and are often dose-dependent. Examples of type A reactions are the orthostatic hypotension with volume depletion that can occur with furosemide (Lasix), a powerful diuretic, or the overgrowth of nonsusceptible organisms that can occur with ampicillin, an antibiotic. Type B reactions are not as predictable as type A reactions. Anaphylaxis is a classic example of a type B reaction; it is unusual, unexpected, life-threatening, and occurs even when a normal therapeutic dose is administered.

Early recognition of adverse drug effects is important so that therapy can be altered as quickly as possible to prevent or minimize injury to the client; therapy is altered by decreasing the dosage or discontinuing the drug, administering an antidote or symptomatic treatment, or both. Additionally, the nurse documenting the reaction in the clinical records should alert other caregivers. The client is advised to alert future caregivers and to carry a medical information wallet card or wear a MedicAlert bracelet warning others that he or she has experienced an adverse effect of a specific drug.

Be alert for adverse drug effects if the client evidences clinical or laboratory findings that are not typical of the

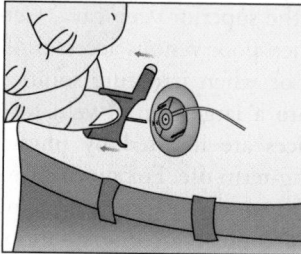

Step 4

FIGURE 5-8 The Quick-set infusion set is a low-profile infusion set with a 90-degree, or "straight-in," soft catheter. The Quick-set comes in 6-mm and 9-mm catheter lengths and two tubing lengths. It disconnects at the infusion site, and a Quick-serter provides optimal placement for insulin absorption.

Courtesy of Medtronic Diabetes, Northridge, CA.

client's disease, if a pathologic sign or symptom occurs at a site that is not involved with the condition being treated, or if a pathologic process occurs that is not in keeping with the condition being treated. If the client exhibits any of these signs or symptoms, review the medication record to see if they are related to one or more of the client's drugs. Issues to be considered in determining causality are: (1) *temporal relationship* (Did the reaction occur at a reasonable time after the drug was administered?); (2) the presence of a positive *dechallenge* (Did the client's reaction diminish or resolve after the drug was discontinued?); (3) the presence of a positive *rechallenge* (Did the client's reaction return when the drug was administered again?); and (4) *lack of a confounding effect* (Can the reaction be explained by a concurrently administered drug or the client's clinical condition?).

Therapeutic drug monitoring requires that the nurse understand the mechanism of action of the drug in relation to the client's health status to clinically determine whether the drug is effective. Monitor clinical indicators at appropriate intervals to assess drug efficacy. For example, in an acute asthmatic episode the nurse monitors vital signs, breath sounds, skin color, sputum, and signs of respiratory dysfunction such as irritability, stridor, nasal flaring, and retractions. A ß₂-agonist drug administered as a bronchodilator is evaluated as effective if respiratory and pulse rate decrease toward a more normal rate and if the client experiences less wheezing and irritability, is relaxed, and expends less effort with the respiratory process. Other signs of respiratory dysfunction also diminish within minutes. In another example, hemoglobin concentration should increase by approximately 0.1 g/dL daily within 2 weeks of starting oral iron therapy for iron deficiency anemia in a client who is not actively bleeding.

Therapeutic drug monitoring may entail determining blood drug levels to determine effective drug dosages and to prevent adverse effects related to toxicity. This is particularly important with drugs such as cardiotonics, antiepileptic drugs, and others, in which the margin of safety within the therapeutic range is narrow. Blood samples may be obtained at the drug's peak level (the highest concentration) and/or at the trough/residual level (the lowest concentration) after a steady state of the drug has been reached in the client. Steady state is generally reached after four to five half-lives of a drug. Peak levels are useful when testing for toxicity, and trough levels are useful to demonstrate the maintenance of a satisfactory therapeutic level. Different laboratories use different units for reporting test results and normal ranges, and often recommend specific times for obtaining samples in relation to drug dosing depending on drug and goals of monitoring. Careful documentation of the precise time the drug was last administered or ingested and the time of the laboratory test is critical for clinicians to accurately interpret drug levels.

Some drugs have organ-specific or system-specific adverse or toxic effects, or potential complications, to which the nurse should be particularly alert:

- *Hepatotoxicity.* Clients receiving drugs that have the potential complication of hepatotoxicity need to be monitored for symptoms of hepatic dysfunction such as anorexia, indigestion, malaise, jaundice, petechiae, ecchymoses, dark urine, clay-colored stools, and increased bleeding tendencies. There is little evidence that drug-induced liver damage can be diagnosed routinely by performing frequent liver function studies before symptoms develop. Liver function tests (serum bilirubin, ALP, ALT, AST, LDH) or a PT test may be ordered as part of a baseline assessment before the drug regimen is started or if clinical symptoms of hepatic dysfunction appear.
- *Nephrotoxicity.* On the other hand, the development of drug-induced nephrotoxicity is usually subtle, and kidney damage may occur before symptoms such as insufficient urine output (less than 30 mL/hr), elevated blood pressure, and dependent edema become evident. When a nephrotoxic drug is given in higher doses or for prolonged periods, routine urinalyses and serum creatinine determinations are helpful in the early detection of toxicity. (See Chapter 35 for formulas for estimating renal impairment from serum creatinine.)
- *Blood dyscrasias.* Many drugs cause blood dyscrasias, a pathologic condition in which any of the constituents of the blood are abnormal in structure, function, or quality. This condition may be caused by a hemolytic effect, in which there is premature destruction of the red blood cells. It may also be caused by bone marrow depression that results in the decreased manufacture and maturation of RBCs, most WBCs, and platelets. Some drugs inhibit platelet aggregation, putting the client at risk for bleeding. In addition to monitoring the client's hematology laboratory reports for these abnormalities, the nurse must have astute assessment skills. Anemia is evidenced by lower than normal levels of hemoglobin, hematocrit, and RBCs, and by a change in the size and hemoglobin content of the RBCs; it may also be noted by fatigue, exertional dyspnea, dizziness, headache, insomnia, pallor, confusion, and cardiac changes in the later stages. Leukopenia, an abnormal decrease in WBCs to fewer than 5000/cm³, is evidenced by fatigue, pallor, weight loss, easy bruising, fever, bone or joint pain, and repeated infections. Thrombocytopenia, a reduction in the number of platelets, may be evidenced as bleeding from small capillaries, such as easy bruising, bleeding gums, nosebleeds, hematuria, melena, or rectal bleeding.
- *Hypotension.* Some drugs, particularly the antihypertensives and CNS depressants, also cause hypotension. This may be evidenced as an abnormally low blood pressure when a client assumes a standing posture. Having the client come to an upright position in slow stages may prevent this effect. Lying, sitting, and standing blood pressures help in monitoring the client's vasomotor status.
- *Electrolyte imbalances.* Some drugs affect electrolyte balances, particularly potassium, which results in either hypokalemia or hyperkalemia. This may occur because the drug contains potassium or because it affects the excretion of potassium, either enhancing its loss from the body or causing it to be retained or spared. Monitor both the serum electrolytes and the

clinical symptoms of the appropriate electrolyte imbalance.

- *Neurologic effects.* There are many adverse neurologic effects of drugs. Some drugs cause CNS depression, which results in dizziness, drowsiness, hypotension, and confusion and progresses to respiratory depression, coma, and death. Other drugs cause CNS stimulation, resulting in nausea, nervousness, tremor, tachycardia, extra systoles, increased blood pressure, diuresis, and visual disturbances. In addition to the drugs known as anticholinergics, many other drugs have antimuscarinic effects. This means the client should be monitored for dry mouth, constipation, urinary retention, confusion, and delirium. Adverse neurologic effects may also be peripheral; drugs with this effect are said to be neurotoxic. The early signs of such peripheral neuropathy are paresthesia (tingling, a "pins and needles" feeling, numbness), motor weakness, limb pain, and decreased deep tendon reflexes. Ototoxicity is the result of a drug's harmful effect on the eighth cranial nerve or on the organs of hearing and balance. The loss of hearing may be reversible or irreversible, and ataxia may also occur.

Remain vigilant in the ongoing monitoring of the client's health status by direct observation and by evaluation of laboratory and diagnostic tests in relation to drug therapy.

Client Education

Updating clients, keeping them informed about their treatment, and providing other necessary information should be an ongoing activity that occurs naturally during any interaction with clients. In any nursing process, teaching should be a part of the plan. The plan may be formal (e.g., a diabetic teaching program), or it may be a simple impromptu discussion based on a question raised by the client.

A strong rationale for teaching clients comes from the many state nurse practice acts that define teaching as a necessary part of nursing, thereby giving it the power of a state mandate: one could be sued for not teaching clients. Although teaching-learning interactions between the client and nurse are among the most necessary and professionally demanding, teaching clients is not as visible as bathing them, measuring their vital signs, or giving them injections. Consequently, teaching may not be seen as important enough to be noted in nursing progress notes. Accreditation agencies, such as the Joint Commission on Accreditation of Healthcare Organizations (JCAHO), recognize the importance of client teaching and look for such documentation during their inspection visits to evaluate agencies that provide health care.

Successful client learning has a direct bearing on successful convalescence at home. Clients need to learn the following about their medications: the names of the medications (should be written down), what they are for, how to recognize the proper effects (in very specific ways), some of the major secondary effects (those that are expected and tolerable, and those that represent toxicity), which symptoms require prescriber notification, ways to prevent or minimize adverse effects, what to do if they miss a dose, how to store the medication, how to take it (e.g., with meals), and whom to call if there is a problem. Clients can be expected to forget many of the instructions; a printed fact sheet or checklist to take home will be helpful to many clients and should augment the verbal explanation. (See Chapter 10 for further discussion of this essential role of nursing.)

Documentation of Drug Administration

Recording the administration of each dose of medication as soon as possible after it is given provides a documented record if there is any question regarding whether the client received the dose. If the administration is not documented, the client may inadvertently receive a second dose from another nurse or nursing student. The busy nurse who "double-pours" (prepares two doses at one time—a "sloppy" practice) may also be tempted to record the second dose at the same time the first dose is recorded. Do not record (chart) medications before they are actually given because something may occur to prevent that dose from being administered; as a result, the client would go unmedicated. The medication record, which is a legal document, would need to be corrected carefully and an incident report filed.

Several different forms are used to record the medications for each client. These forms usually include areas to note each medication's name, date, dose, route, and time of administration, and the initials of the administering nurse (see Figure 5-6). Extra notations may be added in certain instances. For example, when digoxin is given, the apical and radial pulses taken just before administration are noted (e.g., "AP, 78; RP, 76"). If the pulses are found to be outside the normal limits established by that agency, the medication should not be given, the record should be marked "held" and initialed, and the prescriber should be consulted. Clients also have the right to refuse treatment, including medications; despite teaching and counseling, they sometimes do. "Refused" is then noted in the appropriate spot on the medication record, with the reason for the client's refusal. A newer term for refusal being used in some agencies is "declined." A medication may also be recorded as "discarded" or "wasted" if only part of it was administered and the rest had to be discarded (as in a prefilled syringe), or if the medication was dropped or contaminated. If the medication is a controlled substance, its reason for disposal must be documented and fully witnessed; the signatures of two nurses are required on the controlled substance record.

Routine (or continuous) daily medications are recorded on the MAR. Once-only, loading doses, PRN medications, and stat medications should be recorded on the same MAR. Administration of a controlled substance is recorded both on the MAR and on that particular drug's control sheet in the "narcotic book," which includes a running tally of the balance of the controlled substance. A notation is made in the progress notes of the client's chart relating to the assessment of the need for any PRN medication and the evaluation of the client's response to the PRN medication at an appropriate time interval.

The potential for error in drug administration is almost limitless (see also Chapter 4). Some significant mistakes can be rectified if discovered and acted on quickly. Courts tend to look more kindly on the nurse if an error is properly reported and the appropriate actions are taken. Courts generally recognize that nurses are human and that there is the potential for error in clinical practice.

Evaluation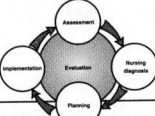

Evaluation of goals follows and, depending on the specific outcomes of care, most often relates to some aspect of drug effects. For individual clients, measure the outcomes and compare them with the criteria in the goals that were written during the planning phase. Broader evaluation is performed through continuous quality initiative committees that critique the quality of nursing care administered to groups of clients and individuals. To perform all functions of the nursing process, nurses must have strong interpersonal, cognitive, and psychomotor skills. Nursing actions are the product of foundational work in the psychosocial, biologic, and physical sciences.

Evaluation, the final step in the nursing process, facilitates the delivery of high-quality nursing care in regard to pharmacotherapeutics. Although planning nursing care and establishing goals, the nurse determines what type of evaluation will occur and when and how it will be performed. Clear and specifically stated goals or outcome criteria make it easy to determine whether the intended outcomes have been achieved or to what degree they have been achieved. Evaluation includes both subjective and objective data. When evaluating nursing care for a client undergoing drug therapy, look at the nursing outcomes and other outcome criteria for the specific nursing diagnoses/collaborative problems. In general, an evaluation of drug therapy includes the following areas:

- Therapeutic response to the drug
- Nontherapeutic responses to the drug, such as adverse effects related to the administered drug itself, the client's health status, or concurrent drug therapy
- Level of client's knowledge related to the medication regimen
- Client's ability to manage the therapeutic regimen (self-medication)

In evaluating a therapeutic response, it is necessary to have a clear understanding of the therapeutic goals. Evaluation may center on a reduction of symptoms, decreased frequency of recurrences, enhanced organ function, elimination of infection, or a multitude of other goals. Clinical observation of the client and monitoring of the appropriate laboratory studies are essential. Evaluation examines a drug's therapeutic response but is also directed toward detecting any response that may be attributed to the drug.

The outcome criteria to be evaluated may also relate to the absence of any adverse effects. An awareness of the pharmacology of the drug used and any potential effects guides this evaluation. For example, outcome criteria related to the therapeutic response for the antiepileptic drug phenytoin (Dilantin) are that the client will demonstrate the following: (1) an absence of or decrease in the frequency or severity of seizures, (2) maintenance of therapeutic serum levels of the drug, and (3) an absence of adverse effects such as ataxia, slurred speech, mental confusion, drowsiness, nystagmus, diplopia, or gingival hyperplasia.

Determine also if educational goals are being met. Often, clients can report back what they have been told yet remain unable to apply this knowledge. Asking hypothetical questions and observing return demonstrations are helpful techniques for evaluating learning. Examples of outcome criteria for client teaching are that the client will do the following:

- State the correct name of the medication
- Identify the medication by its color and shape
- Describe the therapeutic purpose of the medication
- Describe the common adverse effects and how to minimize them
- Identify at least three adverse effects to the drug for which consultation should be immediately sought with the prescriber or other health care professional
- List other drugs that have the potential to interact with the medication
- Demonstrate the proper administration of the medication
- Demonstrate any monitoring techniques associated with the drug, for example, pulse and blood pressure measurements and daily weights

Additionally, evaluate whether the client can effectively manage the therapeutic medication regimen in the home environment. Effective management of the therapeutic regimen refers to following the prescribed regimen correctly. This means that, in addition to the outcome criteria for educational goals, the client will do the following:

- State an intent to practice the self-medication behaviors needed to recover from the illness and prevent a recurrence or complications
- Report less anxiety related to fear of the unknown, fear of loss of control, or misconceptions about his or her medications
- Describe the disease process, causes and factors contributing to symptoms, and the medication regimen for disease and symptom control
- Describe strategies to address complications of the medication regimen should they arise
- Discuss situations that can challenge continued successful management of the medication regimen

Research indicates that at least one fourth of all outpatients fail to follow their prescribed drug therapy correctly. The inability to accomplish any of the previously mentioned outcome criteria indicates ineffective management of the therapeutic regimen. Other behaviors might also be indicators:

- Does the client or family/caregiver continue to speak of nonparticipation in the regimen?
- Have partially used or unused prescriptions been observed?
- Is there persistence or progression of the underlying condition even though the regimen prescribed is an appropriate one?
- Have undesired effects of the drug gone unreported to the health care provider?

In addition to the evaluation by the individual nurse or nursing team of the client's progress toward the goals and expected outcomes of nursing care, health care agencies evaluate the process of medication administration as an important aspect of nursing care provided by that agency. Standards by which to evaluate care are developed from within the health care organization and may also be suggested by external organizations, such as JCAHO. JCAHO is an organization whose mission is to continuously improve the safety and quality of care provided to the public through the provision of health care accreditation and related services that support performance improvement in health care organizations (www.jcaho.org). Within the JCAHO standards for nursing services regarding policies and procedures, guidelines are set forth concerning medication administration; this is done in an effort to ensure safe nursing practice. These guidelines stipulate that the nursing department or service of a health care organization have policies and procedures to govern medication administration and that these should specify, in accordance with applicable law and regulation and pertinent medical staff rules and regulations, who may give orders for drugs; who may accept verbal orders for drugs and when the orders must be authenticated by the prescribing practitioner; who may verify orders for drugs and how this must occur; who may supervise the administration of medications; and who may administer these medications, which medications they may administer, and how these individuals are to be supervised, if necessary. These policies and procedures serve to protect both the client and the nurse by stating the roles and responsibilities of all members of the health care team for the administration of medications. Nursing practice can then be evaluated to determine whether the care provided to clients was in keeping with the policies and procedures of the agency.

The following are suggested indicators for evaluating the administration of medications as part of the nursing quality monitoring process, which may also be known as Total Quality Management (TQM) or Continuous Quality Improvement (CQI):

- The drug is administered in the ordered dose.
- The drug is administered by the ordered route.
- The drug is administered by the ordered site.
- The drug is administered at the ordered rate.
- The drug is administered in the ordered drug form.
- The drug is administered by the ordered schedule.
- The drug is administered using the correct technique.

These indicators may be incorporated into a process of monitoring and evaluation by which nursing professionals examine the care they provide, determine possibilities for improvement of their practice, and take necessary action.

Summary

Nursing process is an appropriate framework for the nurse's role in safely and effectively administering medications and teaching clients to effectively manage their therapeutic regimens.

Professional nurses enhance their decision-making skills by critically reviewing their clients' medication plans and maintaining a strong knowledge base about medications and their indications, mechanisms of action, pharmacokinetics, pharmacodynamics, and dosages.

The quality of nursing assessment relies on the nurse's ability to observe significant cues, to make sound inferences, and to recognize the client's individuality and establish rapport. Thus a nurse can develop a valid diagnosis, establish realistic goals with the client, and formulate an effective nursing plan.

Medication administration is a highly visible, legal function of nurses. Because it depends heavily on the structure and content of a prescriber's orders, conscientious assessment of the drug order becomes a very healthy habit. Professional accountability for all disciplines demands open collaboration on questions about clients' medication orders and plans. Underlying the routine of assessing medication therapy is the major goal of preventing harm. Assessment should emphasize protecting the client from receiving drugs that will complicate a preexisting health condition; will interact, be incompatible, or evoke an allergic response; will not be metabolized or excreted adequately; or will be transferred to a fetus or nursing infant. Creative nursing consists of finding ways to reschedule or space intervals between doses of interactive drugs. Allergic reactions, if anticipated, are usually grounds for a prescriber's decision to change drugs. However, it is often the nurse who notes the offending allergenic substance via a client's history and other data. Again, effective nursing assessment can improve compliance, enhance therapeutic outcomes, and avoid negative secondary effects.

The nursing assessment culminates in the identification of nursing diagnoses (actual, at risk, wellness, or possible) and collaborative problems as potential complications. Although any number of issues is possible within nursing pharmacotherapeutics, eight nursing diagnoses must be considered with every medication to be administered:

1. Risk nursing diagnoses related to the client's preexisting medical conditions, age, and childbearing status
2. Risk nursing diagnoses related to concurrent drug therapy
3. Risk nursing diagnoses related to the client's underlying condition secondary to the ineffectiveness of the drug
4. Risk nursing diagnoses related to the adverse effects of the administered drug
5. Risk for poisoning: drug toxicity

6. Deficient knowledge related to initiation of or change in the medication regimen
7. Noncompliance (specify)
8. Ineffective therapeutic regimen management (individual or family)

Interventions by the nurse to address identified problems may involve collaborative interventions with physicians and other health care providers or interventions that are solely the domain of nurses. Problems falling within the independent nursing domain are best described by the nursing diagnosis, which is a concise statement of a problem that is uniquely addressed by nurses. The potential complications of the pharmacotherapeutic regimen are generally seen as collaborative problems.

After the identification of problems and the formulation of nursing diagnoses and collaborative problems, goals in the form of nursing outcomes and other outcome criteria are established. A specific plan is developed to direct nursing care toward meeting all of the outcomes. The development of goals, and clear planning, form the basis for implementing and evaluating nursing care.

The implementation phase of the nursing process regarding drug therapy begins when the nurse acts to attain the established goals. Nursing interventions are directed at the actual administration of drugs, which includes the preparatory steps and the subsequent recording of drug administration.

The Six Rights of Medication Administration—to ensure the right client, the right medication, the right route, the right dose, the right time, and the right documentation—are reliable criteria for competent, safe, and individualized medication administration. Because nurses are in the position of being on the client care scene and of taking care of clients as no one else does, they are uniquely placed to detect even subtle secondary drug effects, interactions, or incompatibilities.

Evaluation of therapeutic effects and secondary effects, effective management of the prescribed regimen, and client learning follows the implementation phase of the nursing process. This step allows the nurse to determine if nursing outcomes and other outcome criteria were met and measures the effectiveness of nursing care.

✳ Critical Thinking Questions

- As a student, what restrictions are placed on your role in the administration of medications? How will you respond to a prescriber who gives you a verbal order for a medication at the client's bedside?

- You are preparing a client medication with which you are unfamiliar. You search through the drug references on the unit, but information about the drug cannot be found. What actions should you take?

- A hospitalized client expresses curiosity after observing that his medications are administered "in little packages" rather than the "childproof" containers that he is used to receiving from his pharmacy. How would you compare the advantages and disadvantages of the medication delivery systems for your client?

- If one of the adverse effects of the drug you were administering was bone marrow depression, what laboratory results would you monitor to evaluate your client's drug therapy?

- What might be the possible consequences to the client if a client's medication history and medication-taking behaviors are not obtained or are inadequate?

- What nursing actions could be taken to minimize the different types of drug interactions discussed in this text?

- Using information from the drug history of a client, discuss the potential for each of the eight problems within the nursing diagnoses that could be applied to the medications possibly prescribed for that client.

Bibliography

Anderson, D.M., Keith, J., & Novak, P.D. (2002). *Mosby's medical, nursing, & allied health dictionary.* (6th ed.). St. Louis: Mosby.

Brater, D.C. (2004). General principles of drug interactions. *UpToDate, 12*(3).

Carpenito-Moyet, L.J. (2004). *Nursing diagnosis: Application to clinical practice* (10th ed.). Philadelphia: Lippincott, Williams & Wilkins.

Ellis, J.A., et al. (2002). Pain in hospitalized pediatric patients. How are we doing? *Clinical Journal of Pain, 18*, 262-269.

e-LEARNING SUPPLEMENTS

Student CD-ROM
- Final Exam questions
- NCLEX Examination review questions
- Pharmacology animations
- Printable chapter summary

Evolve Website (http://evolve.elsevier.com/mckenry)
- Case study on medication administration and calculation
- Content updates, including information on new drugs
- WebLinks corresponding to this chapter
- Answers to the critical thinking questions in this chapter
- *Elsevier ePharmacology Update* newsletter
- Mosby's Drug Consult Internet Edition
- Supplemental and reference information

Glajchen, M. (2001). Chronic pain: Treatment barriers and strategies for clinical practice, *Journal of the American Board of Family Practitioners, 14*(3), 178-183.

Glover, D.D., Rybeck, B.F., & Tracy, T.S. (2004). Medication use in a rural gynecologic population: Prescription, over-the-counter, and herbal medicines. *American Journal of Obstetrics and Gynecology, 190*(2), 351-357.

Katzung, B.G. (2004). *Basic & clinical pharmacology.* (9th ed.). Stamford, CT: Appleton & Lange.

Lowenthal, D.T., & Parnetti, L. (1996). Drug-food interaction: real, problematic, and potentially harmful. *Consultant, 36*(10), 2149-2152.

Michigan Department of Environmental Quality. (2004). *A remedy for prescription drug disposal.* Lansing, MI: Author.

Mosby's drug consult. (15th ed.) (2005). St Louis: Mosby.

North American Nursing Diagnosis Association. (2002). *Nursing diagnoses: Definitions and classification 2003-2004.* Philadelphia: Author.

Ogden, S.J. (2003). *Calculation of drug dosages* (7th ed.). St. Louis: Mosby.

Stoehr, G.P., Ganguli, M., Seaberg, E.C., Echement, D.A., & Bellle, S. (1997). Over-the-counter medication use in an older rural community: the MoVIES Project. *Journal of the American Geriatrics Society, 45*(2), 158-165.

USP DI: Drug information for the health care professional. (25th ed.) (2005). Greenwood Village, CO: MICROMEDEX Thomson Healthcare.

USP: Quality review: A publication of the USP practitioners' reporting network. (1999). Retrieved April 23, 2005, from http://www.usp. org/pubs/review/rev040 c.htm

Winstein, S.M., Laux, L.F., Thornby, J.I., Lorimer, R.J., Hill, Jr., C.S., Thorpe, D.M., et al. (2000). Physician's attitudes toward pain and the use of opioid analgesics: Results of a survey from the Texas Cancer Pain Initiative. *Southern Medical Journal, 93*(5), 479-487.

6

BIOCULTURAL ASPECTS OF DRUG THERAPY

CHAPTER FOCUS

Health beliefs and treatment outcome are strongly influenced by a client's biologic and cultural background, ethnic practices, and traditions. Effective caring for clients from different cultural groups requires an understanding of the predominant ethnic-specific influences and an assessment of the individual client to determine how those cultural influences affect health needs. Because nearly 2000 cultures and subcultures exist, it is impossible for the nurse to have a working knowledge of all of them. Additionally, research is bringing to light the pharmacogenetic influences on drug response and disease management within different populations. Nurses and other health care professionals should study the predominant cultural groups in their communities, common illnesses for which there is increased risk for certain cultural groups, and significant pharmacogenetic differences between various ethnic and racial groups. This chapter focuses on certain health beliefs and practices and clinically important biologic differences related to selected cultures and pharmacology.

LEARNING OBJECTIVES	• Explore the influence of cultural beliefs on drug therapy.
	• Identify cultural influences on health care.
	• Describe pharmacogenetics in relation to drug activity in the body.
	• Explain the symbolic meaning of drugs to clients.
	• Identify ethnic differences in response to various drug classifications.
	• Use a checklist in preparing a client for discharge.

▲ KEY TERMS
cultural background, p. 103
health beliefs, p. 103
isoenzyme, p. 113
pharmacogenetics, p. 113
pharmacogenomics, p. 114

The **cultural background** of a client is a set of learned values, beliefs, customs, and behaviors of the client; cultural background influences health beliefs and various practices that relate to pharmacology. **Health beliefs** are perceptions of susceptibility to a disease or condition, the consequences of contracting the disease or condition, the benefits of care and barriers to preventive behavior, and the internal or external stimuli that result in appropriate health behaviors. The health beliefs of an individual influence the management of and response to drug therapy. Some similarities exist across cultures in the way the use of drugs is perceived; a primary goal of the appropriate use of medications is to achieve optimal health. Although most individuals share common views regarding life patterns, significant differences occur in values, beliefs, and attitudes. Clients bring to health settings cultural and psychological differences in perceptions of masculine and feminine roles, in rural and urban backgrounds, in ethnic groups, and in social classes that influence drug use. The literature from transcultural nursing and anthropology (see the Bibliography at the end of this chapter) provides valuable insights into various health care beliefs and practices. However, although culture is an essential mediator in people's health status, culture is not the only factor that shapes us. Other factors including environment, economics, genetics, previous and current health status, and psychosocial factors exert considerable influence on our well-being.

Although the information in this chapter provides some background on the various cultures, it is important to avoid stereotyping.

In addition to ethnic differences, there is a fundamental difference between the health beliefs of health care providers (HCPs) and the health beliefs of clients even within the same ethnic group. Although each person enters the health professions with culture-bound definitions of health and illness, these ideas change as the person is socialized into the "health care provider culture." This creates a schism between the provider and the recipient of health care. Comprehensive and appropriate health care can be provided only if HCPs become more sensitive to the traditional health beliefs and practices of clients (Spector, 2004).

Increased cultural awareness takes on even greater importance when the demographic changes occurring in North America are considered. According to the 2000 United States census, whites comprised 75.1% of the population, a change from 1990 in which whites were 80.3% of the population. The ethnic/racial minorities constituted 16.8% of the population in 1980, 19.7% in 1990, and 24.9% in 2000. The 2000 U.S. census distribution of those minorities by percentage are as follows: Hispanic, 12.5%; black or African American, 12.3%; Asian, 4.2%; and American Indian, and Alaska Native, 1.5% (www.census.gov/prod/www.abs.briefs.html). According to the 2001 census in Canada, the total population was 29,639,030 with the visible minority groups comprising 13.4% of the Canadian population and the aboriginal population being 3.3%. Nine percent of the population in Canada was Asian, 2.2% was black, and 0.7% was Hispanic (www.Statcan.ca/English/Pgdb/demo50 a.htm). As the twenty-first century begins, significant changes are occurring in the population of the U.S. and Canada. The white majority is shrinking proportionately, and the black, Hispanic, Asian, Native American, and Canadian aboriginal populations are growing.

Because of these demographic changes, the nurse's practice will be increasingly concerned with the care of ethnic populations. To meet this challenge, the nurse needs to better understand the different health and illness perspectives of diverse cultural groups and practice culturally competent care. The 1999 findings of the Institute of Medicine's (IOM) Report, *Unequal Treatment: Confronting Racial and Ethnic Disparities in Health Care* (Smedley, Stith, & Nelson, 2002) substantiated that need, because it found that:

- Racial and ethnic disparities in health exist and, because they are associated with worse outcomes in many cases, are unacceptable.
- Racial and ethnic disparities occur in a historic and contemporary social and economic inequality, and this discrimination exists in health care.
- Many sources (e.g., health systems, HCPs, clients, utilization managers) may contribute to these disparities.
- Bias, stereotyping, prejudice, and clinical uncertainty on the part of HCPs may contribute to racial and ethnic disparities in health care (Smedley, Stith, & Nelson, 2002).

Although the IOM provided many strategies and recommendations, four are relevant to the content of this chapter: increasing HCPs' awareness of disparities; supporting the appropriate use of interpreters; implementing client education programs to increase clients' knowledge of how to best access care and actively participate in treatment decisions; and integrating cross-cultural education into the education of all current and future health care professionals (Smedley, Stith, & Nelson, 2002). *Healthy People 2010,* a health planning document for the United States, was developed with the expertise of 350 national organizations and 250 public health, mental health, substance abuse, and environmental agencies, has two major goals. The first goal is to increase the quality and years of healthy life of people living in the United States, but also to eliminate health disparities among people of color.

Despite Canada's accomplishments in the field of health promotion, this country, like many other developed nations, also continues to have large disparities in health. These disparities were highlighted in the 1999 *Statistical Report on the Health of Canadians.* It demonstrated that Canada's aboriginal people are at higher risk than the Canadian population as a whole for poor health and early death, and strategies and recommendations for change were proposed in *Toward a Healthy Future* by the Public Health Agency of Canada.

This chapter discusses the nurse's role with clients' drug regimens to assist in minimizing some of these disparities in health care by examining the biocultural aspects of drug therapy. Administering medications effectively and teaching clients self-administration requires an understanding of the predominant cultural influences within the community, assessment of the individual client to determine how these factors influence health needs, and the communication of culturally appropriate interventions. Measuring outcomes of drug regimens requires an understanding of pharmacogenetics of various ethnic and racial groupings of clients.

Cultural Influences on Health Care

Published anthropologic and transcultural studies have offered nurses extensive information on assessing the effect of cultural influences on their clients. Creative cultural measures for improved therapeutics and comfort are available in

Technology Link

Biocultural Aspects of Drug Therapy

The Cross Cultural Health Care Program (www.xculture.org)

Training and resources for HCPs and interpreters.

Diversity Rx (Resources for Cross-Cultural Care) (www.diversityrx.org)

Dedicated to promoting cultural competence in an effort to improve health care standards for ethnically diverse communities.

Ethnomed (http://ethnomed.org)

A guide to ethnic medicine and culture specific information.

Office of Minority Health Resource Center (www.omhrc.gov)

Offers information on minorities and health care by the U.S. Department of Health and Human Services.

The Provider's Guide to Quality and Culture (http://erc.msh.org)

Designed to assist health care organizations in the U.S. in providing high quality, culturally competent services to multiethnic populations.

numerous books and research articles (Andrews & Boyle, 2002; Baker, 1997; D'Vanzo & Geissler, 2002; Giger & Davidhizar, 2004; Leininger, 2002; Spector, 2004) and various internet resources (see the Technology Link box above). Remember that each cultural group has different cultural attitudes toward health, health care, and illness; additionally, within each of these groups exists widely varying health and illness beliefs and practices. In general, this assessment should be known for populations relevant to your area of practice and individualized for each client.

Dr. M. Leininger (2002), a nurse-educator credited as a major voice of the transcultural impetus in nursing, has suggested asking questions such as the following to assess a client's cultural influences: "Could you tell me about yourself and your family?" "How do you keep well?" "What made you become ill?" The client is also likely to respond more readily to therapy if the nurse treats this information with respect and incorporates some of its important aspects into the nursing care plan. Feelings and beliefs will be more openly discussed if the nurse has gained the confidence of the client and family. Box 6-1 provides a comprehensive guide to the assessment of cultural manifestations.

If an illness is mild, the person self-treats the symptoms or, as is often the case, does nothing; gradually the symptoms disappear. If the illness is more severe or is of longer duration, the assistance of a healer of one type or another, usually a physician, is sought. Many cultural groups avoid standard Western medicine until herbal or home remedies are totally ineffective or the illness becomes acute. Such groups may also use both traditional and Western remedies concurrently to validate each other or to enhance the therapy. Haitian, Hispanic, Cuban, Vietnamese, Samoan, Jamaican, Chinese, Native American, and other clients generally follow this practice. Nurses should be aware of any reluctance to seek standard medical care. Such individuals should be counseled on appropriate ways in which to seek health care when the need arises and to effectively manage their therapeutic regimen when prescribed. Because of the wealth of cross-cultural literature, some basic questions the nurse should ask herself or himself in preparing clients of another culture for self-care are in Box 6-2. Although it is beyond the scope of this text to detail the many existing cultures, some insights will be provided for some of the more populous groups.

Populations of African Descent

Although a number of blacks have emigrated voluntarily from Africa and the various islands of the West Indies and Cape Verde during this century, the majority of African Americans are descendants of the Africans brought to America as slaves. Brought to this continent against their will, those of African heritage endured overwhelming hardships and inhumane treatment during slavery but in most circumstances maintained a family and community awareness. After the Civil War, those in the South were overtly segregated and lived in conditions of hardship and poverty; the people who migrated to the North were subjected to the poverty, racism, and covert segregation of urban life. In health care, it is the Tuskegee story that continues to reverberate through the African American community. The Tuskegee study examined the effects of untreated syphilis in black males for 40 years. Although many African Americans did not know the details of that clinical trial, many have heard the story that "something terrible" happened to African Americans during that study. These stories and documented disparities in health and health care may result in conspiracy beliefs and negative attitudes toward health care (Bird & Bogart, 2003; Watts, 2003; Smedley, Stith, & Nelson, 2002). The nurse who wants to integrate traditional health and illness beliefs with modern practice needs to appreciate the historic problems of the African-American community (Spector, 2004).

Contemporary black Americans are a heterogeneous group that consists of those born in the U.S. and refugees or immigrants from Haiti, the Caribbean, South America, and Africa (Cabral, Freid, Levenson, Amaro, & Zuckerman, 1990). Each group differs in terms of heritage, language, culture, and health beliefs and health practices (Watts, 2003). However, some traditional beliefs about health and illness stem from the African origins of African descendants. In this traditional society, life was considered a process rather than a state and could be influenced by other forces. When healthy, one was in harmony with nature; illness was a state of disharmony. In traditional African belief there was no separation of mind, body, and spirit. Disharmony or illness was the result of the activity of demons and

BOX 6-1 GUIDE FOR THE ASSESSMENT OF CULTURAL MANIFESTATIONS

I. Brief history of the origins of the cultural group, including location

II. Value orientations
  A. Worldview
  B. Code of ethics
  C. Norms and standards of behavior (authority, responsibility, dependability, competition)
  D. Attitudes toward:
    1. Time
    2. Work vs. play/leisure
    3. Money
    4. Education
    5. Physical standards of beauty, strength
    6. Change

III. Interpersonal relationships
  A. Family
    1. Courtship and marriage patterns
    2. Kinship patterns
    3. Childrearing patterns
    4. Family function
      a. Organization
      b. Roles and activities (sex roles, division of labor)
      c. Special traditions, customs, ceremonies
      d. Authority and decision making
    5. Relationship to community
  B. Demeanor
    1. Respect and courtesy
    2. Politeness, kindness
    3. Caring
    4. Assertiveness vs. submissiveness
    5. Independence vs. dependence
  C. Roles and relationships
    1. Number and types
    2. Functions

IV. Communication
  A. Language patterns
    1. Verbal
    2. Nonverbal
    3. Use of time
    4. Use of space
    5. Special usage: titles and epithets, forms of courtesy in speech, formality of greetings, degree of volubility versus reticence, proper subjects of conversation, impolite speech
  B. Arts and music
  C. Literature

V. Religion and magic
  A. Type (modern vs. traditional)
  B. Tenets and practices
  C. Rituals and taboos (e.g., fertility, birth, death)

VI. Social systems
  A. Economics
    1. Occupational status and esteem
    2. Measures of success
    3. Value and use of material goods
  B. Politics
    1. Type of system
    2. Degree of influence in daily lives of populace
    3. Level of individual/group participation
  C. Education
    1. Structure
    2. Subjects
    3. Policies

VII. Diet and food habits
  A. Values (symbolism) and beliefs about foods
  B. Rituals and practices

VIII. Health and illness belief systems
  A. Values, attitudes, and beliefs
  B. Use of health facilities (popular vs. folk vs. professional sectors)
  C. Effects of illness on the family
  D. Health/illness behaviors and decision making
  E. Relationships with health practitioners
  F. Biologic variations

From Andrews, M.M., & Boyle, J.S. (2002). *Transcultural concepts in nursing care* (4th ed.). Philadelphia: J.B. Lippincott.

evil spirits; the goal of prevention was to ward off these spirits, and the goal of therapy was to remove them from the body of the ill person. Several traditional practices were used to meet these goals.

African Americans may be likely to view control over health as the result of a higher power (Holt, Clark, Krueter, Rubio, & Bucholtz, 2001). Barroso et al. (2000) found African-American women more likely to believe in chance or to depend on powerful others for their health (e.g., the pastor, congregational nurses, physicians, and church/family members) (Drayton-Brooks & White, 2004). Many individuals of African descent believe in the power of healers. These healers may rely on the strong religious faith of the people and use prayer and the laying on of hands, or

- Have you used an interpreter (if needed) to facilitate communication concerning future medical care, concerns, appointments, etc.?
- If a prescription is necessary, will the client be able to read the directions? If not, can the prescription be written in the client's native language?
- Ask the client to repeat the explanation of the illness and the plan for treatment to ensure understanding.
- Ask where the client is planning to obtain the prescription.
- Have the client describe what daily activities will occur at the medication times (noon meal, walking the dog, etc.).
- Ascertain whether the client uses herbal treatments, home remedies, or supplements.
- Are you aware of any available support from the client's own cultural community that might help (e.g., religious connections, leaders, friends, family members)?

they may be more traditional healers and use herbs and roots in the treatment of illness. (Table 6-1 lists additional cultural values and culture care meanings and action modes for the African-American culture.) Some individuals of African descent are practicing Muslims and maintain a highly structured lifestyle based on religious beliefs. Muslims believe in self-help and the need for self-discipline, and they highly value life and good health. This belief system fosters the effective management of a therapeutic regimen. Dietary restrictions are similar to a kosher diet—abstinence from pork or pork products, and from beans (e.g., black-eyed, kidney, and lima beans), which are considered to be for animal consumption (Spector, 2004). Alcohol ingestion is not permitted because it is believed to cause illness. Because pork consumption is prohibited, a Muslim who has diabetes should not be administered pork insulin. As with other religions, Islam has various sects that differ in the strictness of their practices.

The practices for health promotion and the treatment of illness in the African-American community are varied and abundant. Proper diet, rest, and a clean environment are considered important for health maintenance. Herb teas and laxatives may be used to keep the body working well. Amulets or bracelets may be worn to protect the wearer from harm; during nursing care precautions should be taken so these items are not removed. In addition to prayer and the laying on of hands, "rooting" may be used as folk medicine. In "rooting" the healer or "root man" determines the cause of the illness and then prescribes a therapeutic regimen of substances and practices. Because "rooting" is a practice derived from voodoo, it is essential to obtain a healer who is stronger than the originator of the "hex" or the cause of illness; the more prestigious the healer, the stronger the medicine. There are also a variety of home

remedies, which are passed from one generation to the next. Remedies for colds and congestion include the following: hot lemon water with honey; hot toddies of tea, honey, lemon, and an alcoholic beverage; the ingestion of Vicks Vaporub; and a body rub with white high-proof rum. The health practices of each client should be determined so the prescribed therapeutic regimen can be individualized to meet that client's needs.

For a number of reasons, folk medicine continues to be used even when African Americans live close to local health services. According to Spector (2004), African Americans may perceive their interaction with the health care system as a degrading and humiliating experience. Although a HCP may not intend to be patronizing or demeaning, the client may feel insulted. Those who use clinics may have long waits and lose time at work, and those who are indigent cannot afford health insurance or the high cost of health care. Although these issues could apply to any health care recipient, "the inherent racism within the health system cannot be denied" (Spector, 2004).

✳ **A.T., a 50-year-old African-American man, is brought to his primary care provider by his wife for a work-related knee injury of 3 years' duration. He has gained 40 pounds since his injury and has been treating the discomfort in his knee with nonsteroidal anti-inflammatory agents. His blood pressure is 172/102 (left arm) and 170/100 (right arm) with a pulse of 80 beats/min and regular during the examination.**
African Americans are far more likely to have high blood pressure than whites. According to the American Heart Association (AHA), approximately 37% of African-American men and women have hypertension and they are far more likely to die from it than white Americans. In 1993, the death rate from hypertension was 30/100,000 for African-American males (361% higher than for white males) and 22.6/100,000 for African-American females (370% higher than for white females). Even though the incidence of hypertension is increased in African Americans, 27% are unaware of their high blood pressure, and 32% are receiving inadequate treatment (Hyman & Pavlik, 2001).

✳ **Are there differences in antihypertensive drug effects in African Americans?**
Both the Antihypertensive and Lipid-Lowering Treatment to Prevent Heart Attack Trial (ALLHAT) and African American Study of Kidney Disease and Hypertension (AASK) trial found there was no truth in the misconception that hypertension is more difficult to control in African Americans. However, the following are differences in antihypertensive drug effects in African Americans:

- Thiazide diuretics and long-acting calcium channel blockers (CCBs) seem to have greater blood pressure–lowering effects than other classes of antihypertensive agents in African-American clients.
- Angiotensin-converting enzyme (ACE) inhibitors may be less effective in lowering blood pressure or may require higher doses. There is an increased inci-

TABLE 6-1 CULTURAL VALUES AND CULTURE CARE MEANINGS AND ACTION MODES FOR SELECTED GROUPS

Cultural Values	Culture Care Meanings and Action Modes
AFRICAN-AMERICAN CULTURE*	
1. Extended family networks	1. Concern for my "brothers and sisters"
2. Religion valued (many are Baptists, Muslim)	2. Being involved with
3. Interdependence with "blacks"	3. Giving presence (physical)
4. Daily survival	4. Family support and "get togethers"
5. Technology valued, e.g., radio, car	5. Touching appropriately
6. Folk (soul) foods	6. Reliance on folk home remedies
7. Folk healing modes	7. Rely on spiritual beliefs with prayers and songs
8. Music and physical activities	
ANGLO-AMERICAN CULTURE (MAINLY U.S. MIDDLE AND UPPER CLASSES)	
1. Individualism—focus on a self-reliant person	1. Stress alleviation by:
2. Independence and freedom	Physical means
3. Competition and achievement	Emotional means
4. Materialism (things and money)	2. Personalized acts:
5. Technology dependent	Doing special things
6. Instant time and actions	Giving individual attention
7. Youth and beauty	3. Self-reliance (individualism) by:
8. Equal sex rights	Reliance on self
9. Leisure time highly valued possible	Reliance on self (self-care)
10. Reliance on scientific facts and numbers	Becoming as independent as possible
11. Less respect for authority and the older adult	Reliance on technology:
12. Generosity in time of crisis	4. Health instruction
	Teach us how "to do" this care for self
	Give us the "medical" facts

Modified from Leininger, M.M. (1991). *Culture care diversity and universality: A theory of nursing.* New York: National League for Nursing Press.
*These findings were from Leininger's study of two southern U.S. villages (1980-1981) and from a study of one large northern urban city (1982-1991) along with other studies by transcultural nurses.
†These findings were from Leininger's transcultural nurse studies (1970, 1984) and other transcultural nurse studies in the U.S. during the past two decades.
‡These findings were collected by Leininger and other contributors in the U.S. and Canada during the past three decades. Cultural variations among all nations exist, and so these data are some general commonalities about values, care meanings, and actions.

dence of angioedema and cough in African Americans compared with whites. They are renal protective in African Americans; but should not be used as monotherapy.

- β-adrenergic blockers are not as efficacious as monotherapy, but are used for post-myocardial infarction (MI) therapy (Coleman, 2005).

✱ A.T. has gained 40 pounds in the last 3 years with a body mass index (BMI) of 34 kg/m² (normal is less than 25). As obesity is a contributing factor in hypertension, he and his wife are provided instruction on the Dietary Approaches to Stop Hypertension (DASH) diet composed of fruits, vegetables, fiber, low fat dairy foods, and meat and poultry with reduced amounts of saturated and total fats. He is encouraged to take acetaminophen rather than nonsteroidal antiinflammatory drugs (NSAIDS), because they may result in sodium and fluid retention, also contributing to hypertension.

He is prescribed a thiazide diuretic, chlorthalidone (Hygroton) 25 mg daily and an ACE inhibitor ramipril (Altace) 5 mg daily. He is given an appointment to return in 3 weeks.

Obesity has been linked to an increase in hypertension, diabetes, coronary artery disease, and cancer. As is seen in the population at large, obesity is common in both African-American men and women (Centers for Disease Control and Prevention [CDC], 2002). The reasons may include many factors such as dietary preferences, perception of ideal body size, lower levels of physical activity, less concern about obesity, less overall health knowledge, less likelihood of receiving health education, and low income (Coleman, 2005). The African-American diet is generally high in saturated fat, salt, and simple sugars. High fat diets are associated with increased risk for hypertension, cardiovascular disease, and stroke. A.T. was recommended a DASH (low fat and low salt) diet that has been found to be successful in lowering systolic and diastolic blood pressure in African Americans (Appel et al., 1997). If the acet-

TABLE 6-1 CULTURAL VALUES AND CULTURE CARE MEANINGS AND ACTION MODES FOR SELECTED GROUPS—*cont'd*

Cultural Values	Culture Care Meanings and Action Modes
MEXICAN-AMERICAN CULTURE†	
1. Value extended family	1. Succorance (direct family aid)
2. Interdependence with kin and social activities	2. Involvement with extended family ("other care")
3. Patriarchal (machismo)	3. Filial love/loving
4. Exact time less valued	4. Respect for authority
5. High respect for authority and the older adult	5. Mother as care decision maker
6. Religion valued (many Roman Catholics)	6. Protective (external) male care
7. Native foods for well-being	7. Acceptance of God's will
8. Traditional folk-care healers for folk illnesses	8. Use of folk-care practices
9. Belief in hot-cold theory	9. Healing with foods
	10. Touching
NORTH-AMERICAN INDIAN CULTURE‡	
1. Harmony between land, people, and environment	1. Establishing harmony between people and environment with reciprocity
2. Reciprocity with "Mother Earth"	2. Actively listening
3. Spiritual inspiration (spirit guidance)	3. Using periods of silence ("Great Spirit" guidance)
4. Folk healers (shamans) (the circle and four directions)	4. Rhythmic timing (nature, land, and people) in harmony
5. Practice culture rituals and taboos	5. Respect for native folk healer, carers, and curers (use of circle)
6. Rhythmicity of life with nature	6. Maintaining reciprocity (replenish what is taken from Mother Earth)
7. Authority of tribal elders	7. Preserving cultural rituals and taboos
8. Pride in cultural heritage and "nations"	8. Respect for elders and children
9. Respect and value for children	

aminophen is effective in controlling A.T.'s knee discomfort, he will be encouraged to begin a walking program with his wife for social support. It is important to include A.T.'s wife as African-American men are less likely than women to seek professional help and engage in preventive and self-care techniques (Courtney, 2000).

Hispanic Americans

Hispanic Americans have their origins in Cuba, Mexico, Puerto Rico, any Central or South American country, or Spain. Mexican Americans constitute the largest group of Hispanic Americans, and their number is rapidly rising because of high birth rates and immigration.

Some Mexican Americans consider health to be the consequence of good luck, whereas others see it as being the result of good behavior. One is expected to maintain health by acting, eating, and working appropriately. Prayer, the wearing of amulets, and herbs and spices are used to prevent illness. Poor health is perceived as being caused by the following:

- An imbalance in the body, embarrassment, envy, anger, fear, fright, excessive worry, turmoil in the family, or improper behavior or improper behavior or violations of moral or ethical codes.
- Environmental or natural conditions such as bad air, germs, dust, excess heat or cold, bad food, or poverty.

- Supernatural causes such as malevolent spirits, bad luck, or the witchcraft of living enemies (who are believed to cause harm out of vengeance or envy) (Molina, Zambrana, & Aguirre-Molina, 1994). See Table 6-1.

According to Spector (2004), imbalance in the body relates to the four aspects of the body: blood, which is hot and wet; yellow bile, which is hot and dry; phlegm, which is cold and wet; and black bile, which is cold and dry. According to the "imbalance" theory, equilibrium can be regained if cold remedies or foods are taken for "hot" illnesses and vice versa. However, perceptions of what foods or medications are hot or cold may vary from client to client because these terms do not refer to temperature but are qualities assigned to particular substances. Cold illnesses are treated with hot medications (e.g., penicillin), or hot foods (e.g., chicken soup, hot tea), but they are not treated with orange juice, fruit, or other cold remedies that are commonly recommended by American HCPs (Molina, Zambrana, & Aguirre-Molina, 1994). It is best to consult with the client for specifics once it is determined that the imbalance theory is part of the client's health belief system.

"Empacho" is an example of a dislocation of a part of the body being a cause of illness. Symptoms of abdominal discomfort, pain and cramping, are thought to be caused by a ball of food clinging to the wall of the stomach and are treated by massaging the spine while prayers are spoken. Although this practice is helpful in many cases, as with many folk practices it may delay the client from seeking medical attention for serious illnesses. "Mal ojo" (evil eye), an example of an illness caused by magic, has symptoms of malaise, lethargy, and headaches and is thought to be the result of being excessively admired by another. The remedy is to locate the admirer to provide care for the affected individual. "Susto" is a state of depression caused by a strong emotional state of fright. This illness involves the loss of soul, which leaves the body and wanders freely. A "curandero," or folk healer, is required to coax the soul back into the body. "Envidia," or envy, as a cause of illness is part of a more universally held belief in peasant cultures of "limited good"—material wealth or achievement comes at the expense of the rest of the community because there is only a certain amount of "good" available. Misfortune, or ill health, is therefore the result of the envy and resentment of neighbors.

The services of a traditional healer may be sought, such as an herbalist or yerbero/curandero. Curanderismo is a relatively well-documented form of holistic folk medicine, however 90% of folk medicine adherents do not directly use the services of a curandero, or lay healer, but obtain their remedies from a hierarchy of lay healers (Healy, 2000). Padilla, Gomez, Biggerstaff, and Mehler (2001) found that 91.3% of their sample of Mexican Americans knew of a curandero, only 29.1% had been to one in their lifetime. This was inversely related to their level of income, level of education, and bilingual language skills. Therapies by the curandero include support for the religious practices, massage, and "cleansings" such as the passing of an unbroken egg or small bundles of herbs over the body of the client. Curanderos are well respected within the Mexican-American community and usually maintain a personal relationship with the client. Mexican Americans may expect to have such a relationship with their HCPs, which may not be met within the established health care system (Spector, 2004) and may account for the continued popularity of curanderismo as a health care modality.

Language and poverty continue to be barriers for many Hispanic Americans in receiving appropriate health care. Despite the fact that Spanish-speaking individuals are one of the largest minority groups, there still are inadequate numbers of Spanish-speaking HCPs. This discrepancy will be remedied when more Hispanic Americans are recruited into the health field and when more HCPs learn to speak Spanish (Spector, 2004).

✳ **J.M., a 34-year-old Mexican-American woman, is accompanied to clinic by her 15-year-old daughter because J.M. speaks no English. She believes that she has developed diabetes as she has the same symptoms as her mother and grandmother had; urinary frequency, thirst, and an increase in appetite with significant weight loss. She is unsure of the exact amount of weight loss as she does not have a scale at home, but has decreased two dress sizes. She is 5'1" and weighs 225 pounds; her BMI is 42.5 kg/m². Her laboratory determinations were** **fasting serum glucose, 410 mg/dL (normal is less than 110 mg/dL) and her hemoglobin A$_{1c}$ (HbA$_{1c}$), 11.2% (normal, 4% to 6%). J.M. is diagnosed with type 2 diabetes and is prescribed glyburide 20 mg daily and referred to the clinic's diabetic education class.**

For Hispanic Americans age 50 years of age or older, approximately 25% to 30% have either diagnosed or undiagnosed diabetes. Diabetes is two to three times more common in Mexican American and Puerto Rican adults than in non-Hispanic whites (National Diabetes Information Clearinghouse, 2001). J.M. has a positive family history of diabetes, obesity, and lab values that are indicative of type 2 diabetes. Her care should take into consideration that Hispanics with diabetes tend to have higher hemoglobin A$_{1c}$ levels, fewer physician visits, greater insulin resistance, and problems with obesity and tend to be less likely to self-monitor their blood glucose (Harris, Eastman, Cowie, Flegal, & Eberhardt, 1999).

The diabetic educator who meets J.M. does not speak Spanish, but has a certified interpreter with her to assist her in the educational setting. She greets J.M. in Spanish and addresses her as Senora Martinez to show respect. J.M. has brought her cousin for support; the inclusion of people in the extended family in care is not uncommon. The educator warmly asks J.M. how her family is and indicates that she is willing to take her time to be attentive and show respect. Hispanic clients expect the provider to exhibit confidence and to be warm and friendly and to take an active interest in clients' lives. She also sits closer than the customary 2 feet away from J.M. so that she will not be perceived as distant, uninterested, and detached. The educator knows that diabetes is considered a "hot" disease and that J.M. may be treating it with "cold" foods to restore harmony and balance. J.M. shares with the educator that she had been seeing her curandero who had encouraged her to see a physician and had been treating her with cactus petal (nopal), aloe vera juice, and bitter gourd—"cold" remedies. The educator recognizes these alternative medications and indicates that they will not be harmful if taken with the prescribed glyburide; however, if she should experience diarrhea, it may be the result of the aloe vera. J.M. is not unusual in her concurrent use of services of a curandero and a physician. J.M. does ask why she cannot get her glyburide from the pharmacist without a prescription as is the custom in her home country. The educator explains that the laws in the two countries are different. In many developing countries, prescriptions are not required; in the United States certain medications are available over-the-counter (OTC) but others, such as her antidiabetic medication, do require a prescription. Because the educator has demonstrated respect for J.M. and her culture, J.M. feels that she can work with this Anglo to meet her health care needs.

Asian American and Pacific Islanders

Although the Asian American and Pacific Islanders (AAPIs) community include people whose origins are in Japan, Korea, Pacific Islands, Vietnam, the Philippines, and the Asian subcontinent, this discussion will focus primarily on Chinese

Americans, who constitute the majority of AAPIs. The AAPI groups are diverse, and they practice many religions, including Catholicism (most Filipinos), Islam (most Indonesians), and Hinduism (many Indians). Both Confucianism and Buddhism influence lifestyles and health practices. They both encourage respect for elders and those in authority. In Buddhism, life is a cycle of suffering and rebirth, so pain and illness may be endured and care-seeking delayed. Taoism originated in China but is practiced by many Taiwanese and Koreans and is based on the premise of balancing natural processes and forces such as yin and yang.

Medicine has been a recorded science in China since the Emperor Huang-ti's writings, *Huang-ti Nei Ching* (The Yellow Emperor's Classic of Internal Medicine), in 1628. Within these writings the universe is seen as an indivisible entity in which man must adapt to the order of nature. This universe has two basic components, yin and yang, which are in opposition and in unison. Yang is the male force, a positive energy that creates light, warmth, and fullness. Yin is female, a negative energy representing darkness, cold, and emptiness. Illness is caused by an imbalance of yin and yang. If yin is too strong, one is nervous, apprehensive, and catches colds easily. Yang must be nurtured because it protects the body against outside forces. The inside of the body is yin, and the outside is yang. The five solid organs, which collect and store secretions—the liver, heart, spleen, lungs, and kidneys—are yin. The six hollow organs, which excrete—the gallbladder, stomach, large intestine, small intestine, bladder, and lymph nodes—are yang. The organs have a complex interrelationship that maintains the balance and harmony of the body.

Traditionally, illness was prevented by wearing amulets to ward off evil spirits, or jade charms, which were believed to bring health. The individual is expected to practice moderation, balancing the yin and yang aspects of the body and taking foods and herbs as supplements to maintain that balance (Chin & Bigby, 2003). The healer in Chinese medicine is the physician, who in ancient times was responsible for not only curing disease but also preventing it. In fact, physicians were paid only when the client was healthy. In the event of illness, physicians were not paid and had to provide the necessary medicines. The traditional Chinese physician uses inspection, particularly of the tongue, from which more than 100 conditions can be determined, and palpation of many different pulse types, in which there are 15 ways of characterizing (Spector, 2004).

The primary methods of traditional Chinese healing are holistic medicine, acupuncture, moxibustion, meditation, and herbal remedies, the purpose of which is to restore the balance of yin and yang. Acupuncture, a practice that has been mainstreamed into allopathic medicine, is a method of producing analgesia or altering the function of a body system by inserting fine, wire-thin needles into the skin at specific sites on the body along a series of lines called meridians. Precise puncture points along the meridians are identified in terms of yin and yang, and are associated with specific symptoms and diseases. Deficiencies of yin give rise to symptoms of dryness (e.g., dry mouth, cough) and heat

(e.g., fever, inflammation), whereas deficiencies of yang give rise to symptoms of poor vitality and strength (e.g., fatigue, impotence) and lack of adequate warmth (e.g., chills) (Chin & Bigby, 2003). Whereas acupuncture is perceived as a cold treatment, moxibustion is based on the therapeutic value of heat and is used for an excess of yin. In moxibustion, pulverized wormwood is heated and placed on the skin over specific meridian points (Spector, 2004).

The purpose of herbal remedies prepared according to specific prescriptions by Chinese herbalists is to restore the balance of yin and yang. In China, these folk remedies usually consist of a single dose of a liquid preparation, therefore taking tablets or capsules on a regular schedule could be confusing to the older Chinese client. Herbalists' instructions allow clients a sense of control, because they can regulate the concentration of herbal broths; AAPI clients lose this autonomy with Western prescriptions. This may be why this group prefers teas and topical remedies, may continue to see an herbalist, or increase or decrease the dosage of their Western medication.

For Chinese Americans, barriers to health care relate to language difficulties and socioeconomics, as with other minorities; barriers may also include their beliefs regarding medical practices. Although immunization and the use of x-ray studies are accepted, intrusive practices such as surgical procedures are seen as contrary to having respect for an intact body and may result in an excess loss of blood that will disrupt the humoral balance within the body (Spector, 2004). Many Asians believe blood is not replenished when it is removed from the body; consequently are reluctant to have blood drawn (Chin & Bigby, 2003).

Hospital food is seen as alien and increases the client's sense of social isolation. Even the common practice of leaving ice water at the client's bedside for the administration of medications is questionable because many Chinese and Chinese Americans believe that cold drinks are unhealthy for the sick; therefore they may avoid this fluid intake. This preference, and any other food preferences, should be discussed with the individual; if medically acceptable, hot tea or other substitutes should be provided. If appropriate, the family should be encouraged to supply the client with preferred foods.

In AAPI cultures, the needs of the family take precedence over individual needs, and health care decisions are made as a family. The ultimate decision may rest with the oldest and/or oldest male and is also based on the family's financial situation and other priorities (Inouye, 1999). Although these findings usually lessen with assimilation, it may mean that for many AAPI clients that client autonomy and client confidentiality have little relevance. Some Asian cultures believe it is important to uphold a public façade, or to "save face" rather than admit a personal weakness. As a result many Asian immigrant women may postpone health exams until the symptoms become unbearable (Inouye, 1999).

Generally there is a great deal of reverence toward physicians and the client will remain quiet, taking the provider's advice without asking questions. Asking questions may be seen as a sign of disrespect. However, if the client and family do not have confidence in the HCP, they may seem to agree with the regimen, but not return for care. They may also believe that unless they are given a medication, the physician has not done anything, and may lose confidence and not return (Mattson, 1995).

Cancer is the leading cause of death in AAPI clients and breast cancer is the most common type.

✱ **M.C., a 44-year-old Chinese American woman, was brought to the clinic by her sister who had emigrated from Taiwan 10 years earlier than the client. M.C. is found to have a 3-cm mass in the upper, outer quadrant of her left breast. The physician indicates to M.C.'s sister, whose English skills are the better of the two, that in addition to getting a mammography, he would like to perform a needle biopsy following the mammogram. Both women nod and accept the x-ray requisition with an appointment in 2 days for the biopsy. M.C. did not keep the appointment, and on further checking, it was determined that the mammography was not done.**

Native Americans

Culturally, the Native Americans' belief system of being in harmony with nature or of maintaining a balance between the body, the mind, and the environment is crucial to health maintenance (Hendrix, 2002). Family is of paramount importance among and within Native American groups. Many traditional Native American communities are face-to-face, kinship, and relational-based.

Illness is perceived as being out of balance because of ill spirits, not following traditional beliefs, or a disruption in nature (see Table 6-1). Because Native Americans do not ascribe to the germ theory, the cause of the illness must be traced back to an action or lack of action on the part of the client, which may not be known to the individual (Wauneka, 1990). Recovery therefore is based on diagnosing the problem and reestablishing the harmony or balance with nature. These are just some of the beliefs held by Native Americans; each tribe (there are well over 200) has specific ideas and practices related to health and illness.

The medicine man is the traditional healer of Native Americans and is considered to be wise in the ways of nature and able to seek out the spiritual causes of illness. Treatments used by medicine men include massage, the application of heat, sweat baths, total immersion in water as an act of purification, and the use of herbal remedies. Because of the belief in harmony with nature, herbs are specifically prescribed and carefully prepared, and meticulous attention is given to the timing and the procedures used for gathering them (Spector, 2004). Again, the personal bond between the healer and client is strong, which is why folk medicine continues to be popular.

The difference between what the HCP and the Native American client believe to be the cause of the illness can constitute a barrier to health care for Native Americans

(Mercer, 1996; Sanchez, Plawecki, & Plawecki, 1996). Additionally, differences in communication styles may lead to misunderstanding. The questioning involved in taking a health or drug history may be seen as intrusive and a demonstration of incompetence because Native Americans believe the diagnosis should be made through observation of nonverbal communication. In most Western cultures maintaining direct eye contact during communication is seen as demonstrating interest in the client; however, this practice may be considered inappropriate by many Native Americans. Because Native Americans have maintained their rich history through an oral tradition, note taking is not viewed favorably; the nurse should rely on memory rather than on notes when in the client's presence.

The Native American community moves at a different pace, it is not fast or slow, but it is a pace built over generations. Waiting and patience are words often used; others are preparedness and being at peace in the present. It is necessary to show a deep respect for each community as a place in which people grow and are nurtured.

As recently as 40 years ago, the rates of cardiovascular disease in Native Americans and Alaska Natives were exceedingly low, because of a history of few cardiovascular risk factors such as diabetes, hypertension, and hyperlipidemia. However, over the last few decades, the incidence and prevalence of these risk factors have risen significantly.

•   •   •

In addition to the various cultural groups briefly discussed, there are white ethnic communities served by the health care delivery system. To describe the health beliefs and practices of all the various cultures is beyond the scope of this text. The student is advised to seek additional information from the current journals and references cited in the Bibliography of this chapter. The nurse should gain knowledge of the various cultural groups within the local area of clinical practice. Local hospitals and other health care settings often hold conferences and maintain reference sources of relevant cultural material for the local communities.

Dietary concerns are also strongly intertwined with cultural beliefs. Many ethnic groups (Italian, Mexican, Cuban, and others) believe that their own foods hasten the recovery process. Therefore one major way in which many private and some public hospitals have recognized the cultural differences in health care is in offering ethnic meals as alternatives to the standard fare. Discussing food preferences and preferred methods of preparation with clients is often very important for their well-being.

Additionally, the nurse should be aware of possible cultural influences on the medicating behaviors of clients. Such information may be used to guide the nurse to ask the right questions during the initial history, to be aware of possible reasons for ineffective management of a therapeutic drug regimen, and to help identify specific areas needing additional client teaching.

The client is always the ultimate source of information on the specific ways in which culture affects the client's participation in health care (Holroyd, Katie, Chun, & Ha, 1997; Wright, Cohen, & Caroselli, 1997). Nurses need to be sensitive to the client's life experiences and adapt their nursing care accordingly. The nurse should be aware of the following two dangerous misperceptions: (1) ethnocentrism, the belief that the HCP's ethnic group is superior to other cultures or ethnic groups; and (2) client stereotyping, the assumption that all persons from a particular culture or ethnic group will have the same response to the same or a similar situation (Villarruel, 1995). These are mistaken beliefs. Ethnocentrism can interfere with the provision of health care to individuals from groups other than the provider, and client stereotyping may limit the provider's objectivity and ability to provide nursing care.

Within each cultural or ethnic group can be a wide range of different responses to the administration of medications and management of the therapeutic regimen. An understanding of the potential cultural or ethnic patterns of a client is helpful as a starting point in caring for the individual, as long as stereotypical conclusions are avoided.

Ethnic and Racial Differences in Drug Response

In addition to differences in health beliefs, values, and attitudes, pharmacologic research in the last 15 years has uncovered significant differences among racial and ethnic groups in their metabolism rates, clinical drug responses, and adverse effects of drugs. A new field, **pharmacogenetics,** has evolved to study the genetic influence on drug response that may occur from inherited metabolic defects or deficiencies. This emerging area of clinical investigation is leading to new, clinically relevant information about drug responses in ethnic and racial minorities. However, genetically determined differences in the response to drugs do exist among individuals, and there are differences in the prevalence of these determinations among different populations. At present, race and ethnicity are imprecise substitute measures of the genetic differences. Prescribers and institutional policy makers should be sensitive to the implications of racial and ethnic differences in drug therapy or these groups may be disadvantaged by institutional pharmaceutical policies or treatment protocols that restrict individual drug therapy. Nurses need to be aware of these differences to better monitor the drug therapy of clients from culturally diverse populations. These differences, where documented by research, will be discussed throughout the text.

Pharmacogenetics is the study of the impact of genetics on drug action. Each person differs in how drugs act at receptors and how drugs are metabolized. Toxic responses to drugs in both the individual and, in the case of a pregnant woman, the fetus are often related to genetically based variation in drug metabolism. This genetic variation appears to remain stable throughout life (Evans & McLeod, 2003). The original study of pharmacogenetics began when it was first noted that similar doses of drugs (e.g., isoniazid [INH], an antituberculosis agent, and succinylcholine, a skeletal muscle relaxant) resulted in dramatically different plasma levels in different populations (Weinshilboum, 2003).

Many disease processes have a genetic basis. Similarly, the effectiveness of drugs on many diseases may vary from client to client based on genetic variation in drug receptors, enzyme function, or other cellular systems. Areas in which this has been studied include oncology (in which tumor response to drug is in part genetically determined), and epilepsy (in which approximately one third of individuals with seizures do not respond adequately to pharmacotherapy). Genetic variation is observed in a number of important sites of drug action (Evans & McLeod, 2003) including the following:

- β_2-adrenergic receptor: an important site of drug action for many pulmonary drugs
- ACE: affecting the treatment of hypertension and heart failure (HF)
- Dopamine receptors: site of action of antipsychotic drugs
- Glycoprotein IIb-IIIa receptors: drug receptors on platelets affecting clotting and bleeding
- Serotonin receptors: site of antidepressants and treatments for nausea and vomiting

The genetic variation may be related to changes in receptor configuration, receptor quantity, or intracellular proteins that interact with the receptors (Johnson & Lima, 2003).

Genetics has a large influence on drug metabolism by a number of the cytochrome P450 isoenzymes (See Chapter 3). An **isoenzyme** is a chemically distinct form of an enzyme. The amount of each of these isoenzymes is genetically determined. Codeine (an opioid analgesic) is metabolized to the pharmacologically active morphine by cytochrome P450 isoenzyme 2D6. An estimated 5% to 10% of the population does not obtain adequate analgesia with codeine; this is most likely a result of inadequate amounts of 2D6 to convert this mildly analgesic codeine to the more effective morphine (Mahgoub, Idle, Dring, Lancaster, & Smith, 1977).

Instead of reduced metabolism, some clients experience very rapid metabolism of drugs by these enzyme systems. The degree of metabolism is related to the number of copies of the gene for each enzyme (Dalen, Dahl, Ruiz, Nordin, & Bertilsson, 1998). Among northern Europeans, multiple copies of the 2D6 gene are infrequently observed; in east African populations, however, frequency has been reported as high as 29% of the population (Aklillu et al., 1996). Commonly used drugs metabolized by 2D6 include the novel atypical antipsychotic aripiprazole (Abilify), the norepinephrine reuptake inhibitor atomoxetine (Strattera) for attention deficit/hyperactivity disorder, the angiotensin ACE inhibitor captopril (Capoten) for hypertension and HF, and the selective serotonin reuptake inhibitor fluoxetine (Prozac) for depression (Lacy, 2004). Differences in expression of 2D6 may explain the variation in response observed to these and other agents among individuals and across populations.

Similar genetic differences have been noted for many of the other cytochrome P450 isoenzymes, including 2C9,

2C19, and 3A4. Those individuals with low expression of an isoenzyme are at higher risk for elevated levels of the affected drug with a standard dose and are more likely to experience toxicity and/or teratogenicity. Such a mechanism is proposed for the fatal central nervous system (CNS) toxicity observed with fluorouracil, a chemotherapeutic agent used to treat certain types of cancers (Tuchman, 1985; Diasio, Beavers, & Carpenter, 1988). Alternatively, those clients with high enzyme levels experience increased drug clearance and reduced pharmacologic response to standard drug doses.

Genetic differences across populations have also been observed with drugs metabolized by Phase II reactions. In Phase II of drug biotransformation, conjugation activities add substances such as glucuronic acid, glycine, sulfate, acetyl, or glutathione to the drug itself. This enzymatic process requires energy and the donor group. One of the first substances studied in pharmacogenetics was the N-acetylation of isoniazid, the antitubercular drug. The rate at which isoniazid is acetylated is genetically determined and isoniazid's biotransformation is a classic example of genetic defect in drug metabolism. Slow acetylation is an autosomal recessive trait and is the result of a relative N-acetyltransferase deficiency. Many individuals of East Asian descent are rapid acetylators and require higher doses of isoniazid to have effective control of tuberculosis (Lin, Han, Lin, & Hardy, 1993).

Drug absorption and drug distribution may also be affected by genetics. Transport proteins like P-glycoprotein are expressed differently based on gene coding. These transport proteins may impact the degree of intestinal absorption and distribution to sites like the brain (Evans & McLeod, 2003).

The genetic differences in metabolism probably explain toxic responses or teratogenic risk for many drugs. Decreased metabolism resulting in increased drug levels, or the use of alternate metabolic pathways with toxic metabolites, accounts for many of these toxic responses. Drugs that are metabolized by enzymes with genetic variation may be two to eight times more likely to result in adverse effects than drugs in which clearance is not a function of genetics (Phillips, Veenstra, Oren, Lee, & Sadee, 2001).

Cytochrome P450 1A1 is an enzyme that is responsible for converting toxins in cigarette smoke to inert substances. Ineffective 1A1 function may harm the fetus by decreasing the effective clearance of cigarette smoke toxins. Lower birth weights are noted for infants born to smoking mothers with variants in that gene compared to smoking mothers who do not have this variant (Wang, 2002). Differences in risk for developing fetal alcohol syndrome for mothers who drink alcohol excessively have been noted based on genetic variants in the gene that encodes for the enzyme that metabolizes alcohol—aldehyde dehydrogenase (McCarver, 1997).

This type of genetic study has significant implications for the future. **Pharmacogenomics** is the new science in which discovery of new drugs is based on genetic knowledge and in which client-specific genetic information may be used to customize drug therapy. Such individualized therapy may result in safer and more effective treatments in the future (Phillips et al., 2001). As the sequencing and relevance of the human genome become better understood, drug therapy will likely be tailored to the client's genetic makeup to improve response and reduce toxicity (Evans & McLeod, 2003; van Gelder, Hesselink, van Hest, Mathot, & van Schaik, 2004).

Although pharmacogenetics may hold great promise to customize future drug therapy with maximal benefit and reduced risk for individual clients, a number of clients are likely to have concerns about how genetic information is used. A focus group of minority residents indicated that cost, discrimination, and privacy are important issues that must be addressed if genetics is used to guide drug therapy (Bevan et al., 2003; Condit, Templeton, Bates, Bevan, & Harris, 2003).

Some of the differences of the pharmacogenetic responses can be seen in groups with common genetic influences. Some examples of common drug classification in which these differences are seen are discussed below.

Analgesics

Some individuals have an inadequate analgesic response to codeine because of a genetic alteration in cytochrome P450 2D6, the enzyme responsible for metabolizing codeine to morphine. Approximately 5% to 10% of the population are poor metabolizers. When Chinese participants were compared with whites in a study using codeine as the analgesic for pain, the Chinese participants were found to be less able to metabolize codeine and required increased dosage adjustments to achieve a therapeutic effect (Burroughs, Maxey, & Levy, 2002). Similar effects may also be observed with oxycodone (OxyContin, others), which is also metabolized to a more active pharmacologic compound by the same 2D6 isoenzyme (Lacy, 2004).

Cardiovascular Medications

Cytochrome P450 2D6 polymorphism is also an important pathway for a number of cardiac medications. It has been reported that individuals of African descent are less responsive to β-blocking agents, especially propranolol (Inderal), nadolol (Corgard), and atenolol (Tenormin). Labetalol (Normodyne), a drug with α- and β-blocking properties, is equally effective in whites and individuals of African descent. Cytochrome P450 2D6 is also important for the metabolism of quinidine (Quinaglute), propafenone (Rythmol), and flecainide (Tambocor) which may affect management of cardiac dysrhythmias (Burroughs et al., 2002).

In general, individuals of African descent respond better to diuretics than to β blockers if only one agent is used. Even among the β-blocking agents, responses vary widely between racial or ethnic groups. For example, Chinese people are considerably more sensitive than whites to the effects of the β blocker propranolol (Inderal) (Zhou, Adedoyin, & Wilkinson, 1990). It was reported that the Chinese population may be twice as responsive to the effects of propranolol on blood pressure and heart rate and also have a greater atropine-induced increase in heart rate than the white population in comparative studies (Burroughs et al., 2002).

Plasma renin levels may also be important in determining a person's response to the β-blocking agents; whites usually have higher levels than individuals of African descent, and this may contribute to the racial difference in drug response (Burroughs et al., 2002).

Central Nervous System Agents

A comparative study between Chinese and Caucasian subjects indicated that the Chinese participants required lower doses of benzodiazepines (diazepam [Valium], alprazolam [Xanax]), tricyclic antidepressants, atropine, and propranolol (Inderal) (Burroughs et al., 2002). When the doses were comparable to those of the whites, an increase in adverse effects occurred in the Chinese subjects.

As a result of pharmacologic research conducted over the last two decades, more consideration is being given to the need to individualize drug therapy for special population groups. When testing and evaluating new drugs, the vast majority of drug manufacturers now include ethnic and racial minorities within the clinical trial groups. This effort is likely to reveal additional drug actions and adverse effects specific to minority groups and may also lead to the discovery of therapies that are of specific advantage to minorities.

Symbolic Meaning of Drugs to Clients

In addition to its pharmacodynamic action, every drug administered to a client has a symbolic meaning and a potential psychological effect. A drug not only alters the function or structure of some part of the body but also may influence the behavior, sense of well-being, and mental state of the client. The responses of clients to symbolism may mimic pharmacologic reactions, adverse effects, or even allergic reactions. A profound reaction may even be observed in clients receiving placebos.

Medications tend to be more effective when individuals believe in their capacity to get well, when they have a strong desire to get well, and when they believe that the health care personnel expect the medication to be effective and say so. Clients' past and present conditioning to drugs, illness, hospitals, nurses, and other health personnel, and their health goals, are determinant factors in the response to drugs. Nurses must remember that among the major deterrents to successful drug therapy are divergent goals of the client and the health care personnel. An accurate appraisal of the client's goal in seeking health advice and therapy is important to planning and implementing an effective plan of care.

Medications may be a symbol of help to the client. This meaning is strengthened and drug effectiveness is enhanced when prescribers and nurses suggest to a client that a particular drug will be helpful or beneficial. Repeated suggestions to the client that the drug is beneficial further reinforce the therapeutic value. This effect is similar to the relief that a mother's kiss brings to her child's pain; the assurance given by the kiss makes the child feel better. Investigations of the effects of drugs on the mind have resulted in the conclusion that some drugs are effective only in the presence of an appropriate mental state.

Drugs may also be viewed as symbols of danger. Clients who are using their illness to meet a need for dependence may interpret a cure as a serious threat to their emotional security. Taking medication may also be objectionable if there is a strong need to exhibit an image of independence; adverse effects may even result. The client may complain of dry mouth, nausea, vomiting, palpitation, fatigue, and other vague feelings of discomfort. The individual may resist taking the medication, refuse to have the prescription refilled, or even throw the drug away.

Many people have ambivalent feelings about taking medications. An expressed desire to regain health may coexist with an unconscious reluctance to give up the secondary gains of the sick role, which can include extra attention and freedom from responsibilities. To retain these benefits, individuals may report secondary drug effects or find reasons why they cannot take the medication.

Clients may harbor unsubstantiated notions about medications. Some may believe a medication is too strong or not needed any longer and therefore may refuse to take the drug, decrease its dose at any one time, or decrease the number of times it is taken. This behavior may be suspected when a drug known to be effective for a specific condition is ineffective in a particular client with that condition.

A client who believes the drug is too weak may take the drug too often, request the drug more often than prescribed, or continue drug therapy for longer than prescribed. However, medications such as analgesics may be inadequately prescribed or administered, thus resulting in this type of behavior. Therefore the drug therapy itself should be reviewed first to eliminate the possibility of undertreatment by the professional staff. Some clients who are self-medicating will increase the amount of drug taken, believing that "if one pill is good, two will be better," and overdose themselves. When the drug therapy as prescribed is determined to be appropriate, the reasons for this behavior should be sought and addressed.

Some fantasies concerning resistance evolve from fears. Individuals tend to fear radioactive drugs such as phosphorus (^{32}P) or iodine (^{131}I) and to fear dependence on drugs that have antidepressant, analgesic, or sedative effects. Although few people today believe in cure-all remedies, some have blind faith in a certain medication and prefer taking that drug rather than making an alteration in their lifestyle.

Clients who believe they are allergic to a certain drug, for real or imagined reasons, are likely to react with fear or panic when administration of that drug is contemplated. A detailed personal history and (when possible) tests for drug allergies should be used to corroborate or refute the client's belief. Rejecting a client's claim of an allergic response without evidence is an unwise assessment of data and is negligent to say the least.

The extent, duration, and intensity of the client's response to medication is influenced by several factors, including the following: the route of administration of a drug, the financial cost of treatment, and the client's conscious and unconscious attitudes toward illness, drugs, physicians, nurses, and other HCPs. Certain medications used in the usual dosages may not be effective when a client is angry, resentful, or hostile.

The illness itself may also affect a client's emotional response to a drug. When the illness is short, the recovery complete, and the medical and drug expense not too great, the client tends to have a positive reaction to drugs, hospitals, and health and nursing personnel. Strong negative reactions toward drugs or health personnel result when clients are falsely reassured of a quick and complete recovery, when drugs are ineffective and/or expensive, or when symptoms of allergy, adverse effects, or overdose occur. Preparing clients for the realistic limitations of drugs, for adverse effects, and for drug expense tends to create reasonable expectations.

With any chronic illness, a client may suddenly rebel against ill health and resist therapy with life-sustaining medications. When this occurs, clients may be testing to see if they are really dependent on the drugs, or they may be attempting a real or symbolic act of self-destruction. A stressful event or decision may be the root cause of this behavior. Exploring the client's underlying fears and concerns is essential, and support, caring, and objective assistance in coping are necessary.

To avoid causing the client unnecessary concern or to deflect time-consuming questions, many HCPs are reluctant to present any negative aspects when teaching clients about drugs. A clear, nonthreatening explanation about the purpose of the medication and its effects (including the most common adverse effects reported) is only the most basic of explanations required by the client. Most clients prefer knowing the potential risks of drug therapy. This knowledge also tends to increase their participation and to engender trust. Litigation could ensue if clients suffer harm from unrecognized secondary effects of a drug because they were not informed. However, the nurse should be aware that some people do not want to know the details of their treatment and that some people are very suggestible.

It is important to *listen intently to what the client says* about the medication, the feelings associated with it, and the condition for which it has been prescribed. With this information the HCP can begin to see the situation from the client's point of view and develop an understanding of the client's motivation to seek health care. Does the individual see the treated condition as a physical threat? How much of a threat? How susceptible is the condition to treatment? How much control does the client want to exert over the condition? How probable is it that such control will reduce the threat adequately? Until these concerns and other personal factors are at least briefly explored, the success of treatment is uncertain.

Effects of Drugs on the Mind

Many common drugs have a secondary effect on the client's CNS and result in altered thought processes and sensory-perceptual alterations. Drugs may interfere with judgment, mood, sense of values, motor ability, and coordination. Certain antihistamines used to treat allergies may decrease alertness and cause drowsiness, depression, and predisposition to accidents. Antihypertensive agents may cause depression. Barbiturates and tranquilizers may induce inattentiveness and confusion and reduce initiative. Drug-induced depression calls for discontinuing or decreasing the dosage of the offending drug. Clients should be monitored for self-destructive tendencies—the pharmacologic literature has abundant examples of clients with drug-induced depression who have attempted suicide.

Self-Treatment

Public interest in self-care management is at an all-time high and is exemplified by the numerous self-care books and clinics that now abound. One of the most effective and inexpensive ways to counteract rising health care costs may be through expanded, educated self-care management. Many people who visit a HCP have already started a self-treatment plan. If these people were also helped to learn when to seek medical supervision and how to follow treatment advice wisely, they would have a still greater potential for regaining good health.

With their commitment to collaboration with the client to further health, nurses can educate clients; pharmacists, physicians, nurse practitioners, and many other health care professionals can also work to educate clients. Consumer information pamphlets abound; they are printed by the Food and Drug Administration (FDA) and others—in large type for the visually impaired, or in various languages—and they offer valuable advice about drug interactions, health foods, and nonprescription pain relievers. Health information, some reliable, some unreliable, is available on the Internet. Clients should be encouraged to obtain Internet information only from government sources, recognized health organizations, and health science schools.

Development of the science of public health has led to the realization that the state of a nation's health does not depend exclusively on the interplay between professional medical practice on the one hand and bacteria, malignancy, and other causes of disease on the other. The influence of the individual's personal attempts at self-treatment or at lifestyle alterations on community health is often ignored or underestimated.

Drugs sold without prescription can induce sleep or wakefulness, relieve pain or tension, or supply the body with vitamins and minerals. Remedies can be purchased for symptoms affecting any part of the body. Sales of prescription and nonprescription (OTC) drugs have made the pharmaceutical industry a continually growing, multibillion-dollar industry. Concern regarding the use complementary/alternative medications and self-medication with OTC medications is not new but continues to be a controversial subject (see Chapters 11 and 12).

Summary

Medications tend to be more effective when clients believe in their own capacity to get well and in the drug itself. A client's response to drug therapy is influenced by past and present experiences with drugs, illness, hospitals, nurses, and other health care personnel, and their own health beliefs and practices. Assessing all of these factors is most important in planning and implementing an effective care plan.

Health beliefs and treatment outcome are strongly influenced by a client's cultural background, ethnic practices, beliefs, and tradition. Providing effective care to clients from different cultural groups requires an understanding of the predominant ethnic-specific influences and an assessment of individual clients to determine how those cultural influences affect health needs. There are also significant differences among racial and ethnic populations in terms of drug metabolism rates, clinical drug responses, and adverse effects to drugs. These can be attributed to genetic differences in individuals, but the current state of the science and clinical application uses race and ethnicity as an imprecise measure of these genetic differences.

Critical Thinking Questions

- What personal experiences or client experiences with drug therapy can you think of that relate to the expectations of a drug's effect on symptoms?
- What do you think are your health benefits related to the use of medications?

Bibliography

Aklillu, E., Persson, I., Bertilsson, L., Johansson, I., Rodrigues, F., & Ingelman-Sundberg, M. (1996). Frequent distribution of ultrarapid metabolizers of debrisoquine in an Ethiopian population carrying duplicated and multiduplicated functional CYP2 D6 alleles. *Journal of Pharmacology and Experimental Therapeutics, 278,* 441-446.

Andrews, M.M., & Boyle, J.S. (2002). *Transcultural concepts in nursing care* (4th ed.). Philadelphia: J.B. Lippincott.

Appel, L.J., et al., for the DASH Collaborative Group. (1997). A clinical trial of the side effects of dietary patterns on blood pressure. *New England Journal of Medicine, 336,* 1117-1125.

Baker, C. (1997). Cultural relativism and cultural diversity: implications for nursing practice. *Advances in Nursing Science, 20*(1), 3-11.

Barroso, J., McMillan, S., Casey, L., Gibson, W., Kaminski, G., & Meyer, G. (2000). Comparison between African-American and white women in their beliefs about breast cancer and their locus of control, *Cancer Nursing, 23*(4), 268-276.

Bevan, J.L., Lynch, J.A., Dubriwny, T.N., Harris, T.M., Achter, P.J., Reeder, A.L., et al. (2003). Informed lay preferences for delivery of racially varied pharmacogenetics. *Genetics in Medicine, 5*(5), 393-399.

Bird, S.T., & Bogart, L.M. (2003). Birth control conspiracy beliefs, perceived discrimination, and contraception among African Americans. *Journal of Health Psychology, 8*(2), 263-276.

Burroughs, V.J., Maxey, R.W., & Levy, R.A. (2002). Racial and ethnic differences in response to medicines: Towards individualized pharmaceutical treatment. *Journal of the National Medical Association, 94*(10), 1-26.

Cabral, H., Freid, L.E., Levenson, S., Amaro, H., & Zuckerman, B. (1990). Foreign-born and U.S.-born black women: Differences in health behaviors and birth outcomes. *American Journal of Public Health, 80*(1), 70-71.

Centers for Disease Control and Prevention, National Center for Health Statistics. (2002). National Health and Nutrition Examination Survey. *Journal of the American Medical Association, 288,* 1723-1727.

Chin, J.L., & Bigby, J. (2003). Care of Asian Americans. In J. Bigby. (Ed.), *Cross-cultural Medicine.* Philadelphia: American College of Physicians.

Coleman, L.T. (2005). Delivering culturally competent care. In Koda-Kimble, M.A., Young, L.Y., Kradjan, W.A., Guglielmo, B.J., Alldredge, B.K., Corelli, R.L. (Eds.), *Applied therapeutics: The clinical use of drugs* (8th ed.). Philadelphia: Lippincott Williams & Wilkins.

Condit, C., Templeton, A., Bates, B., Bevan, J., Harris, T.M. (2003). Attitudinal barriers to delivery of race-targeted pharmacogenetics among informed lay persons. *Genetics in Medicine, 5*(5), 385-392.

Courtney, W.H. (2000). Behavioral factors associated with disease, injury, and death among men: Evidence and implications for prevention. *Journal of Men's Studies, 9*(1), 81-142.

Dalen, P., Dahl, M.L., Ruiz, M.L.B., Nordin, J, & Bertilsson, L. (1998). 10-Hydroxylation of nortriptyline in white persons with 0, 1, 2, 3, and 13 functional CYP2 D6 genes. *Clinical Pharmacology and Therapeutics, 63,* 444-452.

D'Avanzo, C.E., & Geissler, E.M. (2003). *Pocket guide to cultural assessment* (3rd ed.). St. Louis: Mosby.

Diasio, R.B., Beavers, T.L., & Carpenter, J.T. (1988). Familial deficiency of dihydropyrimidine dehydrogenase: biochemical basis for familial pyrimidinemia and severe 5-fluorouracil-induced toxicity. *Journal of Clinical Investigations, 81,* 47-51.

Drayton-Brooks, S., & White, N. (2004). Health-promoting behaviors among African-American women with faith-based support. *Association of Black Nursing Faculty Journal, 13*(5). Available at http://www.findarticles.com/p/articles/mi_mOMJT/is_5_15/ai_n6260852.

Evans, W.E., & McLeod, H.L. (2003). Drug therapy: pharmacogenomics—drug disposition, drug targets, and side effects. *New England Journal of Medicine, 348*(6), 538-549.

Giger, J.N., & Davidhizar, R.E. (Eds.) (2004). *Transcultural nursing: Assessment and intervention* (4th ed.). St. Louis: Mosby.

e-LEARNING SUPPLEMENTS

Student CD-ROM
- Final Exam questions
- NCLEX® Examination review questions
- Pharmacology animations
- Printable chapter summary

Evolve Website (http://evolve.elsevier.com/mckenry)
- Case study on biocultural aspects of drug therapy
- Content updates, including information on new drugs

- WebLinks corresponding to this chapter
- Answers to the critical thinking questions in this chapter
- *Elsevier ePharmacology Update* newsletter
- Mosby's Drug Consult Internet Edition
- Supplemental and reference information

Harris, M.I., Eastman, R.C., Cowie, C.C. Flegal, K.M. & Eberhardt, M.S. (1999). Racial and ethnic differences in glycemic control for adults with type 2 diabetes, *Diabetes Care, 22,* 403-408.

Healy, K.M. (2000). Concepts of alternative healing systems: An overview of Mexican curanderismo. *Perspective on Physician Assistant Education, 11*(1), 51-55.

Healthy People 2010. Retrieved April 28, 2005, from http://www.healthypeople.gov.

Hedeen, A.N., White, E., & Taylor, V. (1999). Ethnicity and birthplace in relation to tumor size and stage in Asian American women with breast cancer, *American Journal of Public Health, 89*(8), 1248-1252.

Hendrix, L.R. (2002). *Health and health care of American Indian and Alaska Native elders.* Stanford, CA: Stanford University.

Holroyd, E., Katie, F.K.L., Chun, L.S., & Ha, S.W. (1997). "Doing the month": an exploration of postpartum practices in Chinese women. *Health Care for Women International, 18*(3), 301-313.

Holt, C.L., Clark, E.M., Krueter, M.W., Rubio, D.M. & Bucholtz, D.C. (2001). Health beliefs and spirituality among African American women: Toward a more effective approach to health communication on breast cancer, Abstract #26810. Presented at the 129th Annual Meeting of the American Public Health Association, October 21-25, 2004, Atlanta.

Hyman, D.J., & Pavlik, V.N. (2001). Characteristics of patients with uncontrolled hypertension in the United States, *New England Journal of Medicine, 345*(7), 479-486.

Inouye, J. (1999). Asian American Health and Disease. In R.M. Huff, & M.V. Kline. (Eds.), *Promoting health in multicultural populations: A handbook for practitioners.* Thousand Oaks, CA: Sage Publications.

Johnson, J.A., & Lima, J.J. (2003) Drug receptor/effector polymorphisms and pharmacogenetics: current status and challenges. *Pharmacogenetics, 13*(9), 525-534.

Lacy, C.F., Armstrong L.L., Goldman M.P., Lance L.L. (2004). *Lexi-Comp's Drug Information Handbook* (12th ed.). Hudson, Ohio: Lexi-Comp.

Leininger, M. (1991). *Culture care diversity and universality: A theory of nursing.* New York: National League for Nursing.

Leininger, M., & McFarland, M.R. (2002). *Transcultural nursing: Concepts, theories, and practices.* New York: John Wiley & Sons.

Levy, R.A. (1993). *Ethnic and racial differences in response to medicines: Preserving individualized therapy in managed care pharmaceutical programs.* Reston, VA: National Pharmaceutical Council.

Lin, H.J., Han, C.Y., Lin, B.K. & Hardy, S. (1993). Slow acetylator mutations in the human polymorphic N-acetyltransferase gene in 786 Asians, blacks, Hispanics, and whites: application to metabolic epidemiology. *American Journal of Human Genetics, 52,* 827-834.

Lipson, J.G., Dibble, S.L., & Miarik, P.A. (1996). *Culture and nursing care: A pocket guide.* San Francisco: UCSF Nursing Press.

Mahgoub, A., Idle, J.R., Dring, L.G., Lancaster, R. & Smith, R.L. (1977). Polymorphic hydroxylation of debrisoquine in man. *Lancet, 2,* 584-586.

Mattson, S. (1995). Culturally sensitive perinatal care for southeast Asians, *Journal of Obstetric, Gynecologic, and Neonatal Nursing, 24*(4), 18-27.

McCarver, D.G., Thomasson, H.R., Martier, S.S., Sokol, R.J. & Li, T.K. (1997) Alcohol dehydrogenase-2*3 allele protects against alcohol-related birth defects among African Americans. *Journal of Pharmacology and Experimental Therapeutics, 283*(3), 1095-1101.

Mercer, S.O. (1996). Navaho elderly people in a reservation nursing home: Admission predictors and culture care practices. *Social Work: Journal of the National Association of Social Workers, 41*(2), 181-189.

Molina, C., Zambrana, R.E., & Aguirre-Molina, M. (1994). The influence of culture, class, and environment in health care. In C. Molina, & M. Aguirre-Molina. (Eds.), *Latino Health in the U.S.: A growing challenge.* Washington, DC: American Public Health Association.

National Diabetes Information Clearinghouse. (2001). Retrieved April 28, 2005, from http://www.diabetes-help.com/what_is_diabetes1%20HISPANICS.htm.

Padilla, R., Gomez, V., Biggerstaff, S.L., & Mehler, P.S. (2001). Use of curanderismo in a public health care system. *Archives of Internal Medicine, 161,* 1336-1340.

Phillips, K., Veenstra, D.L., Oren, E., Lee, J.K., & Sadee, W. (2001). Potential role of pharmacogenomics in reducing adverse drug reactions: A systematic review. *Journal of the American Medical Association, 286*(18), 2270-2279.

Polifka, J.E., & Friedman, J.M. (2002). Medical genetics: 1. Clinical teratology in the age of genomics. *CMAJ Canadian Medical Association Journal, 167*(3), 265-273.

Purnell, L.D., & Paulanka, B.J. (2003). *Transcultural health care: A culturally competent approach* (2nd ed.). Philadelphia: F.A. Davis.

Sanchez, T.R., Plawecki, J.A., & Plawecki, H.M. (1996). The delivery of culturally sensitive health care to Native Americans. *Journal of Holistic Nursing, 14*(4), 295-307.

Smedley, B.D., Stith, A.Y. & Nelson, A.R. (2002). *Unequal treatment: Confronting racial and ethnic disparities in healthcare.* Washington, DC: National Academy Press.

Spector, R.E. (2004). *Cultural diversity in health and illness.* (6th ed.). Upper Saddle River, NJ: Prentice Hall, Inc.

Statistical Report on the Health of Canadians. (1999). Retrieved April 28, 2005, from http://www.hc-sc.gc.ca/english/media/releases/1999/pdf_docs/hofc2ebk2.pdf.

Tuchman, M., Stoeckeler, J.S., Kiang, D.T., O'Dea, R.F., Ramnaraine, M.L. & Mirkin, B.L. (1985). Familial pyrimidinemia and pyrimidinurea associated with severe fluorouracil toxicity. *New England Journal of Medicine, 313,* 245-249.

van Gelder, T., Hesselink, DA., van Hest, RM; Mathot, RA.A., & van Schaik, R. (2004). Pharmacogenetics in immunosuppressive therapy: The best thing since TDM? *Therapeutic Drug Monitoring, 26*(4), 343-346.

Villarruel, A.M. (1995). Mexican-American cultural meanings, expressions, self-care and dependent-care actions associated with experiences of pain. *Research in Nursing and Health, 18*(5), 427-436.

Wang, X., Zuckerman, B., Pearson, C., Kaufman, G., Chen, C., Wang G, et al. (2002). Maternal cigarette smoking, metabolic gene polymorphism, and infant birth weight. *Journal of the American Medical Association, 287,* 195-202.

Watts, R.J. (2003). Race consciousness and the health of African Americans. *Online Journal of Issues in Nursing, 8*(1), Manuscript 3.

Wauneka, A.D. (1990). Helping a people to understand. In P.J. Brink (Ed.), *Transcultural nursing.* Prospect Heights, IL: Waveland Press.

Weinshilboum, R. (2003). Genomic medicine: Inheritance and drug response. *New England Journal of Medicine, 348*(6), 529-537.

Wright, F., Cohen, S., & Caroselli, C. (1997). Diverse decisions: How culture affects ethical decision making. *Critical Care Nursing Clinics of North America, 9*(1), 63-74.

Zhou, H.H., Adedoyin, A., & Wilkinson, G.R. (1990). Differences in plasma binding of drugs between Caucasians and Chinese subjects. *Clinical Pharmacology Therapeutics, 48,* 10.

7

MATERNAL AND CHILD DRUG THERAPY

CHAPTER FOCUS

The effects of pharmaceutical agents vary in clients of different ages. The reasons for these variations are complex. Understanding the rationale behind these effects will help the nurse to administer medications safely and to evaluate the responses to these drugs appropriately. The client's age might also determine special techniques of administering medication to provide greater safety for the client. This chapter discusses special factors relating to the dosing and administration of medications in childbearing clients, breastfeeding clients, neonates (birth to approximately 1 month of age), infants (1 month to 2 years), and children.

LEARNING OBJECTIVES

- Describe special considerations for drug administration to childbearing or breastfeeding women.
- Identify common drugs contraindicated drug pregnancy and lactation.
- Implement nursing activities to reduce the risk of infant exposure to drugs in breast milk.
- Calculate pediatric dosages using body weight and body surface area methods.
- Describe pharmacokinetic alterations related to childbearing clients, breastfeeding clients, or children.
- Administer medications safely and accurately to childbearing clients, breastfeeding clients, or children.

▲ KEY TERMS

carcinogenic, p. 122
fetal alcohol syndrome, p. 124
mutagenic, p. 122
teratogenicity, p. 120

The human life span is a continuum in which development, maturity, and degeneration occur without any distinct demarcation. However, individuals mature and decline and/or have special needs at different ages, at different rates, and under different circumstances. These factors affect the client's response to drug therapy in characteristic ways. Therefore, nursing management of drug therapy needs to be based on both physiologic and psychosocial developmental levels.

Childbearing Clients

Any substance ingested or absorbed by a pregnant woman is likely to reach the fetus by way of maternal circulation or to be transferred to the breastfed neonate by way of breast milk if the substance is in a sufficient concentration and is well distributed. Therefore drugs taken by the mother can cause serious harm to the fetus or neonate. No drug is known to be absolutely safe for the developing embryo, but some oral medications that are inactivated in the mother's stomach or are not absorbed by the maternal gastrointestinal (GI) tract are assumed to be relatively safe. The effects of many drugs and other substances on the fetus are unknown.

Considerations for drug therapy in the childbearing client center on evaluating the risk-benefit ratio of drug use. This ratio is evaluated on the basis of the mother's condition and the effect of the drug(s) on the mother and the developing fetus or nursing infant. In some instances prescription and over-the-counter (OTC) drugs taken during pregnancy have resulted in fetal drug toxicity and **teratogenicity** (the ability to cause fetal abnormalities). Although the possible effect of some medications taken during pregnancy is known, new medications, different drug combinations, or a deficiency in metabolism in the fetus may change a drug previously known to be safe into a hazardous one. The period of greatest danger for drug-induced developmental defects is the first trimester of pregnancy—a time when many women may not realize they are pregnant. As such, all women of childbearing age who could become pregnant should be aware that any drug use may be potentially hazardous to a developing fetus. Self-treatment of minor illnesses is discouraged during pregnancy, and women should be instructed to keep a complete record of all medications consumed during pregnancy (Lowdermilk & Perry, 2004).

Andrade et al. (2004) investigated prescription drug use during pregnancy and found that 64% of the 152,000 women in the study were prescribed drugs other than vitamin and mineral supplements. Nearly 40% received Category C drugs (e.g., drugs for which human safety during pregnancy has not been established), 1.9% received Category D drugs (e.g., positive evidence of fetal risk, but benefits might outweigh the risks), and 0.1% received Category X drugs (e.g., definite fetal risk, with risk outweighing any possible benefit). See the FDA pregnancy safety category discussion in Chapter 2. Additionally, OTC drug use is high and there is also the use of recreational drugs (Black & Hill, 2003; Ebrahim & Gfoerer, 2003; OTC Drugs Can Be Harmful to the Unborn Child, 2000). The use of medication during pregnancy is therefore of utmost concern during the parenting stage of life. Nurses are commonly required to provide accurate information with rationales, discuss available health care options, and support parents' decisions during the childbearing process. Nurses should ensure that the information is current and based on evidence and that the woman understands that the baseline risk for teratogenicity (causing fetal defects) in pregnancy is approximately 3%—even in the absence of any known teratogenic exposure (Katzung, 2004). Health care providers and parents alike may need to make difficult choices on the basis of the benefit-to-risk ratio, which is determined by maternal medication regimens, the benefits to the mother, and the risks to the fetus or neonate. This dilemma illustrates the absolute necessity for nurses to be knowledgeable about medications and highly skilled at retrieving information from reliable sources. Parents should make the final de-

cisions regarding care on the basis of informed, sensitive input from all appropriate health care professionals.

✳ How are drugs taken by the mother transferred to the fetus?

There are multiple physiologic changes during pregnancy that affect the pharmacokinetics of drug action. Pregnancy does not seem to have much effect on drug absorption from the GI tract, but protein binding is decreased for some substances, which increases the amount of drug available for placental transfer. Biotransformation of drugs in the liver is probably delayed in pregnancy, but renal excretion may be more rapid because increased renal blood flow significantly increases glomerular filtration rate (see Chapter 3).

The human placenta is the interface between the mother and fetus in the uterus. Until recently it was generally believed that the uterus provided a protective environment for the fetus. It is now accepted that any chemical substance, including most therapeutic agents, administered to a mother permeates across the placental barrier (Holcberg, Tsadkin-Tamir, Sapir, Huleihel, & Ben Zvi, 2003). At the placental interface, the transfer of drugs and other substances occurs primarily by simple diffusion and partly by active transport. Transfer across the placenta depends on the chemical properties of the drug: its molecular weight, protein-binding capabilities, chemical configuration, and lipid solubility. The potential for transfer to the fetus is proportional to the concentration of the drug in maternal blood and the period of time the drug remains in the maternal bloodstream. Transfer is greater during late gestation because of enhanced uteroplacental blood flow, increased placental surface at the interface, thinner membranes separating maternal blood flow and placental capillaries, and an increased proportion of free drug available to the circulation. Pathologic processes in the placenta, such as inflammation, degeneration, or partial separation, can alter blood flow and thus drug transfer. Although many drugs are transferred across the placenta, not all are dangerous. Most drugs that cross the placenta stabilize in the fetus at a level between 50% and 100% of the maternal level. Some drugs (e.g., diazepam and local anesthetics) stabilize at levels even higher than those of the mother's. However, continued exposure of the fetus to a drug is more important than the rate of placental transport. The placenta itself is a site of drug metabolism. It converts some drugs (e.g., phenobarbital) to harmless metabolites, but it may create toxic metabolites and increase drug toxicity for other drugs (e.g., ethanol). By whichever mechanism, drug transfer can result in significant fetal drug effects. After delivery, drugs accumulated in utero may present problems for the newborn, including withdrawal reactions. Table 7-1 lists drugs associated with neonatal withdrawal symptoms (Wang, 2004; Nordeng, Lindemann, Perminov, & Reikvam, 2001).

✳ L.W. is a 26-year-old woman with epilepsy who would like to start a family. She is healthy except for a history of generalized tonic-clonic seizures that have been well controlled with oral phenytoin 100 mg four times daily. She has been seizure-free for 4 years.

TABLE 7-1 DRUGS ASSOCIATED WITH NEONATAL WITHDRAWAL SYMPTOMS*

| | Withdrawal Symptoms | |
	General	Central Nervous System (CNS)
Alcohol	Irritability, poor sleep pattern, diaphoresis	Crying, hyperactivity, increased sensitivity to sound, hypertonicity, tremor, seizures
Cocaine	Tremulousness, poor sleep pattern	Hypotonia, hyperreflexia
Marijuana		Fine tremor, increased sensitivity to sound, and prominent Moro reflex
Nicotine	Mild increased muscle tone	Fine tremor
Selective serotonin reuptake inhibitors (SSRIs)	Irritability, eating and sleeping difficulties	Excessive crying, shivering, increased tonus, seizures
ANTIHISTAMINES		
diphenhydramine (Benadryl)	Tremulousness	
hydroxyzine (Atarax, Vistaril)	Irritability	Hyperactivity, tremor, jitteriness, shrill cry, hypotonia, seizures
BARBITURATES		
phenobarbital, secobarbital (Seconal)	Irritability, poor sleep pattern, diaphoresis, skin abrasions	Excessive crying, hyperreflexia, increased sensitivity to sound, hypertonicity, tremor, seizures
BENZODIAZEPINES		
chlordiazepoxide (Librium)	Irritability	Tremors
diazepam (Valium)	Hypothermia	Hyperactivity, hypotonia, hypertonia, apnea/tremor, hyperreflexia
OPIOIDS		
codeine heroin meperidine (Demerol) methadone morphine	Irritability, wakefulness, yawning, tearing, fever, diaphoresis, skin excoriations, voracious sucking, poor sleep pattern, hypothermia	Coarse tremors, seizures, twitching Hyperactivity (high-pitched cry), hypertonicity Hyperreflexia, increased sensitivity to sound, photophobia, apneic spells
pentazocine (Talwin)	Respiratory symptoms (stuffy/runny nose, sneezing, tachypnea, respiratory alkalosis), gastrointestinal symptoms (hiccups, salivation, vomiting, diarrhea, failure to thrive)	
propoxyphene (Darvon)	Irritability, fever	Hyperactivity, tremor, high-pitched cry

Data from Nordeng, H., Lindemann, R., Perminov, K.V. & Reikvam, A. (2001). Neonatal withdrawal syndrome after in utero exposure to selective serotonin reuptake inhibitors. *Acta Paediatrics, 90*(3), 288-289 and Wang, M. (2004). Perinatal drug abuse and neonatal drug withdrawal. In D.N. Sheftel, R. Konop, B.S. Carter, & C.L. Wagner. (Eds.). *emedicine* Retrieved May 1, 2005, from http:// www.emedicine.com/ped/topic2631.htm
*Symptoms depend on the drug and frequency of use by mother during pregnancy.

✱ What are the possible fetal effects of drug use during pregnancy?

Drugs crossing the placenta enter the fetal circulation via the umbilical cord. Approximately 40% to 60% of umbilical venous blood enters the fetal liver; the rest directly enters the fetal circulation. A drug passing through the fetal liver may be partially metabolized before entering the fetal circulation. Additionally, a large proportion of the blood returning to the placenta from the fetus may be shunted through the placental tissue, back to the umbilical vein, and into the fetus again.

The effects of drugs in the fetus may be more significant and prolonged than in the mother because of (1) probable immature enzyme drug metabolizing systems or an absence of such systems, and (2) slower excretion rates. In the fetus, drug excretion is accomplished by the kidneys. Waste products are excreted into the amniotic fluid, which is reabsorbed by the mother or swallowed by the fetus. Thus the immature or underdeveloped physiologic mechanisms of the fetus may result in altered drug responses and perhaps toxicity.

Occasionally, various fetal complications such as anemia and syphilis exposure are actively treated by drugs in utero. Corticosteroids are used to stimulate fetal lung maturation when a premature birth is expected (Katzung, 2004). The chosen routes of drug delivery have been either a passive, transplacental approach or direct instillation into the amniotic fluid.

It continues to be well documented that the administration of various drugs before delivery or the continued use of prescription and recreational drugs throughout pregnancy may have toxic and harmful effects on the newborn. The embryo or fetus runs the risk of developing the usual side or toxic effects, just as the mother does. For example, if the mother consumes alcohol, barbiturates, or opioids, the neonate at birth may have the following withdrawal symptoms: hyperactivity, crying, irritability, seizures and, perhaps, sudden death. (See Table 7-1 for a list of drugs that can cause symptoms of withdrawal.)

Medications may be lethal or teratogenic, **mutagenic** (causing genetic mutation), or **carcinogenic** (causing or accelerating the development of cancer). An example of a carcinogenic effect is the precancerous or cancerous cell changes discovered in youths whose mothers took the hormone diethylstilbestrol (DES) during pregnancy (Schrager & Potters, 2004).

Every embryo undergoes a series of precisely programmed steps from cell proliferation, differentiation, and migration to organogenesis. The critical periods for drug effects on the fetus are (1) the first 2 weeks of rapid cell proliferation, when exposure to drugs can be lethal to the embryo, and (2) the third through the tenth weeks of pregnancy, when the axial skeleton, muscles, limbs, and organs are developing most rapidly. Figure 7-1 illustrates the critical periods of human development.

Indirectly, teratogenic drugs may interfere with the passage of oxygen and nutrition through the placenta and affect the most rapidly metabolizing fetal tissues. More di-

rectly, some drugs may alter the normal processes of differentiation of fetal development, such as vitamin A analogue (isotretinoin). Deficiencies of crucial substances appear to play a role in some fetal abnormalities. This may be demonstrated by the fact that an increased intake of folic acid during early pregnancy appears to reduce the incidence of neural tube defects, such as spinal bifida.

An unfortunate example of a teratogenic effect is the abnormal limb development (phocomelia) in many children whose mothers received the drug thalidomide during pregnancy, especially between the third and sixth week of pregnancy. When it was administered beyond the tenth week of pregnancy (after the rapid development of the skeleton), physiologic or behavioral alterations and delays in growth were more likely.

Cocaine abuse by pregnant women has resulted in frequent miscarriages, fetal hypoxia, and low-birth-weight infants. Cocaine exposure in utero has caused fetal tremors, fetal strokes, and an increase in stillbirth rates. Exposed infants are also at high risk for developing congenital heart disease, skull defects, and other congenital malformations. At birth the newborn may exhibit symptoms of withdrawal: increased irritability, increased respiratory and heart rates, diarrhea, irregular sleeping patterns, and poor appetite. Long-term behavioral patterns of infants born to cocaine-abusing women, such as poor attention spans and a decrease in organizational skills, have been reported (Frank, Augustyn, Knight, Pell, & Zuckerman, 2001). In a number of instances the legal system or the courts have intervened to protect the unborn fetus or to punish the mother of a child born with medical complications resulting from cocaine abuse.

In certain situations drugs are necessary during pregnancy and breastfeeding. Some maternal conditions (e.g., hypertension, epilepsy, diabetes, and infection) seriously jeopardize both mother and fetus if left untreated. Although authoritative literature and drug package inserts routinely warn that drugs have not been tested for use in pregnancy, during breastfeeding, or for infants, much empiric and some research data are accumulating. The Food and Drug Administration (FDA) classifies drugs according to their safety for use during pregnancy. This rating is discussed in Chapter 2 and is included in the discussion of specific drugs throughout this text.

A major issue regarding the use of drugs during pregnancy and the neonatal period involves the legal and ethical problems associated with drug research experiments during pregnancy; these problems contribute to the lack of information in this area. Although fraught with ethical dilemmas, well-controlled research is undeniably needed.

Certain categories of drugs are expressly contraindicated during pregnancy or are used only when the risk-benefit situation has been carefully considered and thoroughly discussed with the client. Drugs that are contraindicated with reported teratogenic effects are listed in Table 7-2. Table 7-3 lists selected drugs that are may pose unique risks in pregnancy and that are used only when safer alternatives are not available and the benefit outweighs risk. Some drugs

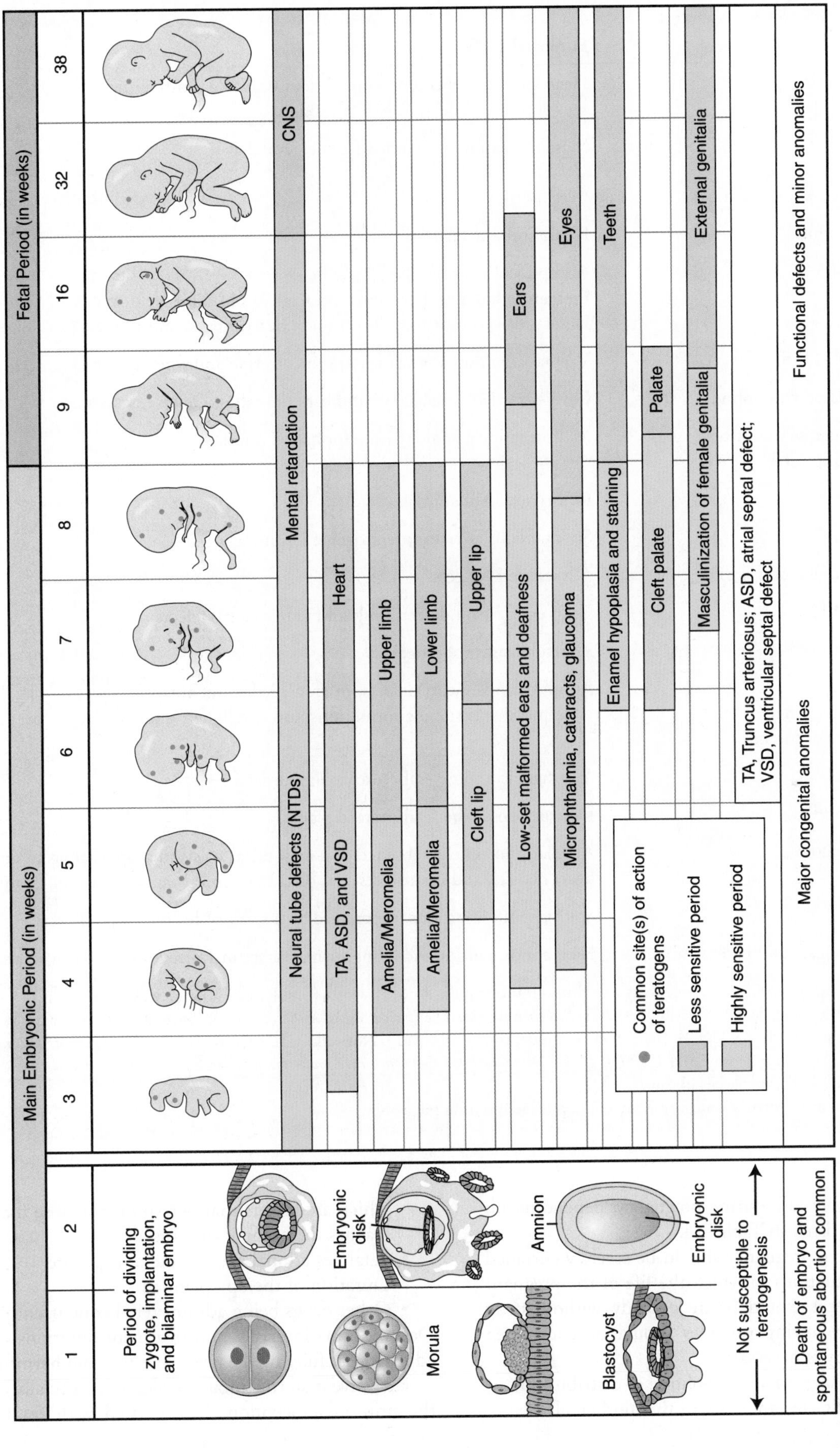

FIGURE 7-1 Schematic illustration of the critical periods in human prenatal development.

Modified from Moore, K.L., & Persaud, T.V.N. (2003). The developing human: Clinically oriented embryology (7th ed.). Philadelphia: W.B. Saunders.

TABLE 7-2 DRUGS THAT ARE CONTRAINDICATED DURING PREGNANCY*

Drug	Potential Defect
alcohol use, chronic	Heart defects, central nervous system (CNS) abnormalities Developmental delay, low birth weight
Androgens: • danazol (Danocrine) • testosterone (Androderm)	Masculinization of external female genitalia
clomiphene (Clomid)	Neural tube defects
cocaine	Abruptio placentae Premature labor and delivery, intracranial bleeding Defects of genitourinary (GU) tract, heart, limbs, and face.
diethylstilbestrol (DES)	Vaginal adenosis, vaginal carcinoma, uterine abnormalities, male infertility
estrogen and related compounds	Cardiovascular defects, eye and ear anomalies, Down's syndrome
HMG-CoA reductase inhibitors (e.g., atorvastatin [Lipitor])	Malformations; anal atresia, esophageal atresia
leflunomide (Arava)	Embryotoxic in animals.
leuprolide (Eligard)	Spontaneous abortion; teratogenic in animals
lysergic acid diethylamide (LSD)	Adverse fetal effects
methotrexate (MTX)	Skull ossification defect, limb and craniofacial defects
misoprostol (Cytotec)	Abortifacient properties
Retinoids: • acitretin (Soriatane) • isotretinoin (Accutane)	Anophthalmia, heart defects, microcephalus, meningomyelocele, skeletal and/or connective tissue malformations; low intelligent quotient (IQ) scores
ribavirin (Rebetol)	Teratogenic and/or embryotoxic in animals
sodium iodide (^{131}I)	Destruction of the fetal thyroid gland
thalidomide (Thalomid)	Amelia, phocomelia, absence of bones, facial palsy, microphthalmos, congenital heart defects, and gastrointestinal (GI) tract and urinary tract abnormalities
vaccines, live	Spontaneous abortions, premature births, possible congenital defects
vitamin A (high doses and parenteral)	Fetal abnormalities, including urinary tract malformations, growth retardation

Data from Young, V.S.L. (2005). Teratogenicity and drugs in breast milk. In M.A. Koda-Kimble, L.Y. Young, W.A. Kradian, B.J. Guglielmo, B.K. Alldredge, & R.L. Corelli (Eds.), *Applied therapeutics: The clinical use of drugs* (8th ed.). Philadelphia: Lippincott Williams & Wilkins; Katzung, B.G. (Ed.). (2004). *Basic & clinical pharmacology* (8th ed.). Norwalk, CT: Appleton & Lange; *Mosby's drug consult* (15th ed.). (2005). St. Louis: Mosby; and *USP DI: Drug information for the health care professional* (25th ed.). (2005). Greenwood Village, CO: MICROMEDEX Thomson Healthcare.

*All drugs classified as Pregnancy Category X are contraindicated during pregnancy.

considered relatively safe during pregnancy, depending on the situation, are listed in Table 7-4.

Drug use during pregnancy should be severely curtailed and limited to situations in which the life of the pregnant woman or the fetus would be in jeopardy without drug treatment. The following variables should be considered when drug therapy is necessary:
- Maternal dosage, maternal volume of distribution, and metabolic clearance rate of the mother, all of which are factors that determine the dose that reaches the embryo or fetus
- Fetal gestational age at time of exposure
- Duration of therapy planned
- Other drugs being administered concurrently

Doses, dosing intervals, and treatment durations should be adjusted carefully by the prescriber to avoid harmful effects.

Excessive maternal intake of alcohol, especially at or near the time of conception, is associated with **fetal alcohol**

TABLE 7-3 SELECTED DRUGS THAT REQUIRE CAREFUL EVALUATION OF RISK/BENEFIT BEFORE USE IN PREGNANCY

Drug/Drug Class	Fetal/Neonatal Effect
Adrenergics • ephedrine • epinephrine	Inguinal hernia, clubfoot, minor anomalies
amiodarone	Fetal hypothyroidism, low birth weight, prematurity, dysrhythmias
angiotensin-converting enzyme (ACE) inhibitors	Renal dysgenesis, defects in skull ossification
angiotensin II-receptor blockers (ARBs)	As for ACE inhibitors
Antiepileptics • carbamazepine • ethosuximide • phenobarbital • phenytoin • valproic acid	 Spina bifida Patent ductus arteriosus, cleft lip/palate and hydrocephalus Fetal/newborn addiction Cleft palate, cleft lip, heart abnormalities, fetal anticonvulsant syndrome* Spina bifida, fetal anticonvulsant syndrome*
Antiinfectives • aminoglycosides • chloramphenicol • fluconazole • metronidazole • quinolones • rifampin • tetracyclines • trimethoprim (TMP)	 VIII cranial nerve toxicity Cardiovascular collapse (gray syndrome) in newborns Defects of central nervous system (CNS), extremities, and cleft palate Oral cleft Erosion of cartilage, arthropathy Hydrocephalus, limb malformations, renal tract defect Stained teeth, bone growth defect Neural tube defect, cardiovascular defects, oral cleft
Antineoplastics • busulfan • hydroxyurea • mercaptopurine	 Anomalous deviation left lobe liver, bilobular spleen, pulmonary atelectasis, pyloric stenosis, cleft palate, corneal opacity Teratogenic/embryotoxic in animals Microphthalmia, corneal opacity, cleft palate, polydactyly, and neonatal anemia
Antithyroid agents: • methimazole • propylthiouracil	 Esophageal atresia, facial and skin dysmorphology, psychomotor delay, and growth restriction Mild hypothyroidism, goiter
aspirin	Adversely affect clotting in newborns
azathioprine	Hydrocephalus, anencephaly, cleft palate, atrial septal defect, and polydactyly
benzodiazepines	Cleft lip/palate, congenital heart disease, defects of the CNS, lung, abdomen, gastrointestinal (GI) tract, and digits
β blockers	Reduced birth weight
codeine	Congenital heart disease, respiratory malformations, genitourinary (GU) tract defects, hydrocephaly, and pyloric stenosis
corticosteroids	Increased risk of oral cleft

Data from Young, V.S.L. (2005). Teratogenicity and drugs in breast milk. In M.A. Koda-Kimble, L.Y. Young, W.A. Kradian, B.J. Guglielmo, B.K. Alldredge, & R.L. Corelli (Eds.). *Applied therapeutics: The clinical use of drugs* (8th ed.). Philadelphia; Lippincott Williams & Wilkins; Katzung, B.G. (Ed.). (2004). *Basic & clinical pharmacology* (8th ed.). Norwalk, CT: Appleton & Lange; *Mosby's drug consult* (15th ed.). (2005). St. Louis: Mosby; and *USP DI: Drug information for the health care professional* (25th ed.). (2005). Greenwood Village, CO: MICROMEDEX Thomson Healthcare.
*Mental and prenatal growth deficiency, microcephaly, fingernail hypoplasia, and craniofacial defects.

Continued

TABLE 7-3 SELECTED DRUGS THAT REQUIRE CAREFUL EVALUATION OF RISK/BENEFIT BEFORE USE IN PREGNANCY—cont'd

Drug/Drug Class	Fetal/Neonatal Effect
ergotamine	Fetal hypoxia
lithium	Ebstein's anomaly
marijuana	Fetal growth retardation
nicotine	Miscarriage Low birth weight and perhaps delay in development
NSAIDs: • ibuprofen • indomethacin • naproxen	 Premature closure of ductus arteriosus Constriction of fetal ductus arteriosus Persistent pulmonary hypertension of the newborn
penicillamine	Pyloric stenosis, inguinal hernia, hyperflexion of hips and shoulders and low set ears
progesterone and related compounds	Cardiac malformations, CNS defects, masculinization of female fetuses, and limb defects
sulfonylureas, oral	Prolonged hypoglycemia
thiazides and related diuretics	Decrease placental perfusion, neonatal thrombocytopenia
Tricyclic antidepressants • amitriptyline • imipramine	 Limb reduction defects Bilateral amelia, polydactyly, diaphragmatic hernia, cleft palate, and adrenal hypoplasia
warfarin	Fetal hemorrhage, optic atrophy, brain abnormalities

syndrome (FAS), which produces congenital anomalies and both growth and mental retardation (Box 7-1). Other very common, potentially dangerous substances during pregnancy include extended-release aspirin (Pregnancy Category D), parenteral vitamin A (category X), and nicotine chewing gum and nicotine transdermal systems (category X and category D, respectively) (*USP DI,* 2005).

A problem with drug use is that the effects on the embryo may occur before the woman is aware she is pregnant. Women of childbearing age who are not using contraceptives and who are sexually active should be prescribed drugs carefully and should be instructed to use OTC medications cautiously. Education and prevention are considered the best therapy.

✳ **L.W. visits her physician to plan for her conception. It is important for her to continue to have good seizure control during her pregnancy. Because she has not had a seizure for 4 years, it is planned to taper her phenytoin dosage over 3 months. If withdrawal turns out not to be an option for her, the fact that she is on monotherapy puts her at less risk for fetal complications. Close monitoring of her phenytoin plasma concentrations will be necessary during pregnancy. After a discussion of the risk of fetal hydantoin syndrome, the possibility of changing L.W.'s medication was considered, but any change would mean that seizure control would need to be achieved before conception. After**

some consideration, L.W. decides to remain on phenytoin during her pregnancy.

✳ **How do nurses manage medication administration with childbearing clients?**
Most nursing goals related to medication administration should be aimed at ensuring that parents know that any foreign substance absorbed by the mother may have life-long effects on the child and family. A balance must be maintained between protecting the individual and promoting the role and formation of the family. To accomplish these goals, it is necessary to be an advocate for the client, establish an environment conducive to the exchange of information, and minimize the parents' feelings of guilt or fear associated with drug administration and the potential impact on the unborn. The following information should be conveyed to the family:

• Both the potential harm to the unborn child resulting directly from substances to which the mother is exposed and the potential risks and benefits to both mother and child if treatment is avoided must be weighed. These decisions must be made with the prescriber whenever exposure to an unfamiliar substance or drug is contemplated.
• OTC medications and other common substances such as aspirin, high-dose or multiple vitamin supplements, alcohol, caffeine, and nicotine may have detrimental effects on the fetus.

TABLE 7-4 SELECTED DRUGS CONSIDERED RELATIVELY SAFE FOR USE IN PREGNANCY

Agent	Recommendations and Cautions*
ANALGESICS	
acetaminophen (Tylenol)	Considered safest analgesic during pregnancy
ANTIASTHMATICS	
budesonide (Pulmicort)	Relatively safe
cromolyn sodium (Gastrocrom Intal)	Relatively safe
ANTICOAGULANTS	
heparin	For use during first trimester; use caution if given during last trimester
ANTIDIABETICS	
insulin	Relatively safe; drug of choice
ANTIEMETICS	
cyclizine (Marezine) dimenhydrinate (Dramamine) ginger (*Zingiber officinale*) meclizine (Antivert) metoclopramide (Reglan) prochlorperazine (Compazine)	For use as necessary for severe nausea or vomiting
ANTIHYPERTENSIVES	
methyldopa (Aldomet)	Safest of antihypertensives during pregnancy (especially as substitute for diuretics in pregnancy for diastolic blood pressure >110 mm Hg in third trimester)
hydralazine (Apresoline)	Safest for hypertensive crises in pregnancy
ANTIINFECTIVES	
cephalosporins	Safe during pregnancy
Macrolides: azithromycin (Zithromax) and erythromycin (E-Mycin)	For use as substitute for penicillin hypersensitivity
metronidazole, systemic (Flagyl)	Not to be used during first trimester
metronidazole, vaginal (Metro Gel)	Use only if clearly needed
nystatin	Relatively safe
penicillin and derivatives	Relatively safe
ANTIULCER AGENTS	
antacids, famotidine (Pepcid AC), nizatidine (Axid), ranitidine (Zantac)	Relatively safe
CARDIAC GLYCOSIDES	
digoxin (Lanoxin)	Relatively safe; maternal plasma levels should be closely monitored
LAXATIVES	
lactulose, magnesium sulfate	Increase fluid intake and fiber in diet, and moderate exercise (walking)

Data from Young, V.S.L. (2005). Teratogenicity and drugs in breast milk. In M.A. Koda-Kimble, L.Y. Young, W.A. Kradian, B.J. Guglielmo, B.K. Alldredge, R.L. Corelli (Eds.). *Applied therapeutics: The clinical use of drugs* (8th ed.). Philadelphia: Lippincott Williams & Wilkins; Katzung, B.G. (Ed.). (2004). *Basic & clinical pharmacology* (8th ed.). Norwalk, CT: Appleton & Lange; *Mosby's drug consult* (15th ed.). (2005). St. Louis: Mosby; and *USP DI: Drug information for the health care professional* (25th ed.). (2005). Greenwood Village, CO: MICROMEDEX Thomson Healthcare.
*Recommendations may change over time; therefore manufacturers' package inserts should always be consulted. No drugs are known to be absolutely safe during pregnancy. The risks and benefits of using many substances, including most drugs not on this list, should be carefully considered by the obstetrician. See drug monographs for specific drug information; see also the Bibliography for sources of information about drugs in this table.

BOX 7-1 ALCOHOL AND THE CHILDBEARING CLIENT: FETAL ALCOHOL SYNDROME

Many people do not consider alcohol to be a drug; thus it may be overlooked as being hazardous if used during pregnancy. The teratogenic effects of intrauterine alcohol exposure on the fetus are well documented. Heavy use of alcohol by the childbearing client has been associated with the following effects on the fetus/infant:

- Facial: ptosis, strabismus, myopia, cleft lip or palate
- Central nervous system (CNS): retardation, impaired coordination, increased irritability during infancy, hyperactivity in childhood
- Growth: slowed
- Cardiac: murmurs, tetralogy of Fallot
- Muscular: Hernias of the groin, umbilicus, or diaphragm

Although a direct relationship between the quantity of alcohol consumed and the severity of fetal alcohol syndrome (FAS) has not been identified, it appears that the fetus is at greatest risk when alcohol consumption is in excess of the liver's capability to detoxify it. Genetics, which affects alcohol metabolism, may also play a role in the risk for fetal alcohol syndrome. The exact mechanism of FAS has not been identified, but studies indicate that counseling to eliminate maternal alcohol intake has a beneficial effect on the health of both the mother and infant. It has been recommended that women discontinue alcohol use at least 3 months before becoming pregnant.

The nurse must be aware of clients who are at risk of FAS and be prepared to provide client education, counseling, and referral.

Data from Young, V.S.L. (2005). Teratogenicity and drugs in breast milk. In M.A. Koda-Kimble, L.Y. Young, W.A. Kradian, B.J. Guglielmo, B.K. Alldredge, R.L. Corelli (Eds.), *Applied therapeutics: The clinical use of drugs* (8th ed.). Philadelphia: Lippincott Williams & Wilkins.

- An obstetrician or pediatrician should evaluate any prescription written by a professional who is not a specialist in the care of pregnant women or nursing mothers. The specialist may need to change the prescription to a safer drug or dosage.
- Close health care supervision is essential if the mother is exposed to a questionable substance. If there is high risk for fetal or infant injury, the parents need ongoing support as they endure the sometimes lengthy wait for manifestation of the effects. If birth defects or toxic effects are present or if invasive diagnostic tests or a therapeutic abortion is to be performed, objective psychological intervention may help parents endure this critical period.

Children

Neonates

Newborns require special consideration because they lack many of the protective mechanisms that allow older children and adults to be relatively resistant to all types of stressors. Their skin is thin and permeable, their stomachs lack acid, and their lungs lack much of the mucus barrier. Peristalsis in the neonate is irregular and may be slow; drug absorption of oral drugs may be unpredictable. GI enzyme activity tends to be lower in the newborn than in the adult. The neonate has a higher percentage of its body weight in water (70% to 75%) than does the adult (50% to 60%); this may affect the distribution of water-soluble drugs. In general, protein binding is decreased in the neonate. Bilirubin may also bind to available plasma protein. Administration of highly plasma protein bound drugs in the neonate may lead to elevated free bilirubin levels (increasing the risk for kernicterus and risk for brain injury) and higher levels of free drug. In the adult this higher concentration of free drug results in faster elimination. The enzymes responsible for drug metabolism may not be fully developed in neonates. This is particularly true for premature infants, who may lack many of the cytochrome P450 isoenzymes required for drug biotransformation. With reduced metabolism and lower glomerular filtration rates in newborns compared with older infants, children, or adults, this ability to prevent toxicity by excreting excess amounts of the drug may not happen, leading to accumulation and toxicity. Neonates regulate body temperature poorly and become dehydrated easily. Their liver and kidneys are immature and cannot manage foreign substances as well as older children and adults. These factors change rapidly after birth. Specific factors affecting medication use in neonates are listed in Table 7-5. To demonstrate how these physiologic changes affect half-lives of drugs for neonates, see Table 7-6.

Breastfed Infants

Almost all forms of drugs in the maternal circulation can be readily transferred to the colostrum and breast milk. Because drugs or their biotransformed products are handled by different pathways in the infant and the fetus, the impact of maternal medications on the infant is likely different from (probably less than) the impact on the fetus. This difference can guide the health care professional in prescribing medications for the breastfeeding woman. Typical nontherapeutic outcomes in the breastfed infant are signs of the drug's usual adverse effects.

Other adverse effects may also occur, such as allergic sensitization to penicillin or gray-brown stains of later-erupting teeth as a result of tetracycline therapy of more than 10 days' duration. Most drug products that reach the neonate via the breast milk have undergone maternal biotransformation and are probably less than the original dose. However, immaturity of the neonate's hepatic and renal systems may limit the capacity for further metabolism and excretion.

TABLE 7-5 PHYSIOLOGIC PROCESSES AFFECTING MEDICATION USE IN NEONATES

Physiologic Process	Neonate	Type of Drugs Affected
ABSORPTION		
Gastric pH	Increases to 6-8 for first 24 hours; then achlorhydria usually occurs for 10-15 days	Acid-labile drugs, such as oral penicillin, are better absorbed. Oral forms of phenobarbital or phenytoin have reduced bioavailability.
Gastric emptying time	Prolonged, usually 6-8 hours	Oral absorption of penicillin is increased; absorption of phenytoin and phenobarbital is decreased.
DISTRIBUTION		
Total body water (TBW) content	75%-79%	Average adults have approximately 60% TBW and 25%-45% fat. There are vast differences in drug distribution across the age span.
Adipose (fat) content	5%-12%	Water-soluble drugs have a larger volume of distribution in newborns, whereas fat-soluble drugs have considerably less. Drug dosage adjustments are largely based on this factor.
Protein binding	Decreased	Highly protein-bound drugs require dosage adjustments to avoid toxicity as a result of increased free drug concentrations in the plasma.
METABOLISM		
Liver metabolism Microsomal enzymes	Decreased Low	Potent or potentially toxic drugs requiring liver metabolism are slowly metabolized; lower dosages are necessary for such drugs, especially chloramphenicol (Chloromycetin) and theophylline, among others.
EXCRETION		
Glomerular filtration Tubular secretion	Decreased Decreased	Drugs excreted by filtration or secretion will accumulate in the neonate; dosage adjustments are necessary, especially with aminoglycosides and digoxin (Lanoxin).

TABLE 7-6 APPROXIMATE HALF-LIVES OF SELECTED DRUGS IN NEONATES AND ADULTS

Drug	Neonatal Age	Neonates $t_{1/2}$ (hours)	Adults $t_{1/2}$ (hours)
acetaminophen		2.2-5	0.9-2.2
diazepam		25-1000	40-50
phenobarbital	0-5 days	200	64-140
	5-15 days	100	
	1-30 months	50	
Phenytoin (low to moderate dosing)	0-2 days	80	12-18
	3-14 days	18	

Modified from Katzung, B.G. (Ed.). (2004). *Basic & clinical pharmacology* (8th ed.). Norwalk, CT: Appleton & Lange.

Data about an infant's capabilities for drug absorption, distribution, metabolism, and excretion are scant and conflicting. In general, the proved benefits of continuing breastfeeding must be weighed on an individual basis against the risks of maternal medication to the infant. The mammary glands are a relatively insignificant route for maternal drug excretion and the drug level in breast milk is usually less than the actual maternal dose, and the infant's actual dose depends largely on the volume of milk consumed. Thus a single measurement of a drug in human milk will not accurately reflect the total dose received by the infant.

The concentration of the drug in maternal circulation depends on the relationship of several factors: dosing and route of administration, distribution, protein binding, and maternal metabolism and excretion. The mammary alveolar epithelium consists of a lipid barrier with water-filled pores; thus it is more permeable to drugs during the colostrum stage of milk production—during the first week of life.

Drug factors that enhance drug excretion into milk are nonionization, low molecular weight, fat solubility, and concentration. Drug distribution and the absorptive processes of the infant's GI tract are estimated to be similar to those in the adult, which means that lipid-soluble substances are well absorbed. The infant's age (thus the amount of drug-containing milk consumed) and the relative immaturity of the infant's important organs have a significant effect on the outcome. The following factors are also relevant: (1) if the drug is fat-soluble, it may be more highly concentrated in breast milk at the end of feedings and at midday; (2) because the infant's total serum protein is lower in comparison to the adult's, more free drug may be available to the circulation; (3) metabolic reactions in the liver of an infant are slower than in the older child, and therefore drug biotransformation may likewise be delayed; and (4) drug excretion is delayed in the neonate because it occurs mainly via the kidneys, in which immature glomerular filtration rates and tubular functioning are maintained for several months. The extreme variability among drug effects and infants' capabilities makes it difficult to decide whether or not the mother should take a drug and whether or not she should breastfeed.

If human milk contains small, fixed amounts of substances absorbed by the mother in a short course of drug therapy, it is usually recommended that breastfeeding be temporarily interrupted and the breasts pumped to remove drug-containing milk. Less often, it is advisable to cease breastfeeding altogether. Dosages and routes may also be changed. It is recommended that certain drugs be avoided while breastfeeding (Table 7-7).

✴ **L.W. delivers a healthy normal girl infant. She decides that she would like to breastfeed.**

✴ **What factors are considered for drug therapy of the breastfeeding woman and their infants?**
A drug is used only if medically necessary and treatment cannot be delayed until the infant is ready to be weaned. In selecting an appropriate drug to prescribe for a breastfeeding mother, the prescriber should consider whether the drug could be given directly to the infant; avoid long-acting formulations; and consider if there are localized routes of administration rather than systemic that would be as effective. Drug effects may be minimized by substituting formula for the midday breastfeeding, because that feeding is highest in fat content and thus is more likely to contain higher amounts of fat-soluble drug products. Breastfeeding mothers who must take medications can take the medication immediately *after* breastfeeding so as much time as possible elapses and the drug can reach a relatively low concentration before the next feeding. Always observe the infant for unusual symptoms (e.g., sedation, irritability, rash, failure to thrive). Provide client education to increase understanding of risk factors. Drugs considered relatively safe during breastfeeding are summarized in Table 7-8.

Therapy with radioactive substances is of short duration; if a diagnostic radioisotope test is to be performed, breastfeeding is interrupted until all radiation is absent from milk samples. Breastfeeding will probably be terminated whenever the drug is so potent that minute amounts may profoundly affect the infant, when the drug has high allergenic potential, when the mother's renal function decreases (which augments drug excretion into breast milk), or when serious pathologic conditions require prolonged administration of high doses of the drug.

Changes in the activity level of the fetus or nursing infant signal dangerous effects resulting from drug administration. Parents should be taught how to assess and report unusual fetal inactivity or infant apathy.

Both health care professionals and clients place a high value on the use of pharmaceuticals to treat minor illnesses. However, many illnesses are self-limited or cause only minor discomforts that end or decrease without medication or with nondrug alternatives (e.g., relaxation techniques rather than tranquilizers). The risk-to-benefit effect of any medication should consider the physiologic, physical, and psychological effects of therapy on both the mother and the child (Schou, 1998).

Another possibility is to delay the mother's pharmacologic therapy until the infant is weaned or to select another drug that can meet the therapeutic goal without interfering with breastfeeding. The age and maturity of the child must also be considered, because the ability of a drug to cause harmful effects diminishes as an infant develops physiologically. The frequency of feedings should also be considered. An infant who depends on breast milk for total nutrition will receive higher doses of drugs than an infant who breastfeeds only once or twice a day and receives other forms of nourishment.

Nonbreastfed Infants

Infant formula feeding is used for the following situations:
- The mother chooses not to breastfeed, *or*
- The mother is advised not to breastfeed because of illness or disease, *or*
- The infant has special formulation needs.

Commercial infant formulas prepared from nonfat cow's milk are available and are generally divided into two cate-

TABLE 7-7 DRUGS TO BE USED WITH CAUTION OR CONTRAINDICATED DURING BREASTFEEDING

The American Academy of Pediatrics Committee on the Transfer of Drugs and Other Chemicals Into Human Milk has suggested that the following drugs be avoided by women who are breastfeeding:

Agent	Effect	Agent	Effect
acebutolol	Hypotension; bradycardia; tachypnea	fluoxetine	Colic, irritability, feeding and sleeping disorders, slow weight gain
alcohol (ethanol), chronic use	Drowsiness, diaphoresis, weakness, decrease in linear growth	haloperidol	Decline in developmental scores
amiodarone	Possible hypothyroidism	heroin	Tremors, restlessness, vomiting, poor feeding
amphetamine	Cause irritability and poor sleep patterns	lamotrigine	Potential therapeutic serum concentrations in infant
antidepressants	Effect unknown but may be of concern	lithium	Significant blood levels in infants
antipsychotics, in general	Effect unknown but may be of concern	marijuana	Very long half life for some components
anxiolytics	Effect unknown but may be of concern	metronidazole	In vitro mutagen
aspirin	Metabolic acidosis	nalidixic acid	Hemolysis in infant with G6PD deficiency
caffeine	Irritability, poor sleeping pattern, maternal intake greater than 2 to 3 cups/day	nitrofurantoin	Hemolysis in infant with G6PD deficiency
chloramphenicol (Chloromycetin)	Possible idiosyncratic bone depression	phencyclidine	Potent hallucinogen
		phenobarbital	Sedation
chlorpromazine	Drowsiness and lethargy in infant; decline in development	primidone	Sedation, feeding problems
cocaine	Central nervous system (CNS) stimulation and intoxication	radioactive compounds	Require temporary cessation of breastfeeding; radioactivity in breast milk
clofazimine	Possible increase in skin pigment	sulfapyridine	Caution in infant with jaundice or G6PD deficiency
cytotoxic drug	Potential for immune suppression; cytotoxic effects in infants unknown	sulfisoxazole	Caution in infant with jaundice or G6PD deficiency
danthron	Increased bowel activity		
ergotamine	Vomiting, diarrhea, seizures		

Modified from Committee on Drugs, 2000-2001, American Academy of Pediatrics. (2001). The transfer of drugs and other chemicals into human milk, *American Academy of Pediatrics, 108(3):*776-789.
G6PD, Glucose-6-phosphate dehydrogenase.

gories: general purpose formulas and special purpose formulas. Select formulas from each category are listed in Table 7-9.

Infant formulas contain essential and minor trace elements as found in human breast milk, plus the three sources of calories (protein, carbohydrate, and lipids) in a balanced proportion to promote growth. Many formulas contain vitamins and minerals, and usually the vitamin K in these formulas is more than is contained in breast milk. Vitamin K is included because it reduces the risk of hemorrhagic disease in the infant. Cow's milk differs from human milk in protein content. The protein (80%) in cow's milk is casein, whereas human milk contains whey protein (70%). Human milk protein (whey) is richer in immunoglobulins, albumin, lysozyme, amylase, transaminase, protease, and lipases; casein provides lesser amounts

of these ingredients. Although the protein in many infant formulas is of a higher quality than cow's milk, some infant formulas may contain bovine whey, a protein that contains β-lactoglobulin. This substance contributes to the development of cow's milk allergies.

Infants can absorb 20% to 50% of the iron they need from breast milk, whereas the iron from infant formulations is only minimally absorbed (4% to 7%). The reason for this difference in absorption is unknown. The Food and Drug Administration (FDA) has issued recommendations that all infant formulations contain at least 0.3 to 0.5 mg/L (the lowest iron level found in human milk) and that the iron be in a bioavailable form. Infants at risk for iron deficiency should be given supplements containing 1 to 2 mg/100 kcal of iron, or approximately 6 to 12 mg/L. Most iron-supplemented infant formulas today contain 12 or 13 mg/L.

TABLE 7-8 SELECTED DRUGS CONSIDERED RELATIVELY SAFE DURING BREASTFEEDING

Agent	Recommendations and Precautions*	Agent	Recommendations and Precautions*
ANALGESICS		isoniazid	Relatively safe; no hepatotoxicity reported in infants
acetaminophen	Relatively safe	ethambutol	No problems reported
butorphanol	With usual dosages, drug levels in breast milk are usually low	**BRONCHODILATORS**	
codeine		theophylline	Irritability
ibuprofen		**CARDIOVASCULAR DRUGS**	
ketoconazole		digoxin	Safe if maternal serum levels are closely monitored
meperidine		methyldopa	Distributed in breast milk; no documented problems in humans
morphine	Relatively safe, but infant may have measurable blood concentration	propranolol	Relatively safe at lower maternal dosages (higher drug levels in breast milk than in maternal bloodstream because of high lipid solubility of drug)
propoxyphene			
ANTIDIABETICS		warfarin	
insulin	Safe; not distributed in breast milk	**DIURETICS**	
ANTIEPILEPTIC DRUGS		spironolactone	Safe
carbamazepine		thiazides	May suppress lactation; avoid in first month of lactation
valproic acid		**GASTROINTESTINAL DRUGS**	
ANTIINFECTIVES		antacids	Relatively safe
amoxicillin		cimetidine	
cefadroxil	Low concentrations distributed into breast milk, no problems reported	**LAXATIVES (EXCEPT DANTHRON)**	
cefazolin		**VACCINES**	
cefoxitin		RhoGAM	Considered safe
ceftriaxone			
ciprofloxacin			
clindamycin			

Modified from Committee on Drugs, 2000-2001, American Academy of Pediatrics. (2001). The transfer of drugs and other chemicals into human milk, *American Academy of Pediatrics 108*(3), 776-789.
*Recommendations may change over time; therefore manufacturers' package inserts should always be consulted by pediatricians and nurses. Most substances should be avoided during the period of breastfeeding. (Details about specific drugs are located under relevant chapter headings in this text.) Consult Bibliography for sources of information.

Drug Administration in Children

Administering medications to children requires special knowledge and approaches. The dosage of a medication may be prescribed, but it is the nurse's responsibility to know the safe dosage range of any medication administered to children. Usually, the most reliable pediatric dosage information is that provided by the manufacturer in the package insert. However, many times such information is not included from the manufacturer, even though studies have been published in the medical literature; this reflects the reluctance of the manufacturers to label their products for pediatric use (Katzung, 2004). Pediatric clients should be given medications that have been appropriately evaluated for their use in that population. Safe and effective pharmacotherapeutics requires the timely development of information on the proper use of drug products in pediatric clients of various ages and, often, the development of pediatric formulations of those products. Drug development programs should usually include the pediatric client population when a product is being developed for a disease or condition in adults and it is

TABLE 7-9 SELECTED EXAMPLES OF INFANT FORMULAS

Product Name/Manufacturer	Indications/Special Features
GENERAL PURPOSE FORMULAS	
Enfamil (Mead Johnson) Good Start (Carnation) Similac (Ross)	Supplement to breastfeeding; combination of cow's milk based proteins and lactose; if not breastfeeding for some infant feedings, use formulations with iron
SPECIAL-PURPOSE FORMULAS	
Alimentum Liquid (Ross)	Severe food allergies, protein sensitivity or maldigestion, or fat malabsorption; corn and lactose free
Pregestimil Powder (Mead Johnson)	Severe malabsorption disorders
SOY FORMULAS	Infants with family history of allergies; lactose, milk, and sucrose free
ProSobee (Mead Johnson)	
Similac Isomil (Ross)	
Alsoy (Carnation)	
INFANT FORMULAS WITH IRON	
Enfamil with Iron (Mead Johnson)	
Similac with Iron (Ross)	
SMA Iron Fortified (Mead Johnson)	
Lofenalac Powder (Mead Johnson)	Low phenylalanine plus iron

BOX 7-2 PEDIATRIC DRUG LABELS

Before 1997, many drugs were released without pediatric dosage information. Earlier FDA regulations requested that drug manufacturers add more complete pediatric dosing information on their drug products, but this was voluntary. In 1997, with a concern that more medical treatments should be available for children, the FDA required pediatric-use information for drugs that might offer improved therapy for children as compared to existing drug therapies. However, it was not until the Pediatric Research Equity Act was signed into law in 2003 that all applications for new ingredients, new indications, new dosage forms, new dosing regimens, and new routes of administration must contain a pediatric assessment unless the sponsor has obtained a waiver or deferral of pediatric studies.

Critical questions that need answers to ensure safe pediatric drug use include the following:

* Are there data about the pediatric use of this drug as the result of well-designed, controlled studies?
* If so, what was the dosage and method of administration?
* Was the drug administered as a single dose or are there long-term exposure studies?
* What was the age of the youngest child or infant who received the drug?
* Were any adverse effects reported? What was the frequency of such effects?

anticipated the product will be used in the pediatric population. A standard medication dosage is nearly nonexistent in pediatrics (Box 7-2); medications are usually ordered according to the weight or body surface area (BSA) of the child. Some pharmaceutical companies continue to supply medications in standard adult-dose strength, and the nurse must be able to calculate the correct pediatric dosage before administering the medication.

In the absence of explicit pediatric dose recommendations, an approximation can be made by any of several methods based on age, weight, or surface area. Although all three methods will be discussed, currently the BSA is pre-ferred. Calculations based on age or weight are conservative and tend to underestimate the required dose.

Age (Young's rule):

$$\text{Dose} = \text{Adult dose} \times \frac{\text{Age (years)}}{\text{Age} + 12}$$

Weight (Clark's rule):

$$\text{Dose} = \text{Adult dose} \times \frac{\text{Weight (kg)}}{70}$$

$$\text{or Dose} = \text{Adult dose} \times \frac{\text{Weight (lb)}}{150}$$

Calculating the pediatric dosage on the basis of weight alone implies that the pediatric client is a small adult, which is not true. The physiologic differences between infants and adults definitely affect the amount of drug needed to produce a therapeutic effect. For example, an infant's body composition is approximately 75% water (adults have 50% to 60%), and infants have a smaller fat content than adults. Therefore water-soluble drugs are generally administered in larger doses (in proportion to body weight) to infants and children than to adults. Rules based on weight, such as Clark's rule, are generally taught and used by students in clinical areas to assess pediatric dosages; this rule has limited usefulness as a guide. For the approximately 75% of drugs that have no established dosage for children, Clark's rule to calculate the pediatric dosage as a fraction of the average adult dosage is too imprecise. However, Clark's rule may be used (mg/kg) when the dosage according to BSA has not been established.

Body Surface Area:

Approximate pediatric dose =

$$\frac{\text{Child's BSA in square meters (from nomogram)} \times \text{Adult dose}}{1.73}$$

Prescribers usually carry a simple slide rule or nomogram, such as the West nomogram (Figure 7-2), or use automated formulas on PDA devices to make rapid BSA conversions from weight and height. It is believed that the larger amount of total body water (TBW) in children—and the percentage of water in body weight and the part of that percentage formed by extracellular water—accounts for the fact that children tolerate or require larger dosages of some drugs on a mg/m² basis.

As a relationship between height and weight, BSA can provide a more precise guide to the maturity of the child's organs and metabolic rate of functioning for effective pharmacokinetics. The dosage should be tailored to the individual child according to the amount of medication per square meter of BSA.

A nurse calculating dosages of digoxin, insulin, barbiturates, and opioids should have the calculations and the prepared medication dose checked by another nurse or a pharmacist before administering the drug. Pediatric dosages are often minute, and thus a slight calculation error may result in a greater proportional error.

✳ What are the nursing management issues in medication administration for children?

Although the previously discussed rules have been devised for converting adult dosage schedules to schedules for infants and children, it must be emphasized that *no rules or charts are* adequate to guarantee safety of dosage at any age, particularly in the neonate. No method takes into account all variables, particularly individual tolerance differences. Astute, accurate nursing observations of how individual children react to drugs can assist in monitoring drugs and dosages.

Administering medications to infants and children is both challenging and frustrating. Giving injections skillfully will enhance safety and help to gain a child's coopera-

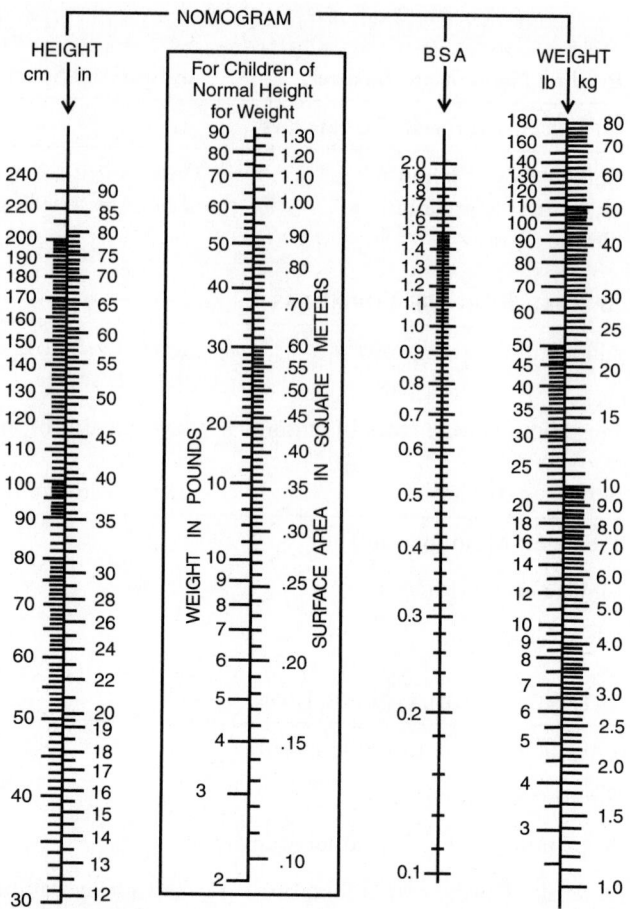

FIGURE 7-2 BSA is indicated where the straight line that connects height (on the left) and weight (on the right) intersects the BSA column or, if client is above average size, from weight alone (enclosed area).

Modified from data of E. Boyd by C.D. West; from Behrman, R.E., & Vaughan, V.C. (Eds.) (2003). *Nelson's textbook of pediatrics* (17th ed.). Philadelphia: W.B. Saunders.

tion. A sound knowledge of growth and development also provides the nurse with information about how a child might be approached, whether reasoning will help or hinder the process, and whether assistance will be needed. The principles of safe administration of medication apply to all age groups, but children differ from adults, and the nurse has added responsibilities when administering a medication to a child (Box 7-3).

Ideally, a child will cooperate more readily with a nurse once a positive relationship has been established. The child may also more easily accept the discomforts of injections and of some oral medications from a nurse who is associated with daily hygiene, feeding, holding, play, and happy times. Additionally, the nurse will feel less guilty when the child associates the nurse with pleasure and comfort most of the time and with discomfort only when it is necessary in order for the child to get well.

When a child is afraid or anxious, his or her natural response is to strike out at the frustration or avoid it. By accepting this behavior as a natural response, the nurse will be

1. Parents are often good sources of information about successful methods or vehicles of giving medications to their children.
2. Try to avoid putting medications in essential foods such as milk, cereal, or orange juice, because the child may refuse to accept that food in the future.
3. Never underestimate a child's reactions. The taste of the medication may not need to be disguised.
4. A sip of cold fruit juice, ice chips, a frozen fruit bar, or a mint-flavored substance before and after the administration of an unpalatable medicine may effectively dull its taste.
5. Sugarless vehicles should be used to disguise the taste of medications given to children who have diabetes or are following a ketogenic diet.
6. Jam and syrup are ideal for suspending drugs that do not dissolve easily in water.
7. Because fruit syrups are usually acidic, they should not be used for medicines that react in an acid medium (e.g., sodium bicarbonate, soluble barbiturates, and penicillin).
8. Nursing time can be saved by recording the most successful method of administering medications and pertinent nursing orders on the child's care plan. This notation also saves the child frustration, fear, and anxiety.

able to deal with it and to be honest when a medication or procedure will be unpleasant or painful. Truthful explanations are essential with children. They have a right to an explanation of any procedure that concerns them. The timing and type of explanation should be geared to the child's ability to perceive and understand. For the child 2 years of age or younger very simple explanations such as "I have some medicine for you to drink" or "I have an injection to give you, and it will hurt a little" are sufficient. Young children may be less resistant to injectable medications if a parent holds and comforts them. In an ambulatory care setting, it is best to have the child all dressed and ready to leave before administering immunizations and other injectables. A brief exposure of the appropriate injection site to determine landmarks, a quick injection, and then an exit from the facility will decrease the child's association of the discomfort of an injection with the clinical setting.

Long explanations to children under 5 years of age do little more than prolong the anticipation and increase anxiety or fear. Telling 4-year-old children to stop kicking, hitting, or performing any other avoidance behavior only conveys to them that they are not understood and that they will receive little or no help with their feelings of frustration about being medicated. Providing the preschool-age child opportunities at play (e.g., to give a doll an "injection" [empty syringe without a needle] or "drops") affords an important outlet and allows the child to work through the trauma of the experience.

Many children are courageous, or like to be considered so, and therefore appealing to their courage is sometimes effective. Children 4 years old or over may choose to hold their own medicine cup or drink unassisted and to take pills from the container without any assistance from the nurse. Children of this age are motivated by social reinforcers, such as being praised for their cooperation or being told that "your job is to stay very still," which enhances their self-esteem and feelings of competence. Helping the child to identify what he or she can do during the procedure will help him or her to cope. Because of the sense of achievement that follows, children may want to save the medicine cups to show their parents. Box 7-4 lists developmental perspectives for administering medications.

Oral Medications Success in administering oral medications usually requires a kind but firm approach and a positive attitude. The nurse should reflect certainty that the child will take the medicine in the choice of words and tone of voice. The nurse might say, "Jimmy, it's time to take your yellow medicine" or "Do you want to take your pill now or with your Jell-O?" Such statements indicate that the child is expected to cooperate and also allow him or her some control over the situation. An unwise approach that conveys doubt on the nurse's part might be "I have your yellow pill, Jimmy. Will you take it for me, please?"

Nurses should be aware of how a medicine tastes so that they can answer questions such as, "Does it taste bad?" or "Will it burn my mouth?" A helpful reply would be, "It tastes like cherry to me. Tell me what it tastes like to you." Often the child will accept the suggestion to taste and find out. However, if the medication has an unpleasant taste, attempting to deceive or lie is as futile and destructive with a child as it is with an adult.

Medications that have a disagreeable taste should be disguised if at all possible. Small amounts of syrup, jam, fruit, and some fruit juices are suitable sweet vehicles for less palatable drugs. Some pills can be crushed and suspended in small amounts of these substances as long as the two substances are compatible. Infants and children swallow many liquid medications more readily if mixed with a sweet substance or diluted with a small amount of water. (If large amounts of water or other substances are used and the child refuses to take all of the mixture, it is difficult to estimate how much medication the child received.) Fortunately, many drugs are available as palatable syrups or in a suspension form well suited for administration to infants and children. Suspensions should be thoroughly agitated to ensure that doses are not offered in unequal concentrations.

To prevent aspiration, exercise caution when giving oral medications to children. Medications must be given to infants slowly and in small amounts to avoid choking. Liquid medications may be administered via a nipple, plastic medicine cup, plastic dropper, or plastic syringe without the needle. Water should be rinsed through the inside of these containers *first* to prevent the medication from sticking, which can cause an inaccurate dose. Glass cups, droppers, or syringes should be avoided because of the obvious danger of them breaking in the

---

BOX 7-4 DEVELOPMENTAL PERSPECTIVES FOR ADMINISTERING MEDICATIONS

GENERAL INTERVENTIONS

- Always come prepared for the procedure with all necessary equipment and assistance.
- For in-hospital administration, ask the parent and/or child if the parent should or should not remain for the procedure.
- Assess comfort methods appropriate for preadministration and postadministration.

INFANTS

- Perform the procedure swiftly, then offer comfort measures (e.g., parent holding, rocking, cuddling, soothing).
- Allow self-comforting measures (e.g., use of pacifier, fingers in mouth, self-movement).

TODDLERS

- Offer a brief, concrete explanation of procedure, and then perform it.
- Accept aggressive behavior (within reasonable limits) as a healthy response.
- Provide comfort measures immediately after the procedure (e.g., touch, holding).
- Help the child to understand the treatment and his or her feelings through playing with puppets or hospital equipment, such as a syringe and water.
- Provide for ways to release aggression with play, such as hammering or water play.

PRESCHOOLERS

- Offer a brief, concrete explanation.
- Provide comfort measures after the procedure (e.g., touch, holding).
- Accept aggressive responses and provide outlets for them.
- Make use of magical thinking; use "ointments" or "special medicines" to make the discomfort go away.
- The role of the parent is very important for comfort and understanding.

SCHOOL-AGED CHILDREN

- Explain the procedure, allowing for some control over body and situation.
- Provide comfort measures.
- Explore feelings and concepts through therapeutic play, drawings of own body and self in the hospital, and the use of books and realistic hospital equipment.
- Set appropriate behavior limits (e.g., okay to cry or scream but not to bite).
- Provide activities for releasing aggression and anger.
- Use this opportunity to teach about the relationship between the medication and body function and structure (e.g., what a seizure is and how medication helps prevent the seizure).
- Offer the complete picture (e.g., need to take medication, relax with deep breaths, medication will help prevent pain).

ADOLESCENTS

- Prepare in advance for the procedure.
- Allow for expression in a way that does not cause the adolescent to "lose face," such as giving the adolescent time alone after the procedure and giving him or her time to discuss the discomfort if he or she wants to verbalize feelings.
- Explore current concepts of self, hospitalization, and illness and correct any misconceptions.
- Encourage self-expression, individuality, and self-care.
- Encourage participation in the procedure to the extent agreed on in advance. Increased participation should be discussed after the procedure.

Modified from Blaber, M. (1990). Related to nursing intervention in pain. *Newington Children's Hospital Manual for Global Pediatric Nursing Assessment* (unpublished).

---

child's mouth. A plastic dropper or syringe is best suited for placing a liquid medication along one side of an infant's tongue. Older infants and toddlers seem to prefer taking their medications from a plastic medicine cup. Children are less likely to aspirate the medication if they are held or placed in a sitting position than if they lie on their backs.

When administering a medication with a dropper or syringe, the nurse may purse the infant's lips with one hand to keep the medicine from running out of the mouth. Droppers and syringes used for medication should be kept clean, should be reserved for only one client's use, and should be rinsed or washed before being returned to the medication bottle.

If the child refuses to cooperate even after being given explanations and encouragement, the nurse may need to ask whether the child will take the medication alone or will need the nurse to give it. Physical coercion is seldom necessary; if used, it should be mild, quick, and firm, because aspiration is a danger. The nurse must not combine force with anger or

resort to force when one nurse has been unable to administer the medication. Careful consideration should be given to factors such as the following: Why does the child resist? Does the child disapprove of only one nurse? Have past experiences with medications given at home or in the hospital frightened the child? Will forcing a medication cause a struggle that will negate the effects of a drug given for sedation? If mild restraint is necessary, explain to the child that this form of treatment is necessary. The child will not cooperate if force is seen as a punishment for an inability to cooperate; often the child loses confidence in all personnel.

Topical Medications Children have a large skin surface area in proportion to total body weight. Their skin, especially the skin of neonates, is particularly thin and permeable and has limited protective oil.

Although adults absorb much more medication through intact skin than was previously believed, the child is at even more risk for systemic medication administration. The discovery that hexachlorophene can cause encephalopathy in newborns and that topically applied boric acid can cause systemic poisoning testifies to the hazard of applying drugs to children's skin, especially for contact that is prolonged or is over broken skin areas. Plain soap and water, not medicated dressings, may be the preferred treatment for abrasions or open lesions.

Subcutaneous Injections There are wide variations in the amounts of subcutaneous fat in children. Neonates have a proportionately smaller amount, with body fat increasing slightly to 23% by 1 year of age. From 1 to 5 years of age the amount of body fat drops to between 8% and 12%; it climbs to approximately 20% when the child reaches 10 years of age. Lipid-soluble drugs have an affinity for fat tissue; less subcutaneous fat means that lower dosages of fat-soluble drugs (e.g., diazepam and barbiturates) are necessary to maintain blood levels. Additionally, less subcutaneous tissue for injections may be available. An alternate route may need to be selected—oral, intramuscularly (IM), or intravenously (IV).

Intramuscular Injections The principles and techniques of administrating IM injections in children are similar to those for adults, except that different muscle groups are used for injection sites as a result of the difference in muscular development at different ages. The younger the child, the less muscle tissue available for IM injections. If repeated injections are necessary, the available sites may become overused, inflamed, or dystrophic; the nurse is therefore required to make a concerted effort to develop systematic plans for rotating sites and inform the rest of the staff about them, or to consult with the prescriber about changing to an oral or IV dosage form.

In the interest of safety, a child should usually be restrained for an injection, and the injection should be given rapidly. Two or more persons should be available for children over 4 years of age, even children who promise to "hold still." An extra sterile needle may be carried in a pocket in case the first needle becomes contaminated when a child moves unexpectedly. Asking the child to wiggle the toes may distract his or her attention from the injection. Because children enjoy trying out each other's beds, the identifying wristband must be checked to ensure proper client identification before giving each medication.

Rectal Administration Several drugs, such as sedatives, aspirin, and antiemetics, are available in suppository form. The rectal route is often advised when oral administration is difficult or contraindicated. Many children perceive use of the rectal route as an extreme invasion of their bodies and anticipate pain as a result. It may help to let them participate (e.g., to insert the suppository). Suppositories made with a cocoa butter base melt rapidly at normal body temperature, releasing the drug for absorption. After inserting a suppository into an infant, the buttocks should be held or taped together for 5 to 10 minutes to relieve pressure on the anal sphincter and thereby help ensure retention and absorption of the medication. Infants and children with diarrhea may easily expel sup-

positories with explosive stools. Similarly, if a child has constipation or a rectum full of stool, the suppository will be surrounded with stool and has little chance of being absorbed.

Health care professionals often divide suppository doses by cutting them. This is a dangerous practice, because all of the medication might be contained in one area of the suppository. If divided doses must be administered, the pharmacist should be contacted for alternate product advice and guidance.

Nose Drops, Eardrops, and Eyedrops Because of the danger of aspiration, aqueous preparations of nose drops are the only safe preparations to use. Many nose drop preparations contain vasoconstrictors, and prolonged or excessive use may be harmful. Infants are nose breathers, and nasal congestion will inhibit their sucking. For this reason, nose drops, if necessary, should be instilled 20 to 30 minutes before feedings.

Before the initial administration of a course of therapy with *eardrops,* assess whether the child has excessive cerumen. If so, it may be necessary to consult with the prescriber about removing it with cerumen softeners or irrigation before instilling the eardrops. Instilling eardrops requires knowledge of anatomic structure, because the auditory canal is shorter and more horizontal in a young child than in an adult.

Eyedrop instillation in children is performed in the same way as with adults except that the head may be stabilized by an assistant. Many eyedrops cause a burning sensation for a few seconds, so if both eyes are to be medicated it is wise to do the second instillation quickly—before the child begins to blink and tear as a reaction to the burning sensation in the first eye. Mild pressure for 30 seconds over the inner canthus next to the nose prevents premature drainage of the medication away from the eye.

Aqueous preparations of nose drops, eardrops, and eyedrops may support the growth of bacteria and fungi. For this reason small volumes of such medications are ordered and should be used for only *one* individual (not shared by family members). The dropper (especially an eyedropper) should not be permitted to become contaminated by touching anything but the medication. To avoid forming a medium for microbiologic growth, the dropper should never be inverted so that medication or water runs into the rubber bulb. A dropper from one medication should not be used to measure and administer another type of medication because droppers are not standardized—not all droppers are manufactured to deliver drops of the same volume. The viscosity of drugs also varies, which affects drop size.

Eyedrops and eardrops are more comfortably tolerated if they are warmed (if not contraindicated) before instillation. To do this, run warm water over the side of the bottle without the label, or immerse the bottle in some warm water in a medicine cup. Carrying the bottle in a pocket for half an hour or so also takes the chill off the drops.

Intravenous Medications The use of IV drug therapy is widespread on most pediatric services for several reasons. In children with vomiting and diarrhea, medications given by mouth may be vomited, and precious time in drug management is lost. Because these children may have poor absorption of drugs and fluids as a result of dehydration or peripheral vascular collapse, drugs administered via the IM route may be equally ineffective. Premature infants are at risk for necrotizing enterocolitis (NEC) and death when administered feedings or oral drugs that have an osmolality greater than that of body fluids. Elixirs of theophylline, phenobarbital, calcium, digoxin, and dexamethasone have osmolalities 10 times greater than body fluids and have been implicated in causing NEC, and analysis shows that the contained additives actually raise the medication's osmolality. Therefore it may be preferable to give premature or physiologically distressed neonates certain high-osmolality drugs by IV administration.

The suggestions in the Medication Safety Alert box below may be helpful to pediatric nurses responsible for the administration of IV drugs. Most older children may be given fluids or drugs intravenously following the same principles and techniques used for adults. The younger and smaller the child, the narrower the margin for error.

Other Factors Influencing Drug Dosages Again, the dosage of most agents is related to the child's age, weight, and height. A child's body systems grow and develop at varying rates, leading to unpredictable primary and secondary effects in pediatric medication administration. One example of secondary effects specific to children is discoloration of teeth and depression of enamel growth with the administration of tetracycline in children under 8 years of age. Although this adverse effect is well documented, the drug is still being prescribed for this age group, according to the FDA. Children receiving long-term adrenocortical steroids experience impaired skeletal growth.

Individual variations are noted in children's responses to digoxin, insulin, opioids, and oral enzyme products; doses require careful titration. Clients with cystic fibrosis (CF) often require increased doses of antimicrobials to achieve similar levels and response to those without CF. Paradoxic responses are noted with a few drugs; the responses may be directly opposite to those expected in adults. Excessive reactivity to atropine by infants may be related to immaturity of the central nervous system (CNS). Because of the complex medicolegal issues involved in experimentation on children, many drugs that are safe and effective for adults have not been tested for use with children, nor have dosages been established.

Summary

Nursing management of medication administration to clients of different age groups requires that the nurse be knowledgeable about growth and development and about the various effects of pharmaceutical agents on clients of different ages. Understanding the rationale behind these effects helps the nurse to administer medications safely and to evaluate client responses appropriately, regardless of the client's age. Childbearing clients, neonates, infants, and children have unique needs related to the accurate and safe administration of medications—needs that are based on their unique physiologic and psychosocial development.

✦ Medication Safety Alert

IV Drug Administration in Children

1. IV drug therapy should be used only if other channels of drug administration are impractical. Pediatric nurses who are skilled in giving medications to children via other routes may be able to influence prescribers' decisions regarding successful routes of drug administration.
2. For small infants a scalp vein or a superficial vein of the wrist, hand, foot, or arm may be most convenient and most easily stabilized. Scalp veins are the most frequent sites for infant infusions; because these veins have no valves, infusions may be in either direction. Older children may receive infusions through any accessible vein.
3. An IV infusion or injection that is too rapid may cause "speed shock," with a rapid fall in blood pressure, respiratory irregularity, blood incoagulability, and even death. Preventive measures include use of the minidropper (note that the milliliter per hour in the order translates to the drops per minute with this tubing), calibrated volume control chambers, and infusion pumps.
4. Total parenteral nutrition (TPN) solutions are usually infused into the vena cava or innominate or subclavian veins approached via the external or internal jugular veins. The inferior vena cava is occasionally entered via the femoral vein.
5. Once a drug is injected intravenously, the action of the drug is relatively irreversible.
6. Drugs must be properly diluted. This caution cannot be emphasized too much.
7. Give the smallest possible dose at the slowest possible rate.

✳ Critical Thinking Questions

- Select one drug, such as phenytoin or warfarin, and discuss the potential risks to the fetus or breastfeeding child in relation to needed benefits to the mother.
- Ms. Leverett, a nursing student, is assigned to care for Sally, a 3-year-old, and Loretta, an 8-year-old, who are sharing the same hospital room. From a developmental perspective, how will her approach to the two children differ when it comes to administering medications?

Bibliography

Andrade, S.E., Gurwitz, J.H., Davis, R.L., Chan, K.A., Finkelstein, J.A., Fortman, K., et al. (2004). Prescription drug use in pregnancy. *American Journal of Obstetrics and Gynecology, 191,* 398-407.

Anderson, D.M., Keith, J., & Novak, P.D. (Eds.) (2002). *Mosby's medical, nursing, and allied health dictionary* (6th ed.). St. Louis: Mosby.

Black, R.A., & Hill, D.A. (2003). Over-the-counter medications in pregnancy. *American Family Physician, 67*(12), 2476-2478.

Drug facts and comparisons (58th ed.). (2005). St. Louis: Facts and Comparisons.

Ebrahim, S.H., & Gfoerer, J. (2003). Pregnancy-related substance abuse in the United States during 1996-1998. *Obstetrics & Gynecology, 101*(2), 374-379.

Frank, D.A., Augustyn, M., Knight, W.G., Pell, T., & Zuckerman, B. (2001). Prenatal cocaine exposure study: Growth, development, and behavior in early childhood following prenatal cocaine exposure. *Journal of the American Medical Association, 285,* 1613-1625

Holcberg, G., Tsadkin-Tamir, M., Sapir, O., Huleihel, M. & Ben Zvi, Z. (2003). New aspects in placental drug transfer. *The Israeli Medical Association Journal, 5*(12), 873-876.

Katzung, B.G. (Ed.). (2004). *Basic & clinical pharmacology* (8th ed.). Norwalk, CT: Appleton & Lange.

Lowdermilk, D.L., & Perry, S. (2004). *Maternity nursing and women's health care.* (8th ed.). St. Louis: Mosby.

Mosby's drug consult (15th ed.). (2005). St. Louis: Mosby.

Nahata, M.C., & Taketomo, C. (2002). Pediatrics. In J.T. DiPiro, et al. (Eds.), *Pharmacotherapy: A pathophysiological approach* (5th ed.). New York: McGraw-Hill.

Nordeng, H., Lindemann, R., Perminov, K.V. & Reikvam, A. (2001). Neonatal withdrawal syndrome after in utero exposure to selective serotonin reuptake inhibitors. *Acta Paediatrics, 90*(3), 288-289.

OTC Drugs Can Be Harmful to the Unborn Child. (2000). *Drug & Therapy Perspectives, 16*(3), 12-14.

Pigarelli, D.L.W., & Kraus, C.K. (2002). Pregnancy and lactation: Therapeutic considerations. In J.T. DiPiro, R.L. Talbert, G.C. Yee, G.R. Matzke, B.G. Wells, & L.M. Posey (Eds.), *Pharmacotherapy: A pathophysiological approach* (5th ed.). New York: McGraw-Hill.

Schou, M. (1998). Treating recurrent affective disorders during and after pregnancy. What can be taken safely? *Drug Safety, 18*(2), 143-152.

Schrager, S., & Potters, B.E. (2004). Diethylstilbestrol exposure. *American Family Physician, 69,* 2395-2400, 2401-2402.

USP DI: Drug information for the health care professional (25th ed.). (2005). Greenwood Village, CO: MICROMEDEX Thomson Healthcare.

Wang, M. (2004). Perinatal drug abuse and neonatal drug withdrawal. In D.N. Sheftel, R. Konop, B.S. Carter, & C.L. Wagner. (Eds.). *emedicine* Retrieved July 26, 2005, from http://www.emedicine.com/ped/topic2631.htm

Wong, D.L, Hockenberry, M.J., Wilson, D., Winkelstein, M.L., & Kleine, N.E. (2003). *Wong's nursing care of infants and children* (7th ed.). St Louis: Mosby.

Young, V.S.L. (2005). Teratogenicity and drugs in breast milk. In M.A. Koda-Kimble, L.Y. Young, W.A. Kradian, B.J. Guglielmo, B.K. Alldredge, & R.L. Corelli (Eds.), *Applied therapeutics: The clinical use of drugs* (8th ed.). Philadelphia: Lippincott Williams & Wilkins.

e-LEARNING SUPPLEMENTS

Student CD-ROM
- Final Exam questions
- NCLEX® Examination review questions
- Pharmacology animations
- Printable chapter summary

Evolve Website (http://evolve.elsevier.com/mckenry)
- Content updates, including information on new drugs
- WebLinks corresponding to this chapter
- Answers to the critical thinking questions in this chapter
- *Elsevier ePharmacology Update* newsletter
- *Mosby's Drug Consult* Internet Edition
- Supplemental and reference information

8

DRUG THERAPY FOR OLDER ADULTS

CHAPTER FOCUS

Older adults represent the fastest growing population in the United States and Canada. An understanding of the physiologic changes that occur with the aging process will help the nurse in safely administering, teaching, and monitoring drug regimens. The goal of drug treatment is to develop strategies to treat or alter a disease process and, if possible, to restore function to older adults. Many of the medication-related problems reported in older adults are preventable, and the nurse and all health care professionals play a vital role in preventing these adverse drug effects.

LEARNING OBJECTIVES

- Describe factors that promote drug misuse in older adults.
- Describe the alterations in pharmacokinetics and pharmacodynamics related to aging.
- Identify potentially inappropriate medication use in older adults.
- Identify the risk factors for ineffective management of the medication regimen by older adults.
- Manage effectively the administration of medications for older adults.

▲ KEY TERMS

polypharmacy, p. 141

The older adult population represents a small but growing proportion of our population today. In the United States, the over 65 age population was 11.4% in 1980, 12.6% in 1990, and 14.4% in 2000 (www.census.gov/prod/www.abs.briefs.html). In Canada, the over 65 age population was 11% in 1986 and 13% in 2001 (www.Statcan.ca/English/Pgdb/demo50a.htm). However, this proportion of the population consumes about 30% of all prescription medications, spending about $3 billion annually (Williams, 2002). Sixty-one percent of older people seeing a physician are taking at least one prescription medication, and most older Americans take an average of three to five medications. These data do not include the use of over-the-counter (OTC) medications or herbal remedies. It is estimated that up to 30% of hospital admissions in older adult clients are

a result of drug-related problems or drug toxic effects. Medication-related problems in the United States cause up to 106,000 deaths annually at an estimated cost of $85 billion (Kohn, Corrigan, & Donaldson, 1999). It has been projected that more than 20% of the population will be 65 years or older by the year 2030. Because older adults are the most rapidly increasing segment of the population, an understanding of age-related alterations in pharmacokinetics and pharmacodynamics is necessary. The increased incidence of chronic diseases in older adults often results in increased numbers of prescriptions, OTC medications, and home remedies (prescribed or self-selected). The age of specialization has in some ways added to this problem, with multiple health care providers usually prescribing a variety of medications—often without discontinuing the drugs the client is currently taking. This practice, the indiscriminate use of numerous medications concurrently, is often referred to as **polypharmacy.**

✴ M.L., an 86-year-old male, is brought to the nursing clinic at the senior citizen center by his daughter with a brown bag of all of his medications. She is concerned that her father takes so many medications and seems to be "napping" most of the time, has lost his appetite, and does not seem to have any energy. M.L. complains that he is constipated and his "plumbing doesn't work as well as it used to." M.L. has a history of atrial fibrillation, heart failure (HF), osteoarthritis, and benign prostatic hypertrophy. A review of the contents of his brown bag found the following: warfarin (Coumadin) 3 mg daily except for Wednesday when it is 2 mg, generic digoxin 0.25 mg daily, tamsulosin (Flomax) 0.4 mg daily, metoprolol (Lopressor) 100 mg daily, furosemide (Lasix) 80 mg twice daily, KCl 40 mEq twice daily and fluoxetine (Prozac) 40 mg daily. In addition to his prescription medications, M.L. takes Extra Strength Tylenol PM (acetaminophen 500 mg and diphenhydramine 25 mg) every night for sleep, milk of magnesia 30 mL daily and loperamide (Imodium) 2 mg on the days his stools are loose. In the bottom of the bag the nurse finds an old prescription for Lanoxin 0.125 mg, which M.L. says he has been taking for the past week because "it made him feel better last time he was sick."

✴ **Why is polypharmacy problematic in the older adult population?**

Polypharmacy and inappropriate prescribing can be a dangerous practice that may increase the risk of drug interactions and adverse effects and the need for, or prolongation of, hospitalization. Lazarou, Pomeranz, and Corey (1998) found that adverse drug effects in older clients led to hospitalizations in 25% of individuals 80 years of age and older. Although the magnitude of problems caused by polypharmacy is enormous, it is often overlooked as being the causative factor. It is important for health care providers to realize that the vast majority of undesirable drug effects resulting from polypharmacy are *preventable.*

Beers et al. (1991) developed explicit criteria for determining inappropriate medication use in nursing home residents. This list, that has become known as the Beers Criteria, has been used to assess the appropriateness of drug regimens of various older adult populations (Hanlon, Ruby, Guay, & Artz, 1992; Beers, 1997; McLeod, Huang, Tamblyn, & Gayton, 1997) and has been updated and refined by a U.S. Consensus Panel of Experts (Fick et al., 2003). Table 8-1 incorporates many of these recommendations.

TABLE 8-1 MEDICATIONS THAT MAY BE INAPPROPRIATE FOR OLDER ADULTS

Drug	Concern
ANTIHISTAMINES	
Anticholinergic antihistamines: • chlorpheniramine (Chlor-Trimeton) • cyproheptadine (Periactin) • dexchlorpheniramine (Polaramine) • diphenhydramine (Benadryl) • hydroxyzine (Vistaril, Atarax) • promethazine (Phenergan) • tripelennamine (PBZ)	Potent anticholinergics; May cause confusion and excessive sedation Should not be used as a hypnotic Use nonanticholinergic antihistamines in the older adult population
ANTIDEPRESSANTS	
Anticholinergic antidepressants: • amitriptyline (Elavil) • doxepin (Sinequan)	Strong anticholinergic and sedation properties; Rarely the antidepressant of choice for the older adult population
fluoxetine (Prozac)	Long half-life with greater risk for CNS stimulation
ANTIDIABETIC AGENTS	
chlorpropamide (Diabinese)	Prolonged half-life in older adults with risk for prolonged hypoglycemia Risk for SIADH

Modified from Fick, D.M., Cooper, J.W., Wade, W.E., Waller, J.L., Maclean, J.R., & Beers, M.H. (2003). Updating the Beers criteria for potentially inappropriate medication use in older adults, *Archives of Internal Medicine, 163*(22), 2716-2724.
CNS, Central nervous system; *GI,* gastrointestinal; *HF,* heart failure; *MI,* myocardial infarction; *NSAID,* nonsteroidal antiinflammatory drug.

Continued

TABLE 8-1 MEDICATIONS THAT MAY BE INAPPROPRIATE FOR OLDER ADULTS—*cont'd*

Drug	Concern
ANTIINFECTIVE	
nitrofurantoin (Macrodantin)	Not effective with renal impairment
ANTIPSYCHOTICS	
mesoridazine (Serentil)	Higher risk CNS and anticholinergic adverse drug effects
thioridazine (Mellaril)	Risk for QT interval prolongation and torsades de pointes
ANXIOLYTICS/SEDATIVES	
Barbiturates used for sedative/hypnotic (exception: phenobarbital for seizure control)	Potential for dependence Greater risk for adverse drug effects than alternative therapies
Benzodiazepines (long acting): • chlordiazepoxide (Librium) • diazepam (Valium) • flurazepam (Dalmane)	Prolonged half-life in older adults Prolonged sedation effects Increased risk for falls
Benzodiazepines (short acting [do not exceed dose in brackets]): • alprazolam (Xanax) [2 mg] • lorazepam (Ativan) [3 mg] • temazepam (Restoril) [15 mg]	Higher doses do not usually provide additional benefit Higher doses associated with increased risk of adverse drug effects
meprobamate (Miltown)	May cause dependence Excessive sedation
CARDIOVASCULAR AGENTS	
amiodarone (Cordarone)	Associated with QT interval prolongation and risk for torsades de pointes. Lack of efficacy in older adults
disopyramide (Norpace, Norpace CR)	Potent negative inotrope with risk for HF Anticholinergic
guanadrel (Hylorel) guanethidine (Ismelin)	May cause orthostatic hypotension Safer alternatives exist
methyldopa (Aldomet)	Risk for bradycardia Increased risk for depression in older adults
nifedipine, short acting (Procardia, Adalat)	Risk for hypotension and constipation
ticlopidine (Ticlid)	No more effective than aspirin as antiplatelet Safer alternatives available
GASTROINTESTINAL (GI) DRUGS	
GI antispasmodic agents: • dicyclomine (Bentyl) • hyoscyamine (Levsin, Levsinex) • propantheline (Pro-Banthine) • belladonna alkaloids (Donnatal) • clidinium-chlordiazepoxide (Librax)	Highly anticholinergic Of uncertain benefit
trimethobenzamide (Tigan)	Extrapyramidal effects (EPS) Among the least effective antiemetics

Modified from Fick, D.M., Cooper, J.W., Wade, W.E., Waller, J.L., Maclean, J.R., & Beers, M.H. (2003). Updating the Beers criteria for potentially inappropriate medication use in older adults, *Archives of Internal Medicine, 163*(22), 2716-2724.
CNS, Central nervous system; *GI,* gastrointestinal; *HF,* heart failure; *MI,* myocardial infarction; *NSAID,* nonsteroidal antiinflammatory drug.

TABLE 8-1 MEDICATIONS THAT MAY BE INAPPROPRIATE FOR OLDER ADULTS—*cont'd*

Drug	Concern
HORMONAL AGENTS	
desiccated thyroid	Risk for cardiac adverse effects
methyltestosterone (Android, Virilon, Testrad)	Potential for prostatic enlargement Potential for cardiac problems
LAXATIVES	
Stimulant laxatives (long term): bisacodyl (Dulcolax) cascara sagrada (Neoloid)	Risk for increased bowel dysfunction considered appropriate in the presence of opioid therapy
mineral oil	Risk for aspiration pneumonia
MUSCLE RELAXANTS AND ANTISPASMODICS	
carisoprodol (Soma) chlorzoxazone (Paraflex) cyclobenzaprine (Flexeril) metaxalone (Skelaxin) methocarbamol (Robaxin) orphenadrine (Norflex) oxybutynin (Ditropan)	Anticholinergic adverse effects Excessive sedation and weakness Often poorly tolerated in older adults
NONSTEROIDAL ANTIINFLAMMATORY DRUGS (NSAIDs)	
indomethacin (Indocin and Indocin SR)	NSAID that produces the most CNS adverse effects.
ketorolac (Toradol)	Significant number of asymptomatic GI pathologic conditions
NSAIDs, long term use of longer half-life, non–COX selective: • naproxen (Naprosyn, Anaprox, Aleve) • oxaprozin (Daypro) • piroxicam (Feldene)	Greater risk for: GI bleeding Renal failure Hypertension HF
OPIOID ANALGESICS	
meperidine (Demerol)	Not as effective as oral analgesics in commonly prescribed dosages; May cause confusion, seizures
pentazocine (Talwin)	Causes more CNS adverse effects than other opioid analgesics (e.g., confusion and hallucinations)
STIMULANTS	
amphetamines anorexic drugs	May cause dependence Cardiovascular risks: hypertension, angina, MI

To minimize the risks associated with the use of multiple medications, inappropriate prescribing, and adverse drug effects in this population, health care providers need to provide continuous drug regimen monitoring, with a primary goal of reducing the number of prescriptions and/or eliminating inappropriate medications and improving the client's quality of life. The nurse needs to understand how drugs affect the aging body to appreciate the risk inherent in medicating older adults.

❋ What physiologic changes of aging contribute to adverse drug effects in the older adult population?

Older adults undergo a variety of physiologic changes that may increase their sensitivity to drugs and drug-induced disease (Figure 8-1). It has been estimated that 70% to 80% of all adverse drug effects in older adults are dose-related. The loss of body weight in many older adults may require initiating therapy at a lower adult dosage or reevaluating dosages of medications already in use. The criterion for

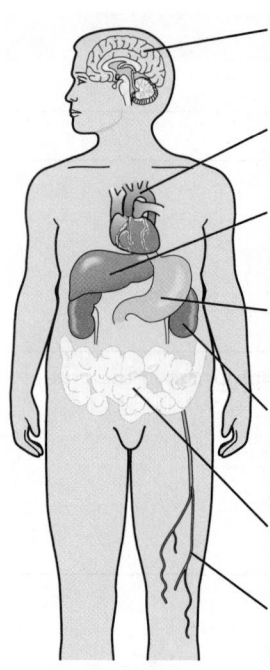

The blood-brain barrier is more easily penetrated by fat-soluble drugs such as the β blockers, which raises the risk of dizziness and confusion.

Reduced baroreceptor response exaggerates the hypotensive effects of antihypertensives and diuretics.

As liver size, blood flow, and enzyme production decline, toxicity can result from the rise in the half-life of drugs such as propranolol, nitrates, and diazepam.

Slower gastric emptying time plus an increase in the pH of gastric juices increases the risk of stomach irritation with drugs such as aspirin.

Decreased renal blood flow and filtration can cause drugs that are cleared through the kidneys—such as furosemide (Lasix) and digoxin (Lanoxin)—to be toxic at normal dosages.

Increased abdominal adipose tissue can lead to toxicity of fat-soluble drugs such as the phenothiazines.

Altered peripheral venous tone exaggerates the hypotensive effects of antihypertensives and diuretics.

FIGURE 8-1 How physiologic changes of aging increase sensitivity to drugs and drug-induced disease.

BOX 8-1 POTENTIAL ALTERED PHARMACOKINETICS IN OLDER ADULTS

ABSORPTION

- Increase in gastric pH
- Altered gastric emptying and intestinal blood flow
- Decrease in first-pass metabolism in the liver

DISTRIBUTION

- Altered body composition (decrease in lean body mass, increase in adipose [fat] stores)
- Decrease in total body water
- Decrease in serum albumin
- Decrease in blood flow and cardiac output

METABOLISM

- Decrease in Phase I metabolic reactions (cytochrome P450 system)
- Decrease in hepatic blood flow and drug metabolism

EXCRETION

- Decrease in renal function (with most persons, a loss of 10% of renal function per decade after 50 years of age)

Modified from Kim, J., & Cooper, A. (2002). Geriatric drug use. In J.T. DiPiro, R.L. Talbert, G.C. Yee, G.R. Matzke, B.G. Wells, & L.M. Posey (Eds.), *Pharmacotherapy: A Pathophysiological Approach* (5th ed.). New York: McGraw-Hill; and Hanlon, J.T., Ruby, C.M., Guay, D. & Artz, M. (2002). Geriatrics. In J.T. DiPiro, R.L. Talbert, G.C. Yee, G.R. Matze, B.G. Wells, & L.M. Posey (Eds.), *Pharmacotherapy* (5th ed.). New York: McGraw Hill.

dosages should be shifted from age to weight. Even though some older adults weigh no more than the average large child, and some weigh a lot less, they are prescribed the larger "adult" dosages; this practice is incorrect.

Alterations in Pharmacokinetics

Pharmacokinetics may be altered in older adults because reduced gastric acid and slowed gastric motility result in unpredictable rates of drug dissolution and absorption (Box 8-1). Changes in absorption may occur when acid production decreases and alters the absorption of weakly acidic drugs such as barbiturates. However, few studies of drug absorption have shown clinically significant changes occurring with advanced age.

Changes in body composition have been noted in older adults and include an increased proportion of body fat and decreased total body water, plasma volume, and extracellular fluid. An increased proportion of body fat increases the body's ability to store fat-soluble compounds such as antipsychotics (e.g., haloperidol [Haldol]), barbiturates (e.g., phenobarbital) and benzodiazepines (e.g., diazepam [Valium]) and thus increases the accumulation of those drugs. Reduced lean body mass affects drug distribution by decreasing the volume in which the drug circulates, thereby causing higher peak levels. The risk of toxicity with hydrophilic or water-soluble drugs increases as total body water decreases. Digoxin (Lanoxin), theophylline (Theo-24), and the aminoglycoside antibacterials (e.g., tobramycin [Nebcin]) are examples of hydrophilic drugs that may accumulate and result in an adverse effect or toxicity.

Decreased serum albumin for highly protein-bound drugs may lead to increased amounts of free drug in the circulation. The anticoagulant warfarin (Coumadin), the antiepileptic drug phenytoin (Dilantin), and the benzodiazepine diazepam (Valium) are a few examples of highly protein-bound drugs.

Drug metabolism in the liver is also affected by aging. Medications that undergo Phase I metabolism (reduction, oxidation, hydroxylation, or demethylation usually involving the cytochrome P450 isoenzymes) may have a decreased metabolism, whereas Phase II (glucuronidation, acetylation, conjugation) is not affected by aging. The half-life of diazepam (Valium) which undergoes extensive Phase I metabolism, increases from 20 hours in a 20-year-old to 90 hours in individuals in their 80s because of the increase in drug volume in the body of the older adult. Other drugs, such as the vasodilating nitrates, barbiturates, β-adrenergic blockers like propranolol (Inderal), and the cardiac dysrhythmic lidocaine may also have decreased hepatic metabolism in older adults (Kim & Cooper, 2002).

Disorders common to older adults, such as HF, may impair liver function and influence biotransformation by decreasing the metabolism of drugs and increasing the risk of drug accumulation and toxicity. Renal function may be impaired because of a loss of nephrons, decreased blood flow, and decreased glomerular filtration rate. A reduction in renal function is also secondary to HF and uncontrolled diabetes mellitus. Decreased renal clearance may cause in-

BOX 8-2 HOW TO ASSESS THE "AT-RISK" OLDER ADULT

1. Interview the client to obtain a complete drug history. Carefully question him or her about disease states, illnesses, current use of medications (e.g., prescribed, OTC, home remedies, herbals, vitamins), drug allergies (description of allergy, time it occurred, intervention used, outcome), and any troubling adverse effects.
2. Make a list of the name, strength, and directions of each medication (prescribed, OTC, and complementary/alternative) taken by the client. Include as needed (PRN) medications, especially if the client reports taking them one or more times per week.
3. Identify all prescribers for this client. This information may be obtained by client interview and should be verified by checking prescription labels.
4. Prescription bottles may also provide additional information to review. For example, check the name(s) of the pharmacy (or pharmacies) that have dispensed medications to the person. If more than one pharmacy is involved, determine the reason why.
5. Check all prescription and OTC drug containers for expiration dates. Ask the client for permission to destroy any expired medications because they have the potential of being ineffective or causing harm.
6. Question clients on their self-medication practices: How do they remember to take their scheduled medications? Do they ever forget to take a dose and, if so, what do they do? Have they ever deliberately stopped their medication (if yes, obtain an explanation why)? Such information will help in evaluating compliance and in determining if the medications are being consumed safely according to the prescribed schedule.
7. Determine whether the client has any limitations that may impair the safe self-administration of medication. Examples include physical impairment, memory loss, health or cultural beliefs, financial constraints, and a lack of social support.

creased plasma drug concentrations and longer half-lives of drugs and active metabolites that the kidney usually excretes. Drugs that are highly dependent on the kidneys for excretion include the aminoglycosides, ciprofloxacin (Cipro), digoxin (Lanoxin), lithium (Eskalith), and numerous other drugs (Kim & Cooper, 2002). Principles of dosage adjustment for clients with renal impairment are presented more fully in Chapter 35.

Therefore careful monitoring of drug regimens is crucial, especially for older adults. Box 8-2 describes how to assess the "at-risk" older adult.

The previously described aging process does not necessarily affect all older adults. For example, with drugs primarily excreted by the kidneys, reduced or impaired renal function may result in drug accumulation and perhaps toxicity. However, up to one third of older adults have little or no "age-related renal insufficiency."

Alterations in Pharmacodynamics

Changes in target organ or receptor sensitivity in older adults may result in a greater or lesser drug effect at these sites. The reason for this alteration is unknown but may be a result of a decrease in the number of receptors at the site or to an altered receptor response to the medication. Older adults often exhibit a decreased response to β-agonists and antagonists, but they have a greater response (central nervous system [CNS] depression) with benzodiazepines, such as diazepam (Valium) (Kim & Cooper, 2002). It has also been reported that the muscarinic receptors in the cortex tend to decrease with aging, and therefore older adults are often very sensitive to anticholinergic medications. The anticholinergic adverse effects of confusion, dry mouth, blurred vision, constipation, and urinary retention are often noted. (See Chapter 21 for additional information on anticholinergic drugs.)

There is also believed to be a loss in responsiveness or an age-related decline in β-adrenergic receptors and dopamine receptors in older adults. The number of receptors may vary or the alteration may be in different areas of the aging body, which may result in altered drug responses or an increased risk for drug-induced Parkinson's disease.

In summary, older adults are perceived to have a greater sensitivity to drugs, especially to medications that act on the CNS. If monitoring and dosage adjustments are not instituted, they may encounter more adverse effects than occur in younger persons.

❋ **How does the ineffective management of the self-medication regimen contribute to adverse drug effects?** The numerous factors that complicate drug therapy regimens may result in improper self-medication, errors in administration, and therapeutic failure (Box 8-3). Detecting medication misuse is an important function of the health care provider, because appropriate interventions may reverse this outcome. A variety of situations may result in medication misuse, which leads to the following questions:

- Does the risk or cost of one or more of the drugs in the client's drug regimen outweigh the benefits? Benefits may be viewed as physiologic responses or as psychological and economic considerations.
- What is the older adult's or primary caregiver's knowledge of the prescribed therapy? Does the client follow a specific medication schedule (by times or hours) and keep track of all medications taken daily? Does the client or primary caregiver know the name of and use for each medication? Can they explain the instructions from the label on each bottle? (See Chapter 10 for a detailed discussion of client education.)
- Can the client open the child-resistant caps on his or her medications? Is the client aware that he or she can request regular caps from the pharmacist?
- Is the client having any difficulty taking the medication, perhaps needing a change in dosage form to facilitate swallowing (e.g., from tablet to liquid)?
- Is the client exhibiting drug adverse effects? Such reactions are often overlooked, and the prescriber may

---

> **BOX 8-3 FACTORS THAT MAY COMPLICATE DRUG THERAPY IN OLDER ADULTS**
>
> Older adults:
> - Are living longer
> - May have one or more chronic diseases
> - May receive prescriptions from two or more prescribers
> - Undergo physiologic changes that may result in altered pharmacokinetics and/or pharmacodynamics
> - May have altered thought processes such as confusion, memory loss
> - May have impaired physical mobility related to arthritis, fatigue
> - May have sensory-perceptual alterations such as impaired vision or hearing
> - May have limited income, which may affect the continuity of drug therapy
> - On the average, use more prescription and OTC drugs than the general population
> - May experience polypharmacy, which has resulted in an increase in the reports of drug interactions and adverse effects

prescribe a new medication for the symptoms rather than discontinue the offending medication.

Behavioral and mental changes are very common symptoms of medication misuse, and therefore the nurse should constantly compare the client's current function with his or her past performance. Consultation with a family member or caregiver is essential. Confusion, increased irritability, disorientation, and agitation are just a few of the changes often caused by medications (Desai, 2003). Physical problems such as increased weakness, falls, and a decrease in physical activity may also be caused by a variety of prescribed medications. Although most individuals can identify an acute drug reaction if it occurs after the start of a new medication, the slower-evolving adverse effects are often more difficult to identify. At times the prescriber may discontinue a potential offending drug and observe the client to see if the adverse effects are alleviated. The prescriber may discontinue a drug that has a long duration of action and substitute a drug that has a shorter duration of action. This, too, helps in preventing the cumulative or additive effects of medications, especially the CNS-acting drugs (e.g., hypnotics, antianxiety agents, antidepressants, opioids, and tranquilizers).

Medications in Older Adults

The potent medications available to treat older adults often have a narrow index between effectiveness and toxicity. Table 8-1 summarizes inappropriate drugs for older adults and indicates drugs that should be avoided entirely in older adults. For example, the three long-acting benzodiazepines (diazepam [Valium], chlordiazepoxide [Librium], and flurazepam [Dalmane]) have been associated with daytime sedation and an increased risk of falls, whereas the antidepressant amitriptyline (Elavil) has been reported to cause the most anticholinergic and orthostatic hypotensive adverse effects as compared with other drugs in this category. Therefore prescribing such medications for older adults increases the risk of inducing adverse effects, and perhaps injury.

Although all systems are altered by the aging process, the CNS, cardiovascular and renal systems appear to be the most affected. To reduce the potential for adverse effects, it has been recommended that CNS-acting medications be started at a fraction of the dose used in young adults (Katzung, 2004). The potential for drug-induced adverse effects declines if the prescriber titrates slowly to the therapeutic effect, the "start low, go slow" approach.

Liu and Christensen (2002) report that the prevalence of inappropriate prescribing remains alarming high for the older adult population in general and for nursing home residents in particular. Prolonged use of oral antibiotics, short-acting benzodiazepines, and histamine-2 (H_2) antagonists, and high dosages of iron products, H_2 antagonists, and antipsychotic medications is also reported. Inappropriate prescribing of psychotropic medications in long-term facilities has resulted in federal legislation Omnibus Reconciliation Acts (OBRA) that has established guidelines for the proper use of such medications in older adults. (See Chapter 19 for additional information.)

The primary responsibility of a health care provider is to reduce or eliminate the potentially adverse risk factors associated with various drug regimens. This can be accomplished with a thorough assessment of the client's health status, current medication regimen, and environmental factors that would influence the accurate and safe administration of medication by the client or the client's caregivers, and implementation of the appropriate interventions, client education, and counseling. (See Chapters 5, 6, and 10 for more information.)

Ideally the prescriber individualizes and simplifies drug therapy for the client. Keeping medications to a minimum with the least frequent dose administration necessary will help to reduce the potential for drug interactions and also improve the client's ability to manage the drug regimen effectively. The nurse should be an advocate for simplification of the client's medication regimen.

✳ **After examining the contents of M.L.'s brown bag and speaking with M.L. and his daughter, the nurse takes M.L.'s apical pulse. He has been taking both digoxin and Lanoxin, a trade name for digoxin, and has anorexia (an early symptom of digoxin toxicity), and his pulse is 42 beats/min. The nurse calls M.L.'s primary care provider (PCP) who requests that M.L. report to the local hospital's emergency department (ED) to have a digoxin serum level drawn. After consultation with the nurse, the PCP indicates that he will review M.L.'s medication regimen for fewer and more appropriate medications. The nurse counsels M.L. and his daughter on better practices of sleep hygiene, indi-**

cating that the Extra Strength Tylenol PM contains a medicine (diphenhydramine with anticholinergic effects of urinary retention) that may increase his urinary symptoms. She plans with them another visit to the senior center to discuss the promotion of better bowel patterns through increasing fluid intake, increasing fiber in the diet, moderate exercise, and weaning from his bowel preparations.

✱ What are the nursing management concerns for medication administration for older adults?

Older adults are at risk for toxicity because of the effects of drugs in the aging body, variables of drug administration, and the effects of polypharmacy. Nurses should make every attempt to simplify the drug therapy plan in view of the effects just outlined and because of the multiplicity of drugs prescribed for older adults and the older adult's potential for occasionally unreliable memories and senses, inadequate financial status, and propensity for developing adverse effects secondary to drugs. Suspect medications as the cause whenever there is a change in an older adult's behavior, particularly restlessness, irritability, and confusion. Alterations in thought processes may be the earliest signs of drug toxicity. Nursing assistants, home health aides, family, caregivers, and others should be encouraged to report to a nurse any change in the client's behavior. Often what passes for senility is drug-induced lethargy or confusion.

In the administration of medications, the older adult may have special needs. Older adults often have dry mucous membranes, which impede swallowing, and thus water should be offered both before and after oral medications (if the client's condition permits). Position older adults upright so that gravity can assist the drug through the esophagus and minimize the possibility of aspiration. Because of diminished sensation, the client may be unaware that the tablet is stuck between the lip and gum, so ask the client for permission to examine his or her mouth to ensure that the medication has been swallowed. Some older adults may have slowed reflexes and a reduced understanding of treatment. It helps to organize the dispensing of medication so that enough time is allowed for clients who require more time and assistance with medications, possibly by medicating them last to prevent being rushed.

With older adults, the selection of sites for injectable medications may present the nurse with a challenge. Because muscle mass declines with age, there may be fewer suitable sites for intramuscular (IM) injection than in younger individuals, and palpating to detect muscles of adequate body and size requires more skill and effort. On the other hand, decreased sensory perception, including pain perception, may make injections less painful.

Physical problems may often interfere with the ability of older adults to comply with prescribed drug regimens. Some may be unable to read labels or locate drugs because of failing eyesight; others, such as clients with arthritis, may have difficulty opening bottles (particularly childproof containers) or handling small pills, and clients with hearing impairments may not hear all of the instructions. The logistics

---

BOX 8-4 CLIENT EDUCATION FOR MEDICATION ADMINISTRATION

1. Review all medications with the client or caregiver to determine drug effectiveness and adverse effects.
2. Have the client (or the caregiver) repeat the name and use for each medication plus the dosing instructions. If necessary, clarify the information.
3. Perform a functional assessment to determine if the client needs a compliance aid or a memory cue to take medications. If a caregiver is not available, determine if one is necessary.
4. Provide a written medication schedule in larger print for the client, which will enhance independent, effective management of therapeutic regimen.
5. If the drug regimen is complicated, discuss possible changes (simplification) with the prescriber. Then recommend ways the client may be able to manage the drug regimen.

---

and economic cost of obtaining drugs may be a deterrent to complying with therapy. Multiple-drug therapy may simply be too complex for the client to manage without assistance. Simplify drug administration and scheduling as much as possible. Dosage schedules and calendars often help the forgetful client. Drug packaging that is easy to use and is clearly labeled, and printed directions and drug information, help to ensure compliance in older adults.

Assess the older adult's functional capabilities to determine the educational requirements for safe and accurate self-administration of medications in the home (Box 8-4). Creativity and skill are essential in devising teaching plans to enhance client compliance with the home medication regimen (see Chapter 10). Discuss prescription, over-the-counter (OTC), and complementary/alternative medications with clients and their family and caregivers; clients and caregivers should be able to describe in detail how and when they take all medications. Frequently reassess the effectiveness of the management of the therapeutic regimen as the older adult's functional capacity changes.

The most important part of the nursing process for older adults may be the nurse's ability to communicate patience, warmth, and understanding and to treat older adults as persons having dignity and the ability to reason, to feel, and to contribute.

Summary

As the older adult population increases, both proportionately and in numbers, it becomes of greater importance to ensure their well-being. The tendency toward polypharmacy in this population requires that the nurse be more astute in assessment, intervention, teaching, and counseling. All older adults have unique physiologic and psychosocial needs. The nursing management of medication administration to older adults requires that the nurse be knowledgeable about the various pharmacokinetic and pharmacodynamic effects of pharmaceutical agents in this population. Understanding the rationales behind these effects will help the nurse to administer medications safely and to evaluate client responses appropriately, regardless of the client's age.

(✱) Critical Thinking Questions

- M.C., a 75-year-old male client states, "I've been taking care of myself, wife, and kids all of my life. I ran this ranch year-round, even when snow was everywhere and the wind blew so hard a body could hardly stand. Why would I drive 112 miles just to see a doctor and get some pills when I can go to the store 20 miles down the road and get some that do the trick just as good?" What approach would you use to provide information about the safe use of OTC medications with this client?

- Mr. Holmes is an 81-year-old client of a home health agency in a rural area of western Massachusetts. He lives alone and still drives himself for shopping, health care provider visits, and other errands. Describe the assessment required to determine if Mr. Holmes is at risk for ineffective management of his medication regimen.

Bibliography

Anderson, D.M., Keith, J., & Novak, P.D. (Eds.) (2002). *Mosby's medical, nursing, and allied health dictionary* (6th ed.). St. Louis: Mosby.

Beers, M.H. (1997). Explicit criteria for determining potentially inappropriate medication use by the elderly: An update. *Archives of Internal Medicine, 157,* 1531-1536.

Beers, M.H., Ouslander, J.G., Rollingher, I., Reuben, D.B., Brooks, J., & Beck, J.C. (1991). Explicit criteria for determining inappropriate medication use in nursing homes. *Archives of Internal Medicine, 151,* 1825-1832.

Desai, A.K. (2003). Use of psychopharmacologic agents in the elderly. *Clinics in Geriatric Medicine, 19,* 679-719.

Fick, D.M., Cooper, J.W., Wade, W.E., Waller, J.L., Maclean, J.R., & Beers, M.H. (2003). Updating the Beers criteria for potentially inappropriate medication use in older adults. *Archives of Internal Medicine, 163*(22), 2716-2724.

Hanlon, J.T., Ruby, C.M., Guay, D. & Artz, M. (Eds.). (1992). Geriatrics. In J.T. DiPiro, R.L. Talbert, G.C. Yee, G.R. Matzke, B.G. Wells, & L.M. Posey (Eds.), *Pharmacotherapy* (5th ed.). New York: McGraw Hill.

Katzung, B.G. (Ed.). (2004). *Basic & clinical pharmacology* (9th ed.). New York: McGraw-Hill.

Kim, J., & Cooper, A. (2002). Geriatric drug use. In J.T. DiPiro, R.L. Talbert, G.C. Yee, G.R. Matzke, B.G. Wells, & L.M. Posey (Eds.), *Pharmacotherapy: A Pathophysiological Approach* (5th ed.). New York: McGraw-Hill.

Kohn, L., Corrigan, J., & Donaldson, M. (Eds.). (1999). *To err is human: Building a safer health care system.* Washington, DC: National Academy Press.

Lazarou, J., Pomeranz, B.H., & Corey, P.N. (1998). Incidence of adverse drug reactions in hospitalized patients. *Journal of the American Medical Association, 279,* 1200-1205.

Liu, G.G., & Christensen, D.B. (2002). The continuing challenge of inappropriate prescribing in the elderly: An update of the evidence. *Journal of the American Pharmaceutical Association, 42,* 847-857.

McLeod, P.J., Huang, A.R., Tamblyn, R.M., & Gayton, D.C. (1997). Defining inappropriate practices in prescribing for elderly people: A national consensus panel. *Canadian Medical Association Journal, 156*(3), 385-391.

Schmader, K.E., Hanlon, J.T., Pieper, C.F., Sloane, R., Ruby, C.M., Twersky, J., et al. (2004). Effects of geriatric evaluation and management on adverse drug reactions and suboptimal prescribing in the frail elderly. *American Journal of Medicine, 116,* 394-401.

USP DI: Drug information for the health care professional. (2005). (25th ed.). Greenwood Village, CO: MICROMEDEX Thomson Healthcare.

Williams, C.M. (2002). Using medications appropriately in older adults. *American Family Physician, 66*(10), 1917-1924.

e-LEARNING SUPPLEMENTS

Student CD-ROM
- Final Exam questions
- NCLEX® Examination review questions
- Pharmacology animations
- Printable chapter summary

Evolve Website (http://evolve.elsevier.com/mckenry)
- Case study on drug therapy for older adults
- Content updates, including information on new drugs
- WebLinks corresponding to this chapter
- Answers to the critical thinking questions in this chapter
- *Elsevier ePharmacology Update* newsletter
- Mosby's Drug Consult Internet Edition
- Supplemental and reference information

9

SUBSTANCE MISUSE AND ABUSE

CHAPTER FOCUS

Despite concerted efforts to educate the public, the misuse and abuse of drugs and alcohol in North American society are widespread. Because of the scope of the problem, this issue has moved to the forefront of health care. No matter what the health care delivery setting, the nurse must be able to recognize and assist clients with substance abuse problems.

LEARNING OBJECTIVES

- Describe the scope of substance abuse.
- Cite etiologic factors of substance abuse.
- Identify the pharmacologic basis of physical drug dependence and tolerance.
- Describe the pathophysiologic changes characteristic of chronic substance abuse.
- Identify the signs, symptoms, and treatment for the overdose of commonly abused drugs.
- Identify the street names for commonly used drugs.
- Summarize nursing management of the care of clients who abuse drugs and other substances.

▲ KEY TERMS

abstinence or withdrawal syndrome, p. 158
addiction, p. 149
drug abuse, p. 149
Drug Abuse Warning Network (DAWN), p. 152
drug misuse, p. 149
hallucinogen, p. 158
metabolic (pharmacologic) tolerance, p. 156

physical dependence, p. 149
pK$_a$, p. 171
predatory drugs, p. 153
psychological dependence, p. 149
receptor site (tissue) tolerance, p. 156
substance abuse, p. 149
tolerance, p. 156

All prescribed or self-administered drugs have the potential to be misused or abused. Although the terms used to describe substance misuse and abuse are interpreted differently, Doering (2002) provided more precise definitions. **Drug misuse** refers to the use of a drug that varies from a socially or medically accepted use. Most of this chapter will focus on substance abuse and drug dependence. **Substance abuse** refers to the use of a psychoactive substance in a manner detrimental to the individual or society but not meeting criteria for substance or drug dependence. Similarly, **drug abuse** refers to the use of drugs that causes physical, psychological, economic, legal, or social harm to the user or others affected by the drug user's behavior. **Physical dependence** is a physiologic state of adaptation to a drug or alcohol in which tolerance to drug effects and development of a withdrawal syndrome in abstinence is usually present. **Psychological dependence** is related to the emotional state of craving a drug for either its positive reinforcing effects or to avoid the negative effects of withdrawal. **Addiction** is a chronic disorder in which compulsive use of the drug results in physical, psychological, or social harm to the user and yet use continues despite that harm.

✳ How widespread is substance abuse?

Substance abuse is neither a new nor a recent phenomenon. It has been known throughout history as one expression of an individual's search for the relief of physical, psychological, social, and economic problems. Contemporary substance abuse has attained prominence as an issue with moral, legal, religious, social, psychological, and medical implications. Substance abuse is not confined to any particular socioeconomic, cultural, or ethnic group. It is a major medical, social, economic, and interpersonal problem that affects individuals across the life span and from all economic backgrounds and urban and rural settings (Cronk & Sarvela, 1997).

In the United States in 2003, the use of illicit drugs (defined as marijuana, cocaine, heroin, hallucinogens, inhalants, or any prescription psychotherapeutic drug used nonmedically) in the past month was estimated at 8.2% of the general population 12 year of age or older. The rate was as high as 20.3% for those aged 18 to 25 years of age. Alcohol use is considerably higher for the same year: 51% for all age 12 years of age or older. Alcohol use peaks at 18 to 25 years of age (61.4%) and is more prevalent in males (National Center for Health Statistics, 2004). In Canada, a 2004 national survey of Canadians' use of alcohol and other drugs found that 79.3% of the 18 years of age and older population were current drinkers (drinking within the last year) and of those 17%, or 13.6% of all Canadians, are considered high-risk drinkers (indicated by an Alcohol Use Disorders Identification Test [AUDIT]). Forty-five percent had used cannabis in their lifetime with 14% using cannabis in the last year. One in 20 Canadians report a cannabis-related concern. Any other drug use, excluding cannabis, in the past year was 3% of those surveyed (Canadian Executive Council on Addictions, 2004). Both of these sets of data are based on household interviews. Such reporting strategies typically underreport the nature of the problem because many individuals are reluctant to reveal such data.

✳ G.M., a 24-year-old nurse, reports for duty on the day shift. During the changeover report with nights, she is loud, belligerent, aggressive, and exhibits other behaviors that indicate that she is impaired and unable to practice nursing safely. The charge nurse calls the Nursing Office. A representative from Nursing Office asks G.M. to accompany her to the emergency department (ED) for a drug screen as per hospital policy and the union contract. She consents to being tested and her tests are positive for alcohol and marijuana. G.M. admits to having a chemical dependency problem, but indicates that she has not diverted any client drugs for her own use. The Board of Nursing is notified and G.M. voluntarily surrenders her license pending an evaluation by an addictionologist and participation in the Board-approved rehabilitation program.

✳ Is substance abuse observed in health care professionals?

Many physicians, nurses, and other health professionals experience alcohol and chemical dependencies. About 10% of doctors and nurses will develop alcohol or other substance abuse problems in their lifetime—the same percentage as is found in the general population (Gjesvold, 2001). Substance abuse by nurses is related to work setting and nursing specialty. Compared with nurses in women's health, pediatrics, and general practice, emergency nurses are 3.5 times as likely to use marijuana or cocaine; oncology and administration nurses are twice as likely to engage in binge drinking; and psychiatric nurses are most likely to smoke. Trinkoff and Storr (1998) examined the prevalence of past-year substance use among registered nurses by specialty. Of the 4438 nurses responding, the prevalence of past-year substance use for all substances combined was 32%. For marijuana/cocaine use, the prevalence was 4%; for prescription drugs, 7%; for cigarette smoking, 14%; and for binge drinking, 16%. Rates varied by specialty, with oncology nurses reporting the highest past-year prevalence for combined substances (42%), followed by psychiatry (40%) and emergency and adult critical care (both 38%). The highest prevalence of marijuana/cocaine use was found with emergency and pediatric critical care nurses (7%) followed by adult critical care nurses (6%). Prescription drug use was less varied across specialties, with oncology, rehabilitation, and psychiatry having the highest prevalence of use. Psychiatry had the highest prevalence of cigarette smoking (23%), followed by emergency and gerontology (both 18%); pediatric critical care nurses were least likely to smoke (8%). Binge drinking was high among oncology, emergency, and adult critical care nurses. In general, substance use among nurses occurred at rates comparable to rates in the general population.

The American Nurses Association has publicly recognized substance abuse as a problem among nurses (American Nurses Association, 1994).

Although the substances most commonly abused by health care professionals are prescription drugs (opioids and benzodiazepines), alcohol, and tobacco, the choice of drug and route of administration vary by profession. Nurses and physicians are more apt to abuse injectable drugs, pharmacists often use multiple oral drugs, dentists have a problem with nitrous oxide addiction, and anesthesiologists and nurse anesthetists commonly abuse fentanyl (Sublimaze) or similar products (Talbot, Gallegos, & Angres, 1998).

Career pressures and easy accessibility to drugs place health care professionals at greater risk for substance abuse. Impaired health care professionals constitute a hazard to their clients' and their own well-being; therefore these problems cannot be ignored, overlooked, or left unreported. It is vital that health agencies be alert to individuals with suspected substance abuse problems on their staffs. Many agencies and most states have mandatory reporting of, and active rehabilitation programs for, impaired health care professionals.

Substance abuse (alcohol and drugs) is considered a "handicap," and such employees may be protected by state and federal employment discrimination laws. The Rehabilitation Act (29 USC, Section 706 [7][B]) states that employers are required to employ these individuals if they can properly perform their job functions and are not a threat to safety or property. Many health care facilities and other businesses have employee assistance programs to help impaired employees with rehabilitation.

✳ What is the role of drug testing?

In an effort to identify persons with alcohol- and drug-related problems, many businesses, government agencies, and health-related facilities perform drug analysis or urine drug tests on their employees under specified conditions. Drug screens may also be part of a preemployment physical examination. A number of testing procedures are available, and it is important to know the analytic techniques used and the purpose and limitations of any tests performed. Urine testing for specific drugs may detect substances used days or even a week before the test (Table 9-1). Such tests give evidence only of use or of prior exposure to a drug; they are not indicative of the individual's pattern of substance abuse or degree of drug dependency.

✳ When G.M. was in the ED to be tested, a blood sample was taken for blood alcohol levels, and a urine sample was taken for a drug screen for drugs of abuse.

A nurse in the ED was designated as the specimen collector. Collectors are required to ensure the specimen is collected from the correct individual, obtain samples, determine if

TABLE 9-1 TIME VS. DRUG DETECTION IN URINE

Drug	Detection in Urine (days)*
Alcohol	Less than 1 day
Amphetamines	Up to 1 day
Barbiturates	Up to 1 day
Benzodiazepines	Up to 2 days
Cocaine	Up to 2 days
Methadone	Up to 3 days
Marijuana Single use Chronic use	 Up to 6 days Up to 29 days
Opioids Short acting	 Up to 1 day
Phencyclidine	Up to 6 days
Phenobarbital	Up to 6 days

Data from Zizzo, W.O., & Zizzo, P.V. (2005). Drug abuse. In M.A. Koda-Kimble, L.Y. Young, W.A. Kradjan, B.J. Guglielman, B.K. Alldredge, & R.L. Corelli (Eds.). *Applied therapeutics: The clinical use of drugs* (8th ed.). Philadelphia: Lippincott, Williams & Wilkins.
*Chronic high doses may extend the time intervals.

certain forms of adulteration have occurred, and establish a chain of custody for the specimen. Because many specimens will be used as evidence in legal proceedings, great care is taken in their collection and maintenance. Identification (ID) is done by using a photo ID or by having the donor sign a certification statement on the specimen's custody and control form. The collector ensures that the room in which the specimen is obtained is "clean" (e.g., contains no toilet bowl cleaners, soaps, the faucets are disabled). The donor is usually allowed to urinate in private, but direct observation may be necessary if the donor appears intoxicated, is suspected of specimen adulteration, or has abused drugs. The temperature of the specimen, measured within 4 minutes of donation, must be between 90° F to 100° F. The specimen is sealed with tamper-resistant tape and initialed on the bottle label and dated by the collector and initialed by the donor. Each bottle has a unique ID number. The specimen may be split into two specimens, one for testing now and one for testing at a later date. Both bottles are labeled as above, and specimen "A" and specimen "B" are designated. Chain of custody forms are maintained for both portions. Chain of custody is a legal term that refers to the ability to guarantee the identity and integrity of the specimen from collection through reporting of the test results. It is used to maintain and document the chronologic history of the specimen and includes name of the individual collecting the specimen, each person or entity subsequently having custody of it, the date the specimen was collected or transferred, employer or agency, specimen number, client's or employee's name, and a brief description of the specimen (Ford, Delaney, Ling, & Erickson, 2001).

Initial positive tests should be confirmed with more specific and accurate tests because false-positive and false-negative results may occur. A second test specific for the agent reported in the screening test is necessary to ensure accuracy. The health care providers interpreting the tests should be familiar with drugs known to cross-react or give a false-positive result with the test in use. For example, diphenhydramine (Benadryl) may test positive in urine for methadone, and phenylpropanolamine (Dexatrim) has been reported to test positive for amphetamines. An alternate, more specific drug test can be ordered if the individual reports taking such medications.

It is beyond the scope of this chapter to explore all aspects of substance abuse in depth. Rather the focus is on the actions of drugs and on the treatment of substance abuse. To achieve a more holistic frame of reference, the nurse is urged to investigate independently other aspects of the complex phenomenon of substance abuse.

✳ What factors increase the risk for substance abuse?

A characteristic common to most drugs that cause dependence is that they are initially taken because the individual believes a desirable pharmacologic effect will result. Because very few drugs or substances without central nervous system (CNS) effects are abused, one of the predominant factors contributing to substance abuse appears to be intrapsychic—a desire to alter one's state of mind. This desire may arise from a number of factors such as curiosity, boredom, peer pressure,

BOX 9-1 THE FOUR CHARACTERISTICS OF SUBSTANCE ABUSE

1. Altered state of consciousness
2. Development of tolerance
3. Rapid onset of action of desired effects
4. Possible abstinence syndrome if drug is discontinued abruptly after extended period of use

multiple and diverse alienation, hedonism (pleasure-seeking behavior), affluence, and the attention paid to substance abuse by the mass media. The person who is dependent on a drug has found something that provides relief from personal problems, and the drug generally is used as a maladjustive coping mechanism or, as evidence of the nursing diagnosis, ineffective coping. More individual or subjective reasons are personal inadequacy or failure, conflicts terminating in tension, feelings of shame, and a predisposition to depression, which may lead to emotional and behavioral problems. All or any combination of these factors may lead to misuse of drugs and substances. The characteristics of substance abuse are listed in Box 9-1.

For decades, opioid dependence was viewed as a problem of motivation, willpower, or strength of character. Through careful study of its natural history and through research at the genetic, molecular, neuronal, and epidemiologic levels, it has been determined that opioid addiction is a medical disorder characterized by predictable signs and symptoms. Other arguments for classifying opioid dependence as a medical disorder include the following:

- Despite varying cultural, ethnic, and socioeconomic backgrounds, there is clear consistency in the medical history, signs, and symptoms exhibited by individuals who are opioid-dependent.
- There is a strong tendency to relapse after long periods of abstinence.
- The opioid-dependent person's craving for opioids induces continual self-administration even when there is an expressed and demonstrated strong motivation and powerful social consequences to stop.
- Continuous exposure to opioids induces pathophysiologic changes in the brain (National Institutes of Health Consensus Statement, 1997).

✴ Which types of drugs are abused?

In 1990, the American Society of Addiction Medicine (ASAM) described alcoholism and other chemical dependencies as "primary, chronic, relapsing diseases with genetic, psychosocial, and environmental factors influencing their development and manifestations" (ASAM, 2005). Treatment centers have evolved to address the biopsychosocial factors associated with substance abuse.

Although all drugs have some abuse potential, the more commonly used chemically active substances are the xanthines and caffeine, which are found in coffee, tea, chocolate, and colas (see Chapter 18). Although the lay public rarely perceives these substances as drugs, they do produce mild stimulant and euphoric effects, and their use may lead to physical dependence. Nicotine and ethyl alcohol (ethanol) are the most commonly misused and abused drugs, and physical and psychological dependence may result. Other CNS drugs such as anticholinergics, steroids, amphetamines, pentazocine (Talwin), and levodopa (Larodopa) may induce altered states of perception, thought, and feelings and drug-induced psychoses as a result of prolonged and concentrated therapeutic use or abuse. Few drugs without CNS effects are misused or abused.

This chapter will review the drugs most commonly reported to the **Drug Abuse Warning Network (DAWN)** as being involved in drug-abuse–related episodes resulting in death. DAWN is a federal agency that monitors the data on medical and psychological problems associated with drug use and changing patterns of substance abuse. Table 9-2 lists the most common drugs related to ED visits. Table 9-3 lists selected drugs commonly abused and symptoms of their abuse.

✴ What patterns of substance abuse emerge?

Substance abuse may take the following forms:

- *Experimental abuse* occurs when individuals use drugs in an exploratory way, after which they accept or reject continuing use of the drugs.
- *Social-recreational substance* abuse may occur only in social contexts. The drugs commonly abused in social situations are alcohol, marijuana, cocaine, nicotine, and caffeine.
- *Episodic substance abuse* refers to the periodic abuse of a drug.
- *Compulsive substance abuse* is characterized by irrational, irresistible, or compelling abuse of a drug.
- *Ritualistic substance abuse* may be related to religious practices.

Polydrug or multiple substance abuse is common. Marijuana, alcohol, and other depressants are often used together and in conjunction with CNS stimulants. Heroin may be used with cocaine, and pentazocine (Talwin) may be used with tripelennamine (PBZ), alcohol, or other depressants.

Cocaine (especially crack cocaine) became popular in the 1980s. Its abuse is seen fairly often. According to ED statistics, cocaine use increased in the 1990s; its use was reported in 37% of ED drug episodes involving men and in 18% of drug episodes involving women.

The 1980s also documented the development of synthetic "designer drugs" produced by illegal laboratories or chemists. The molecular structure of a controlled substance is modified to produce a new variant that mimics the effects of the original drug. The types of drugs most commonly modified and sold are analogues of meperidine (Demerol), fentanyl (Sublimaze), and MDMA (3,4-methylenedioxymethamphetamine, also known as "ecstasy") from the illicit psychedelic agent MDA (3,4-methylenedioxyamphetamine). When "designer drugs" or "club drugs" are identified, the Drug Enforcement Administration (DEA) enacts

TABLE 9-2 ILLICIT DRUG–RELATED EMERGENCY DEPARTMENT VISITS BY CLIENT CHARACTERISTIC: THIRD QUARTER AND FOURTH QUARTER 2003*

Client Characteristics	Selected Drugs							
	Cocaine	Heroin	Marijuana	Stimulants	MDMA (Ecstasy)	GHB	LSD	PCP
	Drug-Related Emergency Department Visits							
Total-Drug Related Visits	**125,921**	**47,604**	**79,663**	**42,538**	**2221**	**990**	**656**	**4581**
GENDER								
Male	78,293	30,205	53,162	25,389	1523	513	616	3377
Female	47,483	17,330	26,340	17,142	698	477	39	1202
Unknown	145	68						
AGE (YEARS)								
0-5		7	7					
6-11			15		1			6
12-17		411	12,202	3739			71	
18-20	7274	2714	11,923	4917	688	274	57	
21-24	11,892	6200	10,230	6096		65		934
25-29	14,765	7724	8806	5833		133		573
30-34	17,922	6216	10,017	6818		60	184	901
35-44	46,175	14,921	17,215	10,062	77	277		516
45-54	21,030	8151	8128	3617	11	5	9	
55-64	2729	1131	957	552				
65 and older	452	104		23				
Unknown	112	25	11	8	10			
RACE/ETHNICITY								
White	62,581	25,209	47,175	31,098	927	847	562	1442
Black	40,184	10,194	17,644	1193	564	9	18	2331
Hispanic	11,264	4515	7574	3364				554
Race/ethnicity NTA	2005	428	1180	756			26	31
Unknown	9887	7258	6092	6127	185		32	223

Retrieved May 1, 2005, from http://dawninfo.samhsa.gov/files/DAWN_ED_Interim2003.pdf

regulations to ban them. Until it is banned, such a substance is legal to make, sell, and use. Once a substance is outlawed, underground chemists often make a new, legal variation of the product, which is sold until a ban against it is established. Therefore "designer drugs" are constantly changing and should be considered potentially dangerous substances. Contaminants have been identified in these products, and overdoses and deaths have been reported with their use.

In addition, in the late 1990s, law enforcement agencies noted a new trend of involving the use of drugs to facilitate robbery or sexual assault. The substances involved in the drugging of victims are called "predatory drugs," and include flunitrazepam (Rohypnol), GHB, and ketamine. These drugs are dangerous because they are odorless; victims are unaware that they have ingested a drug and are rendered incapable of resisting an assault. As a result of memory impairment caused by these substances, the victim may

TABLE 9-3 SELECTED DRUGS COMMONLY ABUSED AND SYMPTOMS OF ABUSE

Drug Category	Street Names	Methods of Use	Symptoms of Use	Hazards of Use
Marijuana/hashish	Pot, grass, reefer, weed, joint, Acapulco gold, hash, hash oil, gram, quarter moon	Most often smoked, can also be swallowed in solid form	Sweet, burnt odor Neglect of appearance Loss of interest, motivation Possible weight loss	Impaired memory, perception, amotivational syndrome Interference with psychological maturation Possible damage to lungs, heart, reproductive and immune systems Psychological and physical dependence
Alcohol	Booze, hooch, juice, brew	Swallowed in liquid form	Impaired muscle coordination, judgment	Heart and liver damage Death from overdose Death from car accidents Addiction Seizures on withdrawal

STIMULANTS

Drug Category	Street Names	Methods of Use	Symptoms of Use	Hazards of Use
Amphetamines* • Amphetamine	Speed, amp, jelly baby, rippers, uppers, pep pills, Bennies	Swallowed in pill or capsule form, or injected into veins	Excess activity Irritability; nervousness Mood swings Needle marks	Loss of appetite Hallucinations, paranoia Seizures, coma
• Dextroamphetamine	Dexies			
• Methamphetamine	Moth, crystal, meth, black beauties			
Cocaine	Coke, blow, snow, toot, white lady, crack, ready rock, candy, nose candy	Most often inhaled (snorted); also injected or swallowed in powder form; smoked	Restlessness, anxiety Intense, short-term high followed by dysphoria	Intense psychological and physical dependence Life-threatening cardiac dysrhythmias, hypertension, hemorrhagic cerebrovascular accident Sleeplessness, anxiety Nasal passage damage Lung damage Death from overdose
Nicotine, also used in combination with other drugs (e.g., cigarettes laced with cocaine and heroin [flamethrowers])	Coffin nail, butt, smoke	Smoked in cigarettes, cigars, and pipes; snuff; chewing tobacco	Smell of tobacco High carbon monoxide blood levels Stained teeth	Cancers of the lung, throat, mouth, esophagus Heart disease, emphysema

Data from Zizzo & Zizzo (2005); Office of National Drug Control Policy (2004); National Institute on Drug Abuse (NIDA) (2004). Commonly abused drugs, street names for drugs of abuse, National Institute on Drug Abuse. Retrieved December 11, 2004 from http://www.nida.nih.gov/DrugsofAbuse.html
*Includes look-alike drugs resembling amphetamines that contain caffeine, phenylpropanolamine (PPA), and ephedrine.

Drug Category	Street Names	Methods of Use	Symptoms of Use	Hazards of Use
DEPRESSANTS				
Barbiturates	Barbs, downers	Swallowed, injected	Drowsiness Confusion Impaired judgment Slurred speech Needle marks Constricted pupils	Infection after parenteral use Addiction with severe, life-threatening withdrawal symptoms Nausea Death from overdose
• pentobarbital	Yellow jackets			
• secobarbital	Red devils			
• amobarbital	Blue devils			
Opioids	Dreamer, junk		Drowsiness Lethargy Needle marks Loss of appetite	Loss of appetite Addiction with severe withdrawal symptoms
• oxycodone HCl	OxyContin; oxy, O.C., killer	Swallowed, snorted, injected		
• Dilaudid, Percodan	Dreamer, junk	Swallowed, injected		
• Demerol, Methadone		Injected into veins, smoked, swallowed		
• Morphine				
• Heroin	Smack, horse, big H, Henry, skag, sh*t, red rock			
• Codeine	Schoolboy			
CLUB DRUGS				
Methylenedioxy-methamphetamine (MDMA); may be combined with other substances of abuse such as heroin or methamphetamine (chocolate chip cookie)	Ecstasy, decadence, elephants, hug drug	Ingested	Muscle tension; involuntary teeth clenching, blurred vision; faintness; chills and sweating	Confusion, depression, sleep disorders, anxiety, paranoia
gamma hydroxy-butyrate (GHB)	liquid ecstasy, somatomax, scoop, Georgia Home Boy, or grievous bodily harm	Ingested	Insomnia, anxiety, tremors, and sweating	Used as a "date rape" drug
ketamine	Special "K", vitamin "K", KitKat, jet	Ingested	Slurred speech, blurred vision, incoordination, sedation, amnesia, dysphoria on withdrawal	Used as a "date rape" drug
flunitrazepam (Rohypnol)	Ropies, roche, rophy, forget pill	Ingested	Slurred speech, blurred vision, incoordination, sedation, amnesia	Used as a "date rape" drug
HALLUCINOGENS				
PCP (phencyclidine)	Angel dust, killer weed, hog, dust, Love Boat	Most often smoked; can also be inhaled (snorted), injected, or swallowed in tablets	Slurred speech, blurred vision, incoordination Impaired memory, perception Confusion, agitation Aggression, violence, psychosis	Anxiety, depression Death from accidents Death from overdose

Continued

TABLE 9-3 SELECTED DRUGS COMMONLY ABUSED AND SYMPTOMS OF ABUSE—CONT'D

Drug Category	Street Names	Methods of Use	Symptoms of Use	Hazards of Use
HALLUCINOGENS—*cont'd*				
LSD	Acid, cubes, purple haze	Injected or swallowed in tablets or on blotter paper	Dilated pupils, elevated body temperature, increased heart rate and blood pressure, sweating, dry mouth	Tremors, sleep disorders, panic, flashbacks
Mescaline	Mesc, cactus	Usually ingested in natural form	Dilated pupils Delusions, hallucinations	Breaks from reality Emotional breakdown
Psilocybin	Magic mushrooms	Usually ingested in natural form	Mood swings	Flashback
INHALANTS				
Gasoline		Inhaled or sniffed, often with use of paper or plastic bag or rag	Poor motor coordination Impaired vision, memory and thought processes Abusive, violent behavior	High risk of sudden death Drastic weight loss Brain, liver, and bone marrow damage
Airplane glue				
Paint thinner				
Nitrites Amyl Butyl	Poppers, locker room, rush, snappers	Inhaled or sniffed from gauze or ampules	Slowed thought Headache	Anemia, death by anoxia

Data from Zizzo & Zizzo (2005); Office of National Drug Control Policy (2004); National Institute on Drug Abuse (NIDA) (2004). Commonly abused drugs, street names for drugs of abuse, National Institute on Drug Abuse. Retrieved December 11, 2004 from http://www.nida.nih.gov/DrugsofAbuse.html

not be aware of the attack until 8 to 12 hours after it occurred and this makes it difficult to obtain a history of the event. As the drugs are metabolized rapidly, there may be little physical evidence that these drugs were used to facilitate an attack (U.S. Drug Enforcement Agency [DEA], 2005). However, the nurse caring for a victim may be required to obtain a urine sample using prescribed procedures and documentation to maintain a chain of custody for the sample. See Box 9-2 for safety tips to avoid predatory drugs.

Concealment of drugs is also problematic among clients. A particularly dangerous practice includes "body packing," or concealing contraband in the body—often to cross borders or smuggle drugs. In such circumstances, very high concentrations of heroin or cocaine are placed in a latex balloon or condom and swallowed or inserted rectally to facilitate transport of the drug. If the storage container ruptures, significant toxicity or death may occur. Such events have been observed in both children and adults (Traub, Kohn, Hoffman, & Nelson, 2003).

BOX 9-2 PROTECTION FROM PREDATORY DRUGS

- Don't accept an open drink from someone you don't know very well.
- Only drink from a can or bottle that you open or a drinks that you have watched poured.
- Don't drink from a punchbowl or other premixed container.
- Watch your drink while you are out, and if you leave to go to the bathroom or dance floor. Have a friend watch your drink.
- Don't drink your drink if it has turned blue or cloudy. Flunitrazepam (Rohytnol) is now made so that it turns blue in a clear liquid or turns a dark drink somewhat cloudy.)

✱ What is dependence?
Psychological and physical dependence on a drug can exist independently or simultaneously. Both psychological and physical dependence can potentially lead to compulsive pat-

TABLE 9-4 SIGNS AND SYMPTOMS OF ACUTE INTOXICATION OF COMMONLY ABUSED GROUP DRUGS

Drug(s) Abused	Signs and Symptoms
Cannabis drugs	Tachycardia and postural hypotension, conjunctival vascular congestion, distortions of perception, dryness of mouth and throat, possible panic
Cocaine	Increased stimulation, euphoria, increased blood pressure and heart rate, anorexia, insomnia, agitation; in overdose, increased body temperature, hallucinations, seizures, death
Opioids	Depressed blood pressure and respirations; fixed, pinpoint pupils; depressed sensorium; coma; pulmonary edema
Barbiturates and other general CNS* depressants	Depressed blood pressure and respirations, ataxia, slurred speech, confusion, depressed tendon reflexes, coma, shock
Amphetamines	Elevated blood pressure, tachycardia, other cardiac dysrhythmias, hyperactive tendon reflexes, pupils dilated and reactive to light, hyperpyrexia, perspiration, shallow respirations, circulatory collapse, clear or confused sensorium, possible hallucinations, paranoid feelings
Hallucinogenic agents	Elevated blood pressure, hyperactive tendon reflexes, piloerection, perspiration, pupils dilated and reactive to light, anxiety, distortion of body image and perception, delusions, hallucinations

*CNS, Central nervous system.

terns of drug use in which the user's lifestyle is focused on procurement and administration of the drug. However, unlike psychological dependence, physical dependence is an adaptive state that occurs after prolonged use of a drug. Discontinuation of the drug causes physical symptoms that are relieved by retaking the same drug or a pharmacologically related drug. Several hypotheses attempt to explain the pharmacologic basis of the physiologic adaptation that occurs in tolerance and physical dependence.

What is tolerance?

Tolerance is the tendency to increase drug doses to maintain the effect formerly produced by a lower dose. Tolerance may exist with either psychological or physical dependence and may be viewed in two ways. Receptor site (tissue) tolerance is a form of adaptation in which the effect produced depends both on the concentration of the drug and on the duration of exposure. The clinical effect of the drug is reduced as the duration of exposure continues because of changes in the number or function of receptors. Metabolic (pharmacologic) tolerance refers to an aspect of drug disposition. Prolonged exposure to a drug can change the body's metabolic response to the drug, increasing drug clearance with repeated ingestion. For example, with prolonged exposure to barbiturates, steady-state blood concentrations fall progressively with continued administration of the same dose. This may be attributed to the inducing effect of the barbiturates on hepatic microsomal enzymes, which increases barbiturate metabolism.

What are the pathologic outcomes of substance abuse?

Physical and psychological dependence on drugs is often associated with debilitated physical states caused by extensive abuse of the drug, which often results in malnutrition, dehydration, and hypovitaminosis. Respiratory complications

such as pneumonia, pulmonary emboli, and abscesses are often associated with neglect, debilitation, and the respiratory depression produced by CNS depressants. The intravenous (IV) administration of illicit drugs often leads to a high incidence of sepsis, hepatitis, infective endocarditis, and acquired immunodeficiency syndrome (AIDS) as a result of using contaminated equipment. Alcohol and drug use also increase risk behaviors associated with accidents and the contraction of sexually transmitted diseases (O'Hara, Parris, Fichtner, & Oster, 1998). Cellulitis, sclerosis of the veins, phlebitis, and skin abscesses may occur. Death from accidental overdose is common.

Overdose is a particularly significant potential danger because illegal drugs are notoriously unreliable in regard to the potency of their active ingredient. The drugs are commonly adulterated (mixed) with various substances such as active substances (e.g., amphetamines, benzodiazepines, hallucinogens) and inactive substances (e.g., lactose, sugars) by the time they reach the user. The risk of toxicity and death exists if an individual who has been using adulterated drugs unknowingly receives pure or stronger drugs. Overdose may also occur when an individual who has been withdrawn from drugs for some time (and has thereby lost accumulated tolerance) injects the previous usual dose, which now is in excess of the tolerance level.

As a consequence of all these factors, the life expectancy of persons who are psychologically dependent on drugs is generally lower than that of nondependent individuals. Table 9-4 presents common drug groups that are abused, along with the signs and symptoms of acute intoxication.

How does culture influence substance abuse?

In various societies certain drugs are accepted as legal and useful, and other drugs may be banned or considered illicit. For example, alcohol, caffeine, and nicotine are widely accepted and commonly used substances in the United States, Canada, and parts of Western Europe. Amphetamines are the major drugs of abuse in Japan, in which increases in personal productivity are desired. Cannabis is considered a legal drug in many parts of the Middle East, but alcohol is usually forbidden. Some Native American tribes use peyote, a hallucinogen (a drug that causes auditory or visual hallucinations), for religious services. In general, such hallucinogens have no accepted therapeutic use in the United States. In the high-altitude areas of the South American Andes mountains (e.g., Peru), coca leaves are brewed as a tea or chewed to decrease the sensation of hunger, increase work performance, and increase a sense of well-being.

The use and acceptance or rejection of a substance depends on the society and its subgroups. When drug substances are considered illicit or illegal and are in short supply, non–law-abiding persons may be motivated to produce and/or sell the banned substances. This activity is usually extremely profitable.

Opioids

✳ **M.L. is 21-year-old white female admitted to the ED with a shallow respiratory rate of 6 breaths/min, blood pressure of 96/54 mm Hg, pinpoint pupils, cyanotic, deeply sedated, and unresponsive to noxious stimuli. She is accompanied by a friend who indicates that M.L. first used heroin 2 months ago, and is now using heroin intravenously on a daily basis. She has one "fresh" track and several healed scars from needle puncture wounds in her antecubital fossa area.**

Opioids, including heroin, are among the most commonly abused types of drugs and often are listed in the top five for drug-related ED episodes. The pharmacologic types of drugs from natural sources (opiate) include the opium alkaloids (heroin, morphine), the semisynthetic group (hydromorphone [Dilaudid], oxymorphone [Numorphan]), and the synthetic group (meperidine [Demerol], levorphanol [Levo-Dromoran], methadone [Dolophine]). Heroin, propoxyphene (Darvon), oxycodone (Percodan, Percocet, OxyContin), and morphine are the opioids most often abused. The term *opioid* is preferred because it refers to both natural and synthetic products that have morphine-like effects.

In general, the opium derivatives can be administered percutaneously, (absorbed through the mucous membranes) by sniffing (*snorting*), by subcutaneous injection (*skin popping*), or by direct IV injection (*mainlining*). The rate of absorption is correspondingly increased, with mainlining producing almost immediate drug effects.

✳ What pharmacologic properties make opioids reinforcing?

Opium derivatives are CNS depressants that probably act on the sensory cortex, on higher centers, and on the thalamus. These drugs do not produce hallucinogenic or psychotomimetic effects. They are particularly likely to lead to physical and psychological dependence because they can relieve pain; change or elevate mood; relieve tension, fear, and anxiety; and produce feelings of peace, euphoria, and tran-

quility. Rapid IV injection produces warm, flushing sensations described as being similar to sexual orgasm followed by a soothing state that seems to be best characterized as a state of complete drive satiation. An individual who is "high" on opioids feels no need to satisfy drives for basic biologic needs and is often described as being "on the nod"— drowsy, content, and euphoric.

✳ How does an acute opioid overdose present?

M.L. presents in a classic pattern. Acute overdose of opioid substances may result in severe pulmonary edema and respiratory depression. These outcomes are dose-dependent and are related to the degree of individual tolerance. What constitutes a lethal dose depends on the individual's tolerance for the drug. Symptoms of overdose occur rapidly in most individuals (see Table 9-4).

Opioid toxicity is manifested in various ways, such as slow, shallow breathing; cold, clammy skin; severe hypoxia; mixed overdose conditions; or severe acidosis. Miosis (pinpoint pupils) is common with most opioids, but mydriasis (dilated pupils) may occur with meperidine overdose. Bradycardia, hypotension, muscle spasm, lethargy, respiratory depression, and urinary retention may also occur, but the toxic effects of meperidine may be more excitatory, causing significant tachycardia. The presence of thrombophlebitis, scarred veins, and puckered scars from subcutaneous injections may help identify the client with opioid toxicity. Opioids tend to delay motility and gastric emptying time; reviving the client may increase peristalsis and further increase absorption of oral forms of the drug, producing a coma cycle. Chronic abuse may result in abscesses, cellulitis, endocarditis, glomerulonephritis, encephalopathy, tetanus, and thrombophlebitis. These conditions are caused by a spectrum of factors that range from injection technique to adulterants in the substance of abuse.

✳ How should M.L. be treated?

The treatment of choice for acute overdose of opioids is administration of an antagonist (e.g., naloxone) and respiratory support (see the Management of Drug Overdose: Opioids box on p. 159).

✳ On receiving naloxone (Narcan) 2 mg intravenously, M.L. became alert within 1 minute and her respirations returned to about 20 breaths/min. She became combative, with restlessness, chills, and gastrointestinal (GI) discomfort. Is this a typical reaction?

Physical dependence on opioids usually is described in relation to heroin or morphine, but the other derivatives manifest similar symptoms. Physical dependence is evident in the marked tolerance that develops with continued use of the drug and in the symptoms of abstinence or withdrawal syndrome experienced by a chemically dependent person who is suddenly deprived of the substance of abuse.

Persons dependent on heroin or morphine often feel satiated, and therefore physical, emotional, and social deterioration commonly occur. The individual may feel little need for food and may become grossly malnourished and weak. A preoccupation with obtaining the drug makes participation in the usual social and vocational aspects of life

Management of Drug Overdose

Opioids

General Approach

- Provide symptomatic and basic supportive care of airway, breathing, and circulation (the "ABCs"). Maintain cardiac output, blood pressure, urinary output, and peripheral perfusion.
- If oral opioids were consumed, charcoal and gastric lavage may be utilized to limit further drug absorption. Emesis is not contraindicated with CNS depressants.

Specific Approach

- If apnea is present, maintain a patent airway, using assisted or controlled respiration and oxygen as necessary.
- When the triad of miotic pupils, coma or stupor, and bradypnea (reparations slowed to a rate of 4 to 6 per minute) appears, the administration of naloxone (Narcan) is indicated and will help to differentiate opioid poisoning from other conditions.
- Naloxone, a pure opioid antagonist, reverses opioids toxicity. The usual adult dose is 0.4 to 2 mg IV, which may be repeated at 2- to 3-minute intervals if necessary until desired response is achieved or 10 mg has been administered. To achieve a "wake-up" response, doses up to 10 mg may be required. If 10 mg of naloxone does not produce any response, it is most likely not an opioid overdose.

- Support blood pressure and maintain respirations after the client responds to naloxone (Narcan). Blood and urine samples should be examined with a multiple drug screen to aid in diagnosis. A positive response to naloxone is characterized by dilation of the pupils (if previously miotic) and an increase in respiratory function, blood pressure, and cardiac rate.
- Children with a known or suspected opioid overdose may receive 0.01 mg/kg of naloxone (Narcan) as the first dose. (Dilute naloxone with sterile water for injection.) If the child does not respond to the first dose, additional IV doses at 2- to 3-minute intervals may be administered.
- Naloxone reverses apnea and coma within minutes and should be titrated to the client's arousal with a respiratory rate in a range of 10 to 20 breaths/min. Continued client monitoring is necessary because additional naloxone (IV bolus or IV infusion) is often necessary to prevent the reemergence of opioid toxicity. Because the elimination half-life of the offending opioid may exceed the short elimination half-life of naloxone, the client should be monitored carefully for at least 4 hours after the last administered dose of naloxone.

Modified from Zimmerman, J.L. (2003). Poisonings and overdoses in the intensive care unit: General and specific management issues. *Critical Care Medicine, 31*(12), 2794-2801.

---

difficult if not impossible. As the drug craving grows, tolerance to the drug also increases, and eventually the motivation for using the drug becomes oriented more to the avoidance of withdrawal symptoms and less to the achievement of euphoria.

In a client who is physically dependent on opioids, the use of naloxone to produce an abrupt and complete reversal of the opioid effects may precipitate an acute abstinence or withdrawal syndrome. Although opioid abstinence syndrome may be reversed by administration of an opioid, doing so in a drug-dependent client is prohibited by law except if he or she has been admitted to the hospital for an emergency procedure or is being detoxified or maintained in an approved federal drug treatment program. Methadone is usually considered the drug of choice in the treatment of this clinical condition.

Withdrawal Symptoms The initial withdrawal symptoms are related to the half-life of the opioid being used. Symptoms of withdrawal from heroin are autonomic in origin and appear within 8 hours after the last dose in physically dependent individuals. These symptoms are less life threatening than those of other substances of abuse and are manifest as restlessness, chills and hot flashes, restless sleep, piloerection on the skin (which gives rise to the term *cold turkey*), rhinorrhea, drowsiness, lacrimation, and mydriasis during the first 24 hours. These symptoms become more severe as withdrawal progresses, and additional symptoms may include sneezing,

yawning, generalized anxiety, abdominal cramps, lower back pain, lower extremity cramps, vomiting, diarrhea, anorexia, diaphoresis, muscular twitching, insomnia, elevated pulse rate, elevated blood pressure, elevated temperature, and a craving for the drug. Occasionally withdrawal symptoms are severe enough to result in cardiovascular collapse.

Depending on the drug used, abstinence syndrome develops within 2 to 48 hours and peaks at 72 hours. Withdrawal that is left untreated may continue for up to 7 to 10 days, after which the physical dependence of the body on the presence of opioids is eventually lost. Psychological dependence continues for a longer period; some authorities claim it continues forever.

❋ Are there nonopioid treatments that can reduce withdrawal symptoms?

Clonidine Treatment Clonidine (Catapres-TTS), a sympatholytic antihypertensive, decreases sympathetic outflow from the CNS by stimulating α_2 receptors in the brain. This produces a decrease in peripheral resistance, heart rate, and blood pressure. Clonidine relieves selected symptoms of acute drug withdrawal (e.g., opioids, nicotine, alcohol) and aids in detoxification. Withdrawal symptoms may be caused by hyperactivity of the noradrenergic pathways of the brain. The nurse should be aware that it takes 2 to 3 days to reach a peak effect when clonidine transdermal patches are used, which is often too late to treat the worst effects of opioid withdrawal. The tablet dosage form offers a quicker and is a more easily titrated method of preventing or reducing unwanted effects.

A clonidine dosage of 5 mcg/kg/day, increasing to 17 mcg/kg/day as necessary, has been used to prevent withdrawal syndrome. The dosage is individualized according to the client's tolerance and the quantity and type of opioid agonist used. The daily dose is administered in equally divided doses over a 24-hour period for approximately 10 days; it is then reduced by 50% on days 11, 12, and 13 and discontinued on day 14 (*USP DI*, 2005).

The sedative and hypotensive effects of clonidine limit its clinical usefulness, and extremely close supervision of the client is necessary to monitor adverse effects and any manipulation of the dosage by the client. The nurse should withhold the dose of clonidine and consult the prescriber if the client's blood pressure is less than 90 mm Hg systolic or 60 mm Hg diastolic. This detoxification process eliminates physical dependence on opioids; nonpharmacologic intervention can be used to address the remaining psychological dependence. Additional information on clonidine is presented in Chapter 27.

✸ **M.L. is stabilized in the ED. A consult with social services is conducted, and arrangements are made to transfer M.L. to a substance abuse treatment center.**

✸ **How is opioid dependence treated?**

Withdrawal Programs In general, opioid withdrawal is difficult, and repeated relapses may be expected. Abrupt and complete withdrawal (cold turkey) can be accomplished, but this procedure is dangerous (especially in clients with a coexisting medical illness), inhumane, and should generally be avoided. Therapeutic withdrawal from an opioid may be somewhat more comfortably achieved by successively tapering the drug's dosage over a period of several days.

The choice of withdrawal program is partly influenced by the following factors: the client's physical condition, the duration of drug dependence, the type and amount of drug being taken, motivations for substance abuse and withdrawal, and whether the individual is also dependent on other drugs, such as alcohol. Depending on these factors, opioid withdrawal may in some instances need to be accomplished in a hospital with close medical supervision.

In identifying the criteria for evaluating opioid withdrawal, it should be noted that recovery from morphine-type dependence is not equated with cure. Therapeutic programs should continue regardless of repeated relapses to substance abuse. Progress in withdrawal may be indicated by progressively longer periods of abstinence from opioids without resorting to the use of other psychoactive drugs or alcohol and by the client's growing confidence in the ability to function effectively without drugs.

Therapeutic Community Programs The ultimate goal of using any medication to treat dependency is to provide relief from the compulsive craving for the drug of abuse. To achieve rehabilitation, the individual needs to turn to more than just another prescribed or illicit medication. A client also needs human dignity, sincerity, compassion, warmth, self-respect, and hope with positive reinforcement. To achieve independence and become a self-sustaining, productive member of the community, the client must be provided with emotional and social support. Many treatment programs do not effectively address these human resources, and treatment failures are the result.

Because persons withdrawing from drugs often cannot make the transition easily, groups of persons who have decided to abstain from drug use can meet or live together in an attempt to support and guide one another. Therapeutic community programs such as Phoenix House and halfway houses have been established to include group psychotherapy and self-help approaches. An additional advantage of such approaches includes physically removing the client from the drug-using lifestyle and drug-using peers. Ultimately, an individual should emerge from such a program with sufficient personal growth and appropriate support systems to be able to manage life satisfactorily without resorting to substance abuse.

Methadone Detoxification and Withdrawal A currently preferred method of withdrawal is by substitution of the abused opioid with methadone. Methadone is a synthetic opioid analgesic that, by virtue of cross-tolerance, permits effective substitution of methadone dependence for heroin dependence. Its effectiveness against heroin dependence results from its ability to forestall the euphoric effects of heroin and the craving for the drug without producing the deleterious physical and mental effects. When properly administered, methadone allows the individual to function adequately without intellectual or emotional impairment.

For adults in detoxification, methadone is taken orally in 15- to 40-mg doses per day, titrated according to client response, until withdrawal symptoms are controlled. Methadone therapy is initiated empirically according to client symptoms. As a general guide, 1 mg of methadone is substituted for 20 mg of meperidine, 4 mg of morphine, or 2 mg of heroin (Jacobson & Jacobson, 2001). (For a review of recommended dosages and dosage adjustments, see current substance abuse references or the references cited in this chapter.)

Regular administration of methadone results in the development of tolerance to methadone and cross-tolerance to heroin. The client does not experience an opioid-induced "rush" and euphoria unless a dose that exceeds the tolerance level is administered. The nurse is aware that some clients might exaggerate their withdrawal symptoms to obtain more methadone. Supportive psychological or psychiatric counseling of clients being treated with methadone may relieve some of the burdens that led to drug dependence. During this phase the methadone may be gradually withdrawn, usually at a rate of 20% reduction or 5-mg increments. Some clients, however, will require life-long methadone therapy. Even with methadone, up to one quarter of clients may continue to use intravenous heroin (van den Brink et al., 2003).

Methadone maintenance programs are controversial and are not always successful. Previous opioid abusers who are unable to negotiate life in a drug-free state may revert to their former dependence or alternative substance abuse or may return to the methadone therapy detoxification.

Methadone Maintenance Maintenance methadone treatment programs in the United States require licensing and approval from both the Food and Drug Administration (FDA) and the state. The ultimate goal of these programs is complete withdrawal from drug dependency, but some clients continue taking methadone for an extended time. Methadone programs can include psychological, vocational, and rehabilitation services in addition to medical support. Approved methadone programs are required to comply with all the requirements in the Federal Methadone Regulations.

Admittance to a methadone maintenance program usually requires evidence of current dependence on morphine-type drugs and at least a 1-year history of opioid dependence. Nurses should be aware that clients with addiction disorders hospitalized with medical conditions other than addiction might require pharmacologic support with methadone or opioids during their stay. Because a cross-tolerance to opioids is common, these clients usually require higher analgesic doses to control pain. Verification of enrollment in an approved methadone maintenance program is usually required to continue methadone during the hospital stay. The hospital pharmacist should be consulted on the regulations and for assistance in such matters.

The nurse should also be aware that treatment centers vary in their methods and drugs used for opioid withdrawal. Some treatment centers report having accomplished withdrawal from opioids through the use of clonidine (Catapres-TTS), whereas others maintain that methadone is the drug of choice.

Methadone dependence does occur. The withdrawal symptoms are less severe but last for a longer period. Methadone withdrawal programs generally include supplemental rehabilitation techniques such as vocational and social rehabilitation. Theoretically, an individual can be withdrawn from methadone maintenance after he or she has functioned for a sufficient period free from other opioids, secured steady employment, and readjusted his or her lifestyle. The pharmacokinetics and pharmacodynamics of methadone are presented in Chapter 14.

Additional Agonist Analgesics Used for Maintenance

Buprenorphine/Naloxone (Suboxone) Buprenorphine is an opioid agonist used for both pain management and opioid dependence. When combined with the opioid antagonist naloxone in low doses, it is used for maintenance therapy in treating opioid dependence. Buprenorphine/naloxone reduced craving and increases success in abstinence programs (Fudala et al., 2003). In the United States, its use is restricted to registered prescribers. Up-to-date information is available at the U.S. Department of Health and Human Services website: http://www.buprenorphine.samhsa.gov/.

Levomethadyl Acetate Treatment Levomethadyl acetate (ORLAAM) is a longer-acting alternative to methadone and is for use only in approved opioid treatment programs. It is similar to methadone and has a longer duration of action.

It is usually given three times a week, such as Monday, Wednesday, and Friday. This product can be dispensed only through approved opioid addiction treatment programs, and it should never be given daily. Because federal regulations do not allow take-home doses of Orlaam, clients who are ill or require hospitalization are usually transferred to methadone on a temporary basis (Jacobson & Jacobson, 2002).

Heroin Maintenance Diacetylmorphine (heroin), a Schedule I drug (see Chapter 2), is a substance with no accepted medical use in the United States. It has been banned because of its high potential for abuse and because of the increasing number of people addicted to heroin. Today it remains one of the top drugs of abuse in the United States and Canada and often is used in combination with cocaine.

Although most countries have banned heroin use, it is legal in some European countries that are experimenting with heroin prescriptions. Physicians are permitted to prescribe heroin and other opioids for persons with a history of intractable dependence, thereby maintaining them and preventing withdrawal symptoms. Prescriptions are issued through designated hospitals or clinics.

The approval of heroin as an analgesic for intractable pain has been proposed and denied numerous times in the United States. Pharmacologically, heroin is a pro-drug—it is converted in the liver to morphine. Opponents of heroin legislation state that legalized heroin is unnecessary because morphine and other opioids are available in the United States.

✳ **What other opioid analgesics have been implicated in substance abuse?**

pentazocine [pen **taz** oh seen]
(Talwin)
Pentazocine (Talwin), an opioid agonist-antagonist, 60 mg IM is considered approximately equivalent to 10 mg IM of morphine. Sharp increases in the incidence of pentazocine substance abuse led the DEA to place it in Class IV under the Controlled Substances Act. The potential for pentazocine to produce psychological and physical dependence is significant even in low doses; infants born to pentazocine-dependent women experience withdrawal immediately after birth. Pentazocine can cause visual hallucinations, feelings of depersonalization, and nightmares.

The CNS effects of pentazocine are similar to those of opioids and include analgesia, sedation, and respiratory depression (reversed by naloxone [Narcan]). In high doses pentazocine causes increases in blood pressure and heart rate. Lung problems in pentazocine abusers have been reported when tablets are crushed, dissolved, and administered intravenously. This may be a result of the talc binders and other particulate matter in tablet dosage forms. The use and reuse of cotton as a filter may result in "cotton fevers," a type of allergic reaction caused by tiny cotton fibers. This syndrome occurs within 30 minutes of the injection, with the client experiencing increased heart rate, hypotension, increased sweating, shaking chills, and fever. These symptoms often resolve in approximately 4 to 24 hours without treatment, but the health care provider should be aware that sepsis, embolism, and other complications are possible. Other potential effects include seizures and ulceration and severe sclerosis of the skin and subcutaneous tissue and muscles caused by subcutaneous or IM injections. "Cotton fevers" may occur with other IV illicit drugs. The combination of pentazocine with other CNS depressants such as barbiturates and alcohol may be lethal.

Clients who abuse pentazocine report that tripelennamine is used to increase the onset of action and prolong the duration of the euphoria produced by pentazocine. This combination is known as *Ts* and blues (T for Talwin and blue for the color of the generic tablet of tripelennamine). Ts and blues are oral tablets that are crushed together, dissolved, and injected either through a cotton filter intravenously (like heroin) or subcutaneously. Abscesses and necrotic tissue that require hospitalization and grafting have resulted.

To discourage abuse, oral pentazocine now contains naloxone with a brand name of Talwin-Nx. The addition of naloxone has no effect on the analgesic properties of oral pentazocine, but if this combination is administered intravenously, the naloxone nullifies or cancels the rush effect of the injected "Ts and blues" combination.

Treatment of pentazocine dependence is gradual reduction of the drug in a controlled environment. The psychotomimetic effects should be observed closely in a controlled environment because they may persist for 5 to 7 days. Additional pharmacokinetic and pharmacodynamic information about pentazocine is presented in Chapter 14.

propoxyphene [proe **pox** i feen]
(Darvon, Novapropoxyn✦)

The use of propoxyphene products in excessive doses, either alone or in combination with other CNS depressants (including alcohol), is a significant cause of drug-related deaths. Because an overdose of propoxyphene, a centrally acting analgesic, may result in fatality, intensive supportive and symptomatic therapy must be instituted immediately.

Clients should be warned not to take propoxyphene in doses higher than those recommended by the manufacturer. The judicious prescribing of propoxyphene is essential for the safe use of this drug. With clients who are depressed or suicidal, consideration should be given to the use of nonopioid analgesics.

Because of its depressant effects, propoxyphene should be prescribed with caution for those whose medical condition requires the concomitant administration of sedatives, tranquilizers, muscle relaxants, antidepressants, or other CNS-depressant drugs. Clients are cautioned against the concomitant use of propoxyphene products and alcohol because of the potentially serious CNS additive effects of these agents. Deaths have occurred as a consequence of the accidental ingestion of excessive quantities of propoxyphene alone or in combination with other drugs. Propoxyphene-related deaths have occurred in individuals with previous histories of emotional disturbances or of misuse of tranquilizers, alcohol, and other CNS-depressant drugs.

The clinical effects of an acute propoxyphene overdose are similar to acute opioid toxicity—coma, respiratory arrest, pulmonary edema, circulatory collapse, and death. Generalized tonic-clonic seizures have also been reported. Propoxyphene is metabolized in the liver to norpropoxyphene, which may be responsible for some of its toxicity. Toxic propoxyphene serum levels are between 0.6 and 10 g/mL; lethal levels are reportedly more than 10 mcg/mL.

Norpropoxyphene has a smaller CNS-depressant effect than propoxyphene but has a greater anesthetic effect on the myocardium—similar to that of amitriptyline and antidysrhythmic drugs such as lidocaine and quinidine. Electrocardiographic monitoring is essential in the management of overdose. The manufacturer recommends contacting a poison control center in all suspected overdose cases for the most current treatment of the overdose.

Propoxyphene has also been abused by parenteral administration of the oral dosage form. Propoxyphene napsylate (Darvon-N, Darvocet-N) is considered a less-toxic propoxyphene formulation because of its delayed absorption orally and its relative insolubility in water. Thus the napsylate dosage form has less abuse potential than propoxyphene hydrochloride.

Propoxyphene is pharmacologically related to the opioids; therefore naloxone may reverse the signs of toxicity. Propoxyphene overdose may be accompanied by seizures and require antiepileptic drugs, and emergence from a coma may require the use of restraints before administering naloxone because of the client's disorientation, agitation, and confusion. Clients need psychological and emotional support during this time. A quiet, calm environment with reduced sensory stimulation may reduce disorientation and agitation. The nurse should use a simple, direct approach and communicate with reality orientation and reassurance.

Alcohol (Ethanol)

✲ **T.S. is a 19-year-old college student admitted to the ED with minor trauma after a motor vehicle accident. She was the driver of the vehicle and appears mildly intoxicated. A blood alcohol level is obtained and noted to be 0.05 (below the legal limit for driving).**

✲ **What is alcohol?**

Although there are many different types of alcohols, the term alcohol usually refers to ethyl alcohol. Methyl, propyl, butyl, and amyl alcohols are examples of other alcohols that are very toxic when taken orally.

ethyl alcohol (ethanol)

Ethyl alcohol is the only alcohol used extensively in medicine and in alcoholic beverages. It is colorless and mixes readily with water; because it lowers surface tension, it is a good solvent for a number of substances. Ethyl alcohol is also referred to as grain alcohol and is the product of the fermentation of a sugar by yeast. Many over-the-counter (OTC) "nighttime" cough and cold remedies contain alcohol (up to 25%, or 50 proof) with antihistamines and may be abused because of their considerable sedative potential. Table 9-5 lists the ethyl alcohol content of various OTC preparations.

✲ **What are the local pharmacologic properties of ethanol?**

Ethyl alcohol may have either a local or a systemic action. Applied topically, ethyl alcohol denatures proteins by precipitation and dehydration. This is the basis for its germicidal, irritant, and astringent effects. It irritates denuded skin, mucous

TABLE 9-5 ETHYL ALCOHOL CONTENT OF OTC PREPARATIONS

Medicinals	Alcohol Content (%)	Alcohol Proof
COUGH-COLD PREPARATIONS		
Daycare	10	20
Formula 44 D	20	40
NyQuil	25	50
Robitussin DM	1.4	2.8
Triaminic Expectorant	5	10
Actifed	0	0
Coricidin	0	0
MOUTHWASH PREPARATIONS		
Cepacol	14.5	29
Listerine	26.9	53.8
Scope	14.3	28.6

Data from San Diego State University, Driving Under the Influence Program (2004).

membranes, and subcutaneous tissue as well. Subcutaneous injection of ethyl alcohol may cause considerable pain and sloughing of tissues. When injected into or near a nerve, it may cause nerve degeneration and anesthesia.

✱ What systemic effects are observed with ethanol?

Contrary to popular belief, ethyl alcohol is not a stimulant but a CNS depressant. What sometimes appears to be stimulation results from the depression of the higher faculties of the brain and represents the loss of inhibitions acquired by socialization. Cardiovascular, GI, and renal effects are also observed.

Central Nervous System Effects Alcohol is thought to interfere with the transmission of nerve impulses at synaptic connections, but how this is accomplished is not known. It causes progressive and continuous depression of the CNS, the sequence being cerebrum, cerebellum, spinal cord, and medulla. Its action is comparable to that of the general anesthetics except that the excitement stage is longer and definite toxic symptoms are present when the anesthetic stage is reached. The margin between the anesthetic stage and the fatal dose is a narrow one.

The action of alcohol varies with the individual's size, tolerance, the presence or absence of extraneous stimuli, the rate of ingestion, and the gastric contents. Small or moderate quantities produce a feeling of well-being, talkativeness, greater vivacity, and increased confidence in mental and physical power. There is a general loss of inhibitions. The finer powers of discrimination, insight, concentration, judgment, and memory are gradually dulled and lost. Large quantities may cause excitement, impulsive speech and behavior, laughter, hilarity and, in some persons, combativeness; others may become melancholy or unduly sentimental. Table 9-6 lists the content of ethyl alcohol in various beverages.

The effects of large quantities of alcohol become apparent when the individual attempts to operate machinery such as an automobile. Visual acuity (especially peripheral vision) is diminished, reaction time is slowed, judgment and self-control are impaired, and the individual tends to be overly self-confident. Drivers under the influence of alcohol take chances they would never take ordinarily. This leads to disaster, as accident statistics reveal.

An individual who is intoxicated usually becomes ataxic, mutters incoherently, has disturbance of the special senses, is often nauseated, may vomit, and may eventually lapse into stupor or coma. Although respiratory neurons are usually not depressed except by large doses of alcohol, rapid ingestion of large quantities (as may be seen with binge drinking) may result in respiratory depression or death.

Cardiovascular Effects Alcohol depresses the vasomotor neurons in the medulla and causes dilation of the peripheral blood vessels, especially those of the skin. This causes a feeling of warmth. Heat is lost from the interior, which accounts for the fact that an intoxicated person may freeze to death more quickly than a nonintoxicated person. Alcohol also depresses the heat-regulating mechanism.

Small doses of alcohol (10 to 25 mL) produce an insignificant increase in pulse rate, which is caused mainly by the effect of excitement and reflex on the GI tract. Larger doses (more than 25 mL) produce the same effect but may be followed by lowered blood pressure (BP) caused by the effect on the vasoconstrictor neurons. Chronic alcoholism may result in cardiomyopathy, hypertension, and a variety of cardiac dysrhythmias, especially atrial fibrillation and flutter. However, over the past two decades, studies have consistently demonstrated an inverse relationship between alcohol consumption and the occurrence of myocardial infarction (MI) and cardiac death, with a J-shaped curve relating alcohol intake to mortality, favoring moderate alcohol drinkers compared with nondrinkers or heavy drinkers (Goldfinger, 2003).

Gastrointestinal Effects The effect of alcohol on the function of the digestive organs depends on the presence or absence of GI disease, the degree of alcohol tolerance, the concentration of the alcohol, and the type and amount of food present. Small doses of alcohol stimulate the secretion of gastric juice that is rich in acid. Salivary secretion is also reflexively stimulated. Large and concentrated doses of alcohol tend to inhibit secretion and enzyme activity in the stomach, but the effect in the intestine seems to be negligible. Chronic alcohol ingestion causes pancreatitis and hepatic cellular damage, which results in fibrosis and scarring, cirrhosis, and/or hepatitis. In addition, gastritis, nutritional deficiencies, and other untoward results have been observed when large quantities of alcohol are ingested over a prolonged period. See Box 9-3 for ethical considerations of the sequelae of substance abuse, such as the need for liver transplantation.

Renal Effects Alcohol produces an increased flow of urine because of the increase in fluid intake. Alcohol also acts as a diuretic through CNS depression and inhibition of the release of antidiuretic hormone (ADH). If the individual has preexisting renal disease, the kidney may be further damaged. Large and concentrated doses of alcohol are thought to injure the renal epithelium

Beverages	Alcohol Content (%)	Alcohol Proof
Beer	4	8
Wine (red/white)	12	24
Brandy	30 to 45	60 to 90
Tequila, whiskey, vodka	45	90
Martini	30	60
Daiquiri, brandy Alexander, margarita (regular size)	15	30

TABLE 9-6 CONTENT OF ETHYL ALCOHOL IN VARIOUS BEVERAGES

BOX 9-3   ETHICAL CONSIDERATIONS IN SUBSTANCE ABUSE: LIVER TRANSPLANTATION IN PEOPLE WITH ALCOHOL-RELATED LIVER DISEASE

With organ transplantation established as a cost-effective and desirable treatment for people with end-stage disease, how are these limited resources allocated? The debate over the rationing of health care is ongoing and increasing. To allocate scarce donor organs is to make judgments about the worthiness of the potential recipients. It would seem that the rationing of donor livers already exists—only 10% of liver transplants are performed on recovering alcoholics, even though alcoholism is the leading cause of liver failure in the United States. The position taken to limit transplantation for alcoholics (even those who are "dry") is that the donor organ is a nonrenewable resource that should be reserved for those whose disease was not a result of their behavior (DeGeest, Dobbels, Martin, Willems, & Vanhaecke, 2000). The argument that survival rates will be lower in recovering alcoholics has been disproved (Dimartini, Weinrieb, & Fireman, 2002).

The negative attitudes of health personnel related to race, gender, socioeconomic level, and substance abuse are well documented as barriers to providing needed care (Jones, Johnson, & McNinch, 1996; Raferty, Smith-Coggins, & Chen, 1995; Todd, Deaton, D'Adamo, & Goe, 2000). Respect for persons, beneficence, compassion, honesty, and justice are cardinal principles of ethics that should guide care of all clients, including persons with substance use disorders. The application of these concepts can help address dilemmas inherent to the difficult situations that accompany addiction, such as consideration for transplantation. The principle of justice suggests that the profession of nursing has an obligation to provide care for acutely ill persons, irrespective of the details of their life circumstances, ethnicity, or diagnosis, and this principle has helped in bringing better services to people with stigmatizing conditions.

CRITICAL THINKING QUESTIONS

* What factors might be involved in the selection process for liver transplantation in recovering alcoholics?
* Would the situation be different for heart transplantation to individuals with unhealthy lifestyles of smoking, overeating, and not exercising?
* If noncompliance is a critical behavioral risk factor in the occurrence of late acute rejection episodes in heart transplant clients, would it be justified to assess this risk in potential transplant recipients given the limited resources available?
* What is the nurse's role in giving comprehensive and individualized care to people in stigmatized groups?

TABLE 9-7   PROGRESSIVE EFFECTS OF ALCOHOL

Blood Alcohol Concentration (mg%)	Changes in Feelings and Personality	Brain Regions Affected	Impaired Activities (continuum)
10-50 mg%	Relaxation Sense of well-being Loss of inhibition	Cerebral cortex	Alertness Judgment
60-100 mg%	Pleasure Numbness of feelings Nausea, sleepiness Emotional arousal	Cerebral cortex + forebrain	Coordination (especially fine motor skills) Visual tracking
110-200 mg%	Mood swings Anger Sadness Mania	Cerebral cortex + forebrain + cerebellum	Reasoning and depth perception Inappropriate social behavior (e.g., obnoxiousness)
210-300 mg%	Aggression Reduced sensations Depression Stupor	Cerebral cortex + forebrain + cerebellum + brainstem	Slurred speech Lack of balance Loss of temperature regulation
310-400 mg%	Unconsciousness Death possible Coma	Entire brain	Loss of bladder control Difficulty breathing Slowed heart rate
410 mg% and greater	Death		

Data from Advisory committee and NIAAA scientists. Retrieved May 1, 2005, from http://science.education.nih.gov/supplements/nih3/alcohol/guide/info-alcohol.htm

What are the pharmacokinetics of ethanol?

Alcohol does not require digestion before absorption. A small amount is absorbed in the stomach, and most is absorbed in the small intestine.

After absorption, alcohol is distributed in every tissue of the body in approximately the same ratio as its water content. Therefore a rough estimate of the quantity consumed may be obtained from an analysis of the blood; the effects of ethanol are correlated with blood levels (Table 9-7).

Approximately 90% of the alcohol is metabolized in the liver. Alcohol dehydrogenase, the liver enzyme, oxidizes alcohol (ethanol) to acetaldehyde; acetaldehyde oxidizes to acetic acid, which is buffered to acetate that eventually oxidizes to carbon dioxide and water. Approximately 90% to 98% of ethanol is metabolized (oxidized) in the liver, with the remainder primarily excreted by the lungs and kidneys. As plasma ethanol levels increase, the hepatic alcohol dehydrogenase pathway becomes saturated, resulting in an increase in the unmetabolized alcohol ratio.

Health care professionals should be aware of the approximate total amount of alcohol in different beverages: 12 ounces of beer = 4 ounces of wine = 1 ounce of whiskey. Therefore alcohol abuse can occur with any alcoholic beverage, depending on the quantity consumed.

How does alcohol interact with other drugs?

Ethanol interacts with many prescription and OTC drugs via both pharmacodynamic and pharmacokinetic mechanisms. Pharmacodynamically, alcohol acts synergistically with other CNS depressants to result in dramatic altered levels of consciousness. The combination of ethanol with benzodiazepines, opioids, barbiturates, or other CNS depressants can lead to coma or even death. Pharmacokinetically, chronic ethanol ingestion often results in altered drug metabolism for many commonly used agents. The degree of altered drug metabolism varies significantly among drugs and clients. Some of the more significant alcohol-drug interactions are presented in Table 9-8.

TABLE 9-8 SELECTED SIGNIFICANT ALCOHOL-DRUG INTERACTIONS

Substances Interacting with Alcohol	Mechanism	Possible Effect(s)
I. antihistamines antidepressants opioid analgesics sedative-hypnotics antianxiety agents antipsychotic drugs	Additive	Enhanced CNS* depressant effects
II. aldehyde dehydrogenase inhibitors A. disulfiram (Antabuse) B. other agents • cefamandole and some other oral second- and third-generation cephalosporins • chlorpropamide (Diabinese) and other oral antidiabetic agents to varying degrees • griseofulvin (Fulvicin) • metronidazole (Flagyl) • procarbazine (Matulane)	Inhibition of aldehyde dehydrogenase in metabolism of alcohol, leading to acetaldehyde accumulation (disulfiram or a "disulfiram-type reaction")	Most severe effects seen with disulfiram and alcohol: flushing, stomach pain, head throbbing, increased heart rate, hypotension, sweating, nausea, and vomiting With antidiabetic agents: mild to severe hypoglycemia
III. phenytoin (Dilantin)	Increase or decrease in liver metabolism	With chronic alcohol abuse: possible decrease in antiseizure effect caused by increased metabolism With acute alcohol use: a possible decrease in metabolism, causing increased serum levels of phenytoin leading to toxicity
IV. nonsteroidal antiinflammatory agents (NSAIDs) • salicylates • COX-1 and COX-2 inhibitors (e.g., ibuprofen)	Additive	Increased gastrointestinal irritability and bleeding
V. nitrates nitroglycerin • nitroglycerin	Additive	Vasodilation leading to hypotension, syncope

*CNS, Central nervous system.

✸ **T.S. is discharged from the ED, but referred to the campus health center to undergo alcohol education counseling about alcohol abuse.**

✸ **How common is alcohol abuse?**
Alcohol is the most commonly used and abused drug in North America. Because of its associated medical conditions, alcohol dependence is often seen by health care providers, occurring in 15% to 20% of primary care and hospital clients (American Society of Addition Medicine, 2004). Binge drinking, defined as consumption of five or more standard drinks on one occasion, is reported at high rates in the United States. Binge drinking has been reported on at least one occasion in 14% of adults over the prior 30 days. Although rates are highest in the 18- to 25-year-old population, it is reported that half of binge drinking occurs among moderate drinkers aged 35 or older (Naimi et al., 2003).

The typical signs of alcohol dependence are changes in drinking patterns, such as the need for early morning drinking, drinking alone, hiding partial or full liquor bottles, or the need to have a drink before performing a potentially stressful event (e.g., job interview, keeping an appointment); personality changes; family discord; job absenteeism; personal appearance neglect; poor eating habits; memory lapses; and blackouts. Table 9-9 provides an overview of the psychophysiologic effects of various levels of blood alcohol concentration, and Table 9-10 lists the clinical manifestations and suggested drug treatment of alcohol withdrawal.

The major objectives for the treatment of alcohol withdrawal include prevention or treatment of complications, and the development of long-term rehabilitation plans. Supportive care includes maintaining a quiet environment, monitoring of health, fluid and electrolyte status, adequate nutrition, thiamine to prevent the development of Wernicke encephalopathy, and antiepileptic drugs if necessary. A sedative drug such as a long-acting benzodiazepine may be necessary for severe withdrawal reactions; its dosage can then be tapered and discontinued. Ethanol administration in lower doses to treat withdrawal is not recommended despite its continued availability in hospitals across North America (Blondell et al., 2003). In selected persons, β-adrenergic blocking agents or clonidine may be used to reduce the sympathetic manifestations of alcohol withdrawal such as increased anxiety, tachycardia, hypertension, and tremors.

✸ **What other alcohols are potentially abused?**
Isopropyl alcohol and methyl or wood alcohol are occasionally ingested either by accident or by intention. These alcohols are toxic when taken internally. When some individuals with alcohol addiction are unable to purchase ethanol (ethyl alcohol), they substitute agents such as isopropyl (rubbing) alcohol, methyl alcohol (antifreeze), or any available substance that might prevent alcohol withdrawal. This is a dangerous practice that can cause severe poisoning and death. Management of the ingestion of these substances is discussed in Chapter 72.

✸ **P.M. is a 42-year-old business executive with a 20-year history of ethanol abuse. He is admitted to the ED with generalized tonic-clonic seizures and intermittent combativeness. He is fearful that the walls are**

TABLE 9-9 PSYCHOPHYSIOLOGIC EFFECTS BASED ON BLOOD ALCOHOL CONCENTRATION

BAC (mg%)*	Psychophysiologic Effect
20	Light and moderate drinkers begin to feel some effects. Approximate BAC is reached after one drink.†
40	Most people begin to feel relaxed.
60	Judgment is mildly impaired. People are less able to make rational decisions about their capabilities (e.g., driving skills).
80	Definite impairment of muscle coordination and driving skills occurs. Person is legally drunk in some states.
120	Vomiting occurs unless this level is reached slowly.
150	Balance and movement are impaired. Equivalent of one-half pint of whiskey is circulating in the bloodstream.
300	Many people lose consciousness.
400	Most people lose consciousness, and some die.
450	Breathing stops; person eventually dies.

From Lewis, S.L., Heitkemper, M.M., & Dirksen, S.R. (2004). *Medical-surgical nursing: assessment and management of clinical problems.* (6th ed.). St. Louis: Mosby.
*Blood alcohol concentration (BAC) is generally recorded in milligrams of alcohol per deciliter (mg/dL) of blood, or milligrams percent (mg%). BAC is determined by how much alcohol is consumed, how fast it is consumed, and the person's weight.
†One drink is 12 ounces of beer, 5 ounces of wine, or 1 ounce of distilled spirits, which provide the same amount of alcohol.

closing in and that the floor is shaking. He indicates that his last drink was 2 days ago.

How is acute ethanol withdrawal manifested?

For individuals with infrequent ethanol ingestion, withdrawal from acute ingestion is often termed a "hangover" and can include headache, malaise, nausea, vomiting, and generalized discomfort. Clients with a history of chronic alcohol ingestion are at risk for acute alcohol withdrawal syndrome and seizures on withdrawal of ethanol. In addition, thiamine (Vitamin B₁) deficiency can be manifest with symptoms of Wernicke-Korsakoff syndrome.

Acute alcohol withdrawal (formerly referred to as delirium tremens or DTs) typically presents 48 to 72 hours into ethanol withdrawal. Clients often experience intense anxiety, confusion, nightmares, sweating, and depression. Hallucinations or panic-type attacks are common in this period as well. The client is often distressed by a sensation of room spinning or floor movement, and is at high risk for falls or injury. Delirium may be mild, moderate, or severe, and is often accompanied by tachycardia and elevated temperatures. Clients with a history of chronic alcohol ingestion who are hospitalized without access to alcohol may begin to exhibit these symptoms as they are being weaned from opioid analgesia following a surgery or admission secondary to an accident. Alcohol withdrawal seizures are not uncommon and usually manifest as generalized tonic-clonic seizure activity.

The thiamine-deficiency syndromes can be potentially life threatening if not treated with thiamine early. Korsakoff psychosis presents as mental confusion and confabulation whereas Wernicke encephalopathy can lead to coma and death without thiamine replacement. Although clients with Wernicke encephalopathy treated with thiamine may still be affected by nystagmus, ataxia, and Korsakoff psychosis.

How should P.M. be treated?

P.M. presents with classic alcohol withdrawal seizures. Treatment consists of parenteral benzodiazepines (often lorazepam [Ativan] and thiamine). These treatments are discussed in greater depth in Chapters 16 and 17.

During short-stay admission in the hospital, P.M. is also diagnosed with clinical depression and is begun on antidepressant therapy. P.M. indicates he is frightened by the events of the prior few days and indicates he is ready to address his alcoholism. The social services unit is consulted and identifies a treatment program placement.

How is alcoholism treated?

Alcoholism is a life-long disease. Successful treatment for alcoholism requires a motivated client and complete abstinence. Behavioral and psychosocial support, as seen with Alcoholics Anonymous (AA), is considered the mainstay of treatment. In many circumstances, alcoholism is compounded by concurrent depression or anxiety. In such cases, clients often report self-treatment of symptoms with alcohol. Treatment of coexisting depression and/or anxiety with antidepressants or anxiolytics can contribute to increased likelihood of success. Occasionally, other drugs are used as adjuncts to treatment, and include disulfiram and naltrexone.

disulfiram [dye **sul** fi ram]
(Antabuse)
Disulfiram is used to sensitize an individual to alcohol by inducing an unpleasant alcohol-disulfiram reaction. This reaction begins with flushing of the face and develops into intense vasodilation of the face, neck, and upper body. Hyperventilation and increased pulse rate may occur. Nausea occurs in 30 to 60 minutes along with facial pallor, hypotension, and copious vomiting. There is usually an intense feeling of discomfort, a pulsating headache, palpitations, dyspnea, syncope, and a constrictive feeling in the neck. The reaction lasts from 30 minutes to several hours—as long as the alcohol is

TABLE 9-10 CLINICAL MANIFESTATIONS OF ALCOHOL WITHDRAWAL SYNDROME WITH SUGGESTED DRUG TREATMENT

Clinical Manifestations	Medications
Minor Withdrawal Syndrome	Benzodiazepines (e.g., chlordiazepoxide [Librium], lorazepam [Ativan])
Tremulousness, anxiety	Thiamine (prevention of Wernicke encephalopathy)
Increased heart rate	Multivitamins (folic acid, B vitamins)
Increased blood pressure	Phenytoin (Dilantin)—for seizures or past history of seizures
Sweating	Magnesium sulfate (if serum magnesium is low)
Nausea	Temazepam (Restoril)
Hyperreflexia	Haloperidol (Haldol) for hallucinations
Insomnia	For acute alcohol withdrawal: may need IV* fluids (do not overhydrate), cooling
Major Withdrawal Syndrome	blanket, well-lighted quiet room, consistent staff, frequent vital signs, check
Disorientation	for hypoglycemia, assessment of any other health problems
Visual/auditory hallucinations	
Increased hyperactivity without seizures	

From Lewis, S.L., Heitkemper, M.M., & Dirksen, S.R. (2004). *Medical-surgical nursing: assessment and management of clinical problems.* (6th ed.). St. Louis: Mosby.
*IV, Intravenous.

being metabolized. It is then followed by drowsiness and sleep. (See Table 9-8 for a list of other drugs that have been reported to cause a disulfiram-type reaction when taken with alcohol.)

Disulfiram inhibits the enzyme aldehyde dehydrogenase. As a result, acetaldehyde cannot be converted to acetate. Acetaldehyde then accumulates and causes the unpleasant toxic effects. Disulfiram has few effects unless the person ingests alcohol.

Indications

Disulfiram is used in the management of chronic alcoholism in conjunction with behavioral support.

Pharmacokinetics/Dosing

Disulfiram is metabolized in the liver. The initial effect may be delayed from 3 to 12 hours because of drug storage in adipose tissue. Studies indicate that up to 20% of a dose remains in the body for up to 6 days. Elimination is via the kidneys, with smaller amounts excreted in the feces and lungs. Because of slow and incomplete absorption and elimination, the effects persist up to 2 weeks after therapy is discontinued. Clients should be instructed not to ingest any substance containing alcohol during this time.

Initially the client is given up to 500 mg PO daily for 7 to 14 days; the maintenance dosage is 250 mg PO daily.

Adverse Effects

The primary adverse effects observed with disulfiram therapy relate to its intended "disulfiram reaction" described above. Psychosis, hepatitis, and hypersensitivity reactions including rash have also been reported. Disulfiram is a category X drug, which must be avoided in pregnancy.

✱ What is the nursing management of disulfiram for P.M.?

Assessment Because of the unpleasant reaction P.M. would experience with the ingestion of alcohol, the nurse reviews his level of understanding of the purpose, procedure, and consequences of disulfiram therapy before he makes a decision about drug therapy. His health history is reviewed for cardiovascular disease, diabetes mellitus, and epilepsy as a disulfiram-alcohol reaction may worsen these conditions; there is a higher rate of hepatotoxicity in clients with existing hepatic dysfunction. It must be ascertained that the client has not ingested alcohol in any form (e.g., beverages, vinegars, sauces, OTC preparations, liniments, colognes, and aftershave lotions) or been treated with paraldehyde in the 12 hours before beginning a disulfiram regimen to prevent an interaction between the alcohol and disulfiram. P.M.'s concurrent drugs are also reviewed for significant drug interaction if he were to begin disulfiram therapy; such as with anticoagulants, antiepileptic drugs, benzodiazepines, isoniazid (INH), and metronidazole. The nature of the client's support services should also be determined.

Nursing Diagnoses While P.M. is taking disulfiram, he is at risk for the following selected nursing diagnoses: risk for injury related to a disulfiram-alcohol reaction (nausea and vomiting, blurred vision, tachycardia, flushing of the face, sweating, headache, dyspnea, and rarely, seizures, loss of consciousness, and death); disturbed sleep pattern related to the CNS effects of the drug (drowsiness); and the potential complications of peripheral neuritis (numbness, tingling, or weakness of the hands and feet), optic neuritis (change in vision), encephalopathy (mental changes) and hepatitis (abdominal discomfort, anorexia, jaundice, dark urine, light stools).

Planning P.M. will not drink alcoholic beverages and not experience adverse effects of the drug while on and after the completion of disulfiram therapy.

Implementation

Monitoring The effectiveness of disulfiram therapy is monitored by assessing the client's abstinence from alcohol use. Observe the client for visual disturbances and eye pain, which might indicate optic neuritis. Tingling or numbness of the hands or feet may indicate the development of peripheral neuritis. Jaundice may indicate a drug-induced hepatotoxicity.

Intervention Written client consent is to be obtained before beginning disulfiram therapy.

Education Caution P.M. that ingesting any form of alcohol while taking disulfiram, and for up to 14 days after the last dose, will cause a very unpleasant response—dizziness, syncope, nausea and vomiting, headache, chest pain, dyspnea, palpitations, tachycardia, profuse sweating, facial flushing, and blurred vision. If the response is severe, seizures, unconsciousness, heart attack, and death can result. The extent of the reaction depends on the dose of the drug and the amount of alcohol ingested. All foods and liquid medications should be checked for the presence of alcohol. Alcohol is available in prescription drugs, OTC drugs, liquid cough-cold analgesic products, foods, flavorings, mouthwashes, salad dressings, vinegars, and other such products. P.M. is to wear a Medic Alert identification while taking the drug and should alert any health care professionals providing care. He is to consult with his prescriber at 6-month intervals for blood and liver function studies or immediately if any of the following occur: chest pain, respiratory difficulty, jaundice, or the ingestion of alcohol.

Evaluation P.M. will abstain from alcohol without experiencing adverse effects of disulfiram. He will effectively manage his therapeutic regimen, including stating food and medication sources of alcohol, wearing a MedicAlert bracelet, and maintaining scheduled appointments with prescriber for monitoring and treatment.

✱ P.M. is eager to regain control of his life, but he expresses concern over the risks of disulfiram therapy. He elects to attend AA, and will use naltrexone 50 mg daily for the first 3 months of abstinence to reduce alcohol cravings.

Naltrexone ([nal **trex** one] [ReVia]) is a longer-acting opioid antagonist, which appears to be effective in the short term in reducing alcohol cravings. The exact mechanism of reducing ethanol cravings is not clear, but may be related to blocking alcohol-induced endorphin activity in the CNS. It is typically dosed at 50 mg daily. Its beneficial effects appear most prominent during the first 3 to 6 months of therapy (Anton et al., 2001; Krystal et al., 2001). The pharmacology of opioid antagonists and nursing management are discussed more fully in Chapter 14.

How can the nurse support P.M. to achieve success?
The importance of compliance with his naltrexone schedule is emphasized and all components of his integrated program of mental and social support, that naltrexone is only intended as a support for these other interventions for the treatment of his alcohol dependence. P.M. will need to visit his prescriber periodically for hepatic function studies and inform all his other health care providers of the use of naltrexone. This will be important should he require any opioids for pain, as the therapeutic effects of these drugs would be ineffective. He is not to attempt to overcome the effects of naltrexone by taking opioids because such actions could lead to coma and death. Although P.M.'s drug of abuse was alcohol, he is to be alerted that he is at risk for developing addictions to any other addicting drugs (Jungnickel, 2005). He is advised to avoid any mood-altering drugs until he discusses their use in advance with his health care provider who understands addiction and P.M.'s recovery.

Cocaine

F.C. is a 23-year-old female with recent escalating cocaine use admitted to the ED with chest pain and tachycardia. The treatment team obtains a urinalysis for a toxicology screen and pregnancy test. The urinalysis is positive for cocaine use and positive for pregnancy.

Which central nervous stimulants are frequently abused in North America?
The primary CNS stimulants abused include cocaine and amphetamine products, especially methamphetamine. Over the past decade, use of MDMA (3,4-methylenedioxymethamphetamine or Ecstasy) has become epidemic in many communities.

Cocaine is a very dangerous substance with a high amount of financial, psychological, and physical control over the user. In Canada and the United States, it is one of the most commonly mentioned drugs resulting in ED visits, second only to alcohol in combination with other substances (DAWN, 2004). It has been estimated that 3.6% of Americans are regular users of cocaine (Bureau of Justice Statistics, 2004).

How does cocaine act?
Although classified as a controlled substance, cocaine is an alkaloid related to the belladonna alkaloids. Topically it has the therapeutic effects of local anesthesia and vasoconstriction; thus it has limited use in a few selected surgical procedures, such as nasal surgery.

Cocaine is a very potent, short-lived CNS stimulant; it is a highly addicting and potentially lethal drug. As a social-recreational drug of abuse, it is popular for its euphoric effects. It also produces increased energy like the amphetamines and may lead to a similar psychotic state with strong elements of paranoia.

The purity of the illicitly produced drug varies greatly because it is often diluted or cut with agents such as amphetamines, boric acid, quinine, mannitol, procaine, and lidocaine. The vasoconstricting effect of cocaine may be responsible for limiting its own absorption. Multiple drugs are often taken with or after cocaine, such as alcohol (84% of users), marijuana (98% of cocaine addicts), heroin, barbiturates, benzodiazepines, and phencyclidine (PCP) (National Institute on Drug Abuse [NIDA], 2004).

How is cocaine administered?
Cocaine may be taken by sniffing (snorting) the white, fluffy crystalline powder (which resembles snow, hence its street name), by direct IV injection, or by smoking the converted base form called "freebase" or crack (transalveolar route). In the United States and Canada, cocaine is usually found as the hydrochloride salt or in the base form. Cocaine hydrochloride is water-soluble and thus can be inhaled (snorted) or injected intravenously. It may be inhaled from a small spoon, rolled dollar bills, a lengthened fingernail, or various other inhalation devices. Sniffing causes vasoconstriction, which limits the amount of cocaine absorbed from the nasal mucosa into the systemic circulation; more intense effects are derived from freebase or crack cocaine.

Freebase and crack cocaine (minus the hydrochloride salt) are essentially the same free alkaloid base; the difference between them is that different solvents are used in the manufacturing process. Freebase is dangerous to make (ether and ammonia are involved) and dangerous to use. The freebase form is heat-resistant, which lends itself to smoking in any form, including "coke pipes." Smoking freebase cocaine produces a more intense effect and is dangerous because of the possibility of administering an excessive dose. The freebase solvents are flammable and may explode during the process, causing further harm to the user.

When dried, freebase cocaine looks like rocks; when smoked, it makes a cracking sound. Therefore the street names of freebase cocaine include "rock," "crack," "gravel," and "ready rock." Freebase cocaine has largely been replaced by crack cocaine, which produces a fast and very intense effect. Crack cocaine is a freebase, but it is made without any volatile chemicals. It has become popular because of its availability in smaller amounts at a much lower cost than freebase cocaine and because its use does not require any elaborate paraphernalia. The cocaine market has thus become affordable to all economic groups.

What are the important pharmacokinetic considerations with cocaine?
Cocaine is rapidly metabolized in the liver; the cocaine abuser may need to use the drug every half hour or less to maintain the high. Cocaine serum levels are not proportional to toxicity, and the elimination half-lives by oral, intranasal, and IV routes are similar (50, 80, and 60 minutes, respectively). Cocaine stimulation of the CNS initially affects the intellect (cognition) and behavior (affective domain).

What are the safety risks with cocaine?
At this time there is no absolute level that is lethal. In determining fatal reactions, the rapidity of the increase in blood level may be as important as the peak blood concentration. Factors other than blood concentration must be examined,

including tolerance, reverse tolerance, previous history of co-caine abuse, individual susceptibility, the presence of other drugs, and medical problems associated with cocaine abuse.

The initial symptoms of cocaine use are restlessness, my-driasis, hyperreflexia, vasoconstriction, tachycardia, hyperten-sion, hallucinations, nausea, vomiting, and muscle spasms. These symptoms may be followed by respiratory failure, seizures, coma, and circulatory collapse. In chronic abusers, a toxic cocaine psychosis (similar to paranoid schizophrenia) is often found and is characterized by hallucinations and para-noid delusions. Skin eruptions (with itching and compulsive scratching) caused by self-inflicted skin irritation are also com-monly observed. Energetic individuals may be prone to out-bursts of violent behavior. Blood in the nose and a perforated nasal septum are often seen in individuals who chronically snort cocaine.

The medical complications associated with cocaine abuse are numerous and vary with the type of cocaine used and the route of administration. The most important ad-verse effects are cardiovascular with a high risk for MI, dys-rhythmias, thrombosis, hypertension, tachycardia, and sud-den death. For clients with chest pain associated with cocaine risk, this is particularly true, and risk for MI or an-other serious adverse effect is highest for the following 12 hours (Weber, Shofer, Larkin, Kalaria, & Hollander, 2003). Other body systems are affected, including respiratory (pul-monary abscesses, lung infections, pulmonary edema and hemorrhage, and pneumonitis); renal (rhabdomyolysis—the release of skeletal muscle contents into the plasma, which results in generalized muscle aches and pains and, in one third of the reports, acute renal failure); and neurologic (seizures, stroke, and intracranial hemorrhage). Psychiatric conditions (psychosis, suicide, delirium, and clinical de-pression) may occur, and miscellaneous other conditions such as septicemia, hepatitis, and human immunodefi-ciency virus (HIV) infection. (See the Management of Drug Overdose: Cocaine box at right.)

✳ How frequent is drug abuse in pregnant women?

Illicit drug use in pregnancy appears to depend on whether the woman is aware of being pregnant. Rates of drug use range from about 2% to 3% for pregnant women and 6% to 7% for nonpregnant women. Although marijuana and alcohol are the most commonly abused agents, cocaine is noted in about 10% of cases. Drug abstinence increases during pregnancy, but relapse postpartum was common (Ebrahim & Gfroerer, 2003).

✳ Given that F.C.'s pregnancy test was positive, what are the risks of cocaine to a fetus?

Cocaine is particularly dangerous in pregnancy. It has been as-sociated with an increased risk of stillbirth, preterm labor, and neonatal complications such as congenital malformations, cerebral infarction and hemorrhage, and sudden infant death syndrome (SIDS). Neonatal complications include acute withdrawal symptoms (increased irritability, tremors, abnor-mal reflexes, tachypnea, and poor eating and sleeping pat-terns) and neurobehavioral delays during the first year of life. Such infants may also be susceptible to cocaine-induced

---

 Management of Drug Overdose

Cocaine

General Approach

- Provide symptomatic and basic supportive care of air-way, breathing, and circulation (the ABCs).
- Prepare for cardiac monitoring with continuous ECG or telemetry.
- Establish an IV line using an isotonic or hypotonic so-lution for the administration of the medications neces-sary to treat the adverse effects induced by cocaine.
- Continuously monitor client's vital signs and core body temperature.
- Avoid or reduce sensory stimulation because it may pro-voke or worsen agitation and paranoid behavior.

Specific Approach

Treat medication complications as necessary:
- For metabolic acidosis, administer sodium bicarbonate.
- For hyperthermia, use external cooling measures such as sponging with cold water, or use a cooling blanket.
- For seizures, administer benzodiazepines (e.g., diazepam [Valium], lorazepam [Ativan]). Benzodiazepines will also help in the management of hypertension and tachycardia commonly seen in cocaine overdose.
- For psychosis, administer antipsychotic therapy (e.g., haloperidol [Haldol])
- For cardiac ischemia, hypertension, and risk for MI, may administer nitroglycerin, aspirin, labetalol (Normodyne), nitroprusside, phentolamine (Regitine). Benzodiazepines are also helpful (see above). If an actual MI is present, use of intravenous antiplatelets, anticoagulants, and/or fibrinolytics may be considered. β-adrenergic blockers without α-blocking activity may result in worsened hy-pertension and are contraindicated in cocaine overdose.
- For cardiac dysrhythmias, antidysrhythmic therapy may be considered.
- Monitor and treat other adverse effects as necessary.

Modified from Zimmerman, J.L. (2003). Poisonings and over-doses in the intensive care unit: General and specific management issues. *Critical Care Medicine, 31*(12), 2794-2801.

---

seizures, cerebral infarction, and potentially a variety of other complications. Long-term sequelae include delays in physical and mental development, SIDS, and learning disabilities (Singer et al., 2004). Such effects have resulted in child-abuse convictions for mothers who used cocaine while pregnant and many states have mandatory reporting laws for the birth of a child to a substance-abusing mother.

F.C.'s pregnancy is considered a high-risk pregnancy and she should receive extensive prenatal care. She is to be re-ferred to a clinic within the community that has experience in working with pregnant women with substance abuse. See Chapter 7 for additional information on pregnancy and care of the client with substance abuse.

⊛ **F.C.'s cardiac symptoms are evaluated with lab and electrocardiogram (ECG) testing for a MI. She has no obvious cardiovascular damage, and is referred to social services for substance abuse treatment and appropriate prenatal care.**

Amphetamines

⊛ **What are the pharmacologic properties of amphetamines?**

Chemically, amphetamines are similar to the natural catecholamines, epinephrine, norepinephrine, and dopamine. They can activate catecholamine receptor sites to increase stimulation and therefore have been classified as sympathomimetic agents. In addition, they increase the release of natural catecholamines and block their reuptake into the neurons, which results in the induction of an artificial "fight-or-flight" response (Zizzo & Zizzo, 2005). Chemically, there are three types of amphetamines—salts of racemic amphetamines, dextroamphetamines, and meth-amphetamines—all of which vary in their degree of potency and peripheral effects. Dextroamphetamine is said to have the fewest peripheral effects, such as hypertension and tachycardia.

Amphetamine abuse has been reported for more than 50 years. After declining for a while, its use has now increased (see Table 9-2). In the United States, it was the fourth-ranking cause of drug-related admissions to EDs in 2002 (DAWN, 2004). (See Table 9-3 for street names of and additional information about amphetamines.)

The amphetamines are usually abused because they produce mood elevation, reduction of fatigue, and a sense of increased alertness. They do not create extra physical or mental energy but instead promote the expenditure of present resources, often to the point of hazardous fatigue. IV injection of amphetamines results in marked euphoria—an orgasmic feeling known as a "rush" that is accompanied by a sense of great physical strength and clear thinking. The person feels little or no need for rest, sleep, or food and may continually engage in vigorous activity that the user may perceive as exhilarating and creative. To an observer, however, the individual appears inefficient and is performing repetitive behaviors, which is common during an amphetamine high. Tolerance to these effects is noted with continued use, however, and may lead to escalating self-administered dosing.

Termination of the drug's effect may result from exhaustion, fright, or an inability to obtain more drugs. Drug withdrawal is followed by long periods of sleep, and on awakening the individual often feels hungry, extremely lethargic, and profoundly depressed. This phenomenon is known as "crashing." Suicide risk is quite possible during this period.

⊛ **What are the important pharmacokinetic aspects of amphetamines?**

Oral amphetamines are absorbed from the GI tract and concentrate in the brain, kidneys, and lungs. They are metabolized in the liver and excreted via the kidneys. Amphetamines are a basic drug with a **pKa** (the point at which half the drug amount in the body is ionized and half is nonionized) of 9.9; therefore a urine pH of 7 or more extends the

half-life to approximately 20 hours. A urine pH of 5 reduces the half-life to 5 to 6 hours. Persons who abuse amphetamines are usually aware of the prolonged effect they can achieve by alkalizing their urine. Prescribers are also aware that acidifying the urine to a pH of 4.5 to 5.5 will enhance amphetamine excretion.

⊛ **What are the clinically significant adverse effects of amphetamines?**

The stimulant properties of amphetamines can cause dramatic cardiorespiratory effects such as tachycardia, dyspnea, chest pain, and hypertension. The person may panic because these signs and symptoms are also those of a MI. To deal with these disturbing symptoms, individuals often use depressants or "downers" such as large amounts of alcohol, marijuana, benzodiazepines, barbiturates, or heroin to offset the overstimulation effect (Zizzo & Zizzo, 2005).

Acute toxic amphetamine effects can be very serious. In addition to the signs and symptoms mentioned previously, seizures and circulatory collapse have been reported. Detoxification and the use of conventional therapies for medical complications are necessary in the treatment of the acute toxicity.

Amphetamines may also contribute to hallucinations, but there is conflicting evidence regarding the cause of amphetamine psychosis. It is important to differentiate the origin of psychosis, including underlying mental illness or paranoid, delusional, or aggressive symptoms secondary to sleep deprivation

Amphetamine and stimulant use related to the treatment of attention deficit hyperactive disorder (ADHD) does not appear to be associated with increased risk for future substance abuse, and in fact may be associated with reduced risk for future abuse potential (Wilens, Faraone, Biederman, & Gunawardene, 2003). (See the discussion in Chapter 18.) Amphetamine use outside of the legitimate use in the treatment of ADHD, however, is often problematic. The health care professional should be aware that the use of amphetamines (especially methamphetamine) is on the increase, with much of it being made by illicit laboratories in the United States. Crystal methamphetamine (known as "ice" or "crystal meth") is gaining popularity because a high usually results in less than a minute when these crystals are heated and the vapor inhaled (Zizzo & Zizzo, 2005). In some instances, individuals who use oral amphetamine also smoke methamphetamine concurrently to vastly increase the intensity of effect. Methamphetamine serum levels after smoking produce elevated plasma levels and a high that can persist for 12 hours, whereas the smoking of freebase cocaine rapidly peaks and is rapidly eliminated because it has a half-life of approximately 1 hour. The toxicity resulting from the combination of smoking and oral administration produces an enhanced and potentially dangerous effect. (See the Management of Drug Overdose: Amphetamines/MDMA box on p. 172.)

MDMA

⊛ **J.B. is a 17-year-old high school senior who presents to the ED with friends in a nonresponsive state,**

Management of Drug Overdose

Amphetamines/MDMA

General Approach

- No specific antidote is available to treat amphetamine/MDMA overdose.
- Psychotic symptoms usually occur within 36 to 48 hours after a single large overdose. These symptoms usually clear in approximately 1 week.
- Treatment is mainly supportive and symptomatic.

Specific Approach

- Activated charcoal is the preferred method of treatment, particularly if the overdose is discovered within 1 to 2 hours. Gastric lavage and saline cathartics are also sometimes used.
- The person should be closely monitored because of the potential for hypertension, hyperpyrexia, and seizures.
- To increase renal excretion of amphetamines, an osmotic diuretic such as mannitol is occasionally used.
- After the acute episode, the amphetamine abuser will need intensive counseling, and perhaps desensitization techniques, on a long-term basis to overcome the craving and relapses common with the abuse of this stimulant drug.

  Dehydration may be treated with intravenous hydration and electrolyte management.

  Agitation may be treated with benzodiazepines like lorazepam (Ativan).

  Psychosis may be treated with antipsychotics like haloperidol (Haldol).

  Hypertension or cardiac dysrhythmias are less common, but treatment would be similar to that observed with the treatment of cocaine (See the Management of Drug Overdose: Cocaine box on p. 170). As with cocaine overdose, β-adrenergic blockers without α-blocking effects are avoided.

Modified from Zimmerman, J.L. (2003). Poisonings and overdoses in the intensive care unit: General and specific management issues. *Critical Care Medicine, 31*(12), 2794-2801.

BP 138/45 and heart rate of 165 beats/min. He is diaphoretic, skin is cool, and he is not responsive to painful stimuli. Naloxone 2 mg is administered with no change in level of consciousness. His friends indicate he was at a rave party and was alert, active, and "dancing up a storm." A toxicology screen is obtained and is positive for MDMA.

✱ What are the pharmacologic properties of MDMA?

At low to moderate doses, MDMA reduces inhibition and a strong sense of well-being by stimulating CNS release of serotonin. The onset of action is often observed within 30 to 60 minutes of oral ingestion, and continues for up to 4 hours. A period of alertness or mild agitation is also common for up to 8 hours after ingestion of low to moderate

doses. A "crash" or dramatic period of depressed mood is often observed 4 to 12 hours after dosing, and may prompt users to redose to avoid this effect. Unfortunately, tolerance to the euphoric effects often develops quickly. Post-MDMA depression can last up to 5 days after use, and appear more common among frequent or high dose administration.

MDMA (Ecstasy) was first studied in the early 1900s by the German pharmaceutical company, Merck. Currently, its use has skyrocketed among teens and young adults. It is often taken in the context of rave parties in which crowds, sometimes thousands of participants, dance to hard, rapidly pounding music accompanied by psychedelic videos, smoke, fog, fire, and sparks.

✱ What are the important pharmacokinetic principles of MDMA?

MDMA is rapidly absorbed orally, and is metabolized by cytochrome P450 2D6. It may interact with other hepatically metabolized drugs. In addition, for individuals with diminished 2D6 activity, pronounced MDMA effects may occur.

✱ What are the risks for MDMA?

MDMA poses a number of potential risks. In the United States, MDMA is classified as a schedule I drug (considered high-abuse potential and no legitimate medical use). Since MDMA is obtained illicitly, doses are not standardized, and tablets may contain a number of other agents or contaminants. Variation in dose or contaminants may result in toxic responses.

Repeated MDMA use has resulted in long-term memory impairment. The risk for Parkinson's disease or eventual paralysis has also been suggested.

Individuals under the influence of MDMA often act in uninhibited ways. It is not unusual for judgment to be impaired with engagement in risky behavior. When used in the context of rave parties, users often dance for extended periods of time and may become dehydrated and hyperthermic. Numerous reports of significant dehydration and hyperthermia have been noted, with clients presenting in unconscious states, tachycardia, hypotensive. The risk for rhabdomyolysis, disseminated intravascular coagulation, and death are possible.

✱ J.B. is treated with saline and electrolyte infusions, requires ventilator support, and is diagnosed with muscle breakdown and acute renal dysfunction. After a 5-day hospital course, J.B. is discharged with improving renal function.

✱ What other agents are commonly abused?

A number of other substances are abused including cannabis (marijuana/hashish), sedatives (barbiturates, benzodiazepines), hallucinogens (including mescaline, psilocybin, and phencyclidine), inhalants, and anabolic steroids. Although not representing classic abuse, intentional drug overdose with nonopioid analgesics like acetaminophen or aspirin are relatively common. Each will be discussed briefly in the following sections.

Cannabis Drugs (Marijuana/Hashish)

Efforts to control marijuana use in youth may be an important strategy to reduce future substance abuse. Whether cannabis represents a "gateway" drug to more dangerous drug use has been hotly debated. Recent evidence suggests however, that early marijuana use may in fact increase risk for later abuse of alcohol or other agents by two- to fivefold (Lynskey et al., 2003).

The cannabis drugs are derived from the leaves, stems, fruiting tops, and resin of both female and male hemp plants (*Cannabis* sativa). The potency of the active ingredient, tetrahydrocannabinol (THC) is greatest in the flowering tops of the plant and seems to vary according to the climatic conditions under which the plant is grown.

Both the availability of more potent species and varieties of marijuana ad the increase in use among young adolescents (12 to 14 years of age) require a new attitude of concern toward the substance. The potency of THC in marijuana varies, with the typical leaf containing 3%. When carefully cultivated, imported marijuana may contain as much as 6% to 13% THC (Zizzo & Zizzo, 2005). Marijuana grown under scientifically controlled conditions is often much more potent than the domestic variety smoked in the past.

Preparations Marijuana and hashish are the most common forms of cannabis in use. *Hashish* refers to the powdered form of the plant's resin, which contains 7% to 12% THC (Zizzo & Zizzo, 2005). Other forms of cannabis used in such countries as Jamaica, Mexico, Africa, India, and the Middle East include *ganja, bhang,* and *charas,* which corresponds to American marijuana. *Kif* is used in Morocco, whereas in South Africa a cannabis drug called *dagga* is often used.

Marijuana plants contain hundreds of different chemicals. Approximately 100 chemicals have been isolated and are generally termed *cannabinoids.* Of these, only THC (delta-9-tetrahydrocannabinol) and CBD (cannabidiol) have been studied in humans to identify their pharmacologic effects. Although many questions remain unanswered, it is believed the major psychoactive ingredient in cannabis is THC.

Dronabinol (Marinol or THC) is a synthetic cannabinoid available for the treatment of cancer chemotherapy-induced nausea and vomiting that is not responsive to standard therapies. Both products have a high potential for abuse and are therefore closely regulated under the Federal Controlled Substances Act (Schedule II).

Administration Cannabis drugs may be absorbed when administered by oral, subcutaneous, or pulmonary routes, but they are most potent when inhaled. Either the pure resin or the dried leaves of the cannabis plant may be smoked in pipes or cigarettes (joints). Because the smoke is acrid and irritating, some users prefer to smoke marijuana through a water pipe. The smoke is inhaled deeply and retained in the lungs as long as possible to achieve maximal saturation of the absorbing surface. Powdered hashish and marijuana may also be mixed with foods, a mode of administration that delays the drug's absorption. The effects sought by individuals who use this substance are mental relaxation and euphoria. The sedative-hypnotic effects of smoking are rapid and generally last 2 to 3 hours, whereas the effects of the orally ingested drugs may not begin for several hours. Hashish oil injected intravenously has a high incidence of mortality.

Pharmacology All of the cannabis drugs seem to act as CNS depressants. They depress higher brain centers and consequently release lower centers from inhibitory influences. Although some controversy exists regarding their classification, the cannabis drugs are not opioids but are legally classified as controlled substances. They are more commonly classified as sedative-hypnotic-anesthetics or psychedelic (capable of altering perception, thought, and feeling) drugs. Like the sedative-hypnotics, they appear to depress the ascending reticular activating system. As the dose increases, their effects proceed from relief of anxiety, disinhibition, and excitement to anesthesia. If the dose is high enough, respiratory and vasomotor depression and collapse may occur.

The potency of marijuana varies with plant strain and cultivation, but the cigarettes usually produce moderate to intense psychopharmacologic effects that peak in 15 minutes and last 1 to 4 hours. The drug has intoxicating, mind-altering properties. It induces an anxiety-free state characterized by a feeling of well-being. Perceptions of time and space are distorted. Ideas flow freely and disconnectedly; interruptions in thought that are blanks or gaps similar to an absence seizure may occur. The individual may experience palpitations, loss of concentration, light-headedness, and floating sensations followed by weakness, tremors, postural hypotension, incoordination, and ataxia. Hallucinations can occur with high doses of the drug.

Dissociative phenomena are also reported; research suggests that impaired decision making and psychometric performance are related to marijuana use. The drug experience is highly subjective; the novice may not perceive the presence of an altered state of consciousness until sensitized to it by colleagues. Factors that influence the psychological and behavioral effects of marijuana include drug dose, the user's personality, the user's expectations of the effects of the drug, the environment, social influences, and life experiences.

The adverse effects of marijuana use include immediate tachycardia and delayed bradycardia, delayed hypotension, conjunctival vascular congestion (red eyes), dry mouth and throat, delayed GI disturbances, possible vasovagal syncope, and enhanced appetite and flavor appreciation. The more serious adverse effects are psychological and may relate to marijuana itself or the addition of other drugs to marijuana. These effects include fear, panic (especially among first-time or naive users), paranoia, disorientation, memory loss, confusion, and a variety of perceptual alterations. Marijuana has been known to precipitate acute psychotic reactions and toxic psychoses in poorly organized personalities. It has also been associated with long-term anxiety, schizophrenia, and depression with regular use (Arseneult et al., 2002; Patton et al., 2002; Rey & Tennant, 2002; Zammit, Allebeck, Andreasson, Lundberg, & Lewis, 2002). The incidence of adverse effects appears to be highest in novice users of the drug.

Pharmacokinetics The peak plasma level of THC after smoking one marijuana cigarette is reported to occur within minutes. THC is metabolized in the liver, with the major route of elimination being bile and feces. Only trace amounts of the unmetabolized THC are detected in the urine.

Marijuana may affect the metabolism of other drugs in the liver or compete with other drugs for protein-binding sites in the plasma; ethyl alcohol, barbiturates, amphetamines, cocaine, opioids, and atropine are some of the reportedly affected drugs.

Withdrawal Symptoms Physiologic withdrawal symptoms have been reported with discontinued use of marijuana. Minor discomfort may pass in several days, but insomnia, anxiety, irritability, and restlessness may persist for weeks. Craving for the drug can recur intermittently for months after the drug is stopped. In general, nonpharmacologic interventions and an exercise program are preferred over substitution of another drug product.

Sedatives

Barbiturates and Nonbarbiturates Reports of the use and abuse of barbiturates and nonbarbiturate sedative-hypnotics have declined greatly in recent years, probably as a result of the availability of newer agents that have greater safety and effectiveness profiles. It has been suggested that treatment of abuse and addiction to these agents should be similar to the interventions reviewed for alcohol and benzodiazepine abuse. (See Table 9-3 for barbiturate information.) See Chapter 16 for a discussion of sedative-hypnotics.

Benzodiazepines (diazepam, alprazolam, lorazepam) Benzodiazepines are commonly prescribed for anxiety or insomnia. Although they are not considered street or illegal drugs, misuse, abuse, and drug dependency have been reported, especially with diazepam (Valium), alprazolam (Xanax), and lorazepam (Ativan).

Benzodiazepine withdrawal syndrome is more likely to occur if the drug has been taken regularly for more than 3 months, if the drug dose consumed was higher than recommended, if clients have a history of substance abuse or if the drug is discontinued abruptly. Withdrawal symptoms from short-acting benzodiazepines occur within 1 to 2 days and from long-acting benzodiazepines in 5 to 7 days. Symptoms include increased anxiety and irritability, twitching, aching, muscle weakness, tremors, headache, nausea, anorexia, depression, lethargy, blurred vision, sleep disturbance, hypersensitivity to stimuli (light, touch, sound), and hyperreflexia. Delirium, psychosis, and seizures are rare but have been reported.

Management of benzodiazepine dependence should include gradual drug withdrawal. If the individual is dependent on a short-acting benzodiazepine, a switch to a long-acting benzodiazepine is recommended for the withdrawal process. Withdrawal symptoms occur more frequently and are more severe in individuals who suddenly withdraw from short-acting benzodiazepines, whereas the use of a long-

---

BOX 9-4 CLASSIFICATION OF BENZODIAZEPINES

SHORT-ACTING (HALF-LIFE LESS THAN 12 HOURS)

alprazolam (Xanax)

oxazepam (Serax, Apo-Oxazepam✦)

triazolam (Halcion)

MEDIUM-ACTING (HALF-LIFE 12 TO 12 HOURS)

estazolam (ProSom, Nuctalon)

lorazepam (Ativan, Apo-Lorazepam✦)

temazepam (Restoril)

LONG-ACTING (HALF-LIFE LONGER THAN 24 HOURS)

chlordiazepoxide (Librium, Novopoxide✦)

clonazepam (Klonopin)

diazepam (Valium, Apo-Diazepam✦)

flurazepam (Dalmane, Novoflupam✦)

quazepam (Doral)

---

acting benzodiazepine is associated with less prominent withdrawal symptoms (Box 9-4). In general, a 10% to 25% reduction in the benzodiazepine dosage every 1 to 2 weeks is recommended. Titration schedules and dosage reductions may vary, but the time frame is usually within 1 to 4 months. In very difficult withdrawals, the addition of an antiepileptic drug or a β-adrenergic blocker (e.g., propranolol [Inderal]) may help to reduce withdrawal symptoms.

Flumazenil (floo **may** zuh nil)(Romazicon) is a benzodiazepine receptor antagonist that is administered intravenously for the treatment of benzodiazepine toxicity. Although it appears to have no pharmacologic effects of its own, it has been reported to be associated with seizures, cardiac dysrhythmias, and other serious adverse effects in clients receiving benzodiazepines or in those with mixed drug overdoses (particularly with tricyclic antidepressants). Therefore in high-risk clients the smallest effective dose should be used with close monitoring (*Drug Facts and Comparisons*, 2005). (See Chapter 16 for benzodiazepine pharmacokinetics, additional pharmacologic information, treatment of benzodiazepine overdose, and nursing management of benzodiazepine therapy.)

Hallucinogens

Classifications of the most common hallucinogenic agents include lysergic acid diethylamide or lysergide (LSD) and its variants, mescaline, psilocybin, and PCP. A number of psychoactive hallucinogenic drugs have been used as adjuncts to religious services or were used experimentally on college campuses in the 1960s. LSD, dimethyltryptamine (DMT), PCP, mescaline, psilocybin, MDMA (3,4-methylenedioxymethamphetamine, also known as Ecstasy), and MDA, drug similar to

MDMA, are examples of the drugs that can produce distortions in perception or thinking at very low doses.

LSD (lysergide)

LSD is a very potent and illicit hallucinogen that is usually available in doses of approximately 200 mcg. It causes a central sympathomimetic effect within 20 minutes of oral administration—hypertension, dilated pupils, hyperthermia, tachycardia, and enhanced alertness. The psychoactive effects occur in approximately 1 to 2 hours and have been described as heightened perceptions, distortions of the body, and visual hallucinations. The effect on mood is unpredictable and ranges from euphoria to severe depression and panic.

Unpleasant experiences with LSD are rather common. Clinically, evidence of impaired judgment in the toxic state is common and well known; such behavior is demonstrated, for example, by LSD users attempting to stop traffic with their bodies. Altered states of consciousness may cause psychosis or trigger a latent psychosis into activity. Feelings of acute panic and paranoia during a toxic LSD psychosis can result in homicidal thoughts and actions. Toxic delirium, with altering and alternating levels of consciousness, follows toxic psychosis; the experience generally resolves in a stage of exhaustion in which the user feels "empty," is unable to coordinate thoughts, and is depressed. Suicide is a definite risk during this time.

Significant unfavorable reactions induced by LSD include prolonged, delayed, and recurrent reactions such as depression and long-term schizophrenic or psychotic reactions. Recurrent reactions have been described as flashback phenomena and refer to the transient, spontaneous repetition of a previous LSD-induced experience that is unrelated to renewed administration of the drug. Flashbacks occur in 15% to 77% of LSD users. A bad "trip" (anxiety or panic reaction) on LSD is likely to be a paranoid experience, and tendencies toward violence can be characteristic of LSD intoxication.

The treatment for "bad trips" has not changed over the years. A "talk-down" approach in a quiet, relaxed environment is often used. This helps to reassure the individual that he or she is safe and that the drug effects will dissipate in a few hours. If talking down cannot help the panic, then drug therapy with an oral benzodiazepine might be considered. The use of phenothiazines, especially chlorpromazine (Thorazine) is avoided because such agents can potentiate the panic reaction, induce postural hypotension, and perhaps induce anticholinergic toxicity. In any case, the administration of medication is recommended only as an adjunct to crisis intervention psychotherapy, which consists of directing the person's attention away from perceptions that produce panic and providing reassurance that the experience will dissipate and that no permanent harm has been done. Flashbacks are treated as acute drug-induced episodes.

The practice of administering massive doses of tranquilizers, applying restraints, and isolating such individuals should be avoided. The client's dramatically heightened awareness of the environment and distorted perceptions may render these measures traumatic rather than therapeutic.

Pregnant women should be especially cautioned against taking LSD. Because lysergic acid is the base of all ergot alkaloids, it has uterine stimulant properties that can adversely affect a pregnancy.

mescaline [**mes** kah leen]

Mescaline is the chief alkaloid extracted from mescal buttons (flowering heads) of the peyote cactus; it produces subjective hallucinogenic effects similar to those of LSD. It is usually ingested in the form of a soluble crystalline powder that is either dissolved into teas or capsulated. The usual dose of mescaline is 300 to 500 mg.

Prodromal abdominal pain, nausea, vomiting, and diarrhea characterize the effects of mescaline doses up to 500 mg, and these are followed by vivid and colorful visual hallucinations. After oral ingestion, a syndrome of sympathomimetic effects is encountered and includes anxiety, hyperreflexia, static tremors, and psychic disturbances with vivid visual hallucinations. The half-life of mescaline is approximately 6 hours, and it is excreted in the urine.

psilocybin [sye loh **sye** bin]

Psilocybin is a drug derived from Mexican mushrooms and produces subjective hallucinogenic effects similar to those of mescaline but of shorter duration. A hallucinogenic dysphoric state begins within 30 to 60 minutes after the ingestion of 5 to 15 mg psilocybin. A dose of 20 to 60 mg may produce effects lasting 5 or 6 hours. The mood is pleasant to some users, and others experience apprehension. The individual using psilocybin has poor critical judgment capacities and impaired performance ability. Hyperkinetic compulsive movements, laughter, mydriasis, vertigo, ataxia, paresthesia, muscle weakness, drowsiness, and sleep are also seen.

PCP (phencyclidine)

PCP is a hallucinogen with a history of the most serious adverse effects; more suicides, assaults, and murders appear to result from its use. It was developed in the late 1950s as an anesthetic for dissociative anesthesia, a cataleptic state in which the person appears to be awake but is detached from the surroundings and unresponsive to pain. The drug was withdrawn from human use after hallucinogenic effects were noted in clients emerging from this anesthetic. It is, however, used in veterinary practice, and this use is the origin of one of its street names, "hog" (Katzung, 2004).

Pharmacokinetics

PCP is rapidly metabolized in the liver to inactive metabolites. The ingestion of large amounts results in high concentrations of the unmetabolized drug in urine. PCP is lipophilic and has a half-life of 30 to 60 minutes in small doses and from 1 to 4 days in larger doses. The pK_a of the drug is 8.5. The "ion trapping" of the drug into extravascular areas, which are more acidic than the serum, is thought to be a major cause of prolonged toxicity. Recirculation of the drug, secretion into the acidic gastric fluid, and reabsorption in the small intestine may also account for the prolonged toxicity and offers a key to the management of the toxicity of overdose. These observations have led to treatment using urine acidification with diuresis and continuous gastric drainage in severe intoxication to enhance elimination. Urinary excretion is enhanced when the urine is acidified with ascorbic acid to a pH of 5.5 or less. The fact that PCP may be found in adipose tissue may indicate that the long-term effects are related to its lipophilic nature. PCP is possibly released during a nutritional fast, and the resulting symptoms are interpreted as a flashback.

Effects

In humans, the common peripheral signs of PCP use include flushing, profuse sweating, nystagmus, diplopia, ptosis, analgesia, and sedation. Other effects of PCP are as follows:

- A state similar to alcohol intoxication with ataxia and generalized numbness of the extremities
- Psychological effects that usually proceed in three stages: change in body image and feelings of depersonalization; perceptual distortions (visual or auditory); and discomforting feelings of apathy, estrangement, or alienation
- Disorganization of thought and derealization that is greater than with LSD
- Impairment of attention span, motor skills, and sense of body boundaries, movement, and position
- Hallucinations that can recur unpredictably for days, weeks, or months
- Increased risk for violence directed to self and/or others

PCP is similar to ketamine in producing stages of anesthesia. In addition, excitation, paranoid behavior, self-destructive acts (because the sensation or feeling of pain is absent), horizontal and vertical nystagmus, tachycardia, hypertension, seizures, increased reflexes, muscle rigidity, respiratory depression, and coma with open eyes may ensue. PCP is a strong sympathomimetic and hallucinogenic dissociative anesthetic agent. Because the drug is now classified as a controlled substance, penalties for illegal manufacture have been enacted and enforced.

Some investigators claim that the effects of PCP mimic schizophrenia more accurately than those of other psychotomimetics or

Management of Drug Overdose

PCP

General Approach

- The clinical symptoms and signs of PCP intoxication are dose related. The waxing and waning of these signs may be related to the pharmacokinetics of enteric reabsorption of the alkalized (nonionized) PCP with the recirculation and redistribution of the agent, as described earlier.
- The health care professional should be aware of these signs because this time period constitutes the greatest threat for both the client and the health care professional.
- The client often has alternating periods of paranoia, auditory and/or visual hallucinations, assaultive behavior, terror, rotary nystagmus, and hyperactivity followed by a calm demeanor, blank stare, or withdrawn period.
- During the acute intoxication phase, the client is unable to process incoming sensory stimuli. Acute PCP overdose typically resolves in 48 hours, but chronic abuse symptoms may last up to 10 days.

Specific Approach

- Treatment is primarily symptomatic.
- Keep client in a dark room with minimal sensory stimulation and protection from self-inflicted injury. Do not attempt to talk down the PCP-anxious individual because it may provoke more serious anxiety or agitation.
- Diazepam (Valium) or haloperidol (Haldol) has been used for its antianxiety and antipsychotic effects, respectively.
- The use of PCP causes a wide range of subjective effects that require careful monitoring of the client. Be aware that prolonged and severe behavioral disturbances may progress to respiratory and cardiovascular emergencies as serum levels of the drug change.

hallucinogenics. Like the symptoms of schizophrenia, the effects of PCP are reduced by sensory deprivation. Currently no chemical antidote exists for inhibiting the effects of PCP. Keeping the user quiet and away from sensory stimuli may decrease the intensity of some of the effects. The pressor effects of PCP may cause hypertensive crisis, intracerebral hemorrhage, seizures, coma, and death. (See the Management of Drug Overdose: PCP box on p. 176).

Inhalants

Volatile hydrocarbons and aerosols are other substances of abuse. Representatives of this group include toluene, xylene, benzene, gasoline, paint thinner, typewriter correction fluid, lighter fluid, airplane glue, and nitrous oxide.

Volatile hydrocarbons are often used as propellants in aerosol products. When sniffed (inhaled), these agents may produce a rapid general CNS depression with marked inebriation, dizziness, floating sensations, exhilaration, and intense feelings of well-being that are at times exhibited as reckless abandon, disinhibition, and feelings of increased power and aggressiveness similar to those seen with alcohol intoxication. Inhalation may result in bronchial and laryngeal irritation,

transient euphoria, headache, giddiness, vertigo, ataxia, and renal tubular acidosis, especially with glue sniffing. At high doses, confusion, coma, and blood dyscrasia occur. Depression may follow these early excitatory effects.

Chronic toluene abuse leads to hepatic and renal toxicity, and death from cardiac dysrhythmia and respiratory failure has been reported. Recovery from lower doses may be seen in 15 minutes to a few hours. Inhalant use is no longer limited to young children and preteens. Inhalants are widely used in 12 to 17 years of age, with equally common use by both genders. The nurse in the pediatric setting may be the first health care professional to become aware of a problem with inhalants in a child or adolescent.

Butyl nitrite is a clear, yellow liquid sold as a room deodorizer under trade names such as Rush, Bolt, and Bullet. This substance is sold in drug paraphernalia shops and adult bookstores and by mail order. The opened container is placed under the nose; the individual inhales deeply and becomes dizzy, feels faint, and possibly loses consciousness. This rush lasts less than 1 minute and may include a headache, perspiration, and flushing, all caused by rapid vasodilation. It strongly resembles the effects achieved from amyl nitrite (a prescription smooth muscle relaxant and vasodilator). Amyl nitrite is sometimes abused to heighten a sexual orgasm in both partners. Both butyl nitrite and amyl nitrite lower blood pressure and reduce the heart's oxygen consumption. They diminish sexual inhibition and by their physiologic action may prolong sexual intercourse (Katzung, 2004).

Inhaled nitrite abuse has been implicated as being associated with or as being a contributory factor in the development of opportunistic infections and Kaposi sarcoma in immunosuppressed persons. The nitrites themselves are not considered a major risk factor, but individuals who use amyl nitrite and other nitrite products tend to have more sexual partners and could be at a higher risk of developing infections.

The development of tolerance also occurs with inhalants. For example, persons starting with one tube of glue sniffing per day may eventually increase to three, four, or more tubes per day to maintain the effect. In economically depressed populations, inhalants are often the first drug of abuse used.

Anabolic (Androgenic) Steroids

Anabolic-androgenic steroids are synthetic formulations produced from testosterone, the male hormone. Young people take these agents to increase strength and body weight, to look good, and to improve their chances of winning in sports. Box 9-5 lists the major effects of anabolic steroids. Unfortunately, men and women of all ages who are involved in athletic activity use anabolic steroids. Use is estimated in up to 80% of weight lifters and bodybuilders, and its use overall in competitors is approximately 50%. The abuse of these drugs is widespread and has been documented in young school-age students, in older persons, and in both males and females. The use of anabolic steroids in growing athletes may result in:

- Acceleration of maturation
- Early epiphyseal closure

BOX 9-5 MAJOR EFFECTS OF ANABOLIC STEROIDS

ANDROGEN-TYPE EFFECTS

- Increased growth and development of the seminal vesicles and prostate gland
- Increased body and facial hair
- Increased production of oil from the sebaceous glands
- Deepening of the voice
- Increased sexual interest and desire
- Enhancement of abstract and spatial dimension thinking ability
- Increased aggression

ANABOLIC-TYPE EFFECTS

- Increased organ and skeletal muscle mass
- Increased calcium in bones
- Increased retention of total body nitrogen
- Increased hemoglobin concentration
- Increased protein synthesis

LONG-TERM ADVERSE EFFECTS

- Gastric ulcers
- Liver complications:
  - Increase in liver enzymes
  - Liver failure
  - Benign liver neoplasm
  - Hepatocellular carcinoma
- Hyperglycemia (hyperinsulinemia)
- Prostatic enlargement (possible increased risk for prostatic cancer)
- Decrease in glycoproteins (FSH and LH) with:
  - Decreased spermatozoa
  - Decreased testosterone levels
  - Reduction in testicular size
- Reduction in high density lipoprotein (HDL)
- Increased platelet aggregation, with risk for increased cardiovascular disorders

Data from Greydanus, D.E., & Patel, D.R. (2000). Sports doping in the adolescent athlete, *Asian Journal of Paediatric Practice, 4,* 9-14.

BOX 9-6 MAJOR ADVERSE EFFECTS TO ANABOLIC STEROIDS

FEMALES

- Oily skin; acne
- Decrease in breast size, ovulation, lactation, or menstruation
- Hoarse and deep voice tone (usually irreversible)
- Clitoral enlargement
- Unusual hair growth and/or male-type baldness (usually irreversible)

MALES

Prepuberty

- Increased size of penis' number of erections, and secondary male characteristics

Postpuberty

- Priapism (continuing erections), difficult/increased urination
- Increased breast size (gynecomastia)
- Testicular atrophy, oligospermia, impotence

BOTH GENDERS

- Hypercalcemia
- Edema of the feet or legs
- Jaundice, liver impairment
- Liver carcinoma (rare)
- Urinary calculi
- Hypersensitivity
- Insomnia
- Iron deficiency anemia
- Nausea, vomiting, anorexia, stomach pains

- Shortened ultimate adult height
- Increase in tendon injuries

Since 1984 many organizations have publicly denounced or banned the use of anabolic steroids, including the American College of Sports Medicine, the American Medical Association, the National Collegiate Athletic Association, the International Olympic Committee, and the U.S. Power Lifting Federation. Many states have also passed laws to ban or limit the selling of such products.

Nevertheless the debate continues over the use of these agents. Anabolic steroids have been prescribed, especially for underweight persons and for athletes seeking an edge in the competitive field. Many anabolic steroidal preparations are available and are used orally and parenterally. Athletes often use the drugs in amounts far in excess of the recommended dosages. This misuse led to the withdrawal of ana-

bolic steroid products from the market in 1982. "Stacking" drugs or taking multiple anabolic steroids at one time is practiced by a number of athletes. This usually includes taking very large doses of the agent on an 8-week cycle schedule while following a regular strenuous exercise program (perhaps on isolated muscle groups) and consuming a high-protein diet. The long-term effects of such a schedule have not been studied, but documented short-term effects include increased aggressive behavior and some masculinization in females.

The disqualification of Olympic athletes for using steroids, in addition to the many undesirable and harmful effects reported from their usage, has led to an increase in the regulation of this category of drugs. In 1991, all anabolic steroids were placed in the Schedule III controlled substances category. Some states have even further restricted the availability of these drugs for nontherapeutic usage or are considering doing so. Despite decades of awareness of the use of anabolic steroids, questions of use and effects in sports persist (MacAuley, 2004). The general public should be informed of the serious health problems associated with short-term and long-term consumption of anabolic steroids (Box 9-6).

Nonopioid Analgesics (acetaminophen, aspirin, ibuprofen)

Acetaminophen (Tylenol), aspirin, and ibuprofen (Motrin, Advil) are OTC drugs readily available in many outlets in the United States and Canada. These same ingredients may also be contained in additional combination formulations and sold with or without a prescription. Thus the potential for intentional and nonintentional drug overdose exists with this category of drugs.

Overdoses from nonopioid analgesics are commonly seen in EDs. The DAWN reports that 82% of OTC analgesic overdose reports in the United States in 2002 are associated with acetaminophen, alone (20%) or in combination, with ibuprofen and aspirin accounting for 11% and 5%, respectively. Approximately 58% of the overdoses occur in children under 6 years of age. (See Chapter 11 for additional information on this drug category.)

✳ What is the role of the nurse in substance abuse prevention and management?

Because substance abuse transcends the boundaries of economics, social class, race, and ethnic background, all clients have the potential to abuse substances or be affected by someone who does. Great diversity exists among substances that may be abused and the manner in which they are abused. The role of the nurse may involve prevention, detection, treatment, and rehabilitation. Preventive nursing roles both inside and outside the health care agency environment include the following:

- Education on addiction as it is manifested in relation to a substance or behavior, including the recreational misuse of substances such as alcohol and drugs
- Identification of individuals at high risk for the development of addictions, such as children of alcoholics and individuals who have been involved in a wide range of drug experimentation
- Identification of early signs and symptoms of addiction
- Activities to effect social change, such as networking and supporting legislation and policy directed toward reducing the incidence of addiction and its consequences to society
- Use of knowledge about alcohol, tobacco, food, and drug use and abuse in the comprehensive health teaching of clients receiving nursing care
- Use of knowledge of compulsive and dependent behaviors as the basis for health maintenance teaching

Health care providers, including nurses, have a high rate of substance abuse and related problems. Nurses must be aware of the potential for drug or substance abuse among themselves and other health care providers and be alert to recognize and deal with this problem should it arise. Many health care agencies and most states and provinces have substance abuse rehabilitation programs specifically for health care professionals.

Although the nurse plays an essential role in the prevention of substance abuse, many times the initial contact with the client is in the acute setting during acute drug intoxication and withdrawal. Signs of acute intoxication differ according to the substance abused and may have various manifestations. In addition, identification of the problem may be complex if multiple drugs are used.

Alcohol and drug overdose and intoxication may be life-threatening. The immediate goals are to stabilize and maintain vital functions and minimize damage. Supportive treatment is combined with specific treatment once the drug has been identified. This is a time of acute psychological stress for the client, and the nurse must remember to treat the whole client, not just a physiologic system. It is also a time of crisis during which the client and family may be especially receptive to intervention and long-term treatment of the problem.

Each nurse must evaluate his or her own feelings about and responses to substance abuse. Some nurses tend to react with disgust or disdain; this type of behavior often increases a client's low self-esteem and results in ineffective lectures and scare tactics. Another common response of the nurse is that of "enabler"—someone who shields the client from the consequences of substance abuse or unintentionally encourages continued substance abuse. The most effective response is to recognize and confront the problem directly. Nurses must acknowledge that substance abuse often results in death if left untreated. Appropriate treatment can often help individuals with addiction disorders overcome their problems and restore them to productive lives without dependence on harmful substances or drugs. Simply addressing the problem and providing an avenue for assistance can often begin the process of recovery, which might not start at that time but months or years later.

The role of the nurse is to intervene with clients for the treatment of substance abuse. The five areas of nursing interventions are (1) identification of the problem with an abused substance, (2) communication about the problem, (3) education regarding substance use and abuse, (4) counseling the individual, family, and significant others, and (5) referral for treatment and aftercare. This approach is useful for intervention with clients abusing alcohol and other substances.

Assessment Assessment includes both physical and psychological signs and symptoms of substance abuse. Observe closely both verbal and nonverbal responses to questions because an element of denial may often be ascertained in clients who abuse substances. The client's nonverbal responses may provide additional information and either contradict or reinforce what is verbally stated.

Physical assessment includes assessing vital signs, pupillary signs, and skin (especially for needle marks or "tracks" and abscesses that are often seen with injected substance abuse), and collecting data on nutrition, elimination, and sleep patterns. Diagnostic tests may be used to detect drugs or their metabolites in the blood or urine. Be aware of the possibility of false-positive results.

Past medical history of the client may include prior treatment of substance abuse or a history of drug-related illness such as hepatitis, abscesses, or bacterial endocarditis. Alcohol-related problems should be considered in clients with any of the following medical diagnoses: cellulitis, gastritis, ulcers, pancreatitis, cirrhosis, pneumonia, tuberculosis, peripheral neuropathy, seizure disorders, cerebellar degeneration, depression, suicide attempt, injuries from accidents or victimization, anemia, or malnutrition. A thorough drug history for current or past use of OTC, prescribed, or social/recreational drugs should be obtained and should include the frequency, magnitude, and circumstances of drug use and abuse, and the development of withdrawal symptoms if drug use was stopped.

Table 9-11 uses Gordon's Function Health Patterns to provide examples of selected clinical data that may indicate substance abuse. A further assessment is needed if a cluster of data indicates possible substance abuse.

One of the simplest and most widely used screening tools is the CAGE questionnaire (Krizik, 2004; Mersey, 2003; Miller & Brady, 2004). It was designed for use with alcohol addiction but can be modified for substance abuse. It can be verbally incorporated into the process of taking every client's history by asking the following:
- Have you ever felt the need to **C**ut down your drinking (use of drugs)?
- Have you ever felt **A**nnoyed by criticism of your drinking (drug use)?
- Have you ever had **G**uilt feelings about drinking (drug use)?
- Have you ever taken a morning **E**ye opener (required a drug fix to get on with your day's activities)?

This assessment addresses common reactions to abuse, including concern for harm, hypersensitivity to criticism, perception of guilt in the harm the abuse does to others, and the occurrence of habituation or tolerance that requires a repeated dose to prevent early withdrawal symptoms (Mersey, 2003).

Nursing Diagnosis The following selected nursing diagnoses/collaborative problems may be identified in a client with substance abuse problems: risk for injury and falls related to substance abuse and abrupt withdrawal; denial related to inability to tolerate consciously the consequences of substance abuse, ineffective coping related to inability to meet role expectations, inadequately learned coping behaviors, or a social life that revolves around substance use; risk for self-directed/other-directed violence related to social isolation, hopelessness, or depression; ineffective health maintenance related to substance dependency, inadequate diet, poor lifestyle habits, impaired perception, poverty, or inability to communicate needs; ineffective therapeutic regimen management related to lack of resources (financial, social, personal) or mistrust of health personnel; powerlessness; and the potential complication of withdrawal syndrome.

Planning During therapy for substance abuse, the client will do the following:
- Remain without injury related to substance abuse and abrupt withdrawal.
- Use alternative coping mechanism instead of denial.
- Will have fewer or no violent responses.
- Will verbalize intent to engage in health maintenance behaviors.
- Make decisions and follow through with appropriate actions to end substance abuse.
- Describe strategies to address progression or complications of substance abuse.

Implementation

Monitoring Assessment of the effectiveness of the client's therapy is focused on how the client has tolerated the withdrawal period and developed new coping strategies. After the withdrawal period, the client must decide to remain drug free and maintain a healthy lifestyle. Relapses may occur and should not be viewed as the nurse's failure; the goal of treatment is longer and longer periods of sobriety/substance-free status and shorter and less frequent relapses. Participation by the client in long-term support from the appropriate agencies is essential in helping to remain drug free. Ultimately the decision to use and abuse drugs remains with the client.

Intervention Physical and/or psychological withdrawal symptoms may follow the abrupt cessation of drug or substance use. Interventions include monitoring vital signs, administering medications (if prescribed for treatment of withdrawal), and providing supportive nursing care. Clients who abuse substances often have nutritional deficiencies and other health problems, which should be corrected. Promotion of adequate nutrition, safety, rest, and orientation are general nursing interventions during this time. Rehabilitation begins during the withdrawal period and is continued in an attempt to avoid relapse.

Use a straightforward and receptive approach with clients who are abusing substances. Therapeutic communication should be focused on increasing self-esteem and confronting manipulative behavior although teaching effective coping mechanisms and problem solving. A client cannot restructure a manner of thinking, feeling, and acting until he or she achieves a new self-image. Many individuals who abuse substances suffer from the deprivation of basic needs such as physical closeness and emotional openness, which may in part be caused by the dissolution of basic family relationships. Such deprivation affects individual needs and the expectations of what one is entitled to in these meaningful relationships. A lack of fulfillment of these needs leads to a pronounced disequilibrium. Substance abuse affects all members of the family. Family members often enable the alcoholic or substance abuser to continue the abuse pattern by denying the problem. An open, caring, nonjudgmental discussion of the problem with the client and family members can have a positive effect on client outcomes.

A multidisciplinary approach is often best for these clients because they commonly have many health, personal, and social problems that must be addressed. Referral to appropriate agencies (e.g., AA, Alateen, Cocaine Anonymous, Narcotics Anonymous, Al-Anon, Rational Recovery, and Adult Children of Alcoholics) will assist in the follow-up care of these clients and their family members and will provide much needed support and encouragement.

TABLE 9-11 Nursing Assessment for Substance Abuse and/or Dependence

Functional Health Pattern	Client Data That May Indicate Substance Abuse/Dependence
Health perception-health management	Choices of daily living that are ineffective for meeting the goals of a treatment or prevention program Leaving the hospital against medical advice Stated desire to decrease substance abuse Boasting of ability to tolerate large amounts of substances Frequent changing of health care providers Appearance older than stated age
Nutritional-metabolic	Malnutrition Irregular meal pattern Poor dental hygiene Frequent heartburn, anorexia, nausea Skin lesions (rash, ulcers, bruises, needle marks)
Elimination	Recurrent diarrhea Chronic constipation
Activity-exercise	Fatigue, decreased energy Loss of interest in nonsubstance-seeking activities Poor hygiene Smelling of alcohol or other substances Heavy smoking
Sleep-rest	Insomnia Diminished response to sleep or pain medication
Cognitive-perceptual	Mental confusion Memory loss Poor judgment Diminished reality testing Blackouts Hallucinations Seizures
Self-perception–self-concept	Denial of problem
Role-relationship pattern	Social life that revolves around substance use Poor fiscal management Marital problems Neglect of vulnerable individuals in home Verbalized inability to meet role expectations Unemployment or excessive absenteeism from work Repeated minor injuries on and off the job
Sexuality-reproductive	Impotence
Coping-stress tolerance	Binge drinking/drug bingeing Negative behaviors: hostility, aggression, lying, paranoia Depression Chronic complaints of anxiety/stress Frequent hospitalization Suicide attempts
Values-belief	Lack of belief in future Lack of realistic goals Lack of belief system (religious or philosophic)

Modified from Bennett, E.G., & Woolf, D.S. (1991). *Substance abuse: Pharmacologic development and clinical perspectives* (2nd ed.). Albany, NY: Delmar Publishers.

Technology Link

Substance Misuse and Abuse

American Outreach Association Educational Material for Children (www.americanoutreach.org)

This site provides educational material for children, parents, and teachers regarding substance abuse.

Canadian Center on Substance Abuse (www.ccsa.ca/)

This site provides objective, evidence-based information and advice that will help decrease the health, social, and economic harm associated with substance abuse and addiction.

National Council on Alcohol and Drug Dependence (NCADD) (www.ncadd.org/)

This organization offers education and information on alcohol and drug abuse, a list of prevention and treatment programs in the United States, publications, and other resources.

The National Center on Addiction and Substance Abuse at Columbia University (www.casacolumbia.org/)

This site reviews the social and economic costs of substance abuse; reviews what works for prevention, treatment, and law enforcement; lists research programs; and more.

National Institute on Drug Abuse (NIDA) (www.nida.nih.gov/)

This organization provides research, training, and information on the prevention and treatment of drug abuse.

Education Assist the client in developing effective coping mechanisms and "nondrug strategies" to deal with stress. Information should be provided in a factual, nonjudgmental way. Education of the client and family should include content about drugs and abused substances, such as signs and symptoms, effects on the body, progression of the condition, health problems associated with substance abuse, and psychosocial effects of substance abuse. General treatment options and the types and location of specific treatment facilities within the community should be discussed. See the Technology Link box above for Internet resources.

Evaluation The client will experience minimal or no effects of withdrawal, verbalize an understanding of substance abuse and treatment, identify barriers to health maintenance, use problem-focused coping skills, evidence positive coping without abused substances, experience no violent behaviors, relate less anxiety related to fear of the unknown and fear of loss of control, and successfully manage the therapeutic regimen.

Summary

Although substance abuse is not a new phenomenon, the dimension of the problem for society is significant. Substance abuse is a common denominator across cultural, ethnic, and socioeconomic populations and affects every aspect of life. As a consequence, the nurse needs to be familiar with drugs that have a potential for abuse—not only in their therapeutic use but also in their street forms. This knowledge will enhance the nursing role for the prevention, detection, treatment, and rehabilitation of clients with substance abuse.

The etiology of substance abuse for any given client may vary. The drug must produce a desired effect for it to cause dependence. Currently the commonly abused drugs are opioids and related compounds; antianxiety agents; amphetamines, cocaine, and other CNS stimulants; cannabis; hallucinogens and other mood modifiers; inhalants; and anabolic steroids. In addition, multiple drug use is common, and psychological and physical dependence can exist independently or simultaneously.

Opioids are some of the most commonly abused drugs. Therefore the nurse should be alert to opioid abuse in the general population, and in the health professions. Because the "high" from opioids is characterized by complete drive satiation, the client may exhibit malnutrition and other signs of neglect from ignoring basic biologic needs. Acute overdose of opioids with miotic pupils, stupor, and respiratory depression is considered to be a medical emergency; symptoms may be reversed by adequate amounts of naloxone (Narcan), an opioid antagonist. Treatment of opioid dependence may involve withdrawal with supportive therapy, methadone detoxification and withdrawal, or clonidine treatment followed by either a methadone maintenance program or a therapeutic community program.

Other forms of analgesics such as pentazocine (Talwin) and propoxyphene (Darvon) tend to be abused based on access, fashion, and availability of other substances on the street.

Alcohol is the most common substance of abuse. The ingestion of alcohol does not carry with it the social stigma attached to the abuse of other drugs. However, the chronic abuse of alcohol causes physiologic damage to every body system; its therapeutic use is quite limited. Disulfiram (Antabuse) is used to sensitize the individual to alcohol by causing such an unpleasant response—nausea, headache, palpitations, dyspnea, and intense discomfort—that the use of alcohol is no longer desired.

Benzodiazepines are the antianxiety agents most abused, generally as the result of overprescribing to women and older adults.

Amphetamines and cocaine are the most commonly abused CNS stimulants. Because cocaine is available as "crack" at a much lower cost than other drugs, it is becoming increasingly popular and is much more of a health problem with its strong physical and psychological dependence.

Cannabis drugs are increasingly being used by young teenagers for recreation to produce an anxiety-free state of relaxation and a sense of well-being. Studies indicate that impaired decision making, apathy, and memory loss are related to cannabis use. Psychological and physical dependence develop with chronic use.

Psychedelic drugs and inhalants are also substances for abuse because of their mind-altering properties. Anabolic steroids are abused by individuals who want to improve their appearance or performance in sports.

The nurse has an important role in preventing substance abuse because of his or her knowledge and extent of contact with individuals of all ages and circumstances. Assessment for the detection of substance abuse and intervention in an acute overdose or withdrawal situation are performed in a straightforward and receptive manner. Because of the multiplicity of problems in clients who abuse substances, the nurse may be part of a multidisciplinary team in the provision of support.

✴ Critical Thinking Questions

- Jane Parker is a receptionist for the executive office suite of a large manufacturing firm. She is single, attractive, and enjoys an active social life. A few months ago she began attending parties where cocaine was being used, and she began using cocaine to "fit in" with the crowd. Her coworkers have noticed that she has become edgy, has lost weight, and has been unable to concentrate on her work. One of the executives sends Jane to the company nurse because she "does not look well." As the company's occupational nurse, how could you intervene with Ms. Parker? What activities could the company undertake as part of a substance abuse prevention program?

- Ronald Taylor, 72 years of age, is brought to the hospital after falling off his roof while doing home repairs. He is taken to surgery for an open reduction of a fractured femur. On the third day of hospitalization, Mr. Taylor becomes increasingly irritable and refuses to participate in his physical therapy. He indicates that he wishes to sign himself out of the hospital. The nurse notes from Mr. Taylor's past medical history that he has sustained multiple injuries as the result of minor automobile and home accidents. The nurse begins to consider that Mr. Taylor might abuse alcohol. Why would that be a consideration at this time? As the nurse in question, how will you intervene?

Bibliography

American Nurses Association. (1994). ANA position statement: Drug testing of health care workers. Silver Spring, MD: Author.

American Society of Addiction Medicine (2005). Retrieved July 26, 2005, from http://www.asam.org/ppol/Definition%20of20Alcoholism.htm

Anderson, D.M., Keith, J., & Novak, P.D. (2002). *Mosby's medical, nursing & allied health dictionary* (6th ed.). St. Louis: Mosby.

Anton R.F., Moak, D.H., Latham, P.K., Waid, L.R., Malcolm, R.J., Dias, J.K., et al. (2001). Posttreatment results of combining naltrexone with cognitive-behavior therapy for the treatment of alcoholism. *Journal of Clinical Psychopharmacology, 21*(1), 72-77.

Arseneault, L., Cannon, M., Poulton, R., Murray, R., Caspi, A., & Moffitt, T.E. (2002). Cannabis use in adolescence and risk for adult psychosis: Longitudinal prospective study. *BMJ, 325*, 1212-1213.

Blondell, R.D., Dodds, H.N., Blondell, M.N., Looney, S.W., Smoger, S.H., Sexton, L.K., et al. (2003). Ethanol in formularies of U.S. teaching hospitals. *Journal of the American Medical Association, 289*, 552.

Bureau of Justice Statistics. (2004). Retrieved December 11, 2004 from http://www.ojp/gov/bjs/

Canadian Executive Council on Addictions. (2004). *Canadian addiction survey (CAS): A national survey of Canadians' use of alcohol and other drugs.* (n.d.) Retrieved December 11, 2004 from http://www.ccsa.ca/pdf/ccsa-004804-2004.pdf

Cronk, C.E., & Sarvela, P.D. (1997). Alcohol, tobacco and other drug use among rural/small town and urban youth: A secondary analysis of the monitoring the future data set. *American Journal of Public* Health, *87*(5), 760-764.

DeGeest, S., Dobbels, F., Martin, S., Willems, K., & Vanhaecke, J. (2000). Clinical risk associated with appointment noncompliance in heart transplant recipients. *Progress in Transplantation, 10*(3), 162-168.

Dimartini, A., Weinrieb, R., & Fireman, M. (2002). Liver transplantation in patients with alcohol and other substance use disorders, *Psychiatric Clinics of North America, 25*(1), 195-209.

Doering, P.L. (2002). Substance-Related Disorders: Overview and depressants, stimulants, and hallucinogens. In J.T. DiPiro, et al. (2002). *Pharmacotherapy: A pathophysiological approach* (5th ed.). Stamford, CT: Appleton & Lange.

Drug Abuse Warning Network (DAWN). (2004). *Drug Abuse Warning Network.* Emergency Department Data. Office of Applied Studies, Substance Abuse and Mental Health Services Administration, Rockville, MD: Department of Health and Human Services. Retrieved July 26, 2005, from http://dawninfo.samhsa.gov/old_dawn/

Drug facts and comparisons. (2005). St. Louis: Facts and Comparisons.

Ebrahim, S.H., & Gfroerer, J. (2003). Pregnancy-related substance use in the United States during 1996-1998. Obstetrics & Gynecology, *101*, 374-379.

𝒆-LEARNING SUPPLEMENTS

Student CD-ROM
- Final Exam questions
- NCLEX® Examination review questions
- Pharmacology animations
- Printable chapter summary

Evolve Website (http://evolve.elsevier.com/mckenry)
- Case study on substance misuse and abuse
- Content updates, including information on new drugs

- WebLinks corresponding to this chapter
- Answers to the critical thinking questions in this chapter
- *Elsevier ePharmacology Update* newsletter
- Mosby's Drug Consult Internet Edition
- Supplemental and reference information

Ford, M., Delaney, K., Ling, L. & Erickson, T. (Eds.). (2001). *Clinical toxicology.* Philadelphia: W.B. Saunders.

Fudala, P.J., Bridge, T.P., Herbert, S., Williford, W.O., Chiang, C.N., Jones, K., et al and the Buprenorphine/Naloxone Collaborative Study Group (2003). Office-based treatment of opiate addiction with a sublingual-tablet formulation of buprenorphine and naloxone. *New England Journal of Medicine, 349,* 949-958.

Gjesvold, J. (2001). Health care professionals not immune to drug, alcohol problems. Retrieved May 12, 2004, from http://www.eugene.com/health/substance_abuse_9.shtml

Goldfinger, T.M. (2003). Beyond the French paradox: the impact of moderate beverage alcohol and wine consumption in the prevention of cardiovascular disease. *Cardiology Clinics, 21*(3), 449-457.

Jacobson, A.L., & Jacobson, A.M. (Eds.). (2001). *Psychiatric secrets.* (2nd ed.). Hanley & Belfus.

Jones, J.S., Johnson, K., & McNinch M. (1996). Age as a risk factor for inadequate emergency department analgesia. *American Journal of Emergency Medicine, 14,* 157-160

Jungnickel, P.W. (2005). Alcohol abuse. In M.A. Koda-Kimble, L.Y. Young, W.A. Kradjan, B.J. Guglielmo, B.K. Alldredge, & R.L. Corelli (Eds.), *Applied therapeutics: The clinical use of drugs* (8th ed.). Philadelphia: Lippincott, Williams & Wilkins.

Katzung, B.G. (2004). *Basic & clinical pharmacology* (9th ed.). New York: McGraw Hill.

Krizik, T.J. (2004). The impaired surgical resident. *Surgical Clinics of North America, 84*(6), 1587-1604.

Krystal, J,H., Cramer, J.A., Krol, W,F., Kirk, G.F., & Rosenheck, RA. Veterans Affairs Naltrexone Cooperative Study 425 Group. (2001). Naltrexone in the treatment of alcohol dependence. *New England Journal of Medicine, 345*(24), 1734-1739.

Lynskey, M.T., Heath, A.C., Bucholz, K.K., Slutske, W.S., Madden, P.A., Nelson, E.C., et al. (2003). Escalation of drug use in early-onset cannabis users vs co-twin controls. *Journal of the American Medical Association, 289,* 427-433.

MacAuley, D. (2004). Cheating at Athens: Is it worth it? *British Medical Journal, 329*(7462), 407.

Mersey, D.J. (2003). Recognition of alcohol and substance abuse. *American Family Physician, 67*(7), 1529-32.

Miller, N.S., & Brady, K.T. (2004). Addictive disorders. *Psychiatric Clinics of North America, 27*(4), 661-74.

Mosby's drug consult (15th ed.). (2005). St. Louis: Mosby.

Naimi, T.S., Brewer, R.D., Mokdad, A., Denny, C., Serdula, M.K., & Marks, J.S. (2003). Binge drinking among U.S. adults. *Journal of the American Medical Association, 289,* 70-75.

National Center for Health Statistics. (2004). Use of Selected substances in the past 12 months by persons 12 year of age and over according to age, sex, race, and Hispanic origin: United States: 2002. Retrieved October 31, 2004 from http://www.cdc.gov/nchs/data/hus/tables/2003/03 hus062.pdf

National Institute on Drug Abuse (NIDA) (2004). Commonly abused drugs, street names for drugs of abuse, National Institute on Drug Abuse. Retrieved December 11, 2004 from http://www.nida.nih.gov/DrugsofAbuse.html

National Institutes of Health (NIH). (1997). Consensus statement: Effective medical treatment of opiate addiction. Retrieved May 1, 2005 from http://odp.od.nih.gov/consensus/cons/108/108_statement.htm

Office of National Drug Control Policy (2004). Retrieved July 26, 2005, from http://www.whitehousedrugpolicy.gov/streetterms/

O'Hara, P., Parris, D., Fichtner, R.R., & Oster, R. (1998). Influence of alcohol and drug use on AIDS risk behavior among youth in dropout prevention. *Journal of Drug Education, 28*(2), 159-168.

Patton, G.C., Coffey, C., Carlin, J.B., Degenhardt L., Lynskey M., & Hall W. (2002). Cannabis use and mental health in young people: Cohort study. *British Medical Journal, 325,* 1195-1198.

Raftery K.A., Smith-Coggins R., & Chen A.H. (1995). Gender-associated differences in emergency department pain management. *Annals of Emergency Medicine, 26,* 414-421.

Rey, J.M., & Tennant, C.C. (2002). Cannabis and mental health: More evidence establishes clear link between use of cannabis and psychiatric illness. *British Medical Journal, 325,* 1183-1184.

Singer, L.T., Minnes, S., Short, E., Arendt, R., Farkas, K., Lewis, B., et al. (2004). Cognitive outcomes of preschool children with prenatal cocaine exposure. *Journal of the American Medical Association, 291,* 2448-2456.

Talbott GD, Gallegos KV, & Angres DH. (1998). Impairment and recovery in physicians and other health professionals. In Graham, D.W., & Schultz, T.K. (Eds.). Principles of addiction medicine. Chevy Chase, Maryland: American Society of Addiction Medicine.

Todd, K.H., Deaton, C., D'Adamo, A.P., & Goe, L. (2000). Ethnicity and analgesic practice. *Annals of Emergency Medicine, 35* (1), 11-16.

Traub, S.J., Kohn, G.L., Hoffman, R.S., & Nelson, L.S. (2003). Pediatric "body packing." *Archives of Pediatric Adolescent Medicine, 157,* 174-177.

Trinkoff, A.M., & Storr, C.L. (1998). Substance use among nurses: Differences between specialties. *American Journal of Public Health, 88*(4), 581-585.

U.S. Drug Enforcement Agency. (2005). What are predatory drugs? Retrieved July 26, 2005, from http://www.usdoj.gov/dea/concern/predatory.html.

USP DI: Drug information for the health care professional. (2005). (25th ed.). Greenwood Village, CO: MICROMEDEX Thomson Healthcare.

van den Brink, W., Hendriks, V.M., Blanken, P., Koeter, M.W., van Zwieten, B.J., & van Ree, J.M. (2003). Medical prescription of heroin to treatment resistant heroin addicts: Two randomised controlled trials. *British Medical Journal, 327,* 310-312.

Watson, W.A., Litovitz, T.L., Rodgers, G.C., Youniss, J. Rutherford, R., Borys, D., et al. (2003). 2002 annual report of the American Association of Poison Control Centers toxic exposure surveillance system, *MDConsult* (www.MDConsult.com).

Weber, J.E., Shofer, F.S., Larkin, G.L., Kalaria, A.S., & Hollander, J.E. (2003). Validation of a brief observation period for patients with cocaine-associated chest pain. *New England Journal of Medicine, 348,* 510-517.

Wilens, T.E, Faraone, S.V, Biederman, J., & Gunawardene, S (2003). Does stimulant therapy of attention-deficit/hyperactivity disorder beget later substance abuse? A meta-analytic review of the literature. *Pediatrics, 111,* 179-185.

Zammit, S., Allebeck, P., Andreasson, S., Lundberg, I., & Lewis, G. (2002). Self reported cannabis use as a risk factor for schizophrenia in Swedish conscripts of 1969: Historical cohort study. *British Medical Journal, 325,* 1199-1201.

Zimmerman, J.L. (2003). Poisonings and overdoses in the intensive care unit: General and specific management issues. *Critical Care Medicine, 31*(12), 2794-2801.

Zizzo, W.O., & Zizzo, P.W. (2005). Drug abuse. In M.A. Koda-Kimble, L.Y. Young, W.A. Kradjan, B.J. Guglielmo, B.K. Alldredge, & R.L. Corelli (Eds.), *Applied therapeutics: The clinical use of drugs* (8th ed.). Philadelphia: Lippincott, Williams & Wilkins.

CLIENT EDUCATION FOR SELF-ADMINISTRATION OF MEDICATION

CHAPTER FOCUS

Effective management of a therapeutic regimen requires a major commitment by the client and the family or caregiver. A well-planned teaching program can provide the information needed to safely and accurately self-manage medications in the home setting and enhance compliance with the drug regimen. It can also decrease the number of complications arising from medications by preparing the client to recognize the early signs and symptoms of adverse effects and to report them to the prescriber. Therefore the nurse needs to be not only knowledgeable in pharmacologic content but also skilled in client education.

LEARNING OBJECTIVES

- Assess a client and family regarding the need and readiness to learn how to administer medications.
- Identify the nursing diagnoses of deficient knowledge, noncompliance, and ineffective therapeutic regimen management as they relate to self-administration of medications.
- Identify factors that affect client compliance in the self-administration of medications.
- Write measurable objectives for a client who is learning to self-administer medications.
- Discuss at least three teaching techniques that may increase a client's knowledge of medications.
- Identify four or more safety precautions necessary for a client in self-administering medications.
- Document the client's and the family's learning, including content, method, and progress toward learning goals.

▲ KEY TERMS

compliance, p. 192
deficient knowledge, p. 192
ineffective therapeutic regimen management, p. 192

noncompliance, p. 192
therapeutic seeding, p. 197

✳ Why is client education an important component of the nursing role?

Nurses have been teaching their clients since the advent of the discipline. However, an increasing emphasis has been placed on the role of nurses in supporting clients' abilities for self-care, adaptation to illness, and high-level wellness. Various factors are responsible for this change in emphasis. A growing consumer awareness of health issues and services has prompted consumers to take a greater interest in participating in their own health care. The client is more apt to request information and to request it from the nurse with whom they have contact. Nurses have responded by promoting the client's active involvement in planning and implementing nursing care. In 1972, the American Hospital Association published "A Patient's Bill of Rights," which gave formal recognition to the client's right to know about his or her health status, treatments, alternative methods of treatment, and continuing care requirements. Client education is being recognized as one way of making possible a shorter length of hospital stay. A shorter length of hospital stay has been an important factor in the economic climate since the development of a prospective payment system for health care by the Health Care Financing Administration in 1983, the advent of diagnosis-related groups (DRGs), the development of managed care, and the increasing growth of health maintenance organizations (HMOs), which continue to shorten lengths of stay.

Technology has both extended life expectancy and increased the number of chronically ill individuals. Many older adults or debilitated clients require health teaching to enable them to remain independent. Since 1976, the Joint Commission for the Accreditation of Healthcare Organizations (JC-AHO) has required evidence in the client's clinical record that specific instructions were provided to the client and family regarding medications, diet, and follow-up care. Nurse practice acts have set guidelines and developed standards for the nurse's role in health education. There have been successful lawsuits alleging that nurses provided less than adequate health teaching. But regardless of the environmental and societal issues that reinforce the importance of the nurse's participation in client education, professional nursing's foundation lies in the promotion of wellness-oriented self-care involving comprehensive education and coordination of appropriate resources. These characteristics distinguish nurses as unique from other health care providers and are essential in today's health care system (Sherry, Simmons, Wung, & Zerwic, 2003).

Client education is a process that helps people to learn and incorporate health-related behaviors into everyday life. Learning is defined as a change in behavior, and nurses assist individuals in changing their behavior. Nurses provide health-related information and teach in a way that helps ensure the client's compliance with a therapeutic regimen. At no time is this more important than when educating clients in the self-administration of medications.

Medical research has provided us with potent drugs that can cure and prevent progression of many diseases that once caused significant morbidity and mortality. However when medications are prescribed, most clients take only a portion of their drugs. Between 33% and 94% of drugs are not taken as intended by their prescriber. Many clients will never start or will stop therapy completely within the first year, and only a minority will continue taking their drugs as prescribed. Noncompliance is a significant problem in all client populations, from children to older adults and tends to worsen the longer a client continues on drug therapy (Billups, Malone, & Carter, 2000).

A lack of adherence with prescribed therapeutic regimens has been a concern to health professionals since the time of Hippocrates (Evangelista & Dracup, 2000). This concern per-

sists as reflected in over 14,000 published reports on the topic and investigations of more than 250 possible etiologies for noncompliance found in the research literature (Donovan, 1995). Misuse and noncompliance with drug regimens have been well documented with compliance rates at 52% to 64% with nonpsychiatric drugs (Dolder, Lacro, & Jeste, 2003), 18% to 52% with mood stabilizers (Scott & Pope, 2002), 20% to 58% with drugs for heart failure (Evangelista & Dracup, 2000), 15% to 44% with medications for type 2 diabetes (Rubin, 2005), 54% to 100% with tuberculosis medications (Macintyre, Goebel, & Brown, 2005), 55% in post–kidney transplantation (Vasquez, Tanzi, Benedetti, & Pollak, 2003); and DeKlerk et al. (2003) reported that in clients with rheumatoid arthritis, polymyalgia, and gout there was no evidence of dosing in 10%, 10%, and 15% of the monitored days, respectively. Although a number of factors determine whether or not clients will adhere to a medication regimen, clients must be provided with accurate information on which to base their behaviors.

Because of the shortened length of hospital stays and the increasing time limitations for office visits under HMOs, one of the current trends is to relegate counseling about proper medication administration to the community pharmacist. Many clients have difficulty with this process because of the lack of privacy and the busy environment of the pharmacy setting. Some health care providers are concerned because the pharmacist does not have access to the client's medical history. Johnson, Butta, Donohue, Glenn, and Holtzman (1996) found that only 44% of families were counseled about their child's medication by their pharmacist. Their recommendation was for health care professionals engaged in the client's care to teach the client and/or family safe and accurate medication administration.

The teaching-learning process may be structured along the lines of the nursing process with the first step being assessment—the gathering of facts and information that will assist the nurse in meeting the client's and family's needs for learning. Planning, the next step in the process, begins as soon as a learning need has been identified, with goals being written as outcomes for the client's learning. The implementation phase is the actual communication of information. Evaluation focuses on the client's behaviors and attitudes as a measure of whether or not the client has achieved the learning objectives. As was discussed in Chapter 5, the various components of the nursing process are not always sequential, so the nurse may be required to conduct teaching in the midst of an assessment.

Nursing Assessment

⚙ **What are the important issues for a nursing assessment of the client's needs for education?**

A thorough assessment of the client is essential for educating about medications in the most efficient and effective way. Realistic goals for a client's medicating behaviors are the result of the nurse's accurate assessment. The nurse should conduct a comprehensive assessment regarding the client's response to illness. A comprehensive assessment includes determining the

---

Cultural Considerations

Cultural Expressions of Bodily Awareness among Chronically Ill Filipino Americans

Having an awareness of the client's cultural identity enhances the nurse's ability to work with the client to effectively mange the therapeutic regimen. The portrayal of bodily experience, the connection between how people experience their bodies and how they talk about them, offers clues for illness management, especially for self-monitoring and self-care techniques. Becker (2003) used semistructured interviews with 85 Filipino Americans who had one or more chronic illnesses and who were engaged in efforts to maintain control of illnesses, such as diabetes, hypertension, and asthma. The purpose was to determine whether cultural traditions surrounding bodily awareness, especially the concept of balance and harmony, were relevant to Filipino Americans' perception of signs and symptoms related to chronic illness, and to actions they took to manage their chronic illness. In this study, paying attention to bodily awareness through continuous social interchange strengthened values of self-care and reinforced efforts to monitor illnesses and control them. Awareness of this health value may be used to facilitate client education about how to manage chronic illness in the Filipino American population.

1. Would this study have greater applicability to older rather than younger clients? Why or why not?
2. How would you determine whether your Filipino American client valued bodily awareness?

Modified from Becker, G. (2003). Cultural expressions of bodily awareness among chronically ill Filipino Americans. *Annals of Family Medicine, 1*(2), 113-118.

---

client's competence in self-care and mobility, nutritional status, sleep patterns, and social support mechanisms. The data collected should describe factors influencing the client's ability, motivation, and interest in following health advice. The client's cultural perspectives, health beliefs, and attitudes need to be included in the assessment. (See the Cultural Considerations box above.) All of these factors influence the teaching-learning process for the self-administration of medications. Not all clients need to know everything about their medications, nor are all clients ready to learn about them. However, Czar and Engler (1997) found that content about medications was ranked as one of the three most important learning needs of clients during hospitalization and follow-up clinic visits.

Current Level of Client Knowledge Related to the Therapeutic Regimen

Assessing a client's learning needs means ascertaining what the client already knows: "What medications are you presently taking?" "What is each medication for?" "How often and how much of each medication should you be taking?" "What are the adverse effects of each drug?" "Which of these adverse ef-

fects should you report to your prescriber?" (See Chapter 5 for a medication history form.) If the client knows the answers to these questions, the objective for learning may have been met.

If the client has deficient knowledge, determine a point of reference for learning by validating the client's present level of knowledge. New information is easier to absorb when it can be related to what the client already knows. For example, when teaching about nitroglycerin (an antianginal medication), the nurse might ask the client what is understood about the diagnosis of angina. The nurse can discuss the therapeutic action of the nitroglycerin by using the words the client used to describe the condition. Determine a baseline of data to evaluate what knowledge the client has gained by comparing what was known before and after the learning process.

Be aware of any incorrect knowledge or misunderstanding the client may have. The client's health information may be a collection of folklore, hearsay, handed-down family experience, advertising claims, and misconceptions. Incorrect information needs to be identified and dealt with before the teaching of the correct material can be initiated.

Because of shortened hospital stays, instruction must sometimes be limited to survival content—only the most important information. What will the client need to know about when returning home? What must the client learn to survive until additional information can be obtained? Does the client know whom to call if additional information is needed? Although many nurses prefer to teach some mechanism of action of the client's drug as a foundation for the self-administration of medications, the anxiety and health status of the client sometimes preclude that depth of explanation. Clients who have undergone ambulatory surgery are discharged after having received an array of medications before and during their surgical procedures; as a result, they may have a decreased ability to understand and process information. The types of agents commonly used in these settings (e.g., benzodiazepines, opioid analgesics, and anticholinergics) have been shown to impair the ability of clients to process and recall information.

A client can become easily overwhelmed by highly technical content and lose the essential information needed to take the drug safely and accurately. However, some clients may ask for additional technical information. Hospitalized clients tend to focus on the issues related to hospitalization (e.g., how to administer the insulin injection) rather than on long-term dietary management of their diabetes mellitus. (See the Evidence-Based Practice box on p. 187.) Clients in ambulatory care may have difficulty absorbing all they need to understand about their medications in the brief time of a typically scheduled visit. In-home assessments are beneficial for assessing the client's adherence to the prescribed medication regimen.

Perceptions of Current Health Status Research by Petrie, Weinman, Sharpe, and Buckley (1996) suggests that clients focus their ideas about illness on five themes, which health psychologists call illness perceptions:

- *Identity*: the label the client uses to describe the illness and the symptoms that he or she views as being part of the disease

✦✦✦ Evidence-Based Practice

The Role of Client Education in Diabetic Education

Client education has an important role in diabetic education to reduce complications, optimize quality of life, and improve metabolic control for clients.

The incidence of diabetes mellitus, particularly type 2, is increasing in the general population. Similarly, the incidence of clients with diabetes mellitus who develop end-stage renal disease (ESRD) has increased to 44% in the dialysis facility. McMurray et al. (2002) allocated 83 clients, either to the control group or the study group based on their day of dialysis treatment. All of them were followed for a year. Participants in the study group underwent a diabetes education program and were followed up by a care manager who provided self-management education, diabetes self care monitoring/management, motivational coaching, and foot checks. As a result the following occurred:

- The control group baseline foot risk category worsened from 2.7 to 3.3 ($p < 0.05$) compared to no significant change in the study group (2.2 to 2.0).
- No amputations in the study group vs. five in the control group ($p < 0.05$).
- Ten clients in the control group were hospitalized with diabetes- or vascular-related admissions vs. one client in the study group ($p < 0.002$).
- Hemoglobin A1 c levels declined from 6.9 to 6.3 on the study group, whereas the control group levels were unchanged ($p < 0.005$).
- Diabetes-related quality-of-life scores increased in the study group from 76 to 86 ($p < 0.001$ vs. the control group).
- There was a significant improvement in self-management behavior in all six categories evaluated in the study group vs. the control group.
- Dialysis centers were recognized by the American Diabetes Association to provide diabetes education.

1. The results of this study suggest that behavior change strategies are more effective than didactic methods. Why would that be so?
2. What would be the benefits of this study's approach in other settings with clients with diabetes?

- *Cause:* personal ideas about the cause of the illness
- *Time line*: how long the client believes the illness will last
- *Consequences*: the expected effects and outcomes of the illness
- *Cure or control*: how the client recovers from or controls the illness

Although the research of Petrie et al. examined client participation in rehabilitation regimens following myocardial infarction (MI), their findings could relate to adherence practices with medication regimens. Clients who strongly believed that their illnesses were amenable to cure or control were more likely to participate in rehabilitation programs (adhere to a medication regimen). Clients who anticipated that their illness would have major consequences on their life were slower to recover. Client beliefs may not correspond to professional views of the illness, and health care professionals may not be aware of these differences. The client's meaning or perception of the illness experience is very influential in determining the client's participation with the medication regimen. It is essential that the nurse assess the client's perceptions of illness.

Cognitive Impairment Assess if the client has memory or concentration problems, or loss of the capacity to understand the anticipated outcome of treatment versus no treatment. Deficits in cognition may be overt or may be relatively subtle following stroke, MI, hypoxia, surgery, or other health conditions or procedures. Family members can be assistive in determining whether the client has a history of cognitive problems or whether the client's behavior differs from the usual behavior. If the client would be unable to effectively manage the therapeutic regimen independently, then a caregiver(s) is identified to participate in the learning-teaching process.

Psychopathology Emotional state influences the client's perspective on the world and readiness to learn. Mild anxiety may stimulate the client to learn, whereas severe anxiety may shorten the attention span and be incapacitating. Anxiety may also be associated with the negative interpretation of adverse effects that may lead to nonadherence with the therapeutic regimen. Compared with nondepressed clients, depressed clients are three times more likely to be noncompliant with medical treatment recommendations (DiMattero, Lepper, & Croghan, 2000). Clinical depression found in clients with cardiac conditions over the course of their disease influences a client's energy to make and sustain changes, increases hopelessness, and promotes thoughts that treatment does not matter (Glassman et al, 2002). A high level of anger and hostility is four times as likely in heart transplant clients with persistent medication compliance problems (Frasure-Smith et al., 2000). In clients with renal transplantation, anger was associated with an increased risk for noncompliance (Penkower et al., 2003).

Motivation for Treatment The manner in which a client perceives self-ability to change or control the circumstance has an impact on willingness or ability to adhere to a medication regimen. Feeling pressured by others and conflicted about change is associated with noncompliance; by comparison, intrinsic motivation that involves positive self-related outcomes sustain adherence (Bellg & Rosenson, 2004). The client's perception of self-ability to influence or control life falls along an internal-external continuum. At one end of the continuum a client is internally (self-) oriented; at the other end a client is externally (others- or fate) oriented about health behaviors. Clients with an internal motivation are more apt to be health-oriented and adhere to a medication regimen. Internal motivation may be assessed by listening to client's statements, such as "I forgot to take my medication" (internal responsibility) rather than, "My husband didn't remind me to take my medicine" (external displacement of responsibility). In one instance the client assumes accountability for the actions, and in the other the responsibility is placed elsewhere.

Readiness to Learn Many factors affect the client's readiness to learn (Petrie et al., 1996). (See Box 10-1.) A client goes through various stages in adapting to illness or injury, including developing awareness, reorganization, resolution, and identity change. During the assessment the nurse should be aware of the client's stage of adaptation. Understanding the client's coping strategies will prevent the nurse from attempting to teach information that the client is not ready to learn. Anger, fear, and mistrust of health care personnel may also impede readiness for learning.

Functional Illiteracy Clients who lack functional literacy (lack the ability to read well enough to understand and use information as intended) are also at risk for not following a medication regimen. This also occurs when health care providers use unfamiliar medical terminology when describing disease processes and medical interventions. Health literacy is the ability to understand and act on health information; it is necessary to have the capacity to obtain, process, and understand basic health information and services to make appropriate health decisions. In a study of Medicare recipients, Gazmararian et al. (1999) found that 48% did not understand the written instructions "take medicine every 6 hours," 68% could not interpret a blood sugar value, 27% could not identify their next appointment; and 27% did not understand "take medicine on an empty stomach" (instructions written at a fourth-grade level). When questioned about understanding, the client will most likely indicate an understanding of the material, even if it is not understood. This response may be a result of an inadequate vocabulary or an inability to explain what is not understood. Nearly half of all Americans—90 million people—have difficulty understanding and using health information (Institute of Medicine, 2004).

Traditionally, nurses have used the client's stated last year of schooling to estimate health literacy, but in the Gazmararian et al. study (1999) 27% of the clients who had a high school diploma and 17% of those who had some college education had inadequate or marginal health literacy.

Communication Language barriers exist when there are differences in the primary language spoken by the health

care provider and the client. According to the 2000 census, 18% of U.S. residents speak a language other than English as their primary language (U.S. Census Bureau, 2000). Laws addressing the provision of health services to clients who have limited English proficiency exist at both the federal and the state level; the primary federal law is Title VI of the Civil Rights Act of 1964 (Jacobs & Mutha, 2004).

Whenever possible, nurses should learn the language of the clients with whom they are interacting. If that is not practical, nurses should learn key phrases related to greetings and the health care services provided. Interpreters can also be used, but they should understand health care terminology, have training in transcultural interpretation, know the language of both the health care provider and the client, and respect both cultures (Putsch & Kaufert, 1997). There is a legal mandate for the use of interpreters.

Clients from other cultures may indicate understanding as a sign of respect. For example, in many Asian cultures it is respectful to smile and nod one's head to a person of authority, regardless of the level of understanding. In these instances, the nurse may enlist the assistance of the client's support system—the individuals or group that provide comfort, aid, and information to help him or her cope with life. The support system can consist of family, friends, and members of the community and church or religious groups.

If at all possible, however, the nurse should avoid using family members or visitors as interpreters because the shared information sometimes includes sensitive material. Family members or visitors may modify the interpretation to protect the client from information they believe will cause cultural strain or difficulty for the client and family.

Tripp-Reimer & Afifi (1989) offered the following classic guidelines for working with clients when there is a language barrier:

- Speak slowly (plan the teaching session to last at least twice as long as a typical session).
- Make the sentence structure simple (use active, not passive, voice; use a straightforward subject-verb pattern).
- Avoid technical terms (e.g., use "heart" rather than "cardiac"), professional jargon, and American idioms ("red tape").
- Provide instructional material in the same sequence in which the client should carry out the plan.
- Do not assume you have been understood. Ask the client to explain the protocol; optimally, if appropriate, obtain a return demonstration.

Although these guidelines are suggested for clients with a language barrier, they hold true for most clients.

Nonverbal communication is also important in teaching across cultures. Unspoken cues such as eye contact, distance between speakers, body movements, touch, and silence have cultural components. In general, whites value direct eye contact when speaking. Eye contact provides feedback to ensure understanding of what has been communicated. In some other cultures (e.g., Native American, Asian, and African), direct eye contact is considered disrespectful. Diverting the eyes downward and to one side of the speaker

---

BOX 10-1 FACTORS AFFECTING READINESS TO LEARN

- Pathophysiologic: severity of illness, pain, fatigue, sensory deprivation, physical disabilities
- Treatment-related: complexity of regimen
- Situational: illiteracy, language differences, ineffective coping patterns, financial concerns, home environment
- Maturational: family roles and relationships, health maintenance practices

indicates that a person is listening intently. Nurses need to be observers of nonverbal communication and learn what these cues mean from the client's cultural perspective.

Cultural Issues A cultural assessment should be conducted to elicit the client's beliefs, values, and attitudes about health, illness, medications, and the client role (see Chapter 6) for every client, not just client's that are culturally diverse from the nurse. Health beliefs are particularly important in medication compliance:

- Risk perceptions concerning illness. For example, the perceived threat of cardiovascular disease is often minimized by clients (e.g., clients in their 30s and 40s who believe they are not susceptible to an "old person's disease").
- Perceived benefits of treatment. Clear communication of progress (e.g., changes in blood pressure values and their meaning to the client) is essential. The lack of perceived symptoms in a condition such as hypertension means that the client's understanding of the benefits of treatment is based on the effectiveness of communication with health care providers.
- Barrier beliefs concerning medicines or a specific medication. Clients are often concerned about medication interactions or taking too many medications. They also frequently have misinformation or misunderstandings about treatment (e.g., when my blood pressure is normal, I can quit the medicine). Personal beliefs about "becoming dependent" on medicine or preferences for lifestyle also frequently affect medication compliance (Stretcher & Rosenstock, 1997).

Care should be negotiated between the client and nurse until an agreement is reached for a culturally appropriate and acceptable intervention. Only then will culturally appropriate teaching and learning take place.

Developmental Stage Assess the client's level of development because this will affect the ability to make decisions, to assume responsibility for the result of those decisions, and to manage life. If the client's developmental stage is not accurately assessed, the nurse may misdirect goals and inhibit client learning. Erickson and other researchers have described the physical, emotional, and psychological stages of development and related developmental. Box 10-2 describes Erickson's stages of development.

All individuals pass through the same predictable life stages, but passage through these stages occurs at different rates. Some individuals are ready to accept adult responsibilities at 18 years of age; others may be well past 35 years of age before they are ready to accept responsibility for themselves and others. Although movement through these stages is sequential, clients can fluctuate among stages, often in response to stress. Stressors such as illness and hospitalization may cause the client to regress temporarily to an earlier stage. The client needs to be addressed at his or her current developmental stage rather than at the developmental stage expected for the client's chronologic age. Table 10-1 summarizes changes related to aging and the educational strategies

---

BOX 10-2 ERICKSON'S STAGES OF DEVELOPMENT

Infant (birth to 1 year of age): Trust vs. mistrust. Infant learns to trust self, others, and the environment; learns to love and be loved.

Toddler (1 to 3 years of age): Autonomy vs. shame and doubt. Toddler learns independence; learns to master the physical environment and maintain self-esteem.

Preschooler (3 to 6 years of age): Initiative vs. guilt. Preschooler learns basic problem solving; develops conscience and sexual identity; initiates and imitates activities.

School-age child (6 to 12 years of age): Industry vs. inferiority. School-age child learns to do things well; develops a sense of self-worth.

Adolescent (12 to 18 years of age): Identity vs. role confusion. Adolescent integrates many roles into self-identity through role models and peer pressure.

Young adult (18 to 45 years of age): Intimacy vs. isolation. Young adult establishes deep and lasting relationships; learns to make commitment as spouse, parent, partner.

Middle-aged adult (45 to 65 years of age): Generativity vs. stagnation. Adult learns commitment to community and world; is productive in career, family, civic interests.

Older adult (over 65 years of age): Integrity vs. despair. Older adult appreciates life role and status; deals with loss and prepares for death.

---

to address them. These changes are important in deciding whether the client can self-administer medications accurately. In some instances, responsibility for the administration of medications may need to be delegated to a caregiver.

Sensory Impairment Modify the teaching plan for clients with vision and hearing impairments. Instructions in large print and pill containers with the days of the week printed in Braille are two modifications that may be considered for the visually impaired client. Written instructions are imperative for the hearing impaired; try to keep all written communication simple and straightforward. If the client with a hearing impairment can read lips or speech, make sure to support this activity.

The assessment for teaching-learning is similar to other types of nursing assessment; it is continuous and involves observation, listening and questioning, and other communication skills. The assessment phase can be used to establish rapport and gain the mutual nurse-client respect necessary for the teaching-learning process. Because nurses are seen as having a position of power in relation to the client, they must recognize the need to initiate the educational process. When the client perceives an attitude of sincerity, integrity, and warmth in the nurse, the milieu is set for the client to feel free to ask questions and to discuss all matters, regardless of how personal those issues may be.

TABLE 10-1 EDUCATIONAL STRATEGIES FOR COMMON CHANGES RELATED TO AGING

Changes Related to Aging That May Influence Learning	Educational Strategy
ALTERED THOUGHT PROCESSES	
Slowed cognitive functioning	Slow pace of presentation.
Decreased short-term memory	Provide smaller amounts of information at one time.
Decreased ability to think abstractly	Repeat information frequently.
Decreased ability to concentrate	Use examples to illustrate information.
Increased reaction time (slower to respond)	Decrease external stimuli as much as possible. Allow more time for feedback. Use a variety of methods, such as audiovisuals and practice sessions. Provide written instructions for home use.
ALTERED SENSORY-PERCEPTUAL STATUS	

Hearing
  Decreased ability to distinguish sounds (e.g., words beginning with S, Z, T, D, F, and G)
  Decreased conduction of sound
  Loss of ability to hear high frequency sounds
	Speak distinctly.
	Sit on side of learner's "best" ear.
	Do not shout; speak in a normal voice, but lower its pitch.
	Face the client so that lip-reading is possible.
	Use visual aids to reinforce verbal instruction.
	Reinforce teaching with easy-to-read materials.
	Decrease extraneous noise.

Vision
  Decreased visual acuity
  Decreased ability to read fine detail
  Decreased ability to discriminate among blue, violet, and green; all colors tend to fade, with red fading the least
  Thicker and more yellow lenses of eyes; with decreased accommodation
  Smaller pupils; decreased amount of light reaching retina
  Decreased depth perception
  Decreased peripheral vision
	Ensure that glasses are clean and in place.
	Use printed material with large print.
	Use high-contrast materials, such as black on white.
	Avoid the use of blue, violet, and green in type or graphics; use red instead.
	Use nonglare lighting and avoid contrasts of light (e.g., darkened room with single light).
	Adjust teaching to allow for the use of touch to gauge depth.

Touch and vibration Decreased sense of touch	Increase time for the teaching of psychomotor skills, repetitions, and return demonstrations.
Decreased sense of vibration	Teach client to palpate more prominent pulse sites (e.g., carotid and radial arteries).

Modified from Weinrich, S.P., et al. (1989). Continuing education: adapting strategies to teach the elderly. *Journal of Gerontologic Nursing, 15*(11), 17.

Barriers to Compliance

Cost The financial cost of medicines is a barrier for many clients. However, there are other costs of treatment—the costs of office visits, the cost of laboratory tests, and the costs of morbidity and mortality associated with failure to achieve therapeutic goals. Assess the client's previous experience with purchasing medications, understanding of the benefits of the drug coverage of the current health insurance plan, and the benefits (financial and health) of taking, and the consequences of not taking medications.

Lifestyle Issues Ascertain the client's compliance with previous medication regimens with open-ended questions. If the client indicates that compliance has been an issue in the past, attempt to determine the rationale. Some possible issues for discussion if the client missed or was late taking the medication follow (Kohler, Davies, & Bailey, 2004):

- Running out of medication
- Feeling good and forgetting to take the medication
- Feeling good and deciding that the medication was not needed
- Involvement in an activity and forgetting
- Planned change in normal routine
- Unexpected change in normal routine
- Feeling sick from the medication (adverse effects)
- Feeling that the medicine wasn't working
- Inconvenience of taking medication
- Confusion about what medicine to take or how to take it?

Accurately assessing the problem will assist in working with the client for better adherence. The inconvenience of changing a daily routine to incorporate medications, or the maintenance of a medication schedule while traveling, camping, or on vacation may affect compliance. Medications often require lifestyle changes, (e.g., in alcohol consumption and diet) that may be difficult to implement or maintain.

Assessment of the Medication Regimen

Evaluate the medication regimen for possible barriers to compliance by the client.

Complexity of Medication Regimen Higher numbers of medication doses per day result in discontinuation rates that are higher than regimens with fewer doses per day (Neutel & Smith, 2003; Buring, Winner, & Doering, 1999). Many prescribers are unaware of the extent of client's number of doses a day, even if they have a list of the drugs taken by the client, if the client sees several physicians. It not uncommon for an older adult to see many physicians (e.g., primary care physician, cardiologist, urologist, dermatologist, rheumatologist, and ophthalmologist) resulting in polypharmacy. Consult with the client's primary care physician to attempt to simply the medication regimen if the client is unable to do so. See the Evidence-Based Practice box above. Ask the prescriber about the appropriateness of combination drugs. They may be more expensive or not (one copay vs. two or one trade name drug vs. two generics), but if there is added expense, it may be worth the therapeutic outcome if it increases the client's compliance.

Appropriateness of the Drug Therapy Nurses serve as a safety net in determining the appropriateness of the prescribed drug therapy, and concurrent alternative and complementary and over-the-counter (OTC) medications, that the client may be taking. Liu and Christensen (2002) found that the prevalence of inappropriate prescribing remains alarmingly high, particularly in the older adult. This, despite the focus in recent years on the Institute of Medicine's (IOM) report in 2000 indicating that the death rate attributed to medical error was greater than that of vehicle acci-

 Evidence-Based Practice

Advocate for the Client to Receive the Least Complex Drug Regimen Possible

Nguyen and Achusim (2002) studied medication adherence in an immigrant population of Vietnamese Americans with the intention of discovering root factors for the nonadherence rate within the population. Using a retrospective review of the medication refill rate of all identifiable Vietnamese clients in the outpatient pharmacy information system for one year, it was determined that adherence for different age and gender populations were not significant. The mean compliance rate was 67% and included analgesics and antipyretics, gastrointestinal (GI) drugs, cardiovascular drugs, antidiabetic drugs, antiasthmatic agents, antiinfectives, estrogens, and hormonal contraceptives. Adherence rates decreased with each group of increasing age in which assimilation into the majority culture was less. However, the dominant factor in medication adherence was the total number of refillable prescriptions. The rate of adherence declined in direct relation to the increase in the number of refillable prescriptions. Although cultural differences may play a role in nonadherence, it was not a significant factor; however, further study is required to determine this factor more accurately.

dents, breast cancer, or acquired immune deficiency syndrome (AIDS) (Kohn, Corrigan, & Donaldson, 2000). Although most of the research has been done using older adult populations, these data are significant because of the growing proportion of the population that is older adult. Inappropriate medication in the older adult is not restricted to any health care setting. Golden et al. (1999) determined that 39.7% of nursing home-eligible homebound older adults were affected. Mott & Meek (2000) reported that 14.3% of older adults using a community pharmacy were affected, as were older adults participating in managed care (Fick et al., 2001) and in an academic medical center (Chin et al., 1999). Chin et al. also reported inappropriate use of drugs with older adults in the emergency department (ED)—10.6% during admission, 3.6% during ED stay, and 5.6% during ED discharge. All of these studies used Beers Criteria for inappropriate prescribing for the older adult (see Table 8-1).

Adverse Effect Profile It is evident that clients with chronic and asymptomatic diseases, such as dyslipidemia, hypertension, or asymptomatic type 2 diabetes mellitus, often have problems complying with drug regimens. Clients who do not perceive any physical harm from their disease or immediate benefit from medication may believe therapy is not necessary and may be poorly motivated with treatment (Pearson & Kopin, 2003). On the other hand, clients who are experiencing unpleasant adverse effects of their medications (e.g., nausea, fatigue, dizziness, lightheadedness, activity intolerance, impotence) are also apt to be non-compliant. Allow clients to describe their concerns and provide information to assist them to manage their adverse effects. If this is not possible, encourage them to consult with their prescriber for an alternative medication.

Nursing Diagnosis

⊛ **What are the most common nursing diagnoses involved in client education?**

Three of the most common nursing diagnoses in relation to clients and the self-administration of medications are deficient knowledge, noncompliance, and ineffective therapeutic regimen management. **Deficient knowledge** is the state in which the individual has a deficiency in cognitive knowledge or psychomotor skills regarding the condition or treatment plan; this is somewhat different from noncompliance. **Noncompliance** is the state in which an individual or group desires to comply but is prevented from doing so by factors that deter adherence to health-related advice given by health care professionals. **Ineffective therapeutic regimen management** is a pattern of regulating and integrating into daily living a program for treating illness and the sequelae of illness that is unsatisfactory for meeting specific health goals (Carpenito-Moyet, 2004). These three nursing diagnoses are not always listed for each drug as it is discussed in the text. However, *all* clients undergoing drug therapy, whether administered by the client or a health care provider, should be assessed for the nursing diagnoses of risk for deficient knowledge, noncompliance, and ineffective therapeutic regimen management. Any of these nursing diagnoses might appear in the same fashion: the client's inability to administer medications safely and accurately, a return of the client's symptoms or the occurrence of complications, or inappropriate behavior related to the therapeutic regimen. However, the etiology for each of the nursing diagnoses will be different.

Interventions to enhance compliance and effective therapeutic regimen management focus on client concerns or health beliefs (e.g., concern over possible adverse effects or the cost of the drug), and they are distinctly different than teaching for deficient knowledge. Teaching for deficient knowledge is appropriate when the assessment clearly identifies that the client does not have sufficient or accurate information about the medication regimen and that the deficiency is interfering with the client's ability to self-administer medications. The client may request information, verbalize a misconception, or state the problem (e.g., "I don't understand. . . ."). With noncompliance or ineffective therapeutic regimen management, the client may fail to keep appointments or demonstrate an inability to set or keep mutually agreed on goals. The nurse may be aware of previous appropriate health education from the clinical record or may have performed the teaching and determine that the client did not seem to integrate the content into health-related behaviors. The issue then becomes a matter of noncompliance or ineffective therapeutic regimen management rather than deficient knowledge.

When care is mutually planned by the nurse and client, noncompliance is minimized. **Compliance** is the degree to which clients take medication instructions seriously, concur with them, and follow through. This term can have an offensively controlling ring to it, implying that the prescriber directs the client, who must follow those directions. Some practitioners prefer the term *adherence*, or *effective management of the therapeutic regimen*. However, because compliance is the standard accepted term, it is used here, but "concurrence with therapy" and "adherence to instructions" are synonymous terms.

Why do clients seek medical care and then not follow through with the suggested medication plan at home? There are many reasons—some personal, some social, some psychological, some cultural. Everyone is potentially noncompliant, whether or not they intend to be. As discussed earlier, medication compliance has been estimated to vary between 33% and 94% (Billups, Malone, & Carter, 2000). Some clients never fill the prescription, most take them at unscheduled times, and many stop taking the medication early.

The consequences of not following the medication plan include inexplicable medication failures with continuing symptoms or overdoses. Medications not used may be kept and taken inappropriately later, when health status may differ from original presentation and the potency and chemical activities of the drug may have changed. When confronted with apparent medication failures, prescribers tend simply to increase the drug dosage or change medications instead of investigating for noncompliance with the therapeutic plan.

The following are examples of situations known to foster noncompliance or ineffective management of the therapeutic regimen:

- The client is chronically ill or is undergoing prolonged therapy. In chronic illness, symptoms tend to grow worse and then improve in a cyclic fashion. Clients often do not see any clear causal relationship between taking or not taking the prescribed medication and the waxing and waning of symptoms. Cheng, Kalls, and Feifer (2001) found that over the course of a study of compliance with hypertensive clients that compliance fell from 85% to 64% and drug therapy was suboptimal. It has been shown that routinely reviewing medications with clients and inquiring how they are taken at home will dramatically increase compliance, a "booster" in their education as it were (Awad, 2004). When appropriate, it should be stressed to the client that the medication will need to be taken indefinitely and should not be precipitously discontinued.
- The client is relatively asymptomatic or feels better. Reasons for needing to take all of the drug should be explained. For example, many people are not aware that organisms mutate and that antibiotic medications should be completed as prescribed to ensure their eradication in the first place.
- The medication is expensive or inconvenient to obtain. Prescriptions purchased by generic name and

further explanations of the importance of the medication (e.g., the consequences of not taking the drug) may be effective in remotivating the client.

- The medication instructions are complex and not easily understood. "Take with meals" may mean twice a day to the person who always skips breakfast or before or after meals for others. Written instructions with a picture of the drug taped to them may assist as a reminder when the client is home and has forgotten what was heard in the office or in the hospital when being discharged (Martens, 1998; McKenry, 1999).

- The medication is unwieldy to take because the bottle cap is difficult for arthritic hands or because there are complicated mixing or measuring directions. Measuring cups or droppers can be offered, and the client should be told that easy-to-remove caps can be requested when purchasing the medicine.

- The medicine tastes unpleasant or must be taken at inconvenient times (e.g., during sleep hours, at work) or too many times a day to be feasible. The medication can be mixed with or taken with various liquids that are both pleasant and compatible. After consultation with the prescriber, medication prescriptions can often be changed to higher doses given less frequently or to a sustained-action form if available and if feasible.

- The therapeutic plan contains many different medications, and the drug-taking schedule is complicated. Occasional systematic review of the medications by the prescriber and the nurse, especially in home health care, is necessary to see if the client still needs all of them and to simplify the care plan. Confrontation of the client's habits is necessary when medication containers that should be empty remain full. Written schedules with sample drugs attached are helpful. Small medication boxes with separate compartments for each dosing time are available at pharmacies. The nurse may suggest that the client keep the medication near equipment used at a specific time each day (e.g., a coffee cup or the kitchen table) or associate taking the medication with a specific routine activity (e.g., walking the dog, brushing teeth, or watching the television news).

- Many people wait more than an hour to be seen by their prescriber in the office or clinic setting. Longer waiting periods have been correlated with a distinct drop in following the prescriber's medication instructions. Often the wait is unavoidable, but the situation can be improved if the practitioner is empathic and explains the reason for the delay.

- The client does not understand or accept the illness or disorder, or the explanation of the illness or treatment plan does not fit the client's concepts of illness, health care, or health. Typical of the factors that influence attitudes toward treatment are the extent to which clients believe that (1) they are susceptible to the illness, (2) the illness is serious, and (3) they will benefit from taking action. Therefore giving information is not the entire answer. It helps to seek the active participation of the client in the health and nursing process and to show interest in and respect for client ideas, feelings, and beliefs.

- The client and health care practitioners perceive the problems or goals in divergent ways, yet do not effectively communicate this (Britten, 1996).

- The medication is seen as an artificial additive or contaminant to the body or as a crutch on which dependence should be limited.

- Adverse effects are severe or interfere with functioning in daily activities.

- The client has problems with memory or confusion or has visual or hearing impairments.

The specific nursing diagnosis selected for a particular client will depend on the nurse's astute assessment of the individual situation with the client and family.

Planning

✷ In planning for client education, how are goals established and written?

The next part of the teaching-learning process is planning, which begins once a learning need has been identified. The learning needs are discussed; planning the expected outcomes is a mutual undertaking between the nurse, the client and, where appropriate, the family. The goals of learning for the client's ability to self-medicate are expected outcomes that should result from the teaching-learning interactions. The teaching plan should be included in the written plan of care whether it is a standardized one generated as part of a protocol or is a unique one developed specifically for a client with complex learning needs. The written plan should include the topic, who initiates teaching and when, who reinforces teaching and when, educational materials given, and a comments section for documenting client-caregiver response.

In order for the teaching plan outcomes to clarify what is to be learned and how that learning will be evaluated, the outcome should contain a verb that is measurable (Box 10-3). Although the nurse would like the client to "know" about his or her medications, "understand" how the medication relates to the illness, and "comprehend" what action to take if an adverse effect occurs, these verbs are not appropriate for writing goals because they are neither easily interpreted nor measurable. Terms such as "define," "list," "identify," and "state" are measurable, have fewer interpretations, and are therefore more useful in evaluating the achievement of outcomes for learning. The following are examples of statements that include measurable verbs:

The client will:
- State the major action of digoxin.
- Identify at least three adverse effects of warfarin that should be reported to the prescriber.

BOX 10-3 EXAMPLES OF MEASURABLE AND NONMEASURABLE VERBS

MEASURABLE VERBS

describe	self-administer
discuss	exercise
identify	cough
list	sit
relate	stand
state	walk
verbalize	has an absence of
administer	
demonstrate	
perform	

NONMEASURABLE VERBS

accept	know
appreciate	think
feel	understand

How will you know that the client understands? What behaviors need to be evident for you to observe that he or she appreciates (or accepts, etc.)?

- List the signs and symptoms of hypoglycemia (e.g., tachycardia; palpitations; cool, clammy skin; diaphoresis; irritability; tiredness; hunger; numbness; and blurred vision).

Goals need to be realistic regarding the client's achievements. They can be determined only by assessing with the client his or her ability to achieve the expected outcomes.

Implementation

✳ How is client education implemented?

The most difficult steps of the teaching-learning process have been completed once a learning need has been identified and the expected outcomes have been agreed on by the client and the nurse. The implementation phase consists of conveying the specific information required by the objectives.

Instructional sessions about medications should be integrated throughout the extent of nurse-client interactions and not saved for the day of discharge from the health care agency. Short encounters staggered over the course of the client's length of stay enhance learning because it takes place in small incremental steps rather than in one overwhelming session. One of the most appropriate times to teach the client about medications is as they are being administered. This dialogue will help the client to cue in specific medications at certain times of the day and at particular intervals.

The practice of manual skills is rather straightforward, such as the manipulation of a syringe and vial to self-administer insulin. Nurses are familiar with the practices of

BOX 10-4 GUIDELINES FOR EDUCATING CLIENTS AS CONSUMERS OF DRUGS

1. Be aware that, like prescription medications, complementary/alternative medications and OTC medications are truly drugs and deserve the same care in use.
2. Identify some types of medications that are considered useful for home treatment (see Chapters 11 and 12).
3. Advise the client about safety precautions.
4. Instruct that nonprescription drugs do not usually cure a condition but instead make the symptoms bearable. Treated conditions that persist, recur, or produce unusual reactions should be evaluated by a health care provider.
5. Counsel and instruct the client, when appropriate, about alternate nursing therapies or therapies that accompany drug taking (e.g., instruct about increasing fluids, activity, and roughage to reduce a laxative habit).
6. Warn about certain drugs that can produce physical and psychological dependence (e.g., analgesics, stimulants, and laxatives).

demonstration and return demonstration, but variations exist that can conserve time. A nurse may draw up the insulin and ask the client to complete the injection, may ask the client to direct the procedure, or may coach the client through the procedure. Equipment may be left with the client to allow for practice time without the nurse's presence before a return demonstration is scheduled. Such equipment should be labeled as "practice equipment," and the client should be instructed that this material is contaminated and should not be used for the actual intervention.

The communication of ideas is more complex but just as necessary. Ideas are more easily understood if they are organized in a logical order and if they move from simple to complex. For example, it is helpful for clients to know the therapeutic effect of a drug before learning about its adverse effects. Ideas need to be practiced, too. The application of information is important for clients. Knowing what to do is more helpful than reciting the symptoms of digoxin toxicity. Clients should be asked questions such as, "What will you do if you take your pulse and the rate is below 60 beats/min?"

Providing the client with scenarios in which decisions must be made regarding lifestyle and medications is beneficial. For example, a client who takes disulfiram (Antabuse), a drug that causes vomiting when alcohol is ingested, could be asked, "Suppose you're having dinner at a friend's home and you're asked to have a drink. How will you respond?"

The client can demonstrate commitment to a medication regimen if he or she is able to state to the nurse and family how he or she intends to manage a medication that needs to be taken four times a day within a schedule that includes home, office, and business travel. Assisting the client to identify potential or actual problems with compliance is beneficial, but can be challenging. See Boxes 10-4 and 10-5.

Encourage the client to plan for medication administration and to incorporate this activity into his or her lifestyle. Writ-

Box 10-5 Captain Bob Can't Remember

On her first home care visit to Mr. Robert Stetson, Ms. Staysa, the community health nurse, found a frail 86-year-old man who suffered from hypertension, heart failure, type 2 diabetes, prostate cancer, and anemia. "Captain Bob" (as he preferred to be called), a former charter boat captain, had lost his wife last year and was trying unsuccessfully to self-manage his care at home. His chronic conditions could never be controlled without proper treatment, but he seemed too confused to remember to take his medications. He had difficulty even remembering the time of day. After every nap, he thought it was a new morning and took his morning medications again, if he could find them. He frequently misplaced his medication bottles, substituted OTC medications for prescribed ones, forgot his doctor's instructions, and missed his medical appointments.

Captain Bob required skilled nursing care, but he had already been discharged by one home health agency because of noncompliance. He was, however, determined to stay in his own home with his wife's memories and refused to go to a nursing facility. It was essential that he remember to take his medication or he could never hope to function safely on his own.

Ms. Staysa had been able to assist other clients to remember to take their medications by identifying the medications (Figure 1), color-coding the bottles (Figure 2), or placing the medications in envelopes (Figure 3). That didn't work for Captain Bob because he would put the envelopes or bottles away and forget where they were! Ms. Staysa then bought a partitioned box of transparent plastic. She put each medication in a compartment and labeled the compartment with the day and time the medication should be taken (Figure 4). The system seemed clear enough, but Captain Bob would have difficulty opening the little compartments with his big, rough hands;

would overturn the box, dumping out the contents; or would put the box in a drawer and then forget where he put it.

Ms. Staysa thought perhaps he would do better if each dose of medication was in a separate container. She then gave Captain Bob simple instructions: Read the writing on the envelope, count the number of pills, and take the medicine (Figure 5). This worked better than the previous attempt, but Captain Bob sometimes lost the envelopes or forgot which ones he had already used. Finally Ms. Staysa switched to plastic sandwich bags. She prepared several days' dosages and marked the day and the time that they should be used. She hung the bags from clothespins on a board near the chair that Captain Bob used all day. That way, he could see which bags were empty and which were full. Because the bags were so close to his chair, he had little chance of misplacing them. At last! It seemed they had found a system that worked (see Figures 6 and 7).

Despite his increasing compliance, Captain Bob required close monitoring. Ms. Staysa phoned the captain several days in a row to remind him to take his medicine. Before long, Captain Bob was beginning to anticipate Ms. Staysa's calls—a sign his memory was improving.

Over the course of their interaction, Ms. Staysa involved other community groups to call Captain Bob, a relative to fill the medication bags, and Meals-on-Wheels to provide support and increase his social interactions. Ten months after Captain Bob met Ms. Staysa, his condition had stabilized so that he no longer required skilled nursing visits, needed fewer clinic visits, and needed fewer changes in medication. Although at times he still forgets, is increasingly frail, and still experiences discomfort, Captain Bob has increased his coping skills and continues to live at home.

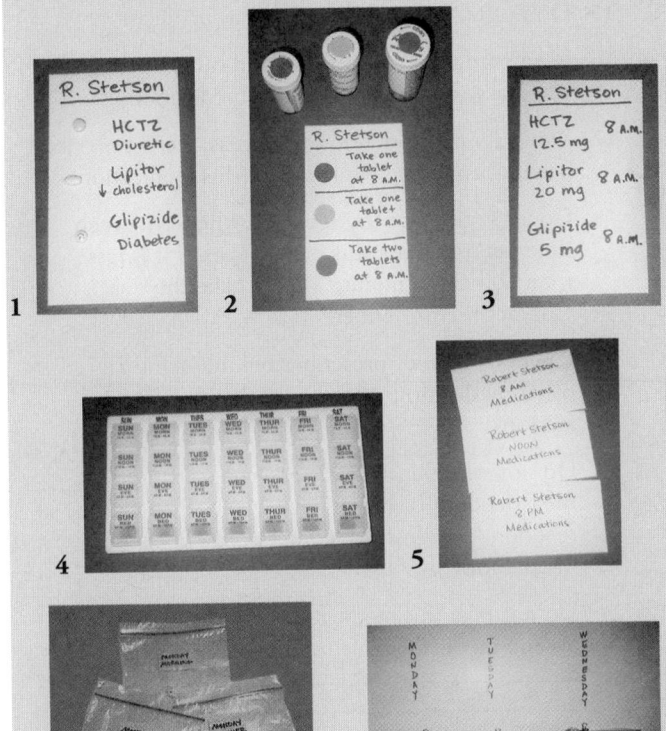

Figure 1. A card with color photographs of pills helps the client identify the medications and gives the reason for taking them. Review the chart frequently with the client and caregivers.

Figure 2. Colored dots on pill containers match the dots on the chart that gives the name of each medicine and informs the client when it is supposed to be taken. Dots can be made with stickers, marking pens, or nail polish.

Figure 3. Individual envelopes with medications and their dosages to be taken at the same time of day are prepared ahead of time.

Figure 4. Partitioned boxes can assist a client to organize medications and take them on time. Pills are placed in different compartments that are labeled according to day of the week and time to be taken.

Figure 5. Medication envelopes can be prepared and labeled in advance for the day and time to be taken.

Figure 6. Plastic see-through storage bags may also be used and labeled in large letters. This makes it easy for the client to see the medication and remember to take it.

Figure 7. A hanging board keeps medication bags within easy reach. All of the day's envelopes are placed in a plastic bag and clipped to the board.

Modified from Smith, J.B. (1986). The patient who can't remember to take her meds. *RN, 49*(9), 38-41.

ten instructions are particularly helpful for the client to refer to once discharged from the health care setting (Figure 10-1). Medication schedules have proven to be particularly helpful in assisting clients with adherence to a medication regimen. A medication calendar may be made by obtaining a calendar with space enough to write in the names of the drugs and the times of the day they should be taken. The medications can be checked off on the calendar as they are taken, and the client will have a home medication record. This method is particularly helpful with clients who are concerned that they may forget or for those clients trying to establish a routine for taking their medications. Having an alarm clock next to the calendar so that it may be reset for the next dose helps to decrease the anxiety related to forgetting a dose. Give the client written information about the medication, including its name, its purpose, its appearance, directions for taking it, the time to take it, what action to take if a dose is missed, and any special precautions related to the drug. The adverse effects should also be written, along with the symptoms that should be reported and to whom they should be reported. In addition to providing information regarding the client's specific medication regimen, the nurse should take the opportunity to educate the client as a consumer of drugs (see Box 10-4).

Develop a repertoire of approaches and materials to be used for client teaching. Relying solely on the client's hearing is not encouraging an optimal learning experience. Include as many of the client's senses in the learning experience as possible. For example, in teaching about medications while administering them, allow the client to hear the reason the drug is indicated for the condition. The pill can also be seen and felt by the client and tasted while taken. During recent years the amount of health teaching materials and the variety of media have proliferated. Audiovisual and other materials such as pamphlets, videotapes, CDs, and DVDs can show the client settings and situations that are beyond the ability of the nurse to present at the bedside, in the clinic, or in the home setting. Computer-generated instructions as part of a standard teaching plan and computer-assisted instructions for some clients have demonstrated success.

Use these supplements to enhance the teaching process. With increasingly short lengths of stay in hospitals or brief encounters in the office, clinic, or home, these adjuncts become more important to include in the nurse's scope of teaching techniques. Select materials according to the appropriateness of content, accuracy, simplicity, and appeal for the client. However, they should never replace individualized in-

MEDICATION CAUTIONS

1. Avoid alcoholic beverages while taking this medication.

2. Swallow these tablets. Do not chew them. Do not take if coating is cracked.

3. Do not drive a car or operate machinery if this medication makes you drowsy. If you have to drive home, wait until you get home to take your first dose.

4. Do not allow this medication to contact the skin, eyes, or clothing.

5. Take this medication on an empty stomach either 1 hour before meals or 2 hours after meals. You may drink water.

6. Do not take this medication with fruit juice.

7. Take this medication _____ hour(s) before meals.

8. Limit caffeine use.

9. Do not take this medication with milk or milk products. You may drink water or juice.

10. Take this medication with at least 8 ounces of water.

11. Take this medication with food to avoid upset stomach.

12. This medication may discolor the urine or stools.

13. Do not take this medication with antacids.

14. Do not take aspirin with this medication.

15. Do not take mineral oil with this medication.

16. Take orange juice, bananas, and other foods high in potassium while taking this medication.

17. Avoid tyramine-rich foods such as cheese, pickled herring, and wine while taking this medication.

18. Count your pulse (by feeling at the wrist) each time before taking this medication. If it is less than 60 beats a minute, do not take the dose. Contact the prescriber.

19. Check with your prescriber before taking any other medications (even over-the-counter medications).

20. Do not take this medication if pregnant or breastfeeding or if you have ever had an allergic reaction to it. Instead, contact prescriber for instructions.

21. Do not take this medication if you have the following medical problems or symptoms:
_____
_____
_____

FIGURE 10-1 Example of a general medication self-instruction sheet for the client, which may be individualized by indicating specific instructions appropriate to the client's therapeutic regimen.

struction, because the client may overlook needed information or be overwhelmed by a comprehensive audiovisual presentation. These various media techniques should facilitate the nurse's role as a teacher rather than act as substitutes.

Bille (1981) recommends the process of **therapeutic seeding** as a teaching approach when clients are unable to express learning needs or concerns. This technique involves mentioning ideas to clients, allowing time to pass so the client has a chance to think about the idea, and then reintroducing the idea. On the second opportunity the client may more easily identify the concept and see it as a learning need. For example, an older female client who has received a prescription for conjugated estrogens may not identify any drug-related learning needs at that time. On the next visit, the nurse may use therapeutic seeding with a statement such as, "Ms. Ackerman, many women who take this medication have expressed concerns about its adverse effects. What concerns do you have about the medication?" If the client states, "I'm not concerned about that," she may be saying, "I'm not ready to hear that information yet." Referring to the comment on the next visit may prepare the way for discussing possible adverse effects and what symptoms to report to the prescriber. Therapeutic seeding allows the client more of an opportunity to negotiate the teaching-learning program.

Practical information about prescription drugs is available to consumers from the American Medical Association, package inserts produced by the pharmaceutical houses, some health care providers, the *USP DI (USP DI, 2005)*, or computerized information sheets from the pharmacy. Most printed information includes the drug's purpose, possible adverse effects, and the best way to take the drug. More than 1000 common drugs are listed annually in the *USP DI*, which is geared partly to those who dispense or administer prescriptions and partly to those who take them. *USP DI* offers jargon-free guidelines for safe and informed self-administration of prescription drugs by generic name. The *USP DI* information is available to consumers from their health practitioners or pharmacists, who can reproduce for distribution a limited number of pages from the *Advice* section.

The client and family need to be active members of the team, especially because much of the convalescent care is shifting from hospital to home. Encourage them to participate whenever and wherever possible in all aspects of the client's care. Family members may be responsible for changing dressings, taking care of drains and intravenous (IV) lines, running complex equipment, and administering parenteral medications. The client's family may be of great support not only in providing assistance but also in easing the transition to home.

Identify which family members are supportive and can assume the ongoing responsibility for care, including the administration of medications. In a crisis, family members tend to gather around the client but may normally live at some distance or return to a daily work schedule when the client is ready to return home. Ensure that the appropriate family members are taught to provide the ongoing care. If the family will not be in attendance at home, it may be more appropriate to provide information to the client's friends, neighbors, or paid care providers regarding the medications.

Although there may be many opportunities to teach family members, the nurse may need to schedule an appointment with them to ensure that they are present to learn the medication regimen and other discharge instructions. The assistance of family members needs to be actively sought and encouraged; some may be hesitant because they are unsure of the part they are to play in the client's care.

Successful teaching programs with clients and families include the following:
- Positive reinforcement or praise for desired behaviors.
- Feedback about progress toward goals.
- Individualization, whereby learning needs are determined for the specific client and the pace of teaching is mutually negotiated.
- Facilitation, in which the nurse assists the client to take action, such as making personalized medication schedules.
- Relevance, making sure that the content and teaching-learning methods are meaningful for the client. Attempt to incorporate these issues into each of the teaching sessions.

There is no single best way to educate clients about self-administering medications (Peterson, Takiya, & Finley, 2003). Using the same approach each time does not take into account the data gathered from the client in the assessment phase of the teaching-learning process. Assessing each individual's learning needs to develop the best teaching approach is the most effective use of nursing resources (Pumilia, 2002). Given the seriousness of client's compliance to medication regimens, additional efforts need to be directed toward developing and testing innovative approaches to assist clients in following treatment prescriptions.

Evaluation

✷ How is client education evaluated?

The Process of Evaluation

Evaluating whether client education has taken place is essential. Some nurses may consider the teaching process complete after handing out a brochure or showing a video. However, the emphasis should be on the client's response—behavioral changes, knowledge, and skills gained as a result of the method and content of the teaching-learning process. The evaluation process should involve assessing the client's progress toward specific goals for self-administration of medication, and the response to the teaching-learning process.

✷ How is the evaluation of client education documented?

Documentation is the final step in the process of client teaching for the self-administration of medications. Unfortunately, JCAHO has found the lack of documentation of the client's and family's knowledge of self-care to be one of the most common nursing deficiencies cited during accreditation audits. Documentation related to education about medications should contain at least three items: the specific content, the method of teaching, and the evaluation of learning.

Although the nursing care plan contains the specific learning goals agreed on by the nursing team and the client, the narrative documentation following the teaching-learning process should indicate the specific content that was covered. This information needs to be recorded in such a way that any other nurse will know enough about what was taught to be able to continue the teaching from that point. The following are appropriate examples: "The need for taking a pulse before a digoxin dose was discussed," "The client was cautioned not to take antacids with the tetracycline," or "The adverse effect of furosemide, hypokalemia and its symptoms, were discussed." A common error of documentation is the statement "Medications taught," particularly in a setting in which the client may have a polydrug regimen, such as in home health care. The following questions are raised: What medications? What about them? What dosing schedule? What adverse effects? What special precautions? Such vague documentation does not support the provision of skilled nursing care and in the home health care setting may provide justification for nonreimbursement for nursing care. Because clients are transitioned from one health care setting to another more often in today's health care environment, documentation becomes even more important. Such data allows the nurse within the client's next health care setting to provide continuity of instruction without repeating previous information or omitting essential learning.

Documenting the method of instruction allows the next nurse to know which teaching techniques were successful for the client's learning. Although "taught" is the most common verb used, it does not explain what or how the material was covered. More appropriate words are "discussed," "demonstrated," or "(a specific piece of literature) was reviewed and given to the client." Documentation may also include the client's characteristics as a learner and any barriers to learning that may have been determined. Recording the "teaching" part of the teaching-learning process leads then to the most important part—recording the "learning" of that process.

Many health care agencies that use a clinical pathway approach to the provision of care and its documentation have also developed teaching pathways to provide a comprehensive approach to client education for specific disease or procedure populations. These teaching pathways serve as a guide to teaching and identifying learning objectives along a designated time line, and they provide consistent documentation (Sciartelli, 1995).

Recording an evaluation of the client's and/or family's learning indicates the achievement of, or progress toward, the learning goals originally established by the client and the nurse. The evaluation documentation includes a description of what occurred, the client's response to the teaching-learning encounter (using his or her own words and behaviors), and the observable or measurable activities of the client and family that would indicate that the instructions were understood. Documentation, as the final step of the teaching-learning process, is essential in recording the client's progress.

Summary

Medications tend to be more effective when clients believe in the drugs and in their capacity to get well. Their past and present conditioning to drugs, illness, hospitals, nurses, and other health care personnel, and their own health beliefs and practices, influence their response to drug therapy. An accurate assessment of these factors is most important to plan and implement an effective client education component for the care plan.

The three most common nursing diagnoses related to the self-administration of medications for which the client is at risk are deficient knowledge, ineffective therapeutic regimen management, and noncompliance. These problems need to be resolved so that the client may accurately and safely self-administer medications.

From the onset of drug therapy, the client should be advised of the purpose of the medication and any possible adverse effects. All information should be presented in a non-threatening and straightforward manner. It is important to listen to what the client has to say about the medication, the feelings associated with the drug and whether these feelings are based on fear or anxiety, and the perception of the condition for which the drug has been prescribed.

Client education plays an important role when the individual needs to follow a prescribed medication plan after discharge. Routinely reviewing medications with clients and inquiring about how medications are taken at home have been shown to increase compliance with a medication plan.

The nurse should make sure that the client thoroughly understands the medication instructions. Written schedules and instructions will remind clients when they are at home and may have forgotten what they heard in the office or on discharge from the hospital.

Documentation of the teaching-learning process for self-administration of medications needs to include content, method, and the client's and the family's progress in relation to the planned objectives for learning.

⊛ **Critical Thinking Questions**

- What type of strategies would you use to determine the educational needs of a client who will eventually self-administer medications at home?

- If your contact time with a client is limited (e.g., an ED setting), what are the most essential elements to get across to the client?

- How would you differentiate between the nursing diagnoses of deficient knowledge and ineffective therapeutic regimen management if you ascertained that the client was not taking his or her medications as prescribed?

- How would you assess the learning needs of and develop a teaching plan for an older adult? A client with a language barrier?

Bibliography

Awad, A.G. (2004). Antipsychotic medications: Compliance and attitudes towards treatment. *Current Opinion in Psychiatry, 17*(2), 75-80.

Babcock, D.E., & Miller, M.A. (1994). *Client education: Theory & practice.* St. Louis: Mosby.

Bellg, A.J., & Rosenson, R.S. (2004). Compliance with lipid altering medications and recommended lifestyle changes, *UpToDate, 12*(3). Bille, D.A. (Ed.) (1981). *Practical approaches to patient* teaching. Boston: Little, Brown & Co.

Bille, D.A. (Ed.) (1981). *Practical approaches to patient teaching.* Boston: Little, Brown.

Billups, S.J., Malone, D.C., & Carter, B.L. (2000). Relationship between drug therapy noncompliance and patient characteristics, health-related quality of life, and health care costs. *Pharmacotherapy, 20*(8), 941-949.

Britten, D.M. (1996). Lay views of drugs and medicine: Orthodox and unorthodox accounts. In S.J. Williams & M. Calnam (Eds.), *Modern* medicine: Lay perspectives and experience. London: U.C.L. Press.

Buring, S.M., Winner, L.H., & Doering, P.L. (1999). Discontinuation rates of Helicobacter pylori treatment regimens: A meta-analysis. *Pharmacotherapy, 19*(3), 324-332.

Carpenito-Moyet, L.J. (2004). *Nursing diagnosis: Application to clinical practice* (10th ed.). Philadelphia: Lippincott, Williams & Wilkins.

Cheng, J.W.M., Kalls, M.M., & Feifer, S. (2001). Patient-reported adherence to guidelines of the Sixth Joint National Committee on Prevention, Detection, Evaluation, and Treatment of High Blood Pressure. *Pharmacotherapy, 21*(7), 828-841.

Chin, M.H., Wang, L.C., Jin, L., Mulliken, R., Walter, J., Hayley, D.C., et al. (1999). Appropriateness of medication selection for older persons in an urban academic emergency department. *Academic Emergency Medicine, 6*, 1232-1241.

Craig, C. (1995). Teaching food-drug interactions. *Journal of Psychosocial Nursing, 33*(2), 44-46.

Czar, M.L., & Engler, M.M. (1997). Perceived learning needs of patients with coronary artery disease using a questionnaire assessment tool. *Heart Lung, 26*(2), 109-117.

De Klerk E., Van Der Heijde, D., Van Der Tempel, H., Urquhart, J. & Van Der Linden, S. (2003). Patient compliance in rheumatoid arthritis, polymyalgia, and gout, *Journal of Rheumatology 30:*44-54.

DiMattero, M.A., Lepper, H.S., & Croghan, T.W. (2000). Depression is a risk factor for noncompliance with medication treatments: Meta-analysis of the effects of anxiety and depression in patient adherence. *Archives of Internal Medicine, 160,* 14, 2101-2107.

Dolder, C., Lacro, J., & Jeste, D. (2003). Adherence to antipsychotic and nonpsychiatric medications in middle-aged and older patients with psychotic disorders. *Psychosomatic Medicine, 65,* 156-162.

Donovan, J. (1995). Patient decision making: The missing ingredient in compliance research. *International Journal of Technology Assessment in Health Care, 11,* 443-455.

Esposito, L. (1995). The effects of medication education on adherence to medication regimens in an elderly population. *Journal of Advanced Nursing, 21,* 935-943.

Evangelista, L.S., & Dracup, K. (2000). A closer look at compliance research in heart failure patients in the last decade. *Progress in Cardiovascular Nursing, 15*(3), 97-103.

Fick, D.M., Waller, J.L., Maclean, J.R., Rodriguez, N.A., Short, L., Heuvel, R.V., et al. (2001). Potentially inappropriate medication use in a Medicare managed care population: association with higher costs and utilization. *Journal of Managed Care Pharmacy, 7,* 407-13.

Frasure-Smith, N., Lesperance, F., Gravel, G., Masson, A., Juneau, M., Talagic, M., et al. (2000). Social support, depression, and mortality during the first year after myocardial infarction, *Circulation, 101*(16), 1919-1924.

Gazmararian, J.A., Baker, D.W., Williams, M.V. Parker, R.M., Scott, T.L., Green, D.C., et al. (1999). Health literacy among Medicare enrollees in a managed care organization. *Journal of the American Medical Association, 281,* 545-551.

Glassman, A.H., O'Connor, C.M., Califf, R.M., Swedberg, K., Schwartz, P., Bigger, J.T., Jr., et al. (2002). Sertraline treatment of major depression in patients with acute myocardial infarction or unstable angina. *Journal of the American Medical Association, 288*(6), 701-709.

Golden, A.G., Preston, R.A., Barnett, S.D., Horente, M., Hamden, K., & Silverman, M.A. (1999). Inappropriate prescribing in homebound older adults. *Journal of American Geriatrics, 47,* 948-953.

Gottlieb, H. (2000). Medical nonadherence: Finding solutions to a costly medical problem. *Drug Benefit Trends, 12*(6), 57-62.

Hanlon, J.T., Shimp, L.A., & Semia, T.P. (2000). Recent advances in geriatrics: drug-related problems in the elderly. *Annals of Pharmacotherapy, 34,* 360-364.

Institute of Medicine. (2004). Health literacy: A prescription to end confusion. The National Academics Press. Retrieved July 26, 2005, from http://nap.edu/books/0309091179/html.

Jacobs, J.P., & Mutha, S. (2004). Legal and regulatory obligations to provide culturally and linguistically appropriate ED services. *Clinical Pediatric Emergency Medicine, 5*(2), 85-92.

Johnson, K.B., Butta, J.K., Donohue, P.K., Glenn, D.J., & Holtzman, N.A. (1996). Discharging patients with prescriptions instead of medications: Sequelae in a teaching hospital. *Pediatrics, 97*(4), 481-485.

Kaplan, N.M. (2004). Patient compliance and the treatment of hypertension, *UpToDate* 12(3).

e-LEARNING SUPPLEMENTS

Student CD-ROM
- Final Exam questions
- NCLEX® Examination review questions
- Pharmacology animations
- Printable chapter summary

Evolve Website (http://evolve.elsevier.com/mckenry)
- Content updates, including information on new drugs
- WebLinks corresponding to this chapter

- Answers to the critical thinking questions in this chapter
- *Elsevier ePharmacology Update* newsletter
- Mosby's Drug Consult Internet Edition
- Supplemental and reference information

Kohler, C.L., Davies, S.L., & Bailey, W. (2004). Enhancing patient adherence to asthma therapy, *UpToDate 12*(3).

Kohn, L.T., Corrigan, J.M., & Donaldson, M.S. (Eds.). (2000). *To err is human: Building a safer heath system.* Washington, DC: National Academy Press.

Kohn, L.T., Corrigan, J.M., & Donaldson, M.S. (Eds.). (2000). *To err is human: Building a safer health system.* Washington, D.C., Academy Press.

Lile, J.L., & Hoffman, R. (1991). Medication-taking by the frail elderly in two ethnic groups. *Nursing Forum, 26*(4), 19-24.

Liu, G.G., & Christensen, D.B. (2002). The continuing challenge of inappropriate prescribing in the elderly: An update of the evidence. *American Journal of the Pharmacists Association, 42*(6), 847-857.

Macintyre, C.R., Goebel, K., & Brown, G.V. (2005). Patient knows best: Blinded assessment of nonadherence with antituberculous therapy by physicians, nurses, and patient compared with urine drug levels. *Preventive Medicine, 40*(1), 41-45.

Martens, K.H. (1998). An ethnographic study of the process of medication discharge education (MDE). *Journal of Advanced Nursing, 27*(2), 341-348.

McKenry, L.M. (1999). *Mosby's patient guide to medications.* St. Louis: Mosby.

McMurray, S.D., Johnson, G., Davis, S., & McDougall, K. (2002). Diabetes education and care management significantly improved patient outcomes in the dialysis unit. *American Journal of Kidney Diseases, 40*(3), 566-575.

Mott, D.A., & Meek, P.D. (2000) Evaluating prescriptions in the elderly: drug/age criteria as a tool to help community pharmacists. *Journal of the American Pharmacists Association, 40,* 166-76.

Neutel, J.M., & Smith, D.H.G. (2003). Improving patient compliance: A major goal in the management of hypertension. *Journal of Clinical Hypertension, 5*(2), 127-132.

Nguyen, N., & Achusim, L.E. (2002). Medication adherence in an immigrant population: Vietnamese Americans. *Drug Benefit Trends, 14*(4), 34-35, 39-48.

Pearson, T., & Kopin, L. (2003). Bridging the gap: Improving compliance with lipid-modifying agents and therapeutic lifestyle changes. *Preventive Cardiology, 6*(4), 204-213.

Penkower, L., Dew, M.A., Ellis, D., Sekeika, S.M., Kitutu, J.M., & Shapiro, R. (2003). Psychological distress and adherence in the medical regimen among adolescent renal transplant recipients. *American Journal of Transplantation, 3*(11), 1418-1425.

Peterson, A., Takiya, L., & Finley, R. (2003). Meta-Analysis of interventions to improve drug adherence in patients with lipidemia. *Pharmacotherapy, 23*(1), 80-87.

Peterson, T., & Kopin, L. (2003). Bridging the treatment gap: Improving compliance with lipid-modifying agents and therapeutic lifestyle changes. *Preventive Cardiology, 6*(4), 204-213.

Petitta, A., Hart, S.M., & Bailey, E.M. (1999). Economic evaluation of three methods of treating urogenital chlamydial infections in the Emergency Department. *Pharmacotherapy, 19*(5), 648-654.

Petrie, K.J., Weinman, J., Sharpe, N., & Buckley, J. (1996). Role of patient's view of their illness in predicting return to work and functioning after myocardial infarction: Longitudinal study. *British Medical Journal, 312*(7040), 1191-1194.

Pumilia, C.V. (2002). Psychological impact of the physician-patient relationship on compliance: A case study and clinical strategies. *Progress in Transplantation, 12*(1), 10-16.

Putsch, R.W., & Kaufert, J.M. (1997). Communication through interpreters in health care: ethical dilemmas arising from differences in class, culture, language and power. *Journal of Clinical Ethics, 8*(1), 88-93.

Redman, B.K. (1997). *The practice of patient education.* (8th ed.). St. Louis: Mosby.

Reichman, L.B., & Lardizabal, A.A. (2004). Adherence to tuberculosis treatment, *UpToDate 12*(3).

Rubin, R.R. (2005). Adherence to pharmacologic therapy in patients with type 2 diabetes mellitus. *American Journal of Medicine, 118*(5), 27S-34S.

Sciartelli, C.H. (1995). Using a clinical pathway approach to document patient teaching for breast cancer surgical procedures. *Oncology Nursing Forum, 22*(1), 131-137.

Scott, J., & Pope, M. (2002). Nonadherence with mood stabilizers: Prevalence and predictors. *The Journal of Clinical Psychiatry, 63*(5), 384-390.

Sherry, D.C., Simmons, B., Wung, S.F., & Zerwic, J.J. (2003). Noncompliance in heart transplantation: A role for the advanced practice nurse. *Progress in cardiovascular Nursing, 18*(3), 141-146.

Stretcher, V.J., & Rosenstock, I.M. (1997). The Health Belief Model: explaining health behavior through expectancies. In K. Glanz, K., B.K. Rimer, & F.M. Lewis (eds.), *Health Behavior and Health Education: Theory, Research and Practice.* San Francisco: Jossey-Bass.

Tripp-Reimer, T. & Afifi, L.A. (1989). Cross-cultural perspectives on patient teaching. *Nursing Clinics of North America, 24*(3), 613-619.

USP DI: Advice for the patient (25th ed.). (2005). Greenwood Village, CO: MICROMEDEX Thomson Healthcare.

U.S. Census Bureau. (2000). DP.2: Profile of selected social characteristics: 2000. Retrieved May 1, 2005, from http://factfinder.census.gov/bf/lang=envtname=DEC2000SF3UDP2geoid+01000US.htm

Vasquez, E.M., Tanzi, M., Benedetti, E. & Pollak, R. (2003). Medication noncompliance after kidney transplantation, *American Journal of Health-System Pharmacist, 60*(3), 266-269.

Williams, M.V. (2002). Recognizing and overcoming inadequate health literacy, a barrier to care. *Cleveland Clinic Journal of Medicine, 69*(5), 415-418.

OVER-THE-COUNTER MEDICATIONS

CHAPTER FOCUS

Over-the-counter (OTC), or nonprescription, drugs are medications that can safely be used to self-treat minor illnesses without the supervision of a licensed health care practitioner, provided that consumers follow directions on the package. Because OTC drugs are widely available and commonly used by clients, nurses need to assess their use as part of every drug history. Nurses' knowledge of nonprescription drugs should be as thorough as that of prescription drugs so they can provide client education regarding potential drug-drug interactions, expected outcomes of their use, and other issues related to OTC drugs. This chapter reviews the regulatory difference between a prescription and an OTC drug and discusses the process involved in changing a drug from prescription to OTC status. General considerations on drug marketing, consumer education for the safe administration of OTC drugs, and selected major OTC drug categories are also discussed.

LEARNING OBJECTIVES	• Compare and contrast the strength, dosing, and other recommendations for prescription and OTC (nonprescription) drugs.
	• Discuss issues related to drug marketing, safety, selection, storage, and administration of OTC medications by the client.
	• Describe how to advise the client on the safe self-administration of selected OTC preparations (e.g., analgesics, antacids, laxatives, cough-cold preparations) as they become available.

▲ KEY TERMS

analgesic, p. 206
antacid, p. 207
antihistamines, p. 212
constipation, p. 208
diarrhea, p. 210
dysmenorrhea, p. 214

laxative, p. 208
perceived constipation, p. 208
premenstrual syndrome (PMS), p. 215

★☞ KEY DRUGS

acetaminophen (Monograph in Chapter 14, p. 274)
aspirin (Monograph in Chapter 14, p. 268)
ibuprofen (Monograph in Chapter 14, p. 269)

✷ What is the role of over-the-counter (OTC) medications?

The general public commonly uses over-the-counter (OTC), or nonprescription, medications to self-treat minor illnesses. Such preparations are readily available in pharmacies, supermarkets, and other nonpharmacy outlets for those who want to avoid the time and expense associated with going to a prescriber. It is reported that Americans visit their physicians for only 10% of their illnesses and injuries, and that 6 out of every 10 medications purchased are OTC medications. The Food and Drug Administration (FDA) indicates that 60% to 95% of all illnesses are initially treated with self-care, including self-treatment with OTC drugs. Glover (2004) reported that 96.5% of rural women in their study self-medicated with OTCs. OTC drugs have a tremendous market; it has been estimated that more than 100,000 such products are available in the United States in various dosages and strengths (Hesselgrave, 1997). These products contain between 700 and 1000 active ingredients.

When used wisely, OTC medications save time and money for the individual and, ultimately, help to reduce overall health care costs. A good example of these cost savings is the use of second generation antihistamines (e.g., loratadine [Claritin]) used for allergies. When they became available as OTC preparations, there was an estimated annual savings to Americans of 4 billion dollars when compared with the medical model of physician visits, prescriptions, and other related costs (Sullivan & Nichol, 2004).

✳ Are there risks associated with the use of OTC medications?

Although OTC medications are generally considered to be safe and effective for consumer use, problems can result. Self-medication requires a self-diagnosis of the signs and symptoms of a clinical condition. In general, the public may consider most illnesses to be minor. However, if a potentially serious condition is self-treated with an OTC medication, the condition may be masked, and professional help for appropriate treatment is delayed. Additionally, OTC drugs may contain potent chemicals, many of which used to be prescription drugs. The trend in the 1990s was to transfer more and more prescription medications to OTC status (Snyder, 1997). The health care professional should be aware that many OTC products (new and old) are capable of producing both desired and undesirable effects, drug interactions, and drug toxicity. This potential problem has been recognized by a current pharmacy law (Omnibus Budget Reconciliation Act, [OBRA]), which mandates that OTC drugs be considered an important part of the client's medical record.

Although the FDA issued regulations that require OTC package labeling to be stated in terms understandable to the average consumer, many consumers believe the labels are confusing; often the print is too small to read. Approximately 35% of Americans read at a 6th to 10th grade level, and an estimated 20% are considered functionally illiterate, reading below a fifth-grade level (Tuijnan, 2000). There is no statistically significant difference in the Canadian findings. Therefore OTC labeling that is difficult to understand and apply may result in unsafe or improper medication use.

In response, the FDA has developed a new, standardized label that OTC manufacturers were required to begin using in 2002, however, there are still significant difficulties with the OTC labeling.

Before simplifying the OTC label, the FDA conducted extensive research on how consumers use OTC drug labels. The readability of OTC drug labels, especially for older Americans, who purchase almost 30% of the nonprescription drugs sold in the United States, is problematic. The FDA also found that consumers thought words like "indications," "precautions," and "contraindications" were too technical and confusing.

Previously, information about product directions, warnings, and approved uses has appeared in different places on the label depending on the OTC product and brand. Finding information about inactive ingredients has also been a challenge for those who may be allergic to an ingredient in a drug product.

Patterned after the Nutrition Facts food label, the new Drug Facts label uses simple language and an easy-to-read format to help people compare and select OTC medicines and follow dosage instructions (Figure 11-1). The following information must appear in this order:

* The product's active ingredients, including the amount in each dosage unit.
* The purpose of the medication.
* The uses (indications) for the drug.
* Specific warnings, including when the product should not be used under any circumstances, and when it is appropriate to consult with a doctor or pharmacist. The warnings section also describes adverse effects that could occur and substances or activities to avoid.
* Dosage instructions addressing when, how, and how often to take the medication.
* The product's inactive ingredients, which is important information for those with specific allergies.

Along with the standardized format, the new drug label uses plain-speaking terms to describe the facts about each OTC drug. For example, "uses" replaces "indications," while other technical words like "precautions" and "contraindica-

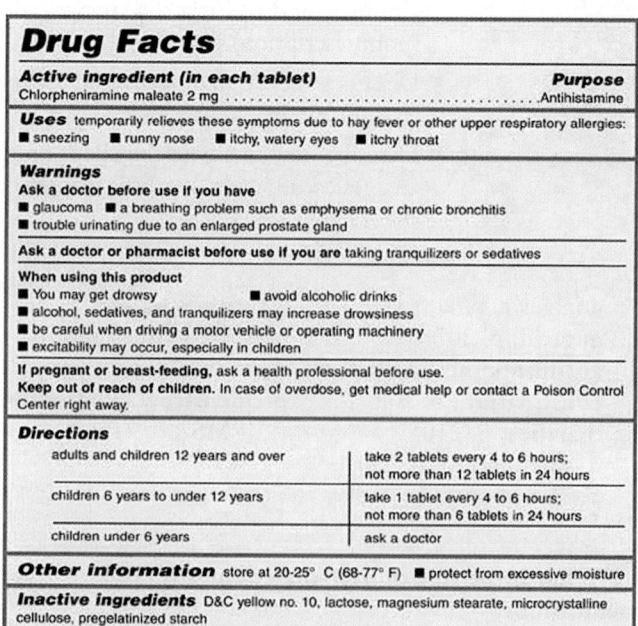

FIGURE 11-1 Sample of new OTC labeling required by the FDA.

tions" have been eliminated. The new label also requires a type size large enough to be easily read and specific layout details—bullets, spacing between lines and clearly marked sections—to improve readability.

✱ How does a drug achieve OTC status?

The FDA regulates and makes decisions about the safety and effectiveness of a drug, its classification as prescription or OTC, and the information printed on the drug labels. Drug substances are subjected to regulation, review, and various study requirements before being released with FDA approval and may be monitored afterward to a limited extent. Medications not considered safe enough for the general public to use without medical supervision are restricted to prescription status only. OTC drugs are defined as safe and effective drugs for self-treatment by the public, assuming that the manufacturer follows good manufacturing practices and consumers follow directions on the label.

At one time many OTC drugs were being marketed without the more current standards of proof of documented safety and effectiveness. In 1972, the FDA established a number of OTC expert advisory panels to review drug categories and make recommendations to the FDA. As a result of this review, many ingredients used in OTC products were removed from the market, including aphrodisiacs, hair growers, hexachlorophene products, and others. These drugs were found to be either ineffective, dangerous, or both. In 1991, the FDA established an OTC Drugs Advisory Committee to assist in review and evaluation and to advise the FDA Commissioner on its findings and recommendations. The Committee may also suggest that prescription drugs be changed to OTC status based on expert findings that the medication is safe and effective for general public use.

The definitions for OTC drug safety and effectiveness include the following:

- *Safety:* The drug product has a low incidence of severe adverse effects and a low potential for harm, assuming that proper instructions and adequate warnings are given on the label.
- *Effectiveness:* When properly used, the drug ingredient will provide relief of the minor symptom or illness in a significant portion of the population.

✱ Can a prescription drug eventually achieve OTC status?

Over the years the FDA has approved nearly 600 prescription drugs for OTC availability. Approximately one third of all new OTC drugs released between 1975 and 1994 were previously prescription medications (Jacobs, 1998). With some products a lower strength of the active ingredient was required in the OTC product, although others retained the same strength as the prescription drug when released in OTC form. Ibuprofen (Motrin IB) was released in a 200-mg strength as an OTC drug; the higher dose tablet strengths, 400- or 800-mg, still require a prescription. The lower strength of ibuprofen is considered to be safe and effective for the self-treatment of a minor illness if the label

instructions are followed. Use of higher strength ibuprofen requires medical supervision and a prescription because it could cause serious adverse effects. Table 11-1 provides examples of prescription drugs that have been reclassified as OTC drugs.

✱ How do regulations for OTC drugs differ from prescription drugs?

In contrast to prescription drugs, OTC medications may be marketed without FDA approval. Monographs of information developed by the OTC drug review identified specific drugs "generally recognized as safe and effective" (GRASE). Any drug manufacturer may produce such products for marketing without prior government approval. The manufacturer has flexibility in package labeling. Although the use of certain approved terminology is required (e.g., heartburn, acid indigestion, and sour stomach for antacids), other terms that have not been approved may also be used as long as they are not false or misleading.

Unlike with prescription drugs, adverse effects of OTC drugs are not required to be reported to the FDA. The manufacturer may substitute one GRASE ingredient in an OTC preparation for another GRASE ingredient without changing the name of the OTC drug and without indicating the change to the public with a warning on the package or label. The only method of determining the ingredients in a product is to check the label before each purchase. This can become problematic when a client or health care provider refers to a brand name OTC product and does not recognize that the brand name product was reformulated with different active ingredients. This often occurs when the safety of one of the active ingredients is called into question (e.g., phenolphthalein—a laxative with potential for cancer; ephedra—an appetite suppressant with cardiovascular risk; phenylpropanolamine—a decongestant and appetite suppressant with cardiovascular risks).

Another important concept to understand is the difference between drug potency and drug effectiveness. As defined in Chapter 5, drug potency is the amount of drug required to produce a desired effect. When drug manufacturers claim their product is more potent than another product, they usually mean that a smaller quantity of the drug is necessary to produce the same effect as the comparison drug. This does not mean the more potent drug is also the more effective drug (unless greater effectiveness has been proven and clearly stated)—it refers only to the amount of drug necessary to produce a desired effect. This terminology is often used and may be misleading if health care providers or consumers do not understand the difference between potency and effectiveness.

OTC analgesics have a number of extra-strength dosage forms that imply greater potency than the regular strength of the same brand or the competitor's usual adult strength (usually 500 mg compared with 325 mg of analgesic). However, if a more potent drug does not have documented proof of greater effectiveness when compared with an equivalent dose of the second drug, then there is no advantage to a "more potent" medication. When the only differ-

TABLE 11-1 PRESCRIPTION DRUGS THAT HAVE BEEN RECLASSIFIED AS OTC DRUGS

Ingredient (Prescription Name)	Year of OTC Status	OTC Name (examples)	Principal Use
brompheniramine (Dimetane, etc.)		Dimetane, Bromphen, etc.	Antihistamine
clemastine (Tavist)	1992	Tavist, etc.	Antihistamine
chlorpheniramine (Chlor-Trimeton, etc.)	1981	Chlor-Trimeton, Aller-chlor, etc.	Antihistamine
cimetidine (Tagamet HB)	1995	Tagamet HB	Heartburn, acid indigestion relief
clotrimazole (Gyne-Lotrimin, etc.)	1989	Lotrimin AF, Zeasorb-AF, etc.	Antifungal
cromolyn (Nasalcrom)	1997	Nasalcrom	Allergy prevention
diphenhydramine (Benadryl)	1985	Benylin Cough, Diphen Cough, etc.	Cough suppression
diphenhydramine (Benadryl)	1982	Nytol, Sominex, etc.	Sleeping aid
famotidine (Pepcid AC)	1995	Pepcid AC	Heartburn, acid indigestion
hydrocortisone (Cort Dome, etc.)	1975+	Cortizone, Dermolate, etc.	Topical for itching and rash relief
ibuprofen (Motrin IB)	1984	Advil, Nuprin, etc.	Analgesic
ketoconazole	1997	Nizoral	Dandruff shampoo
loperamide (Imodium, etc.)	1997	Imodium A-D, Kaopectate II, etc.	Antidiarrheal
loratadine (Claritin)	2002	Claritin, Claritin Reditabs, etc.	Antihistamine
miconazole (Monistat)	1982	Micatin, etc.	Antifungal
naproxen (Naprosyn)	1994	Aleve	Analgesic, antipyretic
nicotine polacrilex	1996	Nicorette	Smoking cessation
nicotine transdermal	1996	Nicotrol, Nicoderm CQ	Smoking cessation
nizatidine (Axid)	1996	Axid AR	Heartburn, acid indigestion relief
omeprazole (Prilosec)	2003	Prilosec OTC	Acid reducer
permethrin (Acticin)	1990	Nix	Pediculicide
pyrantel (Antiminth)	1986	Reese's Pinworm, etc.	Pinworm remedy
sodium fluoride	1980	Fluorigard, ACT, etc.	Dental rinse
tioconazole	1997	Vagistat-1	Anticandidal
triprolidine (Myodil, etc.)	1982	Actifed, Actidil, etc.	Antihistamine

Data from the Consumer Healthcare Products Association (http://www.chpa-info.org/web/advocacy/general_issues/switch/switch_list.pdf); and Rheinstein, P.H. (1997). FDA perspective: Prescription to over-the-counter drug switches. *American Family Physician, 56*(4), 1211-1214.

ence is drug strength, the therapeutic effect expected with either drug is the same; the potential disadvantages in using a more potent drug may include increased costs, adverse effects, and unknown long-term effects.

✸ How can the nurse affect the safe and effective use of OTC medications?

Nurses have a major role in educating consumers for accurate and safe self-administration of OTC medications. Al-

though many of these medications are also found in care settings in which the nurse's role is to administer such drugs, it is important be familiar with OTC medications to best advise clients for safe self-treatment of minor illnesses. The following information about OTC preparations should be shared with clients as an aspect of health promotion in both formal and informal instructional situations. Such teaching is applicable to almost any setting in which the nurse interacts with clients. See the Medication Safety Alert

Taking OTCs Wisely

- Always start by reading the label—all of it.
- Look for an OTC medicine that will treat only the symptoms you have.
- Know what activities, food, and other medications to avoid while taking an OTC.
- When in doubt, ask your pharmacist or primary care provider before you buy or use an OTC medicine.
- Take the medicine EXACTLY as stated on the label.
- Use extra caution when taking more than one OTC drug product at a time.
- Don't combine prescription medicines and OTC drugs without talking to your primary care provider first.
- Make sure that each of your health care providers has a list of all the medicines you are taking.
- Always give infants and children OTC medicines that are especially formulated for their age and weight.
- Don't use OTC medicines after their expiration date.

Modified from National Council on Patient Information and Education. (2004). Retrieved July 27, 2005, from http://www.bemedwise. org/ten_ways/ten_ways.htm.

box above for important safety information to share with clients who take OTCs.

OTC drugs have the image of being very safe and thus not requiring the special precautions necessary to take a prescription drug safely. Nothing could be farther from the truth. As with prescription drugs, OTC products have the potential for being misused, abused, and for inducing adverse effects. They also may be very dangerous if taken in certain disease states or if taken concurrently with other drugs, food, or alcohol. The health care professional needs to be aware of this information before administering or advising about an OTC preparation.

Product ingredients have either proven or questionable effectiveness; a careful check of ingredients is necessary to select the appropriate product in a specific drug category. The consumer should be encouraged to select the proper ingredient for treating a specific symptom. Combination products may contain substances that are not necessary for the person's symptoms. If the individual experiences an adverse effect of the combination drug, it may be difficult to determine the responsible ingredient. Additionally, many different products may have the same active ingredients that may or may not differ in strength, dosage form (liquid, tablet, capsule), or combination. If the ingredients are not carefully checked, an accidental overdose is possible by taking the same ingredient in a number of different products. Nurses should encourage consumers to read labels and select the label containing the same ingredients based on price.

Having the same ingredients in different preparations may allow for product substitution. For example, thousands of antacid products are available throughout the United States that primarily contain only four or five recognized active ingredients. Many OTC antacids are therefore duplicate preparations. A generic product is often as effective as an advertised product, and there is usually little if any advantage in purchasing the more expensive item.

Consumers should check the selected product for tampering. Most products are now packaged in tamper-resistant or tamper-evident packaging, which allows the consumer to detect signs of tampering. If the package is suspect, it should be taken to the pharmacist or store manager. The expiration date should also be checked to ensure that it has not passed.

Consumers should read labels very carefully if they have ever had an allergic or unusual response to any medication, food, or other substance (e.g., yellow dye or sulfites) to ensure that such an ingredient is not included. An individual should use caution if on a special diet (e.g., low-sugar or low-sodium), because many OTC drugs contain more than their active ingredients, and many liquid preparations contain alcohol. A woman who is pregnant or breastfeeding should not take OTC medications without first consulting her health care provider. Individuals with underlying medical conditions such as hypertension or diabetes should read labels carefully to determine whether the medication may be contraindicated with their condition.

Instructions and warnings on the label are to be followed carefully. The individual should be advised to consult with a pharmacist before purchasing an OTC medication if the following is true:

- The person has medical condition(s).
- The person is not familiar with the proper way to select an individual product based on ingredients and cost.
- The package instructions seem unclear.
- The current problem for which he or she is self-medicating is persistent and requires consultation with a health care provider.

Additional situations and conditions that require evaluation by a physician or other health care provider are summarized in Box 11-1. A health care provider should be consulted if the symptoms for which the OTC drug is being taken are not relieved in the time interval indicated on the label. Additionally, OTC medications are drugs that must be reported to a health care provider during a drug history taken during routine health visits.

Unless instructed otherwise, both prescription and OTC medications should be stored in closed containers in a cool, dry place and out of the reach of children. They should not be stored in the bathroom, near sinks, or in damp places because heat, moisture, and strong light may cause deterioration or a loss of medication potency.

All solid-dose medications (tablets and capsules) should be taken with a full glass of water (8 ounces). The individual should be advised to sit up for approximately 15 to 30 minutes after taking a solid-dose medication to help reduce the potential for esophageal irritation or injury. Drinking a small amount of water before taking a tablet or capsule is very helpful for individuals with problems of dry mouth or

Prior to purchasing OTC medications, the following situations or conditions should be evaluated by a physician or other health care provider:

- Child is under 6 months old.
- Infant has diarrhea for over 24 hours.
- The woman is pregnant.

  The individual has the following:

- Oral temperature greater than 39.8° C (102° F) or, the fever has lasted longer than 2 days.
- Cold or flu symptoms for more than 1 week.
- Been vomiting for more than 12 hours.
- Severe abdominal pain or cramps.
- Redness or swelling in a painful site.
- Difficulty breathing.
- A sudden, severe headache, slurred speech, and confusion.
- Visual changes or eye pain.
- Recurrent or persistent pain or fever.
- Severe sore throat for more than 2 days.
- Diarrhea for longer than 2 days.
- Three or more alcohol containing beverages daily.

  The above are selected general guidelines, the nurse should be aware that other criteria may also be applied.

minor problems in swallowing. If the drug is a long-acting medication, it should be swallowed whole. If the medication is in liquid form, the specially marked measuring spoon or other device provided by the manufacturer should be used to measure each dose accurately.

✴ What are the most commonly used OTC drug categories?

A number of drugs are available for OTC purchase, including analgesics, antacids, laxatives, and others. A brief overview of nursing implications for each category will be listed here. Further discussion of each drug can be found in the chapter discussing the use of the particular category of drug.

Analgesics

An **analgesic** is the term used to describe a drug that relieves pain. A number of analgesics are available as OTCs including acetaminophen (Tylenol), aspirin, and the nonsteroidal anti-inflammatory agents (NSAIDs) such as ibuprofen (Advil, Motrin IB), naproxen (Aleve), and ketoprofen (Actron, Orudis-KT). Also available are combinations of one of these analgesics with caffeine for vascular headaches or with decongestants and/or antihistamines and/or cough suppressants or expectorants to relieve pain associated with sinus inflammation, colds, influenza, or allergies. Daily low-dose aspirin is also often part of an antiplatelet regimen for clients at risk for coronary artery disease.

Encourage clients to see their health care provider if pain is not adequately relieved by the occasional use of OTC

analgesics. Also, they should review chronic use of any OTC analgesic with a prescriber. Concerns for acetaminophen use include avoidance of high doses to reduce the risk for hepatotoxicity. The maximum dose for short-term therapy with acetaminophen is up to 4 grams daily. Caution clients that acetaminophen is found in many combination products for cold symptoms, in addition to analgesics, and that a daily intake total should take into account all sources of the drug. Management of acetaminophen overdose is presented in Chapter 14.

Warn clients that aspirin and NSAIDs should be avoided or used under medical supervision if a client has a risk for gastrointestinal (GI) bleeding, renal dysfunction, or asthma. Non-aspirin NSAIDs may also pose a cardiovascular risk and are often avoided for clients with serious cardiovascular disease. Avoid the use of aspirin in children under the age of 17 years of age as a result of the risk of Reye syndrome. Reye syndrome is an acute encephalopathy whose etiology is unknown but its occurrence is associated with the administration of aspirin in children with viral diseases. Although children and adolescents are at increased risk, those age 4 to 12 years of age are at the highest risk. Fortunately, cases of Reye syndrome have declined dramatically over the past two decades as a result of the awareness of aspirin use as a causative factor (McCoy, Sorvillo, & Simon, 2004).

A number of drugs may interact with OTC analgesics (particularly aspirin and NSAIDs) so instruct clients to review their other medications and problem list with the pharmacist or prescriber before use. See Boxes 11-2 and 11-3 for more OTC analgesics cautions. A more complete discussion of these OTC analgesics is presented in Chapter 14.

✴ **Mrs. V.S., an 81-year-old widow, stands in her local pharmacy examining the labels on the bottles of OTC analgesics. She is beginning to experience some mild discomfort of her osteoarthritis and is looking for something safe to take for her "aches and pains." The labels list the same ingredients, but there is such a difference in price, she wonders if there is a difference in quality. The Extra-Strength Tylenol is 500 mg of acetaminophen for $11.99 and the pharmacy's brand for what seems to be the same thing, is $5.99. She wonders if she could just buy the pharmacy's brand instead, but she would feel so disloyal if she didn't buy Tylenol. Mrs. S. sees her neighbor Mr. M., who is a nurse at the local hospital, coming down the aisle. After greeting him, she asks what the difference between the two medications is. Mr. M. assures her that both medications are equivalent strengths of acetaminophen per tablet, but Tylenol is a brand name, and the other is a generic name. Thinking of her limited income, she decides to purchase the pharmacy's package of acetaminophen and passes this helpful hint on to her friends at the seniors' club.**

✴ **In addition to analgesics, what are some other commonly used OTCs?**

Box 11-2 ACETAMINOPHEN AND ASPIRIN OTC WARNINGS

GENERAL PRECAUTIONS FOR BOTH ANALGESICS

- Consult with prescriber before taking any analgesic if you are allergic to an analgesic or have had a severe allergic analgesic reaction such as asthma, swelling, hives, rash, and other symptoms.
- Avoid taking analgesics if you have kidney disease or liver damage, are pregnant or breastfeeding, have taken the analgesics for more than 10 days for pain in an adult or 5 days in a child or 3 days for fever, if pain increases or painful site is inflamed, if new symptoms develop, or if sore throat is very painful or lasts more than 2 days.
- If stomach distress occurs, take analgesic after meals or with food.

ASPIRIN

Special Dosing Information

- Avoid aspirin use with children and teenagers (under 17 years of age) for fever or symptoms of a viral infection, especially flu or chickenpox, without prescriber approval. The use of aspirin in viral illnesses may cause a very serious condition known as Reye's syndrome in children. Symptoms include severe vomiting, weakness, and stupor that may progress into coma, seizures, and even death.
- Stop aspirin use at least 5 to 7 days before a scheduled surgery.
- Never put aspirin products directly on a tooth or gum surface, as they can burn the tissues and cause injury.
- Avoid consumption of aspirin that has a strong, vinegar-like odor, because the odor indicates the aspirin is deteriorating.
- Inform your primary care provider if you have aspirin or salicylate allergy, asthma, nasal polyps, anemia, gout, ulcers or ulcer symptoms, or hemophilia or other bleeding problems.

Box 11-3 OTC NONSTEROIDAL ANTIINFLAMMATORY DRUG WARNINGS

GENERAL PRECAUTIONS

- With NSAIDs, contact the prescriber if the person reports they had a severe allergic reaction to any analgesic, such as asthma, swelling, hives, rash, or any other reaction, because the NSAIDs are capable of causing similar reactions.
- Avoid regular use of NSAIDs with any other OTC analgesics (acetaminophen, aspirin, or other NSAIDs).
- Avoid taking these products for more than 10 days for pain, 3 days for fever, if painful area is inflamed, if pregnant or breastfeeding, if new symptoms occur or current symptoms worsen, or if abdominal pain occurs. Contact prescriber for advice.
- Do not use NSAIDs during the last 3 months of pregnancy because it may adversely affect the fetus or result in complications during delivery.
- Alcohol (especially three or more drinks daily) and many other medications may result in adverse drug interactions. Review all medications with the prescriber or pharmacist before taking an NSAID.
- Avoid use for clients with renal impairment as NSAIDs may induce acute renal failure
- Avoid use for clients with a history of peptic ulcer disease as these agents have a higher risk for inducing GI bleeding for these individuals.
- The older adult may be at particular risk for renal or GI complications with NSAID use and caution is advised.

Antacids and Gastric Acid Suppressors

An orally administered liquid or tablet that buffers, neutralizes, or absorbs hydrochloric acid in the stomach would be considered an antacid. Antacids are primarily used to treat occasional heartburn or sour stomach. Alternatives to antacids are histamine blockers and proton pump inhibitors, which suppress gastric acid secretion and are also indicated for the treatment of gastric and duodenal ulcers and gastroesophageal reflux disease (GERD).

The antacids primarily consist of magnesium, aluminum and/or calcium salts and serve to directly increase gastric pH. Occasionally, simethicone is added to help break up gas bubbles and assist expelling painful gas buildup. The magnesium-containing antacids often lead to diarrhea, whereas aluminum and, to some degree, calcium salts are constipating. Aluminum salts may affect phosphate absorption and be problematic for clients with osteomalacia. Systemic absorption of aluminum may lead to central nervous system (CNS) toxicity for clients with renal failure who cannot eliminate the excessive aluminum levels. The majority of antacids contain 10 mg or less of sodium per recommended adult dose; however, because they are salts, clients on sodium-restricted diets should read ingredient listings carefully. All antacids may interfere with absorption of drugs (most importantly, quinolone antibacterial drugs, like ciprofloxacin [Cipro], and tetracyclines). See Table 11-2 for further adverse effects.

The histamine 2 (H_2) blockers are antagonists at the parietal cell of the gastric mucosa and reduce gastric acidity. They are indicated in low doses for the treatment of occasional gastritis (heartburn) and, at higher doses, for peptic ulcers and GERD. The primary agents available OTC are cimetidine (Tagamet HB), ranitidine (Zantac), and famotidine (Pepcid AC). Although serious adverse effects are rare, they may interfere with drugs metabolized by the cytochrome P450 system and result in fluctuations in response to other prescription and other OTC medications.

The proton pump inhibitors are the latest class of GI agents to achieve OTC status. These highly effective suppressors of gastric acid are used for treating gastritis, peptic ulcer disease, and GERD. Like the histamine blockers, they too may interfere with metabolism of other drugs.

TABLE 11-2 ANTACIDS: ADVERSE EFFECTS

Name	Potential Adverse Effects
ALUMINUM	
aluminum carbonate (Basaljel) aluminum hydroxide (Alterna- GEL, Alu-Cap, Amphojel) aluminum/magnesium compounds (Aludrox, Gaviscon, Maalox, Mylanta)	Constipation (combination products with magnesium reduce this) Phosphate depletion via feces (including weakness, apnea, hemolytic anemia, tetany) Delay in gastric emptying Concretions (nonabsorbable intestinal and renal mineral mass) Encephalopathy from aluminum intoxication (especially with renal insufficiency) Bone demineralization (osteomalacia, osteoporosis)
BICARBONATE	
sodium bicarbonate (Alka-Seltzer, Instant Metamucil)	Systemic alkalosis or sodium overload (elevated plasma pH and carbon dioxide, anorexia, mental confusion) Gastric acid hypersecretion ("acid rebound") Enhanced effects of amphetamines, quinidine, quinine
CALCIUM	
calcium carbonate (Tums)	Milk-alkali syndrome (including metabolic alkalosis, anorexia, nausea, vomiting, confusion, hypercalcemia, possibly renal impairment) Increased potential for calcium stone formation Nephrocalcinosis Gastric acid hypersecretion ("acid rebound") Antagonism of oral digoxin Elevated serum and urine calcium levels Kidney failure Constipation Decreased phosphate levels (if dietary phosphate intake low)
MAGNESIUM	
magnesium hydroxide (Phillips' Milk of Magnesia) magnesium trisilicate	Diarrhea (combination products with aluminum reduce this) Decreased potassium levels (hypokalemia) Increased magnesium levels (hypermagnesemia) in clients with renal failure or severe kidney impairment (causing low blood pressure, nausea, vomiting, respiratory depression, central nervous system depression, coma)

Self-medication with antacids, H_2 blockers, or proton pump inhibitors more frequently than a few times per month may indicate a more serious GI problem for which a health care provider should be consulted (Hoogerwerf & Pasricha, 2001). Additionally, the pharmacist or prescriber should review any other medications the client receives before the client takes one of these GI drugs. These agents are more completely discussed in Chapter 40.

Laxatives

Most laxatives are available for OTC purchase. A **laxative** induces defecation and is used in the prevention and treatment of constipation. **Constipation** is difficult fecal evacu-

ation as a result of hard stool and perhaps infrequent movements. Factors leading to constipation include failure to respond to the normal defecation impulse, insufficient time to permit the bowel to produce an evacuation, inadequate fluid and dietary fiber intake, sedentary habits, and insufficient exercise. **Perceived constipation,** a nursing diagnosis, is the state in which an individual makes a self-diagnosis of constipation and ensures a daily bowel movement through use of laxatives, enemas, and suppositories. In this instance, laxatives may be misused and abused to meet the client's perception of a normal bowel elimination pattern. Focus consumer education on the lifestyle changes necessary to promote a normal bowel elimination pattern for individuals with constipation and perceived constipation.

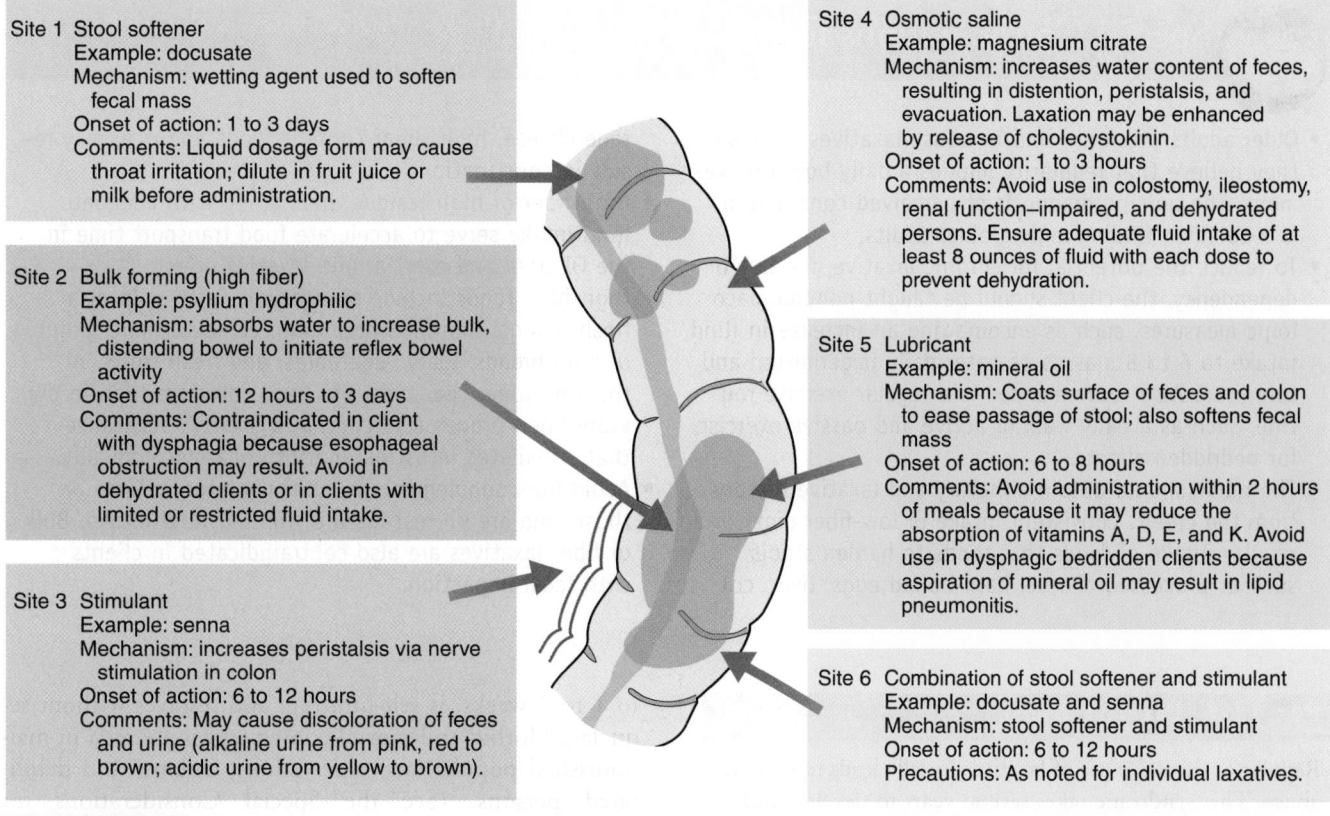

Site 1 Stool softener
Example: docusate
Mechanism: wetting agent used to soften fecal mass
Onset of action: 1 to 3 days
Comments: Liquid dosage form may cause throat irritation; dilute in fruit juice or milk before administration.

Site 2 Bulk forming (high fiber)
Example: psyllium hydrophilic
Mechanism: absorbs water to increase bulk, distending bowel to initiate reflex bowel activity
Onset of action: 12 hours to 3 days
Comments: Contraindicated in client with dysphagia because esophageal obstruction may result. Avoid in dehydrated clients or in clients with limited or restricted fluid intake.

Site 3 Stimulant
Example: senna
Mechanism: increases peristalsis via nerve stimulation in colon
Onset of action: 6 to 12 hours
Comments: May cause discoloration of feces and urine (alkaline urine from pink, red to brown; acidic urine from yellow to brown).

Site 4 Osmotic saline
Example: magnesium citrate
Mechanism: increases water content of feces, resulting in distention, peristalsis, and evacuation. Laxation may be enhanced by release of cholecystokinin.
Onset of action: 1 to 3 hours
Comments: Avoid use in colostomy, ileostomy, renal function–impaired, and dehydrated persons. Ensure adequate fluid intake of at least 8 ounces of fluid with each dose to prevent dehydration.

Site 5 Lubricant
Example: mineral oil
Mechanism: Coats surface of feces and colon to ease passage of stool; also softens fecal mass
Onset of action: 6 to 8 hours
Comments: Avoid administration within 2 hours of meals because it may reduce the absorption of vitamins A, D, E, and K. Avoid use in dysphagic bedridden clients because aspiration of mineral oil may result in lipid pneumonitis.

Site 6 Combination of stool softener and stimulant
Example: docusate and senna
Mechanism: stool softener and stimulant
Onset of action: 6 to 12 hours
Precautions: As noted for individual laxatives.

FIGURE 11-2 Classification of laxatives according to site of action.

Laxatives are usually classified according to their mechanism of action. Some laxatives serve to increase GI peristaltic action, although others soften stool. The choice of laxative depends primarily on whether the client has a hard stool, difficulty in passing stool or both. Laxatives are also indicated for individuals who should not strain during defecation (e.g., coronary artery disease, risk for aneurysm), for clients with hemorrhoids (hard stools exacerbate hemorrhoids), and for individuals preparing for a procedure that requires a clean bowel.

Laxative classifications include the following (Figure 11-2):

- Stool softeners, which reduce the surface tension of stool (e.g., docusate—Colace)
- Agents that enhance bulk and moisture content to stool (e.g., psyllium—Metamucil; methylcellulose—Citrucel)
- Oral saline laxatives that draw water into the intestinal lumen (e.g., magnesium hydroxide [Phillips' Milk of Magnesia]); rectal saline laxatives (e.g., phosphate enemas [Fleet Enema])
- Lubricant laxatives, which coat stool with a water-immersible film (mineral oil)
- Stimulant laxatives, which increase peristalsis (e.g., senna extracts [Senokot], bisacodyl [Dulcolax])
- Osmotic laxatives, which increases fluid accumulation in the bowel (e.g., lactulose [Chronulac; not OTC in United States, but it is OTC in Canada]).

Because constipation is common in children, parents need to be informed about problems associated with indiscrimi-

nate use of laxatives. In children, emotions, environmental changes (new home, new school, new friends), dietary changes, and febrile illnesses may all contribute to or cause constipation. Adding or increasing fluids, vegetables, fruits, and bran products may be very helpful. Malt soup extract is often suggested for infants up to 2 months old. For older children, glycerin suppositories or docusate sodium (Colace) may be appropriate.

The older adult may have an increased incidence of constipation because of multiple illnesses that require a variety of medications, the aging process with its associated decline in physiologic functions, plus a progressive decrease in physical activity (see the Special Considerations for Older Adults box on p. 210). An increase in fluid intake, a moderate exercise program if permitted, and an increase in intake of bran products, vegetables, and fruit will help to correct this problem. Laxative abuse is often reported with this age group. Because there may be many factors contributing to constipation, a complete and thorough history by the health care professional is necessary.

Constipation is commonly reported during pregnancy. It is usually caused by colon compression as a result of an increase in uterine size or a decrease in muscle tone and peristalsis. Vitamins containing iron and calcium are often prescribed for pregnant women, and such products also tend to be constipating. Laxatives used in pregnancy should be limited to emollients or bulk-forming laxatives. Most of the other laxatives have the potential for undesirable effects; for example, castor oil may induce premature labor, mineral oil may decrease absorption of fat-soluble vitamins, and os-

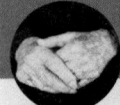

Special Considerations for Older Adults | NONPHARMACOLOGIC LAXATIVE THERAPY

- Older adults often use and/or abuse laxatives because they believe that regularity implies a daily bowel movement. The nursing diagnosis of perceived constipation is a common finding among older adults.
- To reduce the potential for chronic laxative use and/or dependency, the client should be taught nonpharmacologic measures, such as encouraging an increase in fluid intake to 6 to 8 glasses of water daily if permitted and tolerated. Also recommended is a regular exercise routine, such as a daily walk or active and passive exercise for bedridden clients.
- The nurse should obtain a dietary and laxative history from the client. Consistent intake of low-fiber diets or a regular intake of foods that tends to harden stools, such as processed cheese, hard-boiled eggs, liver, cot-

tage cheese, high sugar content foods and rice, may result in constipation.
- High-fiber or high-residue diets along with adequate fluid intake serve to accelerate food transport time in the GI tract and exert a mild laxative effect.
- High-fiber foods include orange juice with pulp or a fresh orange, bran or whole grain cereals, whole grain or bran breads, leafy vegetables, and fresh fruits. Although prunes, bananas, figs, and dates are high in dietary fiber, prunes also contain a laxative substance that stimulates intestinal motility pharmacologically.
- Avoid fiber supplements in nonambulatory clients or those who are on restricted or limited fluid intake. Bulk or fiber laxatives are also contraindicated in clients with fecal impaction.

BOX 11-4 LAXATIVE ABUSE

Regular or excessive use of laxatives usually leads to laxative abuse. This syndrome takes several years to develop and is often undiagnosed. It is often reported among older adults. Laxative abuse may occur in conjunction with eating disorders, such as bulimia or anorexia. Symptoms are similar to other disease states, such as nephritis, diabetes insipidus, ulcerative colitis, or Addison disease. The major complaints on hospital admission are diarrhea and abdominal cramps. More often than not, clients deny excessive laxative usage.

If chronic laxative abuse is not detected and the client is not weaned off the laxative, permanent bowel damage, osteomalacia, and electrolyte imbalance may occur.

motic agents may induce dangerous electrolyte alterations. Advise the childbearing woman about proper diet, adequate fluid intake, appropriate exercise programs, and the importance of discussing the problem with her health care provider for her pregnancy.

Laxatives should not be taken if the individual is experiencing undiagnosed abdominal pain because it may be a result of an inflammatory disorder of the alimentary tract, such as appendicitis, typhoid fever, or chronic ulcerative colitis. If an inflamed appendix causes the pain, a laxative may bring about a rupture of the appendix by increasing intestinal peristalsis. Laxatives are also a classification of drug that may be abused (Box 11-4). A further discussion of the use of laxatives is presented in Chapter 40.

Antidiarrheal Agents

Diarrhea is the frequent passage of loose watery stools (Anderson, 2002). Acute diarrhea is sudden in onset in a previously healthy individual, lasts approximately 3 days

to 1 to 2 weeks, is self-limiting, and resolves without sequelae. Morbid and mortal consequences are seen in malnourished populations, older adults, infants, and debilitated persons. (See the Special Considerations for Children box on p. 211.)

Chronic diarrhea can last for more than 3 to 4 weeks, with the recurring passage of diarrheal stools, fever, anorexia, nausea, vomiting, weight reduction, and chronic weakness. Chronic diarrhea necessitates definitive treatment directed to the organic cause or causes and may include infectious, psychogenic, and neoplastic origins.

The drugs used to treat acute and chronic diarrhea diminish stool water by inhibiting intestinal fluid secretion, increasing intestinal fluid absorption, or inhibiting GI motility. Although these drugs decrease the number, consistency, and fluidity of the stool, there is no absolute clinical evidence that the client experiences an effective antidiarrheal therapeutic benefit. However, the bothersome symptoms that interrupt daily routines are relieved.

OTC antidiarrheal agents include adsorbents and synthetic opioids. Adsorbents coat the walls of the GI tract, absorbing the bacteria or toxins causing the diarrhea, and passing them out with the stools; examples include bismuth salts (Pepto-Bismol) and kaolin/pectin or attapulgite (Kaopectate). Opioid and opioid-related compounds have a direct effect at the opioid receptor in the gut to decrease gastric motility. Although any opioid can slow GI motility, loperamide (Imodium), a synthetic opioid devoid of abuse potential, is the most common OTC agent in this class.

Treatment of diarrhea should include adequate fluid and electrolyte management and antidiarrheal therapy. Although important for all clients, it is particularly critical for infants, young children, and older adults. For diarrhea accompanied by fever, blood, or pus in the stool, or profuse and protracted diarrhea, the health care provider should be contacted.

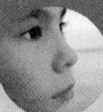 Special Considerations for Children | OTC MEDICATIONS FOR DIARRHEA

- Diarrhea is a common problem in children and may be as a result of a variety of causes, such as intestinal disease, infection, congenital disorder, and food or formula intolerance. In some instances, it may be secondary to antibiotic use.
- Persistent diarrhea can lead to water and electrolyte imbalance. In infants or very young children it can cause cardiovascular collapse and death. Rehydration and correction of electrolyte disturbances is critical in the treatment of diarrhea.
- Although hospitalization may be necessary in severe dehydration, milder cases are often treated with oral replacement therapy. The World Health Organization (WHO) recommends oral rehydration with balanced electrolyte

and glucose solutions (see http://www.WHO.org). Products such as PediaLyte and InfaLyte are formulated to meet WHO recommendations. When Gatorade or a similar product is used, the preparation should be diluted to half-strength with water. Be aware, however, that glucose concentrations over 5% can cause osmotic diarrhea.
- The use of any OTC antidiarrheal product is not usually recommended for preschool children without the specific advice of a physician. Package labeling often provides age-specific dosage instructions; follow such instructions carefully or, preferably, consult first with the prescriber.

Modified from Gilger, M.A. (2003). Approach to the child with acute diarrhea, *UpToDate, 13*(1). Wellesley, MA: UpToDate.

TABLE 11-3 COLDS, ALLERGIC RHINITIS, AND INFLUENZA: SIGNS OR SYMPTOMS

Signs or Symptoms	Common Cold	Allergic Rhinitis	Influenza
Fever	Rare	Absent	Common—sudden onset, may range 102° F to 104° F
Aches and pains	Slight	Absent	May be severe
Sneezing	Usual	Common	Infrequent
Pruritus	Absent or rare	Common	Absent
Cough	Mild-moderate	Uncommon	Common
Headaches	Rare	Can occur	Prominent
Causative	Viruses	Usually allergens	Viruses
Occurrence	Anytime	Usually seasonal	Usually seasonal
Complications	Sinus congestion, earache	Uncommon	Bronchitis, pneumonia

✸ **How effective are OTC cough and cold preparations?**

Cough-Cold/Allergy Preparations

A great number of cough/cold and allergy preparations are available over the counter. Table 11-3 describes the major differences between colds, allergic rhinitis, and influenza (flu). The OTC preparations used to alleviate symptoms of these conditions include antitussives, antihistamines, expectorants, decongestants, and zinc preparations. The use of complementary therapy (e.g., echinacea) is discussed in Chapter 12.

Antitussives Antitussives work to suppress cough. Coughing is defined as a protective reflex for clearing the respiratory tract of environmental irritants, foreign bodies, or accumulated secretions and therefore should not be depressed indiscriminately. In general, only a nonproductive

cough that is dry, irritating, frequent, and prolonged should be treated because it can be exhausting, painful, and taxing to the circulatory system and the elastic tissue of the respiratory system. Antitussive drugs act either by suppressing the cough center in the medulla or by lessening irritation of the respiratory tract peripherally. Stress intake of fluids and inhalation of fully water-saturated vapors (steam) as important means of producing increased amounts of mucus and thinning such secretions. Opioids, including codeine and hydrocodone, are strong cough suppressants, but require a prescription in the United States.

The most common OTC antitussive agent is dextromethorphan, which is administered orally and has an onset of action between 15 and 30 minutes and a duration of activity up to 6 hours. The adverse effects are minimal with the usually recommended doses. Nausea, mild dizziness, and drowsiness have been reported. Significant drug interactions have been reported with CNS depressants and monamide oxidase (MAO) inhibitor medications. The former may result in enhanced CNS depressant effects, and concurrent use with MAO inhibitors may result in increased excitability, tremors, sedation, severe hypertension, intracranial bleeding, hyperpyrexia, and psychosis. Persons taking a MAO inhibitor should not take dextromethorphan.

Another OTC agent with some cough suppressant activity is the antihistamine, diphenhydramine (Benadryl), discussed below under antihistamines.

Antihistamines Antagonists of the histamine 1 receptor (H_1) are commonly referred to as **antihistamines** and are used to relieve symptoms of allergy including allergic rhinitis and watery eyes. The OTC antihistamines related to cold and allergy symptoms include sedating agents such as diphenhydramine (Benadryl), chlorpheniramine (Chlor-Trimeton), and brompheniramine (Dimetane), and the nonsedating loratadine (Claritin). The reduced sedation of loratadine is related to decreased distribution to CNS histamine receptors.

Antihistamines prevent the physiologic histamine effects of sneezing, increased nasal secretions, and itching and watering eyes by preventing histamine from reaching its site of action. The antihistamines of the H_1 type have the greatest therapeutic effect on nasal allergies, particularly on seasonal hay fever and colds with histamine-like symptoms. In allergies, they relieve symptoms better at the beginning of the hay fever season than during its height but fail to relieve the asthma that often accompanies the hay fever. Antihistamines are palliative agents. Their action is comparatively short-lived and provides only symptomatic relief.

Many OTC preparations contain antihistamines, and some contain two or more. Antihistamines may be used in a variety of OTC medications, including antitussive agents, cough-cold products, sleep-inducing products, oral analgesic products, menstrual formulations, and many others. For example, diphenhydramine depresses the cough center in the medulla of the brain (antitussive effect), has antihistamine effects (blocks H_1 receptors), central antimuscarinic effects (antiparkinsonian action), and sedative-hypnotic effects, and it is used to prevent or treat the nausea and vomiting associated with motion sickness. Consumers should check the ingredients of all medications they buy, consume, or administer. Individuals often experience unwanted adverse effects or an accidental overdose because the same product is available in several different medications they are consuming; unfortunately, this fact is often overlooked in a community setting. H_1 antagonists are discussed more fully in Chapter 38.

Expectorants Expectorants are substances that reduce the viscosity of secretions, thus promoting the ejection of mucus or other exudates from the lungs, bronchi, and trachea. In OTC preparations the only expectorant with evidence of safety and effectiveness is guaifenesin (Robitussin). Unless otherwise contraindicated, clients should be encouraged to maintain fluids to also assist with expectoration. A discussion of agents used to clear respiratory secretions is presented in Chapter 37.

Decongestants Decongestant agents are vasoconstricting agents used to shrink engorged nasal mucous membranes in mild upper respiratory tract infections. In OTC products, they are available in oral and nasal preparations.

The oral agents are sympathomimetic amines, and their vasoconstricting properties are not limited to the nasal mucosa. They can also elevate blood pressure in individuals with hypertension, induce cardiac stimulation and dysrhythmias in some people and, depending on the sympathomimetic amine, may increase blood glucose in individuals with diabetes. For this reason, warnings on the labels instruct consumers with hypertension, hyperthyroidism, diabetes mellitus, or ischemic heart disease to contact their prescriber before using the product. The most commonly available oral decongestant is pseudoephedrine (Sudafed). Some combination products also include phenylephrine. Phenylpropanolamine, another historically popular decongestant, was removed from the U.S. market in 2002 related to risks for cerebrovascular accidents. Reported adverse effects of decongestants include CNS stimulation or nervousness, insomnia, restlessness, dizziness, headaches, and increased irritability.

Many drugs are used exclusively as nasal vasoconstrictors or topical decongestants. Because of their wide popular use and lack of serious hazard (when used topically), a large number of preparations have been provided by the pharmaceutical industry for direct sale to the public. The FDA advisory review panel has recommended the following topical nasal decongestant products as safe and effective: ephedrine 0.5%; naphazoline (Privine) 0.05%, 0.025%; oxymetazoline (Afrin 12-Hour Original, Dristan) 0.05%, 0.025%; phenylephrine (Neo-Synephrine) 0.125%, 0.25%, 1%; and xylometazoline (Otrivin) 0.1%, 0.05%. Table 11-4 lists the recommended dosages for topical nasal decongestant products and oral decongestant products. These drugs are adrenergic agents that act on the α receptors of blood vessels in the nasal mucosa to produce vasoconstriction and therefore a decrease in mucosal swelling. Some nasal decongestant products (those containing ephedrine, epinephrine, metaproterenol, and others) also possess β-stimulating effects, which may cause CNS stimulation and perhaps the adverse effect of vasodilation after vasoconstriction.

Nasal decongestants are used to shrink engorged mucous membranes of the nose and to relieve nasal stuffiness. However, consumers tend to use them excessively or too frequently. Excessive use may result in "rebound" engorgement or swelling of the mucous membranes and a paradoxical bronchospasm. Sprays and nose drops are beneficial when used judiciously. However, if an infection is present, there is always the possibility that nasal sprays or drops will spread the infection deeper into the sinuses or to the middle ear. Additives such as preservatives, antihistamines, and detergents are sometimes included in a decongestant preparation. In some cases, reactions may be caused by the additive in the preparation rather than by the decongestant.

Selection of Combination Cough-Cold Preparations Combination OTC products require careful selection because some of these multidrug formulations contain unnecessary

TABLE 11-4 TOPICAL/ORAL NASAL DECONGESTANTS: DOSAGES

Drug/Strength	Adults	Children (6 to 12 years old)
ephedrine, 0.5% (in Va-Tro-Nol and others)	2-3 drops q4h	1-2 drops q4h
naphazoline (Privine and others)		
0.05%	1-2 drops/spray q6h	Not recommended
0.025%	—	1-2 drops q6h
oxymetazoline (Afrin, Allerest, Dristan Long-Lasting and others)*		
0.05%	2-3 drops twice daily	Same as adults
phenylephrine (Neo-Synephrine and others)*		
1%	1-2 drops/spray q4h	Not recommended
0.25%	Same as 1%	1-2 drops q4h
xylometazoline (Otrivin)		
0.1%	2-3 drops/spray q8-10h	Not recommended
0.05%	Same as 0.1%	2-3 drops/spray q8-10h
Oral nasal decongestants (usually combined with other drug products)		
phenylephrine	10 mg q4h	5 mg q4h
pseudoephedrine	60 mg q6h	30 mg q6h

*Other strengths also available.

drugs. Combinations that contain an analgesic or antipyretic agent should be avoided for several reasons. First, there is the risk of masking a bacterial infection. Second, a fixed amount of analgesic or antipyretic is taken with other ingredients on a regular basis, whether needed or not. Third, it would be difficult to identify the offending agent if an adverse effect occurs. If an analgesic/antipyretic is necessary, the proper dose should be selected and administered separately.

When only one drug effect is necessary (e.g., a nasal decongestant, an expectorant, or an antihistamine effect), a therapeutic dose of that single drug entity should be taken. If the individual has several symptoms that need to be addressed, selection of a combination product should be limited to addressing just those symptoms, with few if any additional substances. For example, for cough suppressant and expectorant effects, an OTC product that contains guaifenesin and dextromethorphan (Robitussin DM and many others) may be selected. To treat allergy, nasal congestion, sneezing, and rhinorrhea, an antihistamine and decongestant combination is used, such as triprolidine and pseudoephedrine (Actifed), or many others. For nasal or sinus congestion alone, an oral or a nasal decongestant may be selected, such as pseudoephedrine (Sudafed) or oxymetazoline (Afrin 12-Hour Original). (See Table 11-5 for selected cough-cold combinations.)

✳ **Mr. P.T., a 55-year-old male, comes to the health center for symptoms of an upper respiratory infection.**

Mr. T. also has hypertension, and has had his blood pressure (BP) well controlled with his antihypertensive drug regimen for more than 4 years, but on this visit his BP is 164/94. The nurse asks if his routine has changed at all, but in particular, has he taken anything OTC for his cough and cold. Mr. T. indicated that nothing in his life had changed appreciably, except for "this dang cold." He stated he was taking two capsules of Robitussin Severe Congestion Liqui-Gels every 4 hours during the day and Nytime Cold Medicine Liquid at night because he was so miserable with the head congestion of his cold. Additionally, he was also taking something for his cough, Robitussin Maximum Strength Cough Syrup, when it bothered him. The nurse indicated that the increase in his BP was probably as a result of his OTC medications, because she calculated that Mr. T. had been consuming about 240 mg of pseudoephedrine, a decongestant, every 24 hours. When questioned about reading the label on OTCs, Mr. T. admitted that he had trouble because "the print is so small" and "the words are confusing," so he "didn't do that anymore." Mr. T. was cautioned against using decongestants because of his hypertension and to use antihistamines instead. The nurse provided Mr. T. a list of generic names of antihistamines for him to look for when he has his next cold or to ask the pharmacist about if reading labels was difficult. He was also instructed in the use of steam inhalation to try to help

TABLE 11-5 SELECTED COUGH-COLD COMBINATIONS

Brand Name	Ingredients	Pharmacologic Effect
Robitussin	guaifenesin	Expectorant
Robitussin-CF	guaifenesin, pseudoephedrine, dextromethorphan	Expectorant, decongestant, and cough suppressant
Robitussin-DM	guaifenesin, dextromethorphan	Expectorant, cough suppressant
Robitussin Flu Liquid	dextromethorphan, chlorpheniramine, pseudoephedrine, acetaminophen	Cough suppressant, antihistamine, decongestant, antipyretic
Robitussin-PE	guaifenesin, pseudoephedrine	Expectorant, decongestant
Robitussin Night Relief	pyrilamine, pseudoephedrine, dextromethorphan, acetaminophen	Antihistamine, decongestant, cough suppressant, analgesic, alcohol free
Robitussin PM Cough & Cold Formula	chlorpheniramine, pseudoephedrine, dextromethorphan,	Antihistamine, decongestant, cough suppressant,
Benylin Expectorant	guaifenesin, dextromethorphan	Expectorant, cough suppressant, alcohol and sugar free
Cheracol Syrup	guaifenesin, codeine	Expectorant, cough suppressant, contains alcohol (4.75%)
Cheracol D Cough Formula	guaifenesin, dextromethorphan	Expectorant, cough suppressant, contains alcohol (4.75%)

From *Drug facts and comparisons*. (58th ed.). (2005). St. Louis: Facts and Comparisons.

relieve his congestion; even though there is insufficient evidence regarding its general effectiveness, it might work for him.

✳ Are there OTC drugs available for the common health problems of women?

Women may have a broad range of medical problems that includes nearly all the diseases that affect the male, plus many additional disorders and/or conditions. From puberty on, women may encounter dysmenorrhea and premenstrual syndrome, pregnancy, fertility and family planning, menopause, osteoporosis and the gynecological issues of yeast infections, pelvic inflammatory disease, urinary tract infections, and bacterial vaginosis. Various cancers that primarily affect women include cervical, endometrial, ovarian, and breast cancer. Many of the pharmacological treatments for these disorders will be discussed in the appropriate chapters throughout this textbook. However, many women initially use OTC drugs to prevent or treat a number of conditions. This chapter will specifically address the OTC drugs that women may select for self-treatment prior to visiting their health care provider, such as dysmenorrhea and premenstrual problems, vaginal products, and contraceptives.

✳ What are the symptoms of dysmenorrhea and premenstrual syndrome for which OTC drugs are effective?

Hormonal changes during menstrual cycles may affect the physical and emotional symptoms that women experience during a month. Although most women have mild symptoms, some have symptoms severe enough to compromise their ability to function. Many women with premenstrual syndrome and dysmenorrhea commonly use OTC preparations. An overview of the menstrual cycle is reviewed in Chapter 50, and the hormones and drugs that affect the female reproductive system are discussed in Chapter 51.

Dysmenorrhea is a painful menstruation that usually occurs prior to or during menses and is believed to be a result of uterine contractions and ischemia caused by the release of prostaglandins from the endometrium. This type of dysmenorrhea is also known as primary dysmenorrhea because of its association with the ovulatory cycle. A secondary dysmenorrhea or acquired dysmenorrhea is a painful menses that is caused by other reproductive problems, such as fibroid tumors, endometriosis, pelvic lesions, or infections that require intervention and treatment by a health care provider.

About 10% of women with primary dysmenorrhea have lower abdominal cramps and pain that impairs their functioning for up to 3 days a month. Other symptoms may include headache, nausea, increased irritability, depression, nervousness, fluid retention, constipation or diarrhea, and frequent urination. Depending on the severity of the dysmenorrhea; mild symptoms are treated with acetaminophen with the application of a heating pad or local heat to the abdomen or lower back, whereas moderate to severe primary dysmenorrhea may require a NSAID such as ibuprofen, naproxen, or ketoprofen. The most effective treatment pharmacologically is with the use of NSAIDs (prostaglandin inhibitors), discussed earlier in this chapter.

Table 11-6 OTC Menstrual Products

Product	Ingredient*	Indications
Midol Maximum Strength Cramp Formula	ibuprofen 200 mg	Analgesic
Midol Maximum Strength Menstrual	acetaminophen 500 mg caffeine 60 mg pyrilamine 15 mg	Analgesic Diuretic Antihistamine, antipruritic
Midol Maximum Strength PMS	acetaminophen 500 mg pamabrom 25 mg pyrilamine 15 mg	Analgesic Diuretic Antihistamine, antipruritic
Midol Teen Maximum Strength	acetaminophen 500 mg pamabrom 25 mg	Analgesic Diuretic
Pamprin Multi-Symptom	acetaminophen 500 mg pamabrom 25 mg pyrilamine 15 mg	Analgesic Diuretic Antihistamine, antipruritic
Premsyn PMS	acetaminophen 500 mg pamabrom 25 mg pyrilamine 15 mg	Analgesic Diuretic Antihistamine, antipruritic
Women's Tylenol Multi-Symptom Menstrual Relief	acetaminophen 500 mg pamabrom 25 mg	Analgesic Diuretic

From *Drug facts and comparisons* (58th ed.). (2005). St. Louis: Facts and Comparisons.
*It is important to check package for ingredients because formulations may change without notification.

Premenstrual syndrome (PMS) refers to the physical and mood changes that some women experience in the luteal phase of the menstrual cycle, usually the week prior to menstruation. The symptoms include abdominal bloating, headache, irritability, fatigue, fluid retention, weight gain, and breast tenderness, which may be related to estrogen causing a fluid retention effect in the body. The exact cause of PMS is unknown but theories include alterations in estrogen and progesterone, dysfunction of the serotonin system, endorphin withdrawal, vitamin (B_6) and mineral (magnesium, calcium, zinc) deficiencies and other systemic abnormalities (Casper, 2002). This condition usually improves and/or disappears within a few hours of the onset of menses.

It is important to differentiate PMS from premenstrual dysphoric disorder (PMDD). Premenstrual dysphoric disorder involves significant altered mood with depression, anxiety, and/or irritability that markedly interferes with day-to-day functioning, is closely correlated with at least two consecutive menstrual cycles over the prior 6 months, and is not explained by other pathology (Dell, 2004). PMDD is not responsive to OTC treatments and is typically managed with prescription antidepressants—selective serotonin reuptake inhibitors (SSRIs) such as fluoxetine (Prozac, Sarafem)—for 2 weeks each month. Further discussion is found in Chapter 19.

There is no single treatment for PMS, instead the treatment usually depends on the symptoms that are present. For example, if edema is present, reducing salt intake or taking a mild diuretic may be helpful. For increased irritability, avoiding caffeine products such as coffee, tea, colas, chocolate, etc. may be helpful. For a list of selected menstrual products containing multiple ingredients, see Table 11-6.

The primary ingredients in these products are acetaminophen for pain, a mild diuretic such as pamabrom or caffeine for fluid accumulation and pyrilamine, an antihistamine, antipruritic agent. Caffeine is a xanthine that promotes diuresis by inhibition of the reabsorption of sodium and water in the renal tubules. The dose to produce this effect is 100 to 200 mg every 3 to 4 hours. However, large doses of caffeine can cause GI irritation, nervousness, irritability, tachycardia, anxiety, and insomnia. Therefore, individuals with a history of peptic ulcer disease, insomnia or persons taking other caffeine containing food, beverages, or medications (xanthines, theophylline, etc.) should avoid products containing caffeine. Pamabrom is a theophylline derivative used for diuresis. It is used in doses of 50 mg four times a day.

Many other medications have been evaluated for the treatment of dysmenorrhea and PMS and they have not been classified in Category I (safe and effective). These include the smooth muscle relaxants, antihistamines, sympathomimetics, and herbal preparations.

✷ What topical vaginal products are available OTC?
Vaginal OTC preparations include antifungal, feminine hygiene (antimicrobial), and lubricating products.

✷ What types of vaginal infections can be treated with OTC preparations?
It is important to differentiate fungal or yeast infections, which can be treated with OTC products, from bacterial or

protozoan infections, which require evaluation by a prescriber and treatment with prescription products (Table 11-7).

Vaginal infections primarily include bacterial vaginosis (noninflammatory infection), candidal vulvovaginitis, and trichomoniasis.

Candidal vulvovaginitis is a fungal vaginal infection, most often caused by *Candida albicans*. Symptoms may include a thick white discharge, vaginal erythema, and an intense pruritus. The absence of an offensive discharge odor is helpful in distinguishing a candidal infection from the other vaginal infections. Women are more susceptible to this infection during pregnancy, HIV infection, during use of estrogen-containing hormonal contraceptives, in diabetics, or following treatment with a broad-spectrum antibiotic or immunosuppressant agent.

The OTC antifungal vaginal agents are primarily the imidazole derivatives that include butoconazole (Femstat 3 vaginal cream), miconazole (Monistat 7 cream and suppository), and clotrimazole (Femizole-7, Gyne-Lotrimin, Mycelex-7 and others) (*Drug Facts and Comparisons,* 2005). The change of these drugs from prescription to OTC status in the early 90s saved millions of dollars for the health care system and in convenience of women to self-treat (Lipinsky, 1999). These products are considered to be equivalent, effective, and generally lack any major adverse effect. They produce their effect by inhibiting the cytochrome P450 enzymes in the fungal cell membrane, which results in a decreased synthesis of fungal ergosterol. The reduction of ergosterol results in an increase in methylated sterols that cause damage and loss of normal fungus membrane function. These agents are discussed in Chapters 59 and 65.

These agents are minimally absorbed and adverse effects include vaginal burning, itching, and irritation in less than 1% of women (*Drug Facts and Comparisons,* 2005). If the rare adverse effects of abdominal cramps, headache, hives, urticaria, and allergic reactions occur, the woman should stop the medication and contact her health care provider. If no improvement is noted after 3 days of therapy, or if the symptoms are not completely resolved after the course of therapy or if the symptoms return within 2 months of treatment, then a provider's evaluation is necessary.

Trichomoniasis is caused by *Trichomonas vaginalis* and is considered to be a sexually transmitted infection (STI). It is a disease affecting young women with symptoms usually during or after menstruation although up to 50% of women can be asymptomatic. Symptoms include a white (or yellow, gray, green), foamy vaginal discharge that may contain an odor. Other symptoms may include stomach pain and pruritus (Parent-Stevens & Sagraves, 2005).

Bacterial vaginosis is the most prevalent vaginal infection occurring in women of childbearing age. This infection has been referred to as nonspecific vaginitis, *Haemophilus vaginitis* and *Gardnerella vaginitis* that usually results in an increase in anaerobe bacteria (*Peptostreptococcus, Bacteroides*) and a decrease in *Lactobacillus.* The classic symptom is a vaginal discharge with a fishy odor when the discharge is alkalinized with 10% potassium hydroxide. Unfortunately, vaginosis is often asymptomatic and may increase risk for miscarriage with pregnancy (Klebanoff, 2004).

The usual treatment of bacterial vaginosis and trichomoniasis is with prescription drugs such as, metronidazole vaginal gel (MetroGel Vaginal) and clindamycin (Cleocin) vaginal cream for bacterial vaginosis, although the oral metronidazole is often used to treat trichomoniasis. Treatment of candidal vaginal infections requires the use of antifungal agents. See Chapter 58.

✲ What OTC contraceptives are available?

The most effective forms of birth control are the hormonal contraceptives, discussed in Chapter 51. Nonprescription contraceptive approaches include a variety of natural family planning approaches (rhythm method, basal body temperature method, and others), condoms (female and male), diaphragm, and spermicides. As spermicides are the only pharmacologic agents in this group, this discussion will be limited to them.

Spermicides are vaginal contraceptives that use a surface-active agent to immobilize sperm. The majority of OTC products contain nonoxynol-9 (Delfen, Emko, Encare, K-Y

TABLE 11-7 DIFFERENTIATION OF FUNGAL, BACTERIAL, OR PROTOZOAN VAGINAL INFECTIONS

Fungal/Yeast Infection	Protozoan Infection	Bacterial Vaginosis
Common Pathogen: • *Candida albicans* Contributing Factors: • Often after treatment with antibiotics or corticosteroids • Heat, moisture, and occlusive clothing Presenting Signs/Symptoms: • White curd-like discharge • Vulvovaginal erythema • Intense pruritus • Minimal or no odor	Common Pathogen: • *Trichomonas vaginalis* Contributing Factors: • Transmitted through coitus Presenting Signs/Symptoms: • Pruritus • Variable discharge, may be foamy, yellow-green • Malodorous • Vaginal erythema	Common Pathogens: • Overgrowth of *Gardnerella* and other anaerobes Contributing Factors: • Excessive douching • Heat, moisture, occlusive clothing • Not sexually transmitted Presenting Signs/Symptoms: • Malodorous discharge without obvious vulvitis or vaginitis • Grayish, sometimes frothy discharge • Often asymptomatic

Plus and many others) with only a few products containing octoxynol-9 (Ortho-Gynol✦). These agents are available in the following jelly, cream, film, foam, and suppository dosage forms:

- Jelly and creams—If the vaginal cream or jelly is used without a diaphragm, a product with a high spermicide concentration should be selected. Creams are better lubricants, although the gel product is usually less messy. These agents are effective immediately after application and are usually effective for approximately 60 minutes. It is recommended that douching be delayed for at least 8 hours after intercourse to permit the spermicide time to produce its effect on sperm. Allergic reactions are rare with these products.
- Foam—Foam contraceptives are more effective alone than the other topical vaginal contraceptives because they adhere better and are more evenly distributed to the cervix and vaginal walls. This dosage form is often used as a back up method or in combination with other contraceptives (oral, condoms, IUDs). Foams are effective immediately and similar to the cream and jellies, may be inserted up to an hour before coitus. It is also recommended that douching be delayed for at least 8 hours after intercourse.
- Suppositories—A vaginal suppository is inserted high in the vagina about 10 to 15 minutes prior to coitus. The suppository is activated by the moisture in the vaginal tract and generally, is not recommended because of their low efficacy.
- Film—A vaginal film is placed near the cervix where it is activated by vaginal secretions. It should be inserted approximately 5 minutes before intercourse and is effective for about 2 hours.

Advise women to closely follow labeled directions as they vary from product to product.

Spermicides have a high failure rate, especially during the first year of usage; 6 to 21 failures per 100 woman-years of use (Hardman, 2005). The vaginal foam appears to be the most effective spermicide and if it is used in combination with a condom or diaphragm, the efficacy of the product is increased (Hardman, 2005).

Clients should be educated that spermicides do not protect against sexually transmitted infections, including HIV. Although nonoxynol-9 appears to decrease viral replication of HIV in the test tube, studies have revealed it does not protect against HIV and in fact its use may increase the risk of HIV transmission because of irritation of tissues (Hardman, 2005).

• • •

Other OTC Drugs: A number of other product categories are available OTC; a wide array of topical skin protectants, corticosteroid, antifungal, and antibacterial products are available (see Chapter 65). Complementary and alternative therapies are discussed in Chapter 12, and a review of vitamins is presented in Chapter 67.

Summary

OTC, or nonprescription, drugs are medications that are safe for self-treating the symptoms of minor self-limiting illnesses without the supervision of a health care practitioner. Because these drugs are widely used and readily available, the nurse should be knowledgeable about a client's OTC drug practices and the drugs themselves. In addition to acquiring the skill to elicit information about such practices during the client's drug history, the nurse's knowledge of OTCs will assist in the guidance of clients on the safe self-administration of these medications. The most commonly used types of OTC medications are analgesics, antacids, laxatives, antidiarrheals, cough-cold preparations, and products for women's health.

Clients should be instructed to review the labels of OTC medications carefully before selection to ensure that the ingredients have proven to be safe and effective and are also safe for them to use (check warnings and contraindications). The nurse should advise the client to follow dosing instructions carefully and to be aware that many OTC medications do not contain a comprehensive list of possible drug interactions. Clients taking prescription drugs should consult with their prescriber before taking any OTC medication. OTC preparations that are used wisely can effectively treat many symptoms at a cost savings to the individual and the health care delivery system.

✸ Critical Thinking Questions

- While working at a local health care agency, a home health aide tells you that her two children are home from school with colds. She asks your advice about what type of OTC preparations would be best to use for treatment. How will you respond?
- Mae Stearns, age 72, comes to the physician's office for a routine health visit. While you are updating her health history, she states she has been getting constipated lately. What additional questions will you ask her? What will you say when she asks what type of OTC products for constipation would be most effective for her?

Bibliography

Anderson, D.M. (2002). *Mosby's medical, nursing, & allied health dictionary* (6th ed.). St. Louis: Mosby.

Brass, E.P. (2001). Drug therapy: Changing the status of drugs from prescription to over-the-counter availability. *New England Journal of Medicine, 345*(11), 810-816.

Carpenito-Moyet, L.J. (2004). *Nursing diagnosis: Application to clinical practice* (10th ed.). Philadelphia: Lippincott, Williams & Wilkins.

Casper, R.F. (2002). Epidemiology and pathogenesis of premenstrual dysphoric disorder. *UpToDate.* Wellesley, MA: UpToDate.

Consumer Healthcare Products Association. (2003). Ingredients and dosages transferred from Rx to OTC status by the FDA since 1975. Retrieved May 10, 2005, from http://www.chpa-info.org/web/advocacy/general_issues/switch/switch_list.pdf.

Dell, D. (2004). Premenstrual syndrome, premenstrual dysphoric disorder, and premenstrual exacerbation of another disorder. *Clinical Obstetrics & Gynecology, 47*(3), 568-575.

Drug facts and comparisons. (58th ed.). (2005). St. Louis: Facts and Comparisons.

Fitzgerald, W.L. (1994). Legal control of pharmacy services. In OBRA '90: A practical guide to effecting pharmaceutical care. Washington, DC: American Pharmaceutical Association.

Gittelman, A., Mahabee-Gittens, E.M., & Gonzalez-del-Rey, J. (2004). Common medical terms defined by parents: Are we speaking the same language? *Pediatric Emergency Care, 2*(11), 754-758.

Glover, D.O. (2004). Medication use in a rural gynecologic population: prescription, over-the-counter and herbal medications, *American Journal of Obstetrics & Gynecology, 190*(2), 351-357.

Hardman, J.L. (2005). Contraception. In M.A. Koda-Kimble, L.Y. Young, W.A. Kradian, B.J. Guglielmo, B.K. Alldredge, & R.L. Corelli. (Eds.). *Applied therapeutics: The clinical use of drugs* (8th ed.). Philadelphia: Lippincott Williams & Wilkins.

Hesselgrave, B. (1997). Will managed care embrace Rx-to-OTC product switches? Prescription drugs changing to non-prescription status. *Drug Topics.* 11(141), 13-17.

Hoogerwerf, W.A., & Pasricha, P.J. (2001). Agents used to control gastric acidity and treatment of peptic ulcers and gastroesophageal reflux disease. In J.G. Hardman & L.E. Limbird (Eds.), *Goodman & Gilman's the pharmacological basis of therapeutics* (10th ed.). New York: McGraw-Hill.

Jacobs, L.R. (1998). Prescription to over-the-counter drug reclassification. *American Family Physician.* Retrieved February 29, 2000, from http://home.aafp.org/afp/980501ap/jacobs.html

Klebanoff, M.A., Schwebke J.R., Zhang J., Nansel T.R., Yu, K.F., & Andrews, W.W. (2004). Vulvovaginal symptoms in women with bacterial vaginosis. *Obstetrics Gynecology, 104,* 267-272.

Lipinsky, M.S. (1999). The "prescription to OTC switch" movement: Its effects on antifungal vaginitis preparations. *Archives of Family Medicine, 8*(4), 297-300.

McCoy, L., Sorvillo, F., & Simon, P. (2004). Varicella-related mortality in California, 1988-2000. *Pediatric Infectious Disease Journal, 23*(6), 498-503.

National Council on Patient Information and Education. (2004). Retrieved July 27, 2005, from http://www.bemedwise.org/ten_ways/ten_ways.htm

Parent-Stevens, L., & Sagraves, R. (2005). Gynecologic and other disorders of women. In M.A. Koda-Kimble, L.Y. Young, W.A. Kradian, B.J. Guglielmo, B.K. Alldredge, & R.L. Corelli. (Eds.). *Applied therapeutics: The clinical use of drugs* (8th ed.). Philadelphia: Lippincott Williams & Wilkins.

Snyder, K. (1997). Trends driving switch-hitters: prescription drugs changing to over-the-counter status, *Drug Topic, 11*(141), 89-91.

Spruill, W.J., & Wade, W.E. (2002). Diarrhea, constipation and irritable bowel syndrome. In J.T. DiPiro, R.L. Talbert, G.C. Yee, G.R. Matzke, B.G. Wells, & L.M. Posey (Eds.), *Pharmacotherapy: A pathophysiologic approach* (5th ed.). New York: McGraw-Hill.

Sullivan, P.W., & Nichol, M.B. (2004). The economic impact of payer policies after the Rx-to-OTC switch of second-generation antihistamines. *Value Health, 7*(4), 402-412.

Tuijnan, A. (2000). *International adult literacy survey: Benchmarking adult literacy in America: An international comparative study.* Jessup, MD: United States Department of Education, Education Publications Center.

USP DI: Drug information for the health care professional (25th ed.) (2005). Greenwood Village, CO: MICROMEDEX Thomson Healthcare.

e-LEARNING SUPPLEMENTS

Student CD-ROM
- Final Exam questions
- NCLEX® Examination review questions
- Pharmacology animations
- Printable chapter summary

Evolve Website (http://evolve.elsevier.com/mckenry)
- Interactive concept map on osteoarthritis
- Content updates, including information on new drugs
- WebLinks corresponding to this chapter
- Answers to the critical thinking questions in this chapter
- *Elsevier ePharmacology Update* newsletter
- Mosby's Drug Consult Internet Edition
- Supplemental and reference information

COMPLEMENTARY AND ALTERNATIVE PHARMACOLOGY

CHAPTER FOCUS

Nearly half of Americans use "dietary supplements" (Bennett & Brown, 2000) and one quarter of adults report use of an herb to treat a medical illness within the last year (Bent & Ko, 2004). Individuals are increasingly proactive in promoting their own health and treating their own medical conditions. Eisenberg et al. (1998) found that the percentage of adults using herbs to treat medical conditions rose from 3% in 1990 to 12% in 1997. Use of complementary and alternative medicines (CAMs) among peri- and postmenopausal women has been reported as high as 79% (Mahady, Parrot, Lee, Yun, & Dan, 2003). A recent survey of surgical clients indicated that over half had used herbal medicine at some point in their lives, and over one third used herbal medicine within the past 2 years (Adusumilli, Ben-Porat, Pereira, Roesler, & Leitman, 2004). Although the estimated percentage of adults currently using CAM varies and depends on how the data was collected, it is clear that CAMs are used by a large and growing percentage of the population.

Seven of every ten clients who use alternative therapies do so without the physician's knowledge (Anderson, 1996). Health care professionals should be knowledgeable about alternative options to help guide the client through the array of options and use those that may be of benefit (Flaherty, 2000). This chapter will provide an understanding of the most common complementary and alternative substances taken to prevent and/or treat disease.

LEARNING OBJECTIVES

- Differentiate between allopathic medicine and complementary and alternative therapies.
- Describe the role of the National Center for Complementary and Alternative Medicine in evaluating complementary and alternative therapies.
- Explain the advantages and disadvantages of complementary and alternative therapies.
- Describe specific complementary and alternative therapies that might help or harm.
- Provide consumer information for clients taking complementary and alternative therapies.

▲ KEY TERMS

allopathic medicine, p. 220
complementary and alternative therapies, p. 220
homeopathy, p. 220

✱ How are complementary and alternative therapies different from other drugs?

Treating illness with a natural remedy, such as herbal products, dates back to the earliest records of humankind. All cultures have long histories of folk medicine that include the use of plants and other substances. Throughout history people have methodically and scientifically collected information on herbs and other medicinal materials and have maintained well-defined pharmacopeias. Many remedies of scientific medicine were derived from the herbal lore of native people well into the twentieth century. As medicine evolved in North America, plants continued to be a mainstay of rural medicine. Until the 1940s, textbooks of pharmacognosy—books that characterize plants as proven-by-use medications—contained hundreds of medically useful comments about barks, roots, berries, twigs, and flowers. Many drugs used today, such as aspirin, digoxin, vincristine, curare, and ergot, are of herbal origin.

As twentieth-century technology advanced and created an increasing admiration for technology, simple plant and water mixtures and other folk remedies were discarded by allopathic medicine. **Allopathic medicine** is the dominant medical culture of the Western world, a system of medical therapy in which a disease or abnormal condition is treated with active interventions, such as medical or surgical treatment, intended to bring about effects opposite from those produced by the disease or condition. Many therapies that fall outside of this scientific type of medicine are now considered alternative therapies. **Complementary and alternative therapies** are considered to encompass all health systems, modalities, and practices that are not intrinsic to the politically dominant health system. Although many modalities are considered complementary or alternative (e.g., homeopathy, massage, meditation, therapeutic touch, acupressure, bioelectromagnetic applications), the content of this chapter will focus on herbs and other substances, complementary/alternative medicines (CAMs), taken to promote health, prevent illness, relieve symptoms, and cure disease.

Under the law, manufacturers of dietary supplements are responsible for ensuring safety of their products before they go to market. They are also responsible for determining that the claims on their labels are accurate and truthful. Dietary supplement products are not reviewed by the government before they are marketed, but the Food and Drug Administration (FDA) has the responsibility to take action against any unsafe dietary supplement product that reaches the market. If the FDA can prove that claims on marketed dietary supplement products are false and misleading, the agency may take action against products with such claims (Food and Drug Administration, 2002). The growing interest in herbal and other remedies by North Americans has prompted a reevaluation of their safety, efficacy, and role in health care.

Homeopathy is a system of therapeutics based on the theory that "like cures like"—if a large amount of medicine produced symptoms of a disease, then a small amount may reduce those symptoms. Only the smallest amount of the drug necessary to control the symptoms is prescribed, and only one drug is prescribed at a time. In Europe, homeopathy represents a substantial portion of the over-the-counter (OTC) market (D'Huyvetter & Cohrssen, 2002). European physicians more commonly practice homeopathy, more than 10,000 French and German physicians use homeopathy as part of their practice (Vickers & Zollman, 1999).

Mainstream medical practitioners in North America are trained to prescribe medicines, the compositions of which are well defined and their safety and efficacy have been established in scientifically designed tests and trials. Physicians who have spent years studying physiology and biochemistry tend at best to be uneasy about substances such as herbs, enzymes, and extracts from plant and animal sources. Although traditional healers, homeopathic physicians, and non-Western medical practitioners have administered many of these substances for years to hundreds of thousands of sick people, the composition of each preparation can vary enormously and may not be as effective for some individuals as for others. There is a need for well-designed random controlled trials (RCTs) to prove the efficacy of CAM therapies before there can be greater acceptance by health care providers (Hoffer, 2003).

✱ T.L. is a 28-year-old secretary who calls the office of her physician for general advice regarding a news story she heard that drug supplements are not safe. The office nurse is given the responsibility to respond to her concerns.

✱ How are complementary and alternative therapies evaluated for safety and efficacy?

Many alternative therapies in common use have little scientific data to support their claims. Until recently, the research that has been done was performed in Europe, India, China, and Japan, where herbal and other alternative therapies are more widely accepted. The German E Commission, a German governmental regulatory agency similar to the United States' Food and Drug Administration, was established in 1978 to evaluate the usefulness of herbal products. Although their evaluation process is different than that of the FDA, it evaluated over 300 herbal products and found about two thirds of these products had merit.

In North America, considerable interest has been given to complementary and alternative approaches to mainstream medicine. As public interest has grown, some allopathic prescribers have become interested in learning about alternative treatments, what benefits are claimed, the potential risks, and the physiologic effects of the ingredients. Some prescribers are attempting to submit such substances to the same rigorous study as other pharmaceutical agents.

To support this interest, the Office of Alternative Medicine (OAM) was established at the National Institutes of Health (NIH) in 1992 and became the National Center for Complementary and Alternative Medicine (NCCAM) in 1999. The NCCAM is 1 of the 27 institutes and centers that make up the NIH.

The role of NCCAM is "to explore complementary and alternative healing practices in the context of rigorous science, train CAM researchers, and disseminate authoritative information to the public and professionals" (http://nccam.nih.gov/).

Part of the problem lies in defining CAM therapies. "CAM is a group of diverse medical and health care systems, practices, and products that are not presently considered to be part of conventional medicine—that is, medicine as practiced by holders of MD (medical doctor) or DO (doctor of osteopathy) degrees and their allied health professionals, such as physical therapists, psychologists, and registered nurses. In CAM, **complementary** medicine is used **together with** conventional medicine, and **alternative** medicine is used **in place of** conventional medicine" (http://nccam.nih.gov/).

The NCCAM is attempting not to be exclusionary in nature. It is considering a broad interpretation of alternative therapies including "approaches from nutritional and lifestyle changes to hypnotherapy, acupressure, chelation therapy, and bioelectromagnetic applications such as magnetoresonance spectroscopy and blue light treatment."

In 2003, although NCCAM funding continued to support research in the area of such modalities of acupuncture, massage, yoga, placebo therapy, chiropractic, and Vedic medicine, a significant proportion of the support went for continuing research into ginkgo biloba, ginger, black cohosh, Panax ginseng, garlic, St. John's wort, phytoestrogens, echinacea, and other herbal and antioxidant therapies.

The NCCAM serves as a clearinghouse of information for the alternative health community by sponsoring research and programs for grant writing and clinical research and by maintaining a network within the NIH and other government agencies for collaboration. Although the NCCAM cannot serve as a referral agency or advise individual clients, it does provide information about specific therapies. It also provides contact names for organizations that represent different types of treatments and individual fact sheets on issues and events.

As a result of the establishment of a federal office for alternative therapy, the allopathic medical community is reconsidering its position toward understanding the alternative therapies and their benefits. Many U.S. medical schools now offer courses in alternative therapy, and NCCAM has more than 30 research centers around the United States for the study of complementary and alternative therapies. Nurses should also understand these alternative modalities sufficiently so they can respond to clients' questions or direct them to appropriate sources of information. Given the range of alternative therapies, this chapter will consider only biologically based therapies with a focus on the adult, and only the most commonly used substances will be discussed. There is a lack of good information available regarding the safety and efficacy of many of these therapies for children and for pregnant or lactating women. Use in such clients requires an extra measure of caution.

✳ How are complementary and alternative therapies regulated?

Clients who wish to use alternative therapy need to be aware that currently there is no guarantee about these medications. Under the Dietary Supplement Health and Education Act of 1994, a new category of substances has been created that is distinct from food or drugs. This category includes vitamins, herbs, amino acids, and any other substance sold as a supplement before October 15, 1994. Manufacturers of these remedies are not required to test for standardization, safety, or efficacy, which is routine for regular drugs. As a consequence, there is no way to be sure of the following: (1) the active ingredients, whatever they might be, have actually ended up in the tablets or other dosage form; (2) the ingredient is in a form usable by the body; (3) the dosage is appropriate; (4) there are no other ingredients in the tablets; (5) the tablets are safe; or (6) the next bottle of tablets will have the same ingredients. Figure 12-1 illustrates the lack of standardization of ginseng, one of these alternative products. Similar findings have been observed with other complementary and alternative therapies (Gilroy, Steiner, Byers, Shapiro, & Georgian, 2003).

This lack of standardization also applies to home preparation of herbal remedies. The efficacy of herbal prepara-

Product (listed alphabetically)	Ginseng per capsule*	Ginsenosides per capsule†	Concentration† (percentage ginsenoside)
American Ginseng	250 mg	12.8 mg	
Ginsana (extract)	100	3.0	
Herbal Choice Ginseng-7 (extract)	100	6.5	
KRG Korean Red Ginseng	518	11.5	
Natural Brand Korean Ginseng	648	23.2	
Naturally Korean Ginseng	648	2.3	
Nature's Resource Ginseng	560	10.7	
Rite Aid Imperial Ginseng	250	0.4	
Solgar Korean Ginseng (extract)	520	10.6	
Walgreen's Gin-zing (extract)	100	7.6	

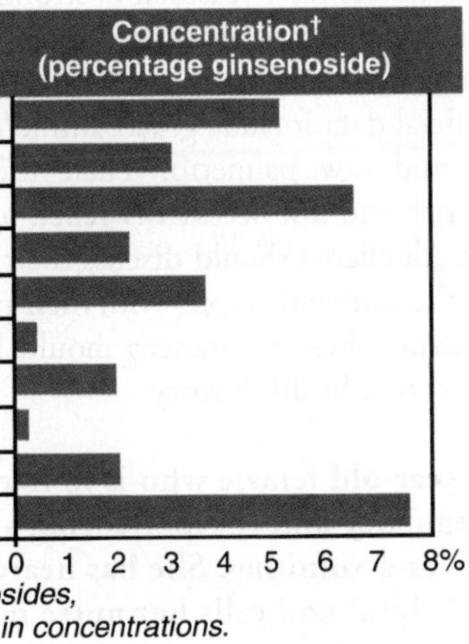

⚹ *According to label*
⊞ *Based on six major ginsenosides. Estimates for two other ginsenosides, if added, would boost totals only slightly and not change variation in concentrations.*

0 1 2 3 4 5 6 7 8%

FIGURE 12-1 Variations of total "ginsenoside" in 10 brands of ginseng. The amounts of ginseng found in the products in this chart were learned as a result of Consumers Union's test, not as reported by the manufacturers or distributors.

tions depends on the ailment and the quality and dose of the preparation used. Efficacy cannot be determined with the home preparation of herbs because the quality and dose of the preparation is unknown. Many herbal preparations, particularly tinctures, may also contain alcohol, which poses a risk for those driving or operating machinery.

There is also concern that complementary and alternative therapies may be harmful. Their use may delay the individual from seeking medical consultation for a condition that warrants allopathic medicine. There is also concern that the preparations have no efficacy and so are a waste of effort and money or that they may actually be toxic. Some Chinese herbal medications have been found to be contaminated with a variety of substances: undeclared prescription drugs such as nonsteroidal antiinflammatory drugs (mefenamic acid, phenylbutazone), benzodiazepines, anticholinergics, corticosteroids, or ephedrine (Ernst, 2002a); aconitine (a family of plants that have medicinal and poisonous properties); heavy metals (mercury, arsenic, lead) (Ko, 1998; Saper et al., 2004); pesticides or other deleterious substances (De Smet, 2002).

In 2003, the FDA proposed expanded oversight of the safety, manufacturing, and labeling of dietary supplements in conjunction with the Federal Trade Commission's role in regulating advertising of these products. In a proposed rule, increased emphasis on utilizing good manufacturing practices in the preparation of dietary supplements would be required, including requirements on facilities that manufacture these products, quality controls in manufacturing, packaging and labeling, and requirements for testing (Taylor, 2003b).

For the remainder of this chapter, agents will be classified according to how beneficial or dangerous therapy is likely to be based on published and unpublished data. Discussion will also include agents in which, despite clear pharmacologic data for clinical effects, the role in therapy is not clear. Finally, discussion will include agents for which evidence is lacking regarding their safe and effective use.

✳ Which commonly used agents are considered potentially beneficial?

A number of substances have reasonably strong evidence to support beneficial physiologic properties and are the subject of further research. Some of the more common agents that have some beneficial data include glucosamine/chondroitin, ginger, ginkgo, and saw palmetto. Their use should be weighed against risk and not necessarily relied on for regular medical therapy. All clients should discuss their use of complementary and alternative therapies with their prescriber. As with any other drug, these substances should be discussed within the context of a health history.

✳ P.L. is a 22-year-old female who is in her first trimester of pregnancy and is experiencing significant morning nausea and vomiting. She has heard that ginger tea may be helpful and calls her nurse midwife for advice.

ginger (*Zingiber officinale* **[sheng jiang])** Ginger is a culinary spice that has been used for medicinal purposes since ancient times. Ginger is recommended to stimulate digestion and to relieve nausea and aches and pains. The presumed active ingredient in ginger is 8-gingerlol, and serves as a functional antagonist at ileal 5-hydroxytryptamine receptors. It improves the digestion of protein, strengthens the mucosal lining of the upper gastrointestinal (GI) tract and therefore protects against ulcers.

Efficacy of Ginger in Postoperative Nausea and Vomiting Use in preventing postoperative nausea and vomiting is conflicting. Phillips, Ruggier, and Hutchinson (1993) studied 120 women presenting for elective laparoscopic gynecologic surgery on a day-stay basis and found ginger to be superior to placebo and equally effective as metoclopramide (Reglan); there was no difference in the requirements for postoperative analgesia, recovery time, and time until discharge. A later study (Eberhart et al., 2003) noted no difference in nausea or vomiting in 184 women undergoing gynecologic laparoscopic procedures who received either placebo, or 300 mg or 600 mg of ginger extract.

Efficacy of Ginger in Nausea and Vomiting of Pregnancy The antiemetic properties of ginger may be considered as an alternative for treating the nausea and vomiting of pregnancy. In one short-term trial, 70 women with pregnancy related nausea and vomiting were randomized to either 1 gram of ginger per day or placebo for 4 days (Vutyavanich, Kraisarin, & Ruangsri, 2001). Nausea symptoms and vomiting episodes were significantly reduced in women who received ginger. No adverse effects on pregnancy were identified in this small study. Other studies have also demonstrated the efficacy of ginger in the nausea and vomiting of pregnancy (Portnoi et al., 2003; Niebyl & Goodwin, 2002). A meta-analysis by Ernst and Pittler (2000) concluded that the studies collectively favored ginger over placebo for the treatment of nausea and vomiting of pregnancy.

Efficacy for Other Indications Antiemetic efficiency as an adjunct to cancer chemotherapy is controversial and requires further research (Boon & Wong, 2004). Lien, Sun, Chen, Hasler, and Owyang (2003) report the reduction of nausea in induced motion sickness.

Adverse Effects No adverse effects have been noted with therapeutic doses, but the potential to inhibit clotting does exist (Heck, DeWill, & Lukes, 2000). There is evidence that ginger modulates the synthesis of eicosanoid (prostaglandins, thromboxanes, and leukotrienes) in ways that reduce abnormal inflammation and clotting. It may be as effective as some of the nonsteroidal antiinflammatory drugs (NSAIDs) while also protecting the stomach lining rather than damaging it as the NSAIDs sometimes do. The antiinflammatory effects of ginger may have an inhibitory effect on skin tumor promotion (Park, Chun, Lee, Less, & Surh, 1998).

Formulations Ginger comes in a variety of forms, from fresh rhizome to candied pieces to encapsulated, dried, and powdered ginger. The average dose is 1 to 4 grams. It is considered to be nontoxic, but some individuals may experience heartburn if large amounts of raw ginger are taken on an empty stomach; it should be taken with food. There is some controversy about the use of ginger in pregnancy because of its abortifacient effects, but this effect has not been documented in humans. A review of the literature found no reason for contraindicating ginger during pregnancy when it is taken at the usual therapeutic dose, although further research is warranted (Borrelli et al., 2005).

✳ **P.S. is a 74-year-old male whose wife has moderately severe Alzheimer's-type dementia. He hears an advertisement on television for a dietary supplement with ginkgo and asks the visiting nurse whether it would help his wife.**

ginkgo (*Ginkgo biloba* L.) The *G. biloba* leaf, its extract, or purified mixtures of ginkgolides are contained in many herbal preparations.

Efficacy of Ginkgo for Memory Enhancement Less well controlled trials (e.g., open label trials in which everyone is aware of who receives treatment) suggest ginkgo is effective for improving memory. More rigorous analyses find limited evidence that ginkgo improved cognitive function over 24 to 26 weeks compared with placebo in people with Alzheimer's disease or vascular dementia (LeBars, Kieser, & Itil, 2000). A review of 50 studies (with meta-analysis of the four strongest studies) identified ginkgo as producing only modest (3%) improvement is cognition for individuals with Alzheimer's-type dementia (Birks, Grimley, & Van Dongen, 2002).

Efficacy of Ginkgo for Intermittent Claudication Clinical data based on double-blind clinical trials using matched client groups with peripheral arterial insufficiency have demonstrated the clinical efficacy of a standardized extract of *G. biloba*. Significant improvements in pain-free walking time and maximum walking distance were achieved (Peters, Kieser, & Holscher, 1998). A meta-analysis (study involving combining data from smaller similar studies) of eight randomized placebo-controlled double-blind trials noted that ginkgo extract resulted in modest, but definite improvement in pain free walking distance with only rare, mild and transient adverse effects (Pittler & Ernst, 2000b).

Adverse Effects Ginkgo leaf extract is usually well tolerated, although occasional bleeding complications are reported as noted above. Mild GI disturbances may be minimized by slowly titrating the ginkgo dose. Contact with and ingestion of the fruit pulp has produced severe allergic reactions and should not be handled or ingested. The seed of the plant also causes severe adverse effects when ingested. Use of ginkgo has also been associated with increased bleeding risk (Rowin & Lewis, 1996), although standardized extracts of ginkgo have not been associated with altered bleeding or coagulation times (Kohler, Funk, & Kieser, 2004).

Formulations Ginkgo products are usually standardized at 24% flavonoids and 6% terpenes. The daily dose of standardized ginkgo leaf extract is 120 to 160 mg.

✳ **L.C. is a 39-year-old postal worker who walks about 7 miles each day covering her postal route. She complains of frequent knee pain and her health care provider diagnoses early osteoarthritis. She is considering starting glucosamine/chondroitin and asks the office nurse for his impression on whether it is beneficial.**

Glucosamine Glucosamine is an amino sugar naturally found in the body and isolated from crab, lobster, and shrimp shells. It is a building block used in the biosynthesis of glycosaminoglycans and proteoglycans, important constituents of articular cartilage. It is often combined with chondroitin for the treatment of osteoarthritis, particularly osteoarthritis of the knee.

Efficacy of Glucosamine for Osteoarthritis Meta-analysis of six well-designed studies evaluating glucosamine in knee osteoarthritis revealed improvement in symptoms (McAlindon, LaValley, Gulin, & Felson, 2000). Glucosamine may alter the pathologic progression of osteoarthritis. In a 3-year evaluation, glucosamine sulfate resulted in significantly less joint space loss compared to placebo in individuals with knee osteoarthritis over 50 years of age (Reginster et al., 2001).

Chondroitin Chondroitin is a large proteoglycan derived from shark cartilage and is responsible for giving cartilage elasticity. Chondroitin is often combined with glucosamine in the treatment of osteoarthritis.

Efficacy of Chondroitin for Osteoarthritis Like glucosamine, meta-analysis of chondroitin has demonstrated improved symptoms in the treatment of knee osteoarthritis (McAlindon et al., 2000). Unlike glucosamine, a 3-year placebo controlled trial of chondroitin sulfate 400 mg three times daily for 3 years in 165 clients with hand osteoarthritis did not reveal any changes in joint space (Verbruggen, Goemaere, & Veys, 2002).

Safety Both glucosamine and chondroitin are considered safe, although glucosamine has been associated with allergic reactions in individuals with shellfish or iodine allergies. However, the latest research suggests that people with seafood allergy usually can take glucosamine without a problem because glucosamine comes from shrimp, crab, and lobster. It comes from the shells, and the allergens are usually in the meat of the seafood. Tell clients to watch for allergic signs, but it is usually safe for seafood-allergic people to use glucosamine (Gray, Hutcheson, & Slavin, 2004). Although theoretical changes in serum glucose have been suggested, glucosamine has not resulted in clinically significant changes when used in clients with diabetes (Tessier, 2002).

Formulations Glucosamine is available as both a hydrochloride and sulfate salt. Most data has been conducted with a dose of glucosamine sulfate 500 mg three times daily. Chondroitin is typically available as a sulfate salt in doses of 400 mg three times daily, and is often combined with glucosamine.

✱ **P.C. is a 78-year-old male with benign prostatic hyperplasia (BPH) with significant nocturia. He awakens on average three times per night to urinate, and finds it difficult to initiate a urine stream. He asks his nurse if there are any nonprescription therapies that might help.**

saw palmetto Saw palmetto inhibits five α-reductase isoenzymes, dihydrotestosterone binding in prostate cells, and α_1-adrenergic receptor antagonism. Among other effects, it reduces cell proliferation in prostatic cells and is used to relieve urinary symptoms for older men with BPH (De Smet, 2002; Zi & Agarwal, 1999).

Efficacy in Urinary Symptoms of Benign Prostatic Hyperplasia A double blind randomized 6-month trial of saw palmetto resulted in moderate improvement in urinary symptoms without significant adverse effects or sexual dysfunction (Gerber, Kuznetsov, Johnson, & Burstein, 2001). Large randomized controlled trials with standard interventions, finasteride, or tamsulosin, suggest similar effects with saw palmetto (Debruyne et al., 2002; Carraro et al., 1996). Systematic reviews have also revealed similar conclusions (De Smet, 2002; saw palmetto/www.usp.org; Ernst, 2002b; Wilt et al., 2001).

Safety Most evaluations identify few if any significant adverse effects with saw palmetto therapy (Gerber et al., 2001). One case report of interoperative bleeding and altered bleeding times related to saw palmetto has been described (Cheema, El-Mefty, & Jazieh, 2001).

Formulations Various formulations for saw palmetto are available, with typical doses in most studies at 160 mg twice daily or 320 mg once daily.

✱ **P.F. is a visiting nurse who is requested by the local senior citizen's group to discuss complementary and alternative therapies that might be dangerous.**

✱ **Which frequently used agents are considered dangerous?**
Over the past few years, more widespread use of complementary and alterative medications has yielded additional data and experience. With additional reports, and more careful FDA scrutiny, some therapies have been identified as dangerous. These include chaparral, comfrey, ephedra, kava, lobelia, and yohimbe.

chaparral Chaparral, a desert shrub, is sold as a tea, tablet, and capsule for its antioxidant properties. Chaparral was removed from the FDA's "generally recognized as safe" list in 1970 after animal studies revealed damage to kidney and lymph organs. Four reports of liver toxicity occurred in 1992, which prompted the FDA to warn against the use of any product containing chaparral (News you can use, 1995). In addition to these U.S. cases, three cases have been reported in Canada (Food and Drug Administration, 1993). The National Nutritional Foods Association has asked its member companies not to carry these products, but chaparral is still being sold and sometimes is an ingredient in combination products.

comfrey Comfrey, an herb, is sold as a tea, tablet, capsule, tincture, poultice, and lotion. It has been linked to a number of cases of liver impairment, and studies with animals demonstrate injury to lung, kidney, and GI tissue. Australia, Canada, Germany, and the United Kingdom restrict the availability of comfrey.

ephedra (ma huang) Ephedra has historically been promoted for energy boosting and weight control. It possesses sympathomimetic activity, which causes vasoconstriction and may increase blood pressure and cause cardiac dysrhythmias. Significant reports of cardiovascular events, cerebrovascular events, and deaths prompted a more close evaluation of the role of ephedra (Shekelle et al., 2003). Reports from poison control centers and reports to the FDA in 2002 and 2003 indicated increasing life-threatening events associated with ephedra (Bent, Tiedt, Odden, & Shlipak, 2003). In early 2003, the FDA issued a regulation prohibiting the sale of ephedra in the United States (*FDA News*, 2004).

kava (*Piper methysticum*) Kava is derived from a Pacific island shrub. When ingested, it produces anxiolytic properties and has an affinity for gamma amino butyric acid (GABA) receptors. It appears to inhibit norepinephrine reuptake, antagonizes dopamine, and inhibits monoamine oxidase (MAO). It does not appear to have action at benzodiazepine or opioid receptors (Assemi, 2001). Although data have identified reductions in anxiety compared to placebo (Pittler & Ernst, 2000a), reports of serious hepatotoxicity and hepatic failure have resulted in removal of this drug from many European markets (Estes et al., 2003).

lobelia (*Lobelia inflata* [Indian Tobacco]) The lobelia leaf yields lobeline sulfate, which acts like nicotine and may be used as antitobacco therapy. It acts as an agonist at nicotine receptors both peripherally and centrally. Lobelia produces behavioral stimulation and depression, cardiac acceleration, peripheral vasoconstriction, and elevated blood pressure. It is contraindicated for use in individuals with unstable cardiovascular conditions such as angina, dysrhythmias, postmyocardial infarction, and hypertension.

yohimbe (*Corynanthe yohimbe*) Yohimbe is a plant product made from the bark of an African tree; it is generally touted as an aphrodisiac for men. Its active ingredient, yohimbine, is used for the treatment of erectile impotence, but neither the United States nor Canada include that as an indication for its use in its package labeling. In some individuals it has caused increased blood pressure and heart rate, dizziness, headache, irritability, or nervousness. Documentation of the usefulness of yohimbe to treat impotence is inconclusive; it is likely unsafe (Jellin, Batz, & Hitchens, 1999).

✴ For which common agents are roles in therapy less clear?

A number of agents produce some beneficial effects, but ongoing evaluation is underway to determine their role in therapy. In some circumstances, data is variable and not consistent (e.g., co-enzyme Q-10, Echinacea, St. John's wort); in others, a clear benefit is observed, but the degree of benefit is relatively small or debated (e.g., garlic, red yeast rice). In some cases, the risk is unclear and may not be worth the benefit (e.g., valerian).

✴ K.P. is a 67-year-old woman with moderately severe heart failure (HF). She is being treated with standard medical therapy, including an angiotensin converting enzyme (ACE) inhibitor and a diuretic to manage fluid balance and improve cardiac functioning. She reads an article in the paper about the wonders of co-enzyme Q10 and asks the office nurse whether she should start taking it.

co-enzyme Q10 Co-enzyme Q10 is a naturally occurring substance in muscle cells and appears to play a central role in mitochondrial oxidative phosphorylation. It also serves as an antioxidant. These actions have prompted extensive study of co-enzyme Q10 in cardiovascular and neurologic conditions in which lipid peroxidation is believed to play a role. Initial studies with Q10 were conducted in Japan in the 1970s and noted that concentrations of coenzyme Q10 are decreased in myocardial cells of clients with advanced heart failure and the degree of Q10 deficiency correlates with the severity of heart failure.

Efficacy of Co-enzyme Q10 in Heart Failure A number of Japanese clinical reports (most uncontrolled) described favorable effects of coenzyme Q10 in HF. Based on this data, the Japanese government approved coenzyme Q10 for the treatment of HF in 1974 (Khatta et al., 2000).

More recent data analysis with more rigorous methodology has resulted in mixed conclusions. A randomized trial of the effect of Q10 on 322 clients with advanced HF noted significantly less pulmonary edema and hospitalization with 2 mg/kg/day therapy for 1 year compared to placebo, but no difference in mortality was observed (Morisco, Trimaro, & Condorelli, 1993). In a randomized, double-blind trial of Q10 200 mg daily had no influence on oxygen consumption, exercise duration, or ejection fraction in 55 clients receiving therapy (Khatta et al., 2000). At this time, these findings are inconclusive to make recommendations on their use for these indications.

Efficacy of Co-enzyme Q10 for Other Indications One study noted decrease in angina in 144 Indian clients who received 120 mg daily for 4 weeks after acute myocardial in-

farction (Singh et al., 1998). Preliminary data suggests that very high dose of Q10 (600 to 1200 mg daily) may offer some benefit for early Parkinson's disease (Shults et al., 2002).

✴ P.L. is a 19-year-old college sophomore who reports to the college health service three weeks into the start of the semester with runny nose, watery eyes, chest congestion, and a cough. She is only mildly febrile, and asks whether she should take *Echinacea* to treat her cold and to prevent future colds.

echinacea (purple cornflower) *Echinacea*, an herb, is used as a general immunity booster. It was one of the most popular plant drugs in North America until the advent of sulfa drugs in the 1930s, and it has remained an active part of folk medicine. In Europe, clinicians use *Echinacea* preparations as preventatives and treatments for colds and flu.

Efficacy of Echinacea to Prevent or Treat Viral Infection
In laboratory tests, *Echinacea* increased the number of immune system cells and developing cells in bone marrow and lymphatic tissue, and it seemed to speed their development into immunocompetent cells.

In more than 350 studies, most of them conducted in Europe, *Echinacea* seems to stimulate the immune system nonspecifically rather than act against specific organisms. A critical review of five of these studies by Melchart et al. (1995) identified only three randomized, placebo-controlled clinical trials of mono-preparations (e.g., preparations in which *Echinacea* was not combined with other substances). Two of these studies determined that an extract of the root of the plant had a positive effect on the symptoms of upper respiratory tract infections, and the other study demonstrated a slight reduction in the risk of infection. There are an additional 15 randomized trials of antineoplastic therapies in the treatment and prevention of infections or in the reduction of undesirable effects; 13 of these studies claim to have positive results (Melchart et al., 1995).

More recent evaluations have not supported the benefits of *Echinacea*. In an evaluation of *Echinacea* in 40 healthy male volunteers age 20 to 40 years, two 14-day treatments of freshly expressed Echinacea juice had no effect of phagocytic activity or polymorphonuclear leukocyte or monocyte activity, and did not influence tumor necrosis factor (TNF)—alpha or interluken-1 (Schwarz et al., 2002). A randomized, double-blind, placebo controlled trial of 1 gram of *Echinacea* six times daily for 10 days in 148 college students with recent onset common cold yielded no significant differences in severity or duration of upper respiratory symptoms (Barrett et al., 2002). In a study of 524 children aged 2 to 11 years, no difference between *Echinacea* and placebo was noted for duration of symptoms, severity, number of days of fever, or parental assessment of infection (Taylor et al., 2003a). No significant difference in rhinovirus infections were noted in an additional evaluation of *Echinacea* in 48 healthy adults (Sperber, Shah, Gilbert, Ritchey, & Monto, 2004).

Safety Reports of significant immunoglobulin E (IgE)-mediated hypersensitivity reactions to *Echinacea* in Australia including anaphylaxis, angioedema, and asthma have raised awareness that serious toxicity with this product is possible (Mullins & Heddle, 2002). A study in 524 children (noted above) identified a higher risk for rash with *Echinacea* compared to placebo (Taylor et al., 2003a). *Echinacea* is contraindicated for progressive diseases such as infectious or autoimmune diseases, including tuberculosis, lupus, multiple sclerosis, acquired immunodeficiency syndrome (AIDS), and infections with human immunodeficiency virus (HIV). The herb may also interfere with immunosuppressive therapy used to treat rheumatoid arthritis and Crohn's disease and to prevent transplanted organ rejection.

✳ **T.S. is an active, nonobese 54-year-old male with moderately elevated cholesterol. His low density lipoprotein (LDL) level is modestly elevated at 135 mg/dL and his high density lipoprotein (HDL) level is low normal at 40 mg/dL. He presents with no cardiovascular history, has a blood pressure of 125/70, is a nonsmoker, and he is not a diabetic. His drug therapy is limited to a multivitamin once daily and occasional use of ibuprofen for headaches. He asks his health care provider whether the addition of garlic or red yeast rice may help his cholesterol. (Also refer to Chapter 31 for a discussion of goal lipid levels and treatments.)**

garlic (*Allium sativum* [da suan]) Garlic has long been used as a flavoring in many of the world cuisines and as a substance with healing properties in many folk medicine traditions. The major component of garlic is alliin; when garlic is crushed, alliin is converted to allicin, the pharmacologically active ingredient. Alliin must be converted to allicin to be effective. Because alliin is unstable in gastric fluid, the best commercial preparations are enteric-coated or capsule forms. The recommended daily dose of alliin is approximately 8 mg, the equivalent of one clove of garlic. Garlic may have a wide range of health benefits, enough to justify its use as a general tonic.

Efficacy for Clients with Hyperlipidemia Garlic has far-reaching effects on the cardiovascular system. It is used primarily to decrease serum cholesterol levels. As Warshafsky, Kamer, and Sivak reported in the *Annals of Internal Medicine* (1993), a meta-analysis of the controlled trials of garlic to reduce hypercholesteremia showed a significant reduction in total cholesterol levels. The best available evidence suggests that garlic, in an amount approximating one half to 1 clove per day, decreased total serum cholesterol levels by approximately 9% in the groups of individuals studied. A meta-analysis of randomized, double-blind, placebo-controlled trials by Stevinson and Ernst (2000) concluded that garlic is superior to placebo in reducing total cholesterol levels. But in a double-blind, placebo-controlled treatment trial, it was found that garlic did not significantly affect plasma lipid levels (Gardner, Chatterjee, & Carlson, 2001).

Efficacy of Garlic for Other Indications In a review of 30 studies of garlic's hypotensive effects, only three of them demonstrated that decrease to be statistically significant (Ackerman et al., 2001). One of the therapeutic actions of garlic includes inhibition of platelet aggregation, which reduces the clotting tendency of blood and may prevent heart attacks and stroke. This effect may account for the many reports in the literature cautioning about an increased risk of bleeding in persons undergoing surgery (Muluk & Macpherson, 2004; Steiner & Lin, 2001). Clients who are taking drugs with anticoagulant effects (e.g., warfarin and aspirin) should be cautioned about garlic dietary supplements (Rozenfeld, Sisca, Callahan, & Crain, 2000).

Garlic also acts as an antiinfective, counteracting the growth of many types of bacteria that cause disease in humans (Ankri & Mirelman, 1999). There is also interest in garlic for its antiviral activity. In one double-blind, placebo-controlled study, Josling (2001) found an allicin-containing garlic supplement beneficial in preventing attack by the common cold virus. But, further research is required before the antiviral activity of garlic can be substantiated.

After reviewing the strengths and weaknesses of 60 studies related to the antitumorigenic effects of garlic, Dorant, van den Brandt, Goldbohn, Hermus, and Sturmans (1993) concluded in the *British Journal of Cancer* that laboratory experiments and epidemiologic studies have not provided conclusive evidence of the preventive activity of garlic. However, study continues into the possible immune enhancing and anticancer effects of its sulfur containing compounds as a preventive against stomach, colon, bladder and other types of cancers (Thomson & Ali, 2003; Kamat & Lamm, 2002; Dong, Lisk, Block, & Ip, 2001; Kyo, Uda, Kasuga, & Itakura, 2001).

red yeast rice (*Monascus purpureus*) The yeast *Monascus purpureus*, when grown on rice and fermented and dried, results in a product that dates back to 800 A.D. in China and is associated with cholesterol-lowering properties. Red yeast rice, prepared and manufactured as Cholestin, demonstrates hydroxymethylglutaryl coenzyme-A (HMG-CoA) reductase inhibition and is pharmacologically similar to the most commonly used class of drugs used for the treatment of elevated cholesterol levels (the "statins") (Hermann, 2002).

Efficacy in Hyperlipidemia A randomized double-blind trial of 2.4 grams per day of Cholestin in 82 clients with elevated LDL (greater than 160 mg/dL) noted reductions of total cholesterol of approximately 15% and LDL cholesterol of 22% (Heber et al., 1999).

Safety Like the commercially available HMG-CoA reductase inhibitors ("statins"), red yeast rice inhibits cytochrome P450 3 A4 activity and is likely to activate a number of clinically significant drug interactions. Further study is warranted (Prasad, Wong, Meliton, & Bhaloo, 2002).

✳ **T.J. is a 43-year-old female who has been feeling "blue" and not sleeping well over the past month. She** hears from a friend that St. John's wort and valerian may help her symptoms, and asks the nurse for advice during a wellness visit.

St. John's wort (Hypericum perforatum) St. John's wort, a flowering perennial plant, has been used medicinally for hundreds of years and has most recently been identified as an effective treatment for mild to moderate depression. Extract of Hypericum, the reference substance for pharmaceutical standardization, is widely used in Europe, especially Germany. It has been used for excitability, neuralgia, and specifically for menopausal neurosis (Newall, Anderson, & Phillipson, 1996).

Efficacy of St. John's Wort in Depression An overview and meta-analysis of randomized clinical trials from 1979 to 1996 concluded that such extracts are more effective than a placebo for the treatment of depressive disorders; however, it is not known whether they are more effective for certain disorders than others (Linde, Ramirez, Mulrow, Pauls, & Weidenhammer, 1996). Since that study, others have presented conflicting results. Some studies have concluded that St. John's wort has results equivalent to those of many antidepressant drugs and has a much more favorable incidence of adverse effects (Szegedi et al., 2005; Lecrubier, Clerc, Didi, & Kieser, 2002; Kalb, Trautmann-Sponsel, & Kieser, 2001; Philipp, Kohnen, & Hiller, 1999), although others have identified no difference between St. John's wort and placebo (Hypericum Depression Trial Study Group, 2002; Shelton et al., 2001). These differences have fueled debate regarding the definition of depression treated, identification of the active ingredient or ingredients, and standardization of preparations used. Additional trials should be conducted to investigate the long-term adverse effects and relative efficacy of different preparations and doses. The NCCAM (2005) indicated that St. John's wort may be useful for treating mild to moderate depression but is of no benefit in treating major depression of moderate severity. In a meta-analysis by Linde et al., the Cochrane Review (2005) concluded that the current evidence regarding St. John's wort extract is inconsistent and confusing, particularly given the pharmaceutical quality of the preparations currently available.

Safety Some individuals experience adverse effects similar to that seen with other antidepressants including restlessness, GI upset, and cardiovascular effects (De Smet, 2002). Delayed hypersensitivity or photodermatitis has been documented for St. John's wort following the ingestion of an herbal tea made from the leaves. Individuals taking this herb should be warned to avoid direct sunlight and to wear SPF 15 sunscreen lotion. In view of the lack of toxicity data and documented photosensitizing activity, excessive use of St. John's wort should be avoided.

Interactions with other drugs are likely. The combination of St. John's wort with other antidepressants can lead to of the potentially fatal serotonin syndrome. St. John's wort is a potent inducer of cytochrome P450 3 A4 and is likely to interact significantly with a great number of drugs, including hormonal contraceptives, medications for HIV disease, cholesterol-lowering drugs ("statins") and many other agents (Markowitz et al., 2003; Zhou, Chan, Pan, Huang, & Lee, 2004).

valerian (Valeriana officinalis) Valerian, an herb, is used for sleep problems and probably has mild sedating and tranquilizing effects. The medicinal use of this plant has been recorded since ancient Greek and Roman times. Although it is an attractive plant with pink and white flowers, even the Roman physician Galen noted its objectionable odor. The root and the rhizome of the plant are used for therapeutic effect. The root contains the volatile oil (valerianic acid) and valepotriate fractions, which have a calming effect (Jellin, Batz, & Hitchens, 1999). Valerian is used extensively in Europe where it is accepted by allopathic medicine. Valerian appears to affect reuptake of GABA and has an affinity for serotonin receptors (Stevinson & Ernst, 2000).

Efficacy in Insomnia Many studies have indicated that valerian not only eases the trouble of falling asleep but also improves the quality of sleep during the night. It seems to offer the benefit of a good night's sleep without the grogginess that accompanies some over-the-counter (OTC) sleep medications. However, valerian has not been found to have any effect on objective measures such as electroencephalogram (EEG) sleep parameters (Newall et al., 1996). A systematic review of nine randomized, double-blind placebo-controlled trials resulted in inconclusive evidence in the role of valerian in the treatment of insomnia (Stevinson & Ernst, 2000).

Safety Valerian is known to produce headache and morning grogginess. Whether valerian can cause dependence similar to other sedative-hypnotics remains unclear (Stevinson & Ernst, 2000). Like many other complementary and alternative preparations, valerian is not recommended for women who are pregnant or lactating because of potential safety concerns.

Formulations It is recommended that the root be chopped into small pieces and steeped until cool before drinking (1 teaspoon of root for each cup of liquid). One to three cups may be consumed each day. Valerian is also prepared in capsule and tincture forms for dosing. It is considered to be nontoxic even when taken over long periods.

✱ For which agents are compelling data lacking?
A number of therapies lack objective standardized data to support use, but early noncontrolled or small studies suggest some potential for benefit.

astragalus (Astragalus membranaceus [huanqi]) Astragalus, an herb, is used as a tonic and for the treatment of colds and influenza. The herbal medicine is derived from the root of the nontoxic Chinese species. Traditional Chinese physicians consider this plant to be a true tonic that helps strengthen debilitated people and increases resistance to disease. In contemporary Chinese medicine *Astragalus* is a chief component of combination therapy to restore immune function in oncology clients undergoing chemotherapy and radiation (Duan & Wang, 2002). Pharmacologic studies in the West support the immune system-enhancing effects of *Astragalus* (Block, 2003). In vitro and in vivo studies of *Astragalus membranaceus* show that it contains active compounds that increase phagocytic activity, stimulate interferon production, and potentiate the effects of biologic response modifiers such as recombinant interleukin. *Astragalus membranaceus* has demonstrated herpes simplex virus-1 (HSV-1)–inhibiting efficacy and low cytotoxicity (Sun & Yang, 2004). Additionally, in vivo animal studies have demonstrated that substances isolated from this herb can reverse immune suppression (Shao et al., 2004; Calis et al., 1997; Yoshida, Wang, Liu, Shan, & Yamashite, 1997). At present, more research is being performed in relation to the therapeutic effects of *Astragalus*.

feverfew (Tanacetum parthenium)

Feverfew has been used for the treatment of headaches since the first century. Parthenolide is considered to be the active component of feverfew for the treatment of migraines. Depending on geographic location, the parthenolide content of feverfew has been found to be highly variable or absent. The recommended daily dose is 125 mg of dried leaves that contain a minimum parthenolide content of 0.2%.

Drug trials conducted to demonstrate the efficacy of feverfew vary in results and may be related to parthenolide content. However, a Cochrane Review in 2004 concluded that there is insufficient evidence from randomized, double-blind trials to suggest an effect of feverfew over and above placebo for preventing migraine and that feverfew presents no major safety issues (Pittler, 2004).

ginseng root (Panax ginseng [ren shen])

The Chinese have used ginseng for more than 3000 years as a tonic, a restorative, and a specific treatment for several ailments. Ginseng has been subjected to extensive study in recent years. Results of clinical research studies demonstrate that ginseng may improve psychological function (Kennedy, Scholey, & Wesnes, 2002; Ellis & Reddy, 2002) and immune function (Scaglione, Weiser, & Alessandria, 2001). Overall it appears to be well tolerated, although caution is advised about concomitant use with some pharmaceuticals, such as warfarin, oral hypoglycemic agents, insulin, and phenelzine (Kiefer & Pantuso, 2003).

Because ginseng has a history of being adulterated or mislabeled, some adverse effects may be because of contaminants; individuals who experience adverse effects should discontinue its use. Headache may be the result of extremely high doses of ginseng. Individuals with hypertension should not use ginseng.

green tea (Camellia simensis)

In general, tea is one of the most popular beverages consumed worldwide. Many individuals consume green tea as a refreshing beverage and a tonic. Studies in Japan, where green tea is the national beverage, indicate an inverse association between the consumption of green tea and various serum markers, which shows that green tea may act protectively against cardiovascular disease (Hirano et al., 2002) and liver disorders. Green tea improves the risk factors for heart disease by hypolipidemic and antioxidant mechanisms and possibly has a fibrinolytic effect (Maron et al., 2003; Vinson & Dabbagh, 1998). Many laboratory studies have demonstrated the inhibitory effects of green tea preparations and tea polyphenols against tumor formation and growth. In an analysis of 31 human studies, Bushman (1998) found that three of five studies reporting on colon cancer found an inverse association and one a positive association. For rectal cancer, only one of four studies reported an inverse association, whereas increased risks were seen in two of the studies. Of ten studies examining the association of green tea and stomach cancer, six suggested an inverse association and three a positive association. Pancreatic cancer studies hint at an inverse association in two of three studies. A strong inverse effect was found with green tea and esophageal cancer. An inverse association was suggested for urinary bladder cancer in two of two studies. Recent epidemiologic studies have supported a protective role of tea against cancers of the urinary tract. This inhibitory activity is believed to be mainly a result of the antioxidative and possible antiproliferative effects of polyphenolic compounds in green tea. Polyphenolic compounds suppress the activation of carcinogens and trap genotoxic agents (Sato, 1999). Further laboratory and epidemiologic study is required to determine the relationship between green tea consumption and human cancer risk. Because green tea is cheap, nontoxic, and readily available, it would be an ideal chemopreventive agent if proven to have a protective effect on bladder cancer development in prospective studies. Green tea, high in vitamin K, is known to interfere with the effects of the anticoagulant warfarin (Coumadin) (Heck, DeWitt, & Lukes, 2000).

hawthorn (Crataegus oxyacantha)

Hawthorn grows as a spiny tree or shrub with thorny, branching stems. Both its blossoms and its berries are used for their therapeutic properties. Hawthorn had a long history of use in Europe before being introduced to this country in the nineteenth century. Because then it has been used as a folk remedy, primarily as a cardiac tonic and a mild diuretic. Its therapeutic properties have long been recognized in Europe. This acceptance has been supported by a 4-year study of hawthorn commissioned by the German Federal Ministry of Health. The study concluded that hawthorn increases cardiac contractility and the rate of blood flow. It was also found to increase both coronary and myocardial circulation by its dilation effect on the coronary arteries. After taking hawthorn, individuals report a reduction in the number of angina attacks and symptom relief (Loew, 1999). A meta-analysis of its use in HF indicated that symptoms such as dyspnea and fatigue improved significantly with hawthorn treatment as compared with placebo. Reported adverse events were infrequent, mild, and transient; they included nausea, dizziness, and cardiac and GI complaints. In conclusion, these results suggest that there is a significant benefit from hawthorn extract as an adjunctive treatment for chronic heart failure (Pittler, Schmidt, & Ernst, 2003).

Hawthorn has been used in combination with digoxin, enhancing the effects of the cardiac glycosides found in digoxin. The dose of digoxin may be decreased if used in conjunction with hawthorn. If clients also take β blockers for their hypertension, which reduce cardiac output, the inotropic effects of hawthorn may cause a slight increase in blood pressure. Individuals with mild to moderate HF may benefit from hawthorn alone. Because of a lack of data, hawthorn cannot be seen as a substitute for the more powerful prescription drugs, but it may complement them and enhance their activity. Clients currently taking cardiac drugs should discuss the use of hawthorn with their prescriber before taking the drug.

milk thistle (Silybum marianum) Evidence exists that milk thistle may be hepatoprotective through a number of mechanisms: antioxidant activity, toxin blockade at the membrane level, enhanced protein synthesis, antifibriotic activity, and possible antiinflammatory or immunomodulating effects (Agency for Healthcare Research and Quality, 2000). Standardized extracts of milk thistle concentrate silymarin, a substance that apparently prevents the membrane of undamaged liver cells from letting toxins enter. Laboratory studies demonstrate that silymarin functions as a potent antioxidant stabilizes cellular membranes, stimulates detoxification pathways, stimulates regeneration of liver tissue, inhibits the growth of certain cancer cell lines, exerts direct cytotoxic activity toward certain cancer cell lines, and may increase the efficacy of certain chemotherapy agents. Human clinical trials have investigated milk thistle or silymarin primarily in individuals with hepatitis or cirrhosis (National Cancer Institute, 2004). Regarding adverse effects, little evidence is available regarding causality, but available evidence does suggest that milk thistle is associated with few, and generally minor, adverse effects. There are no documented contraindications or interactions with other remedies. Although there are no known serious adverse effects, a mild laxative effect is occasionally reported.

✱ **P.S. is an emergency department (ED) nurse responsible for obtaining intake information from clients. She is working with her colleagues to identify a documentation system for drugs and CAMs, and triage clients regarding risks involved. As part of her assessment of risk, she questions her clinical pharmacist regarding how complementary and alternative therapies interact with other medications.**

✱ **What are the nursing management issues related to CAM?**
Complementary and alternative remedies will continue to be used because of strong traditions and because of the desire of clients to increase a sense of control to improve their well-being. The nurse must recognize and clarify his or her own values and beliefs regarding CAMs, to avoid imposing personal health beliefs onto the client and family.

Assessment Explore the use of CAMs during an assessment of the client's concurrent medications. Proactively question clients about the use of complementary and alternative remedies, and document the responses in the health record. For most CAMs, the potential for interactions has yet to be evaluated. Like with allopathic therapies, the mechanisms of interaction can be pharmacokinetic (e.g., ephedra interacting with other stimulants to cause hypertension and cardiac dysrhythmias, bleeding when garlic is used with anticoagulants like warfarin [Coumadin], serotonin syndrome when St. John's wort is given with other serotonergic antidepressants) or pharmacokinetic (e.g., red yeast rice interacting with other agents metabolized by cytochrome P450 3 A4). A number of commonly used CAMs inhibit some of the cytochrome P450 enzymes with unknown clinical significance (Budzinski, Foster, Vandenhoek, & Arnason, 2000). CAMs are subject to the same genetics differences as other medications (see the Special Considerations for Pharmacogenetics box below).

If the client is being admitted for a surgical procedure, a history of the use of CAMs is particularly important. See the Medication Safety Alert box on p. 230.

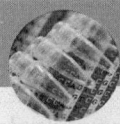 **Special Considerations for Pharmacogenetics** | **COMPLEMENTARY ALTERNATIVE MEDICATIONS**

PHARMACODYNAMICS

Given the genetic variation in pharmacodynamic response with many other drugs, altered action based on genetics would be expected for complementary and alternative therapies. However, little definitive data exists to date.

PHARMACOKINETICS

A number of complementary and alternative medications are metabolized by P450 enzyme systems, which are genetically determined, such as St. John's wort (Markowitz et al., 2003), red yeast rice (Prasad et al., 2002), and *Echinacea* (Budzinski

et al., 2000). Significant variation in P450 3 A4 expression is observed in humans (Wojnowski, 2004).

ADVERSE EFFECTS

Injury to the liver is often related to toxic metabolites produced by altered enzyme systems. Hepatotoxicity associated with herbal preparations may be higher than that observed with other known hepatotoxic agents, and genetic variation in enzyme function has been proposed as a potential mechanism (Estes et al., 2003; Lee, 2003).

Medication Safety Alert

Herbal Medications and Surgical Procedures

The American Society of Anesthesiologists (ASA) recommends that all herbal medications be discontinued 2 to 3 weeks before an elective surgical procedure. If clients are not sure of the contents of the herbal medicine, encourage them to bring the container so that the anesthesiologist can review the contents of the preparation. Although this addresses an issue in elective surgical situations, anesthetic care in emergency settings should be based on a thorough drug history from the client or family member, if possible.

Herbal Remedies That Decrease Platelet Aggregation

- Bilberry
- Don quoi
- Feverfew
- Fish oil
- Flax seed oil
- Garlic
- Ginger
- Ginseng
- Ginkgo biloba
- Grape seed extract

Herbs That Inhibit Clotting

- Chamomile
- Dandelion root
- Dong quoi
- Horse chestnut

Herbs That Potentiate CNS Depression of Anesthesia

- Hops
- Kava kava
- Passion flower
- Valerian

Modified from Kaye, A.D., Kucera, I., & Sabar, R. (2004). Perioperative anesthesia clinical considerations of alternative medicines, *Anesthesiology Clinics of North America, 22*(1), 125-139.

Nursing Diagnosis Nursing diagnoses and potential complications would relate to the anticipated beneficial aspects and the adverse effects of the particular CAM.

Planning The client will experience the following:
- Anticipated beneficial effect
- Absence of adverse effects

Implementation

Monitoring Objective criteria should be determined with the client so that measurable progress or lack of progress can be documented to decrease the power of suggestion regarding the therapeutic effects of the drug (e.g., weekly weights in the case of weight loss medications).

If a serious toxicity is suspected, the client should be able to provide a sample of the remedy for chemical analysis. Encourage clients to purchase products with labels that show the scientific name of the herb, the name and address of the manufacturer, a lot number, the date of manufacture, and an expiration date. This will provide valuable information if there is an adverse effect. Health care providers should report serious adverse effects involving herbal remedies to the FDA MedWatch Program (800-332-1088).

Education The nurse needs to self-educate with scientific proof, including clinical studies, to be able to discuss them adequately with clients. The nurse can then assist the client and family to explore their values and beliefs. This will help the client to make the "right" decisions and will help the nurse to better understand and support the client's choices. The nurse may then incorporate the reasonable components of alternative therapy into the client's therapeutic regimen.

If a client takes or wishes to take a complementary or alternative remedy, he or she should consult with his or her primary health care provider about the benefit or harm that might occur as a result of taking the substance. The prescriber could also provide information on the efficacy of the particular remedy. This consultation would be especially important if the client is taking prescription medications. Any of the complementary and alternative medications may interact with the client's current medication regimen by enhancing or inhibiting its effects or by combining for a toxic effect. Pregnant and breastfeeding women should not take any alternative remedies without the prescriber's approval.

Just as with OTC drugs, consider complementary and alternative remedies as medications, and share information related to their use as current medications in the client's health history.

Advise the client about lifestyle changes that may be more effective than complementary and alternative remedies in accomplishing therapeutic goals. For example, low-fat, high-fiber diet and exercise may be more effective in lowering serum cholesterol levels and less expensive than garlic supplements. Just as with allopathic medications, the therapeutic outcome is enhanced by supportive behavioral changes.

Just as with OTC medications, the client should use single-agent products. This provides for more effective evaluation of the remedy's therapeutic effect and also minimizes the adverse responses that may occur from taking multiple substances. If the client experiences an adverse effect, determination of the causative agent is easier. Make sure that all ingredients and the dose of each are listed on the product label. The product should also be evaluated for standardization; this increases the chance that the contents of the remedy will be consistent from dose to dose.

Teach clients to read labels well and heed warnings on the package. Caution parents to keep these substances out of the reach of children. The client needs to be knowledgeable about the expected actions of the medication; if these actions do not occur in a reasonable time, the drug should be discontinued. Adverse effects should also be known, and the client should discontinue the drug and notify a physician if there is a problem.

Caution clients that commercially available alternative medications may be adulterated because they do not undergo standardized testing for safety and efficacy by the FDA. The role of the nurse is to educate clients regarding the appropriate use or possibly hazardous misuse of complementary and alternative medications.

Evaluation The client will experience the anticipated benefits of the complementary or alternative medication with no adverse effect.

Summary

Many complementary and alternative remedies have been promoted on the basis of anecdotal or subjective accounts—sometimes for hundreds of years—from people who indicate that a particular substance has kept them well or cured their illness. There is no way of knowing what might have been the result if the individual had not taken the remedy; many illnesses are self-limiting, and the placebo effect cannot be discounted. Many of these remedies show promise for further research. Until the same rigorous standard of randomized, double-blind trials is applied to complementary and alternative remedies, consumers need to remain cautious about their use.

✷ Critical Thinking Questions

- How would the cautions previously discussed regarding complementary and alternative remedies differ from the adverse effects of allopathic medicines?
- What are some culturally sensitive strategies that nurses can use to assess and intervene with clients who use CAMs both common and uncommon?

Bibliography

Ackerman, R.T., Mulrow, C.D., Ramirez, G., Gardner, C.D., Morbidoni, L. & Lawrence, V.A. (2001). Garlic shows promise for improving some cardiovascular risk factors. *Annals of Internal Medicine, 161,* 813-824.

Adusumilli, P.S. Ben-Porat, L., Pereira, M., Roesler, D., & Leitman, I.M. (2004). The prevalence and predictors of herbal medicine use in surgical patients. *Journal of the American College of Surgeons, 198(4),* 583-590.

Agency for Healthcare Research and Quality (AHRQ). (2000). *Milk thistle: Effect on liver disease and cirrhosis and clinical adverse effects: A meta-analysis.* Retrieved May 17, 2005, from http://www.ahrq.gov/clinic/epcsums/milktsum.htm

Anderson, L.A. (1996). Concern regarding herbal toxicities: Case reports and counseling tips. *Annuals of Pharmacotherapy, 30,* 79-80.

Ankri, S., & Mirelman, D. (1999). Antimicrobial properties of allicin from garlic. *Microbes Infection, 1(2),* 125-129.

Assemi, M. (2001). Herbs affecting the central nervous system: gingko, kava, St. John's wort, and valerian. *Clinical Obstetrics & Gynecology, 44(4),* 824-833.

Barrett, B.P., Brown, R.L., Locken, K., Maberry, R., Bobula, J.A. & D'Alessio, D. (2002). Treatment of the common cold with unrefined Echinacea. A randomized, double-blind, placebo-controlled trial. *Annals of Internal Medicine, 137(12),* 939-946.

Bennett, J., & Brown, C.M. (2000). Use of herbal remedies by patients in a health maintenance organization. *Journal of the American Pharmaceutical Association, 40(3),* 353-358.

Bent, S., & Ko, R. (2004). Commonly used herbal medicines in the United States: a review. *American Journal of Medicine, 116(7),* 478-485.

Bent, S., Tiedt, T.N., Odden, M.C., & Shlipak, M.G. (2003). The relative safety of ephedra compared with other herbal products. *Annals of Internal Medicine, 138(6),* 468-471.

Bhandari, U., Sharma, J.N., & Zafar, R. (1998). The protective action of ethanolic ginger (Zingiber officinale) extract in cholesterol fed rabbits. *Journal of Ethnopharmacology, 61(2),* 167-171.

Birks J., Grimley E., & Van Dongen M. (2002). Ginkgo biloba for cognitive impairment and dementia. *Cochrane Database Systematic Review, 4,* CD003120.

Block, K.I. (2003). Immune system effects of echinacea, ginseng, and astragalus: a review. *Integrative Cancer Therapy, 2(3),* 247-267.

Boon, H., & Wong, J. (2004). Botanical medicine and cancer: A review of the safety and efficacy. *Expert Opinion in Pharmacotherapy, 5(12),* 2485-2501.

Borrelli, F., Capasso, R., Aviello, G., Pittler, M.H., & Izzo, A.A. (2005). Effectiveness and safety of ginger in the treatment of pregnancy-induced nausea and vomiting. *Obstetrics & Gynecology, 105(4),* 849-856.

Brody, J.E. "Personal health: Modern doctors confirm the ancient wisdom that garlic has many benefits." *New York Times* 27 July 1994.

Budzinski, J.W., Foster, B.C., Vandenhoek, S.. & Arnason, J.T. (2000). An *in vitro* evaluation of human cytochrome P450 3 A4 inhibition by selected commercial herbal extracts and tinctures. *Phytomedicine, 7(4),* 273-282.

Bushman J.L. (1998). Green tea and cancer in humans: a review of the literature. *Nutrition & Cancer, 31,* 151-159.

e-LEARNING SUPPLEMENTS

Student CD-ROM
- Final Exam questions
- NCLEX® Examination review questions
- Pharmacology animations
- Printable chapter summary

Evolve Website (http://evolve.elsevier.com/mckenry)
- Case study on complementary and alternative pharmacology
- Content updates, including information on new drugs
- WebLinks corresponding to this chapter
- Answers to the critical thinking questions in this chapter
- *Elsevier ePharmacology Update* newsletter
- Mosby's Drug Consult Internet Edition
- Supplemental and reference information

Calis, I., Yuruker, A., Tasdenir, D., Wright, A.D., Sticher, O., Luo, Y.D., et al. (1997). Cycloartane triterpene glycosides from the roots of *Astragalus melanophrurius. Planta Medica, 63*(2), 183-186.

Carraro, J.C., Raynaud, J.P., Koch, G., Chisholm, G.D., Di Silverio, F., Teillac, P., et al. (1996). Comparison of phytotherapy (Permixon) with finasteride in the treatment of benign prostate hyperplasia: a randomized international study of 1,098 patients. *Prostate, 29*(4), 231-240, 241-242.

Cheema P., El-Mefty O., & Jazieh A.R. (2001). Intraoperative haemorrhage associated with the use of extract of Saw Palmetto herb: a case report and review of literature. *Journal of Internal Medicine, 250*(2), 167-169.

Cochrane Review. (2005). St. John's wort for depression. Retrieved May 17, 2005, from http://www.cochrane/org/cochrane/revabstr/AB000448.htm.

De Smet, P. (2002). Drug therapy: Herbal remedies. *New England Journal of Medicine, 347*(25), 2046-2056.

Debruyne, F., Koch, G., Boyle, P., Da Silva, F.C., Gillenwater, J.G., Hamdy, F.C., et al. (2002). Comparison of a phytotherapeutic agent (Permixon) with an alpha-blocker (Tamsulosin) in the treatment of benign prostatic hyperplasia: a 1-year randomized international study. *European Urology, 41*(5), 497-507.

D'Huyvetter, K., & Cohrssen, A. (2002). Homeopathy. *Primary Care, 29*, 407-418.

Dong, Y., Lisk, D., Block, E. & Ip, C. (2001). Characterization of the biological activity of gamma-glutamyl-Se-methylselenocysteine: a novel, naturally occurring anticancer agent from garlic. *Cancer research, 61*(7), 2923-2928.

Dorant, E., van den Brandt, P.A., Goldbohn, R.A., Hermus, R.J., & Sturmans, F. (1993). Garlic and its significance for the prevention of cancer in humans: A critical review. *British Journal of Cancer, 67*(3), 424-429.

Duan, P., & Wang, Z.M. (2002). Clinical study of effect of astragalus in efficacy enhancing and toxicity reducing of chemotherapy in patients with malignant tumor. *Zhongguo Zhong Xi Yi Jie He Za Zhi, 22*(7), 515-517.

Eberhart, L.H., Mayer, R., Betz, O., Tsolakidis, S., Hilpert, W., Morin, A.M., et al. (2003). Ginger does not prevent postoperative nausea and vomiting after laparoscopic surgery. *Anesthesia & Analgesia, 96*(4), 995-998.

Eisenberg, D.M., Davis, R.B., Ettner, S.L., Appel, S., Wilkey, S., Van Rompay, M., et al. (1998). Trends in alternative medicine use in the United States, 1990-1997: Results of a follow-up national survey. *Journal of the American Medical Association, 280*(18), 1569-1575.

Eisenberg, D.M., Kessler, R.C., Foster, C., Norlock, F.E., Calkins, D.C., & Delbanco, T.L. (1993). Unconventional medicine in the United States: Prevalence, costs, and patterns of use. *New England Journal of Medicine, 328*(8), 246-252.

Ellis, J.M., & Reddy, P. (2002). Effects of Panax ginseng on quality of life. *Annals of Pharmacotherapy, 36*, 375-379.

Ernst, E., (2002a). Adulteration of complementary herbal medicine with synthetic drugs: A systematic review. *Journal of Internal Medicine, 252*, 107-113.

Ernst, E. (2002b). The risk-benefit profile of commonly used herbal therapies: Ginkgo, St. John's wort, ginseng, echinacea, saw palmetto, and kava. *Annals of Internal Medicine, 136*(1), 42-53.

Ernst, E., & Pittler, M.H. (2000). Efficacy of ginger for nausea and vomiting: A systematic review of randomized clinical trials. *British Journal of Anaesthesia, 84*(3), 367-371.

Estes, J.D., Stolpman, D., Olyaei, A., Corless, C.L., Ham, J.M., Schwartz, J.M., et al. (2003). High prevalence of potentially hepatotoxic herbal supplement use in patients with fulminant hepatic failure. *Archives of Surgery, 138*(8), 852-858.

FDA News. (February 6, 2004). FDA issues regulation prohibiting sale of dietary supplements containing ephedrine alkaloids and reiterates its advice that consumers stop using these products. Retrieved February 24, 2004, from http://www.fda.gov/bbs/topics/NEWS/2004/NEW01021.html

Flaherty, J.H. (2000). The use of complementary and alternative medical therapies among older persons around the world, *Clinics of Geriatric Medicine, 20*(2), 179-200.

Food and Drug Administration News. (2004). Retrieved May 17, 2005, from http://www.fda.gov/oc/initiatives/ephedra/february2004/

Food and Drug Administration. (2002). Retrieved May 17, 2005, from http://www.fda.gov/fdac/features/2002/202 _supp.html

Food and Drug Administration. (1993). From the Food and Drug Administration. *Journal of the American Medical Association, 269*(3), 328.

Food and Drug Administration. (2000). Public Health Advisory: Risk of drug interactions with St. John's wort and indinavir and other drugs. Retrieved May 17, 2005, from http://www.fda.gov/cder/drug/advisory/stjwort.htm.

Gardner, C.D., Chatterjee, L.M., & Carlson, J.J. (2001). The effect of a garlic preparation on plasma lipid levels in moderately hypercholesterolemic adults. *Atherosclerosis, 154*(1), 213-220.

Gerber, G.S., Kuznetsov, D., Johnson, B.C., & Burstein, J.D. (2001). Randomized, double-blind, placebo-controlled trial of saw palmetto in men with lower urinary tract symptoms. *Urology, 58*, 960-964.

Gilroy, C.M., Steiner, J.F., Byers, T., Shapiro, H. & Georgian, W. (2003). Echinacea and truth in labeling. *Archives of Internal Medicine, 163*(6), 699-704.

Gray, H.C., Hutcheson, P.S., & Slavin, R.G. (2004). Is glucosamine safe in patients with seafood allergy? *Journal of Allergy and Clinical Immunology, 114*(2), 459-460.

Heber, D., Yip, I., Ashley, J.M., Elashoff, D.A., Elashoff, R.M., & Go, V.L. (1999). Cholesterol-lowering effects of a proprietary Chinese red-yeast-rice dietary supplement. *American Journal of Clinical Nutrition, 69*(2), 231-236.

Heck, A.M., DeWitt, B.A., & Lukes, A.L. (2000). Potential interactions between alternative therapies and warfarin. *American Journal of Health-System Pharmacy, 57*(13), 1221-1227.

Hepatic toxicity possibly associated with kava-containing products—United States, Germany, and Switzerland, 1999-2002. (2002). *Morbidity & Mortality Weekly Report, 51*, 1065-1067.

Hermann, D.D. (2002). Naturoceutical agents in the management of cardiovascular disease. *American Journal of Cardiovascular Drugs, 2*(3), 173-196.

Hirano R., Momiyama Y., Takahashi R., Taniguchi H., Kondo K., Nakamura H., et al. (2002). Comparison of green tea intake in Japanese patients with and without angiographic coronary artery disease, *American Journal of Cardiology, 90*, 1150-1153.

Hoffer, L.J. (2003). Investigating CAM. *Canadian Medical Association Journal, 168*(12), 1527-1528.

Hypericum Depression Trial Study Group. (2002). Effect of Hypericum perforatum (St. John's wort) in major depressive disorder: A randomized controlled trial. *Journal of the American Medical Association, 287*, 1807-1814.

Jellin, J.M., Batz, F., & Hitchens, K. (1999). *Pharmacist's letter/prescriber's letter natural medicines comprehensive database*. Stockton, CA: Therapeutic Research Faculty.

Josling, P. (2001). Preventing the common cold with a garlic supplement: a double-blind, placebo-controlled survey. *Advanced Therapeutics, 18*(4), 189-193.

Kalb, R., Trautmann-Sponsel, R.D., & Kieser, M. (2001). Efficacy and tolerability of Hypericum extract WS 5572 versus placebo in mildly to moderately depressed patients: a randomized double-blind multicenter clinical trial. *Pharmacopsychiatry, 34,* 96-103.

Kamat, A.M., & Lamm, D.L. (2002). Chemoprevention of bladder cancer. *Urological Clinics of North America, 29*(1), 157-168.

Kiefer, D., & Pantuso, T. (2003). Panax ginseng. *American Family Physician, 68*(8), 1539-1542.

Kennedy, D.O., Scholey, A.B., & Wesnes, K.A. (2002). Modulation of cognition and mood following administration of single doses of Ginkgo biloba, ginseng, and a ginkgo/ginseng combination to healthy young adults. *Physiology & Behavior, 75,* 739-751.

Khatta, M., Alexander, B.S., Krichten, C.M., Fisher, M.L., Freudenberger, R., Robinson, S.W., et al. (2000). The effect of coenzyme Q10 in patients with congestive heart failure. *Annals of Internal Medicine, 132*(8), 636-640.

Ko, R.J. (1998). Adulterants in Asian patent medicines. *New England Journal of Medicine, 339*(12), 847.

Kohler, S., Funk, P., & Kieser, M. (2004). Influence of a 7-day treatment with Ginkgo biloba special extract EGb 761 on bleeding time and coagulation: a randomized, placebo-controlled, double-blind study in healthy volunteers. *Blood Coagulation & Fibrinolysis, 15*(4), 303-309.

Kyo, E., Uda, N., Kasuga, S. & Itakura, Y. (2001). Immunomodulatory effects of aged garlic extract, *Journal of Nutrition, 131,* 3S, 1075S-1079S.

LeBars, P.L., Kieser, M., & Itil, K.Z. (2000). A 26-week analysis of a double-blind, placebo-controlled trial of Ginkgo biloba extract Egb 761 in dementia. *Dementia and Geriatric Cognitive Disorders, 11,* 230-237.

Lecrubier, Y., Clerc, G., Didi, R., & Kieser, M. (2002). Efficacy of St. John's wort extract WS 5570 in major depression: a double-blind, placebo-controlled trial. *American Journal of Psychiatry, 159,* 1361-1366.

Lee, W.M. (2003). Medical Progress: Drug-induced hepatotoxicity. *New England Journal of Medicine, 349*(5), 474-485.

Lien, H.C., Sun, W.M., Chen, Y.H., Hasler, W., & Owyang, C. (2003). Effects of ginger on motion sickness and gastric slow-wave dysrhythmias induced by circular vection. *American Journal of Physiology, Gastrointestinal and Liver Physiology, 284*(3), G481-489.

Linde, K., Ramirez, G., Mulrow, C.D., Pauls, A., & Weidenhammer, D.M. (1996). St. John's wort for depression: An overview and meta-analysis of randomised clinical trials. *British Medical Journal, 313,* 253-258.

Loew, D. (1999). Phytogenic drugs in heart diseases exemplified by Crataegus. *Wiener Medizinische Wochenschrift, 149*(8-10), 226-228.

Mahady, G.B., Parrot, J., Lee, C., Yun, G.S., Dan, A. (2003). *Botanical dietary supplement use in peri- and postmenopausal women.* Menopause, *10,* 65-72.

Markowitz, J.S., Donovan, J.L., DeVane, C.L., Taylor, R.M., Ruan, Y., Wang, J.S., et al. (2003). Effect of St. John's wort on drug metabolism by induction of cytochrome P450 3 A4 enzyme. *Journal of the American Medical Association, 290,* 1500-1504.

Maron, D.J., Lu, G.P., Cai, N.S., Wu, Z.G., Li, Y.H., Chen, H., et al. (2003). Cholesterol-lowering effect of a theaflavin-enriched green tea extract: A randomized controlled trial. *Archives of Internal Medicine, 163,* 1448-1453.

McAlindon, T.E., LaValley, M.P., Gulin, J.P. & Felson, D.T. (2000). Glucosamine and chondroitin for treatment of osteoarthritis: a systematic quality assessment and meta-analysis. *Journal of the American Medical Association, 283*(11), 1469-1475.

Melchart, D., Linde, K., Worku, F., Sarkady, L., Holzmann, M., Jurcic, K., & Wagner, H. (1995). Results of five randomized studies on the immunomodulary activity of preparation of Echinacea. *Journal of Alternative & Complementary Medicine, 1*(2), 145-160.

Morisco, C., Trimaro, B., & Condorelli, M. (1993). Effect of coenzyme Q10 therapy in patients with congestive heart failure: a long-term multicenter randomized study. *Clinical Investigator, 71*(8 Suppl), S134-S136.

Mullins, R.J., & Heddle, R. (2002). Adverse reactions associated with echinacea: the Australian experience [comment]. *Annals of Allergy, Asthma, & Immunology, 88*(1), 42-51.

Muluk, V., & Macpherson, D.S. (2004). Perioperative medication management, II. Wellesley, MA: Up To Date.

National Cancer Institute. U.S. National Institutes of Health. Retrieved July 27, 2005, from http://www.nci.nih.gov/cancertopics/pdq/cam/milkthistle

National Council of Complementary and Alternative Medicine. (2005). St. John's wort and the treatment of depression. Retrieved May 17, 2005, http://nccam.nih.gov/health/stjohnswort/.

Newall, C.A., Anderson, L.A., & Phillipson, J.D. (1996). *Herbal medicine: A guide for health care professionals.* London: The Pharmaceutic Press.

News you can use. (1995). *Alternative & Complementary Therapy,* 1(5), 342.

Niebyl, J.R., & Goodwin, T.M. (2002). Overview of nausea and vomiting of pregnancy with an emphasis on vitamins and ginger. *American Journal of Obstetrics and Gynecology, 186,* S253-S255.

Park, K.K., Chun, K.S. Lee, J.M., Less, S.S., & Surh, Y.J. (1998). Inhibitory effects of (6)-gingerol, a major pungent principle of ginger, on phorbol ester-induced inflammation, epidermal ornithine decarboxylase activity and skin tumor promotion in ICR. *Cancer Letters, 129*(2), 139-144.

Peters, H., Kieser M., & Holscher U. (1998).Demonstration of the efficacy of Gingko biloba special extract EGb 761 on intermittent claudication: a placebo-controlled, double-blind multicenter trail. *Vasa, 27,* 106-110.

Philipp, M., Kohnen, R., & Hiller, K.O. (1999). Hypericum extract versus imipramine or placebo in patients with moderate depression: randomised multicentre study of treatment for eight weeks. *British Medical Journal, 319,* 1534-1538.

Phillips, S., Ruggier, R., & Hutchinson, S. (1993). Zingiber officinale (ginger)—an antiemetic for day case surgery. *Anaesthesia, 48*(8), 715-717.

Pittler, M.H. (2004). Feverfew for preventing migraine, *Cochrane Database of Systematic Reviews (Online:Update Software):* CD002286.

Pittler, M.H., & Ernst, E. (2000a). Efficacy of kava extract for treating anxiety: systematic review and meta-analysis. *Journal of Clinical Psychopharmacology, 20,* 84–89.

Pittler, M.H., & Ernst, E. (2000b). Ginkgo biloba extract for the treatment of intermittent claudication: a meta-analysis of randomized trials. *American Journal of Medicine, 108*(4), 276-281.

Pittler, M.H., Schmidt K., & Ernst E. (2003). Hawthorn extract for treating chronic heart failure meta-analysis of randomized trials. *American Journal of Medicine, 114,* 665-674.

Portnoi, G., Chng, L.A., Karimi-Tabesh, L., Koren, G., Tan, M.P. & Einarson, A. (2003). Prospective comparative study of the safety and effectiveness of ginger for the treatment of nausea and vomiting in pregnancy. *American Journal of Obstetrics and Gynecology, 189*(5), 1374-1377.

Prasad, G.V., Wong, T., Meliton, G., & Bhaloo, S. (2002). Rhabdomyolysis due to red yeast rice (Monascus purpureus) in a renal transplant recipient. *Transplantation, 74*(8), 1200-1201.

Reginster, J.Y., Deroisy, R., Rovati, L.C., Lee, R.L., Lejeune, E., Bruyere, O., et al. (2001). Long-term effects of glucosamine sulphate on osteoarthritis progression: a randomised, placebo-controlled clinical trial. *Lancet, 357*(9252), 251-256.

Rowin, J., & Lewis, S.L. (1996). Spontaneous bilateral subdural hematomas associated with chronic Ginkgo biloba ingestion. *Neurology, 46,* 1775-1776.

Rozenfeld, V., Sisca, T.S., Callahan, A. & Crain, J.L. (2000). Double-blind, randomized, control trial of aged garlic extract in patients stabilized on warfarin therapy (poster presentation). Las Vegas, NV: American Society of Hospital Pharmacists.

Saper, R.B., Kales, S.N., Paquin, J., Burns, M.J., Eisenberg, D.M., Davis, R.B., et al. (2004). Heavy metal content of Ayurvedic herbal medicine products. *Journal of the American Medical Association, 292,* 2868-2873.

Sato, D. (1999). Inhibition of urinary bladder tumors induced by N-butyl-N-(4-hydroxybutyl)-nitrosamine in rats by green tea. *International Journal of Urology, 6,* 93-99.

Saw palmetto. *USP DI: Drug information for the health care professional.* (2002). Retrieved February 24, 2004, from http://www.usp.org

Scaglione, F., Weiser, K., & Alessandria, M. (2001). Effects of the standardized ginseng extract G115® in patients with chronic bronchitis: a nonblinded, randomized, comparative pilot study. *Clinical Drug Investigation,* 21, 41-45.

Schwarz, E., Metzler, J., Diedrich, J.P., Freudenstein, J., Bode, C. & Bode, J.C. (2002). Oral administration of freshly expressed juice of Echinacea purpurea herbs fail to stimulate the nonspecific immune response in healthy young men: results of a double-blind, placebo-controlled crossover study. *Journal of Immunotherapy, 25*(5), 413-420.

Shao, B.M., Xu, W., Dai, H., Hu, P., Li, Z. & Gao, X.M. (2004). A study on the immune receptors for polysaccharides from the root of Astragalus membranaceus, a Chinese medicinal herb. *Biochemistry & Biophysiology Research, 320*(4), 1103-1111.

Shekelle, P.G., Hardy, M.L., Morton, S.C., Maglione, M., Mojica, W.A., Suttorp, M.J., et al. (2003). Efficacy and safety of ephedra and ephedrine for weight loss and athletic performance: a meta-analysis. *Journal of the American Medical Association, 289*(12), 1537-1545.

Shelton, R.C., Keller, M.B., Gelenberg, A., Dunner, D.L., Hirschfeld, R., Thase, M.E., et al. (2001). Effectiveness of St. John's wort in major depression: a randomized controlled trial. *Journal of the American Medical Association, 285*(15), 1978-1986.

Shults, C.W., Oakes. D., Kieburtz, K., Beal, M.F., Haas, R., Plumb, S., et al. and the Parkinson Study Group. (2002). Effects of coenzyme Q10 in early Parkinson disease: evidence of slowing of the functional decline. *Archives of Neurology, 59*(10), 1541-1550.

Singh, R.B., Wander, G.S., Rastogi, A., Shukla, P.K., Mittal, A., Sharma, J.P., et al. (1998). Randomized, double-blind placebo-controlled trial of coenzyme Q10 in patients with acute myocardial infarction. *Cardiovascular Drugs & Therapy, 12*(4), 347-353.

Sperber, S.J., Shah, L.P., Gilbert, R.D., Ritchey, T.W., Monto, A.S. (2004). Echinacea purpurea for prevention of experimental rhinovirus colds. *Clinical Infectious Diseases, 38,* 1367-1371.

Steiner, M., & Lin, W. (2001). Aged garlic extract, a modulator of cardiovascular risk factors: a dose-finding study on the effects of AGE on platelet functions. *Journal of Nutrition, 131*(3S), 980S-984S.

Stevinson, C., & Ernst, E. (2000). Valerian for insomnia: a systematic review of randomized clinical trials. *Sleep Medicine, 1,* 91–99.

Stevinson, C., Pittler, M.H., & Ernst, E. (2001). Garlic for treating hypercholesterolemia: A meta-analysis of randomized clinical trials. *Annals of Internal Medicine, 133*(6), 420-429.

Sun, Y., & Yang, J. (2004). Experimental study of the efficacy of Astragalus membranacues against herpes simplex virus – type 1. *Di Yi Jun Yi Da Xue Xue Ban, 24*(1), 57-58.

Szegedi, A., Kohnen, R., Dienel, A., & Kieser, M. (2005). Acute treatment of moderate to severe depression with Hypericum extract WS 5570 (St. John's wort): Randomised controlled double blind non-inferiority trial versus paroxetine. *British Medical Journal, 330,* 503-507.

Taylor, J.A., et al. (2003a). Efficacy and safety of echinacea in treating upper respiratory tract infections in children: a randomized controlled trial. *Journal of the American Medical Association, 290*(21), 2824-2830.

Taylor, J.M. (2003b). Statement of John M. Taylor, Associate Commissioner For Regulatory Affairs, Food And Drug Administration Before The Committee On Commerce United States Senate, October 28, 2003. Retrieved February 24, 2004, from http://www.Fda.Gov/Ola/2003/Dietarysupplements1028.html

Tessier, E.G. (2002). Glucosamine: an evidence based review of safety and efficacy. Natural Standard Research Database, Volume 1. Boston, MA: Natural Standard. Retrieved July 27, 2005, from http:// www.naturalstandard.com

Thomson, M., & Ali, M. (2003). Garlic [Allium sativum]: a review of its potential use as an anti-cancer agent. *Current Cancer Drug Targets, 3*(1), 67-81.

Verbruggen, G., Goemaere, S., & Veys, E.M. (2002). Systems to assess the progression of finger joint osteoarthritis and the effects of disease modifying osteoarthritis drugs. *Clinical Rheumatology, 21,* 231-243.

Vickers, A., & Zollman, C. (1999). ABC of complementary medicine: homeopathy. *British Medical Journal, 319,* 1115-1118.

Vinson, J.A., & Dabbagh, Y.A. (1998). Effect of green and black tea supplementation on lipids, lipid oxidation and fibrinogen in the hamster: Mechanisms for the epidemiological benefits of tea drinking. *Federation of European Biochemical Societies Letters, 433*(1-2), 44-46.

Vutyavanich, T., Kraisarin, T., & Ruangsri, R.A. (2001). Ginger for nausea and vomiting in pregnancy: randomized, double-masked, placebo-controlled trial. *Obstetrics and Gynecology 97,* 577-582.

Warshafsky, S., Kamer, R.S., & Sivak, S.L. (1993). Effect of garlic on total serum cholesterol: A meta-analysis. *Annals of Internal Medicine, 119*(7 Pt 1), 599-605.

Wilt, T., Ishani, A., Stark, G., MacDonald, R., Mulrow, C. & Lau, J. (2001). Serenoa repens for benign prostatic hyperplasia. *Cochrane Database Systematic Review 2001, 2,* CD001423.

Wojnowski, L. (2004). Genetics of the Variable Expression of CYP3 A in Humans. *Therapeutic Drug Monitoring, 26*(2), 192-199.

Yoshida, Y., Wang, M.Q., Liu, J.N., Shan, B.E., & Yamashite, J. (1997). Immunomodulating activity of Chinese medicinal herbs and Oldenlandia diffuse in particular. *International Journal of Immunopharmacology, 19*(7), 359-370.

Zhou, S., Chan, E., Pan, S.Q., Huang, M., & Lee, E.J. (2004). Pharmacokinetic interactions of drugs with St. John's wort. *Journal of Psychopharmacology, 18*(2), 262-276.

Zi, X., & Agarwal, R. (1999). Silibinin decreases prostate-specific antigen with cell growth inhibition via G1 arrest, leading to differentiation of prostate carcinoma cells: implications for prostate cancer intervention. *Proceedings of the National Academy of Sciences of the United States of America, 96*(13), 7490-7495.

OVERVIEW OF THE CENTRAL NERVOUS SYSTEM

CHAPTER FOCUS

The nervous system coordinates all body functions, and its activities allow the individual to adapt to the internal and external environment. Because of the complexity of this system, the monitoring of pharmacologic interventions can be challenging. Knowledge of the anatomy and physiology of the central nervous system provides a foundation for sound clinical decision making in this area.

LEARNING OBJECTIVES

- Identify the major components of the central nervous system.
- Describe the functions of the components of the central nervous system.
- Identify the structure and function of the blood-brain barrier.
- Describe three major functional systems of the central nervous system.
- Describe the function of the common neurotransmitter substances.

▲ KEY TERMS

acetylcholine, 241
blood-brain barrier, p. 239
brainstem, p. 237
catecholamine, p. 241
cerebellum, p. 237
cerebrum, p. 236
depolarization, p. 239
endorphin, p. 241
extrapyramidal system, p. 240
hypothalamus, p. 237

limbic system, p. 240
medulla oblongata, p. 237
midbrain, p. 237
neurons, p. 238
pons, p. 237
refractory, p. 239
repolarization, p. 239
reticular activating system, p. 240
synapse, p. 238
thalamus, p. 237

The nervous system consists of the central nervous system (CNS) and the peripheral nervous system (PNS) (Figure 13-1). The PNS is discussed in Chapter 20. This chapter reviews the primary areas of the CNS and focuses on the specific areas affected by drug therapy.

✸ How do the CNS and PNS interact for homeostasis?

The CNS is composed of the brain and spinal cord and essentially controls all functions in the body. When a drug is described as having a central action, it means that it has an action on the brain or the spinal cord. The PNS is the network that transmits information to and from the CNS and alerts the CNS to internal and external changes such as muscle tension, blood vessel alterations, pain, fever, sound, smell, taste, touch, and sight. This information is integrated and instructions are relayed to the appropriate cells or tissues for producing the necessary actions and environmental adjustments. Information concerning these actions and ad-

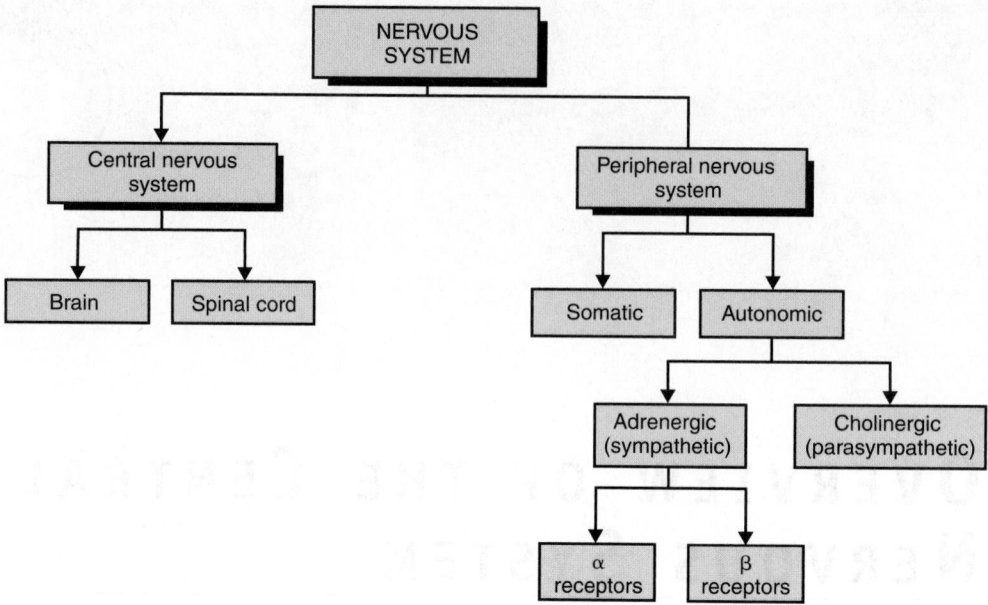

FIGURE 13-1 Overview of the nervous system.

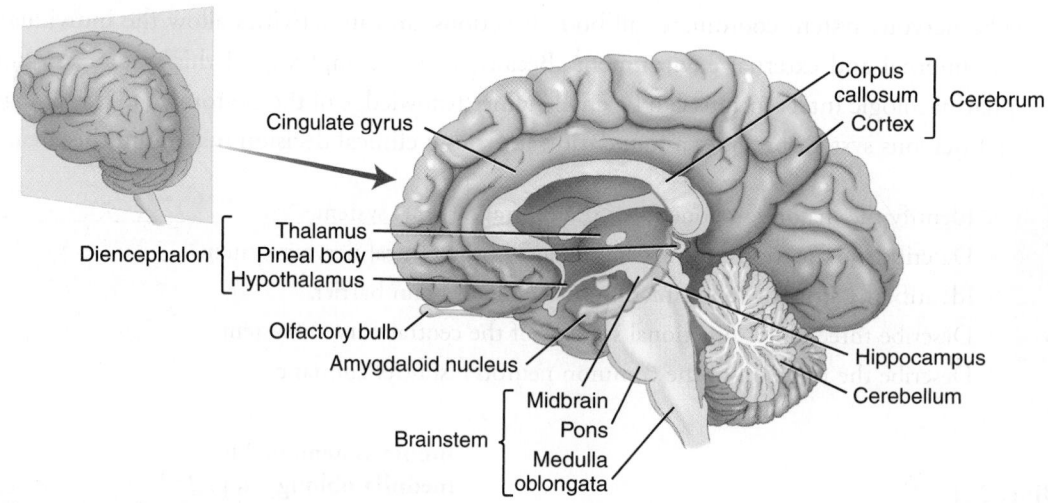

FIGURE 13-2 Divisions of the brain and the limbic system.

justments is fed back to the CNS. This constant feeding of information to the CNS permits continuous adjustments in the instructions sent to various tissues to ensure effective control of body functions.

✳ What are the functions of the major parts of the brain and how are they affected by drugs?

The brain can be physically divided in various ways. A simplified approach is to divide it into its major components: cerebrum, thalamus, pineal body, hypothalamus, midbrain, pons, medulla oblongata, and cerebellum (Figure 13-2).

Cerebrum The **cerebrum,** the largest and uppermost section of the brain, is the highest functional area of the brain. Memory storage and sensory, integrative, emotional, language, and motor functions are controlled in this area. The cerebrum consists of two hemispheres (right and left) and the corpus callosum, the nerve tissues that connect the right and left hemi-

spheres. The outer surface of the cerebrum is the cerebral cortex—or gray matter—of the brain; this surface covers the four lobes into which each hemisphere is divided. These lobes are named for the bones of the skull under which they lie: frontal, parietal, occipital, and temporal. The frontal lobe contains the motor and speech areas. The sensory cortex is located in the parietal lobe, the visual cortex in the occipital lobe, and the auditory cortex in the temporal lobe. Association areas lie near these lobes and act in conjunction with them. In addition, large parts of the cortex are concerned with higher mental activity—reasoning, creative thought, judgment, and memory. These attributes are unique to humans and separate them from other animals.

Drugs that depress cortical activity may decrease the acuity of sensation and perception, inhibit motor activity, decrease alertness and concentration, and even promote drowsiness and sleep. Drugs that stimulate the cortical areas may cause more vivid impulses to be received and greater awareness of the surrounding environment. Increased muscle activity and restlessness may also occur. The specific response brought forth by a drug depends to a large extent on the personality of the individual, the individual's emotional and physiologic state, the specific attributes of the drug, and a host of other factors.

Thalamus The thalamus is composed of sensory nuclei and serves as the major relay center for impulses to and from the cerebral cortex. It also registers sensations such as pain, temperature, touch, and other sensory impulses, and relays this information to the cerebrum.

The thalamus enables the individual to have impressions of pleasantness or unpleasantness, and it also appears to play a part (with the reticular activating system) in arousal or alerting signals. (See Reticular Activating System, p. 240.) Drugs that depress cells in various portions of the thalamus may interrupt the free flow of impulses to the cerebral cortex. This is one way in which pain may be relieved.

Pineal Body The pineal body resembles a small pinecone and appears to be involved in regulating the human body's biological clock. It also produces hormones, such as melatonin. The secretion of melatonin is inhibited by sunlight and is related to sleep and mood disorders.

Hypothalamus The hypothalamus provides a major link between the mind and the body. It lies below the thalamus and is vital for maintaining many body functions and the well-being of the individual. Hypothalamus functions include body temperature regulation, carbohydrate and fat metabolism, and water balance; it is also thought that the appetite center and pleasure or reward centers are located here. There is evidence that a center for sleep and wakefulness also exists within the hypothalamus. Some of the sleep-producing drugs are thought to depress hypothalamic centers.

As part of its integrative role in neurohormonal regulation, neurons in the hypothalamus release hormones that affect the anterior pituitary gland. Growth hormone, hormones that affect sexual glands or functions, thyroid hormones, and the adrenal cortex hormones are under the control of the hypothalamus.

The hypothalamus, along with other specific areas of the brain, is also involved with the control of emotions. Drugs may affect these functions of the hypothalamus. An example is the use of antidepressants to treat the symptoms of depression. The action of antidepressants on the hypothalamus often reverses the symptoms of weight loss, anorexia, decreased libido, and insomnia associated with depression. Other psychotherapeutic agents may cause a number of hypothalamic adverse effects, including breast engorgement, lactation, amenorrhea, appetite stimulation, and alterations in temperature regulation.

Brainstem The brainstem is composed of the midbrain, pons, and medulla oblongata and is the source of 10 of the 12 cranial nerves (Table 13-1); the exceptions are the olfactory and optic nerves, cranial nerves one and two. The medulla, pons, and midbrain contain many important correlation centers (gray matter), as well as ascending and descending pathways (white matter). The midbrain contains nerve tracts to and from the cerebrum and serves as a relay station from higher areas of the brain to lower centers. It is the source of the third (oculomotor) and fourth (trochlear) cranial nerves; some optic fibers are also located here. The pons is the source of the fifth, sixth, seventh, and eighth cranial nerves. It also contains a center that controls involuntary respiratory regulation. Drugs also affect the midbrain and pons as the reticular activating system is stimulated or depressed. The medulla oblongata contains the vital centers: the respiratory, vasomotor, and cardiac centers mediated by cranial nerves IX through XII (glossopharyngeal, vagus, accessory and hypoglossal). Such centers are referred to as vital because they are necessary for survival. Other essential functions also originate here, such as vomiting, hiccupping, sneezing, coughing, and swallowing reflexes.

If the respiratory center is stimulated by a drug, it will discharge an increased number of nerve impulses over nerve pathways to the muscles of respiration. If it is depressed, it will discharge fewer impulses, and respiration will be correspondingly affected. Other centers in the medulla that respond to certain drugs are the cough center and the vomiting center.

Cerebellum The cerebellum, located in the posterior cranial fossa behind the brainstem, contains centers for muscle coordination, equilibrium, and muscle tone. It receives afferent impulses from the vestibular nuclei and the cerebrum, and it plays an important role in the maintenance of posture and voluntary muscular activity. Drugs that disturb the cerebellum, or the vestibular branch of the eighth cranial nerve, may cause dizziness and loss of equilibrium.

✴ What is the role of the spinal cord in the CNS?

The spinal cord, a center for reflex activity, also functions in the transmission of impulses to and from the higher centers in the brain and may be affected by the action of drugs. Ascending sensory tracts conduct impulses up from the peripheral nerves to the brain, and descending motor tracts conduct impulses down from the brain to the peripheral nerves.

A cross section of the spinal cord reveals an internal mass of gray matter enclosed by white matter (Figure 13-3). The butterfly-shaped gray matter is divided into sections, or horns; the afferent (sensory) nerve fibers are located in the dorsal or posterior horn, and the efferent (motor) nerve fibers exit from the ventral or anterior horn. When a pain impulse reaches the dorsal horn, the impulse is transmitted along special tracts (lateral spinothalamic tract) to the thalamus, which then distributes the message to other areas of the brain. The brain responds by means of the descending efferent fiber pathways to inhibit or modify other incoming pain stimuli. (See Chapter 14 for further discussion of the gate control theory.) Small doses of spinal stimulants may increase reflex excitability; larger doses may cause seizures.

TABLE 13-1 CRANIAL NERVES

Cranial Nerve	Type of Nerve	Function*
I Olfactory	Sensory	Smell
II Optic	Sensory	Sight
III Oculomotor	Motor	Movement of eye and eyelid muscles; pupillary constriction
IV Trochlear	Motor	Eye muscle movement for downward and inward motion of eye
V Trigeminal	Motor	Chewing; lateral jaw movement
	Sensory	Sensations of the face, scalp, oral cavity, teeth, and tongue
VI Abducens	Motor	Eye movements
VII Facial	Motor	Facial expressions
	Sensory	Taste
VIII Vestibulocochlear	Sensory	Hearing; equilibrium
IX Glossopharyngeal	Motor	Swallowing; salivation
	Sensory	Taste; throat sensations
X Vagus	Motor	Voice production; swallowing; decrease in heartbeat; increased peristalsis
	Sensory	Gag reflex; sensations of throat, larynx, and abdominal viscera
XI Spinal accessory	Motor	Head and shoulder movements
XII Hypoglossal	Motor	Tongue movements

*Drug effects, toxicity, or both have been reported to affect various cranial nerve functions. For example, ototoxicity (damage to cranial nerve VIII) has been reported with aminoglycoside antibiotics. Vincristine, an antineoplastic agent, may produce ptosis (cranial nerve III), trigeminal neuralgia (cranial nerve VII), facial palsy (cranial nerve V), and jaw pain. Because various medications have the potential to affect the cranial nerves adversely, students should be familiar with the functions of the cranial nerves.

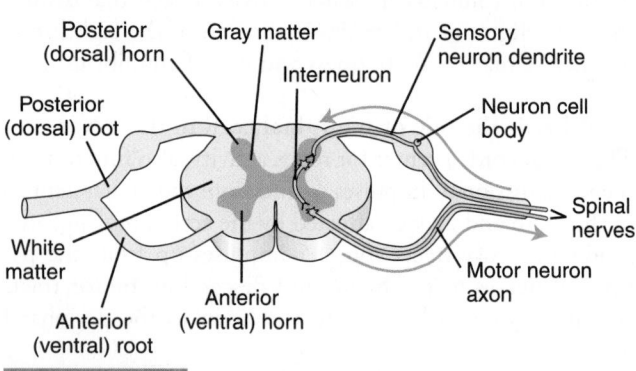

FIGURE 13-3 Cross section of the spinal cord.

✹ What types of cells are found in the CNS?

The two major cell types in the CNS are glial cells and neurons. The functions of the glial cells are not fully understood, but recent studies indicate they are composed of many types of neurotransmitter receptors and ion channels. It is possible that this type of network serves to support and assist neurons in the transfer and integration of information in the CNS and PNS.

Neurons have four basic parts: dendrites, cell body, axon, and axon or nerve terminals (Figure 13-4). The cell body contains the nucleus (genetic information) and the ribosomes, Nissl substance, and endoplasmic reticulum necessary for protein synthesis. The Golgi complex stores, processes, and concentrates the protein, and the mitochondria in the cell body and dendrites provide the production of energy necessary for protein synthesis and lipid metabolism.

Dendrites also contain some neurotransmitter vesicles; thus incoming messages from other neurons are received in the dendrites, processed in the cell body, transported in the axon, and exit via the axon terminal. This process of conveying messages from one cell body to another usually involves electrical or chemical transport of the message across a **synapse,** the junction point between neurons or between a neuron and an effector organ. Most information transmitted in the CNS is the result of alterations in electrical currents. The following paragraphs provide a brief summary of this process; more detailed information can be found in a current anatomy and physiology text.

The electrical properties of nerve cells are generated by various ions, pumps, and channels located in the cell membrane. Figure 13-5 illustrates a nerve cell in the resting state. A membrane difference or potential is caused by changes in the concentration of sodium, potassium, and chloride ions. Pumps are capable of actively moving charged ions from one side of the membrane to the other side, and channels are membrane pores that allow specific ions to pass from one side of the membrane to the other.

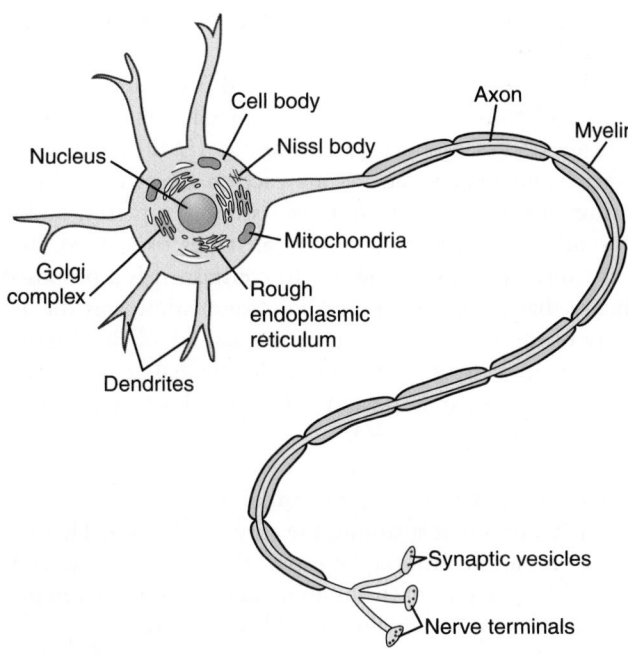

FIGURE 13-4 Structural components of neurons.

Extracellular

Sodium channel (closed at rest) — Sodium-potassium pump (3-for-2 exchange) — Potassium channel (open at rest) — Intracellular passive fluxes (leak current)

Intracellular

FIGURE 13-5 A nerve cell in the resting state. *ADP,* adenosine diphosphate; *ATP,* adenosine triphosphate.

In the resting state, sodium and chloride are found in large amounts outside the cell, and potassium is in high concentration inside the cell. These concentration gradients (the resting membrane potential) are stabilized and maintained by the sodium-potassium ATPase (adenosine triphosphatase) pump, which trades three sodium ions from the intracellular fluid for two potassium ions from the extracellular fluid. The movement and concentration of these ions in and around the cell are the primary determinants that affect the membrane potential of the nerve cells.

During this resting state, the sum of charged ions in the nerve cell result in a net negative charge in the cell as compared to the external cellular environment.

When factors alter the cellular excitability (e.g., chemical or mechanical stimulation), rapid movement of sodium into and potassium out of the cell is observed. This process is often referred to as **depolarization** and produces a net negative intracellular charge to a near neutral or positive charge. This reduction in membrane potential generates an action potential as a result of the changes illustrated in Figure 13-6, and is responsible for the movement of the electrical current to nearby membranes.

The process whereby ions migrate to their original positions observed during rest is referred to as **repolarization**. Repolarization involves the passive transfer of ions across cell membranes, as well as the energy-dependent sodium-potassium ATPase pump (see Figure 13-5). Until the ions reach their original state at rest, the neuron is considered **refractory** or unable to fire.

Drugs can act directly on the ion channel or via receptors that affect ion channels. For example, general anesthetics and ethanol bind to specific receptors that effectively reduce sodium influx to prevent regeneration of action potentials and conduction of nerve impulses. The action of the sodium-potassium pump on cardiac cells is discussed in Chapter 25.

✱ What is the blood-brain barrier?

The **blood-brain barrier** is actually a covering of nerve cells (astrocytes) that encircle the capillary walls of the brain.

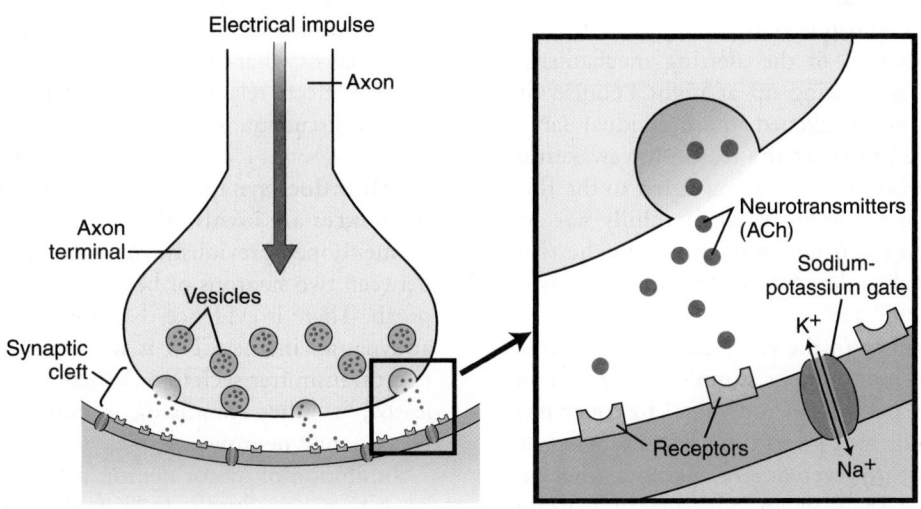

FIGURE 13-6 Nerve cell depolarization.

This covering prevents the passage of many drugs and large molecules into the brain, but it does allow small molecules (e.g., water, alcohol, oxygen, and carbon dioxide), glucose, gases, and lipid-soluble substances to penetrate. Such selective processing allows the brain a degree of security against the toxic effects of some drugs on the CNS. However, the permeation of such substances across the blood-brain barrier increases with large doses or in instances of meningeal inflammation. Current research is studying methods to increase the permeability of the blood-brain barrier to specific therapeutic agents, such as antibiotics or antineoplastic agents needed to treat a localized brain infection or brain tumors.

✳ In addition to the anatomic structures of the CNS, what are the functional systems of the system and how are they affected by drugs?

The three major functional systems of the CNS that are affected by select drug or chemical administration are (1) the reticular activating system, (2) the limbic system, and (3) the extrapyramidal system.

Reticular Activating System The reticular activating system (RAS) is a diffuse system of nuclei in the brainstem that permits two-way communication among the spinal cord, thalamus, and cerebral cortex. The primary functions of the RAS are as follows:

- A consciousness and arousal effect
- An alerting mechanism
- A filtering process that allows for concentration

When stimulated, the gray matter of the pons and the midbrain transmits impulses to the thalamus, which further transmits the impulse to various areas of the cerebral cortex. This results in consciousness or awakening and possibly an arousal effect. Arousal reactions require an external signal, such as a pain stimulus, an alarm clock, or bright lights. The cerebral cortex may signal the RAS or vice versa, but the end result is activation of both areas that may lead to the additional transmission of impulses throughout the body (e.g., skeletal muscle activation). Inactivation of the RAS results in sleep, whereas injury or disease may produce a lack of consciousness or a comatose state.

The primary function of the alerting mechanism is self-preservation (e.g., waking up at night because of a chilly sensation). Once awakened, the individual can assess the situation and discover the reason for awakening, such as the blanket on the bed having fallen to the floor. In this situation the sensation of feeling chilly has activated the RAS and caused the awakening, but the situation must be assessed to determine why the chilliness occurred.

The filter mechanism of the RAS allows for a decrease in the perception of monotonous stimuli that usually surrounds everyone. It permits an individual to concentrate on a specific stimulus at a given time. For example, at a large party where nearly everyone is talking at the same time, a functioning RAS allows an individual to focus on a single conversation or person of interest by filtering out all other conversations. In other words, it permits selective concentration.

Many drugs act on the RAS. Anesthetics dampen its activity and induce sleep, whereas amphetamines stimulate or activate it. Lysergic acid diethylamide (LSD) and certain other hallucinogenic agents may act on the RAS by interfering with its ability to filter out stimuli; a person taking this substance is bombarded by all types of wanted, and sometimes unwanted, stimuli. In contrast, it is a proposed theory that chlorpromazine (Thorazine) stimulates the activity of the RAS and reinstates the activity of the filtering process, making it useful for reducing hallucinations in clients who are psychotic and in individuals experiencing an untoward reaction to LSD.

Limbic System The limbic system is a border of subcortical structures that surround the corpus callosum. This system forms a ring around the top of the brainstem and consists of the portions of the brain remaining after the cerebral hemispheres and cerebellum have been removed.

The limbic system is extremely complex in its functioning. The emotions of anger, fear, anxiety, sexual feelings, pleasure, and sorrow are related to the limbic system. It may work with or inhibit other parts of the brain such as the cerebral cortex, brainstem, or hypothalamus to normalize expressions of emotions, influence their ultimate expression to other than normal, or affect the biologic rhythms, sexual behavior, and motivation of an individual. Learning and memory have been associated with the hippocampus, a component of this system.

Drugs that affect the limbic system are the benzodiazepines and morphine. The benzodiazepines are believed to suppress the limbic system, preventing it from stimulating the RAS and resulting in drowsiness and sleep, especially in clients with anxiety. Morphine is thought to alter subjective reactions to pain in addition to abolishing pain stimuli received by special areas within the limbic system.

Extrapyramidal System The extrapyramidal system is a somatic motor pathway located in the CNS that affects skeletal muscles. This system is associated with posture and the coordination of muscle group movements. Antipsychotic agents that block dopamine receptors may produce adverse effects related to this system. (See Chapter 19 for further discussion of these effects.)

✳ How does synaptic transmission occur and what substances are involved?

As mentioned previously, the synapse is the junction point between two neurons or between a neuron and an effector organ. There is evidence that the transmission of impulses at synapses in the CNS is humoral, occurring through a neurotransmitter secretion. When a neurotransmitter is released, it either stimulates or inhibits the activity of the postsynaptic neurons.

Inhibition of motor neuron activity may be presynaptic or postsynaptic. Studies indicate that presynaptic inhibition occurs in the brain and is widespread at the spinal level, affecting transmission in afferent fibers from skin and muscle. The function of presynaptic inhibition is probably to suppress weak inputs that would otherwise cause unnecessary responses. With this modulation of nerve impulses, less transmitter substance is liberated. The net effect is a limiting or "inhibiting" of impulses to postsynaptic nerve fibers. Inhibition is important for orderly function.

Postsynaptic inhibition may be the result of changes in the membrane permeability of the postsynaptic cells caused by the release of chemical transmitters from presynaptic nerve endings. Upper motor neurons are scattered throughout the cerebral cortex and a number of them are located in the motor cortex. Approximately three-fourths of the nerve fibers from these motor neurons cross to the opposite side at the level of the medulla, descend to the spinal cord, and synapse with interneurons, which, in turn, synapse with the lower motor neurons. Almost all motor neurons of one side are controlled by the motor cortex of the other side. Therefore injury to the motor cortex of the right side of the brain causes paralysis on the left side of the body (left hemiplegia). Although systems other than the upper and lower motor neuron systems are concerned with voluntary movement, the lower motor neurons form the common final pathway for stimuli for voluntary movement.

Some of the neurotransmitters that are discussed in the following sections are acetylcholine, the catecholamines (dopamine, norepinephrine, and epinephrine), serotonin, and neuroactive peptides (enkephalins, endorphins, and dynorphins).

Acetylcholine
Acetylcholine is the best known chemical transmitter of nerve impulses. Not all parts of the CNS contain acetylcholine. Areas with high concentrations of acetylcholine are the motor cortex, thalamus, hypothalamus, and anterior spinal roots; very low concentrations are found in the cerebellum, optic nerves, and dorsal roots of the spine. Acetylcholine can cause cardiac inhibition, vasodilation, gastrointestinal peristalsis, and other parasympathetic effects.

The lower motor neurons release acetylcholine at the neuromuscular junction, causing contraction in striated (voluntary) muscle. The concentration of acetylcholine must be high because a large number of muscle fibers must respond synchronously for striated muscle contraction to occur and because acetylcholine is very rapidly destroyed by the enzyme cholinesterase.

Catecholamines and Related Substances
Dopamine, norepinephrine, and epinephrine (which are neurotransmitters of the catecholamine subclass, a group of sympathomimetic compounds) and the amine neurotransmitter serotonin (5-hydroxytryptamine) are synthesized, stored, and metabolized in the brain. They act directly on sympathetic effector cells by binding to receptors. These substances do not easily penetrate the blood-brain barrier, but their precursors do. The effect of injected catecholamines on the CNS is slight in comparison with the effect on the autonomic nervous system. An increase in catecholamines

and serotonin causes cerebral stimulation. Drugs such as reserpine that release catecholamines and reduce amine concentration in the brain have a depressing or sedative action. Methyldopa lowers the levels of serotonin and norepinephrine; this, too, has a cerebral depressing effect.

Special diagnostic techniques indicate that there are adrenergic (sympathomimetic) and serotoninergic tracts within the CNS. Dopamine is especially concentrated in the basal ganglia. The low level of dopamine at this site in individuals suffering from Parkinson's disease led to the use of its precursor, levodopa, as a therapeutic approach; in many cases the results have been good.

Neuroactive Peptides
Neuroactive peptides may be considered neuromodulators, neurohormones, or neurotransmitters. These peptides may affect neuronal activity by increasing or decreasing the synthesis, release, or breakdown of neurotransmitters, neurohormones, or neuromodulators. The parenteral or intracerebral injection of these components causes potent behavioral effects. A number of these peptides exist in tissues other than the CNS, primarily in the cells of the gastrointestinal (GI) tract.

Enkephalins, endorphins, and dynorphins are three major polypeptides that are found in the brain and each has opioid activity. The concept of internal opiates or natural painkillers developed after studies indicated that enkephalins may bind to the same neuroreceptor membranes as morphine. Enkephalins behave as inhibitory neurotransmitters, allowing modification and control of the perception and emotional aspect of pain. To do this, enkephalins may block opiate receptors in the dorsal horn of the spinal cord by blocking the release of substance P. Substance P, a transmitter of pain impulses in the nerve fibers, has been proposed to be a transmitter for the primary afferent sensory fibers.

Endorphin (from "endogenous morphine") is a general term that includes many peptides in the brain that suppress pain. These peptides are also found in the pituitary gland, the intermediate lobe, and the corticotropin cells of the adenohypophysis. Subgroups of endorphins have been isolated and identified, including β-endorphin, an analgesic substance that is much more potent than enkephalin.

Technology has shown that the brain, pituitary gland, and GI tract each have enkephalins and β-endorphins. These peptides are not found in the same cells. The brain cells containing β-endorphins are different from those that contain enkephalins.

Dynorphin is an endorphin found in the pituitary gland, hypothalamus, and spinal cord. It is the most potent pain-relieving substance discovered; dynorphin is 50 times more potent than β-endorphin and 200 times more potent than morphine.

Naloxone, a potent opioid antagonist, reverses the analgesic effect of opioids. Animal studies demonstrate that if naloxone is administered after enkephalins or endorphins are given, the analgesic effect produced by the polypeptides is reversed. Endorphin release in the body is higher after acupuncture and transcutaneous electrical nerve stimulation, and each effect may be reversed by the use of naloxone.

It has been proposed that the analgesic response associated with the use of a placebo may result from an increased release of endorphins in the body. From peptide research may come pain relievers with fewer adverse effects and minimal to no addiction potential. An increased understanding of mental disorders and addiction mechanisms may also be gained from this research.

Summary

The CNS is composed of the brain and the spinal cord and essentially controls all of the functions of the body. The CNS integrates information received from the peripheral nervous system concerning the internal and external environment of the body and then sends messages to produce the adjustments necessary for maintaining homeostasis.

The cerebrum is the highest functional area of the brain. Drugs that affect the cerebral cortex may decrease mental acuity, consciousness, and motor function by their depressive action or increase muscle activity and restlessness through their stimulating effects. The thalamus relays impulses to the cerebral cortex and also registers pain, temperature, touch, and other sensory impulses. The hypothalamus is a major link between the nervous system and the endocrine system. Ten of the 12 cranial nerves and the involuntary respiratory center originate in the brainstem.

The RAS, limbic system, and extrapyramidal system are the three major functional systems of the CNS. The RAS is responsible for consciousness, filtering, and alerting to stimuli; the limbic system is responsible for learning and memory and for the emotions of anger, fear, anxiety, pleasure, and sorrow; and the extrapyramidal system is responsible for muscle coordination.

The blood-brain barrier prohibits the passage of many drugs into the brain. The respiratory centers, as well as the centers for coughing and vomiting in the brainstem, are highly sensitive to drugs. Medications that disturb the cerebellum cause dizziness and loss of balance. Drugs may also affect the spinal cord, which transmits impulses to and from the brain. The RAS, limbic system, and extrapyramidal system may also be affected by medications.

Neurotransmitters affect the postsynaptic neurons to increase or decrease their activity. The most important of the neurotransmitters are acetylcholine, the catecholamines, serotonin, and the neuroactive peptides. Neurobiologic research is currently demonstrating the increasing importance of understanding more about these substances and, in general, the CNS.

✴ Critical Thinking Questions

- Richard Akers was diagnosed with a tumor in the area of the hypothalamus. What bodily functions could be adversely affected by an abnormal growth in this structure?
- Delores Lightfoot sustained a head injury in an automobile accident. The physician suspects there may be injury to the cerebellum. What symptoms would Delores most likely exhibit if there were cerebellar injury?
- How do neurotransmitters function in synaptic transmission?

Bibliography

Anderson, D.M., Keith, J., Novak, P.D. & Eliot, M.A. (2002). *Mosby's medical, nursing, & allied health dictionary* (6th ed.). St. Louis: Mosby.

DiPiro, J.T., Talbert, R.L., Yee, G.C., Matzke, G.R., Wells, B.G. & Posey, L.M. (Eds.). *Pharmacotherapy: A pathophysiological approach* (5th ed.). New York: McGraw-Hill.

Herlihy, B., & Maebius, N.K. (2003). *The human body in health and illness* (2nd ed.). Philadelphia: W.B. Saunders.

McCance, K.L., & Huether, S.E. (2002). *Pathophysiology: The biological basis for disease in adults and children* (4th ed.). St. Louis: Mosby.

Porth, M.C. (2002). *Pathophysiology—Concepts of altered health states* (6th ed.). Philadelphia: Lippincott Williams & Wilkins.

Thibodeau, G.A., & Patton, K.T. (2003). *Anatomy & physiology* (5th ed.). St. Louis: Mosby.

 e-LEARNING SUPPLEMENTS

Student CD-ROM
- Final Exam questions
- NCLEX® Examination review questions
- Pharmacology animations
- Printable chapter summary

Evolve Website (http://evolve.elsevier.com/mckenry)
- Content updates, including information on new drugs
- WebLinks corresponding to this chapter
- Answers to the critical thinking questions in this chapter
- *Elsevier ePharmacology Update* newsletter
- Mosby's Drug Consult Internet Edition
- Supplemental and reference information

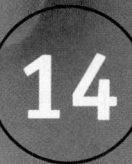

ANALGESICS

Chapter Focus

Pain is a paradox. It is a universal occurrence—everyone experiences pain occasionally in a lifetime. However, everyone's experience is unique and subjective. Only the client is an expert on his or her pain. Because the pain experience is so common with clients, nurses must be knowledgeable about pain and skillful in interventions to prevent and relieve it.

LEARNING OBJECTIVES

- Describe the physiology, characteristics, and types of pain.
- Discuss the myths that interfere with pain management.
- Discuss special considerations for opioid use during pregnancy, labor, delivery, and breastfeeding.
- Discuss special considerations for pain management for clients with substance abuse.
- Discuss special considerations for opioid use in children and older adults.
- Describe the nurse's role in opioid therapy.
- Differentiate among the opioid analgesics, antagonists, and agonist-antagonist agents.
- Describe the relationship between prostaglandin synthesis and nonsteroidal antiinflammatory drug effects in inflammation.
- Discuss the pharmacokinetics, adverse effects, and drug interactions of nonsteroidal antiinflammatory drugs.
- Implement a plan of care for individual clients who require the administration of opioid analgesics, opioid antagonists, and nonsteroidal antiinflammatory drugs.

Pain is a common human problem. Approximately $120 billion dollars is spent each year on treatment, lost revenues, and wages for chronic pain clients in the United States alone. Approximately 28% to 30% of the U.S. population suffers from some chronic pain condition. According to a June 2000 Gallup Survey of "Pain in America," 42% of adults experience pain daily. It is more distressing and disabling than nearly any other client symptom. This is unfortunate, because most **analgesics** (pain-relieving drugs) currently available are safe and effective when properly selected and applied, based on the pharmacokinetics of the drug and the individual client's response. The Joint Commission on Accreditation of Healthcare Organizations (JCAHO), acknowledging that pain is a coexisting condition with many other diseases and injuries, has established standards to make pain management an integral part of all treatment plans, essentially making pain the fifth vital sign.

✳ If analgesics are effective, why do people experience pain?

Effective pain management is a collaborative effort between health care professionals and client and family. However, within this relationship, there are barriers on both the part of health care providers and clients that inhibit effective pain management. Health care professionals often fail to routinely assess and document pain. Because of inadequate training, they may lack knowledge and skills to assess and manage pain appropriately. They also may lack sufficient knowledge to use equianalgesic principles to effectively substitute one analgesic for another when altering a pain management program to meet a client's needs for pain relief. It is not uncommon for health care professionals to have exaggerated concerns related to the adverse effects of opioids, especially about tolerance and addiction. This may be a concern because **opioids** are natural and synthetic chemicals that have opium-like effects but are not derived from opium. As a system's contribution, there may be a lack of practical, effective treatment protocols within the health care agency for pain relief.

Health care professionals may undertreat pain because of their belief in common misconceptions about pain and/or opioids. Some of the myths relating to client pain are the following:

- A client's perception of chronic pain can be correlated with vital sign changes and evidence of injury.
- Clients in pain readily express their pain to health care professionals.
- Clients of certain gender, cultural, ethnic, or socioeconomic backgrounds consistently underreport or overreport their pain.
- Opioids are addictive and a treatment of last resort because of unmanageable adverse effects.
- Older clients and cognitively impaired clients do not perceive pain as intensely as other clients.
- If clients are able to sleep, they are not in very much pain.

- The goal of chronic pain management is to keep the dose of medication as low as possible.
- Clients with a history of substance abuse who require intravenous (IV) opioids should never be allowed to control their own dose of medication (i.e., patient-controlled analgesia [PCA]).
- There is no physiologic basis for the moderation effects of emotions on pain perception.
- Prescribers who liberally treat pain with opioids should fear prosecution and suspension or loss of professional license.

But for their part, clients may also come to the pain experience with their own set of misconceptions, such as the following:

- Severe or chronic pain cannot be effectively controlled.
- Opioids are always addictive and a treatment of last resort ("I must be dying").
- Pain is always evidence of disease progression.
- It is more admirable or socially acceptable to ignore pain.
- Pain is unavoidable result of aging or disease.
- Pain is a deserved punishment (University of Michigan Health System, 2004).

Research continues in the area of pain and the health care professional mythology related to it. Drayer, Henderson, and Reidenberg (1999) found that providers still fear client addiction, expect that clients will exaggerate their pain, and believe there is poor correlation between pain behavior and pain intensity, despite literature that indicates the converse (McCaffery & Pasero, 1999; Salerno & Willens, 1996; Agency for Health Care Policy & Research [AHCPR], 1994). Another area of concern is the influence of personal biases on decisions to administer pain medications. McCaffery and Ferrell (1992) questioned gender effect and bias in pain management. They reported that nurses generally believe there is a difference between male and female pain sensitivity, pain tolerance, and distress, which influences the nurse's assessment of the client's pain and the amount of drug used in treatment. This belief would lead to undertreatment of pain in women.

Cleeland et al. (1994) studied pain treatment in approximately 1300 outpatients with metastatic cancer from 54 cancer treatment centers that ranged from university cancer centers to community based hospitals and oncology programs. The study outcome indicated undertreatment with medication for pain, finding that: (1) women were at a greater risk for being undermedicated for pain, especially those younger than age 50 years; (2) adults older than age 70 years (both genders) often received less potent pain medication, even with reports of significant pain; (3) clinics that service predominantly minority populations were nearly three times more likely to undertreat pain than were centers that service predominantly nonminority populations; (4) there was a vast discrepancy between the physician's and the individual cancer client's estimate of pain severity; and (5) more than half the clients in this study had pain, with 62% reporting pain as interfering with their daily functioning. Although these studies were completed in the last decade, a

Pain Management for African Americans and Caucasian Americans

Studies and research have identified the problems associated with inadequate cancer pain management and the Agency for Health Care Policy and Research (AHCPR) issued *Clinical Practice Guidelines for Acute Pain Management and Cancer Pain Management* (AHCPR, 1994) to help correct this problem. However, additional studies are needed in the area of gender, age, and ethnic and cultural biases in pain management. Culture has been identified as a factor that influences a person's reaction to pain as well as health care use in response to that pain. Green, Baker, and Ndao-Brumblay (2004) descriptively compared health care use and referral in African and Caucasian Americans with chronic pain. They found that African Americans agreed more than Caucasian Americans that ethnicity and culture affected access to health care and pain management. They also tended to agree more than Caucasian Americans that pain medication could not control pain. African Americans were more likely to report that chronic pain was a major reason for financial problems and to make significantly more visits to the emergency room for pain care. In another study, Green, Baker, Sato, Washington, & Smith (2003a) addressed the potential differential effects of chronic pain in black and Caucasian Americans, 18 to 50 years of age. These results showed that on initial assessment black Americans with chronic pain report significantly more pain and sleep disturbance, as well as more symptoms consistent with posttraumatic disorder and depression, than do Caucasian Americans, and that black Americans also experience a higher prevalence of self-identified symptoms, including dizziness, chest pain, and high blood pressure. This study suggests that there may be a significant decrease in the overall physical and emotional health of black Americans with chronic pain. Another study by Green, Baker, Smith, and Sato (2003b) also looked at chronic pain, but with older black and Caucasian Americans. It also suggests that chronic pain adversely affects the quality of life and health status of black Americans to a greater extent than Caucasian Americans.

Critical Thinking Questions

- How could the knowledge of these findings alter your assessment of chronic pain in clients?
- How would you alter your implementation of pain relief measures for a black American with chronic pain?

continuing concern for the influence of gender and race continues to be evident in the literature (Green, Wheeler, & LaPorte, 2003; Weisse, Sorum, & Dominguez, 2003). (See the Cultural Considerations box above.) Client beliefs may also contribute to inadequate management of pain.

Because opioids have the potential for abuse and illegal diversion, federal and state laws strictly monitor and regulate their availability, prescription, and use. Although the intent of federal law is not to interfere with the appropriate prescribing, many states have enacted laws or regulations that limit, restrict, and closely monitor opioid prescribing. As a result, many prescribers are reluctant to prescribe opioids for fear of prosecution and suspension or loss of their professional licenses. Such regulations have resulted in undertreatment of pain, even in clients with severe cancer pain (AHCPR, 1994). In 2001, Gilson and Joranson wrote that physicians are concerned about regulatory investigation, negatively influencing their prescribing of opioid analgesics. However, a Gilson and Joranson 1997 survey of state medical board members contrasted with a 1991 survey, demonstrating that there were important positive changes in attitudes, particularly regarding characteristics of "addiction" and the legality of prolonged prescribing of opioids.

✸ What is pain?

Because of its highly subjective nature, pain is difficult to define. The International Association for the Study of Pain defines pain as "an unpleasant sensory and emotional experience associated with actual or potential tissue damage, or described in terms of such damage" (American Pain Society [APS], 2003). McCaffery, a widely recognized nurse expert in pain assessment and management opined that pain is whatever the person experiencing the sensation says it is, existing whenever that person says it does (McCaffery & Pasero, 1999). The North American Nursing Diagnosis Association (NANDA) defines pain as "the state in which a person experiences and reports the presence of severe discomfort or an uncomfortable sensation . . ." (NANDA, 2005).

Pain involves a subjective sensation and response to actual or potential tissue damage. Pain can be viewed as having two components: (1) the physical component or the sensation of pain, and (2) the psychologic component or emotional response to pain. The physical component of pain involves nerve pathways and the brain. The psychologic component or the emotional response to pain is the product of factors such as an individual's anxiety level, previous pain experience, age, gender, and culture.

A relatively constant pain threshold exists in all persons under normal circumstances. For example, heat applied to the skin at an intensity of 45° to 48° C will initiate a sensation of pain in almost all individuals. However, pain tolerance—the point beyond which pain becomes unbearable—varies widely among individuals and under different circumstances in a single individual. Figure 14-1 shows the factors that affect the pain threshold.

Welk (1991) described an educational model that illustrates pain and suffering and the various issues that influence suffering in a terminally ill client (Figure 14-2).

As this model notes, physical pain is only part of the suffering model and is not interchangeable with suffering. A

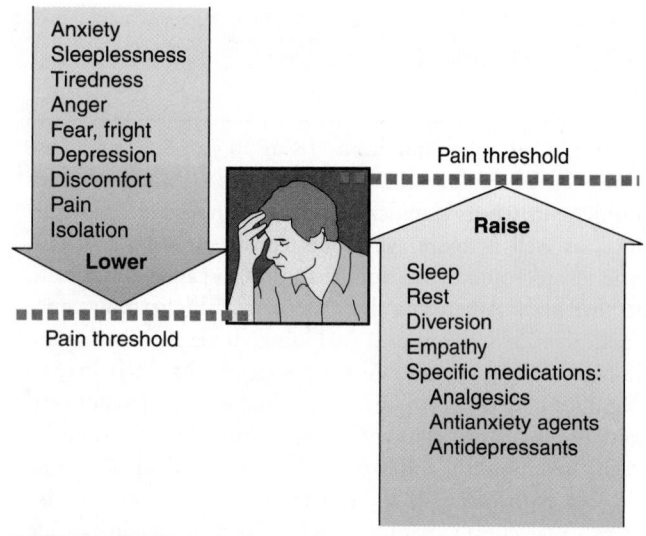

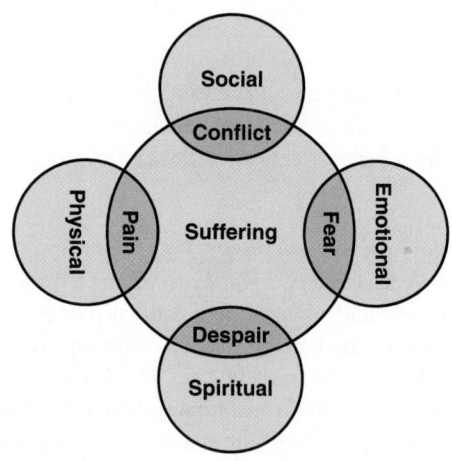

FIGURE 14-2 Education model illustrating pain and suffering.

From Welk, T.A. (1991). An educational model for explaining hospice services. *American Journal of Hospice & Palliative Care, 8*(5), 14-17.

person may be suffering without physical pain or may have physical pain without suffering. Suffering involves multiple issues that prevent a person from living without fear, such as physical pain, emotional fear (e.g., fear of the unknown, fear of dying, fear of dying alone), social conflict (e.g., conflicts with family and friends), and spiritual despair (not necessarily religious, a spiritual dimension to meet an individual client's need). Other persons with persistent, chronic pain may also have factors other than physical pain involved. These factors are often addressed by interdisciplinary teams in hospices and pain management programs.

✱ **J.F. is a 56-year-old female with severe rheumatoid arthritis who is admitted to the hospital for bilateral knee replacement. What type of pain did J.F. experience prior to her surgery? What type of pain can J.F. expect after surgery?**

Pain can be classified in various ways. For example, it may be acute or chronic. **Acute pain,** the presence of severe discomfort or an uncomfortable sensation, lasting from 1 second to

over time	
RESPONSE TO ACUTE PAIN	**ADAPTATION**
(Observable signs of discomfort)	(Decrease in observable signs although pain intensity unchanged)
Physiologic responses	**Physiologic responses**
↑ Blood pressure ↑ Pulse rate ↑ Respiratory rate Dilated pupils Perspiration	Normal blood pressure Normal pulse rate Normal respiratory rate Normal pupil size Dry skin
Behavioral responses	**Behavioral responses**
Focuses on pain Reports pain Cries and moans Rubs painful part ↑ muscle tension Frowns and grimaces	No report of pain unless questioned Quiet, sleeps or rests Turns attention to things other than pain Physical inactivity or immobility Blank or normal facial expression

(PAIN SENSATION)

FIGURE 14-3 Acute pain model vs. adaptation.

Data from McCaffery, M., & Pasero, C. (1999). *Pain: Clinical manual for nursing practice* (2nd ed.). St. Louis: Mosby.

less than 6 months has a sudden onset and usually subsides with treatment (NANDA, 2005). Examples of acute pain include the pain of myocardial infarction, appendicitis, kidney stones, and surgical pain. For J.F., the pain related to knee surgery and knee pain observed during the days after surgery would be considered primarily acute pain. **Chronic pain** may have a sudden or slow onset, can be of any intensity from mild to severe, is constant or recurring, cannot be anticipated or predicted, and has a duration of greater than 6 months (Ackley & Ladwig, 2006). Most likely, J.F. experienced chronic pain related to rheumatoid arthritis prior to surgery, and is likely to continue to have some chronic pain in other joints post surgically. Chronic pain can be difficult to treat, and often requires multiple modes of therapy. Cancer-related pain is a third type of pain that displays elements of both acute and chronic pain (Table 14-1). Acute pain involves physiologic and behavioral responses; the body adapts to pain over time and those physiologic and behavioral responses change with chronic pain (Figure 14-3).

Pain may occur because of actual injury (**somatic pain**) or without obvious tissue damage. Somatic pain may present as **nociceptive pain,** where tissue damage results in peripheral nerve stimulation; because there is typically an inflammatory component, some clinicians refer to this type of pain as **inflammatory pain** (Backonja, 2003). Somatic pain may also present as **neuropathic pain,** where a dysfunction in the central or peripheral nervous system affects nerve conduction in a negative way, often involves neural supersensitivity (Reisman & Pasternak, 2001; Schwartzman, Grothusen, Kiefer, & Rohr, 2001), and is usually responsive to antiepileptic drugs or antidepressants. **Visceral pain** is often considered an additional type of somatic pain that originates in smooth muscle or sympathetically innervated organ systems. Visceral pain is often difficult to localize because it is dull and aching and may

TABLE 14-1 DIFFERENTIATION OF ACUTE, CHRONIC, AND CANCER-RELATED PAIN

	Acute Pain	Chronic Pain	Cancer-Related Pain
Onset	Usually sudden	Variable	Variable
Duration	Hours to days	Months to years	Variable
Characteristics	Generally sharp, localized, may radiate	Dull, aching, persistent, diffuse	Variable, usually persistent
Associated pathology	Present	Unpredictable	Present with worsening as cancer progresses
Prognosis	Predictable	Unpredictable	Usually predictable, progressive course
Associated problems	Anxiety	Depression, negative attitude	Many, especially loss of control
Nerve conduction	Rapid	Slow	Slow
Physiologic response	Elevated blood pressure, heart rate, sweating, pallor	Generally absent	Variable, usually absent
Biologic value of pain	High	Low or absent	Low
Social effects	Few	Profound	Profound
Goals of treatment	Relief of pain; sedation often desirable	Prevention of pain; sedation not desirable	Relief and prevention of pain; sedation often not desirable
Treatment	Drugs have a primary role	Multimodal, behavioral interventions have primary role; drugs secondary role	Multimodal; drugs have a primary role

also be referred (i.e., felt at a site distant from its origin). An example of referred pain is the pain of a myocardial infarction that is felt initially in the arm. For J.F., her pain would be expected to be primarily nociceptive, although there may be elements of neuropathic and visceral pain.

✱ What causes pain?

Nociceptive pain involves tissue injury or inflammation with resultant stimulation of the nociceptors (pain receptors). These nociceptors are afferent peripheral nerve fibers located throughout the body, including the skin, skeletal muscle, joints, and abdominal, thoracic, and cranial cavities. Nociceptive pain typically presents as a throbbing, aching pain observed after trauma to muscles, ligaments, or joints. Many stimuli can activate nociceptors, including tissue trauma, ischemia, and mediators of the resultant inflammatory process. One important mediator is prostaglandin E_2 (PGE$_2$).

Prostaglandins are hormone-like, unsaturated fatty acids that act on local target organs to affect vasomotor tone, capillary permeability, smooth muscle tone, platelet aggregation, endocrine and exocrine functions, and the autonomic and central nervous systems (CNS). They have been referred to as tissue hormones because they are secreted in many different tissues and perform their activity only within a short distance—usually to other cells within the same tissue. They are rapidly metabolized in the bloodstream, resulting in low levels of circulating prostaglandin levels.

At least 16 prostaglandins have been identified and produce a variety of diverse effects. Prostaglandin E_1 is involved

in protecting gastric mucosa from acid. Prostaglandin F is involved in the reproductive system, causes uterine muscle contractions, and has been used to induce labor. Prostaglandins are metabolized from arachidonic acid via the enzymes cyclooxygenase-1 (COX-1) and cyclooxygenase-2 (COX-2). COX-1 appears to be primarily involved in maintaining gastric protection and hemostasis, whereas COX-2 is integral in the synthesis of prostaglandins involved in inflammatory, pain and fever. Therapies that interfere with COX-2 function (e.g., the nonsteroidal antiinflammatory drugs [NSAIDs]) are often quite effective at treating nociceptive pain and have minimal CNS effects (Figure 14-4).

Whereas nociceptive pain is usually the result of tissue inflammation and direct stimulation of intact afferent nerve endings, neuropathic pain is caused by peripheral nerve injury and not by stimulation. Neuropathic pain, like nociceptive pain, may involve inflammation and may even be triggered by nociceptive pain, but the inflammation in neuropathic pain is noted in the nerve itself (Backonja, 2003). Neuropathic pain is also called *paresthesia* and is described as a burning, shooting, and/or tingling sensation, and often persists beyond the expected healing period for the inflamed nerve. It is frequently associated with *dysesthesia*, a common effect of spinal cord injury that also includes numbness. Neuropathic pain caused by cancer tumor invasion or treatment-induced nerve damage may be accompanied by sympathetic nervous system dysfunction. It is also observed with viral infection of the nerve (e.g., genital herpes, herpes zoster), and in many chronic conditions with

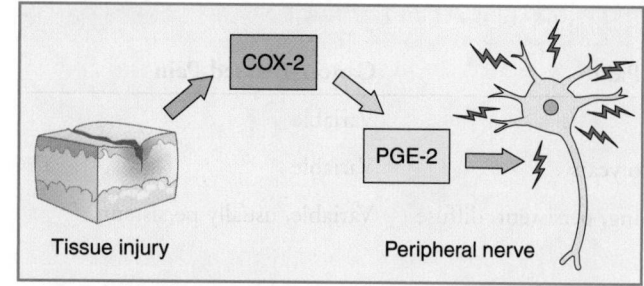

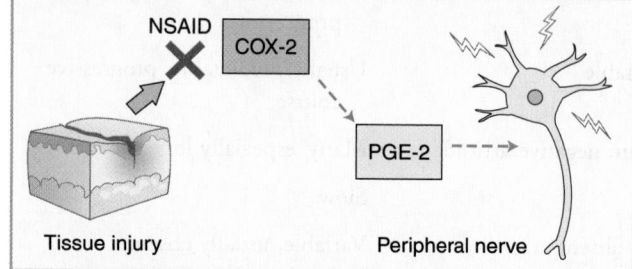

FIGURE 14-4 Model for nociceptive pain. **A,** Tissue injury triggers cyclooxygenase-2 (COX-2) in peripheral tissue to convert arachidonic acid to prostaglandin E₂ (PGE₂), resulting in stimulation of the nociceptor in peripheral nerve to send a signal for pain to the central nervous system. **B,** Nonsteroidal antiinflammatory drug (NSAID) interfering with COX-2–mediated prostaglandin synthesis.

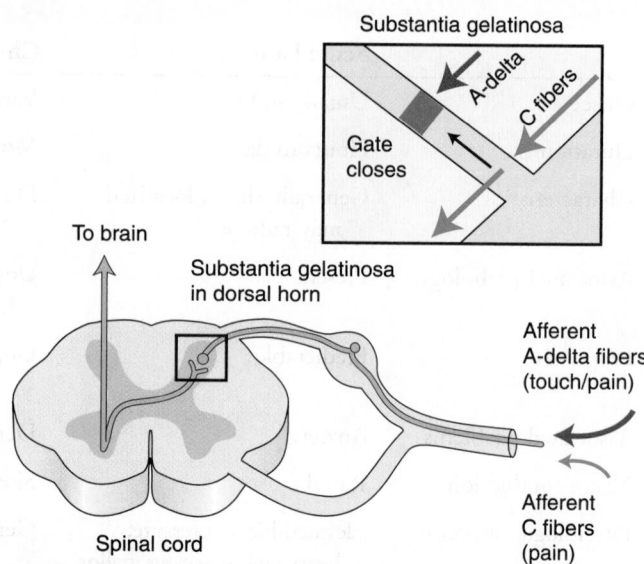

FIGURE 14-5 Gate control theory. Activity from A-delta (large afferent) fibers excites activity in the substantia gelatinosa, thus closing the gate to C fibers, the pain-stimulating fibers.

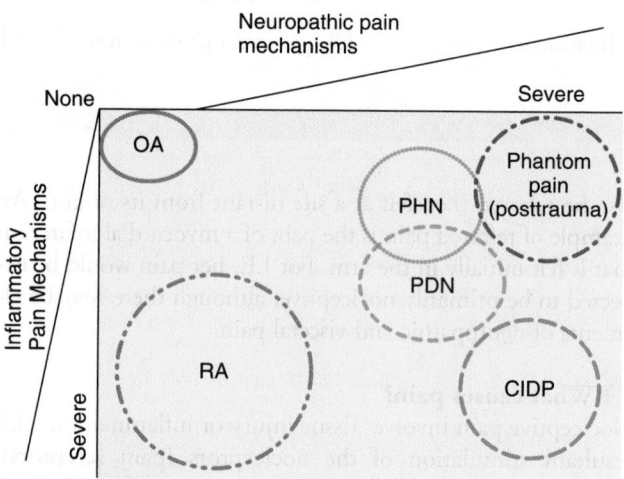

FIGURE 14-6 The hypothetical relationship between inflammatory and neuropathic pain mechanisms. *CIDP,* Chronic inflammatory demyelinating polyneuropathy; *OA,* osteoarthritis; *PDN,* painful diabetic neuropathy; *PHN,* postherpetic neuralgia; *RA,* rheumatoid arthritis.

From Backonja, M. (2003). Defining neuropathic pain. *Anesthesia & Analgesia, 97*(3), 785-790.

neuronal complications (e.g., diabetic neuropathy and sciatic nerve inflammation). Neuropathic pain responds less well to opioid analgesics and often requires adding adjunct medication that has a more direct effect on nerve conduction (e.g., antiepileptic drug, tricyclic antidepressant).

The great variation in the pain experience has prompted much research and has led to the proposal of several theories of pain transmission and pain relief. The gate control theory proposed by Melzack and Wall (1965) attempted to explain modulations in the pain experience (Figure 14-5). This theory proposed that a mechanism in the dorsal horn of the spinal cord (the "spinal gate") can alter the transmission of painful sensations from the peripheral nerve fibers to the thalamus and cortex of the brain, where they are recognized as pain. The "spinal gate" is closed by large-diameter, low-threshold afferent fibers (the fast-acting A-delta fibers) and is opened by small-diameter, high-threshold afferent fibers (the slower-acting C fibers). Descending control inhibition from the brain further influences the "gate." Thus the stimulation of large-diameter fibers will "close the gate" to stop the perception of slower-acting painful stimuli. It is on this theory that many nondrug regimens for pain relief are based, including massage or the use of counterirritants. It is also a foundation of the Lamaze method of "natural childbirth."

Many clients will experience a mix of nociceptive/peripherally inflammatory and neuropathic mechanisms in their expression of pain (Figure 14-6). Successful pain relief is partly related to the extent to which the health care team can establish the nature of the pain and institute targeted therapy. Antiinflammatory drugs and opioids are effective for nocicep-

tive or peripherally inflammatory pain while antiepileptic drugs and antidepressants will target neuropathic pain.

Pain may also have an emotional origin. Psychiatric illness or psychosocial issues (e.g., anxiety and depression, fear of dying) have been known to cause severe pain. Negative emotions facilitate the expression of pain (Rhudy & Meagher, 2001). Individuals with chronic pain are also noted to be significantly more fearful and avoidant of social interactions, suggesting anxiety disorders. In such cases, treatment with a combination of analgesics, psychotherapy,

Date _____

Client's Name _____ Age _____ Room _____

Diagnosis _____ Physician _____

Nurse _____

I. Location: Client or nurse mark drawing

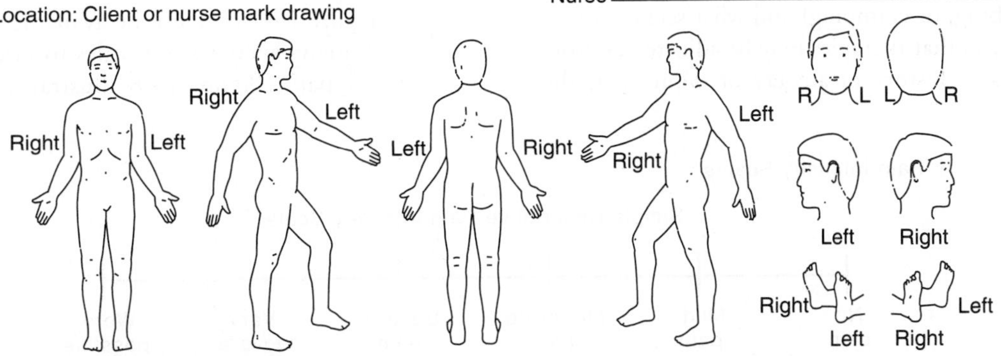

Right   Left   Right   Left   Left   Right   Left   Right   R   L   L   R

Left   Right

Right   Left   Left   Right

II. Intensity: Client rates the pain. Scale used _____
    Present: _____
    Worst pain gets: _____
    Best pain gets: _____
    Acceptable level of pain: _____

III. Quality: (Use client's own words, e.g., prick, ache, burn, throb, pull, sharp) _____

IV. Onset, duration variations, rhythms: _____

V. Manner of expressing pain: _____

VI. What relieves the pain? _____

VII. What causes or increases the pain? _____

VIII. Effects of pain: (Note decreased function, decreased quality of life)
    Accompanying symptoms (e.g., nausea) _____
    Sleep _____
    Appetite _____
    Physical activity _____
    Relationship with others (e.g., irritability) _____
    Emotions (e.g., anger, suicidal, crying) _____
    Concentration _____
    Other _____

IX. Other comments: _____

X. Plan: _____

FIGURE 14-7 Pain assessment tool of M. McCaffery and A. Beebe.

From McCaffery, M., & Pasero, C. (1999). *Pain: Clinical manual for nursing practice* (2nd ed.). St. Louis: Mosby.

and drug therapy of the underlying psychiatric condition may be more successful than using analgesics alone.

How should J.F.'s pain be assessed?

Nurses must use all of their skills to successfully manage the care of clients who are experiencing pain. The nurse often coordinates the implementation of pain management with active client involvement. Some health care agencies have pain teams comprised of anesthetist, psychologist, pharmacist, and nurse (McDonnell, Nicholl, & Read, 2003).

Accurate pain assessment is based on both subjective and objective information. Because "pain" cannot be observed (it is a perception, not an object), a nurse must assess J.F.'s physical and psychologic signs and symptoms. Each person perceives and reacts to pain differently on the basis of physical, emotional, and cultural influences. In particular, cultural background affects the manner in which pain is communicated and various clients may respond differently to the same noxious stimulus. A nurse does not assess pain by the presence or absence of any individual behavior such as crying or moaning, but listens to the client's statement of pain and evaluates each pain episode as unique. With nonverbal clients, the total clinical presentation is assessed.

Assessing J.F.'s pain is the first step toward understanding pain as she experiences it, and provides a basis for positive client-nurse collaboration in its management. Careful documentation provides a baseline to select appropriate nursing interventions and to evaluate the effectiveness of nursing care. Figure 14-7 is an example of a tool from McCaffery and Pasero (1999) that illustrates the essential components for the assessment of pain. It is necessary to determine the *intensity* and *location* of J.F.'s pain. For example, postoperative discomfort cannot be assumed to be "incisional" pain when it is possible that a client may be experiencing pain related to other conditions such as deep vein thrombosis or myocardial infarction. It is vital that the assessment be described in J.F.'s own words, both in terms of the *quality* and *description* of the pain (sharp, dull, burning, radiating, stabbing, or cramping) and what seems to *intensify* or *relieve* it, so that therapies may be adjusted appropriately. If she has a history of anxiety or depression, these should be addressed with drug and nondrug interventions. This assessment information will assist a nurse to determine J.F.'s manner of expressing pain and its effects.

Although a complete pain assessment tool such as the one in Figure 14-7 may not be available in all health care agencies, many agencies use scales to rate the *intensity* or *severity* of pain. Figure 14-8 illustrates several of these

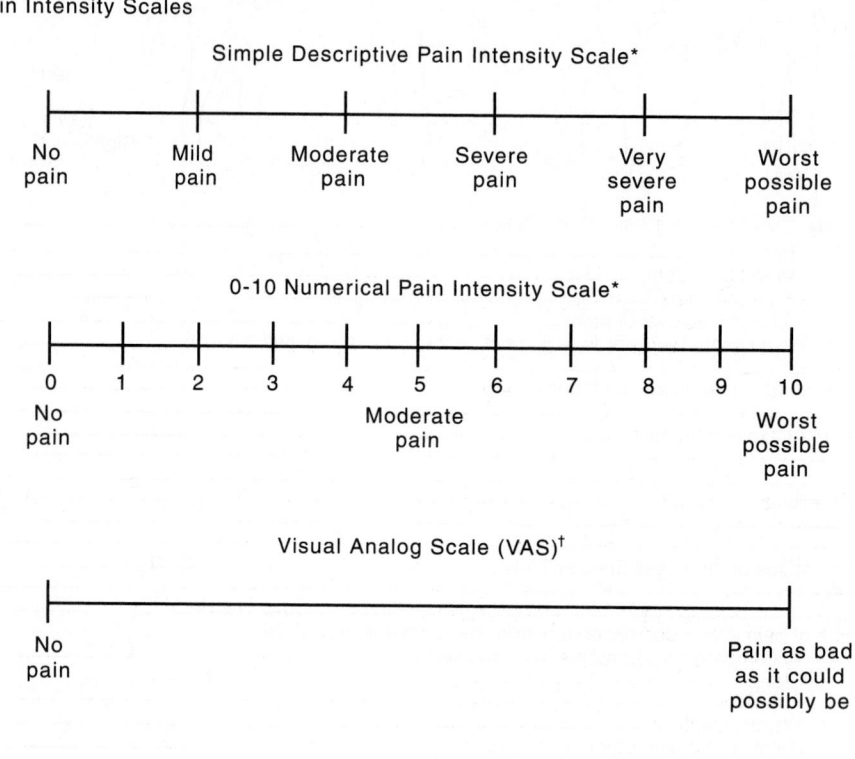

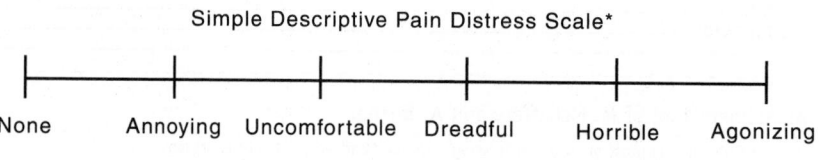

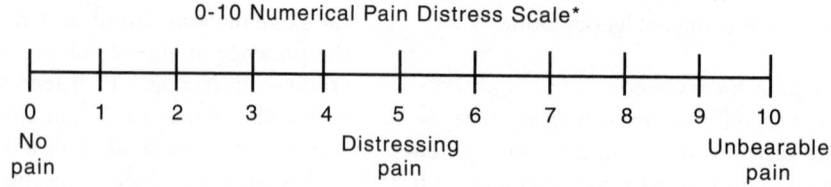

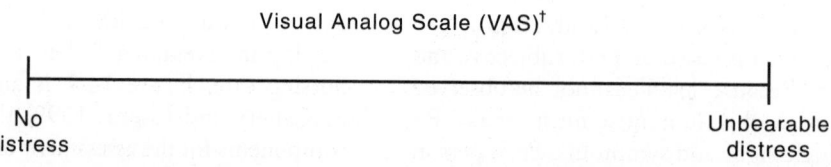

FIGURE 14-8 Scales for rating the intensity and distress of pain. *If used as a graphic rating scale, a 10-cm baseline is recommended. †A 10-cm baseline is recommended for VASs.

From Acute Pain Management Guideline Panel. (1992). *Acute pain management: Operative or medical procedures and trauma. Clinical practice guideline.* AHCPR Pub. No. 92-0032. Rockville, MD: Agency for Health Care Policy and Research, Public Health Service, U.S. Department of Health and Human Services.

scales. If printed scales are not available, ask J.F. to rate the pain on a scale of 0 (no pain) to 10 (unbearable pain); this will provide consistency for the assessment of her perception of the pain. In addition, have her rate the pain at an appropriate time interval after administering an analgesic to evaluate the medication's effectiveness and to titrate the dosage to achieve adequate pain relief without adverse effects.

Pain may bring forth many emotions from a client, such as fear, anger, or impatience. There are a number of physiologic responses to acute pain that are usually sympathetic in nature (e.g., sweating, pallor, restlessness, agitation, and/or increased blood pressure, pulse, or respirations). Of note, increased blood pressure, pulse or respirations may be limited only to the first few hours of acute pain and may quickly return to baseline despite ongoing uncontrolled pain (McCaffery & Pasero, 1999).

J.F. is assessed for the following nursing diagnoses: anxiety, disturbed sleep pattern, activity intolerance, fear, fatigue, self-care deficit, social isolation, ineffective coping, acute pain, or chronic pain.

✲ **The nurse caring for J.F. preoperatively discusses an anticipated pain management plan with her and asks what her expectations are for postoperative pain.** J.F. replies, "I'm pretty used to pain. I've had this arthritis for 15 years. The pain didn't bother me as long as I wasn't moving, but my knees hurt like the devil when I tried to keep up with my grandchildren. I only take the pills the doctor gave me when I've got to go down stairs a lot or if I really want a good night's sleep. This pain scale looks like a good idea, but I really don't want to bother the nurses; I can tough it out. I'm from hardy stock." "Your knees will be painful after surgery but we can keep you comfortable," responds the nurse. "It's important for you to be able to move in order to perform some of the postoperative activities we discussed that will help to prevent complications, such as respiratory problems and deep vein thrombosis. Please let us know when your pain begins; it is easier to relieve the pain when it is in the lower part of the scale than when it becomes extreme."

J.F. needs to be assessed and cleared for any preexisting conditions for which opioid use would be contraindicated: hypersensitivity to the prescribed drug, acute respiratory depression, or diarrhea associated with drug-induced pseudomembranous colitis. These conditions may worsen. Opioids should also be used with extreme caution in conditions such as acute bronchial asthma or any respiratory impairment or chronic disease, increased intracranial pressure (may increase), or severe inflammatory bowel disease (risk of toxic megacolon). See the Pregnancy Safety box above for Food and Drug Administration (FDA) pregnancy safety classifications.

Her concurrent medication regimen is reviewed for the risk of significant drug interactions. See Table 14-2.

The goal for pain management decided upon by J.F. and the nursing staff is that she will experience pain no greater than 3 on a 10-point scale so that she may participate in her therapies with minimum opioid adverse effects.

PREGNANCY SAFETY
ANALGESICS

Category	Drug
B	diclofenac, flurbiprofen, ibuprofen, indomethacin, ketoprofen, meclofenamate, nalmefene, naloxone, naproxen, oxycodone, sulindac
C	All opioid agonists (alfentanil, codeine, fentanyl, heroin, hydrocodone, hydromorphone, levorphanol, meperidine, methadone, morphine, opium, propoxyphene), except oxycodone; buprenorphine, butorphanol, celecoxib, dezocine, diflunisal, etodolac, ketorolac, mefenamic acid, nabumetone, nalbuphine, naltrexone, oxaprozin, pentazocine, piroxicam, salsalate (first trimester), tolmetin, trisalicylate
D	aspirin; all NSAIDs in third trimester or near delivery

Data from *Mosby's Drug Consult* (15th ed.). St. Louis: Mosby.

✲ **How are interventions for pain relief chosen for J.F.?**
In the general population, Gu and Belgrade (1993) reported that nearly 35% of hospitalized medical inpatients identified pain as their major complaint. Despite all of the literature about pain management, the undertreatment with analgesics of clients in pain continues to be well documented (Bostrum, Sandh, Lundberg, & Fridlund, 2004; Ardery, Herr, Hannon, & Titler, 2003; Sloan, Montgomery, & Musick, 1998; Cleeland et al., 1994).

Effective relief of pain requires pharmacologic and nonpharmacologic interventions. Each strategy is targeted based on the type of pain, its mechanisms and presentation, and client comorbidities. For acute nociceptive pain, opioids (like morphine) and cyclooxygenase inhibitors (e.g., NSAIDs and COX-2 inhibitors) are mainstays of therapy. Similarly, for cancer pain, these strategies are used in combination with targeted therapies for neuropathic pain (e.g., antidepressants, antiepileptic drugs) and aggressive psychosocial support. In the management of chronic pain, drug therapy plays an important, but incomplete role; a greater emphasis is placed on psychosocial supports, treatment of underlying anxiety and depression, use of alternative modalities (e.g., physical and occupational therapies, chiropractic manipulations, acupuncture/acupressure, exercise, etc.). Each intervention is customized to a client, with the intervention adjusted based on response and function. A preoperative discussion with a client regarding surgical and postsurgical expectations and a review of client-specific, historically effective interventions will contribute to greater success (Skilton, 2003). For J.F., intravenous (IV) morphine is indicated to treat her nociceptive pain. She will likely benefit from other modalities, including physical therapy, and perhaps COX-2 inhibitors.

✲ **J.F. is treated with morphine during and after surgery to address her pain.**

TABLE 14-2 DRUG INTERACTIONS WITH ANALGESICS

Analgesic Drug	Other Drug	Reaction	Management
Opioids Opioid partial agonists	Central nervous system (CNS) depressants (alcohol, barbiturates, sedative-hypnotics)	Additive CNS or respiratory depression	Avoid concurrent use Monitor respiratory status Monitor mental status
buprenorphine (Buprenex)	Opioid agonists, other partial agonists	Additive respiratory depression, reduced analgesia	Avoid concurrent use
propoxyphene (Darvon)	carbamazepine (Tegretol)	Decreased metabolism of carbamazepine with ↑ levels	Avoid if possible; monitor carbamazepine levels
Opioids, especially meperidine (Demerol)	MAO inhibitors—furazolidone (Furoxone), procarbazine (Matulane), phenelzine (Nardil), tranylcypromine (Parnate)	Risk for hypertension, respiratory depression, muscle rigidity, coma, seizures, hyperpyrexia, death	Avoid combination
Opioid partial agonists; Opioid antagonists—naloxone (Narcan), naltrexone (ReVia)	Chronic opioid use	Induces withdrawal reactions	Avoid unless life-threatening opioid toxicity*
Opioid agonists (especially morphine)	zidovudine (AZT)	↓ Clearance of zidovudine	Avoid if possible; monitor for zidovudine toxicity
tramadol (Ultram)	carbamazepine (Tegretol)	Increased metabolism of tramadol	Monitor response to tramadol; consider need to increase tramadol dose
NSAIDs	anticoagulants (warfarin [Coumadin]), (heparin, low-molecular-weight heparins: enoxaparin, etc.)	↑ Risk for gastrointestinal (GI) hemorrhage	Avoid concurrent use, or use GI cytoprotection
NSAIDs	antihypertensives, diuretics	Edema, hypertension, reduced diuretic effect	Avoid if possible; monitor for edema, hypertension, and response to diuretic/antihypertensive
NSAIDs	cyclosporine (Neoral)	↓ Metabolism of cyclosporine and potential renal toxicity	Avoid concurrent use
NSAIDs	lithium (Lithane, Eskalith)	↑ Lithium levels and risk lithium toxicity	Avoid concurrent use
NSAIDs	methotrexate (Mexate)	↑ Methotrexate levels and toxicity	Adjust methotrexate dose accordingly
NSAIDs	probenecid (Benemid)	↑ NSAID levels with risk for GI or renal toxicity	Avoid combination
NSAIDs	valproate, divalproex (Depakene, Depakote); cefotetan (Cefotan)	↑ Risk of GI bleeding (secondary to platelet effect of valproate and decreased prothrombin time with cefotetan)	Avoid concurrent use, or use GI cytoprotection
indomethacin (Indocin)	zidovudine (AZT)	↓ Clearance of zidovudine	Avoid concurrent use if possible; monitor for zidovudine toxicity

*Exception: Low-dose naloxone is sometimes used to reduce pruritus with epidural morphine.

✳ How does morphine work?

Morphine [**mor** feen] is the prototype opioid analgesic agonist. An opioid (also referred to as an opioid agonist) binds to specific receptors inside and outside the central nervous system (CNS). The primary opioid receptors concentrated in the CNS are mu (μ), kappa (κ), delta (δ), and sigma (σ) receptors. Analgesia is associated with the first three receptors. Research on the delta receptor is limited, and therefore the primary analgesic receptors at this time are the mu and kappa receptors (Figure 14-9). The sigma receptors are primarily associated with psychotomimetic or unwanted effects, such as dysphoria (depression and anguish), hallucinations, and confusion.

Morphine is still obtained from opium poppy because of the difficulty encountered in synthesizing morphine in the laboratory. Because of its superior clinical efficacy, it is considered the analgesic standard to which many other analgesics are compared. In addition to producing analgesia, opioids can alter the perception of and emotional responses to pain because the receptors are widely distributed in the CNS, especially in the spinal and medullary dorsal horn, limbic system, thalamus, hypothalamus, and midbrain. Pain perception is inhibited when these areas are stimulated and this enhances the analgesic effect of morphine.

Morphine is commonly used to treat moderate to severe nociceptive pain. Although morphine is considered the drug of choice for cancer pain, it has additional pharmacologic effects that are useful in treating pulmonary edema, chest pain, and nonproductive cough. Morphine produces peripheral vasodilation, which reduces heart workload, improves cardiac function, reduces pulmonary edema, and reduces anxiety (Salerno & Willens, 1996). Depression of the cough reflex is proposed to occur via a CNS mechanism independent of the opioid receptors (Reisman & Pasternak, 2001).

✳ Just prior to surgery, J.F. receives her first dose of IV morphine by the anesthesiologist and presents with a hives-like reaction shortly after administration.

✳ Is J.F. allergic to morphine? Are there alternative opioids that could be used?

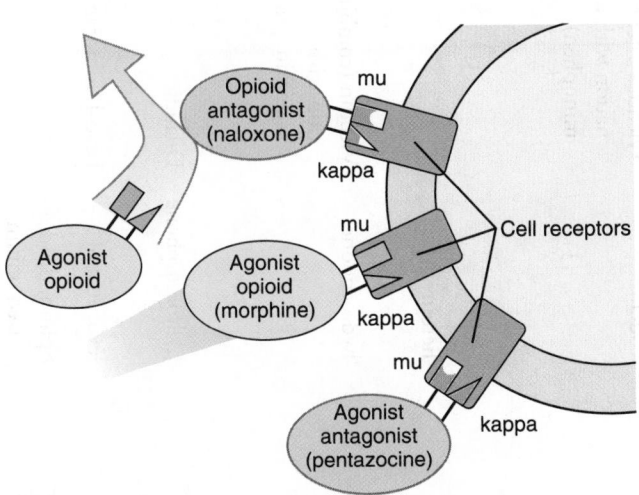

FIGURE 14-9 Receptor interactions of opioids.

Rash secondary to IV or epidural morphine is not uncommon. Often a hives-type reaction is associated with IV or epidural morphine and meperidine; most of the time this is not a true allergy, but instead is a "pseudoallergic reaction" usually secondary to histamine release (Hepner & Castells, 2003), and the reaction is limited to a short-term dermal response. In J.F.'s case, this pseudoreaction does not warrant the avoidance of future morphine use. If a true hypersensitivity to morphine were present (e.g., full immunoglobulin E [IgE] hypersensitivity reaction with wheezing or anaphylaxis), morphine should be discontinued, and other structurally similar opioids should be avoided. The three chemical classes of opioid agonists are phenanthrene derivatives, phenylpiperidine derivatives, and the diphenylheptane derivatives; they are presented in Table 14-3.

Each of the opioid agonists presented in Table 14-3 has subtle differences from morphine, but when used in therapeutically equivalent doses, they are unlikely to produce better analgesia than morphine. They vary in potency, routes of administration, pharmacokinetic profile, and, to some degree, pattern of adverse effects.

Opioid Agonists

Phenanthrene Derivatives

✴ ⬛ morphine [**mor** feen]
(Astramorph, MS Contin, Roxanol, Statex✤)

Indications
As discussed previously, morphine is the classic opioid agonist, and is used for moderate to severe pain. It is also used for chronic cancer pain and, in some circumstances, for chronic noncancer pain. Morphine is also used during myocardial infarction for its analgesic, moderate anxiolytic, and hemodynamic effects. It is also used in low doses for pulmonary edema in palliative care.

Pharmacokinetics/Dosing
Administered IV, morphine demonstrates analgesic properties within 5 to 10 minutes. Morphine exhibits extensive first-pass effect on oral administration, requiring higher oral doses. The chronic administration of morphine affects the extent of first-pass effect. Clients who have not received morphine require oral doses up to six times the IV dose to obtain adequate analgesia whereas for chronic use of morphine, an oral dose three times the effective parenteral dose is adequate. Morphine is extensively metabolized to active and inactive metabolites that are primarily eliminated in the urine. Active metabolites (particularly morphine-6-glucuronide) may accumulate in clients with renal failure and may contribute to central nervous system toxicity in these individuals. Table 14-3 presents the half-life and dosing of morphine for clients who are opioid naive (e.g., those without long-term opioid use). Chronic administration of morphine (as is seen for clients with cancer pain) typically requires higher doses because of tolerance.

Adverse Effects
One secondary effect of morphine is constipation. Decreased peristalsis and reduced production of hydrochloric acid and intestinal secretions is mediated by the binding of morphine to mu and delta receptors in the gastrointestinal (GI) tract (Reisman & Pasternak, 2001). Constipation is typically managed with aggressive laxative regimens. Acute abdominal pain in a client who receives morphine warrants aggressive evaluation for intestinal obstruction. In clients who present to health care providers without a history of opioid use, however, the presence of acute abdominal pain is not a contraindication to use of morphine (Thomas et al., 2003).

Respiratory depression is a potentially serious consequence of morphine therapy. Respiratory depression appears to be related to the binding of morphine at the mu receptor. Decreased respiratory

TABLE 14-3 COMPARISON OF OPIOID AGONISTS

Class	Generic Name	Brand Name	Initial IV Dose*	Initial Oral Dose Immediate Release*	Other Routes of Administration	Half-life (t$_{1/2}$) in hours	How Different From Other Opioid Agonists
Phenanthrene	morphine	Astramorph Roxano SR MS Contin	2.5-10 mg q2-3h	10-30 mg q3h	Epidural, IM, rectal, subcutaneously	2-4	Used for MI, pulmonary edema
	codeine	Tylenol #3 (combination with acetaminophen)	Codeine is rarely used parenterally	15-60 mg q4-6h	IM, subcutaneously	2.5-3.5	Metabolized to morphine via cytochrome P450 (CYP) 2D6, 3A4 For mild to moderate pain only More apt to cause constipation than other opioids; ~10% of population does not metabolize to morphine (see text)
	heroin						Limited therapeutic use in UK, Canada only
	hydrocodone	Vicodin (combination with acetaminophen)	NA	2.5-10 mg q4h		3-4	Lower doses for suppressing cough Used in combination with acetaminophen (be aware of potential for acetaminophen toxicity in combination drugs)
	hydromorphone	Dilaudid	1-4 mg q4-6h	1-4 mg q4-6h	IM, rectal, subcutaneously	1-3	Lower doses for suppressing cough
	levorphanol	Levo-Dromoran	NA	2 mg q6-8h	Subcutaneously	11-16	Longer half-life
	opium, deodorized opium tincture		NA	0.6-1.5 mL/dose			Mix of alkaloids, including morphine; lower dose for diarrhea

	Brand names			Route		Comments
oxycodone	Roxicodone SR, OxyContin, Percocet (with acetaminophen)	NA	10 mg q12h 10 mg q12h 2.5-5 mg q4-6h		2-3	Euphoria and abuse associated with crushed forms of SR product
oxymorphone	Numorphan	0.5 mg q4h	NA	IM, rectal, subcutaneously	1-1.5	Wide variation in client response
Phenylpiperidine						
alfentanil	Alfenta	0.5-3 mcg/kg × 1†	NA	NA		
fentanyl	Sublimaze, Duragesic (patch), Actiq (transmucosal)	0.5-1 mcg/kg × 1‡	NA	Topical patch, transmucosal (buccal) delivery system	2-4	Topical patch for chronic and terminal pain (see text)
meperidine	Demerol	50-100 mg q3-4h Relatively contraindicated for clients older than 65 yr (25 mg q4h sometimes used)	150-300 mg q3-4h (infrequently used because of poor bioavailability)	IM, subcutaneously	2.5-4	Avoid with older adults Avoid use beyond 48 hours Accumulation of normeperidine increases seizure risk (see text)
Diphenylheptane						
methadone	Dolophine	NA	2.5-10 mg q3-8h	IM, subcutaneously	4-48 "Variable"	Dosing for maintenance of opioid dependence: 20-120 mg daily
propoxyphene	Darvon, Darvon-N, Darvocet-N (with acetaminophen)	HCl: 65 mg q3-4h Napsylate: 100 mg q3-4h			8-24	Avoid with older adults; toxic metabolite For mild to moderate pain only

IM, Intramuscularly; *MI*, myocardial infarction; *NA*, not applicable; *SR*, sustained release.

*Opioid naive adult.

†Use typically limited to anesthesiologist during procedures.

‡Parenteral use often limited to anesthesiologists.

drive with morphine is a dose-related phenomenon and involves a reduced response of the brainstem respiratory center to carbon dioxide. This becomes a particularly important consideration for those clients with chronic bronchitis whose respiratory drive is maintained by elevated carbon dioxide levels; for such individuals, morphine can result in complete respiratory arrest. Respiratory depression can also be additive with other CNS depressants (see Table 14-2). Acute treatment of respiratory depression with an opioid antagonist (e.g., naloxone [Narcan]) is required when decreased or shallow opioid-induced respirations are life-threatening.

Other relatively common but undesirable effects of morphine include vertigo, faintness, and light-headedness; confusion; fatigue; sleepiness; nausea and vomiting; rash; increased sweating; and hypotension. Less common adverse effects include dry mouth; headache; anorexia; abdominal cramping; nervousness; increased anxiety; mental confusion; urinary retention or painful urination; visual disturbances; and nightmares. With epidural and IV administration, pruritus secondary to histamine release, as noted above, is common. Among the more serious (but rare) adverse effects reported are seizures; tinnitus; jaundice (hepatic toxicity); facial edema (allergic reaction); breathing difficulties; severe respiratory depression; and excitability (paradoxical reaction seen mainly in children) (*USP DI*, 2005).

Drug Interactions
See Table 14-2.

codeine [**koe** deen]
(Paveral✦, Empracet✦)
Codeine is available in phosphate salts and is marketed three forms: oral tablets, oral solution, and injectable dosage.

Indications
Codeine is not as effective for pain management as morphine and is typically limited to the treatment of mild to moderate pain. It is effective as an antitussive and antidiarrheal, and is often used for this purpose. Codeine is most often given orally and in combination with acetaminophen (e.g., Tylenol #2 [15 mg of codeine], Tylenol #3 [30 mg of codeine], and Tylenol #4 [60 mg of codeine]), but it is occasionally administered parenterally as codeine phosphate.

Pharmacokinetics/Dosing
Codeine is metabolized to morphine by cytochrome P450 2D6 (Eichelbaum, 2003). Approximately 5% to 10% of the population does not experience adequate metabolism to morphine and observes a suboptimal analgesic benefit from codeine. (See the Special Considerations for Pharmacogenetics box below.) See Table 14-3 for dosing and half-life information.

Adverse Effects
Codeine produces similar adverse effects as observed with other opioid agonists with a higher risk for constipation, particularly in older adults (Offerhaus, 1997).

hydrocodone bitartrate [hye droe **koe** done]
(Vicodin, Robidone✦)
Indications
Hydrocodone is marketed in combination with homatropine in the United States. In Canada, Robidone consists of hydrocodone bitartrate only. The combination of hydrocodone and acetaminophen (Vicodin) is commonly used orally to manage moderate to severe pain. When used in combination with acetaminophen, care should be taken to monitor total daily acetaminophen intake in order to avoid liver toxicity. Although the product name is similar in both countries, the formulation is not identical. Hydrocodone bitartrate is also used in lower doses as an antitussive.

Pharmacokinetics/Dosing
See Table 14-3.

Adverse Effects
Similar to morphine.

hydromorphone [hye droe **mor** fone]
(Dilaudid, Dilaudid HP✦)
Indications
Hydromorphone is prescribed for its analgesic and antitussive effects.
Pharmacokinetics/Dosing
Hydromorphone is a semisynthetic opioid that has a faster onset but shorter duration of action than morphine. It is available orally, parenterally and rectally. See Table 14-3.
Adverse Effects
Similar to morphine.

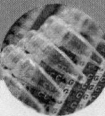
Special Considerations for Pharmacogenetics | ANALGESICS

PHARMACODYNAMICS

Considerable variation in pain response to morphine is noted and likely is influenced by pharmacogenetics (Aubrun, Langeron, Quesnel, Coriat, & Riou, 2003). This may be related in part to genetic variation in the mu opioid receptor. A study measuring pupil response to morphine and its active metabolite morphine-6-glucuronide identified a genetic basis for variation among subjects (Lotsch et al., 2002).

PHARMACOKINETICS

Codeine is metabolized to morphine by the isoenzyme cytochrome P450 2D6 (Eichelbaum, 2003). Approximately 5% to 10% of the population has a genetically determined deficiency of this enzyme (Weinshilboum, 2003). Oxycodone, metabolized by the same isoenzyme to a pharmacologically active compound (Lacy, Armstrong, Goldman, & Lance, 2004), may also be affected in clients with 2D6 deficiency. Morphine metabolism to its glucose-6-glucuronide may also display genetically based variation (Skarke et al., 2004). A possible explanation for the lack of therapeutic

response to opioids in a number of clients may be related to genetically based differences in metabolism.

ADVERSE EFFECTS

Genetic variation in metabolism of acetaminophen may identify individuals who are at higher risk for hepatotoxicity (Court et al., 2001). The tricyclic antidepressants, frequently used for neuropathic pain management, are metabolized by P450 2D6, which has varied expression across populations. For individuals with low potential to metabolize 2D6, risks for life-threatening cardiac dysrhythmias are possible (Flores, Alvarado, Wong, Licinio, & Flockhart, 2004). The metabolism of the COX-2 inhibitors (celecoxib [Celebrex], valdecoxib [Bextra], and rofecoxib [Vioxx]) each differ and involve the P450 enzyme systems (Barkin & Buvanendran, 2004; Kirchheiner et al., 2003). It is possible that pharmacogenetics plays a role in the adverse effect profile of each agent and may account for the higher rates of cardiovascular events with rofecoxib and valdecoxib, prompting their removal from the market.

levorphanol [lee **vor** fa nole]

(Levo-Dromoran)

Indications

Levorphanol is indicated for moderate to severe pain, but is less frequently used because of the risk of drug accumulation.

Pharmacokinetics/Dosing

Levorphanol has a longer analgesic duration of effect than either morphine or meperidine and a half-life of 11 to 16 hours (*Drug Facts and Comparisons*, 2005). Drug accumulation and overdose may result from doses that are too large or too frequent, chronic dosing of children or small adults, or even the use of average dosages in medically compromised clients (see Table 14-3).

Adverse Effects

Similar to morphine, but because of drug accumulation risk, dose-related effects such as respiratory and CNS depression may be more likely.

opium preparations

Opium contains several alkaloids, including morphine and small amounts of codeine and papaverine. The effects of opium result from the presence of morphine in the preparations.

Indications

Paregoric is an antidiarrheal agent. In some instances it has been used to treat neonatal opioid dependence, but this use is controversial. Opium alkaloids injection or opium and belladonna suppositories (B&O Supprettes) are used to relieve moderate to severe pain reported with urethral spasms and have also been prescribed for breakthrough pain between injections of opioids.

Pharmacokinetics/Dosing

Opium tincture contains 10 mg morphine/mL and is used as an antidiarrheal agent. When diluted, it is used for the treatment of neonatal opioid dependence. Camphorated tincture of opium (paregoric) contains 2 mg morphine/5 mL and high concentrations of ethanol (45%). Opium alkaloids hydrochloride injection (Pantopon) contains 20 mg opium alkaloids (*Mosby's Drug Consult*, 2005). This product is available only in Canada. Number 15 A opium and belladonna suppositories (B&O Supprettes) contain 30 mg powdered opium (10% morphine and other alkaloids) and 16.2 mg powdered belladonna alkaloid (the principal belladonna alkaloids are atropine and scopolamine). Number 16 A contains 60 mg powdered opium and 16.2 mg belladonna extract. The adult dosage for opium tincture is 0.3 to 1 mL PO four times daily, to a maximum of 6 mL daily. The dosage for camphorated tincture of opium (paregoric) is 5 to 10 mL PO one to four times daily, with a maximum of 10 mL four times daily. The paregoric dosage for children 2 years of age and older is 0.25 to 0.5 mL/kg body weight one to four times daily.

Adverse Effects

Paregoric contains camphor, which can cause serious toxicity, including seizures and respiratory depression; it also contains benzoic acid, which can displace bilirubin from albumin. Both substances may enhance the typical problems seen in opioid-dependent infants (e.g., seizures and hyperbilirubinemia); therefore many prescribers seem to prefer the use of diluted opium tincture to paregoric.

oxycodone [ox i **koe** done]

(Roxicodone, OxyIR, OxyContin, Supeudol✦)

Indications

Oxycodone is indicated for moderate to severe pain.

Pharmacokinetics/Dosing

Oxycodone is available as Roxicodone and OxyIR, in combination with aspirin (Percodan) or acetaminophen (Percocet, Roxicet, Tylox), and in extended-release dosage form (OxyContin). The suppository dosage form is not available in the United States, but is available in Canada. See Table 14-3 for additional information.

Adverse Effects

Nontherapeutic effects are similar to morphine. Oxycodone may be associated with a greater euphoria than other opioids, which may account for the abuse observed with crushed forms of the sustained action product.

oxymorphone [ox i **mor** fone]

(Numorphan)

Indications

Oxymorphone is a potent analgesic infrequently used for moderate to severe pain, preoperative medication, obstetric analgesia, and as adjunct therapy for the treatment of anxiety caused by dyspnea that results from pulmonary edema associated with left ventricular failure.

Pharmacokinetics/Dosing

It is available in parenteral and rectal suppository dosage forms (see Table 14-3).

Adverse Effects

Oxymorphone causes more nausea, vomiting, and psychic effects (euphoria) than morphine; it may also be less constipating and cause less suppression of the cough reflex than morphine.

Phenylpiperidine Derivatives

fentanyl [**fen** ta nil]

(Sublimaze, Innovar, Duragesic, Actiq)

Indications

Parenteral fentanyl is used for analgesia as a premedication, as an adjunct to anesthesia, and in the immediate postoperative period. Parenteral administration should be restricted to those experienced with this product and with the management of fentanyl-induced respiratory depression (see Chapter 15). The transdermal patch formulation is used for chronic pain management.

Pharmacokinetics/Dosing

The transdermal patch system is available in 25, 50, 75, and 100 mcg/hr dosage forms. The manufacturer publishes an equianalgesic potency chart and a morphine-to-fentanyl conversion chart that should be used to determine the fentanyl dosage. In opioid-naive clients, in adults 60 years of age and older, and in debilitated clients, the starting dose should not be higher than 25 mcg/hr transdermally. Clients who are maintained on a total oral dose of less than 60 to 90 mg daily are more likely to exhibit significant sedation and respiratory depression when transitioned to transdermal fentanyl 25 mcg/hr. Because of the delay in onset and prolonged effect after removal from skin, the use of the fentanyl patch is limited to management of chronic pain as an alternative to the other opioids, especially for clients who have difficulty swallowing.

To use, remove the transdermal system from the package immediately before applying. Do not cut or break the patch. Use water to clean the skin area before application. Do not use soap, oils, lotions, alcohol, or other products because they may alter the absorption of this product. Apply the medication to a dry, flat (hairless) area of the upper torso (front or back). Do not apply to skin that is burned, cut, irritated, very oily, or recently shaved. If the skin area is hairy, cut the hair with scissors. Hold the patch in place for 10 to 20 seconds to be sure it is securely fastened to the client. Then check the patch to make certain skin contact is complete and the edges of the system adhere to the skin. Wash hands after applying the patch. Use large amounts of water in washing, especially if the gel accidentally comes in contact with your skin. Avoid using soap, alcohol, or any other solvent. The patch releases fentanyl continuously by absorption through the skin, which aids in controlling pain around-the-clock, for as long as 72 hours if the dose is adequate.

After application, fentanyl is absorbed and concentrated in the upper layers of skin. Serum levels increase slowly and usually reach a plateau between 12 and 24 hours. During the initial application of the patch, a short-acting analgesic should be prescribed for the first 12 to 24 hours, because peak serum levels usually occur between 24 and 72 hours. Thereafter the person should have an order for a short-acting opioid to manage breakthrough pain.

Because it may take as long as 6 days to stabilize levels of a new transdermal dose, dosage adjustments after the initial 72-hour change should be instituted on an every-6-day schedule. If another system is required after 72 hours, apply it to a new site.

Withdraw the client from the drug gradually. Because the serum level of fentanyl decreases slowly, give half the equianalgesic dose of the new analgesic 12 to 18 hours after removal of the last patch. Fold old patches in half and either flush them down the toilet or put them in a sharps container.

Adverse Effects

Fentanyl and the fentanyl derivatives, sufentanil (Sufenta) and alfentanil (Alfenta), may rarely cause rigidity of chest wall muscles if given rapidly in large doses; this reaction requires supportive respiratory ventilation and perhaps a rapid-acting muscle relaxant. Respiratory depression is dose-related (*USP DI*, 2005).

meperidine [me **per** i deen]
(Demerol)

Meperidine is a semisynthetic opioid that differs from morphine in a few respects. Meperidine is less apt to release histamine than morphine. While data historically suggested that meperidine may be less likely to increase biliary tract pressure than morphine and is perhaps safer for clients with biliary colic or pancreatitis, this is no longer considered an important aspect of the pharmacology of meperidine (Berardi & Montgomery, 2002).

Indications

Meperidine is used for the short-term management of acute moderate to severe pain in clients who are younger and have adequate renal function.

Pharmacokinetics/Dosing

The duration of action of meperidine is shorter than morphine. As such a more frequent dosing schedule is necessary. Meperidine has poor oral bioavailability, requiring oral doses of 150 to 300 mg compared to the 25- to 100-mg parenteral dose. Meperidine may produce a vagolytic effect resulting in tachycardia (a problem for clients with cardiac dysrhythmias or coronary artery disease). Meperidine also can produce a life-threatening hypertensive reaction for those receiving monoamine oxidase inhibitors (MAOIs) concurrently.

Most important clinically is that meperidine is metabolized in the liver to normeperidine, a CNS neurotoxic metabolite. Normeperidine has a half-life between 15 and 20 hours in persons with normal renal function. Prolonged administration, the use of high dosages of meperidine, or the use in older adults or in clients with impaired renal or hepatic function has resulted in normeperidine accumulation. See Table 14-3 for additional information on dosing.

Adverse Effects

In addition to the adverse effects observed with morphine, meperidine produces adverse effects secondary to normeperidine accumulation. Normeperidine-induced CNS toxicity can manifest as significant mood changes such as sadness, anger, restlessness, apprehension, increased irritability, nervousness, tremors, agitation, quivering, seizures, and myoclonus (American Hospital Formulary Service, 2004). Naloxone (Narcan), an opioid antagonist, antagonizes meperidine but not normeperidine and may, in some instances, cause further CNS excitation and seizures. Management of normeperidine toxicity includes stopping meperidine, substituting an alternate opioid such as morphine, and using an antiepileptic drug if seizures occur. For these reasons, meperidine should not be used for more than a 48-hour period, for chronic pain, or in older adults or those with renal dysfunction.

Diphenylheptane Derivatives

methadone [**meth** a done]
(Dolophine, Methadose, Metadol✤)
Indications

Methadone use is primarily limited to the detoxification and maintenance of opioid addiction and for chronic pain management. Methadone dependence is substituted in individuals who are physiologically dependent on heroin, opium, or other opioids. In the United States, methadone use for opioid detoxification or maintenance is primarily limited to authorized licensed methadone clinics. To improve rural access to methadone, individuals who have been successfully maintained for a set period of time may obtain their methadone for detoxification or maintenance from primary care physicians providing a number of criteria are met. In Canada, it is available through specially authorized physicians. When used for detoxification, it is important for the nurse to directly observe administration to avoid the potential for drug diversion. (See Chapter 9 for information on methadone treatment programs.) Because of its relatively long half-life and duration of therapy, methadone has been used to manage chronic pain, and such use does not require the same level of strict federal oversight.

Pharmacokinetics/Dosing

The duration of action for methadone is usually listed at 4 to 6 hours, but with repeated oral dosing the half-life may extend from 22 to 48 hours (perhaps even longer in older adults and in clients with renal dysfunction). Despite this extended half-life, it must be given every 6 to 8 hours when used as an analgesic. However, this long half-life is beneficial when used to prevent withdrawal reactions in detoxification and maintenance programs. See Table 14-3.

Adverse Effects

Similar to morphine, but variable kinetics may increase likelihood for toxicity.

propoxyphene [proe **pox** i feen]
(Darvon)
propoxyphene napsylate
(Novopropoxyn✤)

Propoxyphene is a synthetic analgesic that is structurally related to methadone.

Indications

Propoxyphene is indicated for the treatment of mild to moderate pain. Controlled studies report that propoxyphene alone has no advantage over aspirin, acetaminophen, or codeine in relieving pain (Baumann, 2002). As such, its use has diminished over the past 20 years. Propoxyphene combined with aspirin or acetaminophen usually provides more analgesia than either aspirin or acetaminophen alone.

Pharmacokinetics/Dosing

Norpropoxyphene, a toxic metabolite of propoxyphene, has a long half-life of 30 to 36 hours (*USP DI*, 2005). See Table 14-3.

Adverse Effects

Similar to morphine and codeine. Propoxyphene may cause seizures and cardiotoxicity and therefore should not be used with older adults.

✳ **Upon recovery from surgery, J.F. indicates that the sharp, throbbing pain in her knees is an 8 on a 10-point scale and she is very uncomfortable and getting anxious. Movement aggravates the pain and she is trying to be very still. Her respiratory rate is 24 breaths/min and her heart rate is 110 beats/min. What intervention is appropriate?**

The elevations in respiratory and heart rates are consistent with an autonomic nervous system response to acute pain, and corroborate her discomfort. A continuous infusion of opioids is helpful for the short-term treatment of severe pain (e.g., pain management in the postoperative period) or when other routes of administration may be inappropriate, such as in clients with intractable vomiting or when severe local bruising follows an intramuscular (IM) or subcutaneous injection. IV opioids are also used when other routes have failed to provide satisfactory pain relief, such as for clients with severe pain unrelieved by oral, rectal, or intermittent parenteral opioid dosing.

J.F. and all clients in pain should receive nursing care directed toward reducing pain and enhancing the analgesic effect of medications. A nurse often has significant influence over pain medication through PRN (when needed) prescribing of analgesic medications. As previously mentioned, the greatest abuse of analgesics is underuse that results in failure to adequately relieve or control pain. Analgesics should be used before pain reaches peak intensity and prior to painful events. A PRN order can be used preventively if the nurse assesses a client's needs. For acute intermittent pain, the appropriate dose of analgesic with a rapid onset of action should be used, with dosing on an as-needed or PRN basis. If the order is for "q4h PRN" and a nurse determines that the pain will be fairly constant for the next 24 hours, as in J.F.'s case, the drug may be given at 4-hour intervals and documented in the medication record to be given every 4 hours around-the-clock. This regimen in no way exceeds what the prescriber has specified as long as the client is monitored for sedation, confusion, or respiratory depression (indicating that the frequency or the dose should be decreased), pain relief (suggesting efficacy), and ongoing pain (indicating additional analgesic strategies are re-

quired). With this plan, the blood levels of the analgesic remain steady and there should be no breakthrough pain.

Parenteral opioids are usually given IV or subcutaneous. IM injections are usually avoided because they are usually more uncomfortable and offer no advantage over IV or subcutaneous administration. Opioids may also be administered via epidural or intraspinal infusion (Boxes 14-1 and 14-2).

✦ **The postoperative team elects to initiate patient-controlled analgesia (PCA) morphine for J.F. at a concentration of 1 mg/mL, self-dose of 1 mg (1 mL) IV, a lockout time of 6 minutes, a basal dose of 1 mg/hr IV, and a rescue of 1 mg IV every 20 minutes as needed for breakthrough pain. The 1-hour limit total is 12 mg IV. The PCA is held for respiratory rate less than 10 breaths/min, excessive sedation, or systolic blood pressure (BP) less than 90 mm Hg (or a predetermined score on the agency's sedation scale).**

An alternate method of maintaining serum levels of the analgesic is to use a PCA infusion pump. The PCA infusion pump allows for optimal dosing of opioids compared with PRN and fixed dosing regimens (Figure 14-10). It also pro-

---

BOX 14-1 EPIDURAL ANALGESIA

Epidural analgesia is a therapeutic modality that offers an alternative to traditional methods of pain control. It can be administered as an intermittent injection or a continuous infusion of opioid into the epidural space. The nursing management of clients receiving epidural analgesia to manage postoperative pain is an essential for client comfort and safety. In general, the client should understand the purpose and the benefits of epidural analgesia and provide consent to the modality before surgery.

With the client in a side-lying position, the epidural catheter is inserted, most commonly at the L2 level, by the anesthesiologist. Once the catheter is tested for placement, it is stabilized with an occlusive dressing. It should be taped in such a manner that the tubing does not pull or kink. The anesthesiologist should be notified if the catheter becomes dislodged or the dressing becomes loose or wet. The catheter may be connected to a continuous infusion or capped and should be carefully labeled "for epidural use only." Because some preservatives might be toxic to neural tissue, medications for epidural use must not contain preservatives.

Although rare, respiratory depression can occur with the administration of spinal opioids. The respiratory status of the client receiving intermittent epidural analgesia should be monitored once each hour for the first 12 hours or until the respiratory rate exceeds 12 breaths/min, then every 2 hours for 12 hours, and then every 4 hours for the duration of therapy. With continuous infusion of the analgesic agent, the client should be monitored every hour for the first 24 hours or until the respiratory rate is greater than 12 breaths/min, then once every 4 hours for the duration of therapy. Auscultate respiratory status with stethoscope. Clients with low respiratory rates should be monitored as necessary. Monitor pulse oximetry and arterial blood gases (ABGs) as ordered.

Naloxone, an opioid antagonist, is usually kept in the immediate client environment according to health care agency policy. The anesthesiologist is called immediately if respiratory depression occurs. Naloxone 0.4 mg IV is usually ordered, but this dose may also reverse the analgesic effect of the opioid, and the client will experience pain. Have Ambu bag, oxygen, and suction in working order nearby. Maintain IV access for emergency drugs.

Pruritus is experienced by approximately one-third of all clients receiving spinal opioids. Although the mechanism is unclear, this reaction is believed to occur when epidural opioids produce sensory sensations that are interpreted by the sensory cortex as itching. Low doses of naloxone are administered to relieve the pruritus without concomitant reversal of analgesia. Nausea and vomiting may also be an issue with some clients. Fluid balance monitoring and the assessment of bladder distention should be maintained while the client is receiving epidural analgesia to detect any urinary retention that may occur. Monitor dressing and site every shift.

Using a pain scale, the client's level of comfort should be assessed every 2 to 4 hours for the first 24 hours after surgery. Supplemental parenteral analgesics may be required for "breakthrough" pain. Assess the level of consciousness every 2 hours for the first 24 hours and then every 4 hours for the duration of therapy. Some agencies require a motor and sensory assessment at least every 2 hours and before ambulation. Blood pressure and pulse should be determined before ambulating the client for the first time.

Instruct the client to notify the nurse if pain is experienced and if increased drowsiness and/or leg numbness and weakness occur. Epidural analgesia is not usually continued past the fifth postoperative day.

vides consistent analgesic serum levels within guidelines. Provide J.F. with instructions regarding the PCA pump. The PCA pump provides pain relief that allows J.F. to participate more freely in her care and, hopefully, recover more quickly with fewer adverse effects. J.F.'s anxiety level should decline because she knows when the next dose is being administered. For chronic, continuous pain, the appropriate dosage of analgesic would be titrated to her needs. Dosage titration in many institutions is based on a sedation scale, such as the Richmond Agitation-Sedation Scale (RASS) that has specific criteria based on objective measurement of the client's level of consciousness (Sessler et al., 2002). The analgesic should have as long a duration as feasible and be given around-the-clock to prevent the return of pain. Breakthrough pain is treated using appropriate medications on a PRN basis.

Before starting J.F.'s pump infusion, obtain baseline blood pressure, pain assessment, and respiratory rate, rhythm, and depth. All previous pain medication orders are discontinued. Administer the solution using a microdrip infusion set and an infusion control pump. Figure 14-11 shows a PCA unit commonly used in a hospital setting, most often after surgery. This pump allows J.F. to self-administer a predetermined IV bolus (a quantity of drug introduced into a vein at one time) of an opioid (morphine, fentanyl, hydromorphone) by pressing the pump's activation mechanism. A prescriber orders the analgesic dose and a set lockout interval of 5 to 20 minutes; in this case 6 minutes. The pump is then set to deliver the ordered dose whenever J.F. activates the button. The lockout mechanism prevents an inadvertent overdose or excessive analgesic administration. This pump also records the number of times the button is pushed and the total cumulative dose delivered. The pump may be programmed for continuous administration, client-activated delivery, or clinician-activated delivery. The pump also records all bolus attempts, successful and unsuccessful, made by a client. Thus the nurse and the

prescriber are able to evaluate the appropriateness of the medication therapy and determine when a client is not receiving adequate medication. A portable PCA wrist model may also be used. Because it is lightweight (approximately 15 ounces) and easily worn, it does not impair ambulation in mobile clients.

J.F.'s current pain treatment requirements and degree of pain control determine the initial infusion rate. Adjustments to this rate are based on pain intensity and sedation scales. Monitor J.F.'s potential for respiratory depression every hour for the first 4 hours and routinely thereafter. If

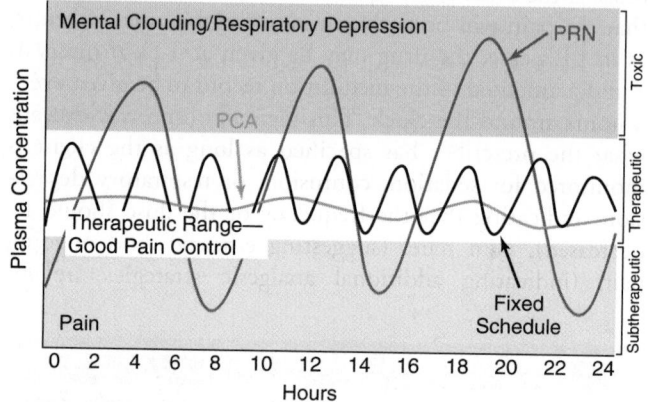

FIGURE 14-10 Impact of various morphine regimens on analgesia and toxicity. *Red line:* Serum drug levels when analgesia is administered on a PRN basis with analgesia relying on less frequently administered but higher doses of morphine. *Black line:* Serum drug levels when a fixed schedule of dosing is used (not PRN). *Green line:* Patient-controlled analgesia (PCA) in which the client receives a regularly scheduled dose of morphine in addition to bolus doses in real time. Subtherapeutic response is found when drug levels are in the peach-colored portion of the graph, therapeutic response in the white area, and toxicity in the light blue area.

BOX 14-2 INTRASPINAL ANALGESIA

Another type of analgesic therapy—continuous intraspinal morphine infusion—reduces the client's pain without diminishing CNS functioning. An implantable infusion device is connected to an implantable catheter that is placed in the epidural and intrathecal space. The system administers the medication continuously and is refilled by injection through a septum into a central chamber of the device. In the home setting, the client and family are taught how to care for the device and how to evaluate the response to the therapy. The device is usually refilled every 2 weeks by a home health care nurse. Bruera and Kim (2003) found that there was prolonged survival and enhanced caregiver quality of life with early application of intraspinal analgesia compared with other forms of analgesia, although most random, controlled studies support intraspinal analgesia late in the client's course of pain. Research is ongoing with this unique method of pain control, which promises relief for clients with intractable pain while increasing quality of life.

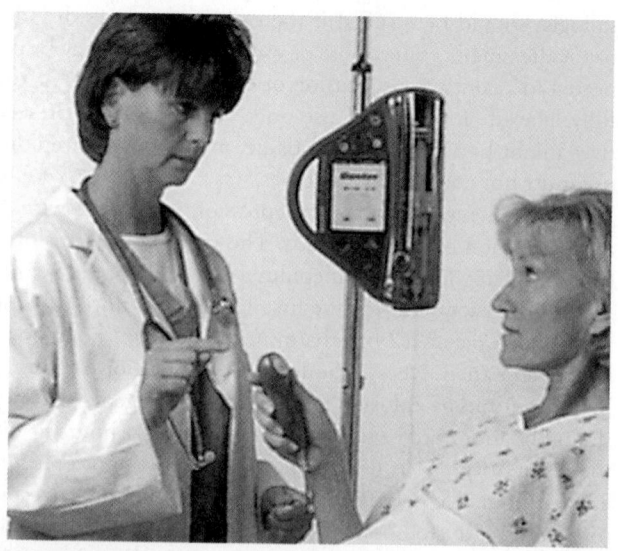

FIGURE 14-11 Example of a PCA unit.

Courtesy of Baxter Healthcare Corporation, Deerfield, IL.

her respiratory rate falls below the established limit, reduce the rate of flow, notify the prescriber, and monitor sedation levels. In the case of significantly suppressed respirations, mechanical ventilation may be preferred to naloxone (Narcan) to relieve the respiratory depression, because naloxone will also diminish or reverse pain relief.

In addition to respiratory rate, monitor J.F.'s orientation, reflexes, bilateral grip strength, level of consciousness, pupil size, bowel sounds, and urinary output. This nursing assessment yields important information required by a prescriber to determine possible adverse drug effects on a client. Signs of opioid overdose are cold and clammy skin, drowsiness, dizziness, restlessness and mental confusion, miosis (pinpoint pupils), and decreasing pulse rate and blood pressure. Oral and injectable opioid analgesics produce unacceptable or undesirable effects such as nausea and vomiting, constipation, urinary retention, cough reflex suppression, and CNS effects. See the Nursing Care Plan below for selected nursing diagnoses related to opioid therapy.

Duramorph, a preservative-free morphine sulfate solution, is commonly prescribed for IV, epidural, or intrathecal use. The risk of inducing respiratory depression is reportedly greater with the intrathecal route than with epidural administration (USP DI, 2005). Although nurses do not usually administer drugs intraspinally, they may be required to fill the drug reservoir of an implanted intraspinal delivery system. Special training of the nurse is required, and the manufacturer's directions should be followed closely.

⭐ **Four hours after the start of PCA morphine, J.F.'s respiratory rate is 12 breaths per minute and she is very groggy. A nurse recognizes that the PCA pump was programmed incorrectly. What action is appropriate?**
Medical errors related to drug delivery devices are surprisingly common. These types of errors can usually be avoided with a combination of clear education on how to use medical devices, regular quality improvement checks on all medical equipment, clear and consistent medical orders, and supportive documentation tools to simplify assessment and management. Many settings use protocols whereby two RNs are required to program PCA pumps. With decreased respirations and level of consciousness, the use of an opioid antagonist should be con-

NURSING CARE PLAN SELECTED NURSING DIAGNOSES RELATED TO OPIOID THERAPY

Nursing Diagnosis	Outcome Criteria	Nursing Interventions
Ineffective airway clearance related to cough reflex suppression	Evidence of good pulmonary ventilation Absence of adventitious lung sounds	Reposition the immobile client frequently. Teach turning, coughing, and deep breathing.
Ineffective breathing pattern: hypoventilation related to CNS depressant effects of drug	Respiratory rate 16-20/min Absence of cyanosis	Assess respiratory rate before administering each dose; if below 12/min, withhold dose. Administer oxygen.* Elevate head of bed. Have opioid antagonist and respiratory support systems nearby during IV administration.
Risk for deficient fluid volume related to nausea and/or vomiting	Absence of and/or decrease in nausea and/or vomiting	Administer prescribed antiemetics. Administer oral analgesics with food. Reduce noxious environmental stimuli. Apply cool cloth to the face. Provide small, frequent meals.
Constipation	Evidence of client's normal bowel patterns	Assess client's bowel status. Increase fluid consumption. Instruct in high-fiber diet. Encourage ambulation. Obtain an order for a stool softener and/or a bulk-forming laxative. Provide relaxed environment for elimination.
Urinary retention	Evidence of urinary status without urgency and/or retention	Increase fluid intake to about 2500 mL daily, unless contraindicated. Administer sitz bath. Provide relaxed environment for elimination. Suggest a dose reduction or switch to alternative therapy.
Risk for injury related to sensory/perceptual alterations	Absence of injury	Assist to ambulate. Caution against driving and other hazardous activities. Caution against taking alcohol and other CNS depressants concurrently.

*Administration of oxygen may be contraindicated for clients with CO_2 retention, such as those with chronic bronchitis. For such clients, more aggressive respiratory support may be required.

Medication Safety Alert

Analgesics

The Institute for Safe Medication Practices (ISMP) has identified a number of issues related to safety with the use of analgesics, including the following:

- Acetaminophen dosing with combination products (e.g., orders for acetaminophen plus orders for combination products with acetaminophen such as oxycodone/acetaminophen, hydrocodone/acetaminophen) leading to client acetaminophen intake greater than 4 g daily and hepatotoxicity
- Assessing pain without assessing level of sedation and respiratory status
- Dangerous abbreviations:
  - DPT: Demerol, promethazine, Thorazine vs. diphtheria, pertussis, tetanus vaccine
  - MSO₄: MgSO₄ vs. morphine sulfate vs. magnesium sulfate
- Dosing and labeling confusion with liquid and rapidly dissolving acetaminophen formulations
- Interchange of tincture of opium (10 mg/mL morphine) for paregoric (2 mg/5 mL and 45% ethanol)
- Patient-controlled analgesia (PCA): errors risking client safety include:
  - Inappropriate client selection
  - Inadequate client education
  - Inadequate lockout periods
  - Inadequate staff training
  - Inadequate monitoring
  - Drug product mix-ups
  - Inappropriate programming of pump
  - Flaws in pump design
  - Dose calculation errors
- Polypharmacy orders given in rapid sequence (e.g., moderate dose of opioid if moderate pain, high dose for severe pain, where inadequate time to evaluate response to the first order occurs)
- Sound-alike names:
  - Toradol vs. Foradil
  - Hydroxyzine vs. hydralazine

For more information, see the ISMP website: http://www.ismp.org

---

sidered as a last resort. A discussion of safety is presented in the Medication Safety Alert box above. The management of drug overdose of opioids is presented in Chapter 9.

Opioid Antagonists

Opioid antagonists bind to opioid receptors and competitively displace the opioid analgesics from their receptor sites. As such, these agents reverse the effects of opioid agonists such as morphine and heroin. Naloxone is the prototype opioid antagonist. Naltrexone and nalmefene are also opioid an-

tagonists. Nalmefene is a chemical analogue of naltrexone and at full dosages has a longer duration of action than naloxone. Nalmefene and naloxone are administered parenterally, whereas naltrexone is available as an oral drug.

Antagonists block opioid effects and can precipitate withdrawal symptoms in individuals who are physically dependent on opioids. These products are used to reverse the adverse or overdose effects of opioids (codeine, diphenoxylate, fentanyl, heroin, hydromorphone, levorphanol, meperidine, methadone, morphine, oxymorphone, opium derivatives, and propoxyphene) and most partial agonists (agonist-antagonist drugs such as butorphanol, nalbuphine, and pentazocine).

Respiratory depression induced by nonopioids (e.g., barbiturates), CNS depression, or disease progression does not usually respond to opioid antagonist drug therapy. It has also been reported that larger drug dosages are necessary to antagonize the effects of buprenorphine, butorphanol, nalbuphine, and pentazocine. However, a buprenorphine overdose may not respond to the opioid antagonists or, at best, may only partially respond (*USP DI,* 2005).

In an opioid analgesic overdose, naloxone and naltrexone reverse respiratory depression, sedation, miosis (constriction of pupils), and euphoric effects; they may also reverse the psychotomimetic effects of the agonist-antagonist analgesics (pentazocine and others). The drugs are believed to work at all three receptor sites, but their greatest activity is at the mu receptors (see Figure 14-9).

⬛ naloxone hydrochloride [nal **ox** one]
(Narcan)
Naloxone is inactivated orally but is very effective parenterally.
Indications
Naloxone is used for partial or complete reversal of CNS and respiratory depression associated with opioid agonists and partial agonists as discussed above.
Pharmacokinetics/Dosing
Naloxone has an onset of action is 1 to 2 minutes (IV) and 2 to 5 minutes (IM or subcutaneous). The half-life is between 60 and 100 minutes. Duration of action depends on the dose administered and the route of administration. Usually the IM dose results in a prolonged effect. Naloxone is widely distributed throughout the body and also crosses the placenta. It is metabolized in the liver and excreted via the kidneys.

The adult dose of naloxone is 0.4 to 2 mg as single dose or 0.1 to 0.2 mg for postoperative opioid depression. Naloxone may be diluted with sterile water for injection if a larger volume is needed (*USP DI,* 2005). For continuous infusion, 2 mg of naloxone may be diluted in 500 mL of normal saline or 5% dextrose injection. Because naloxone is shorter acting than most opioids, repeat naloxone injections or continuous infusion is necessary to prevent the recurrence of respiratory depression.
Adverse Effects
Adverse effects include nausea, vomiting, dizziness, hypertension, tachycardia, sweating, nervousness, abdominal cramps or pain, headache, weakness, joint and muscle pain, insomnia, hallucinations, confusion, mood alterations, tinnitus, and fever.

naltrexone [nal **trex** one]
(ReVia)
Indications
Naltrexone is indicated for adjuvant treatment in detoxified, opioid-dependent clients. It is also used in the management of ethanol dependence.

Pharmacokinetics/Dosing

Absorption is rapid, but it undergoes an extensive first-pass metabolism in the liver to the major metabolite 6-β-naltrexol, which also has opioid antagonist effects. Peak serum concentration is reached in 1 hour; the elimination half-life for naltrexone is 4 hours, and approximately 13 hours for the metabolite. The duration of action is dose dependent. Excretion is via the kidneys.

Treatment with naltrexone is started cautiously, usually 25 mg PO with close monitoring for withdrawal signs and symptoms for approximately 1 hour. The balance of the daily dose is given if no withdrawal effects occur. The maintenance dosage is usually 50 mg PO daily.

Adverse Effects

Similar to naloxone.

nalmefene [**nal** mah feen]

(Revex)

Indications

Similar to naloxone.

Pharmacokinetics/Dosing

Nalmefene has an onset of action of 2 to 5 minutes (IV) or 5 to 15 minutes (IM or subcutaneous). Time to peak levels is 90 minutes by subcutaneous injection and 2.3 hours by IM injection; therefore the time to peak effect and duration of action is dependent on the dose and route of administration. Nalmefene is metabolized in the liver and excreted primarily by the kidneys.

The adult dose to manage an opioid overdose is 0.5 mg/70 kg of body weight (IV); a second dose of 1 mg/70 kg can be given 2 to 5 minutes later. To reverse postoperative opioid depression, the dosage is 0.25 mcg/kg (IV) at 2- to 5-minute intervals, as necessary.

Adverse Effects

Similar to naloxone.

✳ What is a nurse's role in the administration of opioid antagonists?

Nurses administer opioid antagonists as emergency treatment of opioid overdose and as maintenance therapy for former opioid-addicted individuals. An understanding of opioid analgesics and opioid antagonists is necessary to provide nursing care to these clients.

Assessment Observe clients carefully. Abrupt and complete reversal of opioid effects will produce an acute abstinence syndrome or withdrawal in clients who are physically dependent. Consequently, opioid antagonists should either not be administered or administered with extreme caution to a client known or suspected to be physically dependent on opioids (including newborns of dependent mothers). Use naloxone cautiously in clients with preexisting ventricular irritability because ventricular tachycardia and fibrillation may occur. Naltrexone is contraindicated in clients with acute hepatitis or hepatic failure because there is an increased risk of hepatotoxicity.

A baseline assessment includes the symptoms for which the opioid antagonist is being administered, such as sedation, hypotension and respiratory depression.

Nursing Diagnosis Nursing diagnoses associated with the administration of opioid antagonists are: altered comfort related to withdrawal symptoms (anxiety, irritability, body aches, diarrhea, tachycardia, runny nose, sweating, yawning, anorexia, nausea, vomiting, trembling, shivering) and the potential complication of decreased cardiac output related to the cardiovascular effects (tachycardia, hypotension, hyper-

tension) of the drug. In addition to these symptoms, the neonate may also experience seizures with naloxone.

Planning The client will experience relief from the symptoms of opioid overdose without withdrawal symptoms.

Implementation

Monitoring Continued nursing observation is necessary for the client who has responded to naloxone; doses should be repeated as necessary, since the duration of action of some opioids exceeds the duration of action of naloxone. Monitor closely for airway obstruction and maintain suction equipment at the bedside until the client is recovered. Monitor vital signs, particularly respirations, minimally every 5 minutes until the client is stable. The respiratory rate should increase within 1 to 2 minutes of the first dose. Administration of the IV drug should be titrated according to a client's response. The client should probably be admitted to an intensive care unit until the effects of the drug have completely abated. Clients should be observed for a day or longer regardless of the apparent recovery.

Intervention In addition to opioid toxicity, naltrexone is indicated for the treatment of opioid dependency and addiction. When used as such, it should be as an adjunctive measure to a comprehensive drug rehabilitation program involving counseling and psychotherapy. Naltrexone therapy should not be started until the client has been completely detoxified as evidenced by being opioid free for 7 to 10 days, having no withdrawal symptoms, and a negative urinalysis for opioids or naloxone challenge test. If, in an emergency situation, an opioid analgesic is required for a client receiving naltrexone therapy, it should be administered in a hospital setting where careful monitoring is available. Because high doses of the analgesic are required to overcome the effects of naltrexone, the client is at risk for prolonged respiratory depression and circulatory collapse. Naltrexone does not cause physical or psychologic dependence.

To verify abstinence from opioids, as is frequently done before naltrexone therapy, a naloxone challenge test may be done. This test should not be done in the presence of withdrawal symptoms (body aches, diarrhea, gooseflesh, sneezing and runny nose, irritability, diaphoresis, trembling and weakness, abdominal cramping, tachycardia, nausea and vomiting) or opioids in the urine. If administered IV, give one-fourth of the total dose and observe the client for 30 seconds for withdrawal symptoms. If none occurs, give the remainder of the dose and observe the client for 20 minutes. If administered subcutaneously, give the full dose and observe the client for 45 minutes for withdrawal symptoms. If withdrawal symptoms occur, repeat the test at 24-hour intervals until the absence of opioid dependence is confirmed. Remember that naloxone has no effect on respiratory depression caused by nonopioid drugs. If the client has taken multiple drugs, naloxone will reverse only the activity of the opioids.

Education When opioid antagonists are used in emergency treatment, focus client education on assisting the client to cope with the immediate situation. Keep the client informed of what is to occur and help the client cooperate with treatment procedures, even when the client appears unresponsive. Discuss the dangers of drug abuse or dependence at some time after emergency treatment. Compliance with long-term naltrexone therapy is improved if someone other than the client (health care provider or family member) administers the naltrexone.

With naltrexone, stress the importance of the need to maintain other parts of the rehabilitation program (counseling sessions, support group meetings, etc.); regular visits to the prescriber for hepatic function studies to detect hepatotoxicity; notifying other health care providers of naltrexone use; and carrying an identification indicating the use of this drug. Alert the client not to take opioid medications for pain relief, diarrhea, or cough because they will not be effective. Caution the client not to take large doses of opioids to overcome the effects of the drug because that may result in coma and death. The drug should not be shared with others, including those dependent on opioids.

Evaluation After administration of antagonists, evaluate for development of opioid withdrawal syndrome in a possible opioid-dependent client. When naltrexone is used to maintain an opioid-free state in former opioid-addicted individuals, follow-up evaluations are needed to reinforce and ensure compliance. With the use of nalmefene and naloxone in the reversal of opioid toxicity, the respiratory rate and volume will increase to normal parameters for the client, and the blood pressure will return to normal if it has been depressed.

✱ **In the case of J.F., it was elected to temporarily stop the PCA infusion and allow her respirations and level of consciousness to improve. Although the IV administration of naloxone would result in increased respirations and level of consciousness almost immediately, it would also likely reverse the analgesic effects of morphine and contribute to unnecessary anxiety. Because her circumstances are not life-threatening and she is closely monitored, naloxone was not administered. Once respirations and level of consciousness improved, her PCA pump was reprogrammed and restarted. Pain for J.F. improves postoperatively, and on day two, she is converted from IV PCA morphine to oral morphine. Her PCA morphine intake for the past 24 hours has been 1 mg/hr continuously and an average of 2 mg used every 2 hours for breakthrough pain. The PCA is discontinued and she starts on oral morphine 15 mg or 5 mg subcutaneously every 6 hours as needed for pain. Is this an appropriate regimen?**
Morphine may be administered orally, intramuscularly, intravenously, subcutaneously, epidurally, intrathecally, and rectally. Table 14-3 describes the pharmacokinetics, dosage, and administration of morphine. Morphine is distributed widely in body tissues. Morphine exhibits a high first-pass effect accounting for the higher oral dose to achieve a similar effect as lower doses administered parenterally. It is metabolized in the liver primarily to morphine-3-glucuronide

(M3G) and morphine-6-glucuronide (M6G), an active metabolite, and it is excreted primarily via the kidneys. The half-life of morphine is relatively short; if used for intermittent dosing, it should be dosed at least every 3 hours. Although the dose appears appropriate for J.F., the interval should be shortened to every 3 hours PRN. At the present 6-hour interval, it would be expected that she would develop significant pain before her next dosing opportunity, which would contribute to cyclic pattern of pain, leading to increased anxiety and discomfort, which contributes to a greater perception of pain.

Sustained-action formulations of morphine (e.g., MS Contin) are available for regular administration, usually for individuals with chronic pain. They are appropriate for every 8- or 12-hour dosing to maintain consistent levels of morphine in the system, but do not have an appreciable effect over the first hour or two of dosing. If used, they should be supplemented with an immediate-release morphine product to address breakthrough or immediate pain.

✱ **Three days after surgery, J.F. is noted to have a fecal impaction. Is this related to the morphine?**
Constipation secondary to opioids is often profound. Health care team members should diligently anticipate and manage constipation for clients on morphine. Morphine-induced constipation routinely requires concurrent use of stimulant laxatives or combination laxative regimens (see Chapters 11 and 40). Increase J.H.'s fluid intake to 1500 to 2000 mL daily. As she returns to a normal diet, her diet should include 15 to 25 g of fiber daily. Assist her to the bathroom promptly so that she may respond to GI urges. As her mobility increases, this will also assist in maintaining normal elimination patterns.

✱ **While being assisted to the bathroom, J.F. voices concerns about becoming "addicted" to morphine. How should the nurse respond to her concerns?**
As discussed earlier, the greatest abuse with opioid analgesics is not inducing addiction but the fear of inducing addiction. Health care providers and the general public are overly concerned about the potential of inducing addiction as a result of using opioid analgesics to treat pain. This is unfortunate because addiction related to opioid use for acute pain management is very rare in clinical practice, and the fear of inducing addiction or even respiratory depression in a client with severe pain is not an acceptable reason for undertreatment. However, "pseudoaddiction" refers to clients who are inadequately treated for pain and, as a result, develop a pattern of drug-seeking behaviors to achieve pain control (Weissman & Haddox, 1989). This pattern is often mistaken for opioid addiction. The concepts of addiction are more fully discussed in Chapter 9.

Tolerance, or the need to increase the dosage of an analgesic to maintain the desired effect, is sometimes mistaken by clients for addiction. Tolerance is not usually seen in opioid-naive clients (clients who have never used opioids before) with severe acute or chronic pain resulting from trauma, tumor growth, or postsurgical pain. An increase in pain in such individuals is usually a result of disease progression or complications. **Physical dependence** is an adaptive physiologic condition observed after chronic administration where tolerance to drug effect is observed and a withdrawal syndrome is noted with prolonged abstinence (American Pain Society, 2003).

If careful assessment, prescribing, and monitoring are done during opioid use, respiratory depression is a very unlikely effect (Box 14-3). Although very large amounts of opioids are often necessary to control pain in clients who have advanced cancer or are terminally ill, doses of these agents are titrated to effect, and selective tolerance to respiratory depression and sedation develops over time.

When using long-acting morphine to manage chronic noncancer pain, many prescribers institute an agreement or "contract" with a client, specifying the client's willingness to use multiple modalities in treating the pain (i.e., not just relying on the opioid) and agreeing to only obtain analgesics from that prescriber or health team. Such an agreement helps a client to appreciate the multimodal interventions in the treatment of chronic noncancer pain and helps both the client and health care team have confidence that everyone is "on the same page" in exploring and implementing safe and effective plans of treatment.

The risk for addiction to morphine in managing J.F.'s pain is remote. Address her concerns directly, stressing the use of multiple interventions in her recovery process, including receiving adequate analgesia, ongoing disease modification treatments for her rheumatoid arthritis (see Chapter 63), physical therapy, and psychosocial supports. It is also important to share the consequences of unrelieved pain with the client.

✹ What nonpharmacologic interventions will serve to support J.F.'s analgesic therapy?

Nonpharmacologic forms of interventions can serve as adjuncts to analgesic therapy. It is well known that anxiety exacerbates pain and causes muscle tension. Relaxation techniques can be effective in reducing the amount of pain experienced. Simple methods that promote comfort, such as a quiet, pleasant environment or proper body position, may prove very effective. Rhythmic breathing, counting, and purposeful relaxation of muscle groups are among the techniques that nurses can teach J.F. More advanced nonpharmacologic methods include acupuncture, meditation, cognitive behavioral therapy, guided imagery, therapeutic touch, biofeedback, and hypnosis. An example of a highly

---

BOX 14-3 TIME REQUIRED TO PRODUCE MAXIMAL RESPIRATORY DEPRESSION EFFECTS WITH OPIOID ANALGESICS	
ROUTE OF ADMINISTRATION	APPROXIMATE TIMES
IV	Within 7 minutes
IM	Within 30 minutes
Subcutaneous	Within 90 minutes

---

successful relaxation technique for pain control is the psychoprophylactic or "Lamaze" method of rhythmic breathing and focusing to blunt the perception of pain during labor and delivery. These same techniques are useful for the management of many other types of acute pain.

Shifting J.F.'s focus of attention away from the painful stimulus is known as distraction. This technique greatly improves a client's ability to cope with pain. Listening to music, watching television, visiting with friends, and working on a project can be effective distractions as she recovers.

Mood and psychological issues play an important role in a client's perception of pain. This is particularly true for clients with underlying anxiety or depression. Psychotherapy, support groups, prayer, and pastoral counseling can also help in the management of pain (Rabow & Pantilat, 2003).

Asking J.F. what methods of pain relief she has used in the past is important. Reinforcing these methods and supplementing them with new techniques often reduces the need for pain-relieving medications.

✹ Given that J.F. will be using opioids for some time after her surgery, what client education will be essential?

Instructing J.F. in various techniques for relieving pain is an important part of pain therapy—both now following surgery, and in the future because of her chronic arthritic pain. A nurse may know many techniques for dealing with pain and can teach them to clients (e.g., using the PCA, splinting an abdominal incision with a pillow to reduce the discomfort of coughing). Clients receiving drugs for pain relief should be informed of the purpose of the medication because analgesic effects may be enhanced by positive suggestion.

Because orthostatic hypotension (a form of low blood pressure that occurs when a person stands) can occur in ambulatory clients, caution J.F. about rising quickly from a supine position. Opioids can impair mental and physical abilities, so instruct her to use caution when ambulating and to ask for assistance.

If J.F. were to go home on an opioid, she should be taught the proper dosage, correct administration, adverse effects and what to do when they occur, drug interactions (e.g., other opioid analgesics, CNS depressants, cyclic antidepressants, neuroleptics, anxiolytics, ethanol, or sedative-hypnotics, because the combination of any of these can produce CNS depression) and the safe storage of controlled substances. Because of potential CNS depression, she should refrain from ingesting alcoholic beverages while taking opioids.

✹ How will the effectiveness of J.F.'s analgesia be determined?

Evaluation involves reassessing the physiologic responses and J.F.'s perception of pain. Rate the pain using a pain scale before and after treatment to document the response to treatment. Outcomes of J.F.'s opioid therapy would be control of pain in keeping with her wishes, and using decreasing dosages over time without respiratory depression, nausea, constipation, or other nontherapeutic effects.

✪ On day five, J.F. is discharged to a rehabilitation facility for transition care until she can ambulate and perform activities of daily living.

✪ What additional analgesics could be considered for J.F. at discharge?

In addition to the classic opioid agonists noted above, a number of other drugs are used to treat pain. These include the opioid-like drugs, the partial opioid agonists/antagonists (rarely used), and nonopioid analgesics.

Opioid-like Drugs

tramadol [**tram** a dole]
(Ultram)
Tramadol is a central-acting synthetic analgesic that is not chemically related to the opioids. This product appears to bind to the mu opioid receptors and also inhibits the reuptake of norepinephrine and serotonin. Its efficacy is comparable to low-dose codeine.

Indications
Tramadol is indicated for the treatment of moderate to moderately severe pain.

Pharmacokinetics/Dosing
Tramadol is well absorbed orally with an onset of action within 60 minutes, a peak effect in 2 hours, and a half-life of approximately 6 to 7 hours. It is metabolized in the liver to inactive and active metabolites, and is primarily excreted in urine. The usual adult dosage is 50 to 100 mg every 6 hours. The maximum daily dose is 400 mg.

Adverse Effects
Tramadol was initially believed to have less potential for respiratory depression and drug dependency than the opioids. However, in 1996, the manufacturer recognized the risk of seizures, anaphylactoid reactions, and substance abuse associated with tramadol. Consequently, its use is not recommended for persons with a history of opioid allergy, dependence, or a past or present history of addiction.

Drug Interactions
Tramadol increases metabolism of the antiepileptic drug carbamazepine (Tegretol). Tramadol, when dosed with amphetamines, antidepressants, antipsychotics, and MAOIs may increase seizure risk. Such combinations are typically avoided.

Partial Opioid Agonist-Antagonists

Although the exact mechanism of action of **opioid agonist-antagonists** is unknown, these agents have both agonist and antagonist effects on the opioid receptors. For example, buprenorphine (Buprenex) is a partial agonist at the mu receptors. Butorphanol (Stadol), nalbuphine (Nubain), and pentazocine (Talwin) produce agonist effects at the kappa and sigma receptors and may displace agonists (opioids) from their mu receptor sites, thus inhibiting their effects and perhaps inducing a drug withdrawal reaction in clients who are physically dependent on agonist opioids. These drugs should never be used for individuals who receive chronic pain management with opioids, individuals on methadone, or active users of opioids. Dezocine (Dalgan) is a partial agonist at the mu receptor and has some effect at the sigma receptors after high doses.

In general, these drugs are less potent analgesics and have a lower dependency potential than opioids, and withdrawal symptoms are not as severe as those reported with the opioid agonist medications when used in opioid-naive clients. In-

terestingly, women seem to respond to the analgesic effects of these agents to a greater extent than do men (Holdcroft & Power, 2003). This gender difference appears to be related to differences in receptor site binding. The opioid agonist-antagonist agents have pharmacokinetics, adverse effects, and significant drug interactions similar to morphine.

buprenorphine [byoo pre **nor** feen]
(Buprenex)
Buprenorphine dissociates very slowly from the mu receptor, thereby reducing or blocking the effect of concurrent or subsequent dosing with opioid agonist drugs.

Indications
Parenteral buprenorphine is infrequently used to treat moderate to severe pain. More commonly, a sublingual formulation combined with naloxone (Suboxone) is used in management protocols for opioid dependence.

Pharmacokinetics/Dosing
Buprenorphine undergoes extensive first-pass metabolism and dosing can be variable. Refer to other drug references for a more complete discussion.

Adverse Effects
Respiratory depression and other adverse effects of this drug are often difficult to reverse because naloxone is not very effective in treating buprenorphine-induced adverse effects. The primary management of overdose is mechanical assistance of respiration when naloxone is ineffective in reversing respiratory depression (*Drug Facts and Comparisons*, 2005).

butorphanol tartrate [byoo **tor** fa nole]
(Stadol)
Indications
Butorphanol tartrate is indicated for the treatment of moderate to severe pain and as an anesthetic adjunct.

Pharmacokinetics/Dosing
It is administered parenterally (IM or IV) and as a nasal spray.

Adverse Effects
Use caution when administering butorphanol as a preoperative medication for hypertensive clients, because it may increase blood pressure. It should not be administered to clients with acute myocardial infarction because the cardiovascular effects tend to increase the workload on the heart. However, butorphanol may be used with clients with gallbladder disease or gallstones because biliary spasm has not been reported. Butorphanol may elevate cerebrospinal fluid (CSF) pressure; therefore it should be used with caution in clients with head injuries or preexisting increased CSF pressure.

The safety of using butorphanol in pregnancy before the labor period has not been established. The safety to the mother and fetus after the administration of butorphanol during labor has been established, with clients experiencing no adverse effects other than those observed with commonly used analgesics. This drug should be used with caution in women delivering premature infants. It is also passed on in breast milk.

nalbuphine [**nal** byoo feen]
(Nubain)
Indications
Nalbuphine, an analgesic for moderate to severe pain, is also used preoperatively as an adjunct to anesthesia and for obstetric analgesia for opioid-naive clients.

Pharmacokinetics/Dosing
Onset of action of nalbuphine is 1 to 3 minutes after IV administration and up to 30 minutes after subcutaneous dosing. The elimination half-life is 3 to 5 hours. It is typically dosed 10 to 20 mg every 3 to 6 hours.

Adverse Effects
Similar to butorphanol.

⬛🔳 pentazocine [pen **taz** oh seen]

(Talwin)

Indications

Pentazocine is indicated for the treatment of moderate to severe pain in opioid-naive clients. It is generally avoided in older adults and in those clients with renal impairment.

Pharmacokinetics/Dosing

Pentazocine displays an extensive first-pass metabolism with oral administration. Dosed orally, its duration of action is approximately 4 hours. Dose varies on indication and client age. In the United States, pentazocine oral tablets are combined with naloxone (Narcan) because of the high incidence of pentazocine abuse. Naloxone taken orally is not pharmacologically active, but if this combination is dissolved and injected, naloxone will block the effects of pentazocine that lead to abuse.

Adverse Effects

The analgesic pentazocine is not indicated for pain caused by acute myocardial infarction because of its effects on cardiac function. It increases cardiac workload by increasing systemic and pulmonary arterial pressure, systemic vascular resistance, and left ventricular end-diastolic pressure. It also has a higher incidence of psychotomimetic adverse effects than the majority of other analgesics, thus limiting its usefulness, especially in terminally ill clients or in clients who are already anxious or fearful.

Drug Interactions

Significant drug interactions are the same as those for butorphanol. Subcutaneous administration is to be avoided because of tissue damage at the injection sites; IM sites should be routinely rotated for the same reason.

Nonopioid Analgesics

The nonopioid analgesics are effective for mild to moderate pain and are often combined with opioid analgesics to enhance the control of severe pain. The major drugs in this classification include the cyclooxygenase inhibitors (NSAIDs, salicylates, and COX-2 inhibitors), acetaminophen, and the adjunct analgesics. These agents are used to treat mild to moderate pain, fever, and inflammation caused by rheumatoid arthritis, osteoarthritis, and various other acute and chronic musculoskeletal and soft-tissue inflammation. Recent evidence suggests that NSAIDs such as ibuprofen may be more effective than acetaminophen for the treatment of osteoarthritis (Boureau, Schneid, Zeghari, Wall, & Bourgeois, 2004). NSAIDs are also used to treat metastatic bone pain, usually in combination with an opioid analgesic. The over-the-counter (OTC) dosage forms of these preparations are discussed in Chapter 11, but doses available in these formulations are often too low to adequately treat pain. Aspirin is also prescribed for its antiplatelet effects in reducing the risk of transient ischemic attacks (TIAs), myocardial infarcts, and stroke.

Cyclooxygenase Inhibitors

Aspirin and the NSAIDs peripherally inhibit the cyclooxygenase (COX) enzyme (the first enzyme in the prostaglandin pathway), which results in a reduction of the synthesis and release of prostaglandins (see Figure 14-12). The two identified forms of COX are COX-1 and COX-2. COX-1 is found primarily in the blood vessels, stomach, and kidneys, whereas COX-2 is activated by inflammation induced by the cytokines and inflammatory mediators. The cause of the adverse GI and renal toxicity is believed to be secondary to the inhibition of COX-1, whereas COX-2 inhibition produces the beneficial effects reported with this drug classification.

The selective COX-2 inhibitors have had a checkered history since their introduction to the market in 1999. These drugs were introduced as treatment for rheumatoid arthritis and osteoarthritis and were often used for other inflammatory-based pain. It was initially believed that these agents would be safer than the nonselective COX-1 and COX-2 inhibitors because they are much less apt to inhibit COX-1 (the cyclooxygenase that protects the stomach) and therefore are much less ulcerogenic (Simon et al., 1999). Unfortunately, cardiovascular safety concerns were identified after FDA approval, prompting the removal from the market of rofecoxib (Vioxx) in late 2004 and valdecoxib (Bextra) in early 2005. Cardiovascular events associated with these agents included reports of increased risk for thromboembolic disease, including myocardial infarction and cerebrovascular accidents. The safety of celecoxib (Celebrex), the sole marketed COX-2 inhibitor at the time of this publication, is also undergoing careful scrutiny. Whether these cardiovascular effects are possible with other COX-2 or COX-1/COX-2 inhibitors is under ongoing evaluation. (See the discussion below and the Evidence-Based Practice box on p. 268).

Aspirin affects both COX-1 and COX-2, causing an irreversible inhibition of cyclooxygenase activity; the NSAIDs produce reversible, competitive inhibition of cyclooxygenase (Roberts & Morrow, 2001). Nabumetone (Relafen) is

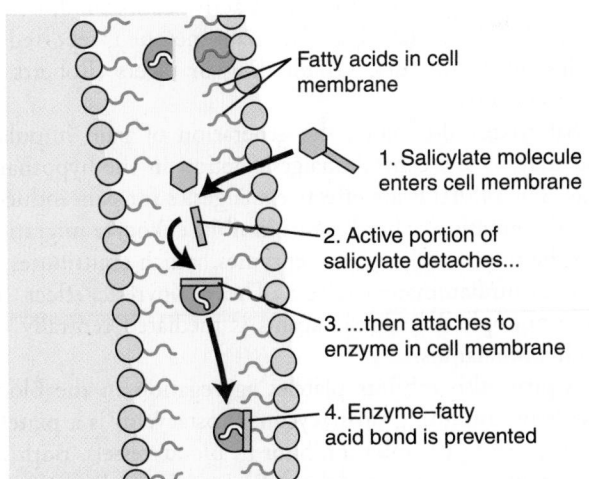

Fatty acids in cell membrane

1. Salicylate molecule enters cell membrane

2. Active portion of salicylate detaches...

3. ...then attaches to enzyme in cell membrane

4. Enzyme–fatty acid bond is prevented

FIGURE 14-12 Inhibition of prostaglandin production by salicylates. Inflammatory diseases and local injuries are often related to an increased production of prostaglandins. Salicylates and NSAIDs act peripherally by entering the cell membrane *(1)*, in the case of salicylates, the active portion detaches *(2)*. Then the NSAID or active portion of the salicylate attaches to the enzyme (cyclooxygenase) in the cell membrane *(3)*. Because this new complex *(4)* cannot react with fatty acids to induce prostaglandin synthesis, inflammation and pain are reduced in the affected area.

Evidence-Based Practice

Cardiovascular Risks of Cyclooxygenase Inhibitors

Clients with cardiovascular conditions require careful monitoring while taking NSAIDs. All NSAIDs (both those that are COX-2 selective, and the older COX-1/COX-2 inhibitors) are associated with edema, hypertension, and the risk for developing heart failure (HF) (Mamdani et al., 2004). Although there has been speculation about the risk for cardiovascular and cerebrovascular events associated with COX-2 inhibitors since their approval by the FDA in 1999, this issue has been highlighted by the recall of rofecoxib (Vioxx) in 2004 and the subsequent recall of valdecoxib (Bextra) in early 2005.

The voluntary removal of rofecoxib from the market by the manufacturer was based on a trial comparing rofecoxib to placebo in clients without cardiovascular disease. This study, which was halted early, indicated that the rate of myocardial infarctions was nearly double in those who received rofecoxib instead of placebo (FDA News, 2004). Earlier data was also suggestive of a greater risk for heart attack with rofecoxib (Bombardier et al., 2000). A meta-analysis of 10 trials published by the end of 2000 suggests that adequate data was available in late 2000 for the removal of rofecoxib from the market (Juni et al., 2004). Such data have raised controversy not only about COX-2 inhibitors but also about the drug approval process through the FDA.

Valdecoxib (Bextra) was removed from the market in April 2005 based on an FDA alert that noted increased cardiovascular and serious dermal risks associated with its use (FDA Alert, 2005). In the same alert, the FDA recommended limiting the use of celecoxib (Celebrex), the sole remaining marked selective COX-2 inhibitor, to "properly selected and informed patients" using "the lowest effective dose for the shortest duration."

Whereas aspirin reduces risk for myocardial infarction by inhibiting thromboxane A_2 and platelet aggregation, the specific inhibition of COX-2 inhibitors may block synthesis of other prostaglandins (e.g., I_2) which may have beneficial antiplatelet and vasodilatory properties (FitzGerald, 2004). The cardiovascular risks associated with the nonselective COX-1/COX-2 inhibitors is less clear. The FDA issued a warning about potential cardiovascular risks with naproxen in late 2004 based on a trial using naproxen in clients with a risk of developing Alzheimer's disease (FDA Statement on Naproxen, 2004). Other data suggest that naproxen and other COX-1/COX-2 inhibitors are relatively safe (Juni et al., 2004). Abrupt withdrawal of chronic use of COX-1/COX-2 inhibitors (e.g., ibuprofen, naproxen) may actually *increase* the risk for myocardial infarction (Fischer et al., 2004), suggesting a cardioprotective effect for these agents while being used.

More careful assessment of the effect on platelet aggregation and myocardial risk for selective COX-2 inhibitors and nonselective COX-1/COX-2 inhibitors is likely over the next few years. In the interim, use of these agents for clients with cardiovascular disease should be carefully scrutinized, and close monitoring for worsening symptoms is warranted.

---

an exception; it is a prodrug that is inactive when ingested and is converted in the liver to its active compound, which primarily inhibits COX-2. Thus nabumetone is reported to be less likely to cause GI bleeding or ulcers (Roberts & Morrow, 2001).

Salicylates also block the generation of pain impulses and may have a central analgesic action in the hypothalamus. The NSAIDs are effective analgesics for pain induced by inflammation. These agents inhibit leukocyte migration and the release of lysosomal enzymes, which contributes to their antiinflammatory effect. The antipyretic effect for these nonopioid analgesic agents is mediated centrally via the hypothalamus.

Aspirin also inhibits platelet aggregation in the blood vessels by inhibiting prostacyclin. Prostacyclin is a platelet aggregation (reversible) inhibitor in blood vessels. Both effects may be dose dependent. Prescription salicylates include controlled-release aspirin 800 mg (ZORprin), salsalate (Disalcid and others), choline magnesium trisalicylate (Trilisate), and magnesium salicylate (Magan). Salsalate is converted to salicylate during absorption from the GI tract and in the liver. Both salsalate and choline magnesium trisalicylate have the advantage of producing little, if any, adverse GI effects, and they do not affect platelet aggregation. The analgesic effects of salsalate are equivalent to aspirin. The magnesium from these combination agents may be absorbed, which may result in systemic toxicity in clients with renal impairment. High-dose salicylate therapy is associated with concentration dependent elimination; once elimination systems are saturated, no further elimination is possible and drug accumulation can occur.

aspirin (ASA) [as pir in]
(Entrophen✦, Novasen✦)

Indications
At low to moderate doses, aspirin is used as prophylaxis for myocardial infarction (MI), stroke, and transient ischemic attacks (TIAs). Higher doses of aspirin are also used to treat mild to moderate pain, inflammation, and fever.

Pharmacokinetics/Dosing
Aspirin is metabolized to the pharmacologically active salicylate in the GI mucosa. Salicylate is metabolized in the liver by pathways that are saturated at high doses. Doses of 75 to 325 mg daily are used as prophylaxis for MI, stroke, and TIA prevention, although doses as high as 650 mg twice daily have been used in clinical trials for stroke prevention. For clients with unstable angina or acute MI, 160 to 325 mg of immediate-release aspirin is crushed or chewed and swallowed with water for a prompt effect. As an analgesic or antiinflammatory agent, doses of 650 mg every 4 to 6 hours are typically used.

Adverse Effects
As with all drugs with antiplatelet action, aspirin poses a risk for bleeding at any site. The risk for GI ulceration with chronic use can be as high as 30%, which is due to aspirin's inhibition of prostaglandin synthesis and antiplatelet effects. Clients with a history of GI bleeding should either avoid aspirin therapy or consider concurrent use of proton pump inhibitors with aspirin use (see Chapter 40). Other risks in-

Management of Drug Overdose

Salicylates and Aspirin

Although less frequently observed than acetaminophen overdose, excessive salicylate ingestion requiring acute management may be seen in clinical practice.

Principles of management and treatment include the following:

- Obtaining an accurate history to estimate time and amount of salicylate ingested. It is also critical to establish if the ingested product was an immediate-release formulation or sustained action/enteric coated and if the ingestion was chronic or acute.
- Use of serum salicylate levels in assessing toxicity and guiding therapy (Lacy et al., 2004). Serum levels are typically monitored every 4 hours for at least 24 hours since concretions (solid mass of drug in the GI tract) are common with salicylate overdose. Serum level monitoring continues until a significant drop in two sequential levels is observed:
  - Levels between 250 and 400 mcg/mL: nausea, vomiting, tinnitus, sweating, diarrhea, tachycardia
  - Levels greater than 400 mcg/mL: respiratory alkalosis, hemorrhage, mental status changes, seizures, tetany, risk cardiovascular collapse, respiratory failure, coma
  - Levels may not be reliable for assessing toxicity for use of ingestion of large quantities of delayed-release salicylates
- Multiple doses of activated charcoal are used as primary decontamination intervention. Gastric lavage may also be used in severe cases.
- Hyperventilation is a classic sign of salicylate toxicity and often results in respiratory alkalosis with a compensatory metabolic acidosis and dehydration. Gastrointestinal bleeding is also possible.
- Careful monitoring of electrolytes (particularly potassium), acid-base balance, prothrombin time (PT/INR), partial thromboplastin time (PTT), and anion gap is routine in management. Fluid and electrolyte and acid/base management is a critical component of care.
- Severe cases may require respiratory support, hemodialysis, and sodium bicarbonate (Roberts & Morrow, 2001).

---

clude hypersensitivity reactions, bronchospasm (particularly for clients with a prior history of asthma and/or nasal polyps), and liver and renal toxicity. Aspirin must be avoided in children and adolescents because of the risk for Reye's syndrome. See the Management of Drug Overdose box above regarding symptoms and management of salicylate and aspirin overdose.

Drug Interactions
Angiotensin-converting enzyme (ACE) inhibitors may be less effective when administered with higher doses of aspirin. Aspirin and methotrexate may result in elevated methotrexate levels. Concurrent use of aspirin with other antiplatelet drugs or anticoagulants or fibrinolytics may increase bleeding risk, but this combination has been used successfully for a number of high-risk clients to prevent or manage thromboembolic events.

Approximately 20 different NSAIDs are now available in the United States and Canada. Although aspirin is also an NSAID, the term *NSAID* most commonly refers to the newer aspirin substitutes on the market. The NSAIDs have analgesic, antipyretic, and antiinflammatory effects, and the indications for each NSAID may vary according to specific testing and clinical data submitted to the FDA for approval.

The NSAIDs are indicated for the treatment of acute or chronic rheumatoid arthritis, osteoarthritis, ankylosing spondylitis, and other rheumatic diseases; mild to moderate pain, especially when the antiinflammatory effect is also desirable (such as after dental procedures, obstetric and orthopedic surgery, and soft-tissue athletic injuries); fever; nonrheumatic inflammation; and dysmenorrhea. For conditions where inflammation is a major component (e.g., gout, renal colic/kidney stones), NSAIDs are often considered first-line therapy in pain management (Holdgate & Pollock, 2004). Most NSAIDs are well absorbed orally, highly bound to plasma proteins, and are hepatically metabolized. Although topical application of NSAIDs for the

treatment of osteoarthritis has been studied, it is not yet an accepted practice (Lin, Zhang, Jones, & Doherty, 2004; Bookman, Williams, & Shainhouse, 2004).

✱⬛ ibuprofen [eye byoo **proe** fen]
(Motrin, Advil, Apo-Ibuprofen✚, Novoprofen✚)
Ibuprofen is a nonselective inhibitor of both COX-1 and COX-2.
Indications
Ibuprofen is indicated for the treatment of mild to moderate pain, inflammatory diseases, fever management, and dysmenorrhea.
Pharmacokinetics/Dosing
Ibuprofen is well absorbed orally with analgesic and antipyretic effects observed in the first 30 to 60 minutes. Ibuprofen is highly bound to plasma proteins, and is eliminated via hepatic metabolism. Table 14-4 describes the dosing.
Adverse Effects
Like other nonselective COX inhibitors, ibuprofen poses a risk for gastrointestinal bleeding. It may also result in renal failure in clients with preexisting moderate renal impairment. Other adverse effects include edema, hypertension (usually modest), and GI discomfort.

✱⬛ celecoxib [se le **koks** ib]
(Celebrex)
Celecoxib is a selective inhibitor of COX-2 and may result in GI bleeding. Cardiovascular risks for this drug classification have prompted similar agents to be removed from the market. Efficacy as an analgesic and antiinflammatory is comparable to the nonselective agents.
Indications
Celecoxib is indicated for the treatment of osteoarthritis and rheumatoid arthritis in clients who have not responded to other agents and who do not have a history of cardiovascular disease. It is also used in the treatment of acute pain and dysmenorrhea in selected individuals.
Pharmacokinetics/Dosing
Celecoxib is well absorbed orally. Like many other NSAIDs, it is highly bound to albumin. It is eliminated by hepatic metabolism. See Table 14-4 for more information on pharmacokinetics and dosing.

TABLE 14-4 COMPARISON OF CYCLOOXYGENASE (COX) 1 AND 2 INHIBITORS

Class	Generic Name	Brand Name	Onset of Action (hr)	Half-life (hr)	Usual Adult Dose	Risk of Upper GI Bleeding*	Comments
Acetic Acid Derivatives	diclofenac	Voltaren†	0.5	1.2-2	50 mg three to four times daily	4.6	Less effect on platelets than other NSAIDs, but may increase risk for bone marrow suppression
	etodolac	Lodine†	0.5	6-7	200-400 mg three to four times daily	2.2	
	indomethacin	Indocin†	0.5	4-6	25-50 mg two to four times daily	5.2	Higher risk for GI bleeding and renal dysfunction; available as a suppository
	ketorolac	Toradol	IM: 10 min	4-6	15-30 mg IM/IV q6h; 10 mg PO q4-6h	NA (considered high risk by other sources)	*Limited to 5 days due to high risk for GI bleeding and renal dysfunction;* IM use often avoided
	nabumetone	Relafen	Variable	22	500-1000 mg daily divided in one or two doses	3.4	Converted to active metabolite (6-MNA); may have lower risk for GI bleed
	sulindac	Clinoril	Variable	8	150-200 mg twice daily	NA	Fewer reports of renal toxicity than other NSAIDs
	tolmetin	Tolectin	Variable	5	200-600 mg three times daily	NA	Increased reports anaphylactic reactions
Fenamates	meclofenamate	Meclomen	1	2-3	50 mg three to four times daily	NA	Less effect on platelets than other NSAIDs; may cause an increase in sodium retention
	mefenamic acid	Ponstel	Variable	2	250 mg four times daily	2.7	Less effect on platelets but reports of prolonged prothrombin times
Oxicams	piroxicam	Feldene	2-4	24	20 mg daily or 10 mg twice daily	6.2	Contraindicated in renal impairment; potentially higher risk for GI bleeding
	meloxicam	Mobic	4-5	20-29	7.5-15 mg daily	NA	

Category	Generic	Brand			Dose		Comments
Propionic Acid Derivatives	flurbiprofen	Ansaid	Variable	5.7	100 mg daily to three times daily	4.6	Available as postsurgical ophthalmic preparation
	ibuprofen	Motrin, Advil	0.5	2	300-800 mg three to four times daily	2.5	Available in tablet, liquid, and OTC formulations; less GI bleeding than aspirin
	ketoprofen	Orudis†	Variable	1.5-5	27-75 mg three to four times daily	3.3	May have higher risk for sodium retention and renal dysfunction
	naproxen	Naprosyn, Aleve	1	13	250-500 mg twice daily	4	Available in tablet, liquid, and OTC formulations
	oxaprozin	Daypro	Variable	21-25	600 mg daily to twice daily	NA	Increased half-life with age and chronic dosing; May have higher risk for perioperative bleeding
Salicylates	acetylsalicylic acid, aspirin	Bayer Aspirin	0.5	Variable: 2.4-19	650 mg q4-6h	NA	Most commonly used for its antiplatelet effects in coronary artery disease and for transient ischemic attacks; may use salicylate levels in monitoring high-dose therapy
	diflunisal	Dolobid	1	8-12	250-500 mg two to three times daily	NA	Fluid retention more commonly observed
	salsalate	Disalcid	Variable	7-8	1 g twice daily to three times daily	NA	
	trisalicylate	Trilisate	Variable	Variable: 2-30	500-1500 mg two times daily	NA	May use salicylate levels in monitoring high-dose therapy
Selective COX-2 Inhibitors	celecoxib	Celebrex	1-3	11	Osteoarthritis: 200 mg daily or 100 mg twice daily. Rheumatoid arthritis: 100-200 mg twice daily	NA, lower than COX-1 and COX-2 inhibitors	Cardiovascular risk? See the Evidence-Based Practice box, p. 268

Modified from Garcia Rodriguez, L.A., & Hernandez-Diaz, S. (2001). Relative risk of upper gastrointestinal complications among users of acetaminophen and nonsteroidal anti-inflammatory drugs. *Epidemiology 12*, 570–576.

NA, Data not available.

*Upper GI Complication Relative Risk Assessment where risk of 3 would represent a three-fold risk for complication.

†Extended-release formulations also available.

Adverse Effects
The cardiovascular risk of the COX-2 selective inhibitors is under evaluation (see the Evidence-Based Practice box on p. 268). Celecoxib is less likely to produce gastrointestinal bleeding compared with nonselective cyclooxygenase inhibitors. Like other NSAIDs, it can induce renal insufficiency, edema, and mild elevations in blood pressure.

✳ **At the rehabilitation facility, J.F. receives oxycodone 5 mg/acetaminophen 325 mg (Percocet) one to two tablets every 4 hours PRN pain × 1 week, docusate 100 mg/casanthranol 30 mg (Peri-Colace) two PO twice daily for constipation × 1 week, and celecoxib 200 mg (Celebrex) twice daily as an ongoing order.**

✳ **What are the nursing considerations with administration of NSAID therapy to J.F.?**

Assessment One of the most significant adverse effects of the NSAIDs, particularly those that inhibit COX-1, is the risk for gastric or duodenal ulcers, particularly for older adults. The agents vary in the degree of GI bleeding and these differences are reflected in Table 14-4 (Garcia Rodriguez & Hernandez-Diaz, 2001). Assess J.F. for a history of gastric or duodenal ulcers because these drugs should generally be avoided. If they are used in such individuals, the risk for bleeding is reduced when COX-2 selective agents are chosen. If a COX-1 or COX-2 inhibiting drug is chosen, lower doses and concurrent cytoprotective therapy reduce risk, for example treatment for active *Helicobacter pylori* infection, or use of a proton pump inhibitor or misoprostol (Cytotec); refer to Chapter 41 (Hawkey & Langman, 2003). Ongoing monitoring for GI bleeding is warranted, including evaluating any reports of gastric pain or upset, coffee grounds emesis, black or tarry stools, and hypotensive states with reflex tachycardia.

Another risk of any COX-1 or COX-2 inhibitor for which to assess J.F. is renal insufficiency. Among the prostaglandin synthesis that is inhibited by these agents is a prostaglandin that helps maintain renal blood flow. For individuals with moderate to severe preexisting renal impairment, the institution of COX inhibitors can lead to decreased renal perfusion and acute renal failure. This renal failure may present with elevated serum creatinine and blood urea nitrogen levels and may or may not include a change in urine output. Most clinicians avoid the use of these agents in individuals with a creatinine clearance below 30 mL/min and carefully monitor for changes in renal function for individuals with creatinine clearances below 50 mL/min (see Chapter 35).

A third area of risk and controversy is the use of these drugs in individuals with a history of cardiovascular disease. All COX inhibitors have reportedly resulted in elevations in blood pressure and/or fluid retention for some clients who take them. Usually these changes are modest, but occasionally are more significant and include the risk for inducing heart failure (Mamdani et al., 2004). This may be a concern for individuals with preexisting hypertension or heart failure, or who experience elevations in blood pressure or edema related to the use of these drugs. In addition, there is some concern that the available NSAIDs and COX-2 inhibitors may be associated with a modest increase in risk for coronary events, such as myocardial infarction (Gajraj, 2003). The removal from the market of rofecoxib (Vioxx) in late 2004 and valdecoxib (Bextra) in 2005 focused attention on this issue. While the risk is unknown, quantification of this risk is ongoing, and J.F. should review any concerns with her prescriber. If used, it is important to instruct J.F. to monitor daily her weight and blood pressure. See the Evidence-Based Practice box on p. 268.

Establish J.F.'s allergies before administering NSAIDs. The anaphylactoid reaction may be life-threatening in individuals with a documented history of allergy or hypersensitivity to aspirin. Clients with the triad of aspirin allergy, nasal polyps, and bronchospastic disease may experience bronchospasm, leading to respiratory failure with the use of NSAIDs. Clients sensitive to one NSAID may also be sensitive to other NSAIDs. The NSAIDs are contraindicated in individuals when the drugs have caused asthmatic symptoms, rhinitis, urticaria, nasal polyps, angioedema, or bronchospastic events. Diclofenac is contraindicated for clients with a history of or active blood dyscrasias or bone marrow depression because these conditions will be precipitated or worsen.

NSAIDs should be used with caution in older adults, who are more prone to the upper GI, hepatic, and renal effects of these agents. See the Special Considerations for Older Adults box on p. 273.

Review the client's current medication regimen for the risk of significant drug interactions; see Table 14-2 for those drugs of concern.

Although not relevant for J.F., a woman who is pregnant or intends to become pregnant while using an NSAID should notify her health care provider, because these drugs may interfere with maternal and infant blood clotting and prolong the duration of pregnancy and parturition. They may prematurely lead to closure of the patent ductus arteriosus in the fetus if administered during the third trimester of pregnancy. There is a correlation between the use of NSAIDs and an increase in the incidence of stillbirths and neonatal deaths in humans. If a mother intends to breastfeed, alert her that salicylates are detected in the breast milk and are cleared from the body more slowly by infants. See the Pregnancy Safety box on p. 251 for the FDA classification of the various NSAIDs.

J.F.'s baseline assessment before NSAID therapy includes blood pressure, temperature, pulse, respirations, adventitious lung sounds, orientation, complete blood cell count (CBC), clotting times, renal and hepatic function tests, stool guaiac, and a detailed description of her pain.

Nursing Diagnosis While J.F. is receiving NSAID therapy, she has the potential for the following nursing diagnoses: constipation; diarrhea; acute pain or chronic pain related to ineffective dosage of the NSAID; disturbed sensory perception evidenced by visual changes, tinnitus, or dizziness; excess fluid volume (periorbital edema, peripheral edema, respiratory rales); ineffective protection related to hypoprothrombinemia; and ineffective health maintenance related to insufficient knowledge of contraindications, potential hazards, or signs and symptoms of bleeding. The potential complications of seizures, acute renal failure, myocardial infarction, hemorrhage, and GI ulcers and perforation exist with the administration of NSAIDs.

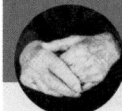

Special Considerations for Older Adults | NONSTEROIDAL ANTIINFLAMMATORY DRUGS

Among individuals taking NSAIDs, the incidence of perforated peptic ulcers and/or bleeding is more common in older adults than in younger adults, with serious consequences occurring more often in this older age-group. The risk for HF, hypertension, and myocardial infarction may also be higher in older adults.

Clients with renal impairment may be at increased risk for NSAID-induced liver or renal toxicity and often require a dosage reduction to prevent drug accumulation.

Clinicians have recommended that clients age 70 years or older be started at one-half the usual adult dosage with close monitoring and careful dosage increases. The dosage increase should be based on the client's therapeutic response and lack of signs and symptoms of toxicity. Specific drug warnings include the following:

- *Flurbiprofen* (Ansaid) may result in elevated peak serum levels in women who are between 74 and 94 years of age. This serum level has not been documented in older

men (*USP DI*, 2005). Therefore older women may need a lower dosage to produce a therapeutic response.
- *Indomethacin* (Indocin) is responsible for a higher incidence of CNS adverse effects, especially confusion, in older adults.
- The use of *naproxen* (Naprosyn) in older adults results in a higher proportion of unbound (free) naproxen, which may not be reflected by the total serum level. The steady-state concentration of unbound naproxen may be nearly double that of a younger adult, which may result in an increase in adverse effects, even with a normal serum level range. The nurse should be aware of this potential because the prescriber may need to be notified about the possible need for a dosage reduction.
- *Oxaprozin* is more likely to cause a significant decrease in renal function, adverse GI effects, or a decrease in hemoglobin in clients older than age 60 years, than in younger clients.

Planning While taking NSAID therapy, J.F. will:

- Experience pain relief at an acceptable level for her with minimal adverse effects.
- Effectively manage her therapeutic regimen including demonstrating nonpharmacologic measures to minimize her pain and NSAID adverse effects, and identifying signs and symptoms of adverse effects and reporting to her health care provider appropriately.
- Collaborate with the health team in maintaining scheduled visits for monitoring and treatment.

Implementation

Monitoring While implementing J.F.'s care, monitor her pain and mobility of affected areas periodically. Clients require close monitoring of their prothrombin time if they are receiving concomitant anticoagulant therapy or if they have other intrinsic hemostatic coagulation defects. Clients taking other NSAIDs should have hematologic determinations only if symptoms of blood dyscrasias occur. Precipitation of acute renal failure may occur in clients with preexisting diminished sodium excretion, heart failure, cirrhosis, hypertension, or renal disease.

Monitor fluid intake and output and other symptoms of fluid volume excess (weight gain, edema, increased blood pressure) with the administration of NSAIDs.

Intervention NSAID doses are taken 30 to 60 minutes before meals or 2 hours postprandially to reach the appropriate blood level more readily. Administer with a full glass of water and have J.F. remain in an upright position for 15 to 30 minutes to minimize the risk of tablets becoming lodged in the esophagus, which may cause

esophageal irritation. Administration with a meal followed by a full glass of water will also aid in preventing gastric upset.

Education Advise J.F. to maintain contact with her prescriber for periodic determinations of white blood cells (WBCs), hemoglobin, and/or hematocrit.

If J.F. had a clinical problem such as erosive gastritis, ulcers, bleeding disorders, mild diabetes, or gout, or if she was receiving anticoagulant drugs, she should be alerted to discuss NSAID use with her prescriber. The effect of edema caused by these agents should be considered in individuals with diseases such as heart failure and hypertension. Alcoholic beverages produce a synergistic effect with NSAIDs in causing GI bleeding.

Instruct J.F. that if she omits a scheduled dose, she should not double the next dose but should resume the usual dosing interval. The analgesia provided by NSAIDs is subject to a ceiling effect; higher than recommended dosages will not provide more therapeutic effect in the treatment of pain not associated with inflammation.

Discuss with J.F. the most common adverse effects, which, however, are not always an indication of excessive dosage and should be reported to the prescriber. Inform her that if a skin rash, itching, visual disturbances, edema, persistent headache or heartburn, chest pain, or dark stools occur, she should immediately notify the prescriber. A therapeutic alternative may need to be evaluated.

Some individuals have drowsiness and dizziness and should be cautioned about performing tasks with which the NSAID would interfere. The problem of morning stiffness in affected joints may be overcome by taking the last dose as late as possible in the evening.

Caution J.F. not to use any OTC analgesics concurrently with the NSAID unless the prescriber specifically recommends them. Compliance may be an issue for some NSAIDs because the time until effectiveness is lengthy (e.g., 2 weeks with indomethacin).

Because photosensitivity occurs with diflunisal and ibuprofen, advise clients to avoid the use of sun lamps and prolonged exposure to the sunlight.

Ibuprofen is available without prescription in the 200-mg strength for self-medication. Clients using ibuprofen as an OTC medication should report to their health care provider if their symptoms do not improve, if fever persists for more than 3 days, or if swelling or redness occurs in the painful area.

Evaluation Positive outcomes for NSAID therapy are that J.F. reports increased comfort and increased range of motion and ability to perform activities of daily living. There is decreased or absence of joint swelling, redness, and warmth. J.F. will not experience any untoward effects of NSAID therapy. If a NSAID is administered as an antipyretic, the temperature will be within normal limits.

Other Analgesics

◼✱🄫 acetaminophen [a seet a **min** oh fen]
(Tylenol, Abenol❦, Atasol❦)
Acetaminophen appears to produce its analgesic effect by inhibiting prostaglandin synthesis in the CNS (predominant effect) and peripherally. Although the exact mechanisms of action are unknown, the antiinflammatory effects are minimal. Like the cyclooxygenase inhibitors, acetaminophen also reduces fever via action in the hypothalamus, but is less effective than ibuprofen at reducing fever in children (Perrott, Piira, Goodenough, & Champion, 2004).

Indications
Acetaminophen is indicated for mild to moderate pain and is commonly used in the treatment of fever.

Pharmacokinetics/Dosing
The duration of action of acetaminophen is approximately 4 to 6 hours. It undergoes hepatic metabolism, but at doses above 4 g daily, a hepatotoxic metabolite (acetyliminoquinone) accumulates and can produce hepatic necrosis. The typical adult dose is 650 mg every 4 hours or 1000 mg every 6 hours not to exceed 4 g daily (maximum of 2 g daily if client has a history of alcoholism). Clients may unwittingly ingest more than 4 g daily when using cough/cold or opioid/acetaminophen combination products and should be alerted to the risk for poisoning.

Adverse Effects
Acetaminophen overdose is often fatal secondary to hepatotoxicity and must be treated as a medical emergency (see the Management of Drug Overdose box on p. 275). See Chapter 11 for more detail on acetaminophen. Blood dyscrasias (including hemolytic anemia) and renal dysfunction are rare, but possible consequences of acetaminophen use.

Adjuvant Medications

Adjuvant (coanalgesic) medications are used in combination with other analgesics to enhance pain relief or to treat symptoms that exacerbate pain; in some instances they are used alone to treat specifically identified pain. Adjuvant analgesic medications include a variety of medications such as antiepileptic drugs, antidepressants, antihistamines, corticosteroids, local anesthetics, antidysrhythmics, psychostimulants, clonidine, and capsaicin. Antiepileptic drugs, antidepressants, anesthetics, and occasionally antidysrhythmics are prescribed alone or in combination with opioids for neuropathic pain.

Corticosteroids are beneficial for cancer pain that originates in a fairly restricted area, such as in the intracranial region, alongside a nerve root, or in pelvic, neck, or hepatic areas. Dexamethasone (Decadron) is prescribed for an increase in intracranial pressure and for relief of pain caused by pressure on a nerve. Corticosteroids may also relieve pain by suppressing the release of prostaglandins, thereby inhibiting the inflammatory process.

The antihistamine hydroxyzine (Vistaril) is reported to have some analgesic properties. It also has anxiolytic and sedative effects, which may be useful in some clients. Psychostimulants, such as methylphenidate (Ritalin) and dextroamphetamine (Dexedrine), potentiate opioid analgesia and also help to increase alertness or reduce persistent, opioid-induced sedation in some clients. The analgesic effects are postulated to occur centrally and in the descending spinal inhibitory pathways. Opioid-induced cognitive impairment in clients with cancer or acquired immunodeficiency syndrome (AIDS) has improved with the administration of a psychostimulant drug (Escalante, 2004).

The usual approach to opioid-induced persistent sedation is to reduce the opioid dosage and increase daily drug frequency. The opioid should be switched if the client does not respond appropriately with this method. If the sedation problem persists with these alternative strategies, a psychostimulant may be added to the opioid regimen (AHCPR, 1994).

Additional useful adjuvant analgesics include clonidine (Catapres, epidural Duraclon) and capsaicin. Clonidine is a centrally acting, α_2-adrenergic agonist that has been used for the treatment of pain associated with complex regional pain syndrome (CRPS), diabetic neuropathy, postherpetic neuralgia, spinal cord injury, phantom pain, and pain in cancer clients who are opioid tolerant (Reuben, 2004).

Capsaicin, an alkaloid found in chili peppers, is formulated into a topical cream (Zostrix) that is effective in the treatment of neuralgia, skeletal/muscle, and arthritic pain (Mason, Moore, Derry, Edwards, & McQuay, 2004). On application it causes an initial release and then a depletion of substance P from nerve fibers, which results in a decrease in pain transmission.

Complementary and alternative therapies for specific conditions associated with pain are available with varying evidence to support their use. These include agents to treat osteoarthritis (e.g., glucosamine, chondroitin) and are discussed in Chapter 12.

✱ **J.F. has orders for physical therapy at home and a follow-up appointment with her rheumatologist.**

✱ **What options are available for the rheumatologist to consider in treating rheumatoid arthritis?**
In addition to the drugs discussed above for pain management, other modalities may be used to specifically treat the ongoing inflammatory process of rheumatoid arthritis. Unlike the analgesics, these disease-modifying agents may de-

⚙ Management of Drug Overdose

Acetaminophen (Tylenol)

Assessment

- Symptoms of acetaminophen overdose occur in four phases, can be latent, and may last for up to 14 days.
  - *Phase 1 (2 to 24 hours after ingestion)*: Anorexia, nausea, vomiting, sweating, abdominal pain or cramping, and diarrhea.
  - *Phase 2 (24 to 72 hours after ingestion)*: Symptoms may appear improved. Right upper quadrant pain, hepatomegaly, oliguria or acute tubular necrosis may be present. Modestly elevated liver transaminases and bilirubin levels and elevated prothrombin time may be observed, indicating early hepatic injury.
  - *Phase 3 (72 to 96 hours after ingestion)*: Nausea and vomiting, malaise, jaundice, confusion, somnolence, and even coma may be noted. Dramatic elevations in liver enzymes and prothrombin time may be observed.
  - *Phase 4 (6 to 7 days after ingestion)*: Depending on the amount of acetaminophen ingested and the treatment instituted, resolution of hepatic damage may be noted. Often liver function tests return back toward the normal range. Not all clients have resolution, and fatal hepatic failure may occur in untreated clients.

Treatment

- Activated charcoal is the preferred method for decontamination. Gastric lavage is also employed in some cases.
- Treatment is based on acetaminophen levels 4 hours postingestion. For ingestion of immediate-release formulations of acetaminophen, the Rumack-Matthew nomogram shown at right is typically utilized.
- When hepatotoxicity is possible or likely, sequential doses of acetylcysteine are administered orally every 4 hours for a total of 18 doses. Acetylcysteine interferes with the metabolic process that results in the formation of hepatotoxic metabolite of acetaminophen during overdose. Acetylcysteine is most effective if administered within 8 hours of ingestion, but benefit may be observed if initiated up to 24 hours after ingestion. The dose of acetylcysteine is 140 mg/kg initially (loading dose) followed by 17 doses of 70 mg/kg every 4 hours.

- Acetylcysteine is an orally administered liquid. It is often associated with nausea and vomiting with oral ingestion because of the sulfa-like smell. Adherence can be improved by preparing the drug with juice or a carbonated beverage in a paper cup with a lid and straw to help the client not smell the drug on ingestion. If emesis occurs within the first hour of acetylcysteine administration, the dose should be repeated. It is often administered with antiemetics such as metoclopramide (Reglan) or ondansetron (Zofran).

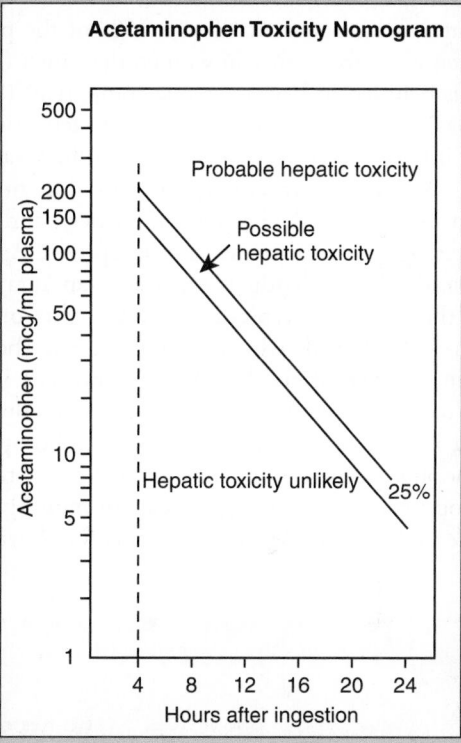

Rumack-Matthew nomogram for predicting hepatotoxicity post ingestion of immediate release formulations of acetaminophen.

Reprinted from Smilkstein MJ, Bronstein, A.C., Linden, C., Augenstein, W.L., Kulig, K.W., & Rumack, B.H. (1991). Acetaminophen overdose: A 48-hour intravenous N-acetylcysteine treatment protocol. *Ann Emerg Med, 20*(10), 1058, with permission from American College of Emergency Physicians.

---

lay the progression of, or even halt or moderately reverse pathology observed in rheumatoid arthritis. Unfortunately, these drugs often have serious adverse effects and their prescribing is typically limited to a rheumatologist. Included in this group are the antimalarial agents (discussed in Chapter 60); gold salts and penicillamine (see Chapter 63); chemotherapeutic agents, such as methotrexate, azathioprine, cyclophosphamide (discussed in Chapter 56); immunosuppressants used in transplantation medicine, such as cyclosporine (discussed in Chapter 63); and the immunologic agents, such as adalimumab (Humira), etanercept (Enbrel), infliximab (Remicade), and leflunomide (Arava), which are also discussed in Chapter 63.

✴ **P.S. is a 26-year-old mother of two who reports severe headaches about twice per month over the last 3 months. Each headache lasts 2 to 4 hours, and typically presents with photophobia (aversion to light), phonophobia (aversion to sound), and nausea. What assessments and treatment options are appropriate?**
Headache is a common malady that is associated with varying degrees of discomfort, may include significant disruption in daily activities or ability to work, and occasionally signals serious underlying illness. Assessment of the symptoms, duration, timing, and triggers are important in establishing headache type and potential for rare but serious pathology, including intracranial tumors, meningitis, in-

tracranial hemorrhage, glaucoma, carbon monoxide poisoning, or hypertension.

The most frequent types of headaches are tension-type, migraine, cluster headache, and headache secondary to medication overuse. Each type of headache responds to different interventions.

Tension-type headaches are the most prevalent type, accounting for up to 80% of headaches. The attacks typically last a few hours and are described as a band-like pressure around the head. They are often triggered by stress. Treatments effective for tension-type headache include the NSAIDs, aspirin, and acetaminophen. Regular exercise also helps. For tension headaches not responsive to these interventions, the use of low doses of tricyclic antidepressants or antiepileptic drugs may be considered.

Migraine affects between 2% and 15% of the population, is seen more frequently in women than men (3:1 ratio), and is believed to have a genetic component (Steiner & Fontebasso, 2002). Migraine involves the activation and release of inflammatory substances that produce vasodilation and plasma extravasation. Triggers for migraine include menses, stress, depression and anxiety, and, occasionally, estrogens or hormonal contraceptives. Approximately one-third of individuals experience an aura in advance of the migraine (typically flashing lights or other change in visual fields), which is observed for about 30 minutes in advance of the headache. Symptoms include moderate to severe pain (which may be unilateral or throbbing) that is often accompanied by nausea, photophobia, and phonophobia. Symptoms may last for hours to days, and may occur on a regular (e.g., weekly or monthly) basis (Steiner & Fontebasso, 2002). Treatments for aborting an existing migraine headache include NSAIDs, acetaminophen, metoclopramide (Reglan) (discussed in Chapter 40), ergot alkaloids (see Chapter 21) and the triptans. Prophylaxis of migraines is typically reserved for clients with a history of frequent migraines over a period of at least 4 to 6 months; prophylactic interventions include β-adrenergic blockers, such as atenolol or propranolol (see Chapter 22), an antiepileptic drug such as valproate (Depakote, Depakene) (see Chapter 17), tricyclic antidepressants (see Chapter 19), and methysergide (see Chapter 22). Even the angiotensin receptor blockers (e.g., candesartan, which is discussed in Chapter 27) may have a role in migraine prophylaxis (Tronvik, Stovner, Helde, Sand, & Bovim, 2003).

The triptans bind to serotonin $(5-HT)_1$ receptors, producing vasoconstriction, which is effective in aborting a migraine headache. The benefits of the triptans in improving acute symptoms of migraine are offset by the risk of their inducing vasospasm or vasoconstriction. As such, these agents are contraindicated for clients with coronary artery disease (e.g., angina, history of myocardial infarction); they are also potentially problematic for individuals with atherosclerosis and hypertension. A strict limit of daily dosing is important to prevent serious vasoconstrictive complications. Dosage adjustment may be required for those with renal or hepatic insufficiency. Sumatriptan represents the prototype drug of the class. Table 14-5 lists the available triptans.

sumatriptan [soo ma **trip** tan]
(Imitrex)
Indications
Sumatriptan is indicated for the acute treatment of migraine headache.

TABLE 14-5 TRIPTANS FOR MIGRAINE HEADACHE

Generic	Brand	Routes of Administration	Adult Dose (normal renal/ hepatic function)	Maximum Daily Dose (per 24 hours)
almotriptan	Axert	Oral	6.25-12.5 mg PO × 1	25 mg PO
eletriptan	Relpax	Oral	20-40 mg PO × 1	80 mg PO
frovatriptan	Frova	Oral	2.5 mg PO × 1	7.5 mg PO
naratriptan	Amerge	Oral	1-2.5 mg PO × 1	5 mg PO
rizatriptan	Maxalt Maxalt MLT	Oral, sublingual	5-10 mg PO/sublingual × 1 (5 mg PO/sublingual if taking β blocker)	30 mg PO/sublingual (15 mg if taking β blocker)
sumatriptan	Imitrex	Oral, subcutaneous, nasal	25-100 mg PO × 1 6 mg subcutaneously × 1 5-20 mg × 1 nasal spray	200 mg PO *or* 12 mg subcutaneously *or* 40 mg nasal spray
zolmitriptan	Zomig Zomig-ZMT Zomig Nasal Spray	Oral, sublingual Nasal	1.25-2.5 mg PO/sublingual × 1 5 mg nasal spray × 1	10 mg PO/sublingual/ nasal

Pharmacokinetics/Dosing

The onset of effect is observed within 30 minutes of the subcutaneous injection of sumatriptan. The typical oral dose is 25 to 100 mg one time with a single repeat dose at 2 hours. Intranasal dose is 5 to 20 mg one time with a single repeat dose in 2 hours if needed. The subcutaneous dose is 6 mg with a single repeat dose after 1 hour if needed. More than two doses by any route over 24 hours is not recommended.

Adverse Effects

The most serious of adverse effects of sumatriptan is myocardial ischemia, chest pain, and risk for MI. Sumatriptan and other agents in the class are contraindicated for clients with coronary heart disease. Other adverse effects include dizziness, flushing, altered taste (especially with the nasal formulation), nausea/vomiting (particularly with nasal form), and tingling.

Cluster headaches are less frequently observed clinically than tension or migraine headaches, affect men more commonly than women (6:1 ratio), and are often triggered by ethanol ingestion. They occur in episodic form with clusters of headaches noted for a period of 6 to 12 weeks, then remitting for a year or two. Cluster headaches consistently present with unilateral intense pain around the eye, and last for 30 to 60 minutes. Typical analgesics are ineffective in the management of cluster headaches. Acute treatments that offer some relief include the triptans and oxygen. Prophylactic uses of verapamil (a calcium channel blocker; see Chapter 27), corticosteroids (see Chapter 48), lithium (see Chapter 19), ergotamine or methysergide (see Chapter 22) have been somewhat effective (Steiner & Fontebasso, 2002).

Medication overuse headaches occur daily or near daily, and affect up to 5% of the population. They are related to habitual use of medications for headache (NSAIDs, ergotamine, triptans) and are much more common in women than men (5:1 ratio) (Steiner & Fontebasso, 2002). Caffeine withdrawal is also a common cause of headache.

✱ **P.S. presents with classic migraine-type headaches, although she does not describe an aura in advance of headaches. Migraine often occurs for P.S. when she is under stress; no other triggers have been identified, and she does not take estrogens or hormonal contraceptives. She has no history of hypertension or cardiac disease. She reports that neither ibuprofen nor acetaminophen has been successful in helping abort her headaches. She appears a likely candidate for triptan therapy, and is started on intranasal sumatriptan.**

✱ **What nursing implications are appropriate for P.S.?**

Assessment Assess P.S. for the following nursing diagnoses for triptan therapy: acute pain (chest pain, difficulty in swallowing; heaviness, tightness, or pressure in chest and/or neck); altered comfort related to irritation in the nose (burning, discharge, pain, or soreness); nausea or vomiting; anxiety; and the sensory/perceptual alteration of taste perversion. Although P.S. is prescribed intranasal sumatriptan and the risk of acute chest pain and associated symptoms are less than 1% for intranasal and oral routes, contrasted to 13% with subcutaneous administration, her situation still requires medical attention.

Planning While using triptan therapy, P.S. will experience less frequent migraines with minimal or no discomfort and without adverse effects. She will effectively manage her therapeutic regimen and will collaborate with her prescriber for monitoring and treatment.

Implementation

Monitoring After her first inhalation, monitor P.S. closely for chest pain for 30 minutes. Instruct her to report to her prescriber if such pain occurs in the future. If the first dose of sumatriptan does not bring relief, additional doses should not be administered. If the first dose is effective, the drug can be used for breakthrough pain and future occurrences.

Education Sumatriptan is not administered until the occurrence of headache pain. For self-administration, instruct P.S. to clear her nasal passages, release the spray into one nostril. Advise P.S. to lie down and relax in a quiet, darkened room after taking her dose to assist in relieving headache pain. Instruct her that the drug is only to be used for migraines, not other types of headaches. Tolerance may be an issue. P.S. is not to use a course of sumatriptan more often than every 5 to 7 days. If P.S. is using the autoinjector rather than the intranasal spray, instruct her on the use and disposal of the unit. Because P.S. is of child-bearing age, alert her that sumatriptan is a Pregnancy Category C drug, as are all the 5-HT$_1$ receptor agonists.

Evaluation The expected outcome of her drug therapy is that P.S. will experience relief from the migraine attack without having any adverse effects. She will effectively manage her triptan theapy (e.g., administering the drug appropriately, using a darkened room as a supportive measure, reporting breakthrough pain and adverse effects).

✱ **How is pain managed in pregnancy, labor, and delivery?**

Most women experience pain during labor. Ideally, the analgesic used should provide pain relief without interfering with labor and also without increasing the risk or danger to the mother or fetus. Currently, there is no ideal analgesic available for use during pregnancy; consequently, the prescriber should carefully choose the analgesic based on the individual and the prevailing conditions.

Opioid analgesics may increase or decrease the time of labor, and the primary concern with their use is neonatal respiratory depression. These agents cross the placenta to enter fetal circulation, and therefore the dose administered to the mother should be sufficient to reduce the pain and discomfort to a level that can be tolerated by the woman but not large enough to cause respiratory depression in either the mother or fetus. Regional anesthesia, epidurals, and spinals, particularly patient-controlled epidural analgesia, is a common practice. The IV route may also be used. In a primigravida (a woman who is pregnant for the first time), the analgesic medication is usually not administered until the contractions occur approximately every 2 to 3 minutes and the cervix is dilated (3 to 4 cm). A multiparous woman might receive the analgesic slightly earlier (Grant, 2004).

Although meperidine is commonly prescribed for pain during pregnancy, "it is not recommended as a first-line opioid for any type of pain, including perinatal pain" (McCaffery & Pasero, 1999). The partial opioid agonists-antagonists (e.g., nalbufene) are sometimes preferred for obstetric analgesia because they are less likely to induce respiratory depression in the newborn. They are contraindicated in clients receiving chronic opioids, however, because they may precipitate acute opioid withdrawal. Morphine and fentanyl are the most commonly prescribed opioids for newborns. Be aware that although morphine causes more sedation and has less risk of causing chest wall rigidity than fentanyl, the pharmacokinetics of morphine are significantly different in the preterm and term neonate. The preterm neonate has a longer elimination half-life than does the term neonate, and a term infant (younger than 4 days old) has an elimination half-life that is seven times higher than that of an older infant. Dosage adjustments are necessary to avoid drug accumulation and toxicity. McCaffery and Pasero (1999) have a guideline chart for health care professionals on morphine and fentanyl infusion rates for preterm, term, and older infants.

Naloxone (Narcan), an opioid antagonist, should be available to treat the mother or neonate if excessive CNS depression occurs. If an opioid is administered to a woman who is nursing, the next scheduled feeding should be 4 to 6 hours after the opioid is administered to minimize the amount of drug passed to the infant.

A second concern with the use of opioids during pregnancy (particularly in women with a history of substance abuse) is that these agents may lead to physical drug dependence in the fetus and cause severe withdrawal reactions in the neonate after birth. Pregnant women enrolled in methadone maintenance programs may present with fetal distress syndrome in utero and often deliver an underweight baby. See the Pregnancy Safety box on p. 251.

✳ What special issues arise in the pain management of children?

Children are often untreated or inadequately treated for pain. They suffer needlessly because of the many myths and misconceptions about pain and pain management in this population. The assessment of pain in a young child is more difficult and should be based on thorough knowledge of the pain-producing procedure or event and a child's nonverbal behavior. Even when children have the ability to verbalize their feelings, they are often reluctant to express pain, fearing the results (diagnostic test, examination, or injection) may be more painful. Young children are unable to make the connection between the immediate pain from the injection and the pain relief experienced later. Their reaction to the injection may interfere with nursing judgment, resulting in no medication and unnecessary pain for the child (Waters, 1992).

The health care provider should consider giving pain medication to an infant or child for the same circumstances for which it would be given to an adult. Even premature neonates demonstrate mature peripheral, spinal, and supraspinal pain transmission by 26 weeks gestation (Berde & Sethna, 2002). Interestingly, breast milk and glucose solutions each have demonstrated analgesic effects in neonates (Bauer, Ketteler, Hellwig, Laurenz, Versmold, 2004; Carbajal, Veerapen, Couderc, Jugie, & Ville, 2003). Holding and positioning also impact on neonatal perceptions of pain (Johnston et al., 2003). In children younger than 2 years of age with observably increased irritability, anorexia, and loss of interest in play and in whom the assessment of whether the problem is "merely" irritability or pain is unclear, the decision to medicate appropriately is justified. Medicating in this instance should lead to a more comfortable, less anxiety-ridden child. In a child older than 2 years of age, the health care provider should know how a child's age and stage of devel-

0   1   2   3   4   5

1. Explain to the child that each face is for a person who has no pain (hurt, or whatever word the child uses) or has some or a lot of pain.

2. Point to the appropriate face and state, "This face is ..."
   0-"very happy because he doesn't hurt at all."
   1-"hurts just a little bit."
   2-"hurts a little more."
   3-"hurts even more."
   4-"hurts a whole lot."
   5-"hurts as much as you can imagine, although you don't have to be crying to feel this bad."

3. Ask the child to choose the face that best describes how much pain he has. Be specific about which pain (e.g., "shot" or incision) and what time (e.g., now? earlier? before lunch?).

FIGURE 14-13 Scale for rating intensity of pain with pediatric clients.

Modified from Wong, D. (2003). *Whaley & Wong's nursing care of infants and children* (7th ed.). St. Louis: Mosby.

opment influences the ability to perceive and communicate the experience. The approach to the child should be individualized, and the child's words and gestures for communication should be used. Figure drawings may help a child to point out "where it hurts." More graphic scales may be used with children to rate the intensity of their pain (Figure 14-13). Assess also for other signs of discomfort, such as restlessness, decreased activity, anorexia, whining, and crying. Consult the parents regarding the child's pain status, because they are most familiar with the child. When in doubt, assume that pain is present and consult with the prescriber for "around-the-clock" pain coverage.

As with adults, pain is best managed if the child is medicated before the pain becomes severe. To decrease the possibility of the child denying pain to avoid an injection, the nurse may administer analgesics by an alternative route. Children find suppositories and liquid formulations more acceptable than injections. Assist the child in associating the medication with pain relief by indicating that it will make him or her "feel better," and then check whether the medication has been effective, reminding the child that he or she probably "feels better" because of the medication.

Local anesthetics are a safe and often effective modality in children. Lidocaine and bupivacaine (see Chapter 15) can be used to provide local or regional pain relief. Topical formulations of lidocaine and prilocaine (EMLA) and tetracaine gel are often applied prior to minor surgical procedures or procedures involving needles.

Peripheral, nonopioid therapies are commonly used as first-line interventions for mild to moderate pain. Appropriately dosed acetaminophen (Tylenol), given orally or rectally, is safe and effective for pain and fever reduction. Ibuprofen (Motrin) is available as an oral tablet or liquid formulation for the same indications, and is rarely associated with adverse GI effects in children (Berde & Sethna, 2002). Avoid giving aspirin and salicylates to children because of the risk of potentially fatal Reye hepatic en-cephalopathy. This syndrome typically presents with nausea, vomiting, rash, and a change in mental status, and is more likely with concurrent varicella, influenzae, or other viral infection (Beers & Berkow, 1999-2003).

Opioid analgesics are indicated in children for the treatment of postoperative pain, pain caused by sickle crisis, and cancer pain. Newborns and infants younger than the age of 6 months may be more likely to develop respiratory depression with opioids, but this can be carefully managed in acute care settings with the concurrent use of pulse oximetry and direct observation (Berde & Sethna, 2002). Patient-controlled analgesia has been used with success in children as young as 6 years of age (Berde & Sethna, 2002). Oral transmucosal fentanyl (Actiq), a lozenge on a stick, may be an appropriate alternative for select children; this formulation bypasses the first-pass metabolic process of fentanyl and results in effective analgesia for short-term procedures.

Guidelines for the administration of medications to children are found in Chapter 7. Table 14-6 lists dosing data for analgesics in children and adolescents.

How does pain management in older adults differ from pain management in other populations?
Approximately half of community-dwelling older adults, and as many as 80% of nursing home residents, are believed to suffer from pain (Horgas, 2003). Sources of this pain include chronic inflammatory states (e.g., rheumatoid and osteoarthritis, peripheral vascular disease), chronic disease (osteoporosis, coronary artery disease), and postsurgical and cancer pain.

Analgesic dosing in older adults usually requires dosage and dosing interval adjustments according to the client's therapeutic response and the development of adverse effects (increased pain, confusion, excessive untoward CNS effects, respiratory depression). Older adults reportedly have enhanced medication responses and may not tolerate side or adverse drug effects as well as younger clients. Older adults

TABLE 14-6 ANALGESIC DOSES IN CHILDREN OLDER THAN 2 YEARS OF AGE

Drug	Parenteral Dose Less Than 60 kg	Parenteral Dose Greater Than or Equal to 60 kg	Oral Dose Less Than 60 kg	Oral Dose Greater Than or Equal to 60 kg
acetaminophen	N/A	N/A	10-15 mg/kg q4h	650-100 mg q4h (not >4000 mg daily)
ibuprofen	N/A	N/A	5-10 mg/kg q6h	400-600 mg q6h
naproxen	N/A	N/A	5-6 mg/kg q12h	250-375 mg q12h
codeine	NR	NR	0.5-1 mg/kg q3-4h	30-60 mg q3-4h
morphine	0.1 mg/kg q2-4h	5-8 mg q2-4h	0.3 mg/kg q3-4h	15-20 mg q3-4h
oxycodone	N/A	N/A	0.1-0.2 mg/kg q3-4h	5-10 mg q3-4h

Modified from Berde, C.B., & Sethna, N.F. (2002). Drug therapy: Analgesics for the treatment of pain in children. *New England Journal of Medicine, 347*(14), 1094-1103.
N/A, not applicable; NR, not recommended.

often have multiple medical problems and may have additional medications prescribed for them (polypharmacy). Thus it is important to carefully assess, evaluate, and closely monitor the older adult to reduce the potential for undertreatment or overtreatment and adverse effects. Pain rating and sedation scale monitoring are the standard approach to titrate dosing of analgesics in all clients, including older adults. Height, weight, and body surface area are not accurate measurements for dosing analgesics in older adults.

Older adults often report pain differently than younger persons, often because of physiologic, psychologic, and cultural differences (AHCPR, 1994). Cognitive impairment, dementia, and confusion may add to the barriers for pain assessment. Because traditional approaches are limited in this population, pain assessment and management require close supervision and the monitoring of daily functioning and quality of life as outcomes. In the past, lower dosages of analgesics were often recommended for older adults, but this approach should not be the rule. Although age is not a significant factor in determining analgesic dosage, it is important in establishing the frequency of drug dosing. Because liver or kidney impairment may reduce drug clearance, less frequent drug dosing may be necessary. Both dosage and drug frequency should be carefully titrated to the individual's response to the analgesic medication. The presence of adverse effects influences drug dosage and drug frequency.

Specific analgesics that are considered inappropriate for use in older adults include propoxyphene (Darvon products), indomethacin (Indocin), pentazocine (Talwin), and meperidine (Demerol) (Chutka, Takahashi, & Hoel, 2004). These agents are more toxic in older adults and much safer analgesics are available. The use of NSAIDs must also be carefully assessed, with close monitoring for GI, renal, and cardiovascular toxicity (Briggs, 2003). The use of standard NSAIDs (e.g., ibuprofen) with concurrent proton pump inhibitors may reduce the risk for gastric or duodenal complications (Chan et al., 2002).

The aging process may also influence the route of analgesic administration. Older adults may have a diminished circulatory process, which results in slower absorption of drugs administered IM or subcutaneously. Administering additional doses in such a situation may result in unpredictable or increased drug absorption, which increases the potential for adverse effects.

Use care in working with older adults who are experiencing pain. Older adults may be less likely to ask for pain medication because they accept pain as a part of old age, do not want to be a "bother," or deny discomfort as a cultural and ethnic issue. Assess nonverbal communication, such as irritability, anorexia, decreased activity, a tendency to cry easily, or object gripping. Decreased activity resulting from pain increases the risk of complications of immobility. The stress of the pain experience leads to fatigue and anxiety and reduces the older adult's diminished physical and psychologic resources. If in doubt, assume pain is present and intervene appropriately. Because an older adult may be taking many drugs concurrently, health care providers should be aware of specific drug interactions with analgesic therapy.

✱ **How does pain management in clients with dependency differ from pain management in other populations?**
Chemical dependency is a common, chronic disease that affects up to 25% of clients seen in primary care practices (Jones, Knutson, & Haines, 2003). In an emergency situation, the immediate need is to relieve a client's pain; this may require greater-than-normal dosages of opioids. An opioid-tapering regimen is instituted within 24 hours after the analgesic dose is stabilized. The first step in this process is opioid consolidation (Reisner & Koo, 2005). A longer-acting opioid analgesic will minimize pain and analgesia fluctuation. One method is to add up a client's total opioid use daily during the last several weeks, if known, and then convert to an equivalent dose of either methadone or sustained release morphine. Or an arbitrary dose of oral methadone, such as 5 mg every 6 hours may be started and all of a client's current analgesics could be discontinued. If this dosage is insufficient, a temporary increase may be necessary. Such clients benefit from a long-term and multidisciplinary approach including behavioral therapy and dosage adjustments. The opioid dose can be decreased approximately 10% every 3 to 5 days without inducing withdrawal symptoms (Reisner & Koo, 2005).

Pain as an Issue of End-of-Life Care

✱ **S.F., an 82-year-old male with advanced prostate cancer and metastasis to the bone, has elected palliative care at home with the home hospice team.**

✱ **How does the approach to pain management for palliative care differ from the approach to pain management for other clients?**
Many physicians and nurses have been educated in the medical and scientific advances or the technologically sophisticated approach to medicine. When these approaches (often referred to as therapeutic techniques) fail to cure or contain an advanced disease stage, health care professionals often abandon, ignore, or pay less attention to an individual with an unfavorable prognosis and no known cure. Such persons are referred to as terminally ill, and their care is primarily palliative, end-of-life care. Despite the well-accepted approach of palliative care, its implementation varies significantly across different regions of North America (Wennberg et al., 2004).

End-of-life care requires an organized approach of palliative and supportive care for dying individuals and their families. The need for a comprehensive, multidisciplinary approach of total care for the dying person evolved in the hospice movement in the United States. Total palliative care has been defined as the provision of medical, nursing, psychosocial, and spiritual services for clients and their families both during illness and during bereavement (Woodruff, 1993).

The following two quotes best describe the key issues involved in caring for these clients:

- In our system, it is easier to get open-heart surgery than Meals on Wheels, easier to get antibiotics than eyeglasses, and certainly easier to get emergency care aimed at rescue than to get sustaining, supportive care (Lynn, 2001).

- Good care of the dying person means making the body as comfortable as possible so that the client can prepare for death mentally and spiritually. It will mean allowing the client to live as fully as possible up until he dies (Favaro, 2002).

End-of-life care must address and expand on these issues.

Physical Issues The physical issues present during the end-of-life stage can be extensive. Some of the most common physical problems include pain, dyspnea, constipation, nausea and vomiting, myoclonus, and delirium. Refractory dyspnea at rest, in particular, is responsive to low-dose morphine, and results in improved comfort, less breathlessness, and improved sleep (Abernethy et al., 2004). The dying person may also experience anorexia and dehydration, which is of greater concern to the family than to the individual. Favaro (2002) states that it is common for clients to stop eating when preparing to die. There is a gradual decrease in eating habits, with meats generally being refused first, then vegetables, then a preference for softer foods, then liquids only. Although this is quite difficult for the family to accept, it should be accepted that it is permissible not to eat.

Because health care professionals should be knowledgeable about the proper use of pharmacology or drug therapy in end-of-life care, this section is devoted to the pharmacologic aspects of palliative care.

Pain Pain is a common symptom identified in persons with cancer, with 20% to 50% reporting pain at the time of diagnosis and approximately 33% reporting pain during therapy (Hammack & Loprinzi, 1994). If left uncontrolled, pain typically causes physical and mental distress that results in disabling of the individual. The impact of uncontrolled pain also has a significant negative effect on friends and family (Riley, 2003). Pain assessment is the most important aspect in developing a treatment plan. The health care provider must be aware that many factors can cause pain and that the key to proper treatment is determination of the cause whenever possible. One should never assume that increased pain always results from advancement of the underlying disease process. Bone fractures, nerve injuries or compression, arthritis or inflammatory pain, or pain secondary to severe constipation may be overlooked and thus improperly treated in this population. Whenever possible, treat the cause of the pain.

The use of analgesics provides many pharmacologic approaches available to treat pain. Treatment should be individualized and, whenever necessary, aggressive. Fear of inducing opioid addiction is of little or no concern.

Be aware that persons unable to report pain may also be in severe pain. When nonverbal pain signs are overlooked, the client will be undertreated. Some nonverbal signs and symptoms of pain may include increased irritability, decreased activity, whining or crying easily, tight gripping of an object, restlessness, anxiety, or favoring (protecting) of a body area. An around-the-clock trial of analgesics for 24 to 48 hours may be considered with an evaluation to see if the signs and symptoms decrease.

Pain Management As illustrated in Figure 14-14, many health care agencies have protocols that use different initial regimens of analgesics based on the client's level of pain. The World Health Organization recommends a three-step approach to pain management (www.who.int/cancer/palliative/painladder/en/) and most facilities use these guidelines. An example of such a guideline is as follows:

PAIN DESCRIPTION	NUMERICAL RATING	THERAPEUTIC RECOMMENDATION
"Mild pain"	1-3/10	Nonopioid analgesic taken on regular schedule, not PRN, such as acetaminophen 1000 mg q6h or ibuprofen 600 mg q6h
"Moderate pain"	4-6/10	Add an opioid, use on a schedule, not PRN, such as acetaminophen 325 mg/codeine 60 mg q4h or acetaminophen 325 mg/oxycodone 5 mg q4h
"Severe pain"	7-10/10	Change to a more potent opioid; administer on a regular schedule, such as morphine 15 mg q4h, morphine controlled release 60 mg q8h, or hydromorphone 4 mg q4h

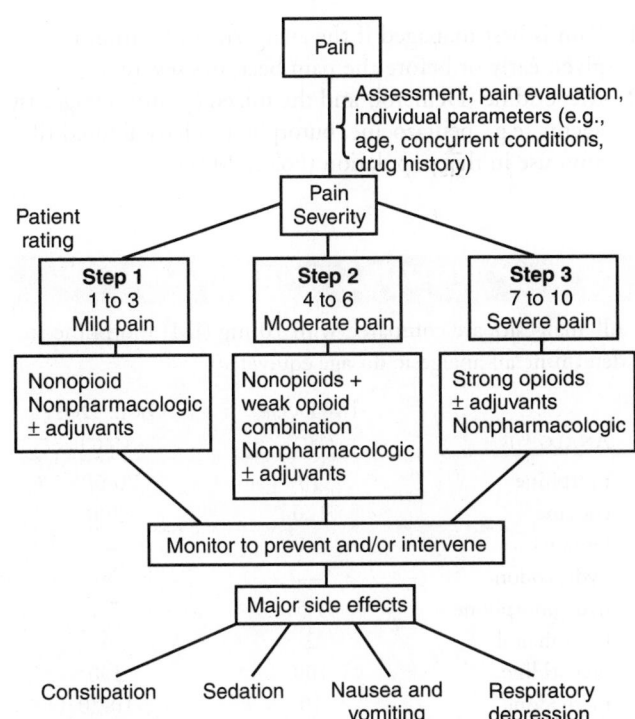

FIGURE 14-14 Sample pharmacologic chart for the management of pain. Although pain and its management are highly individualized, many health care agencies have algorithms or "stepped" approaches for pain management, including the World Health Organization.

From Salerno, E., & Willens, J.S. (1996). *Pain management handbook: An interdisciplinary approach.* St. Louis: Mosby.

Adjuvant analgesics are also added based on client need; these include antidepressants for neuropathic pain, antiepileptic drugs for neuropathic, lancinating, or tic-like pain; glucocorticoids or steroids for tumor-related pain or tumor infiltration in nerve or bone; and local anesthetics for neuropathic pain not responsive to antidepressants or antiepileptic drugs.

Drug Selection The selection of an analgesic depends on the level of the client's pain. The proper drug may be selected with the use of a pain scale (0 [no pain] to 10 [severe pain]). When a sustained-release dosage form is used around-the-clock, a shorter-acting analgesic (whenever possible, the same analgesic) should also be prescribed for breakthrough pain. Frequent use (twice daily or more) of the rescue drug indicates the need to increase the dose of the long-acting around-the-clock opioid with a continuance of the immediate release analgesic on a PRN basis. The calculated rescue dose is often 5% to 15% of the total daily dose of the sustained-release analgesic administered every 2 to 4 hours as necessary (Favaro, 2002).

Opioid Analgesic Equivalency All analgesics are compared with 10 mg IM of morphine to determine an analgesic dosage equivalent. Equianalgesic information (i.e., the dose of one drug that produces approximately the same analgesic effect as the dose of another drug) is very useful information for the health care provider (Box 14-4).

Analgesic Tips for Palliative Care

1. Pain is best managed if the analgesic medication is given early or before the pain becomes severe.
2. Meperidine (Demerol) and the mixed agonist-antagonist agents (e.g., pentazocine, butorphanol) have limited (if any) use in this population (Foley, 2001).

3. Nonpharmacologic approaches (e.g., relaxation exercises, imagery, biofeedback, music therapy) and adjuvant drugs are used in conjunction with the opioid analgesics. These techniques and medications can be very helpful.
4. Myoclonus (muscle spasms, tremors, jerking of extremities) first requires an assessment for underlying causes (e.g., renal or hepatic failure, hyponatremia, hypercalcemia, hypoxia). It may also be induced by high-dose opioids, which may require the prescriber to switch to a different opioid analgesic. The addition of a benzodiazepine such as clonazepam (Klonopin) may also be helpful (Collins & Cheong, 2001).
5. The following interventions may be considered for severe dyspnea (Foley, 2001):
   a. Place the client in an upright position and leaning forward, with the arms supported by a bed table *or*
   b. Use oxygen in hypoxemic individuals *or*
   c. Use small doses of oral or IV morphine *or*
   d. In some instances, a benzodiazepine also may be helpful
6. Children and older adults are often untreated or inadequately treated for pain. Pain assessment and management requires close supervision and monitoring.
7. Information regarding pain management is changing every day. See the Technology Link box below for online sites to consult frequently.

BOX 14-4 ANALGESIC EQUIVALENCY CHART

All analgesics are compared with 10 mg (IM) morphine to determine an analgesic dosage equivalent.

ANALGESIC	IM DOSE (MG)	ORAL DOSE (MG)
morphine	10	20-60*
codeine	120	200
fentanyl	0.1	—
hydrocodone	—	30
hydromorphone	1.5	7.5
levorphanol	2	4
meperidine	100	300
methadone	10	10-20
oxycodone	20	30
oxymorphone	1	—

Modified from American Pain Society. (2003). *Principles of analgesic use in the treatment of acute pain and cancer pain* (5th ed.). Glenview, IL: American Pain Society.

*For a single dose or intermittent use. Chronic administration may decrease oral dose to 30 mg equivalent.

Technology Link

Analgesics

American Chronic Pain Association (www.theacpa.org)

A support system that provides education and self-help group activities for persons with chronic pain.

American Pain Foundation (www.painfoundation.org)

This is an online resource for people with pain, their families, friends, caregivers, and the general public. This site is devoted to client information and advocacy, and provides many links to additional resources.

American Pain Society (www.ampainsoc.org)

This organization's site provides current information on standards, policies, and research related to pain management.

Mayo Clinic (www.mayohealth.org)

This site offers a wide variety of medical information. A pain management search on this site provides a long list of articles on pain.

National Hospice and Palliative Care Organization (www.nhpco.org)

This organization is devoted to improving end-of-life care. The site provides information on hospices in the United States, educational and conference programs, and more.

Additional Drugs Used in End-Of-Life Care In addition to pain management, many other conditions may require medications within an end-of-life context. The majority of the following agents are discussed elsewhere in this text. Box 14-5 presents examples of drugs commonly used within an end-of-life context. The nurse should be aware that drug dosages may range widely depending on the client's condition, stage of disease, and individual requirements (Collins & Cheong, 2001; Foley, 2001).

Summary

Pain continues to be a worldwide health problem. It disables and distresses more people than any other symptom and is the most common reason for seeking health care.

Few things that a nurse does are more important than alleviating pain. The attitudes, fears, and biases of clients, families, and caregivers contribute to the unnecessary undertreatment of pain. The nurse must have the skill and knowledge to assess accurately and to intervene effectively in the relief of the pain of the clients in the nurse's care.

Morphine and other opioid agonists were the earliest medications used for pain relief and are still among the more effective. However, the nurse needs to be alert to the toxic symptoms resulting from inappropriate use of these analgesics. Naloxone, nalmefene, and naltrexone are opioid antagonists used for the reversal of opioid toxicity. Opioid agonist-antagonists are also used for pain relief.

NSAIDs are used to treat the signs and symptoms of inflammation, fever, and pain. Since the mid-1970s these as-

---

BOX 14-5 SUPPORTIVE DRUGS COMMONLY USED IN END-OF-LIFE CARE

These drugs do not, in and of themselves, provide analgesia. Instead they are useful in addition to analgesics in managing comorbid presentations commonly seen with pain or adverse effects associated with analgesic regimens.

ANXIETY

- hydroxyzine* (Atarax, Vistaril) 25 mg three times daily
- lorazepam (Ativan) 0.5-1 mg three times daily

ORAL *CANDIDA*

- clotrimazole (Mycelex) one troche 5 times daily for 2 weeks
- fluconazole (Diflucan) 200 mg PO × 1 then 100 mg daily
- nystatin (Mycostatin) suspension 4-6 mL, or troches, four times daily

CONSTIPATION

Stool Softeners

- docusate (Colace, Surfak) 100 mg one to three times daily

Stimulant Laxatives

- senna or sennosides (Senokot) 2-4 tablets once or twice daily
- bisacodyl (Dulcolax) 5 mg 1-3 tablets daily
- See Chapter 11 for additional laxatives. The reader should also be aware that clients receiving large doses of opioid analgesics may require larger dosages of laxatives than listed.

DEPRESSION

- citalopram (Celexa) 20-40 mg once daily
- fluoxetine (Prozac) 20-40 mg once daily
- sertraline (Zoloft) 50-150 mg once daily
- If sleep disturbance is significant with depression, then amitriptyline* (Elavil) 50-150 mg at bedtime *or* doxepin* (Sinequan) 50-150 mg at bedtime *or* trazodone (Desyrel) 50 mg at bedtime; lower doses of tricyclic antidepressants may be used for neuropathic pain.

DIARRHEA

- diphenoxylate* (Lomotil) 5 mg four times daily
- loperamide (Imodium) 2-4-mg dose according to package insert

SLEEP DISTURBANCE

- Many anxiolytic benzodiazepines are effective hypnotic agents. When a client is receiving a benzodiazepine such as lorazepam during the day and a hypnotic drug is necessary, an equivalent dose of the same drug may be considered. For example, 1 mg of lorazepam is considered to be approximately equivalent to 15 mg flurazepam (Dalmane) or 15 mg temazepam (Restoril). Refer to Chapter 16 for additional information.

MUSCLE SPASMS

- baclofen (Lioresal) 5-20 mg three times daily
- diazepam (Valium) 5 mg three times daily
- tizanidine (Zanaflex) 4-8 mg three times daily

NAUSEA, VOMITING, AND OTHER GASTROINTESTINAL DISTURBANCES

- dicyclomine* (Bentyl) 20 mg four times daily
- meclizine* (Antivert, Bonine) 25 mg four times daily
- metoclopramide (Reglan) 10 mg four times daily
- prochlorperazine (Compazine) 5-10 mg four times daily
- promethazine (Phenergan) 25 mg three times daily
- scopolamine* 0.4 mg PO as ordered or scopolamine* transdermal patch applied behind ear every 3 days (often used to dry excessive pulmonary secretions)

PEPTIC ULCERS/GASTROESOPHAGEAL REFLUX

- omeprazole (Prilosec) 20 mg at bedtime
- famotidine (Pepcid) 20 mg at bedtime
- metoclopramide (Reglan) 10 mg four times daily

*Agents with potentially significant and additive antimuscarinic/anticholinergic properties.

pirin substitutes have become quite popular for the treatment of mild to moderate pain and for the antiinflammatory treatment of arthritis. Although widely available, these agents are not without adverse GI, hepatic, and renal effects. The COX-2 inhibitors have reduced gastrointestinal risk, but renal and possible cardiovascular risks persist with these agents.

Disease-modifying drugs used in the treatment of arthritis, are much slower acting and much more toxic than the NSAIDs. Specific therapies targeted at headache, particularly the triptans, often pose cardiovascular risks, requiring that their use be carefully assessed and limited.

The approach to end-of-life care, like other pain-relieving strategies, requires clear assessment and planning. The primary focus is on comfort for the client. It involves an aggressive, multisymptom management approach with drug and nondrug strategies to alleviate physical, emotional, and spiritual discomfort.

✴ Critical Thinking Questions

- Tyrone Scali, age 42 years, comes to the emergency department after a fall while playing tennis, and is diagnosed with a sprained ankle. The health care provider wraps Mr. Scali's ankle with an elastic bandage and advises him to elevate the ankle and keep it at rest. He is given a prescription for aspirin 650 mg PO every 4 hours PRN for pain. Before instructing the client about aspirin therapy, you review his health history, looking for what data that might contraindicate the use of aspirin?

- Sarah Smith, age 53 years, has just returned to the general surgical unit from the postanesthesia care unit following thyroidectomy. Her surgeon has prescribed morphine sulfate 2 to 4 mg IV every 2 hours PRN for postoperative pain. She requests pain medication for "a stabbing pain" in her throat. What assessments are critical before administering the analgesic?

- Robert Staysa, age 85 years, has osteoarthritis that is causing pain in his back, hips, and knees. His physician prescribes ibuprofen 400 mg PO four times daily. Why would ibuprofen be prescribed rather than a low-dose opioid analgesic? Given his age, the client is most at risk for what adverse effect of NSAID therapy?

Bibliography

Abernethy, A.P., Currow, D.C., Frith, P., Fazekas, B.S., McHugh, A. & Bui, C. (2003). Randomised, double blind, placebo controlled crossover trial of sustained release morphine for the management of refractory dyspnea. *British Medical Journal, 327,* 523-526.

Ackley, B.J. & Ladwig, G.B. (2006). *Nursing diagnosis handbook* (7th ed.). St. Louis: Mosby.

Agency for Health Care Policy and Research (AHCPR), Public Health Service. (1994). *Clinical practice guideline: Management of cancer pain.* Rockville, MD: Department of Health and Human Services.

American Hospital Formulary Service. (2004). *AHFS: Drug information '04.* Bethesda, MD: American Society of Hospital Pharmacists.

American Pain Society. (2003). *Principles of analgesic use in the treatment of acute pain and cancer pain* (5th ed.). Glenview, IL: American Pain Society.

Anderson, D.M., Keith, J., & Novak, P.D. (Eds.). (2002). *Mosby's medical, nursing, and allied health dictionary* (6th ed.). St. Louis: Mosby.

Ardery, G., Herr, K., Hannon, B.J. & Titler, M.G. (2003). Lack of opioid administration in older hip fracture patients. *Geriatric Nursing, 24*(6), 353-360.

Aubrun F., Langeron, O., Quesnel, C., Coriat, P., & Riou, B. (2003). Relationships between measurement of pain using visual analog score and morphine requirements during postoperative intravenous morphine titration. *Anesthesiology, 98*(6), 1415-1421.

Backonja, M. (2003). Defining neuropathic pain. *Anesthesia & Analgesia, 97*(3), 785-790.

Bajwa, Z.H. & Warfield, C.A. (2004). Pharmacologic therapy of cancer pain. In B.D. Rose (Ed.). Wellesley, MA: UpToDate.

Barkin, R.L., & Buvanendran, A. (2004). Focus on the COX-1 and COX-2 agents: Renal events of nonsteroidal and anti-inflammatory drugs—NSAIDs. *American Journal of Therapeutics, 11*(2), 124-129.

Bauer, K., Ketteler, J., Hellwig, M., Laurenz, M. & Versmold, H. (2004). Oral glucose before venipuncture relieves neonates of pain, but stress is still evidenced by increase in oxygen consumption, energy expenditure, and heart rate. *Pediatric Research, 55*(4), 695-700.

Baumann, T.J. (2002). Pain management. In J.T. DiPiro, R.L. Talbert, G.C. Yee, G.R. Matzke, B.G. Wells, & L.M. Posey (Eds.), *Pharmacotherapy: A pathophysiologic approach* (5th ed.). New York: McGraw-Hill.

Beers M.H., & Berkow R. (1999-2003). *The Merck manual of diagnosis and therapy* (17th ed.). Retrieved November 9, 2003, from: http://www.merck.com/mrkshared/mmanual/home.jsp

Berardi, R.R., & Montgomery, P.A. (2002). Pancreatitis. In J.T. DiPiro, R.L. Talbert, G.C. Yee, G.R. Matzke, B.G. Wells, & L.M. Posey (Eds.), *Pharmacotherapy: A pathophysiologic approach* (5th ed.). New York: McGraw-Hill.

e-LEARNING SUPPLEMENTS

Student CD-ROM
- Final Exam questions
- NCLEX® Examination review questions
- Pharmacology animations
- Printable chapter summary

Evolve Website (http://evolve.elsevier.com/mckenry)
- Case study on analgesics
- Content updates, including information on new drugs
- WebLinks corresponding to this chapter
- Answers to the critical thinking questions in this chapter
- *Elsevier ePharmacology Update* newsletter
- Mosby's Drug Consult Internet Edition
- Supplemental and reference information

Berde, C.B., & Sethna, N.F. (2002). Drug therapy: Analgesics for the treatment of pain in children. *New England Journal of Medicine, 347*(14), 1094-1103.

Bombardier, C., Laine, L., Reicin, A., Shapiro, D., Burgos-Vargas, R., Davis, B., et al.: VIGOR Study Group. (2000). Comparison of upper gastrointestinal toxicity of rofecoxib and naproxen in patients with rheumatoid arthritis. *New England Journal of Medicine, 343,* 1520-1528.

Bookman, A.A., Williams, K.S., Shainhouse, J.Z. (2004). Effect of a topical diclofenac solution for relieving symptoms of primary osteoarthritis of the knee: A randomized controlled trial. *Canadian Medical Association Journal, 171,* 333-338.

Bostrum, B., Sandh, M., Lundberg, D., & Fridlund, B. (2004). Cancer-related pain in palliative care: Patients' perceptions of pain management. *Journal of Advanced Nursing, 45*(4), 410-419.

Boureau F., Schneid, H., Zeghari, N., Wall, R., & Bourgeois, P. (2004). The IPSO study: Ibuprofen, paracetamol study in osteoarthritis. A randomised comparative clinical study comparing the efficacy and safety of ibuprofen and paracetamol analgesic treatment of osteoarthritis of the knee or hip. *Annals of the Rheumatic Diseases, 63*(9), 1028-1034.

Briggs, E. (2003). The nursing management of pain in older people. *Nursing Standard, 17*(18), 47-55.

Bruera, E., & Kim, H.N. (2003). Cancer pain. *Journal of American Medical Association, 290,* 2476-2479.

Carbajal, R., Veerapen, S., Couderc, S., Jugie, M., & Ville, Y. (2003). Analgesic effect of breastfeeding in term neonates: Randomised controlled trial. *British Medical Journal, 326,* 13-15.

Chan, F.K., Hung, L.C., Suen, B.Y., Wu, J.C., Lee, K.C., Leung, V.K., et al. (2002). Celecoxib versus diclofenac and omeprazole in reducing the risk of recurrent ulcer bleeding in patients with arthritis. *New England Journal of Medicine, 347,* 2104-2110.

Chutka, D.S., Takahashi, P.Y., & Hoel, R.W. (2004). Inappropriate medications for elderly patients. *Mayo Clinic Proceedings, 79*(1), 122-139.

Cleeland, C.S., Gonin, R., Hatfield, A.K., Edmonson, J.H., Blum, R.H., Stewart, J.A., et al. (1994). Pain and its treatment in outpatients with metastatic cancer. *New England Journal of Medicine, 330,* 592-596.

Collins, P. & Cheong, S. (2001). *Improving care at end of life: Essential issues, self-study.* Miami: Baptist Health Systems of South Florida.

Court, M.H., Duan, S.X., von Moltke, L.L., Greenblatt, D.J., Patten, C.J., Miners, J.O., et al. (2001). Interindividual variability in acetaminophen glucuronidation by human liver microsomes: Identification of relevant acetaminophen UDP-glucuronosyltransferase isoforms. *Journal of Pharmacology & Experimental Therapeutics, 299*(3), 998-1006.

Drayer, R.A., Henderson, J., & Reidenberg, M. (1999). Barriers to better pain control in hospitalized patients. *Journal of Pain & Symptom Management, 17*(6), 434-440.

Drug Facts and Comparisons. (58th ed.). (2005). St. Louis: Facts and Comparisons.

Eichelbaum, M. (2003). In search of endogenous CYP 2D6 substrates. *Pharmacogenetics, 13*(6), 305-306.

Escalante, C.P. (2004). Cancer-related fatigue: Assessment and treatment. In B.D. Rose (Ed.). Wellesley, MA: UpToDate.

Favaro, M.K.A. (2002). *Pharmacology: An introductory text* (9th ed.). Philadelphia: W.B. Saunders.

FDA Alert for Healthcare Professionals: Valdecoxib. (2005, April 7). Retrieved May 1, 2005 from http://www.fda.gov/cder/drug/InfoSheets/HCP/valdecoxibHCP.pdf.

FDA News. (2004, September 30). *FDA issues public health advisory on Vioxx as its manufacturer voluntarily withdraws the product* (P04-95). Retrieved November 13, 2004, from http://www.fda.gov/bbs/topics/news/2004/NEW01122.html.

FDA Statement on Naproxen. (2004, December 20). Retrieved May 1, 2005, from http://www.fda.gov/bbs/topics/news/2004/NEW01148.html.

Fischer, L.M., Schlienger, R.G., Matter, C.M., Jick, H., & Meier, C.R. (2004). Discontinuation of nonsteroidal anti-inflammatory drug therapy and risk of acute myocardial infarction. *Archives of Internal Medicine, 164,* 2472-2476.

FitzGerald, G.A. (2004). Coxibs and cardiovascular disease. *New England Journal of Medicine, 351,* 1709-1711.

Flores, DL, Alvarado, I., Wong, M.L., Licinio, J., Flockhart, D. (2004). Clinical implications of genetic polymorphism of CYP2 D6 in Mexican Americans. *Annals of Internal Medicine, 140*(11), 939.

Foley, K. (2001). Pain and symptom control in the dying ICU patient. In J.R. Curtis & G.D. Rubenfeld (Eds.), *Managing death in the ICU.* London: Oxford University Press.

Gajraj, N.M. (2003). Cyclooxygenase-2 inhibitors. *Anesthesia & Analgesia, 96*(6), 1720-1738.

Garcia Rodriguez, L.A., & Hernandez-Diaz, S. (2001). Relative risk of upper gastrointestinal complications among users of acetaminophen and nonsteroidal anti-inflammatory drugs. Epidemiology, 12, 570–576.

Gilson, A.M., & Joranson, D.E. (2001). Controlled substances and pain management: Changes in knowledge and attitudes of state medical regulators, *Journal of Pain and Symptom Management, 21*(3), 227-237.

Grant, G.J. (2004). Management of pain during labor and delivery. In B.D. Rose (Ed.). Wellesley, MA: UpToDate.

Green, C.R., Baker, T.A., & Ndao-Brumblay, S.K. (2004). Patient attitudes regarding healthcare utilization and referral: A descriptive comparison in African- and Caucasian Americans with chronic pain. *Journal of the National Medical Association, 96*(1), 31-42.

Green, C.R., Baker, T.A., Sato, Y., Washington, T.L., & Smith, E.M. (2003a). Race and chronic pain: A comparative study of young black and white Americans presenting for management. *Journal of Pain, 4*(4), 176-183.

Green, C.R., Baker, T.A., Smith, E.M. & Sato, Y. (2003b). The effect of race in older adults presenting for chronic pain management: A comparative study of black and white Americans. *Journal of Pain, 4*(2), 82-90.

Green, C.R., Wheeler, J.R., & LaPorte, F. (2003). Clinical decision making in pain management: Contributions of physician and patient characteristics to variations in practice, *Journal of Pain, 4*(1), 29-39.

Gu, X., & Belgrade, M.J. (1993). Pain in hospitalized patients with medical illness. *Journal of Pain and Symptom Management, 8*(1), 17-21.

Hammack, J.E., & Loprinzi, C.L. (1994). Use of orally administered opioids for cancer-related pain. *Mayo Clinic Proceedings, 69,* 384-390.

Hawkey, C.J., & Langman, M.J.S. (2003). Non-steroidal anti-inflammatory drugs: Overall risks and management. Complementary roles for COX-2 inhibitors and proton pump inhibitors. *Gut, 52*(4), 600-608.

Hepner, D., & Castells, M.C. (2003). Anaphylaxis during the perioperative period. *Anesthesia & Analgesia, 97*(5), 1381-1395.

Holdcroft, A., & Power, I. (2003). Management of pain. *British Medical Journal, 326*(7390), 635-639.

Holdgate, A., & Pollock, T. (2004). Systematic review of the relative efficacy of non-steroidal anti-inflammatory drugs and opioids in the treatment of acute renal colic. *British Medical Journal, 328,* 1401-1404.

Horgas, A.L. (2003). Pain management in elderly adults. *Journal of Infusion Nursing, 26*(3), 161-165.

Johnston, C.C., Stevens, B., Pinelli, J., Gibbins, S., Filion, F., Jack, A., et al. (2003). Kangaroo care is effective in diminishing pain response in preterm neonates. *Archives of Pediatric & Adolescent Medicine, 157,* 1084-1088.

Jones, E.M., Knutson, D., & Haines, D. (2003). Common problems in patients recovering from chemical dependency. *American Family Physician, 68*(10), 1971-1978.

Juni, P., Nartey, L., Reichenbach, S., Sterchi, R., Dieppe, P.A., Egger, M. (2004). Risk of cardiovascular events and rofecoxib: Cumulative meta-analysis. *Lancet, 364,* 2021-2029.

Kirchheiner, J., Stormer, E., Meisel, C., Steinbach, N., Roots, I., Brockmoller, J. (2003). Influence of CYP2 C9 genetic polymorphisms on pharmacokinetics of celecoxib and its metabolites. *Pharmacogenetics, 13*(8), 473-480.

Lacy, C.F., Armstrong, L.L., Goldman, M.P., & Lance, L.L. (2004). *Lexi-Comp's drug information handbook* (12th ed.). Hudson, OH: Lexi-Comp.

Lin, J., Zhang, W., Jones, A., & Doherty, M. (2004). Efficacy of topical non-steroidal anti-inflammatory drugs in the treatment of osteoarthritis: Meta-analysis of randomised controlled trials. *British Medical Journal, 329,* 324-326.

Lotsch, J., Skarke, G., Grosch, S., Darimont, J., Schmidt, H., & Geisslinger, G. (2002). The polymorphism A118 G of the human mu-opioid receptor gene decreases the pupil constrictory effect of morphine-6-glucuronide but not that of morphine. *Pharmacogenetics, 12*(1), 3-9.

Lynn, J. (2001). Travels in the valley of the shadow. In P. Collins & S. Cheong (Eds.), *Improving care at end of life: Essential issues, self-study.* Miami: Baptist Health Systems of South Florida.

Mamdani, M., Juurlink, D.N., Lee, D.S., Rochon, P.A., Kopp, A., Naglie, G., et al. (2004). Cyclo-oxygenase-2 inhibitors versus non-selective non-steroidal anti-inflammatory drugs and congestive heart failure outcomes in elderly patients: A population-based cohort study. *Lancet, 363,* 1751-1756.

Mason, L., Moore, R.A., Derry, S., Edwards, J.E., & McQuay, H.J. (2004). Systematic review of topical capsaicin for the treatment of chronic pain. *British Medical Journal, 328,* 991-994.

McCaffery, M., & Ferrell, B. (1992). Pain control discussion, *Nursing 22*(8), 48.

McCaffery, M., & Pasero, C. (1999). *Pain: Clinical manual for nursing practice* (2nd ed.). St. Louis: Mosby.

McDonnell, A., Nicholl, J., & Read, S.M. (2003). Acute pain teams and the management of postoperative pain: A systematic review and meta-analysis. *Journal of Advanced Nursing, 41*(3), 261-273.

Melzack, R., & Wall, P.D. (1965). Pain mechanisms: A new theory. *Science, 150,* 971-979.

Mosby's drug consult. (15th ed.). (2005). St. Louis: Mosby.

North American Nursing Diagnosis Association (NANDA). (2005). *Nursing diagnoses: Definitions & classification 2005-2006.* Philadelphia: Author.

Offerhaus, L. (Ed.). (1997). *Drugs for the elderly* (2nd ed.). Copenhagen: World Health Organization Regional Office for Europe.

Peat, S. (1995). Providing pain relief for the surgical patient. *Care of Critical Illness, 11*(1), 16-19.

Perrott, D.A., Piira, T., Goodenough, B. & Champion, G.D. (2004). Efficacy and safety of acetaminophen vs ibuprofen for treating children's pain or fever: A meta-analysis. *Archives of Pediatric & Adolescent Medicine, 158,* 521-526.

Rabow, M.W., & Pantilat, S.Z. (2003). Care at the end of life. In L.M. Tierney, Jr., S.J. McPhee, & M.A. Papadakis (Eds.), *Current medical diagnosis & treatment.* (42nd ed.) New York: Lange Medical Books/McGraw-Hill.

Reisman, T., & Pasternak, G. (2001). Opioid analgesics and antagonists. In J.G. Hardman & L.E. Limbird (Eds.), *Goodman & Gilman's the pharmacological basis of therapeutics* (10th ed.). New York: McGraw-Hill.

Reisner, L., & Koo, P.J.S. (2005). Pain and its management. In M.A. Koda-Kimble, L.Y. Young, W.A. Kradjan, B.J. Guglielmo, B.K. Alldredge, & R.L. Corelli. (Eds.), *Applied therapeutics: The clinical use of drugs* (8th ed.). Philadephia: Lippincott Williams & Wilkins.

Reuben, S.S. (2004). Preventing the development of complex regional pain syndrome after surgery. *Anesthesiology, 101*(5), 1215-1224.

Rhudy, J.L., & Meagher, M.W. (2001).The role of emotion in pain modulation. *Current Opinion in Psychiatry, 14*(3), 241-245.

Riley, J. (2003). Freedom from pain goes a long way to a "good death." *British Medical Journal, 327*(7408), 235.

Roberts, L.J., & Morrow, J.D. (2001). Analgesic-antipyretic and antiinflammatory agents and drugs employed in the treatment of gout. In J.G. Hardman & L.E. Limbird (Eds.), *Goodman & Gilman's the pharmacological basis of therapeutics* (10th ed.). New York: McGraw-Hill.

Salerno, E. & Willens, J.S. (1996). *Pain management handbook.* St. Louis: Mosby.

Schwartzman, R.J., Grothusen, J., Kiefer, T.R., & Rohr, P. (2001). Neuropathic central pain: Epidemiology, etiology, and treatment options. *Archives of Neurology, 58*(10), 1547-1550.

Sessler, C.N., Gosnell, M.S., Grap, M.J., Brophy, G.M., O'Neal, P.V., Keene, K.A., et al. (2002). The Richmond Agitation-Sedation Scale: Validity and reliability in adult intensive care unit. *American Journal of Respiratory and Critical Care Medicine, 1666,* 1335-1344.

Simon, L.S., Weaver, A.L., Graham, D.Y., Kivitz, A.J., Lipsky, P.E., Hubbard, R.C., et al. (1999). Anti-inflammatory and upper gastrointestinal effects of celecoxib in rheumatoid arthritis: A randomized control trial. *Journal of the American Medical Association, 282*(20), 1921-1928.

Skarke, C., Langer, M., Jarrar, M., Schmidt, H., Geisslinger, G., Lotsch, J. (2004). Probenecid interacts with the pharmacokinetics of morphine-6-glucuronide in humans. *Anesthesiology, 101*(6), 1394-1399.

Skilton, M.D. (2003). Post-operative pain management in day surgery. *Nursing Standard, 17*(38), 39-44.

Sloan, P.A., Montgomery, C., & Musick, D. (1998). Medical student knowledge of morphine for the management of pain. *Journal of Pain & Symptom Management, 15*(6), 359-364.

Steiner, T.J., & Fontebasso, M. (2002). Headache. *British Medical Journal, 325*(7369), 881-886.

Thomas, S.H., Silen, W., Cheema, F., Reisner, A., Aman, S., Goldstein, J.N., et al. (2003). Effects of morphine analgesia on diagnostic accuracy in emergency department patients with abdominal pain: A prospective, randomized trial. *Journal of the American College of Surgeons, 196,* 18-31.

Tronvik, E., Stovner, L.J., Helde, G., Sand, T., & Bovim, G. (2003). Prophylactic treatment of migraine with an angiotensin II receptor blocker: A randomized controlled trial. *Journal of the American Medical Association, 289,* 65-69.

USP DI: Drug information for the health care professional (25th ed.). (2005). Greenwood Village, CO: MICROMEDEX Thomson Healthcare.

University of Michigan Health System. (2004). Pain management: Staff development & education. Part 4: Acute pain management staff education. Retrieved February 15, 2004, from www.med.umich.edu/pain/apainmgt.htm

Warfield, C.A., & Bajwa, Z.H. (Eds.). (2004). *Principles and practice of pain management* (2nd ed.). New York: McGraw-Hill.

Waters, L. (1992). Pharmacologic strategies for managing pain in children. *Orthopedic Nursing, 11*(1), 34.

Weinshilboum, R. (2003). Genomic medicine: Inheritance and drug response. *New England Journal of Medicine, 348*(6), 529-537.

Weisse, C.S., Sorum, P.C., & Dominguez, R.E. (2003). The influence of gender and race on physicians' pain management decisions. *Journal of Pain, 4*(9), 505-510.

Weissman, D.E., & Haddox, J.D. (1989). Opioid pseudoaddiction: An iatrogenic syndrome. *Pain, 36*(3), 363-366.

Welk, T.A. (1991). An educational model for explaining hospice services. *American Journal of Hospice Palliative Care, 8*(5), 14-17.

Wennberg, J.E., Fisher, E.S., Stukel, T.A., Skinner, J.S., Sharp, S.M. & Bronner, K.K. (2004). Use of hospitals, physician visits, and hospice care during last six months of life among cohorts loyal to highly respected hospitals in the United States. *British Medical Journal, 328,* 607-610.

Woodruff, R. (1993). *Palliative medicine.* Melbourne, Australia: Asperula.

15

ANESTHETICS

CHAPTER FOCUS

Advances in modern surgical technique would not be possible without the developments that have occurred in anesthesia. These agents protect the client from the trauma of surgical pain and provide the surgeon the time and exposure to the surgical field necessary to accomplish sophisticated procedures. Nursing during the perioperative period involves three distinct phases: preoperative, intraoperative, and postoperative. Although the care the nurse provides in each of these phases varies in its approach, the ultimate goal is the safety and well-being of the client.

LEARNING OBJECTIVES

- Describe common general anesthetic agents.
- Identify the significant physiologic changes observable in a client at each stage of anesthesia.
- List the common drugs that interact with anesthetic agents and the possible result of concomitant use.
- Identify disease and risk factors that can alter a client's response to anesthesia.
- Describe nursing measures to prevent or treat common postoperative complications.
- Explain the use and adverse effects of local anesthetics.
- Apply the nursing process to a client receiving general or local anesthetic agents.

▲ KEY TERMS

balanced anesthesia, p. 289
caudal anesthesia, p. 305
conduction (block) anesthesia, p. 305
conscious sedation, p. 294
dissociative anesthesia, p. 295
general anesthesia, p. 288
infiltration anesthesia, p. 304
local anesthesia, p. 288

neuroleptanalgesia, p. 296
regional anesthesia, p. 288
saddle block, p. 305
spinal anesthesia, p. 305

✳ KEY DRUGS

halothane, p. 291
ketamine, p. 295
lidocaine, p. 303
thiopental sodium, p. 294

✳ What are anesthetics?

Anesthetics are central nervous system (CNS) depressants used to induce a loss of sensation, especially the sensation of pain. There are two major categories of anesthesia: general and regional/local. **General anesthesia** induces a state of unconsciousness and varying amounts of analgesia, amnesia, muscle relaxation, and loss of reflexes (sensory and autonomic). This state is achieved with intravenous (IV) or inhalation routes of drug administration. The use of general anesthesia typically requires the health care team to provide respiratory support throughout the duration of general anesthetic action.

Regional or local anesthesia blocks pain sensations in specific areas of the body without loss of consciousness. In general, the effect of regional anesthesia is related to the target nerve and its distribution in the body, whereas local anesthesia is a blockade of the nerves in the infiltrated tissues. Local anesthesia may be achieved topically or by setting up a field block in an area that encircles the surgical field (infiltration anesthesia). Spinal, epidural, caudal, and nerve block anesthesia have been referred to as both regional and local anesthesia.

This chapter first examines general anesthetics, how they work, their role in clients undergoing invasive procedures, and issues pertinent to nursing care of clients receiving such agents. Next, the role of local anesthetics and nursing implications for these modalities are discussed.

How do general anesthetics work?

General anesthesia is the absence of sensation and consciousness and is induced by inhalation or IV injection of various anesthetic agents. It is an important mode of therapy, especially for surgical procedures. A general anesthetic alters the CNS to produce varying degrees of analgesia, depression of consciousness, amnesia, skeletal muscle relaxation, and reflex reduction.

At concentrations that produce anesthesia, general anesthetics affect all excitable tissues of the body. They vary widely in their individual effects and in the concentration necessary for each to produce a given state of anesthesia. Although many theories of anesthesia have been proposed, none satisfactorily explains the basic mechanisms of action. Indeed, different anesthetics may have different modes of action, and no single theory may suffice.

The pattern of depression is similar for all general anesthetics—irregular and descending. Initially, an anesthetic produces a loss of the perception of sight, touch, taste, smell, awareness, and hearing. Unconsciousness is usually produced. The medullary centers are depressed last, which is fortunate because these are the vital centers concerned with heart action, blood pressure, and respiration. The two classes of general anesthetics are inhalation anesthetics (gases or volatile liquids) and IV agents.

A combination of drugs is necessary to produce all of the desired effects sought with anesthesia. Analgesia, muscle relaxation, unconsciousness, and amnesic effects are not produced safely by a single anesthetic. **Balanced anesthesia** involves the induction of anesthesia with a combination of drugs, each for its own specific effect, rather than with a single drug that has multiple effects. For example, anesthesia may be induced by premedicating with a short-acting barbiturate or benzodiazepine, and then with an opioid analgesic and a neuromuscular blocker, followed by an anesthetic gas administered by the anesthetist. The specific drugs and dosages depend on the procedure being performed and the client's physical condition and response to the medications. The advantage of balanced anesthesia is a lower reported incidence of postoperative nausea, vomiting, and pain.

What are the stages of anesthesia?

General anesthesia generally consists of four stages, which vary with the choice of anesthetic, speed of induction, and skill of the anesthetist. Not all stages occur with all anesthetics. The current practice of administering an IV anesthetic before administering an inhalation anesthetic promotes rapid transition from consciousness to surgical anesthesia, and the early stages of anesthesia are not seen. However, if the drug is given slowly enough, all stages are usually observed. All stages are most easily seen when an inhalation anesthetic is used as the only anesthetic. Signs of anesthesia, first described by John Snow in the mid-1800s and later outlined as four stages by Guedel in the 1920s, are presented in Table 15-1 and described in the following

TABLE 15-1 GUEDEL'S STAGES OF ANESTHESIA

Stage	Alternative Nomenclature	Key Features	Nursing Management
Stage 1: Analgesia	Induction	Analgesia/numbness Loss of senses Auditory/visual hallucinations	Maintain tranquil environment
Stage 2: Excitement		Exaggerated reflexes Client may struggle Periods of apnea Vomiting or incontinence may occur Reduced with use of balanced anesthesia	Maintain airway Protect against aspiration
Stage 3: Surgical Anesthesia	Plane 1	Eye movement stops	Maintain airway Protect against aspiration
	Plane 2	Partial intercostal paralysis Divergent pupil dilation	
	Plane 3	Complete intercostal paralysis	
	Plane 4	Diaphragmatic paralysis	
Stage 4: Medullary Paralysis	Toxicity	Respiratory arrest Vasomotor collapse	Resuscitation

paragraphs. Although these stages are still used to this day, not every individual follows these stages precisely (Evers & Crowder, 2001).

Stage 1: Analgesia This stage begins with the onset of anesthetic administration and lasts until loss of consciousness. Smell and pain are abolished before consciousness is lost. The client may experience vivid dreams and auditory or visual hallucinations. Speech becomes difficult and indistinct. Numbness spreads gradually over the body, and the body feels stiff and unmanageable. Hearing is the last sense lost.

Before the anesthetic is administered, restraining straps are put in place and the client is covered for warmth and modesty. The nurse ensures a quiet and tranquil environment because even low voices and equipment sounds may be interpreted as excessively loud and may be counterproductive to the anesthetic for the client.

Stage 2: Excitement During this stage, reflexes are still present and may be exaggerated, particularly with sensory stimulation such as noise. A client may struggle, shout, laugh, swear, or sing. Autonomic activity, muscle tone, eye movement, and rapid and irregular breathing increase. Irregular respirations may cause uneven absorption of the anesthetic; a period of apnea followed by a few deep breaths may produce a high concentration of anesthetic in the blood. Vomiting and incontinence sometimes occur in this stage. The client should not be stimulated, or touched, during this stage except for safety reasons.

Stage 2 varies greatly with individuals and depends on (1) the amount and type of premedication, (2) the anesthetic agent used, and (3) the degree of external sensory stimuli. Since the advent of balanced anesthesia, the signs and duration of this stage have been reduced. Stages 1 and 2 constitute the stage of induction.

Stage 3: Surgical Anesthesia This stage is divided into four planes of increasing depth of anesthesia. The character of the respirations, eyeball movement, pupil size, and the degree to which reflexes are present determine the plane the client is experiencing. As a client moves into plane one, the respiratory irregularities of the second stage usually disappear and respirations become full and regular. Respiration becomes shallower and more rapid as anesthesia deepens. Increased abdominal breathing follows paralysis of the intercostal muscles; finally, only the diaphragm is active. A loss of reflexes occurs in a cephalocaudal direction—from the head downward. The eyelid reflex is lost and the eyeballs, which initially exhibit a rolling movement, gradually move less and then cease to move. If the pupils were reflexively dilated in the second stage, they normally now constrict to their approximate size in natural sleep; their reaction to light becomes sluggish. The pupils dilate as plane 4 is approached.

The client's face is calm and expressionless and may be flushed or even cyanotic. The musculature becomes increasingly relaxed as the reflexes are progressively abolished. Most abdominal surgery cannot be performed until the abdominal reflexes are absent and the abdominal wall is soft. Body temperature is lowered as the anesthetic state contin-

ues. The pulse remains full and strong. Blood pressure may be elevated slightly, but in plane four the blood pressure drops and the pulse weakens. The skin, which was warm, now becomes cold, wet, and pale.

Most surgical procedures are performed in plane two or in the upper part of plane three. The anesthetist closely monitors each phase of anesthesia and gives approval to begin the procedure when the client has reached the appropriate plane for surgery. This approval is obtained before preparing the skin, surgically draping the client, and proceeding with surgery.

Stage 4: Medullary Paralysis (Toxic Stage) This stage is characterized by respiratory arrest and vasomotor collapse. Respiration ceases before the heart action. This stage may be reversed by reducing the gaseous agent to lighten the anesthetic state.

Within the operating room, the nurse is part of the surgical team in providing resuscitative measures; the necessary drugs, equipment, and supplies; and other assistance as necessary.

✵ What are inhaled anesthetics?

Inhalation, or volatile, anesthetics are gases or liquids that can be administered by inhalation when mixed with oxygen. These can effect a concentration in the blood and brain to depress the CNS and cause anesthesia. Inhalation anesthetics have the following characteristics:

- They are complete anesthetics and thus can abolish superficial and deep reflexes.
- They provide for controllable anesthesia, because depth of anesthesia is easily varied by changing the inhaled concentration.
- Allergic reactions to these agents are uncommon.
- Rapid recovery can occur as soon as administration ceases because the anesthetic is excreted in expired air.

✵ Which inhaled anesthetics are used clinically?

Ether and chloroform (as volatile liquids) and cyclopropane and nitrous oxide (as gases) were commonly used over the years, but only nitrous oxide is clinically still in use today. Chloroform is hepatotoxic, and ether and cyclopropane are highly flammable; these agents have been replaced by safer anesthetics. In 1956, halothane (Fluothane), a nonflammable agent, largely replaced the older volatile liquids. However, halothane is associated with hepatic dysfunction and failure. Since then, newer, less toxic, volatile liquids have been developed: desflurane (Suprane), enflurane (Ethrane), isoflurane (Forane), methoxyflurane (Penthrane), and sevoflurane (Ultane).

Gases

nitrous oxide [**nye** trus **ok** syde]
Indications
Nitrous oxide, an anesthetic gas, is the most commonly used agent for analgesia during dental surgery, minor surgery, and obstetric procedures. It is often combined with other anesthetics to enhance its effects and is used extensively in major surgery.

Pharmacokinetics/Dosing

Nitrous oxide is excreted 100% unchanged through the lungs. For general anesthesia, the recommended dose is 70% with 30% oxygen inhalation for induction, and 30% to 70% with oxygen for maintenance.

Adverse Effects

Nitrous oxide administration may result in postoperative nausea, vomiting, or delirium. The gas has no known significant drug interactions. At the termination of anesthesia, the rapid movement of large amounts of nitrous oxide from the circulation into the lungs may dilute the oxygen in the lungs. This dilution may result in a phenomenon known as diffusion hypoxia. To prevent this, the anesthetist usually administers 100% oxygen to clear nitrous oxide from the lungs. During recovery the nurse administers humidified oxygen by mask and encourages the client to breathe deeply to promote ventilation.

Volatile Liquid Anesthetics

✶▀▔ halothane [hal uh thayn]
(Fluothane)
Indications
Halothane is used primarily as a general anesthetic.

Pharmacokinetics/Dosing

Table 15-2 details the pharmacokinetics of halothane.

Adverse Effects

Postoperative nausea and vomiting may occur in many clients and may be more common if nitrous oxide is used to supplement other anesthetics. A rare complication of halothane is liver damage (halothane hepatitis). Although the mechanism is not known, some experts believe the liver damage to be caused by a hypersensitivity-type reaction to a metabolite of halothane. The diagnosis is made on the clinical findings of unexplained fever, eosinophilia, rashes, and abnormal liver function tests within 2 weeks of exposure, especially after a repeat exposure. The syndrome is more common in older or obese clients and is not seen in children. See Table 15-2 for more detail.

Drug Interactions

Halothane is the only volatile anesthetic agent that sensitizes the myocardium to the effects of catecholamines (epinephrine, norepinephrine, or dopamine) or sympathomimetic agents (e.g., ephedrine, metaraminol). These agents may produce serious cardiac dysrhythmias in the presence of halothane. Levodopa, a drug used in the treatment of Parkinson's disease and which pharmacologically increases the quantity of dopamine in the CNS, should be discontinued at least 6 to 8 hours before halothane is administered.

TABLE 15-2 VOLATILE LIQUID ANESTHETIC AGENTS

| Agent | Pharmacokinetics | | | MAC (%) | Toxicity | Adverse Effects |
	Absorption	Metabolism	Excretion			
halothane (Fluothane)	By lungs	~20% by liver	~80% unchanged by lungs; remainder via kidneys as halothane or metabolite	0.75	Risk of halothane hepatitis (see text)	↓BP Cardiovascular depression ↓Body temperature ↓Respirations Malignant hyperthermia Emergence delirium: shivering, trembling, confusion, hallucinations, nervousness, excitability
desflurane (Suprane)		<0.2% by liver	Lungs	7.3	Airway irritation Severe laryngospasm Cough	
enflurane (Ethrane)		~2.5% by liver	~80% unchanged by lungs; remainder via kidneys as enflurane or metabolite	1.68		
isoflurane (Forane)		<1% by liver	Lungs	1.15		
methoxyflurane (Penthrane)		~50% by liver	~35% unchanged by lungs; remainder via kidney as methoxyflurane and metabolites	0.16	Nephrotoxicity (dose-related secondary to metabolite)	
sevoflurane (Ultane)			Lungs	2.1	Bradycardia, hypotension	

BP, Blood pressure; *MAC*, minimum alveolar concentration (percent in oxygen) that prevents movement in 50% of clients exposed to painful stimuli. May need higher concentration in some clients.

desflurane [des **floo** rayn]

(Suprane)
Released in the early 1990s, desflurane is an alternative to halothane and isoflurane. It produces a more rapid induction of and emergence from anesthesia than other volatile gases.

Indications
See halothane.

Pharmacokinetics/Dosing
See Table 15-2.

Adverse Effects
The use of desflurane has been associated with a moderately high incidence of airway irritation, coughing, and laryngospasm. For this reason it is not indicated for anesthesia induction in children, although it is approved for anesthesia maintenance in infants and young children.

enflurane [en **floo** rayn]

(Ethrane)

Indications
Enflurane is indicated for the induction and maintenance of general anesthesia.

Pharmacokinetics/Dosing
It is only slightly metabolized in the body. Its clinical effects are similar to those of halothane, but it is less potent.

Adverse Effects
Enflurane may cause seizures when given at high concentrations; therefore it is not recommended for use with clients who are seizure prone, such as those with epilepsy or head injuries. Also see Table 15-2.

isoflurane [eye soe **floo** rayn]

(Forane)

Indications
Isoflurane is indicated for the induction and maintenance of general anesthesia.

Pharmacokinetics/Dosing
Isoflurane undergoes an extremely low degree of metabolism. Until the release of desflurane, isoflurane was promoted as having a more rapid action than the other inhalation agents and causing less cardiovascular depression.

Adverse Effects
See Table 15-2.

methoxyflurane [me thox i **floo** rayn]

(Penthrane)

Indications
Methoxyflurane is used for anesthesia and analgesic effects and is a potent anesthetic agent used for obstetric analgesia.

Pharmacokinetics/Dosing
Methoxyflurane is given in concentrations of 0.3% to 0.8%. Methoxyflurane is highly metabolized; a by-product of its metabolism is free fluoride, which is toxic to the kidney (nephrotoxic). Because of the potential for dose-related nephrotoxicity with methoxyflurane, its use is limited to minor surgical procedures and obstetrics, where lower doses are effective.

Adverse Effects
Nephrotoxicity as described above. Also see Table 15-2.

sevoflurane [sev oh **floo** rayn]

(Ultane)

Indications
Sevoflurane is an inhalation general anesthetic indicated for induction and maintenance during surgery.

Pharmacokinetics/Dosing
The induction dose is individualized, but the usual adult inhalation dose is from 0.5% to 3% when administered alone or combined with nitrous oxide. Sevoflurane was released in 1995 and has a faster uptake, distribution, and rate of elimination than isoflurane and halothane. When compared with desflurane, it has a slower uptake and distribution but a similar rate of elimination.

Adverse Effects
Bradycardia and hypotension are dose-related effects of sevoflurane. Also see Table 15-2.

✺ What alternatives to inhaled agents are available for general anesthesia?

A number of intravenously administered anesthetic agents are available for the induction or maintenance of general anesthesia, for the induction of amnesia, and as an adjunct to inhalation-type anesthetics. They are seldom used alone for anesthesia except for short procedures such as electroconvulsive therapy (ECT), cast application or removal, and hypnosis. The major groups of IV anesthetic agents include ultrashort-acting barbiturates, the benzodiazepines, short-acting opioids, and other short-acting agents that are not represented in these three classes. IV anesthetics reduce the amount of inhalation anesthetic required, making them valuable in allaying emotional distress in those clients who dread having a tight mask placed over their face while they are fully conscious. Box 15-1 lists the advantages and disadvantages of IV anesthetics. Table 15-3 compares the commonly used intravenously administered anesthetics.

Ultrashort-Acting Barbiturates

These agents are among the most commonly used IV anesthetics. They are very-fast-acting CNS depressants that produce hypnosis and anesthesia without analgesia, control seizures, and are commonly used with other agents in a balanced anesthesia regimen.

Their exact mechanism of action for anesthesia, antiseizure effects, or the reduction of intracranial pressure (an

BOX 15-1 ADVANTAGES AND DISADVANTAGES OF INTRAVENOUS ANESTHETICS	
ADVANTAGES	DISADVANTAGES
Rapid induction of unconsciousness	Swelling, pain, ulceration, tissue sloughing, and necrosis if drug infiltrates tissue
Amnesia	Thrombosis and gangrene if arterial injection
Prompt recovery with minimal doses	Hypotension, laryngospasm, respiratory failure from overdose or prolonged administration
Simplicity of administration	
No irritation of mucous membranes	
No hazard of fire or explosion	
Less occupational exposure	

TABLE 15-3 INTRAVENOUSLY ADMINISTERED GENERAL ANESTHETICS

Agent	Typical Adult Dose Range for Induction*	Onset	Duration	Adverse Effects
BARBITURATE				
thiopental sodium (Pentothal)	3-5 mg/kg	30-60 sec	5-30 min	Respiratory depression Bradycardia Hypotension Paradoxical excitation Confusion Pain at injection site
BENZODIAZEPINE				
midazolam (Versed)	0.5-2 mg slow IV over 2-3 min	1-5 min	Variable, 30 min to 2+ hr	Respiratory depression Hypotension Paradoxical excitation Confusion Pain at injection site
diazepam (Valium)	2-10 mg slow IV over 2-3 min	1-10 min	Variable, with more pronounced "hangover"	
lorazepam (Ativan)	1-4 mg slow IV over 2-5 min	1-10 min	Variable	
OPIOID				
alfentanil (Alfenta)	0.5-75 mcg/kg	Almost immediate	30-60 min	Respiratory depression Bradycardia Hypotension Paradoxical excitation Confusion Nausea/vomiting
fentanyl (Sublimaze)	0.5-50 mcg/kg	Almost immediate	30-60 min	
remifentanil (Ultiva)	0.5-1 mcg/kg	1-3 min	Variable	
sufentanil (Sufenta)	1-30 mcg/kg	1-3 min	Variable	
GENERAL ANESTHETIC				
etomidate (Amidate)	0.2-0.6 mg/kg over 30-60 sec	1 min	3-5 min	Nausea/vomiting Pain at injection site Muscle/eye movements
propofol (Diprivan)	0.5-2.5 mg/kg over 10-60 sec	10-50 sec	3-10 min	Apnea Hypotension Pain at injection site Anaphylaxis
DISSOCIATIVE ANESTHETIC				
ketamine (Ketalar)	1-2 mg/kg	1-2 min	5-15 min	Hypertension Tachycardia ↑ Intracranial pressure Hallucinations Muscle movements Abuse potential

Modified from Lacy, C.F., et al. (2004). *Lexi-Comp's drug information handbook* (12 th ed.). Hudson, OH: Lexi-Comp.
*Dose varies widely based on degree of anesthesia desired and if other concurrent CNS depressants administered. Doses for conscious sedation may be below this range. Use of general anesthesia requires respiratory support.

indication for thiopental) is unknown, but several theories have been proposed. General anesthesia with ultrashort-acting barbiturates is believed to result from suppression of the reticular activating system.

✱ thiopental sodium [thye oh **pen** tal]
(Pentothal)

Indications

Intravenous general anesthesia.

Pharmacokinetics/Dosing

Barbiturates are distributed rapidly throughout the body and across the blood-brain barrier because of their high lipid solubility. The onset of action for these barbiturates is generally rapid (20 to 60 seconds). When administered as a single moderate dose, the duration of action is short because of a rapid redistribution of the drug from the brain to fat deposits in the body (e.g., 5 to 30 minutes). While the elimination half-life is moderately long at 3 to 12 hours, this is not predictive of duration of action with single doses because the duration of action is related to redistribution of drug in and out of the CNS. Multiple doses or continuous infusion of these ultrashort-acting barbiturates may result in saturation of the drug in fat deposits, and, ultimately, a slow rate of drug release and prolonged duration of action. Barbiturates are extensively metabolized in the liver and excreted by the kidneys. Doses vary for the induction of general anesthesia and the resultant duration of action. Thiopental is individually dosed according to the client's response.

Adverse Effects

The most common adverse effects during the recovery period are shivering and trembling. Nausea, vomiting, prolonged somnolence, and headache are less commonly reported. Serious effects reactions include emergence delirium (increased excitability, confusion, and hallucinations), cardiac dysrhythmias (tachycardia, bradycardia, or myo-cardial depression), allergic response (bronchospasm, rash, hives, hypotension, and edema of eyelids, lips, or face), respiratory depression, and thrombophlebitis.

Careful assessment and close monitoring are required when IV barbiturates are used in combination with other CNS depressants, which may result in enhanced depression effects, as well as with diuretics, antihypertensive agents, and calcium-blocking drugs, because hypotension may occur.

methohexital sodium [meth oh **hex** i tal]
(Brevital)

Indications

Similar to thiopental.

Pharmacokinetics/Dosing

Similar to thiopental. Methohexital requires 1 to 2 mg/kg for induction and has a duration of action of 5 to 7 minutes.

Adverse Effects

Similar to thiopental.

Benzodiazepines

Benzodiazepines are most often used for conscious sedation where full anesthesia is not required such as during endoscopy, or as a premedication or adjunct in balanced anesthesia. **Conscious sedation** provides analgesia, relieves anxiety, and/or provides amnesia following the administration of a CNS depressant drug and/or analgesic. Benzodiazepines have multiple pharmacologic properties, including sedation, anxiolysis, antiseizure, and modest skeletal muscle relaxation, via their action at specific benzodiazepine receptors. Unlike opioids, however, benzodiazepines do not possess analgesic properties; therefore concurrent analgesics (usually opioids) are often used. Midazolam causes a decrease in cerebrospinal fluid (CSF) pressure

and thus may be selected for anesthesia induction in clients with intracranial lesions. These agents also induce amnesia at higher doses. This is an advantage for clients who are undergoing painful or uncomfortable procedures because it diminishes recall of traumatic events while under the influence of the agent. A common intravenously administered benzodiazepine is midazolam, which is presented in the following monograph. Diazepam and lorazepam, both used intravenously as part of anesthesia, are presented in Chapter 16. The mechanism of action and other uses of benzodiazepines are more fully discussed in Chapters 16 and 17.

midazolam [**mid** ay zoe lam]
(Versed)

Indications

Midazolam is indicated for preoperative and conscious sedation, intensive care unit (ICU) sedation and as an adjunct to general anesthesia.

Pharmacokinetics/Dosing

Benzodiazepines differ primarily in their water/lipid solubility, and in their onset and duration of action. Compared with the barbiturates, benzodiazepines have a slower onset of CNS effects and a more prolonged postanesthetic recovery period. Midazolam is water soluble and is less irritating at the injection site; midazolam becomes more lipid soluble in the body and readily crosses the blood-brain barrier. Midazolam has a rapid onset and short duration of action. Midazolam is metabolized in the liver and produces pharmacologically active metabolites.

Adverse Effects

To prevent excessive apnea, these agents are administered slowly (e.g., IV over 2 to 3 minutes). The concurrent use of benzodiazepines with alcohol or CNS depressants may result in hypotension, respiratory depression, or respiratory and cardiac arrest. A reduction in drug dosage and close monitoring are indicated if such drugs are used concurrently. Debilitated clients and those 55 years and older require a smaller than normal midazolam dose administered at a slower rate (*USP DI*, 2005). If CNS depressants are used concurrently, the midazolam dose is reduced by at least 50%.

Short-Acting Opioids Used in General Anesthesia

Fentanyl and short-acting derivatives of fentanyl (sufentanil [Sufenta], alfentanil [Alfenta], remifentanil [Ultiva]) are commonly used as adjuncts to general anesthesia. The role of topical fentanyl in the treatment of chronic pain is presented in Chapter 14.

fentanyl [**fen** ta nil]
(Sublimaze)

Indications

Fentanyl is a rapid-acting opioid used as adjunct medication for balanced anesthesia. They are commonly used with other general anesthetics (including the inhaled agents) for optimal induction and maintenance of anesthesia.

Pharmacokinetics/Dosing

Information on the dosage and administration of these drugs appears in Table 15-3. Fentanyl crosses the blood-brain barrier and is rapidly distributed to various tissues. It is highly protein bound and has a triphasic half-life, that is, a distributive phase, a redistributive phase, and an elimination phase. It is metabolized in the liver and excreted by the kidneys.

Adverse Effects

The effects and adverse effects of fentanyl and related agents are discussed in depth in Chapter 14. The most commonly reported adverse effects when fentanyl is used as an adjunct to anesthesia are drowsiness, hypotension, bradycardia, and respiratory depression (allergic reaction). Less common reactions are chills, nausea, vomiting, increased weakness, dizziness, constipation, depression, pruritus, muscle spasms, and increased excitability (paradoxical reaction). Rarely, chest wall rigidity has been reported with rapid IV administration. Seizures have also been reported.

Other Short-Acting General Anesthetics

etomidate [eh **toe** mi date]
(Amidate)
Indications
Etomidate is a short-acting, nonbarbiturate hypnotic used for the induction of general anesthesia. It is reported to decrease the activity of the reticular formation in the brainstem in animals. Because it has minimal cardiac and respiratory effects, it may be advantageous for the client with impaired cardiac function, respiratory function, or both. Etomidate is used intravenously for induction of general anesthesia and also supplements subpotent anesthetic agents (nitrous oxide in oxygen) for short procedures.

Pharmacokinetics/Dosing
Etomidate induces hypnosis within 1 minute and has a duration of action between 3 and 5 minutes. To reduce recovery time in adults, a 0.1 mg IV dose of fentanyl (Sublimaze) is often administered 1 or 2 minutes before anesthesia induction, thus reducing the amount of etomidate needed. Etomidate is metabolized in the liver and excreted by the kidneys.

Adverse Effects
The adverse effects most commonly reported during the recovery period are nausea and vomiting, hypotension, hypertension, and dysrhythmias. Breathing difficulties are reported less often. Involuntary muscle movements have been reported, especially when fentanyl is not given before induction with etomidate. Pain at the injection site is also reported. A client is monitored for enhanced CNS depression when etomidate is given with other CNS depressants. *Special warning*: Etomidate can suppress the production of steroid hormones in the adrenal gland (e.g., cortisol), which can result in temporary gland failure. Electrolyte imbalance, hypotension, and shock may result. Seriously ill or postoperative clients may need adrenal cortex supplementation.

propofol [**proe** poe fol]
(Diprivan)
Indications
Propofol is a rapidly acting, nonbarbiturate hypnotic used for the induction and maintenance of general anesthesia. It is also used for ICU sedation.

Pharmacokinetics/Dosing
It has a rapid onset of action (within 40 seconds), and the duration of effect is only 3 to 5 minutes. Its redistribution from the brain to other body tissues explains the short effect. The elimination half-life is 3 to 12 hours. Because of the fat solubility of propofol, it is available as an emulsion in soybean fat. As with other emulsions, it should not be used if the components of the emulsion have separated. This preservative-free, milky looking product is capable of supporting rapid bacterial growth; strict sterile technique and immediate use following drug preparation is essential to prevent administration of a contaminated product.

Adverse Effects
Propofol is a respiratory depressant and may produce apnea and cardiac depression depending on the dose, rate of administration, and concurrent drugs administered. Bradycardia and hypotension may also occur frequently. Nausea, vomiting, and involuntary muscle movement are commonly reported.

★▀▀ ketamine hydrochloride [**keet** a meen]
(Ketalar)
Ketamine is a rapid-acting nonbarbiturate IV anesthetic and is often referred to as a dissociative anesthetic. It is a derivative of phencyclidine, a psychotomimetic drug of abuse. As with the barbiturates, keta-mine acts on the midbrain within the reticular formation. It produces analgesia and amnesia, but not muscular relaxation. The mechanism of action is not fully known. Ketamine blocks the afferent transmission of impulses associated with the affective-emotional aspect of pain perception, and it may also suppress spinal cord activity. Ketamine produces a **dissociative anesthesia**, an anesthesia characterized by analgesia and amnesia without the loss of respiratory function or pharyngeal and laryngeal reflexes. It produces a cataleptic state in which the client appears to be awake but is detached from his or her environment and is unresponsive to pain. The client's eyelids usually do not close; nystagmus (rapid, involuntary oscillation of the eyeballs) is common, and slight involuntary and purposeless movements may occur.

Because ketamine increases the secretions of the salivary and bronchial glands, the administration of an anticholinergic agent (e.g., atropine) may be necessary. Ketamine may increase blood pressure, muscle tone, and heart rate. Respirations are usually not depressed. After recovery, the client has no recall of events that occurred while under the influence of ketamine.

Indications
Ketamine is best suited for short diagnostic or surgical procedures that do not require skeletal muscle relaxation. It is also used to induce anesthesia before the administration of general anesthetics and as an adjunct to low-potency anesthetics, such as nitrous oxide.

Pharmacokinetics/Dosing
When ketamine is given intravenously, the onset of anesthesia occurs within 30 seconds. When administered intramuscularly, the onset of action occurs within 3 to 4 minutes. The duration of action is 5 to 10 minutes for an IV dose of 2 mg/kg body weight or 12 to 25 minutes for an intramuscular (IM) dose of 10 mg/kg body weight. Ketamine is metabolized in the liver. Termination of anesthetic action occurs with redistribution from the CNS and liver biotransformation. Ninety percent is excreted in the kidneys. The recommended adult dose for anesthesia induction is 1 to 2 mg/kg body weight IV or 5 to 10 mg/kg body weight IM. The recommended rate for maintenance is 10 to 50 g/kg body weight by infusion at a rate of 1 to 2 g/min. As with any anesthetic, the dosage needs to be carefully assessed and individualized.

Adverse Effects
The most commonly reported adverse effects of ketamine include hypertension and increased pulse rate and an emergence reaction, such as a distortion in body image, delirium, explicit dreams, illusions, and dissociative-type experiences. Flashbacks of vivid dreams with or without illusions may occur weeks later in some clients. Because of these effects, ketamine should be avoided in anyone with a history of mental health problems. Less commonly reported adverse effects include hypotension, bradycardia, respiratory depression, and vomiting. No significant drug interactions have been reported.

In recent years, ketamine has become a common drug of abuse. Street names for the drug include "Special K," "Vitamin K," and "K." Its use is popular because of the dissociative effects experienced by individuals under its influence. Unfortunately, abusers unaware of the degree of anesthesia or the nature of the drug effect may unwittingly experience respiratory arrest, deep levels of anesthesia or coma, or alarming dissociative reactions without adequate support. See Chapter 9 for a further discussion of this use of ketamine as well as its use as a predatory drug.

dexmedetomidine [deks med e **toe** mi deen]
(Precedex)
Dexmedetomidine is a selective α_2-adrenergic receptor agonist with sedative and hypotensive properties. Agents affecting the adrenergic nervous system are more fully discussed in Chapter 22.

Indications
Dexmedetomidine is indicated for sedation in intubated and mechanically ventilated clients who are being managed in an ICU setting. Use should not extend beyond 24 hours.

Pharmacokinetics/Dosing
Given IV, dexmedetomidine produces rapid sedative and hypotensive action. It is metabolized by cytochrome P450 2A6, primarily in the liver, and has a short half-life of 6 minutes.

Adverse Effects

Because of significant potential for hypotension and cardiac dysrhythmias, dexmedetomidine use is limited to the settings where continuous cardiovascular, respiratory and CNS monitoring can be maintained.

Other Drugs

droperidol [droe **per** i dole]
(Inapsine)

Droperidol is a dopamine-blocking drug with sedative, tranquilizing, and antiemetic properties, and a prolonged duration of action. It is chemically similar to haloperidol (Haldol) and discussed in greater depth in Chapter 19. Droperidol has historically been used with other drugs to produce neuroleptanalgesia, a state characterized by quiet, reduced motor activity and anxiety, indifference to surroundings, and the ability to respond to commands. The risk for prolonged QT interval and cardiac dysrhythmias with droperidol has greatly reduced this practice.

Indications

Droperidol is used as an antiemetic and as an adjunct to anesthesia. Because of its potential to produce life-threatening ventricular dysrhythmias, its use is limited to circumstances when other therapies are not effective.

Pharmacokinetics/Dosing

The typical dose of droperidol is 0.625 to 2.5 mg IV or 2.5 mg IM. The onset of action for droperidol, when given either IV or IM, is between 3 and 10 minutes, with a peak effect at 30 minutes. The duration of action is 2 to 4 hours. Alteration of consciousness may persist up to 12 hours. Droperidol is metabolized in the liver and excreted by the kidneys.

Adverse Effects

In addition to prolonged QT interval on electrocardiography, other reported adverse effects for droperidol are hypotension, hypertension, dystonia, increased hyperexcitability, anxiety, and sweating. Less commonly reported effects include bronchospasm, emergence delirium (hallucinations), chills, shivering, depression, and nightmares. The risk for respiratory depression is higher when used in combination with an opioid analgesic, making careful monitoring necessary.

✳ How are some of the undesirable adverse effects of general anesthesia managed?

Various medications are used as preanesthetic agents, or as adjuncts to anesthesia, to reduce the undesirable effects produced by apprehension or by the induction and maintenance of anesthesia. As discussed earlier, opioid analgesics not only reduce anxiety and provide analgesia but because of their additive effects also allow for a reduction in the dose of anesthetic administered. Morphine and meperidine (Demerol) are among the more commonly used opioid analgesics; they are discussed in depth in Chapter 14.

The use of general anesthetics may increase the risk of aspiration of gastric contents because of depressed protective reflexes. This risk, although small (e.g., 2 to 10 cases of aspiration per 10,000 surgical cases conducted) (Ng & Smith, 2001), can result in significant pulmonary toxicity. To avoid this toxicity, the clinical team may elect to identify higher-risk clients, and consider the aggressive use of agents to reduce postoperative nausea and vomiting or to alter gastric contents or pH. Aggressive management of postoperative nausea and vomiting can be achieved with a number of agents, including those that affect serotonin receptors (e.g., ondansetron [Zofran], dolasetron [Anzemet]). Antimus-

carinic/anticholinergic agents may be used prior to surgery to inhibit secretions and to reduce the likelihood of vomiting; although the preoperative use of anticholinergics is not associated with improved outcomes related to pulmonary aspiration and is not recommended (American Society of Anesthesiologists [ASA], 1999). Antimuscarinics that may be used include atropine, scopolamine, and glycopyrrolate (Robinul). Agents that alter the pH of gastric contents include the proton pump inhibitors (e.g., omeprazole [Prilosec]) and the histamine blockers (e.g., famotidine [Pepcid]). Their use prior to surgery is not routine, but is considered for those individuals who have other conditions that justify their concurrent use (e.g., risk for upper gastrointestinal bleeding or gastroesophageal reflux) (ASA, 1999). Each of these agents is discussed in Chapters 21 and 40.

✳ What other drug therapies are used during surgery?

Two other drug classes commonly used during surgical procedures are neuromuscular blockers, to reduce or eliminate muscle movement during delicate surgery, and antibacterial drugs, to reduce the risk of intraoperative infections. The prophylactic use of antibacterial drugs during surgery is discussed in Chapter 59.

The administration of neuromuscular blockers provides surgeons with easier access to and increased visualization of the surgical site and prevents inadvertent client movement during the procedure. Examples of neuromuscular blockers include atracurium (Tracrium), cisatracurium (Nimbex), doxacurium (Nuromax), mivacurium (Mivacron), pancuronium (Pavulon), pipecuronium (Arduran), rocuronium (Zemuron), and vecuronium (Norcuron). Because all muscles, including respiratory muscles, are impacted by these agents, airway support is vital prior to their use. In addition to use during surgery, these drugs may be used to assist muscle relaxation during intubation, and for clients who are "fighting the vent" while on respirators. All of these agents will suppress or halt skeletal muscle activity, but they possess no analgesic, amnesic, anxiolytic, or antiepileptic action. With muscle relaxation, the ventilated client may appear comfortable and relaxed, but unless the client is receiving other medications (e.g., opioid analgesics, benzodiazepines, or other anesthetics), the client is likely to be very anxious and uncomfortable. Consequently, it is critical to administer analgesics for pain and benzodiazepines or other anesthetics that affect level of consciousness and memory prior to and during treatment with neuromuscular blockers. The neuromuscular blockers are discussed more fully in Chapter 21.

✳ What significant drug interactions exist with the drugs used during anesthesia?

Among the risks facing a surgical client is an unexpected drug interaction that occurs during preparation for or during anesthesia. Anesthetists must always be familiar with the interactions between anesthetic drugs and the maintenance drug therapies used in a wide range of illnesses. A serious drug interaction may be underway before surgery, and the surgical anesthesia may complicate the interaction. A critical analysis of the client's drug regimen (prescribed, over-the-counter, and alternative/complementary medications) should be performed in relation to the anesthetic drugs and preanesthetic drugs to be used.

Although it is the anesthetist's responsibility to obtain the preoperative drug history, a nurse should be aware of all the medications a client has taken in the 2- to 3-week preoperative period so that the nurse can assess the risk for injury related to concurrent drug therapy. Various pharmacologic classes of medication may result in adverse effects in clients anesthetized for surgery. For example, drugs affecting coagulation/clotting, such as heparin and warfarin, are usually discontinued 48 hours (aspirin, 7 days) before surgery to reduce the increased risk of hemorrhage. CNS depressants such as opioids and hypnotics not prescribed as part of the anesthetic process may increase the risk of enhanced CNS-depressant effects.

Antidysrhythmics such as propranolol hydrochloride may induce decreased cardiac output, decreased heart rate, and bronchospasm. Quinidine, procainamide, and lidocaine may reduce cardiac conduction, increase peripheral vasodilation, and potentiate neuromuscular blocking agents.

Selected antihypertensive agents such as guanethidine (Ismelin) and methyldopa (Aldomet) deplete the synthesis or storage of norepinephrine in the sympathetic (adrenergic) nerve endings and may result in severe hypotension when combined with anesthetics and analgesics. Prescribers may consider reducing or stopping such medications before surgery.

When used as long-term therapy, corticosteroids usually produce adrenal gland suppression, which may result in hypotension during surgery. Because the stress of anesthesia and surgery usually increases the need for and release of endogenous cortisol, it is recommended that corticosteroid dosages be increased in the perioperative period.

Cholinesterase inhibitors (e.g., echothiophate iodide [Phospholine Iodide] and demecarium bromide [Humorsol]) and exposure to organophosphate insecticides may prolong succinylcholine blockade. Extended apnea and death have been reported with this combination. It is generally recommended that cholinergic eyedrops be stopped approximately 2 weeks before elective surgery.

Antibiotics—particularly aminoglycoside antibiotics (e.g., amikacin [Amikin], gentamicin [Garamycin], tobramycin [Nebcin])—may potentiate the neuromuscular blocking agent or cause neuromuscular blockade. A reduction in the dosage of the neuromuscular blocking agent may be necessary, along with careful titration or careful dosing of the drug according to the client's response. Clients with myasthenia gravis, Parkinson's disease, or other neuromuscular disorders must be monitored carefully.

Complementary/alternative preparations may also interact with general anesthetics, anticoagulants, or other modalities used during surgery. The ASA recommends that all herbal medications be discontinued 2 to 3 weeks before an elective surgical procedure (Kaye, Kucera, & Sabar, 2004). See the Medication Safety Alert box on p. 230 in Chapter 12 for the rationale for specific herbal prepara-

tions. If discontinuation of the medicine is not possible, as in an emergency, a careful history is important.

Many other drugs have the potential to induce an unwanted effect intraoperatively or postoperatively. Concurrent administration of various drugs with anesthetic agents requires close supervision and monitoring of a surgical client. As a general guideline, a drug that is needed for treatment preoperatively should be continued through surgery (e.g., insulin for clients with type 1 diabetes mellitus). Drugs that may be suspended temporarily without harming a client's health are discontinued before surgery for a period at least five times the half-life of the drug. Drugs having significant interactions with anesthetic agents are replaced, when possible, with an alternative medication before surgery.

✱ Are there certain populations for whom we should take special precautions in relation to anesthetics?

Many disease states and risk factors can alter a client's response to anesthesia. The preoperative nursing assessment of risk for injury related to anesthesia includes a client's health status with other factors, such as acute and chronic medical conditions.

Alcoholism Clients with a history of active ethanol abuse may have a variety of associated disease states, including liver dysfunction, pancreatitis, gastritis, and esophageal varices. The anesthetic requirements for these clients may be increased because of an increase in liver-metabolizing enzymes and the development of cross-tolerance. Such clients are monitored closely during the postanesthetic period for alcohol withdrawal syndrome, because its onset may be delayed with the administration of medications for pain relief. Pharmacologic intervention with a benzodiazepine (e.g., lorazepam [Ativan]) may be required to prevent the occurrence of withdrawal symptoms.

Obesity Clients who are overweight or obese may have cardiac insufficiency, respiratory problems, atherosclerosis, hypertension, or an increased incidence of diabetes, liver disease, or thrombophlebitis. Obtaining the desired depth of anesthesia and muscle relaxation may be problematic. With prolonged administration of fat-soluble anesthetic agents, there is delayed recovery as a consequence of the saturation of fat depots. In general, fat-soluble anesthetics, especially those with toxic metabolites such as methoxyflurane (Penthrane), should be avoided.

Smoking Clients who smoke usually have an increasingly rigid arterial vascular system, adrenal gland stimulation, and perhaps lung disease (e.g., bronchitis, emphysema, or carcinoma). Postoperative complications are therefore much more common in smokers than in nonsmokers. Smoking also increases the client's sensitivity to neuromuscular blockers.

Pregnancy See the Pregnancy Safety box on p. 298 for the Food and Drug Administration rating of anesthetic drug safety during pregnancy. Before any drug is used, the expected drug benefits should be considered against the pos-

Category	Drug
B	desflurane, levobupivacaine, lidocaine, prilocaine, methohexital, enflurane, propofol, ropivacaine, sevoflurane
C	alfentanil, articaine, bupivacaine, chloroprocaine, droperidol, etomidate, fentanyl, halothane, isoflurane, ketamine, mepivacaine, methoxyflurane, nitrous oxide, procaine, remifentanil, sufentanil, tetracaine, thiopental sodium
D	diazepam, lorazepam (parenteral), midazolam

Data from *Mosby's drug consult* (15th ed.). (2005). St. Louis: Mosby.

BOX 15-2 WASTE ANESTHETIC GASES AS OCCUPATIONAL HEALTH HAZARD

Chronic exposure of health care providers in the operating room to waste anesthetic gases (WAGs) may present a significant occupational health hazard. The effects of exposure to WAGs include dizziness, lightheadedness, nausea, fatigue, irritability, and depression. Difficulty with cognition, perception, and motor skills place workers and others at risk. Studies demonstrate an increased incidence of birth defects, spontaneous abortions, and infertility among workers exposed to nitrous oxide, as well as among their spouses. In addition, neurologic, hepatic, and renal disorders have been seen in the chronically exposed. Health care providers should protect themselves by ensuring anesthesia equipment is functioning properly and client masks fit well, and by avoiding the area within a foot of the client's mouth and nose when the breath contains exhaled anesthetic agents. Health care providers should be active in establishing exposure monitoring programs to detect unsafe levels caused by faulty equipment and unsafe practices (Occupational Safety and Health Administration [OSHA], 2004).

sible risk to the fetus. Box 15-2 describes the risks of waste anesthetic gases to health care providers. For descriptions of the pregnancy safety categories, see Chapter 2.

Young Age The physical characteristics of neonates may predispose them to upper airway obstruction or laryngospasm during anesthesia induction or resuscitation. A small mandible and neck, a narrow cricoid ring, a large body water compartment with a high extracellular water turnover rate, immaturely functioning liver and kidneys, and a rapid metabolic rate all contribute to the need for careful consideration of infants or children. Drug dosages and administered fluids must be carefully calculated using the body weight or surface area of the child. Halothane and nitrous oxide are commonly used in pediatrics because the

incidence of hepatitis in children is considered rare after the use of halothane. Neonates are usually more sensitive to the nondepolarizing neuromuscular blockers.

Advanced Age Aging results in a generalized decline in organ function (approximately 1% per year after age 30 years), the existence of chronic disease processes, or both. The complexity of drug treatment increases as the number and complexity of illnesses increase with age; this results in a greater potential for drug interactions and adverse effects. In general, an increased and prolonged drug effect is seen in older adults. Mortality rates for older clients undergoing major surgery may be four to eight times higher than for younger clients.

✳ **What is the role of nursing in managing the care of a client undergoing general anesthesia?**
Nursing during the perioperative period encompasses three distinct phases: preoperative, intraoperative, and postoperative. These phases are a continuum, but nursing care during each phase differs in its approach to the client and the goals for health outcomes.

✳ **R.S., a 70-year-old man, was admitted to the hospital the afternoon before his scheduled elective abdominal aortic aneurysm repair. During the preoperative nursing assessment, his blood pressure was 158/100 mm Hg, and he stated he has hypertension that is poorly controlled, although he is taking propranolol 80 mg twice daily. He also indicated that he has "diet-controlled diabetes." He denies any other medication use within the last 2 weeks, including over-the-counter drugs and complementary/alternative preparations. This was the first time R.S. has ever had surgery and he is highly anxious. He has no allergies and no one in his family has had an adverse response to anesthesia.**

Preoperative Phase

A major responsibility of a nurse during the preoperative period is to complete a focus assessment—the acquisition of selected or specific data as determined by the nurse and the client or family, or as directed by a client's condition (Carpenito-Moyet, 2004). In the assessment of R.S., his age, hypertension, aneurysm, diabetes, and anxiety are important issues. Although general health data are gathered during admission of a client to a health care agency, it is important to focus on those factors that will influence a client's experience with anesthetic agents to allow optimal anesthesia to be achieved without adverse effects. The nurse has identified R.S.'s, underlying acute and chronic conditions and the medications he has recently taken or is currently taking.

The nurse has also assessed his experience with previous surgeries to allay anxiety and to identify risk factors to prevent adverse effects, particularly malignant hyperthermia. Malignant hyperthermia is a condition characterized by often-fatal hyperthermia. It is important to ask if the client or a family member has ever had problems with anesthesia, because this condition is associated with an autosomal dominant trait.

Because R.S. is hospitalized the night before surgery, a sedative or hypnotic may be administered to ensure a sound and restful sleep. The timing of the administration of this medication provides an opportunity to assist R.S. to gain insight into his anxiety regarding the anticipated surgical procedure. Many clients have anxieties regarding the experience of anesthesia, such as a fear of not waking up, having pain during surgery, talking while they are anesthetized, or having nausea and vomiting after surgery. The nurse can minimize the client's anxieties by ensuring that R.S. and his family are well-informed about the perioperative routine and the anesthetic agents to be used.

The surgeon or the anesthetist can best answer questions about the rationale for a particular agent or method of anesthesia. Very few clients talk while anesthetized, and those who do are generally unintelligible. However, R.S. may have other valid concerns that need to be discussed to ensure that there is informed consent for the anesthesia. He can be reassured that he will have close surveillance throughout the surgical procedure and in the immediate postoperative period. If R.S. persists in his fears regarding anesthesia or surgery, he will need consultation with the surgeon and/or the anesthetist before undergoing final preparation for surgery. Unless allayed, severe anxiety or fear affects both the autonomic and central nervous systems and may cause detrimental physiologic and psychological reactions. An anxious client may resist relaxation and "fight" the anesthetic. In such a case, a greater amount of anesthetic would be required, and toxic levels of drugs might be administered inadvertently. Preoperative teaching regarding postoperative events (e.g., parenteral fluids, dressings, nasogastric tubes, indwelling catheters, pain management), and counseling by a nurse help to alleviate a client's anxiety. This preoperative counseling may be managed by a case manager or by preoperative visits to the hospital, particularly with day or short-stay surgeries.

In addition to R.S.'s preanesthetic medications, explain all preoperative care activities to him. Most clients are unfamiliar with the procedures involved in the perioperative experience. Alert R.S. that he will "wake up" or recover from the anesthetic in a different place from his room, a postanesthetic care unit. Teach R.S. about the necessity for postoperative coughing, deep breathing, frequent turning, and the use of incentive spirometer. These activities help to prevent the postoperative complications of general anesthetics, such as hypostatic pneumonia and atelectasis. Preoperative teaching promotes cooperation when R.S. is asked to do these activities, which often cause discomfort after a surgical procedure.

The ASA supports a fasting period of 2 hours for clear liquids for all clients, 6 hours for a light meal (tea and toast), and for infants, 4 hours for breast milk and 6 hours for infant formula and nonhuman milk (ASA, 1999). This procedure helps prevent aspiration if vomiting occurs as a response to anesthesia. In clients where hydration is an ongoing concern, IV fluids may be ordered by a physician during this period.

Be mindful of R.S.'s drug history during the preoperative preparation. Withholding his propranolol because he is to have nothing by mouth (NPO) prior to surgery has the physiologic effect of abrupt withdrawal and may cause perioperative infarction and death (Shammash et al., 2001). Because most medications are well-tolerated through surgery and do not interfere with anesthetic administration, most drugs should be continued through the morning of surgery unless relatively unnecessary (e.g., vitamins) or contraindicated (e.g., herbal products). In particular, antihypertensive, antiseizure, and antipsychotic medication should be given unless specifically contraindicated (Mercado & Petty, 2003). Consult with the primary prescriber regarding rescheduling any drugs that are of concern, the time of administration, changing the route of administration of the standing medication, or both. Although a parenteral form of propranolol is available, R.S. (who is NPO for surgery) may be allowed to take his oral medications with a small amount of water (30 to 60 mL).

Premedicating clients such as R.S. is less common now than in the past. A client's age, weight, physical condition, and level of anxiety; the anesthetic method selected; and the duration and type of surgery are considered. Not including drugs in the preoperative preparation may be appropriate for some clients, whereas others may need aggressive pharmacologic intervention to produce the desired preoperative state. Because he is scheduled for major surgery, R.S. has been prescribed midazolam to provide sedation and anxiolysis.

Opioid analgesics, barbiturates, or benzodiazepines (anxiolytics are most commonly used) are administered before R.S. is taken to surgery to promote serenity and amnesia, to smooth induction, and to decrease the amount of anesthetic required to produce anesthesia. It is important to administer preoperative medications at the exact time ordered. If given too close to the time of administration of the general anesthetic, they may achieve their full effect during anesthesia and cause severe respiratory depression or hypotension.

Because the time needed to complete specific surgical procedures varies, it is impossible for many preoperative medications (other than the first cases of the day in the operating room) to be ordered for a specific time. For cases after the first of the day, the preoperative medication is ordered "on call" to the operating room or, in some cases, may be given in the preoperative holding area.

All of the physical tasks involved with R.S.'s preparation for surgery (e.g., signing surgical permits, final voiding before surgery, obtaining vital signs) should be accomplished before the preoperative medication is administered. The consent for anesthesia, surgery, or both is not considered valid if a client has received sedation before signing. Once the medication is administered, the nurse places R.S. on bed rest with the side rails up and the call light within reach. This decreases stimulation, enhances the action of the medication, and enhances client safety.

Intraoperative Phase

The nurse has a highly specialized role within the operating room. Nursing responsibilities include the maintenance of safety, physiologic monitoring, and psychological support of R.S.; however, the nurse's role related to the administration of anesthetic agents is to support the anesthesiologist or the nurse anesthetist administering the anesthetic. The role of the nurse anesthetist, who assumes direct responsibility for the administration of anesthetics, requires a formal certification program for advanced practice within that specialty.

The operating room nurse monitors R.S. for factors that may result in hypotension, nerve injury, or malignant hyperthermia. Hypotension may result from an excess of nonvolatile drugs that depress the vasomotor center. When opioids are given, the nurse assesses R.S.'s pain thoroughly and records his vital signs. Although opioids may increase hypotension, severe pain can also increase heart rate and blood pressure. In such cases, an opioid may both alleviate pain and normalize blood pressure.

The operating room nurse must also be on the alert for nerve injury, which may follow spinal anesthesia or malpositioning during general anesthesia. The brachial, radial, ulnar, and perineal nerves are the nerves most likely to be injured. The operating room nurse is responsible for ensuring that R.S. is positioned properly to prevent injury from nerve damage. Having knowledge of proper positioning for the particular surgical procedure is essential.

A rare but very dangerous adverse effect of inhaled, fat-soluble anesthetics is malignant hyperthermia—an emergency situation in which a client's temperature suddenly escalates. A client may die if this condition is not treated appropriately and promptly. Individuals susceptible to malignant hyperthermia have an underlying muscle disorder, which is an autosomal dominant trait. See the Special Considerations for Pharmacogenetics box below. The use of neuromuscular blocking agents is also associated with this adverse effect, especially when used with the inhalation anesthetics. The onset of this condition may be more abrupt with concurrent use of succinylcholine.

With malignant hyperthermia, body temperature may increase as much as 1° C (1.8° F) every 5 minutes, reaching reported highs of 43° C (109.4° F). Although the condition is relatively rare, occurring in 1 in 50,000 surgical clients, it is a life-threatening condition with a mortality rate of 30% to 40%. The operating room team, within which the nurse has a key role, should have a preplanned course of action, including the availability of dantrolene sodium, a central-acting skeletal muscle relaxant (see Chapter 23 for drug monograph); a complete change of anesthesia circuit; hyperventilation with 100% oxygen; methods to lower body temperature rapidly; and other symptomatic treatment. Dantrolene sodium has been used prophylactically and in the treatment of this disorder.

Postoperative Phase

The major objective of the immediate postoperative period is to help R.S. recover from the effects of the anesthetic and the surgery safely, comfortably, and as quickly as possible.

Assessment A general postoperative assessment of R.S. includes the following:

- Airway and breathing: adequacy of the airway and airway reflexes (gag, cough, swallow); type of airway in place; rate and quality of respiration; breath sounds; ability to cough and deep breathe; amount and method of oxygen administered and the time it was initiated
- Circulation: pulse rate, peripheral pulses, blood pressure readings, cardiac monitor pattern, skin color, and temperature
- Metabolic state: skin integrity and turgor, temperature, urine output, type and rate of IV fluids administered
- General: location, condition, and output from drains and catheters; muscle strength and response; bowel sounds; status of the surgical incision; pain; level of consciousness; ability to communicate

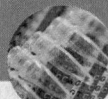 Special Considerations for Pharmacogenetics | Anesthetics

Pharmacodynamics

The mu opioid receptor displays genetically based variation (Lotsch et al., 2002), and likely results in altered drug response across populations. This may affect clients who receive opioids (e.g., fentanyl, morphine) as adjuncts to anesthesia. Genetic differences in the mouse model suggest differences in response to anesthetic gasses (Quinlan et al., 2002), but the implications for humans is unclear. Pharmacodynamic variation believed to correlate with the RYR1 gene has been reported in the study of halothane (Chang & Altman, 2004).

Pharmacokinetics

Transfer of volatile anesthetics across alveolar membranes varies based on genetic influences in the rat model (Stekiel et al., 2004) and may have implications for humans. Intraindividual differences in midazolam metabolism via cytochrome P450 3A4-5 is also thought to be genetically based (Chang & Altman, 2004).

Adverse Effects

The risk for malignant hyperthermia, the rare but life-threatening adverse reaction to general anesthetics, is likely to be genetically linked (Sei et al., 2004). Identification of clients at risk through genetics may reduce the potential for developing this serious complication (Girard et al., 2004).

Nursing Diagnosis A client such as R.S. who is receiving a general anesthetic may experience the following nursing diagnoses/collaborative problems: ineffective airway clearance related to inadequate cough and tenacious secretions; ineffective breathing pattern related to excess or cumulative effects of drugs administered during anesthesia induction; risk for aspiration related to nausea and vomiting, gastrointestinal distention, medication and anesthesia, stimulation of the vomiting center or chemoreceptor trigger zone, or anoxia during anesthesia; impaired physical mobility related to fear of pain; hypothermia; disturbed sensory perception; and the potential complications of urinary retention, incisional pain, abdominal distention or paralytic ileus, shock and thrombophlebitis (IV anesthetics).

Planning Before receiving the general anesthetic, R.S. will:
- Describe what to expect in the recovery phase of anesthesia.

Following general anesthesia, R.S. will:
- Follow the instructions he received preoperatively related to his postoperative care.
- Collaborate with the plan of care to minimize the risk of complications related to anesthesia.
- Not experience injury related to anesthesia.

Implementation

Monitoring At frequent intervals, the frequency of which are determined by R.S.'s condition, evaluate his status as in the initial assessment on the previous page.

The recovery phase for volatile anesthetic agents is generally short and there is no analgesia residue; thus the postoperative analgesia phase is short and R.S. will experience pain. In addition, shivering and tremors may be observed postoperatively.

Intervention Neuromuscular blocking agents such as succinylcholine and tubocurarine can cause hypoventilation. It is critically important to maintain a patent airway until R.S. has fully responded in the postoperative period. Nursing measures include encouraging him to deep breathe and cough frequently. Changing his position to prevent pooling of pulmonary secretions can help to improve ventilation and prevent atelectasis. R.S. (as well as most clients who received a general anesthetic) will receive supplemental oxygen until he is fully recovered from anesthesia. Mobilization and alternating the contraction and relaxation of muscles help to promote circulation.

Postoperatively, the nurse can administer a prescribed antiemetic and position R.S. on his side to prevent aspiration. R.S. should not be given anything by mouth until peristalsis returns. Normal bowel sounds and progression to an appropriate diet are the desired health outcomes.

Use caution when changing R.S.'s position during the recovery phase. In addition to vasodilation, compensatory vasoconstriction mechanisms are depressed, which may result in a significant drop in blood pressure with position changes (postural hypotension). Administer oxygen as ordered during the immediate recovery period to compensate for the respiratory depression caused by anesthetic agents and for the body's increased oxygen needs from shivering. Analgesic medications provide relief from immediate postoperative pain. Because of the combined effects of the CNS depressants (e.g., residual anesthetic agents and analgesics), remember that any sedative or analgesic probably needs to be decreased to one-half to one-fourth of the usual dose for the first dose after surgery. See Chapter 14 for a discussion of pain management. Measures to prevent heat loss from vasodilation include using warm blankets, covering the head with a blanket, and using a hyperthermic automatic blanket.

Detecting impending shock early and instituting the proper therapy may prevent, or at least modify, its severity. Note the rate, volume, and rhythm of the pulse, as well as R.S.'s color and skin temperature. A rapid, thready, weak pulse; cyanosis or extreme pallor; cold, clammy skin; and low blood pressure are characteristic signs of shock. Check for bleeding at the surgical site; hemorrhagic shock may occur if R.S. loses blood postoperatively. Postoperative shock also may result from extensive surgical trauma, prolonged operating time, prolonged deep anesthesia, or even inadequate anesthesia. Keep resuscitative equipment within the immediate environment when general (inhalation or IV) anesthetic agents are administered. Take care to avoid extravasation of the drug into the tissues during IV injection; pain, swelling, ulceration, and necrosis may occur. Intraarterial injection of IV anesthetics may result in tissue necrosis and gangrene.

Education Although R.S. will stay in the hospital after surgery, increasing numbers of surgeries are being performed at ambulatory surgical centers, and client-family teaching for the client returning home after same-day surgery is necessary to help the client recover more fully from anesthesia and the surgery. In addition to providing specifics regarding the surgical procedure and its relevant postoperative care, prepare R.S. for experiencing some degree of psychomotor impairment and sensory-perceptual alterations during the first 24 hours following anesthesia. If R.S.'s surgery had been a day surgery, he would be cautioned against attempting tasks that require alertness and coordination, such as driving. Instruct clients to avoid using alcohol or other CNS depressants within the first 24 hours of anesthesia unless prescribed by the health care provider.

Evaluation R.S. will effectively maintain his airway and will have an effective cough, gag reflex, normal respiratory rate and depth, and normal breath sounds. Temperature, blood pressure, and pulse will be within normal limits. He will experience no postoperative pain or an acceptable level of postoperative discomfort. There will be no evidence of a thromboembolic event secondary to IV anesthetic agents. His urinary output will be more than 30 to 50 mL/hr without complaints of urgency or bladder fullness and he will be oriented to person, time, and place and respond to verbal commands after his general anesthesia experience.

TABLE 15-4 LOCAL ANESTHETICS: METHOD OF ADMINISTRATION AND THERAPEUTIC USE

Method	Tissue Affected	Preparation Used	Examples of Drugs Used	Therapeutic Use
Topical	Sensory nerve endings in mucous membranes and dermis	Solution Ointment Cream Powder	cocaine benzocaine ethyl aminobenzoate bupivacaine	Relief of pain or itching Examination of conjunctivae
Infiltration	Sensory nerve endings in subcutaneous tissues or dermis	Injection	lidocaine procaine prilocaine chloroprocaine mepivacaine	Minor surgery
Block	Nerve trunk	Injection	lidocaine procaine prilocaine chloroprocaine mepivacaine	Dental and limb surgery Sympathetic block
Spinal (subarachnoid block)	Spinal roots	Injection	procaine tetracaine lidocaine	Abdominal surgery Surgery of the lower extremities Muscle relaxation

✷ **J.M., a 7-year-old boy, is scheduled for a minor procedure that is anticipated to last 30 minutes. He is brought to the ambulatory surgical suite with his parents. He is frightened of "needles" and is extremely apprehensive about his parents leaving. The anesthetist decides to administer ketamine IM.**

Ketamine produces a dissociative state or conscious sedation; J.M. will not appear to be asleep but will have excellent analgesia and be compliant should his cooperation be required during the procedure. Instruct his parents that his stare and random movement are consequences of the ketamine. Respiratory depression is rare, but protect J.M. from visual, tactile, and auditory stimuli during emergence from ketamine to decrease the possibility of psychic effects. Up to 50% of unpremedicated clients report dreams and hallucinations as the drug wears off, and these can occur up to 24 hours after the administration of ketamine. Disturbing responses may be alleviated with diazepam, although J.M. is at lower risk because of his age, the dose, and the route of administration. Keep environmental stimulation to a minimum during recovery to reduce the risk of an emergent reaction. Do not arouse J.M. until he awakens on his own.

Because of psychomotor impairment, caution J.M.'s parents against outside play or other hazardous activities for 24 to 48 hours. If J.M. were older, he would be warned against alcohol ingestion for at least 24 hours after recovery from ketamine. The expected outcome of ketamine administration is that J.M. will experience effective anesthesia, and his safety will be maintained. Sensory-perceptual alterations associated with ketamine will be minimized or absent.

✷ **What alternatives exist to general anesthesia?**
Local anesthesia refers to the direct administration of an anesthetic agent to tissues to induce the absence of sensa-

tion in a portion of the body. Unlike with general anesthesia, consciousness is not depressed. Local anesthetic agents may be applied to an area or injected into tissues, where they produce their effect in the immediate area only; hence the term local anesthesia. Local anesthetic drugs may also be injected around a nerve or nerve trunk (spinal, epidural) to produce anesthesia in a large region of the body. This is referred to as regional anesthesia.

Surface or Topical Anesthesia

The use of surface, or topical, anesthetics is restricted to mucous membranes, damaged skin surfaces, wounds, and burns. The anesthetic is applied in the form of a solution, ointment, gel, cream, or powder to paralyze afferent nerve endings and produce a loss of sensation. Topical anesthetics do not penetrate unbroken skin. Topical anesthesia is used to relieve pain and itching and to anesthetize mucous membranes of the eye, nose, throat, or urethra for minor surgical procedures. Cocaine in a 4% to 10% solution historically has been a widely used agent for topical anesthesia but is used infrequently today.

Local anesthesia may also be achieved by freezing. Low temperatures in living tissues produce diminished sensation. This form of anesthesia is sometimes used for minor surgical procedures. Tissues that are frozen too intensely for too long may be destroyed. Ethyl chloride is a local anesthetic that can be used to produce this effect, but it is not used extensively.

Local Anesthetics

Local anesthetics are used to abolish pain sensation in a particular part of the body (Tables 15-4 and 15-5). The basic mechanism of action of these drugs is unknown, but most act

TABLE 15-5 PROPERTIES OF COMMONLY USED LOCAL ANESTHETICS

	Procaine	Cocaine	Benzocaine	Lidocaine	Tetracaine	Mepivacaine
Trade names	Novocain	—	Americaine Hurricaine	Xylocaine	Pontocaine	Carbocaine
Potency	—	2-3 times that of procaine	Very low	Twice that of procaine	10 times that of procaine	Twice that of procaine
Onset of action	2-5 min	1 min	Immediate	2-5 min	3-10 min	Less rapid than procaine
Duration	30 min-1 hr	30 min-1 hr	15-20 min	1-3 hr	1 to more than 3 hr	1-3 hr
Dose	0.25%-2%, depending on method of administration 10% for spinal anesthesia Not used topically	1%-4% topically	5%-20% ointment topically	0.5%-4% for injection; 2% and 5% topically	1% topically; 0.15%-0.25% for injection	1%-2% solution
Toxicity	Least toxic of all local anesthetics	More toxic than procaine when injected subcutaneously	Relatively nontoxic	See procaine	More toxic than procaine, but toxic effects are rare because of low dosage used	Twice that of procaine; less than lidocaine
Precautions	Overdose of rapid injection may cause CNS stimulation	Not recommended for infiltration, nerve block, or spinal anesthesia Repeated use causes psychological dependence	Suitable for topical use only Sensitization may develop	When administered rapidly or in large doses, may cause seizures and hypotension	Drug interaction with cholinesterase inhibitors and sulfonamides	Combined with vasoconstrictor to delay drug absorption and prolong duration Avoid in pregnancy—may cause constriction of uterine artery

by stabilizing or elevating the threshold of excitation of the nerve cell membrane without affecting resting potential (blockage of sodium channels). This action is a result of the reduction of membrane permeability to all ions, thus preventing depolarization and the transmission of nerve impulses.

Table 15-5 presents some commonly used local anesthetics and their properties. Benzyl alcohol, an aromatic alcohol of low potency, is used topically with procaine to extend procaine's duration of action. The choice of local anesthetic for a particular procedure depends on the duration of drug action desired. Procaine, cocaine, and benzocaine are considered short-acting; lidocaine and mepivacaine, intermediate-acting; and tetracaine, long-acting. Vasoconstrictors such as epinephrine and norepinephrine are used with the local anesthetic to decrease systemic ab-

sorption and prolong the duration of action of the anesthetic. They are not used for nerve blocks in areas with end arteries (fingers, toes, ears, nose, and penis) because ischemia may develop, resulting in gangrene. Lidocaine is considered the prototype local anesthetic.

✱■■ lidocaine [lye doe kane]
(Xylocaine, Xylocard✦, Zilactin-L)
Indications
Lidocaine is used as a local anesthetic. It is also used systemically to treat ventricular dysrhythmias; see Chapter 26.
Pharmacokinetics/Dosing
Topically or locally applied lidocaine has limited distribution to other tissue sites. Doses used topically or for local injection vary based on formulation and procedure. Topical patch lidocaine is often dosed at the site of pain for up to 12 hours during a 24-hour pe-

riod. Pharmacokinetics and dosing of intravenous lidocaine for dysrhythmias are presented in Chapter 26.

Adverse Effects
Adverse effects following the topical application of lidocaine are usually limited to localized hypersensitivity reactions. Use during spinal anesthesia may be associated with headache or hypotension. Central nervous system and cardiovascular effects are usually limited to the use of higher IV doses in the treatment of cardiac dysrhythmias (see Chapter 26).

A number of local anesthetic agents cannot be injected. However, because they are absorbed slowly, they can be used safely on open wounds, ulcers, and mucous membranes. Occasionally they cause dermatitis and allergic sensitization, in which case they are discontinued. The ester-type local anesthetics (cocaine, procaine, tetracaine, and benzocaine) are metabolized to para-aminobenzoic acid (PABA) metabolites, which are mainly responsible for allergic reactions in some clients. The amide anesthetics (lidocaine, mepivacaine, bupivacaine, prilocaine) are not metabolized to PABA derivatives, and therefore allergic reactions induced by these anesthetics are very rare (Katzung, 2004).

Topical anesthetics for skin disorders are used primarily to relieve pruritus, discomfort, pain, and soreness; the indications for mucous membranes are similar. These anesthetics are poorly absorbed through intact skin, but absorption is increased through mucous membranes and skin breaks and sores (e.g., abrasions, trauma, and ulcers); this leads to the possibility of systemic involvement. When they are used in the oral cavity (mouth and pharynx), interference with swallowing may occur and puts a client at risk for aspiration. Assess a client for a returning gag reflex by gently touching the back of the pharynx with a tongue blade. Withhold all foods and fluid until the reflex returns.

Local anesthetics are capable of abolishing all sensation, but pain fibers are affected first, probably because they are thinner, unmyelinated, and more easily penetrated by these drugs. Loss of pain is followed in sequence by a loss of response to cold, warmth, touch, and pressure. Most motor fibers also can be anesthetized when an adequate concentration of the drug is present over a sufficient time.

Parenteral local anesthetics have complete systemic absorption, which is decreased by the addition of a vasoconstrictor such as epinephrine. Onset of action is a function of the anesthetic technique used, the type of block desired, dosage, and the pKa of each anesthetic (negative logarithm of ionization constant of an acid, or the pH at which equal concentrations of the acid and conjugate base forms of a substance are present). The time it takes for a drug to reach a peak concentration depends on the type of block but ranges from 10 to 30 minutes.

Reactions to Local Anesthetics Local anesthetics produce vasodilation by acting directly on blood vessels and by anesthetizing sympathetic vasoconstrictor fibers. This action can cause rapid absorption of the drug; when the rate of absorption exceeds the rate of elimination, toxic effects can occur. Epinephrine or other vasoconstrictor drugs are used to prolong local anesthetic effects and to decrease the

rate of absorption and incidence of toxic effects by allowing more time for metabolic degradation. The dosages of vasoconstrictors must be carefully determined to prevent ischemic necrosis at the injection site. Because local anesthetics are potentially toxic drugs, a client's age, weight, physical condition, and liver function must be taken into account when determining drug dose. Most reactions to local anesthetics result from overdose, rapid absorption into the systemic circulation, or individual hypersensitivity or allergic response.

Central Nervous System At first the CNS may be stimulated and cause anxiety, restlessness, confusion, dizziness, tremors, and even seizures. Depression may then occur, and unconsciousness and death may ensue.

Cardiovascular System Myocardial depression, bradycardia, and hypotension can occur because of smooth-muscle relaxation and inhibition of neuromuscular conduction. The client suddenly becomes pale, feels faint, and experiences a drop in blood pressure. Cardiac arrest can be the result of a cardiovascular reaction.

Anesthetics containing a vasoconstrictor are used with caution in clients receiving drugs that may change blood pressure, such as monoamine oxidase inhibitors, phenothiazines, and tricyclic antidepressants. Such a combination may produce severe hypotension or hypertension. Cardiac dysrhythmias occur when catecholamine vasoconstrictors (e.g., epinephrine) are used in clients receiving cyclopropane, halothane, or trichloroethylene.

Allergic Reaction True allergic reactions are said to be uncommon. Sometimes a reaction is thought to be allergic when really it is caused by overdose. Nevertheless, allergic reactions can occur and may be relatively mild (hives, itching, skin rash) or acutely anaphylactic.

Allergic reactions are characteristically manifested by cutaneous lesions, urticaria, or edema and may result from factors such as hypersensitivity, idiosyncrasy, or diminished tolerance. These rare allergic reactions are usually limited to the ester type of anesthetics. The most important risk with local anesthetics is dose-related CNS toxicity, which may progress from sleepiness to seizures.

Small test doses are often given to gauge the extent of the client's sensitivity to the anesthetic agent. The anesthetic agent chosen, its concentration, the rate of injection, and physical and emotional factors in a client all influence reactions to local anesthetics.

Regional Anesthesia

Anesthesia by injection is accomplished with either infiltration or conduction (spinal, caudal, or saddle block).

Infiltration anesthesia is produced by injecting dilute solutions (0.1%) of an agent into the skin and then subcutaneously into the region to be anesthetized. The sensory nerve endings are anesthetized. Epinephrine is often added to the solution to intensify the anesthesia in a limited region and to prevent excessive bleeding and systemic effects. Repeated injections prolong the anesthesia as long as needed. This method of administration is used for minor surgery such as incision and drainage or excision of a cyst.

Conduction (block) anesthesia involves a loss of sensation, especially pain, in a region of the body. This type of anesthesia is produced by injecting a local anesthetic into the vicinity of a nerve trunk to inhibit the conduction of impulses to and from the area supplied by that nerve (the region of the surgical site). The injection may be made at some distance from the surgical site. A single nerve may be blocked, or the anesthetic may be injected where several nerve trunks emerge from the spinal cord (paravertebral block). A more concentrated solution is required because of the thickness of nerve trunk fibers. This method of anesthesia is often used for foot and hand surgery.

Spinal anesthesia is a type of extensive nerve block that is sometimes called a subarachnoid block. The anesthetic solution is injected into the subarachnoid space and affects the lower part of the spinal cord and nerve roots.

For low spinal anesthesia, a client is placed in a flat or Fowler position. A solution with a specific gravity greater than that of the CSF is used, because the solution tends to diffuse downward. For high spinal anesthesia, Trendelenburg position with the head sharply flexed is used along with an anesthetic solution that is of lower specific gravity than the CSF (which tends to diffuse upward) or the same specific gravity as the CSF (which may diffuse upward or downward, depending on position used). Solutions with the same specific gravity as the CSF act primarily at the site of injection.

The onset of spinal anesthesia usually occurs within 1 to 2 minutes after injection. The duration of anesthesia is 1 to 3 hours depending on the anesthetic used. Spinal anesthesia is used for surgical procedures on the lower abdomen, inguinal area, and lower extremities. It may be the method of choice for clients with severe respiratory problems or with liver, kidney, or metabolic disease. Marked hypotension, decreased cardiac output, and respiratory inadequacy tend to occur during anesthesia and are considered disadvantages of this method of anesthesia.

Headache is the most common postoperative complaint and may be accompanied by hearing or seeing difficulties. Headache may be postural and occur only in the head-up or sitting or standing position. This symptom is the result of the opening in the dura made by the large spinal needle, which may persist for days or weeks, permitting a loss of CSF and decreasing CSF pressure. These symptoms are usually alleviated when CSF pressure returns to normal. Paresthesias such as numbness and tingling may occur after spinal anesthesia; these sensations are usually limited to the lumbar or sacral areas and disappear within a relatively short time. The success and safety of spinal anesthesia depend primarily on the skill and knowledge of the anesthetist.

Caudal anesthesia is produced by injecting an anesthetic solution into the caudal canal, the sacral part of the vertebral canal containing the cauda equina (the bundle of spinal nerves that innervates the pelvic viscera). It is used in obstetrics and for pelvic or genital surgery. The advantage over spinal anesthetics is that caudal anesthetics do not have direct access to the spinal cord and medullary centers. Thus the respiratory muscles and blood pressure are not directly affected, and undesirable effects are less likely to occur.

Saddle block anesthesia is sometimes used in obstetrics and for surgery involving the perineum, rectum, genitalia, and upper parts of the thighs. A client sits upright while the anesthetic is injected after a lumbar puncture and then remains upright for a short time, until the anesthetic has taken effect. The name saddle block is used because the body parts that become anesthetized are those that contact a saddle when riding.

Injectable Local Anesthetics Table 15-5 lists the injectable local anesthetics. In general, the onset of action for an anesthetic is the result of drug concentration and the targeted nerve-tissue area. The potency and duration of anesthetic action increase with lipid solubility of the drug. Table 15-5 provides further information on metabolism, indications, and pharmacokinetics.

Adverse Effects The adverse effects of injected local anesthetics generally require medical intervention. Cyanosis caused by methemoglobinemia is one of the most common adverse reactions reported with an epidural block or high spinal injection. It has been reported with all local anesthetics but is most prevalent with prilocaine. Symptoms may include weakness, breathing difficulties, increased heart rate, dizziness, or collapse.

Other reactions reported with an epidural block or high spinal injection include diaphoresis, hypotension, bradycardia or irregular heart rate, pale skin color (cardiovascular depression), diplopia, seizures, tinnitus, increased excitability, shivering, involuntary shaking (caused by stimulation of CNS), nausea, and vomiting.

The effects most commonly reported with ester compounds include skin rash and an allergic reaction manifested by edema of the face, lip, mouth, or throat. Anaphylaxis and severe hypotension have been reported but are rare.

With central nerve block anesthesia, the most common adverse effects are in the form of neuropathies or neurologic effects, including headaches. Other adverse effects include paresthesia or paralysis of the lower legs, breathing difficulties, severe hypotension, bradycardia, and backache. Some clients report a reduction or loss of sexual functions, bladder control, or bowel movements.

Meningitis-type effects are most often reported with spinal anesthesia. These effects include headaches, nausea, vomiting, and a stiff or sore neck.

Allergic effects manifested by dental anesthesia are numbing or tingling of the lips and mouth and edema of the lips or mouth. Sympathomimetic or adrenergic effects are reported with epinephrine or other vasoconstrictors. These most commonly include hypertension, shaking, increased anxiety or nervousness, tachycardia, headache, and chest pain.

Significant Drug Interactions Significant drug interactions with injectable local anesthetics are limited. However, this does not preclude a variety of unexpected responses, thus indicating the need for close observation.

Prior or concurrent administration of CNS depressant drugs may result in additive CNS depression effects. Dosages should be adjusted and monitored closely. When combined with local anesthetics, vasoconstrictor agents such as epinephrine, norepinephrine, or phenylephrine may cause impaired circulation of the area, resulting in sloughing of tissue. Ischemia resulting in gangrene may develop if vasoconstrictor agents are used for end arteries, such as toes or fingers. Extreme caution is advised.

✳ **H.T., a 60-year-old, 5'10", 102-kg man, is undergoing a herniorrhaphy. His medical history is positive for type 1 diabetes mellitus for 49 years, hypertension, and angina. The anesthesiologist chooses to provide regional anesthesia with a spinal rather than administer general anesthesia.**

General anesthesia is not always necessary for more localized surgery. With H.T.'s medical diagnosis and obesity, regional anesthesia would be appropriate. Regional anesthesia differs from general anesthesia in that the client may experience the following nursing diagnoses: risk for injury related to the loss of sensation, and decreased cardiac output related to an adverse response to the drug, and the potential complication of an allergic reaction.

The goals for H.T.'s care are the same as for a general anesthetic but the outcome criteria would also relate to the recovery of sensation in the area affected by the regional anesthesia. During and after the administration of a local anesthetic, monitor H.T. for signs of pain, allergy, and other adverse effects. Minimal monitoring parameters for H.T. are blood pressure, heart rate and rhythm, respiratory rate, skin condition, and mental status. It is especially important to monitor hypertension and cardiac status for dysrhythmias when a local anesthetic containing a vasoconstrictor such as epinephrine is administered.

Protect H.T. from trauma to the anesthetized portion of the body because the perception of pain and pressure, the body's normal protective mechanism, has been diminished or obliterated. Pressure from side rails and other objects normally perceived and avoided by the client may cause injury. After his spinal anesthetics, keep H.T. well hydrated and have him remain lying down for up to 12 hours to minimize the risk of spinal headache.

The expected outcome of H.T.'s regional anesthesia is that he will experience an effective sensory block without experiencing any adverse effects of the drug.

Role of the Nurse for Topical Anesthesia Topical anesthetic agents are prepared in a variety of forms—creams, lotions, sprays, foams, and suppositories—and unlike other anesthetic agents, nurses often administer topical local anesthetics and instruct clients in their self-administration.

With local anesthetic ointments and creams, thoroughly cleanse and dry the area before applying. When the suppository form of an agent is used, chill the drug in the refrigerator for 30 minutes, remove the wrapper, and moisten the suppository with water or a lubricant for insertion. Instruct the client in the use of the provided applicator for the rectal aerosol foam preparation. Avoid using the rectal aerosol foam if bleeding hemorrhoids are present.

Some local anesthetics may cause paralysis of the upper respiratory tract when used topically in the nose or throat; this may lead to aspiration. Measure the preparation accurately and apply it with a cotton swab; swishing should be used for application to the mouth and gums and gargling for application to the throat. Do not allow the local anesthetic to be swallowed unless this has been specifically cleared with the prescriber. Caution the client not to inhale while using the topical aerosol or spray dosage forms. After inducing local anesthesia of the nasopharyngeal area, test for adequacy of a gag reflex by touching the back of the throat with a tongue depressor or swab. To prevent aspiration, withhold food or drink until this reflex returns. Because of the variability in response, be sure each client is able to swallow before food is offered. Advise the client not to chew gum while the anesthetic is in effect, because there is a risk of biting the tongue or buccal mucosa.

For local anesthetics to be self-administered, instruct a client to use the preparation exactly as prescribed—not to use a larger amount and not to use it more often or for a longer period of time.

Summary

Anesthetic agents are invaluable in limiting pain and suffering. These agents allow surgical procedures and other painful therapies to be performed by either altering consciousness or interfering with the conduction of impulses to the pain centers of the CNS.

There are two major categories of anesthesia: general and regional (or local). General anesthesia may be achieved either intravenously or by inhalation. Regional anesthesia is obtained by injecting an anesthetic drug near a nerve trunk or into a specific site. Local anesthesia may be accomplished with either topical application or infiltration of the surgical area. Because no anesthetic agent produces analgesia, muscle relaxation, unconsciousness, and amnesic effects with perfect safety, a combination of agents is generally used, each for its specific effect; this technique is called balanced anesthesia.

Although nurses do not administer general anesthetics unless they are certified nurse anesthetists, they may be called on to assist the physician to a degree, depending on the clinical setting. It is also necessary for the nurse to have an understanding of the effects of anesthetic agents in order to provide appropriate nursing care in the perioperative period. In the preoperative period, the emphasis of the nurse is on thorough assessment and preparation of the client to alleviate anxiety and to minimize the potential for physiologic injury intraoperatively and in the postoperative period. Immediately after surgery, the need is to help the client to recover from the effects of the anesthetic safely, comfortably, and as quickly as possible. Common postoperative complications for which the nurse should be alert are hypotension, nausea and vomiting, hypoventilation, oliguria, nerve injury, paralytic ileus, thrombosis, shock, atelectasis, hypothermia/hyperthermia, and malignant hyperthermia.

Inhalation therapy can be administered by gases or volatile liquids. Because these agents are primarily exhaled and excreted through the lungs, their anesthetic effect can be rapidly reversed if respiration is maintained satisfactorily.

IV anesthetic agents are used to induce amnesia, to induce and maintain general anesthesia, and as adjuncts to inhalation anesthetics. Because of the risk of respiratory and cardiovascular depression, a client's vital signs need to be closely monitored, and resuscitation equipment must be nearby when these agents are administered.

Consciousness is not depressed with local anesthesia, but a portion of the body is rendered insensitive to pain. Because the perception of pain and pressure is a protective mechanism of the body, the observations of the nurse are important to ensure that the client does not aspirate (if topical anesthesia has been used in the nose and throat) or that tissue damage does not occur through trauma to anesthetized parts of the body.

The role of the nurse in the administration of anesthetics is generally not a direct one, but one in which assessment and protection of the client take priority.

✳ Critical Thinking Questions

- Mrs. Clarke, age 42 years, was admitted to the hospital for an abdominal hysterectomy. While you are reviewing the preoperative routine with her on the night before surgery, she asks why she should get an injection before she goes to the operating room. How do you respond?

- Differentiate between the three regional block anesthesias: caudal, saddle, and spinal. Identify a client situation in which each would be the regional block of choice?

- What are the additional nursing observations required if a client receives a local anesthetic with epinephrine rather than one without epinephrine?

Bibliography

American Society of Anesthesiologists Task Force on Preoperative Fasting and the Use of Pharmacologic Agents to Reduce the Risk of Pulmonary Aspiration. (1999). *Practice guidelines for preoperative fasting and the use of pharmacologic agents to reduce the risk of pulmonary aspiration: Application to healthy patients undergoing elective procedures.* Retrieved May 26, 2005, from http://www.asahq.org/publicationsAndServices/NPO.pdf

Anderson, D.M., et al. (Eds.). (2002). *Mosby's medical, nursing, & allied health dictionary* (6th ed.). St. Louis: Mosby.

Carpenito-Moyet, L.J. (2004). *Nursing diagnosis: Application to clinical practice* (10th ed.). Philadelphia: Lippincott Williams & Wilkins.

Chang, J.T., & Altman, RB. (2004). Extracting and characterizing gene-drug relationships from the literature. *Pharmacogenetics, 14*(9), 577-586 and linked supplemental website http://bionlp.stanford.edu/genedrug/gene_drug_predictions.html (as cited December 2, 2004).

Crenshaw, J.T., & Winslow, E.H. (2002). Preoperative fasting: Old habits die hard. *American Journal of Nursing, 102*(5), 36-44.

Donnelly, A.J., & Golembiewski, J.A. (2005). Perioperative care. In M.A. Koda-Kimble, L.Y. Young, W.A. Kradjan, B.J. Guglielmo, B.K. Alldredge, & R.L. Corelli. (Eds.) *Applied therapeutics: The clinical use of drugs* (8th ed.). Philadelphia: Lippincott Williams & Wilkins.

Drug facts and comparisons (58th ed.). (2005). St. Louis: Facts and Comparisons.

Evers, A.S., & Crowder, C.M. (2001). General anesthetics. In J.G. Hardman, A.G. Gilman, & L.E. Limbird, *Goodman & Gilman's the pharmacological basis of therapeutics* (pp. 337-365). New York: McGraw Hill.

Girard, T., Treves, S., Voronkov, E., Siegemund, M., & Urwyler, A. (2004). Molecular genetic testing for malignant hyperthermia susceptibility. *Anesthesiology, 100*(5), 1076-1080.

Katzung, B.G. (2004). *Basic and clinical pharmacology* (9th ed.). New York: McGraw Hill.

Kaye, A.D., Kucera, I., & Sabar, R. (2004). Perioperative anesthesia clinical considerations of alternative medicines. *Anesthesiology Clinics of North America, 22*(1), 125-139.

Lacy, C.F., Armstrong L.L., Goldman M.P., Lance L.L. (2004). *Lexi-Comp's drug information handbook* (12th ed.). Hudson, OH: Lexi-Comp.

Lotsch, J., Zimmermann, M., Darimont, J., Marx, C., Dudziak, R., Skarke, C., et al. (2002). Does the A118 G polymorphism at the [mu]-opioid receptor gene protect against morphine-6-glucuronide toxicity? *Anesthesiology, 97*(4), 814-819.

Mercado, D.L., & Petty, B.G. (2003). Perioperative medication management. *The Medical Clinics of North America, 8,* 41-57.

𝒆-LEARNING SUPPLEMENTS

Student CD-ROM
- Final Exam questions
- NCLEX® Examination review questions
- Pharmacology animations
- Printable chapter summary

Evolve Website (http://evolve.elsevier.com/mckenry)
- Case study on anesthetics
- Content updates, including information on new drugs

- WebLinks corresponding to this chapter
- Answers to the critical thinking questions in this chapter
- *Elsevier ePharmacology Update* newsletter
- Mosby's Drug Consult Internet Edition
- Supplemental and reference information

Mosby's drug consult. (15th ed.). (2005). St. Louis: Mosby.

Ng, A., & Smith, G. (2001). Gastroesophageal reflux and aspiration of gastric contents in anesthetic practice. *Anesthesia & Analgesia, 93*(2), 494-451.

Occupational Safety and Health Administration, U.S. Department of Labor. (2004). Retrieved May 26, 2005, from http://www.osha.gov/SLTC/wasteanestheticgases/index.html.

Phipps, W.J., Monahan, F.D., Sands, J.K., Marek, J.F., & Neighbors, M. (2003). *Medical-surgical nursing: Health and illness perspectives* (7th ed.). St. Louis: Mosby.

Quinlan, J.J., Ferguson, C., Jester, K., Firestone, L., & Homanics, G.E. (2002). Mice with glycine receptor subunit mutations are both sensitive and resistant to volatile anesthetics. *Anesthesia & Analgesia, 95*(3), 578-582.

Sei, Y., Sambuughin, N., Davis, E.J., Sachs, D, Cuenca, P.B., Brandom, B.W., et al. (2004). Malignant hyperthermia in North America: Genetic screening of the three hot spots in the type I ryanodine receptor gene. *Anesthesiology, 101*(4), 824-830.

Shammash, J.B., Trost, J.C., Gold, J.M., Berlin, J.A., Golden, M.A., & Kimmel, S.E. (2001). Perioperative beta-blocker withdrawal and mortality in vascular surgical patients. *American Heart Journal, 141*(1), 148-153.

Stekiel, T., Contney, S., Bosnjak, Z.J., Kampine, J.P., Roman, R.J., & Stekiel, W.J. (2004). Reversal of minimum alveolar concentrations of volatile anesthetics by chromosomal substitution. *Anesthesiology, 101*(3), 796-798.

USP DI: Drug information for the health care professional (25th ed.). (2005). Greenwood Village, CO: MICROMEDEX Thomson Healthcare.

ANTIANXIETY, SEDATIVE, AND HYPNOTIC DRUGS

16

CHAPTER FOCUS

Anxiety and sleep disorders are common health problems across the life span. Anxiety with apprehension, tension, or uneasiness related to anticipated danger is often a normal and beneficial response to a situation. However, excessive anxiety can interfere with daily functioning. As a group, the anxiety disorders affect approximately 15% of the population. During the course of a year, 35% of adults report episodes of insomnia, making it by far the most common sleep disorder. The antianxiety, sedative, and hypnotic drugs discussed in this chapter, along with supportive nonpharmacologic nursing care, should enable clients to increase their psychological and physiologic comfort.

LEARNING OBJECTIVES

- Describe the physiology and stages of sleep.
- Differentiate between antianxiety, sedative, and hypnotic drug effects.
- Explain specific nursing interventions when using antianxiety, sedative, and hypnotic agents in children and older adults.
- Identify the characteristics of commonly used benzodiazepines and barbiturates.
- Formulate an appropriate plan of care for a specific client receiving an antianxiety, sedative, or hypnotic agent.

▲ KEY TERMS

amnesic effect, p. 317
antianxiety or anxiolytic
  agents, p. 313
anxiety, p. 309
hypnotics, p. 313

insomnia, p. 310
non-REM sleep,
  p. 310
REM sleep, p. 310
sedatives, p. 313

✸ KEY DRUGS

diazepam, p. 320
flumazenil, p. 321
lorazepam, p. 319
zolpidem, p. 321

The agents discussed in this chapter are often categorized according to the degree of central nervous system (CNS) suppression, and are broadly referred to as anxiolytics, sedatives, hypnotics, and/or anesthetics based on the extent of their effect along this continuum from inducing calm to loss of consciousness. Any one agent may be considered in more than one of these categories depending on its dose.

✳ What is anxiety?

Anxiety is a state or feeling of apprehension, uneasiness, agitation, uncertainty, and fear resulting from the anticipation of some threat or danger, usually of psychic origin, whose source is generally unknown or unrecognized. It is usually a normal psychological and physiologic response to a personally threatening situation, such as a threat to health, body, loved ones, job, or lifestyle. It has two components: mental features (e.g., worry, fear, difficulty concentrating) and physical symptoms (e.g., racing heart, shortness of breath, trembling, pacing). In general, normal anxiety stimulates the person to take a purposeful or deliberate action to counteract or offset the anxiety-producing state. Help is necessary when excessive anxiety interferes with daily functioning and a person is unable to cope with a persistently stressful situation.

There are a number of conditions for which anxiety is a major component. These are classified by fourth edition of the *Diagnostic and Statistical Manual of Mental Disorders* as panic disorder, generalized anxiety disorder (GAD), phobic disorders (including social anxiety disorder), obsessive-compulsive disorder (OCD), posttraumatic stress disorder (PTSD), and acute stress disorder. Each of these conditions has different presenting symptoms, and treatment strategies. Panic disorder is characterized by very brief periods of intense apprehension or terror accompanied by dyspnea, dizziness, sweating, trembling, and palpitations that overcome an individual, often without warning. GAD manifests as a global anxious state existing for 6 months or more with symptoms ranging from mild, chronic tenseness, with feeling of timidity, fatigue, apprehension, and indecisiveness, to more intense states of restlessness and irritability with physical symptoms of tremor, sustained muscle tension, tachycardia, increased respiration, and profuse perspiration. OCD involves obsessions (recurrent, persistent and intrusive thoughts, ideas, and feelings generally inappropriate to the circumstance) and compulsions (behaviors or mental actions as an attempt to alleviate the obsession) that cause marked distress, consume considerable time, or significantly interfere with a client's occupational, social, or interpersonal functioning. A phobic disorder is an obsessive, irrational, and intense fear of a specific object, such as spiders (arachnophobia) or water (hydrophobia); of an activity, such as meeting strangers (xenophobia) or leaving the familiar setting of home (agoraphobia); or of a physical situation, such as heights (acrophobia) or closed spaces (claustrophobia), accompanied by symptoms of acute anxiety. Posttraumatic stress disorder (PTSD) is characterized by an acute emotional response to a traumatic event or situation involving severe environmental stress, such as a natural disaster, serious vehicular accident, or military combat. Behavioral interventions and environmental changes are commonly used modalities to treat these conditions. Drug therapy for these conditions may include the antianxiety drugs (e.g., the benzodiazepines) but more often involves other drug therapy (e.g., antidepressants, which are discussed in Chapter 19). Table 16-1 further differentiates each of these conditions.

✳ What is insomnia?

Insomnia refers to an altered pattern of falling asleep, staying asleep or both. Each year, about a third of the general population experience insomnia to some degree, and it constitutes the most common of sleep disorders. To better understand insomnia, it is helpful to review the normal physiology of sleep.

Physiology of Sleep

Sleep is a recurrent, normal condition of inertia and unresponsiveness during which an individual's overt and covert responses to stimuli are markedly reduced. During sleep a person is no longer in sensory contact with the immediate environment and stimuli that bombard the senses of sight, hearing, touch, smell, and taste during the waking hours. Such factors no longer attract attention or exert a controlling influence over voluntary and involuntary movements or functions. It is not difficult to understand that everyone needs to escape from constant stimuli.

Research has shown that sleep is not one level of unconsciousness but consists of two basic stages that occur cyclically:

* Nonrapid eye movement (non-REM) sleep
* Rapid eye movement (REM) sleep

The stages of sleep are based on electrical activity that can be observed in the brain with an electroencephalogram (EEG). The EEG provides graphic illustrations of brain waves, which are an indication of the electrical activity occurring in the brain (Figure 16-1).

During sleep an individual moves through the four stages of **non-REM sleep.** These first four stages are characterized on the EEG by alpha waves, which are slow and of low amplitude; stage 4 is considered the deepest level of non-REM sleep. The individual then moves through the fifth stage of sleep, **REM sleep,** which is characterized by rapid eye movement, dreaming, and delta waves on the EEG; these sleep-wake cycles vary across the life span (Figure 16-2). Alternating periods of REM and non-REM sleep occur throughout the night (McCance & Huether, 2002). It should be kept in mind that REM sleep is not synonymous with light sleep. It takes a more powerful stimulus to arouse a person from REM sleep than from synchronous slow-wave sleep.

The dynamic physiologic equilibrium of the body continues to be maintained even during sleep. Depression of physiologic functions occurs during deep, nondreaming sleep, whereas an increase in functions occurs during dreaming. It is known that the following occurs during nondreaming sleep:

* Blood pressure falls by 10 to 30 mm Hg
* Pulse rate is slowed
* Metabolic rate is decreased
* Gastrointestinal tract activity is slowed
* Urine formation is slowed
* Oxygen consumption and carbon dioxide production are lowered
* Body temperature is decreased slightly
* Respirations are slower and shallower
* Body movement is minimal

Dreaming sleep tends to increase most of these parameters. Body movements are more noticeable—turning, jerking, moving the arms and legs, talking, crying, or laughing—and eye movements are visible under the closed lids.

Sleep research indicates that there are psychological and physiologic reasons for the body to maintain equilibrium

TABLE 16-1 PSYCHIATRIC CONDITIONS WITH ANXIETY AS A COMPONENT

Condition	Presenting Symptoms	Treatment Alternatives
Panic disorder	Brief period of intense fear or discomfort in which 4 or more of the following develop abruptly and reach peak within 10 minutes: • Palpitations, pounding or accelerated heart rate • Trembling or shaking • Sensations of shortness of breath or smothering • Feeling of choking • Chest pain/discomfort • Nausea • Dizziness • De-realization or depersonalization • Fear of losing control or going crazy • Fear of dying • Paresthesias • Chills or hot flashes	Behavioral therapy SSRI antidepressants Tricyclic antidepressants Benzodiazepines β-adrenergic blockers
Generalized anxiety disorder (GAD)	Excessive anxiety or worrying more days than not for at least 6 months. Anxiety or worrying is associated with 3 or more of the following: • Restlessness • Fatigue • Difficulty concentrating • Irritability • Muscle tension • Sleep disturbance	Behavioral Benzodiazepines Buspirone
Obsessive-compulsive disorder (OCD)	Obsessions: • Recurrent or persistent thoughts, impulses or images that are experienced that are intrusive and inappropriate and cause marked anxiety or distress. • The thoughts, impulses, or images are not simply excessive worries about real-life problems. • The person attempts to ignore, suppress such thoughts, impulses, or images, or to neutralize them with some other thought or action. • The person recognizes that the obsessive thoughts, impulses, or images are a product of his or her own mind. Compulsions: • Repetitive behaviors or mental acts that the person feels driven to perform in response to an obsession or according to rules that must be applied rigidly. • The behaviors or mental acts are aimed at preventing or reducing distress or preventing some dreaded event or situational however, these behaviors or mental acts are not connected in a realistic way with what they are designed to prevent.	Tricyclic antidepressants (clomipramine) SSRIs Benzodiazepines
Phobias	• Marked or persistent fear of one or more social or performance situations in which the person is exposed to unfamiliar people or possible scrutiny by others. • Individual fears that he or she will act in a way that will be embarrassing or humiliating. • Feared social situations are avoided or else endured with intense anxiety or distress. • Significant impairment to social and occupational functioning.	Behavioral therapy SSRIs Benzodiazepines
Posttraumatic stress disorder (PTSD)	• Distressing, intrusive, and recurrent recollections of a traumatic stressor. • Individual fears that he or she will act in a way that will be embarrassing or humiliating. • Feared social situations are avoided or else endured with intense anxiety or distress. • Significant impairment to social and occupational functioning.	Behavioral therapy SSRIs Other antidepressants Atypical antipsychotics Prazosin (Peskind, Bonner, Hoff, & Raskind, 2003).

Modified from American Psychiatric Association (2000). *Diagnostic and statistical manual of mental disorders, fourth edition, text revision.* Washington, DC: American Psychiatric Association.

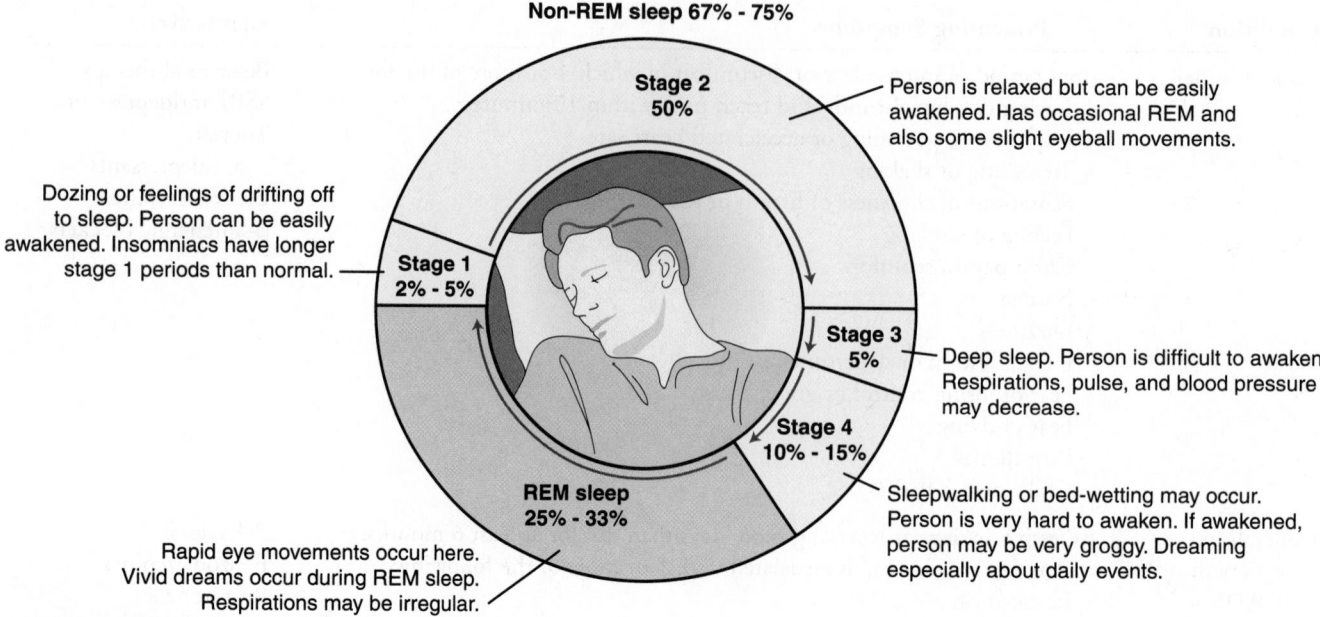

Non-REM sleep 67% - 75%

Stage 2
50%

Person is relaxed but can be easily awakened. Has occasional REM and also some slight eyeball movements.

Dozing or feelings of drifting off to sleep. Person can be easily awakened. Insomniacs have longer stage 1 periods than normal.

Stage 1
2% - 5%

Stage 3
5%

Deep sleep. Person is difficult to awaken. Respirations, pulse, and blood pressure may decrease.

Stage 4
10% - 15%

REM sleep
25% - 33%

Sleepwalking or bed-wetting may occur. Person is very hard to awaken. If awakened, person may be very groggy. Dreaming especially about daily events.

Rapid eye movements occur here. Vivid dreams occur during REM sleep. Respirations may be irregular.

FIGURE 16-1 Stages of sleep.

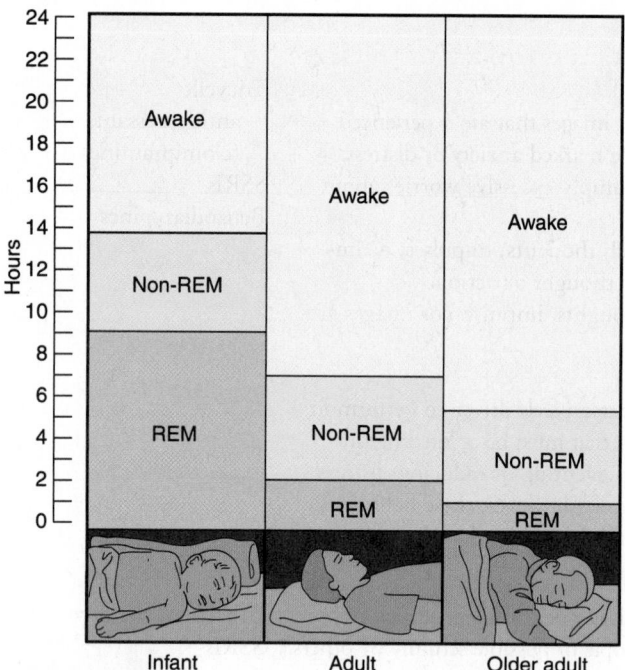

FIGURE 16-2 Sleep-wake cycles across the life span. During infancy and young childhood, REM sleep predominates, but REM sleep declines and stabilizes at about 1 year of age. Awake time starts to increase during young adulthood. Older adults have a longer wake time while trying to get to sleep, and more frequent, brief arousals.

between the various stages of sleep. Studies show that when individuals are deprived of deep sleep, they become physically uncomfortable, tend to withdraw from their friends and society, become less aggressive and outgoing, and manifest concern over vague physical complaints and changes in bodily feelings. The overall impression made by persons de-

prived of deep sleep is that of a depressive and hypochondriac reaction.

Dream sleep is also important. Many psychologists and psychiatrists believe that wish fulfillment finds expression in dreams and that potentially harmful thoughts, feelings, and impulses are released through dreams so there is no interference with the functioning of the personality during waking hours.

Studies indicate that subjects deprived of dreaming sleep (awakened every time they attempt to dream, as evidenced by rapid eye movements) experienced a variety of undesirable effects afterward. During waking hours these individuals became less integrated and less effective and exhibited signs of confusion, suspicion, and withdrawal. They appeared anxious, insecure, and irritable; had greater difficulty concentrating; had a marked increase in appetite with a definite weight gain; and were introspective and unable to derive support from other people.

It is also known that the longer dream deprivation continues, the greater the increase in attempts to dream until the individual begins to dream almost on falling asleep. When subjects are finally allowed to dream, a marked increase in dreaming is noted for the entire night, and as much as 75% of the night may be spent in dreaming. This amount diminishes for each succeeding recovery night until the individual reestablishes his or her normal sleep pattern.

Research shows that deep sleep takes priority over dreaming sleep when there has been prolonged sleep deprivation. In other words, deep sleep needs are met first, after which dreaming sleep needs are met. The body then attempts to reestablish the normal equilibrium between the sleep stages.

Each individual establishes his or her own normal sleep pattern, which may vary from night to night and is influenced by the individual's emotional and physical state. For

BOX 16-1 CAUSES OF INSOMNIA

HEALTH-RELATED

- Chronic pain disorders (e.g., osteoarthritis, metastatic disease)
- Respiratory problems (e.g., asthma, chronic obstructive pulmonary disease)
- Neurologic problems (e.g., Parkinson's disease, nocturnal myoclonus)
- Cardiovascular problems that cause dyspnea
- Endocrine problems (e.g., hyperthyroidism, degenerative disease)
- Lower urinary tract problems (e.g., benign prostatic hyperplasia and detrusor instability that cause urinary frequency)
- Gastrointestinal problems (e.g., gastroesophageal reflux disease, constipation)
- Pruritic skin conditions
- Sleep apnea

PSYCHIATRIC

- Anxiety
- Major depression
- Dementia

DRUG USE

- See Table 16-2

PRIMARY SLEEP DISORDERS

- Excessive arousal and wakefulness
- Poor sleep hygiene related to lifestyle
- Sleep state misperception: achievement of adequate sleep but not perceived by client

Modified from Arcangelo, G., & Peterson, A.M. (Eds.). (2001). *Pharmacotherapeutics for advanced practice.* Philadelphia: Lippincott Williams & Wilkins.

most individuals, any disturbance in the sleep pattern will cause insomnia. Because drugs affect physical and emotional states, they also influence an individual's sleep pattern. Box 16-1 lists selected causes of insomnia.

✳ What is the role of drug therapy in the treatment of anxiety or insomnia?

Nondrug interventions should always be considered in the treatment of both anxiety and insomnia. Environmental and dietary changes, evaluation of the use of concurrent drugs that may be stimulating, and the use of biofeedback and behavioral modalities are often effective in correcting the problem. Table 16-2 outlines substances associated with anxiety or insomnia; their use should be addressed before instituting drug therapy. In the case of insomnia, sleep patterns can be improved by instituting good sleep hygiene practices, as outlined in Table 16-3.

Agents discussed in this chapter are often categorized according to degree of CNS suppression, and are broadly referred to as anxiolytics, sedatives, hypnotics, and/or anesthetics based on the extent of effect. An agent may be considered in more than one category depending upon dose.

The antianxiety or anxiolytic agents reduce feelings of excessive anxiety, such as apprehension, fear, nervousness, worry, or panic, and are used when non-drug interventions are not effective or are inappropriate for the degree of symptoms present. Sedatives reduce nervousness, excitability, or irritability by producing a calming or soothing effect; these agents are generally considered more sedating than the anxiolytics. Hypnotics are used to induce sleep. The major difference between a sedative and a hypnotic is the degree of CNS depression induced. A small dosage may be used for a sedative effect, and larger dosages may be used for hypnotic effects. Anesthetics, as discussed in Chapter 15, produce significant CNS depression beyond that observed with sedatives and are generally reserved for use by those trained in anesthesia and when airway management can be assured.

⬡ Complementary and Alternative Considerations

Melatonin

Melatonin is a hormone synthesized in the body by the pineal gland and secreted into the blood and cerebrospinal fluid. It regulates the body's circadian rhythm, endocrine secretions, and sleep patterns. It may be useful for treating circadian rhythm sleep disorders related to jet lag (Arendt, 2003; Spitzer et al., 1999) but the International Consensus Conference on the Treatment of Insomnia indicates that melatonin has no established place in the treatment of insomnia (Stimmel & Dopheide, 2000). Advise consumers selecting melatonin that the safety and efficacy of melatonin has not been clearly established and that its purity is not regulated by the Food and Drug Administration (FDA). Although the usual doses of 0.5 to 5 mg are usually well tolerated, its adverse effects include sleepiness, headache, and nausea (Kryger, Roth, & Dement, 2000).

Among the first sedative/hypnotics were ethanol and the opioid derivatives where the secondary effects of sedation were used to advantage. Valerian, kava kava, and melatonin are natural substances that have long been used as sedatives; see the Complementary and Alternative Considerations box above for additional information on melatonin; safety and efficacy issues for valerian and kava kava are discussed in Chapter 12. Potassium and sodium bromides were used in the early twentieth century but are no longer considered safe and effective. A myriad of other sedative agents, including methaqualone (Quaalude), meprobamate (Miltown), glutethimide (Doridan), methyprylon (Noludar), and ethchlorvynol (Placidyl) have been largely replaced with safer and more effective alternatives as well. The primary categories of anxiolytic/sedative/

TABLE 16-2 AGENTS ASSOCIATED WITH ANXIETY OR INSOMNIA

Category	Item	Drug/Chemical
Foods	Coffee/tea/soft drinks	caffeine
	Cocoa	theobromine
Antidepressants	SSRIs*	fluoxetine (Prozac), others
	Other antidepressants	bupropion (Wellbutrin, Zyban)
Antipsychotics	Dopamine antagonists	haloperidol (Haldol), others (akathisia)
Cough/cold	Decongestants	pseudoephedrine (Sudafed, others)
Dietary aids	Stimulants to reduce appetite	ephedra (no longer on market) Various OTC products
Drugs of abuse	Psychostimulants	amphetamines, cocaine, others
	Hallucinogens	LSD, PCP, Ecstasy, ketamine, others
Endocrine treatments	Thyroid supplements	levothyroxine (Synthroid), others
	Corticosteroids	prednisone, prednisolone, others
Hypertension/cardiovascular	β blockers*	propranolol (Inderal), others
	Centrally acting alpha agents	methyldopa (Aldomet), clonidine (Catapres)
Late-day fluids → nocturia	Diuretics late in day	furosemide (Lasix), others
Parkinson's disease treatment	Dopamine agonists	levodopa (Sinemet), others
Psychostimulants	CNS stimulants	amphetamines, methylphenidate (Ritalin), others
Withdrawal	Benzodiazepine withdrawal	diazepam (Valium), others
	Opioid withdrawal	heroin, morphine, others
	Barbiturate withdrawal	phenobarbital, others
	SSRI withdrawal	fluoxetine (Prozac), others
	Tricyclic antidepressant withdrawal	amitriptyline (Elavil), others
	Ethanol withdrawal	ethanol

CNS, Central nervous system; *LSD*, lysergic acid diethylamide; *PCP*, phencyclidine; *SSRI*, selective serotonin reuptake inhibitor.
*Degree of anxiety varies with individual and condition treated; may be used to treat some conditions with anxiety as component.

hypnotic agents in use today include the benzodiazepines, the benzodiazepine-like drugs and the serotonergic drug, buspirone (BuSpar). To a lesser extent, barbiturates, antihistamines, and chloral hydrate (Noctec) are used in specific circumstances. The remainder of this chapter categorizes drugs based on pharmacologic action or class in lieu of the previously mentioned categories of anxiolytics, sedatives, hypnotics, and anesthetics.

❋ How do benzodiazepines work?

Benzodiazepines do not exert a general CNS depressant effect. Instead a wide range of selectivity is seen with various members of this class. Some general pharmacologic properties of this class include muscle relaxant, antianxiety, antiseizure, and hypnotic effects.

At least two benzodiazepine receptors have been identified: BZ_1 and BZ_2. The BZ_1 receptors are primarily located in the cerebellum and are believed to mediate the antianxiety and sedative effects. BZ_2 receptors are found in the basal ganglia and hippocampus and are associated with muscle relaxation and cognitive effects (memory and sensory functions).

Benzodiazepines potentiate the effects of the inhibitory neurotransmitter gamma-aminobutyric acid (GABA) by binding to BZ_1 and BZ_2 receptors in the brain and spinal cord. This increases the effect of GABA on chloride influx and results in hyperpolarization of the cell membrane and nerve inhibition. See the Special Considerations for Pharmacogenetics box on p. 315 for issues with anxiolytics/sedatives.

The limbic system, which is associated with the regulation of emotional behavior, contains a highly dense area of

TABLE 16-3 PRINCIPLES OF GOOD SLEEP HYGIENE

Principle	Explanation
Go to bed only when sleepy	Going to bed when wide awake may lead to excessive tossing and turning before falling asleep. Consider a warm, decaffeinated drink before bed.
Environment of bedroom should evoke pleasant/restful thoughts	Avoid bringing work or nonpleasure reading to bed. Avoid eating in bed and excessive environmental stimulation in the room (e.g., television). Consider addition of "white noise" (sound machine emulating rainfall, water movement, etc.) to room. Keep the bedroom slightly cool; warm rooms and excessively cold rooms disturb sleep. Keep the room darkened. Write down recurrent thoughts and disturbing thoughts that interfere with sleep and consider a plan of action to solve the problem.
Do not remain in bedroom for extended periods in a wakeful, agitated state	If not asleep in 15-20 min, consider moving to another room and engage in a relaxing activity (e.g., reading, meditation).
Use regular sleep schedule	Going to bed and waking up the same time each day strengthens circadian cycling. Avoid daytime naps.
Avoid late-day stimulation	Avoid ethanol, caffeine, theobromine-containing foods, or smoking, especially late in day. Taking 30 min before bedtime to relax helps sleep onset. Write down things that need to be done the next day and clear your mind. Avoid eating a heavy meal late in the day. Exercise earlier in the day, not just before bed. Engage in calming activity before bed (e.g., reading, meditation). Get as much outside light in the morning and during the day as possible.

Modified from Cohen, L., Tessier, E., & Germain, M. (2003). Neuropsychiatric complications. In H.R. Brady & C.S. Wilcox (Eds.), *Therapy in nephrology and hypertension* (2nd ed.). St. Louis: Mosby.

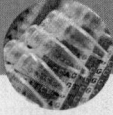 Special Considerations for Pharmacogenetics | ANXIOLYTICS/SEDATIVES

PHARMACODYNAMICS

Function at GABA, benzodiazepine, and serotonin receptors purportedly displays genetic variation in animals (Belzung, 2001; Belzung, Le Guisquet, & Griebel, 2000). These receptors appear to play important roles in anxiety and its treatment. However, the clinical impact of these findings in humans remains unclear but may account for differences among individuals in response to benzodiazepines (Rodgers, 2001).

PHARMACOKINETICS

The benzodiazepines and related agents are extensively metabolized by the cytochrome P450 enzyme systems. Examples of genetically based differences in metabolism include diazepam, midazolam, and zaleplon:

- diazepam (Valium): 3%-5% of whites and 13%-23% of Asians have little or no cytochrome P450 2C19 (CYP2C19) activity and are poor metabolizers of diazepam (Blaisdell et al., 2002; Tassaneeyakul et al., 2002).
- midazolam (Versed): Metabolism of midazolam is affected by cytochrome P450 3A4 for which there is con-

siderable interindividual variation. The extent of impact on midazolam clearance is probably low, however (Floyd et al., 2003).

- zaleplon (Sonata): Peak serum concentration of zaleplon was 37% higher in Japanese individuals. The effects of race on pharmacokinetics among other ethnic groups are not well defined (*USP DI*, 2005). These genetic differences in part explain variation in drug levels across populations.

Variation in barbiturate metabolism is also related to genetic markers for CYP2B6 and 2C19 (Kobayashi et al., 2004).

ADVERSE EFFECTS

Given the clear link between a number of benzodiazepines and varied clearance base on genetic predisposition (Chang & Altman, 2004), it is likely that a number of individual adverse effects observed with benzodiazepines in some clients is pharmacogenetic in nature.

benzodiazepine receptors in the amygdala that appear to correspond to the specific antianxiety effects of certain drugs. Two subtypes of GABA receptors have also been reported: GABA-A and GABA-B. The BZ_1 and BZ_2 receptors are associated with the GABA-A receptor subtype. GABA-A also has binding sites for alcohol, barbiturates, and some anesthetic agents, which may explain the cross-tolerance observed with these agents and the rationale for the use of benzodiazepines and barbiturates in the treatment of alcohol withdrawal syndrome (Marx, Hockberger, & Walls, 2002).

✳ What are the advantages of benzodiazepines over other agents?

The benzodiazepines are among the most widely prescribed drugs in clinical medicine, primarily because of their advantages over the older agents (e.g., barbiturates, meprobamate, and alcohol). Their popularity probably results from their anxiolytic and hypnotic dose-related effects, which have the following advantages: (1) lower fatality rates with acute toxicity and overdose, (2) lower potential for abuse compared with barbiturates, (3) more favorable adverse effect profiles, and (4) fewer potentially serious drug interactions reported when administered with other medications.

✳ What are the indications for benzodiazepines?

The most common indications for benzodiazepines include anxiety disorders, alcohol withdrawal, preoperative medication, insomnia, seizure disorders, and neuromuscular disease. They are also used to induce amnesia during cardioversion and endoscopic procedures as discussed in Chapter 15.

Anxiety Disorders Alprazolam (Xanax), chlordiazepoxide (Librium), clorazepate (Tranxene), diazepam (Valium), halazepam (Paxipam), lorazepam (Ativan), oxazepam (Serax), and prazepam (Centrax) are the benzodiazepines used as antianxiety agents. In addition, alprazolam (Xanax), lorazepam (Ativan), and oxazepam (Serax) are used as adjunct medications to treat anxiety associated with depression.

The root cause of anxiety should be determined and appropriately treated, with benzodiazepines used to treat acute symptoms. Long-term use of benzodiazepines may be appropriate in some circumstances, but other long-term interventions (e.g., antidepressants for OCD, panic disorder, and social phobias; buspirone for GAD; behavioral or environmental changes) should be instituted when appropriate.

Alcohol Withdrawal The benzodiazepines are the drugs of choice for the treatment of acute alcohol withdrawal (Marx et al., 2002). The medications most often used for this syndrome are chlordiazepoxide (Librium), clorazepate (Tranxene), diazepam (Valium), and lorazepam (Ativan). These drugs are very useful for the acute agitation, tremors, and other symptoms of acute alcohol withdrawal. Their use in acute situations is often in conjunction with a protocol for managing withdrawal symptoms. The revised Clinical Institute Withdrawal Assessment for Alcohol (CIWA-Ar) scale is one of the most widely accepted tools to evaluate alcohol withdrawal and is often incorporated into the proto-

col for benzodiazepine use (Jaeger, Lohr, & Pankratz, 2001).

✳ **R.W., a 29-year-old man, is brought to the emergency department by ambulance after a single-car vehicular accident. Physical examination reveals multiple contusions and a possible fractured femur. His blood ethanol level on admission was 280 mg/dL. When contacted by telephone, his wife reported that R.W. had a history of heavy drinking, had been "on a bender" for the past 3 weeks, and had missed several days of work during that time. Twelve hours after admission, R.W. begins to sweat profusely, appears anxious and agitated, and has a coarse hand tremor. He complains of nausea. His pulse is 120 beats/min.**

Treatment for alcohol withdrawal includes supportive therapy such as fluids and electrolytes and thiamine. For those with mild symptoms, this may be all that is required. However, the symptoms of withdrawal run a continuum from autonomic hyperactivity, anxiety, and delirium tremors to seizures. Those clients with more severe symptoms are managed with benzodiazepine therapy to control withdrawal symptoms.

Although guidelines for the management of alcohol withdrawal have been generally accepted, they may vary slightly depending on the health care agency's protocol. Jaeger and colleagues (2001) developed a symptom-triggered therapy for alcohol withdrawal based on the use of the CIWA-Ar (http://www.ogp.med.va.gov/cpg/SUD/SUD_CPG/ModuleA/appA_App4.htm) and benzodiazepine dosages based on those assessments. However, this process requires staff skilled in using the symptom-trigger approach. Where these are not available, a time-based management process can be used, as long as the doses are individualized for breakthrough withdrawal symptoms. See Table 16-4 for a sample protocol.

Other drugs may be used as adjuncts; clonidine and β blockers have been helpful with adrenergic responses during withdrawal.

✳ **R.W. was provided with supportive care and benzodiazepine therapy was initiated with lorazepam. He recovered from alcohol withdrawal without incident and was referred to an outpatient alcohol treatment program.**

Panic Disorders Panic disorders are most often treated with other modalities, including the use of behavioral therapy, β_2-adrenergic blockers, and antidepressants. Alprazolam (Xanax) is approved by the FDA for the treatment of panic disorders and may be part of a treatment plan for some individuals. Clonazepam (Klonopin) has also been studied in the management of panic disorders.

Preoperative Medication Parenteral lorazepam (Ativan), midazolam (Versed), and occasionally diazepam (Valium) are used preoperatively to reduce anxiety and to help induce general anesthesia. These three drugs are also used for endoscopic procedures to decrease anxiety and tension. These

TABLE 16-4 SAMPLE OF ORAL DOSING CONSIDERATIONS FOR BENZODIAZEPINES IN ACUTE ALCOHOL WITHDRAWAL

SYMPTOM-TRIGGERED REGIMEN

Administer one of the following medications every hour when CIWA-Ar is greater than 8 to 10:
- Chlordiazepoxide, 50-100 mg
- Diazepam, 10-20 mg
- Lorazepam, 2-4 mg

FIXED-SCHEDULE REGIMEN

- Chlordiazepoxide, 50 mg q6h × 4 doses, then 25 mg q6h × 8 doses
- Diazepam, 10 mg q6h × 4 doses, then 5 mg q6h × 8 doses
- Lorazepam, 2 mg q6h × 4 doses, then 1 mg q6h × 8 doses

Provide additional medication as needed when symptoms are not controlled (i.e., CIWA-Ar greater than 8 to 10).

Data from College of Pharmacy, University of Illinois at Chicago. (200%). Retrieved May 5, 2005, from http://www.uic.edu/pharmacy/services/di/index.htm.
CIWA-Ar, Clinical Institute Withdrawal Assessment—Alcohol, revised.

agents also produce an anterograde **amnesic effect,** a loss of memory about the procedure, which is a clear advantage for clients undergoing uncomfortable or potentially traumatic interventions. Such use is discussed in greater depth in Chapter 15.

Sleep Disorders The short-term use of benzodiazepines for insomnia is indicated when nondrug interventions are unsuccessful and the degree of insomnia interferes with a client's level of functioning. Estazolam (ProSom), nitrazepam (Mogadon), and temazepam (Restoril) are usually prescribed for sleep disorders such as insomnia. Concerns with their use include worsening or masking underlying sleep apnea, tolerance with chronic use, habituation, and withdrawal upon discontinuation. These agents also differ in onset and duration of action; the longer-acting agents, such as flurazepam (Dalmane), may be associated with significant morning hangover effects, whereas the shorter-acting agents, such as triazolam (Halcion), may result in early morning awakening, memory loss, and/or agitation/hallucinations.

Seizure Disorders Clonazepam (Klonopin) is available orally as an antiepileptic drug in treating primarily myoclonic seizures. Parenteral diazepam (Valium) and lorazepam (Ativan) are indicated for intractable, repetitive seizures such as status epilepticus. Midazolam (Versed) has also been used for controlling seizures, although this is not an FDA-approved indication. Benzodiazepines are generally not used for the long-term management of seizures as efficacy wanes over weeks or months of continuous use. Chapter 17 presents a more complete discussion of the role of benzodiazepines in controlling seizures.

Neuromuscular Disease Other skeletal muscle relaxants, such as methocarbamol (Robaxin) and baclofen (Lioresal) are more commonly used to treat skeletal muscle spasms related to acute or chronic musculoskeletal conditions. Benzodiazepines, however, may be useful as adjunct therapy for the treatment of skeletal muscle spasms caused by muscle or joint inflammation or spasticity resulting from upper motor neuron dysfunction, such as cerebral palsy and paraplegia. Diazepam (Valium) is the most commonly used benzodiazepine for this purpose because of its long duration of action.

✳ How do benzodiazepines differ pharmacokinetically?

While all benzodiazepines appear to have similar action at benzodiazepine receptors, they differ widely in their pharmacokinetic profile. Oral benzodiazepines are readily absorbed from the gastrointestinal (GI) tract. Clorazepate (Tranxene) and diazepam (Valium) are the most rapidly absorbed drugs in this class. The more rapidly absorbed benzodiazepines usually produce a more prompt and intense onset of action.

Most of the benzodiazepines are lipid-soluble (lipophilic) (e.g., diazepam [Valium]) and are widely distributed in the body and brain. Diazepam is also highly bound to plasma protein. Benzodiazepines accumulate in the adipose tissues of the body because of their lipid solubility. This saturation of storage sites accounts for greater blood concentration and longer action with repeated use; it also explains the prolonged action of benzodiazepines after they have been discontinued.

The GI tract and the liver are the sites of cytochrome P450 metabolism for benzodiazepines. The acid environment of the stomach is the site of conversion of clorazepate (Tranxene) to its active form, desmethyldiazepam, a long-acting metabolite (30 to 100 hours). Prazepam (Centrax, which is not available in the United States) also undergoes metabolism in the stomach and liver to the active metabolite desmethyldiazepam. Chlordiazepoxide (Librium), diazepam (Valium), and flurazepam (Dalmane) are converted to active metabolites, notably desmethyldiazepam (*USP DI,* 2005). The long-acting benzodiazepines and their active metabolites are more apt to accumulate, especially in older adults, resulting in an increased risk for falls and hip fractures (*USP DI,* 2005).

Benzodiazepines such as lorazepam (Ativan) and oxazepam (Serax) that do not undergo cytochrome P450 metabolism, tend to have inactive metabolites and shorter durations of action. These agents are often preferred in older adults and in those individuals with liver disease.

The injectable benzodiazepines include chlordiazepoxide (Librium), diazepam (Valium), lorazepam (Ativan), and midazolam (Versed). The onset of the antiseizure, antianxiety, and muscle relaxant effects of these agents after intravenous (IV) administration is approximately 1 to 5 minutes. Onset of action is approximately 15 to 30 minutes after intramuscular (IM) injection. Table 16-5 gives a pharmacokinetic overview of selected benzodiazepine drugs.

TABLE 16-5 COMPARATIVE PHARMACOKINETICS OF BENZODIAZEPINES

Agent	Typical Adult Dose	Elimination Half-life	Time to Peak Effect	Active Metabolite?	Comments
SHORT-ACTING BENZODIAZEPINES					
alprazolam (Xanax)	0.25-0.5 mg PO two to three times daily	12 hr	1.5 hr	Yes	Withdrawal symptoms frequently observed if dosed less than twice daily Anecdotal reports of more habituation because of short half-life
midazolam (Versed)	1 mg IV over 2-3 min	1.9 hr	Immediate IV 45 min PO	Yes	Use typically limited to conscious sedation and adjunct to anesthesia Available airway support recommended with use
oxazepam (Serax)	10-30 mg PO three to four times daily*	8.2 hr	3 hr	No	Used typically for anxiety, alcohol withdrawal Metabolites inactive Often used for older adults or those individuals with liver disease
triazolam (Halcion)	0.125-0.5 mg PO at bedtime PRN	2.9 hr	1.3 hr	Yes	Use typically limited to insomnia Reports of early morning withdrawal, confusion
INTERMEDIATE-ACTING BENZODIAZEPINES					
estazolam (ProSom)	1-2 mg PO at bedtime PRN	10-24 hr	2 hr	Yes	Use typically limited to insomnia
lorazepam (Ativan)	0.5–2 mg PO q6-8h* 1-4 mg PO at bedtime PRN	14 hr	1.2 hr	No	Commonly used for insomnia, anxiety, alcohol withdrawal, adjunct to anesthesia, status epilepticus Metabolites inactive Often used for older adults and those with liver disease
temazepam (Restoril)	7.5-30 mg PO at bedtime	8 hr	1.5 hr	No	Use typically limited to insomnia
LONG-ACTING BENZODIAZEPINES					
chlordiazepoxide (Librium)	5-25 mg PO three to four times daily*	24-48 hr	~2 hr	Yes	Use typically limited to alcohol withdrawal
clonazepam (Klonopin)	0.25-0.5 mg PO two to three times daily	23 hr	2.5 hr	Yes	Use limited to anxiety, panic disorder, seizure control Wide variation in dose response observed
clorazepate (Tranxene)	7.5-50 mg PO daily*	93 hr	45 min	Yes	Used for anxiety, EtOH withdrawal, partial seizures
diazepam (Valium)	2-10 mg PO two to four times daily 5-20 mg IV × 1	43 hr	1.3 hr (PO)	Yes	Used for anxiety, skeletal muscle relaxation, status epilepticus Rectal, IV for seizures
flurazepam (Dalmane)	15-30 mg PO at bedtime	Active metabolite: 47-100 hr	0.5-1 hr	Yes	Use limited to insomnia Typically avoided in older adults because of hangover effect

Data from Charney, D.S., Mihic, S.J. & Harris, R.A. (2001); Epocrates Rx Version 7.0 as updated November 17, 2004.
EtOH, Ethyl alcohol; *IV*, Intravenous; *PO*, by mouth; *PRN*, as needed.
*Higher doses often used for EtOH withdrawal protocols.

❋ What are the adverse effects of benzodiazepines?

Benzodiazepines are Schedule IV substances with the potential for psychological and physical dependence. The most common adverse effects of benzodiazepines include drowsiness, hiccups (especially with midazolam [Versed]), lassitude, and loss of dexterity. Less common adverse effects include dry mouth, nausea, vomiting, headaches, constipation, abdominal cramping, unsteadiness, dizziness, and blurred vision. Inform the prescriber if adverse effects continue, increase, or disturb the client. Other adverse effects include increased behavioral problems, which are seen mostly with children (anger, decreased ability to concentrate). Paradoxical neurologic reactions are rare, but include insomnia, increased excitability, hallucinations, and apprehension. In addition, a client may experience pruritus, skin rash, sore throat, elevated temperature, increased bruising or bleeding episodes, mental depression, hepatitis, confusion, mouth or throat sores, and muscle weakness. Clients using midazolam (Versed) have reported muscle tremors, tachycardia, shortness of breath, or breathing difficulties. Contact the prescriber if adverse effects occur because medical intervention may be necessary.

❋ What benzodiazepines are available and how do they differ from each other?

A number of different benzodiazepines are available in the United States and Canada. Differences in pharmacokinetics and dosing are outlined in Table 16-5. A brief discussion of the more commonly used agents is presented below.

Short-Acting Benzodiazepines

alprazolam [al **pray** zoe lam]
(Xanax, Apo-Alpraz✸, Novo-Alprazol✸)
Indications
Alprazolam is used as an antianxiety and antipanic agent.
Pharmacokinetics/Dosing
Accumulation is minimal after multiple doses, and elimination rapidly follows termination of therapy. See Table 16-5.
Adverse Effects
In some clients, rapid decreases in dosage or an abrupt discontinuation of therapy has resulted in seizures, delirium, and withdrawal reactions. The risk of seizures is greatest within 1 to 3 days of abrupt discontinuation. To reduce or avoid the potential for these adverse effects, alprazolam should be gradually tapered at 3- to 5-day intervals (dosing at least three times daily) until discontinued.

midazolam [**mid** ay zoe lam]
(Versed)
Used as a component of balanced anesthesia; see p. 294, Chapter 15.

oxazepam [ox **a** ze pam]
(Serax, Apo-Oxazepam✸)
Indications
Oxazepam is indicated for anxiety associated with mental depression and for the treatment of acute alcohol withdrawal symptoms.
Pharmacokinetics/Dosing
The metabolism of oxazepam does not involve the cytochrome P450 system, and it does not have an active metabolite. Drug accumulation is minimal during multiple-dose therapy, and the drug is rapidly eliminated when discontinued. Because of its rapid clearance, ox-

azepam is often considered a preferred agent to use in older adults and in individuals with hepatic insufficiency. See Table 16-5.
Adverse Effects
Similar to other oral benzodiazepines.

triazolam [trye **ay** zoe lam]
(Halcion, Apo-Triazo✸)
Indications
Triazolam is an infrequently used sedative-hypnotic because of its adverse-effect profile.
Pharmacokinetics/Dosing
See Table 16-5.
Adverse Effects
A number of reports of anterograde amnesia (Mintzer & Griffiths, 2003), more profound reductions in REM sleep and a relatively high rate of paradoxical rage reactions have all been reported with triazolam. Although each type of reaction is possible with all of the benzodiazepines, the rates of such reactions with triazolam have rendered it less popular.

Moderate-Acting Benzodiazepines

estazolam [es ta **zoe** lam]
(ProSom)
Indications
Estazolam is similar to the other hypnotic benzodiazepines. It is indicated for the short-term treatment of insomnia.
Pharmacokinetics/Dosing
It is widely distributed in the body and easily crosses the blood-brain barrier. (See Table 16-5.)
Adverse Effects
Similar to other oral benzodiazepines. It has an intermediate to long half-life and is less likely to cause rebound insomnia after drug withdrawal.

⭐ lorazepam [lor **a** ze pam]
(Ativan, Apo-Lorazepam✸, Novo-Lorazem✸)
Indications
Lorazepam is among the most commonly used benzodiazepines. It is indicated for use as an antianxiety agent, sedative-hypnotic, amnesic, antitremor agent, adjunct skeletal muscle relaxant, antiepileptic drug (parenteral only), antiemetic in cancer chemotherapy (parenteral only), and for the treatment of acute alcohol withdrawal symptoms and tension headaches.
Pharmacokinetics/Dosing
Like oxazepam, the metabolism of lorazepam does not involve the cytochrome P450 systems and it does not have an active metabolite. Because of its rapid clearance, lorazepam is considered a preferred agent for use with older adults and with individuals with hepatic insufficiency. Lorazepam must be mixed with an equal amount of a compatible diluent (dextrose 5% in water [D_5W] solution, normal saline [NS], sterile water for injection) immediately before IV use. It may be infused directly into a vein or through IV tubing. Infusion rates are not to exceed 2 mg/min. Intraarterial injection should be avoided because it can cause arteriospasm and gangrene. IM lorazepam is injected undiluted into deep muscle mass. The tablet dosage form may be administered orally or sublingually. See Table 16-5 for comparative pharmacokinetics.
Adverse Effects
Similar to other benzodiazepines.

temazepam [te **maz** e pam]
(Restoril, Apo-Temazepam✸, Novo-Temazepam✸)
Indications
Temazepam is indicated as a sedative-hypnotic.

Pharmacokinetics/Dosing
Only minimal accumulation occurs during multiple doses, and elimination is rapid when therapy is discontinued. The slow absorption pattern of temazepam means that it usually takes 1 to 2 hours to reach effective blood levels. Its effectiveness for inducing sleep can be enhanced with proper scheduling of its administration—1 to 1.5 hours before bedtime. (See Table 16-5.)

Adverse Effects
Similar to other benzodiazepines.

Long-Acting Benzodiazepines

The long-acting benzodiazepines may achieve their prolonged duration of action secondary to either a prolonged elimination half-life and/or production of an active metabolite or metabolites that prolong the duration of effect. Many of these agents also have a strong affinity for body tissues and are displaced from those tissues slowly after the drug is discontinued. Long-acting benzodiazepines have the advantage of having less withdrawal phenomenon upon abrupt withdrawal after chronic use. A disadvantage for these agents, however, may be a sense of grogginess or hangover.

chlordiazepoxide [klor dye az e **pox** ide]
(Librium, Libritabs, Apo-Chlordiazepoxide❦, Novopoxide❦)
Indications
Chlordiazepoxide was one of the first benzodiazepines to be developed and used clinically. Besides its use as an antianxiety agent, chlordiazepoxide is also used as a sedative-hypnotic, an antitremor drug, an antipanic agent (parenteral), and for the relief of acute alcohol withdrawal symptoms. It has also been used to treat tension headaches.

Pharmacokinetics/Dosing
Parenteral IV administration is preferred to IM injection, because IM absorption is slow and erratic. IV administration should be slow, over a period of at least 1 minute. Be careful not to use the IM diluent when preparing a solution for IV administration, because the IM diluent tends to form air bubbles.

When preparing a chlordiazepoxide solution for IM administration, use only the manufacturer's diluent, and administer the drug deeply into the muscle. Mixing the drug with sodium chloride or sterile water for injection will cause pain on injection. Use solutions immediately after reconstitution, and discard any unused solution. Because the long-acting metabolites remain in the bloodstream for several days, monitor the client for cumulative effects of the drug. (See Table 16-5.)

Adverse Effects
Similar to other benzodiazepines.

clonazepam [kloe **na** zi pam]
(Klonopin, Clonapam❦, Rivotril❦)
Indications
Clonazepam is used as an antiepileptic drug and for the treatment of panic disorders. When used as an antiepileptic drug, clients receiving long-term therapy should avoid abrupt withdrawal because this may result in seizures. However, tolerance develops after a few months of therapy, resulting in a loss of antiseizure activity in up to 30% of clients (*USP DI*, 2005). While dosage adjustments may restore the efficacy of clonazepam as an antiepileptic drug, its long-term use as an antiepileptic drug is typically reserved for circumstances where alternative therapies have not been successful.

Pharmacokinetics/Dosing
Clonazepam administered concurrently with carbamazepine may result in a decrease in the serum levels and half-life of clonazepam. (See Table 16-5.)

Adverse Effects
Similar to other benzodiazepines. Clients receiving combination antiseizure therapies should be monitored closely.

clorazepate [klor **az** e pate]
(Tranxene, Novo-Clopate❦)
Indications
Clorazepate is used as an antianxiety agent, sedative-hypnotic, antiepileptic drug, and for the relief of acute alcohol withdrawal symptoms.

Pharmacokinetics/Dosing
When given orally, it is one of the most rapidly absorbed benzodiazepines. (See Table 16-5.)

Adverse Effects
Similar to other benzodiazepines.

⬛✶⌐ diazepam [dye **az** e pam]
(Valium, Apo-Diazepam❦, Vivol❦)
Indications
Diazepam is considered the prototype benzodiazepine. It is used as an antianxiety agent, sedative-hypnotic, antiepileptic drug, skeletal muscle relaxant, antitremor agent, and antipanic agent. It is also indicated for the treatment of acute alcohol withdrawal, status epilepticus, tension headache, temporomandibular joint disorders, and as a preoperative medication. Parenteral diazepam also has an amnesic indication.

Pharmacokinetics/Dosing
IV administration should be accomplished slowly, at least 1 minute for each 5 mg, to prevent apnea, hypotension, bradycardia, or cardiac arrest. IV injection should be made into a large vein, not small veins such as those found on the back of the hand and wrist.

Diazepam is not compatible with aqueous solutions. Continuous IV infusion is not recommended because diazepam may precipitate in the infusion bag and be adsorbed by the plastic infusion bags and tubing. If direct IV injection is not possible, the drug should be slowly injected through an infusion port as close as possible to the point of the needle or cannula insertion. Glass infusion sets and polyethylene/polypropylene plastic syringes are recommended for the administration of diazepam emulsion. Use a diazepam emulsion within 6 hours of opening the ampule, and do not dilute it or mix it with other solutions.

Diazepam is also available in a rectal gel dosage form (Diastat) for use primarily as an antiepileptic drug. A diazepam oral solution is also available (Diazepam Intensol, PMS-Diazepam❦) (*USP DI*, 2005). This variety is very useful in helping the health care provider to select a proper diazepam dosage form for an individual client. Refer to Chapter 17 for more discussion on the use of diazepam as an antiseizure therapy. For comparative pharmacokinetics, see Table 16-5.

Adverse Effects
Similar to other benzodiazepines.

flurazepam [flure **az** e pam]
(Dalmane, Apo-Flurazepam❦)
Indications
Once very popular, flurazepam is now infrequently used as a sedative-hypnotic because of its long duration of action, morning hangover effects, and increased risk for falls. Although the sleep pattern will improve the first night, instruct the client that 2 to 3 nights might be required before flurazepam becomes fully effective.

Pharmacokinetics/Dosing
Elimination is slow; metabolites remain in the body for several days, which may produce unwanted daytime carryover effects that result in poor coordination and drowsiness, and is particularly hazardous for older adults. The effects may be overcome by using lower doses and administering the medication every other evening. The client must be warned of the sustained effect of the active metabolites. (See Table 16-5.)

Adverse Effects
Similar to other benzodiazepines, but the long half-life of active metabolite may account for excessive "hangover" effect the following day.

Pharmacokinetics/Dosing

Reversal of benzodiazepine-induced sedation requires an initial IV dose of flumazenil, 0.2 mg injected over 15 seconds. This dose may be repeated at 1-minute intervals up to a maximum of 1 mg. The same initial dose is given for a benzodiazepine overdose, usually over 30 seconds; additional doses of 0.3 mg and, if necessary, 0.5 mg may be given at 1-minute intervals up to a maximum of 3 mg of flumazenil. Refer to the current package insert for additional dosing information. The antagonistic effects of flumazenil occur within 1 to 2 minutes, a peak effect occurs in 6 to 10 minutes, and the duration of action is approximately 1 to 3 hours, depending on the dose of benzodiazepine consumed. Because most benzodiazepines have a half-life longer than 1 hour, repeated injections of flumazenil are necessary. Flumazenil is metabolized in the liver and excreted by the kidneys.

Adverse Effects

Because flumazenil will reverse the effects of benzodiazepines acutely, the risk for seizures is very real in clients who have received long-standing benzodiazepine therapy, have an underlying seizure history, or have ingested an overdose of drugs known to lower seizure threshold (e.g., antidepressants, antipsychotics). Other adverse effects include headache, visual disturbance, excess sweating, increased anxiety, nausea, light-headedness, and pain at the injection site (which can be significantly decreased by infusing the drug through a freely running IV solution into a large vein). Cardiac dysrhythmias have also been reported with the use of flumazenil. Use caution when giving flumazenil to clients who are known to use benzodiazepines chronically, because moderate to severe withdrawal symptoms may occur.

What are the alternatives to benzodiazepines?

There are a number of alternatives to benzodiazepines, including the benzodiazepine-like drugs, the serotonergic agent buspirone, the antihistamine hydroxyzine, the alcohol derivative chloral hydrate, and the barbiturates. The alternative therapies of kava kava and valerian are discussed in Chapter 12.

Benzodiazepine-like Drugs

Over the past decade, three newer agents that act at GABA receptors and are similar in action to benzodiazepines have been released. They differ from benzodiazepines in that tolerance to their sedative effect is much less likely to occur.

zolpidem tartrate [**zole** pi dem]
(Ambien)

Zolpidem tartrate was the first of a new class of drugs referred to as nonbenzodiazepine hypnotics. It is more selective than the benzodiazepines in its binding to GABA receptors. The benzodiazepines bind to omega$_1$, omega$_2$, and omega$_3$ GABA receptors, but zolpidem binds only to omega$_1$ receptors. Therefore only some of the pharmacologic properties of zolpidem are similar to those of the benzodiazepines; zolpidem lacks the antiseizure, muscle relaxant, and antianxiety properties associated with the benzodiazepines.

Indications
Zolpidem is used for the short-term treatment of insomnia.

Pharmacokinetics/Dosing
Zolpidem is rapidly absorbed orally, has a rapid onset of action, and reaches a peak serum level in 30 minutes to 2 hours. Absorption is improved if taken on an empty stomach. It is metabolized in the liver into inactive metabolites and is excreted via the kidneys (48% to 67%) and feces (29% to 42%). The adult dosage is 10 mg at bedtime. A 5-mg initial dose is recommended for older, debilitated clients and for individuals with hepatic insufficiency. No dosage has been established for clients younger than 18 years of age.

Management of Drug Overdose

Benzodiazepines

One of the advantages of benzodiazepines over other sedative hypnotics is that they rarely produce respiratory depression when they are the sole CNS depressant used. In the event that a benzodiazepine overdose is suspected or known, the client should be carefully monitored to maintain respiratory status. Usually supportive care is all that is required.

Occasionally, use of the benzodiazepine receptor antagonist flumazenil (see below) is considered, but only in cases in which benzodiazepines are the only ingested agent in a client without risk for seizure activity. Use of flumazenil in clients with a seizure history and/or multisubstance overdose may result in seizures that are difficult to treat.

Do the benzodiazepines interact significantly with other drugs?

Significant drug interactions, such as enhanced CNS depressant effects, may occur when benzodiazepines are used in combination with alcohol and CNS depressants, opioid analgesics, anesthetics, or tricyclic antidepressants. Close monitoring is necessary because the dosage of one or both drugs may need to be adjusted. Concurrent administration of benzodiazepines with zidovudine (AZT), an antiviral drug, may inhibit zidovudine metabolism, leading to an increased potential for accumulation and toxicity. If used concurrently, monitor the client closely for adverse effects.

Most of the benzodiazepines are metabolized by cytochrome P450 enzymes and interact with other drugs that have impact on these systems. The systemic antifungal drugs ketoconazole (Nizoral), itraconazole (Sporanox), and fluconazole (Diflucan) are among the drugs that are likely to increase most benzodiazepine levels via these enzyme systems. The benzodiazepines that are not metabolized by the cytochrome P450 systems include lorazepam (Ativan) and oxazepam (Serax), and are unlikely to experience fluctuations in levels when concurrently administered with other drugs.

Benzodiazepines are relatively safe in overdose when other CNS depressants are not involved. See the Management of Drug Overdose box above.

flumazenil [floo **may** ze nil]
(Romazicon)
The mechanism of action for flumazenil is competition with the benzodiazepines at the binding site of the GABA-benzodiazepine receptor.

Indications
Flumazenil, a benzodiazepine-receptor antagonist, is indicated for the treatment of a benzodiazepine overdose or to reverse the sedative effects of benzodiazepines following surgical or diagnostic procedures. This drug will not reverse the effects of opioids or other nonbenzodiazepine drugs. Although flumazenil can reverse the sedative effects of benzodiazepines, reversal of benzodiazepine-induced respiratory depression and amnesia have not been demonstrated (*USP DI,* 2005). Therefore, management of hypoventilation must include establishing an airway, ventilation assistance, and interventions to support circulation (*USP DI,* 2005).

Adverse Effects

Adverse effects include ataxia, depression, hypersensitivity reaction, rash, hypotension, nightmares, anterograde amnesia, drowsiness, dizziness, vertigo, dry mouth, nausea, vomiting, headache, tiredness, double vision, and diarrhea.

zaleplon [**zall** eh plon]
(Sonata, Starnoc✢)

Zaleplon is similar to zolpidem in its action.

Indications

Zaleplon is available for short-term management of insomnia.

Pharmacokinetics/Dosing

It is extensively metabolized by first-pass metabolism with only 30% of the oral dose reaching systemic circulation. Peak plasma levels are achieved about 1 hour after oral ingestion. The usual dose is 5 to 10 mg at bedtime.

Adverse Effects

Similar to zolpidem.

eszopiclone [es zoe **pik** lone]
(Lunesta)

Eszopiclone is similar to zolpidem and zaleplon and binds to GABA receptors to produce sedation.

Indications

Eszopiclone is indicated for the short-term treatment of insomnia.

Pharmacokinetics/Dosing

Eszopiclone is well absorbed orally and is extensively metabolized by cytochrome P450 3A4 and 2E1 with an elimination half-life of approximately 6 hours in healthy adults and 9 hours in adults over 65 years of age. The typical adult dose is 2 or 3 mg at bedtime. An initial dose of 1 mg at bedtime is recommended for older adults.

Adverse Effects

Altered taste, headache, and excessive somnolence appear to be the most commonly reported adverse effects of eszopiclone. Pulmonary infections have also been reported at higher rates with eszopiclone use.

Serotonergic Anxiolytics

buspirone [**byoo** spye rone]
(BuSpar, Buspirex✢, Bustab✢)

Buspirone is not related pharmacologically to the other medications discussed in this chapter. Its exact mechanism of action is unknown, but the drug has a high affinity for serotonin receptors and a moderate affinity for D_2 dopamine receptors in the CNS. It does not affect GABA, nor does it have any significant affinity for the benzodiazepine receptors.

Indications

It is indicated for the treatment of anxiety disorders as an alternative to the benzodiazepines, but usually with less sedation.

Pharmacokinetics/Dosing

Although buspirone is very well absorbed, it undergoes extensive first-pass metabolism in the liver. Protein binding is high (95%). The onset of effect may take 1 to 2 weeks, with full effect often not noted for 3 to 6 weeks. Clients may not notice any effects during this time because the medication does not cause muscle relaxation or sedation. The half-life (elimination) is between 2 and 3 hours after a single 10- to 40-mg dose. Buspirone is metabolized in the liver with one active metabolite. It is excreted in the urine and feces. The recommended dosage for adults is 5 mg by mouth (PO) two or three times daily, increased by 5 mg daily every 2 to 3 days, until the desired response is achieved. Many clients respond to doses of 10 mg three times daily. The maximum dosage is 60 mg daily. No dosage has been established for persons younger than 18 years old.

Adverse Effects

Adverse effects include headache, nausea, increased nervousness, faintness, tinnitus, abdominal distress, insomnia, nightmares, increased weakness, dry mouth, blurred vision, muscle pain or spasms,

and decreased ability to concentrate. Rare adverse effects include chest pain, tachycardia, muscle weakness, paresthesia, sore throat, elevated temperature, depression, and confusion.

Antihistamine Anxiolytics

hydroxyzine [hye **drox** i zeen]
(Atarax, Vistaril, Apo-Hydroxyzine✢, Novohydroxyzine✢)

Hydroxyzine, a piperazine antihistamine, is an antianxiety agent, sedative-hypnotic, antihistamine, and antiemetic. The antianxiety effect may be caused by the suppression of activity in selected subcortical areas of the CNS, but its full mechanism of action is unknown. Its antihistamine and sedative effects are a result of competition with histamine at H_1 receptor sites. The antiemetic, anti-motion sickness, and antivertigo effects of hydroxyzine may be the result of central anticholinergic activity and decreased vestibular stimulation and labyrinthine function. Hydroxyzine may also have an effect on the chemoreceptive trigger zone.

Indications

Hydroxyzine is used in the treatment of anxiety, as a sedative, and in the treatment of pruritus. Unlabeled uses include the treatment of motion sickness and nausea/vomiting, and the management of ethanol withdrawal symptoms. Hydroxyzine is often a preferred agent in the management of acute anxiety for clients with a history of substance abuse since hydroxyzine is not associated with dependency.

Pharmacokinetics/Dosing

Hydroxyzine is absorbed well. Onset of action occurs 15 to 30 minutes after an oral dose. The duration of effect is 4 to 6 hours when the drug is given orally, and the half-life is 20 to 25 hours. Hydroxyzine is metabolized in the liver and excreted by the kidneys. One active metabolite of hydroxyzine is cetirizine, a pharmacologically active histamine$_1$ receptor antagonist with reduced central nervous system distribution marketed as Zyrtec.

The recommended adult dosage of hydroxyzine is 25 to 100 mg PO, three to four times daily as necessary. For the management of generalized anxiety disorder, lower doses (e.g., 12.5 mg in the morning and midday and 25 mg at bedtime) are effective and are associated with less sedation. The dose for adults with insomnia is 50 to 100 mg at bedtime. When administered to children as an antianxiety agent or sedative-hypnotic, the dosage is 0.6 mg/kg body weight PO. For antihistaminic or antiemetic effects in adults, the dosage is 0.5 mg/kg body weight PO every 6 hours PRN. The parenteral adult dosage is 25 to 100 mg IM every 4 to 6 hours if necessary. When used in children as an antiemetic or adjunct to opioid medication, the dosage of hydroxyzine is 1 mg/kg body weight IM as a single dose.

Adverse Effects

Adverse effects include sedation, which usually disappears after a few days of therapy or when the dosage is reduced, and anticholinergic effects such as dry mouth, blurred vision, and constipation. The use of hydroxyzine is generally avoided in older adults due to excessive sedation and anticholinergic effects. Adverse effects are rarely reported but include skin rash and trembling or seizures (in dosages higher than recommended).

✷ **R.S., a 75-year-old man, complains to his nurse practitioner of having trouble sleeping, feeling nervous, and worrying constantly. His wife passed away last year and he resides with his daughter. R.S. was a handyman until he retired 15 years ago. With his diminished vision, he cannot do the woodworking he enjoyed in the past, and his osteoarthritis limits his gardening. He tends to spend his days in front of the television or engaged in light housekeeping chores in his little apartment attached to his daughter's house. Doing "the bills" and negotiating his physician's appointments are stressful and were tasks his wife always** did. R.S. has mild right-sided heart failure, macular degeneration, and osteoarthritis. His current medications include atorvastatin (Lipitor), furosemide (Lasix), potassium chloride, and warfarin, and he self-medicates with acetaminophen (Tylenol) for sleep. He drinks one cup of coffee in the morning and a gin and tonic or two in the evening to calm down when he feels he has had a stressful day. R.S. denies a history of psychiatric illness but states he has always been an active person and somewhat "edgy."

The nurse practitioner performs a complete physical and laboratory workup, with a thorough medical and psychiatric history, to exclude possible reversible causes, before making a diagnosis of generalized anxiety disorder. Medical illness in general, and especially in older individuals such as R.S., is associated with anxiety. Successfully managing the illness will often relieve anxiety, but other interventions may also be necessary, such as short-term anxiolytic drugs or nonpharmacologic measures. R.S.'s medications would not seem to contribute to his anxiety; however, his use of alcohol to self-manage his anxiety, although not excessive, may produce a cycle of dependency during which withdrawal can increase his anxiety. The loss of a spouse may cause profound anxiety, but this is usually self-limiting, lessening over a period of months. The onset of a chronic anxiety state often occurs during a stressful period. Whereas short-term therapy can be beneficial during acute stress, management of a primary anxiety disorder usually requires extended treatment.

The nurse practitioner ensures that R.S.'s medical conditions are controlled, and treats him for generalized anxiety disorder. She offers him support with psychotherapy, cognitive-behavioral therapy (reducing negative thoughts), relaxation training, and meditation to relieve his anxiety and improve his coping skills. Unfortunately, R.S.'s health plan has limited mental health benefits for such therapies, so the nurse practitioner instructs him in relaxation therapy and beginning meditation, and prescribes buspirone 5 mg twice daily with a return to the office in 2 weeks for follow up.

✳ One month later, R.S. reports that he is feeling in better spirits. He has decided to start using a cookbook to increase the variety of foods he has been eating and to do something "different." The only symptom that he has noticed is dry mouth, which he has been treating with frequent sips of water and sugarless hard candies.

Alcohol Derivatives

The CNS depressant effects produced by choral hydrate are believed to be caused by its active metabolite, trichloroethanol, but its exact mechanism of action is unknown.

chloral hydrate [**klor** al **hye** drate]
(Somnote, PMS-Chloral Hydrate✷)
Indications
Chloral hydrate is indicated as a sedative and as a hypnotic. Chloral hydrate is unique among the sedatives in that it has minimal impact on EEG readings, making it an ideal sedative for conscious sedation before EEG evaluations for seizure potential.

Pharmacokinetics/Dosing
The oral and rectal forms of choral hydrate are rapidly absorbed. The onset of action of a hypnotic dose occurs within 30 minutes, and the half-life is approximately 7 to 10 hours. It is metabolized in the liver and erythrocytes to its active metabolite, trichloroethanol; further liver metabolism is to inactive metabolites. It is excreted by the kidneys. The chloral hydrate elixir is difficult for clients, particularly children, to ingest because of the unpleasant taste and odor. Unless it is administered as a preoperative medication, make the elixir more palatable by mixing it with fruit juice or some type of chilled fluid (e.g., ginger ale), or administer capsules after meals with 8 ounces of fluid to decrease gastric irritation. Chill suppositories in the refrigerator for ease of administration. Client safety is essential. Assist the client with ambulation if there are signs of somnambulism, confusion, or dizziness. The adult hypnotic dosage is 0.5 to 1 g PO or rectally 15 to 30 minutes before bedtime. The daytime sedative dosage is 250 mg three times daily, after meals

Adverse Effects
Adverse effects include nausea, abdominal distress, ataxia, dizziness, drowsiness, confusion, excitability (paradoxical reaction), hallucinations, and skin rash.

Barbiturates

The barbiturates were once the most commonly prescribed class of medications for hypnotic and sedative effects. With only a few exceptions, they have been largely replaced by the benzodiazepines. Phenobarbital is generally considered the prototype drug for this classification, but it is presented more fully in Chapter 17 with other antiseizure drugs.

The barbiturates are classified according to the duration of their action as long-, intermediate-, short-, and ultra-short-acting drugs. Long-acting barbiturates require more than 60 minutes for onset and peak over a period of 10 to 12 hours. Long-acting barbiturates are used for treating epilepsy and other chronic neurologic disorders, as well as for sedation in clients with high anxiety. Intermediate-acting barbiturates have an onset of 45 to 60 minutes and peak in 6 to 8 hours. Intermediate-acting barbiturates are used as sedative-hypnotics.

The short-acting drugs produce an effect (onset) in a relatively short time (10 to 15 minutes) and peak over a relatively short period (3 to 4 hours). Short-acting barbiturates are used for treating insomnia, for preanesthetic sedation, and in combination with other drugs for psychosomatic disorders.

Ultrashort-acting barbiturates like thiopental sodium are used as IV anesthetics. They act rapidly and can produce a state of anesthesia in a few seconds. See Chapter 15 for further discussion.

The mechanism of action for barbiturates is nonselective depression of the CNS. High doses of barbiturates may induce coma and, potentially, death. Barbiturates similar to the benzodiazepines appear to enhance systems that use GABA as an inhibitory transmitter. In addition, barbiturates may also decrease excitatory neurotransmitter effects. The ascending reticular formation receives stimuli from all parts of the body and relays impulses to the cortex (thus promoting wakefulness and alertness); barbiturate depression of the ascending reticular formation decreases cortical stimuli, thus reducing the need for wakefulness and alertness. Unlike benzodiazepines, however, they will produce a dose-related respiratory depression, and are fatal in overdose.

With barbiturates, the extent of effect varies from mild sedation to deep anesthesia, depending on the drug selected, method of administration, dosage, and reaction of the individual's nervous system. The barbiturates are not regarded as analgesics and cannot be depended on to produce restful sleep when insomnia is caused by pain. However, when a barbiturate is combined with an analgesic, the sedative action seems to reinforce the action of the analgesic and to alter a client's emotional reaction to pain.

All barbiturates depress the motor cortex of the brain when used in large doses. Phenobarbital and mephobarbital (Mebaral) exert a selective action on the motor cortex even in small doses. This explains their use as antiepileptic drugs. Therapeutic doses have little or no effect on medullary centers, but large doses, especially when administered IV, depress the respiratory and vasomotor centers.

Barbiturates are commonly used as adjuncts to anesthesia and for treatment of seizure disorders; several are indicated for the treatment of insomnia. However, the benzodiazepine drugs have generally replaced these agents. Barbiturates are indicated for only short-term treatment of insomnia because they tend to lose their effectiveness in 14 days or less.

Barbiturates have been used for their sedative effects in treating anxiety and nervousness. However, for daytime use the benzodiazepines have largely replaced the barbiturates, primarily because they produce less drowsiness and ataxia.

Short-acting barbiturate anesthetics such as thiopental (Pentothal) and methohexital (Brevital) are used to induce anesthesia for selected surgical procedures. Short-acting barbiturates such as pentobarbital (Nembutal) may be used for their preanesthetic effect to reduce anxiety and facilitate anesthesia induction. Diazepam (Valium) and other benzodiazepines are often used as preanesthetic agents to help with anesthesia induction, to reduce anxiety, and to induce an amnesic effect.

Antiepileptic Drug Barbiturates are also used as second-line agents to prevent or control convulsive seizures associated with tetanus, strychnine poisoning, meningitis, eclampsia, and epilepsy. They may be prescribed alone or in conjunction with other antiepileptic drugs. Phenobarbital is used in the treatment of epilepsy (generalized tonic-clonic) and for seizures induced by fever. Mephobarbital (Mebaral) may be an alternative agent for phenobarbital.

Hyperbilirubinemia Although not approved for the treatment of hyperbilirubinemia, phenobarbital (oral and injectable) is often used to lower bilirubin concentrations to prevent or treat this condition in neonates and in clients with congenital nonhemolytic unconjugated hyperbilirubinemia.

Barbiturates are readily absorbed after oral, rectal, and parenteral administration. The soluble sodium salts are absorbed faster than the free acids. Most of the barbiturates undergo change in the liver before being excreted by the kidney. The longer-acting barbiturates are metabolized more slowly than the rapidly acting barbiturates. The slower a barbiturate is altered or excreted, the more prolonged the action. Cumulative effects result if excretion is slow and administration is prolonged.

Adverse effects of barbiturates include ataxia, drowsiness, dizziness, hangover effect, nausea, vomiting, insomnia, constipation, restlessness, faintness, headache, night terrors, hypersensitivity reaction (e.g., skin rash, exfoliative dermatitis, sore throat, fever, edema, serum sickness, apnea, bronchospasm, urticaria, and Stevens-Johnson syndrome). Stevens-Johnson syndrome is a severe, occasionally fatal, inflammatory disease of children and young adults. It is characterized by fever, bullae of the skin, and ulcers of the mucous membranes of the mouth, nose, eyes, and genitalia.

Clients of any age, but especially older or debilitated clients, may exhibit confusion, disorientation, and mental depression as a result of barbiturate use. A paradoxical reaction (increased excitability) may occur in children, older adults, or debilitated clients. Long-term barbiturate use may result in osteomalacia and rickets (bone pain or aching, anorexia, myalgia, loss of weight), which can be minimized with vitamin D supplementation. Abstinence syndrome (see Chapter 9) may be seen after abrupt withdrawal of long-term therapy, as well as seizures in clients with epilepsy; dosages should be tapered slowly. Toxic signs include very severe confusion and persistent irritability. Acute toxic effects of barbiturates may include bradycardia, confusion, respiratory problems (apnea, laryngospasm), ataxia, extreme weakness, and visual disturbances.

Instruct clients on long-term barbiturate antiseizure therapy to increase their intake of folic acid (green leafy vegetables, liver, asparagus, nuts, whole-grain cereals) and vitamin D (saltwater fish, especially salmon, sardines, and herring, organ meats, fish-liver oils, egg yolk). Also caution them about the concurrent use of alcohol, other CNS depressants, and herbals, such as kava kava and valerian. Women taking an estrogen-containing oral contraceptive may experience a decrease in contraceptive effects because barbiturates enhance the metabolism of estrogen. The prescriber may need to consider a nonhormonal birth control method or progestin-only oral contraceptive.

Special Circumstances

✲ **Are anxiolytics/sedatives/hypnotics safe for use in pregnancy?**
Most of these drugs are avoided during pregnancy because of their detrimental effect on the developing fetus. Buspirone and zolpidem are among the safer agents for use in pregnancy (see the Pregnancy Safety box on p. 325).

✲ **Are these drugs safe for use in children?**
The use of antianxiety, sedative, or hypnotic agents in children is limited. Because young children are much more sensitive to the CNS depressant effects of this classification of drugs, counseling and psychotherapy are usually tried first. Paradoxical reactions (reactions contrary to the expected reaction) have been reported with the use of barbiturates in

both children and older adults. These reactions include increased excitability, hostility, confusion, hallucinations, and perhaps an acute elevation of body temperature. Sedation may be indicated for particular situations if the drug and dosage are carefully selected for the individual child (e.g., for the treatment of severe anxiety associated with an acute attack of asthma, as an adjunct preanesthetic agent, or in the treatment of convulsive disorders). Close monitoring and assessment by a health care provider is required. See the Special Considerations for Children box below.

✳ **What issues should be considered when using sedatives/hypnotics with older adults?**

✳ **H.R., a 70-year-old woman, has a history of being unable to sleep and of pacing at night. She has just been placed in a nursing home by her family, who can no longer provide her care. Four weeks prior to her admission, she fell and broke her right hip. H.R. had a hip replacement and uses a walker to ambulate. Her sleep problems continue.**

A common concern of older adults is insomnia—difficulty falling asleep, difficulty staying asleep, or early morning awakening. Older adults have more fragmented sleeping patterns—they go to bed earlier, wake up earlier, and may take multiple daytime naps. This may be partly responsible for the changes in sleep pattern stages reported in this age group, such as a progressive decline in REM sleep (Asplund, 1999). Age-related physiologic changes may also contribute to the reported changes in sleep patterns. Many other factors may result in sleep disturbances, such as retirement, death of a close friend or spouse, social isolation, and increased use of medications (see Box 16-1). The three most common reasons for not being able to maintain sleep are respiratory difficulties, pain, and muscle or leg cramps; these underlying issues require treatment. The prevalence of insomnia increases with age and occurs nearly twice as often in women as in men (Miller, 2004). Older women are more apt to take hypnotic medications, and sleep deprivation in women is more likely to result in mood alterations.

H.R. is not unusual. Although they make up approximately 12% of the population, older adults consume between 35% and 40% of all sedative-hypnotics prescribed. The newer short-acting hypnotics zaleplon and zolpidem (both selective for the type-1 GABA-A benzodiazepine receptor) have minimal withdrawal effects and appear to be safer in the older client. If hypnotics are prescribed for older clients, they should be started at the lowest dose that will be clinically effective and have the fewest adverse effects, and for a short period of time. Some hypnotic agents, particularly the longer-acting forms, may have multiple adverse effects in the older client. These effects range from hypersomnolence and a tendency to be accident-prone to disrupted sleep structure (reduced REM sleep). See the Special Considerations for Older Adults box on p. 326.

✳ **As with any client, H.R. needs a thorough assessment to understand the etiology of her sleep disorder before a course of treatment is determined.**

PREGNANCY SAFETY
ANTIANXIETY, SEDATIVE, AND HYPNOTIC DRUGS

Category	Drug
B	buspirone, methohexital, zolpidem
C	chloral hydrate, flumazenil, hydroxyzine, pentothal, thiopental, zaleplon
D	amobarbital, benzodiazepines (alprazolam, clonazepam, clorazepate, chlordiazepoxide, diazepam, lorazepam, oxazepam, midazolam), mephobarbital, meprobamate
X	estazolam, flurazepam, hydroxyzine (first trimester), quazepam, temazepam, triazolam
Unclassified	other benzodiazepines, estazolam

Data from *Mosby's drug consult* (15th ed.). (2005). St. Louis: Mosby.

Special Considerations for Children | ANTIANXIETY AGENTS AND SEDATIVES

- Young children are more susceptible to the CNS-depressant effects of the benzodiazepines. In neonates, profound CNS depression may result because of the lower rate of drug metabolism by the immature liver.
- Because buspirone (BuSpar) use has not been studied sufficiently in persons younger than age 18 years, it is not recommended for use in this age group.
- Although diazepam (Valium) may be used in infants age 6 months and older, this drug and other benzodiazepines should not be used to treat a hyperactive or psychotic child.

- To reduce or minimize potential adverse CNS-depressant effects, carefully follow the manufacturer's dosage instructions and, whenever possible, avoid concurrent administration of other CNS-depressant types of drugs.
- Monitor child for excessive sedation, lethargy, and lack of coordination; if any of these effects are present, dosage adjustments may be necessary.
- Paradoxical reactions with the use of barbiturates have been reported in both children and in older adults. (See description under Are These Drugs Safe for Children?, p. 324.)

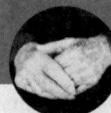

Special Considerations for Older Adults | INSOMNIA AND HYPNOTICS

- Sleep latency increases even though REM and stage 4 sleep may be absent in the older client. Sleep disturbance is a frequent concern of older adults.
- Evaluate the individual for preexisting health conditions because various illnesses, such as arthritic pain, hyperthyroidism, cardiac dysrhythmia, and paroxysmal nocturnal dyspnea, may alter sleep patterns.
- Hypnotics should be reserved to treat acute insomnia and, when prescribed, limited to short-term or intermittent use to avoid the development of tolerance and dependency.

- A hypnotic with a short duration of action is preferred. When longer-acting hypnotics are given, daytime sedation, ataxia, and memory deficits may result.
- Encourage the older client to use nonpharmacologic approaches to promote sleep.
- Be aware that older adults, children, and persons with CNS dysfunction may experience a paradoxical reaction (CNS stimulation) to hypnotics and antihistamines.

Assessment Determine H.R.'s sleep habits and how a good night's sleep is usually ensured. In this case, it also would be important to know what H.R. did at home before her fall. Such a history includes the following information:

- Environmental control, which includes ventilation, lighting, and noise (Does she prefer an open window, night light, soft music?)
- Physical care (Does she prefer a shower or bath before retiring? Does a back rub help?)
- Food (Does she prefer to snack before retiring? What foods does she like?)
- Before bed activities (Does she engage in quiet recreation, such as reading, before sleep?)
- Current sleep pattern (This may be assessed by the use of various sleep history mnemonics shown in Box 16-2.)
- Desired sleep pattern (How does the client's current sleep pattern differ from what the client desires?)

Various problems may cause the client to have insomnia. These include circadian rhythm irregularities, sleep apnea, restless leg syndrome, intake of alcohol or caffeine, use of various medications (see Box 16-1), and poor sleep hygiene, which is characterized by irregular bedtimes, daytime napping, and strenuous exercise or heavy eating just before bedtime. If the client's disturbed sleep pattern is a result of discomfort or pain at night, an analgesic or an increased dose of analgesic may be indicated at bedtime. Joint pain or stiffness that results in insomnia will usually respond to acetaminophen or a nonsteroidal antiinflammatory drug such as ibuprofen (Motrin).

It is important to determine H.R.'s general health status because older adults, as well as children, are more sensitive to the effects of sedative-hypnotics. Clients with hepatic or renal dysfunction require smaller or less frequent doses.

Obtain a thorough drug history when admitting H.R. to the nursing home and include the use of prescription, herbal, and over-the-counter (OTC) sleep preparations. This will ascertain if H.R.'s drug regimen is contributing to her sleep problems, as well as assess for drug interactions, which generally involves the use of alcohol or other CNS depressants. If H.R. brought sleep medications from home, remove these as well as all other medications for safety.

BOX 16-2 SLEEP HISTORY MNEMONICS

The following mnemonics may assist the nurse in identifying important factors in sleep assessment.

BEARS

B	Bedtime
E	Excessive daytime sleepiness
A	Awakenings
R	Regularity and duration of sleep
S	Snoring

I SNORED

I	Insomnia
S	Snoring
N	Not breathing
O	Obese/older
R	Restorative sleep
E	Excessive daytime sleepiness
D	Drugs/alcohol

REST

R	Restorative sleep
E	Excessive daytime sleepiness, tiredness, fatigue
S	Snoring nightly
T	Total sleep time

Data from Sleep Research Laboratory, University of Chicago. (2004). Sleep history mnemonics. Retrieved February 21, 2004, from http://sleepmed.bsd.uchicago.edu/SleepMnemonics.html.

✳ **H.R. is a fairly typical new resident to a nursing home, trying to cope with various medical problems and adjusting to a new life situation. The physician determines that her insomnia is difficulty falling asleep and maintaining sleep. She is medically stable and has** no major psychiatric diagnosis. For situational anxiety she was prescribed lorazepam on arrival. H.R.'s nursing notes describe her as taking 1- to 2-hour naps two to three times a day and awakening two to three times per night to urinate. She is taking the following medications: ibuprofen 400 mg PO every 8 hours, omeprazole 20 mg PO at bedtime, lorazepam 0.5 mg three times daily, hydrochlorothiazide 12.5 mg daily, potassium chloride 20 mEq daily, Senokot 1 tablet every morning and at bedtime. Zolpidem tartrate 10 mg has just been ordered for her insomnia.

The nurse is concerned with H.R.'s disturbed sleep pattern since her admission to the nursing home and has reservations about the addition of the zolpidem for sleep. One nap a day is often normal for older adults and does not interfere with sleeping through the night. H.R.'s napping is excessive and may keep her from resting well at night. Lorazepam, although prescribed for anxiety, does have sedative action and an intermediate half-life of 10 to 20 hours. Consultation with the physician results in H.R.'s lorazepam dosage being adjusted to 0.5 mg in the morning and 1 mg at bedtime and the zolpidem order being cancelled. Concurrent consumption of two or more benzodiazepine or benzodiazepine-like agents, even for daytime anxiety and bedtime insomnia, is considered inappropriate therapy. Using one benzodiazepine to accomplish both purposes is preferred because (1) the effectiveness is usually equivalent, (2) the drug will be better tolerated and controlled by a client, and (3) the therapy is less expensive. The nurse also discovered that H.R. has been "pocketing" her hydrochlorothiazide to take later in the day, so she won't have to take so many pills at once, which contributes to her nocturia. A plan of care is developed to improve H.R.'s sleep hygiene in keeping as close as possible to her past successful modalities.

Nursing Diagnosis When it is necessary to prescribe sedative-hypnotics, there is the risk for the following nursing diagnoses/collaborative problems: disturbed sleep pattern related to continuation of a client's underlying problem; disturbed thought processes (confusion); risk for falls related to the CNS effects of the drug (daytime sedation, dizziness, incoordination, ataxia); and the potential complication of paradoxical stimulation (increased irritability, hyperactivity).

Planning While on sedative therapy, H.R. will:
- Remain free of sleep deprivation.
- Remain free of falls and other adverse effects (e.g., confusion, rebound insomnia, hangover, respiratory depression, addiction).
- Implement measures for good sleep hygiene.

Implementation

Monitoring Have H.R. keep a written "sleep diary" to help evaluate the effectiveness of the medication. The diary should include foods eaten and activities engaged in before sleep, bedtimes, waking times, naps, and medication administration. Review the diary to help identify the success

of therapy or continued areas of poor sleep hygiene. Monitor for symptoms of overdose (e.g., inappropriate sleepiness, slurred speech, confusion, and respiratory depression) and tolerance (e.g., continuing and increasing anxiety and insomnia).

Intervention Because nurses are in a strategic position to influence a client's sleep through direct administration of a drug or client education, it cannot be stressed enough to exercise caution when decisions are made about giving or repeating at bedtime or as needed (PRN) order for a sleeping medication. Immediately administering a sleeping medication when H.R. indicates she is unable to sleep may do her more harm than good. Use alternative methods of relaxing her. Try using supportive nursing measures (e.g., a back rub, reduction of environmental stimuli, relaxation therapy, or a warm drink) either alone, before administering a hypnotic, or together with the drug.

If H.R. is experiencing pain or depression, these should be treated in addition to the insomnia. If a client is depressed or has a history of attempted suicide, precautions should be taken to prevent hoarding of sedative-hypnotics. Ensure that each dose is swallowed.

Many interruptions for various aspects of care can do nothing but further alter H.R.'s sleep pattern. Every effort should be made not to disrupt a sleeping client. If at all possible, other medications are scheduled before sedative-hypnotics are given. Take her vital signs before she falls asleep.

Because H.R. can become physically and psychologically dependent on sedative-hypnotic drugs, gradually taper the lorazepam dosage to avoid an abstinence syndrome reaction. Some hypnotics are used on a long-term basis, but this is not recommended. Intermittent nightly use of the drug is suggested to reduce or avoid the development of tolerance. For example, if H.R. has one or two nights of "good" sleep (as defined by her), it may be possible to omit the drug the next night.

To preclude ataxia or excessive sedation in H.R., the initial dose is small and increments may be added gradually according to H.R.'s response. Until the effects of the new dosage of lorazepam are known, caution H.R. about ambulating unassisted or unsupervised. If she were a community-based client, she would need to be cautioned against driving a car, operating machinery, or participating in any activity that may be dangerous until the effects of the drug are known. Although H.R. may deny feeling sleepy the next day, activity performance may show a definable impairment because serum levels of some of these drugs are retained. Excessive doses of benzodiazepines may result in incontinence, a loss of the ability to ambulate, or confusion in older adults who were previously continent, ambulatory, and alert.

Education Instruct H.R. that nonpharmacologic approaches to promote sleep will enhance the effectiveness of any agent prescribed (see the Complementary and Alternative Considerations box on p. 313). Clients and their families need to be taught ways to promote restful sleep without resorting to OTC sleep aids such as Sominex, Nytol, Sleep-Eze, or Unisom. Explain to H.R. that sedative or hypnotic drugs taken in combination with alcohol, antihistamines, antianxiety agents, antidepressants, or antipsychotic agents will produce an enhanced CNS depressant effect. In addition, the antimuscarinic/anticholinergic effects of antihistamines or tricyclic antidepressants may increase the risk for delirium. This combination should be avoided.

Evaluation The expected outcome of sedative-hypnotic therapy for H.R. is that she will report feeling rested and wakeful without residual drowsiness or "drug hangover" during the daytime or other adverse effects of the sedative-hypnotic regimen.

• • •

Appropriate therapy for insomnia should be limited to identification of the cause and treatment of the specific problem. Careful selection of drugs and dosages is necessary to avoid producing excessive CNS depression in older adults. The aging process may be associated with physiologic alterations, including a decline in metabolism and in many organ functions, especially liver and kidney functions. Because drug half-lives may be extended, agents with shorter half-lives and no active metabolites may be safer for older adults. Monitor older adults for paradoxical reactions (e.g., increased excitability, rage, hostility, confusion, and hallucinations), that have been reported with the barbiturates and, in rare instances, the benzodiazepines. The appearance of such adverse effects requires immediate discontinuance of the medication and consultation with the prescriber. (See Chapter 8 for additional information on inappropriate drug use in older adults.)

Barbiturates should be avoided in older adults because enhanced CNS depression, confusion, ataxia, and paradoxical reactions are commonly reported. The short-acting benzodiazepines are usually the agents of choice for treating insomnia in older adults and are much safer than the barbiturates, which are less effective anxiolytic and hypnotic agents. Studies indicate that long-acting benzodiazepines are associated with a greater risk of delirium and hip fractures (Jacobson & Jacobson, 2001). Therefore oxazepam (Serax), lorazepam (Ativan), and temazepam (Restoril), which have short to intermediate half-lives, are usually recommended for older adults who require a benzodiazepine.

It has been reported that many anxiolytic benzodiazepines may also be very effective hypnotic agents. Clients receiving a daytime benzodiazepine (e.g., alprazolam [Xanax], diazepam [Valium], or lorazepam [Ativan]) who also require temporary use of a hypnotic drug may be prescribed an equivalent hypnotic dose of the anxiolytic agent. For example, 0.5 mg alprazolam, 5 mg diazepam, and 1 mg of lorazepam are considered equivalent to 15 mg flurazepam (Dalmane), 15 mg temazepam (Restoril), or 0.25 mg triazolam (Halcion).

When possible, prescribers often suggest that older adults limit their intake of hypnotics to three or four times

per week, which allows clients to select the nights on which they need to take their medication. This schedule usually results in enhanced effectiveness, less daytime drowsiness or sedation, and a decreased potential for inducing tolerance to the medication. Regular and careful assessment, monitoring, and reevaluation of the need for hypnotics are highly recommended. See the Technology Link box above for additional sources of information on anxiolytics, sedatives, and hypnotics.

❊ Which therapies are most appropriate for an individual with a substance abuse history?
Individuals with a history of substance abuse often have concurrent anxiety, often in the context of other psychiatric conditions. For anxiety in conjunction with panic attacks, OCD, or social phobias, primary therapy with antidepressants is usually in order. For generalized anxiety disorder, many clinicians would consider the use of buspirone on a long-term basis, and a nonbenzodiazepine such as hydroxyzine, for short-term management.

With the exception of the management of alcohol withdrawal syndromes, benzodiazepines are not typically used for individuals with substance abuse. Benzodiazepines have a potential for habituation and are Schedule IV substances per the Drug Enforcement Agency of the United States. Similarly, barbiturates are Schedules II though IV substances and their use is limited to circumstances where other modalities are not effective.

Summary

When a client is unable to cope with a persistently stressful situation because excessive anxiety interferes with daily functioning, an antianxiety agent may be prescribed. Benzodiazepines are the most commonly used drugs in this group. Before their advent, sedatives were used to reduce nervousness or irritability by producing a soothing effect. Hypnotics are used to induce sleep. Sedatives and hypnotics differ only in the degree of CNS depression.

Benzodiazepines are among the most commonly prescribed drugs for a variety of disorders: anxiety disorders, alcohol withdrawal, preoperative medication, neuromuscular disease, and sleep and seizure disorders. Barbiturates, previously more widely used, have been largely replaced by the benzodiazepines. However, barbiturates are still indicated as hypnotic, antianxiety, anesthetic induction, preanesthetic, antiepileptic, and antihyperbilirubinemic agents in limited circumstances.

Benzodiazepines do not exert a general CNS depressant effect, and their wide range of selectivity of action allows their use for a variety of conditions—as antiepileptic drugs, hypnotics, muscular relaxants, and antianxiety agents. Conversely, barbiturates are used for mild sedation to deep anesthesia. A barbiturate is not an analgesic, but when administered with an analgesic it reinforces analgesic effects and alters the client's emotional response to pain.

Sleep is important for humans, and both REM sleep and non-REM sleep are essential for good mental health. Antianxiety, sedative, and hypnotic drugs may be prescribed to assist with sleep.

Children and older adults are much more sensitive to the CNS depressant effects of these drugs. Children usually respond better to counseling and psychotherapy than to antianxiety agents. Because of a decline in organ function, older adults are more effectively treated with shorter-acting benzodiazepines. Both groups of clients are at greater risk for paradoxical reactions than the general population.

The nurse's role in sedative-hypnotic therapy is to assess the extent of the client's sleep pattern disturbance, its cause, and the client's previous methods of coping with it. Nonpharmacologic nursing interventions to induce sleep should be used in place of or as adjuncts to a sedative-hypnotic agent. Client education should focus on good sleep hygiene and safe self-administration, emphasizing that performance may be impaired because blood levels of some of these drugs are retained. Effectiveness will be indicated by client reports of feeling rested without residual drowsiness during the day.

Although antianxiety, sedative, and hypnotic drugs create many of the same responses within the client, the nurse must be knowledgeable about the specific agents used. Because these agents exert CNS effects, the nurse needs to be aware that the client may be at risk for injury, sensory-perceptual alterations, self-concept disturbance, and further sleep pattern disturbance. As with all medications, clients and their families may experience a knowledge deficit related to their drug therapy.

⊛ Critical Thinking Questions

- What factors need to be included in an education plan for a client who is taking benzodiazepines? What if the client were a young, married woman? An older adult? An Asian client? A child?
- What nonpharmacologic nursing measures should accompany the administration of a sleep medication?
- What actions might a nurse take if a client experiences altered comfort at night as well as insomnia?

Bibliography

Anderson, D.M. (2002). *Mosby's medical, nursing, & allied health dictionary* (6th ed.). St. Louis: Mosby.

Arendt, J. (2003). Importance and relevance of melatonin to human biological rhythms. *Journal of Neuroendocrinology, 15*(14), 427-431.

Asplund, R. (1999). Sleep disorders in the elderly. *Drugs Aging, 14*(2), 91-103.

Belzung, C. (2001). The genetic basis of the pharmacological effects of anxiolytics: A review based on rodent models. *Behavioural Pharmacology, 12,* 451–460.

Belzung, C., Le Guisquet, A.M., & Griebel, G. (2000). [beta]-CCT, a selective BZ-[omega]1 receptor antagonist, blocks the anti-anxiety but not the amnesic action of chlordiazepoxide in mice. *Behavioural Pharmacology, 11,* 125–131.

Blaisdell, J., Mohrenweiser H., Jackson J., Ferguson S., Coulter S., Chanas B., Xi, T., Ghanayem, B. & Goldstein J. (2002). Identification and functional characterization of new potentially defective alleles of human CYP2C19. *Pharmacogenetics, 12*(9), 703-711.

Chang, J.T., & Altman, R.B. (2004). Extracting and characterizing gene-drug relationships from the literature. *Pharmacogenetics, 14*(9),

ℓ-LEARNING SUPPLEMENTS

Student CD-ROM
- Final Exam questions
- NCLEX® Examination review questions
- Pharmacology animations
- Printable chapter summary

Evolve Website (http://evolve.elsevier.com/mckenry)
- Case study on antianxiety, sedative, and hypnotic drugs
- Content updates, including information on new drugs

- WebLinks corresponding to this chapter
- Answers to the critical thinking questions in this chapter
- *Elsevier ePharmacology Update* newsletter
- *Mosby's Drug Consult* Internet Edition
- Supplemental and reference information

577-586, and linked supplemental website http://bionlp.stanford.edu/genedrug/gene_drug_predictions.html (as cited December 2, 2004).

Charney, D.S., Mihic, S.J., & Harris, R.A. (2001). Hypnotics and sedatives. In J.G. Hardman, L.E. Limbird, & A.G. Gillman (Eds.), *Goodman & Gillman's the pharmacologic basis of therapeutics* (10th ed.). New York: McGraw-Hill.

Curtis, J.L., & Jermain, D.M. (2002). Sleep disorders. In J.T. DiPiro, R.L. Talbert, G.C. Yee, G.R. Matzke, B.G. Wells, & L.M. Posey (Eds.), *Pharmacotherapy: A pathophysiologic* approach (3rd ed.). New York: McGraw Hill.

Dopheide, J.A., & Stimmel, G.L. (2005). Sleep disorders. In M.A. Koda-Kimble, L.Y. Young, W.A. Kradjan, B.J. Guglielmo, B.K. Alldredge, & R.L. Corelli (Eds.), *Applied therapeutics: The clinical use of drugs* (8th ed.). Philadelphia: Lippincott Williams & Wilkins.

Drug facts and comparisons. (58th ed.). (2005). St. Louis: Facts and Comparisons.

Epocrates Rx, version 7.0 as cited via www.epocrates.com and updated November 17, 2004.

Floyd, M.D., Gervasini, G., Masica A.L., Mayo G., George, A.L., Bhat, K., et al. (2003). Genotype-phenotype associations for common CYP3A4 and CYP3A5 variants in the basal and induced metabolism of midazolam in European- and African-American men and women. *Pharmacogenetics 13*(10), 595-606.

Jacobson, J.L., & Jacobson, A.M. (Eds.). (2001). *Psychiatric secrets* (2nd ed.). Philadelphia: Hanley & Belfus.

Jaeger, T.M., Lohr, R.H., & Pankratz, V.S. (2001). Symptom-triggered therapy for alcohol withdrawal syndrome in medical inpatients. *Mayo Clinic Proceedings, 76*(7), 695-701.

Jungnickel, P.W. (2001). Alcohol abuse. In M.A. Koda-Kimble, L.Y. Young, W.A. Kradjan, B.J. Guglielmo, B.K. Alldredge, & R.L. Corelli (Eds.), *Applied therapeutics: The clinical use of drugs* (8th ed.). Vancouver, WA: Applied Therapeutics.

Kobayashi, K., Morita, J., Chiba, K., Wanibuchi, A., Kimura, M., Irie, S., et al. (2004). Pharmacogenetic roles of CYP2C19 and CYP2B6 in the metabolism of R- and S-mephobarbital in humans. *Pharmacogenetics, 14*(8), 549-556.

Kryger, M.H., Roth, T., & Dement, W.C. (Eds.). (2000). *Principles and practice of sleep medicine* (3rd ed.). Philadelphia: W.B. Saunders.

Leger, D., Laudon, M., & Zisapel, N. (2004). Nocturnal 6-sulfatoxymelatonin excretion in insomnia and its relation to the response to melatonin replacement therapy. *American Journal of Medicine, 116,* 91-95.

Marx, J., Hockberger, R., & Walls, R. (2002). *Rosen's emergency medicine: Concepts and clinical practice* (5th ed.). St. Louis: Mosby.

McCance, K.L., & Huether, S.E. (2002). *Pathophysiology: The biological basis for disease in adults and children* (4th ed.). St. Louis: Mosby.

Miller, E.H. (2004). Sleep disorders and women. *Clinical Cornerstone, 6,* 1B.

Mintzer, M.Z., & Griffiths, R.R. (2003). Triazolam-amphetamine interaction. Disassociative effect on memory versus arousal. *Journal of Psychopharmacology, 17*(1), 17-29.

Mosby's drug consult. (15th ed.). (2005). St. Louis: Mosby.

Peskind, E.R., Bonner, L.T., Hoff, D.J., & Raskind, M.A. (2003). Prazosin reduces trauma-related nightmares in older men with chronic posttraumatic stress disorder. *Journal of Geriatric Psychiatry and Neurology, 16*(3), 165-171.

Rodgers, R.J. (2001). Anxious genes, emerging themes. Commentary on Belzung "The genetic basis of the pharmacological effects of anxiolytics" and Olivier et al. "The 5-HT 1A receptor knockout mouse and anxiety". *Behavioural Pharmacology, 12*(6-7), 471-476.

Spitzer, R.L., Terman, M., Williams, J.B., Terman, J.S., Malt, U.F., Singer, F., et al. (1999). Jet lag: Clinical features, validation of a new syndrome-specific scale, and lack of response to melatonin in a randomized, double-blind trial. *American Journal of Psychiatry, 156*(9), 1392-1396.

Stimmel, G.L., & Dopheide, J.A. (2000). Sleep disorders: focus on insomnia. *U.S. Pharmacist 25,* 69-80.

Tassaneeyakul, W., Tawalee, A., Tassaneeyakul, W., Kukongviriyapan, V., Blaisdell, J., Goldstein, J., et al. (2002). Analysis of the CYP2C19 polymorphism in a North-eastern Thai population. *Pharmacogenetics, 12*(3), 221-225.

USP DI: Drug information for the health care professional (25th ed.). (2005). Greenwood Village, CO: MICROMEDEX Thomson Healthcare.

Vij, S., & Gentili, A. (2002). Geriatric sleep disorder. Retrieved February 17, 2004, from www.emedicine.com/med/topic3179.htm

17

ANTIEPILEPTIC DRUGS

CHAPTER FOCUS

After stroke, epilepsy is the second most common neurologic disease in North America; it affects 1 of 50 children and 1 of 100 adults. As with other chronic disorders, nurses play a key role in assisting clients to manage their epilepsy effectively. This chapter provides information about antiepileptic medications as a basis for that role.

Epilepsy is a brain disorder in which clusters of neurons in the brain sometimes signal abnormally. In epilepsy, the normal pattern of neuronal activity becomes disturbed, causing strange sensations, emotions, and behavior, or sometimes seizures, muscle spasms, and loss of consciousness. Epilepsy has many possible causes. Anything that disturbs the normal pattern of neuron activity—from illness to brain damage to abnormal brain development—can cause seizures. Epilepsy may develop because of an abnormality in brain wiring, an imbalance of neurotransmitters, or some combination of these factors. Having a seizure does not necessarily mean that a person has epilepsy. Only when a person has had two or more seizures is he or she considered to have epilepsy (National Institute of Neurological Disorders and Stroke, 2003).

Although nearly 70% of seizures do not have an identifiable cause (**primary or idiopathic epilepsy**), approximately 30% have an underlying cause (**secondary epilepsy**) that is treatable (e.g., head injury, cerebrovascular infarct or hemorrhage, infection, brain tumor, drug toxicity, or a metabolic imbalance). Seizures appear to be more common with other comorbidities, including cerebral palsy and mental retardation (Sirven, 2002).

Seizures occasionally result in injury (most often minor head contusions or lacerations) and on rare occasions (particularly with status epilepticus), can be life-threatening.

Status epilepticus, a state of acute prolonged seizure activity or recurrent generalized tonic-clonic seizures that last at least 30 minutes without an intervening stay of consciousness, is a clinical emergency. An alarming 10% to 20% mortality rate results from anoxia during this state. The major cause of status epilepticus is noncompliance with the drug regimen; other causes include cerebral infarction, central nervous system (CNS) tumor or infection, trauma, or low blood concentration of calcium or glucose.

✳ How is an antiepileptic drug selected for a client?

The choice of an appropriate antiepileptic drug depends on accurate diagnosis and classification of the seizure type. A complete medical history, laboratory tests, a neurologic exam, and an electroencephalogram (EEG) are necessary for classification. Computerized tomography and magnetic resonance imaging may detect anatomic defects or locate small focal brain lesions. Identifying specific seizure types is critical to the development of a treatment plan. Box 17-1, on the International Classification of Seizures, lists the terminology currently used with epileptic seizures.

Once a seizure type is identified, pharmacotherapy is selected based on efficacy for that seizure type. Because there may be more than one effective drug, adverse effects, interactions, and adherence issues are also considered.

Antiepileptic Therapy

✳ What is the goal of antiepileptic therapy?

The goal of therapy with antiepileptic drugs (AEDs) is to prevent further seizures without adverse effects for the client. Although secondary seizures usually respond to correction of the underlying condition and perhaps short-term use of AEDs, primary recurrent seizures require long-term AED therapy. Antiepileptic drugs, to date, do not have an effect on the pathogenesis of epilepsy; that is, they will not cure or reduce the risk for seizures once the drug is withdrawn (Schachter, 2002). There is also debate as to whether AEDs alter the risk of temporary or long-term impairment of cognition associated with repeated seizure activity. Therapy with AEDs is associated with moderate risk, including uncomfortable side effects, risks to the fetus when used during pregnancy, significant drug interactions, and, occasionally, life-threatening adverse effects. Accordingly, the decision to use revolves around evaluation of the risk for seizures (e.g., injury, impact on lifestyle, ability to work, go to school, drive), the risk of AEDs, the benefit of seizure control, and the benefit of not taking AEDs. The risk for motor vehicle crashes for example, appears highest for individuals who have had a seizure within the prior 3 months (Drazkowski et al., 2003), and most states or provinces require a seizure-free period of 3 to 12 months before allowing clients to drive. Limitations that driving restrictions may have on earning capacity, completion of education, or activities of daily living may be profound for clients, and must always be considered in the decision to treat seizure activity. Optimal AED therapy may completely control seizures in 60% to 90% of clients. The result depends,

---

BOX 17-1 INTERNATIONAL CLASSIFICATION OF SEIZURES

PARTIAL SEIZURES (SEIZURES BEGINNING LOCALLY)

- Simple partial seizures (no impairment of consciousness)
  Motor symptoms (a single body part, e.g., finger or extremity, may jerk, and such movements may end spontaneously or spread over the entire musculature)
  Somatosensory (tingling) or special sensory symptoms (hallucinations of sight, hearing, or taste)
  Autonomic symptoms (sweating, flushing, abnormal epigastric sensations)
  Psychic (personality changes)
- Complex partial seizures
  Impaired consciousness at outset
  Simple partial followed by impaired consciousness
- Partial seizures evolving to generalized tonic-clonic (GTC)

GENERALIZED SEIZURES (CONVULSIVE OR NONCONVULSIVE)

- Absence seizures (brief loss of consciousness for a few seconds)
- Myoclonic seizures (unaltered consciousness, isolated clonic contractions)
- Clonic seizures (various dysrhythmic contractions in the body)
- Tonic seizures (sustained contractions of large muscle groups)
- Generalized tonic-clonic seizures (alternating tonic-clonic movements)
- Atonic seizures (brief, generalized seizures in which the person's head drops or he or she falls to the ground—epileptic drop attacks)

UNCLASSIFIED SEIZURES (AVAILABLE DATA INCOMPLETE, INADEQUATE, OR LACKS CLASSIFICATION STATUS [SUCH AS NEONATAL SEIZURES])

---

most importantly, upon the choice of the appropriate AED, individualization of dosing, and client compliance (McAuley & Lott, 2005).

In some clients, AEDs are associated with excellent seizure control with minimal adverse effects; in other clients, AEDs are associated with troublesome adverse effects and only moderate control of seizure activity. Evaluation of the risk and benefit of therapy requires excellent communication among the client, family and interdisciplinary team, usually including a neurologist. Often, careful adjustment of drugs or doses can tip the balance and allow for better seizure control with fewer adverse effects.

Secondary seizures usually respond to correction of the underlying condition and perhaps short-term use of AEDs, but primary recurrent seizures require long-term AED therapy. The primary goal of drug therapy is to control or prevent the recurrence of seizure activity.

⊛ How is antiepileptic therapy determined for a particular client?

The choice of AED for an individual client is a function of seizure type, client comorbidity and tolerance, and the drug's adverse effect/drug interaction profile. The major drugs used in the treatment of partial seizures and generalized tonic-clonic seizures are carbamazepine (Tegretol), phenytoin (Dilantin), and valproate (valproic acid [Depakene], divalproex [Depakote]). Carbamazepine and phenytoin are effective for partial seizures and generalized tonic-clonic seizures, but are not effective for myoclonic seizure activity and may actually worsen absence seizure activity. Valproate is effective for generalized tonic-clonic seizures, myoclonic, atonic and absence seizures; it is somewhat less effective for partial seizures. Phenytoin is the oldest nonsedating antiepileptic drug, but its use is diminishing as newer drugs with fewer adverse effects are developed. Carbamazepine and valproate have been approved as AEDs since the 1970s. Beginning in 1993, after a latent period when no new AEDs became available, several new AEDs have been introduced in the United States, including the miscellaneous AEDs—felbamate (Felbatol), gabapentin (Neurontin), lamotrigine (Lamictal), levetiracetam (Keppra), tiagabine (Gabitril), topiramate (Topamax), and zonisamide (Zonegran). Most newer AEDs are primarily effective for partial seizures, although they may have some benefit in generalized seizure types, particularly lamotrigine. Although the new AEDs are not chemically similar to one another, they are a welcome addition to the treatment options for epilepsy. They also create a dilemma because their individual places and their optimal use in the treatment of various forms of epilepsy are evolving. Lamotrigine and valproic acid are used for absence seizures, and clonazepam and valproic acid are the drugs of choice for atonic seizures. Tables 17-1 and 17-2 present a review of the drugs of choice. The antiepileptic drugs are described individually later in the chapter. The drug treatment goal is to attain maximum seizure control with minimal medication adverse effects. The AED or combination of such drugs prescribed depends on the type of seizure, whether the client is having more than one type of seizure, and whether the seizures are difficult to control. Finding the appropriate regimen for each client takes time.

⊛ How do AEDs work in the body to prevent seizures?

Although the exact mode and site of action of these drugs are complex and incompletely understood, a major mechanism of action appears to be stabilization of the cell membrane by altering cation transport, especially sodium, potassium, and calcium. Carbamazepine, phenytoin and valproate block

TABLE 17-1 DRUGS FOR TYPE OF SEIZURE OR EPILEPSY

Seizure Type	First Choice	Second Choice
Complex partial and secondary generalized seizures	carbamazepine, phenytoin, lamotrigine, levetiracetam, oxcarbazepine, topiramate, zonisamide	gabapentin, valproic acid, phenobarbital
Absence seizures	lamotrigine, valproic acid	ethosuximide
Myoclonic seizures	lamotrigine, valproic acid	topiramate, zonisamide
Primary generalized tonic-clonic seizures	lamotrigine, valproic acid	phenobarbital, phenytoin, felbamate
Atonic seizures	clonazepam, valproic acid	lamotrigine, felbamate

Modified from Sirven, J.I. (2002). Antiepileptic drug therapy for adults: When to initiate and how to choose. *Mayo Clinic Proceedings, 77*(12), 1367-1375.

TABLE 17-2 INDICATIONS FOR PARENTERAL USE OF ANTIEPILEPTIC DRUGS

Parenteral Drug	Use
barbiturates, especially phenobarbital, also amobarbital, pentobarbital sodium, and secobarbital sodium	Eclampsia, status epilepticus, severe recurrent seizures, tetanus, antiepileptic drug toxicity, other convulsive states
phenytoin	Status epilepticus, seizure during neurosurgery
magnesium sulfate	Severe toxemias of pregnancy (preeclampsia and eclampsia)
benzodiazepines such as diazepam, lorazepam, clonazepam	Status epilepticus, severe, recurrent seizures, alcohol withdrawal seizures

voltage-sensitive sodium channels of neurons, inhibiting neuronal firing. Valproate is also thought to increase concentrations of the inhibitory neurotransmitter, gamma-aminobutyric acid (GABA). Thus they suppress seizures by stabilizing cell membrane excitability and reducing the spread of seizure discharge. Although the mechanism of action of the newer AEDs is not exactly known, it is thought that they, too, suppress synaptic activity. Thus the two main pharmacologic effects of AEDs are to:

- Increase motor cortex threshold to reduce its response to incoming electric or chemical stimulation; and
- Depress or reduce the spread of a seizure discharge from its focus or origin by depressing synaptic transport or decreasing nerve conduction.

✱ What is the nurse's responsibility for the management of antiepileptic therapy?

Although the nurse's responsibilities in AED therapy may vary with the specific drug (these will be addressed with each drug), there are many similarities in the nursing care provided to all clients with AED therapy. A client being prescribed AED therapy is treated most effectively with a holistic approach. In addition to effectively managing the therapeutic regimen, this client has many special problems, including the fear of sudden loss of physical and emotional control and the stigma of seizures. In recent years, emphasis has been placed on public education about epilepsy to dispel the myths associated with it. The person with epilepsy needs information about the seizure condition and its management, along with psychosocial support from the nurse. The client should understand that the condition can be controlled or modified with medication.

The clinical effectiveness of AED therapy varies with the drug's pharmacokinetics, mechanism of action, and serum levels achieved with scheduled drug dosing. AEDs may exhibit varying blood levels in different clients even if the same dose is administered. This variation results from a complex of interrelated factors including individual absorption, metabolism, distribution, and excretion, which may be caused by genetic and/or environmental factors; concomitant ailments, such as renal or hepatic dysfunction; concurrent medication; diet; client compliance; and physical status. The dosing of certain drugs needs to be adjusted in order to obtain optimal therapeutic effects, and this dosage may vary widely for clients.

Therapeutic dosage ranges are intended to serve as rough guides to therapy; they are not inflexible limits. The ranges provide a point from which the dosage of a drug may be individualized to account for the extremes in variation to response and adverse effects. The client beginning AED therapy should have serum levels measured to establish individual level/dose ratio. This level tends to be a constant measure for an individual; however, it varies considerably among clients. Although the time required to reach a steady serum level is generally about four to five times the half-life of a drug, the usual time for serum level measurement is 1 month after initiating therapy, because levels measured much earlier may be lower than the steady-state level finally achieved.

The **serum half-life** of a drug (the time required for the drug serum level to drop 50% of its initial value when no additional drug is administered) is a function of its rate of excretion and depends on the client's age, pharmacogenetics, concurrent drug therapy, and hepatic or renal function. Most antiepileptic drugs are metabolized via cytochrome P450 enzyme systems. As discussed in Chapter 3, such metabolism is typically reduced in the neonate, is accelerated in young children, and levels off in adults; metabolism is also greatly impacted by genetic predisposition to produce specific cytochrome P450 isoenzymes, and by concurrently administered drugs that are also metabolized by these systems. See the Special Considerations for Children and Special Considerations for Older Adults boxes on p. 335.

✱ With AED therapy, are there special considerations for pregnancy and lactation?

Because many AEDs have the potential for teratogenicity, pregnancy is a time for special concern for the woman with epilepsy. Pregnant women with epilepsy constitute 0.5% of all pregnancies (Nulman, Laslo, & Koren, 1999). Epilepsy may worsen during pregnancy, and status epilepticus increases in frequency during gestation and labor. Many of the commonly used AEDs are established teratogens (see the Pregnancy Safety box on p. 336). Some AEDs appear in breast milk. Emotional stress (psychological, occupational, physiologic, marital, economic) may influence seizure frequency. With proper preconceptual, antenatal, and postpartum care, up to 95% of child-bearing clients with epilepsy have favorable outcomes (Nulman et al., 1999). See the Evidence-Based Practice box on p. 336.

More than one million female Americans are affected by epilepsy. Seizures during pregnancy increase complication risk by two- to threefold (Liporace & D'Abreu, 2003). In addition, pregnancy itself may increase seizure frequency in approximately 25% of women. Many seizures in pregnant women are related to preeclampsia or eclampsia for which the treatment is magnesium (speculated to be related to magnesium's ability to improve cerebral perfusion) (Greene, 2003).

Unfortunately, AEDs are associated with fetal malformations and increased risk for perinatal mortality. The older therapies (e.g., phenytoin, carbamazepine, valproate, phenobarbital) are all associated with teratogenicity, and the mechanisms include production of toxic metabolites, inducing folic acid deficiency, ischemia, or hypoxia. Major congenital anomalies include cardiac defects, spina bifida, and cleft lip or palate where the risk is highest during the first trimester of pregnancy.

Quantifying the risk of treatment versus nontreatment may be difficult, but the risks are reduced with careful drug selection and timing during pregnancy. Use of more than one AED increases risk. Risk appears lower when pregnant women are treated with AEDs (uncontrolled seizures appear to increase risk), lower with monotherapy (compared to the use of multiple drugs) (Pennell, 2003), and lower with maintenance of lower drug levels (Liporace & D'Abreu, 2003). Risks with the newer AEDs are currently being eval-

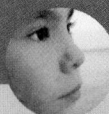

Special Considerations for Children | ANTIEPILEPTIC DRUGS

- Up to 25% of children do not respond adequately to currently available AEDs (Jarrar & Buchhalter, 2003).
- Isolated febrile seizures in children with normal development generally do not cause neurological injury and typically do not require treatment (Jankowiak & Malow, 2003).
- The young client (under age 23) is more susceptible to gingival hyperplasia, especially with phenytoin. Gingivitis or gum inflammation usually starts during the first 6 months of drug therapy, although severe hyperplasia is unlikely in dosages under 500 mg daily. A dental program of teeth cleaning and plaque control started within 7 to 10 days of initiating drug therapy helps to reduce the rate and severity of this condition.
- Coarse facial features and excessive body hair growth are more frequently reported in young clients.
- Impaired school performance is reported with long-term, high-dose, phenytoin therapy (especially at high or toxic serum levels).
- Chewable phenytoin tablets are not indicated for once-daily administration.
- If skin rash develops with use of phenytoin or lamotrigine, discontinue drug immediately and notify prescriber.

- Be aware that neonates whose mothers received phenytoin during pregnancy may require vitamin K to treat hypoprothrombinemia.
- Behavioral changes are more likely to occur in children with carbamazepine.
- Children receiving valproic acid, especially those up to 2 years old, those receiving multiple antiepileptic drugs, or those with organic brain disease or mental retardation, are at a greater risk for developing serious hepatotoxicity. This risk decreases with advancing age.
- During valproate therapy, one metabolite (valproylcarnitine) can lead to carnitine deficiency in children, prompting supplemental carnitine use in pediatric populations.
- Chronic use of clonazepam (Klonopin) for seizure disorders may result in impaired physical or mental functions in the developing child, which may not become apparent until years later.

Data from *USP DI: Drug information for the health care professional* (25th ed.). (2005). Greenwood Village, CO: MICROMEDEX Thomson Healthcare.

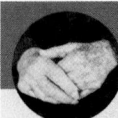

Special Considerations for Older Adults | ANTIEPILEPTIC DRUGS

- Since much seizure activity in older adults is associated with concurrent drugs or comorbidity (e.g., cerebrovascular disease, dementias, etc.), treatment often includes evaluation of non-antiepileptic drug therapy as part of good care. Cerebrovascular accident risk may be considerably higher in older clients with new onset seizure activity compared to other older individuals (Cleary, Shorvon, & Tallis, 2004).
- Older individuals are at greater risk for fractures. Antiepileptic medications have demonstrated a trend in increased risk for fractures of the hip and other bones (Ensrud et al., 2003).
- Older clients are more susceptible to carbamazepine-induced confusion or agitation, AV heart block, SIADH, and bradycardia than younger clients.
- If skin rash develops with the use of phenytoin, discontinue drug immediately and notify the prescriber.
- Debilitated clients or persons with renal or liver disease have a greater risk of developing toxicity with the

AEDs. Lower doses of the AEDs will help to avoid adverse effects.
- Older adults tend to metabolize AEDs more slowly; thus drug accumulation and toxicity may occur. Monitor closely because dosage adjustments (lower doses) may be necessary.
- Administer intravenous doses at a rate slower than the recommended rate for an adult. The rate of administration of phenytoin for individuals over 65 years of age should be 5 to 10 mg/minute up to a maximum of 25 mg/minute.
- Serum albumin levels may be lower in older clients, thus resulting in decreased protein binding of bound drugs, such as phenytoin and valproic acid. Monitor closely because lower drug doses may be necessary.

Data from *USP DI: Drug information for the health care professional* (25th ed.). (2005). Greenwood Village, CO: MICROMEDEX Thomson Healthcare. *AV,* Arteriovenous; *SIADH,* syndrome of inappropriate secretion of antidiuretic hormone.

Evidence-Based Practice

Using Single, Rather Than Multiple, Antiepileptic Drugs to Reduce Neonatal Risks

Researchers in Canada analyzed mostly prospective data from all 414 women with prepregnancy diagnoses of epilepsy who delivered in a tertiary referral center and from 81,759 women without epilepsy. Deliveries occurred from 1978 to 2000.

Women with epilepsy had significantly higher risks than did women without epilepsy for only three complications: antenatal hypertension (but not preeclampsia), induced labor, and fetal cardiovascular malformation. Of women with epilepsy, 83.5% received antiepileptic drugs during pregnancy. Children of women with epilepsy who used multiple antiepileptic drugs had higher rates of major congenital malformations (9.1%) than did children of mothers with epilepsy who used single drugs (6.2%); children in the multiple-drug group also had higher rates of cardiovascular anomalies (3.9% vs. 2.3%) and microcephaly (2.6% vs. 0.8%). Corresponding rates for children of women without epilepsy were 4.5%, 0.7%, and 0.5%, respectively.

Antenatal seizures occurred in 137 pregnancies (33%). Women who had seizures within 2 years of the index pregnancy were significantly more likely than women who had less recent seizures to have antenatal (54.1% vs. 9.4%), intrapartum (2.7% vs. 0%), or postpartum (6.5% vs. 1.9%) seizures; however, pregnancy seizures were not linked with pregnancy complications. The overall miscarriage rate was not available.

These data show that most women with epilepsy can have good obstetric and neonatal outcomes with appropriate care during pregnancy. Using single, rather than multiple, antiepileptic drugs appears to reduce neonatal risks substantially.

Data from Richmond, J.R., Krishnamoorthy, P., Andermann, E., & Benjamin, A. (2004). Epilepsy and pregnancy: An obstetric perspective. *American Journal of Obstetrics & Gynecology, 190,* 371-379.

PREGNANCY SAFETY ANTIEPILEPTIC DRUGS

Category	Drug
A	magnesium sulfate
C	acetazolamide, carbamazepine, ethotoin, felbamate, gabapentin, lamotrigine, levetiracetam, mephenytoin, succinimides, tiagabine, topiramate
D	barbiturates, clonazepam, clorazepate, diazepam, paramethadione, phenytoin (particularly high risk for cleft palate if administered during weeks 6-12 of pregnancy), primidone, valproate, valproic acid, divalproex (neural tube defects, particularly during the first 4-6 wks of pregnancy, and cardiac, facial and skeletal defects)

Data from *Mosby's drug consult.* (15th ed.). (2005). St. Louis: Mosby.

---

uated, but many of these agents can be effective as monotherapy (Beydoun & Kutluay, 2003).

Maintaining adequate vitamin intake (especially vitamins D, K, and folic acid) is critical to reduce fetal risk. Principles of management during pregnancy by the health care team are as follows:

1. Preconception
   - Consider medication reduction or discontinuation
   - Establish lowest effective dose of medicine
   - If valproic acid is the drug of choice, split dosing to three to four times a day or use long-acting formulations
   - Obtain baseline free- and total-drug levels
   - Counsel client about the risks of seizure medications and the need for additional tests
   - Refer client for genetic counseling
   - Initiate folate supplement: prenatal vitamin with 1 mg of folic acid and an additional 1 mg folic acid tablet
2. During pregnancy
   - Encourage regular visits and counseling
   - Suggest client register with AED pregnancy registry: 1-888-233-2334
   - Encourage avoidance of sleep deprivation
   - Encourage AED compliance
   - Monitor free and total AED levels, and adjust as needed
   - Have client continue taking folate and prenatal vitamins
   - Administer vitamin K, 10 mg daily orally in last month of pregnancy
   - Client may have a cesarean section if neural tube defect is present
3. Delivery
   - Ensure administration of AED(s)
   - Administer vitamin K to neonate
4. Postpartum
   - Follow AED levels closely; reduce dose as needed
   - Encourage avoidance of sleep deprivation
   - Give client advice about breastfeeding
   - Discuss child care concerns

Many AEDs enter breast milk in varying concentrations. In general, most women with epilepsy can safely breastfeed, provided that the child is monitored for adverse effects.

✹ What is the prognosis for clients on AED therapy?
Most clients respond well to antiepileptic medication, although some require multiple drugs for good control, and about half of those with partial complex seizures require two or more drugs. A few individuals never achieve adequate control despite adequate trials of multiple medications (Nguyen & Spencer, 2003).

An epilepsy diagnosis no longer implies a lifetime of drug therapy. Studies indicate that AEDs may be withdrawn from selected clients who are seizure-free for at least 2 years. In long-term studies, seizures recurred in 12% to 36% of the clients monitored for up to 23 years, after complete drug withdrawal. Risk factors that help predict seizure recurrence after drug withdrawal include an onset of seizures after 12 years of age; a family history of seizure activity; a range of 2 to 6 years before seizures were finally controlled; having had a large number of seizures before control (more than 30) or a total of more than 100 seizures; an abnormal EEG that was documented even with therapy; the presence of an organic neurologic disorder; moderate to severe mental retardation; and perhaps the withdrawal from phenytoin or valproate drugs which appear to have a higher rate of seizure recurrence than other drugs (McAuley & Lott, 2005). More than 90% of seizure recurrences occur within the first year of withdrawal, and most occur during the withdrawal period or shortly thereafter. Fewer seizures occur when the withdrawal is planned or gradual (usually over months) or when the dose is reduced to minimal maintenance therapy. There is some data to suggest children may tolerate withdrawal of antiepileptic drugs over a period as short at 6 weeks.

Nursing Management of AED Therapy

✹ What are the most important assessment issues for the nurse caring for a client with AED therapy?
Along with a general assessment of preexisting health status that includes baseline blood, renal and hepatic studies, and concurrent medication regimen because of the potential drug interactions, assessment of the client with a seizure disorder includes data specific to the seizures. These data include the number of seizures within a specific time, precipitating events or activities, presence of sensations or perceptions experienced by a client before a seizure, an aura, and the character of the client's seizures.

Assess the presence or absence of an aura and its nature. It may also be helpful to evaluate the ability of the client to describe it (somatic, visceral, psychic). It can also be useful to note the presence or absence of a cry. The onset of seizure should be assessed for site of initial body movements, deviation of head and eyes, chewing and salivation, posture of body, and sensory changes.

After the onset of a seizure it is important to note if tonic and clonic phases are present and, if so, their characteristics. Characteristics include movements of body as the seizure progresses, skin color, airway clearance, pupillary changes, incontinence, and duration of each phase.

The nurse should assess duration of each phase of the seizure, behavior during the postictal (sleep) phase, ability to remember anything about the seizure, orientation, pupillary changes, headache, and any injuries present. Finally, an accurate picture should be formed of the duration of the entire seizure, level of consciousness, and length of unconsciousness if applicable. Because the nurse is often not present when a seizure occurs, family, friends, or other witnesses may provide valuable information about the seizure.

The nurse should assess the client's understanding and management of the AED regimen. One of the most common causes of seizure exacerbations is ineffective management of medications by the client. A number of studies suggest that up to 50% of clients do not take their AEDs regularly (Asawavichienjinda, Sitthi-Amorn, & Tanyanont, 2003; Gomes & Maia, 1998; Ogunniyi, Oluwole, & Osuntokun, 1998). Many clients do not understand the concepts of steady blood levels and half-life. Some clients use the drugs as they would aspirin, taking extra doses when they are afraid they might have a seizure. Some are afraid of the harm they think that their medications could cause, whereas others are concerned about becoming addicted to the drugs. The nurse should assess the client's use of medications as an attempt to gain control and provide information to allow the client to manage the therapeutic regimen effectively.

✹ What nursing diagnoses are commonly found with AED therapy?
In addition to the selected nursing diagnoses presented in the Nursing Care Plan on p. 338, the client receiving AED therapy should be assessed for the following nursing diagnoses related to side/adverse effects:
- Activity intolerance related to antiepileptic-induced weakness
- Altered bowel elimination (constipation or diarrhea) related to gastrointestinal (GI) effects
- Impaired comfort related to headache, nausea and vomiting, or dermatologic effects
- Ineffective protection related to drug-induced blood dyscrasias
- Acute confusion
- Disturbed body image related to hydantoin-induced enlargement of the facial features (hirsutism, alopecia, or gynecomastia [in males])
- Excess fluid volume related to carbamazepine-induced water intoxication
- Risk for injury related to client's underlying seizure activity (effectiveness/ineffectiveness of AED coverage)
- Risk for injury related to the CNS, visual, or hypotensive effects of the drug
- Impaired home maintenance management related to drug-imposed restrictions on driving and other activities
- Impaired skin integrity related to drug-induced rash

The potential collaborative problems are gingival hyperplasia (phenytoin), cognitive impairment, behavioral effects,

NURSING CARE PLAN SELECTED NURSING DIAGNOSES FOR THE CLIENT ON ANTIEPILEPTIC MEDICATIONS

Nursing Diagnosis	Outcome Criteria	Nursing Interventions
Deficient knowledge related to newly prescribed or altered AED therapy	• The client will describe: the seizure condition; how drug therapy relates to the condition; how and when to take the medications; common drug interactions; safety precautions; common adverse effects and which of these warrant reporting; storage requirements of the drugs. • The client will verbalize less anxiety related to fear of the unknown, loss of control, and misconceptions.	• Assess learning needs and learning readiness. • Plan with the client and family for the achievement of realistic goals. • Provide information to meet outcome criteria.
Ineffective management of therapeutic regimen: AED	• The client will self-administer therapeutic regimen medications safely and accurately. • The client will describe or demonstrate life style changes appropriate to epilepsy.	• Determine the client's reasons for inaccuracies of dosing and use appropriate teaching/counseling interventions. • Provide needed AED information concerning rationale for the specific client's seizure status. • Discuss the increased possibility of seizures with ineffective management of the regimen.
Risk for injury related to effects of AED therapy	• The client will maintain AED therapy without untoward adverse effects, reactions, and toxicity.	• Administer drug safely and accurately. • Observe client for drowsiness, ataxia, behavioral changes, slurred speech, mental confusion, vertigo, and excessive sedation (see drug monographs for drug-specific adverse effects). • Instruct client about symptoms to be reported. • Explain the importance of Medic Alert card/tag. • Discourage self-altering of medication regimen. • Caution against activities requiring coordination and alertness until responses to drugs are known.

allergic reaction, blood dyscrasias, and hepatotoxicity with other AEDs.

✴ In implementing nursing activities with clients with AED therapy, what special monitoring is required?

For Efficacy Seizure status as described previously in assessment. The number and severity of seizures should decrease. The most common medical test to evaluate seizure activity is the EEG, a recording of electrical activity generated by the brain made by placing electrodes on the scalp. Monitoring the results of EEGs will indicate the client's progress by decreased seizure activity of the brain. Subjective data to be obtained include the client's understanding of and reaction to the convulsive disorder and drug therapy.

For Toxicity
• CNS symptoms, such as level of consciousness, gait, vision, confusion, impaired cognition and memory, and decreased attention span may occur.
• Bone marrow suppression may occur with symptoms of leukopenia, anemia, and thrombocytopenia, as well as hepatotoxicity. Liver function and blood studies should be monitored. Clients with existing suppressed immune systems have a higher risk for leukopenia.
• Monitor for the occurrence of the nursing diagnoses previously discussed.

AED Serum Levels (for Efficacy and/or Toxicity) Therapeutic alternatives are selected (monotherapy or polytherapy) that best control the client's seizure. Many AEDs have known optimal serum therapeutic ranges, the level of med-

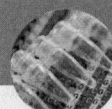

Special Considerations for Pharmacogenetics | ANTIEPILEPTICS

PHARMACODYNAMICS

Early evidence suggests that epilepsy unresponsive to antiepileptic drugs may have a genetic basis. Individuals with multidrug resistance in epilepsy express variation in a gene that codes for a glycoprotein involved in pumping drug across cell membranes (Siddiqui et al., 2003). Better understanding the genetic basis of epilepsy may contribute to improved treatment options (Glauser, 2002).

PHARMACOKINETICS

The amounts of cytochrome P450 enzymes that metabolize antiepileptic drugs are genetically predetermined. Genetic differences in phenytoin, phenobarbital, and carbamazepine metabolism may account for increased or decreased drug metabolism (Anderson, 2004; *USP DI,* 2005). Currently, there is no clinical test available to evaluate the degree of cytochrome P450 activity in a client. As such, expect that a typical dose may occasionally result in unexpected toxicity (because of reduced metabolism) or subtherapeutic response (because of increased metabolism).

ADVERSE/TERATOGENIC EFFECTS

Antiepileptic drugs or their metabolites may produce adverse effects for the client or toxicity to the developing fetus. Genetically determined pathways that slow clearance of the antiepileptic drug or that involve a toxic metabolite may explain why some individuals, but not others, experience toxicity. Given the degree of metabolism with antiepileptic drugs, genetics may play an important, but yet to be determined role in toxicity and teratogenicity (Holmes, 2002; Patsalos, 2000).

---

ication needed to control seizures. Therapeutic drug monitoring includes correlating results of serum concentrations with the client's clinical response. This monitoring has reduced the need for polydrug AED therapy and added greater efficiency in drug selection for each client. Pharmacogenetics may also influence the client's response to AEDs. (See the Special Considerations for Pharmacogenetics box above.)

Increased AED serum levels may signal impending toxic effects. Generally, adverse effects are more serious at higher serum levels. Maintaining a serum level within the therapeutic range is a challenge for some clients (see the Special Considerations for Children and Special Considerations for Older Adults boxes on p. 335). The challenge surfaces when other drugs are added or deleted from the client's regimen, the client ineffectively manages the medication regimen, a hepatic or renal system dysfunction occurs, or undesirable drug effects cause the client to withdraw from drug therapy. Fully informing clients about drug therapy and the need to maintain therapeutic concentrations may reduce therapeutic failures caused by adverse effects or the client's ineffective management of the medication regimen.

✱ What nursing interventions are important with AED therapy?

Although AEDs are usually given orally, there are a few parenteral forms. These are reserved for occasions when the parenteral form is the best choice of therapy. Table 17-2 lists these occasions and the parenteral drugs indicated for each. AEDs should be administered intravenously (IV) in emergency situations (such as status epilepticus) because of slow absorption from intramuscular injection sites.

AEDs should be administered using as long an interval as possible between doses while considering their half-life. To maintain a therapeutic serum concentration and im-

prove compliance, AEDs that have an elimination half-life of 24 hours or more are generally administered only once a day. The daily dose may be administered at bedtime to overcome the sedation seen with peak levels of AEDs.

In nonemergency situations, changes in AED therapy are best done by altering one drug at a time. The nurse and the client must be aware that each time a new AED is started, or the dose of a drug is increased or decreased, it takes four to five half-life intervals to achieve the total therapeutic effect of the new regimen. This time interval allows the concentration of the new drug to reach steady state or the drug being discontinued to decrease by 95% of its concentration.

When serum levels of antiepileptics are ordered, they should be scheduled more than 8 hours after the last dose of a once-daily medication is given. In most circumstances, plasma levels of drugs are obtained as trough levels before the first dose of the day. Some data exist for evaluating antiepileptic safety and efficacy with saliva levels, but this has not been a widespread practice (Grim et al., 2003). A discussion of the principles of therapeutic drug monitoring (blood levels of drugs) is presented in Chapters 3 and 5.

✱ What are important points of client education with AED therapy?

Instruct the client to adopt a moderate lifestyle, follow an appropriate diet, and get sufficient rest and exercise. The client should avoid stressful situations, and if this is not possible, should notify the prescriber for dosage adjustment in ongoing stressful conditions. Caution against drinking alcohol and taking over-the-counter (OTC) medications (see specific drugs for interactions or effects). Explain that some antiepileptics take days or weeks to reach an effective level in the body and that regular AED administration is necessary to prevent seizures. A missed dose may result in a seizure in a few days, and taking an extra dose will not prevent an impending seizure. Although the client may be seizure-free for some time and may perceive that a "cure" has occurred, the medication dose should not be decreased or stopped without consulting the prescriber. Instruct the client to consult with the prescriber if the client thinks the AED regimen should be modified because of adverse effects or anticipated pregnancy. Provider contact for supervision and laboratory tests is important. Contact the prescriber if bruising, bleeding, sore throat, or other symptoms of blood dyscrasias occur. During initiation or change of therapy, avoid activities that require coordination and alertness, such as using power tools, or situations that might be hazardous, such as swimming or ladder climbing, until response to the drug therapy has been determined.

Medications should be stored at home away from light and heat and out of the reach of children, since overdosage is especially dangerous in children. Outdated and discontinued medications should be safely discarded.

The family should keep a daily record of the number and type of seizures that occur during drug therapy. This is one measure of the efficacy of the medication(s) and will help the prescriber determine if increased dosage or an additional agent may be needed.

Instruct the client and family in seizure precautions, and the importance of wearing a Medic Alert pendant or bracelet obtainable at local pharmacy or www. 911 medicalalert.com. A valuable resource for both the nurse and the client is the Epilepsy Foundation of America (located at 4351 Garden City Drive, Landover, MD 20785; www.epilepsyfoundation.org).

✱ How does the nurse evaluate AED therapy?

Evaluate the client's progress on AED therapy by determining the client's achievement of the outcome criteria and the response to nursing interventions. The client should experience a decrease in or absence of seizure activity and maintain therapeutic blood levels of the drug without experiencing any adverse effects of the drug. And as with all drugs, the client should administer the drug safely and accurately when managing his or her own medication regimen.

Antiepileptic Drugs

The three key AEDs—carbamazepine, phenytoin, and valproate—are discussed below followed by a concise review of the other drugs in this classification which indicates their differences from the key drugs. Tables 17-3 and 17-4 help differentiate these agents based on pharmacokinetics, drug interactions, dosing, and differentiating features.

✱▪▪ carbamazepine [kar bam **az** eh peen]
(Tegretol, Apo-Carbamazepine✦)
Carbamazepine is chemically related to tricyclic antidepressants such as imipramine.

The exact mechanism of action of carbamazepine is unknown; however, it is thought to act to block voltage-sensitive sodium channels, inhibiting neuronal firing.

Indications
Carbamazepine is a drug of choice for simple partial and complex partial seizures. It is often used for generalized tonic-clonic seizures, but may worsen control of absence seizures. It is also used for neuropathic pain (including trigeminal neuralgia), bipolar affective disorder, migraine headache prophylaxis.

Pharmacokinetics/Dosing
Carbamazepine is relatively well absorbed orally and extensively metabolized via P450 3A4 and other enzymes. Carbamazepine 10,11-epoxide is a pharmacologically active metabolite that may contribute to CNS toxicity. Carbamazepine is a potent enzyme inducer and will increase metabolism of other drugs and itself. It is not uncommon to observe carbamazepine levels decline with consistent intake during the first few weeks of therapy related to this "autoinduction" effect. The typical adult dose is usually started at 100 to 200 mg twice daily with doses increased every few days to avoid gastrointestinal upset. Adult doses may be as high as 400 mg or 600 mg four times daily, based on response and drug levels. Carbamazepine is available as immediate release, an oral suspension, and as a sustained-action tablet. The sustained-action tablet should not be crushed or broken. See Table 17-3 for a more complete discussion.

Adverse Effects
The more common adverse effects of carbamazepine and its metabolite include CNS toxicity (drowsiness, double or blurred vision, ataxia), nausea and vomiting, and osteomalacia. Also seen are modest declines in leukocyte count, skin rash, and mild elevations in liver enzymes. The syndrome of inappropriate secretion of antidiuretic hormone (SIADH), evidenced by fluid retention and low serum sodium levels, is a relatively common dose-related effect. Severe, but rare effects include blood dyscrasias and Stevens-Johnson syndrome.

Drug Interactions
Carbamazepine interacts with many other agents metabolized by the P450 system, including hormonal contraceptives, corticosteroids, methadone, and other antiepileptics. See Table 17-4 for a more complete listing.

✱ L.G. is a 17-year-old female high school student. As she was leaving for school, she abruptly got up from the breakfast table and began to walk clumsily toward her bedroom; she ran into a number of pieces of furniture and did not respond to her mother's questions. She suddenly fell to the floor and experienced a generalized tonic-clonic seizure that lasted for about 2 minutes. She was taken to the hospital. On arrival in the emergency department, L.G. appeared confused and sleepy. Her physical examination and blood studies were within the normal range. An EEG had abnormal findings with focal epileptiform discharges in the right temporal area. In the hospital, a second seizure occurred much like the first. On questioning, L.G. indicates that she has no memory of what occurred during the seizure, only "a funny feeling with flashes of light" in her head before the seizure.

Assessment It was determined that L.G. experienced complex partial seizures progressing to secondarily generalized tonic-clonic seizures. Given the anticipated limitation of her age-appropriate activities, the potential benefits of AED therapy outweighed the risks.

Carbamazepine and phenytoin are both considered first-line therapy for the type of seizures that she experienced;

Text continued on p. 349

TABLE 17-3 PHARMACOKINETICS/DOSING AND DIFFERENTIAL FEATURES OF ANTIEPILEPTIC DRUGS

Name	Pharmacokinetics	Therapeutic Plasma Levels Adults (mcg/mL)	Serum Half-Life (hours)	Typical Adult Dose for Seizure Management	Typical Pediatric Dose for Seizure Management	How Different from Other AEDs
FIRST-LINE THERAPIES FOR SEIZURE CONTROL						
carbamazepine (Tegretol, Carbatrol)	Oral absorption: >70% Plasma protein binding: 75% Elimination: hepatic (CYP 3A) Induces CYP 2C9, CYP 3A Active metabolite: 10, 11-epoxide	5-12	10-25	800-1600 mg PO per day divided two to four times daily Sustained action: 400-600 mg PO twice daily	20-30 mg/kg PO per day divided two to four times daily	First-line agent for partial or generalized seizures Autoinduction—induces its own metabolism Only available orally Initiate at low dose to reduce GI upset
phenytoin (Dilantin)	Oral absorption: >90% (variable with enteral feedings) Plasma protein binding: 90%-95% (decreased with ↓ albumin, uremia, valproate use) Elimination: >90% hepatic (CYP 2C9, 2C19) (saturable elimination process with higher levels) Induces CYP 2C, 3A	10-20 Free: 1-2 (free levels used with low albumin, uremia, valproate use)	At low levels: 22 At high levels no true half-life	300-400 mg PO per day divided one to three times daily	5-8 mg/kg PO per day divided one to three times daily; do not exceed adult dose range	First-line agent for partial or generalized seizures Pharmacokinetically unique Dose formulation/tube feeds may affect absorption Highly bound to plasma albumin Higher levels result in "saturation" kinetics and predispose to toxicity IV form is irritating and should run no faster than 50 mg/min
valproate (valproic acid, divalproex, Depakene, Depakote)	Oral absorption: <90% Plasma protein binding: ~90% Elimination: >95% hepatic Inhibits CYP 2C9	50-125 (levels above 100 ↑ risk thrombocytopenia)	10-20	10-15 mg/kg PO per day divided two to three times daily up to 60 mg/kg/day	10-15 mg/kg PO per day divided two to three times daily up to 60 mg/kg/day	First-line agent for broad range of seizure types, including absence seizures Fewer significant drug interactions Commonly used for bipolar affective disorders and migraine prophylaxis Available orally and intravenously

Modified from Bazil, C.W. & Pedley, T.A. (2003). Clinical pharmacology of antiepileptic drugs. *Clinical Neuropharmacology, 26*(1), 38-52; Epocrates Rx, version 7.0 as cited via www.epocrates.com and updated November 17, 2004; Johannessen, S.I., Battino, D., Berry, D.J., Bialer, M., Kramer, G., Tomson, T., et al (2003). Therapeutic drug monitoring of the newer antiepileptic drugs. *Therapeutic Drug Monitoring, 25*(3), 347-363; Lacy, C.F., Armstrong, L.L., Goldman, M.P., & Lance, L.L. (2004). *Lexi-Comp's drug information handbook* (12th ed.). Hudson, OH: Lexi-Comp; LaRoche, S.M., & Helmers, S.L. (2004). The new antiepileptic drugs: Scientific review. *Journal of the American Medical Association, 291*(5), 605-614; McNamara, J.O. (2001). Drugs effective in the therapy of the epilepsies. In J.G. Hardman, A.G. Gilman, & L.E. Limbird (Eds.), *Goodman & Gilman's the pharmacological basis of therapeutics.* New York: McGraw Hill; Thummel, K.E., & Shen, D.D. (2001). Design and optimization of dosage regimens: Pharmacokinetic data. In J.G. Hardman, A.G. Gilman, & L.E. Limbird (Eds.), *Goodman & Gilman's the pharmacological basis of therapeutics.* New York: McGraw Hill. *CYP,* Cytochrome P450; *PO,* by mouth.

continued

TABLE 17-3 PHARMACOKINETICS/DOSING AND DIFFERENTIAL FEATURES OF ANTIEPILEPTIC DRUGS—cont'd

SECOND-LINE/ADJUNCT THERAPIES FOR SEIZURE CONTROL

Name	Pharmacokinetics	Therapeutic Plasma Levels Adults (mcg/mL)	Serum Half-Life (hours)	Typical Adult Dose for Seizure Management	Typical Pediatric Dose for Seizure Management	How Different from Other AEDs
acetazolamide (Diamox)	Oral absorption: limited data Elimination: 70%-100% renal Dose adjusted for renal insufficiency	Not used	Limited data	4-30 mg/kg PO per day divided into four doses daily, not to exceed 250 mg four times daily	4-30 mg/kg PO per day divided into two to four doses daily, not to exceed 250 mg four times daily	Second-line agent for generalized or absence seizures Tolerance develops quickly, so it is limited to short-term use Used orally
clonazepam (Klonopin, Rivotril)	Oral absorption: >90% Plasma protein binding; ~85% Elimination: hepatic (CYP 3A)	Levels not typically used clinically	18-28	0.5-5 mg PO three times daily	Initial dose: 0.01-0.03 mg/kg PO per day divided into three equal doses daily Doses may be increased by 0.25-0.5 mg per day every third day, up to a maximum of 0.1-0.2 mg/kg/day, not to exceed adult dose	Tolerance to the antiseizure effects may limit long-term benefit
ethosuximide (Zarontin)	Oral absorption: >90% Plasma protein binding: 0% Elimination: ~65% hepatic, ~25% renal	40-100	Adults: 56-60 Children: 30-36	250 mg PO twice daily to maximum of 750 mg twice daily	15-40 mg/kg PO per day divided into two doses daily	For absence seizures only Fewer interactions with other drugs Only orally available
felbamate (Felbatol)	Oral absorption: >80% Plasma protein binding: ~25% Elimination: ~50% hepatic, ~40%-50% renal	Not typically used clinically	19-24	1200-3600 PO per day divided three or four times daily	15-45 mg/kg PO per day divided three to four times daily	Significant risk for bone marrow suppression Use limited to clients with poor seizure control on other agents
gabapentin (Neurontin)	Oral absorption: 60% (↓ with increased dose) Plasma protein binding: <5% Elimination: 64%-68% renal Dose adjustment for renal insufficiency	4-16 Not typically used clinically	5-8	300-1200 mg PO three times daily	Age 3-4 yr: 40 mg/kg PO per day divided three times daily 5-12 yr: 25-35 mg/kg PO per day divided three times daily	Not as effective an antiepileptic as other agents Renally eliminated, requiring dose adjustment in renal dysfunction Most commonly used in the treatment of neurogenic pain

Drug	Pharmacokinetics			Dose		Comments
lamotrigine (Lamictal)	Oral absorption: >90% Plasma protein binding: 55% Elimination: 90% hepatic, 10% renal	4-16 Not typically used clinically	12-60	With valproate: 25-200 mg PO twice daily Without valproate: 50-250 mg PO twice daily	Age 2-12 yr: With valproate: 1-3 mg/kg PO per day divided one to two times daily (initiate at much lower doses); maximum daily dose: 200 mg Without valproate: 5-15 mg/kg PO per day divided one to two times daily (initiate at much lower doses); maximum daily dose: 400 mg	High risk for Stevens Johnson syndrome, particularly at high doses or with concurrent valproate use Significant pharmacokinetic interactions with many other AEDs
levetiracetam (Keppra)	Oral absorption: ~100% Plasma protein binding: <10% Elimination: ~65% renal Dosage adjustment required for renal insufficiency	5-45 Not typically used clinically	6-8	500-1500 mg PO q12h	Age 4-16 yr (unlabeled use): 10-60 mg/kg PO per day divided twice daily	Second-line adjunct therapy for partial-onset seizures Unlabeled use in bipolar illness
oxcarbazepine (Trileptal)	Oral absorption: variable (high first-pass metabolism) Plasma protein binding: 40% (active metabolite) Elimination: >90% hepatic Induces CYP 3A4/5; inhibits: CYP 2C19 Active metabolite: 10-hydroxycarbamazepine	10-35 (active metabolite) Not typically used clinically	8-10 (active metabolite)	300-1200 mg twice daily	*Initial dose for monotherapy:* 8-10 mg/kg PO per day divided into two doses daily Doses are then typically increased by 5 mg/kg PO per day every 3 days to a weight-based daily maximum *Monotherapy daily max:* 20-24.9 kg: 600-900 mg daily; 25-34.9 kg: 900-1200 mg daily; 35-44.9 kg: 900-1500 mg daily; 45-49.9 kg: 1200-1500 mg daily; 50-59.9 kg: 1200-1800 mg daily; 60-69.9 mg daily; 1200-2100 mg daily; 70 kg and above: 1500-2100 mg daily	Second-line therapy for partial seizures in adults and children older than age 4 yr Chemically similar to carbamazepine Blood levels of the drug are not routinely monitored

Continued

TABLE 17-3 PHARMACOKINETICS/DOSING AND DIFFERENTIAL FEATURES OF ANTIEPILEPTIC DRUGS—*cont'd*

SECOND-LINE/ADJUNCT THERAPIES FOR SEIZURE CONTROL—*cont'd*

Name	Pharmacokinetics	Therapeutic Plasma Levels Adults (mcg/mL)	Serum Half-Life (hours)	Typical Adult Dose for Seizure Management	Typical Pediatric Dose for Seizure Management	How Different from Other AEDs
					Adjunct treatment daily maximum: 20-29 kg: 900 mg daily 29.1-39 kg: 1200 mg daily Over 39 kg: 1800 mg daily	
phenobarbital (Barbital, Luminal)	Oral absorption: >90% Plasma protein binding: 45%-50% Elimination: usually >90% hepatic (CYP 2C9, 2C19), variable renal depending on urine pH Induces CYP 2C, 3A	15-40	100	60 mg PO two to three times daily or 120-240 mg daily at bedtime Status epilepticus: 10-20 mg/kg IV; initial and total dose based on availability of airway support, response, and plasma levels; total loading doses as high as 30 mg/kg IV have been used in adults and children	Younger than 2 mo: 3-5 mg/kg PO/IV per day divided one to two times daily 2 mo-2 yr: 5-8 mg/kg PO/IV per day divided one to two times daily Older than 2 yr: 3-5 mg/kg PO/IV per day divided one to two times daily Status epilepticus: 10-20 mg/kg IV (see adult comments)	Second-line agent for partial or generalized seizures Schedule IV controlled substances Highly sedating and often interfere with intellectual information processing Available intravenously and orally
primidone (Mysoline)	Oral absorption: 60%-80% Plasma protein binding: 99% Elimination: metabolized to phenobarbital and PEMA	Children: 7-10 Adults: 5-12 Phenobarbital levels also monitored	10-12 PEMA: 15 Phenobarbital: 100	Titrate up to 750-1500 mg PO per day divided into three or four doses daily	Neonates: 12-20 mg/kg PO per day divided two to four times daily Younger than 8 yr: titrate up to 10-25 mg/kg/day up to adult dose Older than 8 yr: adult dose	It is metabolized to phenobarbital It is more sedating than most other AEDs

Drug	Pharmacokinetics	Therapeutic Serum Level	Half-Life	Adult Dosage	Pediatric Dosage	Clinical Concerns
tiagabine (Gabitril)	Oral absorption: ~90% Plasma protein binding: 95% Elimination: >90% hepatic (CYP 3A4)	Not typically used clinically	5-13	Initial dose: 4 mg PO once daily; increase total daily dose by 4-8 mg per day at weekly intervals up to adult maintenance dose of 32-56 mg PO per day divided two to four times daily; doses in excess of 4 mg per day should be divided into two to four doses per day; lower doses are used for clients who are not receiving enzyme-inducing antiepileptic drugs.	Older than 12 yr: 4-32 mg PO per day divided two to four times daily	Adjunct therapy for partial seizures in adults and children older than age 12 yr; Best taken with food; Metabolism and dose highly influenced by other enzyme-inducing AEDs (carbamazepine, phenytoin, phenobarbital, primidone)
topiramate (Topamax)	Oral absorption: >70% Plasma protein binding: ~15% Elimination: <30% hepatic, >70% renal; Dosage adjustment for renal insufficiency; Inhibits CYP 2C19	4-10	19-25	200 mg PO twice daily	Age 2-16 yr: 5-9 mg/kg/day PO divided twice daily	Maintaining fluid intake is important to prevent kidney stone formation
zonisamide (Zonegran)	Oral absorption: NA Plasma protein binding: 40% Elimination: 70% hepatic (CYP 3A4)	10-40 Not typically used clinically	63	100-600 mg PO per day divided one to two times daily	Age 16-17 yr: Adult dose; Children and adolescents (not FDA approved): 12 mg/kg PO per day divided one to two times daily, not to exceed adult dose	Adjunct therapy for partial seizures in adults and children 16 years of age or older; Safety and efficacy below 16 years of age not established

PEMA, Phenylethylmalonamide; *NA,* not available.

Continued

TABLE 17-3 PHARMACOKINETICS/DOSING AND DIFFERENTIAL FEATURES OF ANTIEPILEPTIC DRUGS—cont'd

Name	Pharmacokinetics	Therapeutic Plasma Levels Adults (mcg/mL)	Serum Half-Life (hours)	Typical Adult Dose for Seizure Management	Typical Pediatric Dose for Seizure Management	How Different from Other AEDs
TREATMENTS FOR ACUTE SEIZURE CONTROL/STATUS EPILEPTICUS						
diazepam (Valium, Diastat Rectal)	Rectal absorption: 90% Plasma protein binding: 98% Elimination: >90% hepatic (active metabolites)	0.3-0.5 Levels not typically used clinically	20-50 Active metabolite: 50-100	Rectal: 0.2 mg/kg p.r. × 1 IV: 5-10 mg × 1 over 2-5 min May repeat every 10-15 min to a maximum of 30 mg	Rectal: Age 2-5 yr: 0.5 mg/kg p.r. × 1 Age 6-11 yr: 0.3 mg/kg p.r. × 1	Lorazepam is first-line agent given intravenous for status epilepticus Class IV controlled substance Tolerance to the antiseizure effects are more pronounced, rendering them typically used for acute management only
lorazepam (Ativan)	Plasma protein binding: 85% Elimination: >90% hepatic (inactive metabolites)	0.03-0.75 Not typically used clinically	9-19	Status epilepticus: 0.1 mg/kg (typically 4-8 mg) IV over 2-5 min	Status epilepticus: 0.1 mg/kg IV over 2-5 min, not to exceed adult dose	See previous page
fosphenytoin (Cerebyx)	Metabolism: converted to phenytoin Elimination: as with phenytoin	Monitor phenytoin levels (see above)	fosphenytoin: 15 min phenytoin: see above	As with phenytoin; see text May also be given IM	As with phenytoin; see text May also be given IM	Converted to phenytoin Less irritating to vein than phenytoin Typical drug cost is 20 times that of phenytoin
phenytoin (Dilantin)	See p. 341	See p. 341	See p. 341	Status epilepticus: 15-20 mg/kg IV × 1 no faster than 50 mg/min See text re: renal failure or concurrent phenytoin use	Same as adult dose	IV form cardiotoxic if rate faster than 50 mg/min IV form irritating to vein; administer via central line or large-bore peripheral line
magnesium sulfate	Intravenous effect: immediate Elimination: renal (100%) If renal impairment, monitor magnesium levels closely	Per normal serum magnesium levels Adults: 1.2-2 mEq/L Children: 1.2-1.6 mEq/L	NA	Toxemia in pregnancy: 4-5 g (32-40 mEq) IV in 250 mL of D₅W or normal saline administered over 30 min or 1-4 g/hr by continuous infusion	20-100 mg/kg IV diluted in D₅W or normal saline administered over 30-60 min	Use as antiepileptic drug primarily limited to toxemia of pregnancy or magnesium deficiency Also used for treatment of premature labor and for ventricular dysrhythmias (particularly torsades de pointes) It is administered IV and must be diluted before administration

D_5W, Dextrose 5% in water; *p.r.*, by way of rectum.

TABLE 17-4 ANTIEPILEPTIC DRUG INTERACTIONS*†

AED	AED at Left Increases Levels of	AED at Left Decreases Levels of	Drugs That Increase Level of the AED at Left	Drugs That Decrease Level of AED at Left
carbamazepine	clomipramine	alprazolam clonazepam lozapine doxycycline ethosuximide felbamate haloperidol hormonal contraceptives **lamotrigine** phenytoin theophylline tiagabine topiramate valproate warfarin zonisamide	cimetidine diltiazem erythromycin fluoxetine grapefruit juice isoniazid ketoconazole propoxyphene valproate verapamil zonisamide	cisplatin doxorubicin felbamate phenytoin rifampin theophylline
ethosuximide		hormonal contraceptives **lamotrigine**	valproate	carbamazepine
felbamate	carbamazepine epoxide phenobarbital phenytoin valproate	carbamazepine hormonal contraceptives	gabapentin valproate	carbamazepine phenytoin
gabapentin	felbamate		cimetidine	antacids
lamotrigine	carbamazepine epoxide	valproate	sertraline **valproate**	**carbamazepine** **ethosuximide** **oxcarbazepine** **phenobarbital** **phenytoin** **rifampin**
levetiracetam	phenytoin			
oxcarbazepine	phenytoin	hormonal contraceptives itraconazole ketoconazole **lamotrigine**		phenobarbital phenytoin

Modified from Bazil, C.W., & Pedley, T.A. (2003). Clinical pharmacology of antiepileptic drugs. *Clinical Neuropharmacology, 26*(1), 38-52; Epocrates RxPro™, version 6.11, www.epocrates.com, updated September 12, 2003; Johannessen, S.I., Battino, D., Berry, D.J., Bialer, M., Kramer, G., Tomson, T., et al. (2003). Therapeutic drug monitoring of the newer antiepileptic drugs. *Therapeutic Drug Monitoring, 25*(3), 347-363.
*This is a list of common interactions. Other drugs not listed here may produce clinically significant interactions in selected clients.
†Drugs listed in **bold** have more significant interactions.

Continued

TABLE 17-4 ANTIEPILEPTIC DRUG INTERACTIONS—*cont'd*

AED	AED at Left Increases Levels of	AED at Left Decreases Levels of	Drugs That Increase Level of the AED at Left	Drugs That Decrease Level of AED at Left
phenobarbital		bupropion calcium channel blockers clozapine felbamate fluconazole haloperidol hormonal contraceptives itraconazole **lamotrigine** oxcarbazepine phenytoin theophylline topiramate warfarin zonisamide	felbamate **valproate**	thioridazine phenytoin
phenytoin		carbamazepine corticosteroids desipramine digoxin doxycycline estrogens furosemide hormonal contraceptives **lamotrigine** oxcarbazepine phenobarbital quinidine rifampin theophylline tiagabine **topiramate** valproate warfarin zonisamide	amiodarone chloramphenicol chlorpromazine diazepam disulfiram felbamate fluoxetine imipramine isoniazid methylphenidate oxcarbazepine paroxetine sertraline thioridazine topiramate trazodone valproate	carbamazepine phenobarbital sucralfate
tiagabine		valproate		**carbamazepine** **phenobarbital** **phenytoin**
topiramate	phenytoin	digoxin hormonal contraceptives		**carbamazepine** **phenobarbital** **phenytoin** valproate
valproate	benzodiazepines carbamazepine ethosuximide ethyl alcohol felbamate lamotrigine **phenobarbital** phenytoin warfarin	topiramate	chlorpromazine cimetidine erythromycin felbamate	carbamazepine lamotrigine phenytoin tiagabine
zonisamide	carbamazepine		erythromycin fluconazole itraconazole	carbamazepine phenobarbital phenytoin

given her age and the anticipated long-term use of an AED, however, carbamazepine has a better profile for L.G. It is less sedating, has less cosmetic effects (facial coarsening, gingival hyperplasia, hirsutism), and less risk of cognitive impairment than phenytoin.

Contraindications to carbamazepine therapy would be sensitivity to the drug or to tricyclic antidepressants; it would also be contraindicated if L.G. had absence, atonic, or myoclonic seizures because of the possibility of the seizures becoming more generalized with use of the drug. Although not an issue with L.G., other preexisting conditions for which there might also be concern for the use of carbamazepine would be for clients with AV heart block, blood disorders, and bone marrow depression because of the risk of exacerbation of these conditions. The risks and benefits of carbamazepine should also be considered for the client with one or more of the following health conditions: active alcoholism (potentiates CNS depression), behavioral disorder (may activate latent psychosis), cardiac damage or coronary artery disease, glaucoma (may be exacerbated), or renal or hepatic impairment. L.G.'s pregnancy status should also be confirmed before initiating therapy because carbamazepine is teratogenic and the risk and benefit of seizure control with carbamazepine should be carefully assessed.

L.G.'s concurrent medication regimen should be reviewed to detect any significant drug interactions. Carbamazepine is a significant enzyme inducer affecting the metabolism of many other drugs (see Table 17-4 for a summary of drug interactions with carbamazepine and other drugs). Carbamazepine significantly increases metabolism of vitamin D (Liporace & D'Abreu, 2003; Fitzpatrick, 2002) and so to prevent osteomalacia, an increased intake of vitamin D (total 800 to 1200 units daily) and calcium (total 1000 to 1500 mg elemental daily) may be advised for L.G.

Blood studies (complete blood count, serum iron, liver function studies, blood urea nitrogen, and electrolytes), urinalysis, physical examination, ophthalmic examination, and electrocardiogram (ECG) should be done before beginning L.G.'s carbamazepine therapy.

Nursing Diagnosis In addition to the nursing diagnoses for any AED therapy, L.G. or any client receiving carbamazepine should be evaluated for the following nursing diagnoses/collaborative problems: risk for injury related to CNS toxicity (blurred or double vision, nystagmus) and skin photosensitivity; excess fluid volume related to SIADH; acute confusion; diarrhea or constipation; altered comfort (headache, nausea and vomiting, aching joints and muscles); and the potential complications of cardiovascular effects (dysrhythmias, heart failure), Stevens-Johnson syndrome, systemic lupus erythematous-like syndrome, and blood dyscrasias.

Planning During carbamazepine therapy, L.G. will:
- Experience a decrease in the frequency and severity of seizures.
- Experience minimal or no adverse effects associated with carbamazepine drug regimen.

- Comply with therapy.
- Effectively manage the therapeutic regimen, including identification of therapeutic and adverse effects of carbamazepine.
- Collaborate with health team for follow-up care and the appropriate reporting of adverse carbamazepine effects.

Implementation

Monitoring Carbamazepine therapy should be initiated gradually to avoid nausea, vomiting, and excessive sedation. These adverse effects, as well as the level of seizure activity, are monitored as the dose is increased so that dosage adjustments may be made.

To determine *efficacy*, the nurse monitors frequency, intensity, duration, presentation, and time of day of seizures. To monitor for *toxicity*, the nurse assesses the following:
- Level of consciousness, gait, vision
- Because hematologic toxicity usually occurs early in carbamazepine therapy, complete blood counts should be done monthly during the first 2 to 3 months of therapy and annually thereafter
- Bleeding, bruising, sore throat (bone marrow suppression)
- Daily weight (if fluid retention, may be SIADH)
- Plasma carbamazepine concentrations may be helpful; the target should be 6 to 12 mcg/mL. Occasionally, plasma carbamazepine 10,11-epoxide levels (an active metabolite of carbamazepine) may be obtained if CNS toxicity is suspected.

Intervention Carbamazepine should be administered with meals to GI irritation.

Education The importance of compliance with drug therapy should be stressed with L.G. and all clients taking this drug; in clients with epilepsy, abrupt withdrawal of the drug can precipitate a seizure. Regular visits to the prescriber are necessary to monitor carbamazepine therapy.

Clients may experience drowsiness during the initial therapy; caution L.G. about this so that she can avoid hazardous activity. L.G. needs to avoid the use of alcoholic beverages and other CNS depressants while taking carbamazepine, as alcohol will increase the sedation and incoordination drug effects. She should report to the prescriber any signs of hematologic dysfunction such as easy bruising, bleeding, sore throat or mouth, or malaise. Because of possible skin photosensitivity, L.G. should use sunblock products and avoid unprotected exposure to the sun and the use of tanning beds or booths.

Because carbamazepine is a hepatic enzyme inducer, it can cause breakthrough bleeding in women taking hormone contraceptives. Tell L.G. that it may interfere with the effectiveness of estrogen-containing hormone contraceptives, so other birth control measures may need to be used if she is sexually active. L.G. should be aware that carbamazepine is Pregnancy Category C and if she believes she is pregnant, she should notify her prescriber immediately.

Carbamazepine is also excreted in breast milk, so its use in nursing mothers should be evaluated by the prescriber.

Evaluation The expected outcome is that L.G. will have decreased severity and frequency of seizures, have plasma carbamazepine concentrations of 6 to 12 mcg/mL, and be without adverse effects of the drug.

✷ **L.G.'s carbamazepine dosage was increased gradually over 2 months and stabilized at 400 mg twice daily. Her complex partial seizures decreased over that time and she had no generalized tonic-clonic seizures. After about 6 seizure-free weeks, she again began experiencing 1 seizure a week. Her trough serum carbamazepine concentration was 5 mcg/mL. How might these changes in her health status be explained?**

As with all medications, noncompliance may be a consideration when therapeutic regimens become ineffective. Having ruled this out, these changes are characteristic of carbamazepine to induce hepatic cytochrome P450 and so stimulate its own metabolism. Autoinduction can significantly decrease the drug's half-life and will necessitate an increase in dosage to be effective.

✷▛ **phenytoin** [**fen** i toy in]
(Dilantin)
Phenytoin acts to block voltage-sensitive sodium channels, stabilizing neuronal membranes at the cell body, axon, and synapse and so inhibiting neuronal firing, limiting the spread of neuronal or seizure activity.

Indications
Phenytoin, a hydantoin, is a drug of choice for simple partial and complex partial seizures. It is also often used for generalized tonic-clonic seizures, and as a second line agent for status epilepticus. It often worsens control of absence seizures. It is also indicated for neuropathic pain and digoxin-induced ventricular dysrhythmias.

Pharmacokinetics/Dosing
The pharmacokinetics of phenytoin are complicated and often not easily predictable for an individual client, and may be particularly true for older clients (Birnbaum et al., 2003). The oral absorption of phenytoin is variable based on formulation, and not all generic forms of phenytoin are considered interchangeable (Burkhardt et al., 2004). Phenytoin is highly bound to plasma proteins, and phenytoin is easily displaced by urea (as seen in renal failure) or other protein-bound drugs, including valproate. Phenytoin is metabolized by P450 2C9 and 2C19, which can become saturated at normal to higher doses. This dose-dependent metabolism, referred to as Michaelis-Menten kinetics or zero-order kinetics (see Chapter 3), can result in accumulation of phenytoin and toxicity with very slight increases in dose. With low doses of phenytoin, the half-life of phenytoin is approximately 24 hours. At higher levels, however, the drug can accumulate and under such conditions, no true half-life can be determined. Instead, at blood levels typically above 20 mg/L (considered the upper end of the therapeutic blood level), the drug often persists in the blood at elevated levels considerably longer than expected. Table 17-3 presents the pharmacokinetics of phenytoin. The typical oral adult dose of phenytoin is often in the range of 4 to 6 mg/kg/day (sodium extended dose daily or divided every 12 hours; other formulations divided every 8 to 12 hours). Dosing in young children is often 8 to 10 mg/kg/day divided every 8 hours. A number of oral dosage forms are available, including 30- and 100-mg extended-release sodium (Dilantin Kapseals) containing 92% phenytoin, 50 mg tablet (Dilantin Infatab) containing 100% phenytoin,

and two concentrations of oral suspension (30 mg/5 mL and 125 mg/5 mL) (Dilantin Suspension) containing 100% phenytoin. Each of these doses has varying bioavailability and are not considered interchangeable. Refer to Table 17-3 and consult package labeling for more information.

The IV dose is very irritating and must be administered at rates below 50 mg/min to avoid the risk for life-threatening cardiac dysrhythmias. The IV dose for adults in status epilepticus with normal renal function and who have not yet received any phenytoin is 18 mg/kg IV at 25 to 50 mg/min. This dose is often reduced by 50% for clients in renal failure (e.g., 9 mg/kg IV at 25 to 50 mg/min) because of urea displacing phenytoin from plasma-albumin binding sites. If the client has received phenytoin already, the above doses are prorated based on existing phenytoin plasma concentration. See Box 17-2 and package labeling for additional information.

Adverse Effects
The more common adverse effects of phenytoin include sedation, ataxia, and mental dulling, particularly at higher serum concentrations. Very high levels can result in nystagmus (eye twitching) or diplopia, and may actually increase seizure risk. Chronic administration of phenytoin can lead to osteomalacia (bone thinning), gingival hyperplasia, hirsutism (abnormal hair growth), and folate deficiency. Coarsening of facial features (especially in children), bone marrow suppression, and peripheral neuropathies have been reported with phenytoin use. IV phenytoin is very irritating to the vein, leading to significant phlebitis. Rapid IV administration of phenytoin (greater than 50 mg/min) is associated with life-threatening cardiac dysrhythmias and must be avoided. Rarely, phenytoin is associated with Stevens-Johnson syndrome.

Drug Interactions
As with many other antiepileptics, phenytoin is associated with a number of significant drug interactions, which are highlighted in Table 17-4.

fosphenytoin [foss **fen** i toy in]
(Cerebyx)
Fosphenytoin, a prodrug of phenytoin, was formulated to avoid the problems associated with IV administration of phenytoin (i.e., pain and burning at the site of administration). This product is rapidly converted to phenytoin in the body and has the same pharmacologic profile as phenytoin. Fosphenytoin is approximately 20 times more expensive than standard phenytoin injection, its benefits appear limited, and its routine use has been questioned (Touchette & Rhoney, 2000).

Indications
Fosphenytoin is indicated as an alternative to IV phenytoin for short-term treatment acute treatment of seizures and status epilepticus.

Pharmacokinetics/Dosing
Fosphenytoin is rapidly converted in the body to phenytoin with a conversion half-life of approximately 15 minutes when administered intravenously. The usual adult dose for intravenous use is based on phenytoin equivalents and is identical to intravenous phenytoin dosing. Medical errors have resulted from dosing errors related to this product. See Box 17-2, Table 17-3, and package labeling for more complete information.

Adverse Effects
The major adverse effect of intravenous fosphenytoin is cardiovascular collapse, hypotension, and dysrhythmia. Once converted to phenytoin, adverse effects are as noted for that drug.

✷ **T.J. is a 20-year-old male college student who plays team rugby and works 20 hours per week in the campus landscaping and ground maintenance department. T.J. was diagnosed as having epilepsy. He experiences approximately three generalized tonic-clonic seizures monthly. He has been unable to tolerate carba-**

mazepine because of nausea and acute confusion despite low serum carbamazepine levels. The decision is made to place him on phenytoin therapy.

 How does the initiation of phenytoin therapy for T.J. vary from carbamazepine and why?

Because of T.J.'s active lifestyle, gaining quicker control of his seizure activity by a loading dose of phenytoin is beneficial. This would allow therapeutic serum concentrations to be reached more rapidly. However, phenytoin exhibits dose-dependent pharmacokinetics, so the usual concepts of "clearance" and "half-life" are meaningless. At low to moderate doses/levels, phenytoin displays classic concentration-dependent elimination (first order) with a half-life of approximately 24 hours. At high doses/levels, the drug displays non–concentration-dependent elimination (zero order) with no true half-life; as a result of "saturation" of systems that metabolize the drug, drug accumulation and toxicity are probable.

Medication Safety Alert

Phenytoin Suspension

Enteral Administration

When using the suspension form of phenytoin, shake the container vigorously before measuring out the dose in a graduated or exact measuring device (oral syringe). Children and other clients with enteral tube feedings have been undermedicated and later overmedicated from the same container because of inadequate shaking of the container.

Note that the 100-mg capsule of phenytoin sodium contains only 92% phenytoin and is not equivalent to two 50 mg phenytoin chewable tablets (Dilantin Infatab) that contain 100% phenytoin. For clients closely regulated on a set phenytoin dosage, a change of dosage form may over- or undermedicate them.

Nasogastric Tube Administration

Administration of phenytoin suspension without dilution or follow-up irrigation of the nasogastric tube after the phenytoin is given prevents adequate absorption and leads to a significant decrease in plasma concentrations of phenytoin. Until further research is performed, it is recommended that the phenytoin suspension be diluted before administration and that the nasogastric tube be irrigated with 20 mL of fluid (D₅W, normal saline) before and after administration. A significant decrease in the absorption of oral phenytoin may occur when phenytoin is administered to clients receiving enteral feedings. If the client is receiving an enteral feeding, consistent scheduling of the drug and enteral feeding is essential and serum concentrations of phenytoin should be monitored frequently. Doses of phenytoin may require adjustment.

In all dosage forms, abrupt withdrawal may precipitate status epilepticus.

 What would nursing management of T.J.'s phenytoin therapy include?

Assessment Before beginning T.J.'s drug therapy, nursing management of T.J.'s phenytoin regimen includes assessing for preexisting conditions for which phenytoin might be contraindicated, such as a known sensitivity to the drug, impaired cardiac function (parenteral administration may affect ventricular automaticity and cause ventricular dysrhythmias), impaired immune system (potential for increased leukopenia), or porphyria (risk for exacerbation.). It is also necessary to obtain a history of concurrent drugs taken. There are clinically significant pharmacokinetic drug interactions among the antiepileptic drugs (see Table 17-4). Given his age and student status, question him especially about his use of alcohol. Chronic alcohol use speeds up the metabolism of the drug, apparently by enzyme induction, and leads to cross-tolerance that makes normal dosages of phenytoin inadequate. In addition, alcohol withdrawal itself significantly increases the risk for seizures. Phenytoin increases the metabolism of vitamin D (Fitzpatrick, 2002) and may increase the risk of osteomalacia. Because phenytoin is an enzyme inducer, monitor T.J. closely whenever his phenytoin dosage is altered or another drug is added or deleted from his drug regimen. As with all clients on AEDs, T.J.'s assessment will include a baseline of his seizure activity and any neurologic symptoms.

Nursing Diagnosis The following nursing diagnoses/collaborative problems may be identified for T.J.: risk for injury related to his underlying seizure activity and inadequate therapeutic serum levels of phenytoin; disturbed body image related to the coarsening of facial features, hirsutism, alopecia, and gynecomastia (as a male); powerlessness related to chronicity of seizure disorder therapy; and the potential complications of cognitive impairment, blood dyscrasias, hepatotoxicity, and gingival hyperplasia.

Planning During phenytoin therapy, T.J. will:
- Experience a decrease in the frequency and severity of seizures.
- Experience minimal or no adverse effects associated with phenytoin drug regimen.
- Comply with phenytoin therapy.
- Effectively manage the therapeutic regimen, including identification of the therapeutic and adverse effects of phenytoin.
- Collaborate with health team for follow-up care and the appropriate reporting of adverse phenytoin effects.

 Given that T.J. was an ambulatory client, an oral loading dose of 6 mg/kg every 8 hours × 3 followed by 300 mg daily was prescribed for T.J. with serum concentrations drawn on the third day and weekly thereafter.

 What will the monitoring of T.J.'s phenytoin therapy entail?

BOX 17-2 PARENTERAL ADMINISTRATION OF PHENYTOIN/FOSPHENYTOIN

The IM route is not recommended for phenytoin because muscle tissue is more acidic than the phenytoin solution, and it crystallizes when given intramuscularly. The absorption of these crystals is slow and erratic, and pain and necrosis may occur at the injection site. The IM route is not recommended for the treatment of status epilepticus because therapeutic plasma levels of phenytoin cannot be readily achieved for up to 24 hours.

IV administration may be administered by direct IV injection into a large vein through a large-gauge needle or IV catheter, not to exceed the rate of 50 mg/min. More rapid administration may result in cardiovascular irregularities, hypotension, or CNS depression related to its propylene glycol diluent. IV administration should be monitored with a cardiac monitor and blood pressure readings. Extravasation should be avoided because it may result in irritation and extensive sloughing of local tissue.

To prevent these phenytoin tissue reactions, the drug may be administered by intermittent injection. This may be accomplished providing (1) the drug is admixed only with no more than 50 mL of 0.9% sodium chloride injection, (2) the final concentration is between 1 and 10 mg per mL, (3) the admixture is accomplished immediately before beginning the infusion, (4) the infusion is completed within an hour, (5) all tubing is flushed before and after the infusion with 0.9% sodium chloride injection, and (6) a 0.45- to 0.22-micron filter is placed on the line.

Fosphenytoin, a prodrug of phenytoin, may be administered more rapidly by intravenous administration, is not as irritating to tissues and veins, and may be administered intramuscularly. These advantages are offset by fosphenytoin's considerable expense, and no demonstrated advantage in the management of status epilepticus (Manno, 2003). The dosing of fosphenytoin is always expressed in terms of phenytoin sodium equivalents (PEs); 75 mg of fosphenytoin sodium is essentially equivalent to 50 mg of phenytoin sodium. Some clients complain of burning and pain at the IV injection site, but less so than with phenytoin. Because of the alkalinity of the hydantoins, burning and pain raise suspicion of a poorly seated needle, extravasation, or a fluid load that is being infused too quickly into a small vein. Restart the infusion into a large vein, using a larger-gauge needle. Although less caustic than phenytoin, IV infusion of fosphenytoin still necessitates continuous monitoring of the client's ECG, blood pressure, and respiration. Because the effect of the drug is not immediate, other interventions, such as the concurrent administration of a benzodiazepine, is usually necessary in status epilepticus.

Implementation

Monitoring To monitor for efficacy, the nurse should monitor for frequency, intensity, duration, presentation, and time of day of seizures. To assess for adverse drug effects or toxicity, the nurse should monitor for the following:

- Level of consciousness (dizziness, confusion, hallucinations), gait (clumsiness, ataxia), vision (blurred or double), slurred speech, fatigue
- Bleeding, bruising, sore throat (bone marrow suppression)
- Dental status for gingival hyperplasia
- Plasma drug levels:

A trough drug level is usually drawn before the morning dose. The expected total phenytoin level is 10 to 20 mg/L, and the expected free phenytoin level is 1-2 mg/L (ideal for monitoring individuals with hypoalbuminemia, concurrent highly protein-bound drugs, or uremia).

Intervention Although not applicable to T.J., there are concerns related to the oral suspension form of the drug when given by the enteral route; see the Medication Safety Alert box on p. 351 for additional discussion. Box 17-2 presents information about parenteral dosing of either phenytoin or fosphenytoin.

✳ What education will T.J. require specific to phenytoin therapy?

Phenytoin may be taken with meals to decrease gastric distress.

T.J. will need instructions for safe and accurate self-administration, such as the importance of Medic Alert identification, regular administration to prevent seizures, and prescriber and lab visits for the monitoring of therapy. Phenytoin may also cause drowsiness or vision problems, particularly early in therapy, so caution T.J. about his activities. The drug also may interact with other drugs, OTC preparations, and complementary/alternative products.

One adverse effect of the hydantoins is gum hyperplasia; it is therefore important to emphasize proper oral hygiene. T.J. should brush frequently, floss, and massage his gums. This tissue overgrowth is usually greater and more apparent anteriorly than posteriorly, and T.J. may have body image concerns. A program of professional dental prophylaxis and an aggressive program of plaque control will assist T.J. to minimize hyperplasia. T.J. should inform his dentist that he is taking hydantoins so that the dentist will monitor for periodontal problems.

Advise T.J. of possible skin changes. An erythematous-type rash with or without fever should be reported immediately to the prescriber. Instruct T.J. to notify the prescriber if bruising, bleeding or sore throat occurs. Hirsutism, or the excessive growth of body and facial hair, is reported in some clients. This alteration in body image may be more troublesome to young women, but requires supportive care with any client.

To prevent osteomalacia, T.J. may consider increasing his intake of vitamin D (total 800 to 1200 units/day) and calcium (total 1000 to 1500 mg elemental/day). Because calcium supplements may decrease phenytoin absorption by approximately 20%, he will need to space these medications 1 to 3 hours apart.

T.J. should avoid changing drug brands, because the bioavailability of phenytoin may vary. Generic phenytoin and Dilantin (Parke-Davis) are not the same. Dilantin capsules are the only extended form of phenytoin sodium available. The extended form can be used for once-daily dosing and for clients who are stabilized on a 300-mg divided dose. Most other forms of phenytoin are prompt acting and are not intended for once-daily dosing. Generic phenytoin capsules and the chewable tablets from Parke-Davis are prompt-acting forms of the drug. It is important that this information be explained clearly to T.J. and his family.

✷ How will T.J.'s phenytoin therapy be evaluated?

The expected outcome of hydantoin therapy is that T.J. will experience decreased or no seizure activity, maintain a serum level within the therapeutic range (e.g., phenytoin 10 to 20 mcg/mL, or free phenytoin level of 1 to 2), demonstrate an absence of or minimal adverse effects to phenytoin, and self-administer the drug safely and accurately. Occasionally, individuals with intractable seizures require a slightly higher-than—"normal" therapeutic range to achieve successful control; monitoring for adverse effects is even more essential for these individuals.

●   ●   ●

valproate

✷▄▀ valproic acid
(Depakene)
divalproex
(Depakote)

The mechanism by which valproic acid exerts its antiseizure effects has not been fully established. Its activity may be related to direct or indirect increase or enhancement of brain levels of the inhibitory neurotransmitter GABA. By competitive inhibition it may prevent the reuptake of GABA by glial cells and axonal terminals. It may also block voltage-sensitive sodium channels, inhibiting neuronal firing. It also appears to modulate calcium current at the calcium T channel. Valproic acid and divalproex are the available oral forms of valproate, which is available as an IV medication. Divalproex consists of two linked valproic acid molecules; this configuration results in slightly longer duration of action with fewer adverse effects.

Indications

Valproate was used in the late 1960s in Europe and was approved in the United States in 1978 for the treatment of absence seizures. Now valproate is indicated for use as sole and adjunctive therapy in the treatment of absence seizures and as adjunctive therapy in clients with multiple seizure types. It is also used for the treatment of bipolar affective disorder and migraine prophylaxis.

Pharmacokinetics/Dosing

Valproic acid is rapidly absorbed orally, often resulting in more rapid peak plasma levels, and occasionally transient level-dependent adverse effects. Divalproex is enteric coated and is more slowly absorbed. However, the extent of absorption of controlled-release formulations is similar to other formulation, resulting in similar dosing. Valproate is highly plasma protein bound (~90%), but its binding is concentration dependent. With higher drug concentrations, the level of free drug increases. For example, at concentrations up to 150 mg/L, valproate is approximately 70% plasma protein bound. The high rate of plasma protein binding contributes to interactions with other highly protein bound drugs (specifically phenytoin). Adult dosing for both valproate and divalproex is usually in the range of 15 to 60 mg/kg/day divided twice daily to three times daily. A once-daily, long-acting oral formulation (Depakote ER) is also available. Childhood dosing is similar, but this drug is typically avoided in

children younger than age 2 years because of a risk for serious hepatotoxicity. An IV formulation is available for short-term use. See Table 17-3 for a pharmacokinetic overview of valproate.

Adverse Effects

Among the more common adverse effects of valproate are nausea, vomiting, gastrointestinal distress (lessened if dosed with food), sedation, dizziness, insomnia, elevated plasma ammonia levels (usually asymptomatic unless concurrent hepatic disease), and thrombocytopenia (bleeding, bruising). Weight gain is common with valproate. Less frequently observed are alopecia, pancreatitis, elevated liver function tests, and, rarely, Stevens-Johnson syndrome.

Drug Interactions

Valproate has fewer significant drug interactions than other antiepileptics but still interacts with a number of agents. (See Table 17-4.)

✷ S.H., an 8-year-old girl, has begun to have generalized tonic-clonic seizures. Upon careful history taking, it was discovered that she had been having absence seizures for some time, which had gone undiagnosed. Because valproate is effective for both types of seizures, the physician has prescribed this AED at 15 mg/kg/day.

✷ What issues related to valproate therapy will be of concern for S.H.?

Assessment There are no specific issues for S.H. In other clients, however, hepatic disease contraindicates the use of valproate therapy, because there have been some instances of fatal hepatotoxicity with the use of this drug. It is also recommended that caution be used in clients with suppressed immune systems (potential for leukopenia), blood dyscrasias, organic brain disease, hypoalbuminemia, thrombocytopenia, and renal function impairment. Baseline evaluation of mental and neurologic status, bleeding time, blood cell counts, and renal and hepatic function studies are recommended. Concurrent drug therapy should be assessed because of valproate's drug interaction potential.

Nursing Diagnosis S.H. has the potential for the following nursing diagnoses/collaborative problems related to valproate therapy: risk of injury related to visual effects (double vision, nystagmus); imbalanced nutrition: less than body requirements related to anorexia, indigestion, and nausea and vomiting; diarrhea; and the potential complications of hepatotoxicity, adverse ophthalmologic effects, pancreatitis (abdominal pain, nausea and vomiting), cognitive impairment, and thrombocytopenia (unusual bruising or bleeding).

Planning During valproate therapy, S.H. will:
- Experience a decrease in the frequency and severity of seizures.
- Experience minimal or no adverse effects associated with valproate drug regimen.
- Comply with valproate therapy.
- Effectively manage the therapeutic regimen with her parents, including identification of therapeutic and adverse effects of valproate.

- Collaborate with health team and with her parents for follow-up care and the appropriate reporting of adverse valproate effects.

✱ **Two months later, S.H.'s dosage was increased to eradicate occasional absence seizures; her trough valproate serum level was 67 mcg/mL at that time. She was followed with monthly visits in which all her lab work was normal and her clinical presentation was normal. In her fifth monthly follow-up visit, S.H. is seizure-free, both for absence and generalized tonic-clonic seizures with a dosage of 500 mg of divalproex twice a day with meals. Her valproate plasma level is 100 mcg/mL. However, her alanine aminotransferase (ALT) was 24 international units/mL and her aspartate aminotransferase (AST) was 38 international units/mL; norms for these tests are 6 to 14 and 7 to 17 international units/mL, respectively. All other lab tests were normal: alkaline phosphatase (ALP), lactate dehydrogenase, bilirubin, prothrombin time (PT), and serum albumin. Her physical examination was negative, as it has been, for scleral icterus, jaundice, abdominal discomfort, or other signs of liver dysfunction.**

✱ **How do these lab results and signs and symptoms relate to S.H.'s health status and valproate therapy?**
Serious hepatotoxicity related to valproate therapy is extremely rare (McAuley & Lott, 2005). It usually occurs in children younger than 2 years of age with severe, difficult-to-control seizures who are taking multiple AEDs. Hepatic damage occurs early in therapy and is evidenced by anorexia, vomiting, lethargy, edema, and jaundice. These symptoms frequently appear before changes in laboratory indicators. Lab findings would change across the board with elevations of ALT, AST, ALP, total bilirubin, serum ammonia, prolonged PTs, and thrombocytopenia.

S.H. has experienced asymptomatic elevations in liver enzymes that commonly occur during the first 6 months of valproate therapy. These are not associated with severe valproate-induced hepatotoxicity. Because she is responding well to valproate therapy and not experiencing significant clinical findings, there will probably be no change in her drug therapy at this time, but her liver function will be monitored closely.

✱ **What monitoring will be essential for S.H.'s valproate therapy?**
For drug efficacy, the nurse will monitor the frequency, intensity, duration, presentation, and time of day of seizures. To assess the adverse effects of the drug, the nurse will monitor the following:
- More common adverse effects
  Dose related: nausea, vomiting, gastrointestinal distress (lessened if dosed with food), sedation, dizziness, insomnia, elevated plasma ammonia levels (usually asymptomatic unless concurrent hepatic disease), thrombocytopenia (bleeding, bruising) (not always correlated with dose)

  Not dose related: Weight gain (often significant), thinning of hair, essential tremor, elevated liver enzymes
- Less common adverse effects
  Dose related: Confusion
  Not dose related: Hepatic dysfunction (jaundice, scleral icterus, nausea, vomiting, lethargy), acute pancreatitis, Stevens-Johnson syndrome

Plasma drug levels are usually drawn as a trough level before the morning dose. The expected therapeutic ranges are as follows:
- For seizure control: 50-100 mg/L
- For bipolar affective disorder: 40-125 mg/L

✱ **What instruction will be essential for S.H. and her parents at this time?**
Instruct S.H. and her parents that she should take her doses with food to reduce GI adverse effects, and to swallow the medication whole, not to chew the tablet or capsule, because it will irritate her mouth and throat. Combining this drug with alcohol, such as in cough and cold remedies, or other CNS depressants, can potentiate sedation. Valproate may also interact with other drugs, OTC preparations, or natural products. Stress the importance of regular administration to prevent seizures (or, in the case of other clients, to control bipolar disorder or migraine headaches).

Tell S.H.'s parents to report to the prescriber if visual disturbances, rash, or diarrhea occur. Valproate may cause liver dysfunction; therefore they should report signs of liver dysfunction (e.g., spontaneous bleeding and bruising, light-colored stools, jaundice, and protracted vomiting) to the prescriber immediately. S.H. should continue to undergo liver function studies at least every month for the first 6 months of therapy, which is when hepatotoxicity is most likely to occur. S.H. and her parents need to know that valproate may cause drowsiness, particularly early in therapy.

Because of the long-term nature of her health problem, S.H. and her parents could benefit from additional information about living with a seizure disorder. See the Technology Link box on p. 355 for links to websites about epilepsy that may be helpful to this family.

✱ **How will S.H.'s valproate therapy be evaluated?**
The expected outcome of valproate therapy is a decrease in the frequency and severity of seizures with a predose serum valproate concentration of at least 50 mcg/mL, and absence of adverse effects of the drug.

✱ **What other agents are available as antiepilepsy drugs?**
Benzodiazepines
The benzodiazepines used in the treatment of seizures include clonazepam (Klonopin), diazepam (Valium), lorazepam (Ativan), and occasionally midazolam (Versed). As a classification, these drugs are CNS depressants; they produce effects ranging from mild sedation to coma, depend-

ing on the dose. This action may be the result of benzodiazepines enhancing or facilitating the action of GABA, a major inhibitory neurotransmitter of the CNS. These drugs appear to suppress the spread of seizure activity produced by foci in the cortex, thalamus, and limbic areas, and increase the seizure threshold.

Clonazepam (Klonopin) is a long-acting drug used to treat absence seizures and myoclonic seizure disorders. It has been used alone but more often is prescribed as an adjunct to other AEDs in establishing seizure control. Diazepam (Valium) may be used parenterally for status epilepticus and for severe recurrent convulsive seizures. The oral dosage form of diazepam is not effective for maintenance control but has been used as an adjunct for short-term treatment in convulsive disorders. Diazepam is not effective alone, and it is recommended for short-term (7 to 14 days) adjunctive therapy (*USP DI*, 2005). Parenteral lorazepam (Ativan) has been used to treat status epilepticus as part of a multidrug approach with support of the client's vital functions (*USP DI*, 2005). See Table 17-3 for a pharmacokinetic overview of benzodi-

azepines, and Chapter 16 for the adverse effects and nursing management of the benzodiazepines.

The dosage of the benzodiazepines is usually individualized for each client and is increased with caution to avoid adverse effects. A lower dosage with a slow increase is prudent in older adults, debilitated persons, and persons taking other CNS depressant–type medications.

Other Agents

✱◼◻ ethosuximide [eth oh **suks** i mide]
(Zarontin)

Ethosuximide is classified as a succinimide. Succinimides produce a variety of effects, such as increasing the seizure threshold and reducing the EEG spike-and-wave pattern of absence seizures by decreasing nerve impulses and transmission in the motor cortex. Related agents include methsuximide (Celontin) and phensuximide (Milontin).

Indications
Ethosuximide is first-line drug therapy for the treatment of absence seizures.

Pharmacokinetics/Dosing
Ethosuximide is administered orally as a syrup or capsule. The typical dose in children is 7.5 to 20 mg/kg twice daily (15 to 40 mg/kg/day). Table 17-3 discusses the pharmacokinetics of ethosuximide.

Adverse Effects
Adverse effects associated with the succinimides include headache, epigastric pain, anorexia, hiccups, nausea, vomiting, rash, pruritus, mood changes, agranulocytosis and, rarely, Stevens-Johnson syndrome.

Nursing Management
Nursing management unique to ethosuximide is assessment for blood dyscrasias before therapy is initiated because of the drug's adverse hematologic effects, and hepatic and renal dysfunction assessment because changes may occur in these organs. In addition to the nursing diagnoses/collaborative problems discussed previously for AED therapy, the client receiving succinimide therapy has the potential for the following: ineffective protection related to the development of blood dyscrasias (agranulocytosis, thrombocytopenia), the potential complications of Stevens-Johnson syndrome and systemic lupus erythematosus (muscle aches, swollen glands, sore throat, fever, skin rash). To prevent epigastric distress, the succinimides can be taken with milk, food, or antacids.

Although blood dyscrasia is rare with the succinimides, when it does occur, it may result in gingival bleeding, delayed healing, and an increase in the number of client infections. Dental work should be deferred until blood counts are within the normal range. The client may need to modify his or her dental hygiene with cautious use of toothbrushes and dental floss. The client should alert other health care providers about the succinimide regimen if surgery, dental work, or emergency medical care is required. Adverse personality changes can occur while taking this medication; stress to the client the importance of reporting any behavioral changes to the prescriber.

✱◼◻ phenobarbital [fee noe **bar** bi tal]
(Barbita, Luminal)

Barbiturates, especially phenobarbital, have been used for many years for the treatment of generalized tonic-clonic and partial seizures, but they are less commonly used now that there are newer agents with less sedative effects. This class of medications is relatively inexpensive and efficacious. Barbiturates are nonselective depressants of the CNS that can produce all levels of CNS mood alteration from mild sedation or hypnosis to deep coma. As AEDs, they are thought to act by depressing synaptic neurotransmission and by increasing the threshold for electrical stimulation of the motor cortex.

Indications
Phenobarbital is primarily used in the management of generalized tonic-clonic, partial, and febrile seizures. Preventing and/or treating

hyperbilirubinemia observed in neonates is an unlabeled indication. It has historically been used as a sedative, but has been largely replaced by the safer benzodiazepines.

Pharmacokinetics/Dosing
Phenobarbital is well absorbed orally with sedative effects observed within the first 30 to 60 minutes. Phenobarbital is primarily metabolized and displays a long duration of action with a half-life in adults between 50 and 140 hours. Between 20% and 50% of phenobarbital is eliminated unchanged in the urine. It is typical daily oral adult dose for the prevention of seizures is 120 to 240 mg daily at bedtime, but lower doses are used for clients with renal impairment. It is available in oral and intravenous forms, with IV administration usually reserved for the management of status epilepticus. (See Table 17-3.) Seizure control and the absence of toxic effects should indicate an optimal blood concentration of phenobarbital. A serum concentration of 10 to 40 mcg/mL is usually desired.

Adverse Effects
Sedation/somnolence and confusion are the most commonly observed adverse effects. Other effects include nausea, vomiting, dose-related respiratory depression, and apnea. See Chapter 16 for a more complete discussion of the use of barbiturates.

Drug Interactions
See Table 17-4.

Nursing Management
See Chapter 16.

acetazolamide [a seat a **zole** a mide]
(Diamox, Apo-Acetazolamide✦)
Acetazolamide is a carbonic anhydrase inhibitor that retards abnormal, paroxysmal, and excessive discharge from CNS neurons although the exact mechanism of action is unknown. It has been theorized that inhibiting carbonic anhydrase in the CNS may result in an increase in carbon dioxide that slows neuronal activity. Systemic metabolic acidosis may also play a part in its action. Tolerance to the antiseizure effects of acetazolamide develops within weeks, rendering its use limited to short-term management. See Chapter 33 for a more complete discussion of this drug.

Indications
Acetazolamide is usually prescribed for the treatment of open-angle glaucoma. It is used in combination with other AEDs as adjuvant treatment for absence seizures, generalized tonic-clonic seizures, mixed seizures, and myoclonic seizure patterns. It is also used to treat edema, and to prevent or treat acute mountain sickness.

Pharmacokinetics/Dosing
The dosage of acetazolamide for AED therapy in adults and children is 4 to 30 mg/kg/day by mouth (PO) (the initial dosage is usually 10 mg/kg/day) in four divided doses (usually a total of 375 to 1000 mg daily). Sustained-released formulations are not recommended for use in the treatment of epilepsy. See Table 17-3 and Chapter 33 for more complete information.

Adverse Effects
Adverse effects include weakness, diarrhea, malaise, anorexia, nausea or vomiting, paresthesia, increased urination, and weight loss.

Nursing Management
For the nursing management of acetazolamide therapy, see Nursing Management of AED Therapy, p. 337, and the drug monograph in Chapter 33.

felbamate [**fel** ba mate]
(Felbatol)
The mechanism of action of felbamate is unknown, but it has some properties in common with the other AEDs; it increases seizure threshold and reduces the spread or progression of a seizure.

Indications
Felbamate is an oral antiepileptic agent used only as adjunct therapy for those clients who do not respond adequately to other AEDs or if the epilepsy is so severe as to make the risk of aplastic anemia

or liver failure acceptable. It is also indicated for Lennox-Gastaut syndrome in children, a condition of a variety of generalized seizures that appears in the first 5 years of life.

Pharmacokinetics/Dosing
Felbamate is well absorbed orally and eliminated in the urine as inactive metabolites and unchanged drug. See Table 17-3 for additional pharmacokinetic and dosing information.

Adverse Effects
The major risk for felbamate is aplastic anemia that limits its use to high-seizure-risk clients who have not responded to other therapy. Other adverse effects include somnolence, fatigue, gastrointestinal complaints, palpitations, depression, anxiety, weight gain, blurred vision, and hepatic dysfunction. Stevens-Johnson syndrome has also been noted.

Drug Interactions
See Table 17-4.

Nursing Management
The nursing management associated with felbamate is discussed earlier in the chapter under Nursing Management of AED Therapy, p. 337. However, unique to felbamate, the client should be assessed for the following nursing diagnoses/collaborative problems: disturbed sleep patterns (daytime sedation); activity intolerance related to malaise and flu-like symptoms; disturbed thought processes (agitation, aggressive reactions); imbalanced nutrition: less than body requirements related to anorexia, nausea, and vomiting; constipation; and the potential complications of blood dyscrasias, hepatic dysfunction, and Stevens-Johnson syndrome. Shake the oral suspension thoroughly before administering.

primidone [**prim** i done]
(Mysoline, Apo-Primidone✦)
Indications
Primidone is used for the control of generalized tonic-clonic, psychomotor, or focal epileptic seizures, as the only agent or as adjuvant therapy.

Pharmacokinetics/Dosing
Primidone and its metabolites, phenobarbital and phenylethylmalonamide (PEMA), contribute to antiseizure activity. The mechanism of action is unknown, but primidone and its metabolites appear to have active antiseizure effects and raise the seizure threshold. Table 17-3 discusses the pharmacokinetics and dosing of primidone.

Adverse Effects
See phenobarbital, p. 355.

Drug Interactions
See phenobarbital and Table 17-4.

Nursing Management
The nursing management associated with primidone is as for other AEDs discussed earlier in the chapter under Nursing Management of AED Therapy, p. 337.

gabapentin [**ga** ba pen tin]
(Neurontin)
The mechanism for its antiseizure action for gabapentin is unknown. Although the chemical structure of gabapentin is similar to that of the neuronal inhibitor GABA, it does not have strong affinity for GABA receptors.

Indications
Gabapentin is an antiepileptic used primarily for the treatment of neuropathic pain and for the treatment of adult partial seizures with or without secondary generalization. It was tested in clients with refractory partial seizures and was reported to reduce seizure frequency significantly. It may also be useful in the management of restless leg syndrome (Silber et al., 2004) and chronic daily headache (Spira & Beran, 2003).

Pharmacokinetics/Dosing
Gabapentin is moderately well absorbed as an oral drug, lacks binding to plasma proteins, and is eliminated renally for the most part. Dosage must be adjusted for clients with renal dysfunction. See Table 17-3 for more pharmacokinetic and dosing information.

Adverse Effects

The major adverse effects of gabapentin are somnolence, ataxia, and fatigue. Other effects include gastrointestinal upset, weight gain, tremor, and bone marrow suppression.

Drug Interactions

See Table 17-4.

Nursing Management

The nursing management associated with gabapentin is as for other AEDs discussed earlier in the chapter under Nursing Management of AED Therapy, p. 337. However, the client receiving gabapentin should be assessed for the following nursing diagnoses/collaborative problems: disturbed sleep patterns (daytime somnolence, 19% of clients); risk for falls (dizziness, ataxia, 12.5% to 17%); fatigue (11%); and the potential complications of depression, vision disturbances, nystagmus, myalgia, tremor, and peripheral edema. For clients who cannot tolerate oral capsules, the contents of the capsule may be sprinkled over soft foods immediately before use. The medicine degrades quickly and should be taken immediately after being prepared. Clients taking gabapentin three times daily should not allow more than 12 hours to pass between doses.

lamotrigine [la moe **trih** jeen]

(Lamictal)

Lamotrigine is chemically unrelated to other AEDs and its mechanism of action is unknown. It is believed that lamotrigine stabilizes seizures by inhibiting voltage-sensitive sodium channels, thus stabilizing neuronal membranes and inhibiting the release of the excitatory neurotransmitters (glutamate, aspartate) believed to have a role in the development and spread of epileptic seizures (*Drug Facts and Comparisons*, 2005).

Indications

Lamotrigine is indicated as adjunct therapy for the treatment of partial seizures in adults (16 years of age and older). It is also used in the management of bipolar illness.

Pharmacokinetics/Dosing

Lamotrigine is well absorbed orally and is eliminated by hepatic and renal mechanisms. Concurrent use of valproate greatly increases half-life, whereas concurrent use of carbamazepine or phenytoin greatly decreases half-life (see drug interactions). As such, dosing is variable and based on concurrent drug therapy. See Table 17-3 for more information.

Adverse Effects

Lamotrigine is associated with a relatively high rate of central nervous system effects including dizziness, headache, ataxia, and somnolence. Diplopia, blurred vision, and nausea are also frequently observed. Of greatest concern are hypersensitivity reactions with potentially life-threatening Stevens-Johnson type rash, which requires hospitalization. This reaction is more likely with high doses or concurrent use of valproate. Any rash observed for a client receiving lamotrigine requires immediate medical evaluation.

Drug Interactions

Lamotrigine interacts significantly with carbamazepine, phenytoin, and valproate as discussed above. See Table 17-4 for more information on drug interactions.

Nursing Management

The nursing management associated with lamotrigine is as for other AEDs discussed earlier in the chapter. However, unique possible nursing diagnoses related to its adverse effects are as follows: risk for injury related to CNS toxicity (dizziness, ataxia, confusion, depression, increased seizures, or nystagmus); disturbed sleep patterns (drowsiness); anxiety; impaired skin integrity (rash); hyperthermia; and the potential complications of vision abnormalities (diplopia, blurred vision), angioedema, blood dyscrasias, and hypersensitivity syndrome (jaundice, dark urine, flu-like symptoms, swollen lymph nodes, and fatigue). Instruct the client undergoing lamotrigine therapy to notify the health care provider if a skin rash occurs or seizure activity increases.

levetiracetam [leave ty rah **see** tam]

(Keppra)

Levetiracetam is unrelated to other AEDs, and its mechanism of action is unknown. It does not seem to interact with known mecha-

nisms involved in inhibitory or excitatory neurotransmission (*Drug Facts and Comparisons*, 2005).

Indications

Levetiracetam is an AED indicated for the treatment of partial-onset seizures in adults. An unlabeled indication for levetiracetam is in the management of bipolar disorder.

Pharmacokinetics/Dosing

Levetiracetam is well absorbed orally and eliminated in the urine as both unchanged drug and inactive metabolites. Typical adult dose ranges from 500 mg twice daily to 2000 mg twice daily. Dosage adjustment is required for renal insufficiency. See Table 17-3 for further information regarding pharmacokinetics and dosing.

Adverse Effects

The primary adverse effects of levetiracetam include sedation, headache, muscle weakness, and bone marrow suppression. Hallucinations, psychosis, and increased risk for infection have also been noted.

Drug Interactions

See Table 17-4.

magnesium sulfate [mag **nees** ee um]

Magnesium sulfate has a depressant effect on the CNS. In addition, it prevents or controls seizures by blocking peripheral neuromuscular transmission, which reduces acetylcholine release at the myoneural junction, which decreases the sensitivity of the motor endplate and lowers the excitability of the motor membrane.

Indications

Magnesium sulfate has three major indications. As an AED, it is used in the prevention and control of seizures related to acute nephritis in children and seizures related to toxemias of pregnancy (Box 17-3). As a uterine relaxant, it is used in the treatment of uterine tetany and to inhibit contractions of premature labor. It is also used as replacement therapy for magnesium deficiency.

Pharmacokinetics/Dosing

When magnesium sulfate is administered for the treatment of toxemia of pregnancy, the drug crosses the placenta, with fetal blood levels approximately equal to maternal blood levels, and produces similar effects in the neonate and in the mother. Decreased reflexes, muscle tone, blood pressure, and respiratory depression may be seen if the mother received magnesium shortly before delivery. It is recommended that magnesium sulfate not be administered during the 2 hours before delivery, if possible. For seizures caused by toxemia in pregnancy, the dosage is 4 to 5 g (32 to 40 mEq) IV in 250 mL of D_5W or normal saline administered over 30 minutes. Administer intramuscular (IM) doses of up to 10 g (maximum of 5 g in each buttock). (See Table 17-3.)

Adverse Effects

The primary adverse effects of magnesium sulfate infusion include hypotension and risk for asystole with rapid infusion. Elevated magnesium levels are associated with CNS depression, respiratory depression, heart block, diarrhea, and depressed neuronal reflexes. See the Management of Drug Overdose box on p. 358.

Nursing Management

Assessment

The nursing management of a client undergoing magnesium sulfate therapy is somewhat different than management of a client using another AED because of its specific indication of toxemia of pregnancy and the mechanism of action. Magnesium sulfate is not used in the presence of heart block, significant heart damage, or renal failure (creatinine clearance less than 20 mL/min). Exercise caution with clients with severe renal function impairment because of the risk of hypermagnesemia and magnesium toxicity. A baseline assessment includes blood pressure and respiratory rate determination, deep tendon reflexes, ECG for cardiac function, renal function determinations (especially urine output), and serum magnesium levels.

Nursing Diagnosis

The client undergoing magnesium sulfate therapy is assessed for the following nursing diagnoses/collaborative problems: risk for injury related to hypotension and electrolyte imbalances (hypermagnesemia); activity intolerance related to hypotonia; and the potential complication of cardiac dysrhythmias and respiratory paralysis.

Planning

During magnesium sulfate therapy, the client will experience:

- Absence of seizures.
- Minimal or no adverse effects associated with magnesium sulfate regimen.

Implementation

Monitoring

While magnesium sulfate is being administered, monitor seizure activity and vital signs every 15 minutes. Respirations should be at least 16 breaths/min before each parenteral dose. Monitor intake and output; urinary output should be at least 100 mL in the 4 hours before each dose. Closely monitor the client for development of magnesium toxicity. The ECG should be monitored continuously during IV administration. Serum magnesium determinations may be obtained as clinically indicated. Normal average serum magnesium concentrations are 1.6 to 2.6 mEq/L. The following are approximate serum concentrations (mEq/L) indicative of hypermagnesemia:

- 4 to 7: therapeutic range, mild depression of deep tendon reflexes

BOX 17-3 TOXEMIA OF PREGNANCY (PREECLAMPSIA AND ECLAMPSIA)

Toxemia of pregnancy is a syndrome of elevated blood pressure, edema, and proteinuria, which occurs in approximately 5% of all pregnancies in North America. The syndrome is described in clinical terms because its cause is unknown. Preeclampsia is another term for the syndrome. Depending on the severity of symptoms, preeclampsia may be classified as mild (may be treated at home), or severe (requires hospitalization for monitoring and treatment). If the disease progresses, seizures will occur and the syndrome is classified as eclampsia, which is derived from a Greek word used to describe seizures. Sensory changes that occur in severe preeclampsia and eclampsia include headache, epigastric pain, blurred vision, and hyperreflexia. Therapeutic goals for the treatment of toxemia of pregnancy are control of blood pressure, prevention of seizures, maintenance of renal function, and provision of optimal conditions for the fetus. Treatment is symptomatic because the only "cure" for toxemia is delivery of the baby. Seizures may still occur up to 48 hours after delivery, necessitating continued therapy in the immediate postpartum period.

Management of Drug Overdose

Magnesium Sulfate

Signs of hypermagnesemia, which may begin at a serum concentration at or above 5 mEq/L, include flushing, hypotension, sweating, depressed reflexes, reduced respiratory rate, hypothermia, flaccid paralysis, circulatory collapse, slowed heart rate, and CNS depression.

Treatment includes artificial respiration, calcium gluconate IV (5 to 10 mEq of calcium) injected slowly to reverse respiratory depression and heart block. In reduced renal function, dialysis may be necessary.

- 5 to 10: depression of deep tendon reflexes; prolonged PQ interval or widened QRS interval on ECG
- 8 to 10: loss of deep tendon reflexes
- 10 to 13: respiratory paralysis
- 15: altered cardiac conduction
- 25: cardiac arrest

The patellar reflex or knee jerk is an indication of CNS depression from magnesium. The patellar reflex should be checked before beginning therapy and before each dose. The disappearance of the reflex indicates excessive serum levels of magnesium and the dose should be withheld.

Intervention

Approximately one-third of dietary-ingested magnesium is absorbed from the gastrointestinal tract. With IV administration, the onset of action is immediate, and the duration of action is approximately 30 minutes. With IM administration, the onset of action is approximately 1 hour, and the duration of action is 3 to 4 hours. See the Management of Drug Overdose box below. Extreme care must be taken to avoid overdose and toxic serum concentrations of magnesium. IV infusions should be administered with a computerized regulating or controlling device. A calcium salt that can be administered intravenously (calcium gluconate, calcium gluceptate, or calcium chloride) should be available when parenteral magnesium is administered.

Education

The client should report muscle weakness and other adverse effects of magnesium as soon as they are experienced.

Evaluation

The client will not experience seizures related to toxemia of pregnancy, her magnesium serum concentrations will remain in the therapeutic range (4 to 7 mEq/L), and she will not experience hypotonia, cardiac dysrhythmias, or respiratory paralysis.

oxcarbazepine [ox car **bay** zeh peen]
(Trileptal)

Oxcarbazepine is chemically related to carbamazepine. Its antiepileptic mechanism of action is unknown, but it does block the voltage-sensitive sodium channels which results in the stabilization of hyperexcited neural membranes, inhibition of repetitive neuronal firing, and synaptic impulses (*Drug Facts and Comparisons*, 2005).

Indications

Oxcarbazepine (Trileptal) is used as monotherapy to treat partial seizures in adults and as adjunctive therapy for children (ages 4 to 16 years) with epilepsy and adults with partial seizures.

Pharmacokinetics/Dosing

Oxcarbazepine is well absorbed orally. It is a prodrug that is converted to an active metabolite (10-monohydroxy derivative). This active metabolite is further metabolized to inactive metabolites that are eliminated in the urine. See Table 17-3 for dosing and further pharmacokinetic data.

Adverse Effects

This drug is better tolerated than carbamazepine and, unlike carbamazepine, does not induce its own metabolism. Like carbamazepine, it can cause drug-induced SIADH with hyponatremia; consequently, monitoring of serum sodium concentrations is important. Adverse effects include dizziness, somnolence, ataxia, diplopia, blurred vision, nystagmus, nausea, vomiting, and abdominal pain.

Drug Interactions

See Table 17-4.

Nursing Management

The nursing management associated with oxcarbazepine is as for other AEDs discussed earlier in the chapter under Nursing Management of AED Therapy, p. 337.

tiagabine [tye **ah** gah been]
(Gabitril)

The mechanism of action of tiagabine is unknown, but it is thought to enhance the activity of GABA, the major inhibitory neurotransmitter in the CNS.

Indications

Tiagabine is prescribed as an adjuvant for the management of partial seizures in adults and children older than 12 years of age.

Pharmacokinetics/Dosing

Tiagabine is well absorbed orally when taken with food, is highly bound to plasma proteins, and is eliminated by hepatic metabolism involving P450 3A4. The typical adult dose is titrated from 4 mg daily up to 56 mg daily divided in two to four doses. Refer to Table 17-3 for more information.

Adverse Effects

Tiagabine most commonly produces dizziness, sedation, nausea, and muscle weakness. It may also result in confusion, depression, rash, nystagmus, diarrhea, and tremor. Tiagabine, even at low doses, has the potential to induce seizure activity and status epilepticus when used in clients with mental illness who do not have epilepsy (FDA Public Health Advisory, 2005).

Drug Interactions

See Table 17-4.

Nursing Management

The nursing management associated with tiagabine is as for other AEDs discussed earlier in the chapter under Nursing Management of AED Therapy, p. 337. However, unique possible nursing diagnoses/collaborative problems related to its adverse effects are as follows: risk for injury related to the CNS effects of the drug (ataxia, confusion, difficulty in concentrating, memory impairment, weakness); disturbed sleep patterns (drowsiness, insomnia); nausea; diarrhea; impaired skin integrity (rash); and the potential complications of nystagmus, flu-like syndrome, tremor, and myalgia. Tiagabine should be taken with food.

topiramate [toe **pyre** a mate]
(Topamax)

Although the exact mechanism of action for topiramate is unknown, it has three properties that may contribute to its antiseizure characteristics. First, it appears to have a sodium channel blocking action, thus blocking the repetitive depolarization of neurons; second, it potentiates the activity of the inhibitory neurotransmitter GABA; and third, it antagonizes the ability of kainate (a receptor agonist) to activate an excitatory glutamate receptor (*Drug Facts and Comparisons*, 2005).

Indications

Topiramate is indicated for adjunct therapy for partial-onset and tonic-clonic seizures in adults, in children 2 to 16 years of age, and in clients older than 2 years of age with Lennox-Gastaut syndrome. Topiramate may also be effective in the treatment of migraine headache (Brandes et al., 2004). Its role in the treatment of diabetic neuropathic pain is under study with conflicting data to date (Raskin et al., 2004; Thienel, Neto, Schwabe, & Vijapurkar, 2004).

Pharmacokinetics/Dosing

Topiramate is well absorbed orally and is metabolized by P450 2D6 and 3A4 to three active metabolites. The elimination half-life is genetically determined based on variation in P450 activity. Refer to Table 17-3 for dosing and pharmacokinetic information.

Adverse Effects

The adverse effects of topiramate include dizziness, sedation, ataxia, confusion, nausea, nystagmus, diplopia, and an increased risk for infections. Other adverse effects include muscle weakness, gastrointestinal upset, anorexia, flu-like symptoms, and hyperchloremic metabolic acidosis. There is a relatively high risk for developing kidney stones with topiramate; this risk may be reduced with adequate hydration.

Drug Interactions

See Table 17-4.

Nursing Management

The nursing management associated with topiramate is as for other AEDs discussed earlier in the chapter under Nursing Management of AED Therapy, p. 337. Some nursing diagnoses specific to the adverse effects of topiramate are as follows: impaired verbal communication (speech problems); acute confusion; risk for injury related to the CNS effects of the drug (ataxia, weakness, psychomotor slowing); imbalanced nutrition: less than body requirements (anorexia, weight loss); fatigue; impaired oral mucous membrane (gingivitis); and the potential complications of vision disturbances, dysmenorrhea, renal stones, and leukopenia. The client undergoing topiramate therapy has to maintain an adequate fluid intake to minimize the risk of renal stone formation. Caution should be taken with activities that require alertness. The client should use alternative contraception methods if using oral estrogen-containing contraceptives. Avoid breaking topiramate tablets because of the bitter taste.

✱⌐ zonisamide [zoe **nis** a mide]
(Zonegran)

Although the exact mechanism of action of zonisamide is unknown, it is thought to stabilize neuronal membranes and suppress seizure activity.

Indications

Zonisamide is used as an adjunct for the treatment of partial seizures in adults.

Pharmacokinetics/Dosing

Zonisamide is metabolized to metabolites that may be pharmacologically active. It is excreted in the urine as both unchanged drug and as metabolites. See Table 17-3 for dosing and pharmacokinetic information.

Adverse Effects

Sedation, irritability, ataxia, confusion, nausea, abdominal pain, and paresthesias are among the more common adverse effects of zonisamide.

Drug Interactions

See Table 17-4.

Nursing Management

The nursing management associated with zonisamide is as for other AEDs discussed earlier in the chapter under Nursing Management of AED Therapy, p. 337.

Status Epilepticus

✱ K.E., a 22-year-old, 80-kg college student, has been brought to the emergency department. Although recently diagnosed as having idiopathic epilepsy, he has been well-controlled, seizure-free for generalized tonic-clonic seizures for the past 3 months, on 200 mg PO three times daily of carbamazepine. Just prior to his being transported to the emergency department, he experienced two tonic-clonic seizures in the dormitory. On his arrival, in a semiconscious state, his vital signs are blood pressure 190/100 mm Hg, pulse 120 beats/min, respirations 22 breaths/min, and temperature 37° C (98.6° F). As soon as his vital signs are completed, K.E. begins another seizure.

✱ **Does K.E. meet the diagnostic criteria for status epilepticus?**

Status epilepticus (SE) is considered a life-threatening emergency characterized by more than 30 minutes of continuous seizure activity or two or more sequential seizures without a full return to consciousness. Such seizure activity is associated with neuronal damage and loss of cerebral autoregulation. It is estimated that status epilepticus is a likely event at some point in 5% of adults with epilepsy and between 10% and 25% of children with epilepsy. Mortality is reported to be as high as 20%, and is correlated highly with other comorbidities (e.g., stroke, trauma) and advanced age

(Manno, 2003). Continuous electrical seizure activity on EEG without motor manifestations has also been described. Although relatively rare, manifestations may include changes in cognition or behavior, or may present as severe neurologic deficits or coma (Shneker & Fountain, 2003).

❀ How will AEDs be used in the management of K.E.'s status epilepticus?

The overriding goal in the management of SE is to ensure ventilation and to eliminate all seizure activity as quickly as possible. K.E. is positioned on his side to allow for drainage of saliva and to prevent aspiration until such time as his seizure lessens enough to ensure safe placement of an airway. An IV line is inserted to obtain blood chemistries, AED serum concentrations, and toxicology screens, as well as provide access for AEDs.

Agents used for the management of SE include benzodiazepines, phenytoin/fosphenytoin, and barbiturates (Figure 17-1).

Benzodiazepines, specifically lorazepam or diazepam, are considered the first drugs of choice for SE. Lorazepam (Ativan) given IV at a dose of 0.1 mg/kg or diazepam (Valium) 0.15 mg/kg intravenously has been well studied. Lorazepam at this dose resulted in seizure control within 20 minutes in 65% of participants in a large U.S. Department of Veterans Affairs (VA) study (Treiman et al., 1998), and is advocated by most clinicians as the first drug of choice. Baseline vital signs are obtained before parenteral forms of diazepam (Valium) or lorazepam (Ativan) are given. After administration, K.E. is observed at bed rest for decreases in respiratory rate, heart rate, and blood pressure—for at least 3 hours for diazepam and 8 hours for lorazepam.

Diazepam (Valium) is insoluble in water; each milliliter of the parenteral form contains 40% propylene glycol, 10% ethyl alcohol, 5% sodium benzoate/benzoic acid as buffers, as well as 1.5% benzyl alcohol as a preservative. If this ratio is altered, the diazepam becomes insoluble. If direct IV injection is not possible, diazepam may be injected through

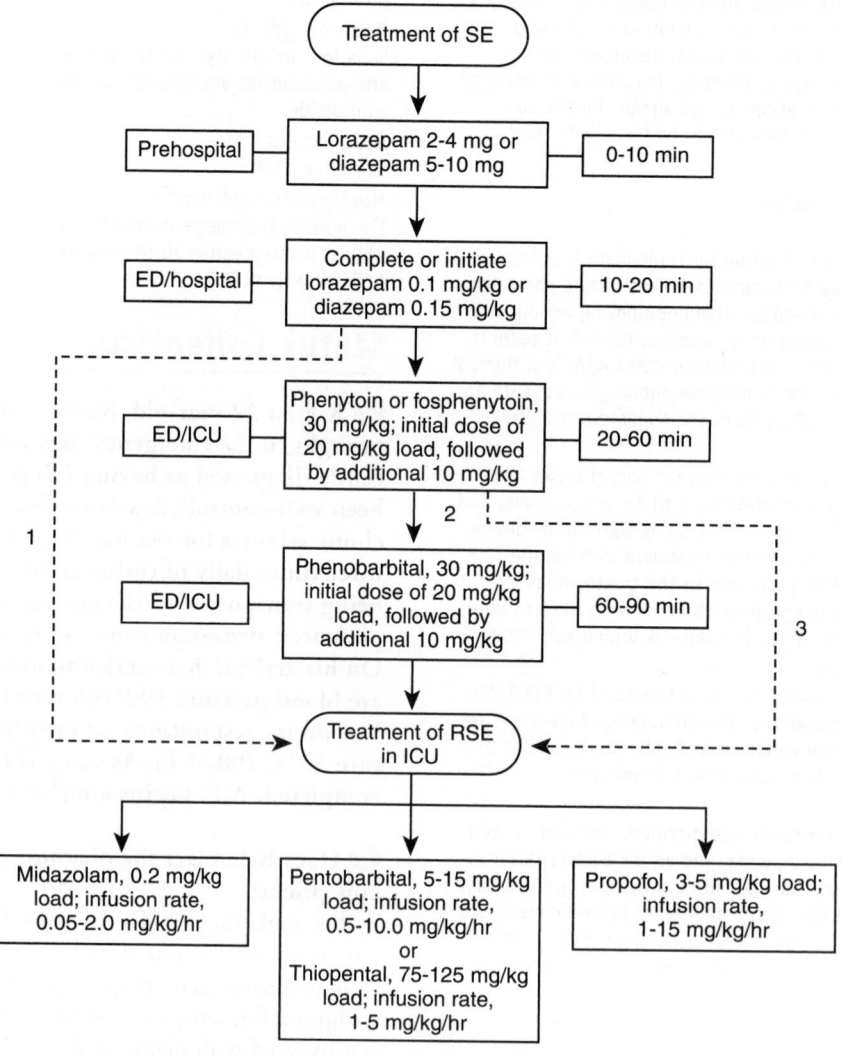

Note: All medications administered intravenously.

FIGURE 17-1 Status epilepticus algorithm. *ED,* Emergency department; *ICU,* intensive care unit; *RSE,* resistant status epilepticus; *SE,* status epilepticus.

From Manno EM. (2003). New management strategies in the treatment of status epilepticus. *Mayo Clinic Proceedings, 78*(4), 508-518.

the infusion tubing as close to the insertion point as possible. Inject slowly, at least 1 minute for each 5 mg.

Lorazepam (Ativan) must be diluted with a compatible diluent immediately before IV use. It may be infused directly into a vein or through IV tubing. To prevent apnea, infusion rates should not exceed 2 mg/min.

Because of the short-lived effect of IV benzodiazepine administration, seizures that are brought under prompt control may recur. Be ready to readminister the drug. Benzodiazepines are not for maintenance; once seizure control is achieved, agents useful in long-term seizure control should be considered. Tonic status epilepticus has been precipitated in some clients treated with IV diazepam for absence seizure status or absence seizure variant status.

Exercise extreme care when administering benzodiazepines (especially by the IV route) to older adults, very ill clients, or clients with compromised pulmonary reserve because of the possibility of apnea and cardiac arrest. Monitor respirations every 5 to 15 minutes and before each IV dose. Resuscitative equipment should be available because of possible hypotension, tachycardia, and respiratory depression.

The efficacy and safety of parenteral diazepam has not been established for neonates 30 days of age or younger. Prolonged CNS depression has been reported in neonates, probably as a result of the inability to biotransform diazepam into inactive metabolites.

The benzoate in the injectable form has been reported to displace other drugs and bilirubin from the plasma protein binding sites, causing jaundice. To minimize the occurrence of thrombophlebitis after IV injection of diazepam, the vein can be flushed with 1 mL of saline per milligram of diazepam.

If benzodiazepines are given along with an opioid, the dosage of the opioid should be reduced. As controlled substances, the nurse is responsible for proper documentation of distribution and use of these drugs.

If benzodiazepines are not effective within 5 to 7 minutes, additional therapy is recommended. Traditional algorithms have recommended initiation of phenytoin or fosphenytoin at doses of 18 to 20 mg/kg load, at rates not to exceed 50 mg/min for phenytoin or 150 mg PE/min for fosphenytoin, with additional follow-up dosing if response is inadequate. ECG monitoring is recommended during K.E.'s infusion. In general, older adults, seriously ill clients, debilitated clients, or clients with renal function impairment should receive a lower dose at a much slower rate of administration. Clients who are maintained on phenytoin should receive a pro-rated dose based on serum levels. Monitor blood pressure and cardiac function closely. The dose-related adverse effects increase with the rapidity at which the client is dilantinized to the therapeutic range. To proceed cautiously and slowly is clinically prudent. Bilateral and vertical nystagmus develops at levels of 15 mg PE/kg body weight administered at 150 mg PE/min; tinnitus, pruritus, ataxia, drowsiness, and diplopia are also seen at this level.

IV phenobarbital has also historically been recommended if benzodiazepines or phenytoin are ineffective (see Figure 17-1). Given the time delay with sequencing phenytoin and phenobarbital, and newer evidence suggesting ir-reversible changes in brain function with prolonged seizure activity, some advocates are recommending changes in management to consider those who fail initial benzodiazepine therapy as having refractory SE and to initiate aggressive general anesthetic strategies in a critical care setting. Such strategies include the use of midazolam (Versed), short-acting barbiturates (pentobarbital, thiopental), or propofol (Diprivan). In such circumstances, an airway must be managed and vasopressor support may be required (refer to Chapter 15 for a more complete discussion of these agents). An additional management approach is to initiate these anesthetic agents while infusing phenytoin to avoid excessive delay in controlling SE (Manno, 2003).

Summary

Epilepsy, a symptom of a brain disorder rather than a disease itself, occurs in only a small percentage of the population. Epileptic seizures have various causes and are classified by symptoms. The nurse needs to be particularly observant in the assessment and documentation of seizures. The drugs used for the treatment of seizures are also varied and include barbiturates, hydantoins, succinimides, and benzodiazepines. The therapy for each client is individualized by taking into account a complex of interrelated factors, such as the pharmacokinetics of the drug in an individual, concurrent ailments and medications, diet, physical status, and compliance with the regimen. The nurse uses a holistic approach, not only to manage the client's physical symptoms but also to provide psychosocial support. For these clients, moderation in rest, exercise, diet, and avoidance of stress is important. The most common nursing diagnoses for clients receiving AED therapy are deficient knowledge, ineffective management of therapeutic regimen, and risk for injury related to the adverse effects of these drugs. An important evaluation factor is the effectiveness of the regimen in controlling and minimizing seizures.

⊛ **Critical Thinking Questions**

- Why is assessment essential in determining a therapeutic antiepileptic medication regimen for a client?

- Mrs. Curtis and her husband have decided to start a family. She is 24 years of age and has been taking phenytoin since childhood for a seizure disorder; she would like to discontinue the medication before getting pregnant. What criteria will be involved in deciding whether to wean Mrs. Curtis from her medication?

Bibliography

Anderson, D.M., Keith, J., Novak, P.D. & Eliot, M.A. (2002). *Mosby's medical, nursing, & allied health dictionary* (6th ed.). St. Louis: Mosby.

Anderson, G.D. (2004). Pharmacogenetics and enzyme induction/inhibition properties of antiepileptic drugs. *Neurology, 63*(10 Suppl. 4), S3-S8.

Asawavichienjinda, T., Sitthi-Amorn, C., & Tanyanont W. (2003). Compliance with treatment of adult epileptics in a rural district of Thailand. *Journal of the Medical Association of Thailand, 86*(1), 46-51.

Bazil, C.W., & Pedley, T.A. (2003). Clinical pharmacology of antiepileptic drugs. *Clinical Neuropharmacology, 26*(1), 38-52.

Beydoun, A., & Kutluay, E. (2003). Conversion to monotherapy: Clinical trials in patients with refractory partial seizures. *Neurology 60*(11 Suppl. 4), S13-S25.

Birnbaum, A., Hardie, N.A., Leppik, I.E., Conway, J.M., Bowers, S.E., Lackner, T., et al. (2003). Variability of total phenytoin serum concentrations within elderly nursing home residents. *Neurology, 60*, 555-559.

Brandes, J.L., Saper, J.R., Diamond, M., Couch, J.R., Lewis, D.W., Schmitt, J., et al.; MIGR-002 Study Group. (2004). Topiramate for migraine prevention: A randomized controlled trial. *Journal of the American Medical Association, 291*, 965-973.

Burkhardt, R.T., Leppik, I.E., Blesi, K., Scott, S., Gapany, R.S., & Cloyd, J.C. (2004). Lower phenytoin serum levels in persons switched from brand to generic phenytoin. *Neurology, 63*, 1494-1496.

Carpenito-Moyet, L.J. (2004). *Nursing diagnosis: Application to clinical practice* (10th ed.). Philadelphia: Lippincott Williams & Wilkins.

Cleary, P., Shorvon, S., & Tallis, R. (2004). Late-onset seizures as a predictor of subsequent stroke. *Lancet, 363*, 1184-1186.

Drazkowski, J.F., Fisher, R.S., Sirven, J.I., Demaerschalk, B.M., Uber-Zak, L., Hentz, J.G., et al. (2003). Seizure-related motor vehicle crashes in Arizona before and after reducing the driving restriction from 12 to 3 months. *Mayo Clinic Proceedings, 78*, 819-825.

Drug facts and comparisons. (58th ed.). (2005). St. Louis: Facts and Comparisons.

Epocrates RxPro™, version 6.11, www.epocrates.com, updated September 12, 2003.

Epocrates Rx, version 7.0 as cited via www.epocrates.com and updated November 17, 2004.

Ensrud, K.E., Blackwell, T.,. Mangione, C.M., Bowman, P.J., Bauer, D.C., Schwartz, A., et al. (2003). Study of Osteoporotic Fractures Research Group. Central nervous system active medications and risk for fractures in older women. *Archives of Internal Medicine, 163*(8), 949-957.

FDA Public Health Advisory. (February 18, 2005). Seizures in patients without epilepsy being treated with Gabitril (tiagabine). Retrieved May 15, 2005, from http://www.fda.gov/cder/drug/advisory/gabitril.htm.

Fitzpatrick, L.A. (2002). Secondary causes of osteoporosis. *Mayo Clinic Proceedings, 77*(5), 453-468.

Glauser, T.A. (2002). Advancing the medical management of epilepsy: Disease modification and pharmacogenetics. *Journal of Child Neurology, 17*(Suppl. 1), S85-S93.

Gomes, M.M., & Maia, F.H.S. (1998). Medication-taking behavior and drug self-regulation in people with epilepsy. *Arquivos de Neuro-Psiquiatria, 56*(4), 714-719.

Greene, M.F. (2003). Magnesium sulfate for preeclampsia. *New England Journal of Medicine, 348*(4), 275-276.

Grim, S.A., Ryan, M., Miles, M.V., Tang, P.H., Strawsburg, R.H., de-Grauw, T.J., et al. (2003). Correlation of levetiracetam concentrations between serum and saliva. *Therapeutic Drug Monitoring, 25*(1), 61-66.

Holmes, G.L. (2002). The interface of preclinical evaluation with clinical testing of antiepileptic drugs: role of pharmacogenomics and pharmacogenetics. *Epilepsy Research, 50*(1-2), 41-54.

Jankowiak, J., & Malow, B. (2003). Seizures in children with fever: Generally good outcome. *Neurology, 60*(2), E1-E2.

Jarrar, R.G., & Buchhalter, J.R. (2003). Therapeutics in pediatric epilepsy, part 1: The new antiepileptic drugs and the ketogenic diet. *Mayo Clinic Proceedings, 78*(3), 359-370.

Johannessen, S.I., Battino, D., Berry, D.J., Bialer, M., Kramer, G., Tomson, T., et al. (2003). Therapeutic drug monitoring of the newer antiepileptic drugs. *Therapeutic Drug Monitoring, 25*(3), 347-363.

Lacy, C.F., Armstrong, L.L., Goldman, M.P., & Lance, L.L. (2004). *Lexi-Comp's drug information handbook* (12th ed.). Hudson, OH: Lexi-Comp.

LaRoche, S.M., & Helmers, S.L. (2004). The new antiepileptic drugs: Scientific review. *Journal of the American Medical Association, 291*(5), 605-614.

Liporace, J., & D'Abreu, A. (2003). Epilepsy and women's health: Family planning, bone health, menopause, and menstrual-related seizures. *Mayo Clinic Proceedings, 78*(4), 497-506.

Manno, E.M. (2003). New management strategies in the treatment of status epilepticus. *Mayo Clinic Proceedings, 78*(4), 508-518.

McAuley, J.W., & Lott, R.S. (2005). Seizure disorders. In M.A. Koda-Kimble, L.Y. Young, W.A. Kradjan, B.J. Guglielmo, B.K. Alldredge, & R.L. Corelli (Eds.), *Applied therapeutics: The clinical use of drugs.* Philadelphia: Lippincott Williams & Wilkins.

McNamara, J.O. (2001). Drugs effective in the therapy of the epilepsies. In J.G. Hardman, A.G. Gilman, & L.E. Limbird (Eds.), *Goodman & Gilman's the pharmacological basis of therapeutics.* New York: McGraw Hill.

National Institute of Neurological Disorders and Stroke. (2003). NINDS epilepsy information page. Retrieved September 20, 2003, from www.ninds.nih.gov/health_and_medical/disorders/epilepsy.htm

Nguyen, D.K., & Spencer, S.S. (2003). Recent advances in the treatment of epilepsy. *Archives of Neurology, 60*(7), 929-935.

 e-LEARNING SUPPLEMENTS

Student CD-ROM
- Final Exam questions
- NCLEX® Examination review questions
- Pharmacology animations
- Printable chapter summary

- WebLinks corresponding to this chapter
- Answers to the critical thinking questions in this chapter
- *Elsevier ePharmacology Update* newsletter
- *Mosby's Drug Consult* Internet Edition
- Supplemental and reference information

Evolve Website (http://evolve.elsevier.com/mckenry)
- Case study on antiepileptic drugs
- Content updates, including information on new drugs

Nulman, I., Laslo, D., & Koren, G. (1999). Treatment of epilepsy in pregnancy. *Drugs 57*(4), 535-544.

Ogunniyi, A., Oluwole, O.S., & Osuntokun, B.O. (1998). Two-year remission in Nigerian epileptics. *East African Medical Journal, 75*(7), 392-395.

Patsalos, P.N. (2000). Antiepileptic drug pharmacogenetics. *Therapeutic Drug Monitoring, 22*(1), 127-130.

Pennell, P.B. (2003). The importance of monotherapy in pregnancy. *Neurology, 60*(11 Suppl. 4), S31-S38.

Raskin, P., Donofrio P.D., Rosenthal N.R., Hewitt D.J., Jordan D.M., Xiang J., et al.; CAPSS-141 Study Group. (2004). Topiramate vs placebo in painful diabetic neuropathy: Analgesic and metabolic effects. *Neurology, 63*, 865-873.

Richmond, J.R., Krishnamoorthy, P., Andermann, E., & Benjamin, A. (2004). Epilepsy and pregnancy: An obstetric perspective. *American Journal of Obstetrics & Gynecology, 190*, 371-379.

Schachter, S.C. (2002). Drug-mediated antiepileptogenesis in humans. *Neurology, 59*(9 Suppl. 5), S34-S35.

Shneker, B.F., & Fountain, N.B. (2003). Assessment of acute morbidity and mortality in nonconvulsive status epilepticus. *Neurology, 61*, 1066-1073.

Siddiqui, A., Kerb, R., Weale, M.E., Brinkmann, U., Smith, A., Goldstein, D.B., et al. (2003). Association of multidrug resistance in epilepsy with a polymorphism in the drug-transporter gene ABCB1. *New England Journal of Medicine, 348*, 1442-1448.

Silber, M.H., Ehrenberg, B.L., Allen, R.P., Buchfuhrer, M.J., Earley, C.J., Hening, W.A., et al.; for the Medical Advisory Board of the Restless Legs Syndrome Foundation (2004). An algorithm for the management of restless legs syndrome. *Mayo Clinic Proceedings, 79*(7), 916-922.

Sirven, J.I. (2002). Antiepileptic drug therapy for adults: When to initiate and how to choose. *Mayo Clinic Proceedings, 77*(12), 1367-1375.

Spira, P.J., & Beran, R.G., for the Australian Gabapentin Chronic Daily Headache Group. (2003). Gabapentin in the prophylaxis of chronic daily headache: A randomized, placebo-controlled study. *Neurology, 61*, 1753-1759.

Thienel, U., Neto W., Schwabe S.K., & Vijapurkar U.; Topiramate Diabetic Neuropathic Pain Study Group. (2004). Topiramate in painful diabetic polyneuropathy: Findings from three double-blind placebo-controlled trials. *Acta Neurol Scand, 110*, 221-231.

Thummel, K.E, & Shen, D.D. (2001). Design and optimization of dosage regimens: Pharmacokinetic data. In J.G. Hardman, A.G. Gilman, & L.E. Limbird (Eds.), *Goodman & Gilman's the pharmacological basis of therapeutics.* New York: McGraw Hill.

Touchette, D.R., & Rhoney, D.H. (2000). Cost-minimization analysis of phenytoin and fosphenytoin in the emergency department. *Pharmacotherapy, 20*(8), 908-916.

Treiman, D.M., Meyers, P.D., Walton, N.Y., Collins, J.F., Colling, C., Rowan, A.J., et al. (1998). Veterans Affairs Status Epilepticus Cooperative Study Group. A comparison of four treatments for generalized status epilepticus. *New England Journal of Medicine, 339*, 792-798.

USP DI: Drug information for the health care professional (25th ed.). (2005). Greenwood Village, CO: MICROMEDEX Thomson Healthcare.

18

Central Nervous System Stimulants

Chapter Focus

The central nervous system (CNS) stimulants may produce dramatic effects, but their therapeutic usefulness is limited because of their multiple actions and adverse effects. Continuous use and misuse of these drugs (especially amphetamines) can result in the development of tolerance, dependence, and abuse. Large doses of the CNS stimulants may precipitate convulsive seizures, coma, and exhaustion. Although the number of drugs that stimulate the CNS is large, only a few of these drugs are actually used for this purpose. The nurse needs to be knowledgeable about both the therapeutic uses and the nontherapeutic effects of CNS stimulant drugs, which are commonly abused in our society.

Learning Objectives

- Identify the characteristics of attention deficit hyperactivity disorder, its subtypes and the drug treatment for this condition.
- Define the terms *analeptic* drug and *anorexiant* drug.
- Describe common CNS stimulant drugs and the indications for their use.
- Identify common physical and psychologic changes attributable to CNS stimulants.
- List caffeine-containing food and beverages, along with their approximate caffeine content.
- Implement an appropriate plan of care for the client receiving CNS stimulant drugs.

▲ Key Terms

amphetamines, p. 364
analeptics, p. 364
anorexiants, p. 364
attention deficit hyperactivity disorder, p. 369
narcolepsy, p. 371

Key Drugs

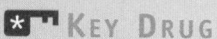

dextroamphetamine/amphetamine, p. 366
caffeine, p. 375
atomoxetine, p. 368

What agents are considered stimulants?

Stimulants increase neuronal activity in the CNS. The classification of a stimulant depends on where in the nervous system it exerts its major effects—on the cerebrum, the medulla and brainstem, or the hypothalamic and limbic regions. **Amphetamines** are mainly stimulants of the cerebral cortex; **analeptics** primarily affect the centers in the medulla and the brainstem; and **anorexiants** suppress the appetite, perhaps by a direct stimulant effect on the satiety center in the hypothalamic and limbic regions. CNS stimulants act by increasing neuronal discharge or by blocking an inhibitory neurotransmitter. These drugs may also affect the autonomic nervous system and result in changes in cardiovascular and other organ systems.

✱ What are the common uses of stimulants?

Amphetamines were once commonly prescribed for obesity and to counteract an overdose of CNS depressants, but such use today is considered obsolete. Although amphetamines do suppress appetite, tolerance develops to the anorexic effect usually before the weight reduction goal is reached, and weight often returns to baseline when drug is discontinued. Treatment of severe CNS depression with stimulants is also discouraged because close monitoring and supportive measures have been found to be quite successful without producing undesirable adverse effects. With their narrow therapeutic index between effectiveness and toxicity, CNS stimulants may induce cardiac dysrhythmias, hypertension, seizures, and violent behavior. Thus the CNS stimulants and newer stimulant-like agents with similar pharmacology are used primarily for the treatment of attention deficit hyperactivity disorder (ADHD) and narcolepsy. Alternative newer stimulant-like agents, including the drug sibutramine (Meridia), have been used in place of the older stimulants when appetite suppression is a goal.

✱ What is the mechanism of action of stimulants?

The classic stimulants amphetamine, amphetamine/dextroamphetamine (Adderall), methylphenidate (Concerta, Metadate, Methylin, Ritalin), dexmethylphenidate (Focalin), pemoline (Cylert), and phentermine (Adipex-P) work as adrenergic agonists in the CNS and also exhibit peripheral effects. These stimulants act to stimulate CNS neuronal discharge by the release of norepinephrine in the neuron. Norepinephrine activates neurons in the reticular formation of the brain. This increases attentiveness and wakefulness. At higher doses, these stimulants release of dopamine and serotonin (5-hyroxytryptamine or 5 HT) in the neuron (Figure 18-1). These agents stimulate the respiratory center, lessen CNS depression with other drugs, and result in increased alertness, elevation of mood, and moderate improvement in mental and physical performance. They may also precipitate seizures in high doses with clients predisposed to seizure activity. Their action at increasing norepinephrine and/or dopamine may explain their ability to suppress appetite, but tolerance to this effect is noted rapidly with repeated use (Hoffman, 2001). With the exception of atomoxetine (Strattera) discussed below, all of these stimulants are controlled drugs; pemoline (Cylert) and phentermine (Adipex-P) are U.S. Food and Drug Administration (FDA) Schedule IV substances; the remaining agents are FDA Schedule II.

Peripheral effects of amphetamine, dextroamphetamine, methylphenidate, and dexmethylphenidate include increased systolic and diastolic blood pressure. At high doses, cardiac dysrhythmias may occur. These agents may result in constriction of the urinary bladder sphincter, increased uterine tone, and variable effects on gastrointestinal (GI) motility (Hoffman, 2001). Cautious use in individuals with hypertension, cardiac conditions, urinary retention, and GI conditions is warranted. These drugs are considered category C in pregnancy, and their use is typically not recommended unless the benefit clearly outweighs the risks. Pe-

moline (Cylert) exhibits fewer peripheral effects and has a Pregnancy Category B rating.

The stimulant-like drugs sibutramine (Meridia) and diethylpropion (Tenuate) work to inhibit reuptake of norepinephrine and dopamine (Figure 18-2). They produce similar effects to the stimulants above and are FDA Schedule IV substances. Modafinil (Provigil) is also a stimulant-like drug; it is unrelated to other stimulants and is primarily used for narcolepsy. It inhibits the reuptake of dopamine. Modafinil is also an FDA Schedule IV substance (Rxlist, 2004b).

Atomoxetine (Strattera) represents a newer approach in the treatment of ADHD. Its action appears similar to sibutramine and diethylpropion, but appears to be selective for the presynaptic norepinephrine transporter (Rxlist, 2004a). Unlike the other stimulant-like drugs, it is not an FDA controlled substance and is not officially considered a stimulant. Atomoxetine appears to have less CNS stimulatory effects than amphetamines and methylphenidate, and a lower likelihood for peripheral effects. Cardiac dysrhythmias have been reported, but appear to be more common in adults compared to children and adolescents (Rxlist, 2004a).

Individual client responses to CNS stimulants may be modified by the client's genetic make-up. See the Special Considerations for Pharmacogenetics box on p. 366.

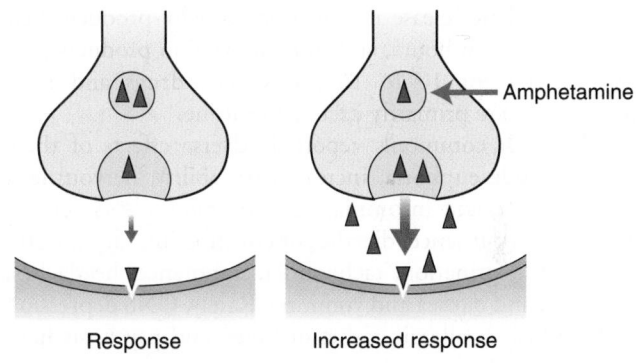

Response   **Increased response**

▲ Catecholamines
(norepinephrine, dopamine, and serotonin)

FIGURE 18-1 Effect of amphetamines on CNS neuron.

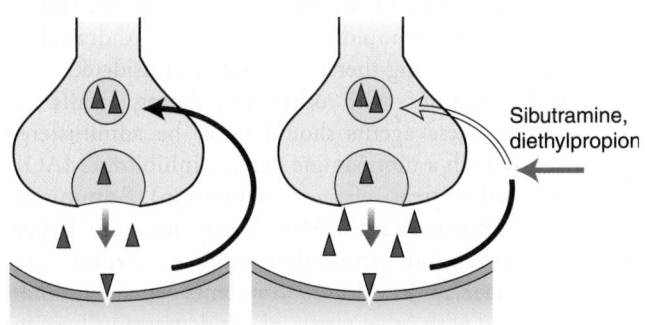

▲ Catecholamines
(norepinephrine, dopamine, and serotonin)

FIGURE 18-2 Action of sibutramine and diethylpropion on CNS neuron. Atomoxetine acts in a similar manner and is specific for norepinephrine only.

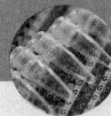 Special Considerations for Pharmacogenetics | STIMULANTS

PHARMACODYNAMICS

Response to methylphenidate (Ritalin) is related to the genetic expression of the norepinephrine transporter gene [G1287 A] (Yang et al., 2004) and the dopamine transporter gene [SLC6 A3] (Roman et al., 2002). Catechol-*O*-methyl transferase (COMT) activity, responsible for degradation of norepinephrine and other monoamine neurotransmitters, has reduced activity in approximately 25% of the white population (Zhu, 2002). These factors may account for altered physiologic response to stimulants.

PHARMACOKINETICS

A number of stimulants and related agents, including atomoxetine (Strattera), dextroamphetamine (in Adderall), and methyl-phenidate (Ritalin), are metabolized extensively by cytochrome P450 2D6 (Lacy et al., 2004). Reduced clearance of MDMA (3,4-methylenedioxymethamphetamine) is expected in the 7% to 10% of the population who are deficient in 2D6 activity (de la Torre et al., 2004), which may explain variation in levels and response across populations.

ADVERSE EFFECTS

The altered clearance of MDMA and other related designer drugs secondary to population variation in 2D6 activity may explain the neurotoxicity, serotonin syndrome, and other complications observed with these agents (Maurer et al., 2004). Given similar metabolic pathways for other stimulants, genetics is likely to play a role in the risk for adverse effects with stimulant therapy.

❋ How are the stimulants and stimulant-like drugs similar?

As a group, these drugs are rapidly absorbed when taken orally, are lipid soluble, and cross the blood-brain barrier. The immediate-release formulations usually produce their effects for 4 to 6 hours, and sustained-action products produce effects for 10 to 16 hours. The drugs and their metabolites are primarily excreted in urine.

The most commonly reported adverse effects of these drugs include euphoria, increased irritability, nervousness, hypertension, and insomnia. Less common adverse effects are visual disturbance, diarrhea or constipation, dry mouth, difficulty in urination, tachycardia, impotence, headaches, sweating, and nausea and vomiting. Rarely, CNS depression and confusion, allergic rashes or hives, and psychosis have been reported.

Acute withdrawal from these agents typically manifests as feelings of restlessness and anxiety. This can be observed on discontinuation of these drugs, but may also be observed at the end of the dosing interval for shorter-acting agents. Any client with rebound anxiety or restless behavior shortly before the next dose should be evaluated for withdrawal effects, and longer acting therapy should be considered.

Drug interactions with other stimulating agents are problematic. These agents should never be administered concurrently with a monoamine oxidase inhibitor (MAOI) (typically used to treat refractory depression). Administration of a stimulant with a MAOI may result in hyperpyrexia, hypertension, cardiac dysrhythmias, seizures, cerebral hemorrhage, and/or death. Stimulants generally should also be avoided with other classes of antidepressants because of excessive stimulation effects and potential for altered metabolism/increased levels of one or both drugs. Concurrent use with other vasoconstrictive drugs (e.g., agents to treat migraine headaches, decongestants) can exacerbate hypertension and risk for coronary events.

❋ How do the stimulant and stimulant-like drugs differ?

In addition to differences in mechanisms of action as noted above, these drugs vary in indication, dose, drug interactions, and abuse potential. Key drugs are presented here; Table 18-1 lists the differences among available agents.

Agents That Stimulate Release of Catecholamines

✦⌐ dextroamphetamine and amphetamine
[dex troe am **fet** a meen and am **fet** a meen]
(Adderall, Adderall XR)

Indications

The amphetamines are among the first of the modern stimulants available on the market, and are indicated for ADHD and narcolepsy. They have historically been used for obesity, and are occasionally used for minimal brain dysfunction in children and as an antidepressant. They are FDA Schedule II drugs.

Pharmacokinetics/Dosing

Different formulations of amphetamine or dextroamphetamine/amphetamine salt combinations are available. The brands Adderall and Adderall XR contain a mixture of two dextroamphetamine and two amphetamine salts to provide pharmacokinetic profile with both immediate and more prolonged action throughout the day. Peak levels are typically seen at about 3 hours with the immediate-release form and at about 7 hours with the extended-release form of the drug. Half-lives of amphetamine salts are in the range of 10 to 13 hours for adults and 9 to 11 hours for children. The typical dose of Adderall XR in children older than age 6 years is 5 to 10 mg once daily in the morning with the dose increased up to 30 mg daily based on response.

Adverse Effects

Reports of 12 unexplained deaths between 1999 and 2003 with the use of Adderall XR prompted its removal from the Canadian market by Health Canada in early 2005 (FDA Alert, 2005). A history of cardiac structural abnormalities was noted in five cases, and elevated levels were cited in two cases. The FDA recommends not using this agent in clients with structural cardiac abnormalities.

TABLE 18-1 COMPARISON OF STIMULANTS AND STIMULANT-LIKE DRUGS

Agent	Indication	Mechanism of Action	Typical Adult Daily Dose†	FDA Schedule	Comments
amphetamine/ dextroamphetamine (Adderall, Adderall XR)	Narcolepsy ADHD*	Stimulates NE, 5-HT, DA release	5-30 mg	II	
dexmethylphenidate (Focalin)	ADHD		2.5-20 mg	II	
dextroamphetamine (Dexedrine)	ADHD Narcolepsy Obesity Adjunct*		5-40 mg	II	
methylphenidate (Concerta, Metadate CD, Metadate ER, Methylin, Methylin ER, Ritalin, Ritalin LA, Ritalin SR)	ADHD Narcolepsy*		10-60 mg	II	
pemoline (Cylert) (United States only)	ADHD Narcolepsy*		37.5-112.5 mg	IV	Risk of hepatic failure Obtain informed consent
phentermine (Adipex-P)	Obesity		15-37.5 mg	IV	PHEN-FEN combo associated with PPH
diethylpropion (Tenuate, Tenuate SR)	Obesity	Inhibits NE/DA reuptake	75 mg	IV	
sibutramine (Meridia)	Obesity		10-15 mg	IV	
modafinil (Provigil)	Narcolepsy Multiple sclerosis*	Inhibits DA reuptake	100-400 mg	IV	May have ↑ cardiovascular risk
atomoxetine (Strattera)	ADHD	Inhibits NE reuptake	40-100 mg	Prescription, but not a scheduled drug	Dose reduction for hepatic insufficiency

DA, Dopamine; *5-HT*, 5-hydroxytryptamine (serotonin); *NE*, norepinephrine; *PHEN-FEN*, phentermine and fenfluramine; *PPH*, primary pulmonary hypertension.
*May not be FDA approved for all formulations.
†Dose may vary by indication. With sustained-action products, the full dose may be given once daily in AM; other formulations may require splitting the total dose into two or three doses during the day.

Additional adverse effects of amphetamines are similar to other stimulants. Anorexia, abdominal pain, insomnia, and emotional lability are among the more commonly observed adverse effects.

methylphenidate [meth ill **fen** i date]
(Concerta, Metadate CD, Metadate ER, Ritalin, Ritalin LA, Ritalin SR)
Indications
Methylphenidate is indicated for the treatment of ADHD and narcolepsy. It is occasionally used in the treatment of depression in older adults or the medically ill, although this is not an official FDA-approved indication for use. Although historically it has been used to manage obesity, this is no longer considered an appropriate use.
Pharmacokinetics/Dosing
Methylphenidate is available in a number of immediate- and sustained-release formulations. It is well absorbed orally, and metabolized via cytochrome P450 2D6 to active metabolites with an elimination half-life of approximately 2 to 4 hours. Specific dose is based on indication, client's age, and formulation used.
Adverse Effects
Methylphenidate shares an adverse effect profile with other stimulants. Among the more common effects are nervousness and insom-

TABLE 18-2 BODY MASS INDEX CALCULATOR*

BMI	19	20	21	22	23	24	25	26	27	28	29	30	31	32	33	34	35
Height (inches)								Body Weight (pounds)									
58	91	96	100	105	110	115	119	124	129	134	138	143	148	153	158	162	167
59	94	99	104	109	114	119	124	128	133	138	143	148	153	158	163	168	173
60	97	102	107	112	118	123	128	133	138	143	148	153	158	163	168	174	179
61	100	106	111	116	122	127	132	137	143	148	153	158	164	169	174	180	185
62	104	109	115	120	126	131	136	142	147	153	158	164	169	175	180	186	191
63	107	113	118	124	130	135	141	146	152	158	163	169	175	180	186	191	197
64	110	116	122	128	134	140	145	151	157	163	169	174	180	186	192	197	204
65	114	120	126	132	138	144	150	156	162	168	174	180	186	192	198	204	210
66	118	124	130	136	142	148	155	161	167	173	179	186	192	198	204	210	216
67	121	127	134	140	146	153	159	166	172	178	185	191	198	204	211	217	223
68	125	131	138	144	151	158	164	171	177	184	190	197	203	210	216	223	230
69	128	135	142	149	155	162	169	176	182	189	196	203	209	216	223	230	236
70	132	139	146	153	160	167	174	181	188	195	202	209	216	222	229	236	243
71	136	143	150	157	165	172	179	186	193	200	208	215	222	229	236	243	250
72	140	147	154	162	169	177	184	191	199	206	213	221	228	235	242	250	258
73	144	151	159	166	174	182	189	197	204	212	219	227	235	242	250	257	265
74	148	155	163	171	179	186	194	202	210	218	225	233	241	249	256	264	272
75	152	160	168	176	184	192	200	208	216	224	232	240	248	256	264	272	279
76	156	164	172	180	189	197	205	213	221	230	238	246	254	263	271	279	287

Data from http://www.nhlbi.nih.gov/guidelines/obesity/bmi_tbl.htm.

*Body mass index is a means to evaluate degree of obesity in objective terms and correlates weight and height. **Underweight:** below 18.5; normal: 18.5-24.9; **overweight:** 25.0-29.9; **obesity class I:** 30.0-34.9; **obesity class II:** 35.0-39.9; **obesity class III:** 40+.

nia. Other potentially concerning effects include tachycardias, dysrhythmias, urticaria or rash, and hypersensitivity reactions.

Agents That Affect Reuptake of Catecholamines

atomoxetine [a toe **mox** e teen]
(Strattera)

Atomoxetine differs from other stimulants and stimulant-like drugs in that its mode of action is related to the inhibition of reuptake of norepinephrine. Although its use requires a prescription, it is not an FDA controlled substance and to date, abuse has not been reported.

Indications

Atomoxetine is indicated for the treatment of ADHD. It is being investigated for its role in treating depression, but this is not an FDA-approved indication for use.

Pharmacokinetics/Dosing

Atomoxetine is well absorbed orally, but the beneficial effect from therapy may not be observed during the first few weeks of therapy. The typical initial dose for children (6 years and older) and adolescents is 0.5 mg/kg/day. Approximately 2% to 7% of the population are poor metabolizers of atomoxetine because of reduced activity of cytochrome P450 2D6 and may require significantly lower doses. Similarly, the antidepressants fluoxetine (Prozac) and paroxetine (Paxil) may inhibit the metabolism of atomoxetine and result in levels 5- to 10-fold higher than without these agents. Dose adjustments are required for clients with hepatic insufficiency.

Adverse Effects

The FDA published a warning about the risk for serious hepatotoxicity with atomoxetine in December 2004. The potential for liver failure requiring transplantation or leading to death is a concern with the use of this agent. Early warning signs include pruritus,

jaundice, dark urine, abdominal tenderness, and unexplained "flu-like" symptoms (U.S. Food and Drug Administration, 2004b). Other adverse effects include headache, insomnia, xerostomia, nausea and vomiting, and anorexia. Adults may be more likely to observe cardiac dysrhythmias, hypertension, orthostatic hypotension, or erectile dysfunction.

sibutramine [sye **byoo** tra meen]
(Meridia)

Sibutramine is a norepinephrine and dopamine reuptake inhibitor in the CNS.

Indications

Sibutramine is indicated for the management of obesity when the body mass index (BMI) is greater than 30 kg/m² or greater than 27 kg/m² if other risk factors (e.g., hypertension, diabetes) are present. (Table 18-2 is a BMI calculator.) Like other agents used for obesity management, it should be used in conjunction with a reduced calorie diet and other lifestyle modifications.

Pharmacokinetics/Dosing

Sibutramine is well absorbed orally, highly plasma protein bound, and metabolized extensively by cytochrome P450 3A4. The typical adult dose is 10 mg daily with titration up to 15 mg after 4 weeks if needed and tolerated.

Adverse Effects

Common adverse effects with sibutramine include headache, insomnia, xerostomia, rhinitis and constipation. Tachycardia, dysrhythmias, nervousness, and gastrointestinal upset have also been reported.

Drug Interactions

As with other stimulants, attention to drug interactions is important, with the avoidance of antidepressants and vasoconstrictive agents warranted.

TABLE 18-2 BODY MASS INDEX CALCULATOR—*cont'd*

BMI	36	37	38	39	40	41	42	43	44	45	46	47	48	49	50	51	52	53	54
Height (inches)									Body Weight (pounds)										
58	172	177	181	186	191	196	201	205	210	215	220	224	229	234	239	244	248	253	258
59	178	183	188	193	198	203	208	212	217	222	227	232	237	242	247	252	257	262	267
60	184	189	194	199	204	209	215	220	225	230	235	240	245	250	255	261	266	271	276
61	190	195	201	206	211	217	222	227	232	238	243	248	254	259	264	269	275	280	285
62	196	202	207	213	218	224	229	235	240	246	251	256	262	267	273	278	284	289	295
63	203	208	214	220	225	231	237	242	248	254	259	265	270	278	282	287	293	299	304
64	209	215	221	227	232	238	244	250	256	262	267	273	279	285	291	296	302	308	314
65	216	222	228	234	240	246	252	258	264	270	276	282	288	294	300	306	312	318	324
66	223	229	235	241	247	253	260	266	272	278	284	291	297	303	309	315	322	328	334
67	230	236	242	249	255	261	268	274	280	287	293	299	306	312	319	325	331	338	344
68	236	243	249	256	262	269	276	282	289	295	302	308	315	322	328	335	341	348	354
69	243	250	257	263	270	277	284	291	297	304	311	318	324	331	338	345	351	358	365
70	250	257	264	271	278	285	292	299	306	313	320	327	334	341	348	355	362	369	376
71	257	265	272	279	286	293	301	308	315	322	329	338	343	351	358	365	372	379	386
72	265	272	279	287	294	302	309	316	324	331	338	346	353	361	368	375	383	390	397
73	272	280	288	295	302	310	318	325	333	340	348	355	363	371	378	386	393	401	408
74	280	287	295	303	311	319	326	334	342	350	358	365	373	381	389	396	404	412	420
75	287	295	303	311	319	327	335	343	351	359	367	375	383	391	399	407	415	423	431
76	295	304	312	320	328	336	344	353	361	369	377	385	394	402	410	418	426	435	443

✱ **A.L. is an 8-year-old male in the second grade of school. He is always interrupting his teacher, jumping out of his seat in class, fidgeting, and butting into other children's games. At home, he runs around recklessly and is seemingly uncontrollable. A.L.'s parents wonder why he will not listen and they are concerned because his grades in school are dropping.**

During the past two decades the prevalence of ADHD and its pharmacologic treatment has increased dramatically in the United States (Robison, Sclar, Skaer, & Galin, 1999). **Attention deficit hyperactivity disorder (ADHD)** is a syndrome characterized by distractibility, a short attention span, impulsive behavior, hyperactivity, and/or learning and behavior disabilities. There are three subtypes of ADHD: those with both inattention and hyperactivity-impulsivity; those with predominantly hyperactivity-impulsivity; and those with predominantly inattentive type. Recognition of the latter type is often missed and therefore, undertreated. Improper functioning of the neurotransmitter systems (noradrenergic, dopaminergic, and serotonergic) has been implicated in this syndrome (Saklad & Sherr, 2001). Stimulant medications and newer agents with similar pharmacology (atomoxetine [Strattera]) tend to decrease distractibility and hyperactivity, resulting in an increased attention span (Berman, Douglas, & Barr, 1999; Sunohara et al., 1999). The accurate diagnosis of ADHD is critical before the initiation of drug therapy. Box 18-1 presents the diagnostic criteria of ADHD.

The onset of ADHD usually occurs between the ages of 3 and 7 years, with boys affected more often than girls by a 4:1 to 9:1 ratio (Saklad & Sherr, 2001). Parents of children with ADHD often have ADHD or comorbid conditions such as anxiety, depression, and obsessive-compulsive disorder, which may affect how ADHD in the child is managed (Chronis et al., 2003). While medication is usually unnecessary until the child enters the school setting, early professional intervention and behavioral counseling to establish regular schedules and sleep patterns can be of significant benefit.

ADHD may persist into adulthood. In one report of young adults who had ADHD in childhood, 31% still had the full syndrome. Adults with ADHD may have a higher incidence of substance abuse, antisocial personality disorders, anxiety, and depression when compared with a control group. Children treated with stimulants are reported to have a better outcome in adulthood (Saklad & Sherr, 2001). Management of this disorder requires a behavioral modification program, with the use of pharmacologic therapy as an adjunct if necessary.

It seems ironic that stimulants improve symptoms of ADHD. Their action in the cerebral cortex appears to improve the ability of individuals with ADHD to better focus on tasks and filter out extraneous stimuli.

Approximately 15% to 20% of children with ADHD either do not respond to stimulant drugs or their symptoms actually increase. Such individuals often also have symptoms of anxiety or depression, and primary treatment of those conditions with antidepressants may be indicated. Clonidine (Catapres) has been used, especially for persons with both ADHD and Tourette syndrome; this product should not be used for children with ADHD and depression because it can worsen the condition (Saklad & Sherr, 2001).

BOX 18-1 DIAGNOSTIC CRITERIA FOR ATTENTION DEFICIT HYPERACTIVITY DISORDER (ADHD)

The diagnosis of ADHD must meet all of the following criteria:

A. Either 1 or 2.
1. Six or more of the following symptoms of inattention for at least 6 months, which are maladaptive:
   • Fails to give close attention or careless mistakes in schoolwork or work.
   • Difficulty sustaining attention in talk or play.
   • Does not seem to listen when spoken to directly.
   • Does not follow through on instructions and fails to finish schoolwork or tasks.
   • Difficulty organizing tasks or activities.
   • Avoids engaging in tasks requiring sustained mental effort.
   • Often loses things necessary for tasks or activities.
   • Is easily distracted by extraneous stimuli.
   • Forgetful.
2. Six or more of the following symptoms of hyperactivity-impulsivity for 6 months, which are maladaptive:
   • Fidgets with hands or feet.
   • Leaves seat in class or other situations where remaining seated is expected.
   • Runs about or climbs excessively (or in adults, subjective feeling of restlessness.)
   • Difficulty in playing or engaging in leisure activities quietly.
   • Often "on the go" or acts as if "driven by a motor."
   • Talks excessively.
   • Blurts out answers before questions have been completed.
   • Difficulty awaiting turn.
   • Interrupts or intrudes on others.
B. Some symptoms present before the age of 7 years.
C. Some impairment of symptoms is present in two or more settings.
D. Clear evidence of clinically significant impairment in social, academic or occupational functioning.
E. Symptoms do not occur exclusively during a course of or accounted for by other mental illness.

Three subtypes of ADHD are commonly observed:
• **ADHD, Combined Type:** Criteria for both inattention and hyperactivity-impulsivity are observed for the past 6 months.
• **ADHD, Predominantly Inattentive Type:** Criteria for inattention, but not hyperactivity-impulsivity, is observed for the past 6 months.
• **ADHD, Predominantly Hyperactive-Impulsive Type:** Criteria for hyperactivity-impulsivity, but not inattention, is observed for the past 6 months.

Data from American Academy of Pediatrics. (2000). Clinical practice guideline: Diagnosis and evaluation of the child with attention-deficit/hyperactivity disorder. *Pediatrics, 105*(5), 1158-1170; and Center for Disease Control and Prevention. (2004). Retrieved March 30, 2004, from http://www.cdc.go/ncbddd/adhd/symptom.htm.

✱ **A thorough evaluation finds no other appropriate medical diagnosis and that A.L. is on no other medications. A.L. indicates he frequently forgets his homework, loses pieces to puzzles and games, and hates to sit and read. While in the office, he is not inattentive, but is easily distracted by people passing in the hallway when the door is ajar.**

✱ **Is A.L. a candidate for pharmacotherapy?**

Based on initial presentation, A.L.'s behaviors and school performance appear to be consistent with ADHD. It is decided to begin A.L. on a course of methylphenidate 5 mg in the morning, with an additional dose to be added at noon if necessary. Other strategies also are discussed with his parents, such as family therapy, parent training, social skills training, academic skills training, and behavioral therapy to be used with the medication.

✱ **What is the nursing management for A.L.'s pharmacotherapy?**

Assessment A.L.'s assessment determines that he does not have any preexisting health conditions that might preclude methylphenidate therapy or require additional surveillance. He also is on no other medications. A baseline assessment includes an evaluation of A.L.'s growth and development status, complete blood counts, and blood pressure determination.

Nursing Diagnosis Once methylphenidate therapy has begun, A.L. is assessed for the following nursing diagnoses/collaborative problems: disturbed sleep patterns; disturbed thought processes (confusion); imbalanced nutrition: less than body requirements related to its anorexiant effects (especially in children); anxiety; situational low self-esteem related to school performance; and the potential complications of mental depression and altered cardiac output (hypertension, tachycardia) related to the cardiovascular effects of methylphenidate.

Planning While A.L. is using CNS stimulants, he will:
• Maintain normal body weight.
• Continue normal growth and development.
• Demonstrate less distraction and improved school performance.
• Experience minimal or no adverse effects of the CNS stimulant (e.g., sleep deprivation, anorexia, palpitations).
• Report any adverse symptoms to his parents.

Implementation

Monitoring A.L. is monitored for weight loss from appetite suppression because of the drug's anorexiant effects. Chart his growth and development with each visit. Pulse rate will determine cardiovascular status. Obtain his perceptions of his progress—how things have changed for him.

Intervention Some children respond better to the immediate-release methylphenidate and dosage varies based on the child's schedule of activities (e.g., a noon dose for an afternoon music lesson). The timing of these agents is important to assure improved control of symptoms during the waking day, but also not interfere with sleep patterns. Most clinicians now strive for once-daily morning dosing of extended-release or longer-acting agents; such dosing achieves good control, may improve adherence to therapy, and does not interfere with sleep. Such dosing also will not require A.L. to bring medicine to school, which can reduce stigma associated with ADHD, and does not place him in the dilemma of transporting a controlled substance back and forth to school. The sustained-release form lasts up to 8 hours and causes more lunchtime anorexia. Dosages should be calculated for each client based on response to methylphenidate. Extended-release dosage forms are used only after the initial therapy has established the appropriate dosage for A.L. To prevent insomnia, administer the last daily dose of the non–extended-release form several hours before bedtime. Children in particular should be assessed on a regular basis for physical growth, because normal weight gain may be suppressed. When the symptoms of ADHD improve, it may be possible to interrupt drug therapy during times of low stress. The client may be given medication-free weekends, holidays, or vacations. The drug is also discontinued periodically to reassess therapeutic need, which is indicated by the return of symptoms. Long-term therapy should be accompanied by repeated medical examinations and tests for complete blood counts and platelet counts.

Education A.L. and his parents are instructed for him to take the medication on an empty stomach 30 to 45 minutes before eating. Extended-release forms should be swallowed whole, not crushed, broken, or chewed. Do not increase the dosage if the medication seems less effective. Regular visits with A.L.'s prescriber are needed to monitor progress of the drug therapy. Withdrawal must be gradual if A.L. takes large doses over an extended period. He is not to stop taking the medication without checking with the prescriber, because there is a risk for depression on withdrawal. Careful supervision is therefore required during withdrawal. Tolerance and psychologic dependence have occurred with long-term use, and abnormal behavior and psychotic episodes have been observed.

In adults, methylphenidate is used cautiously in clients with a history of drug dependence, alcoholism, or other mental health issue. Those who abuse substances have used it as a substitute for amphetamines.

Evaluation The expected outcome of A.L.'s methylphenidate therapy is that he will demonstrate clinical improvement. He will have an increased attention span with a decreased restlessness, improved classroom behavior, improved peer relations, and improved self-esteem, and will be able to sleep without difficulty and not evidence any adverse effects.

✴ What are important considerations with stimulant and stimulant-like drug use in ADHD?

It is well known that individuals with ADHD are at higher risk for substance abuse. Most of the stimulants are controlled drugs. Atomoxetine (Strattera) is a prescription drug with stimulant-like properties, but is not considered a controlled substance, nor is it considered to possess a high abuse potential. Although many families will be concerned that the use of a controlled substance in youth may contribute to the risk for substance abuse, there is relatively strong evidence to support the observation that their use *reduces* by twofold the risk of developing a substance abuse problem for individuals with ADHD (Wilens et al., 2003).

Stimulants have the potential to suppress growth in children and adolescents. It has been a long-standing practice to institute stimulant-free periods (e.g., 1 or more weeks of no stimulants) during holidays to allow for growth spurts. This practice has been debated, with growth suppression only noted in individuals experiencing significant nausea and vomiting and in individuals using high-dose stimulants (Kramer, Loney, Ponto, Roberts, & Grossman, 2000). Clinicians using these agents typically follow growth patterns carefully, and may consider a drug-free period when children are significantly below their peers in growth pattern. Because these agents are also associated with reduced appetite, monitoring weight and eating patterns is important.

There are less long-term data on the use of stimulants in children younger than age 6 years despite increasing use in this population (Greenhill et al., 2003). More studies are required to solidify the role of these agents in very young children.

✴ Which stimulants are used in treating narcolepsy?

Narcolepsy is a condition characterized by excessive drowsiness and uncontrollable sleep attacks during the daytime. In addition, the client may exhibit a sleep paralysis (inability to move that occurs immediately on falling asleep or on awakening), cataplexy (stress-induced, generalized muscle weakness), and hypnologic illusions or hallucinations (vivid auditory or visual dreams occurring at the onset of sleep). CNS stimulants are useful in controlling daytime drowsiness and excessive sleep patterns. The amphetamines methylphenidate and modafinil (Provigil) have been used for narcolepsy. Pemoline (Cylert) has also been used for this purpose, although it is not FDA approved for narcolepsy.

✴ L.D. is a 44-year-old, 62-inch female who weighs 260 pounds. She is otherwise in reasonably good health. She has tried many diets and arrives at clinic seeking a prescription for appetite control.

✴ What is the role of stimulants in the management of obesity?

L.D. presents with a BMI of 42 (obesity class III). Obesity is a risk factor for a number of conditions, including type 2 diabetes mellitus, cardiovascular disease, and a number of cancers. Obesity also significantly increases risk for complications in pregnancy (Cedergren, 2004). Every attempt to encourage weight loss to improve her health status should be made. Before drug therapy is instituted, however, a complete medical history should be obtained, including an evaluation of which types of diets have not been successful. Stimulant therapy should be avoided if there is a history of substance abuse or mental illness (e.g., mania, psychosis). The presence of existing cardiovascular disease may also be problematic with some stimulant therapy. Even though L.D. is considered in the most significant obesity class, many clinicians would consider the institution of a dietary and exercise plan with strong social supports before starting drug therapy. Other controllable cardiovascular risk factors should also be addressed (e.g., smoking, cholesterol management, hypertension). Although L.D. has been on many diets in the past, it is not clear from the little information presented whether she has had adequate support. In addition, if drug therapy is considered, it is only successful when concurrent dietary, exercise, and behavioral supports are in place.

Anorexiants (appetite-suppressant drugs) are considered only for those with a BMI greater than 30 kg/m² (see Table 18-2) or greater than 27 kg/m² if they have two or more risk factors (e.g., hypertension, diabetes, high cholesterol) and have failed to lose weight on a program of diet, exercise, and behavioral therapy. The exact mechanism of action as anorexiants is unknown, but these agents appear to act on the satiety center in the hypothalamus and limbic areas of the brain. As appetite suppressants, they are recommended as an adjunct to other medications (e.g., GI lipase inhibitors such as orlistat [Xenical]) and other regimens (e.g., physical exercise, behavior modification, restriction of caloric intake).

A number of over-the-counter (OTC) and complementary/alternative medicines also have been used as appetite suppressants. Ephedra (ma huang) has historically been a popular dietary supplement used to promote weight loss. Its cardiovascular risk profile in conjunction with serious injury and death related to its use resulted in its being banned from sale in many areas (U.S. Food and Drug Administration, 2003). Studies of its safety raise further concerns about ephedra. Bent, Tiedt, Odden, and Shlipak (2003) found that although ephedra-products make up less than 1% of all dietary supplement sales, these products account for 64% of adverse effects associated with dietary supplements. Another case-controlled study (Morgenstern et al., 2003) concluded that the rate of hemorrhagic (bleeding) strokes among ephedra users was statistically significantly higher than among nonusers, for people who take doses above 32 mg daily (a low to moderate dose).

Other formulas have historically used phenylpropanolamine, a sympathomimetic that also has been removed from the market secondary to cardiovascular risk (U.S. Food and Drug Administration, 2004a). Many OTC "diet pills" contain mixtures of herbal extracts, vitamins, and, often, caffeine. Evidence to support their safety and efficacy is generally lacking.

Tolerance to the appetite-suppressant nature for most of these drugs commonly develops with ongoing use. The use of stimulants routinely demonstrates only modest weight loss beyond that of placebo, and weight loss often returns to baseline after the drugs are discontinued. In addition, long-term safety of these agents is not demonstrated. Agents with an FDA indication for obesity include diethylpropion (Tenuate), phentermine (Adipex-P), and sibutramine (Meridia). Dextroamphetamine (Dexedrine) has also occasionally been used for this purpose despite its lack of FDA approval in obesity.

⚙ **L.D. will be working with a nurse from the agency's weight management team. Initially, they will meet weekly to discuss L.D.'s progress, to give instruction and support. Once supports are in place, she will be considered as a candidate for sibutramine 10 mg daily.**

Assessment Anorexiant drugs are used to treat the nursing diagnosis of imbalanced nutrition: more than body requirements. The initial work with L.D. will determine the causative factors for obesity that results from the ingestion of calories in excess of metabolic need; these can include sedentary lifestyle, lack of nutritional knowledge, or increased food intake related to stress, low self-esteem, or boredom. Nursing interventions can be planned according to the specific etiologic factor for which the anorexiant drug therapy serves as a short-term adjunct. A realistic goal for L.D.'s weight loss is 1 to 2 pounds per week, but some clients with obesity will tend to have a greater weight loss than this, at least initially. It is important to stress the daily goals of good nutrition, modified behaviors, and exercise, and that the long-term goal of weight loss will be forthcoming. The health benefits of the loss of even 10% of her weight should be emphasized.

In general, anorexiants are contraindicated for clients with agitated states, arteriosclerotic disease, cardiovascular disease (particularly clients with dysrhythmias), cerebral ischemia, glaucoma, moderate to severe hypertension, hyperthyroidism, and psychosis because anorexiant therapy may worsen their condition. Clients who have a history of substance abuse or dependence may develop a dependence on anorexiants.

Review L.D.'s current medication regimen for the risk of significant drug interactions, such as those that may occur when anorexiants are taken concurrently with alcohol (increases the risk for adverse CNS reactions such as confusion, dizziness, and fainting); antihypertensive agents (decreases the antihypertensive effects); other CNS stimulants (combined use increases CNS stimulant effects such as confusion, dizziness, and fainting); and MAOIs (may result in hypertensive crisis).

Anorexiant drugs should be administered with caution to clients with diabetes, because the need for insulin may be decreased as a result of the concomitant dietary regimen; monitor blood glucose levels closely.

L.D.'s baseline assessment should include height and weight, vital signs, lifestyle issues related to obesity, knowledge level of the therapeutic regimen, and mental status.

Nursing Diagnosis Once L.D. begins anorexiant therapy, be alert for the following nursing diagnoses/collaborative problems: disturbed sleep patterns and disturbed thought processes (depression) related to CNS effects; impaired comfort related to dry mouth, rash, headache, or GI or urinary effects; situational low self-esteem related to changes in sexual desire or decreased sexual ability; and the potential complication of altered cardiac output related to the cardiovascular effects of CNS stimulants.

Planning While L.D. is taking anorexiant therapy, she will:

- Lose 1 pound or more of body weight each week.
- Effectively manage her therapeutic regimen by implementing behavioral changes, such as increased exercise, balanced nutrition, and others, to support her medication.
- Identify adverse effects of the anorexiant and which are reportable to the health care provider.
- Collaborate with the health team for monitoring and follow-up care.

Implementation

Monitoring Monitor L.D.'s weight on an ongoing basis. Adverse effects of anorexiant drugs usually relate to overstimulation such as nervousness, restlessness, insomnia, and anxiety. Monitor blood pressure and pulse to assess whether she is experiencing an adverse effect of the drug. Tolerance is a common occurrence with anorexiants, and L.D. should be assessed for possible habituation and addiction.

Intervention Because anorexiant drugs are to be used only for a short time, the emphasis is on a total weight-reduction program that includes a suitable diet, an appropriate exercise regimen, and behavior modification related to the cause of the overeating.

Preparations administered daily should be administered in the morning to decrease insomnia. Avoid administering anorexiant drugs within 4 to 6 hours of anticipated sleep times (10 to 14 hours for extended-release or long-acting dosage forms). After prolonged high dosages, the drug should be discontinued gradually to avoid withdrawal symptoms and a rebound increase in appetite.

Education Instruct L.D. to consult her prescriber if the drug seems to be less effective than desired; she should not self-regulate the dosage. Instruct her to avoid caffeine-containing beverages, which will increase the effects of the stimulant anorexiant drugs. Also caution her that these drugs may impair her ability to perform tasks that require physical coordination and alertness. Teach L.D. ways to minimize the side effect of unpleasant taste in and dryness of the mouth with mouth rinses, ice chips, chewing gum, and sugarless candies.

Table 18-1 provides the usual adult dosage and the federal Controlled Substances Act schedule for each anorexiant medication. The lower numbers on the scale of II to IV note the agents with the greatest abuse potential. See the Management of Drug Overdose box for amphetamines on p. 172 in Chapter 9.

Evaluation The expected outcome of her anorexiant therapy is that L.D. will experience decreased appetite with accompanying weight loss; she will also be able to sleep without difficulty and not experience any other adverse effects to

the drug. L.D. will effectively manage her therapeutic regimen so as to continue with weight loss after her anorexiant is discontinued.

✸ What stimulant drugs are used for other indications?

doxapram [**dox** a pram]
(Dopram)
Doxapram is a parenterally administered central respiratory stimulant that results in increased tidal volume and respiratory rate.

Indications
Doxapram use is typically limited to postanesthesia care and management of drug overdose where respiratory depressants are involved and antagonists are not available (e.g., barbiturate overdose). Occasionally, it is also used for very short periods of time (e.g., 1 to 2 hours) for clients with chronic obstructive pulmonary disease (COPD) and elevated carbon dioxide levels.

Pharmacokinetics/Dosing
Administered as a single dose intravenously, doxapram has an onset of action within 20 to 40 seconds, peak effect over 1 to 2 minutes, and duration of effect of 5 to 12 minutes.

Adverse Effects
Adverse effects include flushing, disorientation, bronchospasm or cough, elevated blood pressure, elevated intracranial pressure, and an increased risk for cardiac dysrhythmias.

Nursing Management
Assessment
The client's assessment includes a determination of other conditions for which doxapram may be contraindicated, such as seizure disorders (because of the risk of drug-induced seizures) and cardiovascular disorders (because of the vasopressor effects of the drug). Doxapram is also contraindicated if the client has incompetence of the ventilatory mechanism as a result of airway obstruction, pneumothorax, or flail chest, because these conditions may be worsened.

Obtain a baseline pulse, blood pressure, and deep tendon reflexes, and monitor those indicators at frequent intervals to avoid overdose; the rate of the infusion is adjusted on the basis of these assessments. Arterial blood gases should be analyzed before initiation of therapy (as a baseline) and every 30 minutes during the 2-hour period of infusion to avoid the possibility of respiratory acidosis when doxapram is administered to clients with COPD.

Nursing Diagnosis
When doxapram is administered, the client is at risk for ineffective breathing patterns related to anesthesia-induced respiratory depression (for which doxapram is prescribed); risk for aspiration; risk for injury related to the vasopressor effects of the drug; and the potential complication of drug-induced seizures.

Planning
During doxapram therapy, the client will experience:

- Improved arterial blood gases to within the normal range.
- No adverse effects of doxapram therapy.
- Full alertness with a return of pharyngeal and laryngeal reflexes.

Implementation
Monitoring
Doxapram hydrochloride has a narrow margin of safety. Observe for early signs of toxicity, such as increased blood pressure and pulse rate, dysrhythmias, dyspnea, and increased skeletal response with increased deep tendon reflexes and spasticity. A mild to moderate increase in blood pressure is expected. Because narcosis may recur, close monitoring of the client is necessary until full alertness and pharyngeal and laryngeal reflexes have been maintained for 1 hour. Monitor the intravenous (IV) site frequently for extravasation and thrombophlebitis.

Intervention
Before administering doxapram to clients with respiratory depression, a patent airway should be established and an adequate oxygen supply ensured in an attempt to prevent aspiration. Because IV ad-

ministration tends to cause hemolysis, only diluted solutions should be administered and at a slow rate of infusion. Various injection sites should be used to avoid extravasation and to decrease local tissue reaction and thrombophlebitis. Doxapram is a temporary measure to correct acute respiratory insufficiency. Mechanical assistance with ventilation is safer, more reliable, and effective for long-term (more than 2 hours) therapy. Discontinue if the client develops sudden hypotension or dyspnea.

Evaluation

The expected outcome of doxapram therapy is that the client's respirations will be within normal limits compared with baseline, and that the cough and gag reflex will return. The arterial carbon dioxide of a client with COPD will be within normal limits as compared with baseline.

✱ **What other drugs have stimulant properties?**

Many prescription, OTC, and complementary/alternative medications, as well as agents contained in food, have properties that may mimic to some degree the stimulants discussed in this chapter. Caffeine (in coffee, tea, soft drinks, and a number of OTC products), theobromine (in cocoa), and theophylline (a bronchodilator used in asthma management) are all members of the pharmaceutical class methylxanthines and possess CNS and peripheral autonomic system stimulation. Caffeine is discussed in greater detail below. OTC decongestants, including pseudoephedrine (Sudafed), commonly produce CNS stimulation, as well as vasoconstriction and tachycardia. Many of the treatments for Parkinson's disease are stimulating and result in CNS agitation. Complementary/alternative medicines that may heighten CNS activity include ephedra (as discussed briefly above), ginkgo, and ginseng root; see Chapter 12. Table 16-2, p. 314, lists stimulating substances.

✱ **M.P. is a 29-year-old advertising executive who recently began stopping at the local gourmet coffee/espresso bar before work, during breaks, and after work to pick up a large coffee. Since she started her coffee routine, she notices fewer headaches, but she reports feeling her heart pound and feeling "on edge." She admits that she must interrupt meetings to go to the bathroom. She thought the coffee might be problematic, but when she tried to cut back, she felt "washed out" and had headaches.**

Caffeine is a stimulant found in many beverages, foods, OTC drugs, and prescription drugs (Table 18-3). It is probably the most commonly used stimulant worldwide. Many persons do not consider caffeine to be a drug, but it can produce many therapeutic and adverse effects. For example, a large daily intake of caffeine-containing products may increase alertness but may also induce insomnia and heart dysrhythmias in some persons, especially older adults. A withdrawal syndrome of increased irritability, headache, and increased weakness has been reported when individuals using more than 600 mg of caffeine per day (see Table 18-3) decrease or eliminate this intake. Caffeine is also implicated in many adverse health effects, such as cancer, fibrocystic breast disease, and birth defects. There is also a relationship between caffeine intake and hypertension (Sav-

oca, Evans, Wilson, Harshfield, & Ludwig, 2004). Assessment of caffeine intake should be a routine part of the nursing drug history. This includes caffeine intake from foods and beverages as well as from medications.

✱ **How does caffeine affect the body?**

The mechanisms of action for caffeine were previously postulated to be an increase in cyclic adenosine monophosphate levels by blocking the enzyme phosphodiesterase. However, newer studies indicate that the effects of caffeine are primarily a result of antagonism of the central adenosine receptors (adenosine is a neurotransmitter that is structurally similar to caffeine). Because caffeine has an effect on many body functions, both its short-term and possible long-term effects are of concern.

Central Nervous System Effects Although all levels of the CNS may be affected, regular doses of caffeine (100 to 150 mg) stimulate the cortex to produce increased alertness and decreased motor reaction time to both visual and auditory events. Drowsiness and fatigue generally disappear. Larger doses may affect the medullary, vagus, vasomotor, and respiratory centers, resulting in slowing of the heart rate, vasoconstriction, and an increased respiratory rate. Studies attribute such effects to competitive blockade of adenosine receptors.

Analgesic Adjunct, Vascular Effects Caffeine constricts cerebral blood vessels, resulting in decreased cerebral blood flow and oxygen tension in the brain. Thus caffeine is used in analgesic products and in combination with ergotamine to enhance pain relief and, perhaps, to hasten the onset of action. When caffeine is given with ergotamine, the enhanced effect is believed to be the result of better absorption of ergotamine in the presence of caffeine.

Respiratory Stimulant Effects Although the mechanism of action is not clearly defined, caffeine appears to stimulate the medullary respiratory center. Thus it may be useful for the treatment of apnea in preterm infants and for Cheyne-Stokes respiration in adults.

Cardiovascular Effects Caffeine stimulates the myocardium, increasing both the heart rate and the cardiac output. This effect is antagonistic to that produced on the vagus center; consequently, a slight slowing of the heart may be observed in some individuals, and an increased rate may be observed in others. The latter effect usually predominates after large doses. Overstimulation may cause tachycardia and cardiac irregularities.

Depending on the dose, caffeine may cause an increase in systemic vascular resistance, which can cause an increase in blood pressure. This effect may be secondary to sympathetic nervous system stimulation and blockage of adenosine-induced vasodilation.

Because of its suspected potential for causing dysrhythmias, it is recommended that clients avoid using caffeine if they have symptomatic cardiac dysrhythmias or palpita-

TABLE 18-3 CAFFEINE CONTENT IN SELECTED PRODUCTS

Item	Caffeine per Tablet/Serving
OTC ANALGESICS	
Anacin	32 mg
Cope	32 mg
Excedrin Extra Strength	65 mg
Vanquish Caplets	33 mg
PRESCRIPTION ANALGESICS	
Cafergot	100 mg
Fiorinal	40 mg
Wigraine	100 mg
MENSTRUAL MEDICATIONS	
Midol Maximum	60 mg
HOT BEVERAGES	
Brewed coffee, Grande (Starbucks)*	550 mg/16 oz
Brewed coffee, automatic drip	60-180 mg/5 oz
Brewed coffee, percolator	40-170 mg/5 oz
Brewed espresso, double (Starbucks)*	70 mg/2 oz
Brewed tea, United States	20-90 mg/5 oz
Caffe Latte (Starbucks)*	35 mg/8 oz
Brewed decaffeinated coffee	2-5 mg/5 oz
SOFT DRINKS	
Mountain Dew	54 mg/12 oz
Coca-Cola	45 mg/12 oz
Diet Coke	45 mg/12 oz
Pepsi Cola	38 mg/12 oz
Ginger ale	0

*Data from Nutrition Action. (2004). Caffeine: The inside scoop. Retrieved February 17, 2004, from http://www.cspinet.org/nah/caffeine/caffeine_corner.htm.

tions or are in the recovery phase of acute myocardial infarctions.

Musculoskeletal Effects Caffeine affects voluntary skeletal muscles, stimulating them to increase the contractual force and decrease muscle fatigue.

Gastrointestinal Effects Caffeine increases the secretion of pepsin and hydrochloric acid from the parietal cells. Caffeine also decreases tone of the lower esophageal sphincter and contributes to symptoms of gastroesophageal reflux (GERD). For this reason, coffee is restricted in clients who have a gastric or duodenal ulcer or suffer from GERD.

Renal Effects Caffeine produces a mild diuretic effect by increasing renal blood flow and glomerular filtration rate and by decreasing the reabsorption of sodium and water in the proximal tubules.

Additional Effects Caffeine also increases metabolic activity, inhibits uterine contractions, transiently increases glucose levels by stimulating glycogenolysis, and increases catecholamine levels in plasma and urine.

caffeine [kaf feen]
Indications
Caffeine is used in the treatment of fatigue or drowsiness and as an adjunct to analgesics to enhance pain relief, particularly headache pain.
Pharmacokinetics/Dosing
Its absorption is good and it is distributed to all body compartments. It crosses the blood-brain barrier, enters the CNS, and crosses readily through the placenta. Caffeine is metabolized in the liver. In adults, caffeine is metabolized to theophylline and theobromine, whereas in the neonate, only a small portion is metabolized to theophylline. The half-life is 3 to 7 hours in adults and 65 to 130 hours in neonates. In adults, caffeine is excreted by the kidneys, with only 1% to 2% excreted unchanged; in neonates it is excreted by the kidneys, with approximately 85% excreted unchanged. The adult dosage of caffeine is 100 to 200 mg by mouth (PO), repeated in 3 to 4 hours, if necessary, to a maximum of 1000 mg daily. The extended-release dosage form (200 to 250 mg) has the same recommendations as the tablets. With the exception of its use in neonatal apnea, caffeine is not recommended for use in children younger than 12 years of age (*Drug Facts and Comparisons*, 2005).
Adverse Effects
Adverse effects of caffeine include increased nervousness or jittery feelings and irritation of the GI tract, resulting in nausea. More common adverse effects in neonates include abdominal swelling or distension, vomiting, body tremors, tachycardia, jitters, or nervousness.
Signs of overdose are increased temperature, headache, increased irritability and sensitivity to pain or touch, increased urination, confusion, dehydration, abdominal pain, agitation, muscle twitching, nausea and vomiting, tinnitus, insomnia, and seizures. See the Management of Drug Overdose box on p. 376.

M.P. is displaying classic symptoms of caffeine ingestion, and on discontinuation, caffeine withdrawal. The advent of coffee bars may contribute to increased caffeine ingestion due to both the stronger coffee brew, higher caffeine intakes per fluid ounce, and larger serving sizes of coffee. M.P. may benefit from slow tapering of coffee (e.g., consider incrementally substituting decaffeinated beverages for her usually coffee) and should be educated on caffeine content of commonly used foods and OTC products.

Management of Drug Overdose

Caffeine

- Clients should be observed for anxiety, tachycardia, hypertension, and ECG changes.
- Institute symptomatic and supportive measures according to the individual client's requirement.
- Maintain fluid and electrolyte balance, ventilation, and oxygenation.
- For hemorrhagic gastritis, administer antacids or agents to suppress gastric acid secretion (e.g., proton pump inhibitors); for seizures, administer IV diazepam, phenobarbital, or phenytoin.

PREGNANCY SAFETY
CENTRAL NERVOUS SYSTEM STIMULANTS

Category	Drug
B	diethylpropion, pemoline
C	amphetamine, atomoxetine, caffeine, dexmethylphenidate, dextroamphetamine, methylphenidate, modafinil, phentermine, sibutramine

Data from *Mosby's drug consult* (15th ed.). (2005). St. Louis: Mosby.

Because M.P. is of childbearing age it is of particular importance for her to know that the FDA has warned women to avoid or to decrease caffeine consumption during pregnancy (see the Pregnancy Safety box above). Studies in humans have shown that heavy caffeine use by pregnant women may increase the risk of spontaneous abortion and intrauterine growth retardation (*USP DI*, 2005). Nurses in various settings should instruct women who are pregnant or of childbearing age to avoid drugs and sodas containing caffeine. Women who continue to drink coffee during their pregnancy should be encouraged to drink decaffeinated coffee and to limit their coffee intake to less than 300 mg per day. Women who drink tea should decrease the brewing time or select a decaffeinated brand or herbal tea. The best solution would be to substitute fruit and vegetable juices or water for beverages that contain caffeine.

Caffeine passes into breast milk and may accumulate in nursing infants. Research suggests that infants may appear jittery and have trouble sleeping when nursing mothers consume large amounts of caffeine. Breastfeeding mothers should be advised to limit their intake to one or two caffeine-containing beverages per day.

Caffeine-containing medications and beverages may interfere with sleep when taken close to bedtime. Caffeine is not intended to replace sleep and should not be used for that purpose. Clients with a hypersensitivity to caffeine should be alerted to its combination with analgesics (acetaminophen, aspirin, and phenacetin) for the treatment of headache. Because the adverse CNS reactions to the drug are increased in children, these same combination preparations should not be given to children.

Summary

The CNS stimulants have limited use in practice today. Although used in the past to treat obesity, their use has been discouraged because of their narrow therapeutic index and because of the rapid development of tolerance before the achievement of significant weight reduction. The prime indications for CNS stimulants are ADHD and narcolepsy. When used for their anorexiant effect, they are an adjunct to a regimen of diet and exercise. Because stimulation of the CNS occurs, clients may experience a sleep pattern disturbance, altered thought processes, sexual dysfunction, and altered comfort related to side effects such as dry mouth, headache, rash, and GI or urinary effects. Caffeine, although not often thought of as a drug, is also a CNS stimulant, and the nurse should take an active role in educating clients about its effects.

Critical Thinking Questions

- Herbert Poulin, a client with type 1 diabetes, has been prescribed amphetamine sulfate for short-term treatment of exogenous obesity. He asks why he needs to be on a total weight reduction program in addition to anorexiant therapy. What do you tell him? What would be included in such a program? Will the amphetamine affect his management of his diabetic regimen? What other information should you provide to him?

- The instructor of your health education class has given you the topic of caffeine habituation to present to the student group. What would you consider to be the most relevant information for your college-age group? How would you present this topic?

Bibliography

American Academy of Pediatrics. (2000). Clinical practice guideline: Diagnosis and evaluation of the child with attention-deficit/hyperactivity disorder. *Pediatrics, 105*(5), 1158-1170.

Anderson, D.M. (Ed.). (2002). *Mosby's medical, nursing, & allied health dictionary* (6th ed.). St. Louis: Mosby.

Bent, S., Tiedt, T.N., Odden, M.C. & Shlipak, M.G. (2003). The relative safety of ephedra compared with other herbal products. *Annals of Internal Medicine, 138*, 468-471.

Berman, T., Douglas, V.I., & Barr, R.G. (1999). Effects of methylphenidate on complex processing in attention-deficit hyperactivity disorder. *Journal of Abnormal Psychology, 108*(1), 90-105.

Cedergren, M.I. (2004). Maternal morbid obesity and the risk of adverse pregnancy outcome. *Obstetrics & Gynecology, 103*, 219-224.

Centers for Disease Control and Prevention. (2004). Attention-deficit/hyperactivity disorder: Symptoms of ADHD. Retrieved March 30, 2004, from www.cdc.gov/ncbddd/adhd/symptom.htm

Chronis, A.M., et al. (2003). Psychopathology and substance abuse in parents of young children with attention-deficit/hyperactivity disorder. *Journal of the American Academy of Child & Adolescent Psychiatry, 42*(12), 1424-1432.

de la Torre, R., Farre, M., Roset, P.N., Pizarro, N., Abanades, S., Segura, M., et al. (2004). Human pharmacology of MDMA: Pharmacokinetics, metabolism, and disposition. *Therapeutic Drug Monitoring, 26*(2), 137-144.

Drug facts and comparisons. (58th ed.). (2005). St. Louis: Facts and Comparisons.

FDA Alert. (February 2005). Alert for healthcare professionals: Adderall and Adderall XR (amphetamine) sudden deaths in children. Retrieved May 17, 2005, from http://www.fda.gov/cder/drug/InfoSheets/HCP/adderalHCP.htm.

Greenhill, L.L., Jensen, P.S., Abikoff, H., Blumer, J.L., Deveaugh-Geiss, J., Fisher, C., et al. (2003). Developing strategies for psychopharmacological studies in preschool children. *Journal of the American Academy of Child & Adolescent Psychiatry, 42*(4), 406-414.

Hoffman, B.B. (2001). Catecholamines, sympathomimetic drugs and adrenergic receptor antagonists. In J.G. Hardman, L.E. Limbird, A.G. Gillman (Eds.), *Goodman & Gilman's the pharmacological basis of therapeutics* (10th ed.). New York: McGraw-Hill.

Konofal, E., Lecendreux, M., Arnulf, I., Mouren, M.C. (2004). Iron deficiency in children with attention-deficit hyperactivity disorder. *Archives of Pediatric and Adolescent Medicine, 158,* 1113-1115.

Kramer, J.R., Loney, J., Ponto, L.B., Roberts, M. & Grossman, S. (2000). Predictors of adult height and weight in boys treated with methylphenidate for childhood behavior problems. *Journal of the American Academy of Child and Adolescent Psychiatry, 39*(4), 517-524.

Lacy, C.F., Armstrong, L.L., Goldman, M.P., & Lance, L.L. (2004). *Lexi-Comp's drug information handbook* (9th ed.). Cleveland: Lexi-Comp.

Maurer, H., Kraemer T., Springer D., & Staack R.F. (2004). Chemistry, pharmacology, toxicology, and hepatic metabolism of designer drugs of the amphetamine (Ecstasy), piperazine, and pyrrolidinophenone types: A synopsis. *Therapeutic Drug Monitoring, 26*(2), 127-131.

Morgenstern, L.B., Viscoli, C.M., Kerman, W.N., Brass, L.M., Broderick, J.P., Feldmann, J.L., et al. (2003). Use of ephedra-containing products and risk for hemorrhagic stroke. *Neurology, 60,* 132-135.

Mosby's drug consult. (15th ed.). (2005). St. Louis: Mosby.

Nutrition Action. (2004). Caffeine: The inside scoop. Retrieved February 17, 2004, from http://www.cspinet.org/nah/caffeine/caffeine_corner.htm

Robison, L.M., Sclar, D.A., Skaer, T.L., & Galin, R.S. (1999). National trends in the prevalence of attention deficit/hyperactivity disorder and the prescribing of methylphenidate among school-age children: 1990-1995. *Clinical Pediatrics, 38*(4), 209-217.

Roman, T., Szobot, C., Martins, S., Biederman, J., Rohde, L., & Hutz, M.H. (2002). Dopamine transporter gene and response to methylphenidate in attention-deficit/hyperactivity disorder. *Pharmacogenetics, 12*(6), 497-499.

Rxlist. (2004a). Atomoxetine HCl. Retrieved February 16, 2004, from http://www.rxlist.com/cgi/generic3/strattera_cp.htm

Rxlist. (2004b). Modafinil. Retrieved February 16, 2004, from http://www.rxlist.com/cgi/generic2/modafinil_cp.htm

Saklad, J.J., & Sherr, J.D. (2001). Psychiatric disorders in children, adolescents, and people with developmental disabilities. In M.A. Koda-Kimble, L.Y. Young, W.A. Kradjan, B.J. Guglielmo, B.K. Alldredge, & R.L. Corelli (Eds.), *Applied therapeutics: The clinical uses of drugs* (7th ed.). Philadelphia: Lippincott Williams & Wilkins.

Savoca, M.R., Evans, C.D., Wilson, M.E., Harshfield, G.A., & Ludwig, D.A. (2004). The association of caffeinated beverages with blood pressure in adolescents. *Archives of Pediatric & Adolescent Medicine, 158,* 473-477.

Sunohara, G.A., Malone, M.A., Rovet, J., Humphries, T., Roberts, W., & Taylor, M.J. (1999). Effect of methylphenidate on attention in children with attention deficit hyperactivity disorder (ADHD): ERP evidence. *Neuropsychopharmacology, 21*(2), 218-228.

U.S. Food and Drug Administration. (2003). FDA announces plans to prohibit sales of dietary supplements containing ephedra. Retrieved February 16, 2004, from http://www.fda.gov/oc/initiatives/ephedra/december2003/

U.S. Food and Drug Administration. (2004a). Phenylpropanolamine (PPA) information page. Retrieved February 16, 2004, from http://www.fda.gov/cder/drug/infopage/ppa/default.htm

U.S. Food and Drug Administration. (2004b, December 17). *FDA talk paper—New warning for Strattera T04-60.* Washington, DC: Food and Drug Administration. Retrieved December 27, 2004, from http://www.fda.gov/bbs/topics/ANSWERS/2004/ANS01335.html

USP DI: Drug information for the health care professional (25th ed.). (2005). Greenwood Village, CO: MICROMEDEX Thomson Healthcare.

Wilens, T.E., et al. (2003). Does stimulant therapy of attention-deficit/hyperactivity disorder beget later substance abuse? A meta-analytic review of the literature. *Pediatrics, 111*(1), 179-185.

Yang, L, Wang, Y.F., Li, J., & Faraone, S. (2004). Association of norepinephrine transporter gene with methylphenidate response. *Journal of the American Academy of Child & Adolescent Psychiatry, 43*(9), 1154-1158.

Zhu, B.T. (2002). Catechol-O-methyltransferase (COMT)-mediated methylation metabolism of endogenous bioactive catechols and modulation by endobiotics and xenobiotics: importance in pathophysiology and pathogenesis. *Current Drug Metabolism, 3,* 321–349.

e-LEARNING SUPPLEMENTS

Student CD-ROM
- Final Exam questions
- NCLEX® Examination review questions
- Pharmacology animations
- Printable chapter summary

Evolve Website (http://evolve.elsevier.com/mckenry)
- Case study on central nervous system stimulants
- Content updates, including information on new drugs

- WebLinks corresponding to this chapter
- Answers to the critical thinking questions in this chapter
- *Elsevier ePharmacology Update* newsletter
- *Mosby's Drug Consult* Internet Edition
- Supplemental and reference information

19

PSYCHOTHERAPEUTIC DRUGS

CHAPTER FOCUS

Providing nursing care for clients receiving psychotherapeutic agents can be challenging. Nursing responsibilities include not only planning, implementing, and evaluating drug therapy, but doing so via a meaningful therapeutic relationship with the client. Whether the setting is an acute psychiatric facility, a skilled nursing facility, or a community environment, the nurse's knowledge base of psychotherapeutic drugs provides for direct care and for teaching and counseling the client and caregivers about safe and accurate self-administration of these agents.

This chapter reviews medications used to treat psychoses and affective disorders, especially schizophrenia (antipsychotic agents), depression (antidepressants), and bipolar disorder (lithium and others). To enhance understanding of this chapter, it is necessary to review the functional systems of the central nervous system (CNS), such as the reticular activating system, the limbic and extrapyramidal systems, and the action of acetylcholine and the catecholamines. (See Chapter 13 for a review of the physiology and functions of the CNS.)

LEARNING OBJECTIVES

- Describe the use of drug therapy in psychiatry.
- Identify the common psychotropic drugs.
- Differentiate key agents among the typical and atypical antipsychotic drugs.
- Differentiate key class differences among the tricyclic, second-generation monoamine oxidase inhibitors and selective serotonin reuptake inhibitor antidepressant drugs.
- Describe the agents used in treating bipolar disorder with a focus on lithium.
- Describe the nursing management of the common adverse effects of psychotherapeutic agents.
- Implement appropriate plans of care for clients who require the administration of psychotherapeutic agents.

▲ KEY TERMS

affective disorders, p. 396
antidepressants, p. 380
antimanic agents, p. 380
antipsychotics, p. 380
bipolar disorders, p. 397
depression, p. 396
endogenous depression, p. 396
exogenous depression, p. 396
major depression, p. 397
mania, p. 396
mood stabilizers, p. 380
neuroleptic, p. 380
tardive dyskinesia, p. 385

⌨ KEY DRUGS

chlorpromazine, p. 380
clozapine, p. 389
fluoxetine, p. 406
haloperidol, p. 383
imipramine, p. 397
lithium, p. 409
mirtazapine, p. 402

The Central Nervous System

A holistic view of human beings and their experience no longer allows the health care practitioner to separate the functions of the mind from the functions of the body. The CNS is responsible for consciousness, behavior, memory, recognition, learning, and more highly developed attributes, such as imagination, abstract reasoning, and creative thought. In addition, it serves to coordinate vital regulatory functions such as blood pressure (BP), heart rate, respiration, salivary and gastric secretions, muscular activity, and body temperature.

The interrelationships among the various circuits in the brain produce patterns of behavior that can be modified by external situations or internal autonomic adjustments. This allows the individual to adapt to changes in both the external and the internal environments.

Autonomic Regulation

The sympathetic and parasympathetic nervous systems play an important role in the production of behavior; these systems are discussed in Chapter 20. An understanding of these mechanisms is the basis for learning the actions and adverse effects of the drugs that affect mood and behavior.

Biochemical Mechanisms

The functions of the CNS depend on the actions of certain neurotransmitters located in the brain and peripheral tissues. These neurotransmitters are stored in inactive forms; at the right moment, nerve impulses release the free forms of these substances to stimulate the transmission of appropriate reactions. A neurotransmitter exerts its action by interacting with a receptor (a specialized protein), which is located on the outermost part of the postsynaptic cell and produces both electric and biochemical changes within the postsynaptic cell.

Better understanding of CNS neurotransmitters and their sites of action have played a major role in the understanding and treatment of mental illness. Much of this understanding is related to advances in neuroimaging, which have pinpointed action of individual neurotransmitters with specific neuropsychiatric pathology. The CNS neurotransmitters of primary importance in mental health include norepinephrine, serotonin and dopamine. Others, including acetylcholine, histamine, and gamma-aminobutyric acid (GABA) also play a role in neuropsychiatric status.

High concentrations of norepinephrine are found in the hypothalamus, medulla, limbic system, and cranial nerve nuclei. Tyrosine and dopamine are normal constituents in the brain, and are precursors of norepinephrine synthesis. Areas rich in serotonin include the hypothalamus, pineal gland, midbrain, and spinal cord. An alteration of norepinephrine and/or serotonin levels in the nervous system is associated with changes in mood and behavior. These two neurotransmitters appear to play an important role in depression, and most of the available antidepressant drugs augment their action.

Dopamine is found in high concentrations in the striatum and caudate nucleus. Dopamine exerts widespread inhibitory and excitatory effects on a wide variety of centrally mediated functions such as sleep, arousal, affect, and memory. The relationship of dopamine to the major psychoses has received much attention. There are a variety of dopamine receptors in the brain, especially in the basal ganglia and limbic areas; D_1 and D_2 are the primary receptors involved with the antipsychotic agents. Although both receptors are involved with movement disorders in the basal ganglia, blockade of the D_2 receptors results in short-term reversible and potentially long-term irreversible movement disorders and account for major adverse effects observed with the typical antipsychotic agents.

Drug Therapy in Psychiatry

Drugs play an important role in contemporary approaches to psychiatric care. Drug therapy reduces or alleviates symptoms and allows the client an opportunity to participate more easily in other forms of treatment. Drugs modify behavior, and other therapies (e.g., psychotherapy) can shape behavior and produce a more lasting change. Any enduring effects on behavior are more likely to result from the client's concurrent interaction with the environment. Because incoming information must be translated into biochemical changes before it can affect nervous system function, environmental transactions and drugs may affect similar pathways before influencing behavior. Depending on their nature and direction, the effects of drugs can be additive, potentiating, or antagonistic. The environment may potentiate the effectiveness of the drug or detract from it.

In general, prescribers select psychotherapeutic agents on the basis of the diagnostic category: schizophrenia, bipolar disorder, or depression. In most cases, a psychiatric diagnosis is established or presumed based on evaluation of symptoms and use of standardized diagnosis categories. (See the *Diagnostic and Statistical Manual IV–R*, which can be found by logging on to http://www.appi.org.) Choice of drug is based on evidence that supports the use of the agent or class of agents for individuals with that condition or those symptoms. As with all pharmacotherapy, the risk of a drug should always be evaluated in light of the projected benefit. Differences in therapeutic advantages and adverse effect profiles must be carefully evaluated in determining an optimal drug regimen.

The nurse is pivotal in assessing and documenting psychiatric symptoms and responses to drugs that are an integral part of safe and effective pharmacologic therapy. Nursing management of psychotherapeutic agents focuses on monitoring the client's behavioral and affective responses to the medications, the client's knowledge of the drug therapy, the presence and extent of expected adverse effects, the client's response to dosage adjustments and supportive nursing interventions, and the potential for or existence of drug or food interactions. Knowing the action of drugs also assists health care professionals in understanding the interpersonal responses that occur in the therapeutic relationship with the client.

Psychotherapeutic Agents

A number of agents that influence CNS neurotransmitter actions are discussed in this chapter. This chapter focuses primarily on **antipsychotics** or **neuroleptics** (agents that affect cognitive thought processes and affect dopaminergic receptors), **antidepressants** (agents that primarily elevate mood or affect by increasing norepinephrine or serotonin levels at the nerve synapse), and **antimanic agents** or **mood stabilizers** (agents that affect nerve transmission to stabilize mood).

Antipsychotics

The population of the United States doubled between 1900 and 1950; during this time, the population in public mental hospitals quadrupled. The average length of confinement was usually years, and the trend was definitely toward an annual increase in clients admitted to such institutions. Client and employee injuries caused by combative or abusive clients led to the common use of physical restraints and client isolation.

Before the development of the antipsychotic agents, the treatment of mentally ill clients consisted of either being isolated (i.e., hidden in cellars or attics in their homes) or, if they came to the attention of local authorities, being transferred to jails or homes for the insane. Actual therapies used before the advent of the antipsychotic agents were water or ice pack therapies, straitjackets or other physical restraints, shock therapy with insulin or electricity, lobotomy, and the use of a few drugs such as paraldehyde, chloral hydrate, and the barbiturates.

The era of antipsychotics was ushered in with the release of chlorpromazine (Thorazine) ▮▮ in the early 1950s. Chlorpromazine belongs to a class of drugs referred to as phenothiazines. Antipsychotics are also referred to by the outmoded term "major tranquilizers." These agents block dopaminergic receptors in the CNS and, while not curative, for the first time, allowed adequate symptom control (Box 19-1) to make community living a realistic opportunity for many with significant psychosis-related conditions. The use of the antipsychotic drugs proved to be a revolutionary force in the psychiatric field. The duration of institutionalization has decreased from years to months for many clients; other clients live at home and are treated at community mental health centers. The reported incidence of injuries has declined, and many large public mental health facilities have closed.

The antipsychotics fall into two broad categories: the earlier typical agents, including chlorpromazine (Thorazine) and haloperidol (Haldol), and the newer atypical agents including clozapine (Clozaril) and olanzapine (Zyprexa). Aripiprazole (Abilify) represents a novel approach with dopaminergic agonist-antagonist activity and is discussed separately. While the newer atypical agents have

---

> ### BOX 19-1 POSITIVE AND NEGATIVE SYMPTOMS IN SCHIZOPHRENIA
>
> Clients with schizophrenia present with a wide variety of symptoms that are categorized as positive or negative. Most antipsychotic agents produce an effect on the following positive symptoms: agitation, anxiety, hallucinations, poor hygiene and dress, hyperactivity, delusions, paranoia, and hostility, whereas the negative symptoms of flat affect, social inadequacy, diminished speech patterns, judgment, insight, and others are usually less responsive to drug therapy.
>
> The target symptoms are used as monitoring parameters to evaluate the individual's response to the medication. The atypical antipsychotic drugs (e.g., clozapine, risperidone, olanzapine) appear to be more effective than older typical neuroleptic agents against negative symptoms, although one analysis noted little difference in symptom control between the typical agent haloperidol and the atypical olanzapine (Rosenheck et al., 2003).

largely replaced the older typical antipsychotics, both are discussed here. Table 19-1 presents selected agents.

✱ **J.T. is a 19-year-old male who presents to the emergency department (ED) with his mother. He exhibits hallucinations and combative behavior. According to his history, his behavior has been described as bizarre over the past few weeks, but has escalated to a point that it presents a health and safety issue to J.T. and his family. The mental health crisis team at the ED evaluates J.T.'s status, finds no illicit drug or alcohol use, and recommends an initial dose of haloperidol (Haldol) 4 mg intramuscularly (IM).**

✱ **What are the important differences among the typical antipsychotics?**
The older typical antipsychotics serve as dopaminergic antagonists at both D_1 and D_2 receptors in the CNS (Figure 19-1).

The typical antipsychotics are represented by a number of classes, including (1) aliphatic phenothiazines (e.g., chlorpromazine [Thorazine]); (2) piperidine phenothiazines (e.g., thioridazine [Mellaril]); (3) piperazine phenothiazines (e.g., fluphenazine [Prolixin]); (4) the butyrophenones (e.g., haloperidol [Haldol]); (5) the thioxanthenes (e.g., thiothixene [Navane]); and (6) the dihydroindolones (e.g., molindone [Moban]).

While the chemical class helps predict therapeutic and adverse effects, a more useful classification scheme for the typical antipsychotics is based on affinity for D_2 receptors and are stratified as low-potency (requiring higher doses), moderate potency (midrange dosing), and high potency (using lower dosing). The basis for classification is the quantity of medication necessary to produce an equivalent effect when compared with other agents in the same category. For example, 100 mg of chlorpromazine (Thorazine) is considered to be approximately equivalent to 50 mg of mesoridazine (Serentil) or 2 mg haloperidol (Haldol). Thus

TABLE 19-1 ANTIPSYCHOTICS

Agent	Chemical Class	Typical Oral Adult Daily Dose (mg)*	EPS Risk	TD Risk	Anticholinergic	Sedation	Cardiovascular Risk	Comment
TYPICAL ANTIPSYCHOTICS								
chlorpromazine (Thorazine)	Aliphatic phenothiazine	200-800	Moderate	High	Moderate	High	Moderately high (orthostatic hypotension)	
fluphenazine (Prolixin)	Piperazine phenothiazine	0.5-20	High	High	Low	Low	Low	Long-acting injectable decanoate form available
haloperidol (Haldol)	Butyrophenone	1-15	High	High	Low	Low	Moderate	Long-acting injectable decanoate form available
loxapine (Loxitane)	Dibenzepin	60-100	High	High	Low	Moderate	Low	
mesoridazine (Serentil)	Piperidine phenothiazine	100-400	Low	High	High	High	High (prolonged QT interval)	
molindone (Moban)	Dihydroindolone	50-100	High	High	Low	Low	Low	
perphenazine (Trilafon)	Piperazine phenothiazine	16-24	High	High	Low	Low	Low	
pimozide (Orap)	Diphenyl-butylpiperidine	1-10	High	High	Moderate	Moderate	Moderate (prolonged QT interval)	
thioridazine (Mellaril)	Piperidine phenothiazine	200-800	Low	High	High	High	High (prolonged QT interval)	
thiothixene (Navane)	Thioxanthene	10-30	High	High	Low	Low	Moderate (orthostatic hypotension)	

EPS, Extrapyramidal side effect; *TD*, tardive dyskinesia.
*Doses beyond this amount are of questionable benefit based on maximum effective dose as demonstrated by Davis & Chen, 2004.

Continued

TABLE 19-1 ANTIPSYCHOTICS—cont'd

Agent	Chemical Class	Typical Oral Adult Daily Dose (mg)*	EPS Risk	TD Risk	Anticholinergic	Sedation	Cardiovascular Risk	Comment
ATYPICAL ANTIPSYCHOTICS								
clozapine (Clozaril)	Dibenzodiazepine	300-450	Low	Low	High	High	High	Controls positive and negative symptoms (see Box 19-1) Often effective in refractory cases See text for significant adverse effects, including bone marrow suppression, seizures, drooling Every 1-2 week WBC counts required
olanzapine (Zyprexa)	Dibenzodiazepine	5-10	Low	Low	High	High	High	Controls positive and negative symptoms Risk of weight gain and development of diabetes mellitus
quetiapine (Seroquel)	Dibenzodiazepine	300-500	Low	Low	Moderate	Moderate	Moderate	Controls positive and negative symptoms
risperidone (Risperdal)	Benzisoxazole	1-6	Low (↑ if >6 mg)	Low (?↑ if >6 mg)	Low	Low	Low	Controls positive and negative symptoms ↑EPS for doses greater than 6 mg daily
ziprasidone (Geodon)	Benzisoxazole	40-120	Low	Low	Low	Moderate	Moderate (prolonged QT interval)	Controls positive and negative symptoms
NOVEL ANTIPSYCHOTICS								
aripiprazole (Abilify)	Class not yet established	10-30	Low	Low	Low	Low Moderate	Moderate high	Controls positive and negative symptoms Partial agonist/antagonist activity may explain unique profile

WBC, White blood cell.

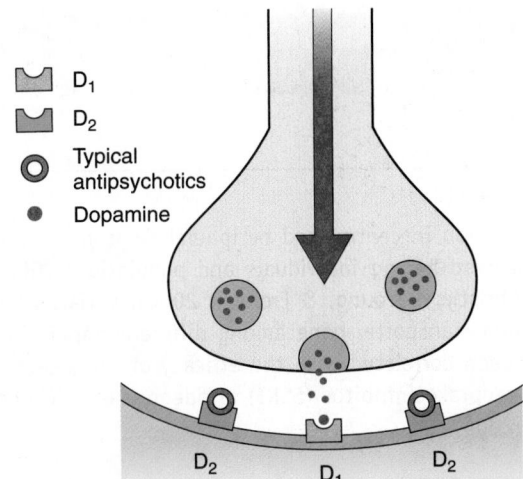

FIGURE 19-1 Typical antipsychotics act to block postsynaptic dopamine receptors. Typical antipsychotics have a greater affinity to D_2 receptors than to D_1 receptors.

chlorpromazine is a low-potency agent; mesoridazine, an intermediate-potency agent; and haloperidol, a high-potency agent (see Table 19-1 for typical adult doses). The student is cautioned not to confuse potency with effectiveness; potency refers to the quantity of a drug necessary to produce an equivalent effect as compared with another drug in the same classification. Effectiveness measures the therapeutic response to various agents, which, depending on the individual drugs being studied, can range from less effective, to equivalent in effectiveness, to more effective.

Although the exact mechanism of action for the typical antipsychotic effects is unknown, their major therapeutic and adverse effects result from dopamine blockade in specific areas of the CNS. There may be variation in response to antipsychotics from client to client based in part on pharmacogenetic differences observed with these agents (see the Special Considerations for Pharmacogenetics box on p. 384). These drugs also produce an α-blocking effect (hypotension); most inhibit or block dopamine at the chemoreceptor trigger zone and peripherally inhibit the vagus nerve in the gastrointestinal (GI) tract (antiemetic effect). In addition, they produce an antianxiety effect by depressing the brainstem reticular system. As a group, they increase the release of prolactin, which infrequently results in gynecomastia (breast swelling) and galactorrhea (milk secretion).

✱⬛ haloperidol [ha loe **per** i dole]
(Haldol, Haldol Lactate, Haldol Decanoate, Apo-Haloperidol✳, Novo-Peridol✳, Peridol✳)
Haloperidol is among the more frequently used of the older typical antipsychotics.

Indication
Haloperidol is used in the treatment of schizophrenia, psychosis, for the control of tics associated with Tourette syndrome (Box 19-2), in the treatment of severe behavioral problems in children, and for emergency sedation in delirium or severe agitation. It is also used as an antiemetic in the treatment of nausea and vomiting.

Pharmacokinetics/Dosing
Haloperidol, like other typical antipsychotics, is well absorbed orally and has an onset of action between 30 and 60 minutes. The onset

---

BOX 19-2 ANTIPSYCHOTICS AND TOURETTE SYNDROME

Tourette syndrome, a rare CNS disorder that results in involuntary, rapid, and repetitive motor movements of muscle groups, is usually accompanied by involuntary vocalizations. Tourette syndrome is more common in males, usually appearing before age 14 years, and may present initially as tics (facial grimaces and blinking). Other symptoms include vocal tics or noises (e.g., grunting, barking, shouting, sniffing, and compulsive swearing [coprolalia]) and movement disorders (involuntary, purposeless movements). The symptoms may peak and wane throughout the individual's life. The individual's intellectual functions are normal. Although there is no cure for Tourette syndrome, antipsychotic medications have produced dramatic improvement in some clients.

of action after IM administration of the lactate (immediate-release) form is within 30 minutes. Haloperidol is metabolized to pharmacologically inactive compounds that are eliminated in the urine and feces. The elimination half-life of haloperidol is approximately 20 hours. The typical oral adult dose ranges from 0.5 mg twice daily to 5 mg three times daily. Doses above 10 mg daily have questionable efficacy for most clients, but some clients may require 30 mg daily or more. Single doses of 2 to 5 mg IM or intravenously (IV) of the immediate-release parenteral formulation of haloperidol lactate (Haldol Lactate) are typically used for acute management. Lower doses are often used in older or debilitated clients.

Use of long-acting haloperidol decanoate (Haldol Decanoate) by IM injection results in a prolonged duration of action of approximately 3 weeks. This product should not be confused with the shorter-acting parenteral formulation. Haloperidol decanoate is generally reserved for circumstances where infrequent dosing is advantageous, the client has tolerated shorter-acting dose forms, and a daily dose has been established. This formulation is often used for clients who do not adhere to conventional therapy. In such circumstances, a number of ethical issues must be addressed (Box 19-3). The typical dose of the decanoate formulation is 10 to 20 times the daily oral dose administered IM every 4 weeks, with the dose titrated to effect.

Adverse Effects
The typical antipsychotics, including haloperidol, are associated with a great number of adverse effects, including orthostatic hypotension, extrapyramidal side effects (EPS) including parkinsonian tremors, dystonic reactions, and akathisia. Other adverse effects include sedation, seizures, amenorrhea, galactorrhea, gynecomastia, sexual dysfunction, urinary retention, jaundice, blurred vision, heat stroke, and neuroleptic malignant syndrome. Chronic use poses the risk for tardive dyskinesia. Haloperidol can also prolong QT interval on electrocardiogram (ECG) and increase the risk of the life-threatening dysrhythmia torsades de pointes. Most of these adverse effects are discussed more completely in the following paragraphs.

✱ **Twelve hours after receiving his first dose of haloperidol, J.T. complains of neck stiffness. He has difficulty in speaking with a subjective sensation that his tongue is "thick." On observation, his eyes appear to have rolled back in his head, his face is twisted to one side, and his neck appears arched and drawn backward.**

✱ **Are J.T.'s symptoms drug related?**

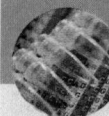

Special Considerations for Pharmacogenetics | **ANTIPSYCHOTICS AND ANTIDEPRESSANTS**

ANTIPSYCHOTICS

Pharmacodynamics

Variation in dopamine receptor subtypes where antipsychotics act may be genetically determined. Binding of atypical antipsychotics and the likelihood for elevations in prolactin levels (a commonly observed effect of these agents) is proportional to the genetic marker for the D_2 receptor [DRD2] (Young et al., 2004). Whether the DRD2 or other markers are predictive of genetically based variation in response to antipsychotics remains to be seen (Malhotra, Murphy, & Kennedy, 2004).

Pharmacokinetics

Genetic variation in metabolism of haloperidol, thioridazine, and clozapine has been reported (Chang & Altman, 2004). Aripiprazole, which is metabolized by both cytochrome P450 2D6 and 3A4 (Lacy, Armstrong, Goldman, & Lance, 2004) is likely to also display varying pharmacokinetics across populations. The clinical significance of these finding is not clear, but may explain the observation that some clients respond to lower doses of antipsychotics whereas other clients require higher doses for adequate response.

Adverse Effects

The risk for tardive dyskinesia (TD) has been correlated with variations in the genetic marker for the D_3 receptor [DRD3] and the cytochrome P450 1A2 isoenzyme, an isoenzyme responsible for metabolism of some antipsychotics, including haloperidol (Malhotra et al., 2004). It is currently unclear whether these markers could be clinically useful to identify individuals at high risk for TD.

Similarly, the risk for developing extrapyramidal side effects (EPS) with typical antipsychotic use is related to cytochrome P450 2D6 expression. Individuals with reduced capacity to metabolize drugs via 2D6 appear to be at higher risk for EPS (Schillevoort et al., 2002).

ANTIDEPRESSANTS

Pharmacodynamics

Genetic variation in central and peripheral serotonin receptors is observed among individuals and populations (Glatt, Tampilic, Christie, DeYoung, & Freimer, 2004). Variations in the serotonin transporter gene among different populations have also been correlated with the efficacy of the selective serotonin reuptake inhibitor (SSRI) antidepressants (Malhotra et al., 2004).

Pharmacokinetics

The polymorphic expression of cytochrome P450 2D6 is highly variable across populations, and explains the wide range of plasma and tissue levels observed with standard doses of many of the antidepressants, including the tricyclics, paroxetine, and fluoxetine. This may explain differences observed in both therapeutic response and toxicity for these agents (Malhotra et al., 2004).

Adverse Effects

Accumulation of a number of antidepressants may be secondary to the significant variation noted in 2D6 activity, which is genetically determined. Among the agents metabolized by this enzyme are many of the tricyclic antidepressants, including amitriptyline, desipramine, imipramine, and nortriptyline. Cardiac dysrhythmias secondary to toxic levels of desipramine have been correlated with 2D6 polymorphism in Mexican Americans (Flores, Alvarado, Wong, Licinio, & Flockhart, 2004).

Differences in metabolism of bupropion (Wellbutrin, Zyban) related to polymorphism of cytochrome P450 2B6 is also noted (Kirchheiner et al., 2003). This may contribute to the risk for seizures in clients who are display reduced metabolic clearance of the drug.

Adverse effects of the typical antipsychotics are significant, uncomfortable, and often adversely affect ongoing adherence to therapy. A major grouping of acute adverse effects of this class of drugs involves antagonistic activity of D_2 receptors in the extrapyramidal tracts and are referred to as a group as extrapyramidal side effects (EPS). Three distinct (and often overlapping) EPS presentations include acute dystonic reactions, akathisia, and parkinsonian symptoms (Box 19-4).

Acute dystonic reactions typically present within 24 to 48 hours of an initial dose or dose increase and are more often observed in the high-potency/low-dose typical agents. Symptoms classically present as oculogyric crisis (eyes roll back in the head), trismus (facial twisting to one side), a protruding and fixed tongue, and opisthotonus (neck arching and stiffness). J.T. presents with a classic dystonic reaction.

Akathisia usually presents as an internally sensed motor restlessness, where clients feel "wound up." It often appears as restlessness, with inability to focus and continuous arm and leg movement. It is most commonly observed in younger clients, and may appear early in therapy (within the first few months). Unfortunately, this motor restlessness may be mistaken for an increase in underlying psychosis, and result in an increase in the dose of the offending agent. Such an action only serves to worsen the akathisia.

A third acute presentation of EPS is drug-induced parkinsonism. This presents in a manner similar to symptoms seen in someone with idiopathic Parkinson's disease, and includes a coarse (3 cycles per second) tremor that worsens on activity, shuffling gait, drooling, a masked look to the face, and muscle rigidity. Common to drug-induced parkinsonism is cogwheel rigidity where passive movement

BOX 19-3 ETHICAL AND LEGAL CONSIDERATIONS IN THE USE OF PSYCHOTROPIC DRUGS

The use of psychotropic drug therapy raises a number of ethical and legal considerations. This is particularly true for antipsychotic drugs, which are associated with significant adverse effects. In many circumstances, the client may not be in a position to fully understand the risks and benefits of therapy. It is important for the mental health team to apply the principles of biomedical ethics to each case.

Four basic principles of biomedical ethics are beneficence, nonmaleficence, autonomy, and justice described below:

1. **Beneficence:** "Do good."
   * Does the intervention help the client?
     Does the drug reduce morbidity or mortality?
     Does the drug improve symptoms?
2. **Nonmaleficence:** "Do no harm."
   * What is the risk of the intervention to the client?
     What are the short-term adverse effects of drug therapy?
     What are the long-term adverse effects of drug therapy?
3. **Autonomy:** "Empower the client."
   * Who makes the decision for the intervention?
     Is the client competent to make decisions?
     Is the client fully informed of the risks and benefits of therapy?

4. **Justice:** "Is it fair for everyone?"
   * What impact does the intervention have on others?
     Does treatment or lack of treatment pose a risk to the health and safety of others?
     Does the cost of the intervention deprive someone else of care or intervention?

Balancing each of these competing aspects is often a difficult, but necessary process in determining when drugs are used, which drugs are selected, how the decision is made, and what is important to monitor. In addition to the above questions, the team must ask if the symptoms warrant drug therapy, which agents are most effective, which agents pose the least risk for the client, how much decision making is made by the client, and what health and safety issues arise if the client is not treated.

The significant adverse effect profiles of antipsychotics may pose an increased legal risk for prescribers and other team members. The risks of these agents (e.g., tardive dyskinesia with typical antipsychotics, bone marrow suppression with clozapine, risk for diabetes mellitus with olanzapine) have prompted many clinicians to obtain informed consent for use of their use.

The nurse should be an active participant in these decisions and function as the client's advocate.

---

of the wrist or elbow of the affected individual by an examiner results in ratchet-like or on-off-like movement.

Treatment of EPS includes avoiding future use of the offending drug, if possible, and use of drugs with anticholinergic (specifically antimuscarinic) properties. Acute dystonic reactions are very distressing to clients. They are typically treated with a drug with antimuscarinic activity (e.g., IM or IV administration of the antihistamine, diphenhydramine [Benadryl]). Treatment of drug-induced parkinsonism includes treatments with other longer-acting antimuscarinics, including benztropine (Cogentin) and trihexyphenidyl (Artane). Unfortunately, these antimuscarinic agents have their own adverse effects, including dry mouth, urinary retention, constipation, and occasionally confusion. Refer to Chapter 21 for a more complete discussion of antimuscarinic agents.

✴ **J.T. is treated with parenteral diphenhydramine (Benadryl) and his symptoms resolve over the next few hours. He expresses concern that the health care team was trying to poison him, and he has heard that drugs like haloperidol (Haldol) can cause long-term movement problems.**

✴ **How likely are long-term movement problems to result from antipsychotic use?**
Paranoid delusions are common with a number of psychiatric conditions, but the adverse-effect profiles of the typical antipsychotics are troublesome and may serve to reinforce paranoid perceptions for clients who do not yet have a full therapeutic response to the antipsychotics.

Although a number of long-term adverse effects may occur with chronic use of the typical antipsychotics, **tardive dyskinesia (TD)** has raised the gravest concern. This is a syndrome of abnormal involuntary muscle movements related to long-term blockade of D_2 receptors. The exact mechanism of how dopamine blockade can lead to TD is not clear, but may involve dopamine supersensitivity, depletion of GABA, neurologic oxidative stress, or some other process (Goldberg, 2002). Genetics has also been proposed as a risk for developing TD (see the Special Considerations for Pharmacogenetics box on p. 384). TD is characterized by involuntary perioral movements such as lip smacking, lip puckering, tongue darting, and jaw movements (see Box 19-4). Also commonly observed is difficulty swallowing, and choreoathetoid (worm-like) movements of the hands, arms, neck, torso, legs, and feet. It is more likely to occur with higher doses of typical agents for long periods of time (e.g., greater than 6 months). Significant EPS early in therapy may signal increased risk for TD. Older women also appear to be at higher risk for developing the condition.

Although there is some data that high-dose vitamin E may offer some improvement in symptoms, there is no reliable treatment for tardive dyskinesia. As such, early identification and prevention are critical. Box 19-5 presents a standardized screening tool for TD.

Other Adverse Effects of Antipsychotics In addition to EPS and TD, other significant adverse effects as a consequence of using the typical agents are possible. Below is a listing of possible adverse effects and considerations for use of these agents.

BOX 19-4 NEUROMUSCULAR ADVERSE EFFECTS OF NEUROLEPTICS

EXTRAPYRAMIDAL SIDE EFFECTS (EPS)
Akathisia

Description
- Motor restlessness is present; client is unable to sit or stand still and feels an urgent need to move, pace, rock, or tap foot.
- Akathisia may also appear as apprehension, irritability, and general uneasiness, and may be mistaken for agitation.
- This condition is more common in females than males; it usually occurs within 5 to 30 days (up to 90 days) of starting drug therapy.

Treatment
- Lower the dosage of the neuroleptic agent, switch to a different drug, or administer an antiparkinson drug such as benztropine (Cogentin).

Dystonia

Description
- This is an acute reaction that requires immediate intervention.
- The client exhibits muscle spasms of the face, tongue, neck, jaw, and/or back.
  There is hyperextension of the neck and trunk and arching of the back.
  The tongue may protrude; also present are facial grimaces, exaggerated posturing of the head, neck, or jaw, and difficulty swallowing and/or talking.
  The client may have oculogyric crisis, manifesting as a fixed upward gaze and/or eye muscle spasms. This may be accompanied by excessive salivation.
- It is usually seen after large doses of neuroleptics, typically within 1 hour to 1 week of initiation of drug therapy. It occurs more often in males than females.

Treatment
- Depending on the severity of the reaction, consider:
  Lowering neuroleptic dosage;
  Administering either benztropine (Cogentin) or diphenhydramine (Benadryl) IM or IV

Drug-Induced Parkinsonism

Description
- Symptoms are similar to Parkinson's disease, with a shuffling gait, drooling, tremors, and increased rigidity (cogwheel). Bradykinesia (slow movements) and akinesia (immobility) are also reported.
- Drug-induced parkinsonism is often dose related, may occur at any time with typical antipsychotic therapy, and is seen in both males and females.

Treatment
- Add an antiparkinson drug such as benztropine (Cogentin) or diphenhydramine (Benadryl).
- The prescriber can switch client to a neuroleptic that is less likely to induce this effect.

TARDIVE DYSKINESIA (TD)

Description
- Presenting features include:
  Facial: grimacing or scowling expression, facial tics, arching of the eyebrows
  Ocular: blinking, eyelid spasms (blepharospasm)
  Oral/buccal: lip smacking, lower-lip thrusting, sucking, puffing of cheeks, chewing of the cheeks (the inside of the mouth should be checked for this)
  Lingual/masticatory: lateral jaw movements, tongue protrusion or thrusting such as "fly catching movements," tongue in lip or cheek resulting in an observable bulge in the specific area

Anticholinergic Effects Many of the lower-potency/higher-dose typical agents have an affinity for the muscarinic acetylcholine receptors in the autonomic nervous system (ANS) (see Chapter 21) and result in sedation, dry mouth, constipation, dry skin, urinary retention, blurred vision, tachycardia, and inhibited ejaculation. Older individuals may be more sensitive to these effects, and may also display some confusion related to anticholinergic activity of the drug.

Bone Marrow Suppression While most commonly observed with the atypical antipsychotic clozapine (Clozaril) (see later), the typical agents may also cause a decrease in white blood cell production. This effect is most likely to occur during the first 1 to 3 months of therapy.

Cardiovascular Effects The typical agents may display both cardiac and vascular effects. Cardiac effects include changes in electrical conduction that might predispose to serious cardiac dysrhythmias. One significant concern is the prolongation of the QT interval on the ECG, which predisposes to life-threatening ventricular dysrhythmias, including torsades de pointes. A common vascular change involves the affinity these agents have for α-adrenergic receptors in blood vessels; this effect is particularly noted with the low-potency/high-dose agents and results in orthostatic hypotension with resultant risk for syncope and/or reflex tachycardia.

Endocrine Changes Changes in glucose levels (particularly for individuals with diabetes mellitus), weight gain, breast enlargement (secondary to changes in prolactin levels), and syndrome of inappropriate secretion of antidiuretic hormone, manifest by low serum sodium levels, have all been implicated with antipsychotic therapy.

Liver Toxicity All of the antipsychotics can, on rare occasions, induce liver injury and jaundice. Chlorpromazine is the most frequently implicated antipsychotic for abnormal changes in liver function.

BOX 19-4 NEUROMUSCULAR ADVERSE REACTIONS OF NEUROLEPTICS—*cont'd*

Systemic effects: foot tapping; rocking from side to side; arms, hands, and fingers possibly displaying a jerking and/or a writhing motion (choreoathetoid motion); pelvic thrusting motions

- Tardive dyskinesia typically manifests after 6 months or more of typical antipsychotic therapy. Symptoms may be masked by increased dose of typical antipsychotics, but the underlying condition will actually worsen over time with the use of higher doses.
- Risk of tardive dyskinesia is highest with D_2 blockers (typical antipsychotics) and may be as high as 20% of those clients who receive ongoing therapy. The risk of inducing tardive dyskinesia increases with the total dose administered and the length of treatment. Older women appear to be at highest risk.

Treatment
- Prevention is vital because the condition might be irreversible.
- Decreasing or discontinuing the antipsychotic agent, if possible, is the recommended procedure.
- Vitamin E may help, but there is no universally effective treatment for TD.

NEUROLEPTIC MALIGNANT SYNDROME

Description
- Client presents with very rigid muscle tone and fever secondary to severe muscle injury.
- Altered mental status, joint pain, tachycardia, tachypnea and sweating are also commonly seen.
- Neuroleptic malignant syndrome almost always presents in the first week to month of starting an antipsychotic or D_2 blocking drug (e.g., metoclopramide).

Treatment
- Discontinue offending drug.

- Supportive nursing and medical care, often in the intensive care setting, is required.
- Dantrolene may be used when significant fever and muscle injury is noted. Benzodiazepines, amantadine, bromocriptine, and electroconvulsive therapy may also be considered.
- Recovery usually requires 7 to 10 days, but may be longer if long-acting agents such as IM haloperidol decanoate were used.

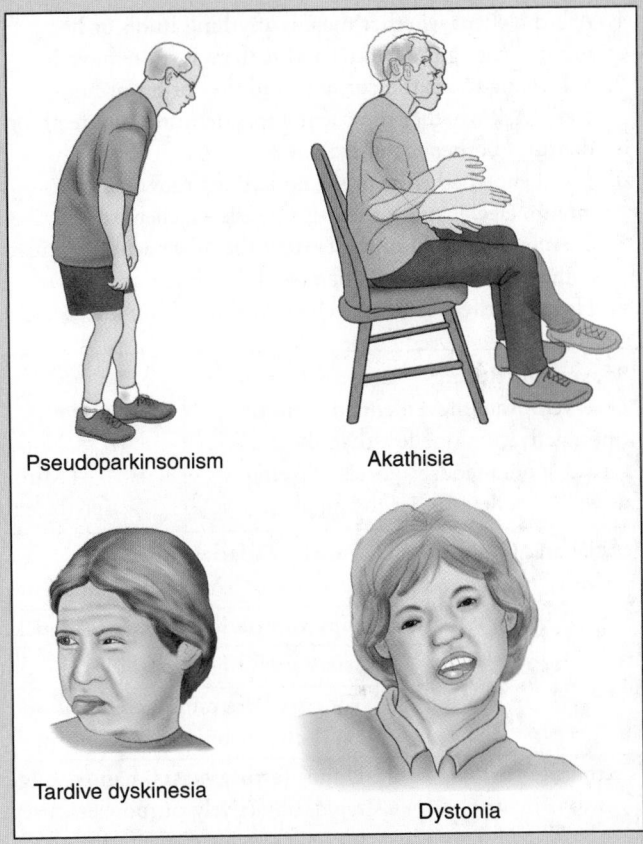

Pseudoparkinsonism

Akathisia

Tardive dyskinesia

Dystonia

Neuroleptic Malignant Syndrome While rare, this life-threatening syndrome is manifested by excess heat production related to increased muscle contraction. It is characterized by hyperpyrexia (elevated temperature), altered consciousness, dramatically increased muscle tone (described as "lead-pipe" rigidity), joint pain, and autonomic nervous system effects, including tachycardia, tachypnea, elevated BP, and diaphoresis. Elevations in urinary myoglobin, increased white blood cell (WBC) counts, and elevated blood creatinine phosphokinase and liver enzymes (alanine aminotransferase, aspartate aminotransferase) levels are usually seen. Its early recognition and management is critical (see Box 19-4).

Ocular Toxicity Blurred vision is common early in the course of therapy with antipsychotics. In addition, light sensitivity, changes in accommodation, eye pain, and pigmentary retinopathy are all possible complications of all the antipsychotics.

Seizures At usual doses, the typical antipsychotics rarely cause seizures. However, for individuals with a preexisting seizure history, or in overdose situations, this risk is real.

Skin Reactions Allergic skin reactions may occur with any of the antipsychotics, but is most likely to be observed during the first 3 months of therapy. Manifestations include maculopapular rashes and photosensitivity, and protection from sun exposure is recommended when any of these agents are used.

✳ **With appropriate symptom control, J.T. could remain living at home. J.T. is considered a candidate for long-term antipsychotic therapy by the mental health crisis team.**

✳ **What considerations are made in choosing antipsychotics for J.T.?**
If J.T.'s diagnosis warrants the use of an antipsychotic agent, the prescriber will try to match the therapeutic advantages

Box 19-5 Screening for Tardive Dyskinesia

The Abnormal Involuntary Movement Scale (AIMS), developed by National Institute for Mental Health researchers, is the standard screening and rating tool for TD in the United States.

PROCEDURE FOR USING THE AIMS RATING TOOL:

Either before or after completing the examination procedure, observe the client unobtrusively, at rest (e.g., in waiting room). The chair to be used in this examination should be a hard, firm one without arms.

1. Ask the client whether there is anything in his or her mouth (e.g., gum, candy) and if there is, to remove it.
2. Ask client about the current condition of his or her teeth. Ask whether the client wears dentures. Do teeth or dentures bother the client now?
3. Ask client whether he or she notices any movements in mouth, face, hands, or feet. If yes, ask the client to describe the movement and to what extent the movement currently bothers the client or interferes with his or her activities.
4. Have the client sit in the chair with hands on knees, legs slightly apart, and feet flat on floor. (Look at entire body for movements while in this position.)
5. Ask client to sit with hands hanging unsupported. If male, between legs; if female and wearing a dress, hanging over knees. (Observe hands and other body areas.)
6. Ask client to open his or her mouth. (Observe tongue at rest within mouth.) Do this twice.
7. Ask client to protrude his or her tongue. (Observe abnormalities of tongue movement.) Do this twice.
8. *Ask client to tap his or her thumb with each finger as rapidly as possible for 10 to 15 seconds; first with the right hand, then with the left hand. (Observe facial and leg movement.)
9. Flex and extend client's left and right arms (one at a time). (Note any rigidity and rate.)
10. Ask client to stand up. (Observe in profile. Observe all body areas again, hips included.)
11. *Ask client to extend both arms outstretched in front with palms down. (Observe trunk, legs, and mouth.)
12. *Have client walk a few paces, turn, and walk back to chair. (Observe hands and gait.) Do this twice.

Movement Ratings: Rate highest severity observed. Rate movements that occur upon activation one less than those observed spontaneously. Circle movement as well as code number that applies.	Code: 0 = None 2 = Mild 1 = Minimal, 3 = Moderate may be extreme normal 4 = Severe	Rater: Date:	Rater: Date:
Facial and Oral Movements	1. **Muscles of facial expression,** e.g., movements of the forehead, eyebrows, perioral area, cheeks, including frowning, blinking, smiling, grimacing	0 1 2 3 4	0 1 2 3 4
	2. **Lips and perioral area,** e.g., puckering, pouting, smacking	0 1 2 3 4	0 1 2 3 4
	3. **Jaw,** e.g., biting, clenching, chewing, mouth opening, lateral movement	0 1 2 3 4	0 1 2 3 4
	4. **Tongue:** Rate only increases in movement both in and out of mouth, NOT the inability to sustain movement. Darting in and out of mouth	0 1 2 3 4	0 1 2 3 4
Extremity Movements	5. **Upper (arms, wrists, hands, fingers):** Include choreic movements (i.e., rapid, objectively purposeless, irregular, or spontaneous), athetoid movements (i.e., slow, irregular, complex serpentine). DO NOT INCLUDE TREMOR (i.e., repetitive, regular, rhythmic)	0 1 2 3 4	0 1 2 3 4
	6. **Lower (legs, knees, ankles, toes),** e.g., lateral knee movement, foot tapping, heel dropping, foot squirming, inversion and eversion of foot	0 1 2 3 4	0 1 2 3 4
Trunk Movements	7. **Neck, shoulder, hips,** e.g., rocking, twisting, squirming, pelvic gyrations	0 1 2 3 4	0 1 2 3 4
Global Judgments	8. **Severity** of abnormal movements overall	0 1 2 3 4	0 1 2 3 4
	9. **Incapacitation** caused by abnormal movements	0 1 2 3 4	0 1 2 3 4
	10. **Client's awareness** of abnormal movements: Rate only client's report No awareness 0 Aware, moderate distress 3 Aware, no distress 1 Aware, severe distress 4 Aware, mild distress 2	0 1 2 3 4	0 1 2 3 4
Dental Status	11. Current problems with teeth and/or dentures?	No Yes	No Yes
	12. Are dentures usually worn?	No Yes	No Yes
	13. Edentulous?	No Yes	No Yes
	14. Do movements disappear in sleep?	No Yes	No Yes

Modified from State of Connecticut, Department of Mental Retardation. (2002). DMR Medical Advisory 2000-2: Monitoring for abnormal involuntary movements (tardive dyskinesia). Retrieved August 29, 2005, from http://www.dmr.state.ct.us/publications/centralofc/hcs_ma 2000-2.htm; and Public Health Service, Alcohol, Drug Abuse, and Mental Health Administration, National Institute of Mental Health. (2000). Abnormal Involuntary Movement Scale (AIMS). Retrieved August 29, 2005, from http://www.dmr.state.ct.us/publications/centralofc/images/hcs_ma2000-2_c.pdf.
*Activated movements.

of a particular drug to J.T.'s symptoms. As with J.T., the client's prior experience with antipsychotics is also an important consideration.

After establishing the need for drug therapy, the prescriber decides what agent or combination of agents is best suited for the client's total health needs. This requires an intimate knowledge of the behavioral actions, pharmacologic effects, and potential adverse effects of the agents used, as well as an awareness of the many individual and environmental factors present (Stahl, 1999).

The additional effects or side-effects profile of a drug is a useful tool in helping the prescriber select an appropriate antipsychotic agent (see Table 19-1). Continuous nursing and medical evaluations based on observation of the client for the therapeutic and adverse effects of the drug are necessary. Nurses play an important role in the evaluation and assessment of client response to drug therapy. They should be aware of the criteria the prescriber uses in selecting psychotherapeutic drugs and of the expected effects of the drug so they can observe and report on the client's progress.

Given the significant acute dystonic reaction seen with J.T. after administration of haloperidol, alternatives to the typical antipsychotics should be considered.

✳ What are the advantages of the atypical antipsychotics?

The atypical antipsychotic agents include the dibenzodiazepines (e.g., clozapine [Clozaril], olanzapine [Zyprexa], and quetiapine [Seroquel]) and the benzisoxazoles risperidone (Risperdal) and ziprasidone (Geodon). These agents have diverse effects and are essentially different from the typical antipsychotic agents discussed in this chapter. Compared with the typical antipsychotics, the atypical antipsychotics have more specific antagonism of the D_1 receptor with lower affinity for the D_2 receptors. They also bind to the serotonin (5-HT_2) receptor (Baldessarini & Tarazi, 2001). In addition to the beneficial effects on the "positive" symptoms of schizophrenia (e.g., hallucinations, bizarre behavior), the atypical agents also appear to be more effective in controlling "negative" symptoms often observed (e.g., flat affect, lack of motivation). Aripiprazole (Abilify) is a novel, newer agent classified as a quinolinone, with partial agonist-antagonist activity at multiple receptors.

As a group, these agents display reduced activity at the D_2 receptor. This pharmacologic property results in a low potential for EPS and TD. This property alone is responsible for these newer agents often to be considered preferable to the older typical agents. Unfortunately, these newer agents are not devoid of adverse effects. Each agent poses unique and significant adverse effects that are important to consider when choosing an agent (Nasrallah & Newcomer, 2004). Because of the diversity of their adverse effect profiles, each is discussed separately.

✳▥ clozapine [**kloe** zah peen]
(Clozaril)
Clozapine was the first of the new atypical antipsychotics. It differs from the other neuroleptics by being active at the limbic dopamine receptors, affecting both receptors but with less affinity for D_2; thus it is less apt to induce extrapyramidal side effects. It binds more to

5-HT_2, α_1, and histamine (H_1) receptors than to dopamine receptors. These differences compared to the typical and some of the other atypical agents account for the success of clozapine when other antipsychotics have failed to adequately controlled symptoms.

Indications
Because clozapine has the potential for causing agranulocytosis, a potentially life-threatening effect, it is reserved for treatment-resistant schizophrenia or for when adverse effects to other drugs preclude their continued use (*USP DI*, 2005). Treatment resistance is defined as the client not responding to an appropriate course of standard antipsychotic agents after trying at least two antipsychotic medications. Other adverse effects also render clozapine use problematic.

Pharmacokinetics/Dosing
Clozapine is rapidly absorbed orally and is distributed extensively throughout the body, including crossing the blood-brain barrier. It reaches peak serum levels in approximately 2.5 hours; the average steady-state serum level is 319 ng/mL. The duration of action is 4 to 12 hours; it is metabolized in the liver, and excreted by the kidneys (50%) and in the feces (30%).

Treatment with clozapine is closely monitored, with the manufacturer recommending that only weekly supplies be dispensed and that weekly WBC testing be performed. The adult dosage is 25 mg once or twice daily, increased by 25 to 50 mg/day until 300 to 450 mg/day is reached by the end of the second week of therapy. Thereafter, dosage increases should not exceed 100 mg once or twice a week. The maximum daily dose is 900 mg (*Mosby's Drug Consult*, 2005; *USP DI*, 2005).

Adverse Effects
Adverse effects of clozapine vary from mild to serious. Bone marrow suppression, although rare, is considered the most serious, and requires weekly or biweekly monitoring of WBC counts. Among the other serious reactions are seizures and orthostatic hypotension. Additional effects include constipation, dizziness, sedation, headache, hypersalivation, nausea, vomiting, weight gain, tachycardia, hypotension, fever, agitation, akathisia, EPS, impotency, insomnia, and neuroleptic malignant syndrome (NMS). Many of these effects are dose related; dosing must be carefully titrated upward on a daily basis from an initial low dose; any significant interruption in therapy (e.g., longer than 48 hours) typically will require retitration from low doses to avoid many of these serious adverse effects. The following are the most serious of the adverse effects:

- Bone marrow suppression: The risk for serious blood dyscrasias (agranulocytosis, thrombocytopenia, etc.) is approximately 4 per 1000 clients exposed (Freedman, 2003). Because of the effect of clozapine on myeloproliferation, it is essential that the client's WBC be determined at the start of therapy, at weekly intervals, and for 4 weeks after the last dose. Therapy should not be initiated if the WBC is less than 3500/mm³ and should be discontinued any time the WBC substantially declines from the baseline WBC or falls below 3000/mm³. Ongoing monitoring for any signs or symptoms of infection is appropriate whenever clozapine is used.
- Seizures: Seizures occur in approximately 3% of clients receiving clozapine. The risk is greatest when doses are advanced rapidly, or when interrupted therapy is resumed at higher doses.
- Orthostatic hypotension: orthostasis with resultant reflex tachycardia is common with clozapine. It is most dramatic after dosage increases, and is best managed with adequate client education to avoid rapid standing after prone position, and care after meals and at bedtime (Box 19-6).
- Weight gain with risk for hyperglycemia and type 2 diabetes mellitus: Clozapine appears to pose a significant risk for weight gain, hyperglycemia, and development of type 2 diabetes mellitus. This effect is also observed with other atypical agents, particularly olanzapine (Bess & Cunningham, 2004; Leslie & Rosenheck, 2004).

olanzapine [oh **lan** zah peen]
(Zyprexa)
Olanzapine is at least equal to, if not more effective than, the typical antipsychotic agents (Buckley, 1999). Like clozapine, it produces

little EPS and is not believed to cause TD. It is also more effective than the typical antipsychotics against the negative symptoms of psychosis (see Table 19-1). Although its exact mechanism of action is unknown, its effectiveness is thought to result from its dopamine and serotonin type 2 blocking effects. Olanzapine is an antagonist at many CNS neurotransmitter receptor sites, which may be associated with its other adverse effects, such as sedation (histamine) and orthostatic hypotension (α_1).

Indications
Olanzapine is indicated for the treatment of schizophrenia and psychosis, and for management of acute mania for clients with bipolar disorder. There is some data to support its use in the management of chronic pain.

Pharmacokinetics/Dosing
Olanzapine is available as both a standard oral tablet (Zyprexa) and as a rapidly disintegrating tablet (Zyprexa, Zydis) that quickly dissolves in saliva. Both formulations are well absorbed. Olanzapine is highly bound to plasma proteins and is extensively metabolized on first pass through the liver via cytochrome P450 1A2 and 2D6. Its elimination half-life in adults is typically 21 to 54 hours, but is shorter in smokers and longer in older adults. The adult dose of olanzapine is typically 5 to 10 mg once daily, although doses as high as 30 mg daily have been used.

Adverse Effects
Adverse effects include dizziness, constipation, somnolence, dry mouth, GI distress, weight gain, EPS, peripheral edema, and rash. Of greatest concern with olanzapine is weight gain and the propensity to trigger type 2 diabetes mellitus in predisposed clients; in one assessment (Koro et al., 2002), this risk was estimated as four times more likely with olanzapine than with most other antipsychotic agents, although a lower estimate was reported by other researchers (Leslie & Rosenheck, 2004). This risk appears highest during the first 2 years of therapy. This serious risk for weight gain and diabetes mellitus raises a number of therapeutic and ethical questions to consider for clinicians who select antipsychotic therapy (see Box 19-3). Olanzapine is also associated with an increased risk of aspiration pneumonia and prolactin-based breast cancers in women with a history of breast cancer.

quetiapine [kwe tye **ah** peen]
(Seroquel)
Indications
Quetiapine is used in the treatment of schizophrenia, mania, bipolar disorder, and psychosis. It is also used in the treatment of autism in children.

Pharmacokinetics/Dosing
Quetiapine is hepatically metabolized primarily via cytochrome P450 3A4 to inactive metabolites. The usual initial adult dosage of quetiapine is 25 mg twice daily, increased as necessary by 25 to 50 mg. Most clients achieve good symptom control at 300 to 500 mg daily. The maximum daily dose is 800 mg.

Adverse Effects
Like olanzapine, quetiapine has a low potential for EPS and TD. With the exception of risk for developing diabetes mellitus, the side-effect profile and risks are similar to olanzapine.

risperidone [ris **per** ih done]
(Risperdal)
Risperidone blocks serotonin and dopamine receptors and is associated with improved positive and negative symptoms of schizophrenia.

Indications
Risperidone is used in the treatment of psychosis, bipolar disorder, mania, and Tourette syndrome. It is also used in the treatment of autism in children and adolescents. It is not approved for the treatment of clients with dementia-related psychosis (FDA Public Health Advisory, April 2005).

Pharmacokinetics/Dosing
Risperidone is available as a standard oral tablet (Risperdal), a rapidly dissolving tablet (Risperdal-M-Tab), an oral solution, and a long-acting IM formulation (Risperdal Consta). The oral solution can be mixed with water, low-fat milk, decaffeinated coffee, or orange juice, but is incompatible with cola, tea, and grapefruit juice. Risperidone taken orally reaches peak serum levels in 1 to 2 hours and is metabolized by cytochrome P450 2D6 and 3A4 to an active metabolite (9-hydroxyrisperidone). The adult dosage of risperidone is 1 mg twice daily, increasing as necessary according to client response. In older adults, the dosage is 0.5 mg twice daily.

The long-acting IM formulation is typically dosed at 25 mg every 2 weeks with doses titrated to effect every 4 weeks up to a maximum of 50 mg every 2 weeks. As with haloperidol decanoate, long-acting IM therapy is typically reserved for clients who tolerate oral therapy, and benefits of IM therapy outweigh risk (see also Box 19-3). Concurrent oral risperidone is often required for the first few weeks of IM therapy.

Adverse Effects
Unlike the other atypical agents, risperidone can produce significant EPS at higher doses (e.g., doses greater than 6 mg/day). It is unclear if higher doses of risperidone increase risk for TD compared to the other atypical agents, but most responders of risperidone have good symptom control at the lower end of the dosing range. Other adverse effects of risperidone include fatigue, cough, dry mouth, increased dreaming, nausea, weight gain, insomnia, visual changes, sexual dysfunction, and anxiety.

ziprasidone [zi **pra** si done]
(Geodon)
Ziprasidone, like risperidone, blocks serotonergic and dopaminergic receptors.

Indications
Ziprasidone is used to treat schizophrenia and Tourette syndrome.

Pharmacokinetics/Dosing
Ziprasidone is highly protein bound. Its elimination half-life is 10 to 24 hours. The initial adult dosage of ziprasidone is 20 mg twice daily with food, increasing as necessary to a maximum of 80 mg twice daily. An immediate-release injectable formulation is available for IM use.

Adverse Effects
Ziprasidone may induce sedation, respiratory disorders, and some risk for EPS. When first marketed, there was considerable concern for risk of prolongation of the QT interval on ECG and it was believed to increase risk for life-threatening ventricular dysrhythmias; this has since been disputed (Roden, 2004; Teich, 2003).

aripiprazole [ah rih **pip** rah zole]
(Abilify)

Aripiprazole is a novel newer antipsychotic that differs pharmacologically from other agents. Similar to other antipsychotics, it serves as a dopamine antagonist at postsynaptic D_2 receptors, but also appears to have partial agonist activity. It serves as a dopamine agonist at presynaptic dopamine receptors and the interplay of agonist/antagonist activity appears to modulate the side-effect profile. Less data exist for its efficacy in treating psychosis compared to other available agents.

Indications

Aripiprazole is used in the treatment of psychosis and schizophrenia. Its role in the treatment of mania and bipolar disorder has been debated (Jagadheesan & Muirhead, 2004).

Pharmacokinetics/Dosing

Aripiprazole is metabolized by cytochrome P450 2D6 and 3A4; an individual with a genetic predisposition for reduced function of these enzymes (see the Special Considerations for Pharmacogenetics box on p. 384), or an individual receiving concurrent drug therapy that inhibits these enzymes (e.g., azole antifungals, some of the selective serotonin reuptake inhibitors such as fluoxetine or paroxetine), may display added sedation or orthostasis. Concurrent use of carbamazepine (Tegretol) may result in reduced levels of aripiprazole. The typical dose range for aripiprazole is 10 to 30 mg daily.

Adverse Effects

Aripiprazole produces little EPS and probably has a low potential for TD with routine doses. Like other agents that have antagonist activity at α_1-adrenergic receptors and histamine$_1$ receptors, it is associated with orthostatic hypotension and sedation. Worsening of psychosis has been reported with its use (Reeves & Mack, 2004). Neuroleptic malignant syndrome is also associated with its use (Chakraborty & Johnston, 2004).

✷ **The treatment team decides to provide inpatient care for J.T. Although J.T. had significant adverse effects with haloperidol (Haldol), his hallucinations and combative behavior appeared to improve. The team initiates quetiapine (Seroquel) 25 mg twice daily.**

✷ **What are the nursing implications for J.T.?**

In managing the nursing care of a client who is receiving antipsychotic drug therapy, such as J.T., a comprehensive perspective is essential.

Assessment Before starting antipsychotic drug therapy, and with his hospital admission, J.T. should undergo a complete history and physical assessment. Of particular importance is a neurologic examination and documentation of orientation, affect, and cognition as a baseline assessment. It is important to obtain a baseline assessment of pulse and BP in the sitting, standing, and lying positions. Ensure that a complete blood count and hepatic and renal function studies are completed.

Assess J.T. for preexisting health conditions that contraindicate the use of a particular agent or conditions that would require cautious use and special monitoring interventions. Antipsychotic agents may cause a number of cardiovascular effects, including hypotension (caused by α-adrenergic blockade), tachycardia (anticholinergic effect), myocardial depressant effects, and electrocardiographic alterations that affect the ST interval and T wave, and widen the QRS complex. The most cardiotoxic agents are chlorpromazine (Thorazine) and thioridazine (Mellaril). Other antipsychotics such as quetiapine (Seroquel) or risperidone (Risperdal) have fewer cardiotoxic effects and therefore may be the preferred agent for clients with cardiovascular disease.

Antipsychotic agents are contraindicated in clients who are comatose or have severe cardiovascular disease or severe CNS depression. They are administered with caution to clients with alcoholism because they may potentiate CNS depression and liver impairment, and may place the client at higher risk of heat stroke. With decreased metabolism by the liver, there may be increased sensitivity to CNS effects and Reye syndrome in children and adolescents (see the Special Considerations for Children box below). Clients with the following disorders may find their symptoms in-

---

Special Considerations for Children | PSYCHOTHERAPEUTIC AGENTS

- Children are at a greater risk of developing neuromuscular or extrapyramidal side effects, especially dystonias. Monitor closely if antipsychotic agents are administered.
- Pediatric clients with chickenpox, CNS infections, measles, dehydration, gastroenteritis, or other acute illnesses will be at special risk of developing adverse effects and possibly Reye syndrome. Avoid use of phenothiazine antiemetic therapy in such clients.
- The tricyclic antidepressants are usually not recommended for the treatment of depression in children younger than 12 years old. However, some agents, such as amitriptyline (Elavil) and imipramine (Tofranil), have been used in children older than 6 years of age for major depressions. Several of these agents are also used in the treatment of enuresis and attention deficit disorder. Be aware that children are very sensitive to an acute overdose, which should always be considered very serious and potentially fatal. Adolescents often require a decreased dose because of their sensitivity to this drug category. Also see the Evidence-Based Practice box on Safety of Antidepressants in Children and Adolescents on p. 401.
- Adverse effects reported in children receiving the tricyclic antidepressants include changes in ECG patterns, increased nervousness, sleep disorders, complaints of tiredness, hypertension, and mild stomach distress.
- Lithium may decrease the bone density or bone formation in children. If necessary to use, monitor closely serum levels and for signs of toxicity.

Data from *USP DI: Drug information for the health care professional* (25th ed.). (2005). Greenwood Village, CO: MICROMEDEX Thomson Healthcare.

creased: blood dyscrasias, cardiovascular disease, glaucoma, hepatic impairment, Parkinson's disease, urinary retention, and chronic respiratory disorders. Antipsychotic drugs should be used cautiously in clients with a history of seizure disorders because of their action in reducing the seizure threshold. Adequate antiepileptic therapy needs to be maintained. The risk of administering these drugs to pregnant women should be weighed against the expected therapeutic outcome (see the Pregnancy Safety box below).

An ophthalmologic examination is recommended before the onset of antipsychotic agent therapy. The examination includes measurement of visual acuity with and without refraction, a color vision test, a slit-lamp study of the fundus, and examination of the visual fields.

Before beginning antipsychotic therapy, J.T.'s drug history should be obtained. If J.T. were older, he might experience unusual adverse drug reactions as compared with younger persons (see the Special Considerations for Older Adults Box below).

Review J.T.'s current medication regimen for the risk of significant drug interactions. Monitor him closely if his regimen includes any drug for which anticholinergic and/or hypotensive effects are the intended purpose or an adverse effect of the drug, as these symptoms will be additive. These additive effects will also occur with extrapyramidal-inducing medications. Alcohol and other CNS depressant drugs may result in enhanced CNS depression, respiratory depression, and increased hypotensive effects. The antipsychotic drug dosage should be reduced to one-fourth to one-half the usual dosage and titrated according to client response. Concurrent alcohol use may increase the risk of inducing heat stroke. Antipsychotic agents block α-adrenergic receptors, thus the administration of epinephrine to treat phenothiazine-induced hypotension may result in severe hypotension. With the α receptors blocked, epinephrine stimulates β receptors, which can result in tachycardia and severe lowering of BP. Avoid concurrent use or a potentially serious drug interaction may occur. If hypotension necessitating drug intervention occurs, norepinephrine or phenylephrine (Neo-Synephrine) may be administered. Concurrent use with the antipsychotic agents may render levodopa ineffective in controlling Parkinson's disease and lithium enhances the risk for EPS.

PREGNANCY SAFETY
PSYCHOTROPIC DRUGS

Category	Drug
B	bupropion, clozapine, maprotiline
C	amitriptyline, amoxapine, clomipramine, desipramine, doxepin, fluoxetine, fluphenazine haloperidol, isocarboxazid, loxapine, mirtazapine, molindone, nefazodone, olanzapine, perphenazine pimozide, phenelzine, protriptyline, quetiapine, risperidone, sertraline, thiothixene, tranylcypromine, trimipramine, venlafaxine
D	imipramine, lithium, nortriptyline

Data from *Mosby's drug consult* (15th ed.). (2005). St. Louis: Mosby.

Special Considerations for Older Adults | PSYCHOTHERAPEUTIC AGENTS

- Older adults tend to have higher serum levels of the antipsychotic and antidepressant drugs because of changes in drug distribution resulting from a decrease in lean body mass, less total body water, less serum albumin, and (usually) an increase in body fat. Therefore, these clients require a lower drug dose and a more gradual drug dose titration than the younger adult client.
- Older clients are more prone to have orthostatic hypotension, anticholinergic adverse effects, EPS, and sedation. They should be carefully evaluated before starting such potent medications, and if the antipsychotic agents are necessary, close supervision and the prescribing of the lowest dose possible is recommended.
- The older adult client generally should receive half the recommended adult dose. The client with organic brain syndrome should only receive 33% to 50% of the usual adult dose with increases in dosage at 7- to 10-day periods. When clinical improvement is noted, attempts at tapering and discontinuing the drug should be instituted.

- The tricyclic antidepressants may cause increased anxiety in the older client. If the client has cardiovascular disease, the use of the tricyclic antidepressants increases the risk of inducing dysrhythmias, tachycardia, stroke, heart failure, and myocardial infarction.
- The treatment of behavioral disorders in older clients with dementia with atypical (second-generation) antipsychotic medications is associated with increased mortality (FDA Public Health Advisory, April 2005).
- Lithium is more toxic in the older client; therefore, lower lithium dosages, a lower lithium serum level, and very close monitoring is critical in this age group. Older adults are more prone to develop CNS toxicity, lithium-induced goiter, and clinical hypothyroidism than is the average adult. Generally, excessive thirst and elimination of large volumes of urine may be early adverse effects of lithium toxicity frequently seen in older adults.

Data from USP DI: *Drug information for the health care professional* (25th ed.). (2005). Greenwood Village, CO: MICROMEDEX Thomson Healthcare.

Nursing Diagnosis The following nursing diagnoses/ collaborative problems may be identified in J.T. while he is undergoing antipsychotic therapy: disturbed sleep pattern (drowsiness), impaired comfort related to dry mouth; constipation and urinary retention related to the antimuscarinic effects; impaired skin integrity (rash); ineffective protection related to bone marrow depression; and the potential complications of allergic reaction, heat stroke, hepatotoxicity, Reye syndrome, akathisia, dystonia, EPS, NMS, and persistent TD. (See the Nursing Care Plan below for a description of the more common nursing diagnoses.)

NURSING CARE PLAN SELECTED NURSING DIAGNOSES RELATED TO ANTIPSYCHOTIC MEDICATION ADMINISTRATION

Nursing Diagnosis	Outcome Criteria	Nursing Interventions
Constipation related to anticholinergic effects of the drug	• The client will maintain his or her usual bowel elimination pattern, select foods high in fiber from the daily menu, maintain a fluid intake of 2500 mL daily, and increase activity as allowed.	• Assess client's usual bowel elimination pattern; monitor and record bowel movements. • Instruct client to establish a routine for bowel elimination, select foods high in fiber, maintain fluid intake of 2500 mL/day, perform isometric abdominal strengthening exercises unless contraindicated, and increase activity as allowed.
Impaired comfort related to dry mouth	• The client will maintain a healthy oral cavity as evidenced by pink, moist, intact mucosa.	• Provide ice chips, sugarless candies, and frequent mouth hygiene if dry mouth occurs.
Risk for injury related to increased sensitivity to the sun, visual effects, and the development of dizziness, hypotension, extrapyramidal effects, and TD	• The client will not experience sunburn, falls, or symptoms of EPS or TD.	• Monitor blood pressure at appropriate intervals; keep client in recumbent position for 30 min after injection; provide assistance with ambulation if sedation, dizziness, orthostatic hypotension, or visual changes occur. • Instruct client to change position from recumbent to upright slowly. • Alert client to hypersensitivity to sun and instruct about sunscreen use, protective covering, and sunglasses. • Monitor for and instruct client in the early signs of TD (facial tics, grimacing, blinking, lip smacking, tongue protrusion, writhing motions of the arms, hands, and fingers) and EPS (akathisia, dystonia, and parkinsonism). Report immediately.
Deficient knowledge related to newly prescribed or altered psychotherapeutic agents	• The client will describe his or her condition, how the drug therapy relates to the condition, how and when to take the medications, common drug interactions, common adverse effects and which of these warrant reporting, and drug storage requirements. • The client will demonstrate less anxiety-related behaviors related to fear of the unknown, loss of control, and misconceptions.	• Assess learning needs and learning readiness. • Plan with the client and family for the achievement of realistic goals. • Provide information to meet outcome criteria.
Ineffective therapeutic regimen management	• The client will demonstrate self-administration of medications safely and accurately.	• Determine the client's reasons for ineffective management of therapeutic regimen, and make appropriate teaching/counseling interventions. • Discuss the increased possibility of the return of symptoms with ineffective management of therapeutic regimen.

EPS, Extrapyramidal side effects; *TD,* tardive dyskinesia.

Planning While on antipsychotic drug therapy, J.T. will:
- Experience improved thought processes without hallucinations.
- Demonstrate appropriate behaviors and social interactions.
- Remain compliant with therapy.
- Effectively manage his therapeutic regimen, including appropriate reporting of adverse drug effects to a health care provider and implementation of other measures supportive of the drug regimen.

Implementation

Monitoring In the past, many clients said to be resistant to antipsychotic therapy were found to be noncompliant with the prescribed therapy. Although this is not an issue with J.T. in an in-house setting, it may be in other settings. Many psychotic clients deny their illness or associate medication use with dependence or weakness. Clients who are refractory to antipsychotic medications should be reviewed for the following:

- *Compliance.* The drug order may be switched to a liquid or rapidly dissolving formulation to be administered in a supervised setting.
- *Inadequate dosage.* The prescriber should adjust the dosage according to J.T.'s clinical response. An inadequate dosage, partial compliance, or the development of drug tolerance may result in an inadequate response to the medication.
- *Questionable oral bioavailability.* Although this is not known to be a common possibility, it is a variable to consider. The prescriber may switch from an oral solid dosage form to a liquid formulation and also adjust the dosage as necessary according to J.T.'s response or development of adverse effects. Switching to or adding another antipsychotic agent may also be considered, as in J.T.'s case.

Observe J.T. for orthostatic hypotension, especially if his drugs need to be administered parenterally at any time; monitor his BP before and after injections. Alert the prescriber if orthostatic (postural) hypotension occurs and causes severe difficulties or serious hazards. The prescriber may then institute one of the following remedial measures: (1) a change to another drug that does not produce this adverse effect with such frequency, (2) a reduction of dosage, or (3) a discontinuation of medication for 24 hours with a gradual reinitiation of the drug dosage as tolerated.

Complete blood counts are drawn periodically. Be alert to signs of blood dyscrasias: decreased white cells, platelets, and red cells. Monitor for other symptoms of agranulocytosis such as sore throat, fever, or weakness; this usually occurs between weeks 4 and 10. The antipsychotic drug is usually discontinued when these symptoms appear; withhold the dose and notify the prescriber as soon as possible.

Contact the prescriber about possible ocular changes, (decreased vision, brownish coloring of vision, impaired night vision, and pigment deposits on the fundus). These changes may be related to dosage levels or therapy duration. Clients receiving long-term or moderate- to high-dose therapy should have periodic ophthalmologic examinations.

Observe J.T. for neuroleptic extrapyramidal adverse effects (see Box 19-4). In particular, monitor the client closely for early signs of TD, which usually appear as small, worm-like motions of the tongue. Because there is no known effective treatment for TD, the drug should be discontinued immediately and the prescriber notified (see Box 19-4). Monitor J.T. for dystonic reactions, neck spasms, eye rolling, dysphagia, and seizures.

Also monitor J.T. for NMS (hyperthermia, dehydration, cardiovascular instability, hypoxemia, and muscular rigidity). Therapy is essentially symptomatic and supportive, and the drug is discontinued immediately.

Because of the anticholinergic effects of the antipsychotic drugs, monitor J.T. for signs and symptoms of urinary hesitancy or retention, constipation, prostatic hypertrophy, narrow-angle glaucoma, or respiratory problems. Hepatic function tests are performed periodically. Observe J.T. for yellow skin, nausea, flu-like symptoms, and rash. The drug should be discontinued immediately when these symptoms occur.

Monitor J.T. for weight gain; this may be an issue of noncompliance for some clients. Assist with appropriate dietary instruction.

To demonstrate the efficacy or inefficacy of the drug, observe J.T. and note if the mental status has changed from the baseline assessment. Routine attempts at drug withdrawal should be considered for most clients receiving a psychotropic medication (Cohen-Mansfield et al., 1999).

Intervention Although not necessary with J.T., rapid neuroleptization or high-dose antipsychotic therapy is appropriate in certain cases. For instance, aggressive treatment is used in clients with acute psychosis who may exhibit dangerous and/or destructive behaviors. IM therapy with a high-potency antipsychotic agent (e.g., haloperidol [Haldol]) is usually given, often on an hourly schedule, until the desired effects are achieved. If a client will take an oral medication, high-dose oral therapy may be substituted. Because of the half-life of the IM doses, the first oral dose is often delayed until 12 to 24 hours after the last IM dose.

Long-acting injections are often useful in antipsychotic therapy. Depot fluphenazine enanthate (Prolixin Enanthate), fluphenazine decanoate (Prolixin Decanoate), haloperidol decanoate (Haldol Decanoate), and long-acting IM risperidone (Risperdal Consta) are available for clients who are persistently noncompliant, do not understand the need for taking medications, or have a high frequency of relapses (psychotic episodes).

In most cases, concurrent treatment with more than one neuroleptic agent is not indicated. If the client does not respond to a particular drug, the dosage of that drug is usually increased or a different drug is prescribed. Occasionally a client may respond best to a combination of two drugs from different classes. However, the potentiation and lowered margin of safety of such combinations require greater precautions for client safety.

The administration of large doses over a prolonged time may lead to anticholinergic psychoses or TD. Maintenance dosages should be periodically evaluated for a possible dosage reduction or the cessation of drug therapy. Clients with pre-existing renal or hepatic disease may require a reduced dosage.

A special dropper should be used for oral, liquid haloperidol (Haldol) administration; a precipitate will form if it is diluted with tea or coffee. If dilution is desired, use at least 60 mL of diluent (water, apricot or grape juice) and mix it just before administration to prevent precipitation. Undiluted haloperidol oral solution may irritate the mucous membranes. Haloperidol tablets may be taken with food or a full glass of water to decrease GI irritation.

For clients on high or long-term dosages, gradual reduction of the antipsychotic over several weeks will help to prevent withdrawal symptoms of nausea, vomiting, irritability, trembling, and transient dyskinetic signs. The only rationale for abrupt withdrawal of long-term antipsychotic therapy is the occurrence of severe adverse effects.

Education If J.T. complains of dizziness, light-headedness, or palpitations, he may be experiencing orthostatic hypotension. This can easily be confirmed by comparing his BP in the prone and standing positions. Instruct him to rise slowly from the recumbent position and to sit on the edge of the bed for a few minutes before attempting to stand. Explaining orthostatic hypotension also may help J.T. to understand this experience, and support and reassurance may be necessary to allay his anxiety.

Caution J.T. against driving, operating dangerous machinery, or performing tasks that require absolute precision, motor coordination, and mental alertness when he is discharged on these medications. Tolerance to drowsiness develops as therapy continues. Clients should be told that it may take several weeks before the antipsychotic medication can treat the disorder effectively.

To prevent photosensitivity, advise J.T. to stay out of the sun and to use sunscreen lotion or wear protective clothing to prevent solar erythema, or assist him by providing the necessary protective measures. Exposure to light also increases the possibility of ocular changes; therefore instruct him to wear sunglasses.

Caution J.T. that dry mouth can be a bothersome adverse effect of antipsychotic therapy and can contribute to the development of caries, gum disease, and oral candidiasis. Review the use of proper oral hygiene with him. For older clients, xerostomia may affect the fitting of full dentures; a referral should be made for dental care for this and other dental problems.

Haloperidol and other antipsychotics affect the regulation of body temperature; alert J.T. to avoid heat stroke by using caution walking in hot, humid weather, or using saunas, hot tubs, and steam baths.

Instruct J.T. to avoid alcohol and other CNS depressants because they increase the CNS depressant effects of the antipsychotic agents. Using these drugs concurrently with

medications that cause extrapyramidal reactions will increase the frequency and severity of the extrapyramidal effects. Encourage J.T. to consult with his prescriber before taking any over-the-counter (OTC) drugs; this will help to prevent serious drug interactions.

Evaluation The expected outcomes of antipsychotic therapy are that J.T. will be able to perform activities of daily living independently, without experiencing adverse effects of the drugs, and that he will self-administer his medication safely and accurately.

❁ **L.F. is a 78-year-old woman who has just been placed in a long-term care facility. She has had difficulty in adjusting to her new surroundings, has become agitated, and frequently paces the corridors. The attending physician starts a new order for quetiapine (Seroquel) 25 mg twice daily PRN for agitation.**

❁ **What are the important legal and ethical issues involved in using antipsychotics for controlling behavior in the long-term care residents?**
In April 2005, the Food and Drug Administration (FDA) issued a warning regarding increased mortality associated with the use of atypical antipsychotics in older adults with dementia and behavioral disorders. This warning was based on an evaluation of 15 studies involving over 5,000 clients in which one or more of the atypical antipsychotics olanzapine, aripiprazole, risperidone, and quetiapine were used. The mortality rate was 1.6- to 1.7-fold higher in clients receiving these drugs compared with those receiving placebo. Causes of death included heart failure, sudden death, and infection. It is unclear if the older typical antipsychotics pose a similar increased risk (*FDA Public Health Advisory,* April 2005).

Despite their mortality risk, these agents are associated with some improvement in agitation, hallucinations, delusion, sleep disturbance, wandering, and verbal or physical aggression associated with dementia (Lee et al., 2004). Ongoing use would therefore be expected to continue to some extent, but such use may potentially be inappropriate.

Inappropriate prescriptions also expose older adults to an increased risk of adverse or serious drug reactions or falls, which often are detrimental to the client's cognitive and functional health status. As such, a careful evaluation of the risks, benefits, and legal and ethical considerations in their use is warranted. Refer back to the overview of ethical considerations in the use of psychotropic medications in Box 19-3. Studies of these practices have resulted in regulations governing Medicare and Medicaid recipients in long-term care facilities.

The Omnibus Budget Reconciliation Act (OBRA) Long-Term Care Requirements Act for long-term care facilities was implemented in 1992. Although this act applies to all drugs that a client receives, attention is focused on the major CNS drug categories: antipsychotics, antianxiety agents, sedatives, hypnotics, and benzodiazepines. The law requires review of the indication, dosage (including duplicate-type drug orders), duration, and monitoring parameters of a drug to determine if the drug is being given in the presence of adverse effects.

Before antipsychotic drugs can be prescribed for a skilled nursing facility resident, an appropriate specific condition must be documented, such as schizophrenia, schizoaffective disorder, delusional disorder, psychotic mood disorder, acute psychotic episode, brief reactive psychosis, schizophreniform disorder, atypical psychosis, Tourette syndrome, or Huntington disease. All of these diagnoses are organic mental syndromes that have associated psychotic or agitation features. Agitation features are defined as (1) specific behaviors that can be quantitatively and objectively documented (e.g., biting, kicking, scratching), cause the client to present a danger to the client or others, and actually interfere with the nursing staff's ability to provide care to the client, or (2) the presence of psychotic symptoms (delusions, hallucinations, or paranoid behavior) that are not a result of a previously mentioned disorder but cause the client extreme distress. To treat the symptoms of hiccups, nausea, vomiting, or pruritus, short-term therapy of 1 week is permissible.

OBRA regulations are intended to eliminate or reduce the inappropriate prescribing of these potent medications for behaviors that may be controlled by nonpharmacologically. For example, insomnia, pacing, wandering, restlessness, crying spells, screaming episodes, deficient memory, uncooperativeness, nervousness, or depression alone would not warrant the use of an antipsychotic agent. For these medications to be prescribed, such symptoms would need to be associated with an appropriate diagnosis as mentioned previously. However, there is still concern for the shift to the use of newer psychotropic agents in the post–Health Care Financing Administration era in a population where close monitoring may not be readily available.

In addition, with the care of older, frail individuals shifting to the community setting, there is concern for the lack of regulatory oversight relating to prescribing practices for this group. Golden et al. (1999), revealed a high prevalence of psychotropic medications and inappropriate drug use among older homebound residents—a group that is at the highest risk for adverse drug reactions and interactions. Psychotropic drug treatment without access to psychotherapeutic support is not appropriate for older clients in the community (Stevens, Katona, Manela, Watkin, & Livingston, 1999).

In the case presented above, the use of quetiapine for L.F. appears initially inappropriate until other environmental and supportive interventions were implemented. In addition, a specific evaluation of the behavior in the context of a psychiatric diagnosis for which antipsychotics are a recognized treatment is in order. Use of an antipsychotic might be considered, even in the absence of such a diagnosis, if the target symptoms pose a significant risk to health and safety, are regularly measured and evaluated, and the response to the drug therapy is observed and documented to be beneficial and outweigh the risks of therapy. Ongoing evaluation of the client for short and long-term adverse effects is also indicated.

Affective Disorders

Affective disorders, or mood disturbances, include **depression** (the most common affective disorder) and **mania** or elation. Clinical depression is quite common in the general population; mania less so. Bipolar disorder presents as fluctuating symptoms with prolonged periods (typically months) of depression that eventually shift to mania or vice versa.

No single factor has been identified as the cause of affective disorders. Psychiatrists who believe in psychosocial factors will probe to identify stressful events or mental conflicts that preceded the onset of depression, whereas others who adhere to biologic factors tend to explain affective disorders by the monoamine theory (i.e., catecholamine [norepinephrine, dopamine, epinephrine] and indolamine [serotonin] levels in the CNS). Many practitioners today believe that both psychosocial and biologic factors lead to a common pathway resulting in an affective disorder.

Many factors are involved with affective disorders, including genetics, psychosocial events (divorce, death of a mate), physiologic stress (illness, infection, childbirth), and personality traits. Any combination of these factors may also affect the biochemical mechanisms of the CNS, which lends weight to the theory that affective disorders have a common pathway.

Centrally acting monoamines, especially norepinephrine and serotonin, are theorized to be the cause of depression and mania. A deficiency in central norepinephrine is associated with depression, whereas an excess of norepinephrine is believed to be related to mania. Serotonin imbalance is also noted in depression, eating disorders, anxiety, and bipolar disorders. The imbalance may be related to altered receptor function, a deficiency in available serotonin, or both.

Depression

Over the years many classifications of depression have been used, such as the time of life that depression occurred (childhood, adolescence, or older adulthood), or the reason for the depression, such as exogenous (reactive) depression or endogenous depression. **Exogenous** (reactive or secondary) **depression** is often a person's response to a loss (a loss of pleasure or interest in activities and everyday living caused, perhaps, by the loss of a loved one or the presence of a debilitating illness) or disappointment (not meeting one's expectations, or the loss of a job, pet, friend). Postpartum depression, classically noted within 6 weeks to 6 months after delivery, is often unrecognized or not diagnosed (Stowe, Hostetter, & Newport, 2005). This is usually referred to as "the blues," or normal depression, and it often remits in several months without the use of antidepressant medications. The mobilization of support systems and, if necessary, psychotherapy are useful adjuncts in exogenous depression. Unipolar or **endogenous depression** is characterized by the absence of external causes. This type of depression may be caused by genetic determination and biochemical alterations (Katzung, 2004). Antidepressant medications are very useful in treating this type of depression.

The current classification of depressive disorders has eliminated the use of these terms. Instead, major affective disorders are defined as **bipolar disorders** (mixed type and manic) and **major depression** as unipolar (single episode or recurrent episodes), along with atypical affective disorders that include depression. Psychiatrists have debated over whether the newer classification is an improvement over the previous types of classification, because it is important for the clinician to have a diagnostic framework from which to work.

Criteria for major depression include the presence of mood changes (sadness, despondency, anxiety, crying spells, guilt feelings, self-pity, pessimism, loss of interest in life and social activities); psychological symptoms (low self-esteem, poor concentration, hopeless or helpless feelings, suicidal tendencies, increased focus on death); physiologic manifestations (sleep disturbances that may range from insomnia to hypersomnia, decreased interest in sex, complaints of fatigue, loss of energy, menstrual dysfunction, headaches, palpitations, constipation, loss of appetite, and weight loss or weight gain); and thinking alterations (a decrease in concentration or attention span, complaints of poor memory, confusion, delusions relating to health, persecution, or religion, and hallucinations if the client is also psychotic). Cognitive impairment, in particular, is often an early manifestation of depression in older adults (Vinkers, Gussekloo, Stek, Westendorp, & van der Mast, 2004). Mood variations are usually diurnal and are often worse in the morning.

Both psychotherapy and pharmacotherapy are used to treat depression. Reduction of environmental stressors and milieu therapy is also helpful. Electroconvulsive shock is an alternative for severe depression refractory to other modalities (The UK ECT Review Group, 2003). Psychotherapy involves three phases, including an initial session or sessions to clarify diagnostic issues, a second phase that focuses on problem resolution, and a third phase aimed at defining gains. The second and third phases vary in the amount of time to complete, and take months and/or years (Hollander, 2001). The combination of drug and other therapies may provide additional benefit beyond single-modality interventions.

Given the cost associated with implementation of psychotherapy, drug therapy for depression has become more popular. There are four major categories of antidepressant drugs; these are the tricyclic antidepressants (TCAs), the second-generation antidepressants, the monoamine oxidase inhibitors (MAOIs), and the selective serotonin reuptake inhibitors (SSRIs). Occasionally, stimulants such as methylphenidate are used to treat depression in older adults (see Chapter 18). There is probably little difference in efficacy of agents to treat depression across class, although the SSRIs are better tolerated in most clients (MacGillivray et al., 2003). Adequate treatment of depression is also associated with improved pain management for clients with chronic pain (Lin et al., 2003), and may be beneficial for clients with concurrent ethanol abuse (Nunes

& Levin, 2004). Use of antidepressants is associated with reduced risk for suicide in older men and women, but may be higher in youth and adolescents (Hall et al., 2003) (also see the Evidence-Based Practice box on p. 401). These classes are discussed below and presented in Table 19-2. St. John's wort, a complementary/alternative therapy used to treat mild to moderate depression and associated with significant drug interactions (Markowitz et al., 2003), is discussed in Chapter 12.

Antidepressants

Tricyclic Antidepressants TCAs were the first available antidepressants used in western medicine, becoming available in the mid-twentieth century. The first of these agents was amitriptyline (Elavil). Amitriptyline blocks both serotonin and norepinephrine at presynaptic CNS nerve terminals, resulting in increased levels of both serotonin and norepinephrine in the synaptic cleft. The increased availability of neurotransmitter to the postsynaptic neurotransmitter receptors is believed to account for the antidepressant activity of these agents.

In addition to the direct effects on norepinephrine and serotonin, these agents have multiple effects at other receptors, including antimuscarinic (anticholinergic at the muscarinic receptor), α-adrenergic tissue, and cardiac tissue. The effects at the serotonin receptor are believed to account for sedation, whereas effects at the muscarinic receptor account for dry mouth, urinary retention, constipation, and tachycardia. α-adrenergic blockade by these agents induces orthostasis. TCAs can cause life-threatening cardiac dysrhythmias, particularly in overdose. Tricyclics may also increase the risk for seizures. These drugs have a high incidence of sexual dysfunction, including loss of libido, difficulty in maintaining an erection for men, and decreased libido and or inability to have an orgasm for both men and women.

The tricyclic antidepressants are considered very dangerous in overdose with significant antimuscarinic (anticholinergic) activity, cardiac dysrhythmias and seizures being the most problematic (see the Management of Drug Overdose box on p. 402). Given safer alternative antidepressants, these drugs are rarely used as first-line therapy for depression, and stringently avoided for individuals with suicidal ideation.

Other indications for TCAs include treatment of neuropathic pain (typically responsive to low doses (see Chapter 14), obsessive-compulsive disorder (clomipramine [Anafranil]), and nocturnal enuresis (imipramine [Tofranil]). The tricyclic antidepressants can be categorized as tertiary amines (such as amitriptyline) or secondary amines. The tertiary amines include clomipramine, doxepin, imipramine, and trimipramine. The secondary amines are amoxapine, desipramine, nortriptyline, and protriptyline. Each of these agents blocks reuptake of serotonin and norepinephrine to varying degrees (see Table 19-2).

★▀ **imipramine** [im **ip** ra meen]
(Tofranil, Tofranil-PM, Apo-Imipramine✦)
Imipramine is often considered the prototypical TCA.

Continued on p. 401

Table 19-2　Antidepressants

Agent	Typical Adult Daily Dose (mg)	NE Reuptake Inhibition	Serotonin Reuptake Inhibition	Antimuscarinic	Sedation	Orthostatic Hypotension	GI Upset	Weight Gain	Comment
Tricyclic Tertiary Amine									
amitriptyline (Elavil)	50-300	Moderate	High	High	High	Moderate	Low	High	Also used for chronic pain
clomipramine (Anafranil)	100-250	Moderate	High	Moderate-high	Moderate-high	Moderate	Low	High	Primarily used for OCD
doxepin (Adapin, Sinequan)	75-150	Low	Moderate	Moderate	Moderate-high	Moderate	None	High	
imipramine (Tofranil)	50-150	Moderate	Moderate-high	Moderate-high	Moderate	Moderate-high	Low	High	Also used for nocturnal enuresis, ADHD
trimipramine (Surmontil)	75-150	Low	Low	Moderate-high	Moderate-high	Moderate	None	High	
Tricyclic Secondary Amine									
desipramine (Norpramin)	50-150	High	Low-moderate	Low	Low-moderate	Low-moderate	None	Low	Also used for chronic pain Active metabolite of imipramine Risk for fatalities higher than other TCAs (Amitai & Frischer, 2004)
nortriptyline (Aventyl, Pamelor)	30-150	Moderate	Moderate	Moderate	Moderate	Low	None	Low	Also used for chronic pain
protriptyline (Vivactil)	15-60	Moderate	Low	Moderate	Low	Low-moderate	None	None	

Drug (Brand)	Dosage range									Comments
SECOND-GENERATION TETRACYCLIC										
amoxapine (Asendin)	100-400	Moderate-high	Moderate	High	Moderate	Moderate	Low	None	Moderate	
maprotiline (Ludiomil)	100-225	Moderate	Low	Moderate	Moderate-high	Moderate-high	Moderate	None	Moderate	
mirtazapine (Remeron)	15-45	Very low	Very low	Moderate	Moderate-high	Moderate	Moderate	None	Moderate-high	Antagonist at postsynaptic 5-HT$_2$ receptor
SECOND-GENERATION PHENYLPIPERAZINE										
nefazodone (formerly Serzone)	300-600	Very high	Very high	Very low	Low	Low	None	Low	None	Risk for hepatotoxicity Brand name product removed from market in 2004; generic formulation may be available
SECOND-GENERATION TRIAZOLOPYRIDINE										
trazodone (Desyrel)	150-300	Moderate-high	None	None	Very high	Moderate-high	Moderate-high	Low	Moderate	25-200 mg at bedtime typically used as nighttime sedative to treat insomnia
SECOND-GENERATION AMINOKETONE										
bupropion (Wellbutrin, Zyban)	300-450	Very low	Very low	Very low	None (often stimulating)	Very low	Very low	Low	None	Increases seizure risk 150 mg two times daily used as adjunct for smoking cessation Inhibits dopamine reuptake
SECOND-GENERATION PHENETHYLAMINE										
venlafaxine (Effexor)	75-375 (XR: 75-225)	Moderate-high	Moderate-high	Very low	Very low	Very low	Very low	Moderate-high	None	Dose dependent

Modified from Hollander, E. (Ed.). (2001). *Professional's handbook of psychotropic drugs.* Springhouse, PA: Springhouse; Lacy, C.F., Armstrong, L.L., Goldman, M.P., & Lance, L.L. (2004). *Drug information handbook* (10th ed.). Cleveland: Lexi-Comp; Amitai Y., & Frischer H. (2004). Excess fatality from desipramine and dosage recommendations. *Therapeutic Drug Monitoring, 26*(5), 468-473.

ADHD, Attention deficit hyperactivity disorder; *GI,* gastrointestinal; *NE,* norepinephrine; *OCD,* obsessive-compulsive disorder; *TCA,* tricyclic antidepressant.

Continued

TABLE 19-2 ANTIDEPRESSANTS—*cont'd*

Agent	Typical Adult Daily Dose (mg)	NE Reuptake Inhibition	Serotonin Reuptake Inhibition	Antimuscarinic	Sedation	Orthostatic Hypotension	GI Upset	Weight Gain	Comment
THIOPHENEPROPYLAMINE									
duloxetine (Cymbalta)	40-60	High	High	Very low	Very low	Very low	Moderate-high	None	
SELECTIVE SEROTONIN REUPTAKE INHIBITORS (SSRI)									
citalopram (Celexa)	20-60	Very low	Very high	Very low	Very low	Very low	Moderate-high	None	
escitalopram (Lexapro)	10-20	Very low	Very high	Very low	Very low	Very low	Moderate-high	None	
fluoxetine (Prozac)	20-60	Very low	Very high	Very low	Very low	Very low	Moderate-high	None	
fluvoxamine (Luvox)	100-300	Very low	Very high	Very low	Very low	None	Moderate-high	None	
paroxetine (Paxil)	20-50	Very low	Very high	None	Very low	None	Moderate-high	Low	
sertraline (Zoloft)	50-150	Very low	Very high	None	Very low	None	Moderate-high	None	
MONOAMINE OXIDASE INHIBITORS (MAOIs)									
phenelzine (Nardil)	15-90	NA	NA	Low	Low	Moderate	Low	Moderate-high	Significant drug interactions and dietary restrictions; see text
tranylcypromine (Parnate)	10-40	NA	NA	Low	Low	Moderate	Low	Moderate	

NA, Not applicable.

Safety of Antidepressants in Children and Adolescents

Psychotropic drug use, including use of antidepressants, is commonplace in children and adolescents for the treatment of depression, obsessive-compulsive disorder, and other conditions. Rates of psychotropic drug prescriptions approach that observed with adults (Zito et al., 2003). There is considerable controversy about the safety of antidepressants in this population, however.

The older tricyclic antidepressants have been used for many years in children. As with adults, these agents pose significant risks for life-threatening cardiac dysrhythmias. These risks are more likely with higher doses and in overdose, but may be observed in typical doses, and appear to be highest for desipramine (Amitai & Frischer, 2004). Other dose-related adverse effects, including anticholinergic effects, seizure risk, and orthostatic hypotension have also rendered the tricyclics unfavorable agents, particularly for clients who have suicidal ideation and may elect to ingest large amounts of the drug in a suicide attempt.

The newer SSRIs, such as fluoxetine, were welcomed as safer alternatives to the tricyclics, and widespread use in children has been observed over the past decade. Of the available SSRIs, only fluoxetine is U.S. Food and Drug Administration (FDA) approved for childhood depression, and it alone among the group appears to be effective for major depression in children (Whittington et al., 2004). Combining it with cognitive behavioral therapy to treat depression improves the therapy response rate when compared to the response rate for drug alone (March et al., 2004). Unfortunately, despite widespread use of fluoxetine and other SSRIs, concerns for increased risk of suicide and other adverse effects associated with their use have surfaced in youth, particularly during the first few weeks of therapy (Jureidini et al., 2004; Jick, Kaye, & Jick, 2004). Asking depressed adolescents about suicidal thoughts does not increase the likelihood of suicidal ideation (Gould et al., 2005).

The FDA evaluated 24 trials of various classes of antidepressant; the trials included more than 4400 clients. This review identified the doubling of risk for suicide attempt (4% among users of antidepressants and 2% for those receiving placebo) (FDA Public Health Advisory, October 15, 2004). This assessment prompted the FDA to alter labeling of all antidepressants (SSRIs, tricyclics, atypicals, and MAOIs) to include the following (*FDA Public Health Advisory*, October 2004):

- "Antidepressants increase the risk of suicidal thinking and behavior (suicidality) in children and adolescents with major depressive disorder and other psychiatric disorders.
- "Anyone considering the use of an antidepressant in a child or adolescent for any clinical use must balance the risk of increased suicidality with the clinical need.
- "Clients who are started on therapy should be observed closely for clinical worsening, suicidality, or unusual changes in behavior.
- "Families and caregivers should be advised to closely observe the client and to communicate with the prescriber.
- "A statement regarding whether the particular drug is approved for any pediatric indication(s) and, if so, which one(s)."

Assessment of antidepressant use in children is likely to continue over the next decade in attempts to identify which agents offer the greatest benefits with lowest risk for this population.

Indications

Imipramine is indicated for the relief of symptoms of depression. It is also used to treat nocturnal enuresis in children, attention deficit hyperactive disorder, and panic disorder, and in lower doses, chronic and neuropathic pain.

Pharmacokinetics/Dosing

Imipramine is metabolized by cytochrome P450 2C19, 2D6, and other isoenzymes to active metabolites, including desipramine (itself a marketed TCA under the brand name Norpramin). The half-life in adults is between 6 and 18 hours. The adult dose for depression is 25 mg three times daily up to 150 mg/day. Occasionally doses as high as 300 mg/day have been used. Doses of 10 to 25 mg daily at bedtime are used for pain management in older adults, with increases up to antidepressant doses if required and tolerated. The typical dose used for nocturnal enuresis in children older than 6 years of age is 10 to 25 mg/day, with doses up to 50 to 75 mg used, depending on age and weight. The therapeutic range for imipramine and its active metabolite desipramine are 150 to 250 ng/mL and 150 to 300 ng/mL, respectively.

Adverse Effects

As indicated above, TCAs have a significant adverse-effect profile, including significant antimuscarinic and cardiovascular effects. Imipramine in particular is associated with significant antimuscarinic action, including dry mouth, urinary retention, constipation, and tachycardia. Other effects include risk for cardiac dysrhythmias (particularly with high doses or overdose, and may be higher with the metabolite desipramine [Amitai & Frischer, 2004]), orthostatic hypotension, hypertension, and sexual dysfunction. Acute withdrawal from chronically administered TCA therapy may be associated with withdrawal symptoms as noted in Box 19-7 on p. 403.

Drug Interactions

Imipramine interacts with a great number of drugs. Box 19-8 on p. 404 presents its pharmacodynamic and pharmacokinetic interactions.

Second-Generation Antidepressants Like the older TCAs, the second-generation antidepressants primarily affect reuptake of neurotransmitters (norepinephrine and/or serotonin and/or dopamine). They are generally associated with a reduced risk for cardiac dysrhythmias and weight gain compared with the TCAs, but other adverse effects vary considerably. These agents are presented in Table 19-2. Given their diversity, selected agents are briefly discussed in greater detail.

bupropion [byoo **pro** pi on]
(Wellbutrin, Zyban)

The mechanism of action for bupropion (Wellbutrin, Zyban) is unknown, but it weakly blocks the reuptake of dopamine, serotonin,

✦ Management of Drug Overdose

Tricyclic Antidepressants

Although less frequently used since SSRI antidepressants became available, tricyclic antidepressants are used for pain management and as second-line therapy for depression. Tricyclic antidepressant (TCA) overdose can be life threatening, resulting in serious adverse effects such as heart block, cardiac dysrhythmias and profound tachycardia, hypotension, life-threatening seizures, and coma. Risk for death with overdose is considered between 6 and 16 times that of other antidepressants (Amitai & Frischer, 2004). Because the condition of the client can decline rapidly, tricyclic antidepressant overdose must be treated aggressively.

Signs and Symptoms

The signs and symptoms of a TCA overdose may vary in severity depending on numerous factors, including the amount ingested and absorbed, the age of the individual, and the interval between ingestion and initiation of a treatment modality. Any acute overdose or unwarranted ingestion of a TCA in children or adults must be considered serious and potentially fatal.

CNS abnormalities include agitation, ataxia, choreoathetoid movements, drowsiness, hyperactive reflexes, muscle rigidity, restlessness, stupor, seizures, and coma. Cardiac abnormalities may include dysrhythmia, ECG evidence of impaired conduction (including widened QRS complex), signs of heart failure, and tachycardia. Quinidine-like adverse effects are common in poisonings with TCAs.

Treatment

Treatment of tricyclic overdose is a medical emergency requiring careful cardiac and neurologic monitoring. Symptomatic and supportive measures are instituted according to the individual client's requirement. They may include the following:

- Activated charcoal with or without gastric lavage is the recommended strategy for decontamination. Ipecac use is contraindicated.
- Sodium bicarbonate is routinely used to treat QRS widening, lower seizure risk, and to increase urine pH, which facilitates ion trapping of the drug in the urine.
- Close monitoring of cardiovascular functioning for at least 5 days. Cardiac dysrhythmias have occurred up to 6 days after massive TCA doses, which may require treatment with antidysrhythmic therapy.
- Maintenance of body temperature and respiratory and cardiac functions.
- Administration of antiepileptic drugs such as diazepam (Valium), phenytoin (Dilantin)/fosphenytoin (Cerebyx), and phenobarbital, control seizures.
- Be aware that hemodialysis, peritoneal dialysis, forced diuresis, and exchange transfusions are not successful in treating a TCA overdose (*USP DI*, 2005).

and norepinephrine. These actions are not only associated with improved symptoms of depression, but also assist a motivated client who is attempting smoking cessation to be successful.

Indications
Bupropion is indicated for the treatment of depression, and as an adjunct to smoking cessation. It is also occasionally used in the management of attention deficit hyperactive disorder.

Pharmacokinetics/Dosing
The usual dose for depression is in the range of 300 to 450 mg daily. When used in conjunction with a behavioral support program, bupropion at doses of 300 mg daily for 8 to 12 weeks reduces cravings for cigarettes and is associated with approximately twice the success rate of quitting smoking as placebo.

Adverse Effects
Bupropion has fewer anticholinergic effects and rarely produces the hypotension, weight gain, or sexual dysfunction associated with other antidepressants. However, it can cause agitation, insomnia, tremors, and dose-related seizures. Because of the stimulating nature of bupropion, it is not recommended for individuals who have anxiety as a component of their depression. The drug is generally avoided for individuals with a history of seizures or eating disorders.

✦ mirtazapine [mir **taz** ah peen]
(Remeron)
Mirtazapine acts to inhibit presynaptic norepinephrine and serotonin reuptake, but also has effects at the postsynaptic serotonin 2 receptor.

Indications
Mirtazapine (Remeron) is considered by many a second-line agent for depression when other interventions have not been successful.

Pharmacokinetics/Dosing
Mirtazapine is extensively metabolized by cytochrome P450 1A2, 2D6, and 3A4. The usual adult dose is 15 mg at bedtime (7.5 mg in older adults), with doses increasing up to 45 mg/day if required. Reduced doses are recommended for renal or hepatic dysfunction.

Adverse Effects
Mirtazapine may be associated with a higher risk for seizures than many other antidepressants (with the possible exception of bupropion discussed above). Although rare, agranulocytosis has been reported and is potentially life-threatening. Careful monitoring for sore throat, fever, stomatitis, or other signs of infection is appropriate.

trazodone [**tray** zoe done]
(Desyrel)
Trazodone (Desyrel) blocks serotonin reuptake and also produces changes in the binding at serotonin receptors.

Indications
Trazodone is rarely used for the treatment of depression and more commonly used in low doses to treat insomnia.

Pharmacokinetics/Dosing
Trazodone is hepatically metabolized via cytochrome P450 3A4 and other isoenzymes. The typical adult dose for sedation is 25 to 50 mg at bedtime with a maximum dose of 200 mg at bedtime.

BOX 19-7 DURATION OF ANTIDEPRESSANT THERAPY AND ANTIDEPRESSANT WITHDRAWAL SYNDROMES

DURATION OF ANTIDEPRESSANTS

Clients who are first diagnosed with depression often are concerned about taking drugs for a prolonged period of time. The duration of antidepressant therapy is partly dependent on response to initial therapy, age of first episode, and whether the depression is recurrent. The following table offers an approach to identifying the appropriate duration of antidepressant therapy for most clients.

Duration of Antidepressant Therapy for Major Depression

	AGE AT FIRST EPISODE (YEARS)		
	<39	40-49	>50
First episode	6-9 months	6-9 months	Indefinitely
Second episode	6-9 months	4-5 years	Indefinitely
Second episode with complications	4-5 years	Indefinitely	Indefinitely
Third or subsequent episode	Indefinitely	Indefinitely	Indefinitely

DISCONTINUATION OF ANTIDEPRESSANTS

Halting antidepressant therapy is often associated with uncomfortable symptoms, which vary slightly by agent. Below are symptoms of withdrawal that are pronounced for 1 to 3 weeks after abrupt discontinuation of antidepressants. When possible, antidepressants should be tapered to avoid or minimize these effects.

Symptoms of Tricyclic Withdrawal

- Sleep disturbance
- Nightmares
- Malaise
- Nausea
- GI upset
- Irritability

Symptoms of SSRI Withdrawal

- Dizziness
- Nausea
- Tremor
- Anxiety
- Palpitations
- Light-headedness

Antidepressant dose for adults is usually 50 to 100 mg three times daily.

Adverse Effects
Trazodone has few, if any, anticholinergic effects, and thus has minimal effects on cardiac conduction. The prescriber should still exercise caution in using this drug in clients with a history of cardiac disease, because several cases of ventricular dysrhythmia have been reported with its use. Trazodone is very sedating; this explains its use in insomnia. Caution should be exhibited when used concurrently with other agents affecting serotonin action because of the risk of serotonin syndrome (Box 19-9). Trazodone can cause gastric distress and postural hypotension early in treatment, especially in older adults, as well as priapism in younger clients (Finley, Laird, & Benefield, 2001).

Monoamine Oxidase Inhibitors The MAOIs include phenelzine (Nardil) and tranylcypromine sulfate (Parnate) and are indicated as second- or third-line antidepressants for the treatment of depression that does not respond to other, safer antidepressants. These agents have numerous drug interactions with prescription and OTC medications, caffeine, and foods and beverages containing tyramine (see Box 19-8). The major adverse effect with these agents is the occurrence of a sudden and possibly very severe hypertension that can progress fatality if left untreated.

Monoamine oxidase (MAO), an enzyme found in nerve terminals, the liver, and the brain, is necessary for the inactivation and degradation of tyramine, catecholamines, serotonin, and various medications. MAOIs interfere with this inactivation, which may result in a potentiation of vasopressor effects and serious adverse effects. Two types of MAO enzymes have been identified and named: MAO-A and MAO-B. MAO-A appears to have a preference for serotonin and is located throughout the body, with high concentrations located in the human placenta. MAO-B is found mainly in human platelets. Approximately equal amounts of both types are found in the liver and brain. The MAOIs currently in use for depression are nonselective. Selegiline (Eldepryl) is a MAO-B inhibitor used primarily in the treatment of Parkinson's disease (see Chapter 23).

The MAOIs are capable of blocking or diminishing the activity of MAO, resulting in a net increase in brain amine levels. Current research indicates that the MAOIs produce desensitization of the α_2, β, and serotonin receptors (downregulation). During early clinical trials of MAOIs as antide-

BOX 19-8 DRUG INTERACTIONS WITH PSYCHOTROPICS

PHARMACODYNAMIC INTERACTIONS

Serious or potentially serious complications are possible with any of the psychotropic agents, especially when drugs with additive adverse effects (e.g., sedation, antimuscarinic properties, orthostatic hypotension, decreased seizure threshold) are combined. Combinations of drugs with serotonergic action may increase risk for serotonin syndrome (see Box 19-9).

Antipsychotic Interactions

The additive effects of multiple agents with sedative, anticholinergic/antimuscarinic properties, orthostasis, seizure risk, or prolongation of QT interval may result in negative client outcomes.

The effect of most antipsychotics on α-adrenergic receptors may render the administration of epinephrine in an emergency situation ineffective and result in further lowering of blood pressure.

MAOI Interactions

MAOIs present a major risk for interactions with foods and other drugs, and can lead to hypertensive crisis. When dosed with tyramine-containing foods or sympathomimetic drugs, the MAOIs can precipitate dramatic elevations in blood pressure accompanied with severe headache, stiff neck, retro-orbital pain, and flushing.

Food Interactions with MAOIs Foods rich in tyramine should be avoided while on an MAOI. The following is a guide to dietary restrictions with MAOIs:

Avoid

- Aged cheeses
- Broad beans
- Herring
- Yeast

Restrict

- Beer
- Snails
- Processed meats
- Liver
- Raisins
- Sauerkraut
- Ripe avocado
- Sardines
- Anchovies
- Fermented foods
- Canned figs
- Coffee
- Licorice
- Soy sauce

Up to 2 oz/day Acceptable

- Sour cream
- Cottage cheese
- Mild Swiss cheese
- Chocolate
- Yogurt
- American cheese
- Wine (avoid Chianti, sherry)

Drug Interactions with MAOIs Concurrent drugs that have activity in the sympathetic nervous system should also be avoided for individuals on MAOIs and include the following:

- Amphetamines
- Appetite suppressants
- Asthma inhalants
- Buspirone
- Carbamazepine
- Cocaine
- Cyclobenzaprine (Periactin)
- Decongestants
- Dextromethorphan
- Dopamine
- Ephedrine
- Epinephrine
- Guanethidine
- Levodopa
- Meperidine (Demerol)
- Methyldopa
- Methylphenidate (Ritalin)
- Other antidepressants
- Reserpine
- Stimulants
- Sympathomimetics
- Tryptophan

Lithium Interactions

Because sodium and lithium are similar chemically, the kidney often considers them as interchangeable. In situations where sodium levels are depleted (e.g., sweating, decreased salt intake, diarrhea, diuretics), the kidney actively reabsorbs more lithium, with lithium toxicity becoming more likely. Early lithium toxicity often causes diarrhea, which only serves to further exacerbate sodium loss and additionally contribute to lithium toxicity.

Concurrent use of nonsteroidal antiinflammatory agents (e.g., ibuprofen [Advil]) may also increase the risk for lithium toxicity via renal mechanisms.

PHARMACOKINETIC INTERACTIONS

A number of the antidepressants and antipsychotics are metabolized by the cytochrome P450 system and may induce or inhibit metabolism of other drugs. In addition, the psychotropic drug levels themselves may be affected by other agents that impact on these enzyme systems. The two most common enzyme systems that metabolize antidepressants are cytochrome P450 2D6 and 3A4. Combinations of drugs that are affected by the same enzyme system may result in altered levels (either higher or lower) of other concurrently administered drugs. The significance of the interaction in part depends on the client's genetically derived enzyme function, and the degree to which the drug is metabolized by more than one enzyme. A partial list of common drugs that affect these systems are listed in the following sections.

2D6

Psychotropic
Antidepressants

amitriptyline	**duloxetine**	**paroxetine**
amoxapine	**fluoxetine**	sertraline
citalopram	imipramine	trazodone
clomipramine	maprotiline	trimipramine
desipramine	mirtazapine	venlafaxine
doxepin	nortriptyline	

Antipsychotics

aripiprazole	**haloperidol**	quetiapine
chlorpromazine	olanzapine	risperidone
clozapine	**perphenazine**	**thioridazine**

BOX 19-8 DRUG INTERACTIONS WITH PSYCHOTROPICS—cont'd

<u>Other Drugs</u>

amiodarone	donepezil	ondansetron
amphetamine	**doxorubicin**	oxycodone
betaxolol	encainide	papaverine
captopril	flecainide	pentazocine
carvedilol	**fluphenazine**	propranolol
celecoxib	hydrocodone	**propoxyphene**
chlorpheniramine	**labetalol**	**quinidine**
cimetidine	lidocaine	**ranitidine**
codeine	loratadine	**ritonavir**
cyclophosphamide	meperidine	selegiline
delavirdine	**methadone**	tamoxifen
dextromethor-	metoclopramide	tiagabine
phan	metoprolol	timolol
diltiazem	mexiletine	tramadol
diphenhydramine	molindone	**valproic acid**
dolasetron	morphine	**vinblastine**

3A4

Psychotropic
Antidepressants

amoxapine	**fluoxetine**	**sertraline**
bupropion	**fluvoxamine**	trazodone
citalopram	imipramine	venlafaxine
clomipramine	**nefazodone**	
escitalopram	**St. John's wort**	

Antipsychotics

aripiprazole	clozapine	risperidone
chlorpromazine	**haloperidol**	ziprasidone

Other Drugs

acetaminophen	amlodipine	**azithromycin**
alfentanil	**amprenavir**	budesonide
alprazolam	**anastrozole**	caffeine
amiodarone	atorvastatin	**cannabinoids**

carbamazepine	granisetron	**quinine**
chlordiazepoxide	**grapefruit juice**	**ranitidine**
cimetidine	*griseofulvin*	*rifabutin*
cisapride	hydrocortisone	*rifampin*
clarithromycin	**indinavir**	**ritonavir**
clofibrate	**isoniazid**	salmeterol
clonazepam	isradipine	**saquinavir**
clorazepate	**itraconazole**	sibutramine
clotrimazole	**ketoconazole**	sildenafil
cocaine	losartan	simvastatin
codeine	lidocaine	sirolimus
cortisone	loratadine	*sulfinpyrazone*
cyclophosphamide	lovastatin	tacrolimus
cyclosporine	methadone	tamoxifen
dapsone	**metronidazole**	temazepam
delavirdine	midazolam	terfenadine
dexamethasone	montelukast	theophylline
diazepam	**nelfinavir**	tiagabine
diltiazem	*nevirapine*	tolcapone
disulfiram	**nicardipine**	tolterodine
dolasetron	nifedipine	tretinoin
doxycycline	nimodipine	triazolam
enalapril	**norfloxacin**	*troglitazone*
erythromycin	**omeprazole**	**verapamil**
estradiol	ondansetron	vinblastine
ethinyl estradiol	*oxcarbazepine*	vincristine
ethosuximide	pantoprazole	warfarin
etoposide	*phenobarbital*	**zafirlukast**
felodipine	*phenytoin*	zaleplon
fentanyl	pioglitazone	zidovudine
finasteride	pravastatin	**zileuton**
fluticasone	prednisone	zolpidem
gemfibrozil	*primidone*	zonisamide
glucocorticoids	**propoxyphene**	
glyburide	**quinidine**	

Modified from Lacy, C.F., Armstrong, L.L., Goldman, M.P., & Lance, L.L. (2004). *Drug information handbook* (10th ed.). Cleveland: Lexi-Comp; Markowitz, J.S., Donovan, J.L., DeVane, C.L., Taylor, R.M., Ruan, Y., Wang, J.S., et al. (2003). Effect of St. John's wort on drug metabolism by induction of cytochrome P450 3A4 enzyme. *Journal of the American Medical Association, 290,* 1500-1504.
Drugs in **BOLD** are more likely to inhibit the metabolism of other drugs metabolized by the same enzyme system.
Drugs in *ITALICS* are more likely to induce metabolism of other drugs metabolized by the same enzyme system.
Drugs in ***BOLD ITALICS*** either induce or inhibit metabolism of other drugs metabolized by the same enzyme system.

pressants, orthostatic hypotension was encountered as a common but inconsistent adverse effect. Many MAOIs were then produced and studied specifically as antidepressant and antihypertensive agents.

MAOIs can increase the concentration of all central amines, although different effects on the individual amines are possible. For example, some MAOIs may increase dopamine or norepinephrine concentrations to a more extensive degree than serotonin concentrations, whereas other MAOIs may raise the level of serotonin to a greater degree than those of norepinephrine and dopamine. The increase in amine concentration is associated with behavioral hyperactivity (amphetamine-like psychomotor stimulation with large

doses) and, in some cases, with the exacerbation of psychotic symptoms. Antiphobic and antidepressant activities are seen with lower doses. In general, these compounds are most effective in reversing the dysphoric state and its attendant vegetative disturbances in clients with depressive syndromes.

Therapeutic doses of MAOIs take from days to weeks to produce a maximal therapeutic effect. MAOIs produce an irreversible inactivation of MAO by forming a stable complex with the enzyme; recovery from the effect of MAOIs thus depends on enzyme regeneration, which may occur over several weeks. Inhibition occurs only with very high doses and may be responsible for some of the toxic effects of MAOIs.

BOX 19-9 SEROTONIN SYNDROME

Serotonin syndrome is a hyperserotonergic state that develops rapidly (within hours or days of adding a serotonergic drug). Complications include seizures, disseminated intravascular coagulation, respiratory failure, and hyperthermia. If not adequately identified and controlled, it can be fatal. It mimics malignant hyperthermia and neuroleptic malignant syndrome. It is often seen with the combination of SSRIs and MAOIs, SSRIs and other serotonergic antidepressants, or MAOIs and other sympathomimetic drugs.

DIAGNOSIS

Medications that affect the metabolism, synthesis, or reuptake of serotonin may result in serotonin accumulation and the serotonin syndrome. This syndrome is characterized by mental status changes (confusion, restlessness, anxiety, disorientation), ataxia, myoclonus, tremors, rigidity, hypertension, and autonomic dysfunction.

Diagnosis of serotonin syndrome requires at least three of the following:

- Mental status changes (confusion, hypomania)
- Hyperreflexia
- Shivering
- Diarrhea
- Fever
- Agitation
- Myoclonus
- Diaphoresis
- Tremor
- Incoordination

Symptoms usually occur within 2 to 72 hours up to several weeks after beginning the administration of a serotonergic drug. Other causes that may cause similar symptoms need to be ruled out, such as infection, metabolic disorders, or the start or increase of a neuroleptic agent before the onset of this syndrome. The most common drug combinations that cause this syndrome include an MAOI with SSRIs, TCAs, tryptophan, lithium, and dextromethorphan.

TREATMENT

In mild cases, discontinue the serotonergic agent and provide supportive treatment as necessary. The symptoms may resolve within 24 hours.

Severe cases require discontinuing the offending drug and providing supportive care, but symptoms may be prolonged, and in some cases, fatal. Diazepam (Valium), propranolol (Inderal), methysergide (Sansert), cyproheptadine (Periactin), mechanical ventilation, and skeletal muscle relaxants like dantrolene have been used for severe cases.

DRUGS THAT AFFECT SEROTONIN

- Serotonin agonist: buspirone (BuSpar).
- Inhibits serotonin metabolism: MAOIs (tranylcypromine [Parnate], phenelzine [Nardil]) and MAO-B inhibitor (selegiline [Eldepryl]).
- Increases serotonin synthesis or release: methylphenidate (Ritalin), lithium, and tryptophan.
- Inhibits serotonin reuptake: antidepressants such as amitriptyline (Elavil), nortriptyline (Aventyl), doxepin (Sinequan), imipramine (Tofranil), and clomipramine (Anafranil). The SSRIs include paroxetine (Paxil), fluoxetine (Prozac), sertraline (Zoloft), and fluvoxamine (Luvox). An opioid meperidine (Demerol) and miscellaneous drugs such as dextromethorphan (DM), trazodone (Desyrel), and venlafaxine (Effexor) may also cause this effect.

---

phenelzine [**fen** el zeen]
(Nardil)

Indications
Phenelzine is typically reserved for refractory depression not responsive to other modalities.

Pharmacokinetics/Dosing
Phenelzine is well-absorbed orally, is metabolized hepatically and eliminated in urine as both metabolites and unchanged drug. The onset of action is observed over 2 to 4 weeks, and duration of effect and interaction potential persists for at least 2 weeks after discontinuation of therapy. Typical adult dose is 15 mg three times daily with doses titrated up to a maximum of 90 mg/day if needed and tolerated. Dose used in older adults starts at 7.5 mg once daily and is slowly increased to 15 to 60 mg/day as tolerated.

Adverse Effects
Orthostatic hypotension is often noted with phenelzine therapy. Combinations with sympathomimetics, caffeine, tyramine-containing foods, or other interacting drugs can lead to significant hypertension, tachycardia, dysrhythmias, and hyperpyrexia, and is potentially fatal.

Interactions
Extensive interactions with serious consequences are possible (see Box 19-8).

Selective Serotonin Reuptake Inhibitors The SSRIs are safer and as effective as the other antidepressants. These agents selectively block the reuptake of serotonin in the presynapses. Their safety profiles in adults are considered preferable to other antidepressants, particularly in the treatment of depression among those with cardiovascular disease (Berkman et al., 2003). Fluoxetine (Prozac) represents the prototype of the class and has been in widespread use for over a decade. Other SSRIs include fluvoxamine (Luvox), paroxetine (Paxil), sertraline (Zoloft), and citalopram (Celexa), and are presented in Table 19-2. With the exception of fluvoxamine, SSRIs are used to treat depression, and most are useful in the management of obsessive-compulsive disorder, panic attacks, and social phobias.

---

fluoxetine [floo **oks** e teen]
(Prozac, Prozac Weekly, Rapiflux, Sarafem, Novo-Fluoxetine♣)

Indications
Fluoxetine is used to treat depression, panic disorder, obsessive-compulsive disorder, bulimia nervosa, and premenstrual dysphoric disorder.

Pharmacokinetics/Dosing
Fluoxetine is well-absorbed orally with an onset of antidepressant activity seen within the first 4 to 6 weeks of therapy. Fluoxetine differs from the other SSRIs in that its metabolite (norfluoxetine) is pharmacologically active. Metabolism occurs via the cytochrome P450 systems, primarily via 3A4 but also via 2D6, so interactions with other drugs metabolized by these systems are possible (see Box

19-8). The adult dose of fluoxetine ranges from 10 to 80 mg daily based on indication and response. The typical dose for depression is 20 to 60 mg daily, whereas a 20 to 80 mg dose range is typical in the treatment of obsessive-compulsive disorder. The long-acting metabolite allows for a once-weekly formulation (Prozac Weekly) at 90 mg once every week, although fluctuations in levels may be observed over the week-long dosing interval.

Adverse Effects

The adverse effect profile of fluoxetine and the other SSRIs differs from the TCAs in that the SSRIs have minimal antimuscarinic and cardiovascular effects. They are considered safe in overdose, which has contributed to their first-line status in the treatment of depression. Adverse effects include GI complaints (nausea, cramping) and sexual dysfunction (seen in up to 75% of individuals receiving full therapeutic doses). Other adverse effects include insomnia (minimized if dosed in the morning), anorexia, and weight loss. Discontinuation of SSRIs is associated with a classic withdrawal response of dizziness, nausea, and agitation. Fluoxetine and other SSRIs used late in pregnancy may contribute to neonatal SSRI withdrawal syndrome in the newborn, which may include seizures, irritability, and tremors (Moses-Kolko et al., 2005; Sanz, De-las-Cuevas, Kiuru, Bate, Edwards, 2005) (see Box 19-7; also see the Evidence-Based Practice box on p. 401).

Use in Pregnancy

The SSRI antidepressants appear to be relatively safe in pregnancy (Källén, 2004), with the high doses correlated with lower birth rates (Hendrick et al., 2003), or development of delayed fine motor coordination (Casper et al., 2003). Antidepressant withdrawal syndromes observed in adults (see Box 19-7) or respiratory distress may also be observed postpartum in neonates (Koren, 2004). Also see the Pregnancy Safety box on p. 392 for pregnancy ratings of psychotropics.

Drug Interactions

All of the serotonergic agents have the potential to produce serotonin syndrome, a rare, but life-threatening event manifested by changes in autonomic nervous system responses. Combinations of the SSRIs with other antidepressants (particularly trazodone, amitriptyline, clomipramine, the MAOIs, or St. John's wort) appear to pose a higher risk for this condition. Refer to Box 19-9 for a further discussion of serotonin syndrome. Multiple interactions are noted with the SSRIs and are presented in Box 19-8.

✱ **K.P. is a 21-year-old woman who visits the student health center because she is feeling blue and getting behind in her studies. She states "I'm feeling overwhelmed" and "I've thought about dropping out of school." Her physical exam is unremarkable and all her laboratory values are within normal limits. K.P. takes no drugs except for an occasional ibuprofen and denies using alcohol or other recreational drugs. When interviewed, she states that she has been feeling increasingly depressed and cries for no reason. She has lost all interest in her old pastimes (hiking and bike riding), has stopped dating, and watches TV all of the time. She wakes up in the middle of the night and is unable to fall back to sleep until morning, and then she wants to sleep all day. K.P. has no energy during the day and has difficulty focusing on her studies. K.P. is an appropriately dressed female who appears sad but who is alert and coherent. She is oriented to time, place, and person, and her intelligence is estimated to be above average. K.P. denies hearing voices or other hallucinations, but does admit to "thinking about ending it all" without specific plans. K.P. is diagnosed with a major depressive disorder with melancholic features.**

✱ **What are the options for K.P.'s treatment?**

K.P. is at some risk for suicide, but she does not relate a detailed plan at present. It is decided that she will be monitored closely by her friends, family members, and a therapist during the first few weeks of pharmacologic therapy. There are essentially four categories of drugs for the treatment of depression: SSRIs, TCAs, MAOIs, and the miscellaneous drugs (e.g., bupropion, mirtazapine, nefazodone, venlafaxine). Because the potential effectiveness of all currently available antidepressants are comparable, there are other considerations to the selection of an antidepressant.

K.P. indicates that she does not know of a first-degree relative with depression. If there was a relative who had undergone a successful course of antidepressant treatment without significant adverse effects, the drug that the relative had received would be a desirable first choice. Because K.P. knows of no such first-degree relative and because K.P. has no preexisting illness and does not currently use any medications, those are not considerations in the drug of choice. Selection often depends on the adverse effect profile of the individual drugs; see Table 19-2. Because K.P. is female and a young adult, a drug associated with significant weight gain would not be a desirable choice. Other issues are convenience of dosing, cost, risk of teratogenicity for women of childbearing age, and K.P.'s preference.

After reading about her choices, K.P. expresses concern over the possible weight gain and the increased risk of suicide with the TCAs and the dietary concerns associated with the MAOIs, she believes that an SSRI would be a drug with which she could be compliant. See the Technology Link box on p. 408 for some online information for clients. Luckily, her health plan covers the expense of the drug. SSRIs also are usually dosed once daily, and K.P. feels the once-daily dosing will be easier for her to manage. She recognizes that sexual dysfunction is common with SSRIs, but figures "I'm not dating anyway."

✱ **K.P. is prescribed sertraline (Zoloft) 50 mg PO daily and makes an appointment to return in a month.**

The nurse informs K.P. that it may be a few weeks before she begins to experience therapeutic benefit from the medication, but benefit is often observed sooner with SSRIs than with the older TCAs. In the meantime, she will see a therapist through the student health center's mental health department. Initially, she will feel an increase in her energy levels, so she needs to report any suicide ideation to her therapist, should it occur. Although the SSRIs have a lower side-effect profile than other antidepressants, the nurse reviews some ways that K.P. can manage her therapy more effectively. Nausea is common but tends to diminish after the first week. However, SSRIs can cause some GI irritation for a couple of hours after taking them. K.P. should always take the medication after a meal or with a snack, particularly during the first week. She may also experience diarrhea in the first week, but this, too, will likely resolve. Although K.P. already has an altered sleep pattern, this may worsen in the first week of therapy; however, her sleep pattern will improve over time. Dry mouth can be managed with sugarless hard candy, ice chips, or small frequent sips of water. Caution K.P. that she may experience dizziness or drowsiness while on the medication, so caution her about driving or performing tasks that require alertness or judgment until the effects of the drug are known. Avoid the use of alcohol. Check with the prescriber before discontinuing the SSRI therapy; gradual reductions in dosage may be needed.

✱ **After 3 months of her SSRI therapy, K.P. feels as though she is "cured." She is doing well in school and is looking forward to a biking tour with her new boyfriend during spring break. K.P. wants to know for how long she will have to take the medication.**
The duration of antidepressant therapy varies from individual to individual. In serious and recurrent depressions, indefinite prophylactic maintenance may be indicated (see Box 19-7). Most experts advise that single or initial episodes of depression should be provided maintenance therapy of at least 6 months, and possibly 1 year, before discontinuation of medication is attempted. Depression tends to be a recurrent disorder, and many studies suggest that longer treatment is superior to shorter treatment in the prevention of relapse. Serious long-term adverse effects of antidepressants have, fortunately, not appeared (Majeroni & Hess, 1998).

✱ **K.P. is satisfied to continue her SSRI therapy for now with reconsideration of that decision at 9 months of therapy. However, she is concerned with her lack of interest in sex given that she has a new boyfriend and they are planning a trip together.**

Unfortunately, K.P. has been on sertraline long enough to determine that her sexual dysfunction is not a symptom of her depression but an adverse effect of her SSRI therapy. Sexual dysfunction (decreased sexual desire or ability) is a frequent effect of SSRI therapy. In men, erectile dysfunction secondary to SSRIs is responsive to sildenafil (Viagra) or similar agents (Nurnberg et al., 2003). In some instances, the client's dose could be decreased, but K.P.'s dose is relatively low. Rothschild (1995) found that some individuals taking sertraline and paroxetine reported a significant improvement in their sexual functioning without a return to depressive symptoms by discontinuing the dose of sertraline after the Thursday morning dose and taking the Sunday dose at noon. K.P. indicated she would try that schedule but would be careful not to become noncompliant the rest of the week.

✱ **K.P. has been on her SSRI therapy for a year. She has had a full therapeutic response, but after a discussion with her prescriber about whether to continue or discontinue her SSRI therapy, K.P. decides she would like to come off of the sertraline.**
Although K.P. is on a relatively low dosage of sertraline, it is decided to taper her dosage over several weeks to minimize the risk of withdrawal and relapse (see Box 19-7). Abrupt withdrawal of any antidepressant that has been taken for an extended time (e.g., longer than 2 months) is accompanied by withdrawal symptoms. Symptoms of withdrawal from SSRI therapy are associated with headache, dizziness, anxiety, and flu-like symptoms. The risk of relapse is relatively low in the first month off medication, but will often return during the second and third month; the risk of relapse is highest during the first 6 months (Finley et al., 2001).

✱ **J.O. is a 55-year-old woman and a professor of history at a local university. She has had increasing difficulty getting to sleep. This past week, she missed a number of committee meetings and an appointment with the dean to discuss student complaints about her teaching. This morning she skipped her lecture at the university and went to a nearby shopping mall instead. While she was there she booked a trip around the world and purchased more than $7000 of clothing at a department store. When she went to pay for her purchases, she was told that her credit card had reached its limit. J.O. began to shout, "How dare you treat the ambassador to China this way!" and became disruptive. The police were called and J.O. was admitted for psychiatric evaluation. On arrival at the facility, J.O. insists "I don't need to see a doctor. I'm going to be late; my private jet is to take off within the hour!" She is dressed in a sequined chiffon evening dress and gold lamé stiletto heels with matching bag. Her makeup is overdone with heavy rouge and eye shadow and bright red lipstick. Although oriented to time, place, and person, she is unable to keep her seat. Her speech is pressured and loud; she often fails to complete sentences. She demands to be released: "The president is waiting for me; he wants me to be his new vice president. I must get to Washington!"**

✳ What are the presenting symptoms of mania?

Mania is characterized by the presence of speech and motor hyperactivity, reduced sleep requirements, flight of ideas, grandiosity, elation, poor judgment, aggressiveness, and, possibly, hostility. The manic state is seen with recurrent manic symptoms with little or no depression, whereas bipolar affective disorders have both an acute manic phase and a hypomanic state or alternating periods of mania and depression.

✳ What treatments are available for mania?

Counseling, psychotherapy, and drug therapy are useful for the treatment of bipolar disorders. Valproate (valproic acid [Depakene]/divalproex [Depakote]) and lithium (Eskalith) are considered the drugs of choice for mania. Carbamazepine (Tegretol) is also used in cases where valproate or lithium is ineffective or contraindicated. Valproic acid and carbamazepine, commonly used in mental health, are antiepileptic agents that are reviewed in Chapter 17. In acute manic states, atypical antipsychotics such as olanzapine (Zyprexa) or quetiapine (Seroquel) are often used on a short-term basis.

✴ 🏴 lithium [lith ee um]
(Eskalith, Lithobid, Eskalith CR, Cibalith-S, Carbolith✤)

The mechanism of action for lithium has not been established. It is theorized that lithium accelerates the presynaptic destruction of catecholamines (serotonin, dopamine, and norepinephrine), inhibits transmitter release at the synapse, and decreases postsynaptic receptor sensitivity with the result that the presumed overactive catecholamine systems in mania are corrected.

Sodium in the cells has been reported to increase by as much as 200% in manic clients. Lithium and sodium are both actively transported across cell membranes, but lithium cannot be pumped out of the cell as effectively as sodium. Thus lithium may stabilize cell membranes.

The third possible mechanism of action is lithium blockade of the inositol triphosphate and diphosphate system in the CNS, that is, its effects on the second messengers necessary for α-adrenergic and muscarinic transmission. At the current time, the latter is the most accepted theory (Katzung, 2004).

Indications
Lithium is indicated for the treatment of bipolar illness, and it is being investigated for use in posttraumatic stress disorder, conduct disorder in children, and aggression management.

Pharmacokinetics/Dosing
Lithium is available in a number of dose forms, including lithium carbonate capsules (Eskalith, Carbolith), lithium carbonate tablets (Eskalith, Lithane), lithium carbonate extended-release tablets (Lithobid, Eskalith CR), and lithium citrate syrup (Cibalith-S). With the exception of the slow-release dosage form, lithium is completely absorbed in 6 to 8 hours and has a half-life of 24 hours in adults, 18 hours in adolescents, and up to 36 hours in older adults. Time to peak serum levels is 30 minutes for syrup, 1 to 3 hours for capsules/tablets, and 4 hours for extended-release tablets. Therapeutic serum levels for the treatment of bipolar disorder are 0.8 to 1.2 mEq/L for acute mania and 0.5 to 1 mEq/L for maintenance. A clinical response is usually reported in 1 to 3 weeks. Lithium is not metabolized and is primarily excreted unchanged by the kidneys. The usual adult dosage of lithium for acute mania is 300 to 600 mg three times daily, adjusted according to the client's response and tolerance up to a maximum dosage of 2.4 g/day. The maintenance dosage is 300 mg three or four times daily. Older adults usually require a lower dosage. The dosage for children up to 12 years old is 15 to 20 mg/kg in two or three divided doses, adjusted according to response.

Adverse Effects
Lithium is considered a narrow therapeutic index drug, with toxicity developing rapidly. Dose-related adverse effects of lithium include hand tremors (slight), thirst, nausea, increased urination, diarrhea, tachycardia, increased weakness, weight gain, respiratory difficulties (on exertion), fainting, and irregular pulse rate. Early signs of toxicity include diarrhea, anorexia, muscle weakness, nausea, vomiting, tremors, slurred speech, and drowsiness. The vomiting and diarrhea observed early in lithium toxicity can lead to sodium depletion and further increase the potential for seriously elevated lithium levels. Later signs are blurred vision, seizures, severe trembling, confusion, ataxia, and increased urine production.

Drug Interactions
Lithium levels are greatly impacted by interventions that affect sodium balance. See Box 19-8 for further discussion and interacting drugs.

✳ Because J.O. previously responded to lithium, it is likely she will respond to lithium again. She is started at a dosage of 300 mg three times daily. The goal for drug management of her acute condition is a serum level between 0.5 and 1.2 mEq/L. Because lithium has a slow onset of action, J.O.'s medication can be adjusted with twice-weekly serum levels until her manic episode resolves. Short-term use of quetiapine will also be considered.

Assessment J.O.'s initial assessment ensures that she does not have a preexisting illness for which lithium is contraindicated, such as a history of leukemia because the leukemia may be reactivated. In addition, lithium may exacerbate cardiovascular disease, and CNS conditions such as epilepsy and parkinsonism. Severe infection with prolonged sweating, diarrhea, or vomiting may necessitate a reduction in the lithium dosage to prevent toxicity caused by dehydration. Delayed lithium excretion resulting from renal insufficiency may also lead to toxicity.

Review J.O.'s current medication regimen for the risk of significant drug interactions. The following identifies possible interactions when lithium is given concurrently with specific drugs:

- Nonsteroidal antiinflammatory analgesics: decreases lithium excretion leading to increased lithium levels and toxicity
- Antithyroid drugs (e.g., calcium iodide, potassium iodide, or iodinated glycerol): enhances the hypothyroid goitrogenic effects of lithium or these medications
- Chlorpromazine (Thorazine): reduces the absorption of chlorpromazine and possibly other phenothiazines and may lead to treatment failure
- Diuretics: decrease lithium excretion, resulting in an increased lithium level and toxicity
- Haloperidol (Haldol): associated with irreversible neurologic toxicity
- Molindone (Moban): may result in neurotoxicity

A baseline assessment should include documentation of J.O.'s symptoms, weight, BP, ECG, electrolytes, renal and thyroid function determinations, and WBC and differential count.

Nursing Diagnosis While J.O. is receiving lithium therapy, she has the potential for the following selected nursing diagnoses/collaborative problems: diarrhea; risk for imbalanced fluid volume; impaired comfort (thirst, anorexia, nausea, vomiting); disturbed sensory perception (confusion); risk for poisoning (overdose); and the potential complications of hypothyroidism, hypovolemia, and electrolyte imbalance.

Planning While J.O. is receiving lithium therapy, she will:

- Not experience injury related to her illness or lithium therapy.
- Experience improved thought processes with no delusional perceptions.
- Demonstrate appropriate behaviors and social interactions.
- Experience improved sleep patterns and nutritional habits.
- Remain compliant with therapy.
- Effectively manage her therapeutic regimen, including appropriate reporting of adverse drug effects to a health care provider, adequate fluid intake and other measures supportive of the drug regimen.

Implementation

Monitoring Assess J.O.'s history of manic episodes, their occurrence and degree of severity, and the cyclic appearance of the pattern. Family intervention for treatment is essential when manic-depressive symptoms appear.

Serum lithium determinations are recommended once or twice weekly during J.O.'s manic phase and until she is stabilized; testing is performed every 2 to 3 months while she is in remission. Test samples are drawn just before the morning dose of lithium, when there is maximum stabilization of the serum concentrations. Serum lithium levels above 1.5 mEq/L produce toxic reactions.

Monitor J.O.'s WBC and energy level for tiredness. Monitor the ECG for changes and the BP for hypotension. Weigh her daily and check for indicators of edema. Monitor the findings of electrolytes (hyponatremia, hypercalcemia, and hypophosphatemia) and renal and thyroid (hypothyroidism) studies. Monitor renal function using urinalysis, blood urea nitrogen, and serum creatinine.

Intervention Administer lithium after meals to prevent laxative action and to decrease gastric upset, tremors, or weakness by prolonging the absorption rate. Dilute the syrup in juice before administration. Do not mix it with or administer it at the same time as any other medication that contains a basic form. Ensure J.O. has an adequate fluid intake of 2.5 to 3 L daily and sufficient sodium intake.

Education J.O.'s compliance, cooperation, and commitment to adhere strictly to therapy are essential to lithium therapy. The family should be advised, in language they can understand, of all the ramifications of therapy, including the effects related to serum level. Discuss the overt clinical signs of lithium toxicity with J.O., her family, or closest companion. Instruct J.O. to avoid changes of sodium in her diet, avoid situations with excessive sweating unless she has adequate salt replacement, and be alert to diarrhea (a sign of early lithium toxicity), which further depletes sodium and hastens lithium toxicity.

If diarrhea, vomiting, tremors, mild ataxia, lack of coordination, drowsiness, or muscular weakness appear, J.O. is to discontinue therapy and notify the prescriber promptly. Advise her of facilities where prompt and accurate serum lithium determinations can be obtained.

Discuss with J.O. and family the importance of a normal diet because sodium-depleted states (e.g., decreased sodium intake, sweating, vomiting, diarrhea) all result in increased reabsorption of lithium in the kidney and can lead to rapidly escalating lithium levels and toxicity.

A fluid intake of 2500 to 3000 mL daily during the initial stabilization period is essential. Instruct J.O. to avoid fluid depletion; coffee, tea, and cola intake should be limited because of the diuretic effect, and exercise, saunas, and exposure to hot weather should be avoided. Advise her to seek the assistance of a health care provider for illnesses that cause diaphoresis, vomiting, or diarrhea.

Advise J.O. that it is necessary to take the medication consistently—initially because it takes 1 to 3 weeks for improvement of the condition and thereafter even though the symptoms may abate. Assess carefully for compliance to the regimen, particularly if she has had an increase in weight. Weight gain is a major cause of noncompliance, especially in female clients. Stress the importance of regular visits to the prescriber for the monitoring of serum lithium levels.

Impairment of alertness may occur, so alert J.O. to avoid activities that require coordination and close attention until the response to therapy has been determined.

Evaluation The expected outcomes of lithium therapy is that J.O. will demonstrate improved mental status behaviors without experiencing adverse effects of lithium and effectively manage her therapeutic regimen.

Summary

Emotions, and therefore behaviors, are the result of a final, unified effect of the CNS, autonomic regulation, and biochemical mechanisms. Because of their ability to modify these processes, drugs are important adjuncts to the treatment of psychiatric disorders. However, it is essential that antipsychotic drugs be prescribed only for appropriate, specific disorders to assist the client to cope more effectively with the environment and better use nonpharmacologic therapies.

Since the advent of tranquilizers in the early 1950s, institutionalization for psychiatric disorders has decreased, not only in terms of duration for the individual client, but also as the only setting for psychiatric care. As a result of the administration of psychotherapeutic agents, most clients are now treated at community mental health centers and at home.

Typical antipsychotics, including the phenothiazine derivatives constitute a major group of drugs which treat the symptoms of psychosis. Although the exact mechanism of their antipsychotic effect is not known, a primary effect is dopamine blockade in specific areas of the CNS. A major role for nursing with the typical antipsychotics is the assessment of the client for the development of adverse effects, because many of them are debilitating and irreversible. Because many clients are treated in the community, health teaching for the safe and accurate self-administration of these medications is essential. Atypical antipsychotic agents have largely replaced the earlier typical antipsychotics, and include olanzapine, quetiapine, risperidone and ziprasidone. Clozapine, also an atypical antipsychotic, is generally reserved for refractory cases because of the potential for serious bone marrow suppression. Aripiprazole represents a newer approach to treating the symptoms of psychosis by modulating neurotransmitter receptors with partial agonist/antagonist agents.

Antidepressant therapy is used for the treatment of affective disorders, or mood disturbances, and increasingly for anxiety states. The older TCAs have become second-line to the newer second-generation antidepressants and SSRIs with fewer significant adverse effects. The MAOIs are reserved for severe or atypical depression unresponsive to other modalities. Lithium and valproic acid are considered the drugs of choice for bipolar disorder. There is no ideal psychotherapeutic agent, because all of them produce undesirable side effects or adverse effects. The nurse's teaching role is important for safe and accurate self-administration of these agents and for the assessment of the untoward effects of the drugs.

✳ Critical Thinking Questions

• Mrs. Thomas, age 84 years, has been admitted to an extended-care facility and has become increasingly combative over the first 3 days. One of the nursing assistants has indicated that she does not want to be assigned to care for Mrs. Thomas because she is afraid of her. As the nurse on the unit, you must decide whether or not Mrs. Thomas meets the criteria for an antipsychotic medication to be prescribed to a resident of an extended-care facility. What do you do?

• Barbara Walton has a bipolar disorder for which she has been prescribed lithium 300 mg PO two times daily. On a recent visit to the clinic, her lithium blood level was 1.7 mEq/L. What action should you take?

• Mr. Shapiro's depression has been treated unsuccessfully with TCAs and SSRIs. The prescriber is going to try to treat him with MAOIs. During the drug history, Mr. Shapiro lists the following dietary intake for the previous day: breakfast—black coffee, bran cereal with skim milk and a sliced banana on top; lunch—diet soda, bologna sandwich, and potato chips from the local lunch wagon; and dinner—salad, spaghetti, a little red wine, and garlic bread. He also stopped on the way home from work and had "a couple of beers with the guys." What instruction will you provide to assist Mr. Shapiro in managing his therapeutic regimen effectively?

Bibliography

Amitai, Y., & Frischer, H. (2004). Excess fatality from desipramine and dosage recommendations. *Therapeutic Drug Monitoring, 26*(5), 468-473.

Anderson, D.M., Keith, J., & Novak, P.D. (Eds.). (2002). *Mosby's medical, nursing, and allied health dictionary* (6th ed.). St. Louis: Mosby.

Baldessarini, R.J., & Tarazi, F.I. (2001). Drugs and the treatment of psychiatric disorders: Psychosis and mania. In J.G. Hardman, L.E. Limbird, & A.G. Gilman (Eds.), *Goodman & Gilman's the pharmacological basis of therapeutics* (10th ed.). New York: McGraw-Hill.

Berkman, L.F., Blumenthal, J., Burg, M., Carney, R.M., Catellier, D., Cowan, M.J., et al. (2003). Effects of treating depression and low perceived social support on clinical events after myocardial infarction: The Enhancing Recovery in Coronary Heart Disease Patients (ENRICHD) randomized trial. *Journal of the American Medical Association, 289,* 3106-3116.

Bess, A.L., & Cunningham, S.R. (2004, April 1). Dear health care provider [Letter]. Retrieved December 2, 2004, from http://www.fda.gov/medwatch/SAFETY/2004/Clozaril-deardoc.pdf

Borovicka, M.C., & Love, R.C. (2005). Mood disorders II: Bipolar disorders. In M.A. Koda-Kimble, L.Y. Young, W.A. Kradjan, & B.J. Guglielmo, B.K. Alldredge, & R.L. Corelli (Eds.), *Applied therapeutics: The clinical use of drugs* (8th ed.). Philadelphia: Lippincott Williams & Wilkins.

Buckley, P.F. (1999). The role of typical and atypical antipsychotic medications in the management of agitation and aggression. *Journal of Clinical Psychiatry, 60*(Suppl. 10), 52-60.

Casper, R.C., Fleisher, B.E., Lee-Ancajas, J.C., Gilles, A., Gaylor, E., DeBattista, A., et al. (2003). Follow-up of children of depressed mothers exposed or not exposed to antidepressant drugs during pregnancy. *Journal of Pediatrics, 142,* 402-408.

ℓ-LEARNING SUPPLEMENTS

Student CD-ROM
• Final Exam questions
• NCLEX® Examination review questions
• Pharmacology animations
• Printable chapter summary

Evolve Website (http://evolve.elsevier.com/mckenry)
• Case study on psychotherapeutic drugs
• Interactive concept map on depression

• Content updates, including information on new drugs
• WebLinks corresponding to this chapter
• Answers to the critical thinking questions in this chapter
• *Elsevier ePharmacology Update* newsletter
• *Mosby's Drug Consult* Internet Edition
• Supplemental and reference information

Chakraborty, N., & Johnston, T. (2004). Aripiprazole and neuroleptic malignant syndrome. *International Clinical Psychopharmacology, 19*(6), 351-353.

Chang, J.T., & Altman, R.B. (2004). Extracting and characterizing gene-drug relationships from the literature. *Pharmacogenetics, 14*(9), 577-586, and linked supplemental website http://bionlp.stanford.edu/genedrug/gene_drug_predictions.html (as cited December 2, 2004).

Cohen-Mansfield, J., Lipson, S., Werner, P., Billig, N., Taylor, L., & Woosley, R. (1999). Withdrawal of haloperidol, thioridazine, and lorazepam in the nursing home: A controlled, double-blind study. *Archives of Internal Medicine, 159*(15), 1733-1740.

Davis, J.M., & Chen, M. (2004). Dose response and dose equivalence of antipsychotics. *Journal of Clinical Psychopharmacology, 24*(2), 192-208.

Drug facts and comparisons (58th ed.). (2005). St. Louis: Facts and Comparisons.

FDA Public Health Advisory. (April 11, 2005). Deaths with antipsychotics in elderly patients with behavioral disturbances. Retrieved May 24, 2005, from http://www.fda.gov/cder/drug/advisory/antipsychotics.htm.

FDA Public Health Advisory. (October 15, 2004). *Suicidality in children and adolescents being treated with antidepressant medications.* Retrieved December 2, 2004, from http://www.fda.gov/cder/drug/antidepressants/SSRIPHA200410.htm

Finley, P.R., Laird, L.K., & Benefield, W.H. Jr. (2001). Mood disorders I: Major depressive disorders. In M.A. Koda-Kimble, L.Y. Young, W.A. Kradjan, & B.J. Guglielmo, B.K. Alldredge, & R.L. Corelli (Eds.), *Applied therapeutics: The clinical use of drugs* (7th ed.). Vancouver, WA: Applied Therapeutics.

Flores, D.L., Alvarado, I., Wong, M.L., Licinio, J., & Flockhart, D. (2004). Clinical implications of genetic polymorphism of CYP2D6 in Mexican Americans. *Annals of Internal Medicine, 140*(11), 939.

Freedman, R. (2003). Drug therapy: Schizophrenia. *New England Journal of Medicine, 349*(18), 1738-1749.

Glatt, C.E., Tampilic, M., Christie, C., DeYoung, J., & Freimer, N.B. (2004). Re-screening serotonin receptors for genetic variants identifies population and molecular genetic complexity. *American Journal of Medical Genetics, 124B*(1), 92-100.

Goldberg, R.J. (2002). Tardive dyskinesia in elderly patients: An update. *Journal of the American Medical Directors Association, 3*(3), 152-161.

Golden, A.G., Preston, R.A., Barnett, S.D., Llorente, M., Hamdan, K., & Silverman, M.A. (1999). Inappropriate medication prescribing in homebound older adults. *Journal of the American Geriatric Society, 47*(8), 948-953.

Gould, M.S., Marrocco, F.A., Kleinman, M., Thomas, J.G., Mostkoff, K., Cote, J., et al. (2005). Evaluating iatrogenic risk of youth suicide screening programs: A randomized controlled trial. *Journal of the American Medical Association 293*, 1635-1643.

Hall, W.D., Mant, A., Mitchell, P.B., Rendle, V.A., Hickie, I.B., & McManus, P. (2003). Association between antidepressant prescribing and suicide in Australia, 1991-2000: Trend analysis. *British Medical Journal, 326*, 1008-1011.

Hendrick, V., Smith, L.M., Suri, R., Hwang, S., Haynes, D., & Altshuler, L. (2003). Birth outcomes after prenatal exposure to antidepressant medication. *American Journal of Obstetrics and Gynecology, 188*, 812-815.

Hollander E. (Ed.). (2001). *Professional's handbook of psychotropic drugs.* Springhouse, PA: Springhouse.

Jagadheesan, K., & Muirhead, D. (2004). Aripiprazole for acute bipolar mania. *American Journal of Psychiatry, 161*(10), 1926-1927.

Jick, H., Kaye, JA., & Jick, S.S. (2004). Antidepressants and the risk of suicidal behaviors. *Journal of the American Medical Association, 292*, 338-343.

Jureidini, J.N., Doecke, C.J., Mansfield, P.R., Haby, M.M., Menkes, D.B., Tonkin, A.L. (2004). Efficacy and safety of antidepressants for children and adolescents. *British Medical Journal, 328*, 879-883.

Källén, B. (2004). Neonate characteristics after maternal use of antidepressants in late pregnancy. *Archives of Pediatrics & Adolescent Medicine, 158*, 312-316.

Katzung, B.G. (Ed.). (2004). *Basic and clinical pharmacology* (9th ed.). New York: McGraw-Hill.

Kirchheiner, J., Klein, C., Meineke, I., Sasse, J., Zanger, U., Murdter, T., et al. (2003). Bupropion and 4-OH-bupropion pharmacokinetics in relation to genetic polymorphisms in CYP2B6. *Pharmacogenetics, 13*(10), 619-626.

Koren, G. (2004). Discontinuation syndrome following late pregnancy exposure to antidepressants. *Archives of Pediatrics & Adolescent Medicine, 158*, 307-308.

Koro, C.E., Fedder, D.O., L'Italien, G.J., Weiss, S., Magder, L.S., Kreyenbuhl, J., et al. (2002). Assessment of independent effect of olanzapine and risperidone on risk of diabetes among patients with schizophrenia: Population based nested case-control study. *British Medical Journal, 325*, 243-245.

Lacro, J. (2005). Schizophrenia. In M.A. Koda-Kimble, L.Y. Young, W.A. Kradjan, & B.J. Guglielmo, B.K. Alldredge, & R.L. Corelli (Eds.), *Applied therapeutics: The clinical use of drugs* (8th ed.). Philadelphia: Lippincott Williams & Wilkins.

Lacy, C.F., Armstrong, L.L., Goldman, M.P., & Lance, L.L. (2004). *Drug information handbook* (10th ed.). Cleveland: Lexi-Comp.

Lee, P.E., Gill, S.S., Freedman, M., Bronskill, S.E., Hillmer, M.P., Rochon, P.A. (2004). Atypical antipsychotic drugs in the treatment of behavioural and psychological symptoms of dementia: Systematic review. *British Medical Journal, 329*, 75-78.

Leslie, D.L., & Rosenheck, R.A. (2004). Incidence of newly diagnosed diabetes attributable to atypical antipsychotic medications. *American Journal of Psychiatry, 161*, 1709-1711.

Lin, E.H., Katon, W., Von Korff, M., Tang, L., Williams, J.W. Jr., Kroenke, K., et al. (2003). Effect of improving depression care on pain and functional outcomes among older adults with arthritis: A randomized controlled trial. *Journal of the American Medical Association, 290*, 2428-2434.

MacGillivray, S., Arroll, B., Hatcher, S., Ogston, S., Reid, I., Sullivan, F., et al. (2003). Efficacy and tolerability of selective serotonin reuptake inhibitors compared with tricyclic antidepressants in depression treated in primary care: Systematic review and meta-analysis. *British Medical Journal, 326*, 1014-1017.

Majeroni, B.A., & Hess, A. (1998). The pharmacologic treatment of depression, *Journal of the American Board of Family Practitioners, 11*(2), 127-139.

Malhotra, A., Murphy, G., & Kennedy, J.L. (2004). Pharmacogenetics of psychotropic drug response. *American Journal of Psychiatry, 161*(5), 780-796.

March, J., Silva, S., Petrycki, S., Curry, J., Wells, K., Fairbank, J., et al. (2004). Fluoxetine, cognitive-behavioral therapy, and their combination for adolescents with depression: Treatment for Adolescents with Depression Study (TADS) randomized controlled trial. *Journal of the American Medical Association, 292*, 807-820.

Markowitz, J.S., Donovan, J.L., DeVane, C.L., Taylor, R.M., Ruan, Y., Wang, J.S., et al. (2003). Effect of St. John's wort on drug metabolism by induction of cytochrome P450 3A4 enzyme. *Journal of the American Medical Association, 290*, 1500-1504.

Mosby's drug consult (15th ed.). (2005). St. Louis: Mosby.

Moses-Kolko, E.L., Bogen, D., Perel, J., Bregar, A., Uhl, K., Levin, B., et al. (2005). Neonatal signs after late in utero exposure to serotonin reuptake inhibitors: Literature review and implications for clinical applications. *Journal of the American Medical Association, 293,* 2372-2383.

Nasrallah, H.A., & Newcomer, J.W. (2004). Atypical antipsychotics and metabolic dysregulation: Evaluating the risk/benefit equation and improving the standard of care. *Journal of Clinical Psychopharmacology, 24*(Suppl. 1), S7-S14.

Nunes, E.V., & Levin, F.R. (2004). Treatment of depression in patients with alcohol or other drug dependence: A meta-analysis. *Journal of the American Medical Association, 291,* 1887-1896.

Nurnberg, H.G., Hensley, P.L., Gelenberg, A.J., Fava, M., Lauriello, J., Paine, S. (2003). Treatment of antidepressant-associated sexual dysfunction with sildenafil: A randomized controlled trial. *Journal of the American Medical Association, 289,* 56-64.

Reeves, R.R., & Mack, J.E. (2004). Worsening schizoaffective disorder with aripiprazole. *American Journal of Psychiatry, 161*(7), 1308.

Roden, D.M. (2004). Drug therapy: Drug-induced prolongation of the QT interval. *New England Journal of Medicine, 350*(10), 1013-1022.

Rosenheck, R., Perlick, D., Bingham, S., Liu-Mares, W., Collins, J., Warren, S., et al. (2003). Effectiveness and cost of olanzapine and haloperidol in the treatment of schizophrenia: A randomized controlled trial. *Journal of the American Medical Association, 290,* 2693-2702.

Rothschild, A.J. (1995). Selective serotonin reuptake inhibitor–induced sexual dysfunction: Efficacy of a drug holiday. *American Journal of Psychiatry 152,* 1514-1518.

Sanz, E.J., De-las-Cuevas, C., Kiuru, A., Bate, A., Edwards, R. (2005). Selective serotonin reuptake inhibitors in pregnant women and neonatal withdrawal syndrome: A database analysis. *Lancet 365,* 482-487.

Schillevoort, I., de Boer, A., van der Weide, J., Steijns, L.S., Roos, R.A., Jansen, P.A., et al. (2002). Antipsychotic-induced extrapyramidal syndromes and cytochrome P450 2D6 genotype: A case-control study. *Pharmacogenetics, 12*(3), 235-240.

Stahl, S.M. (1999). Selecting an atypical antipsychotic by combining clinical experience with guidelines from clinical trials. *Journal of Clinical Psychiatry, 60*(Suppl. 10), 31-41.

Stevens, T., Katona, C., Manela, M., Watkin, V., & Livingston, G. (1999). Drug treatment of older people with affective disorders in the community: Lessons from an attempted clinical trial. *International Journal of Geriatric Psychiatry, 14*(6), 467-472.

Stowe, Z.N., Hostetter, A.L., Newport, D.J. (2005). The onset of postpartum depression: Implications for clinical screening in obstetrical and primary care. *American Journal of Obstetrics and Gynecology, 192,* 522-526.

Teich, J. (2003). Side effects of ziprasidone. *American Journal of Psychiatry, 160*(7), 1355-1356.

The UK ECT Review Group. (2003). Efficacy and safety of electroconvulsive therapy in depressive disorders: A systematic review and meta-analysis. *Lancet, 361,* 799-808.

USP DI: Drug information for the health care professional (25th ed.). (2005). Greenwood Village, CO: MICROMEDEX Thomson Healthcare.

Vinkers, D.J., Gussekloo, J., Stek, M.L., Westendorp, R.G., & van der Mast, R.C. (2004). Temporal relation between depression and cognitive impairment in old age: Prospective population based study. *British Medical Journal, 329,* 881-883.

Whittington, C.J., Kendall, T., Fonagy, P., Cottrell, D., Cotgrove, A., & Boddington, E. (2004). Selective serotonin reuptake inhibitors in childhood depression: Systematic review of published versus unpublished data. *Lancet, 363,* 1341-1345.

Young, R., Lawford, B.R., Barnes, M., Burton, S.C., Ritchie, T., Ward, W.K., et al. (2004). Prolactin levels in antipsychotic treatment of patients with schizophrenia carrying the DRD2*A1 allele. *British Journal of Psychiatry, 185,* 147-151.

Zito, J.M., Safer, D.J., DosReis, S., Gardner, J.F., Magder, L., Soeken, K., et al. (2003). Psychotropic practice patterns for youth: A 10-year perspective. *Archives of Pediatrics & Adolescent Medicine, 157,* 17-25.

20

OVERVIEW OF THE AUTONOMIC NERVOUS SYSTEM

CHAPTER FOCUS

The autonomic nervous system (ANS) regulates the functions of internal viscera such as the heart, blood vessels, digestive organs, and reproductive organs. About one-third of drugs used in clinical practice have either primary or secondary effects on these systems. An understanding of this chapter will help the nurse to predict general responses to a variety of stimuli, explain responses to changes in the environment, understand symptoms that result from ANS dysfunction, and know how drugs affect the ANS.

LEARNING OBJECTIVES

- Describe the reflex control system.
- Explain the major differences between the parasympathetic and sympathetic divisions of the autonomic nervous system.
- Name the primary neurotransmitters for the parasympathetic and sympathetic divisions of the autonomic nervous system.
- State the primary disposition of the neurotransmitters following release from their respective nerves.
- Identify the three basic characteristics of the autonomic nervous system.

▲ KEY TERMS

adrenergic, p. 419
autonomic nervous system, p. 414
catecholamines, p. 420
cholinergic, p. 419
feedback control mechanism, p. 415
muscarinic receptors, p. 420
neuroeffector junction, p. 419

neurohumoral transmission, p. 419
neurotransmitter, p. 419
nicotinic receptors, p. 420
reflex arc, p. 415
somatic nervous system, p. 422
synaptic junction, p. 419

The **autonomic nervous system (ANS)** functions primarily as a regulatory or self-governing system for maintaining the internal environment of the body at an optimal level (homeostasis). This system automatically controls the function of smooth muscle, cardiac muscle, and glandular secretions. Digestion of a meal, maintenance of the pressure of circulating blood, bladder control, involuntary respiration, and many other processes are internally regulated by the ANS.

✳ How does the ANS control involuntary body systems?

The nervous system is the important control and communication system within the body. It collects information

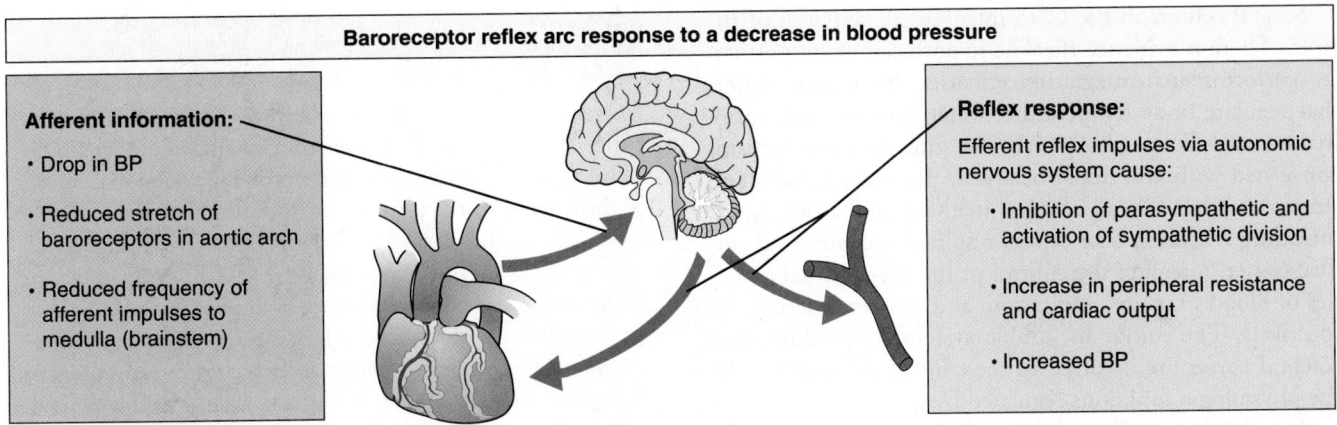

Baroreceptor reflex arc response to a decrease in blood pressure

Afferent information:

- Drop in BP

- Reduced stretch of baroreceptors in aortic arch

- Reduced frequency of afferent impulses to medulla (brainstem)

Reflex response:

Efferent reflex impulses via autonomic nervous system cause:

- Inhibition of parasympathetic and activation of sympathetic division

- Increase in peripheral resistance and cardiac output

- Increased BP

FIGURE 20-1 Baroreceptor reflex arc response to a decrease in blood pressure.

about conditions inside and outside of the body. The simplest means by which the nervous system responds to environmental change is through the action of the reflex arc. The **reflex arc** is an automatic motor response to sensory stimuli. In any reflex, a nerve fiber conducts a nerve impulse; these impulses form the basis of communication of information through the nervous system.

The reflex arc consists of two major functional processes: sensory input and motor output. The first component of the reflex arc is the receptor, which detects environmental changes such as temperature, pressure in blood vessels, and distention in the viscera. These changes are responsible for producing a stimulus in the receptor. Information from the sensitized receptor is transmitted as a nerve impulse along the *afferent neuron* to the central nervous system (CNS), the site of integration. The CNS then issues instructions as an altered motor nerve impulse along the *efferent neuron* to the effector, which produces the appropriate action of muscles and glands.

The information carried *to* the CNS (sensory input) and instructions sent *from* the CNS (motor output) constitute a feedback control mechanism. Information fed back to the CNS from a receptor is modulated so that nerve impulses may vary in frequency and pattern according to the degree of activity required of the effector. The control of visceral function is involuntary; the feedback mechanism must include all the components of a control system essential for performing the reflex act. Consequently, reflex action functions as a **feedback control mechanism,** operating from a receptor to an effector. Its purpose is to prevent extreme changes in function that may create a disturbance in the internal environment.

A good example of feedback control is the blood pressure-regulating reflex (Figure 20-1). Again, the sequence of events follows the pattern of the reflex arc. The carotid sinus in the carotid artery and the aortic sinus in the aortic arch serve as pressure receptors (baroreceptors) that are highly sensitive to stretch; the degree of wall stretching is determined by the amount of pressure within these vessels. Any decrease in blood pressure stimulates the baroreceptors, and this information is conveyed as nerve impulses along the afferent neuron to the vasomotor center in the medulla.

The medulla is the CNS site for integration of blood pressure regulation. After the appropriate neuronal connections have been made, an increase in sympathetic discharge is conducted along the efferent neuron to the effectors, which produces constriction of arteriolar smooth muscles. This constriction causes an increase in blood pressure. Changes in cardiac function to increase cardiac output are also triggered.

✱ What is the relationship of the ANS to other components of the nervous system?

The nervous system is classified on the basis of the reflex arc. The two main divisions are the CNS and the peripheral nervous system (PNS). The CNS consists of the brain and spinal cord and performs the important integrative functions from the peripheral sources. The PNS has two divisions: (1) the somatic nervous system, which innervates voluntary or skeletal muscles; and (2) the ANS, which influences the involuntary activities of smooth muscles, cardiac muscles, and glands. The afferent fibers of both systems are the first link in the reflex arc; they carry sensory information to the CNS. After integration at various levels in the brain, the outflow from the CNS is conducted along either the somatic efferent system or the autonomic efferent system. Both of these systems constitute the final link in the reflex arc (Figure 20-2).

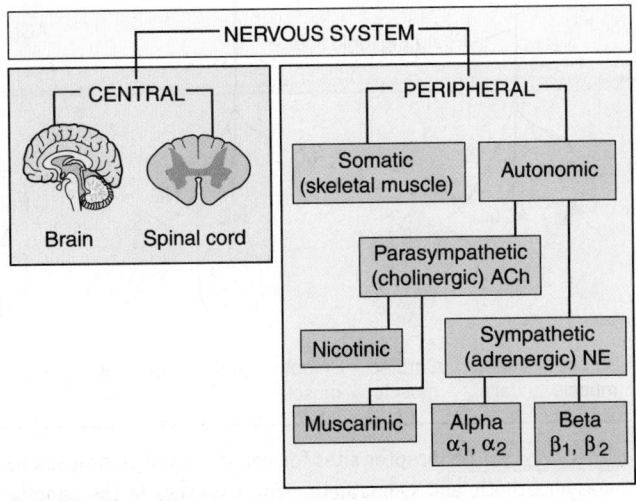

NERVOUS SYSTEM

CENTRAL

Brain   Spinal cord

PERIPHERAL

Somatic (skeletal muscle)   Autonomic

Parasympathetic (cholinergic) ACh

Nicotinic   Sympathetic (adrenergic) NE

Muscarinic   Alpha α_1, α_2 Beta β_1, β_2

FIGURE 20-2 Divisions of the nervous system.

Several centers in the CNS integrate all activities of the ANS. There is evidence that the hypothalamus, in particular, performs such integrating activities. It contains centers that regulate body temperature, water balance, and carbohydrate and fat metabolism. It also integrates mechanisms concerned with emotional behavior, the waking state, and sleep. A series of "vital centers" in the medulla oblongata, including the vasomotor center, respiratory center, and cardiac center, integrate the control of the life-essential activities of blood pressure, respiration, and cardiac function, respectively. The midbrain, limbic system, cerebellum, and cerebral cortex are involved in the control of the ANS and the physiologic functions regulated by it.

The ANS is organized into two subdivisions: (1) the parasympathetic system and (2) the sympathetic system (Box 20-1). The anatomic arrangement of each system consists of two motor nerves, a preganglionic nerve and a postganglionic nerve; a ganglion (group of nerve cell bodies) connects the two neurons (Figure 20-3).

✴ How do the parasympathetic and sympathetic nervous systems differ?

These systems differ physiologically and anatomically. These differences allow for the use of drugs that serve to augment or to slow down aspects specific receptors in each system.

BOX 20-1 AUTONOMIC NERVOUS SYSTEM TERMINOLOGY

Over the years various terms have been used to describe the diversion of the ANS. The anatomic names are sympathetic and parasympathetic; the corresponding functional terms, which relate to the primary neurotransmitters for each system, are adrenergic and cholinergic, respectively. In general, these terms are used interchangeably (i.e., sympathetic or adrenergic and parasympathetic or cholinergic nervous systems). It is important to understand the terms *parasympathomimetic* and *sympathomimetic*, which mean to mimic or produce an effect similar to the activation of either system. The terms *parasympatholytic* or *sympatholytic* imply a blocking of the effects normally seen when either system is activated. The term *anticholinergic* is synonymous with the term *parasympatholytic*.

ANATOMIC NAME	FUNCTIONAL NAME	PRIMARY NEUROTRANSMITTER
Sympathetic	Adrenergic	Norepinephrine
Parasympathetic	Cholinergic	Acetylcholine

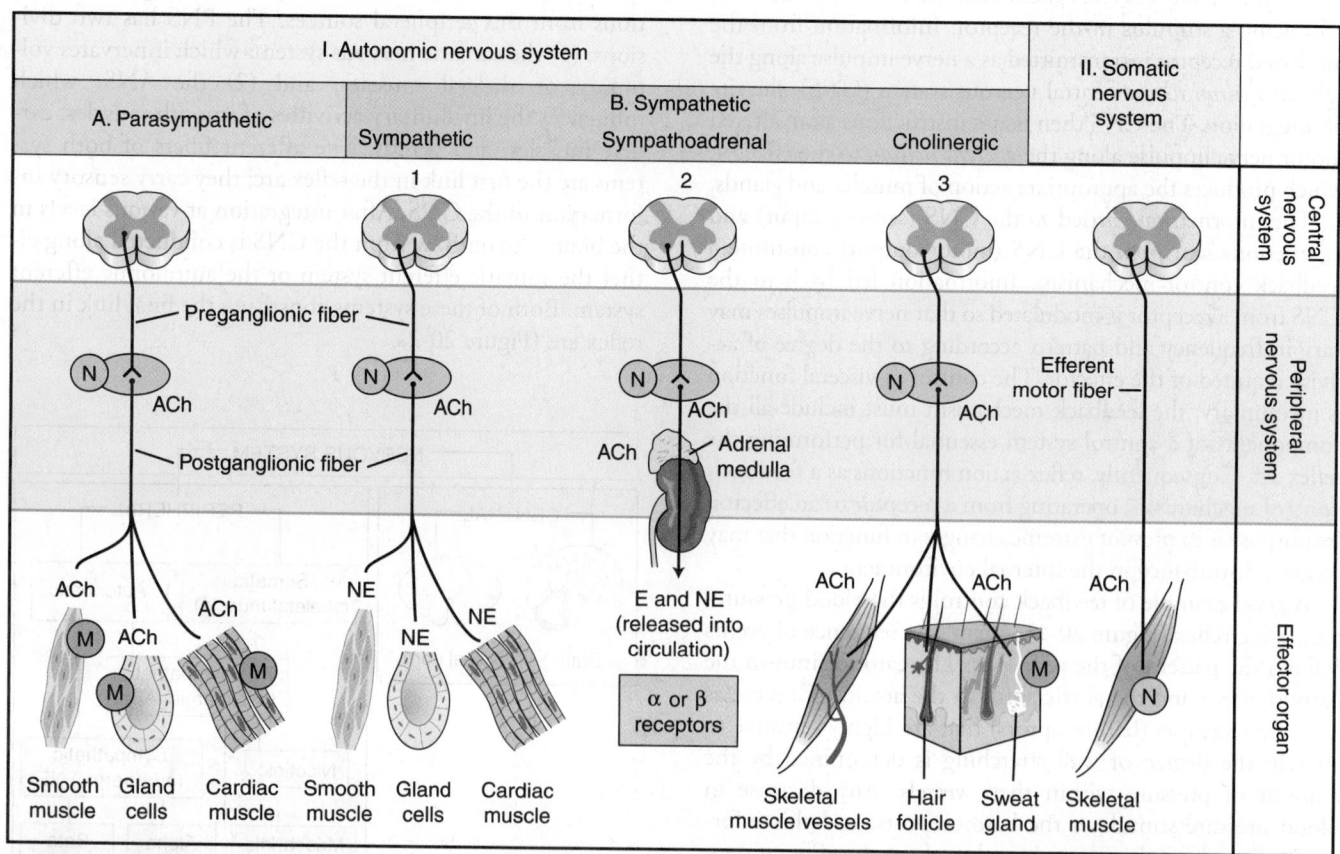

FIGURE 20-3 Receptor sites for neurohumoral transmission. I, Autonomic nervous system, where preganglionic fibers of both parasympathetic and sympathetic nerves synapse in the ganglia. II, Somatic motor nervous system. *ACh,* Acetylcholine; *E,* epinephrine; *M,* muscarinic receptors; *NE,* norepinephrine; *N,* nicotinic receptors.

Physiologic Differences The parasympathetic system and the sympathetic system innervate many of the same organs simultaneously; the opposing actions of these two systems balance one another. The parasympathetic system, otherwise known as the system of "rest and digestion," functions mainly to conserve energy and restore the resources of the body. Its functions include cardiac deceleration, a rise in gastrointestinal activity associated with increased digestion and absorption, and an increase in excretion. In contrast, the sympathetic system mobilizes the organism during emergency and stress situations, and is called the "fight or flight" system. Its functions involve the expenditure of energy and increases in blood sugar concentration, heart activity, and blood pressure (Table 20-1 and Figure 20-4).

Anatomic and Pharmacologic Differences The preganglionic fibers of the parasympathetic (cholinergic) system emerge with cranial nerves III, VII, IX, and X, and at the sacral spinal levels from about S3 through S4. The tenth cranial nerve, or vagus nerve, has extensive branches that supply fibers to the heart, lungs, and almost all of the abdominal organs.

The sympathetic (adrenergic) system is also called the thoracolumbar system because its preganglionic fibers originate in the spinal cord from the thoracic segment at level T1 to the lumbar segment at level L2 (see Figure 20-4 and Table 20-2).

✱ **How is the nerve impulse transmitted?**
There is general agreement that information in the nervous system is transmitted both electrically and chemically. This phenomenon occurs because nerve cells have two special characteristics:
1. Conduction of electrical signals, and
2. Intercellular connections with other nerve cells and with innervated tissues such as muscles and glands.

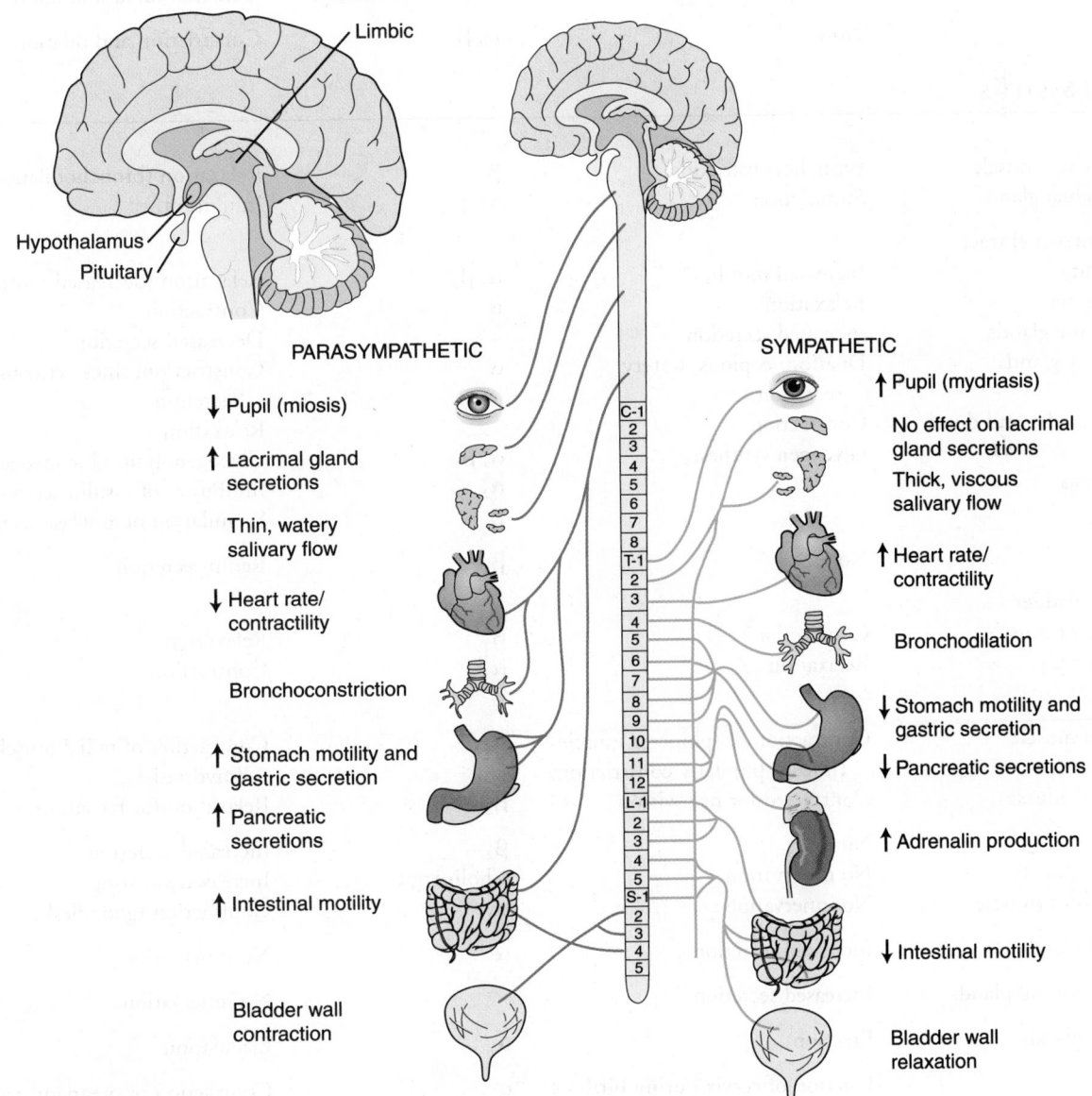

FIGURE 20-4 Diagram of the autonomic nervous system.

TABLE 20-1 EFFECTOR ORGAN RESPONSES TO AUTONOMIC NERVE IMPULSES

Effector Organs	Response to Parasympathetic (Cholinergic) Impulses	Response to Sympathetic (Adrenergic) Impulses	
		Receptor	Response
CARDIOVASCULAR SYSTEM			
Heart			
Sinoatrial node	Decreased heart rate	β_1, β_2	Increased heart rate
Atrioventricular node	Decreased conduction velocity	β_1, β_2	Increased automaticity and conduction velocity
Ventricles	No innervation	β_1, β_2	Increased force of contraction and conduction velocity
Arterioles (smooth muscle)			
Coronary	Constriction	α_1, α_2, β_2, dopaminergic	Constriction and dilation
Skin and mucosa		α_1, α_2	Constriction
Skeletal muscle	No innervation	Cholinergic	Dilation
Cerebral		α_1	Slight constriction
Mesenteric	None	α, β_2, dopaminergic	Constriction and dilation
Renal	None	α, β_2, dopaminergic	Constriction and dilation
Veins	None	α, β_2	Constriction and dilation
OTHER SYSTEMS			
Lung			
Bronchial muscle	Bronchoconstriction	β_2	Relaxation (bronchodilation)
Bronchial glands	Stimulation	α_1, β_2	Inhibition
Gastrointestinal tract			
Motility	Increased motility	α, β_2	Relaxation (decreased motility)
Sphincters	Relaxation	α	Contraction
Exocrine glands	Increased secretion	—	Decreased secretion
Salivary glands	Dilation: copious, watery secretion	α	Constriction: thick, viscous secretion
Gallbladder and ducts	Contraction		Relaxation
Liver	Glycogen synthesis	α, β_2	Glycogenolysis, gluconeogenesis
Pancreas		α_2	Inhibition of insulin secretion
		β	Stimulation of amylase secretion
Kidney	None	β_2	Renin secretion
Urinary bladder			
Detrusor muscle	Contraction	β_2	Relaxation
Sphincter	Relaxation	α_1	Contraction
Eye			
Radial muscle	Contraction of sphincter muscle (miosis, pupillary constriction)	α_1	Contraction of radial muscle (mydriasis)
Iris			
Ciliary muscle	Contracted for near vision	β_2	Relaxation for far vision
Skin	None	β_2	Increased secretion
Sweat glands	No innervation	Cholinergic	Increased sweating
Pilomotor muscle	No innervation	α_1	Contraction (gooseflesh)
Lacrimal glands	Increased secretion	α	No innervation
Nasopharyngeal glands	Increased secretion		No innervation
Male sex glands	Erection	α_1	Ejaculation
Uterus	Dilation of cervix during birth	α	Contraction of pregnant uterus
		β_2	Relaxation of pregnant and non-pregnant uterus

TABLE 20-2 DIFFERENTIATING CHARACTERISTICS BETWEEN THE PARASYMPATHETIC AND SYMPATHETIC NERVOUS SYSTEM

Characteristic	Parasympathetic Nervous System	Sympathetic Nervous System
Origin	Craniosacral	Thoracolumbar
Structure innervation	Cardiac muscle Smooth muscle Glands Viscera	Cardiac muscle Smooth muscle Glands Viscera
Ganglia	Near the effector (vagus, atria of heart)	Near CNS
Length of fibers	Preganglionic (long) Postganglionic (short)	Preganglionic (short) Postganglionic (long)
Ratio of preganglionic to postganglionic fibers	Branching is minimal (1:2); very discrete, fine responses	High degree of nerve branching (1:11, 1:17)
Response	Discrete	Diffuse
Ganglion transmitter	Acetylcholine	Acetylcholine
Transmitter substance (postganglionic nerve endings)	Acetylcholine	Norepinephrine (most cases); epinephrine and norepinephrine (adrenal medulla) Acetylcholine for sweat glands and blood vessels of skeletal muscles
Blocking drugs (postganglionic nerve endings)	Cholinergic blocking agents (atropine)	Adrenergic blocking agents α: phentolamine β: propranolol

The passage of a nerve impulse or an action potential along a nerve fiber or a muscle fiber is called conduction. The presence of a specific chemical at the intercellular connections determines the type of information a neuron can receive and the range of responses it can yield in return. The passage of a nerve impulse across a **synaptic** or **neuroeffector junction** with the use of a chemical is called **neurohumoral transmission.**

Although each nerve fiber may conduct an impulse along the neuron, it is solely the chemical substance called the **neurotransmitter** or neurohormone that permits the action potential of a neuron to cross (1) the synaptic junction from one neuron to another neuron, or (2) the neuroeffector junction from a neuron to an effector organ. In this mechanism, the arrival of an action potential at a nerve terminal starts the release of the neurotransmitter. This hormone or mediator then acts as a messenger by which nerve cells communicate information to the structures they innervate. The neurotransmitter exerts its influence primarily at the junctional spaces (synaptic junction or neuroeffector junction) to facilitate the transmission of impulses to their final destination. Many drugs may also act selectively at these junctions to supplement or inhibit the action of the neurotransmitter.

⚹ **What are the common neurotransmitters?**
The neurohormones acetylcholine and norepinephrine are responsible for neurohumoral transmission. Nerves that

contain acetylcholine are called **cholinergic** neurons and are involved in cholinergic transmission. Nerves that contain norepinephrine or epinephrine (from the adrenal medulla) are known as **adrenergic** neurons and are associated with adrenergic transmission.

In neurohumoral transmission, the sequence of events includes (1) biosynthesis, (2) storage, (3) release, (4) action, and (5) inactivation of the mediator (Figures 20-5 and 20-7). Many autonomic drugs affect one of these individual events, and it is essential to understand the basic mechanisms involved in this complicated process. These drugs have been useful in treating many persons afflicted with autonomic disorders.

How does cholinergic transmission occur?
Transmission of acetylcholine across the synapse involves the steps of synthesis, storage, release, action, and inactivation.

Synthesis and Storage Acetylcholine is synthesized in the cytoplasm of the nerve terminal from acetyl coenzyme A and choline in the presence of choline acetylase (Figures 20-5, *A,1* and 20-6). Once synthesized, the acetylcholine is stored in packets called synaptic vesicles or granules, which are located in the nerve terminal (see Figure 20-5, *A, 2*).

Release and Action The arrival of an action potential at the nerve ending causes the vesicle to approach the membrane and release the acetylcholine molecules into the synap-

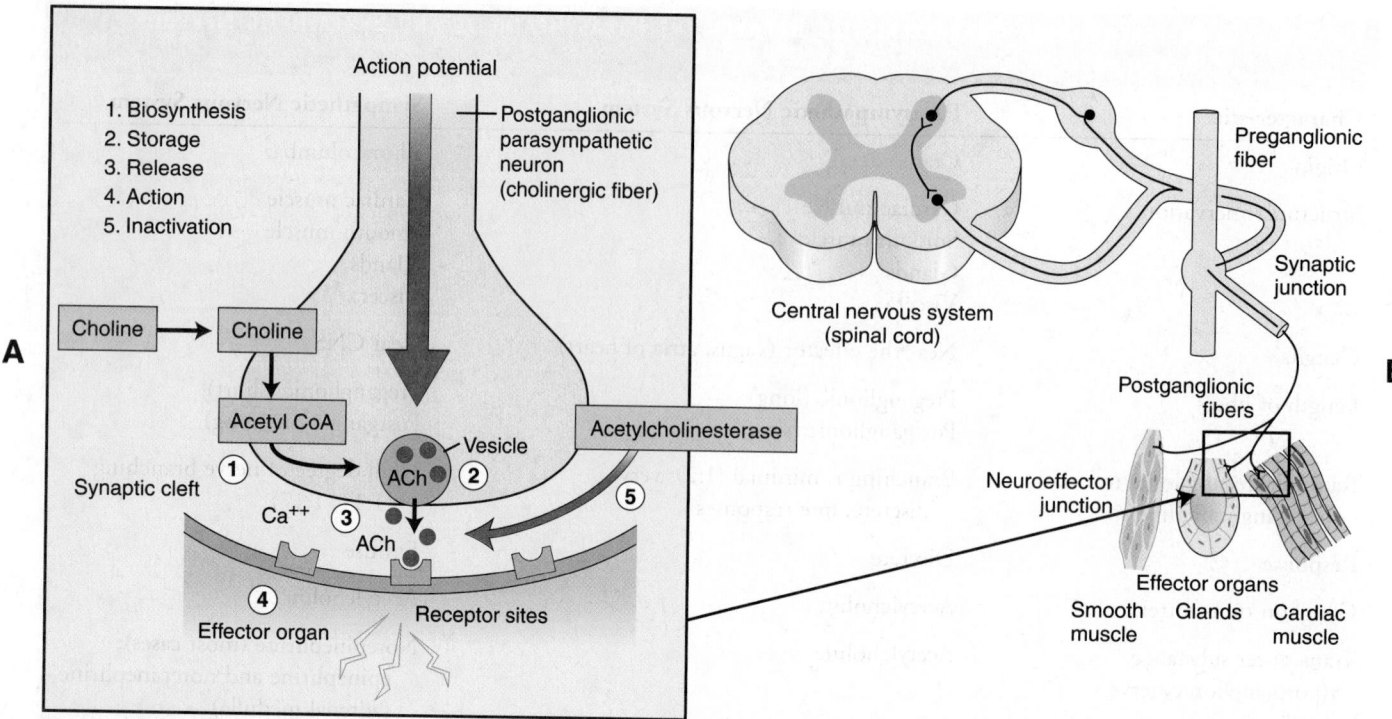

FIGURE 20-5 Cholinergic transmission. **A,** Diagram of parasympathetic postganglionic neuron, showing steps in cholinergic transmission at the neuroeffector junction. **B,** Representation of the relationship between a neuron in the CNS, a neuron in a peripheral ganglion, and an effector organ supplied by the parasympathetic nerve.

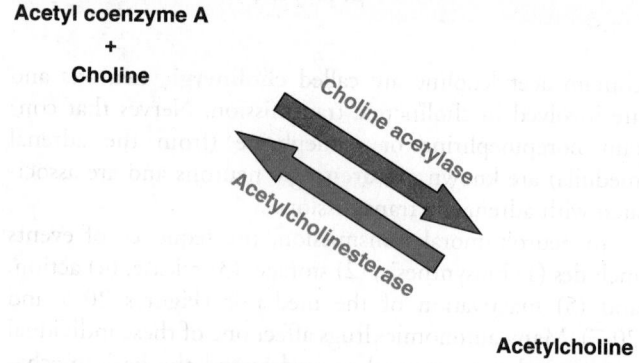

FIGURE 20-6 Formation and deactivation of acetylcholine.

tic cleft or space. Calcium ions must be present for an efficient release. Once free, the acetylcholine diffuses across the synaptic or junctional cleft and attaches itself to specialized receptors (postjunctional sites) on the membrane of the next neuron or neuroeffector. The binding of acetylcholine to the receptor increases the permeability of the membrane to sodium and potassium ions; the depolarizing action that results leads to the excitation or inhibition of neural, muscular, or glandular activity (see Figure 20-5, *A, 3*).

The cholinergic receptor sites that are stimulated by acetylcholine are either nicotinic or muscarinic. **Nicotinic receptors** appear in the ganglia of both parasympathetic and sympathetic fibers, the adrenal medulla, and the skeletal (striated) muscle supplied by the somatic motor system. **Muscarinic receptors** (postganglionic sites) are located in the smooth muscle, cardiac muscle, and glands of the parasym-

pathetic fibers and the effector organs of the cholinergic sympathetic fibers. Figure 20-3 shows nicotinic and muscarinic receptors.

Inactivation Once acetylcholine has exerted its effect on the postjunctional sites (Figure 20-5, *A, 4*), the excess amount is inactivated rapidly by the enzyme acetylcholinesterase. The metabolites formed in this reaction are chemically inactive and are the same compounds from which acetylcholine is formed. Figures 20-5, *A, 5,* and 20-6 show inactivation of this neurohormone as a reverse action.

✱ How does adrenergic transmission differ from cholinergic transmission?
Very similar steps are observed with adrenergic transmission as with cholinergic transmission. The chemicals involved include the catecholamines. **Catecholamines** are a group of chemically related compounds: norepinephrine (noradrenalin), epinephrine (adrenalin), and dopamine. All of these compounds are involved in some aspect of adrenergic transmission.

Synthesis and Storage The catecholamines produced by the sympathetic nervous system include norepinephrine and epinephrine. The complex pathway for the synthesis of these neurotransmitters is mediated by different enzymes located in the postganglionic nerve terminals and in the chromaffin cells of the adrenal medulla.

The formation of norepinephrine is initiated by tyrosine, an amino acid derived from proteins in the diet. When tyrosine enters the cytoplasm of the nerve terminal, it is converted into dopa, which, in turn, is decarboxylated into

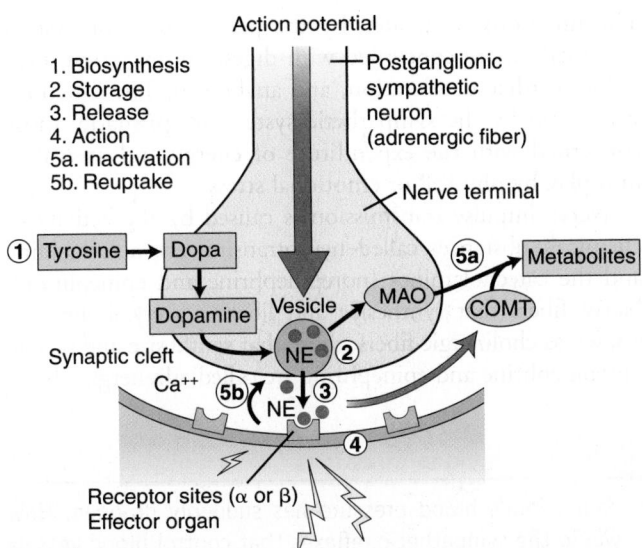

1. Biosynthesis
2. Storage
3. Release
4. Action
5a. Inactivation
5b. Reuptake

Action potential

Postganglionic
sympathetic
neuron
(adrenergic fiber)

Nerve terminal

① Tyrosine → Dopa

Dopamine

Dopamine

Vesicle

MAO

⑤a Metabolites

COMT

NE ②

Synaptic cleft

Ca++

⑤b NE ③

④

Receptor sites (α or β)
Effector organ

FIGURE 20-7 Adrenergic transmission at the neuroeffector junction. *COMT,* Catechol *O*-methyltransferase; *MAO,* monoamine oxidase; *NE,* norepinephrine.

dopamine. Dopamine is taken up into the storage vesicles, or granules, where it is transformed into the neurotransmitter norepinephrine by the enzyme dopamine β-hydroxylase. Figure 20-7, *1,* shows the steps of the process of synthesis for adrenergic transmission.

In the adrenal medullary gland, the enzyme methyltransferase converts norepinephrine to epinephrine. On stimulation, both epinephrine and norepinephrine are released from the adrenal medulla and are carried by the circulation to all parts of the body.

Release The arrival of an action potential at the nerve terminal of the postganglionic fibers causes the vesicles to fuse with the cell membrane and release the stored supply of norepinephrine into the junctional cleft. Calcium ions must be present to enhance the release of norepinephrine from the vesicles. The free form of norepinephrine then diffuses across the cleft to the receptor sites on the postjunctional membrane of neuroeffector cells (smooth muscle, cardiac muscle, or glands) (see Figure 20-7, *3*).

Action Once the norepinephrine combines with either the α or β receptor sites on the membrane of the neuroeffector cells, a series of chemical and electrical events produces either an excitatory or an inhibitory effect (Figure 20-7, *4*). The α receptor activation is primarily responsible for an excitatory response, although it results in intestinal relaxation. By contrast, β receptor activation is usually inhibitory except in the myocardial cells, where norepinephrine produces an excitatory effect.

The adrenergic receptor sites that are stimulated by the endogenous catecholamines—norepinephrine, epinephrine, and dopamine—are classified as α and β receptors. Both classes have two subtypes. The α receptors are identified by neuronal location: (1) α_1 sites are located on the postsynaptic effector cells, and (2) α_2 sites appear on the presynaptic nerve termi-

nals, controlling the amount of norepinephrine release that operates through a negative feedback mechanism. By contrast, the β receptors are designated by organ location: (1) β_1 receptors are located primarily in the heart, and (2) β_2 receptors appear in the smooth muscle of the bronchioles, arterioles, and various other visceral organs in the body. These receptors are discussed further in Chapter 22. At least five types of dopamine receptors have been identified in the CNS. D_1 and D_2 receptors are associated with the antipsychotic medications and movement disorders, such as Parkinson's disease. Stimulation of D_2 receptors is primarily responsible for antiparkinson drug activity; the D_1 receptors may play a similar, but smaller, role in this area.

Inactivation Once norepinephrine has performed its adrenergic function, its action must be rapidly stopped to prevent prolongation of its effects, which could lead to a loss of regulatory control of visceral function. The inactivation of norepinephrine occurs by (1) enzymatic transformation, (2) reuptake of the norepinephrine into nerve terminals, and (3) diffusion (see Figure 20-7, *5a, 5b*).

Catecholamines are metabolized by two enzymes, monoamine oxidase (MAO) and catechol *O*-methyltransferase (COMT). MAO, which is stored in the mitochondria of sympathetic neurons, metabolizes free norepinephrine within the cytoplasm of the nerve terminal. COMT, which is located outside the neuron or at the synaptic cleft, participates in the inactivation or metabolism of norepinephrine outside the neuron.

The mechanism of norepinephrine reuptake plays a more significant role than enzymatic transformation in catecholamine inactivation. In the reuptake process, norepinephrine is removed by the active transport ("amine pump") from the junctional sites (synaptic and neuroeffector junctions) and is returned to the sympathetic nerve terminal and storage vesicles. In this way, an adequate supply of norepinephrine is provided by reuptake, as well as by the process of synthesis.

A small portion of norepinephrine released at the synaptic cleft may be picked up by the circulation and metabolized elsewhere in the body. This is known as the diffusion process.

✴ **What is the interplay of the autonomic neurotransmitters in the peripheral nervous system?**
The location and chemical differences between the autonomic transmitters were identified many years ago. In the ANS, all of the preganglionic fibers originate in the CNS and synapse with the ganglia of the postganglionic fibers. The terminals of all the preganglionic fibers release acetylcholine and interact with nicotinic receptors in the membrane of the postganglionic fibers or the adrenal medulla.

In the parasympathetic system the terminals of the postganglionic fibers also release acetylcholine and interact with muscarinic receptors in the membrane of the smooth muscle, cardiac muscle, and glands.

There are three types of postganglionic neurons in the sympathetic nervous system (see Figure 20-3):
- The sympathetic neuron, the major type, releases norepinephrine and activates either α or β receptors

in the membrane of the smooth muscle, cardiac muscle, and glands.

- An example of the sympathoadrenal neuron, in which the preganglionic fiber synapses with a modified sympathetic ganglion, is the adrenal medulla. This gland releases mostly epinephrine and a small amount of norepinephrine, which are secreted into the circulation and carried to all parts of the body.
- The cholinergic sympathetic neuron releases acetylcholine and stimulates muscarinic receptor sites on the sweat glands to produce sweating and on the blood vessels in skeletal muscle to increase vasodilation and enhance blood flow.

In the **somatic nervous system** (often referred to as the sensory nervous system), a single neuron, the efferent or motor fiber, releases acetylcholine and interacts with the nicotinic sites on the skeletal muscle membrane. The autonomic drugs play an important role by enhancing or inhibiting physiologic activity at these sites of neurohumoral transmission (see Figure 20-3 and Table 20-2).

Summary

A basic knowledge of the anatomy and physiology of the ANS is essential to the nurse's understanding of the pharmacology of autonomic drugs. This knowledge will help the nurse to predict the effects of drugs that stimulate or block autonomic function.

The primary function of the ANS is to control and integrate the many physiologic tasks necessary to preserve internal homeostasis, emergency mechanisms, and repair. Its activities are integrated by a number of centers within the CNS: the hypothalamus, medulla oblongata, midbrain, limbic system, cerebellum, and cerebral cortex. The ANS innervates the smooth muscles, cardiac muscles, and glands. It is composed of two divisions: parasympathetic and sympathetic. The actions of the parasympathetic and sympathetic divisions oppose and balance each other as follows:

- Although both systems are present in the body, only one is predominant at any given time.
- If an ANS function is blocked, the opposite effect will take precedence.
- Drugs are available to stimulate or block either system.

The functions stimulated by the parasympathetic system are chiefly those concerned with digestion, excretion, near vision, cardiac deceleration, and anabolism. The functions stimulated by the sympathetic system are primarily those concerned with the expenditure of energy and are called into play by physical or emotional stress.

Nerve impulse transmission is caused by the activity of chemical substances called neurotransmitters: acetylcholine and the catecholamines (norepinephrine and epinephrine). Nerve fibers that synthesize and liberate acetylcholine are known as cholinergic fibers; those that synthesize and secrete norepinephrine and epinephrine are called adrenergic fibers.

✱ Critical Thinking Questions

- Your client's blood pressure has suddenly dropped. How would the sympathetic reflexes that control blood vessels respond (1) to a sudden decrease in blood pressure or (2) to a sudden increase in blood pressure?
- Clients with diabetes mellitus may develop autonomic neuropathy (i.e., degeneration of the ANS nerves). Which component of the ANS is involved with the following symptoms:
  - Lack of pain with a heart attack?
  - Constipation?
  - Impotence?
  - Decreased pupillary response to light?

Bibliography

Anderson, D.M., Keith, J., & Novak, P.D. (Eds.). (2002). *Mosby's medical, nursing, and allied health dictionary* (6th ed.). St. Louis: Mosby.

Guyton, A.C., & Hall, J.E. (2000). *Textbook of medical physiology* (10th ed.). Philadelphia: W.B. Saunders.

Hardman, J.G., & Limbird, L.E. (Eds.). (2001). *Goodman and Gilman's the pharmacological basis of therapeutics* (10th ed.). New York: McGraw-Hill.

Herlihy, B., & Maebius, N.K. (2003). *The human body in health and illness* (2nd ed.). Philadelphia: W.B. Saunders.

McCance, K.L., & Huether, S.E. (2002). *Pathophysiology: The biological basis for disease in adults and children* (4th ed.). St. Louis: Mosby.

Thibodeau, G.A., & Patton, K.T. (2003). *Anatomy and physiology* (5th ed.). St. Louis: Mosby.

e-LEARNING SUPPLEMENTS

Student CD-ROM
- Final Exam questions
- NCLEX® Examination review questions
- Pharmacology animations
- Printable chapter summary

Evolve Website (http://evolve.elsevier.com/mckenry)
- Content updates, including information on new drugs
- WebLinks corresponding to this chapter

- Answers to the critical thinking questions in this chapter
- *Elsevier ePharmacology Update* newsletter
- *Mosby's Drug Consult* Internet Edition
- Supplemental and reference information

Drugs Affecting the Parasympathetic Nervous System and the Neurotransmitter Acetylcholine

21

Chapter Focus

The parasympathetic component of the autonomic nervous system (ANS) innervates various organs and acts on the heart, gastrointestinal (GI) tract, urinary bladder, and respiratory tract. In conjunction with the sympathetic component of the ANS, the parasympathetic system works to control body functions that occur without conscious thought. Drug therapy associated with this system can influence autonomic processes by mimicking acetylcholine at receptor sites, or it can inhibit the breakdown of acetylcholine at these same sites, prolonging its action. Drugs that act at sites outside of the parasympathetic nervous system but impact acetylcholine are also clinically important. The nurse needs to be knowledgeable about such drugs because they are used across a wide variety of human conditions and clinical settings.

Learning Objectives

- Differentiate between the muscarinic and nicotinic actions of acetylcholine.
- Compare the adverse effects of cholinergic, cholinergic blocking, and synthetic antispasmodic agents.
- Explain the physiologic effects of the belladonna alkaloids.
- Explain the physiologic effects of nicotine.
- Describe the action of agents that act at the ganglion including nerve gas poisons.
- Describe the action of neuromuscular blockers.
- Implement the nursing management of clients receiving agents that affect acetylcholine action and the parasympathetic nervous system.

✳ How are drugs that affect the autonomic nervous system classified?

Autonomic drugs may mimic, intensify, or block the effects of the parasympathetic and sympathetic divisions of the autonomic nervous system. They are divided into the following groups:

- **Cholinergic (parasympathomimetic)** drugs (e.g., bethanechol) act like mediators of the parasympathetic nervous system.
- **Cholinergic blocking (parasympatholytic, anticholinergic, or antimuscarinic)** drugs (e.g., atropine) block the action of the parasympathetic nervous system.
- **Adrenergic (sympathomimetic)** drugs (e.g., norepinephrine) act like mediators of the sympathetic nervous system (see Chapter 22).
- **Adrenergic blocking (sympatholytic)** drugs (e.g., propranolol, a β-blocking agent) block the action of the sympathetic nervous system (see Chapter 22).

✳ What actions do cholinergic drugs have?

Cholinergic drugs, or parasympathomimetic drugs, work to mimic the actions of acetylcholine in the autonomic nervous system (ANS). As discussed in Chapter 20, acetylcholine plays an important role in the transmission of nerve impulses in both the parasympathetic and sympathetic divisions of the ANS.

Acetylcholine has two major actions on the nervous system: (1) it has stimulant effects on the ganglia, adrenal medulla, and skeletal muscle; and (2) it has stimulant effects at postganglionic nerve endings in cardiac muscle, smooth muscle, and glands. The first action resembles the effects of nicotine, such as tachycardia, elevated blood pressure, and peripheral vasoconstriction; this is referred to as the **nicotinic effect** of acetylcholine. The second action of acetylcholine at the postganglionic nerve endings is like that of muscarine (an alkaloid obtained from the toadstool *Amanita muscaria*): intense vomiting, diarrhea, nervousness, severe stomach pains, labored respiration, slow and irregular pulse, delirium, and even fatality. Symptoms will mimic an intense parasympathetic stimulation. This is referred to as the **muscarinic effect** or cholinergic effect of acetylcholine. (See Figure 20-3 p. 416, for a review of nicotine and muscarinic sites.)

Although acetylcholine is important physiologically, it has no therapeutic value because (1) its actions are very brief because of rapid hydrolysis by acetylcholinesterase, and (2) no selective purpose can be achieved through its use because it has several sites of action. Cholinergic fibers are widespread. Nicotinic sites are present in the skeletal muscle. Muscarinic sites are present in the heart, spleen, uterus, vas deferens, colon, and vessels of the skin.

Cholinergic drugs are agents that bring about effects in the body similar to those produced by acetylcholine. These agents are also called parasympathomimetics because they mimic the action produced by stimulation of the parasympathetic nervous system. Drugs typically have action predominately at either the nicotinic or at the muscarinic sites, but not both. Cholinergic drugs may be obtained from natural (plant) or synthetic sources. The synthetic drugs are more stable and have a more selective action on particular organs.

The two groups of cholinergic drugs available are (1) direct acting and (2) indirect acting. **Direct-acting cholinergic drugs** combine directly with the cholinergic receptors in postsynaptic membranes innervated by parasympathetic neurons and evoke effects similar to those produced by acetylcholine. By contrast **indirect-acting cholinergic drugs** don't affect the receptors directly, but instead act primarily on the enzyme inhibiting the action of cholinesterase (acetylcholinesterase), that normally degrades acetylcholine. This results in an accumulation of acetylcholine at all sites where it is liberated (see Figure 20-5, *A, 5,* p. 420). By rendering this enzymatic action ineffective, anticholinesterase drugs cause a prolonged and intensified cholinergic response at the various effector sites.

✳ What constitutes an ideal cholinergic agent?

The ideal cholinergic or anticholinesterase drug has the following characteristics:

- Limited action on one particular structure or organ and is not active at other sites
- Effective when administered orally
- More stable and less easily inactivated than drugs currently available

TABLE 21-1 PROMINENT CHOLINERGIC AND ANTICHOLINESTERASE DRUGS

Generic Name	Indications	Usual Adult Dosage (24 hours)	Usual Route of Administration
bethanechol (D) (Urecholine)	Urinary retention/neurogenic bladder	10-50 mg PO three to four times daily	Oral
		5 mg subcutaneously three to four times daily	Subcutaneously
neostigmine bromide (I) (Prostigmin)	Myasthenia gravis, reversal of neuromuscular blockade, urinary retention	15 mg q3-4h	Oral
neostigmine methylsulfate (I) (Prostigmin)		0.5 mg (dose variable)	IM or subcutaneously
physostigmine (I) (Antilirium)	Anticholinergic toxicity, reversal of neuromuscular blockade	0.5-2 mg (maximum)	IM or IV
pilocarpine (D)	Glaucoma	1-2 drops, 0.5%-4% solution four times daily	Topical (eye)
pyridostigmine (I) (Mestinon)	Myasthenia gravis	Highly variable 60-120 mg q3-8h	Oral

D, Direct acting; *I*, indirect acting; *IM*, intramuscularly; *IV*, intravenously.

• Produces a therapeutic effect with minimal adverse effects

Although this ideal drug is not yet available, progress is being made.

Cholinergic drugs used primarily to lower intraocular pressure include pilocarpine and carbachol; these are discussed in Chapter 42. Table 21-1 lists the prominent cholinergic and anticholinesterase drugs.

✱ How are the cholinergic agonists differentiated?

The clinical utility of cholinergic agonists depends on the degree of activity at nicotinic versus muscarinic sites. The following sections review direct-acting nicotinic ganglionic agonists (e.g., nicotine), indirect-acting nicotinic agonists at the skeletal muscle (e.g., edrophonium, physostigmine), and indirect-acting muscarinic agonists at involuntary smooth muscle (e.g., bethanechol).

Nicotinic Agonists at the Ganglion

The major neurotransmitter of all autonomic ganglia is acetylcholine. Nicotinic agonists act at the ganglion for both the sympathetic and parasympathetic nervous systems (Figure 21-1, *A* and *B*). Because postganglionic fibers produce specific effects on smooth muscle, cardiac muscle, and glands (see Figure 20-3), nonselective drugs that stimulate reactions in this area can produce a broad range of pharmacologic effects. The primary agent involved at these sites is nicotine.

Nicotine may produce a variety of complex and often unpredictable effects in the body. Many actions are dose related, with generally small doses inducing activation or stimulation of a response and larger doses producing a decreased or depressed response. Because nicotine acts on

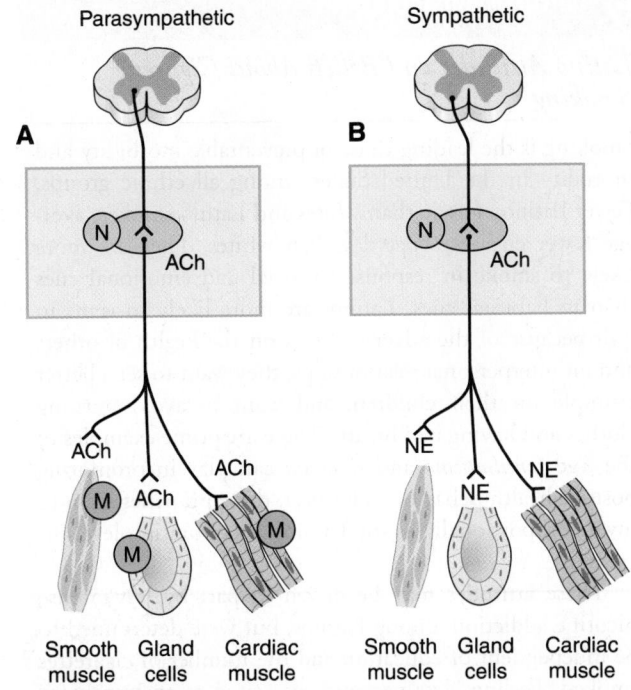

FIGURE 21-1 Nicotinic agonist action at the ganglion in the parasympathetic nervous system **(A)** and the sympathetic nervous system **(B)**. *Ach,* Acetylcholine; *M,* muscarinic receptors; *N,* nicotinic receptors; *NE,* norepinephrine.

multiple systems, the ultimate response may be the sum of its stimulation and depressant actions.

Nicotine temporarily stimulates all sympathetic and parasympathetic ganglia in the ANS. This is followed by depression, which tends to last longer than the period of stimulation. Its effects on skeletal muscle are similar to its effects

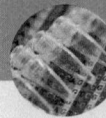

Special Considerations for Pharmacogenetics | NICOTINE

PHARMACODYNAMICS

Genetic variation in dopamine receptors (specifically D_2) and dopamine β-hydroxylase correlate with the efficacy of nicotine replacement therapy (NRT) in clients who are attempting smoking cessation (Johnstone et al., 2004). Tyrosine hydroxylase, an enzyme involved in dopamine synthesis, is also genetically determined. It is proposed that a gene marker for this enzyme may predict the likelihood of future smoking and nicotine addiction (Anney, Olsson, Lotfi-Miri, Patton, & Williamson, 2004). Other genetic markers, including that for cytochrome P450 2E1*1D and monoamine oxidase, also correlate with smoking dependence (Howard, Ahluwalia, Lin, Sellers, & Tyndale, 2003; Ito et al., 2004). Whether these findings will allow for client-specific prediction of who is at higher risk for nicotine addiction and who is likely to succeed with NRT remains to be seen.

PHARMACOKINETICS

An association exists between the extent of individual cytochrome P450 2A6 activity and smoking status. This isoenzyme is responsible for the metabolism of nicotine to an inactive metabolite. In a study of white Americans, those with less 2A6 activity (slower metabolizers of nicotine) were less likely to be smokers than those with higher 2A6 activity. (Schoedel, Hoffmann, Rao, Sellers, & Tyndale, 2004). Among smokers, those who more slowly metabolize nicotine also tend to smoke fewer cigarettes.

ADVERSE EFFECTS

Given the genetic variation in metabolism of nicotine noted above, it is likely that adverse effects vary, at least in part, as a result of genetic makeup. This, however, requires further study.

Cultural Considerations

Latino Attitudes and Beliefs About Cigarette Smoking

Smoking is the leading cause of preventable morbidity and mortality in the United States among all ethnic groups. Fewer Latinos smoke than whites and Latino smokers average fewer cigarettes per day than whites. They are more likely to smoke in response to social and emotional cues than to habitual cues. Latinos are more likely to want to quit because of the adverse effects on the health of others and on interpersonal relationships; they want to set a better example for their children, and want to avoid burning clothes and having bad breath. These are prime examples of the role *familialismo* and *simpatia* can play in promoting positive health behaviors. However, these priorities seem to invert proportionally as the Latinos' acculturation level increases.

These attitudes may be driven in part by less-intense nicotine addiction among Latinos, but were determined to be independent of education and the number of cigarettes smoked. Feeling "less nervous" was cited as an important reason to continue smoking. Less importance was placed on the adverse effects on one's own health and on remaining thin. These findings can be taken into consideration when developing a smoking cessation program or even during office-based counseling. For example, the nurse should appeal to the Latino's sense of family in formulating strategies of smoking cessation.

Data from Perez-Stable, E.J., Marin, G., & Posner, S.F. (1998). Ethnic comparison of attitudes and beliefs about cigarette smoking. *Journal of General Internal Medicine 13*(3), 167-174.

on the ganglia—a depressant phase follows stimulation. During the depressant phase, nicotine exerts a curare-like, or neuromuscular blocking action, on skeletal muscle.

Nicotine stimulates the central nervous system (CNS), especially the medullary centers (respiratory, emetic, and vasomotor). Large doses may cause tremors and seizures. Stimulation is followed by depression. Death may result from respiratory failure, although it may result more from the curare-like action of nicotine on nerve endings in the diaphragm rather than the action on the respiratory center.

The actions and effects of nicotine on the cardiovascular system are complex. Heart rate is commonly slowed at first but later may be accelerated above normal. Nicotine usually produces an increase in heart rate and blood pressure; in general, the cardiovascular effects result from stimulation of the sympathetic ganglia and adrenal medulla along with the release of catecholamines from the sympathetic nerve endings (Corelli & Hudmon, 2005). Nicotine also has an antidiuretic action. Repeated administration of nicotine causes tolerance. The genetic makeup of the individual also influences nicotine dependence and effects (see the Special Considerations for Pharmacogenetics box above).

nicotine [**nik** o teen]
(Nicotrol NS, Nicotrol Inhaler, Nicorette✤)
Indications
Nicotine is used to help reduce nicotine withdrawal symptoms as an aid to smoking cessation. A discussion of smoking cessation and nicotine products used as part of smoking cessation are discussed in Box 21-1. Nicotine itself has no therapeutic use but is of great pharmacologic interest and toxicologic importance.
Pharmacokinetics/Dosing
Nicotine is readily absorbed from the gastrointestinal (GI) tract, respiratory mucous membrane, and skin. Dosage formulations include gum/lozenge (typically 2 to 4 mg nicotine per piece), oral inhaler (4 mg

BOX 21-1 NICOTINE PRODUCTS AND SMOKING CESSATION

Tobacco is the single greatest cause of disease and premature death in America today, and is responsible for more than 430,000 deaths each year. The burning of tobacco can generate approximately 4000 compounds in a gaseous and particle phase, plus 60 carcinogens (Action on Smoking and Health, 2004). Known carcinogens such as tar, formaldehyde, hydrogen cyanide, benzene, and carbon monoxide, among others, have been identified as etiologic factors in a variety of neoplastic diseases (e.g., cancer of the bladder, lung, buccal cavity, esophagus, and pancreas). Other smoking-related illnesses include pulmonary emphysema, chronic bronchitis, coronary heart disease, and myocardial infarction. Of considerable importance is the fact that smokers absorb sufficient nicotine to exert a variety of effects on the autonomic nervous system. In general, nicotine is believed to be a contributing factor in peripheral vascular disease such as thromboangiitis obliterans (Buerger disease). It may cause spasms of the peripheral blood vessels, thus reducing blood flow through the affected vessels. Vasospasm in the retinal blood vessels of the eye is thought to cause serious vision disturbances and is associated with tobacco smoking.

Passive smoking (involuntary smoking, secondhand smoke) refers to the inhalation of cigarette smoke by nonsmokers. Even though this exposure is less concentrated than inhaled smoke, the health risks and/or harmful effects to the nonsmoker can be significant. Reports from the U.S. Surgeon General and the Expert Committee on Passive Smoking indicate that (1) environmental smoke can cause lung cancer in healthy nonsmokers, (2) children of smoking parents often have a greater incidence of respiratory tract symptoms and infections than children from a nonsmoking family, (3) environmental smoke may be a risk factor in cardiac disease, and (4) studies have linked environmental smoke exposure to cancers other than lung cancer (Action on Smoking and Health, 2004).

In addition, the fetus of a mother who smokes may have a low birth weight and increased congenital abnormalities. Children of parents who smoke have an increased incidence of sudden infant death syndrome, an increased incidence of otitis media, respiratory infections, and allergic reactions, as well as an increased likelihood of becoming smokers. Smoking by women is still prevalent and may be higher and even increasing within some cultural groups as they become acculturated (see the Cultural Considerations box on p. 426).

 Management of Drug Overdose

Nicotine

Signs and Symptoms

- Nicotine overdose often presents with increased saliva flow, nausea and vomiting, abdominal cramps, diarrhea, confusion, cold sweat, headache, fainting, hypotension, hypertension, fever, tachycardia, prostration and collapse. In severe cases, seizures may occur. Fatalities, when they occur, usually result from respiratory failure.

General Approach

- *Nicotine gum.* Activated charcoal is typically administered for decontamination. Gastric lavage may also be used with large ingestions or in high-risk cases.
- *Transdermal system.* Remove the patch and flush the area with water. Do not use soap because it may enhance nicotine absorption. If the patch was swallowed, administer an activated charcoal system and repeat for as long as the patch is in the GI tract. Monitor for the passage of the patch in stool.

Specific Approach

- Treat medical complications as necessary, as shown by the following examples:
  Provide respiratory support and interventions for respiratory failure.
  Treat hypotension and cardiovascular collapse aggressively.
  Use antiepileptic drugs (benzodiazepines or barbiturates) for seizures.
  Use atropine for excessive bronchial secretions.
- Closely monitor for adverse effects, including the risk for choking, aspiration with vomiting, and gastrointestinal obstruction, and treat appropriately as necessary.

which at times has led to the death of farm workers. Because nicotine is a major ingredient in tobacco products, both acute toxicity (with the ingestion of such products by small children) and chronic toxicity are well documented. Short-term adverse effects include tachycardia, headache, nausea, vomiting, excessive salivation, and insomnia. Transdermal systems may be associated with pruritus or erythema. Other adverse effects include belching, increased appetite, sore mouth or throat, constipation, coughing, and dizziness or light-headedness. Transdermal patches may cause pruritus and/or erythema under the patch, a generalized rash, nausea, dizziness, myalgias, coughing, difficulty in sleeping, and nightmares. Adverse effects with nicotine gum include injury to the mouth, teeth, or dental work. See the Management of Drug Overdose box above.

Drug Interactions

Many drugs are reported to interact with nicotine. Ingredients other than nicotine in tobacco smoke probably account for the altered drug metabolism and drug interactions observed in smokers.

nicotine delivered from a 10-mg cartridge), nasal spray (0.5 mg per spray), and transdermal systems (delivering between 7 and 21 mg of nicotine over 16 to 24 hours). Plasma levels are achieved most rapidly with the intranasal formulation, and most evenly with the transdermal forms. It is widely distributed to body tissues and breast milk. Nicotine is hepatically metabolized to cotinine, which possesses modest pharmacologic activity. The half-life of nicotine is approximately 4 hours.

Adverse Effects

Nicotine has both short- and long-term toxic effects that are extremely important to the health care professional. Nicotine toxicity has resulted from the misuse of insecticides containing nicotine,

✷ **J.R., a 47-year-old man, visits his primary care center for his annual physical examination. His past medical history is unremarkable, except for mild hypertension that is controlled with medication. The nurse** reviews health promotion issues with him, and J.R. expresses concern that he has been unable to stop smoking. He has a 50-pack-year history and still smokes a pack a day. He admits that he has tried several methods to quit smoking on his own without success, but now feels the time is right for him.

Besides having the most prolonged contact with clients and their families in a variety of settings, nurses have the knowledge and skill to teach them the hazards of smoking and to aid in the selection and referral to a comprehensive smoking-cessation program. Nurses make a difference in smoking cessation, increasing quitting success rates in both hospital and nonhospital settings (Rice & Stead, 2004). Nursing-led interventions for smoking cessation increase by 50% the chances of successfully quitting (Rice & Stead, 2004). *Helping Smokers Quit: A Guide for Nurses,* has been developed by the Health and Human Services Agency for Healthcare Research and Quality (AHRQ) in collaboration with Tobacco Free Nurses and uses the "5 A's" approach to cessation intervention: Ask, Advise, Assess, Assist, and Arrange.*

J.R. has a significant smoking history. A "pack year" is equivalent to smoking one pack of cigarettes a day for one year. This means that at some point in his life, J.R. has smoked more than a pack a day.

Tobacco dependence is a chronic condition that often requires repeated intervention. The AHRQ has guidelines for nurses and other health care professionals relating to smoking cessation (www.ahcpr.gov/path/tobacco.htm). Effective treatments exist that can produce long-term or even permanent abstinence, and are associated with reducing mortality risk (Nicholas et al., 2005). Every client who uses tobacco should be offered at least one of these treatments. Clients such as J.R. who are willing to try to quit using tobacco should be provided with treatments that are identified as effective in the AHRQ guidelines. It is essential that nurses consistently identify, document, and treat every tobacco user who is seen in a health care setting.

Numerous effective pharmacotherapies for smoking cessation now exist. These should be used with all clients who are trying to quit smoking, except in the presence of contraindications. The AHRQ has identified five first-line pharmacotherapies that reliably increase long-term smoking abstinence rates: bupropion (sustained-release), nicotine gum, nicotine inhaler, nicotine nasal spray, and nicotine patch. Two second-line pharmacotherapies, clonidine and nortriptyline, were identified as efficacious and may be considered by clinicians if first-line pharmacotherapies are ineffective. These drugs are discussed in other chapters, but nicotine replacement therapy (NRT) is discussed here. NRT is both clinically effective and cost-effective relative to other medical and disease-prevention interventions (see the Evidence-Based Practice box on p. 429).

✱ **The nurse refers J.R. to the community smoking-cessation program where, in addition to NRT, he joins** a support group with others trying to quit smoking. At his next office visit, he reports "that it has not been an easy road," but he has been "without a cigarette for 3 months."

The epidemiology of tobacco use has continued its 50-year evolution from an equal opportunity addiction to a behavior that now affects primarily the most socioeconomically disadvantaged members of society. For example, in 1999, among those with masters, professional, or doctoral degrees, only 8.5% used tobacco. Conversely, 44.4% of those with only a high school General Educational Development degree used tobacco. Individuals living below the poverty level had a significantly higher smoking rate (33.1%) than did those living at or above the poverty level (24.4%). Recently, college students demonstrated an exception to the above epidemiologic observation. A 1999 survey of nationally representative 4-year colleges found that 45.7% of students reported use of a tobacco product in the past year and 32.9% reported that they were current users, indicating a particular need for assessment and intervention in this population. Nearly 25% of adult Americans currently smoke, and 3000 children and adolescents become regular users of tobacco every day. The U.S. Public Health Service publication Tracking Healthy People 2010 set a national goal of reducing tobacco use to 12% or less among adults by the end of this decade (Fiore, Hatsukami, & Baker, 2002).

The societal costs of tobacco-related death and disease approach $100 billion each year. However, more than 70% of all current smokers have expressed a desire to stop smoking; if they successfully quit, the result will be both immediate and long-term health improvements (Fiore et al., 2000).

Nicotine replacement therapy is available in a nicotine gum (Nicorette), lozenge (Commit), transdermal systems or patches (Nicoderm CQ, Nicotrol), inhaler (Nicotrol Inhaler), and nasal spray (Nicotrol NS) for use in smoking-cessation programs. All are indicated for adjunct treatment of nicotine dependence and are to be used in conjunction with a behavioral modification program. With all NRT, the client is to stop smoking and/or using smokeless tobacco products before beginning NRT, and only one NRT modality is used at a time. Nicotine replacement products should not be used during pregnancy. NRT should be combined with a supervised program for smoking cessation that includes education, counseling, and psychological support (Johnson, Budz, Mackay, & Miller, 1999).

Nicotine resin in the form of chewing gum provides a source of nicotine for the nicotine-dependent client undergoing acute cigarette withdrawal. The client chews a stick of gum for 30 minutes when there is a strong urge to smoke, up to maximum of 30 pieces of gum per day. The client then gradually reduces the number of pieces of gum chewed over 2 to 3 months.

Various nicotine transdermal systems (patches) are also available to aid withdrawal from smoking. Nicoderm CQ is worn for 24 hours a day; Nicotrol was formulated to be worn for 16 hours a day. Nicotrol was designed to mimic the individual's natural smoking pattern, which usually produces higher nicotine serum levels during the day and lower nicotine levels overnight. Theoretically, a decrease in

---

*For free copies of Helping Smokers Quit: A Guide for Nurses, contact AHRQ's Publication Clearinghouse at (800) 358-9295 or e-mail at ahrqpubs@ahrq.gov.

Evidence-Based Practice

Systematic Review of Nicotine Replacement Therapy

Assess every client's smoking history, and if positive, offer counseling and/or referral for smoking cessation.

The Cochrane Collaboration* published a critical review of 123 studies where NRT was compared to placebo, different formulations or doses, or no treatment, and where follow up was for at least 6 months. Nicotine replacement therapy studied included inhalers, tablets, chewing gum, transdermal patches, and/or nasal spray.

Abstinence from smoking after 6 months was more likely with all of the commercially available forms of NRT. NRT increases quit rates approximately 1.5- to 2-fold regardless of setting. The likelihood for quitting appears higher with the use of nasal spray, inhaled nicotine, and sublingual tablet or lozenge than with gum or transdermal patch, but all forms were associated with improved quit rates.

The use of NRT should be preferentially directed to smokers who are motivated to quit and have high levels of nicotine dependence. There is little evidence about the role of NRT for individuals who smoke fewer than 10 to 15 cigarettes a day. The choice of which form of NRT to use should reflect client needs, tolerability, and cost considerations. Patches are likely to be easier to use than gum or nasal spray in primary care settings. Eight weeks of patch therapy is as effective as longer courses, and there is no evidence that tapered therapy is better than abrupt withdrawal. Wearing a patch only during waking hours is as effective as wearing it for 24 hours a day. If gum is used, it may be offered on a fixed dose or on an ad-lib basis. For highly nicotine-dependent smokers who failed with 2-mg gum, 4-mg gum should be offered. There is no current evidence to suggest that routine use of a nicotine patch in doses higher than 22 mg/24 hours or of combinations of different forms of NRT are more effective in achieving long-term abstinence than standard-dose monotherapy. The effectiveness of NRT appears to be largely independent of the intensity of additional support to the smoker. Because all the trials of NRT reported so far have included at least some form of brief advice to the smoker, this represents the minimum of what should be offered to ensure its effectiveness. Provision of more intense levels of support, although beneficial in facilitating the likelihood of quitting, is not essential to the success of NRT. There is minimal evidence that a repeated course of NRT in smokers who have relapsed after recent use of nicotine patches will result in a small additional probability of quitting. NRT does not lead to an increased risk of adverse cardiovascular events in smokers with a history of cardiovascular disease. Finally, marketing claims by manufacturers of NRT products should reflect these points and avoid the possible misunderstanding by health professionals and members of the public that any of these products alone offers a magical cure for the smoking habit.

Critical Thinking Questions

- Given this critical review of the literature for evidence-based practice, what assessments of your client would you complete before starting smoking cessation therapy?
- Based on your assessment, what NRT would you recommend and why?

Data from Silagy, C., Lancaster, T., Stead, L., Mant, D., & Fowler, G. (2004). Nicotine replacement therapy for smoking cessation (Cochrane Review). *Cochrane Database of Systematic Reviews, 4,* and Silagy, C., Mant, D., Fowler, G., & Lancaster, T. (2001). Nicotine replacement therapy for smoking cessation (Cochrane Review). *The Cochran Library, 1.*
*Systematic evidence-based evaluations of existing literature are conducted by a number of researchers and practitioners. The Cochrane Collaboration is an international not-for-profit organization that supports such evidence-based reviews and publishes data via its website, www.cochrane.org, or via other electronic media/medical library services.

---

nicotine serum levels during the night will not affect the client's sleeping patterns. A potential disadvantage is that this drug-free period may result in an early morning craving for a cigarette. Nicotine transdermal systems in combination with cognitive-behavioral therapy are more effective in adolescents than nicotine gum (Moolchan et al., 2005):

Brand Name	Dosage per Patch*	Recommended Duration of Use
Nicotrol Step 1	15 mg/16 hr/day	6-8 weeks
Nicotrol Step 2	10 mg/16 hr/day	2 weeks
Nicotrol Step 3	5 mg/16 hr/day	2 weeks
Nicoderm Step 1	21 mg/24 hr	6 weeks
Nicoderm Step 2	14 mg/24 hr	2 weeks
Nicoderm Step 3	7 mg/24 hr	2 weeks

Data from *Drug facts and comparisons* (58th ed.). (2005). St. Louis: Facts and Comparisons.

Nicotine nasal sprays are comparable in efficacy to the gum and patches but have a faster onset of action. They administer 1 mg of nicotine per two sprays to the nasal membrane; the maximum dosage is 5 mg/hr or 40 mg/day. The nicotine inhaler is used in a similar manner with between 5 and 16 inhalations used daily. The U.S. Food and Drug Administration recommends that the spray be used for at least 3 months but for no longer than 6 months because it is possible to become dependent on the spray. Similar caution is recommended for use of the inhaler.

Refer to nicotine monograph on p. 426 for pharmacokinetics and adverse effects. See the Management of Drug Overdose box on p. 427 for other symptoms and for treatment of overdose.

✱ What is the role of the nurse in smoking cessation?

Assessment Before initiating NRT, assess a client's smoking history and cardiovascular status because the action of catecholamine on the heart will result in increased heart rate and blood pressure. Temporomandibular joint disorder might also be aggravated by chewing nicotine gum. Nicotine smoking-cessation therapy is contraindicated in pregnant women because it may cause fetal harm. Smoking will decrease the effects of acetaminophen, caffeine, oxazepam (Serax), pentazocine (Talwin), propranolol (Inderal), propoxyphene (Darvon), and theophylline (Theo-Dur) because it increases drug metabolism. Smoking cessation will generally reverse this effect. Smoking and nicotine also increase cortisol and catecholamine levels; therefore therapy with the adrenergic agonists or blocking agents may necessitate a dosage adjustment based on the individual's response.

Nursing Diagnosis Clients participating in nicotine replacement smoking-cessation therapy may have any of these nursing diagnoses: risk for injury to mouth, teeth, or dental work related to viscosity of the gum; impaired comfort related to headache, increased watering of the mouth, jaw-muscle ache, fast heartbeat, or sore throat or mouth; ineffective health maintenance related to negative health habits; impaired skin integrity related to localized reaction to the transdermal patch; disturbed sleep pattern (insomnia); and disturbed thought processes (unusual irritability).

Planning During NRT, the client will:
- Maintain compliance with NRT
- Effectively manage the therapeutic regimen with supportive nonpharmacologic measures (e.g., cigarette substitutes [chewing gum], positive activity, and others)
- Cease smoking

Implementation

Monitoring Monitor the client for these nursing diagnoses and for symptoms of nicotine toxicity.

Intervention Maintain supportive contact with client and provide counseling as required.

Education Provide information on the health consequences of smoking. Education of the client for NRT depends on the nicotine vehicle.

Gum A client should discontinue use and consult with the health care provider or dentist if the gum sticks to dental work. Excessive chewing may lead to some temporomandibular joint discomfort. A client may use sugarless hard candies between doses of gum to meet the need for oral stimulation and to relieve oral discomfort. Because an overdose of nicotine can be fatal, particularly in small children, the gum should be kept out of the reach of children. Many pieces chewed at once or in rapid succession may lead to an overdose in an adult; however, the consequences of overdose may be mitigated by the early nausea and vomiting that generally occur with excessive nicotine intake.

Transdermal System The patch is placed on a nonhairy, clean, dry, and intact area of the front or back torso or the outer aspect of the upper arm. It should be removed from its sealed pouch just before application or it will lose efficacy. The protective liner is removed from the sticky side of the patch; touching this side of the patch as little as possible, the patch is applied to the selected skin site. The patch is pressed to the skin with the palm of the hand for approximately 10 seconds to ensure that it sticks well, especially around the edges. The previously used patch is folded in half with the sticky side together and is placed in the newly opened pouch of the replacement patch. The pouch is thrown in the trash, away from children and pets. Nicotine can be very toxic, and the patches contain enough nicotine to poison children and pets. If a child plays with a patch, take it away from the child and contact a poison control center or health center immediately.

Washing hands immediately after patch application is essential because any nicotine on the hands could get into the eyes and cause irritation. The client should apply a new patch every 24 hours, at approximately the same time each day, selecting a different site. Water will not harm the patch; the client may swim, shower, or use a hot tub while wearing a patch. If it should come off, a new patch is to be applied to a new site. In this case the patch may be changed to continue the client's usual 24-hour schedule. The skin under the patch may redden but should not stay red for more than a day after the patch is removed. If the patch site becomes swollen or very red, patches should be discontinued and a prescriber should be consulted.

Nicotine is linked to low-birth-weight infants and to a decrease in fetal breathing movements, possibly as the result of decreased placental perfusion. Consequently, women of childbearing age should be advised to use effective birth control to avoid pregnancy while taking nicotine-based products.

Evaluation Evaluating a client's progress toward smoking cessation should occur at least monthly, and the efficacy of the gum or the transdermal systems in the therapy program should be determined. Treatment should be discontinued if a client is still smoking after 6 months of gum therapy or 4 weeks of transdermal patch therapy, because it is unlikely that this attempt will be successful. With successful nicotine therapy, the client is no longer smoking and denies any adverse effects of the NRT.

Nicotinic Agonists at the Neuromuscular Junction

Agents that stimulate the nicotinic receptors of the neuromuscular junction alter skeletal muscle action (Figure 21-2). Although not limited to action at the neuromuscular junction, physostigmine is used to terminate neuromuscular blocking agents in general surgery, and edrophonium is used to diagnose and treat myasthenia gravis. Organophosphate poisoning and nerve gas exposures also act at the neuromuscular junction (see the Pharmacologic Issues in an Age of Terrorism box on p. 432).

Muscarinic Agonists

Cholinergic drugs that serve to stimulate muscarinic receptors are used to modify involuntary functions innervated by the parasympathetic nervous system (Figure

Somatic

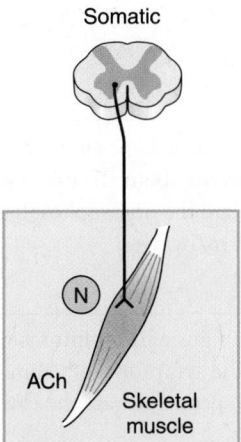

FIGURE 21-2 Stimulation of nicotinic receptors of the neuromuscular junction. *Ach,* Acetylcholine; *N,* nicotinic receptor.

21-3). Bethanechol is a classic example of a muscarinic agonist. Therapeutic uses for muscarinic agonists include the following:

- Stimulating the intestine and bladder postoperatively, thus increasing peristalsis and urination
- Stimulating the bladder for clients with spinal cord injuries and urinary retention
- Lowering intraocular pressure in clients with glaucoma
- Promoting salivation and sweating

✴ **T.L. is a 38-year-old veteran with spinal cord injury and urinary retention secondary to neurogenic bladder. He receives bethanechol (Urecholine) 50 mg three times daily.**

✴ **How does bethanechol work?**

Bethanechol is a synthetic choline ester with actions similar to those of acetylcholine. It produces stimulation of the parasympathetic nervous system. It has predominant muscarinic action with particular selectivity on the detrusor muscle of the urinary bladder and smooth muscle of the GI tract. Hence contraction of the smooth muscle of the bladder is sufficiently strong to initiate micturition and empty the urinary bladder. In the GI tract, the drug stimulates gastric motility, increases gastric tone, and often restores impaired peristaltic activity of the esophagus, stomach, and intestine. It also promotes defecation. Unlike acetylcholine, bethanechol is not destroyed by cholinesterase, making its effects more prolonged than that of the natural neurotransmitter. Therapeutic test doses in normal human subjects have demonstrated little effect on heart rate, blood pressure, or peripheral circulation. However, if a client experiences adverse effects of cholinergic overstimulation (flushing of the skin, headache, severe hypotension, hypothermia, bradycardia, nausea and vomiting, abdominal cramps, bloody diarrhea, shock, or cardiac arrest), atropine is the antidote. The nurse should take caution when T.L. moves from a lying to a sitting or standing position because orthostatic hypotension is a common adverse effect of bethanechol. The expected outcome of bethanechol therapy is that T.L.

Parasympathetic

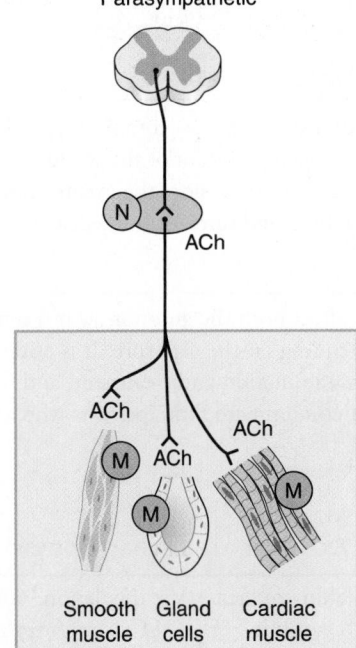

FIGURE 21-3 Cholinergic stimulation of muscarinic receptors in the parasympathetic system. *Ach,* Acetylcholine; *M,* muscarinic receptors; *N,* nicotinic receptors.

will be able to urinate without experiencing urinary retention or any adverse effects of to the drug.

✴🔲 bethanechol [be **than** e kole]
(Urecholine, Duvoid🍁)

Indications

In general, bethanechol has been replaced by more effective drugs, but it is available in the United States for the treatment of postoperative and postpartum nonobstructive urinary retention, and for neurogenic atony of the urinary bladder associated with retention. Although not indicated on its U.S. product labeling, bethanechol has also been used to relieve postoperative abdominal distention and gastric atony or stasis and reflux esophagitis associated with decreased pressure of the lower esophageal sphincter.

Pharmacokinetics/Dosing

Despite being poorly absorbed from the GI tract, bethanechol is effective orally. It is widely distributed to organs innervated by the parasympathetic nervous system. Onset of action is within 30 to 90 minutes of oral administration, peak effect is within 1 hour, and duration of action is up to 6 hours, depending on the dose administered. If given subcutaneously, the onset of action is within 5 to 15 minutes, peak effect is within 15 to 30 minutes, and duration of action is approximately 2 hours. The route of excretion is currently unknown. The typical dose of bethanechol in adults is 10 to 50 mg orally two to four times daily.

Adverse Effects

Bethanechol shares an adverse-effect profile similar to other muscarinic agonists, including tachycardia, flushing, headache, abdominal cramping, diarrhea, nausea, vomiting, salivation, tearing, bronchospasm, and diaphoresis.

✴ **T.L. is able to void more completely since the initiation of bethanechol. However, the nurse notes that T.L. is diaphoretic and flushed and complains of stom-**

Pharmacologic Issues in an Age of Terrorism

Chemical Warfare

Chemical weapons are the most common type of unconventional warfare, which also includes biologic and nuclear weapons. It is estimated that as much as a third of the world's arsenal consists of chemical weapons. Concerns about the use of these agents for terrorist attacks have escalated since the events of September 11, 2001. Among these agents are the organophosphates, VX, and the G agents (sarin, tabun, and soman). Immediate care, including decontamination, could save many lives.

Nerve Agents

Nerve agents affect both the autonomic and central nervous systems. The extent of the signs and symptoms may be localized or systemic, depending on the exposure. It is critical that health care providers recognize the symptoms of chemical agents in order to begin decontamination and treatment, and for their own protection. Many of these agents saturate the clothing as well as the skin, and can contaminate those persons who are treating the victims.

NAME/ SYMBOL	MEANS OF EXPOSURE	LETHAL DOSAGE	RATE OF ACTION	EFFECTS	ANTIDOTES/METHODS OF TREATMENT
Tabun (GA)	Skin contact and/or inhalation	Via inhalation: 400 LCt_{50} mg/min/m^3 Via skin exposure: 1000 LD_{50}	Very rapid Incapacitating effects occur within 1-10 min; lethal effects occur within 10-15 min	Effects seen in eyes (contraction of pupils, pain, dim or blurred vision), nose (runny nose), and airways (chest tightness) Nausea and vomiting also possible Twitching/seizures result when skeletal muscle reached Fluctuations in heart rate Loss of consciousness and seizure activity can occur within 1 min of exposure in cases of exposure to high concentration of agent Eventual paralysis, death	4 steps to management of exposure to nerve agents: decontamination; ventilation; antidotes; supportive therapy Therapeutic drug options: Atropine and pralidoxime chloride (autoinjectors packaged together in kits provided to military personnel) Diazepam, lorazepam (for seizures)
Sarin (GB)	Skin contact and/or inhalation	Via inhalation: 100 LCt_{50} mg/min/m^3 Via skin exposure: 1700 LD_{50}	Very rapid Incapacitating effects occur within 1-10 min; lethal effects occur within 2-15 min		
Soman (GD)	Skin contact and/or inhalation	Via inhalation: 70 LCt_{50} mg/min/m^3 Via skin exposure: 50 LD_{50}	Very rapid Incapacitating effects occur within 1-10 min; lethal effects occur within 1-15 min		
VX	Skin contact and/or inhalation	Via inhalation: 50 LCt_{50} mg/min/m^3 Via skin exposure: 10 LD_{50}	Rapid Incapacitating effects occur within 1-10 min; lethal effects occur within 4-42 hr		
Novichok agents	Novichok 5 estimated to exceed the toxicity effectiveness of VX by 5 to 8 times Novichok 7 estimated to exceed the toxicity effectiveness of soman by 10 times		Very rapid	Assumed to be similar to the effects of other nerve agents listed above	Assumed to be similar to treatment methods for other nerve agents listed above

Modified from http://faculty.ncwc.edu/toconnor/429/429lect18.htm

LCt_{50}, Lethal mass exposure dose; LD_{50}, median lethal dose.

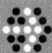 **Pharmacologic Issues in an Age of Terrorism**

Chemical Warfare—cont'd

Essential to recognizing exposure to a nerve agent is the appearance of multiple clients with similar signs and symptoms (Martin & Lobert, 2003). Because many of those affected may not be aware of the initial exposure, a detailed health history is important. The agent should be identified, but this may not be possible. Treatment begins with decontamination, the rapid removal of the agent. It is recommended by the Centers for Disease Control and Prevention (CDC) that health care personnel use chemical protective attire and butyl rubber gloves, as well as a positive-pressure self-contained breathing apparatus if the agent is vapor or liquid. Decontamination of exposed clients must occur before entry into the hospital to avoid contaminating the facility. Clothing is removed as quickly as possible to remove the agent and double bagged and disposed of appropriately. Thorough cleansing of the affected areas with soap and water or a 1:9 solution of household bleach and water. Eyes, mucous membranes, and wounds are flushed with water or normal saline solution (http://www.bt.cdc.gov/planning/personalcleaningfacts.asp).

Recommendations for Emergency Department Management of Nerve Agent Therapy

First responders, paramedics, firefighters, police and nurses will likely be provided with single-dose prefilled autoinjectors containing 2 mg of atropine or 600 mg of pralidoxime chloride for treatment on the scene. See the following table for recommendations for the initial treatment of nerve agent exposure at the hospital. Atropine, an anticholinergic drug, is administered to counteract the muscarinic effects of the nerve agents caused by excessive acetylcholine. Pralidoxime chloride is an adjunct to atropine and should be given as soon as possible to counteract the nicotinic effects. Diazepam is given for seizure prophylaxis or control. Supplemental oxygen, suctioning, and monitoring of vital signs, electrolyte levels, and cardiac rhythm are necessary. Mechanical ventilation may be required. There may be long-term neuropsychological effects of exposure to nerve agents; these may be difficult to distinguish from posttraumatic stress disorder.

| | ANTIDOTES | | |
CLIENT AGE	MILD/MODERATE SYMPTOMS*	SEVERE SYMPTOMS†	OTHER TREATMENT
Infant (age 0-2 yr)	atropine: 0.05 mg/kg IM or 0.02 mg/kg IV 2-PAM Cl: 15 mg/kg IV slowly	atropine: 0.1 mg/kg IM or 0.02 mg/kg IV 2-PAM Cl: 15 mg/kg IV slowly	Assisted ventilation as needed Repeat atropine (2 mg IM or 1 mg IM for infants) at 5- to 10-min intervals until secretions have diminished and breathing is comfortable or airway resistance has returned to near normal
Child (age 2-10 yr)	atropine: 1 mg IM 2-PAM Cl: 15 mg/kg IV slowly	atropine: 2 mg IM 2-PAM Cl: 15 mg/kg IV slowly	
Adolescent (older than age 10 yr)	atropine: 2 mg IM 2-PAM Cl: 15 mg/kg IV slowly	atropine: 4 mg IM 2-PAM Cl: 15 mg/kg IV slowly	Phentolamine for 2-PAM Cl–induced hypertension: 5 mg IV for adults; 1 mg IV for children
Adult	atropine: 2-4 mg IM 2-PAM Cl: 15 mg/kg (1 g) IV slowly	atropine: 6 mg IM 2-PAM Cl: 15 mg/kg (1 g) IV slowly	Diazepam for seizures: 0.2-0.5 mg IV for infants and children younger than age 5 yr; 1 mg IV for children older than age 5 yr; 5 mg IV for adults
Older adults, frail	atropine: 1 mg IM 2-PAM Cl: 5-10 mg/kg IV slowly	atropine: 2 mg IM 2-PAM Cl: 5-10 mg/kg IV slowly	

Modified from Agency for Toxic Substances & Disease Registry (http://www.atsdr.cdc.gov/MHMI/mmg166.pdf).
IM, Intramuscularly; *IV,* intravenously; *2-PAM Cl,* 2-pralidoxime chloride.
*Mild/moderate symptoms include localized sweating, muscle fasciculations, nausea, vomiting, weakness, and dyspnea.
†Severe symptoms include unconsciousness, seizures, apnea, and flaccid paralysis.

ach upset and loose stools. In addition, his pillow is often wet with saliva.

✴ Could T.L.'s symptoms be associated with muscarinic agonist drugs?

Muscarinic agonist drugs such as bethanechol often produce a pattern of effects often remembered with the acronyms "SLUDGE" or "DUMBELS":

SLUDGE

Salivation (or sweating)
Lacrimation
Urination
Diarrhea
Gastrointestinal upset
Eye—miosis (constricted pupil; sometimes remembered as emesis)

DUMBELS

Diarrhea
Urination
Miosis
Bronchoconstriction
Emesis
Lacrimation
Salivation

Most of these effects are dose related, but are not uncommon when any drug serves to increase activity of acetylcholine or mimics the action of acetylcholine at muscarinic receptors. While not commonly observed with usual doses of bethanechol, muscarinic agonists may also serve to decrease heart rate, lower blood pressure and induce bronchospasm. As such, they should be used carefully in individuals with cardiac or respiratory problems. In the case of T.L., his adverse effects may be reduced with the use of a lower dose of bethanechol (e.g., 10 to 25 mg three times daily).

✳ What is the role of the indirect-acting cholinergic drugs?

The indirect-acting cholinergic drugs are anticholinesterases (also referred to as cholinesterase inhibitors); they prolong the effect of acetylcholine by inhibiting the action of the enzyme cholinesterase. Anticholinesterase agents (e.g., neostigmine, physostigmine) exert their influence on both muscarinic and nicotinic sites. They are used to treat myasthenia gravis and glaucoma (see Chapters 23 and 42, respectively). They are also used postoperatively for urinary retention and GI ileus (Thompson, 2005). Physostigmine salicylate is used for anticholinergic substance toxicity and overdose.

Myasthenia gravis is a condition characterized by weakness of the skeletal muscles innervated by the somatic efferent fibers. This disease affects cholinergic transmission, and the anticholinesterase drugs are used because they elevate the concentration of acetylcholine at the myoneural junctions. The prolonged activity of the neurohormone at these sites results in a dramatic increase in muscle strength and function. A more extensive discussion of myasthenia gravis and its treatment is found in Chapter 23. (See also Figure 20-3 for receptor sites for neurohumoral transmission.)

An important group of anticholinesterase inhibitors are the centrally acting agents used to reduce cognitive decline for clients with Alzheimer-type dementia. Agents in this class include donepezil (Aricept), galantamine (Reminyl), rivastigmine (Exelon), and tacrine (Cognex). These agents serve to inhibit the enzymatic degradation of acetylcholine at both central and peripheral sites. SLUDGE-type adverse effects are common with these agents secondary to their ability to increase activity of acetylcholine at peripheral muscarinic sites. A further discussion is found in Chapter 23.

✳ What other uses are there for cholinergic agents?

Unfortunately, agents that act to increase cholinergic action are not limited to therapeutic drugs. A number of toxins and agents used in chemical terrorism can irreversibly bind to and inhibit acetylcholinesterase. Life-threatening muscarinic effects (SLUDGE/DUMBELS) and nicotinic effects (skeletal muscle contraction including contraction of respiratory muscles) are common with these substances. High doses of organophosphates (e.g., accidents involving insecticides) can produce these effects. Nerve gases such as sarin, soman, and tabun are more ominous and can be lethal with relatively low exposures. On March 20, 1995, terrorists re-leased sarin nerve gas at several points in the Tokyo subway system, killing 11 and injuring more than 5500 people.

Treatment for these exposures includes removing the victim from the exposure, preventing exposure to responders and health care personnel, decontamination, administration of antidotes, and supportive care. Two specific types of antidotes are used, including anticholinergics (e.g., atropine [see the Pharmacologic Issues in an Age of Terrorism box on p. 433]) and agents that inactivate the bond between the toxin and acetylcholinesterase (e.g., pralidoxime [Protopam]). A further discussion of pharmacologic issues in an age of terrorism is presented in the Pharmacologic Issues in an Age of Terrorism box on p. 433. Refer to the Technology Link box below for updates.

✳ How are the cholinergic blocking agents differentiated?

Like the agonists at acetylcholine receptors, the antagonists to cholinergic receptors (parasympatholytics) are categorized as either nicotinic or muscarinic blockers. Nicotinic blockers are further differentiated by their site of action (ganglion or neuromuscular junction).

Ganglionic Nicotinic Antagonists

Ganglionic-blocking drugs block the action of acetylcholine on the ganglion cells by competing with acetylcholine at the synapse of the autonomic ganglia in both the parasympathetic and sympathetic systems (Figure 21-4, *A* and *B*). This results in reduced impulse transmission from preganglionic to postganglionic fibers in both parasympathetic and sympathetic nerves. A blockade of sympathetic ganglia abolishes vasoconstrictor tone; the blood vessels dilate and arterial blood pressure falls. Multiple adverse effects are

---

✳✳ Technology Link

Chemical Warfare

Center for Infectious Disease Research & Policy, University of Minnesota (http://www.cidrap.umn.edu/cidrap/content/other/chem/readings/)

Provides selected reading citations for chemical weapon awareness.

Centers for Disease Control and Prevention (http://www.bt.cdc.gov/)

General information on emergency preparedness and response, as well as in-depth information about specific agents.

Medline Plus (http://www.nlm.nih.gov/medlineplus/chemical weapons.html)

A service of the U.S. National Library of Medicine and the National Institutes of Health. A general overview of chemical weapons with details on specific agents.

associated with these agents, including nausea, vomiting, dilated pupils, dry mouth, impotency, tachycardia, angina, and urinary retention. Mecamylamine hydrochloride (Inversine) and trimethaphan camsylate (Arfonad) are two examples of ganglionic blockers. While historically used for severe hypertension, they are no longer in common use.

Neuromuscular Nicotinic Antagonists (Neuromuscular Blockers)

Drugs that block nicotinic receptors at the neuromuscular junction are called neuromuscular blockers (Figure 21-5). These agents are primarily used in surgery or during procedures where voluntary skeletal muscle blockade is desirable. The neuromuscular blocking agents are further characterized as depolarizing and nondepolarizing. The depolarizing agents cause brief excitation to the muscle by allowing opening of ion channels. Initial use is sometimes accompanied by brief muscle contractions. Neuromuscular blockers do not cause any sedation, are not analgesic, and have no effect on cognition. *It is imperative that clients who receive these agents receive respiratory support before and during administration,* because these agents will cause paralysis of respiratory muscles. In addition, clients are likely to be quite anxious and *must receive sedatives and anxiolytics before and during neuromuscular blocker administration to prevent anxiety and to impair memory of the perioperative period.* Neuromuscular blockers must not be confused with skeletal muscle relaxants such as benzodiazepines and baclofen, which relax but do not block muscle action.

The nondepolarizing agents do not produce an initial excitatory effect. There are many more nondepolarizing neuromuscular blockers that prevent muscle contraction. The prototype nondepolarizing agent is curare or tubocurarine, which has historically been used by native South American cultures as dart poisons to cause paralysis to wild animals and simplify capture. Tubocurarine is no longer readily available for clinical use. Among the more common nondepolarizing neuromuscular blockers used today are atracurium (Tracrium), cisatracurium (Nimbex), mivacurium (Mivacron), pancuronium (Pavulon), rocuronium (Zemuron), and vecuronium (Norcuron). See the Pregnancy Safety box on p. 436.

Choice of agent often depends on the drug's duration of action. Short procedures, such as intubation, often can be successfully implemented with the one-time administration of a short-acting succinylcholine. Longer-acting agents are used during surgical procedures, or to allow intubated clients to tolerate mechanical ventilation in intensive care. A peripheral nerve stimulator is often used to monitor the effect of these agents (Box 21-2).

★ ▪▪ succinylcholine [suk sin ill **koe** leen]
(Anectine)
Succinylcholine (Anectine) is a depolarizing neuromuscular blocker that has a quick onset and a short duration of action.
Indications
Succinylcholine is used to facilitate endotracheal intubation and to relax skeletal muscles during surgery.
Pharmacokinetics/Dosing
Succinyl choline is usually administered intravenously, with an onset of action within 30 to 60 seconds, and a duration of action of about 5 minutes after intravenous (IV) administration. It is rapidly metabolized by plasma pseudocholinesterase. The usual dose for facilitating intubation in adults is 1 to 1.5 mg/kg. The pharmacokinetics of succinylcholine and other neuromuscular blockers is presented in Table 21-2.
Adverse Effects
Respiratory paralysis is an expected effect of neuromuscular blockers, and clients must have respiratory support. Adverse effects include bradycardia, excessive salivation, and increased ocular pressure.

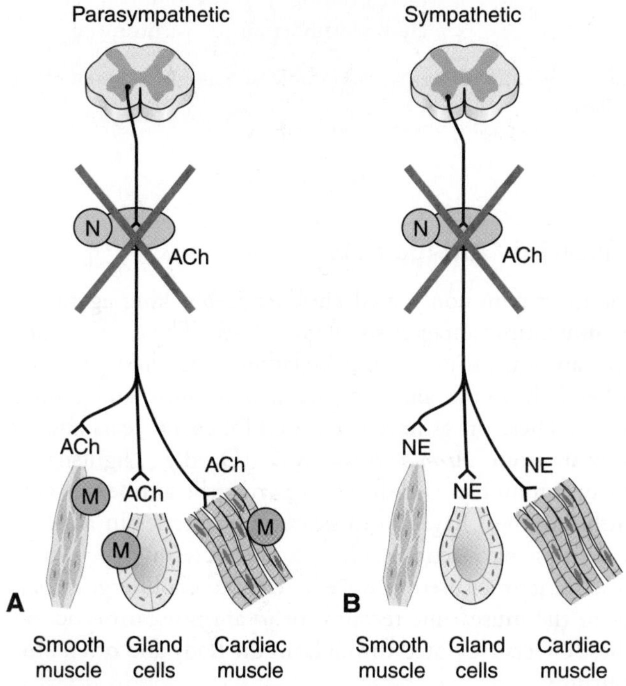

FIGURE 21-4 Ganglionic blocking drugs block the action of acetylcholine at the nicotinic receptor on the ganglion cells. Ganglionic blockers compete with acetylcholine at the synapse of the autonomic ganglia in both the parasympathetic systems **(A)** and the sympathetic system **(B)**. *Ach,* Acetylcholine; *M,* muscarinic receptors; *N,* nicotinic receptors; *NE,* norepinephrine.

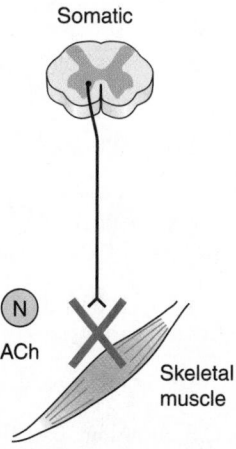

FIGURE 21-5 Nicotinic receptors blockers act at the neuromuscular junction. *N,* Nicotinic receptor.

BOX 21-2 USE OF PERIPHERAL NERVE STIMULATORS IN EVALUATING DOSE AND EFFECT OF NEUROMUSCULAR BLOCKING AGENTS

Neuromuscular blocking agents (NMBAs) are commonly used in many intensive care units to enhance the care of critically ill clients (Murray et al., 2002). Major uses of NMBAs include facilitating endotracheal intubation and mechanical ventilation, decreasing elevated intracranial pressure and tetany, and facilitating diagnostic and therapeutic procedures (Liebelt, 2000). NMBAs have varying onsets of effect, duration, and metabolism. Although their onsets are rapid and their half-lives are short, overdosing may cause prolonged blocking, an inability to wean from the ventilator, a prolonged rehabilitation, and subsequent increased length of hospital stay. Use of a peripheral nerve stimulator (PNS) is essential for the appropriate monitoring and titration of NMBAs by nurses in acute care settings.

The PNS is a small, battery-operated device that sends electrical signals through a nerve to test the capability of that nerve to affect muscular activity (Henderson, 1999). The current output receptacles may consist of metal balls or lead wires. The ulnar nerve is the site usually chosen for measurement.

The most recommended method of monitoring a critical care client under neuromuscular blockage is the train-of-four (TOF). The TOF refers to four series of electrical impulses that are delivered at an ample current. The number of twitches in response to the four stimuli represents the percentage of neuromuscular blockade. For example, four twitches represent less than 75% of blockade; three twitches represent approximately 75% of blockade; two twitches represent 75% to 80% of blockade; one twitch represents 90% blockade; and an absence of twitches represents 100% of blockade. When titrating the NMBA, the goal is to get two twitches or 75% to 80% of blockade. Anything more than two twitches indicates inadequate paralysis and anything less than two indicates that too large a paralytic dose has been administered (Loyola & Dreher, 2003). Titrating the neuromuscular blockade to the lowest effective dose for the least amount of time by using PNS and concurrently monitoring clinical indicators minimizes complications.

TABLE 21-2 NEUROMUSCULAR BLOCKERS

Agent	Onset (minutes)	Half-Life (minutes)	Duration in minutes (bolus dose)
DEPOLARIZING			
succinylcholine (Anectine)	0.5-1	Unknown	4-8
NONDEPOLARIZING			
mivacurium (Mivacron)	1.5-3	2	12-20
atracurium (Tracrium)	2-3	20	20-45
cisatracurium (Nimbex)	2-3	20-30	40-60
rocuronium (Zemuron)	1-1.5	60-70	30-60
vecuronium (Norcuron)	2-3	50-80	20-40
doxacurium (Nuromax)	4-6	100-200	100-160
pancuronium (Pavulon)	3-5	100-170	60-100
pipecuronium (Arduan)	3-5	120-180	60-120
tubocurarine	3-5	100-120	60-90

Modified from Lacy, C.F., Armstrong L.L., Goldman M.P., Lance L.L. (2004). *Lexi-Comp's Drug Information Handbook*, (12th ed.). Hudson, OH: Lexi-Comp.

PREGNANCY SAFETY
NEUROMUSCULAR BLOCKERS

Category	Drug
B	cisatracurium, rocuronium
C	atracurium, doxacurium, mivacurium, pancuronium, pipecuronium, succinylcholine, tubocurarine, vecuronium

Data from *Mosby's drug consult* (15th ed.). (2005). St. Louis, Mosby.

Muscarinic Antagonists

The most commonly used cholinergic-blocking agents are the muscarinic antagonists (Figure 21-6). The classic prototype antimuscarinic is the belladonna alkaloid atropine. Other belladonna alkaloids are hyoscyamine and scopolamine. These drugs have been used for many years and are derived from *Atropa belladonna* (Deadly Nightshade). Many commonly used drugs (e.g., tricyclic antidepressants, antihistamines) have antimuscarinic properties in addition to their primary actions. The less precise term *autocholinergic* is sometimes used; it usually refers to cholinergic blockade at the muscarinic receptor or to antimuscarinic action. These effects are noted throughout the body and often limit their use.

✱ **What are the effects and adverse effects of atropine?**
Atropine is a competitive antagonist at muscarinic receptor sites. It has very little effect on the actions of acetylcholine at nicotinic receptor sites. At autonomic ganglia, where transmission normally involves the action of acetylcholine, relatively high doses of atropine are re-

Parasympathetic

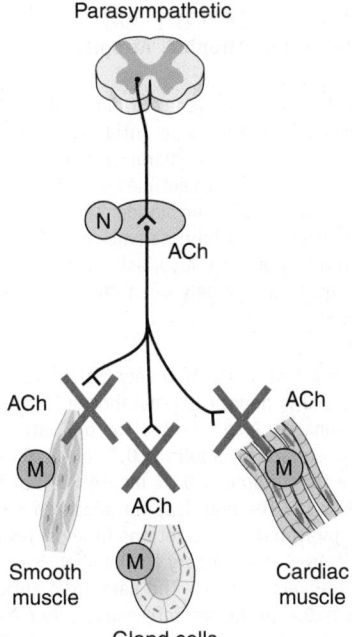

FIGURE 21-6 Receptor activity of cholinergic-blocking agents that are muscarinic antagonists. *Ach,* acetylcholine; *M,* muscarinic receptors; *N,* nicotinic receptors.

PREGNANCY SAFETY CHOLINERGIC AND ANTICHOLINERGIC DRUGS	
Category	Drug
B	atropine, dicyclomine, glycopyrrolate
C	ambenonium, bethanechol, isoflurophate, neostigmine, physostigmine, pilocarpine, pyridostigmine, scopolamine
D	nicotine

Data from *Mosby's drug consult* (15th ed.). (2005). St. Louis, Mosby.

quired to produce even a partial block. At the neuromuscular junctions of the somatic nervous system, where the receptors are exclusively nicotinic, extremely high doses of atropine are required to produce any degree of block. See Figure 20-3 for nicotinic sites on the ganglia or parasympathetic and sympathetic nerve divisions, and for nicotinic sites on effector organs (skeletal muscle) of the somatic motor system.

Atropine can produce a wide range of dose-dependent effects because of a vast distribution of parasympathetic nerves in the body. Small doses depress salivary and bronchial secretions and sweating. Large doses cause mydriasis (dilation of the pupils), inhibit accommodation of the eyes, and increase heart rate by blocking vagal effects of the heart. Larger doses inhibit micturition and decrease the tone and motility of the gut by inhibiting parasympathetic control of both the urinary bladder and the GI tract. Still larger doses are required to inhibit gastric secretion and motility. The major actions are listed here; see also the Pregnancy Safety box above.

Effects on the Eye With atropine, the pupil is dilated (mydriasis), and the ciliary muscle (muscle of accommodation) is relaxed (cycloplegia). The sphincter muscle of the iris and the ciliary muscle are both innervated by cholinergic nerve fibers and therefore are affected by atropine. Because the sphincter muscle is unable to contract normally, the radial muscle of the iris causes the pupil to dilate. Pupil dilation may reduce the outflow of aqueous humor, causing a rise in intraocular pressure. This is a hazardous situation for clients with glaucoma (angle closure). These effects in the eye are brought about by both local and systemic administration of atropine, although the usual single therapeutic dose of oral or parenteral atropine has little effect on the eye. Photophobia occurs after the pupil is dilated; when the drug has reached its full effect, the usual reflexes to light and accommodation disappear.

Ophthalmic preparations should be included in the review of the client's current medications because an ophthalmic preparation may cause systemic effects (*USP DI,* 2005). The systemic absorption of ophthalmic medications resulting in undesirable adverse effects has been reported with atropine and a number of other eye preparations.

Effects on the Skin and Mucous Membranes Because the sweat glands of the skin are supplied by sympathetic cholinergic nerves, atropine decreases or abolishes their activity. This causes the skin to become hot and dry. Furthermore, the flow of secretions from glands lining the respiratory tract is reduced and, as a result, drying of the mucous membranes of the mouth, nose, pharynx, and bronchi occurs. Clients who have been given atropine, particularly for preoperative preparation, often describe having a dry mouth and thirst.

Effects on the Respiratory System Secretions of the nose, pharynx, and bronchial tubes are decreased with the use of atropine. The muscles of the bronchial tubes relax, and the airway widens to ease breathing. Atropine and scopolamine are less effective than epinephrine as bronchodilators and are seldom used for asthma.

Effects on the Cardiovascular System When low doses of atropine are given or an IV dose is administered slowly, the cardiac rate is temporarily and slightly slowed because of the central action of the drug on the cardiac center in the medulla (paradoxical bradycardia). Larger IV doses given rapidly will block the vagal effect on the sinoatrial node and atrioventricular junction and increase heart rate.

Atropine has little or no effect on blood pressure when given in therapeutic doses. This is expected because most vascular beds lack significant cholinergic innervation. Large (and sometimes ordinary) doses cause vasodilation of vessels in the skin of the face and neck. This may result from a direct dilator action or from histamine release. Reddening of the face and neck is seen, especially after large or toxic doses.

Effects on the Gastrointestinal Tract It appears that the amount and character of gastric secretion are little affected by atropine given in ordinary therapeutic doses. The secretion of acid in the stomach is presumably less under vagal control than under hormonal or chemical control. The effect of atropine on the secretion of the pancreas and intestinal glands is not therapeutically significant. Atropine and other belladonna alkaloids decrease tone and peristalsis in the stomach and small and large intestines. Atropine does not affect the secretion of bile but exerts a mildly antispasmodic effect in the gallbladder and bile ducts.

Effects on the Urinary Tract Atropine relaxes the ureter, especially when it has been in a state of spasm. Therapeutic doses decrease the tone of the fundus of the urinary bladder. Atropine relaxes a hypertonic detrusor muscle. It also causes constriction of the internal sphincter, which can produce urinary retention.

Effects on the Central Nervous System Atropine has prominent effects on the CNS and in large doses causes excitement and maniacal behavior. These behavioral effects suggest the existence of important cholinergic pathways and receptors within the CNS.

Small or moderate doses of atropine have little or no cerebral effect. Large or toxic doses cause restlessness, wakefulness, and talkativeness. This condition may develop into delirium and, finally, stupor and coma. The exalted, excited stage has sometimes been called a "belladonna jag." A rise in temperature is sometimes seen, especially in infants and young children. This is probably the result of suppressed sweating rather than action on the heat-regulating center.

Atropine has been used to diminish tremor in Parkinson's disease, perhaps because it reduces cholinergic synaptic transmission. Therapeutic doses of atropine stimulate the respiratory center and make breathing faster and sometimes deeper. When respiration is seriously depressed, atropine is not always reliable as a stimulant; in fact, it may deepen the depression. Large doses stimulate respiration but can also cause respiratory failure and death.

Small doses of atropine stimulate the vagus center in the medulla, causing primary slowing of the heart. The vasoconstrictor center is stimulated briefly and then depressed. Because depression follows soon after stimulation, atropine has been called a borderline stimulant of the CNS.

Topical Effects There is a slight amount of absorption when atropine or belladonna is applied to the skin, especially if it is an alcoholic preparation or in the form of a transdermal patch.

★ atropine sulfate [a troe peen]
(Atropine Sulfate, Isopto-Atropine, Atropisol)

Indications
IV atropine is used in the treatment of bradycardia, arteriovenous block, ventricular asystole, and as an antidote for organophosphate and nerve gas poisoning (see the Pharmacologic Issues in an Age of Terrorism box on p. 432). It is sometimes used in combination with other therapies to reduce bowel or bladder spasm. It has historically been used preoperatively to inhibit salivation and respiratory secretions, as an eye drop to produce mydriasis, and orally to inhibit salivation, but these uses have largely been replaced by agents with less widespread effects.

Pharmacokinetics/Dosing
Atropine is well-absorbed orally, is widely distributed to tissue (including the CNS), and is hepatically metabolized with an elimination half-life of approximately 2 to 3 hours. The oral anticholinergic dosage of atropine sulfate for adults is 0.3 to 1.2 mg every 4 to 6 hours. The dosage for children is 0.01 mg/kg PO (not to exceed 0.4 mg) every 4 to 6 hours. The oral dose for adults to prevent excessive salivation and respiratory tract secretions in anesthesia is 2 mg. The dose should be titrated as necessary to the client's response or to the appearance of adverse effects. The parenteral anticholinergic dosage for adults is 0.4 to 0.6 mg intramuscularly (IM), IV, or subcutaneously every 4 to 6 hours. The pediatric anticholinergic dose is 0.01 mg/kg subcutaneously (not to exceed 0.4 mg); the pediatric dose may be repeated every 4 to 6 hours if necessary. The parenteral dosage for adults to treat bradycardia (dysrhythmia) is 0.4 to 1 mg IV every 1 to 2 hours, up to a maximum of 2 mg; the pediatric dosage for dysrhythmia is 0.01 to 0.03 mg/kg IV.

Adverse Effects
Given the presence of muscarinic receptors throughout the body and the widespread distribution of atropine, it is not surprising that this drug produces numerous undesirable effects. Nontherapeutic responses to atropine include cardiac dysrhythmias, tachycardia, ataxia, delirium, confusion, nervousness, constipation, paralytic ileus, urinary retention, and increased ocular pressure with risk for angle-closure glaucoma. Refer to nursing management issues in the following section.

✴ What are the key nursing issues with the use of atropine?
Although atropine was the first anticholinergic used, its use has been replaced by other agents because of its adverse effects and toxicity related to systemic absorption and excellent CNS penetration. However, it is a classic example of an antimuscarinic agent and the nursing management associated with antimuscarinics and drugs from other classifications with antimuscarinic properties.

Assessment Use atropine with caution in older adults and in children younger than 6 years of age because they are more susceptible to adverse effects such as excitement, sleepiness, or confusion, even when prescribed within the normal dosage range. See the Special Considerations for Older Adults and Special Considerations for Children boxes on p. 439. Anticholinergics should be used with caution in individuals older than 40 years of age because of the risk of precipitating undiagnosed glaucoma. The use of atropine (or belladonna alkaloids) should be avoided in clients with a medical history of severe cardiac disease or tachycardia (increases heart rate), reflux esophagitis (decreased GI motility promotes gastric retention), obstructive disease states in the GI tract or intestinal atony (decreased motility may result in obstruction), urinary retention (aggravates symptoms), prostatic hypertrophy (aggravates symptoms), or myasthenia gravis (aggravates condition by inhibition of acetylcholine). Do not use in clients with open-angle glaucoma (mydriatic effect increases intraocular pressure), ulcerative colitis, or renal or hepatic disease (increases effects of drug). Administer systemic forms carefully to clients with chronic pulmonary disease because bronchial secretions may be sufficiently decreased to result in bronchial plugs. Use with caution in infants and young children and in children with blonde hair and blue eyes, Down's syndrome, spastic paralysis, or brain damage; these individuals tend to be more sensitive to the effects of the drug (*USP DI*, 2005). Review the client's current medication regimen for the risk of significant drug interactions, such as other drugs with anticholinergic properties that would have an additive effect.

Obtain a baseline assessment of the client's vital signs and urinary and bowel status. For older adults and debilitated clients, a mental status assessment is helpful in determining if the client is experiencing any drug-related drowsiness or CNS stimulation. A baseline ECG is required if the drug is used as an antidysrhythmic. A baseline intraocular pressure determination is indicated for clients undergoing long-term therapy.

Nursing Diagnosis The client receiving atropine therapy is at risk for the following nursing diagnoses/collaborative problems: hyperthermia related to the suppression of sweat gland activity; risk for injury related to blurred vision, dizziness, or light-headedness; impaired tissue integrity (irritation at injection site); disturbed thought processes (confusion, agitation); impaired comfort related to dry mouth or increased sensitivity of the eyes to light; urinary retention related to the antimuscarinic effects of the drug; constipation related to decreased motility of the GI tract; and the potential complications of allergic reaction and decreased cardiac output related to the ineffectiveness of the drug.

Planning During atropine therapy, the client will:
- Experience relief from symptoms for which the drug was prescribed.
- Effectively manage the therapeutic drug regimen, including knowledge of the medication, its adverse effects, and which adverse effects are reportable, and compliance with medication schedule.
- Be free of injury related to drug action or adverse effects.

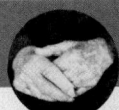

Special Considerations for Older Adults | ANTICHOLINERGIC AGENTS

- Older adults are highly susceptible to anticholinergic adverse effects, especially constipation, dry mouth, and urinary retention (usually in men).
- Avoid using anticholinergic agents in clients with narrow-angle glaucoma or a history of urinary retention.
- Memory impairment has been reported with continuous administration of these agents, especially in older clients.
- When usual adult dosages are administered, some older adults may experience a paradoxical reaction: hyperexcitability, agitation, confusion, and sedation.

- Chronic use decreases or inhibits the flow of saliva, which may contribute to oral discomfort, periodontal disease, and candidiasis.
- Overheating resulting in heat stroke has been reported in persons receiving anticholinergic drugs during vigorous exercise or in periods of hot weather.
- Blurred vision and/or increased sensitivity to light may occur.
- Anticholinergic dosing in older adults should begin with the lowest dosage, with gradual increases until maximum improvement is noted or intolerable adverse effects occur.

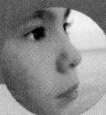

Special Considerations for Children | ANTICHOLINERGIC AGENTS

- Infants and young children are very susceptible to anticholinergic adverse effects.
- Closely monitor children with spastic paralysis or brain damage because they usually have an increased reaction to anticholinergic agents and thus require a dosage reduction.
- Anticholinergics, especially in high doses, may cause a paradoxical-type reaction of increased nervousness, confusion, and hyperexcitability.
- Anticholinergic drugs suppress sweat gland activity. Therefore children receiving these agents in environments where hot weather prevails or temperatures are

high have an increased risk of developing a rapid body temperature increase.
- Dosage adjustments are often necessary for infants and young children and in children with blonde hair, blue eyes, Down's syndrome, spastic paralysis, or brain damage because they usually have an increased response to this drug category. Flushing, increased temperature, irritability, increased pulse, and increased respiratory rate may occur (*USP DI*, 2005).
- Start with low dosages and increase gradually as needed and as tolerated.

Implementation

Monitoring Monitor the client's pulse, which is a sensitive indicator of the response to atropine. Be alert to any change in blood pressure, temperature, or respiration, particularly after IV administration. Electrocardiogram (ECG) recordings are monitored when atropine is used for dysrhythmias. Notify the prescriber of any significant changes. Observe older adults for excitement, agitation, and delirium. Assess for constipation, dryness of mouth and, in older men, urinary retention. Because of the mydriatic effects of atropine, intraocular pressure determinations should be performed at regular intervals for clients undergoing extended atropine therapy.

Intervention Administer oral preparations 30 to 60 minutes before meals. Have physostigmine on hand to treat atropine overdose.

Education Inform client of the possible adverse effects of atropine. Advise the use of sugarless gum and candy, ice, or saliva substitutes to relieve dry mouth. Instruct the client to avoid alcohol and other CNS depressants while taking atropine.

The decreased salivary flow produced by atropine use promotes caries, buccal candidiasis, and periodontal disease. Counsel the client involved in long-term use to follow a consistent dental hygiene program, including semiannual visits to the dentist.

Instruct the client to avoid being exposed to high environmental temperatures, exercising in warm, humid weather, or taking prolonged hot baths; these activities may lead to heat stroke. Children are especially at risk for increased body temperature in hot weather. Any fever must be reported to the prescriber because the medication may need to be discontinued.

Inform the client using an ophthalmic preparation that vision will be impaired for a few days and to wear dark glasses to protect the eyes. The ability to judge distance will also be impaired; driving a car or operating machinery is to be avoided. Signs of local irritation or follicular conjunctivitis may occur after prolonged periods of ophthalmic therapy; in such cases, the drug should be discontinued.

Evaluation The expected outcome of atropine therapy is that the client's ECG will indicate a correction of underlying dysrhythmia without any tachycardia. The client will not experience any adverse effects of the atropine (e.g., constipation or urinary retention). If the drug is taken for an ophthalmic condition, the client will experience therapeutic mydriasis without systemic adrenergic-like effects.

✳ **What other antimuscarinics are in use clinically?**
Common antimuscarinics include scopolamine and hyoscyamine, which are used for motion sickness, bowel irritability, and to dry secretions. Flavoxate (Urispas), oxybutynin (Ditropan), and tolterodine (Detrol) are synthetic antimuscarinics used to treat hyperactive bladder. Other synthetic agents for GI indications include dicyclomine (Bentyl, Bentylol ✚) and glycopyrrolate (Robinul, Robinul Forte). Benztropine (Cogentin) and trihexyphenidyl (Artane), used

to treat parkinsonism and drug-induced extrapyramidal symptoms, are presented in Chapters 19 and 23. Inhaled antimuscarinics for bronchodilation (e.g., ipratropium [Atrovent]) are presented in Chapter 37.

scopolamine [skoe **pol** a meen]
(Transderm-Scop, Transderm-V ✚)
The peripheral effects of scopolamine are similar to atropine, but the CNS effects are different. At therapeutic doses it depresses the CNS and causes drowsiness, euphoria, memory loss, relaxation, sleep, and relief of fear. It does not increase blood pressure or respiration.
Indications
Scopolamine is used to treat irritable bowel syndrome, renal and ureteral colic, and dysrhythmias induced during surgery because of increased vagal stimulation. Because of its depressant action on vestibular function, it is used for motion sickness to prevent nausea and vomiting. It is used as an adjunct medication with general anesthesia to reduce secretions, prevent laryngospasm, and for its sedative (twilight sleep) and amnesic effects.
Pharmacokinetics/Dosing
Administered orally or IM, the onset of action of scopolamine is typically 30 to 60 minutes. The transdermal formulation is effective approximately 4 hours after application. Scopolamine is hepatically metabolized. Dose varies based on indication, with the transdermal patch typically dosed in adults as a 1.5 mg patch, which releases approximately 1 mg over a 72-hour period.
Adverse Effects
Adverse effects of scopolamine are similar to atropine.

✳ **N.D. is a 35-year-old man who has no significant medical history except for motion sickness with air travel. In the past, air travel associated with his job has been managed with dimenhydrate (Dramamine). However, he is getting married and his fiancé has her heart set on a cruise of the Greek Islands for her honeymoon. He is concerned that the dimenhydrate will not be adequate for an extended cruise, so his health care provider prescribes a scopolamine patch.**
For antiemetic or antivertigo effects in adults, a transdermal patch produces an effect for 72 hours. For an antiemetic effect, it should be applied 4 hours before the desired effect is required. Older adults are more sensitive to this drug at the adult dosage; monitor closely for hyperpyrexia, confusion, blurred vision, and ataxia. The transdermal patch is not recommended for children.

Instruct N.D. to wash and dry hands before and after applying the scopolamine patch. He should apply it to the hairless skin area behind the ear, but not over any abrasions or rashes. Alert N.D. that drowsiness and dilated pupils (photophobia and blurred vision) may occur, so that if he rents a car on the islands, he should probably have his wife drive. He will need to wear sunglasses to avoid the effects of photophobia. Alert him to the increased CNS effects that will occur if he uses alcohol or other CNS depressants while wearing the scopolamine patch.

✳ **M.M. is a 62-year-old postmenopausal woman who reports urinary urges frequently and occasional leaking of urine "when she can't make it." Her physical exam reveals atrophic vaginitis without any bladder distention. A residual urine volume was less than 40 mL.**

M.M. is diagnosed with overactive bladder, with symptoms of urinary urgency, frequency, or urge incontinence. Her prescriber begins tolterodine therapy at 4 mg daily in an extended-release form and asks her to return to the office for follow up in 2 weeks.

Bladder control and urinary incontinence are major issues that affect quality of life in older adults. Commonly used anticholinergic medications include oxybutynin (Ditropan) and tolterodine (Detrol, Detrol LA). Although both drugs produce anticholinergic adverse effects (e.g., dry mouth, blurred vision, changes in mental status, constipation), tolterodine appears to have greater affinity for bladder receptors and therefore may produce fewer adverse effects. The adult oral dosage of oxybutynin is 5 mg two to four times daily; and for tolterodine, 2 mg twice daily initially (or 4 mg of sustained-release formulation once daily), lowered to 1 mg twice daily according to response.

The nurse asks M.M. to log her urinary patterns for frequency, urgency, nocturia, incontinence, or distention (if the dosage is too high). She should avoid hazardous activities because dizziness, drowsiness, or abnormal vision (accommodation problems) may occur. Dry mouth may be managed with sugarless hard candies, gum, or ice chips.

Synthetic Substitutes for Atropine

The usefulness of atropine is limited by the fact that it is a complex drug that affects a number of organs or tissues simultaneously. When administered for its antispasmodic effects, it also produces prolonged effects in the eye, causing dilated pupils and blurred vision. It also causes dry mouth and possibly a rapid heart rate. When the antispasmodic effect is desired, other effects become adverse effects that may be distinctly undesirable.

A large number of drugs have been synthesized in an effort to capture the antispasmodic effect of atropine without producing its other effects. These drugs are often used to relieve hypertonicity and hypersecretion in the stomach.

Many products are marketed as antispasmodic and anticholinergic agents, but their formulations are either modifications of a belladonna alkaloid or include one or more of the natural alkaloids as their active ingredients. The pharmacologic properties are similar to the previously reviewed substances and are not repeated here. The more commonly used systemic agents are glycopyrrolate (Robinul) and dicyclomine (Bentyl). Glycopyrrolate is used primarily as a preanesthetic medication to control bronchial, nasal, pharyngeal and salivary secretions. Dicyclomine is indicated for treatment of diarrhea-predominant irritable bowel syndrome in clients for whom other therapy, such as a change in diet and sedation, has not been successful, but its use may be limited because of its antimuscarinic adverse effects.

Summary

Drugs that mimic, intensify, or inhibit the effects of the parasympathetic and sympathetic divisions of the autonomic nervous system are known as the autonomic drugs. They are grouped as cholinergic, cholinergic-blocking, adrenergic, and adrenergic-blocking drugs. The cholinergic (parasympathomimetic) drugs have nicotinic effects that stimulate the ganglia, adrenal medulla, and skeletal muscle, as well as muscarinic effects that stimulate the postganglionic nerve endings in glands and in cardiac and smooth muscle. They are used primarily to stimulate the intestine and bladder postoperatively, to terminate curarization, to lower intraocular pressure, to promote salivation and sweating, to dilate peripheral blood vessels, and to treat myasthenia gravis symptomatically.

Anticholinergic (parasympatholytic) drugs block the muscarinic effects of acetylcholine, which can produce a wide range of pharmacologic effects. They are used to treat illnesses in which spasm is a component, such as irritable bowel syndrome, spastic biliary disorders, and urinary disorders. Because anticholinergics decrease respiratory secretions, they are administered as a preanesthetic drug and to control the excessive salivation of some disorders, such as Parkinson's disease.

The ganglionic drugs are either ganglionic-stimulating or ganglionic-blocking drugs. Nicotine is a ganglionic-stimulating drug. It has no therapeutic use, but the nurse should be knowledgeable about its effects for health teaching purposes. In the 1950s, ganglionic-blocking drugs were used to manage severe and malignant hypertension, but their use has been limited since the advent of more selective and effective antihypertensive drugs in the 1960s. Neuromuscular-blocking agents are used to prevent voluntary muscle movement during procedures or mechanical ventilation; concurrent sedation is required because the neuromuscular-blocking agents possess no analgesic, anxiolytic, or sedating properties.

✳ Critical Thinking Questions

- Nurses in schools and other community agencies are well placed to serve as consultants and counselors to students and to be advocates for smoking cessation. Because children relate better to present than to future consequences of their activities, what would you share with a class of fourth graders about the immediate physiologic consequences of smoking?

- Harry Johnson is receiving dicyclomine 20 mg PO four times daily as part of his treatment for irritable bowel syndrome. He complains of heat intolerance, dry mouth, and constipation. How will you explain these symptoms to him? What instruction will you provide to assist him in managing his therapeutic regimen effectively?

Bibliography

Action on Smoking and Health. (2004). Passive smoking: A summary of the evidence. Retrieved June 23, 2005, from http://www.ash.org.uk/html/passive/html/passive.html.

Agency for Toxic Substances and Disease Registry. (2004). Medical management guidelines (MMGs) for nerve gases: Tabun (GA), sarin (GB), soman (GD), and VX. Retrieved May 2, 2004, from http://www.atsdr.cdc.gov/MHMI/mmg166.pdf.

Anderson, D.M. (Ed.). (2002). *Mosby's medical, nursing, & allied health dictionary* (6th ed.). St. Louis: Mosby.

Anney, R.J.L., Olsson, C.A., Lotfi-Miri, M., Patton, G.C., & Williamson, R. (2004). Nicotine dependence in a prospective population-based study of adolescents: The protective role of a functional tyrosine hydroxylase polymorphism. *Pharmacogenetics, 14*(2)7, 73-81.

Centers for Disease Control and Prevention. *Public health emergency preparedness and response.* Retrieved May 2, 2004, from http://www.bt.cdc.gov

Corelli, R.L., & Hudmon, K.S. (2005). Tobacco use and dependence. In M.A. Koda-Kimble, L.Y. Young, W.A. Kradjan, B.J. Guglielmo, Alldredge, B.K., Corelli, R.L. (Eds.), *Applied therapeutics: The clinical use of drugs* (8th ed.). Philadelphia: Lippincott Williams & Wilkins.

Drug facts and comparisons (58th ed.). (2005). St. Louis: Facts and Comparisons.

Fiore, M.C., Bailey, W.C., Cohen, S.J., Dorfmen, S.F., Goldstein, M.G., Goitz, E.R., et al. (2000). *Treating tobacco use and dependence. Quick Reference Guide for Clinicians.* Rockville, MD: U.S. Department of Health and Human Services. Public Health Service.

Fiore, M.C., Hatsukami, D.K., & Baker T.B. (2002). Effective tobacco dependence treatment. *Journal of the American Medical Association, 288*(14)1, 768-771.

Henderson, C.L. (1999). *Using the peripheral nerve stimulator to guide neuromuscular blocking agent doses. AACN Continuing Education.* Retrieved May 22, 2005, from http://www.aacn.org/aacn/conteduc.nsf/

Howard, L.A., Ahluwalia, J.S., Lin, S.K., Sellers, E.M., & Tyndale, R.F. (2003). CYP2E1*1D regulatory polymorphism: association with alcohol and nicotine dependence. *Pharmacogenetics, 13*(6)3, 321-328.

Ito, H., Hamajima, N., Matsuo, K., Okuma, K., Sato, S., Ueda, R., et al. (2004). Monoamine oxidase polymorphisms and smoking behaviour in Japanese. Pharmacogenetics, 13(2)7, 73-79.

Johnson, J.L., Budz, B., Mackay, M., & Miller, C. (1999). Evaluation of a nurse-delivered smoking cessation intervention for hospitalized patients with cardiac disease. *Heart & Lung, 28*(1), 55-64.

Johnstone, E.C., Yudkin, P.L., Hey, K., Roberts, S.J., Welch, S.J., Murphy, M.F., et al. (2004). Genetic variation in dopaminergic pathways and short-term effectiveness of the nicotine patch. *Pharmacogenetics, 14*(2)8, 83-90.

Lacy, C.F., Armstrong, L.L., Goldman, M.P., Lance, L.L. (2004). *Lexi-Comp's drug information handbook* (12th ed.). Hudson, OH: Lexi-Comp.

Liebelt, E. (2000). Neuromuscular blocking agents. In R. Irwin & J. Rippe (Eds.), *Manual of intensive care medicine.* Sydney: Lippincott Williams & Wilkins.

Loyola, R., & Dreher, H.M. (2003). Management of pharmacologically induced neuromuscular blockade using peripheral nerve stimulation. *Dimensions of Critical Care Nursing, 22*(4)1, 57-164.

Martin, T., & Lobert, S.L. (2003). Chemical warfare: Toxicity of nerve agents. *Critical Care Nurse, 23*(5)1, 15-22.

Moolchan, E.T., Robinson, M.L., Ernst, M., Cadet, J.L., Pickworth, W.B., Heishman, S.J., et al. (2005). Safety and efficacy of the nicotine patch and gum for the treatment of adolescent tobacco addiction. *Pediatrics, 115,* e407-414.

Murray, M., Cowen, J., DeBlock, H., Erstad, B., Gray, A., Tescher, A., et al. (2002). Clinical practice guidelines for sustained neuromuscular blockade in the adult critically ill patient. *Critical Care Medicine, 30*(1), 142-156.

Nicholas, R., Anthonisen, N.R., Skeans, M.A., Wise, R.A., Manfreda, J., Kanner, R.E., et al. for the Lung Health Study Research Group. (2005). The effects of a smoking cessation intervention on 14.5-year mortality: A randomized clinical trial. *Annals of Internal Medicine, 142,* 233-239.

Rice, V.H., & Stead, L.F. (2004). Nursing interventions for smoking cessation. (Cochrane Review). In *The Cochrane Library,* Issue 1. Chichester, U.K.: John Wiley & Sons.

Schoedel, K.A., Hoffmann, E.B., Rao, Y., Sellers, E.M., & Tyndale, R.F. (2004). Ethnic variation in CYP2A6 and association of genetically slow nicotine metabolism and smoking in adult Caucasians. *Pharmacogenetics, 14*(9)6, 615-626.

Silagy, C., Mant, D., Fowler, G., & Lancaster, T. (2001). Nicotine replacement therapy for smoking cessation (Cochrane Review). *The Cochran Library, 1.*

Silagy, C., Lancaster, T., Stead, L., Mant, D., & Fowler, G. (2004). Nicotine replacement therapy for smoking cessation (Cochrane Review). *Cochrane Database of Systematic Reviews, 4.*

Thompson, J.F. (2005). Geriatric urologic disorders. In M.A. Koda-Kimble, L.Y. Young, W.A. Kradjan, B.J. Guglielmo, Alldredge, B.K., Corelli, R.L. (Eds.), *Applied therapeutics: The clinical use of drugs* (8th ed.). Philadelphia: Lippincott Williams & Wilkins.

USP DI: Drug information for the health care professional (25th ed.). (2005). Greenwood Village, CO: MICROMEDEX Thomson Healthcare.

e-LEARNING SUPPLEMENTS

Student CD-ROM
- Final Exam questions
- NCLEX® Examination review questions
- Pharmacology animations
- Printable chapter summary

Evolve Website (http://evolve.elsevier.com/mckenry)
- Case study on drugs affecting the parasympathetic nervous system

- Content updates, including information on new drugs
- WebLinks corresponding to this chapter
- Answers to the critical thinking questions in this chapter
- *Elsevier ePharmacology Update* newsletter
- *Mosby's Drug Consult* Internet Edition
- Supplemental and reference information

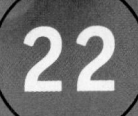

DRUGS AFFECTING THE SYMPATHETIC (ADRENERGIC) NERVOUS SYSTEM

CHAPTER FOCUS

Adrenergic receptors regulate cardiac, arteriolar, bronchial, and gastrointestinal (GI) smooth muscle. Pharmacologic intervention related to these receptors is commonplace and varied. The management of clients who are receiving drugs that affect the sympathetic, or adrenergic, nervous system is routinely a part of clinical practice.

<table>
<tr><td>

LEARNING OBJECTIVES

</td><td>

- Describe the three types of adrenergic drugs.
- Differentiate between α_1-, α_2-, β_1-, and β_2-adrenergic effects.
- Describe the effects of the three naturally occurring catecholamines on the body.
- List common adrenergic drugs and adrenergic blocking agents and their therapeutic and adverse effects.
- Implement the nursing management of clients receiving adrenergic and adrenergic blocking drugs.

</td></tr>
</table>

▲ KEY TERMS

β-adrenergic blocking agents (commonly called "β blockers"), p. 461
calorigenic effect, p. 448
dromotropic effect, p. 447
inotropic effect, p. 447
sympathomimetic drugs, p. 443

KEY DRUGS

dopamine, p. 454
epinephrine, p. 449
norepinephrine, p. 454
prazosin (see monograph in Chapter 27, p. 568)
propranolol, p. 462

✱ How do adrenergic drugs work?

Adrenergic drugs enhance or mimic the effects of sympathetic nerve stimulation. They are also referred to as **sympathomimetic drugs**. These drugs are designed to produce actions similar to those of the neurotransmitters at the postsynaptic effector organs (Figure 22-1) such as increased cardiac output, vasoconstriction of arterioles and veins, and bronchial dilation. Understanding the receptors of the sym-

pathetic (adrenergic) nervous system helps explain the action of the sympathomimetic drugs. Although it is expected that adrenergic responses are the same in all populations, current research demonstrates genetic differences in individuals and some specific populations; see the Special Considerations for Pharmacogenetics box on p. 444.

In the sympathetic nervous system (SNS), the adrenergic receptor cells contain two distinct receptors: α and β.

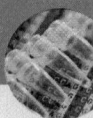 Special Considerations for Pharmacogenetics | **ADRENERGIC AGONISTS AND ANTAGONISTS**

PHARMACODYNAMICS

Variation in the genetic markers for α_1, β_1, and β_2 receptors have been identified and may affect both the pathophysiology and the treatment of heart failure (HF) (Bleumink et al., 2004; Mialet et al., 2003). Genetic variation in β-adrenergic receptors has also been correlated with risk for hypertension (Hopkins & Hunt, 2003). Individuals with an identified genetic markers (ARG389 allele, Thr164 Ile), which code for α- and β-adrenergic receptors, are more responsive to the blood pressure effects of sympathomimetics like dopamine and phenylephrine (La Rosee, Huntgeburth, Rosenkranz, Bohm, & Schnabel, 2004; Dishy et al., 2004). Genetic mapping in the future may guide therapeutic decisions for the management of HF and other cardiac conditions based on adrenergic receptor variation (Kaye et al., 2003).

PHARMACOKINETICS

Polymorphism (generic variation) in the enzymes that metabolize drugs, including adrenergic agonists and antagonists, is well established. Alterations in cytochrome P450 1A2 and 2D6 that affect propranolol and timolol metabolism, respectively, display significant genetic variation (Chang & Altman, 2004), as well as UGT1 A6, which is involved in the metabolism of many β-adrenergic blockers (Nagar, Zalatoris, & Blanchard, 2004). These findings may explain why many Southeast Asians require lower doses of β blockers (Schaefer, Caracciolo, Frishman, & Charney, 2003).

ADVERSE EFFECTS

Differences in response (both therapeutic and adverse) to β_2 agonists (e.g., albuterol) used to treat asthma have been correlated with genetic markers (Small et al., 2004). Dose-related adverse effects related to drug metabolism may be more common in some Asian populations (Schaefer et al., 2003).

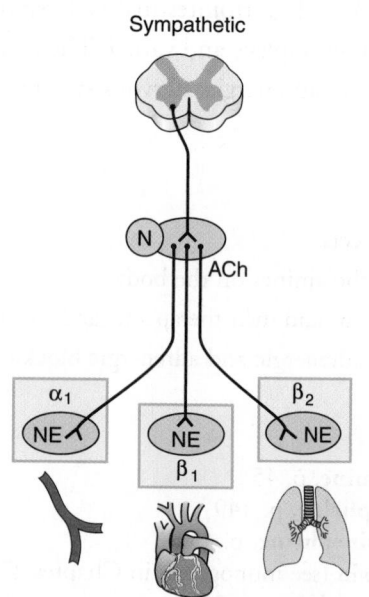

FIGURE 22-1 Site of action of adrenergic drugs. *Ach,* Acetylcholine; *N,* nicotinic receptors; *NE,* norepinephrine.

α Receptors

The α receptors appear in two primary locations. The α_2 receptors are found on the presynaptic nerve terminals, platelets, and smooth muscle and thus are called presynaptic (prejunctional) receptor sites. These are found in both the central and peripheral nervous systems. The presynaptic receptor controls the *amount* of transmitter released per nerve impulse; this can be regulated by a feedback mechanism. When the concentration of transmitter released from the nerve terminal into the synaptic cleft reaches a high level, the presynaptic receptors are stimulated, which pre-

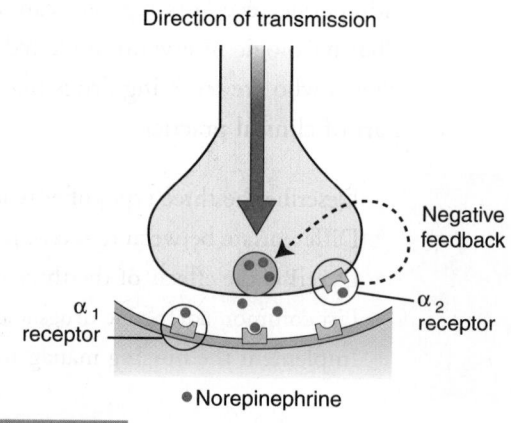

FIGURE 22-2 Site of action of α_1 and α_2 receptors.

vents further release of the transmitter. This type of feedback prevents excessive and prolonged stimulation of the postsynaptic cell. The postsynaptic receptors, which are located on the effector organs, are known as α_1 receptors (in the eye, arterioles, veins, male sex organ, and bladder) (Figure 22-2). The most important α-adrenergic activities in humans are the following:

- Vasoconstriction of arterioles in the skin and splanchnic area, resulting in a rise in blood pressure (BP)
- Pupil dilation
- Relaxation of the gut

β Receptors

The β receptors are subdivided on the basis of their responses to drugs. β_1 receptors are located mainly in the heart, whereas β_2 receptors mediate the actions of cate-

TABLE 22-1 OVERVIEW OF ADRENERGIC RECEPTOR STIMULATION

Receptor	Effect
α_1	Contraction or vasoconstriction of peripheral blood vessels Dilation (contraction) of pupil Increased contractility of heart
α_2	Limit or control of transmitter release Aggregation of platelets Contraction of smooth muscle
β_1	Increased heart rate (chronotropic) Increased contractility of heart (inotropic)
β_2	Dilation of bronchial smooth muscle Relaxation of uterus Activation of glycogenolysis

cholamines on smooth muscle, especially bronchioles and arterial smooth muscle. β-adrenergic activity includes the following:

- Cardiac acceleration and increased contractility (β_1)
- Vasodilation of arterioles supplying skeletal muscles (β_2)
- Bronchial relaxation (β_2)
- Uterine relaxation (β_2)

The effects of both α and β stimulation are the result of their interrelationship at any given time. That is, a change in blood pressure (BP) depends on the degree of vasoconstriction in the skin and splanchnic area (α activity) and the extent of vasodilation in skeletal muscles (β activity), along with changes in heart rate. Large arteries and veins contain both α and β receptors; the heart contains only β receptors. Tables 22-1 and 22-2 present an overview of these receptors.

❋ **How are the sympathomimetic agents classified?**
Sympathomimetic drugs (agonists at the postsynaptic adrenergic receptor) are of three types: (1) direct-acting, (2) indirect-acting, and (3) dual-acting (direct and indirect).

Direct-Acting Adrenergic Drugs

Direct-acting adrenergic drugs work at adrenergic receptors as agonists. The direct-acting sympathomimetic drugs include the naturally occurring catecholamines (dopamine, norepinephrine, and epinephrine) and the synthetic agents isoproterenol and dobutamine.

The three naturally occurring catecholamines in the body—dopamine, norepinephrine, and epinephrine—are synthesized by the sympathetic nervous system (SNS).

Dopamine is a precursor of norepinephrine and epinephrine, but it also has a transmitter role of its own in certain portions of the central nervous system (CNS). Epinephrine is primarily an emergency hormone secreted by the adrenal gland, whereas norepinephrine is an important transmitter of nerve impulses and is an intermediary in epinephrine biosynthesis. These catecholamines are very similar chemically (Figure 22-3). (For more information on adrenergic transmission and catecholamines, see Figure 20-7 and the discussion in Chapter 20.)

The two synthetic sympathomimetics, isoproterenol and dobutamine, are similar chemically to the catecholamines. The subtle chemical differences among the chemical structures of the catecholamines and synthetic agents account for variations in binding capacity at different adrenergic receptors in the body.

Indirect-Acting Adrenergic Drugs

The indirect-acting adrenergic drugs act indirectly on receptors by first triggering the release of the catecholamines, norepinephrine and epinephrine, from their storage sites; these neurotransmitters then activate the α and β receptors. Drugs such as cocaine act primarily in the CNS by this mechanism.

Dual-Acting Adrenergic Drugs

Dual-acting adrenergic drugs have both indirect and direct effects. Dual-acting adrenergic drugs have many and varied uses in medicine, but have been largely replaced by more specific agents. Dual-acting agents include ephedrine, phenylephrine, mephentermine, metaraminol, and methoxamine.

TABLE 22-2 ADRENERGIC RECEPTOR STIMULATION

Effector Organs	Receptor Type	Adrenergic Response
Heart		
Cardiac muscle (atria, ventricles)	β_1	Increased force of contractions (inotropic action)
Sinoatrial node	β_1	Increased heart rate (chronotropic action)
Atrioventricular node	β_1	Increased automaticity and conduction velocity; shortened refractory period (chronotropic action)
Blood vessels		
Arterioles		
Coronary	α_1, β_2, dopaminergic	Constriction, dilation*
Cerebral	α_1	Constriction
Pulmonary	α_1, β_2	Constriction,* dilation
Mesenteric visceral	α_1, β_2	Constriction,* dilation
Renal	α_1, β_2, dopaminergic	Constriction,* dilation
Skin, mucosa	α_1, α_2	Constriction
Skeletal muscle	α_1, β_2	Constriction, dilation
Veins	α_1, β_2	Constriction, dilation
Lung		
Bronchial smooth muscle	β_2	Bronchodilation
Bronchial glands	α_1, β_2	Inhibition
Gastrointestinal tract		
Smooth muscle (motility, tone)	α_1, α_2, β_2	Decreased
Sphincter	α_1	Contraction
Secretion	?	Inhibition
Gallbladder and ducts	—	Relaxation
Liver	β_2	Glycogenolysis
Spleen capsule	α_1, β_2	Contraction,* relaxation
Pancreas: insulin secretion	α_2	Decreased
Adipose tissue	β_1	Lipolysis
Urinary bladder		
Detrusor muscle	β_2	Relaxation
Sphincter	α_1	Contraction
Kidney ureter	α_1	Contraction
Kidney secretion (rennin)	β_1	Increased
Uterus		
Pregnant	α_1	Contraction
Nonpregnant	β_2	Relaxation
Sex organs, male	α_1	Ejaculation
Skin		
Pilomotor muscles	α_1	Contraction
Sweat glands	α_1, cholinergic	Increased secretion
Eye		
Radial muscle, iris (pupil size)	α_1	Contraction—pupil dilation (mydriasis)
Ciliary muscle	β_2	Relaxation for far vision

*Predominant response.

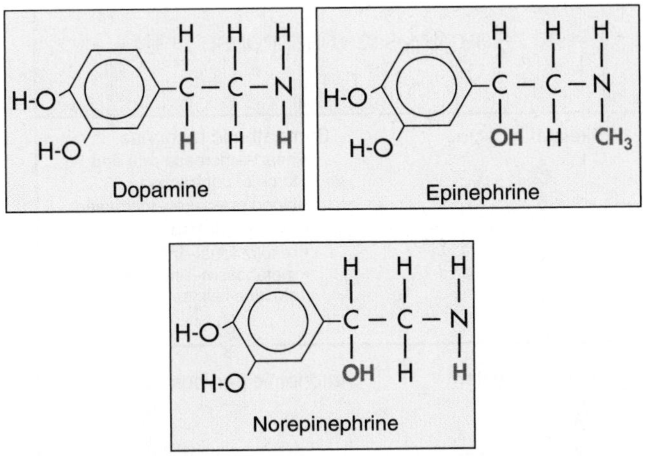

FIGURE 22-3 Chemical structures of the catecholamines.

✳ What are the physiologic and pharmacologic effects of catecholamines?

As catecholamines, epinephrine and norepinephrine are important neurohormones in neural and endocrine integration. They are always present in arterial blood, but the amount varies widely during any one day. Certain physiologic stimuli such as stress and exercise significantly increase blood levels of catecholamine. Studies indicate that the major sources of circulating norepinephrine are stimulated sympathetic nerve endings. Organs such as the heart and blood vessels receive a large fraction of blood and possess large numbers of sympathetic nerve endings; thus they contain the greatest amount of catecholamines. The number of sympathetic nerve endings or adrenergic nerves to various organs determines the magnitude of response of these organs to increased levels or injections of catecholamines.

Cardiac The pharmacologic effects of the catecholamines are essentially a result of their direct effect as agonists on specific α and β receptors (β_1 and β_2). Epinephrine increases heart rate, stroke volume, and cardiac output, whereas norepinephrine does not alter cardiac output and may even slightly decrease heart rate and cardiac output. This effect of norepinephrine is believed to result from its potent vasoconstriction action, which increases resistance to the ejection of blood from the heart. The increased work of the heart to move the blood against increased pressure is "pressure work" rather than "volume work."

Thus the effects of epinephrine and norepinephrine are approximately equivalent on β_1 receptors, but norepinephrine is a more potent agonist at α receptors (vasoconstriction), with little effect on β_2 receptors (vasodilation). Epinephrine is a potent stimulant of α and β receptors, but its peripheral resistance effects may vary depending on the dose and the ratio of α to β receptor response in various areas.

A significant increase in myocardial contraction (positive **inotropic effect**) is the result of the increased influx of calcium into cardiac fibers. Strong myocardial contractions result in more complete emptying of the ventricles and an increase in cardiac work and oxygen consumption. Strong contractions brought about by isoproterenol and epinephrine also increase cardiac output or volume.

Norepinephrine, with its predominantly α-adrenergic activity, may not produce as severe a tachycardia as epinephrine. The increased vasoconstriction and increased BP may cause a reflex bradycardia. Isoproterenol usually produces a tachycardia, because of its direct inotropic and chronotropic effects. Dosage and client variables affect these responses.

An increase in atrioventricular conduction (positive **dromotropic effect**) is another physiologic response. Because epinephrine increases atrioventricular conduction, some cardiologists use it in the treatment of heart block.

Catecholamines may also produce spontaneous firing of Purkinje fibers, which may cause them to exhibit pacemaker activity. This effect may cause ventricular extrasystoles and increase the susceptibility of ventricular muscle to fibrillation. These effects are more likely to occur with epinephrine than norepinephrine.

Vascular The vascular effects of the catecholamines depend on the dose and the vascular bed affected. Low doses of epinephrine may decrease total peripheral vascular resistance and decrease BP via stimulation of β_2 receptors. In large doses, epinephrine activates α receptors in the greater peripheral vascular system, which increases resistance and increases BP. Norepinephrine elevates BP by increasing peripheral resistance and decreasing blood flow through the skeletal muscles. Isoproterenol is not a vasoconstrictor but a pure vasodilator; epinephrine is both a vasoconstrictor and vasodilator, with vasodilation being greater in its overall net effects. For example, during great stress the release of epinephrine from the adrenal medulla constricts blood vessels in the skin and splanchnic areas but dilates those of the skeletal muscles, thus shunting blood to the areas needed for "fight-or-flight" responses.

Renal artery constriction and resistance is greater with epinephrine than with norepinephrine. In large doses, epinephrine may actually stop blood flow through some nephrons and stimulate the release of antidiuretic hormone, thereby reducing urinary excretion.

Central Nervous System In sufficient amounts, epinephrine and isoproterenol can lead to alertness, tremulousness, respiratory stimulation, and anxiety. Norepinephrine is less likely to cause anxiety and tremulousness. The beneficial cerebral effects from epinephrine and norepinephrine in cases of hypotension are thought to result from increased systemic pressure with a resultant improvement in cerebral blood flow.

Smooth Muscle In general, the catecholamines relax nonvascular smooth muscles. When the smooth muscle of the gastrointestinal tract is relaxed, the amplitude and tone of intestinal peristalsis are reduced. Theoretically this may slow the propulsion of food and gastrointestinal (GI) emptying. This effect is rare in humans given therapeutic doses of catecholamines.

In some situations, the smooth muscle of some organs reacts like vascular smooth muscle and contracts. For example, the radial and sphincter muscles of the iris contract,

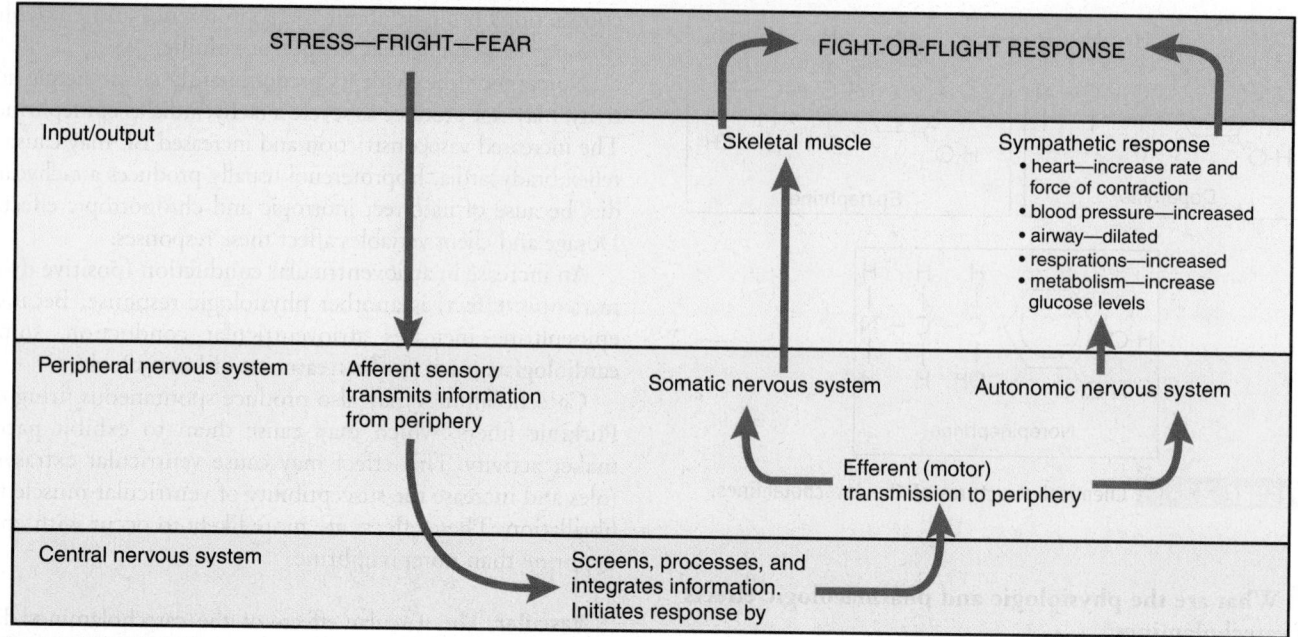

FIGURE 22-4 Nervous system response to severe fright or stress.

and the smooth muscle of the lids may contract, giving rise to the widened, staring eyes seen in sympathetically stimulated individuals.

In the urinary bladder, epinephrine causes trigone and sphincter constriction and detrusor relaxation with a delay in the desire to void.

Catecholamines dilate bronchial smooth muscle. Isoproterenol is a more active bronchodilator than epinephrine, whereas epinephrine is a stronger bronchodilator than norepinephrine.

Glandular As a rule, sympathomimetics decrease secretion and produce a dry mouth. However, epinephrine may increase the amount of viscid saliva excreted. Catecholamines may produce local sweating on the palms of the hands and in the axillary and genital areas. The exact mechanism for these effects is not clear.

Metabolic Epinephrine inhibits insulin secretion. Catecholamines have antagonistic effects on gluconeogenesis, and they decrease liver and skeletal muscle glycogen and increase lipolysis in adipose tissue. The result of these effects is a rise in blood sugar and an increase in free fatty acids. Thus there can be an abundant supply of fuel and energy in response to stress ("fight-or-flight" response) (Figure 22-4).

Catecholamines also have a **calorigenic effect** (capable of generating heat, which increases oxygen consumption) resulting from the sum of the preceding effects. The action of norepinephrine in relation to these effects is weaker than that of epinephrine or isoproterenol.

✱ **P.T. is a 12-year-old male with a history of peanut sensitivity with an anaphylactic response. His pediatrician has ordered self-administered subcutaneous epinephrine (EpiPen) in the event of a peanut exposure. The nurse meets with P.T. and his parents to explain**

Alpha vs. beta effects of sympathomimetics

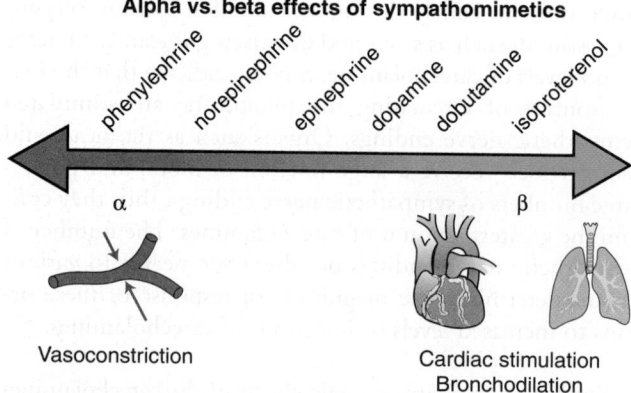

FIGURE 22-5 Comparative activity of sympathomimetics.

the role of epinephrine in the treatment of the symptoms of anaphylaxis.

✱ **Why is epinephrine effective in the treatment of anaphylaxis?**
Major symptoms of anaphylaxis include epiglottal edema, bronchoconstriction, and vasodilation. On a continuum of α to β effects, epinephrine is about central, producing β_1 stimulation to cardiac tissue, β_2 stimulation to the bronchioles causing bronchodilation, and α_1 stimulation to produce vasoconstriction. This combination of effects targets the major symptoms of anaphylaxis more completely than the other catecholamines. Figure 22-5 compares the sympathomimetic agents and their affinity to receptor sites.

✱ **How else are the sympathomimetics differentiated?**
The adrenergic agonists differ in pharmacologic activity, indication, route of administration, and adverse effect profile. Key differences among the agents are presented in the following sections and in Table 22-3.

TABLE 22-3 VASOPRESSOR EFFECTS IN SHOCK

Drug	Receptor Site Effects*			Organ Responses†		
	β_1	β_2	α_1	Kidneys	Cardiac	Blood Pressure
epinephrine	+++	+/++	+++	D	I	D
dobutamine	+++	+	0/+	0	I	—
dopamine	+++	0/+	++	I		0/I
isoproterenol	+++	+++	0	I/D	I	#
norepinephrine	+	0	+++	D	0/D	I

+, Minimal effect; ++, moderate effect; +++, greatest effect; *0*, no effect; *I*, increased; *D*, decreased; #, usual doses maintain or increase systolic pressure.

*Receptor site effects: β_1, inotropic effects; β_2, vasodilation; α_1, vasoconstriction.

†Organ response: *Kidneys*, renal perfusion; *cardiac*, cardiac output; *blood pressure*, blood pressure.

Direct-Acting Sympathomimetics

✶⊓ epinephrine [eh pih **nef** rin]

(Adrenalin)

Epinephrine is an agonist at α_1, β_1, and β_2 receptors.

Indications

Intravenous (IV) and subcutaneous epinephrine are indicated for the emergency treatment of acute anaphylactic shock and severe acute allergic reactions to drugs, animal serums, insect bites, and other allergens to relieve bronchospasm, urticaria, hives, angioneurotic edema, swelling of nasal mucosa, and pulmonary congestion. Epinephrine is also used IV to treat asystole as part of advanced cardiac life support protocols. It is often used in combination with local anesthetics (e.g., lidocaine) to control superficial bleeding from arterioles and capillaries in the skin, mucous membranes or other tissues as part of suturing wounds and to control systemic absorption of the anesthetic. It is used in ocular surgery to control bleeding and to induce mydriasis and conjunctival decongestion. It is also used topically in glaucoma to decrease intraocular pressure. Inhaled forms of racemic epinephrine (AsthmaNefrin, Vaponefrin) are often used for short periods to reduce epiglottal edema commonly associated with croup in children. Inhaled epinephrine to treat bronchospasm is available over-the-counter (OTC) (Primatene Mist), but its use should be discouraged because of the availability of safer products with less cardiovascular stimulation.

Pharmacokinetics/Dosing

Epinephrine should not be given orally because it is rapidly metabolized in the mucosa of the GI tract and liver; serum levels achieved with this route are inadequate. It is well absorbed following intramuscular (IM) or subcutaneous injection.

Epinephrine has a rapid onset of action—from 3 to 5 minutes after inhalation or between 6 and 15 minutes after subcutaneous injection. The duration of action of epinephrine is 1 to 3 hours by inhalation and from 1 to 4 hours after IM or subcutaneous injection. In severe anaphylaxis, asthma, or cardiac arrest, epinephrine doses may need to be repeated every 5 to 20 minutes, depending on the dose used and the client's response. Epinephrine is metabolized in the liver and excreted by the kidneys.

Parenteral dosage forms include epinephrine injection (Adrenalin, EpiPen) and sterile epinephrine suspension (Sus-Phrine). Injectable epinephrine is available in both a 1:1000 (typically for subcutaneous use) and a 1:10,000 solution (often for use in asystole). Epinephrine is also available in solutions for inhalation and ophthalmic administration. Table 22-4 has a more complete discussion of doses and administration of epinephrine.

Adverse Effects

Adverse effects of epinephrine include increased nervousness, restlessness, insomnia, tachycardia, tremors, sweating, increased BP, nausea, vomiting, pallor, weakness, and, with inhalation devices, bronchial irritation and coughing (with high doses), dry mouth and throat, headaches, and flushing of the face and skin.

Nursing Management

Although in the case of P.T. the use of epinephrine in the form of an EpiPen is rather straightforward, epinephrine is the classic sympathomimetic drug and is prescribed for many conditions. The nursing management of a client who is prescribed epinephrine is similar for all the drugs in this classification if administered in a similar dosage form.

Assessment Before administering epinephrine, assess the client for preexisting health conditions for which the drug may be contraindicated or for which a higher level of caution may be indicated. Use epinephrine cautiously in older adults and in those with cardiovascular disease, hypertension, hyperthyroidism, or seizure disorder because the drug may worsen the underlying condition. Clients with coronary insufficiency may develop anginal pain. Clients with diabetes mellitus may require a higher insulin dosage because of epinephrine-induced hyperglycemia.

Administer epinephrine with great caution to clients who are pregnant. Epinephrine is known to cross the placenta, and although appropriate human studies have not been conducted to demonstrate the teratogenic effects seen in rat studies, it may cause anoxia in the fetus. If administered during labor, it may delay the second stage because of the relaxation of uterine muscles. Epinephrine can cause acceleration of the fetal heart rate when given parenterally to maintain maternal BP during delivery; it is contraindicated if the maternal BP is greater than 130/80 mm Hg.

Review a client's current medication regimen for the risk of significant drug interactions, such as those that may occur when epinephrine is given concurrently with the following drugs:

- Systemic anesthetics (e.g., chloroform, enflurane [Ethrane], halothane [Fluothane], methoxyflurane) because these agents may sensitize the heart, increasing the risk of severe dysrhythmias. Monitor closely

TABLE 22-4 EPINEPHRINE: DOSAGE AND ADMINISTRATION

Indication	Adults	Children
PARENTERAL		
Bronchodilator	0.2-0.5 mg subcutaneously every 20 min, up to three doses as needed.	0.01 mg/kg subcutaneously every 15 min for three or four doses, or q4h if needed.
Anaphylaxis	0.3-0.5 mg IM or subcutaneously repeated every 10-20 min as needed for up to three doses.	0.01 mg/kg subcutaneously repeated every 15 min for up to three doses. *Maximum single dose: 0.5 mg*
Cardiac stimulant	IV 0.1-1 mg (base) diluted to 10 mL with sodium chloride injection given to restore myocardial contractility.	0.005-0.01 mg/kg IV; repeat every 5 min or follow with IV infusion at an initial rate of 0.001 mg/kg/min.
Anesthetic (local) adjunct	Intraspinal 0.2-0.4 mg added to anesthetic spinal mixture. With local anesthetic: 1:200,000.	See adult dosage.
AUTOINJECTION		
Autoinjector for emergency self-treatment of anaphylaxis (EpiPen)	0.3 mg IM	*Less than 30 kg:* 0.01 mg/kg/dose up to 0.15 mg *More than 30 kg:* 0.15 mg
SUSPENSION (SUS-PHRINE)		
Bronchodilator	0.5 mg subcutaneously initially, followed by 0.5-1.5 mg q6h as necessary.	0.025 mg/kg subcutaneously. May be repeated in 6 hr. If child weighs less than 30 kg, maximum single dose is 0.75 mg.
INHALATION*		
Bronchodilator 1:100 (1%) solution	Proper dose automatically dispensed by metered nebulizer. Allow 1-5 min between inhalations. Use fewest number of inhalations possible.	
TOPICAL		
Nasal decongestant	1-2 drops (0.1% solution) q4-6h.	
Antihemorrhagic	0.002%-0.1% (1:50,000 to 1:1000) solution of epinephrine applied locally.	

IM, intramuscularly; *IV,* intravenously.
*β$_2$-selective agonists are generally preferred over epinephrine.

because a reduction in epinephrine (sympathomimetics) is usually necessary.
- Local parenteral anesthetics because vasoconstriction and reduced blood supply may result in ischemia and gangrene when used in end artery areas such as fingers, toes, or penis. Use very cautiously in such areas and monitor closely.
- Tricyclic antidepressants because they block reuptake of adrenergic agents in the neuron, increasing the

pressor response to direct-acting agents and decreasing sensitivity to indirect-acting agents.
- β-adrenergic blocking agents, including ophthalmics, as the therapeutic effects of both agents may be inhibited.
- Mucosal-local cocaine because it increases the risk of hypertensive episodes and dysrhythmias and does not provide additional local vasoconstriction.
- Digoxin, quinidine, and other medications that sensitize the myocardium may result in dysrhythmias.

- Monoamine oxidase inhibitors, thyroid hormones, and other sympathomimetic agents because concurrent use may result in dysrhythmias, tachycardia, hypertension, or hyperpyrexia.

A baseline assessment of a client's cardiopulmonary status should be obtained by electrocardiogram (ECG), BP, and auscultation of heart and lung sounds. If used for bronchodilation, arterial blood gases and pulmonary function studies, such as peak expiratory flow (PEF) and spirometry, are to be completed.

Nursing Diagnosis Because of the CNS effects of dizziness or light-headedness, nervousness or restlessness, trembling, and insomnia, evaluate the client with epinephrine therapy for the nursing diagnoses of impaired comfort, disturbed sleep pattern, anxiety, disturbed thought processes, and risk for injury. There also may be impaired comfort resulting from the GI, respiratory, and local effects of the drug. Evaluate for ineffective airway clearance related to the client's preexisting health status to determine the effectiveness of the drug. The cardiovascular effects—headache, hypertension, palpitations, tachycardia, flushing of the face—may indicate the complication of altered cardiac output.

Planning After the administration of epinephrine, the client will:

- Experience relief from the symptoms for which epinephrine was prescribed.
- Effectively manage the therapeutic regimen, including stating the expected benefits, adverse effects, and which effects are reportable to the health care provider.
- Collaborate with health care team by maintaining visits for monitoring and follow-up care.
- Remain compliant with drug therapy.

Implementation

Monitoring Assess a client's vital signs and auscultate the heart and lungs periodically. During IV administration of epinephrine, monitor vital signs, monitor IV site for extravasation, and observe ECG results continuously until stabilized. Depending on a client's condition, intraarterial BP, central venous pressure, pulmonary artery pressure, and pulmonary capillary wedge pressure might also need to be monitored. Measure urine flow and monitor for signs of excess fluid volume such as peripheral edema, sudden weight gain, and distended neck veins. Monitor serum potassium levels because of the risk of hypokalemia. Because epinephrine increases blood glucose levels, observe individuals with diabetes for loss of glycemic control.

Intervention Avoid epinephrine overdose, particularly inadvertent IV administration of the usual subcutaneous doses, which may cause extreme hypertension. Insert IV containing epinephrine in the largest vein available. Cerebrovascular hemorrhage may result, particularly in older adults. Read the labels very carefully; ophthalmic, nasal, and topical solutions of epinephrine must not be injected.

Epinephrine is stored in light-resistant containers. Do not use if the solution is pink or brown in color or contains a precipitate; this color change is caused by oxidation of the drug. Multiple-use vials in which air is injected to withdraw the solution are more prone to this change.

Parenteral Administration Use extreme caution in calculating and preparing doses of epinephrine, noting the strength, dosage, expiration date, and route of administration of the solution. Avoid medication errors by not confusing the 1:1000 with the 1:10,000 solution. Overdose has resulted in fatalities. Use a small syringe (tuberculin syringe) to ensure accuracy in measuring the parenteral injection. Aspirate the syringe before parenteral injection (subcutaneous and IM) to prevent IV injection, which can result in sudden hypertension. Injection sites need to be rotated because repeated local injections may result in necrosis secondary to the vasoconstricting effects of the drug. Massaging the injection site will promote absorption of the drug. Because of this vasoconstriction, administer epinephrine intramuscularly into the anterolateral aspect of the thigh or the deltoid. Do not inject into the buttock; the presence of the anaerobic organism *Clostridium welchii* and reduced oxygen tension within the tissues as a result of the administration of epinephrine creates the potential for gas gangrene. Accidental injection into the hands or feet is to be avoided and requires immediate emergency treatment because it may result in a loss of blood flow to the area.

Epinephrine may be administered intracardially in emergency situations by qualified team members who have experience with this technique. If the client is intubated, the drug can be injected directly into the bronchial tree via the endotracheal tube at the same dose as for IV administration. A 1:1000 solution must be diluted with a 10-mL sodium chloride injection before IV or intracardiac administration.

Inhalation Epinephrine and other β-adrenergic agents are therapeutically interchangeable; allow 4 hours between doses when changing from one to another. Do not administer the doses concurrently.

Nasal Administration To prevent epinephrine from entering the throat, instill nose drops with the head low and in the lateral position. Rinse the nose dropper with hot water to prevent contamination of medication.

Education Take the medication exactly as prescribed and, if required, to take it around-the-clock. The repeated or prolonged use of epinephrine can cause *tolerance* or "epinephrine fastness." The effectiveness of the drug usually returns if withheld 12 hours to several days. Avoid self-medicating with any OTC preparations without consulting with prescriber. The prescriber is to be contacted if tachycardia, shortness of breath, or chest pain is experienced.

Emergency Autoinjection Teach clients with a history of allergic reaction or bronchial asthma how to self-inject epinephrine subcutaneously in case of emergency (Figure 22-6).

DIRECTIONS FOR USE

--Follow these directions *only* when ready to use.

--Never put thumb, fingers, or hand over black tip.

--Do NOT remove gray activation cap until ready to use.

1) Familiarize yourself with the unit.

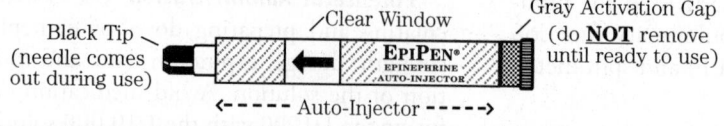

Black Tip (needle comes out during use) — Clear Window — EpiPen® EPINEPHRINE AUTO-INJECTOR — Gray Activation Cap (do **NOT** remove until ready to use)

<----- Auto-Injector ----->

2) Grasp unit, with the black tip pointing downward.
3) Form a fist around the auto-injector (black tip down).
4) With your other hand, pull off the gray activation cap.

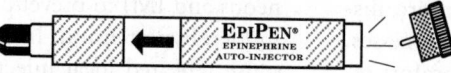

5) Hold black tip near outer thigh.
6) Swing and **jab firmly** into outer thigh so that auto-injector is perpendicular (at a 90° angle) to the thigh.

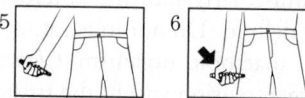

7) Hold **firmly in thigh** for several seconds.

8) Remove unit, massage injection area for several seconds.
9) Check black tip:
   -- if needle is exposed, you received the dose
   -- if not, repeat steps #5-8
10) *Note:* most of the liquid (about 90%) stays in the auto-injector and cannot be reused.

11) Bend the needle back against a hard surface.
12) Carefully put the unit (needle first) back into the carrying tube (*without* the gray activation cap)
13) Recap the carrying tube.
14) See "Immediately After Use" box on right side.

IMMEDIATELY AFTER USE

-- **Go immediately to the nearest hospital emergency room.**
   You may need further medical attention.
-- Tell the physician that you have received an injection of epinephrine (show your thigh).
-- Give your used **EpiPen®/EpiPen® Jr** to the physician for inspection and proper disposal.

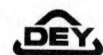

MANUFACTURED FOR DEY,
NAPA, CALIFORNIA 94558, U.S.A.
by Meridian Medical Technologies, Inc.
Columbia, MD 21046, U.S.A.
U.S. Patent No. 4,031,893
03-535-00A 12/00

FIGURE 22-6 Directions for using the EpiPen autoinjector.

Inhalation Instruct the client how to use the metered dose inhaler (see Box 37-2). Instruct the client to measure his or her pulse rate before inhalation therapy. Allow 2 minutes between doses, and do not administer it more frequently than required to relieve symptoms. Excessive repeated use may cause paradoxical bronchospasm. To prevent drug tolerance, caution the client not to overuse the drug.

The prescriber is to be notified if symptoms are not relieved with the usual dosage, because this may be an indication of worsening bronchospasm that requires reassessment of therapy.

The prescriber is to also be notified if the pulse rate increases more than 20 to 30 beats/min over baseline.

A client may expect the symptoms to be relieved in 20 minutes. Instruct the client to rinse his or her mouth with water to prevent mucosal absorption of drug.

Nasal Administration Nasal administration of epinephrine may produce a stinging sensation. Rebound congestion may occur with prolonged use, which may cause rhinitis. Nose drops are not to be used for more than 3 to 5 days.

Ophthalmic Administration Light-headedness, increased perspiration and heart rate, trembling, and pallor are signs of systemic absorption. These symptoms may be avoided by limiting the amount of epinephrine that enters the systemic circulation through the proper instillation of eyedrops. Create a pocket for the solution by gently pinching the skin below the lower eyelid and pulling it away from the eye. Place a drop of the solution into the pocket and hold it open for 1 or 2 seconds to allow the solution to settle. Have the client look down and then gently release the lower eyelid. Press just under the inner corner of the eye for 1 minute. This obstructs the nasolacrimal duct and minimizes the absorption of the drug into the bloodstream.

Administer epinephrine at bedtime or following a miotic to minimize discomfort, blurred vision, and sensitivity to light caused by mydriasis.

Discontinue epinephrine and notify the prescriber if signs of allergy develop (itching, edema of lids, discharge from lids). Headache and stinging of the eyes may occur after initial administration but that these symptoms disappear with continued drug use. Notify the prescriber if these symptoms persist; they may be controlled with a lower dosage. Intraocular pressure determinations should be scheduled periodically.

Brownish pigment deposits caused by oxidation of the drug may occur in the eyelids and conjunctiva or may appear as large dark casts in the lacrimal sac or nasolacrimal duct after long-term use of epinephrine. These deposits, which may be mistaken as foreign objects in the eye, may be removed by irrigation. Instruct clients who wear soft contact lenses to consult with the prescriber regarding the concurrent use of ophthalmic epinephrine instillation, because the medication may discolor the lenses

Evaluation The expected outcomes of epinephrine therapy are that the client's symptoms will be relieved, vital signs will be within the normal range, and the client will not experience any adverse effects of the drug.

✸ **On the last day of class for the school year, the students in P.T.'s class have a potluck lunch. Although it was requested that no peanut products be used in the food's preparation, P.T. begins to "feel funny" about 10 minutes into the meal. When the school nurse arrives, P.T. has tingling and pruritus of both his hands and feet, and appears flushed. He complains of light-headedness and difficulty breathing. The school nurse assists P.T. in injecting himself with his EpiPen in the anterolateral aspect of his thigh and calls 911. His blood pressure is 80/40 mm Hg (normally it is 110/72 mm Hg).**

Anaphylaxis requires quick recognition and aggressive therapeutic interventions because of its life-threatening nature. Epinephrine is the drug of choice for the management of anaphylaxis. The EpiPen is effective in cases in which shock is not present; however, with P.T.'s hypotension it is imperative to obtain further treatment. Vital signs, cardiac and pulmonary function, oxygenation, cardiac output, and tissue perfusion must be assessed and supported. P.T. was stabilized in the emergency department with oxygen and IV fluids to maintain cerebral perfusion and nebulized albuterol (a β agonist) to decrease his bronchospasm, as well as diphenhydramine (an antihistamine) and corticosteroids. His BP returned to normal and his respiratory symptoms resolved. He was transferred to

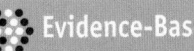
Evidence-Based Practice

Using an EpiPen Autoinjector

Nurses working with clients at risk for anaphylaxis should be familiar with the EpiPen autoinjector for client education and should instruct clients and caregivers in its use.

A survey of EpiPen use in children with a history of anaphylaxis found that many children and their parents did not know how to use an EpiPen and that, often, the physician who prescribed it did not explain its use (Huang, 1998). Another survey of children with a history of anaphylaxis who had a recent anaphylactic reaction found that the prescribed EpiPen was used in only 29% of recurrent anaphylactic reactions and that the majority of parents and children were unfamiliar with its use (Gold & Sainsbury, 2000). In addition, a study of health care professionals indicated that 81% did not have an epinephrine autotrainer to help educate clients, and 75% of these professionals were unable to correctly describe the steps in using the autoinjector (Grouhi, Alshri, Hummel, & Roifman, 1999).

intensive care unit (ICU) for 24 hours of monitoring to ensure his anaphylactic reaction did not reoccur. P.T. was discharged the next afternoon with an oral antihistamine and an oral corticosteroid, detailed instruction on the use of the EpiPen (see the Evidence-Based Practice box above) and instructions to follow up with his primary care provider.

Drugs Used For Circulatory Shock

In any instance of shock, treatment must be directed to the cause. A main concern is the need to improve circulation so that enough oxygen is available for tissue perfusion. Hypoxia that denotes impaired tissue perfusion may result from inadequate pumping action of the heart, decreased blood volume, decreased peripheral resistance of arterial vessels, or an increased size of the venous bed. In hypovolemic shock, sympathomimetic agents are used only as adjuncts to provide temporary support to maintain coronary and cerebral perfusion until volume replacement is completed (*USP DI*, 2005).

During circulatory shock the autonomic nervous system plays an essential compensatory role in an attempt to restore normal circulation. Therefore many sympathomimetic drugs are used to manage this condition. Although there are other agents, the five drugs widely used for circulatory shock are dopamine, epinephrine, and norepinephrine (all of which are vasopressors), as well as dobutamine and isoproterenol (which possess cardiogenic activity). Inamrinone (Inocor), which has positive inotropic and vasodilator effects, can also be used for clients with heart failure who are not responsive to standard therapy. Milrinone (Primacor), an analogue of inamrinone, is also available for short-term use in heart failure (see Chapter 25).

Vasopressors have strong α activity, and dopamine produces less vasoconstriction than epinephrine and norepinephrine. Dobutamine and isoproterenol are important for improving cardiac output because of their capability to stimulate β_1 receptors in the heart. Most of the agents are nonselective β-acting drugs; norepinephrine lacks β_2 activity. With the exception of isoproterenol and inamrinone, all of these agents stimulate α receptors (see Table 22-3).

★⌐🔊 dopamine hydrochloride [**dope** a meen]
(Intropin)

Dopamine is a catecholamine that occurs as an immediate precursor of norepinephrine (see Figure 22-3). It acts both directly and indirectly by releasing norepinephrine. It stimulates dopaminergic receptors, β_1 receptors, and, in high doses, α receptors. Receptor activity is dose dependent and depends on the amount of drug administered.

Unlike norepinephrine, dopamine is unique in low dosages (0.5 to 2 mcg/kg/min) because it acts mainly on dopaminergic receptors to cause vasodilation of the renal and mesenteric arteries. Renal vasodilation may increase renal blood flow, but evidence over the past decade suggests this is not important clinically (Beale, Hollenberg, Vincent, & Parrillo, 2004).

In low to moderate dosages (usually 2 to 10 mcg/kg/min), dopamine acts directly on the β_1 receptors of the myocardium and indirectly by releasing norepinephrine from its neuronal storage sites in the sympathetic neuron. These actions increase myocardial contractility and stroke volume, thereby increasing cardiac output. Systolic BP and pulse pressure may increase with either no effect on or a slight elevation in diastolic BP. Total peripheral resistance usually remains unchanged. Coronary blood flow and myocardial oxygen consumption increase. Heart rate increases only slightly at low dosages.

With higher dosages of dopamine (10 mcg/kg/min or more), α-adrenergic receptors are stimulated, which increases peripheral resistance. As a consequence, a high-dosage level may reduce urinary output, eliminating the benefit of vasodilation because the renal artery becomes constricted. From a therapeutic standpoint, it is important to note that dopamine in low to moderate dosages causes vasodilation in the renal, mesenteric, coronary, and cerebral blood vessels. These vasodilator properties suggest the presence of specific dopamine receptors.

Indications

Dopamine is used as an inotrope in management of acute heart failure, and at higher doses for its vasopressor effects in circulatory shock.

Pharmacokinetics/Dosing

Dopamine must be administered by IV infusion. The drug has a rapid onset of action (2 to 5 minutes) and a short duration of action (5 to 10 minutes); it is widely distributed by the body but does not cross the blood-brain barrier. Dopamine is rapidly metabolized by the liver, kidney, and plasma to inactive substances. It is excreted in the urine.

Short-term use of moderate-dose dopamine (2 to 10 mcg/kg/min) has been used for its inotropic effects in heart failure. Higher-dose dopamine (greater than 10 mcg/kg/min) is useful in treating circulatory shock once fluid imbalances have been corrected. Low-dose dopamine (less than 2 mcg/kg/min) has historically been used to help alleviate inadequate tissue perfusion through the vital splanchnic organ systems. This moderate vasodilation has not been correlated with improved renal function, however, and the practice of instituting low-dose dopamine to prevent renal failure in critical care clients has been largely abandoned (Beale et al., 2004).

Adverse Effects

The adverse effects of dopamine include headaches, nausea, vomiting, angina, respiratory difficulties, decreased BP, or, less commonly, hypertension, irregular or ectopic heartbeats, tachycardia, and palpitations. Like with other vasopressors, the vasoconstrictive effects may lead to local tissue necrosis if administered via a peripheral line.

dobutamine hydrochloride [doe **byoo** ta meen]
(Dobutrex)

Dobutrex is a synthetic catecholamine that acts directly on the heart muscle to increase the force of myocardial contraction. This response is attributed to direct stimulation of the β_1-adrenergic receptors of the heart. At the same time dobutamine produces comparatively little increase in heart rate or peripheral vascular resistance. By enhancing stroke volume, this agent is an effective positive inotropic drug.

Indications

Dobutamine is administered IV for *short-term* inotropic support, such as with heart failure or after cardiac surgery. Because of its minimal influence on heart rate and BP (both are major determinants of myocardial oxygen demand), it is valuable for use in strengthening a decompensated heart in individuals with low cardiac output syndrome. Its beneficial effects include a progressive increase in cardiac output and a decrease in pulmonary capillary wedge pressure (PCWP), thereby improving ventricular contraction. The concurrent use of sodium nitroprusside and dobutamine is sometimes beneficial in clients with heart failure or after an acute myocardial infarction. This combination results in a higher cardiac output and a lower PCWP than when either drug is used alone. Because of the vasodilating effect of nitroprusside, the decrease in peripheral resistance lessens the workload on the heart. Dobutamine is also used as an agent for stress echocardiography (Dhond et al., 1999).

Pharmacokinetics/Dosing

Dobutamine is administered by IV infusion and has an onset of action within 1 to 2 minutes; its plasma half-life is 2 minutes because it is rapidly metabolized by the liver and is excreted in the urine. The adult dosage of dobutamine is by IV infusion, 2.5 to 15 mcg/kg/min. For children, the dosage ranges between 5 and 20 mcg/kg/min.

Adverse Effects

The adverse effects of dobutamine include nausea, headache, angina, respiratory distress, palpitations, increased heart rate and BP, and, occasionally, premature ventricular beats.

★⌐🔊 norepinephrine bitartrate [nor eh pih **nef** rin]
(Levophed)

Norepinephrine is a direct-acting sympathomimetic amine identical to the catecholamine synthesized in the postganglionic nerve endings of the SNS. This agent has a high affinity for the α receptors. Because the blood vessels of the skin and mucous membrane contain only α receptors, norepinephrine produces a powerful constriction in these tissues. In addition, the blood vessels (both arteriolar and venous beds) in the visceral organs, including the kidneys, contain predominantly α receptors. Consequently, norepinephrine causes vasoconstriction and a reduced blood flow through the kidneys and other visceral organs. This agent also modestly activates β_1 receptors in the heart and exerts an increase in the force of myocardial contraction, but cardiac output is usually unchanged due to increased peripheral resistance.

Indications

Norepinephrine is indicated for significant hypotensive states that persist after volume correction. Norepinephrine is used selectively to restore BP in certain acute hypotensive states such as that seen in overwhelming sepsis, sympathectomy, myocardial infarction, pheochromocytomectomy, and blood transfusion reactions. When used to treat hypotension associated with an acute myocardial infarction, an increase in oxygen demand plus the possibility of inducing dysrhythmias may offset the benefits of using the drug to increase BP. Constriction of the venous capacitance vessels, which reduces splanchnic and renal blood flow, may increase the risk for renal or other organ failure.

Pharmacokinetics/Dosing

Norepinephrine is administered only by IV infusion because oral norepinephrine is destroyed in the GI tract and because subcutaneous norepinephrine is poorly absorbed. The onset of action by IV infusion is immediate or rapid, with distribution concentrating mainly in the sympathetic tissues. The duration of action is approximately 1 to 2 minutes and quickly dissipates after discontinuing the IV infusion. The drug is metabolized in the liver and other tissues and by reuptake into the sympathetic nerves; it is excreted by the kidneys.

Stimulation of α and β_1 receptors with norepinephrine is dose related. At low dosages (less than 2 mcg/min), β_1 receptors are stimulated, thus producing an inotropic and chronotropic response. Dosages higher than 4 mcg/min result in stimulation of the α receptors or increased total peripheral resistance.

When norepinephrine is used in the treatment of hypotension in adults, an IV infusion of 0.5 to 1 mcg/min is administered; the dosage is adjusted as necessary to raise and maintain the desired pressure. The maintenance dosage ranges from 2 to 12 mcg/min with dosage adjustments made as necessary to raise and maintain the desired pressure.

Adverse Effects
The adverse effects of norepinephrine include anxiety, dizziness, pallor, tremors, insomnia, headache, pounding heart rate, and perhaps swelling of the thyroid gland in the neck. Like with all the α_1 agonists, significant vasoconstriction may lead to tissue necrosis if administered peripherally and if the IV line becomes dislodged from the vein. Administration via a central line is strongly recommended.

isoproterenol hydrochloride [eye sow pro **tear** en all]
(Isuprel)
isoproterenol sulfate
(Medihaler-Iso)
Isoproterenol is an agonist at β_1 and β_2 receptors. It has minimal activity at α receptors. β_1 receptor activity produces an increase in the force of myocardial contraction and heart rate. Hemodynamically, the β_1 activity of the heart increases cardiac output and venous return to the heart. The β_2 receptor response of the smooth muscle of the bronchi, skeletal muscle, GI tract, and blood vessels of the splanchnic bed causes a relaxation of these organs. Peripheral vascular resistance is reduced, and in normal individuals a significant drop in BP may occur with excessive dosage. It also stimulates insulin secretion and releases free fatty acid.

Indications
Isoproterenol relieves bronchospasm associated with bronchial asthma, pulmonary emphysema, and bronchitis. In generally, however, more specific β_2 agonists are preferred because of the excessive β_1 cardiac stimulation of isoproterenol. It may be used as adjunct therapy in the treatment of cardiogenic shock. However, isoproterenol is no longer used routinely as an inotropic agent. It has been replaced in most clinical settings by newer agents that are less prone to induce ischemia or dysrhythmias (*Mosby's Drug Consult*, 2005).

Pharmacokinetics/Dosing
Isoproterenol is readily absorbed when given parenterally or by inhalation. The absorption of sublingual isoproterenol is erratic and unreliable. Its duration of action is usually up to 2 hours after oral inhalation or subcutaneous administration, and less than 1 hour after IV administration. Isoproterenol is metabolized in the GI tract, liver, and lungs, and is excreted in the urine.

Adverse Effects
The adverse effects of isoproterenol are similar to epinephrine except that inhalation and sublingual dosage forms may induce a pink to red discoloration of saliva (an expected alteration).

✳ **R.C., a 58-year-old man, is transferred to the ICU following a four-vessel coronary artery bypass graft surgery. Two hours after admission to the ICU, his BP begins to decrease and he becomes tachycardic. The ICU team rules out postoperative bleeding, tamponade, and myocardial infarct as the etiology of his cardiogenic shock. It is determined that he is experiencing acute heart failure following trauma to the myocardium, which may take hours to days to resolve. A chest radiograph confirms mild pulmonary edema. His BP**

and cardiac output need to be improved to increase perfusion to vital organs.

An infusion of dopamine is initiated at 3 mcg/kg/min to increase cardiac contraction and cardiac output. Because dopamine is a rapid-acting agent, R.C.'s dose can be reevaluated every 10 minutes, depending on his hemodynamic response. Use an infusion pump with a microdrip for precise regulation of infusion rate. Adjust the IV flow rate to maintain the desired rhythm or BP—usually a systolic pressure of 80 to 100 mm Hg. Monitor ECG patterns and central venous pressure (CVP), as well as urine volume and blood gases. Also monitor pulmonary artery pressure and PCWP. Follow the prescriber's guidelines for titrating flow in relation to heart rate, CVP, BP, ECG changes, and volume of urine flow.

R.C. should be monitored during his dopamine therapy for the following nursing diagnoses/collaborative problems: impaired comfort (nausea, chest pain, palpitations, headache, nervousness); ineffective tissue perfusion related to peripheral vasoconstriction (changes in color, tingling or numbness in fingers or toes); altered cardiac output (hypotension, hypertension, tachycardia); and the potential complications of angina and dysrhythmia.

Monitor R.C.'s respiratory pattern and lung sounds during administration. Observe him for mentation (cerebral circulation), temperature of extremities, and color of earlobes, lips, and nail beds; also monitor for paresthesia.

Discontinue the drug if precordial pain occurs. If the heart rate exceeds 110 beats/min, a slower infusion rate or a temporary discontinuance of the drug may be prescribed. Anticipate the development of ventricular dysrhythmias with doses that cause a heart rate of 130 beats/min.

Inspect the infusion site for extravasation every 10 to 15 minutes. Notify the prescriber immediately if extravasation occurs. Observe R.C. for blanching along the route of the infused vein and for cold, hard swelling around the injection site. Alert R.C. to report immediately any breathing difficulties, headache, chest pain, or discomfort at the infusion site.

The expected outcome of R.C.'s dopamine therapy is that he will demonstrate an improvement in cardiovascular status, with a mean arterial pressure at 75 to 80 mm Hg, apical pulse 110 beats/min or less, PCWP at 12 to 18 mm Hg, urinary output greater than 30 mL/hr, and an absence of adventitious lung sounds.

✳ **R.C. has remained stable for the past 6 hours. It is decided to taper his dosage of dopamine.**
When tapering dopamine, as with any vasoactive agent, R.C. must be stabilized hemodynamically at each new infusion rate for the period that exceeds the time to reach a new steady-state plasma concentration. After each reduction in infusion rate, he must be evaluated for dosage titration in relation to the expected outcomes for his dopamine therapy. Continue to observe R.C. carefully after discontinuing dopamine therapy. The duration of action of this drug is brief, and the beneficial effects of the drug may terminate quickly.

Dual-Acting Sympathomimetics

phenylephrine systemic [fen ill **eh** frin]
(Neo-Synephrine injection)
phenylephrine nasal
(Neo-Synephrine, Alconefrin)

Phenylephrine is a synthetic adrenergic drug chemically related to epinephrine, norepinephrine, and ephedrine. It is primarily a direct-acting agent; its main effects are stimulation of the α receptors, resulting in vasoconstriction and an increase in both diastolic and systolic BPs. The drug has little effect on the β_1 receptors of the heart. Its vasoconstricting action is more prolonged than that of norepinephrine and therefore may be used for acute hypotension that occurs from spinal anesthesia (Table 22-5).

Indications

Parenteral phenylephrine is used for severe hypotension not responsive to fluids. Like the other vasopressors, it is ineffective in treating shock caused by a loss of blood volume. When applied topically to mucous membranes for nasal congestion, phenylephrine reduces rhinorrhea and swelling by constricting the small blood vessels. It is useful in treating sinusitis, vasomotor rhinitis, and hay fever. It is sometimes combined with local anesthetics to slow their systemic absorption and to prolong their action.

Ophthalmic phenylephrine is used to treat glaucoma and to produce mydriasis (see Chapter 42).

Pharmacokinetics/Dosing

Administered IV, phenylephrine produces an immediate effect and has duration of action of 5 to 20 minutes. The drug is metabolized

TABLE 22-5 SELECTED INDIRECT- AND DUAL-ACTING ADRENERGIC DRUG EFFECTS

Receptors Action Sites	Ephedrine (Ephedrine Sulfate)	Phenylephrine (Neo-Synephrine)	Metaraminol (Aramine)
MODE OF ACTION			
α receptors	Stimulates	Stimulates	Stimulates
β receptors	Stimulates More prolonged but less intense action than epinephrine	Not significant	β_1 agonist
EFFECTS			
Cardiovascular			
Myocardium	Variable	Not significant	Some increase in contractility
Pacemaker cells	Not significant	Not significant	—
Coronary vessels	Dilates—increases blood flow	Dilates—increases blood flow	—
Blood pressure	Increases	Increases	Increases
Bronchi	Dilates	Dilates, but less than epinephrine	Not significant
Cerebral effects	Stimulating action	Not significant	—
Blood vessels			
Skeletal muscle	Not significant	Unknown	Not significant
Kidney	Constricts	Constricts	Constricts—decreases blood flow
Gastrointestinal tract	Decreases peristalsis	Decreases motility	Some inhibition
Metabolic	Increase metabolic rate	Some increase in metabolic rate	Not significant
REMARKS			
	Serious dysrhythmias may occur if used with digoxin Can be given orally		
USES			
	Vasopressor Allergic states Nasal decongestant Enuresis Myasthenia gravis	Nasal decongestant Vasopressor Paroxysmal atrial tachycardia Mydriatic	Vasopressor

partially in GI tract tissues and in the liver by the enzyme monoamine oxidase. The route of excretion has not been identified.

The IV injection dosage is 0.2 mg, repeated in 15 minutes if necessary; the IV infusion dosage is 100 to 180 mcg/min until the BP stabilizes, at which point it is reduced to 40 to 60 mcg/min. The adult dosage of phenylephrine for hypotension is 2 to 5 mg subcutaneously (or, rarely, IM) of 1% solution, repeated if necessary.

Adverse Effects

Phenylephrine exhibits fewer adverse effects than epinephrine and has longer-lasting therapeutic effects. Significant vasoconstriction can cause tissue necrosis if extravasation occurs. It has little or no effect on the CNS. Other adverse effects of phenylephrine are uncommon but include anxiety, restlessness, dizziness, tremors, difficulty breathing, pallor, increased weakness, angina, and with the preparations that contain sulfites, allergic reactions (Box 22-1).

ephedrine [e **fed** rin]

Ephedrine has both a direct and indirect sympathomimetic action. It acts indirectly by stimulating the release of norepinephrine from presynaptic nerve terminals and also acts directly on both α and β receptors. Like epinephrine and norepinephrine, ephedrine has positive inotropic and chronotropic activities, but it is a less effective vasoconstrictor. However, it does raise BP and is used for this purpose during spinal anesthesia and in the treatment of orthostatic hypotension.

Indications

Parenteral ephedrine has been used in clients with hypotension unresponsive to fluid replacement, position changes, and specific antidotes in cases of drug overdose, but it has generally been replaced by safer and more effective agents (*USP DI*, 2005). See Table 22-5 for a summary of its effects. Ephedrine is also used as a vasopressor in hypotensive states during spinal anesthesia or after sympathectomy. Ephedrine has been used to produce bronchodilation in the treatment of milder forms of bronchial asthma but, in general, more β_2-selective drugs are preferred (e.g., albuterol, metaproterenol, and terbutaline). It is also used to relieve nasal mucosal congestion.

Box 22-1 SULFITE SENSITIVITY

To improve stability, sulfite is contained in commercially available formulations of the following:

* inamrinone (Inocor)
* dobutamine (Dobutrex)
* dopamine (Intropin)
* epinephrine (Adrenalin)
* metaraminol (Aramine)
* methoxamine (Vasoxyl)
* norepinephrine (Levophed)
* phenylephrine (Neo-Synephrine)

These formulations should not be administered to individuals with a known sensitivity to sulfite agents (sulfur dioxide, potassium or sodium bisulfite, potassium or sodium metasulfite, sodium sulfite).

Symptoms of sulfite sensitivity include the following:

* Skin: clamminess, flushing, pruritus, urticaria, cyanosis
* Respiratory system: bronchospasm, shortness of breath, wheezing, laryngeal edema, respiratory arrest
* Cardiovascular system: hypotension, syncope
* CNS: severe dizziness, loss of consciousness
* Other: anaphylaxis, death

Pharmacokinetics/Dosing

Absorption of this drug is rapid after oral, IM, or subcutaneous administration. The onset of action for bronchodilation occurs within 15 to 60 minutes with the oral dosage form, and within 10 to 20 minutes with the IM dosage form. The duration of action is 3 to 5 hours for the oral dosage form and 30 to 60 minutes for IM or subcutaneous injections of 25 to 50 mg. The vasopressor effects and cardiac responses usually occur within 60 minutes of the parenteral administration of ephedrine. This drug is metabolized in the liver and excreted by the kidneys.

For vasopressor effects, the adult dosage of ephedrine is 25 to 50 mg IM or subcutaneously, repeated if necessary. It may be administered IV if a faster effect is desired. For bronchodilator or decongestant effects, the dosage is 25 to 50 mg PO or 12.5 to 25 mg subcutaneously, IM, or slow IV every 3 or 4 hours as needed. For decongestion, several drops of a 0.5% to 1% ephedrine solution may be applied topically and repeated every 4 hours if necessary.

Adverse Effects

The adverse effects of ephedrine are similar to epinephrine in similar dosage forms. Ephedrine may also cause mood changes and hallucinations. See the Medication Safety Alert box below for information on the hazards of these agents.

⁂ Medication Safety Alert

FDA Prohibits Over-the-Counter Use of Ephedrine Products

A number of plant genera, including ephedra, are known to contain ephedrine alkaloids. *Ma huang* is a common name given to Chinese ephedra, which is used in traditional Chinese medicine. A number of adverse effects associated with ephedrine alkaloid-containing dietary supplements have been reported to the U.S. Food and Drug Administration (FDA), including elevated BP, rapid heartbeat, nerve damage, muscle injury, psychosis, and memory loss. More serious effects have also been reported, including heart attack, stroke, seizure, and death.

The FDA issued a final regulation declaring dietary supplements containing ephedrine alkaloids adulterated under the federal Food, Drug, and Cosmetic Act because these dietary supplements present an unreasonable risk of illness or injury under the conditions of use recommended or suggested in labeling, or if no conditions of use are suggested or recommended in labeling, under ordinary conditions of use. Most dietary supplements containing ephedrine alkaloids are used for weight loss or enhancement of athletic performance.

The FDA concluded that dietary supplements containing ephedrine alkaloids pose a risk of serious adverse events, including heart attack, stroke, and death, and that these risks are unreasonable in light of any benefits that may result from the use of these products. In February 2004, the FDA banned dietary supplements containing ephedrine alkaloids based on the well-known pharmacology of ephedrine alkaloids, peer-reviewed scientific literature on the effects of ephedrine alkaloids, and the adverse events reported in individuals having consumed dietary supplements containing ephedrine alkaloids. Additional information is available at www.cfsan.fda.gov/~lrd/fpephed6.html.

metaraminol [met ah **ram** i nole]
(Aramine)

Metaraminol is a vasopressor agent with both direct (primarily) and indirect effects on the SNS. It acts indirectly by releasing norepinephrine from tissues and storage sites, and directly on α receptors as a neurohormone.

Metaraminol has positive inotropic effects. Because it constricts blood vessels, increases peripheral resistance, elevates both systolic and diastolic BP, and improves cardiac contractility and cerebral, coronary, and renal blood flow, it is used for the treatment of shock. Because metaraminol exhibits β- and α-adrenergic activity, it is often effective in raising BP when α-adrenergic agents are ineffective. This may be because of its ability to bring about more effective venous flow. See Table 22-5.

Indications

Metaraminol is used for acute hypotensive states occurring with spinal anesthesia. It is also administered for the prevention and treatment of acute hypotension associated with surgery, drug-induced reactions, and shock.

Pharmacokinetics/Dosing

This drug is administered only parenterally. The onset of action is within 1 to 2 minutes with IV administration and within 10 minutes with subcutaneous or IM administration. The duration of action is between 20 and 60 minutes; it is metabolized in the liver and excreted in the bile and kidneys.

The adult dosage of metaraminol is 2 to 10 mg subcutaneously or IM to prevent acute hypotension. To avoid cumulative effects, 10 minutes should elapse before additional doses are administered. When metaraminol is given via IV infusion, 15 to 100 mg in 500 mL of sodium chloride injection (0.9%) or 5% dextrose in water is administered at a rate determined by the prescriber to maintain the desired BP response. When given by direct IV injection for severe shock, 0.5 to 5 mg is administered followed by the IV infusion described above. The dosage for children has not been established.

Adverse Effects

Metaraminol does not appear to cause dysrhythmias. In general, it lacks CNS stimulatory effects, and its adverse effects are rare and often related to rapid drug administration. Although similar to norepinephrine in action, it is generally considered a less potent drug.

✱ How are the adrenergic antagonists classified?

The two major classifications of adrenergic blockers are the α-adrenergic blocking agents and the β-adrenergic blocking agents. Within each group are drugs that are typically more specific for location of action (central nervous system versus peripheral nervous system) and receptor subtypes (e.g., α_1, α_2, β_1, or β_2 receptors).

Central-Acting Adrenergic Inhibitors

Although thought of as antiadrenergic drugs, central-acting adrenergic inhibitors are actually central α_2-adrenergic agonists. Central α_2-adrenergic stimulation results in a decreased sympathetic outflow to the heart, kidneys, and peripheral vasculature; this results in decreased heart rate, decreased peripheral vascular resistance, and, as a result, decreased systolic and diastolic BPs. The centrally acting agents clonidine (Catapres), methyldopa (Aldomet), guanfacine (Tenex), and guanabenz (Wytensin) are used primarily as antihypertensives. They are discussed more fully in Chapter 27.

Peripheral Adrenergic Inhibitors

The peripherally active adrenergic inhibitors include guanethidine (Ismelin), guanadrel (Hylorel), and reserpine (Serpalan, Serpasil); they are used for hypertension unresponsive to other modalities. Agents that peripherally block α_1-adrenergic receptors include doxazosin (Cardura), prazosin (Minipress), terazosin (Hytrin), and tamsulosin (Flomax) and are used to manage urinary symptoms for older men with benign prostatic hyperplasia. By blocking α-adrenergic receptors of the bladder neck and proximal urethra, the internal sphincter is relaxed, which improves voiding efficiency in clients with functional outlet obstruction. Doxazosin, prazosin, and terazosin also have significant hypotensive effects and can be used as second-line therapy for hypertension. All of the peripheral adrenergic inhibitors are discussed more completely in Chapter 27.

Phenoxybenzamine and phentolamine are relatively nonselective peripheral α blockers; they antagonize responses mediated by both α_1 and α_2 receptors (Figure 22-7). Hence, they lower BP by preventing norepinephrine from activating α_1 receptors on vascular smooth muscle to produce vasoconstriction.

Because of their unique pharmacology, the ergot alkaloids are considered separately. They are partial α-adrenergic antagonists and produce a spasmogenic effect on vascular smooth muscle, resulting in vasoconstriction. They are primarily used in the treatment of migraine headache.

Each of these agents is discussed in the following sections.

phenoxybenzamine [fen ox ee **benz** ah meen]
(Dibenzyline)

Phenoxybenzamine is a long-acting, irreversible, α-adrenergic blocking agent that abolishes or decreases the receptiveness of α receptors to adrenergic stimuli.

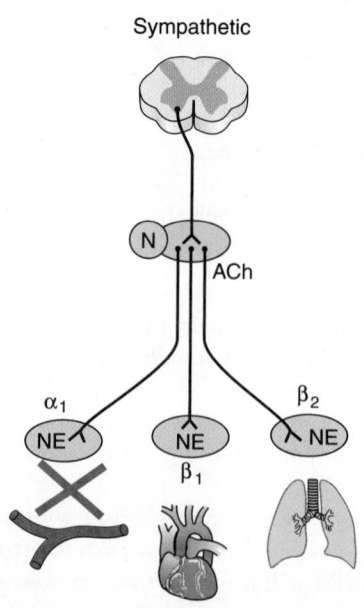

FIGURE 22-7 Site of peripheral α blockers. *Ach,* Acetylcholine; *N,* nicotinic receptor; *NE,* norepinephrine.

Indications

Because phenoxybenzamine competes with the catecholamines, it is also useful in decreasing the BP of clients with pheochromocytoma. It does not block sympathetic impulses on the heart and therefore does not directly impair cardiac output. It is occasionally used to relieve symptoms of benign prostatic hyperplasia, although α_1 blockers such as tamsulosin (Flomax) are more commonly used. Phenoxybenzamine is used in the management of pheochromocytoma prior to surgery, surgery, chronic treatment of individuals with malignant pheochromocytoma, and in individuals for whom pheochromocytoma surgery is contraindicated.

Pharmacokinetics/Dosing

The oral absorption of phenoxybenzamine is variable. The onset of action occurs in 2 hours. This drug can persist for 3 or 4 days because it forms a stable bond with the receptor. The half-life is approximately 24 hours, with metabolism in the liver and excretion in the kidney and bile. The initial adult dosage is 10 mg PO twice daily; the dosage may be increased by 10 mg every other day until the desired effect is noted. The maintenance dosage is 20 to 40 mg two or three times daily. The initial dosage for children is 0.2 mg/kg PO up to a maximum of 10 mg, administered once daily; this dosage may be increased every 4 days until the desired effect is noted. The maintenance dosage for children is 0.4 to 1.2 mg/kg body weight, given in three or four divided doses.

Adverse Effects

The adverse effects of phenoxybenzamine include dizziness (postural hypotension), miosis, tachycardia, nasal congestion, confusion, dry mouth, fatigue, headache, and inhibition of ejaculation.

phentolamine mesylate [fen **toll** ah meen]
(Regitine, Rogitine✽)

Phentolamine is an α-adrenergic blocking agent that competitively blocks α_2 (presynaptic) and α_1 (postsynaptic) receptors. The action occurs at both arterial and venous vessels. This direct relaxation of vascular smooth muscle lowers total peripheral resistance. Phentolamine also decreases pulmonary vascular resistance.

Indications

Phentolamine is used to prevent or control hypertensive episodes in clients with pheochromocytoma. It is also used to reverse the vasoconstrictive action of an overdose or an excessive response to IV administration or extravasation of norepinephrine (Levophed) or dopamine. A subcutaneous injection of phentolamine (Regitine) following extravasation of IV norepinephrine or dopamine prevents tissue necrosis if prompt action is taken.

Pharmacokinetics/Dosing

Parenteral phentolamine is administered IV, and the half-life is approximately 19 minutes. Metabolism and excretion sources are unknown, because only 13% (approximately) of the drug is found in urine after parenteral administration. When phentolamine is used preoperatively, 5 mg IV is administered 1 to 2 hours before surgery; this dose may be repeated if necessary during surgery. As an antiadrenergic preoperative in children, 1 mg IM or IV is administered 1 to 2 hours before surgery and repeated if necessary.

Adverse Effects

The adverse effects of phentolamine include diarrhea, dizziness (postural hypotension), nausea, vomiting, abdominal pain, and tachycardia.

✷ **Before R.C.'s IV dopamine is discontinued in the ICU, he complains of a burning sensation at the infusion site. The nurse notes the site is blanched and cool to the touch without blood return. The physician is notified.**

To prevent sloughing of the skin secondary to infiltration, the affected area of the infusion site is quickly infiltrated by the physician with 5 to 10 mg of phentolamine (Regitine) in 10 to 15 mL of sodium chloride to dilate blood vessels; a fine-gauge needle is used.

Ergot Alkaloids

Ergot is a fungus that grows on rye; when it is hydrolyzed, many of its derivatives dissociate to yield lysergic acid diethylamide (LSD). Ergotamine tartrate is considered the prototype ergot alkaloid. Other ergot alkaloids include dihydroergotamine mesylate (D.H.E. 45), ergoloid mesylates (Hydergine), methysergide maleate (Sansert), and combination products (e.g., ergotamine, belladonna alkaloids and phenobarbital [Bellergal-S, Bellergal✽]). These alkaloids have diverse and somewhat contradictory effects. Ergot alkaloids are partial agonists or antagonists at α-adrenergic receptors. The primary effect of the ergot alkaloids used to treat or prevent migraine and other vascular headaches is α-adrenergic blockade. Only ergoloid mesylates is not used to treat headaches; it is indicated as adjunct therapy to treat dementia symptoms, but this therapy is controversial (USP DI, 2005). A discussion of the management of migraine headache can also be found in Chapter 14 with a discussion of the serotonergic drugs, such as sumatriptan, naratriptan, rizatriptan, and zolmitriptan.

The exact mechanism of action of ergoloid mesylates is unknown, but it may increase nerve cell metabolism, which can result in improved oxygen uptake and cerebral metabolism. Thus lowered neurotransmitter levels may increase to normal. Other ergot alkaloids stimulate smooth muscle, especially of the blood vessels and the uterus, so they decrease the cerebral blood supply.

The early phase of a migraine attack is associated with constriction of the cranial blood vessels. It is characterized by visual symptoms and malaise and appears as a warning or "aura" of an oncoming attack. This is followed by the painful phase of a migraine headache that results in cranial vasodilation. The increase in blood flow in the vessels produces pulsations that appear to be the source of the pain. The ergot alkaloids act as α-adrenergic blocking agents and depress the central vasomotor center. They cause direct vasoconstriction of cranial blood vessels during the vasodilation phase, thereby reducing the pulsation thought to be responsible for the headache.

Ergot alkaloids also possess antiserotonin activity. Abnormalities in serotonin metabolism may play a role in the migraine syndrome. Evidence exists that the drugs that act favorably in alleviating migraine have an influence on serotonin metabolism. Methysergide is a serotonin inhibitor and also acts as a potent vasoconstrictor (see Chapter 39 for information on serotonin). Ergotamine tartrate inhalation is used to abort or reduce a migraine attack, whereas ergotamine, belladonna alkaloids, and phenobarbital are used in combination to prevent vascular headaches. Some of these drugs are used for the treatment of vascular headaches (e.g., migraine and cluster headaches). Dihydroergotamine mesylate or ergotamine tartrate must be given early in the attack; neither drug prevents migraine attacks.

ergotamine tartrate [er **got** ah meen]
(Ergomar✦)
ergotamine tartrate and caffeine
(Cafergot)
ergotamine tartrate inhalation
(Medihaler Ergotamine✦)

Indications
Ergot alkaloids alone or in combination with caffeine are indicated for the acute treatment of migraine headache.

Pharmacokinetics/Dosing
Ergotamine tartrate is slowly and erratically absorbed from the GI tract. Caffeine aids oral absorption. The aerosol dosage form is well absorbed. Rectal suppositories of ergotamine tartrate (available in combination products) produce higher plasma concentrations than the oral dosage form and may be used if other routes are ineffective.

Ergotamine tartrate and its combinations have onset of action within 1 to 2 hours and half-lives of approximately 2 hours. All of the ergot alkaloids are metabolized in the liver and primarily excreted by the kidneys.

The ergotamine dose is 1 to 2 mg PO initially, repeated in 30 minutes if needed; the maximum daily dose is 6 mg no more than twice weekly and at least 5 days apart.

Adverse Effects
The adverse effects of ergot alkaloids include dizziness, nausea, vomiting, headache, diarrhea, pruritus, edema of the lower extremities, and peripheral vasoconstriction or vasospasms (dose related) that may result in cold hands or feet, leg weakness, pain in arms, legs, or lower back. Long-term use of ergot alkaloids (e.g., methysergide) may result in retroperitoneal fibrosis; therefore this product should not be routinely administered for longer than 6 months.

✴ **H.A., a 24-year-old woman, presents to the University Health Center with a 3-month history of left-sided head pain recurring over a period of several months. She had attributed it to the beginning of the stress of graduate school and did not seek medical attention until now. Her headache is always one-sided and associated with nausea, vomiting and photophobia. Sometimes her headaches are preceded by flashes of light and a feeling of faintness. She has been treating them with 400 mg of ibuprofen and a day or two of rest in a dark room. The headaches are becoming more frequent and are beginning to interfere with her classes and study. Her physical and neurologic exams are negative except for the headaches. She takes no medication other than the ibuprofen, except for a multivitamin and calcium carbonate 1200 mg daily.**

Ergotamine tartrate had been the treatment of choice for migraines until the advent of sumatriptan (Imitrex) and other the serotonin receptor agonists. These are described in Chapter 14 and are the most commonly prescribed drugs for migraine. Although *Clinical Evidence* (2004) indicated that ergotamine was likely to be beneficial in the treatment of migraine compared to placebo, it was found less effective than sumatriptan, and on limited evidence, less effective than naproxen, a nonsteroidal antiinflammatory drug (Morillo, 2004). H.A. is tried on a course of zolmitriptan (Zomig) for abortive therapy and is told to return to the University Health Center in 1 month for reevaluation of her drug therapy.

If H.A. did not have drug coverage as part of her student health insurance, the physician may have prescribed ergotamine because of the expense of the triptan class of medications. In this case, H.A.'s assessment of her preexisting health status requires a pregnancy test because ergotamine is not recommended for use during pregnancy due to its oxytocic effects (see the Pregnancy Safety box below). Her concurrent medications, multivitamin and calcium, are not remarkable. Have her maintain a "headache diary" of date, time, precipitating factors, and description of pain, treatment, and length of the migraine attack for continued assessment of her condition.

Receiving ergot alkaloid therapy, H.A. might experience altered comfort related to underlying vascular headache because of ineffectiveness of the drug, a developing tolerance to the drug, dizziness, or nausea; risk for injury related to a decrease in peripheral sensation because of vasoconstriction (paleness, coolness, numbness, or tingling of fingers and toes); excess fluid volume (edema); and the potential complications of CNS toxicity, cardiovascular effects, and pleural or retroperitoneal fibrosis. Nonpharmacologic interventions for pain relief of migraine are used to supplement the medication, such as a quiet environment, relaxation therapy, and other measures specific to her. Tell H.A. to take the initial dose of the ergot alkaloid during the early part of a migraine attack—during the "aura" (visual field defects, paresthesia, and nausea)—and then lie down in a quiet, dark room for several hours. Assure her that the quality of relief is related to the promptness with which the medication is started after the onset of symptoms. Relaxation techniques, adequate rest, and avoidance of stressful situations may alleviate the severity or frequency of attacks.

Because nausea and vomiting may be increased by the administration of ergotamine before headache relief occurs, phenothiazine antiemetics may be required to promote

PREGNANCY SAFETY	
DRUGS AFFECTING THE SYMPATHETIC SYSTEM	
Category	**Drug**
B	acebutolol, dobutamine, pindolol, sotalol
C	atenolol, betaxolol, bisoprolol, carteolol, carvedilol, dopamine, ephedrine, epinephrine, esmolol, inamrinone, isoproterenol, labetalol, mephentermine, metaraminol, methoxamine, metoprolol, milrinone, nadolol, norepinephrine, penbutolol, phenoxybenzamine, phentolamine, phenylephrine, propranolol, timolol
X	dihydroergotamine, ergoloid mesylates, ergotamine tartrate, methysergide

Data from *Mosby's drug consult* (15th ed.). (2005). St. Louis, Mosby.

H.A.'s comfort. Safety measures should be taken to prevent injury to her extremities, and they should be monitored for the ischemic effects of the drug.

Warn H.A. to take ergotamine exactly as prescribed. Prolonged use or overdose can cause circulatory impairment (ergot poisoning), which is evidenced by numbness, tingling sensations, weakness, intermittent claudication, cyanosis of the extremities, muscle pain, and coldness of the extremities. Report such symptoms immediately to the prescriber. If this condition is not corrected, gangrene may develop. Warmth is to be applied, taking care to avoid excessive heat. Severe peripheral vasoconstriction may be treated by administering IV sodium nitroprusside. Discontinuing the drug for 2 to 3 days may relieve these symptoms.

Instruct H.A. to avoid alcohol ingestion because it aggravates the headache. Provide counseling regarding smoking cessation because nicotine increases the peripheral vasoconstrictive effects of the drug. For the same reason, instruct her to avoid exposure to cold. Alert her to the signs and symptoms of infection and tell her to report any signs and symptoms to the prescriber because infection increases sensitivity to the drug.

Because of the possible occurrence of hypertension or hypotension, monitor for fluid volume excess by checking for edema, weighing daily, and maintaining a low salt intake. Position changes from recumbent to upright should be made slowly to avoid dizziness or fainting. Modify activities if dizziness and drowsiness occur as adverse effects. The expected outcome for ergot alkaloid therapy is that H.A. will experience diminished headaches or will not experience any headaches without adverse effects of ergot alkaloid therapy.

How are the β-adrenergic blockers categorized?

β-adrenergic blocking agents inhibit β receptors by competing with the catecholamines at the receptor site. **β-adrenergic blocking agents** are differentiated into two subclasses: β_1 and β_2. Drugs that selectively inhibit only one type of receptor (usually β_1), such as atenolol, are called selective. β_1-selective blocking agents are often referred to as cardioselective blockers because these agents block the β_1 receptors in the heart.

A further differentiation often identifies β-adrenergic blocking agents that have intrinsic sympathomimetic activity (ISA). The ISA property was initially believed to be advantageous when compared with agents that possess only β-blocking effects. It was projected that fewer serious adverse effects would occur with such agents, but the significance of this property has not been proven clinically. ISA causes partial stimulation of the β receptor, but this effect is less than that of a pure agonist. For example, if a client has a slow heart rate at rest, the partial agonists may help to increase the heart rate by their partial agonist property. If a client has a rapid heart rate or tachycardia from exercise, these agents may help to slow down the heart rate secondary to the predominant β-blocking effect. It is believed that the only role for the ISA property might be to treat clients who experience severe bradycardia from the non-ISA medications.

Drugs with ISA properties should not be used to prevent MI because of their partial agonist properties. Figures 22-8 to 22-10 show the sites of action of the β blockers; Table 22-6 presents the classification of β-adrenergic blockers.

What pharmacologic actions are seen with β-adrenergic blockers?

β-adrenergic blocking agents compete with β-adrenergic agonists (e.g., catecholamines) for available β receptor sites located on the membrane of cardiac muscle, smooth muscle of bronchi, and smooth muscle of blood vessels. Cardiac muscle contains β_1 receptors, whereas the smooth muscle sites contain primarily β_2 receptors. Pharmacologically, the β_1-adrenergic blocking action in the heart decreases heart rate, conduction velocity, myocardial contractility, and cardiac output.

The antianginal effects produced by the β blockers are primarily caused by their ability to lower myocardial oxygen requirements. Their antihypertensive actions are not specifically identified, but these effects may result from a decrease in cardiac output, a diminished sympathetic outflow from the vasomotor center in the brain to the peripheral blood vessels, and an inhibition of renin release by the kidney. The result is a decrease in peripheral vascular resistance, which lowers BP.

To prevent a recurrence of a MI, β blockers (without ISA properties) are used for their antidysrhythmic effect plus their ability to decrease the myocardial oxygen demands on the heart. The latter effect may reduce the progression of ischemia and its severity on the heart.

Various mechanisms may be involved in the prevention of vascular headaches, such as prevention of arterial vasodilation, inhibition of platelet aggregation, and increased oxygen release to tissues.

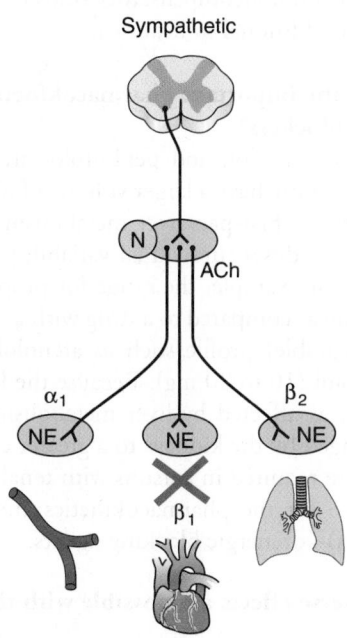

FIGURE 22-8 Site of action of cardioselective β blockers. *Ach*, Acetylcholine, *N*, nicotinic receptor; *NE*, norepinephrine.

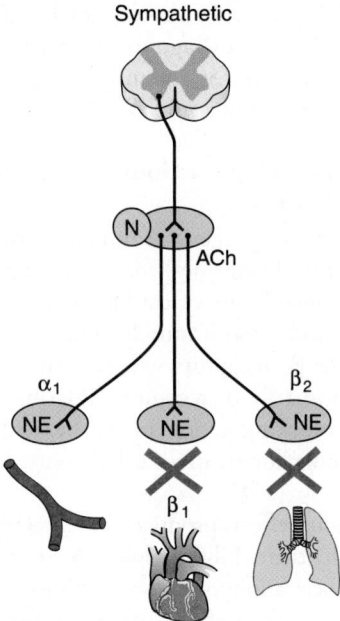

FIGURE 22-9 Site of action of nonselective β blockers with activity at β₁ and β₂ receptors. *Ach,* Acetylcholine, *N,* nicotinic receptor; *NE,* norepinephrine.

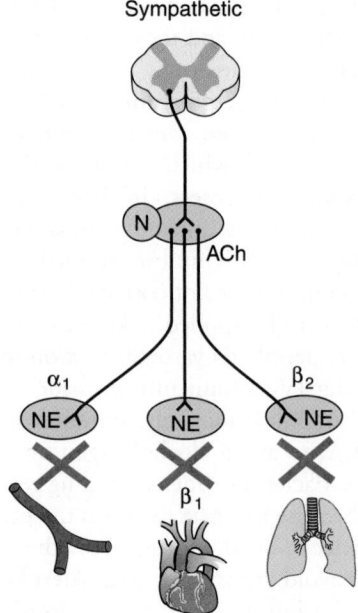

FIGURE 22-10 Site of action of nonselective β blockers with activity at α, β₁, and β₂ receptors. *Ach,* Acetylcholine, *N,* nicotinic receptor; *NE,* norepinephrine.

✳ What are the indications for β blockers?

The β-adrenergic blocking agents are used to treat chronic angina pectoris, hypertension, hypertrophic cardiomyopathy, tremors and anxiety; to prevent and/or treat cardiac dysrhythmias; to prevent a second MI; and to prevent and/or treat vascular headaches; as an adjunct to thyrotoxicosis and pheochromocytoma therapy; and to treat mitral valve prolapse syndrome. Esmolol (Brevibloc) is a parenteral agent indicated for the treatment of supraventricular tachycardia and noncompensatory sinus tachycardia. See Table 22-6 for additional indications.

✳ What are the important pharmacokinetic distinctions with β blockers?

Propranolol, metoprolol, and penbutolol are highly lipid soluble and therefore have a larger volume of distribution in the body, a greater first-pass liver metabolism, and a wider range of effective doses (individual variability) than do the other agents. For example, the range for propranolol is 10 to 640 mg daily as compared to a drug with a less-lipophilic (more water-soluble) profile such as atenolol (50 to 100 mg) or betaxolol (10 to 20 mg). Because the less-lipophilic agents are not as affected by liver metabolism and are excreted unchanged by the kidneys to a greater extent, dosage adjustments are required in persons with renal impairment. See Table 22-6 for the pharmacokinetics and usual adult dosage of the β-adrenergic blocking agents.

✳ What adverse effects are possible with these agents?

The adverse effects of β blockers include drowsiness, weakness, difficulty sleeping, anxiety, nasal congestion, abdominal distress, dizziness, bradycardia, nausea, vomiting, de-

pression, cold hands and feet, sexual dysfunction, and difficulty breathing (bronchospasm).

✳▪ propranolol [proe **pran** oh lole]
(Inderal, Inderal LA, Apo-Propranolol✤)

Propranolol is considered to be the prototype β-adrenergic blocker. Drugs such as propranolol that inhibit both types of receptors are referred to as nonselective β-adrenergic blocking agents and generally have more adverse effects. Propranolol is a competitive antagonist for both β₁ and β₂ receptors.

Indications

Propranolol is used to treat hypertension, angina, cardiac dysrhythmias, essential tremor, pheochromocytoma, and to prevent migraine headaches and myocardial infarction (MI). It has also been used to treat tremors of Parkinson's disease, antipsychotic akathisia, ethanol withdrawal, and aggressive behavior and to manage symptoms of thyrotoxicosis.

Pharmacokinetics/Dosing

On oral administration, propranolol has a high first-pass effect with extensive hepatic metabolism noted. The onset of action is approximately 1 to 2 hours after oral administration, and the duration is about 6 hours. The oral adult dosage range for propranolol varies by indication and ranges from 10 mg once daily up to 160 mg four times daily.

Adverse Effects

The nontherapeutic effects of propranolol are usually predictable based on pharmacologic action and include bradycardia, bronchospasm/wheezing, heart failure, cardiac dysrhythmias (related to arteriovenous nodal blockade or suppression of sinoatrial node), depression, dizziness, confusion, hyperglycemia, sexual dysfunction, and masking of symptoms of hypoglycemia (e.g., blunting tremors, palpitations, sweating).

✳ P.S., a 73-year-old man, has had his hypertension treated successfully for approximately 30 years, first with hydrochlorothiazide (HCTZ) (a diuretic) alone, and then 15 years ago with lisinopril (an angiotensin-converting enzyme inhibitor) 10 mg as the only drug.

TABLE 22-6 COMPARISON OF β-ADRENERGIC BLOCKERS

Agent	Receptor Antagonist	Indications (Non–FDA-Approved Uses)	Typical Oral Adult Dose (Range)	Half-life (hr—Unless Otherwise Noted)	Comment
acebutolol (Sectral)	β₁ (see Figure 22-8)	Hypertension, ventricular dysrhythmias, angina	200 mg twice daily (400-1200 mg daily)	3-8	ISA
atenolol (Tenormin)		Hypertension, angina, post-MI (alcohol withdrawal, supraventricular and ventricular dysrhythmias, migraine prophylaxis)	25-50 mg daily (12.5-100 mg daily)	6-7	
betaxolol (Kerlone)		Hypertension (topical: glaucoma)	5-10 mg daily (5-20 mg daily)	14-22	
bisoprolol (Zebeta)		Hypertension (also, angina, ventricular dysrhythmias, HF*)	5 mg daily (2.5-20 mg daily)	9-12	
esmolol (Brevibloc)		Hypertension, supraventricular dysrhythmias	Varies with indication	9 min	
metoprolol (Lopressor)		Hypertension, angina, prevention of MI, supraventricular dysrhythmias (ventricular dysrhythmias, migraine prophylaxis, aggressive behavior, HF*)	50 mg twice daily (50-450 mg daily)	3-7	
carteolol (Cartrol)	β₁, β₂ (see Figure 22-9)	Hypertension, HF* (angina, cardiomyopathy)	2.5 mg daily (2.5-10 mg daily)	6	ISA
nadolol (Corgard)		Hypertension, angina, prevention of MI, migraine prophylaxis (portal hypertension)	40 mg daily (40-320 mg daily)	20-24	
penbutolol (Levatol)		Hypertension	20-40 mg (20-80 mg)		ISA (Minor)
pindolol (Visken)		Hypertension (ventricular dysrhythmias, akathisia, anxiety, aggressive behavior)	5 mg twice daily (5-60 mg daily)	3-4	ISA
propranolol (Inderal)		Hypertension, angina, pheochromocytoma, essential tremor, tetralogy of Fallot, dysrhythmias, prevention of MI, migraine headache prophylaxis (parkinsonian tremor, alcohol withdrawal, aggressive behavior, acute panic, GI bleeding with portal hypertension)	40 mg twice daily (10-640 mg daily)	3-5	
sotalol (Betapace)		Life-threatening ventricular dysrhythmias (supraventricular dysrhythmias)	80 mg twice daily (80-640 mg daily)	7-18	
timolol (Blocadren)		Hypertension, angina, migraine prophylaxis, prevention of MI (topical glaucoma)	10 mg twice daily (10-60 mg daily)	4	

GI, Gastrointestinal; *HF,* heart failure; *ISA,* intrinsic sympathomimetic activity; *MI,* myocardial infarction.
*Initiate at a low dose for individuals with otherwise stable heart failure.

Continued

TABLE 22-6 COMPARISON OF β-ADRENERGIC BLOCKERS—CONT'D

Agent	Receptor Antagonist	Indications (Non–FDA-Approved Uses)	Typical Oral Adult Dose (Range)	Half-life (hr—Unless Otherwise Noted)	Comment
carvedilol (Coreg)	$\alpha_1, \beta_1, \beta_2$ (see Figure 22-10)	Hypertension, HF* (angina, cardiomyopathy)	3.125-6.25 mg twice daily (6.25-100 mg daily)	7-10	ISA
labetalol (Normodyne)		Severe hypertension (pheochromocytoma, clonidine withdrawal hypertension)	PO: 100 mg twice daily (400-2400 mg daily) IV: 20 mg	6-8	

GI, Gastrointestinal; HF, heart failure; ISA, intrinsic sympathomimetic activity; MI, myocardial infarction.
*Initiate at a low dose for individuals with otherwise stable heart failure.

Two years ago, P.S.'s BP was at 146/74 mm Hg and the prescriber added the HCTZ back into his drug regimen. P.S. was noncompliant with the HCTZ because he felt that it was the cause of "neck and chest discomfort" when he walked and that it did not provide an appreciable change in his blood pressure. On his last routine physical exam, his BP was 168/76 mm Hg and the prescriber noted from P.S.'s daily BP log that his BP has been slowly increasing for some time. To follow up on his "chest tightness," P.S. underwent an exercise stress test that showed a dysrhythmia, which was followed by a coronary angiography with normal findings. His creatinine clearance was slightly elevated for his age and the determination was that P.S. had mild nephrosclerosis secondary to long-term hypertension. To prevent further renal damage, his BP would have to be more closely managed. P.S. was started on atenolol (Tenormin) 100 mg, a β-adrenergic antagonist; valsartan (Diovan), an angiotensin II-receptor antagonist, 160 mg; and HCTZ 12.5 mg daily.

✸ **What are the nursing issues related to β blockers in the case of P.S.?**

Assessment Although P.S. is a remarkable healthy 73-year-old for the most part, his health status is reviewed for preexisting health problems that might contraindicate the use of atenolol. The risk of decreasing myocardial contraction, thus increasing the risk of heart failure, must be considered when selecting a β-blocking agent. Such agents are contraindicated if P.S. were to have heart failure with pulmonary edema, cardiogenic shock, second- or third-degree heart block, and sinus bradycardia (less than 45 beats/min). In addition, atenolol at large doses, blockades β_2 receptors of the bronchial smooth muscle, leading to bronchoconstriction. This effect is particularly hazardous for individuals with a history of allergy, asthma, bronchitis, and emphysema. There is less risk of inducing bronchospasm in these clients when a cardioselective β blocker (β_1 blocker) is used and at lower dosages.

P.S. has a family history of type 2 diabetes mellitus, but does not have the disease. Because β_2-adrenergics blockade

the appearance of the warning signs and symptoms of acute hypoglycemia (sweating, increased heart rate, and anxiety), which is of concern for clients on insulin, these agents should be used with caution in such clients. Exacerbation of depression has been reported in clients with depression or with a history of depression; they should be closely monitored if taking a β-blocking agent.

Review P.S.'s current medication regimen for the risk of significant drug interactions. When β-adrenergic blocking agents are given concurrently with any other medications that therapeutically lower BP or any other medication for which hypotension is an adverse effect, there will be an additive hypotensive effect. Alert P.S. to change position slowly from lying or sitting to sitting upright or standing, to avoid feeling lightheaded. Although there would be the same concern for drugs that cause bradycardia, such as digoxin, this is not an issue with P.S.

Nursing Diagnosis P.S. is at risk for the following nursing diagnoses/collaborative problems with β-adrenergic antagonist therapy: disturbed thought processes (confusion); sexual dysfunction (decreased sexual ability); risk for injury related to dizziness or orthostatic hypotension; ineffective airway clearance (bronchospasm); disturbed sleep pattern (insomnia, drowsiness); activity intolerance related to lethargy and weakness; and the potential complications of mental depression, hepatotoxicity, and altered cardiac output (bradycardia, dysrhythmias, heart failure).

Planning While on β-blocker therapy, P.S. will:
- Experience relief from the symptoms for which the β blocker was prescribed (e.g., a decrease in his BP) without experiencing adverse effects.
- Remain compliant with his drug therapy (not discontinuing it abruptly).
- Effectively manage his therapeutic regimen (e.g., self-monitoring BP, reporting adverse effects appropriately, keeping follow-up appointments for monitoring, using supportive nonpharmacologic measures such as a low-sodium diet, moderate exercise).

Implementation

Monitoring P.S. is to check his apical pulse rate before administering the atenolol; if the pulse is slower than 50 beats/min or the rate is irregular, he will hold taking the drug and call the prescriber immediately. Encourage him to maintain his daily BP log and report significant variations in BP. Low parameters indicate overdose.

To monitor for potential/actual fluid volume excess, have P.S. weigh daily. Fluid retention may cause dyspnea, orthopnea, nocturnal cough, pulmonary rales, distended neck veins, and edema, all of which are signs of impending heart failure. Have him report weight gain and other such symptoms to the prescriber. Given P.S.'s history of manipulating his medications, monitor for adherence to the therapeutic regimen; noncompliance may be an issue related to sexual dysfunction, fatigue, and/or depression.

Intervention Take the apical heart rate before administering a β-adrenergic antagonist. If the pulse is less than 50 beats/min (or other ordered parameter), hold the dose and consult the prescriber.

Education Counsel P.S. not to alter the drug regimen established by the prescriber. β-blocking drugs control, but do not cure, hypertension, making lifetime compliance necessary. The medication should be taken even if he feels well, and he should always have available an adequate supply of drug so that strict compliance is observed. Advise him of the hazards of untreated hypertension, such as his nephrosclerosis or stroke, as with other family members. Emphasize the importance of keeping appointments for periodic laboratory tests. Caution P.S. not to take OTC medications, especially decongestants and cough and cold medications, without consulting his health care provider.

Instruct P.S. to restrict sodium intake to prevent unnecessary fluid retention. Caution him to avoid cold temperatures because there is an increased sensitivity to cold. Painful, cold, and tender hands and feet are a sign of impaired circulation. Palpate peripheral pulses to monitor for a decrease in peripheral circulation. Alcohol ingestion, standing still for long periods, exercise, and hot weather enhance the orthostatic hypotensive effects of the drug. Because drowsiness and dizziness are common adverse effects, caution P.S. about operating a car or hazardous equipment until the drug's effects are known.

Note that β-blocking drugs must be withdrawn slowly to prevent abrupt withdrawal syndrome with tremors, sweating, severe headache, malaise, palpitation, rebound hypertension, life-threatening dysrhythmias, MI (in clients with cardiac problems and angina pectoris), and hyperthyroidism (in clients with thyrotoxicosis). If the drug is to be discontinued, reduce the dosage over a 1- to 2-week period (Box 22-2). To reduce the risk of MI and/or dysrhythmias, advise the client to avoid physical exertion while the drug is being withdrawn.

Evaluation The expected outcome of β-adrenergic blocking drug therapy is that P.S. will experience a BP within

---

BOX 22-2 WITHDRAWAL OF A β-ADRENERGIC BLOCKING AGENT

- Withdraw β-adrenergic blocking agents slowly by tapering or lowering the dose over approximately 14 days.
- Advise the client to avoid vigorous physical exercises or activities during this time to decrease the risk of a reinfarction or cardiac dysrhythmia.
- If withdrawal signs occur (angina or chest pain, sweating, tachycardia, respiratory distress), temporarily reinstitute the β-blocking agent to stabilize the client; then lower the dose slowly with close supervision.

---

normal limits without any adverse drug effects. He will effectively manage his therapeutic regimen.

Summary

Being knowledgeable about drugs that affect the SNS is essential for all areas of nursing practice. Because of the ability of the SNS to produce generalized physiologic responses, drugs that act on this system may affect a wide range of body functions. These agents are described as either adrenergic (sympathomimetic) drugs—those that mimic the effects of sympathetic nerve stimulation—or adrenergic-blocking (sympatholytic) drugs—those that compete with the catecholamines at receptor sites and inhibit adrenergic sympathetic stimulation. The adrenergic drugs can be direct-acting, indirect-acting, or dual-acting (direct and indirect) agents. Knowledge of these agents is essential, because many of them are used to rectify life-threatening situations in which the nurse must act quickly to provide the necessary pharmacologic intervention. Other drugs that act on the sympathetic nervous system are used quite commonly in practice for a wide range of clients.

The adrenergic direct-acting drugs, the catecholamines, interact with and stimulate adrenergic effector cells (α and β receptors). α-adrenergic activity includes vasoconstriction of arterioles in the skin and splanchnic area, which increases BP, pupil dilation, and relaxation of the gut. β-adrenergic activity includes cardiac acceleration and increased contractility, vasodilation of the arterioles of the skeletal muscles, bronchial relaxation, and uterine relaxation. β receptors can be either β_1 receptors, which are located mainly in the heart, or β_2 receptors within the bronchioles and arterial smooth muscle. Understanding the placement of these receptor cells assists the nurse in conceptualizing the activities of the various drugs that affect the sympathetic nervous system.

Epinephrine is a direct-acting catecholamine that stimulates α, β_1, and β_2 receptors. It is considered to be the classic, or standard drug, of this classification because of its long history of use for symptomatic treatment of asthma, emergency treatment of anaphylactic shock and cardiac arrest, local homeostasis, and management of simple, open-angle glaucoma. Isoproterenol is a nonselective β-adrenergic drug.

Norepinephrine, on the other hand, has a high affinity for α receptors. Dobutamine is valuable for individuals with low cardiac output because it directly stimulates the β_1-adrenergic receptors of the heart. Dopamine in low doses acts mainly to cause vasodilation of the renal and mesenteric arteries. All of these drugs are used for the treatment of circulatory shock.

The indirect-acting adrenergic agents act indirectly on receptors by triggering the release of epinephrine and norepinephrine from their storage sites, which then stimulate α and β receptors. Dual-acting adrenergic agents have both indirect and direct effects. Ephedrine has both a direct and an indirect sympathomimetic action and is used more commonly for bronchodilation for milder forms of asthma and as a nasal decongestant. Phenylephrine is also found in many combination cough-cold, antihistamine and decongestant, and ophthalmic preparations. Metaraminol, a dual-acting adrenergic agent, is used primarily for its vasopressor effects with hypotensive clients.

The adrenergic-blocking, or sympatholytic, drugs are also classified by α and β receptors and by their ability to inhibit adrenergic sympathetic nervous stimulation at these sites. There are noncompetitive, long-acting antagonists such as phenoxybenzamine, which is used mainly for vasodilation and inhibition of vasospasm; competitive, short-acting antagonists such as phentolamine, which is used locally to reverse the action of an extravasation of vasoconstricting drugs; and the ergot alkaloids, which are used for the management of vascular headaches. Sumatriptan is also an antimigraine agent but is believed to produce its effects at serotonin receptors; see Chapter 14.

The β-adrenergic blocking agents are differentiated into selective β_1-adrenergic blocking agents such as atenolol and metoprolol, which decrease heart rate, conduction velocity, myocardial contractility, and cardiac output; and the nonselective β-adrenergic blocking agents such as carteolol, nadolol, penbutolol, pindolol, propranolol, sotalol, and timolol. The nonselective β-adrenergic blocking agents affect cardiac muscle and smooth muscle of the bronchi and blood vessels, but are used primarily to treat chronic angina, hypertension, and cardiac dysrhythmias, and to prevent a second MI, vascular headaches, and cardiac dysrhythmias.

Bibliography

Alldredge, B.K. (2005). Headache. In M.A. Koda-Kimble, L.Y. Young, W.A. Kradjan, B.J. Guglielmo, B.K. Alldredge, & R.L. Corelli (Eds.), *Applied therapeutics: The clinical use of drugs.* (8th ed.) Philadelphia: Lippincott Williams & Wilkins.

Anderson, D.M., Keith, J., & Novak, P.D. (Eds.), (2002). *Mosby's medical, nursing, and allied health dictionary* (6th ed.). St. Louis: Mosby.

Beale, R.J., Hollenberg, S.M., Vincent, J.L., & Parrillo, J.E. (2004). Vasopressor and inotropic support in septic shock: An evidence-based review. *Critical Care Medicine, 32*(11 Supple.), S455-S465.

Bleumink, G.S., Schut, A.F., Sturkenboom, M.C., Deckers, J.W., van Duijn, C.M., Stricker, B.H. (2004). Genetic polymorphisms and heart failure. *Genetics in Medicine, 6*(6), 465-474.

Bosker, G. (2004). *Textbook of primary and acute care medicine: Principles, protocols, pathways* (2nd ed.). Atlanta: Thomson American Health Consultants.

Chang, J.T., & Altman, R.B. (2004). Extracting and characterizing gene-drug relationships from the literature. *Pharmacogenetics, 14*(9), 577-586, and linked supplemental website http://bionlp. stanford.edu/genedrug/gene_drug_predictions.html (as cited December 2, 2004).

Dhond, M.R., Donnell, K., Singh, S., Garapati, S., Whitley, T.B., Nguyen, T., et al. (1999). Value of negative dobutamine stress echocardiography in predicting long-term cardiac events. *Journal of the American Society of Echocardiography, 12*(6), 471-475.

Dishy, V., Landau, R., Sofowora, G.G., Xie, H.G., Smiley, R.M., Kim, R.B., et al. (2004). β_2-Adrenoceptor Thr164Ile polymorphism is associated with markedly decreased vasodilation and increased vasoconstrictor sensitivity *in vivo. Pharmacogenetics, 14*(8), 517-522.

Drug facts and comparisons (58th ed.). (2005). St. Louis: Facts and Comparisons.

Gold, M.S., & Sainsbury, R. (2000). First aid anaphylaxis management in children who were prescribed an epinephrine autoinjector devise (EpiPen). *Journal Allergy & Clinical Immunology, 106*(1), 171-176.

Grouhi, M., Alshri, M., Hummel, D., & Roifman, C.M. (1999). Anaphylaxis and epinephrine auto-injector training: Who will teach the teachers? *Journal of Allergy & Clinical Immunology, 104*(1), 190-193.

Hoffman, B.B. (2001). Catecholamines, sympathomimetic drugs, and adrenergic receptor antagonists. In J.G. Hardman & L.E. Limbird (Eds.) *Goodman & Gilman's The pharmacological basis of therapeutics* (10th ed.). New York: McGraw-Hill.

Hopkins, P., & Hunt, S.C. (2003). Genetics of hypertension. *Genetics in Medicine, 5*(6), 413-429.

Huang, S.W. (1998). A survey of EpiPen use in patients with a history of anaphylaxis. *Journal of Allergy & Clinical Immunology, 102*(3), 525-526.

✳ Critical Thinking Questions

- Sean Murphy is admitted to the emergency department with a massive MI. His BP has dropped to 80/40 mm Hg, his pulse has increased to 128 beats/min, and his skin is cool and moist. The physician indicates that Mr. Murphy is in cardiogenic shock and orders an infusion of dopamine, 10 mcg/kg/min. How will this dose affect adrenergic receptors? What would you expect to occur as a result of Mr. Murphy receiving this infusion? As the nurse, what should you be monitoring? What action should you take if the infusion infiltrates?

- Mrs. Melanie Freedman is 43 years old and has a history of migraine headaches. She has tried a number of therapies without success, so ergotamine tartrate (Ergomar✤) is prescribed for her. Mrs. Freedman calls the clinic and indicates that she vomits each time she takes the drug. As the nurse, how should you respond to Mrs. Freedman's comment?

- Dr. Harry Lewis, a 56-year-old university professor, is admitted to the hospital with atrial tachycardia. He is started on propranolol (Inderal), 30 mg four times daily. Dr. Lewis also has diabetes mellitus. What nursing interventions will you take?

Kaye, D.M., Smirk, B., Williams, C., Jennings, G., Esler, M., & Holst, D. (2003). β-Adrenoceptor genotype influences the response to carvedilol in patients with congestive heart failure. *Pharmacogenetics, 13*(7), 379-382.

La Rosee, K., Huntgeburth, M., Rosenkranz, S., Bohm, M., & Schnabel, P. (2004). The Arg389Gly β1-adrenoceptor gene polymorphism determines contractile response to catecholamines. *Pharmacogenetics, 14*(11), 711-716.

Mialet Perez, J., Rathz, D.A., Petrashevskaya, N.N., Hahn, H.S., Wagoner, L.E., Schwartz, A., et al. (2003). Beta 1-adrenergic receptor polymorphisms confer differential function and predisposition to heart failure. *Nature Medicine, 9*(10), 1300-1305.

Morillo, L. (2004). Migraine headache. In F. Godlee (Ed.), *Clinical evidence: The international source of the best available evidence for effective health care.* London: BMJ.

Mosby's drug consult (15th ed.). (2005). St. Louis: Mosby.

Nagar, S., Zalatoris, J., & Blanchard, R. (2004). Human UGT1A6 pharmacogenetics: Identification of a novel SNP, characterization of allele frequencies and functional analysis of recombinant allozymes in human liver tissue and in cultured cells. *Pharmacogenetics, 14*(8), 487-499.

Saseen, J.J., & Carter, B.L. (2005). Essential hypertension. In M.A. Koda-Kimble, L.Y. Young, W.A. Kradjan, B.J. Guglielmo, B.K. Alldredge, & R.L. Corelli (Eds.), *Applied therapeutics: The clinical use of drugs.* (8th ed.). Philadelphia: Lippincott Williams & Wilkins.

Schaefer, B.M., Caracciolo, V., Frishman, W., & Charney, P. (2003). Gender, ethnicity, and genes in cardiovascular disease. Part 2: Implications for pharmacotherapy. *Heart Disease, 5*(3), 202-214.

Small, K.M., Brown, K.M., Theiss, C.T., Seman, C.A., Weiss, S.T., & Liggett, S.B. (2003). An Ile to Met polymorphism in the catalytic domain of adenylyl cyclase type 9 confers reduced β2-adrenergic receptor stimulation. *Pharmacogenetics, 13*(9), 535-541.

USP DI: Drug information for the health care professional (25th ed.). (2005). Greenwood Village, CO: MICROMEDEX Thomson Healthcare.

Young L.Y., Koda-Kimble, M.A., Young, L.Y., Kradjan, W.A., Guglielmo, B.J., Alldredge, B.K., & Corelli, R.L. (Eds.). (2005). *Applied therapeutics: The clinical use of drugs* (8th ed.). Philadelphia: Lippincott Williams & Wilkins.

e-LEARNING SUPPLEMENTS

Student CD-ROM
- Final Exam questions
- NCLEX® Examination review questions
- Pharmacology animations
- Printable chapter summary

Evolve Website (http://evolve.elsevier.com/mckenry)
- Case study on drugs affecting the parasympathetic nervous system

- Content updates, including information on new drugs
- WebLinks corresponding to this chapter
- Answers to the critical thinking questions in this chapter
- *Elsevier ePharmacology Update* newsletter
- *Mosby's Drug Consult* Internet Edition
- Supplemental and reference information

23

DRUGS FOR SPECIFIC DYSFUNCTIONS OF THE CENTRAL AND PERIPHERAL NERVOUS SYSTEMS

CHAPTER FOCUS

Because dysfunctions of the central and peripheral nervous systems are often progressive and incapacitating, appropriate assessment, intervention, and evaluation are important measures for nursing. This chapter discusses Parkinson's disease, myasthenia gravis, dementia, Alzheimer's disease, and skeletal muscle relaxants.

LEARNING OBJECTIVES

- Identify the two neurotransmitters that centrally affect motor function and balance.
- Explain the neurotransmitter balance theory in Parkinson's disease.
- Describe the actions and key adverse effects of medications used to treat Parkinson's disease, myasthenia gravis, dementia, and Alzheimer's disease.
- Describe the physiology of muscle movement and motor nerve response.
- Compare the manifestations of the spinal and cerebral types of muscle spasticity.
- Compare the actions and key adverse effects of central-acting and direct-acting skeletal muscle relaxants.
- Summarize the drug interactions associated with skeletal muscle relaxants.
- Implement the nursing management of clients who have drug therapy prescribed for the treatment of Parkinson's disease, myasthenia gravis, dementia, Alzheimer's disease, and muscle spasm/spasticity.

The personal tragedy of the progressive nature of Parkinson's disease, myasthenia gravis, dementia, and Alzheimer's disease, as well as the emotional distress of family members and the increasing cost of care to families and society, challenge health care providers to develop and manage rational pharmacologic treatments. Because there are currently no "cures," drug therapy attempts to minimize the symptoms of these conditions.

Skeletal muscle spasticity can also be debilitating, but skeletal muscles are affected by many pharmacologic substances. Their effects may occur at the neuromuscular junction or at different levels in the central nervous system (CNS), that is, at the brain or spinal cord. This chapter also discusses these agents.

Parkinson's Disease

✳ **S.T. is a 72-year-old retired farmer who reports to his health care provider accompanied by his wife. He exhibits a coarse tremor, stiff muscles and joints, and stooped posture, and his facial features lack expression. His current medication is limited to atenolol (Tenormin) 25 mg daily for hypertension. The health care team recommends a consult with a neurologist to rule out Parkinson's disease.**

✳ **What are the important features of Parkinson's disease?**

Parkinson's disease is a progressively debilitating disorder of the CNS. This condition is characterized by resting tremor, bradykinesia (abnormal slowing of all voluntary movements and speech), forward flexion of the trunk, muscle rigidity, and weakness. It usually occurs in persons who are between the ages of 50 and 80 years. In the United States, at least 500,000 people are believed to suffer from

Parkinson's disease, and about 50,000 new cases are reported annually. These figures are expected to increase as the average age of the population increases. The disorder appears to be slightly more common in men than women. The average age of onset is about 60 years. Both prevalence and incidence increase with advancing age; the rates are very low in people younger than age 40 years and rise among people in 70- and 80-year-old age groups. Parkinson's disease is found worldwide (National Institute of Neurological Disease and Stroke, 2004).

Although the cause is unknown, viral influences and environmental contaminants are suspected. Genetic factors may also play a role in the development of Parkinson's disease and its treatment (see the Special Considerations for Pharmacogenetics box below). The correct balance of dopamine and acetylcholine is important in regulating posture, muscle tone, and voluntary movement (Figure 23-1). In Parkinson's disease, there is a disorder of the extrapyramidal system in the brain, especially the basal ganglia area. Degeneration of the dopamine-producing neurons in this area produces a dopamine-acetylcholine imbalance, a progressive loss of dopamine (inhibitory neurotransmitter), and an increase in acetylcholine (excitatory neurotransmitter). Other neurotransmitters (e.g., norepinephrine and serotonin) are also decreased in the brain of a person with Parkinson's disease. This condition can also be induced by the use of designer drugs (Box 23-1).

The use of drug therapy is aimed at correcting the dopamine-acetylcholine imbalance by administering exogenous dopamine in the form of a precursor, levodopa; stimulating dopamine receptors within the corpus striatum through the use of dopamine agonists; or inhibiting the major metabolic pathways in the brain responsible for the degradation of levodopa and its metabolites (Ernst, Gottwald, & Gidal, 2005). Two classes of drugs are used in the treatment of Parkinson's disease: (1) drugs with central

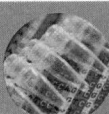

Special Considerations for Pharmacogenetics | ANTIPARKINSON'S/ALZHEIMER'S DEMENTIA TREATMENTS/ SKELETAL MUSCLE RELAXANTS

PHARMACODYNAMICS

Although early in development, genetic markers for a number of CNS diseases may help identify those individuals who may be more responsive to pharmacotherapy for Parkinson's disease, Alzheimer's dementia, and other conditions (Galvin & Ginsberg, 2004; Wang, Si, Liu, & Yu, 2003; Morris, 2003; Drozdzik et al., 2003). Variation in response to ropinirole in the treatment of Parkinson's disease may be attributed to pharmacodynamic differences (Cristina et al., 2003). Response to donepezil and tacrine may also be affected by genetics (Chang & Altman, 2004). Skeletal muscle strength, size and contractility is genetically determined (Thompson et al., 2004). It is likely that response to skeletal muscle relaxants also has a genetic basis.

PHARMACOKINETICS

Differences in the metabolism of carisoprodol (Soma) have been noted to be genetically based (Bramness et al., 2003). This is likely to be true for other drugs metabolized by the cytochrome P450 enzyme system, including the skeletal muscle relaxant cyclobenzaprine and the treatments for Alzheimer's dementia, such as donepezil, galantamine, and tacrine.

ADVERSE EFFECTS

Genetic variation in catechol-O-methyltransferase (COMT) activity may explain different responses and potential adverse effects seen across populations with entacapone or tolcapone used in the treatment of Parkinson's disease (Poewe, 2004).

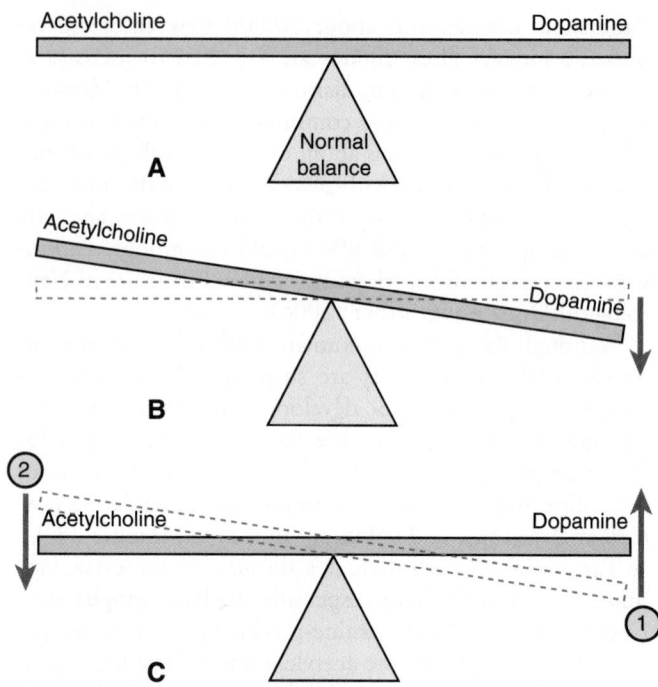

FIGURE 23-1 Central acetylcholine/dopamine balance. **A,** Normal "balance" of acetylcholine and dopamine. **B,** In Parkinson's disease, a decrease in dopamine results in an acetylcholine/dopamine imbalance. **C,** Drug therapy in Parkinson's disease aims at increasing the dopamine level, which restores the acetylcholine/dopamine balance toward normal by (1) increasing the supply of dopamine or (2) blocking or lowering acetylcholine levels.

anticholinergic activity (anticholinergics and antihistamines), and (2) drugs that affect brain dopamine levels or mimic dopamine to enhance dopaminergic action.

✸ **S.T. is evaluated by the neurologist and is determined to have early Parkinson's disease. The neurologist is considering initiating the anticholinergic drug, benztropine (Cogentin).**

✸ **What is the role of anticholinergic drugs in the treatment of Parkinson's disease?**

Symptoms of Parkinson's disease caused by an excess of cholinergic activity are muscle rigidity and muscle tremor. The muscle rigidity or increased tone appears as "ratchet resistance," or "cogwheel rigidity," in which the affected muscle moves easily, then meets resistance or remains fixed in the new position. The muscle tremors appear to have a "to-and-fro" movement caused by the sequence of contractions of the agonistic and antagonistic muscles involved. The tremors are usually worse at rest and are commonly manifested as a "pill-rolling" motion of the hands and a bobbing of the head. Anticholinergics are most useful for younger clients who present primarily with tremors and are early in the course of this disease.

Drugs that inhibit or block the effects of acetylcholine are referred to as **anticholinergic drugs**. The belladonna alkaloids, atropine and scopolamine, were the first centrally

---

Designer drugs, or chemical variations of illegal or controlled substances, are an ever-increasing problem in North America. Such products may not be illegal but generally are produced to induce the psychoactive effects of selected illegal products. Often the user consumes an unknown substance that may or may not be the desired product. Reports indicate that methyl-phenyl-tetrahydropyridine (MPTP), a chemical produced as an analogue of meperidine in clandestine laboratories, has been sold on the streets as heroin, cocaine, or a contaminant of other products.

MPTP has reportedly induced a degenerative CNS disorder characterized by tremors and muscle paralysis similar to the symptoms of Parkinson's disease. In a number of cases, the paralysis has been permanent, even after one-time use.

active (i.e., crossing the blood-brain barrier) anticholinergic agents used to treat parkinsonism and for many years were the only drugs available for such treatment. These drugs have been supplanted by synthetic anticholinergics, which were developed in an effort to produce drugs as effective as the belladonna drugs but with fewer adverse effects. In this group, benztropine is the key drug.

The anticholinergic agents used in the treatment of mild Parkinson's disease and as an adjunct to dopamine replacement include benztropine (Cogentin), biperiden (Akineton), procyclidine (Kemadrin), and trihexyphenidyl (Artane). Anticholinergic agents block central cholinergic excitatory pathways, returning the dopamine/acetylcholine balance in the brain (especially in the basal ganglia) to normal. The effects of the anticholinergic agents include decreased salivation and relaxation of smooth muscle with a decrease in tremors. Decreased rigidity and akinesia (in nearly 50% of clients) are also reported.

These anticholinergic agents that readily cross the blood-brain barrier can produce some improvement in functional capacity. The usefulness of these drugs is limited because of their adverse effects and their tendency to be less effective with continued use. Some anticholinergics are also used to control extrapyramidal reactions, such as rigidity, **akinesia** (difficulty in or lack of ability to initiate muscle movement), tremor, and **akathisia** (restlessness and agitation), that are caused by antipsychotic drugs such as the phenothiazines; see Chapter 19. Chapter 21 has a more complete discussion of anticholinergic drugs. Table 23-1 summarizes information about these agents. Benztropine is considered the prototype of the group.

✸◻ **benztropine** [benz **troe** peen]
(Cogentin, Apo-Benztropine✦)
Indications
Benztropine is indicated for use as an antidyskinetic, for treatment of tremor in Parkinson's disease, and for treatment of drug-induced extrapyramidal symptoms (EPS) associated with typical antipsychotic drug use (see Chapter 19).

TABLE 23-1 AGENTS FOR PARKINSON'S DISEASE

Agent	Typical Oral Adult Dose	Important Adverse Effects	Comments
ANTICHOLINERGICS			
benztropine (Cogentin)	0.5 mg at bedtime up to 2 mg three times daily	Dry mouth Blurred vision Urinary retention Confusion Hallucinations	Efficacy limited to tremor Avoid in older adults Contraindicated if medically complex
biperiden (Akineton)	1 mg at bedtime up to 4 mg four times daily		
trihexyphenidyl (Artane)	1 mg three times daily up to 15 mg daily		
DOPAMINE PRECURSOR			
carbidopa-levodopa (Sinemet)	carbidopa-levodopa 25 mg/100 mg three times daily with titration to effect	Nausea Vomiting Orthostatic hypotension Dyskinesias Hallucinations	Peripheral effects improved if ≥75 mg carbidopa daily Bioavailability of CR product is variable and often requires increase in dose by approximately 20% Unlabeled use: restless leg syndrome
DOPAMINE REUPTAKE BLOCKER (↑ DOPAMINE RELEASE)			
amantadine (Symmetrel)	100 mg twice daily	Confusion Livedo reticularis Visual hallucinations	Adjust dose for renal impairment Tolerance may develop
ERGOT DOPAMINE AGONISTS			
bromocriptine (Parlodel)	1.25 mg twice daily up to 30 mg three times daily	Dizziness Dyskinesias Hallucinations Headache Nausea Orthostatic hypotension Somnolence	May need to decrease Sinemet if add-on therapy Other uses include: acromegaly, hyperprolactinemia, neuroleptic malignant syndrome, Tourette's syndrome
pergolide (Permax)*	0.05 mg daily up to 1.5 mg three times daily		
NONERGOT DOPAMINE AGONISTS			
pramipexole (Mirapex)	0.125 mg three times daily up to 1.5 mg three times daily	Dizziness/sedation Dyskinesias Hallucinations Headache Nausea Orthostatic hypotension Syncope (ropinirole)	May be better tolerated than ergot dopamine agonists Pramipexole: Dosage adjustment needed for renal dysfunction
ropinirole (Requip)	0.25 mg three times daily up to 8 mg three times daily		
MONOAMINE OXIDASE INHIBITOR TYPE B			
selegiline (Eldepryl)	5 mg twice daily	Dysrhythmias Dizziness Dyskinesias Hallucinations Headache Nausea Orthostatic hypotension	Doses >10 mg daily may interact with tyramine-containing foods Increased MAOI effects with concurrent desipramine, paroxetine, sertraline

COMT, Catechol-*O*-methyltransferase; *CR,* controlled release; *MAOI,* monoamine oxidase inhibitor.
*Peroglide was voluntarily removed from the market in March 2007.

Continued

TABLE 23-1 AGENTS FOR PARKINSON'S DISEASE—cont'd

Agent	Typical Oral Adult Dose	Important Adverse Effects	Comments
COMT INHIBITORS			
entacapone (Comtan)	200 mg with each dose of carbidopa-levodopa up to 1600 mg daily	Agitation Dizziness Dyskinesias Hallucinations Headache Insomnia/vivid dreams Nausea Orthostatic hypotension Syncope	Only used with carbidopa-levodopa Use typically limited to clients with "on-off" response to carbidopa-levodopa May require a decrease of approximately 25% in carbidopa-levodopa dose when initiated
tolcapone (Tasmar)	100 mg three times daily up to 200 mg three times daily		
COMBINATION THERAPY			
carbidopa-levodopa/ entacapone (Stalevo)	Tablets: 12/50/200 25/100/200 37.5/150/200 Dosed one tab q3-8h	See individual agents	Use limited to clients who have been titrated on individual agents

COMT, Catechol-*O*-methyltransferase; *CR*, controlled release; *MAOI*, monoamine oxidase inhibitor.

Pharmacokinetics/Dosing

The onset of oral benztropine is 1 to 2 hours and within minutes after intramuscular (IM)/intravenous (IV) administration. The duration of effect is between 6 and 48 hours. Benztropine is metabolized hepatically. The adult dosage of benztropine for Parkinson's disease is 1 to 2 mg PO daily, adjusted as necessary; for drug-induced EPS, the dosage is 1 to 4 mg PO, IM, or IV once or twice daily. The maximum dosage is 6 mg daily.

Adverse Effects

The adverse effects of anticholinergic drugs such as benztropine include blurred vision, mydriasis, constipation, dry skin, anhidrosis, urinary hesitancy, pain on urination, nausea, vomiting, photophobia, drowsiness, xerostomia, and dysphagia.

✴ **What would the nurse assisting S.T. and his family to manage his anticholinergic therapy include in his care?**

Assessment Because S.T. is 72 years of age, he is at risk for developing health problems caused by the anticholinergic effects of these agents, such as dryness of the mouth and constipation, and because he is male, urinary retention (see the Special Considerations for Older Adults box on p. 439 in Chapter 21). Older adults may respond to the usual doses of anticholinergic agents with agitation, confusion, and altered thought processes (hallucinations and psychotic-like symptoms). The anticholinergics block the actions of acetylcholine, which supports many functions of the brain (including memory); as a result, S.T., if he has existing memory problems, may become more impaired with continued use of anticholinergics.

Preexisting health status is also of concern with anticholinergics. Assess S.T. for a history of or current partial or complete intestinal obstruction because anticholinergic activity decreases the tone and motility of the gastrointestinal (GI) tract, necessitating caution. Also assess him for a predisposition to prostatic hypertrophy, urinary retention, or other obstructive uropathy because these conditions may be precipitated or exacerbated. With the use of anticholinergics, S.T.'s heart rate may be increased, and this should be carefully considered before administering drugs with anticholinergic properties if he has preexisting tachycardia or other cardiac dysrhythmias. Assess S.T. for chronic pulmonary disease because the resultant decrease in bronchial secretions caused by anticholinergics may lead to bronchial mucous plugs.

Because he is older than 40 years of age, S.T.'s intraocular pressure will be measured to ensure ST is not at risk for glaucoma. The mydriatic effect of anticholinergics increases intraocular pressure, which may precipitate an acute episode of closed-angle glaucoma or necessitate an adjustment in the therapy of clients with open-angle glaucoma.

Review S.T.'s current medication regimen and lifestyle for the risk of significant drug interactions, such as those that may occur when anticholinergic agents are given concurrently with alcohol and CNS depressants (results in enhanced CNS depressant effects); antacids (may reduce the absorption of anticholinergic agents); and other anticholinergic or other antimuscarinic medications (may result in enhanced anticholinergic effects).

A baseline assessment of S.T. includes his mobility status and other symptoms related to the parkinsonism for which the anticholinergic agent is being prescribed.

Nursing Diagnosis Once S.T. begins dyskinetic therapy with anticholinergic drugs, assessment should relate to the potential development of a number of nursing diagnoses/collaborative problems related to the drug. There may be disturbed sensory perception related to the effects of the drug on vision and somatosensory function, especially at his age. Older adults are also more at risk for disturbed thought processes (confusion and hallucinations) and are at risk for falls and other injury related to the CNS effects of the drug. There may be anxiety, disturbed sleep pattern (extreme drowsiness or insomnia), constipation because of the GI effects, or urinary retention. There may be impaired comfort related to xerostomia, blurred vision, rash, or the GI and genitourinary effects of the anticholinergics. Potential complications include decreased cardiac output (dysrhythmias), extrapyramidal symptoms, and increased intraocular pressure.

Planning While S.T. is on anticholinergic therapy for parkinsonism, he will:
- Remain free of injury related to the illness or the medication.
- Remain independent for as long as possible.
- Maintain as normal as possible bladder and bowel patterns.
- Remain compliant to drug regimen.
- Effectively manage, with his caregiver, the therapeutic regimen, including reporting adverse drug effects appropriately to the health care provider and using nonpharmacologic measures supportive to the drug regimen.
- Collaborate with the health team in keeping appointments for monitoring and continued care.

Implementation
Monitoring Check S.T.'s vital signs at office visits, and report changes in cardiac status. Dysrhythmias have been noted as a result of anticholinergic agents, but these effects are dose related.

Especially monitor S.T. for difficulty in starting his urinary stream because of his age. Older adults are more sensitive to anticholinergic agents and require dosages smaller than the usual adult dosage. Monitor closely for agitation, lethargy, sleepiness, and altered thought processes.

Observe S.T. for **xerostomia,** a reduction in the volume of saliva. This symptom is important and should be reported, not only because extreme dryness of the mouth is usually a discomfort to the client, but also because the severity of xerostomia limits the amount of drug that can be administered. After xerostomia, the progression of adverse effects is usually interference with visual accommodation and difficulty in urination.

Intervention To begin, the dosages of S.T.'s therapy are low and may increase every 5 to 6 days until a therapeutic level is obtained. Except in emergencies, the drug is withdrawn in the same manner—gradually. Sudden withdrawal may cause vomiting, lassitude, and excessive sweating and salivation. Tolerance may develop if the therapy is prolonged, which might require an increase in dosage. The dosage is titrated according to S.T.'s symptoms. If another antiparkinson agent is to be substituted for the initial drug, the dosage of the first drug should be gradually decreased while the substitute is gradually increased. Oral dosage forms of anticholinergic agents may be taken with or immediately after meals to minimize heartburn.

Education Instruct S.T. and his caregiver to check with a pharmacist or prescriber for drug interactions before taking any other drugs, including over-the-counter (OTC) drugs. He should avoid CNS depressants such as alcohol, barbiturates, and opioids while taking anticholinergic agents.

Alert S.T. that anticholinergic agents impair physical and mental functioning (i.e., they cause drowsiness, blurred vision, and confusion) and to use caution when driving or operating machinery. Caution him about the dangers of heat exhaustion and advise him to avoid exercising in warm weather because of the decreased ability to perspire. Instruct S.T. to change positions slowly if orthostatic hypotension is a problem. Advise him to use sugarless hard candy, gum, mouthwash, or ice chips to relieve dryness of the mouth. Instruct him in the necessity of a high-fiber diet and increased fluid intake to minimize the adverse effect of constipation along with gradual increases in activity and the establishment of an elimination routine.

Counsel S.T. to have annual ophthalmic examinations; these determinations are of particular importance because increased ocular tension may occur with the anticholinergic agents.

Evaluation The expected outcome of anticholinergic therapy for S.T.'s parkinsonism is that he will demonstrate improved mobility with a reduction in muscular rigidity and tremor and will not experience any adverse effects of the drug.

✳ **After review with the neurologist, S.T. is started on the dopaminergic drug carbidopa-levodopa (Sinemet).**

✳ **What is the role of dopaminergic drugs in Parkinson's disease?**
Although preliminary data suggest that levodopa therapy may slow the progression of Parkinson's disease (Fahn et al., 2004), dopaminergic agents are not considered curative. Instead they offer some degree of symptom control. Three classifications of drugs affect brain dopamine: those that release dopamine, those that increase brain levels of dopamine, and dopaminergic agonists. The drugs of choice in the treatment of Parkinson's disease are those that in-

crease brain levels of dopamine. The other two classifications are used as adjuncts or when the usual therapy is contraindicated.

The drugs that affect brain dopamine have their major effect on the akinesia seen in Parkinson's disease. Akinesia, difficulty or the lack of ability in initiating muscle movement, is caused by decreased levels of brain dopamine in Parkinson's disease. The client with akinesia exhibits a mask-like facial expression, impairment of postural reflexes, and, eventually, an inability to self-care. Drugs are used to increase the levels of dopamine in the brain, thus creating a balance between dopamine and acetylcholine in the brain, especially in the basal ganglia area.

Drugs That Increase Levels of Dopamine in the Brain

Two agents that are directly converted to dopamine in the CNS are levodopa and the combination of carbidopa-levodopa (Sinemet). Levodopa is considered the prototype agent, although it is most often combined with carbidopa to reduce peripheral adverse effects.

▨▛ levodopa [**lev** oh dope ah]
(L-Dopa, Dopar, Larodopa)
A small percentage of levodopa crosses the blood-brain barrier intact. It is decarboxylated to dopamine, stimulates dopamine receptors, and helps to balance the dopamine-acetylcholine concentrations.
Indications
Levodopa is indicated for the treatment of Parkinson's disease (idiopathic, postencephalitic, symptomatic, or parkinsonism associated with cerebral atherosclerosis).
Pharmacokinetics/Dosing
Levodopa is absorbed by active transport, with approximately 30% to 50% reaching the systemic circulation. It is distributed to most body tissues; the CNS receives less than 1% of the dose because of peripheral metabolism. The enzyme decarboxylase converts levodopa (95%) to dopamine in the stomach, intestines, and the liver. Levodopa has a half-life of 1 to 3 hours.

Improvement is usually seen within 2 to 3 weeks, although some clients may require levodopa for up to 6 months to obtain a therapeutic effect. Peak concentration is achieved in 1 to 3 hours. The duration of action is up to 5 hours per dose. The drug is excreted by the kidneys.

For adults and children 12 years of age and older, the dosage of levodopa (Dopar, Larodopa) is 250 mg PO two to four times daily, increased by 100 to 750 mg daily at 3- to 7-day intervals until a therapeutic response is achieved. The maximum dosage is 8 g daily. Older adults and postencephalitic clients may require lower dosages because they are more sensitive to this medication. The dosage for children younger than 12 years of age has not been established.
Adverse Effects
The adverse effects of levodopa include anxiety, nervousness, confusion (especially in older adults), constipation, nightmares, difficulty with urination, depression, orthostatic hypotension, mood changes, increased aggressiveness, irregular heart rate, severe nausea or vomiting, and choreiform and involuntary movements of the body (face, arms, hands, tongue, head, and upper body) (Ernst et al., 2005).

If S.T. is prescribed levodopa without the carbidopa, provide him with dietary counseling regarding the ingestion of protein and pyridoxine (B$_6$). Proteins are metabolized into amino acids, which may compete with levodopa for transport to the brain and make the response to levodopa unpredictable. Rather than restrict S.T.'s protein intake, it would be divided in equal parts to be taken over the entire day. Vitamin compounds and foods high in pyridoxine (e.g., pork, beef, liver, ham, egg yolks, avocado, beans, sweet potato, dry skim milk, and oatmeal) may decrease the effects of levodopa and should be avoided. Dietary teaching for all clients with Parkinson's disease should include the necessity of a high-fiber diet and increased fluid intake to minimize the adverse effect of constipation with the drug, along with gradual increases in activity and the establishment of an elimination routine. Other eating difficulties may arise if S.T. has full dentures; some clients experience difficulty retaining their dentures while undergoing levodopa therapy.

carbidopa-levodopa [**kar** bih dope ah/**lev** oh dope ah]
(Sinemet, Sinemet CR)
Sinemet and Sinemet CR (controlled or extended release) are combinations of levodopa with carbidopa, a dopa decarboxylase inhibitor. Carbidopa competes for the enzyme dopa decarboxylase, thus slowing the peripheral breakdown of levodopa. Unlike levodopa, carbidopa does not cross the blood-brain barrier, thus it does not interfere with the intracerebral transformation of levodopa to dopamine. Because carbidopa prevents much of the peripheral conversion of levodopa to dopamine, the incidence of systemic adverse effects of levodopa, such as nausea, vomiting, and cardiac dysrhythmias, is decreased. The CNS effects of levodopa are a greater risk with this combination because more levodopa is reaching the brain to be converted to dopamine.
Indications
Carbidopa-levodopa is indicated for the treatment of idiopathic, postencephalitic, and symptomatic Parkinson's disease. (See the previous section for the pharmacokinetics of levodopa.) An unlabeled use is in the management of restless leg syndrome.
Pharmacokinetics/Dosing
Between 40% and 70% of an oral dose of carbidopa is absorbed. Carbidopa is distributed widely within many body tissues, with the exception of the CNS. The metabolism of the drug is insignificant. It is excreted by the kidneys.

The addition of carbidopa to levodopa reduces the required dose of levodopa to approximately 20% to 25% of the original dose. The available carbidopa-levodopa combination dosage forms include 10/100 (10 mg of carbidopa and 100 mg of levodopa), 25/100 (25 mg of carbidopa and 100 mg levodopa), and 25/250 (25 mg of carbidopa and 250 mg of levodopa). Bioavailability of the controlled-release product is variable and often requires an increased dose when converting from the immediate-release product. Older adults and postencephalitic clients may be more sensitive to carbidopa-levodopa and may require a lower dosage.
Adverse Effects
The adverse effects of carbidopa-levodopa are similar to those for levodopa, although this combination is less likely to produce constipation, changes in heart rate, or nausea/vomiting. Eyelid spasms or closing may be an early sign of drug overdose. Mental or mood changes may also occur earlier and may be dose related.

Drug interactions are the same as for levodopa, with the exception of the pyridoxine interaction. The interaction between levodopa and pyridoxine does not occur in the presence of carbidopa.

Dopamine-Releasing Drugs

amantadine [a man **ta** deen]
(Symmetrel, Endantadine✚, PMS-Amantadine✚)
Amantadine is a synthetic antiviral compound that augments dopamine release. Although the exact mechanism of its action is

not completely known, amantadine may release dopamine and other catecholamines from neuronal storage sites. It also blocks the uptake of dopamine into presynaptic neurons, thus permitting the peripheral and central accumulation of dopamine. Amantadine may also give a client a sense of well-being and elevated mood. It is less effective than levodopa but produces more rapid clinical improvement and causes fewer untoward reactions.

Indications
Amantadine is indicated for use as an antidyskinetic (treatment of Parkinson's disease) and as an antiviral (systemic agent) against influenzae type A infection.

Pharmacokinetics/Dosing
Amantadine is well absorbed; it is not metabolized. It has a half-life of 11 to 15 hours. Peak serum levels are reached within 2 to 4 hours, with the onset of antidyskinetic action within 48 hours. A steady state is reached within 2 to 3 days with daily drug administration; the drug serum level is 0.2 to 0.9 mcg/mL. Levels above 1 mcg/mL are considered toxic. Amantadine is excreted by the kidneys. The adult dosage for antidyskinetic action is 100 mg PO once or twice daily. The maximum dosage is 400 mg daily. Older adults are given 100 mg daily to start, titrating to two or three times daily as necessary. Dosage reduction is recommended for clients with renal impairment.

Adverse Effects
The adverse effects of amantadine include impaired concentration, dizziness, increased irritability, anorexia, nausea, nervousness, reddish-blue mottling (livedo reticularis, usually seen with chronic therapy), confusion, hallucinations, mental or mood variations, orthostatic hypotension, and difficult urination. Symptoms of overdose include severe confusion, insomnia, nightmares, and seizures.

Dopaminergic Agonists

The dopamine agonists used to treat Parkinson's disease include the ergot alkaloids, bromocriptine (Parlodel) and pergolide (Permax), and the nonergot dopamine agonists, pramipexole (Mirapex) and ropinirole (Requip).

Ergot Dopamine Agonists

Bromocriptine is an ergot alkaloid derivative marketed as the first agonist of dopamine receptor activity. It activates postsynaptic dopamine receptors, stimulating the production of dopamine and correcting dopamine/acetylcholine imbalances in the brain. Pergolide is a dopamine agonist, usually used in conjunction with levodopa or carbidopa-levodopa to treat the signs and symptoms of Parkinson's disease. It is more potent and longer acting than bromocriptine, and directly stimulates both D_1 and D_2 receptors. In combination therapy, the dose of levodopa or carbidopa-levodopa is often reduced. Up to 75% of clients who did not respond to levodopa did improve with the addition of pergolide. In addition, clinical fluctuations reported in clients receiving carbidopa-levodopa may be reduced; that is, the "on" period was prolonged, whereas the "off" period was decreased in most of the clients studied (Box 23-2) (Ernst et al., 2005).

bromocriptine [brom oh **krip** teen]
(Parlodel, Apo-Bromocriptine✤)
Indications
Bromocriptine is indicated as an antidyskinetic, a growth hormone suppressant, an antihyperprolactinemic, and a prophylactic for lactation after a loss of pregnancy in the second or third trimester.

BOX 23-2 ON-OFF SYNDROME

On-off syndrome refers to a complication following prolonged levodopa therapy (2 years or more). During therapy, the client fluctuates from being symptom free ("on") to demonstrating full-blown Parkinson's symptoms ("off"). These effects may last from minutes to hours and may be a result of a decrease in the delivery of dopamine centrally, an alteration in sensitivity of the dopamine receptors, a variation in the amount and rate of drug absorption, interference with dopamine metabolites, or a combination of effects.

Treatment may require more frequent administration of levodopa or carbidopa-levodopa, and perhaps the addition of bromocriptine, a direct-acting dopamine agonist. Some clients may demonstrate an improved response to the drug therapy following a drug holiday (drug withdrawal) of several days to a week. This may be because of the reestablishment of dopamine receptor sensitivity to levodopa, which is usually only temporary. Because many individuals worsen during the drug-free period, this approach should be instituted in a hospital or highly monitored setting (Ernst et al., 2005).

Pharmacokinetics/Dosing
Approximately 28% of a dose is absorbed, but only 6% reaches systemic circulation. The half-life of bromocriptine is biphasic: alpha (or distribution), 4 to 4.5 hours; beta (or elimination), 15 hours. The onset of activity from a single dose used for antiparkinsonism is 30 to 90 minutes, with a peak concentration reached in 2 hours. This drug is metabolized in the liver. Metabolites of bromocriptine are excreted primarily in bile. The adult dosage for antidyskinetic effects is 1.25 to 2.5 mg PO daily, titrated as necessary. The maintenance dosage ranges from 2.5 to 40 mg daily in divided doses. The dosage for children younger than 15 years of age has not been established.

Adverse Effects
The adverse effects of bromocriptine include drowsiness, headache, nausea, hypotension, and, less commonly, confusion, hallucinations, and uncontrolled movements of the body, face, tongue, arms, hands, and head.

pergolide* [**purr** go lide]
(Permax)
Pergolide stimulates dopamine receptors in the nigrostriatal area. However, unlike bromocriptine, its action is independent of dopamine synthesis or dopamine storage sites. It also inhibits prolactin secretion.

Indications
Pergolide is indicated as an adjunct treatment for Parkinson's disease.

Pharmacokinetics/Dosing
It is well absorbed, and serum protein binding is high (approximately 90%). This drug is excreted by the kidneys. The recommended dosage of pergolide for adults and older adults is 0.05 mg PO daily for 2 days, increased by 0.1 to 0.15 mg every 3 days over the next 12 days. Thereafter the dosage can be increased by 0.25 mg every 3 days until the maximum therapeutic effect is reached. Doses should be divided and given three times daily. The maximum dosage is 5 mg daily. The dosage for children has not been established.

---

*Peroglide was voluntarily removed from the market in March 2007.

Adverse Effects

The adverse effects of pergolide include stomach distress/pain, constipation, light-headedness, sedation, hypotension, cold-type symptoms, nausea, lower back pain, confusion, dyskinesia (e.g., uncontrollable body movements), and hallucinations. Somnolence of sudden onset has been reported by the manufacturer (Lilly Pharmaceuticals, 2003).

Nonergot Dopamine Agonists

Pramipexole and ropinirole are nonergot dopamine receptor agonists. Although their exact mechanism of action is unknown, they are postulated to stimulate dopamine receptors in the striatum (Hobson, Pourcher, & Martin, 1999). There is conflicting data regarding the ability of these agents to be neuroprotective and modify the course of Parkinson's disease (Pan, Le, & Jankovic, 2004; Schapira & Olanow, 2004).

pramipexole [pram ih **pex** all]
(Mirapex)

Indications

Pramipexole is used in the treatment of Parkinson's disease.

Pharmacokinetics/Dosing

Pramipexole is rapidly absorbed orally and reaches peak serum levels in 1 to 2 hours. The half-life of pramipexole is 8 hours (12 hours in older adults). It is not metabolized and is primarily excreted unchanged in the urine. The adult dosage of pramipexole ranges from 0.375 to 4.5 mg daily in divided doses.

Adverse Effects

The adverse effects of pramipexole include nausea, constipation, dizziness, sedation, dyskinesia, hallucinations, confusion, and dystonia. Ropinirole has a higher reported incidence of dizziness, sedation, nausea, vomiting, stomach pain, and dyspepsia (Korczyn et al., 1999).

ropinirole [roh **pin** ih role]
(Requip)

Indications

Ropinirole is used in the treatment of Parkinson's disease.

Pharmacokinetics/Dosing

Ropinirole is well absorbed after oral administration with a peak effect observed within 1 to 2 hours. Ropinirole is extensively metabolized, with only 1% to 2% excreted unchanged by the kidneys. Its half life is 6 hours. The adult dosage of ropinirole is 0.25 to 1 mg three times daily, with dosages adjusted weekly as necessary.

Adverse Effects

Similar to pramipexole.

Monoamine Oxidase Inhibitors

There are two types of monoamine oxidase (MAO) in the body: MAO-A is necessary to metabolize norepinephrine and serotonin, and MAO-B metabolizes dopamine. Selegiline (sometimes called deprenyl) irreversibly inhibits MAO-B, thus preventing the breakdown of dopamine. As a result, it enhances or prolongs the antiparkinson effect of levodopa, which may result in a lowering of the daily dose of levodopa. Its role in the treatment of early Parkinson's disease remains under debate (Ives et al., 2004).

selegiline [sell **eh** geh leen] (also referred to as deprenyl)
(Eldepryl, Novo-Selegiline✦) (SD-Deprenyl)

Indications

Selegiline is used in combination with levodopa or carbidopa-levodopa to treat Parkinson's disease.

Pharmacokinetics/Dosing

Selegiline is well-absorbed orally, reaches peak serum levels in 30 minutes to 2 hours, and has three active metabolites (with half-lives of 2 to 20 hours). It readily crosses the blood-brain barrier and is excreted slowly via the kidneys. The usual adult dosage of selegiline is 5 mg at breakfast and lunch.

Adverse Effects

The adverse effects of selegiline include dry mouth, nausea, vomiting, insomnia, dizziness, stomach distress or pain, dyskinesia, and mood alterations. Higher doses may interact with tyramine-containing foods and produce serious adverse effects, including significant hypertension. See Chapter 19 for MAO inhibitor interactions.

Antiparkinsonism Adjunct Medication

Adjuncts to standard therapy are often used to achieve better control of symptoms for clients with Parkinson's disease. Such agents include the catechol-*O*-methyltransferase (COMT) inhibitors entacapone (Comtan) and tolcapone (Tasmar). Although their exact mechanism of action is unknown, these agents inhibit COMT, which results in a more sustained serum level of levodopa. COMT is responsible for metabolizing catecholamines such as dopamine, norepinephrine, and epinephrine; consequently, its inhibition affects levels of levodopa that may result in a more constant dopaminergic effect in the brain and may lead to an improvement in the symptoms of Parkinson's disease (Rivest, Barclay, & Suchowersky, 1999). The effects of these drugs are selective and reversible. To avoid CNS toxicity of levodopa, doses of concurrent levodopa or carbidopa-levodopa- often require a dosage reduction when COMT inhibitors are initiated. Such CNS toxicity may be due to genetic variation (see the Special Considerations for Pharmacogenetics box on p. 469).

entacapone [en tah cah **pone**]
(Comtan)

Indications

Entacapone is used as an adjunct drug to the carbidopa-levodopa (Sinemet) combination for the treatment of Parkinson's disease in individuals who have signs and symptoms of end-of-dosage or drug-wearing-off effects. The usual adult dosage is a 200-mg entacapone tablet administered with each carbidopa-levodopa dose, to a maximum of 8 doses daily (*Mosby's Drug Consult*, 2005).

Pharmacokinetics/Dosing

Entacapone is rapidly absorbed and highly plasma-protein bound. With this drug, the elimination half-life of levodopa is extended from 1.3 hours to 2.4 hours. It is metabolized in the liver and excreted by the kidneys (10%) and in the feces (90%).

Adverse Effects

Significant adverse effects of entacapone include nausea, diarrhea or, to a lesser degree, constipation, stomach pain, dyskinesia, hyperkinesia or hypokinesia, and dizziness.

✱◻ tolcapone [toll cah pone]

(Tasmar)

Indications

Tolcapone is an adjunct treatment drug used in combination with levodopa and carbidopa to treat the symptoms of Parkinson's disease. The risk for life-threatening hepatotoxicity limits its use to second-line therapy.

Pharmacokinetics/Dosing

Tolcapone is rapidly absorbed orally (administer on an empty stomach for best results) and is very highly protein bound (greater than 99%). It reaches peak serum levels in approximately 2 hours, has a half-life of 2 to 3 hours, is metabolized in the liver, and is excreted by the kidneys (60%) and feces (40%). The usual adult dosage for antiparkinson effects is 100 to 200 mg three times daily in conjunction with carbidopa-levodopa therapy. The maximum daily dose is 600 mg.

Adverse Effects

Hepatotoxicity has prompted the removal of tolcapone from the market in other countries. Other adverse effects of tolcapone include constipation, gastric distress, increase in dream time, sweating, and dry mouth. Adverse effects that require medical attention include orthostatic hypotension, diarrhea, dizziness, anorexia, dyskinesia, hallucinations, headache, insomnia, syncope, chest pain, confusion, dyspnea, hematuria, and upper respiratory infection.

✱ **J.T., a 60-year-old male, is begun on carbidopa-levodopa (Sinemet) 10/100 three times daily for parkinsonism. Over the first few days, he reports nausea and dizziness on rising.**

✱ **Can these effects be related to J.T.'s carbidopa-levodopa therapy?**

The peripheral effects of levodopa commonly include GI complaints and orthostatic hypotension. To obtain the peripheral inhibitor effect of carbidopa, a minimum of 75 mg (range: 75 to 100 mg) daily is necessary. Saturating peripheral dopa decarboxylase requires between 75 and 100 mg daily of carbidopa (Ernst et al., 2005). Nausea and vomiting are reported in clients receiving dosages of carbidopa lower than 75 mg daily. Three combination dosage forms are available to permit greater flexibility in prescribing sufficient amounts of both levodopa and carbidopa for the client. The manufacturer recommends that not more than 200 mg daily of carbidopa be prescribed. As with levodopa alone, the decarboxylation to dopamine replaces the missing brain dopamine and restores a balance to dopamine-acetylcholine concentrations.

✱ **J.T.'s dose of carbidopa-levodopa (Sinemet) is changed to 25/100 three times daily at 7:00 AM, 1:00 PM, and 7:00 PM. Improvement in nausea and dizziness are noted with the change. Both J.T. and his significant other note fluctuations in movements throughout the day with early morning stiffness, improved movement by 8 AM, and agitation and flailing movements at 9 AM. Just before his 1:00 PM dose, J.T. is very stiff.**

✱ **Are these fluctuations in movement expected?**

The time course of action of each of the dopaminergic agents, including carbidopa-levodopa, is usually predictable

PREGNANCY SAFETY DRUGS AFFECTING BRAIN DOPAMINE	
Category	**Drug**
B	bromocriptine, pergolide
C	amantadine, ambenonium, benztropine, biperiden, carbidopa-levodopa, edrophonium, entacapone, levodopa, neostigmine, pramipexole, procyclidine, pyridostigmine, ropinirole, selegiline, tolcapone, trihexyphenidyl

Data from *Mosby's drug consult* (15th ed.). (2005). St. Louis: Mosby.

based on timing of dose and pharmacokinetics of the agent. The stiffness noted before each dose is a commonly observed manifestation of Parkinson's disease. This phenomenon is commonly referred to as "end-of-dose" symptoms, and should be differentiated from "on-off syndrome" (see Box 23-2). The agitation and choreiform movements seen shortly after dosing are related to dopaminergic hyperactivity. The agitation may include confusion or even psychosis and often is problematic to manage. The flailing movements may be similar to tardive dyskinesia (see Chapter 19).

Finding the balance between poor control of parkinsonian symptoms and adverse effects of the dopaminergic drugs is often a challenge. Careful monitoring of symptoms throughout the day, and subtle adjustment of drugs and dosage are typically required when drug therapy is first implemented. This evaluation of drug response is a continuous process for all clients with Parkinson's disease and usually requires caregiver education and participation. Table 23-1 compares agents used in the treatment of Parkinson's disease. The Pregnancy Safety box above lists the pregnancy risk categories of these various drugs affecting dopamine in the brain.

✱ **The formulation and dose of carbidopa-levodopa (Sinemet) for J.T. is changed based on his symptoms throughout the day. His immediate-release carbidopa-levodopa is discontinued. Carbidopa-levodopa continuous release (Sinemet CR) 25/100 is initiated at 7:00 AM, 1:00 PM, and 7:00 PM.**

✱ **What additional education is appropriate for J.T. and his caregivers?**

J.T. should take his carbidopa-levodopa before meals because food impedes its action. Nausea and vomiting occur in 80% of clients early in levodopa therapy, but tolerance develops with continued use of the drug.

If orthostatic hypotension is a problem, J.T. should change to the upright position slowly to minimize his risk for injury related to falls. It may also be minimized with the use of elastic stockings. If J.T. were in a care facility, his blood pressure (BP) would be taken daily.

Alert J.T. that the prescriber should be notified if symptoms of overdose develop (involuntary muscle twitching and involuntary winking) or if involuntary movement of the face, mouth, tongue, and head occur with prolonged therapy, so that his dosage may be adjusted. Caution him that an "on-off" syndrome may occur with prolonged therapy (see Box 23-2). Compliance is essential, because full withdrawal of the drug may worsen parkinsonian symptoms, depression, and immobility, as well as increase the risk of thromboembolic disease.

Periodic visits to the prescriber are essential for monitoring. Levodopa increases the risk for various conditions in predisposed clients, including skin lesions, peptic ulcer, dysrhythmias, urinary retention, glaucoma, aggravation of pulmonary conditions such as asthma and chronic obstructive pulmonary disease, and psychiatric disturbances. J.T. needs to consult his prescriber before taking OTC and other medications.

The expected outcome of his antiparkinson therapy is that J.T. will demonstrate an improvement in mobility with a decrease in muscular rigidity and tremor without experiencing adverse effects of the drug.

✳ **T.F. is a 74-year-old female with advanced Parkinson's disease who lives at home with her husband. She has been stabilized on carbidopa-levodopa (Sinemet CR) 50/200 twice daily at 7:00 AM and 4:00 PM for the past 3 years. Her symptoms of Parkinson's disease have worsened to the point that she requires assistance in ambulation and can only minimally participate in activities of daily living. She is also moderately agitated throughout the day and displays periods of confusion.**

✳ **What is the role of other dopaminergic agents for T.F.?**
Because dopaminergic treatments for Parkinson's disease only provide symptomatic relief, it is important to establish which agents can offer improved symptom control with minimal adverse effects. Striking that delicate balance becomes more difficult when managing advanced Parkinson's disease. Amantadine typically offers only modest improvement of symptoms and may contribute to worsening confusion. Bromocriptine and pergolide can typically be more effective in improving Parkinson's symptoms, but will probably worsen cognition and agitation. Similarly, the nonergot agonists, such as ropinirole or pramipexole, can improve bradykinesias, but with increased confusion or agitation. The COMT inhibitors, such as entacapone and tolcapone, and the MAO-B inhibitor selegiline have similar limitations, and a modest dosage reduction of carbidopa-levodopa would be recommended if use of any of these inhibitors is considered.

✳ **T.F. is started on bromocriptine 1.25 mg twice daily at 7:00 AM and 4:00 PM and doses are increased to 5 mg twice daily over the next 2 weeks. Three weeks into therapy, T.F. falls during ambulation. Her husband reports to the visiting nurse that she is combative and agitated, and remains awake most of the night.**

✳ **What are the next steps for the visiting nurse?**
The visiting nurse's continuing assessment of T.F.'s health status would include BP determinations, as well as a de-

scription of her motor and mental status. Her BP should be closely monitored; 1% to 5% of clients have symptomatic hypotension. In addition to advising caregivers to avoid sudden position changes with T.F. so as to minimize her risk for falls related to orthostatic hypotension, her environment should be assessed to enhance safety in mobility. Small rugs, excessive furniture, and other environmental safety hazards should be remedied. Handrails and other assistive devices should be in place, if not already provided.

Other common adverse effects include constipation, nausea, nasal congestion, and tingling or pain in the fingers and toes when exposed to cold. These effects occur in 30% to 60% of the clients being treated with bromocriptine for Parkinson's disease. The most common adverse effects occur when the client first begins therapy; most of these effects are dose related and seldom occur with doses less than 20 mg daily. However, because of T.F.'s age, these symptoms may occur at lower dosages. Her dosage has been initiated at a low level and gradually increased, but may need to be titrated more carefully to maximize its antiparkinson effects and minimize orthostatic hypotension.

Teach T.F.'s caregivers to prevent or minimize her constipation by increasing dietary fiber, increasing fluid intake to 1500 mL daily, assisting her to perform moderate exercise daily, and establishing a regular time of day for bowel elimination. Advise her caregivers to limit her exposure to cold or have her wear protective clothing to prevent discomfort of the fingers and toes.

Regular dental examinations are advised because bromocriptine inhibits salivation and will increase T.F.'s risk of discomfort, caries, and periodontal disorders.

With the administration of bromocriptine, clients with a history of or predisposition to psychiatric disorders may experience symptoms such as insomnia, confusion, and agitation. This is distressing for clients and their families. T.F. is started on risperidone (Risperdal) an atypical antipsychotic agent, at 0.5 mg twice daily for the management of these symptoms.

Myasthenia Gravis

✳ **What are the key features of myasthenia gravis?**
Myasthenia gravis is a progressive, incurable disease characterized by the loss of or a decrease in acetylcholine receptors; it is caused by an autoimmune process and results in skeletal muscle weakness and fatigue. Because of its involvement with the production of antibodies, the thymus gland is believed to play a role in the development of myasthenia gravis. Nearly 15% of all clients with myasthenia gravis have a thymoma, or a tumor of the thymus gland.

Symptoms of myasthenia gravis usually become worse with exertion and are less noticeable with rest. Stress, infection, menses, surgery, and other factors may also increase the symptoms. The most common early reported symptoms are ptosis and diplopia. Dysarthria, dysphagia, and limb weakness, especially of the upper extremities, also occur in the advanced stages. The client may complain of hand weakness or of shoulder fatigue after shaving or combing the hair; the client may find it difficult to open doors or kitchen jars, or to perform repetitive tasks such as lawn work or playing the piano (Figure 23-2). The most serious effects of myasthenia gravis are dysphagia and respiratory muscle weakness; these effects may result in aspiration pneumonia or respiratory failure.

✱ How is myasthenia gravis treated?

Treatment of this disease can include thymectomy, cholinesterase inhibitors, plasmapheresis and, at times, corticosteroids. The mainstay of therapy is cholinesterase-inhibitor drugs, such as anticholinesterase drugs.

Peripheral Acetylcholinesterase Inhibitors

The peripheral **acetylcholinesterase inhibitors** (also referred to as cholinesterase inhibitors or anticholinesterase agents) are drugs that enhance cholinergic action by blocking the effect of acetylcholinesterase at peripheral sites. As discussed in Chapter 21, these drugs act by inactivating or inhibiting cholinesterase at the sites of acetylcholine transmission, thus permitting the accumulation of acetylcholine (Figure 23-3). The peripheral cholinesterase inhibitors include neostigmine, edrophonium, pyridostigmine, and ambenonium. Neostigmine is considered the prototype peripheral cholinesterase inhibitor. Edrophonium and pyridostigmine are also used clinically. Because of their ability to increase the amount of acetylcholine at the myoneural junction, the cholinesterase inhibitors are primarily used for the diagnosis and treatment of myasthenia gravis and for their local effects in the eye (see Chapter 42). These drugs are also used for urinary retention and paralytic ileus, and as an antidote for the curariform effects of the nondepolarizing neuromuscular blockers, such as tubocurarine (Tubarine) and pancuronium (Pavulon).

Ambenonium (Mytelase) is a slowly reversible cholinesterase inhibitor that can accumulate at cholinergic synapses and produce increased, prolonged effects. Because of the narrow margin between the first appearance of adverse effects and serious toxicity, ambenonium is usually reserved for clients who have not responded adequately to neostigmine or pyridostigmine or for clients who are hypersensitive to the bromide component in both drugs.

Table 23-2 compares the peripheral acetylcholinesterase inhibitors. Other inhibitors of acetylcholinesterase that act in the CNS are used in the treatment of Alzheimer's dementia and are discussed later in the chapter.

✱⌐ neostigmine [nee oh **stig** meen]
(Prostigmin)
Indications
Neostigmine is used to diagnose and treat myasthenia gravis, to reverse the effects of neuromuscular blockers, and to prevent and treat postoperative bladder distention and urinary retention.

Pharmacokinetics/Dosing
Neostigmine is poorly absorbed orally, although an oral formulation is occasionally used for myasthenia gravis. Given IM or subcutaneously, it is effective within 20-30 minutes, within 4-8 minutes after IV administration. The duration of action is approximately 1 to 2 hours after IV and 2 to 4 hours after IM or subcutaneous administration. Neostigmine is metabolized mainly in the liver and is excreted in the kidneys. Adult dosing of neostigmine is 0.5 to 2.5 mg IV for reversal of neuromuscular blockers, or 15 to 30 mg PO every 3 to 4 hours for the treatment of myasthenia gravis.

Adverse Effects
The adverse effects of neostigmine and the other anticholinesterase agents include nausea, vomiting, diarrhea, abdominal cramps, increased sweating, drooling, increased urge to urinate, pinpoint pupils, eye watering, and increased bronchial secretions. Overdose effects include blurred vision, severe diarrhea, increased salivation, increase in bronchial secretions, severe nausea or vomiting, respiratory difficulties, severe abdominal pain, bradycardia, increased weakness, ataxia, confusion, slurred speech, and muscle weakness.

✱ A.O., a 70-year-old male, reported to his primary care provider that he has had increasing difficulty with his hobby of watercolor painting because his arms fa-

Ocular ptosis and/or diplopia

Facial muscle weakness

Dysarthria

Neck flexor weakness

Shoulder girdle weakness

Dysphagia

Respiratory muscle weakness

Forearm weakness

Hand weakness

Lower limb weakness

FIGURE 23-2 Signs, symptoms, and implications of myasthenia gravis.

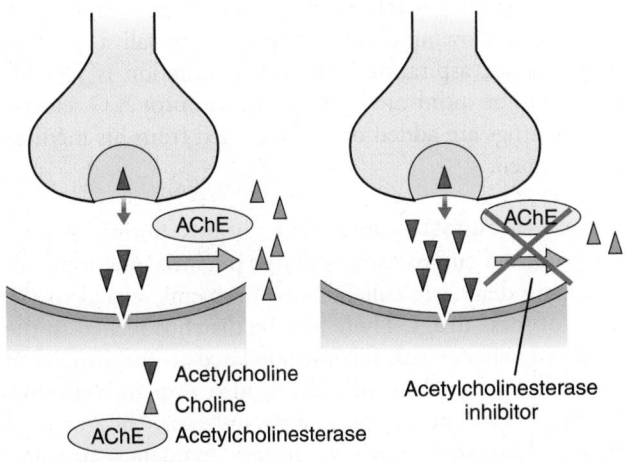

Acetylcholine
Choline
AChE Acetylcholinesterase
Acetylcholinesterase inhibitor

FIGURE 23-3 Site of action of acetylcholinesterase inhibitors.

TABLE 23-2 PERIPHERAL ACETYLCHOLINESTERASE INHIBITORS

Agent	Indication	Onset	Duration	Typical Adult Dose
neostigmine (Prostigmin)	Diagnose myasthenia gravis Treat myasthenia gravis Reverse NMBs Prevent/treat bladder distention	IV: 4-8 min IM: <30 min PO: 45-75 min	2-6 hr	Treatment of myasthenia gravis: 15-30 mg PO q3-4h Reversal of NMBs: 0.5-2.5 mg IV × 1
edrophonium (Tensilon)	Diagnose myasthenia gravis Reverse NMB	IV: 30-60 sec IM: 2-10 min	10-30 min	Diagnosis of myasthenia gravis: 1-2 mg IV Reversal of NMBs: 10 mg IV × 1, repeated up to four times
pyridostigmine (Mestinon)	Treat myasthenia gravis Reverse NMB	IV: 2-5 min IM: <15 min PO: 30-60 min	IV/IM: 2-4 hr PO: 3-12 hr	Treatment of myasthenia gravis: 60-120 mg q3-8h Reversal of NMBs: 10-20 mg IV × 1
ambenonium (Mytelase)	Treat clients with myasthenia gravis who are not tolerating other agents	PO: 10-30 min	PO: 3-8 hr	Treatment of myasthenia gravis: 2.5-5 mg q8h titrated up to 75 mg four times daily if needed

IV, Intravenously; *IM,* intramuscularly; *NMB,* neuromuscular blocker; *PO,* orally.

tigue easily and his vision has begun to blur. He was referred to a neurologist for diagnostic studies, including the diagnostic use of edrophonium; the diagnosis was myasthenia gravis. His anticholinesterase drug therapy is initiated with neostigmine.

✱ **What are the significant nursing management issues with acetylcholinesterase inhibitors?**

Assessment Assess neuromuscular status (ptosis, diplopia, speed of movement, extremity strength) before administering the drug. Observe for subtle changes in A.O.'s speech and facial expression. Ptosis increases and the ability to swallow decreases early, because more weakness occurs with an increase in the nicotinic effects. Other assessments include testing the gag reflex, rating voice quality, and observation of swallowing ability using water or saliva alone to assess risk for aspiration. Pulmonary function is variable and should be monitored frequently. Monitor A.O. closely if other drugs are added or discontinued from his medication regimen.

Nursing Diagnosis Once A.O. begins antimyasthenic therapy, also focus assessment on the potential development of nursing diagnoses/collaborative problems related to the effects of these drugs. There may be diarrhea related to the muscarinic effects; risk for injury related to the visual and CNS effects, especially in older adults; impaired comfort (increased watering of the mouth and eyes); or impaired urinary elimination, such as urinary frequency, urgency, and incontinence. The increase in bronchial secretions may result in ineffective airway clearance. A.O.'s comfort may

also be impaired because of rash, GI effects, or muscle weakness.

Planning While taking acetylcholinesterase inhibitor drugs, A.O. will:
- Remain free of injury related to the illness or the medication (e.g., aspiration).
- Remain independent for as long as possible.
- Remain compliant with the drug regimen.
- Effectively manage, with his caregiver, the therapeutic regimen, including reporting adverse drug effects appropriately to the health care provider and using nonpharmacologic measures supportive of the drug regimen.
- Collaborate with the health team in keeping appointments for monitoring and continued care.

Implementation

Monitoring When treatment is initiated, observe A.O. closely for signs of toxic effects. Keep atropine sulfate and equipment for respiratory support on hand. Observe for cholinergic effects on an ongoing basis when these drugs are used. The time of onset of weakness indicates whether the weakness is caused by overdose or underdose. If the weakness begins approximately 1 hour after drug administration, overdose is a possibility. If it occurs after 3 or more hours, the weakness is usually caused by underdose. Also monitor BP, pulse, pulse oximetry, respirations, movement of the respiratory muscles, respiratory rate, tidal volume, and inspiratory force.

Check vital capacity by asking A.O. to take a deep breath and count as high as possible without taking another breath; most people can count as high as 40 or 50. All these observations are important because symptoms usually seen in respiratory distress, such as nasal flaring and intercostal or suprasternal retractions, may not occur because of muscle weakness. The dosage, route of administration, and frequency of the medication depend on A.O.'s clinical response, the remissions and exacerbations of the disease, and the stresses experienced by him.

Intervention There is no fixed dosage that will relieve A.O.'s symptoms. Different muscles will respond to the same dose with different levels of improvement. The dose and the medication schedule should be the minimal amount needed to provide maximal improvement in the muscles necessary for swallowing and breathing with the fewest adverse effects. A.O. will be on a demand schedule, usually taking the dose before meals or strenuous activity. The medication must be taken or given on time, or A.O. may be too weak to swallow and have poor control of his illness. Instruct A.O. to take the medication as ordered, using an alarm clock for precise timing of doses if necessary. He should keep an adequate supply of medications on hand and his family should also understand the timing of doses. The drugs should be administered on time because they are rapidly metabolized. A delay of 15 to 20 minutes in administration may begin to impair the muscles involved in swallowing and respiration. Around-the-clock therapy is often necessary. Be especially alert to the route of administration because the oral dosage is 30 times greater than parenteral dosages.

Anticholinesterase agents are initiated at a dosage less than that required to produce A.O.'s maximum strength; the dosage is gradually increased at intervals of 48 hours or more according to the severity of the disease and his response to the drug. Oral dosage forms may take several days to produce any change. If the last dosage increment does not produce a corresponding increase in his muscle strength, the dosage needs to be reduced to its previous level. Because it is essential that the smallest dosage for maximum result be used, it is crucial that the nurse assess and document A.O.'s health status.

The drugs administered for myasthenia gravis are best given with food or milk to decrease adverse muscarinic effects, such as abdominal cramping, nausea, and vomiting. However, if dysphagia is a problem, the medication should be administered 30 to 45 minutes before meals, and a rest period from the time of medication until mealtime should be provided to allow for peak muscle strength for eating. Serving frequent, regular, soft foods and encouraging A.O. to take small bites of food with frequent rest intervals may enhance his ability to eat. The main meal should be served at the time of day when he has the most strength.

Be prepared for crisis intervention with medications—edrophonium and neostigmine for a myasthenic crisis, and atropine for a cholinergic crisis. Basic resuscitative equipment should be available: suction catheters, Ambu bag, oxygen, and intubation tray.

Education A.O. and his family should maintain a diary for as long as possible to identify factors that aggravate his symptoms and increase his need for medication. This will help them to be aware of what events, such as emotional stress or infection, worsen the symptoms and how A.O. responds to medication. Teach him to observe for the therapeutic effects of the drug: a decrease or absence of ptosis; improved chewing, swallowing, and speech; increased skeletal muscle strength; and less fatigue. He should plan activities to take advantage of the peak effectiveness of the drug. When stabilized, A.O. can be taught to recognize the muscarinic effects (diaphoresis, salivation, slowed heart rate, and decreased BP) and modify the medication dosage or take atropine if needed. Atropine sulfate, 0.4 mg PO every 4 to 6 hours, may be administered either before or concurrently with anticholinesterase agents to prevent adverse effects such as excessive secretions or bradycardia. The greater control A.O. has over the therapeutic regimen, the less will be his feeling of powerlessness in the face of a devastating and debilitating disease.

Evaluation The expected outcome of anticholinesterase therapy is that A.O. will demonstrate greater muscle strength and an increased ability to swallow, chew, and speak without experiencing adverse effects of the drug.

Dementia

✱ **What are the important considerations for the care of clients with dementia?**

Dementia, a progressive mental disorder characterized by chronic personality disintegration, confusion, and deterioration of intellectual capacity and impulse control, affects 3% to 16% of Americans older than age 65 years. Alzheimer's disease accounts for approximately 50% to 60% of dementia cases; vascular dementia (including multiinfarct dementia, formerly known as cerebrovascular arteriosclerosis), Pick's disease, Parkinson's disease dementia, and other forms account for the balance. It has been estimated that irreversible dementias occur in approximately 90% of persons with dementia (Williams, 2005).

Drugs, emotion, metabolic or endocrine alterations, nutrition, trauma, infection, alcoholism, and systemic illness may cause reversible dementias. The medications most associated with this type of dementia include anticholinergic agents, cardiac drugs, selected antihypertensives, and psychotropics. Box 23-3 lists selected, potentially reversible causes of dementia.

The syndrome of dementia usually develops slowly. Early signs include depression, loss of ability to concentrate, and increased anxiety, irritability, and agitation. Weight loss (in excess of 5 kg) over time is also a predictor of earlier dementia (Stewart et al., 2005). Intellectual ability is usually the first to decline, then recent memory (e.g., names of acquaintances or recent events); this is followed by the loss of orientation to time, place, and person. Personal habits will change. The person may become loud or obscene, or some personality characteristics that were present might become magnified.

BOX 23-3 POTENTIALLY REVERSIBLE CAUSES OF DEMENTIA

DRUGS, CHEMICALS, OR TOXINS

Bromides
Mercury
Drugs such as butyrophenones (e.g., haloperidol), phenothiazines (chlorpromazine), diuretics, sedatives, alcohol

EMOTIONAL PROBLEMS

Depression
Chronic alcoholism

METABOLIC DISORDERS

Hyperglycemia
Hypopituitarism
Hyperparathyroidism
Hypoparathyroidism
Hypothyroidism

EYE/EAR DEPRIVATION

Blindness
Deafness

NUTRITIONAL DEFICITS

Vitamin B_{12} deficiency
Folic acid deficiency
Niacin deficiency

ACUTE TUMORS/TRAUMA

Subdural hematoma
Brain metastasis
Brain tumors

INFECTIONS AND/OR FEVER

Viral infections
Bacterial (tuberculosis)
Bacterial (endocarditis)
Syphilis

ARTERIOSCLEROTIC EVENTS

Vascular occlusion
Stroke

Data from Kasper, D.L., Braunwald, E., Fauci, A.S., Kasper, D.L., Hauser, S.L., Longo, D.L., et al. (Eds.). (2004). *Harrison's principles of internal medicine* (15th ed.). New York: McGraw-Hill.

Helplessness, total dependency, and a loss of manual skills may occur next. In the final stages, the person may be bedridden and experience loss of sphincter control. Eventually the person will die, usually as a result of bronchopneumonia.

The prescriber should first rule out all possible reversible causes of dementia. Approximately one third of older adults treated for dementia receive concurrent drugs that likely worsen the symptoms of dementia (Carnahan, Lund, Perry, & Chrischilles, 2004). Treatment should be instituted to try to prevent or reduce the ongoing damage and to support the client and family in managing this disease process. Drug treatment is indicated only for symptom control; for example, antidepressants can be used for severe depression. Antipsychotics, although historically used for clients with Alzheimer's-type dementia, do not improve agitation and are associated with cognitive decline (Ballard et al., 2005). Atypical antipsychotics have also been associated with increased mortality risk when used to treat behavioral disorders for older clients with dementia (FDA Public Health Advisory, 2005). Elevated risk also may be noted for the older typical antipsychotics. Risk for heart failure, sudden death, and pneumonia account for the majority of increased death risk with atypical antipsychotic drug use in this population. Supportive care should include proper nutrition, moderate exercise if permitted, vitamins if indicated, and the use of environmental aids in a consistent fashion, such as night lights and daily calendar reminders. The efficacy of complementary and alternative therapies (specifically ginkgo and vitamin E) has been debated and is unclear (Morris, 2003). Ginkgo is discussed in Chapter 12.

How is Alzheimer's disease differentiated from other forms of dementia?

Alzheimer's disease is a presenile dementia characterized by confusion, memory failure, disorientation, restlessness, speech disturbances, and hallucinosis; tragically, this condition is incurable. Alzheimer's disease is the most common form of dementia in older adults, accounting for 60% to 80% of dementia cases, and is estimated to affect more than 4 million Americans. Between 2.4 and 3.1 million spouses, relatives, and friends take care of people with Alzheimer's disease. The cost of caring for one person with this disorder at home or in a nursing home is more than $47,000 a year (Shadlen & Larson, 2004).

Clinically, a progressive decline in intellectual functions is noted, such as memory loss, a loss of logical thinking or judgment, time and space disorientation, and an increased tendency to wander as a result of progressive disorientation. In older adults, early cognitive impairment may be a symptom of undiagnosed depression (Vinkers, Gussekloo, Stek, Westendorp, & van der Mast, 2004). Profound memory loss, personality changes, hyperactivity, hostility, and paranoia may occur as the disease progresses. This middle phase in Alzheimer's disease is also characterized by the presence of aphasia (loss of speech or ability to express oneself), apraxia (loss of complex or intentional movements), and anomia (loss of ability to remember the names of persons and objects). In the terminal phase, nearly all higher mental functioning is lost, and the client needs assistance with activities of daily living; as a result, the client requires continuous nursing care.

In this final period clients may be unable to speak intelligibly, walk, sit up in bed, eat or groom themselves, smile,

TABLE 23-3 STAGES OF COGNITIVE DECLINE IN ALZHEIMER'S DISEASE

Stage	Clinical Phase	Symptoms
1	Normal	No change in cognition
2	Very mild	Forgets object location; some deficit in word finding
3	Mild (early confusion)	Early cognitive decline in one or more areas, memory loss, decreased ability to function in work situation, name-finding deficit, some decrease in social functioning, recall difficulties, anxiety
4	Moderate	Unable to perform complex tasks such as managing personal finances, planning a dinner party, concentrating, and knowing current events
5	Moderately severe (early dementia)	Usually needs assistance for survival, reminders to bathe, help in selecting clothes, and other daily functions; may be disoriented as to time and recent events, but this can fluctuate; may become tearful
6	Severe (dementia)	Needs assistance with dressing, bathing, and toilet functions (e.g., flushing); may forget names of spouse/family/caregivers and details of their personal life; may be generally unaware of their surroundings; incontinence of urine and feces may occur; central nervous system disturbances such as agitation, delusions, paranoia, obsessive anxiety, and the potential for violent behavior may increase
7	Very severe (late dementia)	Unable to speak (speech limited to five words or less); may scream or make other sounds; unable to ambulate, sit up, smile, or feed self; unable to hold head erect; ultimately slips into stupor or coma

Data from Alzheimer's Association. (2005). Stages of Alzheimer's disease. Retrieved September 1, 2005, from http://www.alz.org/AboudAD/Stages.asp.

or recognize simple objects or familiar persons. Table 23-3 summarizes the stages of cognitive decline.

In the terminal or last phase of Alzheimer's disease, the client wants to touch or examine all objects with the mouth (hyperorality), exhibits a decrease or loss in emotions, may be bulimic, and may also have a compulsion to touch everything in sight. Insomnia, nighttime wandering, and restlessness have also been reported. The progressive deterioration of brain cells may lead to increased dependency for all needs, decreased mobility to the point of being bedridden and, eventually, death.

Researchers are still searching for the cause of Alzheimer's disease, and many theories have been proposed. Theories under study include (1) a deficiency in acetylcholine, a major neurotransmitter, and perhaps other neurotransmitters in the brain; (2) a slow virus or infection that attacks selected brain cells; (3) genetic predisposition; (4) autoimmune theory—the theory that the body fails to recognize host tissue and attacks itself; and (5) beta-amyloid protein accumulation in the CNS (Williams, 2005).

❂ How is Alzheimer's disease treated?

Current pharmacotherapy is directed toward improving cognitive functioning or limiting disease progression and providing symptom control. Unfortunately, current medication regimens do not cure or prevent Alzheimer's disease.

The reversible acetylcholinesterase inhibitors donepezil (Aricept), galantamine (Reminyl), rivastigmine (Exelon), and tacrine (Cognex) are often associated with modest improvement or stabilization of symptoms of mild to moderate

Alzheimer's disease (Trinh, Hoblyn, Mohanty, & Yaffe, 2003). These agents are similar to the peripheral acetylcholinesterase inhibitors (e.g., neostigmine) discussed earlier in the chapter, but appear to demonstrate more CNS activity. Use of memantine (Namenda), a newer agent affecting CNS glutamate, shows some promise in reducing symptoms of moderate to severe dementia of the Alzheimer's type (Morris, 2003). To date, there is no data to demonstrate that any intervention slows the progression of the disease (Selkoe, 2004). The ergoloid mesylates have historically been used to treat early dementia, but their use is controversial in Alzheimer's disease with some reports of worsening of cognitive ability and behaviors (USP DI, 2005).

For depression, antidepressants with a low anticholinergic profile, such as desipramine (Norpramin) or trazodone (Desyrel, Trazon) have been used. The dosages should start at one-third to one-half the usual adult dosage for clients with Alzheimer's disease and increase slowly as necessary.

In general, the antianxiety agents, especially those with a short to intermediate half-life (e.g., lorazepam [Ativan], oxazepam [Serax], or alprazolam [Xanax]), are selected for clients who exhibit severe anxiety. However, if such agents are used to treat agitation in clients with dementia (or, specifically, Alzheimer's disease), the potential for retrograde amnesia or inducing a paradoxical reaction is present. Such clients may respond with an increase in activity, restlessness, and agitation. Consequently, it is important for the prescriber to differentiate between agitation and anxiety. Determine if the etiology of the agitation could be secondary to a urinary tract infection, constipation, dehydration, or other condition before medicating. If the benzodiazepine antianxiety agents are used, they should be closely monitored because symptoms change with time. Short-term use or a reevaluation at least every 3 to 6 months is necessary.

✱ How are the reversible acetylcholinesterase inhibitors differentiated?

The four centrally acting, reversible acetylcholinesterase inhibitors associated with slowing the progression of Alzheimer's disease are donepezil, galantamine, rivastigmine, and tacrine (Table 23-4). They may also have some modest benefit in the treatment of vascular dementia (Wilkinson et al., 2003) and of dementia associated with Parkinson's disease (Emre et al., 2004), although the cost-benefit ratio has been debated (Courtney, 2004) and they are not particularly effective for clients with modest cognitive impairment (Salloway et al., 2004). These agents act as centrally acting cholinesterase inhibitors and all possess longer durations of action than physostigmine. They are associated with slower rates of de-

cline in the mini-mental status evaluation when compared with placebo. This effect is observed clinically for at least 1 year (Morris, 2003). With the exception of rivastigmine, each of these agents is metabolized by cytochrome P450 enzyme systems and may be prone to drug interactions that can be influenced by genetics (see the Special Considerations for Pharmacogenetics box on p. 469). Because tacrine has a higher risk for hepatotoxicity and requires routine testing of serum alanine aminotransferase for liver toxicity, its use has been largely replaced with the other agents in this class.

Although each of the cholinesterase inhibitors has the potential to produce these GI effects, rivastigmine is more likely than other agents to cause nausea, vomiting, anorexia, and weight loss, especially with rapid dose increases. Consequently, it is recommended that dose titration proceed slowly to reduce the possibility of inducing severe vomiting. Interruption in dosing for more than a few days usually necessitates a slow retitration to dose to avoid these effects.

Donepezil is considered the prototype agent in the class.

TABLE 23-4 AGENTS FOR TREATMENT OF ALZHEIMER'S DEMENTIA

Agent	Mechanism	Typical Adult Dose	Half-life (hours)	Comments
donepezil (Aricept)	Reversible acetylcholinesterase inhibitor for mild to moderate Alzheimer's disease	5 mg at bedtime, may increase to 10 mg after 4-6 weeks	70	Metabolized by cytochrome P450 2D6 and 3A4
galantamine (Razadyne, Reminyl)		4 mg twice daily × 4 weeks, then 8 mg twice daily × 4 weeks, then 12 mg twice daily	6-8	Metabolized by cytochrome P450 2D6 and 3A4. If dose interrupted for ≥3 days, restart at 4 mg twice daily and slowly increase to maximum tolerated dose. ↓ dose with renal or hepatic insufficiency
rivastigmine (Exelon)		1.5 mg twice daily × 2 weeks, then 3 mg twice daily × 2 weeks, then 4.5 mg twice daily × 2 weeks, then 6 mg twice daily	1.5	Higher risk for nausea, vomiting, anorexia, and weight loss. If dose interrupted for ≥2 days, consider restart at 1.5 mg twice daily and slowly increase to maximum tolerated dose
tacrine (Cognex)		10 mg four times daily with titration every 6 weeks up to 40 mg four times daily	2-4	Rarely used due to hepatotoxicity risk. Monitor alanine aminotransferase weekly for first 18 weeks, then every 3 months. Avoid if hepatic insufficiency
memantine (Namenda)	N-methyl-D-aspartate receptor antagonist for moderate to severe Alzheimer's disease	5 mg daily × 1 week, then 5 mg twice daily × 1 week, then 5 mg AM and 10 mg PM × 1 week, then 10 mg twice daily	60-80	Minimal adverse effects. Benefit may be modest

✱⟅⟆ donepezil [doe **neh** peh zil]
(Aricept)
Indications
Treatment of mild to moderate dementia of the Alzheimer's type.
Pharmacokinetics/Dosing
Donepezil is well-absorbed orally. The elimination half-life is considerably longer for donepezil than for the other agents (see Table 23-4). Donepezil is metabolized by cytochrome P450 2D6 and 3A4 systems, and may be involved in interactions with other drugs metabolized by these systems.
Adverse Effects
All of these agents, including donepezil, should be dosed with food because they have the potential to cause nausea, vomiting and loss of appetite. Other frequently observed adverse effects include diarrhea, headache, ataxia, and muscle aches.

✱ How does memantine affect Alzheimer's disease?
Memantine is a newer agent that offers some promise in the treatment of late-stage Alzheimer's disease (Reisberg et al., 2003), and may offer additional benefit for clients on cholinesterase inhibitors (Tariot et al., 2004).

Glutamate is an amino acid believed to be correlated with the development of Alzheimer's disease. Memantine binds to *N*-methyl-D-aspartate (NMDA) receptors and inhibits the action of glutamate. To date, there are no data to suggest that the action of memantine is neuroprotective or slows the progression of the disease.

memantine [me **man** teen]
(Namenda)
Indications
Memantine is used in the symptomatic management in moderate to severe Alzheimer's dementia.
Pharmacokinetics/Dosing
Memantine is administered orally and has a relatively long half-life of 60 to 80 hours. It is partially metabolized to three relatively inactive metabolites, with unchanged drug and its metabolites eliminated in the urine. It is initially dosed at 5 mg daily, with weekly increases by 5 mg a week, to an ultimate dose of 10 mg twice daily.
Adverse Effects
While adverse effects are not common with this agent, there have been infrequent reports of dizziness, hypertension, and, rarely, exacerbation of heart failure, stroke, or transient ischemic attacks.

✱ M.S., a 65-year-old woman, complains of increasing memory problems over the past 3 years. She has started to "lose" things around the house, forget appointments, and fail to pay some important bills. Her physical exam and laboratory tests are within normal limits. M.S. is diagnosed as being in the early stages of Alzheimer's disease.
Because M.S. is in the early stages of Alzheimer's disease, a cholinesterase inhibitor may be prescribed, but it is unlikely that she will receive dramatic or long-lasting results from such drugs. Donepezil may be given as a single daily dose in the evening, increasing compliance and minimizing adverse effects of nausea and headache. Monitor M.S. for cholinergic adverse effects, such as nausea, diarrhea, headache, dizziness, and insomnia. Assess her for the therapeutic effects of the drug; improvement in memory, orientation, and ability to concentrate on complex tasks. Her dose may be increased in 4 to 6 weeks if improvement is not noticeable.

In the pharmacologic management of clients with Alzheimer's disease, care needs to be taken to provide for their safety and comfort. In older adults, most medications prescribed for the treatment of Alzheimer's disease are excreted and metabolized less efficiently than in younger clients. Smaller dosages are required to produce the desired effect. The nurse's assessment and documentation of subtle changes in the client's health status will allow prescribers to individualize medication dosages more closely. Drugs that compromise respiratory function or cause depression, confusion, or sleep alterations, are avoided.

In many ways, Alzheimer's disease remains a perplexing illness. In addition to providing appropriate care, keep abreast of medical and nursing research, be committed to conducting nursing studies on the care of clients with Alzheimer's disease, and share ideas about effective nursing interventions with colleagues.

Skeletal Muscle Relaxants

Most muscle strains and spasms are self-limited and respond to rest, physical therapy, and short-term skeletal muscle relaxants. Spasticity (a form of muscular hypertonicity with increased resistance to stretch) as the result of stroke, closed head injuries, cerebral palsy, multiple sclerosis, spinal cord trauma, and other neurologic disorders requiring the long-term use of skeletal muscle relaxants, will challenge the nurse's rehabilitative skills and knowledge. In both short- and long-term care, the nurse's role is not only to administer medications but also to provide comfort and rehabilitative measures in collaboration with physical therapists and other members of the health care team.

✱ What are the key issues in the pathophysiology and management of skeletal muscle spasticity?
Skeletal muscles are striated (striped) muscles attached to the skeleton. They are usually under voluntary control, and they produce body movements, maintain body position against the force of gravity, and counteract environmental stressors such as wind. A muscle is made of numerous muscle cells or muscle fibers. Each muscle cell is connected to only one motor nerve fiber, but each nerve fiber is connected to several muscle cells. Consequently, stimulation of one nerve fiber causes stimulation and activation of a group of muscle cells. The region where a motor nerve fiber makes functional contact with a skeletal muscle fiber (synaptic contact) is known as the neuromuscular junction.

Skeletal muscle spasms result when there is an involuntary contraction of a muscle or group of muscles that is accompanied by pain or limited function. Most skeletal muscle spasms are caused by local injuries, but some may result from low calcium levels or epileptic myoclonic seizures. Each type of spasm is treated according to its cause.

Skeletal muscle spasticity is characterized by skeletal muscle hyperactivity and occurs when gamma motor neurons (which tonically control muscle spindle contractile activity) become hyperactive. There are two primary types of muscle spasticity: spinal and cerebral. Spinal spasticity can be identified by a marked loss of inhibitory influences with hyperactive tendon stretch reflexes, clonus (alternate contraction and relaxation of muscles), primitive flexion withdrawal reflexes, and a flexed posture. Varying degrees of spasticity of the bladder and bowel can also be seen. Cerebral spasticity has less reflex excitability, increased muscle tone, and no primitive flexion withdrawal reflexes or flexed posture. Dystonia, an impairment of muscle tone, may also be present in individuals with cerebral spasticity.

Muscle spasticity is most commonly seen in clients with CNS injuries and strokes. Moderate to severe spasticity can be seen in two-thirds of clients with multiple sclerosis. Individuals with cerebral palsy and rare neurologic disorders can also have muscle spasticity, but it is seen less commonly in these instances.

Acute skeletal muscle injuries are usually self-limiting and can be treated with rest; physical therapy; immobility with the use of casts, neck collars, crutches, or arm slings; or whirlpool baths. Antiinflammatory drugs may be used for tissue damage and edema.

Central skeletal muscle relaxants are used mainly for conditions in which muscle spasms do not quickly respond to other forms of therapy. Such conditions include musculoskeletal strains and sprains, trauma, and cervical or lumbar radiculopathy as a result of degenerative osteoarthritis, herniated disk, spondylosis, or laminectomy.

Central-acting and direct-acting skeletal muscle relaxants are the drugs of choice in the treatment of muscle spasticity. These drugs include the central-acting agents baclofen (Lioresal) and diazepam (Valium), as well as the direct-acting agent dantrolene (Dantrium). These agents should *not* be confused with the neuromuscular blockers like curare or pancuronium that are used in surgery to prevent movement, produce total muscle blockade, and result in paralysis of respiratory muscles (see Chapter 21). Instead, the drugs discussed here are used to treat uncomfortable muscle spasms and serve to relax, but not block, skeletal muscle activity. These agents are more effective in the treatment of spinal spasticity than cerebral spasticity. For spasticity of skeletal muscle origin, diazepam and a host of other central-acting agents (also discussed below) may be effective, whereas baclofen, other centrally acting agents, and dantrolene appear to be of little use (Turturro, Frater, & D'Amico, 2003). Optimal response cannot be achieved in the treatment of either condition unless physical therapy is given concurrently.

✳ How do the skeletal muscle relaxants differ?

The exact mechanism of action of the skeletal muscle relaxants is unknown. For the majority of these agents, action results from CNS depression in the brain (brainstem, thalamus, and basal ganglia) and spinal cord resulting in the relaxation of striated muscle spasm. Removing the CNS depressant action from the central-acting skeletal muscle re-

laxants is not currently possible. As a result, these drugs create the adverse effects of drowsiness, blurred vision, lightheadedness, headache, and feelings of weakness, lassitude, and lethargy; such effects make long-term use of these drugs undesirable. Table 23-5 presents the most commonly used skeletal muscle relaxants.

✳▪ baclofen [bak low fen]
(Lioresal, Kemstro, Liotec✦)
Baclofen, a gamma-aminobutyric acid inhibitory neurotransmitter, inhibits the transmission of monosynaptic and polysynaptic reflexes. It is considered a prototype skeletal muscle relaxant. Although its exact mechanism of action is unknown, it is a spasmolytic agent at the spinal level, where it inhibits transmission. Baclofen may reduce pain in spastic clients by inhibiting the release of substance P in the spinal cord (Katzung, 2004).

Indications
Baclofen is used in the treatment of spasticity resulting from multiple sclerosis or from injuries to the spinal cord.

Pharmacokinetics/Dosing
Absorption is generally good but may vary with different individuals. The time to peak concentration is 2 to 3 hours. The onset of action is variable and may occur in hours or weeks. Baclofen has a half-life of 2.5 to 4 hours and a therapeutic serum level of 80 to 400 ng/mL. Baclofen is metabolized in the liver and excreted by the kidneys. The adult dosage of baclofen is 5 mg PO three times daily, increased by 5 mg per dose every 3 days until the desired response is achieved; the dosage is not to exceed 80 mg daily. The dosage for children has not been determined. To reduce drowsiness and confusion, the intrathecal administration of baclofen is now relatively common for chronic administration.

Adverse Effects
The adverse effects of baclofen include transient drowsiness, vertigo, confusion, sleepiness, weakness, and nausea.

A number of other central-acting skeletal muscle relaxants are available, including carisoprodol, chlorzoxazone, cyclobenzaprine, metaxalone, methocarbamol, orphenadrine, and tizanidine. The exact mechanism of action of these drugs has not been determined, but it is believed that the muscle relaxant effects of many of these drugs may be related to CNS depressant activity. Carisoprodol interferes with nerve transmission in the descending reticular formation and spinal cord, whereas chlorzoxazone produces its effects in the spinal cord and subcortical brain areas. In addition to skeletal muscle relaxant effects, orphenadrine is also an analgesic. Tizanidine acts primarily as an α_2-adrenergic agonist that affects alpha motor neurons in the CNS and the spinal cord. These drugs are used in adjunct treatment for skeletal muscle spasms, along with rest and physical therapy. Enhanced CNS depressant effects may occur when a skeletal muscle relaxant is given with alcohol, CNS depressants, or opioid analgesics. Monitor closely because the dosage of one or both drugs should be reduced. Also see the Special Considerations for Pharmacogenetics box on p. 469.

Although the mechanism of action for diazepam is unknown, it appears to act primarily by inhibiting afferent spinal polysynaptic (and possibly monosynaptic) pathways. It may also directly suppress muscle function at the neuro-

TABLE 23-5 SKELETAL MUSCLE RELAXANTS

Agent	Typical Oral Adult Dose	Important Adverse Effects	Comments
BENZODIAZEPINE			
diazepam (Valium)	2 mg twice daily up to 10 mg four times daily	See Chapter 16	See Chapter 16
CENTRAL-ACTING SKELETAL MUSCLE RELAXANTS			
baclofen (Lioresal, Kemstro)	5 mg three times daily up to 20 mg four times daily	Drowsiness Dizziness Hypotension Nausea Psychiatric disturbances	Intrathecal administration via implanted pump is available to reduce CNS adverse effects
carisoprodol (Soma)	350 mg three to four times daily	Drowsiness Dizziness Nausea Paradoxical stimulation Psychiatric disturbances Hypotension/syncope Xerostomia (cyclobenzaprine/ tizanidine) Rare: Anaphylaxis Liver toxicity	Typically for short-term (e.g., 7- to 21-day) use (IV forms of methocarbamol, orphenadrine should not be used for more than 3 days) Additive CNS depression with ethanol or other CNS depressants Carisoprodol interacts with fluconazole, gemfibrozil, omeprazole, ticlopidine via CYP 2C19 Cyclobenzaprine interacts with amiodarone, ciprofloxacin, fluvoxamine, ketoconazole, rofecoxib via CYP 1A2 Not recommended for older adults because of the adverse effect profile
chlorzoxazone (Parafon Forte)	250 mg three times daily up to 750 mg four times daily		
cyclobenza-prine (Flexeril)	5 mg three times daily up to 20 mg three times daily		
metaxalone (Skelaxin)	800 mg three times daily up to 800 mg four times daily		
methocar-bamol (Robaxin)	500 mg three times daily up to 1500 mg three times daily		
orphenadrine (Norflex) (Over-the-counter in Canada)	100 mg twice daily		
α₂-ADRENERGIC AGONIST			
tizanidine (Zanaflex)	2 mg three times daily up to 12 mg three times daily	Hypotension Sedation Xerostomia Bradycardia/syncope Insomnia Confusion	Tizanidine interacts with oral contraceptives; food increases rate of absorption
DIRECT SKELETAL MUSCLE RELAXANT			
dantrolene (Dantrium)	25 mg daily up to 100 mg four times daily (dose for malignant hyperthermia: 2.5 mg/kg up to a maximum cumulative dose of 10 mg/kg)	Drowsiness/dizziness Rash Diarrhea/vomiting Respiratory depression	Metabolized by CYP 3A4 with multiple potential drug interactions Agent of choice for malignant hyperthermia Unlabeled use: neuroleptic malignant syndrome

CNS, Central nervous system; *CYP*, cytochrome P450; *IV*, intravenous.

muscular synapse. Diazepam is used in the treatment of skeletal muscle spasm caused by reflex spasm or local pathologic conditions such as inflammation of muscle and joints or secondary to trauma. It is also used to treat spasticity caused by upper motor neuron disorders (cerebral palsy and paraplegia), athetosis, tetanus, and stiff-man syndrome (to overcome the widespread chronic muscular rigidity, pain, and skeletal muscle spasms). It is typically dosed at 2 to 10 mg twice daily to four times daily in adults for the treatment of muscle spasms. Refer to Chapter 16 for a more complete discussion of the pharmacology, indications, pharmacokinetics/dosing, and adverse effects of benzodiazepines.

dantrolene [**dan** troe leen]
(Dantrium)

Unlike the centrally acting agents, dantrolene acts directly on the skeletal muscles to relax them by inhibiting the release of calcium from the sarcoplasmic reticulum to the myoplasm. This results in a decreased muscle response to the action potential and decreased muscle contraction. As an antispastic agent, the direct effect of dantrolene on skeletal muscle dissociates the excitation-contraction coupling. This effect is probably induced by the interference with calcium ion release from the sarcoplasmic reticulum. Dantrolene reduces both monosynaptic- and polysynaptic-induced muscle contractions. These actions account for its use in both the treatment muscle spasm and of malignant hyperthermia (see Chapter 15).

Indications
Dantrolene is used for the prophylaxis and treatment of malignant hyperthermia (see Chapter 15) and spasticity, especially upper motor neuron disorders (e.g., multiple sclerosis, cerebral palsy, spinal cord insults, and cerebrovascular accident).

Pharmacokinetics/Dosing
Dantrolene is available orally and parenterally. The oral absorption of this drug is fair. When used to treat the spasticity of upper motor neurons, the onset of action is 1 week or more. The oral form of this drug has a half-life of 8.7 hours (100-mg dose); the IV half-life is 4 to 8 hours. The time to peak concentration is 5 hours (oral dose). It is metabolized in the liver and excreted by the kidneys.

Adverse Effects
The adverse effects of dantrolene include diarrhea, dizziness, sleepiness, uncomfortable feelings, unusual fatigue, muscle weakness, nausea, vomiting, severe diarrhea, respiratory difficulty, and respiratory depression.

Nursing Diagnosis Once C.C. begins taking tizanidine, a central-acting skeletal muscle relaxant, the nurse's assessment will consider the potential development of a number of nursing diagnoses/collaborative problems related to the effects of the drug. Because of the CNS effects of the drug, the client may experience disturbed thought processes (confusion), activity intolerance related to weakness, and a risk for injury related to hypotension, drowsiness, dizziness, or syncope. With overdose, the potential complications of seizures and respiratory depression also exist.

Planning While taking skeletal muscle relaxant therapy, C.C. will:
- Experience minimal muscle spasm without adverse effects of the drug.
- Remain as independent as possible.
- Remain compliant with drug regimen.
- Effectively manage, with his caregiver, the therapeutic regimen, including reporting adverse drug effects appropriately to the health care provider and using nonpharmacologic measures supportive of the drug regimen.
- Collaborate with the health team in keeping appointments for monitoring and continued care.

Implementation

Monitoring Monitor liver function tests (aspartate aminotransferase, alanine aminotransferase) closely during the first 6 months of therapy, usually 1, 3, and 6 months after baseline, and periodically thereafter. Monitor C.C.'s BP and pulse to monitor his risk for hypotension or bradycardia.

Education Inform C.C. that his mental alertness, judgment, and physical coordination may be affected. Alert him that alcohol and other CNS depressants will increase the CNS effects of these drugs. Because many clients experience postural hypotension with central-acting skeletal muscle relaxants, he should be cautioned about changing his position in keeping with his physical limitations.

✱ **C.C., a 20-year-old male college student, sustained a T3-T4 spinal cord injury a year ago in a car accident. He has been hospitalized for recurrent urinary tract infection. He has difficulty sleeping because he has severe muscle spasms in his lower extremities. Tizanidine (Zanaflex) 4 mg has been prescribed at bedtime to reduce his muscle spasticity.**

Assessment The nurse obtains a baseline assessment of C.C.'s spasticity: the frequency, location, and severity, and the factors that exacerbate and ameliorate the spasm. Thereafter C.C.'s dose can be titrated slowly over 2 to 4 weeks based on his clinical response to the tizanidine. Determine BP and pulse, and liver and renal function as a baseline.

PREGNANCY SAFETY SKELETAL MUSCLE RELAXANTS	
Category	**Drug**
B	cyclobenzaprine
C	baclofen, carisoprodol, chlorphenesin, chlorzoxazone, dantrolene, metaxalone, methocarbamol, orphenadrine, tizanidine
D	diazepam

Data from *Mosby's drug consult* (15th ed.). (2005). St. Louis: Mosby.

Evaluation The expected outcome of central-acting skeletal muscle relaxant therapy is that C.C. will demonstrate increased comfort, decreased involuntary movement and muscle tonicity, and an increased range of motion without experiencing adverse reactions to the drug. C.C. will effectively manage his therapeutic drug regimen.

For pregnancy category information regarding skeletal muscle relaxants, see the Pregnancy Safety Box on p. 488.

Summary

The major CNS-neuromuscular disorders discussed in this chapter—Parkinson's disease, myasthenia gravis, dementia, Alzheimer's disease, and muscle spasticity—are progressive and often incapacitating syndromes. Pharmacologic therapy is essential for symptom control, which allows the client to function as independently as possible for as long as possible.

Clients with Parkinson's disease require correction of the disorder's imbalance of dopamine and acetylcholine. For this reason, the client is treated with drugs that have central anticholinergic activity—anticholinergics and antihistamines—and drugs that affect dopamine levels to enhance dopaminergic mechanisms. Because the condition is debilitating and long-term, clients and caregivers require support and education to maintain compliance with the medication regimen.

Myasthenia gravis is characterized by skeletal muscle weakness and fatigue, and is also progressive and incurable. The anticholinesterase drugs are central to the treatment of this disorder.

Drug therapy is not as specific for dementia and Alzheimer's disease. The reversible acetylcholinesterase inhibitors are used to treat early Alzheimer's disease while the role of NMDA receptor modulators in middle- to late-stage disease is evolving. Low doses of antipsychotic drugs have historically been used in both disorders to control severe agitation, delusions, and hallucinations, but their safety for this use has been questioned.

Pharmacologic agents administered as skeletal muscle relaxants affect skeletal muscle at the neuromuscular junction or at different levels in the CNS, such as the spinal cord or the brain. The effects of the central-acting skeletal muscle relaxants result from CNS depression in the brain and spinal cord. Direct-acting skeletal muscle relaxants affect striated muscle to dissociate the excitation-contraction coupling and thus reduce monosynaptic- and polysynaptic-induced muscle contractions. Although most skeletal muscle spasm is the result of local injury, other instances may be of a more systemic nature; the treatment of each type of spasm is related to its cause.

An essential part of the nurse's role is to identify the subtle changes in the client's health status in any of the discussed conditions, which enables the prescriber to individualize the medication regimen and sustain the highest quality of life for the client.

✴ Critical Thinking Questions

- Mrs. Ross has been diagnosed with myasthenia gravis, for which she has been prescribed pyridostigmine syrup. Her most distressing symptom is a mild dysphagia. How could the nurse best manage Mrs. Ross' drug therapy?

- Mrs. Kelly brings her 72-year-old husband to the clinic for a periodic assessment of his Alzheimer's disease and the effectiveness of his drug therapy. Formulate a line of inquiry to elicit information from Mrs. Kelly that will assist you in determining the effectiveness of her husband's drug therapy.

- In evaluating the effectiveness of skeletal muscle relaxant therapy for a client with spasticity, what would constitute an appropriate assessment of the client's status?

- What would be essential to include in a teaching plan for a client who will be self-administering muscle relaxant therapy?

Bibliography

Anderson, D.M., Keith, J., & Novak, P.D. (Eds.). (2002). *Mosby's medical, nursing, and allied health dictionary* (6th ed.). St. Louis: Mosby.

Ballard, C., Margallo-Lana, M., Juszczak, E., Douglas, S., Swann, A., Thomas, A., et al. (2005). Quetiapine and rivastigmine and cognitive decline in Alzheimer's disease: Randomised double blind placebo controlled trial. *British Medical Journal, 330,* 874-877.

𝑒-LEARNING SUPPLEMENTS

Student CD-ROM
- Final Exam questions
- NCLEX® Examination review questions
- Pharmacology animations
- Printable chapter summary

Evolve Website (http://evolve.elsevier.com/mckenry)
- Case study on drugs affecting the parasympathetic nervous system

- Content updates, including information on new drugs
- WebLinks corresponding to this chapter
- Answers to the critical thinking questions in this chapter
- *Elsevier ePharmacology Update* newsletter
- *Mosby's Drug Consult* Internet Edition
- Supplemental and reference information

Bramness, J.G., Skurtveit, S., Fauske, L., Grung, M., Molven, A., Morland, J., et al. (2003). Association between blood carisoprodol:meprobamate concentration ratios and CYP2C19 genotype in carisoprodol-drugged drivers: Decreased metabolic capacity in heterozygous CYP2C19*1/CYP2C19*2 subjects? *Pharmacogenetics, 13*(7), 383-388.

Carnahan, R.M., Lund, B.C., Perry, P.J., & Chrischilles, E.A., (2004). The concurrent use of anticholinergics and cholinesterase inhibitors: Rare event or common practice? *Journal of the American Geriatrics Society, 52,* 2082-2087.

Chang, J.T., & Altman, R.B. (2004). Extracting and characterizing gene-drug relationships from the literature. *Pharmacogenetics, 14*(9), 577-586, and linked supplemental website http://bionlp.stanford.edu/genedrug/gene_drug_predictions.html (as cited December 2, 2004).

Courtney, C., Farrell, D., Gray, R., Hills, R., Lynch, L., Sellwood, E., et al. (2004). Randomised double-blind trial. *Lancet, 363,* 2105-2115.

Cristina, S., Zangaglia, R., Mancini, F., Martignoni, E., Nappi, G., & Pacchetti, C. (2003). High-dose ropinirole in advanced Parkinson's disease with severe dyskinesias. *Clinical Neuropharmacology, 26*(3), 146-150.

DiPiro, J.T., Talbert, R.L., Yee, G.C., Matzke, G.R., Wella, B.G., & Posey, L.M. (Eds.). (2002). *Pharmacotherapy: A pathophysiologic approach* (5th ed.). New York: McGraw-Hill.

Drozdzik, M., Bialecka, M., Mysliwiec, K., Honczarenko, K., Stankiewicz, J., & Sych, Z. (2003). Polymorphism in the P-glycoprotein drug transporter MDR1 gene: A possible link between environmental and genetic factors in Parkinson's disease. *Pharmacogenetics, 13*(5), 259-263.

Drug facts and comparisons (58th ed.). (2005). St. Louis: Facts and Comparisons.

Emre, M., Aarsland, D., Albanese, A., Byrne, E.J., Deuschl, G., De Deyn, P.P., et al. (2004). Rivastigmine for dementia associated with Parkinson's disease. *New England Journal of Medicine, 351,* 2509-2518.

Ernst, M., Gottwald, M.D., & Gidal, B.E. (2005). Parkinson's disease. In M.A. Koda-Kimble, L.Y. Young, W.A. Kradjan, B.J. Guglielmo, B.K. Alldredge, & R.L. Corelli (Eds.), *Applied therapeutics: The clinical use of drugs* (8th ed.). Philadelphia: Lippincott Williams & Wilkins.

Fahn, S., Oakes, D., Shoulson, I., Kieburtz, K., Rudolph, A., Lang, A., et al. (2004). Levodopa and the progression of Parkinson's disease. *New England Journal of Medicine, 351,* 2498-2508.

FDA Public Health Advisory. (April 2005). Deaths with antipsychotics in elderly patients with behavioral disturbances. Retrieved June 23, 2005, from http://www.fda.gov/cder/drug/advisory/antipsychotics.htm.

Galvin, J.E., & Ginsberg, S.D. (2004). Expression profiling and pharmacotherapeutic development in the central nervous system. *Alzheimer Disease & Associated Disorders, 18*(4), 264-269.

Hobson, D.E., Pourcher, E., & Martin, W.R. (1999). Ropinirole and pramipexole, the new agonists. *Canadian Journal of Neurological Science, 26*(Suppl. 2), S27-S33.

Ives, N.J., Stowe, R.L., Marro, J., Counsell, C., Macleod, A., Clarke, C.E., et al. (2004). Monoamine oxidase type B inhibitors in early Parkinson's disease: Meta-analysis of 17 randomised trials involving 3525 patients. *British Medical Journal, 329,* 593-596.

Katzung, B.G. (Ed.). (2004). *Basic and clinical pharmacology* (9th ed.). New York: McGraw-Hill.

Korczyn, A.D., Brunt, E.R., Larsen, J.P., Nagy, Z., Poewe, W.H., & Ruggieri, S. (1999). A 3-year randomized trial of ropinirole and bromocriptine in early Parkinson's disease: The 053 study group. *Neurology, 53*(2), 364-370.

Lacy, C.F., Armstrong, L.L., Goldman, M.P., Lance, L.L. (2004). *Lexi-Comp's drug information handbook* (12th ed.). Hudson, OH: Lexi-Comp.

Lilly Pharmaceuticals. (2003, December 15). *Dear health care professional letter. Pergolide.* Retrieved December 22, 2004, from http://www.fda.gov/medwatch/SAFETY/2003/permax_deardoc.pdf

Morris, J.C. (2003). Dementia update 2003. *Alzheimer Disease & Associated Disorders, 17*(4), 245-258.

Mosby's drug consult (15th ed.). (2005). St. Louis: Mosby.

National Institute of Neurological Disease and Stroke. (2004). *NINDS Parkinson's disease information page.* Retrieved June 28, 2005, from http://www.ninds.nih.gov

Pan, T., Le, W., & Jankovic, J. (2004). Slowing Parkinson's disease progression: Recent dopamine agonist trials. *Neurology, 62*(2), 343.

Pharmacist's letter. (2001). *Alzheimer's, 17*(5), 26.

Poewe, W. (2004). The role of COMT inhibition in the treatment of Parkinson's disease. *Neurology, 62*(Suppl. 1), S31-S38.

Reisberg, B., Doody, R., Stoffler, A., Schmitt, F., Ferris, S., Mobius, H.J., et al. (2003). Memantine in moderate-to-severe Alzheimer's disease. *New England Journal of Medicine, 348,* 1333-1341.

Rivest, J., Barclay, C.L., & Suchowersky, O. (1999). COMT inhibitors in Parkinson's disease. *Canadian Journal of Neurological Science, 26*(Suppl. 2), S34-S38.

Salloway, S., Ferris, S., Kluger, A., Goldman, R., Griesing, T., Kumar, D., et al. (2004). Efficacy of donepezil in mild cognitive impairment: A randomized placebo-controlled trial. *Neurology, 63,* 651-657.

Schapira, A., & Olanow, C.W. (2004). Neuroprotection in Parkinson disease: Mysteries, myths, and misconceptions. *Journal of the American Medical Association 291*(3), 358-364.

Selkoe, D.J. (2004). Alzheimer disease: Mechanistic understanding predicts novel therapies. *Annals of Internal Medicine, 140*(8), 627-638.

Shadlen, M.F., & Larson, E.B. (2004). Diagnosis of dementia. *UpToDate.* Wellesley, MA: UpToDate.

Stewart, R., Masaki, K., Xue, Q.L., Peila, R., Petrovitch, H., White, L.R., et al. (2005). A 32-year prospective study of change in body weight and incident dementia: The Honolulu-Asia Aging Study. *Archives of Neurology, 62,* 55-60.

Tariot, P.N., Farlow, M.R., Grossberg, G.T., Graham, S.M., McDonald, S., Gergel, I., et al. (2004). Memantine treatment in patients with moderate to severe Alzheimer disease already receiving donepezil: A randomized controlled trial. *Journal of the American Medical Association, 291,* 317-324.

Thompson, P.D., Moyna, N., Seip, R., Price, T., Clarkson, P., Angelopoulos, T., et al. (2004). Functional polymorphisms associated with human muscle size and strength. *Medicine & Science in Sports & Exercise, 36*(7), 1132-1139.

Tierney, L.M. Jr., McPhee, S.J., & Papadakis, M.A. (2003). *Current medical diagnosis & treatment* (42nd ed.). New York: Lange Medical Books/McGraw-Hill.

Trinh, N.H., Hoblyn, J., Mohanty, S., & Yaffe, K. (2003). Efficacy of cholinesterase inhibitors in the treatment of neuropsychiatric symptoms and functional impairment in Alzheimer disease: A meta-analysis. *Journal of the American Medical Association, 289,* 210-216.

Turturro, M.A., Frater, C.R., & D'Amico, F.J. (2003). Cyclobenzaprine with ibuprofen versus ibuprofen alone in acute myofascial strain: A randomized, double-blind clinical trial. *Annals of Emergency Medicine, 41,* 818-826.

USP DI: Drug information for the health care professional (25th ed.). (2005). Greenwood Village, CO: MICROMEDEX Thomson Healthcare.

Vinkers, D.J., Gussekloo, J., Stek, M.L., Westendorp, R.G, & van der Mast, R.C. (2004). Temporal relation between depression and cognitive impairment in old age: Prospective population based study. *British Medical Journal, 329,* 881-883.

Wang, J., Si, Y.M., Liu, Z.L., & Yu, L. (2003). Cholecystokinin, cholecystokinin-A receptor and cholecystokinin-B receptor gene polymorphisms in Parkinson's disease. *Pharmacogenetics, 13*(6), 365-369.

Wilkinson, D., Doody, R., Helme, R., Taubman, K., Mintzer, J., Kertesz, A., et al. (2003). Donepezil in vascular dementia: A randomized, placebo-controlled study. *Neurology, 61,* 479-486.

Williams, B.R. (2005). Geriatric dementias. In M.A. Koda-Kimble, L.Y. Young, W.A. Kradjan, B.J. Guglielmo, B.K. Alldredge, & R.L. Corelli (Eds.), *Applied therapeutics: The clinical use of drugs* (8th ed.). Philadelphia: Lippincott Williams & Wilkins.

24

OVERVIEW OF THE CARDIOVASCULAR SYSTEM

CHAPTER FOCUS

Although progress has been made in increasing public awareness about the lifestyle changes necessary to promote good cardiovascular health, more than 64 million people in the United States and 8 million in Canada have some type of cardiovascular disorder (Centers for Disease Control and Prevention, 2004; Heart and Stroke Foundation of Canada, 2002). But cardiovascular disease (CVD) is a global issue. More than 15 million individuals die directly or indirectly from CVD, accounting for more deaths annually than any other form of disease globally (Millennium Research Group, 2001). Although CVD contributed to a third of global deaths in 1999, the incidence of CVD is changing (World Health Organization, 2004). Over the past 10 years there has been a significant decrease in mortality rates in many developed countries. Male mortality fell by more than 60% in Japan, and in Australia, Canada, France, and the United States, the rate declined by 50%. However, the economic transitions of urbanization, industrialization, and globalization bring about lifestyle changes that promote heart disease. Whereas in 1999, low- and middle-income countries contributed 78% of CVD deaths, it is expected that by 2010, CVD will be the leading cause of death in developing countries. In developed countries, CVD is a disease of disparities, affecting increasing numbers of minorities and women. CVD is the leading cause of death in American women; 30% of all deaths in females each year are a result of heart disease (Anderson, 2002). Heart disease kills more women each year than cancer, accidents, and diabetes combined. As longevity increases, it can be expected that more people will be living with chronic cardiovascular conditions and coping with the results of acute ones.

As a result, nurses will be not only providing care within acute facilities but also assisting clients to manage their therapeutic cardiovascular regimens effectively in a variety of community and home settings. A thorough knowledge of anatomy and physiology of the cardiovascular system is essential for assessment of the client, interpretation of diagnostic examinations, provision of care, and client teaching.

▲ **KEY TERMS**

The rapid development of science and technology has resulted in new knowledge and a greater understanding of cardiac activity. The resulting electrophysiologic, angiographic, ultrasonographic, and pharmacologic information has permitted greater precision in diagnosing and treating cardiac disease, particularly the dysrhythmias. Along with these advances has come the increased use of electrocardiographic monitoring of acutely ill clients and those with known or suspected cardiovascular disorders. In addition, the nurse's clinical role has expanded and now includes the care of clients on many other types of monitoring equipment. This requires the nurse to recognize and understand abnormal electrocardiographic patterns and, in some cases, to begin therapy, including pharmacologic therapy, to prevent serious complications and unnecessary deaths. To keep their knowledge current and their nursing care therapeutically effective, nurses must understand the electrical and physiologic properties of the heart and the effects that drugs have on cardiac activity.

Microelectrode techniques are increasingly sophisticated and help to provide greater understanding of the electrical properties of cardiac fibers and the causes of various cardiac disorders. Fortunately, these advances have led to the discovery of new drugs that are useful in treating cardiac conditions.

Cardiac drugs largely affect three major tissues of the heart: cardiac muscle (**myocardium**), coronary vessels, and the conduction system. This chapter discusses the normal function of these structures.

The Heart

The heart is a hollow muscular organ that consists of two main pumping chambers: (1) the right ventricle, which is linked with the pulmonary circulation, and (2) the left ventricle, which is connected to the systemic circulation. The cardiac muscle, or myocardium, is the largest and most important structure of the heart. As a contractile muscle, it can adapt its performance under normal conditions by adjusting the cardiac output according to needs of the body.

✳ How does cardiac muscle impact cardiovascular function?

The pumping action of the heart depends on the ability of the cardiac muscle to contract. The myocardium is the thick, contractile, middle layer of the heart, and it is composed of many interconnected branching fibers or cells that form the walls of the two **atria** (the upper chambers of the heart) and the two **ventricles** (the lower chambers of the heart). Each individual myocardial fiber contains a nucleus in the middle and a plasma membrane (cell membrane) called the sarcolemma (Figure 24-1, *2, 3*). The cells form a long fiber by joining end to end, with each cell separated from the other by a plasma membrane called an intercalated disk. This disk is believed to provide sites of low electrical resistance to permit the spread of electrical impulses throughout the cardiac muscle.

Each individual muscle fiber (cell) is part of a group of multiple parallel myofibrils; each myofibril is arranged end-to-end in a series of repeating units called the **sarcomere**—the basic unit of contraction in the heart (see Figure 24-1, *4*). The tremendous energy requirements for cardiac muscle contraction may be seen by the great numbers of mitochondria lined up in long chains between the myofibrils (see Figure 24-1, *3*). Under examination with a light microscope, the sarcomere reveals its most characteristic feature, alternating light A bands and dark I bands. These bands result from the crossing of multiple parallel myofibrils, which are aligned in register with one another (see Figure 24-1, *3*). The darkness of the A bands results from

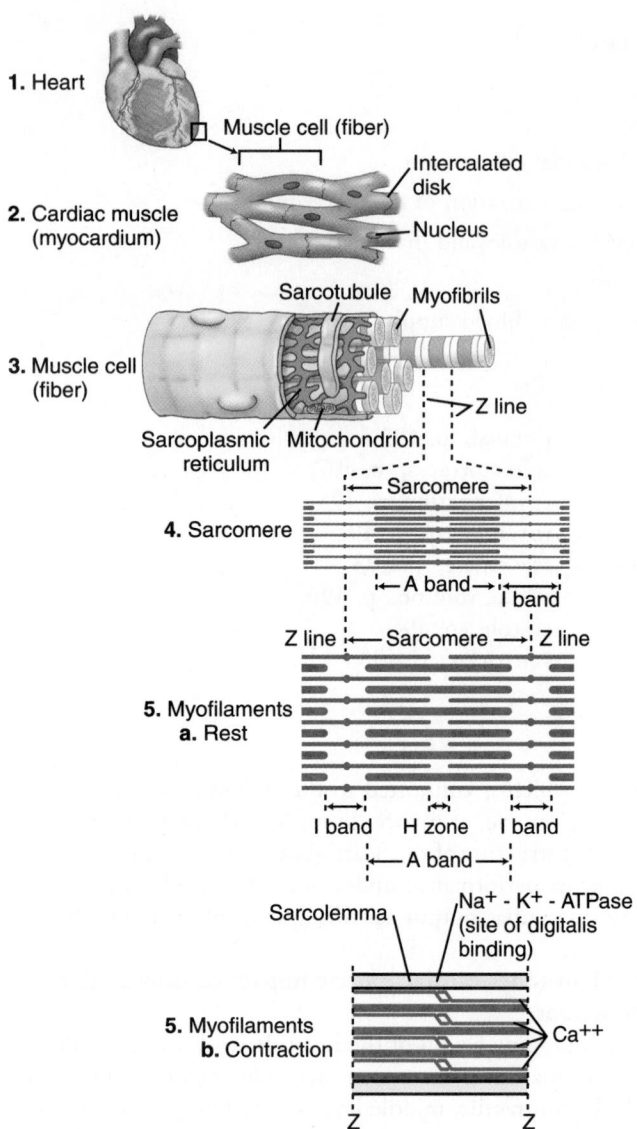

1. Heart

Muscle cell (fiber)

Intercalated disk

2. Cardiac muscle (myocardium)

Nucleus

Sarcotubule Myofibrils

3. Muscle cell (fiber)

Z line

Sarcoplasmic Mitochondrion
reticulum

Sarcomere

4. Sarcomere

A band

I band

Z line Sarcomere Z line

5. Myofilaments
   a. Rest

I band H zone I band

A band

Sarcolemma

Na⁺ - K⁺ - ATPase (site of digitalis binding)

5. Myofilaments
   b. Contraction

Ca^{++}

Z Z

FIGURE 24-1 Structure of the heart and cardiac muscle cell fibers. The heart *(1)* is mainly a muscular organ. The enlargement of the square illustrates a portion of the cardiac muscle (myocardium) *(2)*, which is composed of myocardial cells. Each cell contains a centrally located nucleus and a limited plasma membrane (sarcolemma), which forms the intercalated disk at the termination of each cell. An individual muscle cell (fiber) *(3)* consists of multiple parallel myofibrils. Each myofibril is arranged longitudinally in a series of light and dark repeating units; the content of a unit is called a sarcomere. The sarcomere *(4)* is the unit of muscle contraction. It is composed of two types of bands, the A band and the I band. The I band is divided by the Z line. At the Z line, the sarcolemma invaginates to form the transverse sarcotubules, or T system. An extensive network, called the sarcoplasmic reticulum, encircles groups of myofibrils and makes contact with the sarcotubules. The sarcoplasmic reticulum contains a high concentration of calcium ions. The mitochondria appear in long chains between the myofibrils. Myofilaments of the sarcomere *(5)* include the thin filament (actin) and the thick filament (myosin). The dark appearance of the A band is caused by the myosin and the lighter appearance of the I band by the actin. Here the sarcomere is at rest *(a)*. On contraction *(b)*, the sarcomere shortens so that the thick filaments approach the Z line and the width of the H zone narrows between the thin filaments. Calcium ions are needed for systolic contractions.

the thicker myosin filaments, and the lightness of the I bands reflects the thinner actin filaments.

The sarcomere lies between two successive Z lines of the myofibril. The end unit of the myofibril is the myofilament. At the Z line, the sarcolemma of the muscle fiber interlocks (invaginates) at its end with the sarcomere to form the transverse sarcotubule, or T system, which penetrates deeply into the cell. Internal membranes form an extensive network called the sarcoplasmic reticulum. This structure encircles groups of myofibrils and makes contact with the sarcotubules.

Cross-bridges, which are small projections that extend from the sides of the myosin filament, appear along the entire length of the thick filament. The interaction between the cross-bridges of myosin and the active sites of actin produces contraction. In the sarcomere, the H zone represents the middle, less dense portion of the A band; the myosin filament runs the entire length of this band. The I band is divided by the Z line. The actin filament runs through the entire I band and terminates at the H zone. Figure 24-1, *5a*,

shows this arrangement during rest, and Figure 24-1, *5b*, depicts their arrangement during contraction.

During the past two decades there has been a tremendous increase in the understanding of the fundamental mechanisms governing contraction of cardiac muscle in both normal and pathologic states. However, some aspects of this complicated process remain unknown. Cardiac muscle contraction begins with a rapid change in the electrical charge of the cell membrane. This electrical current spreads to the interior of the cell, where it causes a release of calcium ions from the sarcoplasmic reticulum. The calcium ions then initiate the chemical events of contraction. The overall process for controlling cardiac muscle contraction, called excitation-contraction coupling, involves electrical excitation, mechanical activation, and contractile mechanisms.

✲ What are the key principles of electrical conduction in the heart?

Cardiac muscle contraction begins with electrical excitation or stimulus of the myocardial fiber. The source of electricity

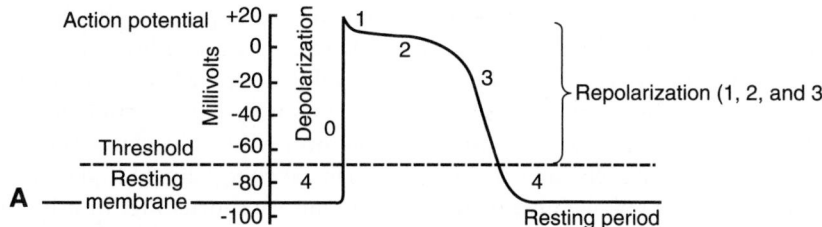

Depolarization

Phase 0—membrane becomes permeable to Na+,
  which flows rapidly into the cell

Repolarization

Phase 1—membrane potential becomes slightly positive because of
  the rapid influx of Na+
Phase 2—slow inward flow of Ca++ and outward flow of K+

Phase 3—rapid outward flow of K+

Resting period

Phase 4—cell membrane actively transports Na+
  outside and K+ inside, returning cell membrane
  to state of polarization

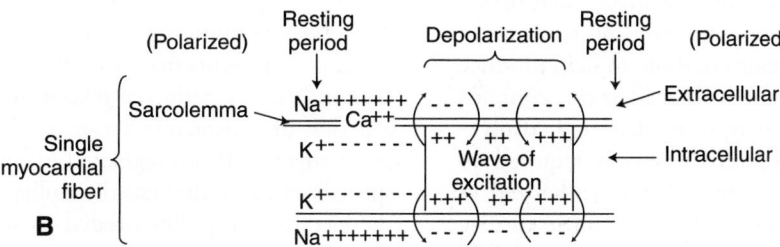

FIGURE 24-2 **A,** Action potential of the ventricle. **B,** Ionic exchanges that occur across the cell membrane of a single myocardial fiber during an action potential.

in the heart is found in the charges of ion concentration—mainly sodium, potassium, and calcium ions—across the cardiac cell membrane of the sarcolemma. The difference in electrical charge, called the **action potential,** produces the rapid ion changes. These changes occur in the membrane of the myocardial cell and result in a self-propagating series of polarization and depolarization. The resting state of an inactive muscle cell in the ventricle is created by the difference in electrical charge across the sarcolemma. In this case, the inside of the cell is negative with respect to the outside of the cell, which is positively charged. Because the sarcolemma separates these opposite charges, the membrane in effect is polarized. At rest, the extracellular environment is rich in sodium ions (Na^+) and the intracellular environment is rich in potassium ions (K^+); calcium ion (Ca^{2+}) concentration is highest in the region of the sarcolemma and where it comes in contact with the sarcotubule (Figure 24-2, *B*).

The cardiac action potential is divided into two stages: depolarization and repolarization. **Depolarization** is the stage in which an electrical impulse results in contraction of the ventricular muscle; it is represented by the QRS complex on the electrocardiogram (ECG). **Repolarization** is the recovery phase after muscle contraction; this stage is represented by the T wave on the ECG. These stages are subdivided into five phases of ionic changes. The resting potential of an inactive myocardial cell is called phase 4; in

this phase, the membrane is polarized with a charge of approximately -90 millivolts (mV). At this voltage the interior of the cell is negative with respect to the exterior, and the membrane cannot be penetrated by ions. Any stimulus that changes the resting membrane potential to a critical value (the threshold) can generate an action potential. (See Figure 24-2, *A,* for the phases of the action potential.)

Threshold may be reached by normal pacemaker activity or by propagation of an electrical impulse from a nearby cell, which opens the sodium channels. The fast inward current of sodium ions (fast channel) results in a membrane that is positively charged to $+20$ mV. This difference in membrane potential results in depolarization and is designated as phase 0 of the action potential. Phase 0 in the ventricular muscle is the contraction phase and is represented by the QRS complex on the surface ECG. Soon after, the repolarization period occurs in three phases. The beginning of phase 1 is the overshoot, and it makes a brief change toward repolarization. Phase 2 is a slow period that forms a plateau with a slow inward current of calcium ions and an outward flow of potassium ions. Calcium ion entry into the cell is essential for the excitation-contraction coupling mechanism.

Phase 3 is accomplished by the rapid efflux of potassium ions from the cell. After repolarization, phase 4 recovery (the resting period) begins. This phase is represented by the

T wave, whereby the cell membrane actively transports sodium ions outside and potassium ions inside, returning the cell membrane to a state of rest or polarization. These cation exchanges require the energy-using transport mechanism of the Na^+-K^+ pump, or Na^+-K^+-ATPase. Adenosine triphosphatase (ATPase) is powered by oxygen and is an enzyme located in the cell membrane or sarcolemma; it furnishes the energy needed for active transport to return sodium ions and potassium ions to their original resting positions at the membrane. Digoxin plays a key role at this site. By binding to the sarcolemma Na^+-K^+-ATPase, digoxin inhibits the return of sodium ions and potassium ions to their resting positions. Consequently, digoxin allows more sodium ions and calcium ions to enter the cell to strengthen myocardial contraction. It is also thought that digoxin toxicity can occur if an excessive amount of these ions appears intracellularly.

✳ How do the changes in ion concentration lead to mechanical activation and cardiac contraction?

The sarcomere is the contractile unit of myocardial tissue. The sarcomere consists of two contractile proteins, actin and myosin. These two filaments combine to help produce cardiac contraction. Myosin, the thicker filament, contains the ATPase enzyme system that is needed to hydrolyze adenosine triphosphate (ATP). Hydrolysis is required to provide the energy for contraction. ATP is synthesized in the mitochondria, which are normally abundant in cardiac muscle. Actin, the thin filament, is involved with calcium ion activity.

Contraction is initiated when the nerve impulse reaches the myocardial cell and travels along the sarcolemma of the muscle fiber. As the depolarization wave spreads along the sarcotubules, it arrives at the sarcoplasmic reticulum to cause the release of its large quantities of calcium ions. These ions then bind to special receptors on the actin filaments. The plateau, which is phase 2 of the action potential, is reached through the slow, inward, calcium current flow (slow channel). *Calcium ion movement is the chief component* that links or couples electrical excitation of the sarcolemma with muscle activation of the myofilaments in the sarcomere. Mechanical activation is finally accomplished when calcium ions bind to troponin, a regulator protein located on the actin filaments. In turn, this mediates the interaction of actin and myosin.

As soon as the actin filaments are activated by the calcium ions, the myosin filaments become attracted to the active sites of the actin filament. This interaction pulls the actin along the immobile myosin filaments toward the center of the A band, thus shortening the sarcomere and producing muscle contraction. In this process, the lengths of individual filaments remain unchanged. The I band narrows as the thick filaments approach the Z line, and the H zone narrows between the ends of the thin filaments when they meet at the center of the sarcomere (see Figure 24-1, *5a, 5b*). The greater the quantity of calcium ions delivered to troponin (a relaxing protein), the faster the rate and numbers of interactions between actin and myosin. The result of this response is the development of tension and an increase in contractility.

ATP is cleaved by myosin ATPase in the presence of magnesium. This reaction releases the energy needed to perform work. The conversion of chemical energy to mechanical energy by ATP plays an essential role in energizing muscle shortening. In other words, it provides energy so the actin-myosin filaments can move and produce muscle contraction. Although this is a somewhat simplified explanation of the contractile mechanism, it illustrates the events important to understanding cardiotonic drug action.

Muscle relaxation depends on removing calcium ions from the sarcomere. The calcium ATPase (located in the walls of the sarcoplasmic reticulum) actively returns calcium ions to the sarcoplasmic reticulum and the sarcolemma, thereby allowing the actin-myosin filaments of the sarcomere to return to their resting positions.

✳ What actions are observed at the tissue and organ level?

The effective pumping action of the heart depends on the regularity of events occurring in the cardiac cycle. Each cycle consists of a period of relaxation (**diastole**) followed by a period of contraction (**systole**). The rhythm and rate of the cardiac cycle are regulated by the **conduction system,** specialized tissue that has the ability to initiate and transmit the electrical impulses needed to stimulate contraction of the cardiac muscle.

The conduction system is made up of the following structures: (1) sinoatrial (SA) node, (2) internodal pathways, (3) atrioventricular (AV) node, (4) bundle of His, (5) right and left bundle branches, and (6) Purkinje fibers. The Purkinje fibers penetrate the endocardium and end in the myocardial cells. The AV node and the His area form the **AV junction,** which extends from the atrial fibers through the AV node to the bifurcation of the bundle of His. When referring to this region, the term *AV junction* is considered to be more accurate than *AV node* (Figure 24-3).

In the normal heart, the SA node initiates the heartbeat. The impulses generated here are conducted through the internodal pathways to the "working" fibers of the atrial myocardium, producing atrial contraction. Electrical conduction is delayed when the impulses move through the AV junction. At the bundle of His, conduction speeds up and the impulses travel through the right bundle branch and the left bundle branch, then through the posteroinferior and anterosuperior fascicles of the left bundle branch. The transmission of impulses at the Purkinje fibers, which consist of tiny fibrils that spread around the ventricles and connect directly with the myocardial cells, is very rapid. The simultaneous depolarization of both ventricles produces ventricular contraction.

The coordinated pumping action of the heart is initiated and regulated by specialized fibers of the conduction system. The individual fibers of this system possess four basic **electrophysiologic properties:** (1) automaticity, (2) rhythmicity, (3) conductivity, and (4) refractoriness.

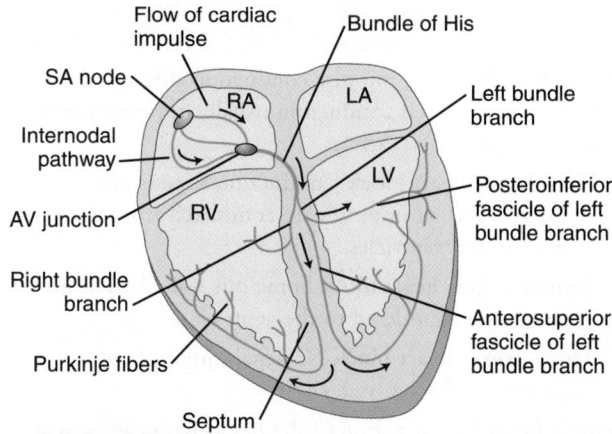

FIGURE 24-3 Conduction system of the heart. The cardiac impulse is initiated at the SA node and is transmitted through the internodal pathways to the two atria, resulting in atrial contraction. The electrical impulse is delayed at the AV node. Conduction speeds up at the bundle of His, with the impulse traveling through the right bundle branch and the left bundle branch and continuing through the posteroinferior fascicle and anterosuperior fascicle of the latter bundle branch. Finally, the arrival of impulses at the Purkinje fibers results in their distribution to all parts of both ventricles where, on excitation, ventricular contraction is produced. *LA,* Left atrium; *LV,* left ventricle; *RA,* right atrium; *RV,* right ventricle.

Automaticity The specialized fibers of the conduction system have the inherent ability to initiate a spontaneous electrical impulse without any external stimuli. This is the most fundamental mechanism of impulse formation. The cells that possess this property of automaticity, the ability to initiate an impulse, are called pacemaker cells. Automaticity is a property of fibers of the conduction system that normally controls heart rhythm.

Pacemaker cells are found in specialized conducting tissues such as the SA node, the AV junction, and the His-Purkinje system. Normally, the impulse of the heart is spontaneously and regularly initiated at the pacemaker cells of the SA node. During late resting potential (phase 4), the membrane of the cell depolarizes itself—spontaneously and gradually—until it reaches threshold and an action potential occurs. The slow depolarization of the membrane in the resting state is called spontaneous diastolic depolarization, or phase 4 depolarization, and defines automaticity. Thus the membrane of pacemaker cells is never truly at rest; this property is attributed to the continuous influx of sodium ions into the interior of the cells, which readily drives the membrane to threshold. The resting potential of automatic pacemaker cells differs from that of the nonautomatic myocardial cells. After full repolarization, the membrane of nonautomatic myocardial cells maintains a steady resting potential until an external stimulus causes it to achieve threshold. However, under pathologic conditions such as myocardial ischemia, nonautomatic myocardial cells do have the potential to exhibit spontaneous depolarization. This explains in part the high rate of cardiac dysrhythmias associated with myocardial infarction.

Rhythmicity The spontaneous excitation of pacemaker cells establishes the normal rhythm of the heart. The regularity of such pacemaking activity is termed rhythmicity. Under normal circumstances, only one functional pacemaker, the SA node, predominates because it has the highest frequency of depolarization. The normal rate of impulse formation is approximately 72 beats/min. If the SA node decreases its impulse formation rate to a rate below that of the AV junction (40 to 60 beats/min), then the AV junction becomes the primary pacemaker of the heart and will drive the heart at approximately 40 beats/min.

Conductivity Conductivity refers to the ability to transmit an action potential or nerve impulse from cell to cell. The property of conductivity therefore exists not only in the cells of the conduction system but also in the cardiac musculature. The speed of impulse conduction varies as it passes from one tissue to another in the heart. It is slowest in the AV junction and fastest in the Purkinje fibers. The significant delay of conduction at the AV junction allows more time for ventricular filling. On the other hand, the rapid depolarization of Purkinje fibers creates an instantaneous spread of impulses from the terminals to the ventricular muscles. Simultaneous activation of the musculature is essential for producing powerful ventricular contraction.

The speed with which electrical activity is spread within the sinus node is quite slow, approximately 0.05 m/sec. The impulse then spreads out rapidly over the atrial musculature at a rate of approximately 1 m/sec. When the impulse reaches the AV node, a delay of approximately 0.05 m/sec occurs to allow for atrial systole and ventricular filling. The impulse then spreads rapidly, at 2 to 4 m/sec, along the right and left bundle branches and Purkinje fibers. This rapid activation of contractile elements evokes a synchronous contraction of the ventricles.

The velocity of conduction is determined by the size of the resting potential of the cell membrane and the rate of rise of phase 0 of the action potential. This defines membrane responsiveness. Antidysrhythmic drugs may affect conduction by slowing the phase 0 depolarization rate, thereby decreasing membrane responsiveness.

Refractoriness Cardiac tissue is nonresponsive to stimulation during the initial phase of systole (contraction). This nonresponsiveness is known as refractoriness and determines how closely together two action potentials can occur. Throughout most of repolarization, the cell cannot respond to a stimulus. The effective refractory period represents that period in the cardiac cycle during which a stimulus, no matter how strong, fails to produce an action potential. Antidysrhythmic drugs can lengthen or shorten the refractory period of cardiac tissues by influencing the level of responsiveness of the cell membrane. A relative refractory period occurs after the effective refractory period and as repolarization nears completion. During this time, a propagated action potential can be elicited if the stimulus is stronger than normally required in diastole. When this happens, the fiber is stimulated to contract prematurely.

✴ How does the autonomic nervous system control cardiac function?

Although the conduction system possesses the inherent ability for spontaneous, rhythmic initiation of the cardiac impulse, the autonomic nervous system has an important role in regulating the rate, rhythm, and force of myocardial contraction of the heart. The heart is innervated by both the parasympathetic and the sympathetic nerves. The vagal nerve fibers of the parasympathetic branch are found primarily in the SA node, atrial muscles, and AV junction, whereas the sympathetic fibers innervate the SA node, AV junction, and the atrial and ventricular muscles.

Vagal stimulation of the heart is mediated by the release of acetylcholine, a neurohormone that acts on the muscarinic receptors to decrease heart rate and is also believed to decrease ventricular contraction. The main effect of acetylcholine on the AV junction is to slow the rate of conduction and lengthen the refractory period. By contrast, sympathetic fiber stimulation is mediated by the release of norepinephrine, which acts specifically on the β_1 adrenergic receptors in the cardiac tissue. Circulating epinephrine from the adrenal medulla may also elicit cardiac responses. By acting on the β-adrenergic receptors, norepinephrine and epinephrine increase both heart rate and the force of myocardial contraction. They also increase conduction velocity and shorten the refractory period of the AV junction. Epinephrine has a very potent effect on the heart. In large doses, its direct effect on the electrophysiologic properties of cardiac tissue can create a number of cardiac dysrhythmias, including ectopic beats, tachycardia, atrial fibrillation and ventricular fibrillation (Box 24-1). Normally the heartbeat is under the continuous influence of both parasympathetic and sympathetic control, with the resting heart rate the result of their opposing influences.

✴ What is the role of the electrocardiogram?

An **electrocardiogram (ECG)** is a graphic representation of electrical currents produced by the heart. Nurses caring for clients on monitoring equipment should be able to detect and interpret changes in the cardiac rate or rhythm, or in the conduction of the wave of electric activity or excitation. The ECG is a useful tool in determining the therapeutic effectiveness of certain drugs. A number of drugs may alter the electric activity of the heart. The ECG may provide the earliest objective evidence of the effectiveness or toxic manifestations of a drug. A knowledgeable and observant nurse can use the information obtained from ECGs to assess the effectiveness of drug therapy for cardiac dysrhythmias.

Electrical activity always precedes mechanical contraction. Immediately after a wave of electrical activity moves through atrial muscle, the muscle contracts and blood flows from the atria into the ventricles. Figure 24-4 illustrates a normal ECG. The P wave is produced by a wave of excitation through the atria (atrial depolarization). The onset of

---

BOX 24-1 COMMON CARDIAC DYSRHYTHMIAS

Heart block Impaired impulse conduction through the heart; the impaired conduction usually occurs between the atria and the ventricles.

  First-degree heart block Conduction time is prolonged, but all impulses are conducted from the atria to the ventricles.

  Second-degree heart block Some but not all atrial impulses are conducted to the ventricles.

  Third-degree heart block No atrial impulses are conducted to the ventricles.

Ectopic beats A contraction of the heart that originates at some place other than the SA node.

Extrasystole "premature beat" A premature contraction of the heart that arises independent of the normal rhythm.

Tachycardia Unusually rapid heart rate (usually faster than 100 beats/min in adult).

Bradycardia Unusually slow heart rate (usually slower than 60 beats/min in adult).

Atrial flutter Extremely rapid rate of atrial contraction; may be 200 to 350 beats/min.

Atrial fibrillation Rapid and uncoordinated contraction of the atria.

Ventricular fibrillation Rapid and uncoordinated contraction of the ventricles; because of the incoordination of contractions, there is little or no effective pumping of blood; death will result if not immediately treated.

---

the P wave follows the firing of the SA node. After the P wave, a short pause or interval (PR interval) occurs while the electrical activity is transmitted to the AV junction, conduction tissue, and ventricles. Depolarization of the ventricles is represented by the QRS complex on the ECG. Repolarization, or recovery, of the ventricles is indicated by the T wave. Atrial recovery or repolarization does not show on the ECG because it is hidden in the QRS complex.

✴ How are the fast and slow channels of cardiac membranes differentiated and how do they relate to cardiovascular function?

A review of the normal physiology of the fast and slow channels that exist in the membrane of the cardiovascular fibers is necessary for understanding the clinical application of calcium channel blockers. The cell membrane is composed of two types of channels that are controlled by "gates." When opened, these gates allow the movement of an inward current of (1) sodium ions through the fast channels, and (2) calcium ions through the slow channels into the cell, depending on the type of fibers involved. These channels appear in the cell membrane of three types of cardiovascular fibers. The heart contains two types: (1) fast-channel fibers, which appear in the myocardial cells of the atria and ventri-

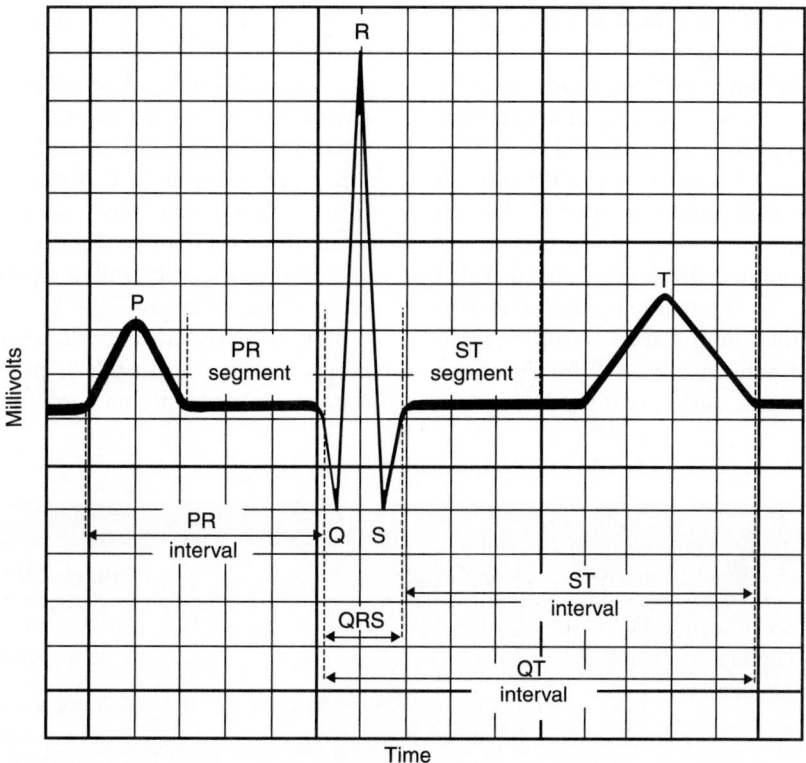

FIGURE 24-4 Representation of the normal ECG. Vertical lines represent time, each square represents 0.04 second, and every five squares (set off by heavy black lines) represents 0.20 second. The normal PR interval is less than 0.20 second; the average is 0.16 second. The average P wave lasts 0.08 second, the QRS complex is 0.08 second, the ST segment is 0.12 second, the T wave is 0.16 second, and the QT interval is 0.32 to 0.40 second if the heart rate is 65 to 95 beats/min. Each horizontal line represents voltage; every five squares equals 0.5 mV.

cles and the Purkinje fibers, and (2) slow-channel fibers, which occur in the SA node and the AV junction. Slow fibers, the third type, are present in the smooth muscle of the coronary and peripheral arterial vessels.

In this mechanism, the role of calcium ions is essential in producing the following three physiologic processes:

- Increasing the strength of myocardial contraction
- Enhancing automaticity and conduction speed (slow-channel fibers)
- Vasoconstriction of coronary arteries and peripheral arterioles (slow fibers)

Calcium ions enter the smooth-muscle cell through slow channels; the rise in free calcium ion concentration is considered to be the primary event in excitation-contraction coupling that is responsible for increasing muscle tone and vasoconstriction. In addition, the activation of smooth muscle can markedly reduce the caliber of small vessels, as is apparent from the "spasm" that may occur in coronary vessels. The calcium channel blockers (specifically vera-pamil, nifedipine, and diltiazem) are capable of blocking the slow calcium ion influx in the smooth muscle of blood vessels, thereby producing relaxation.

The culmination of these cellular and tissue events contributes to the ability of the heart to effectively pump blood to the pulmonary and systemic circulations. This requires effective coordination of electrical and contractile forces to produce a cardiac output that adequately meets body needs.

✱ How is cardiac output determined?

Cardiac output is the volume of blood expelled by the ventricles of the heart; it is equal to the amount of blood ejected at each beat (**stroke volume**) multiplied by the number of beats per minute (**heart rate**). Increased heart rates will increase cardiac output as long as ventricular filling is maintained between beats. Very high heart rates can result in reduced cardiac output when there is inadequate ventricular filling between beats.

Stroke volume, the other major determinant of cardiac output, is affected by three variables: contractility, preload, and afterload. **Contractility** refers to the strength of the muscular contraction of cardiac tissue and can be adversely affected by a number of factors, including myocardial ischemia or infarction, electrolyte disturbance, drugs with negative impact on contractility (referred to as negative inotropes), or infection. In the normal heart, the Frank-Starling relationship holds true. This relationship means that the longer the muscle fibers are at the end of diastole (period of heart relaxation), the more forceful the contraction during systole (the period of contraction). This mechanism applies only when the muscle fiber is lengthened within its physiologic limits.

Preload refers to the amount of blood entering the ventricle before contraction and affects the stretching of the muscle fiber in the ventricle. In a healthy heart, a moderate increase in preload may optimally stretch the muscle fibers of the ventricle and increase stroke volume In heart failure, however, increased preload "overstretches" the ventricle and results in reduced stroke volume (resulting in reduced cardiac output). **Afterload**, the pressure against which the ventricle is pumping blood, is primarily determined by peripheral vascular resistance (e.g., blood pressure). The heart has to work harder when systemic blood pressure is elevated (e.g., high afterload state).

A number of neurohormonal effects are observed which impact on cardiac output. The sympathetic nervous system is activated in reduced cardiac output states, resulting in elevated circulating levels of norepinephrine. While increased heart rate may serve to increase cardiac output, this is often offset by vasoconstriction with increased afterload and altered β_1 receptor sensitivity in the long-term. In the presence of reduced cardiac output, the renin-angiotensin-aldosterone system is activated, resulting in increased salt retention, fluid retention, and vasoconstriction. Endothelins, a set of amino acid peptides, are also released in low cardiac output states such as heart failure, postmyocardial infarction, and ischemia, and may trigger further vasoconstriction, tachycardia, and norepinephrine, aldosterone, and renin release (Kradjan, 2005).

A-type natriuretic peptide is secreted by the atrial tissue; B-type natriuretic peptide is produced in the ventricle in states associated with low cardiac output. These serve to an-

TABLE 24-1 EFFECT OF CARDIAC DRUG GROUPS ON CARDIAC TISSUES

Cardiac Tissue	Physiologic Property	Drug Group	Pharmacologic Action
Cardiac muscle (myocardium)	Force of myocardial contraction (Frank-Starling law)	Cardiac glycosides (e.g., digoxin)	Positive inotropic effect—increases contraction strength
		Angiotensin-converting enzyme inhibitors (e.g., captopril) Angiotensin receptor blockers (e.g., losartan) Diuretics (e.g., furosemide, spironolactone)	Reduce fluid retention, which decreases overstretch of myocardial muscle during ventricular filling (reduced preload)
		Angiotensin-converting enzyme inhibitors (e.g., captopril) Angiotensin receptor blockers (e.g., losartan) Vasodilators (nitrates, hydralazine) Aldosterone antagonist (spironolactone)	Reduce systemic blood pressure, which improves efficiency of ventricle to expel blood (reduced afterload)
		Low-dose β-adrenergic blockers (e.g., carvedilol)	Blunt long-term sympathetic stimulation associated with worsening heart failure
		B-type natriuretic peptide (nesiritide)	Augment neurohormonal response to heart failure with vasodilation; reduce fluid retention
Cardiac conduction system	Automaticity (rhythm and rate) Conductivity	Antidysrhythmic drugs Calcium channel blockers β-adrenergic blockers	Converts to normal sinus rhythm, abolishes dysrhythmia, or controls rate
Coronary arteries	Nutritional blood flow to myocardium and other cardiac structures	Nitrates Calcium channel blockers (e.g., diltiazem) β-adrenergic blockers (e.g., propranolol)	Coronary vasodilation and/or lessens work of the heart
		Antiplatelets (e.g., aspirin) Anticoagulants (e.g., warfarin) Fibrinolytics (e.g., alteplase)	Prevent or treat clot formation in coronary arteries
		Antihyperlipidemics (e.g., lovastatin)	Prevent atherosclerosis and risk for clot formation in coronary arteries

tagonize the effects of the renin-angiotensin-aldosterone system. B-type natriuretic peptide, considered one of a number of "cardiac neurohormones," results in favorable effects, including reduced preload and reduced afterload, and is among the more recent avenues of study in heart failure (Kradjan, 2005).

For individuals with heart failure secondary to low cardiac output, the goals of therapy often include increasing stroke volume by decreasing preload, decreasing afterload, and/or increasing contractility. A number of drugs can achieve these ends, including use of drugs that reduce fluid

retention (e.g., diuretics), reduce preload or afterload (e.g., angiotensin-converting enzyme inhibitors, angiotensin receptor blockers, nitrates, or vasodilators), or increase contractility (e.g., digoxin). These agents are presented in Table 24-1 and discussed in Chapters 25, 27, and 29. Table 24-1 summarizes the physiologic properties of cardiac structures and the drug groups used therapeutically.

What are the key issues involved in coronary vascular supply?

Cardiac tissue has unique demands for a ready supply of oxygenated blood. In cases where oxygen demand is increased (e.g., tachycardia), the integrity and capacity of the coronary arteries are of vital importance. The entire blood supply to the myocardium is provided by the right and left coronary arteries, which arise from the base of the aorta (Figure 24-5). The right atrium and ventricle are supplied with blood from the right coronary artery. The left coronary artery divides into the anterior (descending) branch and the circumflex branch, and supplies blood to the left atrium and ventricle. These main coronary vessels continue to divide, forming numerous branches. The result is a profuse network of coronary vessels. The major arterial vessels are located on the external surface of the ventricles. Arterial branches penetrate the myocardium toward the endocardial surface. Figure 24-6 gives an overview of the heart, blood flow, and valves.

Increased oxygen delivery to the myocardium is supported almost exclusively by increased coronary blood flow. The heart must increase its output when the demand for oxygen and nutrients by body tissues increases At the same

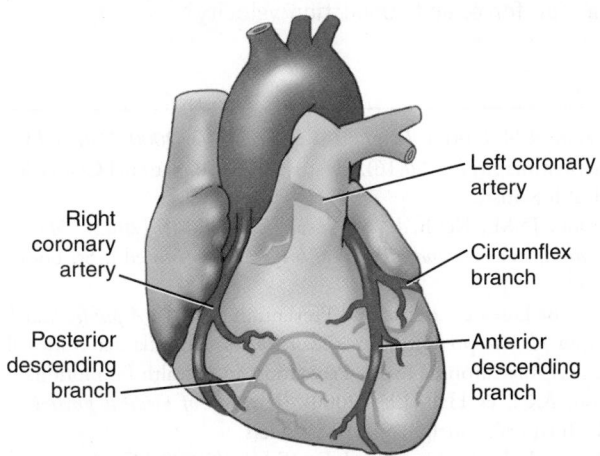

FIGURE 24-5 Coronary blood supply to the heart. Dark-shaded vessels are those located on the external surface of the ventricles; light-shaded vessels show the penetration of arterial branches toward the endocardial surface.

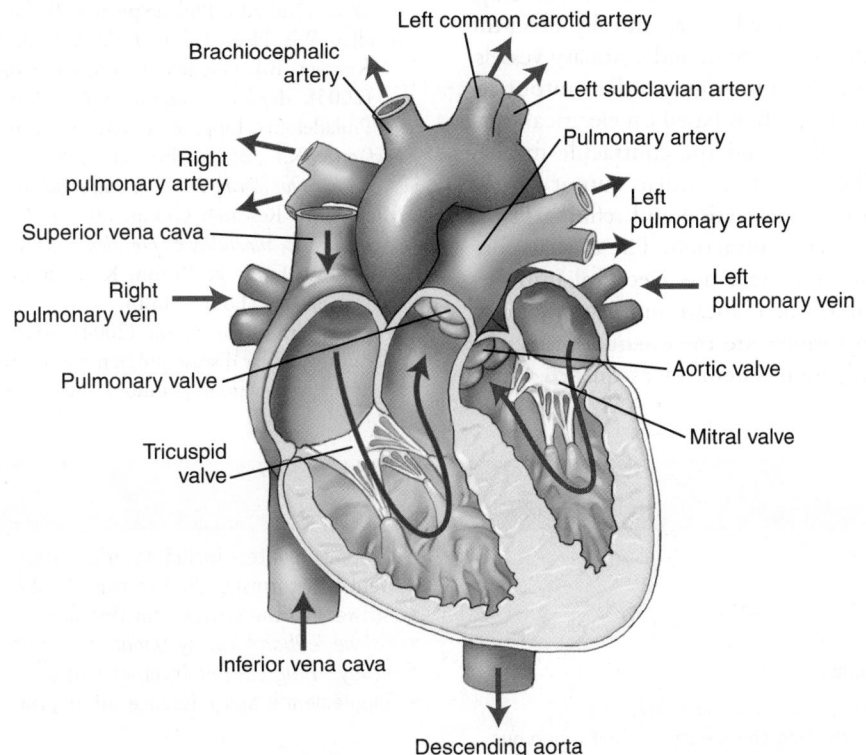

FIGURE 24-6 Overview of the heart, blood flow, and valves.

time, the heart muscle itself must be supplied with enough oxygen and nutrients to replace the energy expended. In other words, a balance must be maintained between energy expenditure and energy restoration. During systole, the myocardial contraction compresses the coronary vascular bed. This restricts oxygenated blood flow to coronary tissue. Coronary perfusion in the left ventricle occurs primarily during diastole, when the ventricles have relaxed and the coronary vessels are no longer compressed. Blood is driven through the coronary arteries by aortic pressure perfusing the myocardium.

A change in heart rate is accomplished by shortening or lengthening diastole. With tachycardia the increased number of systolic contractions per minute reduces the time available for diastole and coronary inflow. An increase also occurs in the metabolic needs of the rapidly beating heart. Coronary dilation normally occurs in an attempt to meet increased metabolic demand and to overcome restricted blood inflow. With bradycardia, the decreased number of systolic contractions per minute prolongs the diastolic period. Resistance to coronary flow and metabolic requirements of the myocardium are reduced.

Myocardial ischemia occurs whenever the delivery of oxygen to the myocardium is inadequate to meet the oxygen consumption needs of the heart. A major cause of ischemia is coronary artery disease, which is caused by atherosclerosis of the coronary arteries.

Summary

It is essential for nurses to understand the electrical and physiologic properties of the heart and the effects of drugs on cardiac activity. The drugs used therapeutically affect the myocardium, the conduction system, and coronary vessels. The action of the myocardium to adjust cardiac output according to the needs of the body is based on electrical excitation, mechanical activation, and the contractile mechanism of myocardial fiber. Effective cardiac output can be achieved only with adequate relaxation and refilling of the cardiac chambers after each contraction. The cardiac conduction system initiates and transmits electrical impulses required for contraction of the myocardium. Automaticity, conductivity, and refractoriness are the essential properties of the fibers of the conduction system. The sequence of cardiac excitation is graphically represented by electrocardiography. The ECG is a useful tool for monitoring cardiac activity to assist nurses in evaluating the effectiveness of a number of drugs used to treat cardiovascular disease.

✳ Critical Thinking Questions

- What is the role of systole and diastole in the cardiac conduction system?
- What are the effects of acetylcholine, norepinephrine, and epinephrine on vagal stimulation of the heart, sympathetic fiber stimulation, heart rate, myocardial contraction force, and conduction velocity?

Bibliography

Anderson, R.N. (2002). *Deaths: Leading causes for 2000. National Vital Statistics Reports 50*(16). Hyattsville, MD: National Center for Health Statistics.

Anderson, D.M., Keith, J., & Novak, P.D. (Eds.). (2002). *Mosby's medical, nursing, and allied health dictionary* (6th ed.). St. Louis: Mosby.

Centers for Disease Control and Prevention. (2004). *A public health action plan to prevent heart disease and stroke.* Atlanta: National Center for Chronic Disease Prevention and Health Promotion.

Guyton, A.C., & Hall, J.E. (2000). *Textbook of medical physiology* (10th ed.). Philadelphia: W.B. Saunders.

Hardman, J.G., & Limbird, L.E. (Eds.). (2001). *Goodman and Gilman's the pharmacological basis of therapeutics* (10th ed.). New York: McGraw-Hill.

Heart and Stroke Foundation of Canada. (2002). Incidence of cardiovascular disease. Retrieved June 29, 2005, from http://www.heartandstroke.ca.

Herlihy, B., & Maebius, N.K. (2003). *The human body in health and illness* (2nd ed.). Philadelphia: W.B. Saunders.

Kradjan, WA. Heart failure. In M.A. Koda-Kimble, L.Y. Young, W.A. Kradjan, B.J. Guglielmo, B.K. Alldredge, & R.L. Corelli (Eds.). (2005). *Applied therapeutics: The clinical use of drugs* (8th ed.). Philadelphia: Lippincott Williams & Wilkins.

McCance, K.L., & Huether, S.E. (2002). *Pathophysiology: The biological basis for disease in adults and children* (4th ed.). St. Louis: Mosby.

Millennium Research Group. (2001). *Global cardiovascular diseases incidences, mortality & prevalence 2001.* Toronto: MRG.

Thibodeau, G.A., & Patton, K.T. (2003). *Anatomy and physiology* (5th ed.). St. Louis: Mosby.

World Health Organization. (2004). Strategic priorities of the WHO cardiovascular disease programme. Retrieved June 24, 2004, from http://www.who.int/cardiovascular_diseases/priorities/en/

e-LEARNING SUPPLEMENTS

Student CD-ROM
- Final Exam questions
- NCLEX® Examination review questions
- Pharmacology animations
- Printable chapter summary

Evolve Website (http://evolve.elsevier.com/mckenry)
- Case study on drugs affecting the parasympathetic nervous system

- Content updates, including information on new drugs
- WebLinks corresponding to this chapter
- Answers to the critical thinking questions in this chapter
- *Elsevier ePharmacology Update* newsletter
- *Mosby's Drug Consult* Internet Edition
- Supplemental and reference information

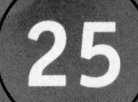

25

AGENTS USED IN THE TREATMENT OF HEART FAILURE

CHAPTER FOCUS

Cardiac glycosides have been used since the first century A.D. for the treatment of the symptoms of heart failure, and digoxin is still commonly prescribed for the treatment of specific cardiac disorders. However, combinations of drugs as well as other inotropic agents are also being used for heart failure therapy. Nurses must be knowledgeable about the administration of these agents and be able to recognize the toxicities that commonly occur with them.

LEARNING OBJECTIVES

- Explain right- and left-sided heart symptoms, including at least three major signs and symptoms.
- Identify the two primary mechanisms of action for digoxin.
- Describe the first symptoms of digoxin-induced dysrhythmias.
- Identify at least three drugs that interact with digoxin and describe the possible effects and the management of any interaction.
- Describe both the fast (rapid) and slow method of digitalization.
- Explore factors that predispose a client to digoxin toxicity.
- Implement the nursing management for the care of clients receiving inotropic agents.

▲ KEY TERMS

chronotropic, p. 504
heart failure, p. 503
digitalization, p. 511
dromotropic, p. 504
inotropic, p. 504

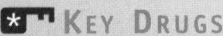 KEY DRUGS

digoxin, p. 510
inamrinone, p. 519
nesiritide, p. 520

Drugs in the digitalis group are among the oldest drugs in use. The effects of digoxin are twofold. It increases the strength of contraction (positive inotrope), and it alters the electrophysiologic properties of the heart by slowing the heart rate (negative chronotrope) and by slowing conduction velocity (negative dromotrope). Digoxin is used both for the treatment of heart failure and to slow conduction through the atrioventricular node in the management of atrial fibrilla-

tion. **Heart failure** (formerly referred to as congestive heart failure or CHF) is an abnormal condition that reflects altered structure and/or function of the ventricle and most often results in reduced cardiac output. The reduced cardiac output observed in heart failure is usually related to reduced stroke volume that may result from reduced ventricular filling or reduced ability of the ventricle to eject blood with each beat. Reduced cardiac output can be a result of many disease states, including pulmonary disease, damaged cardiac valves, dysrhythmias, hypertension, and hyperthyroidism. A number of factors influence the pathogenesis of heart failure, including altered contractility, preload, afterload, and neurohormonal influences (see Chapter 24).

✱ How common is heart failure?

Approximately 23 million people worldwide are afflicted with heart failure (HF), and 2 million new cases of HF are diagnosed each year worldwide. In contrast to other cardiovascular disorders that have actually declined during the past few decades, the incidence of heart failure is on the rise. It is the most rapidly growing cardiovascular disorder in the United States and Canada because of the aging population and better treatment of coronary disease and hypertension (Academic Market Research, 2004). HF is associated with high mortality and morbidity, and so has an enormous impact on public health.

An estimated 4.9 million Americans have HF. It often is the end stage of cardiac disease. Half of the individuals diagnosed with HF die within 5 years of onset. Each year, there are an estimated 400,000 new cases in the United States. The annual number of deaths directly from HF increased from 10,000 in 1968 to 51,546 in 2000 (Figure 25-1), with another 219,000 related to the condition. Whereas the 5-year survival rate following diagnosis is poorer in men than in women, fewer than 15% of women survive more than 8 to 12 years and their 1-year mortality rate is higher than that of men, with 1 in 5 dying during the first year after diagnosis. HF clients are six to nine times more likely than the general population to experience sudden cardiac death. Although prominent in persons 65 years of age and older, HF also afflicts a younger client population. In clients younger than age 65 years, 80% of men and 70% of women who have HF will die within 8 years of onset. Overall, approximately 20% of HF clients will die within 1 year of diagnosis, and 50% will die within 5 years. HF also takes an economic toll. Hospitalization rates associated with HF are extremely high; the American Heart Association reports 999,000 discharges in 2000 with the direct and indirect costs of HF being $24.3 billion for the year. These data stress the need for early detection and management of clients at high risk for HF so as to lessen the devastating effects of HF on both clients and society.

✱ What types of pharmacologic effects do cardiac drugs have on myocardial tissue?

Various medications may directly change the force of myocardial contraction and the rate and rhythm of the heart. Many drugs influence myocardial contraction indirectly via altering fluid balance, blood vessel tone, or other neurohormonal effects. Pharmacologic terms that have specific meaning for the direct actions of drugs on the myocardium include inotropic, chronotropic, and dromotropic effects.

Drugs with an **inotropic** (Gr. *inos,* fiber; *tropikos,* a turning or influence) effect influence myocardial contractility. Drugs with a positive inotropic effect strengthen or increase the force of myocardial contraction (e.g., digoxin, dobutamine, dopamine, epinephrine, and isoproterenol), whereas drugs with a negative inotropic effect weaken or decrease the force of myocardial contraction (e.g., lidocaine, quinidine, and propranolol).

Drugs with **chronotropic** (Gr. *chronos,* time) action affect heart rate. A positive chronotropic effect is produced if the drug accelerates the heart rate by increasing the rate of impulse formation in the sinoatrial (SA) node (e.g., norepinephrine). A negative chronotropic drug has the opposite effect and slows the heart rate by decreasing impulse formation (e.g., acetylcholine).

A **dromotropic** (Gr. *dromos,* a course) effect refers to drugs that affect conduction velocity through specialized conducting tissues. A drug having a positive dromotropic action speeds conduction (e.g., epinephrine), whereas a drug with a negative dromotropic action delays conduction (e.g., verapamil).

✱ What are the key pathophysiologic features of HF?

HF is a myocardial dysfunction resulting in a cardiac output that cannot keep up with body requirements. HF is a complex interrelated response to cardiovascular, hemodynamic and neurohormonal changes (Figure 25-2). To appreciate how cardiac output is determined and is affected by heart rate, preload, afterload, and contractility, refer to Chapter 24, pp. 499 to 501. Classifications of HF are presented below and in Table 25-1.

Infrequently, increased metabolic demand for blood associated with anemia or hyperthyroid states can result in increased cardiac output that cannot keep up with demand. This type of heart failure is termed *high-output HF,* and is not as commonly observed. Most commonly, diminished cardiac output is observed in HF and is secondary to a weakened or poorly compensated heart. This type of HF is often termed *low-output HF.*

Low-output HF may present with symptoms that are predominately related to failure of the left ventricle, right ventricle, or both. With left-ventricular HF, increased hydrostatic pressure in the left ventricle "backs up" into the

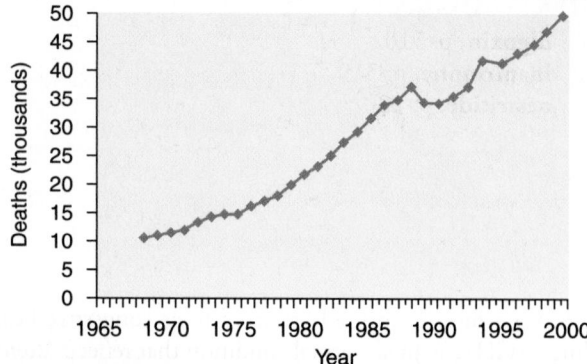

FIGURE 25-1 Deaths from heart failure, United States, 1968-1998. The sharp drop in 1989 is attributed to a change in the type of information recorded on the death certificate.

Data from National Center for Health Statistics. Vital statistics of the United States. Retrieved September 4, 2005, from http://www.cdc/nchs/about/major/dvs/mortdat/htm.

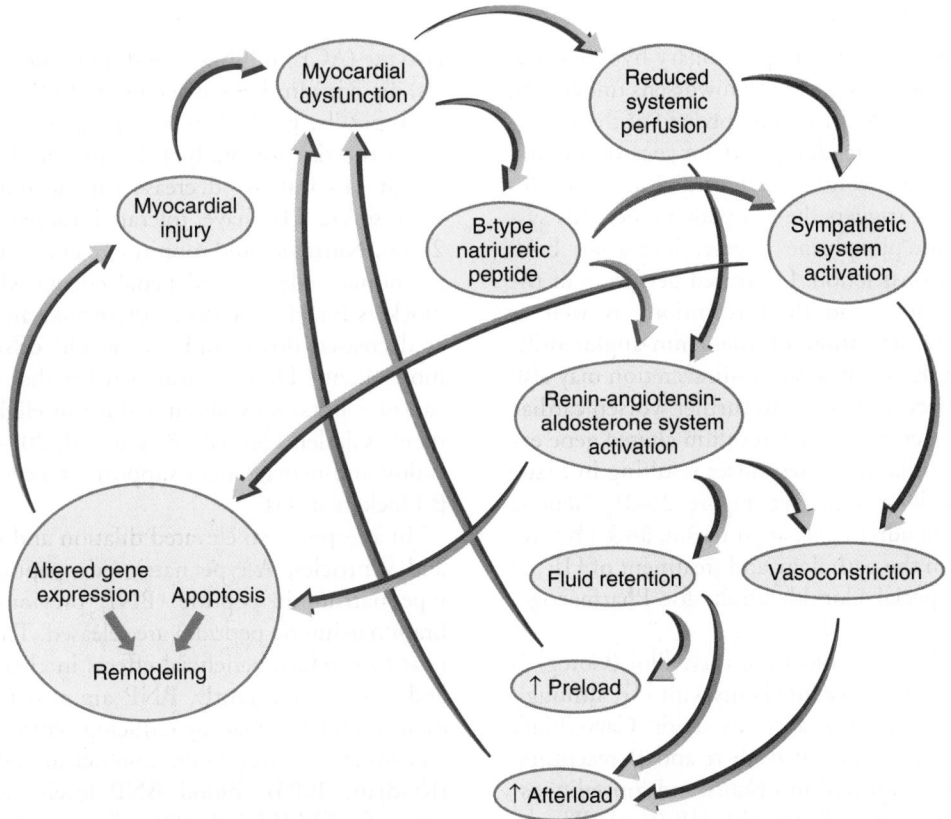

FIGURE 25-2 The progression of heart failure is a complex cascade of events involving cardiac and neurohormonal systems. Brown arrows indicate inhibition.

TABLE 25-1 CLASSIFICATIONS OF HEART FAILURE

| | High-output HF | Low-output HF* | |
		Systolic Dysfunction	Diastolic Dysfunction
Characteristics	Normal: ↑ contractility Normal heart size Normal or ↑ SV Usually ↑ HR ↑ CO	Contractility ↓ Heart size ↑ ↓ SV ↓ CO S₃ heart sound	Normal contractility Normal heart size ↓ SV ↓ CO S₄ heart sound
Frequency	<5%-10% of cases	60%-70% of cases	30%-40% of cases
Contributing factors	↑ Metabolic demands	↓ Contractility ↑ Afterload	Thick left ventricle Stiff left ventricle ↑ Preload
Etiology	Anemias Hyperthyroidism	Myocardial ischemia Hypertension Drugs Heart valve disease Alcoholism	Myocardial ischemia Hypertension Heart valve disease Cardiomyopathy
Goals of treatment	Treat underlying cause	Reduce afterload Increase contractility Reduce preload	Reduce preload Reduce afterload Decrease stiff ventricle (e.g., calcium channel blockers)

Modified from Kradjan, W.A. (2005). Heart failure. In M.A. Koda-Kimble, L.Y. Young, W.A. Kradjan, B.J. Guglielmo, B.K. Alldredge, & R.L. Corelli (Eds.), *Applied therapeutics: The clinical use of drugs* (8th ed.). Philadelphia: Lippincott Williams & Wilkins.

↑, Increased; ↓, decreased; *CO,* cardiac output; *HF,* heart failure; *HR,* heart rate; *SV,* stroke volume.

*May present with predominantly left-sided symptoms, right-sided symptoms, or both.

pulmonary circulation, leading to pulmonary hypertension and pulmonary edema. This state often worsens underlying left-ventricular function by increasing preload of the ventricle, contributing to overstretching of the myocardium, and further reducing stroke volume and cardiac output. Reduced cardiac output triggers the sympathetic nervous system to increase norepinephrine release, increasing both heart rate and vasoconstriction. Decreased perfusion of the kidney triggers sodium and fluid retention, as well as vasoconstriction via activation of the renin-angiotensin-aldosterone system. Excessive vasopressin secretion may also be noted. These effects only serve to further worsen cardiac output in the short-term, and may result in altered gene expression and myocardial tissue responses resulting in tissue remodeling in the long-term (see Figure 25-2). Genetic variation observed in adrenergic, angiotensin, and other receptors important in the pathology and treatment of HF are presented in the Special Considerations for Pharmacogenetics box below.

Of existing β-adrenergic blockers, carvedilol (Coreg) is considered the agent of choice for clients with HF, although metoprolol (Lopressor) may also be used. Carvedilol's unique properties (antagonist at both α and β receptors) may account for the improved morbidity and mortality associated with this agent for clients with HF (Poole-Wilson et al., 2003).

The American College of Cardiology and the American Heart Association recommend β-adrenergic blockers for all stable clients with HF unless such therapy is contraindicated (e.g., asthma). Before initiating therapy, clients should not have evidence of fluid retention nor have recently received an intravenous (IV) inotrope. β blockers are typically used in conjunction with angiotensin-converting enzyme (ACE) inhibitors and other modalities (e.g., diuretics, digoxin) in the management of HF (Hunt et al., 2001).

Typically, β blockers are initiated at very low doses to avoid the risk for bradycardia and fluid retention, both of which can initially decrease cardiac output. Even clients with severe HF have tolerated carvedilol (Krum et al., 2003). Nurses should monitor all clients for slow heart rate, pulmonary edema, and pedal edema when starting on β blockers for HF. However, these risks are low when started at decreased doses, and the benefit offsets these risks for most clients. Despite clear benefits that β blockers in HF can save lives, only about a third of eligible clients receive them (Giesler, Lenihan, & Durand, 2004). Improved education and management support are keys to improve use of β blockers in HF.

In a response to elevated dilation and stretch in the atria and ventricles, A-type natriuretic peptide (ANP) and B-type natriuretic peptide (BNP, previously referred to as brain natriuretic peptide) are released. These substances appear to produce beneficial effects in clients with HF. ANP and, more importantly, BNP are associated with reduced preload and afterload by reducing sympathetic outflow and antagonizing the renin-angiotensin-aldosterone system (Kradjan, 2005). Blood BNP levels are advocated as a screen for HF (Maisel, 2004; Tung et al., 2004).

Sustained pulmonary hypertension of left-sided HF poses an increased afterload to the right ventricle, leading to right-ventricular HF. The reduced right-ventricular stroke volume leads to fluid backup into systemic circulation. The classic symptoms of right-ventricular HF include pedal and peripheral edema, hepatomegaly, and jugular venous distention.

Left-ventricular HF can be related to reduced efficiency of the ventricle to contract *(systolic dysfunction)* or reduced

Special Considerations for Pharmacogenetics | TREATMENT OF HEART FAILURE

PHARMACODYNAMICS

Variation across populations in β₁-adrenergic receptors has been linked to the genetic marker Arg389. Presence of this marker appears to predict responders to β blockers in HF (Mialet Perez et al., 2003). This or other markers may explain the observation of improved outcomes in some black clients (Small, Wagoner, Levin, Kardia, & Liggett, 2002). The ability of the β-blocker atenolol and the angiotensin receptor blocker irbesartan to reduce blood pressure and reduce left-ventricular hypertrophy (a risk for developing HF) is also genetically based (Liljedahl et al., 2004). Genetic variability in angiotensin-converting enzymes, angiotensin receptors, and aldosterone synthesis has also been noted and likely influences response to agents that act at these sites (Bleumink et al., 2004; Chang & Altman, 2004). Generic variation most likely explains the reduced response to angiotensin-converting enzyme inhibitors in blacks (Exner, Dries, Domanski, & Cohn, 2001).

PHARMACOKINETICS

Metabolism of β-adrenergic blockers (e.g., carvedilol, metoprolol) is via the genetically determined cytochrome P450 2D6 isoenzyme. Differences in response may, in part, be a result of genetic variation in metabolism (Evans, 2003; Schaefer, Caracciolo, Frishman, & Charney, 2003). Genetic markers for the metabolism of the angiotensin-receptor blocker losartan has also been reported (Chang & Altman, 2004).

ADVERSE EFFECTS

Angiotensin-converting enzyme inhibitors are more likely to produce cough in women than in men (Schaefer et al., 2003). This finding is believed to be genetically based. Other adverse effects to agents used in HF probably have some basis in genetic variation.

capacity of the ventricle to completely relax and fill with blood between beats, and is termed *diastolic dysfunction.*

With systolic dysfunction, the goals of treatment include decreasing preload, decreasing afterload, and increasing contractility. Treatments include diuretics, vasodilators, agents that interfere with renin-angiotensin-aldosterone, inotropes such as digoxin, and in acute settings, synthetic formulations of BNP.

With diastolic dysfunction, a less-common type of HF, treatments often include reducers of preload and afterload, but may also include negative inotropic drugs that relax the ventricle between beats (e.g., calcium channel blockers). Use of negative inotropes such as calcium channel blockers, while helping diastolic dysfunction, are contraindicated for clients with systolic dysfunction.

On a cellular level, heart failure may be associated with a defect in excitation-contraction coupling, and in some individuals, dysfunction of *contractile proteins* may occur as an additional abnormality. Ineffective calcium pumping by the sarcoplasmic reticulum may alter the normal relaxation process. Furthermore, the mitochondria—*not* the sarcomic reticulum—may act as the dominant calcium uptake storage site. If so, less calcium is available for release from the sarcoplasmic reticulum to activate contraction. Thus the amount of coupling is reduced, and depressed myocardial contractility ensues.

With regard to the dysfunction of contractile proteins in heart failure, attention has been focused on abnormal energy use. Some researchers have shown that the activity of myosin adenosine triphosphatase (ATPase) is decreased. When the activity of this enzyme is reduced in heart failure, the interaction between actin and myosin filaments is reduced in intensity, and thus the force of contractility is lowered.

In summary, the failing heart may show increases in both preload (increased blood volume return to the heart chambers) and afterload (the increased pressure in the aorta that the ventricle muscles must overcome to open the aortic valve and push blood through). The decrease in renal perfusion seen in HF activates the sympathetic and renin-angiotensin-aldosterone (RAA) feedback mechanisms. Sodium and water are then retained, and intravascular volume and blood flow back to the heart increase. In less-serious situations, this is usually enough to maintain arterial blood pressure, and the RAA system is turned off. However, in individuals who have conditions bordering on heart failure, this can produce a frank decompensation or acute heart failure. The increase in circulatory blood volume increases the demands on the heart, which may result in acute pulmonary edema.

✷ What are the principles of treatment of heart failure?

The overall treatment goals for HF primarily include reducing preload and afterload to enhance myocardial contraction. It is necessary to treat any correctable underlying causes of the heart failure, such as hypertension or dysrhythmias. Even correction of sleep apnea improves outcomes for clients with HF (Kaneko et al., 2003). Similarly, it is important to review the client's drug regimen for potential agents that may exacerbate HF (see Box 25-1 and the Special Considerations for Pharmacogenetics box on p. 506). Improper diet has been noted in up to half of clients with HF (Aquilani et al., 2003). Exercise training may also improve outcomes for clients in HF (Piepoli, Davos, Francis, Coats, & ExTraMATCH Collaborative, 2004). Counseling the client and family members on the signs and symptoms of heart failure and the need to adhere to the nonpharmacologic (discussed in nursing management below) and pharmacologic treatments as prescribed, are also fundamental to the management of HF.

Drug therapy is also a combined approach. Table 25-2 presents the drugs used to treat heart failure. Most of these agents are discussed in other chapters. Diuretics are prescribed to reduce the increase in blood volume and edema. An ACE inhibitor (e.g., enalapril, captopril) is usually prescribed for left-ventricular systolic dysfunction. Angiotensin II receptor blockers (ARBs) (e.g., losartan, candesartan) may also be used (Pfeffer et al., 2003). They work to decrease peripheral vascular resistance (afterload), pulmonary capillary wedge pressure (preload), pulmonary vascular resistance, and the secretion of aldosterone. The ACE inhibitors and ARBs are discussed more fully in Chapter 27. Vasodilators, such as nitrates, that pool blood in the extremities and so reduce blood return or preload, as well as arterial vasodilators that decrease arterial resistance and reduce afterload, may also be part of the therapy. Antagonists of aldosterone, including spironolactone (Aldactone) and eplerenone (Inspra) are also effective in HF management (Pitt et al., 2003). A new class of agents, the vasopressin antagonists, may offer some benefit after further study (Gheorghiade et al., 2004).

BOX 25-1 THE ROLE OF β-ADRENERGIC BLOCKERS IN HEART FAILURE

The sympathetic nervous system, when stimulated, typically results in increased heart rate and cardiac output in the short-term. Clients in systolic HF, however, typically experience prolonged sympathetic nervous system stimulation with elevated levels of circulating catecholamines (e.g., epinephrine, norepinephrine). This continuous stimulation leads to vasoconstriction and worsening afterload. The vasoconstriction also contributes to reduced renal perfusion and ultimately triggers the RAA system to retain sodium and fluid (increasing preload), and produces aldosterone triggered vasoconstriction (increasing afterload).

In addition, the chronically elevated catecholamine levels alter β-adrenergic-receptor sensitivity and density, and renders the ventricle less responsive over time to adrenergic stimulation. There appears to be genetic variation in β-receptor-site function (see the Special Considerations for Pharmacogenetics box, p. 506), and it is assumed that this may be an important mechanism for some populations (e.g., black clients) (Small et al., 2002).

TABLE 25-2 DRUG CLASSES USED IN THE MANAGEMENT OF HEART FAILURE

Drug Class	Prototype/Example in Class	Rationale for Use in HF	Chapter Where Drug is Discussed More Fully
Aldosterone antagonist/ potassium-sparing diuretic	spironolactone (Aldactone)	Reduces preload Reduces afterload	33
Angiotensin-converting enzyme inhibitor	captopril (Capoten)	Reduces preload Reduces afterload	27
Angiotensin-receptor blocker	losartan (Cozaar)	Reduces preload Reduces afterload	27
B-type natriuretic peptide	nesiritide (Natrecor)	Reduces preload Reduces afterload	25
β-Adrenergic blocker	carvedilol (Coreg)	Use limited to low dose in otherwise stable clients Reduces adrenergic overstimulation	22
Calcium channel blocker	nifedipine (Adalat, Procardia)	Use limited to diastolic dysfunction HF Increases pliability of ventricle to allow more complete filling	27
Cardiac glycoside*	digoxin (Lanoxin)	Increases contractility	25
Complementary/alternative medication	coenzyme Q10 (ubiquinone)	Increases contractility	12
Inotrope: catecholamine*	dopamine (Intropin)	Use limited to short-term in acute care Increases contractility	22
Inotrope: noncatecholamine*	inamrinone (Inocor)	Use limited to short-term in acute care Increases contractility	25
Loop diuretic	furosemide (Lasix)	Reduces preload	33
Thiazide diuretic	hydrochlorothiazide (Esidrix)	Reduces preload	33
Vasodilator (nitrate)*	nitroglycerin	Reduces preload	28
Vasodilator (nonnitrate)*	hydralazine (Apresoline)	Reduces preload Reduces afterload	27
Vasopressin antagonists (investigational)	tolvaptan (investigational)	Reduces preload Reduces afterload	N/A

HF, Heart failure.
*Often reserved for clients refractory to standard treatment or with other comorbid conditions.

Although it appears counterintuitive, occasionally agents known to acutely worsen HF in the short-term are used to improve HF management long-term. Low doses of β-adrenergic blockers are often used for individuals with stable HF to reduce further morbidity and mortality by affecting the excessive adrenergic stimulation to the heart often seen in HF (Box 25-2). A small subset of individuals who suffer from diastolic dysfunction (where ventricles do not relax enough to allow for adequate ventricular filling) may be treated with calcium channel blockers to allow for increased ventricular filling and therefore improve stroke volume and cardiac output.

Drugs that increase contractility are sometimes used in HF. Among the most common inotropes used in systolic

BOX 25-2 DRUGS THAT MAY PRECIPITATE OR EXACERBATE HEART FAILURE

DRUGS THAT CAUSE SODIUM AND WATER RETENTION OR EXPAND INTRAVASCULAR VOLUME

Albumin

Androgens

Corticosteroids (e.g., cortisone, hydrocortisone, fludrocortisone [Florinef])

Diazoxide (Proglycem, Hyperstat)

Estrogens

Guanethidine (Ismelin)

Mannitol

Methyldopa (Aldomet)

Minoxidil (Loniten)

Nonsteroidal antiinflammatory drugs

Urea

DRUGS THAT INHIBIT MYOCARDIAL CONTRACTILITY (NEGATIVE INOTROPIC OR CARDIOTOXIC AGENTS)

β-blocking agents*

Calcium channel blockers (especially verapamil)†

Disopyramide (Norpace)

Doxorubicin (Adriamycin)

Quinidine

*For more information, refer to Box 25-1.
†Use limited to clients with diastolic HF (Hunt et al., 2001).

HF is digoxin (Lanoxin), which is discussed in this chapter. Limited to critical care settings, the IV inotropes inamrinone (Inocor) and milrinone (Primacor) are also discussed in this chapter. Similarly, nesiritide (Natrecor) is a recombinant form of human BNP used in the management of acute decompensated HF in critical care and is discussed later in this chapter. Dobutamine is used to increase myocardial contractility (see Chapter 22) but its use is also limited to the acute management of HF in critical care. Data supporting the use of coenzyme Q10 in HF varies and is presented in Chapter 12.

How were digitalis glycosides used historically?

The story of the origin of digitalis is interesting in that it was an herbal remedy used for hundreds of years by common people (called "housewife's recipe"). Digitalis is derived from the biennial flower foxglove (see Figure 1-1). Farmers and housewives prepared the remedy for dropsy (fluid accumulation). More than 400 years ago, Dr. Leonhard Fuchs recommended that physicians use it "to scatter the dropsy, to relieve swelling of the liver, and even to bring on

menstrual flow" (Silverman, 1942). Dr. Fuchs was a botanist-physician, and at that time the medical profession paid little attention to a "mere flower picker."

In the mid-1700s, a female client shared an old family recipe for curing dropsy with Dr. William Withering. Dr. Withering used this recipe for his dropsy clients and, after spending 10 years studying digitalis, published his conclusions in *An Account of the Foxglove.* This remarkable publication stressed instructions that are still valid today—the necessity of individualizing dosage according to the client's response. Digitalis was finally admitted to the *London Pharmacopoeia* in 1722 (Silverman, 1942). While many digitalis formulations historically have been used, only digoxin (Lanoxin) remains in widespread use.

What are the pharmacologic properties of digoxin?

Digoxin possesses positive inotropic action, negative chronotropic action, and negative dromotropic action.

Positive Inotropic Action The main function of digoxin is inotropic action. The increased myocardial contractility is associated with more efficient use of available energy. If the failing heart is enlarged, the positive inotropic action of digoxin can cause the myocardium to beat more forcefully, thereby increasing cardiac output and decreasing oxygen use. The improved pumping action of the heart in individuals with HF may reach levels that approach normal because the net effect is not only reduced heart size, but also decreased venous pressure to relieve edema.

Although the positive inotropic mechanism is not precisely known, one theory asserts that digoxin is bound to sites on the myocardial cell membrane (sarcolemma), where it inhibits the action of the membrane-bound Na^+-K^+-ATPase enzyme. Normally this enzyme hydrolyzes adenosine triphosphate to provide the energy needed by the Na^+-K^+ pump to release Na^+ and to transport K^+ into the cardiac cell during repolarization. By binding specifically to Na^+-K^+-ATPase, digoxin inhibits the active transport of Na^+ and K^+ (see Figure 24-1, 5b). Intracellular Na^+ accumulates, which stimulates the release of large quantities of free calcium ion from the sarcoplasmic reticulum. The free calcium ion is essential for linking the electrical excitation of the cell membrane to the mechanical contraction of the myocardial cell, a mechanism known as excitation-contraction coupling.

More free calcium ion produces a greater degree of coupling of actin and myosin to form actinomyosin, which results in more forceful myocardial contraction with a concomitant increase in cardiac output. Inhibition of Na^+-K^+-ATPase activity is projected to be the mechanism by which digoxin increases myocardial contraction without causing increased oxygen consumption. (See "Myocardial Contraction" in Chapter 24.)

Negative Chronotropic and Negative Dromotropic Actions Digoxin has negative chronotropic effects (decreased heart rate) and negative dromotropic effects (slowed conduction velocity) because it can alter the following three electrophysiologic properties of cardiac tissues:

- *Automaticity.* Cardiac tissue has the inherent ability to initiate and propagate an impulse without external stimulation. This property affects the rate and rhythm of the heart. Low to moderate doses of digoxin slow the heart rate because the SA node depolarizes less frequently. On the other hand, toxic concentrations of digoxin can directly increase automaticity. This increases the rate of both action potentials and spontaneous depolarization. This is one of the mechanisms responsible for digoxin-induced ectopic pacemakers. Toxic doses of digoxin may significantly increase impulse formation in latent or potential pacemaker tissue, causing dysrhythmia.

- *Conduction velocity.* All concentrations of digoxin decrease conduction velocity. Atrioventricular (AV) conduction velocity is slowed both by the direct action of digoxin and by increased vagal action. The electrocardiogram (ECG) shows a prolonged PR interval, and in toxic doses the drug can lead to increased heart block (Figure 25-3).

- The *refractory period* effects of digoxin vary in different parts of the heart (see Figure 25-3). If the refractory period in the ventricles is reduced, nearly toxic amounts of digoxin are required. A prolonged refractory period occurs in the AV conduction system, which is very sensitive to digoxin action. This action is partly direct and partly caused by increased vagal tone. Toxic doses of digoxin may prolong the refractory period and depress conduction in the AV conduction system until complete heart block may occur. A shortened digoxin-related QT interval, however, equates with reduced refractory period for the ventricles, and may explain ventricular dysrhythmias associated with digoxin overdose.

digoxin (di **joks** in)
(Lanoxin)

Indications
Digoxin is used to treat heart failure and to slow ventricular rates in atrial fibrillation and atrial flutter.

Pharmacokinetics/Dosing
The bioavailability of digoxin is approximately 60% to 80% with tablets, 70% to 85% with the elixir, and 90% to 100% with the capsule dosage form. Digoxin may undergo some metabolism by gut bacteria, which may account for variation in bioavailability among clients. Approximately 50% to 70% of the drug is eliminated as unchanged drug in the urine, with the remainder as active metabolites. Digoxin has a relatively long half-life of approximately 38 hours, but the elimination half-life may be particularly prolonged with renal insufficiency.

Adverse Effects
A number of adverse effects are noted with digoxin, most of which are dose related. Serious adverse effects include heart block, bradycardia, ventricular fibrillation, and other serious cardiac dysrhythmias, many of which can be more serious in the presence of electrolyte imbalance. Other adverse effects include nausea, vomiting, diarrhea, dizziness, visual disturbances, rash, hallucinations, confusion, dizziness, and delirium.

Drug Interactions
A number of drugs interact with digoxin, including other drugs that slow conduction through the AV node (e.g., β blockers, diltiazem, verapamil), drugs that can result in elevated digoxin levels (e.g., amiodarone, quinidine, azole antifungals, erythromycin), and drugs that reduce gastrointestinal absorption if dosed at the same time (e.g., antacids, bile acid sequestrants such as cholestyramine).

✱ How is digoxin used in the management of heart failure?
A heart in failure is no longer capable of supplying body tissue with adequate oxygen and nutrients or of removing metabolic waste products. Historically, digoxin has been widely used as a positive inotrope to increased myocardial contractility. The increased force of systolic contraction causes the ventricles to empty more completely. A slower

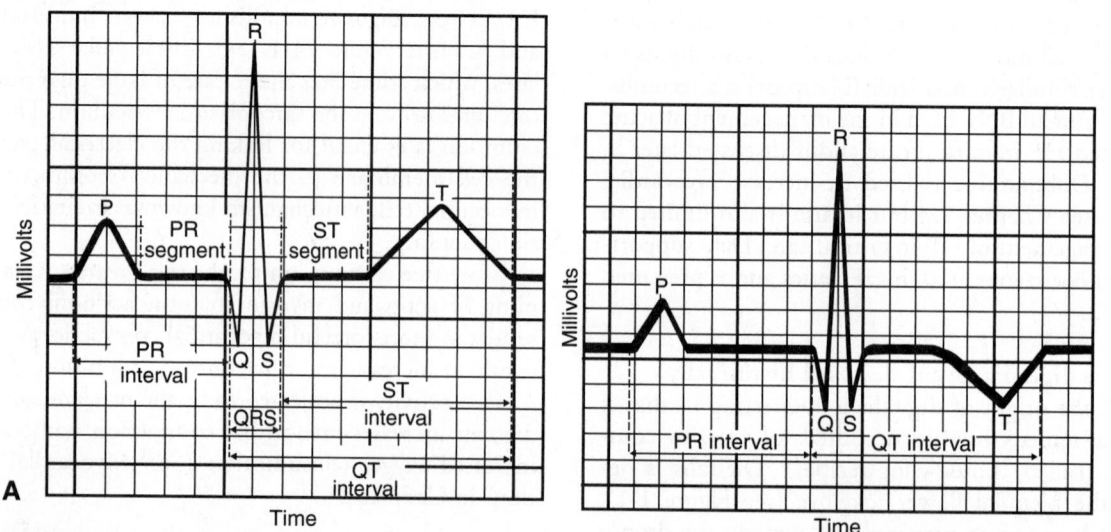

FIGURE 25-3 Effects of digoxin on ECG. **A,** Representation of normal ECG. **B,** Representation of the typical effects of digitalization on the electric activity of the heart as shown on the ECG. Note the prolonged PR interval, the shortened QT interval, and the T-wave inversion.

heart rate permits more complete filling, which results in the following:

- Venous pressure falls, and the pulmonary and systemic congestion and their accompanying signs and symptoms are either diminished or eliminated.
- Coronary circulation is enhanced, myocardial oxygen demand is reduced, and the supply of oxygen and nutrients to the myocardium is improved.
- Heart size is often decreased toward normal.

These effects are seen at the lower end of the dosing range and are correlated with serum levels of 0.8 to 2 ng/mL. Some cardiac glycosides have a true, but mild, diuretic effect. However, marked diuresis in a client with edema primarily results from improved heart action, improved circulation to all body tissues, and improved tissue and organ function, including renal function. When digoxin is effective, the client is noticeably improved and has an increased sense of well-being.

Over the past decade, there has been ongoing debate regarding the role of digoxin in the management of HF. The ACE inhibitors and ARBs have clearly improved morbidity and mortality for many clients with HF (McMurray et al., 2003; Packer et al., 1999). Similarly, the β-adrenergic blockers have reduced mortality in individuals with stable HF (Pritchett & Redfield, 2002). Digoxin has been associated with improvement in some symptoms, but has yet to demonstrate a mortality benefit (Dec, 2003). For clients stabilized on digoxin for HF, its withdrawal is associated with worsening symptoms (Rathore, Curtis, Wang, Bristow, & Krumholz, 2003).

✱ How is digoxin used in the management of atrial fibrillation?

During atrial fibrillation several hundred impulses originate from the atria, but only a fraction of them are transmitted through the AV junction. Figure 25-4 shows the ECG pattern of atrial fibrillation. Digoxin is ideal for slowing the ventricular rate because it increases the refractory period of the AV junction and slows conduction at this site. Higher doses are often required to achieve this effect, with a therapeutic serum level typically at 1.5 to 2.5 ng/mL. It is important to know that the purpose of using digoxin in atrial fibrillation is to slow the ventricular rate to reduce the possibility of inducing ventricular tachycardia. It also may prevent or eliminate cardiac failure. Digoxin *does not* convert the fibrillating atria into normally contracting ones.

An alternative to digoxin in the management of rapid ventricular response to atrial fibrillation is the use of the calcium channel blockers diltiazem (Cardizem) and verapamil (Calan) (discussed in Chapter 27). To reduce the risk for thromboembolic events associated with atrial fibrillation, the anticoagulant warfarin (Coumadin) is often used concurrently.

✱ T.F. is a 68-year-old male with new onset of atrial fibrillation (first symptoms within the past 24 hours) and long-standing HF. He has been maintained for the past 18 months on the diuretic furosemide (Lasix) 40

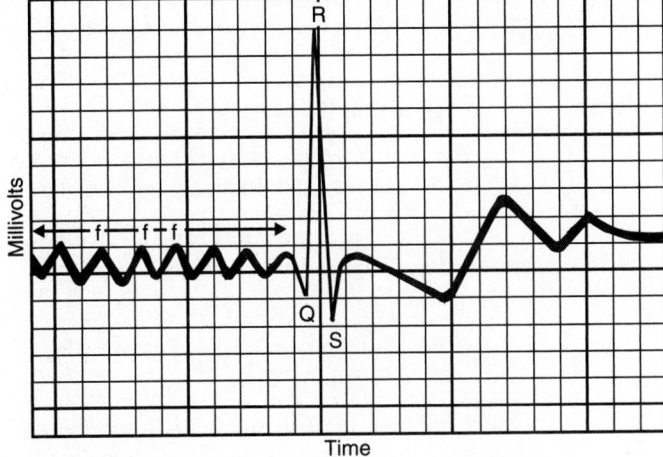

FIGURE 25-4 Atrial fibrillation as seen on ECG.

mg daily and the ACE inhibitor lisinopril (Prinivil, Zestril) 10 mg daily. His health care provider elects to initiate digoxin therapy.

✱ How should digoxin therapy be dosed?

The maintenance dosage of digoxin for adults is usually 0.125 mg or 0.25 mg orally (PO) daily with the higher end of dosing used in the management of atrial fibrillation. The process of initiating a client on digoxin therapy is often referred to as **digitalization**. Digitalization is the saturation of body tissues with enough digoxin to improve the signs and symptoms of heart failure or atrial fibrillation. Although nomograms and formula calculations are available to estimate digoxin dosage based on lean body weight and renal function, most prescribers still prescribe digoxin according to the client's body weight (Table 25-3). However, digoxin has a very narrow therapeutic index (the therapeutic dose is very close to the toxic dose; see Chapter 3 for detailed discussion). Many clients experience digoxin toxicity, so it is vital for the nurse to monitor T.F. for, and to teach him to watch for, signs and symptoms of improvement and of drug toxicity. Drug serum levels should also be monitored. There are essentially two methods of digitalization: the rapid (fast) method, which requires hospitalization of the client, and the slow method, which is usually prescribed in an ambulatory setting.

The rapid digitalization (loading) method is reserved for clients who are in acute distress from heart failure. If the client has not previously received any digoxin, IV digoxin is given in divided doses over a 24-hour period. The goal of treatment is to obtain the maximum therapeutic effect of the digoxin as rapidly as possible. With this method, the drug toxicities quickly become evident, while the client is in the controlled environment of the hospital unit. An advantage is that the toxicities can be easily correlated to a specific drug concentration. For example, the prescriber decides to administer a total IV dose of 1 mg of digoxin. Digoxin may be prescribed as 0.5 mg IV now and 0.25 mg IV every 6 hours for two doses (for a total of 1 mg). The nurse is expected to observe the client for signs of improvement. If the

TABLE 25-3 **DIGOXIN (LANOXIN, LANOXICAPS): DOSAGE AND ADMINISTRATION**

Route	Dosage Range	
	Digitalizing (Loading)	**Maintenance**
IV	Adults: 0.4-0.6 mg (400-600 mcg) initially, then 0.1-0.3 mg (100-300 mcg) q6-8h as needed	0.125-0.5 mg (125-500 mcg) daily as a single dose or in divided doses daily
	Children: give in the following divided doses: ½ dose at once, remainder in fractional doses at 4- to 8-hr intervals:	
	Premature infant, rapid: 15-25 mcg/kg (0.015-0.025 mg/kg)	20%-30% of loading dose daily in divided doses
	Full-term infant, rapid: 20-30 mcg/kg (0.02-0.03 mg/kg)	20%-35% of loading dose daily in divided doses
	Infant (1-24 months), rapid: 30-50 mcg/kg (0.03-0.05 mg/kg)	25%-35% of loading dose daily in divided doses
	Children: 2 to 5 years of age: 25-35 mcg/kg (0.025-0.035 mg/kg) 5 to 10 years of age: 15-30 mcg/kg (0.015-0.03 mg/kg) Older than 10 years of age: 8-12 mcg/kg (0.008-0.012 mg/kg)	25%-35% of loading dose in divided doses two or three times daily
Oral tablet	Adults: Rapid: 0.75-1.25 mg (750-1250 mcg) divided into two or more doses, each administered at 6- to 8-hr intervals Slow: 0.125-0.5 mg (125-500 mcg) once daily for 7 days	0.125-0.5 mg (125-500 mcg) once daily
	Children: 2 to 10 years of age: 0.03-0.04 mg/kg (30-40 mcg/kg) in divided doses q6-8h	20%-30% of digitalizing dose daily
Oral capsule	Adults: Rapid: 0.4-0.6 mg (400-600 mcg), followed by 0.1-0.3 mg (100-300 mcg) q6-8h as necessary Slow: 0.05-0.35 mg (50-350 mcg) daily in two divided doses; repeat dose for 1-3 weeks to reach steady-state serum levels Children: See current literature, because dosages vary according to age	0.05-0.35 mg (50-350 mcg) PO once or twice daily, as necessary

IV, Intravenously; *PO,* orally.

client demonstrates digoxin toxicity after the 1-mg dose, the prescriber will know that this person is not able to tolerate a 1-mg total dose and in the future will avoid any dosage regimen that might reach this level.

As in T.F.'s case, and in general, the slow method of digitalization is used in less-acute situations in the ambulatory setting. The length of time before T.F. reaches full digitalization is much longer than with the rapid method. A daily oral maintenance dose of digoxin is prescribed, with the client not reaching full digitalization until approximately the fifth half-life of the drug. Digoxin, which has a 36-hour half-life, takes approximately 7 days for digitalization.

The advantages of the slow method include the following: (1) T.F. may be treated on an outpatient basis, (2) it is a safer method, (3) close monitoring is not required, and (4) the doses may be taken orally. The disadvantages of the slow method are as follows: (1) the extended length of time be-

fore T.F. is digitalized, and (2) the difficulty in determining when digoxin toxicity occurs, because the onset of symptoms may be very gradual. Loading doses of digoxin are usually unnecessary (Hunt et al., 2001).

✽ **In addition to his furosemide and lisinopril, T.F. is started on the anticoagulant warfarin (Coumadin) with the dose monitored by the anticoagulation clinic and digoxin 0.375 mg once daily for 5 days, then 0.25 mg daily. On day 6 of therapy, T.F. presents to his health care provider with anorexia, nausea, diarrhea, and complains of seeing a yellowish green halo around the florescent lighting of the examining room. His apical pulse is 55 beats/min. Could these effects be attributed to digoxin?**

Because digoxin has a narrow therapeutic index, clients can become quickly toxic on this drug. This is particularly important for T.F. and other clients with atrial fibrillation who must be maintained at higher levels to control ventricular response, those with renal insufficiency, and those who recently had dosage adjustments.

Common dose-related adverse effects of the digoxin include anorexia, nausea, bradycardia, visual disturbances manifest by yellow vision, stomach pain, and dysrhythmias. A loss of appetite is usually the first sign of toxicity; nausea, vomiting, and abdominal distress usually occur several days after the anorexia. Confusion or changes in mental status can also be related to digoxin use, particularly in older adults.

✳ **T.F. is evaluated with an ECG, which shows bradycardia and a prolonged PR interval but no ventricular dysrhythmias. His serum digoxin level is 0.28 ng/mL. His serum creatinine is 1.9 mg/dL, and his estimated creatinine clearance is 36 mL/min. His serum potassium level is 5.1 mEq/L. How should his case be managed?**

Digoxin toxicity can be serious and requires an assessment of cardiovascular risk. Obtaining an ECG is important to rule out dysrhythmias. The dysrhythmias seen with digoxin toxicity are premature ventricular beats, paroxysmal atrial tachycardia with AV block, progressing AV blocks, and ventricular dysrhythmias such as ventricular tachycardia (*USP DI*, 2005). Other drugs that slow heart rate or AV nodal conduction can also contribute to digoxin-induced dysrhythmias. Such drugs include β-adrenergic blockers (e.g., propranolol), calcium channel blockers (specifically diltiazem and verapamil), and some of the antidysrhythmics (e.g., amiodarone, procainamide).

Concurrent drugs that alter the pharmacokinetics of digoxin may also contribute to the risk of digoxin toxicity. A number of other drugs, including the antidysrhythmic drug amiodarone (Cordarone), diltiazem (Cardizem), itraconazole (Spectazole), and erythromycin may result in toxic levels of digoxin.

Alternately, decreased digoxin levels can result from hyperthyroid states, the use of thyroid supplements (e.g., levothyroxine [Synthroid]), and concurrent administration of antacids, bulk laxatives (psyllium [Metamucil]), or cholesterol-binding resins (e.g., cholestyramine [Questran]). If the dose of digoxin is adjusted to account for one of these factors, and the factor is changed (e.g., antacid use is discontinued), digoxin toxicity may result unless the digoxin dose is lowered accordingly.

Electrolyte assessment is important because alterations in calcium, magnesium, and particularly potassium levels can predispose to life-threatening ventricular dysrhythmias in the presence of elevated digoxin levels. Other drugs can significantly affect electrolyte levels. Of note, the loop diuretics (e.g., furosemide [Lasix]), such as T.F. is taking, and thiazide diuretics (e.g., hydrochlorothiazide [Hydrodiuril]) commonly result in *hypo*kalemia. Agents that are correlated with *hyper*kalemia include the potassium-sparing diuretics (e.g., triamterene [an ingredient in Dyazide and Maxzide]) and spironolactone [Aldactone]), the ACE inhibitors (e.g., lisinopril [Prinivil], captopril [Capoten]) and the ARBs

(e.g., losartan [Cozaar]). Serum potassium levels will be important to monitor for T.F. because he is taking both lisinopril and furosemide.

Although digoxin serum levels are of limited value in establishing therapeutic response, they are often helpful as an indicator of toxicity (Box 25-3). Age-related renal or hepatic impairment and a decreased volume of distribution seen in older adults may predispose to digoxin toxicity.

✳ **T.F.'s digoxin toxicity is assessed for the use of the antidote digoxin immune Fab, which would be titrated according to his serum digoxin level.**

For clients with symptomatic ventricular dysrhythmias, significant hyperkalemia in the presence of digoxin toxicity, or other life-threatening manifestations of digoxin toxicity, digoxin immune Fab (Digibind) is used (Box 25-4).

digoxin immune Fab
(Digibind)
Digoxin immune fab binds and makes complex molecules with digoxin in the serum. These molecules are excreted by the kidneys. As more tissue digoxin is released into the serum to maintain equilibrium, it is bound and removed by this product, which results in lower levels of digoxin in serum and body tissues.

BOX 25-3 DETERMINING SERUM DIGOXIN CONCENTRATION

The therapeutic serum digoxin concentration is dependent on indication. For HF management, the typical therapeutic range is 0.8 to 2 ng/mL. For dysrhythmias, the therapeutic range is 1.5 to 2.5 ng/mL. For many clients, serum levels do not clearly distinguish between toxic and nontoxic states. Many clients with digoxin toxicity may manifest symptoms with dosages less than 2 ng/mL (Kradjan, 2005). As such, serum levels should be used as a guide with careful evaluation of the client.

CRITERIA FOR DETERMINING DIGOXIN LEVELS

1. Suspected toxicity
2. Questionable or unreliable client adherence to therapy
3. Client not responding to typical doses
4. Presence of impaired renal function
5. Use of drugs that are known to interact with digoxin (e.g., quinidine, calcium channel blockers, amiodarone)
6. Confirmation of an unusual or seriously abnormal digoxin serum level

TIMING OF DIGOXIN LEVELS

With the exception of determining immediate toxicity, digoxin levels should be obtained as trough levels (immediately before the next scheduled dose). Because digoxin is slow to distribute from the blood to the tissues, obtaining levels within 4 hours of an IV dose or within 6 hours of an oral dose will result in unreliable levels of questionable clinical significance.

BOX 25-4 DIGOXIN TOXICITY

Almost every type of dysrhythmia can be produced by digoxin toxicity. The type of dysrhythmia produced varies with the age of the client and other factors. Premature ventricular contractions and bigeminal rhythm (2 beats and a pause) are common signs of digoxin toxicity in adults, whereas children tend to develop ectopic nodal or atrial beats. Digoxin-induced dysrhythmias are caused by depression of the SA and AV nodes of the heart. This results in various conduction disturbances (first- or second-degree heart block or complete heart block). Digoxin may also cause increased myocardial automaticity, producing extrasystoles or tachycardias.

Nurses must be aware of the predisposing factors to digoxin toxicity. The presence of any of the following factors in clients indicates the need for close observation for the signs and symptoms of digoxin intoxication:

1. *Potassium loss.* Hypokalemia (low potassium levels) can increase digoxin cardiotoxicity. Because potassium inhibits the excitability of the heart, a depletion of body or myocardial potassium increases cardiac excitability. Low extracellular potassium is synergistic with digoxin and enhances ectopic pacemaker activity (dysrhythmias). The following are causes of potassium loss:
   a. Hypokalemia occurs if large amounts of body fluids are lost as a result of vomiting, diarrhea, or gastric suctioning.
   b. The use of various diuretic agents (carbonic-anhydrase inhibitors, ammonium chloride, furosemide, and thiazide preparations) induces potassium diuresis along with sodium and water diuresis.
   c. Poor dietary intake or severe dietary restrictions that decrease electrolyte intake can cause a loss of potassium.
   d. Adrenal steroids cause potassium loss and sodium retention.
   e. Surgical procedures associated with severe electrolyte disturbances (e.g., abdominoperineal resection, colostomy, ileostomy, colectomy, and ureterosigmoidostomy) can cause potassium loss.
   f. The use of potassium-free IV fluids can cause hypokalemia.
2. *Hyperkalemia.* Elevated potassium levels may also predispose to cardiac dysrhythmias and digoxin toxicity. Potential causes of hyperkalemia include renal insufficiency, increased dietary or IV potassium, ACE inhibitors, angiotensin receptor blockers, and potassium-sparing diuretics.
3. *Hypercalcemia.* Excess calcium in the presence of digoxin may cause sinus bradycardia, AV conduction block, and ectopic dysrhythmia.
4. *Pathologic conditions.* Kidney, liver, and severe heart disease are major factors in digoxin toxicity. Approximately 80% of digoxin is excreted by the kidneys.

Indications
Digoxin immune Fab is an antidote for severe digoxin toxicity.

Pharmacokinetics/Dosing
Digoxin immune FAB is administered IV. The onset of action takes place in less than 1 minute, and the half-life is 15 to 20 hours. Initial signs of improvement in digoxin toxicity can be seen in 15 to 30 minutes after administration but can take up to several hours. Dysrhythmias and hyperkalemia are usually reversed first; reversal of the inotropic effect may take several hours. This drug is excreted in the kidneys. Digoxin levels after administration are often elevated, but are not correlated with toxicity because the digoxin bound to the Fab fragment is not available to bind to tissue receptors.

The dosage of digoxin immune Fab in adults may be calculated based on the amount of digoxin consumed, or it may be based on steady-state serum levels. Usually a 38-mg dose for injection will bind approximately 0.5 mg of digoxin. The formulas in Box 25-5 may be applied to determine the dose of the antidote.

Adverse Effects
Close monitoring is necessary because the withdrawal of digoxin may result in a decrease in cardiac output, HF, and hypokalemia. An increase in ventricular rate may be seen in persons with atrial fibrillation. No significant drug interactions have been reported.

BOX 25-5 FORMULAS FOR DIGOXIN IMMUNE FAB (OVINE)

For digoxin tablets, oral solution, or intramuscular injection:

$$\text{Dose (mg)} = \frac{\text{Dose ingested (mg)} \times 0.8}{0.5} \times 38$$

For digoxin capsules, or IV digoxin:

$$\text{Dose (mg)} = \frac{\text{Dose ingested (mg)}}{0.5} \times 38$$

When the amount of digoxin ingestion is unknown and the steady-state serum level is unavailable, 760 mg of digoxin immune Fab (ovine) is usually administered because it is reportedly sufficient to treat most life-threatening ingestions. A common strategy is to administer 380 mg and observe for client response, with an additional 380 mg administered if needed.

⚜ In the case of T.F., digoxin immune Fab is not indicated. His digoxin dose is withheld for 2 days, and he returns to clinic for follow-up electrolytes and digoxin level assessment. If he remains therapeutically responsive to digoxin without toxicity, his dose will likely be reduced to 0.125 mg daily with a follow up of serum electrolyte, renal function, and digoxin serum level determinations. Because of T.F.'s experience with digoxin toxicity, his physician suggests that he enroll in the local hospital's nurse-managed HF program.

⚜ What are the nursing management issues with T.F.'s digoxin therapy?

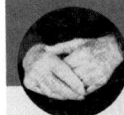

Special Considerations for Older Adults | DIGOXIN

- The administration of digoxin, one of the most commonly prescribed drugs in the world, must be closely monitored; the treatment dose is approximately 60% of the toxic dose. Older adults often have a reduced tolerance for digoxin; thus lower dosages may be necessary to reduce the potential for drug toxicity because of an age-related decrease in renal function and decreased volume of distribution because of decreased muscle mass (*USP DI*, 2005).
- Early toxic signs often include anorexia, nausea, and vomiting; difficulty with reading, which may appear as visual alterations such as green and yellow vision, double vision, or seeing spots or halos; headaches; dizziness; fatigue; weakness; confusion; depression; increased nervousness; and diarrhea. Decreased libido and impotency are reported in approximately 35% of males as a result of the estrogen-type effects of digoxin. Breast enlargement and breast tenderness also are reported in males.
- Be aware that exercise reduces serum levels of digoxin because of increased uptake in skeletal muscles. The nurse must be cognizant of the physical activity of clients who are taking digoxin.
- Laxatives, which are commonly taken by older adults (e.g., bisacodyl [Dulcolax, Fleet Laxative]), may reduce the absorption of digoxin (Lanoxin). Do not administer these drugs concurrently. Dietary bran fiber may affect digoxin bioavailability; have clients take digoxin 1 hour before or 2 hours after having bran.

Assessment T.F.'s health status is assessed for underlying conditions (e.g., a toxic effect from a previous administration of the drug) for which digoxin might be contraindicated. Except for T.F.'s age, the following conditions are not relevant in his case, but digoxin is to be used cautiously when these conditions are noted.

- *Dysrhythmias.* Dysrhythmias may be caused by underlying heart disease or reflect digoxin intoxication; the drug should be withheld if the latter occurs.
- *Progression of AV Block.* Incomplete AV block may progress to advanced or complete heart block in digitalizing clients; this means that heart failure may need to be managed by other measures.
- *Conduction Disorders.* The condition of clients with Wolff-Parkinson-White or sick sinus syndrome may worsen.
- *Ventricular Dysrhythmias.* Clients with premature ventricular contractions or ventricular tachycardia are at risk for exacerbation with the administration of digoxin glycosides.
- *Myocardial Pathology.* Clients with acute myocarditis or myocardial infarction or ischemic heart disease are at higher risk for digoxin-induced dysrhythmias because of their increased sensitivity to the effects of the drug.
- *Clients with Electronic Cardiac Pacemakers.* These clients require careful titration of their dosage because they may demonstrate symptoms of toxicity at dosages usually tolerated by other individuals.
- *Electrolyte Imbalances.* Hypokalemia and hypomagnesemia increase the risk of digoxin toxicity. Exercise great caution in giving the drug to clients with hypercalcemia and hyperkalemia to avoid digoxin-induced dysrhythmia, principally heart block. Hypocalcemia may decrease the effectiveness of digoxin; calcium supplementation may be necessary.

- *Renal Dysfunction.* Clients with renal impairment or acute glomerulonephritis may have reduced excretion and so a greater risk of toxicity.
- *Myxedema, Severe Pulmonary Disease, or Carotid Sinus Hypersensitivity.* These conditions may predispose the client to the toxic effect of digoxin.
- *Older Adults.* Because of their smaller body mass (i.e., lean body weight) and frequent renal impairments, older adults must be given digoxin cautiously. Digoxin has been identified as a cause of drug-induced cognitive impairment in older adults (Rubenstein & Josephson, 2002). See the Considerations for Older Adults box above.

T.F.'s current medication regimen is reviewed for the risk of significant drug interactions, such as those that may occur when digoxin is given concurrently with the following drugs:

- Antacids: may decrease digoxin absorption 25% to 35%
- Antidiarrheal adsorbents (e.g., kaolin, pectin), cholestyramine (Questran), colestipol (Colestid), or large quantities of dietary fiber (bran): may reduce the absorption of digoxin, resulting in a decreased therapeutic response
- Indomethacin (Indocin): renal excretion of digoxin is reduced, leading to increased serum levels and possible toxicity
- Magnesium sulfate injection: may cause alteration in cardiac conduction and heart block may result
- Potassium-depleting drugs, such as amphotericin B (parenteral), corticosteroids, or potassium-depleting diuretics: have the potential to induce hypokalemia and can result in digoxin toxicity
- Drugs that predispose to hyperkalemia, such as potassium salts, angiotensin-converting enzyme (ACE) inhibitors, angiotensin receptor blockers, and

potassium-sparing diuretics are not recommended in digitalized clients with severe heart block
• Amiodarone: may increase serum levels of digoxin
• Drugs that slow AV junction conduction, such as β-adrenergic blockers, calcium channel blockers, or some antidysrhythmics: may have additive effects in slowing AV junction conduction
• Quinidine: may result in increased serum levels of digoxin
• Spironolactone (Aldactone): may increase the half-life of digoxin
• Sucralfate (Carafate): decreases the absorption of digoxin

T.F.'s baseline assessment should include the following: weight; blood pressure, pulse pressure and any postural change in blood pressure; apical pulse rate and rhythm; apical-radial pulse deficit; heart sounds; jugular vein distention; edema; lung sounds; capillary refill time; skin color and temperature; urinary output; determination of the presence of chest discomfort (pain or pressure), shortness of breath, syncope, fatigue, nausea, and perception of heart rate ("skipping beats"); level of consciousness and anxiety; cardiac enzymes; hepatic function studies, serum electrolyte levels, blood urea nitrogen (BUN), and creatinine levels; and ECG.

Nursing Diagnosis While T.F. is taking digoxin, he is at risk for the following selected nursing diagnoses/collaborative problems: ineffective tissue perfusion, cardiopulmonary, related to the pathophysiologic influence of heart failure; impaired comfort (headache, nausea, vomiting); disturbed sensory perception (halos of green-yellow light around objects); diarrhea; disturbed thought processes (confusion); risk for injury related to adverse drug effects (electrolyte imbalance, drowsiness, fainting); deficient knowledge related to first-time use of digoxin; and the potential complications of allergic reaction, mental depression, digoxin toxicity, and dysrhythmias.

Planning While T.F. is receiving digoxin therapy, he will:
• Exhibit improved cardiac output.
• Experience an improved ECG.
• Remain free of the adverse effects of digoxin.
• Effectively manage his therapeutic regimen, including pulse-taking, daily weights, compliance with digoxin, appropriate reporting of adverse effects to the prescriber, and maintaining a sodium-restricted diet

Implementation

Monitoring Because altered cardiac output may occur in relation to the positive inotropic effects of the drug, measure T.F.'s apical pulse for 1 minute before drug administration. Note the rate, rhythm, and quality of pulse. If the pulse is 60 beats/min or slower, or if a dysrhythmia that had not previously occurred is noted, withhold the drug and report immediately to the prescriber. In children, monitoring is somewhat different. Measure the apical pulse 1 minute before administering the drug. Consult with the prescriber to determine the child's apical rate at which the drug should be withheld. The baseline rate is usually higher in children than in adults (see the Special Considerations for Children box below).

Because T.F. is receiving digoxin for atrial fibrillation, take the apical and radial pulse for 1 minute before the administration. Determine whether there is a pulse deficit (apical pulse minus radial pulse).

During digitalization, check the parameters as described in the following paragraphs. Observe T.F. for a positive response to digitalization. An increase in cardiac output reflects a more effective cardiac function, which includes improvement in the rate and rhythm of heartbeat and in respiration, diuresis, weight reduction (e.g., decrease in edema), and a feeling of well-being.

Know therapeutic digoxin serum levels and normal potassium, calcium, and magnesium ion serum levels. A fall in potassium serum levels enhances the effect of digoxin and the risk of digoxin toxicity. T.F. is also taking

---

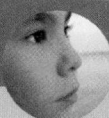

Special Considerations for Children | DIGOXIN

• Early signs of HF include tachycardia (especially during rest and minimum activity), increased fatigue and irritability, a sudden weight gain, respiratory distress, and profuse scalp sweating, especially in infants.
• Individualize dosing with very close monitoring, especially in infants. Be extremely careful in calculating digoxin doses; a placement error of one decimal point can increase the dose 10-fold. Double check all calculations with another health care professional (nurse, pharmacist, or physician).
• Common signs of digoxin toxicity in children include nausea, vomiting, anorexia, bradycardia, and dysrhythmias. As a general rule, digoxin is not given if the pulse

is below 90 to 110 beats/min in infants and young children or below 70 beats/min in older children. Specific guidelines for age of the client are specified by the prescriber. If the child is monitored by an ECG, obtain a rhythm strip to attach to include in the chart for rate and rhythm analysis, such as prolongation of the PR interval and dysrhthmias.
• Give digoxin on a regular time schedule, either 1 hour before or 2 hours after feedings.

Data from Wong, D.L., Hockenberry-Eaton, M., Wilson, D., Winkelstein, M.L., Kline, N.E., & Hockenberry-Eaton, E. (2003). *Wong's nursing care of infants and children* (7th ed.). St. Louis: Mosby.

furosemide, a potassium-depleting diuretic that promotes renal potassium excretion and lowers serum potassium levels, and an ACE inhibitor (lisinopril) that may result in hyperkalemia. Monitor his serum potassium levels closely. Observe him for symptoms of hypokalemia, such as drowsiness, hypoperistalsis, mental depression, paresthesia, muscle weakness, anorexia, depressed reflexes, orthostatic hypotension, and polyuria. Because of his age, also monitor his serum BUN and creatinine levels as evidence of renal function, and monitor the use of drugs that may affect renal perfusion (furosemide, lisinopril).

If T.F. were on an ECG monitor, observe the rhythm strip for digoxin-induced dysrhythmias. Dysrhythmias that might indicate digoxin toxicity are atrial tachycardia with AV block, progressing AV blocks, accelerated junctional rhythms, and ventricular dysrhythmias, including ventricular bigeminy and ventricular tachycardia (Braunwald, Zipes, & Libby, 2001). Discontinue the drug if drug intox-

ication occurs. A digoxin serum level is ordered by the prescriber if toxicity is suspected (see Box 25-4). Be aware that the range of the therapeutic index of digoxin is extremely narrow.

Observe T.F.'s food intake. Anorexia is almost always the first sign of toxicity; nausea and vomiting, sometimes with abdominal discomfort and increased salivation, usually occur 1 to 2 days after the anorexia.

Monitor intake and output. Delayed or diminished renal excretion of digoxin can lead to toxicity. Weigh T.F. daily, preferably before breakfast, to monitor for an alteration in fluid balance. A sudden weight gain is an early sign of fluid retention. Monitor him for signs and symptoms of excess fluid volume, such as dependent edema (pedal or sacral), basilar crackles in the lungs, and jugular distention. Monitor T.F. for excessive sodium intake from diet and drugs, including over-the-counter medications and food supplements (Table 25-4).

TABLE 25-4 SODIUM CONTENT OF SELECTED PRESCRIPTION AND OVER-THE-COUNTER MEDICATIONS

Medications	Sodium/Unit	Sodium/Maximum Daily Dose (Adult)
ANTIBIOTICS		
ticarcillin injection (Ticar)	120-150 mg/g	2.9 to 3.6 g/24 g
ampicillin sodium (Polycillin-N, Omnipen-N, and others)	62-78 mg/g	1 to 1.2 g/16 g
Cephalosporins		
cefamandole nafate (Mandol)	77 mg/g	0.9 g/12 g
ceftriaxone sodium (Rocephin)	83 mg/g	0.33 g/4 g
cephradine injection (Velosef)	136 mg/g	1 g/8 g
OVER-THE-COUNTER MEDICATIONS		
Alka-Seltzer Effervescent Pain Reliever and Antacid Tablets	0.5 g/tablet	
Alka-Seltzer, Lemon-Lime	506 mg/tablet	
Alka-Seltzer, Original	567 mg/tablet	
Bell/Ans	144 mg/tablet	
Bromo-Seltzer powder	0.76 g/capful	
Eno Powder✤	0.8 g/teaspoon	
Rolaids	53 mg/tablet	
Soda Mint Tablets	90 mg/tablet	
FOOD SUPPLEMENTS		
Ensure	844 mg/L	
Meritene	880-1078 mg/L	
Osmolite	549 mg/L	
Sustacal	924-940 mg/L	

Box 25-6 Tips for Sodium-Restricted Dining

Although it is important for the client to know which foods to avoid, emphasize foods that the client can enjoy.

- Eliminate the saltshaker. Don't salt before you taste.
- Use less salt in cooking. In most recipes, salt can be reduced or, in many cases, omitted without compromising the flavor. Use more herbs and spices, such as onion and garlic powder. Also, low-sodium bouillon can add extra flavor, as can wine, vinegar, lemon or lime juice.
- Use low-salt recipes. There are many low-sodium cookbooks available, as well as many low-salt recipes available online.
- Eat more fruits and vegetables. Use less-prepared foods—the less processing, the less sodium. Grill or roast entrees. Use oil and vinegar rather than prepared salad dressings.
- Choose lower-sodium foods. Look for foods labeled sodium free, low sodium, reduced sodium, unsalted, and no salt added.
- Read the label. Know how much sodium is in each serving. If the label says 150 mg sodium per ¼ cup and you eat ½ cup, you're consuming twice as much sodium.
- Be alert to "salty" terms such as brine, cured, marinated, pickled, and smoked.

High-Sodium Foods (Should Be Avoided in the Diet)

Meat, Poultry, Fish, and Other Meat Substitutes

- Ham, Canadian bacon, bacon, luncheon and cured meats, frankfurters, sausages, scrapple, pepperoni, dried beef, chipped beef, corned beef, pastrami, lox, smoked salmon
- Canned and processed foods, such as canned meat, chicken, tuna sardines, herring, anchovies, caviar, regular peanut butter, and frozen T.V. dinners.
- Soy protein products, such as marinated tofu or miso

Dairy

- Cheese, particularly processed cheeses such as American cheese, blue cheese, Roquefort parmesan cheese, feta cheese, cottage cheese

Main Dish Items

- Commercially prepared main entrees, including most frozen dinners or frozen main entrees; pot pies; canned main entrees such as hash, stew, chili; entrees with seasoning mixes such as macaroni and cheese
- Most Asian foods such as Chinese, Japanese foods made with teriyaki or soy sauce, East Indian, Thai, and Vietnamese unless prepared without added sauces containing salt or sodium products; many Asian restaurants will cook food without monosodium glutamate (MSG) if requested
- Most Mexican foods such as tacos, enchiladas, burritos, tamales
- Pizza, lasagna, manicotti, ravioli, quiche, soufflés, blintzes, cheese rarebit

Grains, Cereals, Soups, and Snack Foods

- Cereals: instant hot cereals, cold cereals containing 200 mg or more of sodium

- Salted snack foods: salted pretzels, salted crackers and chips, salted popcorn
- Baked goods: cakes, cookies, pies, pastries, sweet rolls, doughnuts, pancakes and waffles, biscuits and muffins
- Grains: rice or noodles with seasoning packets or sauces such as Ramen noodles; rice pilaf; instant potatoes; stuffing mix
- Soups: canned broth soups, commercially prepared stews, bouillon cubes, and instant or dried soups

Vegetables

- Sauerkraut or other vegetables prepared in brine; olives; pickles; relish; vegetables packed with sauces or seasonings; salted mixed vegetable juice (V-8); regular tomato juice; regular spaghetti sauce; tomato sauce or tomato paste; frozen peas; and lima beans
- Canned vegetables, including beans
- Potatoes: au gratin, scalloped, packaged with sauces and seasoning mixes

Spices, Condiments, and Sauces

- Spices/seasonings: salt, seasoning salts such as garlic, onion and celery salt, meat tenderizers, MSG and bouillon.
- Sauces: soy sauce; teriyaki sauce; Worcestershire sauce; steak sauce; barbecue sauce; smoke-flavored sauces; gravies; marinades; pasta sauces such as marinara, spaghetti, and alfredo; chili sauce; cocktail sauce; tomato puree and tomato sauce
- Condiments and dressings: pickle relish, catsup, mayonnaise, commercial and packaged salad dressings

Food Additives

It is important to read labels when packaging food. Sodium is often added to food in other forms besides salt such as the following:

- MSG as a flavor enhancer
- Baking soda and baking powder: found in many baked goods
- Disodium phosphate: found in quick-cooking cereals and processed cheeses
- Sodium alginate: used in many chocolate milks and ice creams
- Sodium benzoate: used as a preservative in many condiments such as relishes, sauces, and salad dressings
- Sodium hydroxide: used in food processing for softening and loosening skins of olives and certain fruits and vegetables
- Sodium nitrite: used in curing meats and sausages
- Sodium propionate: used in some breads and cakes to inhibit mold growth and in pasteurized cheese
- Sodium sulfite: used to bleach certain fruits such as maraschino cherries and glazed or crystallized fruits to be artificially colored; as a preservative in some dried fruits such as prunes

Note: You should check with your doctor or dietitian before using salt or salt substitutes.

Intervention Digoxin may be given IV, intramuscularly (IM), or orally. When given IV as an undiluted digoxin (0.25 mg/mL), administer it slowly at 0.25 mg/min. Rapid administration is avoided to prevent pulmonary edema. Digoxin may also be administered in diluted form. Administer IV digoxin with caution to clients with hypertension because it causes a temporary increase in blood pressure. IM injection of digoxin is generally limited to clients with no IV or enteral access because it is painful, because the bioavailability of the IM injected drug is low, and because the absorption is unpredictable, especially in clients with severe heart failure, edema, and poor tissue perfusion. However, if an IM injection of digoxin is ordered, administer it deep into the large muscle mass and follow with massage.

Maintenance doses of digoxin may be given orally if the client can tolerate food; otherwise IV injections are required. *Do not* administer the oral preparation with meals that have high fiber content. Studies show that digoxin binds with the fiber, thereby reducing the amount of medication available for absorption from the gut. Advise T.F. to take the drug 1 hour before or 2 hours after meals.

Education Instruct T.F. to take digoxin at the same time each day, precisely as prescribed. Doses should not be skipped, and they should not be doubled if missed. Inform him that digoxin and Lanoxin are the same drug, although there is a difference in bioavailability. Instruct T.F. not to change the brand of drug when a prescription is refilled because of the difference in bioavailability. In some cases, clients were prescribed digoxin and Lanoxin, each by a different prescriber, leading to an overdose. If using an elixir form of the drug, the dose should be determined using the special dropper that comes with the preparation. Caution T.F. not to take other medications without prior approval of the prescriber.

Instruct T.F. to restrict his sodium intake to 2 g or less daily. See Box 25-6 for tips regarding sodium-restricted dining. See Table 25-4 for the sodium content of selected over-the-counter medications and food supplements.

He should report a weight gain of 2 pounds a day. Caution him to avoid licorice because it can induce sodium and water retention and to limit alcohol consumption one drink per day. Fluid intake and exercise should be discussed with the prescriber.

Advise T.F. to carry medical identification and to alert health care professionals unfamiliar with his drug regimen that he is taking digoxin.

Teach T.F. how to take his own pulse, and recommend taking the pulse before each dose of medication. The dose should be withheld and the prescriber notified if the pulse is below 60 or above 110 beats/min and/or is erratic or if he experiences anorexia, diarrhea, nausea, vomiting, sudden weight gain, or apparent edema. Visual disturbances, such as blurred vision or green or yellow halos around objects, should also be reported to the prescriber.

Online information is also available for clients. (See the Technology Link box at right.) These links would be applicable for clients with any cardiovascular disease.

Evaluation The expected outcome of T.F.'s digoxin therapy is that he will demonstrate an improved rhythm on the ECG and clinical improvement, such as an absence of S$_3$ and basilar crackles and dependent edema, improved activity tolerance, decreased cardiomegaly on radiographic studies, and an increased sense of well-being without experiencing digoxin toxicity or other adverse effect of digoxin.

Are there any other agents used to treat HF?
Two inotropes, inamrinone (Inocor IV) and milrinone (Primacor), are available for IV use in the management of acute HF. Their use is typically limited to the critical care setting in the management of the postcardiac surgery client. Nesiritide (Natrecor) is a formulation of B-type natriuretic peptide to treat seriously decompensated HF. A brief description of each follows.

inamrinone [in **am** rih none]
(Inocor)
The mechanism of action of inamrinone has not been fully identified. Inamrinone increases the force and velocity of myocardial tissues, resulting in a positive inotropic effect. Experiments indicate that inamrinone inhibits phosphodiesterase activity, which in turn

Technology Link

Cardiac Glycosides

American Heart Association (www.americanheart.org)

This site has information on a variety of cardiovascular conditions, such as heart failure, high blood pressure, dysrhythmia, and others. It contains client education materials along with a discussion of treatment options. Material is presented in English and Spanish. There is a section for children with age-appropriate literature. Professional information is also included.

Mayo Clinic (www.mayoclinic.com)

This easy-to-navigate site has a wealth of material for hundreds of health conditions. The client material is approached from a "Get the Basics," "Explore Treatments," and "Take Control," perspective. The site has interesting interactive quizzes on the health topics that are selected and includes recipes for a variety of special diets.

National Heart, Lung, and Blood Institute (www.nhlbi.gov/index.htm)

The site provides an A-Z index for diseases and conditions for client information. There are also educational tutorials for a variety of health topics. Unfortunately, the Latino Cardiovascular Health Resources section is in English. For the health professional, practice guidelines, continuing education and health information is available, as well as resources for researchers.

increases the concentration of cellular cyclic adenosine monophosphate (cAMP) and cardiac contractility. Inamrinone appears to produce a direct relaxant effect on the vascular smooth muscle (vasodilation) and to reduce preload and afterload. Older references may refer to this drug as amrinone. The official generic name has been changed to inamrinone to help reduce confusion with sound-alike agents such as amiodarone.

Indications
Inamrinone is used to treat HF in individuals who do not respond to standard therapies, such as digoxin, diuretics, and vasodilators.

Pharmacokinetics/Dosing
Administered IV, the time to peak action of inamrinone is within 10 minutes. The duration of effect is dose related. If 0.75 mg/kg is administered, the duration of action is approximately 30 minutes. If 3 mg/kg is administered, the duration of action is approximately 120 minutes. When administered for HF, the half-life is between 5 and 8.3 hours. This drug is metabolized in the liver and excreted primarily via the kidneys. The adult dosage of inamrinone is 0.75 mg/kg IV slowly over 2 to 3 minutes, repeated in 30 minutes if necessary. The maintenance dosage by IV infusion is 5 to 10 mcg/kg/min, individualized according to response. The maximum dosage is 10 mg/kg/day; in several reports, dosages up to 18 mg/kg/day were given for short time periods.

For neonates and infants, the initial dosage is 3 to 4 mg/kg in divided doses; the maintenance dosage is 3 to 5 mcg/kg/min for neonates and 10 mcg/kg/min for infants. (See the Pregnancy Safety box below for pregnancy safety categories of the Food and Drug Administration.)

Adverse Effects
The adverse effects of inamrinone are infrequent and include nausea, vomiting, abdominal pain, fever, taste alterations, hypotension, dysrhythmias, chest pain, and thrombocytopenia. The inotropic effects of inamrinone are additive to those of digoxin.

milrinone [**mil** rih none]
(Primacor)
Milrinone is a selective inhibitor of cAMP isozymes in cardiac and vascular muscle; it improves cardiac function, contractility, and vasodilation without increasing myocardial oxygen consumption and heart rate. It is a positive inotrope and vasodilator with very little chronotropic activity.

Indications
Milrinone is indicated for the short-term treatment of HF.

Pharmacokinetics/Dosing
When administered IV, milrinone has a half-life of 2.5 hours and a duration of action between 3 and 6 hours. It is excreted by the kidneys.

Interactions
Significant drug interactions have not been reported, but its administration with other hypotension-producing drugs may have an additive effect. A chemical interaction (precipitate) has been reported when furosemide (Lasix) was administered via an IV line containing a milrinone infusion. This procedure should be avoided.

Adverse Effects
Significant adverse effects of milrinone include headaches, hypoten-

PREGNANCY SAFETY		
DIGOXIN AND OTHER DRUGS		
Category	**Drugs**	
C	digoxin, digoxin immune Fab (ovine), inamrinone, milrinone, nesiritide	

Data from *Mosby's drug consult* (15th ed.). (2005). St. Louis: Mosby.

sion, ventricular dysrhythmias, and, rarely, angina and thrombocytopenia. Inotropic effects are additive to those of digoxin. See current guidelines for dosing recommendations.

nesiritide [ni **sir** i tide]
(Natrecor)
Nesiritide is a recombinant formulation of BNP. Elevated BNP levels are noted for clients in HF, and are believed to offset the negative effects of sympathetic and RAA system effects observed in these individuals (Doust et al., 2005). BNP binds to vascular smooth muscle resulting in vasodilation. Such effects are believed to reduce preload and afterload which are beneficial in HF. Concerns regarding the safety of nesiritide surfaced in early 2005. Increased 30-day mortality rates have been reported with the use of the drug (Sackner-Bernstein, Kowalski, Fox, & Aaronson, 2005). In a "Dear Physician/Patient Advocate" letter (Scios, 2005), the manufacturer also identified increased mortality associated with the use of nesiritide and is pursuing additional evaluation of drug safety. In light of these findings, most clinicians have limited the use of this agent to very-high-risk clients in whom benefit outweighs risk.

Indications
Nesiritide is used to treat HF in clients who have significantly decompensated acute failure with symptoms at rest.

Pharmacokinetics/Dosing
Nesiritide is administered IV with an onset of action seen within 15 minutes. Reduced blood pressure is observed for up to 3 hours. It is metabolized by vascular enzymes, and eliminated in the urine. The typical adult dose is an IV bolus of 2 mcg/kg bolus, followed by an infusion of 0.01 mcg/kg/min. Refer to prescribing information for more detail on dosing and monitoring.

Adverse Effects
Among the most significant adverse effects of nesiritide are hypotension, ventricular dysrhythmias, and renal insufficiency. These effects may be correlated with the increased 30-day mortality associate with nesiritide. Other adverse effects include headache, dizziness, nausea, hypersensitivity reactions, and back pain.

Summary

Inotropic drugs, such as digoxin, increase the strength of cardiac contraction and alter the electrophysiologic properties of the heart by slowing conduction velocity; this accounts for their therapeutic properties in the treatment of heart failure. Clients may be hospitalized for rapid digitalization—the saturation of the body tissues with enough digoxin to cause the signs and symptoms of heart failure to improve—or may receive digitalization at a slower rate prescribed in an ambulatory setting. Because the therapeutic index of the drug is so narrow in either case, the nurse has the responsibility to monitor the client closely for signs of toxicity and also to teach the client about the therapeutic and nontherapeutic effects of the drug. The nurse must be aware of the predisposing factors to digoxin toxicity and assist the client to recognize them. Hypokalemia and hyperkalemia are the most common risk factors for digoxin toxicity. Digoxin immune Fab (ovine) for injection is used as an antidote for severe digoxin toxicity.

Inamrinone and milrinone are miscellaneous agents administered parenterally for their positive inotropic effects; nesiritide is a recombinant formulation of BNP. They may be used to treat HF in individuals who do not respond to standard therapies.

The nurse has a major assessment and educational role with clients using positive inotropes and other cardiovascular drugs because many clients take these drugs on a long-term, if not a lifetime, basis. It is important that clients not only take their medications accurately, but that they also be knowledgeable about them so as to minimize the risk for injury inherent in their administration.

✳ Critical Thinking Questions

- What electrolyte imbalances affect the development of digoxin toxicity? In what way?
- Mrs. Stacy, a 74-year-old client with chronic HF, is leaving the hospital with a medication regimen that includes digoxin, furosemide, and potassium supplements. What instructions are essential to include in a teaching plan to enable Mrs. Stacy to self-administer her medications safely and accurately?

Bibliography

Academic Market Research. (2004). Retrieved May 9, 2005, from www.academic.marketresearch.com/product/display.asp?productid+729795&curl=&surl=&view=ab&prid-1111111

American Heart Association. (2002). *Heart disease and stroke statistics—2003 update.* Dallas, TX: Author.

Anderson, D.M., Keith, J., & Novak, P.D. (Eds.). (2002). *Mosby's medical, nursing, and allied health dictionary* (6th ed.). St. Louis: Mosby.

Aquilani, R., Opasich, C., Verri, M., Boschi, F., Febo, O., Pasini, E., et al. (2003). Is nutritional intake adequate in chronic heart failure patients? *Journal of the American College of Cardiology, 42,* 1218-1223.

Bleumink, G., Schut, A.F., Sturkenboom, M.C., Deckers, J.W., van Duijn, C.M., & Stricker, B.H. (2004). Genetic polymorphisms and heart failure. *Genetics in Medicine, 6*(6), 465-474.

Braunwald, E., Zipes, D.P., & Libby, P. (2001). *Heart disease: A textbook of cardiovascular medicine* (6th ed.). Philadelphia: W.B. Saunders.

Burstein, J.M., Yan, R., Weller, I., & Abramson, B.L. (2003). Management of congestive heart failure: A gender gap may still exist: Observations from a contemporary cohort. *BMC Cardiovascular Disorders, 3,* 1-4.

Chang, J.T., & Altman, R.B. (2004). Extracting and characterizing gene-drug relationships from the literature. *Pharmacogenetics, 14*(9), 577-586 and linked supplemental website http://bionlp.

stanford.edu/genedrug/gene_drug_predictions.html (as cited December 2, 2004).

Dec, G.W. (2003). Digoxin remains useful in the management of chronic heart failure. *Medical Clinics of North America, 87,* 317-337.

Doust, J.A., Pietrzak, E., Dobson, A., Glasziou, P. (2005). How well does B-type natriuretic peptide predict death and cardiac events in patients with heart failure: Systematic review. *British Medical Journal, 330,* 625-633.

Drug facts and comparisons (59th ed.). (2005). St. Louis: Facts and Comparisons.

Evans, W.E. (2003). Pharmacogenomics: Marshalling the human genome to individualise drug therapy. *Gut 52*(Suppl. II), ii10-ii18.

Exner, D.V., Dries, D.L., Domanski, M.J., & Cohn, J.N. (2001). Lesser response to angiotensin-converting enzyme inhibitor therapy in black as compared with white patients with left ventricular dysfunction. *New England Journal of Medicine, 344,* 1351-1357.

Gheorghiade, M., Gattis, W.A., O'Connor, C.M., Adams, K.F. Jr., Elkayam, U., Barbagelata, A., et al. (2004). Effects of tolvaptan, a vasopressin antagonist, in patients hospitalized with worsening heart failure: A randomized controlled trial. *Journal of the American Medical Association, 291,* 1963-1971.

Giesler, G., Lenihan, D.J., & Durand, J.B. (2004). The update on the rationale, use and selection of beta-blockers in heart failure. *Current Opinion in Cardiology, 19*(3), 250-253.

Heart failure. Retrieved June 29, 2005, from www.nhlbi.nih.gov/health/dci/Diseases/Hf/HF_whatis.html.

Hunt, S.A., Baker, D.W., Chin, M.H., Cinquegrani, M.P., Feldman, A.M., Francis, G.S., et al. (2001). ACC/AHA guidelines for the evaluation and management of chronic heart failure in the adult: Executive summary. *Journal of the American College of Cardiology, 38*(7), 2101-2113.

Johnson, J.A., Parker, R.B., & Patterson, J.H. (2002). Heart failure. In J.T. DiPiro, R.L. Talbert, G.C. Yee, G.R. Matzke, B.G. Wella, & L.M. Posey (Eds.), *Pharmacotherapy: A pathophysiologic approach* (5th ed.). New York: McGraw-Hill.

Kaneko, Y., Floras, J.S., Usui, K., Plante, J., Tkacova, R., Kubo, T., et al. (2003). Cardiovascular effects of continuous positive airway pressure in patients with heart failure and obstructive sleep apnea. *New England Journal of Medicine, 348,* 1233-1241.

Kradjan, W.A. (2005). Heart failure. In M.A. Koda-Kimble, L.Y. Young, W.A. Kradjan, B.J. Guglielmo, B.K. Alldredge, & R.L. Corelli (Eds.), *Applied therapeutics: The clinical use of drugs* (8th ed.). Philadelphia: Lippincott Williams & Wilkins.

Krum, H., Roecker, E.B., Mohacsi, P., Rouleau, J.L., Tendera, M., Coats, A.J., et al. (2003). Effects of initiating carvedilol in patients with severe chronic heart failure: Results from the COPERNICUS study. *Journal of the American Medical Association, 289,* 712-718.

ℓ-LEARNING SUPPLEMENTS

Student CD-ROM
- Final Exam questions
- NCLEX® Examination review questions
- Pharmacology animations
- Printable chapter summary

Evolve Website (http://evolve.elsevier.com/mckenry)
- Case study on drugs affecting the parasympathetic nervous system

- Content updates, including information on new drugs
- WebLinks corresponding to this chapter
- Answers to the critical thinking questions in this chapter
- *Elsevier ePharmacology Update* newsletter
- *Mosby's Drug Consult* Internet Edition
- Supplemental and reference information

Liljedahl, U., Kahan, T., Malmqvist, K., Melhus, H., Syvanen, A.C., Lind, L., et al. (2004). Single nucleotide polymorphisms predict the change in left ventricular mass in response to antihypertensive treatment. *Journal of Hypertension, 22*(12), 2321-2328.

Maisel, A. (2004). FACC updated algorithms for using B-type natriuretic peptide (BNP) levels in the diagnosis and management of congestive heart failure. *Critical Pathways in Cardiology: A Journal of Evidence-Based Medicine, 3*(3), 144-149.

McMurray, J., Ostergren, J., Pfeffer, M., Swedberg, K., Granger, C., Yusuf, S., et al. (2003). Effects of candesartan in patients with chronic heart failure and reduced left-ventricular systolic function taking angiotensin converting-enzyme inhibitors: The CHARM-Added trial. *Lancet 362,* 767-771.

Mialet Perez, J., Rathz, D.A., Petrashevskaya, N.N., Hahn, H.S., Wagoner, L.E., Schwartz, A., et al. (2003). β_1-Adrenergic receptor polymorphisms confer differential function and predisposition to heart failure. *Nature Medicine, 9,* 1300-1305.

Mosby's drug consult (15th ed.). (2005). St. Louis: Mosby.

National Center for Health Statistics. Vital statistics of the United States. Retrieved September 4, 2005, from http://www.cdc.gov/nchs/about/major/dvs/mortdat/htm.

Packer, M., Poole-Wilson, P.A., Armstrong, P.W., Cleland, J.G., Horowitz, J.D., Massie, B.M., et al. (1999). Comparative effects of low and high doses of the angiotensin-converting enzyme inhibitor, lisinopril, on morbidity and mortality in chronic heart failure. *Circulation, 100,* 2312-2318.

Pfeffer, M.A., Swedberg, K., Granger, C.B., Held, P., McMurray, J.J., Michelson, E.L., et al. (2003). Effects of candesartan on mortality and morbidity in patients with chronic heart failure: The CHARM-Overall programme. *Lancet, 362,* 759-766.

Piepoli, M.F., Davos, C., Francis, D.P., Coats, A.J., & ExTraMATCH Collaborative. (2004). Exercise training meta-analysis of trials in patients with chronic heart failure (ExTraMATCH). *British Medical Journal, 328,* 189-192.

Pitt, B., Remme, W., Zannad, F., Neaton, J., Martinez, F., Roniker, B., et al. (2003). Eplerenone, a selective aldosterone blocker, in patients with left ventricular dysfunction after myocardial infarction. *New England Journal of Medicine, 348,* 1309-1321.

Poole-Wilson, P.A., Swedberg, K., Cleland, J.G., Di Lenarda, A., Hanrath, P., Komajda, M., et al. (2003). Comparison of carvedilol and metoprolol on clinical outcomes in patients with chronic heart failure in the Carvedilol Or Metoprolol European Trial (COMET): Randomised controlled trial. *Lancet, 362,* 7-13.

Pritchett, A.M., & Redfield, M.M. (2002). β-Blockers: New standard therapy for heart failure. *Mayo Clinic Proceedings, 77*(8), 839-846.

Rathore, S.S., Curtis, J.P., Wang, Y., Bristow, M.R., & Krumholz, H.M. (2003). Association of serum digoxin concentration and outcomes in patients with heart failure. *Journal of the American Medical Association, 289*(7), 871-878.

Rubenstein, L.Z., & Josephson, K.R. (2002). The epidemiology of falls and syncope. *Clinical Geriatric Medicine, 18*(2), 144-158.

Sackner-Bernstein, J.D., Kowalski, M., Fox, M., & Aaronson, K. (2005). Short-term risk of death after treatment with nesiritide for decompensated heart failure: A pooled analysis of randomized controlled trials. *Journal of the American Medical Association, 293,* 1900-1905.

Schaefer, B.M., Caracciolo, V., Frishman, W.H., & Charney, P. (2003). Gender, ethnicity, and genes in cardiovascular disease. Part 2: Implications for pharmacotherapy. *Heart Disease, 5*(3), 202-214.

Scios, Inc. (May 6, 2005). Dear Physician/Patient Advocate letter re: Natrecore (nesiritide). Fremont, CA: Scios. Available at http://www.fda.gov/medwatch/SAFETY/2005/natrecor_hcp.pdf.

Silverman, M. (1942). *Magic in a bottle.* New York: Macmillan.

Small, K.M., Wagoner, L.E., Levin, A.M., Kardia, S.L., & Liggett, S.B. (2002). Synergistic polymorphisms of beta$_1$- and alpha$_{2C}$-adrenergic receptors and the risk of congestive heart failure. *New England Journal of Medicine, 347*(15), 1135-1142.

Tung, R.H., Garcia, C., Morss, A.M., Pino, R.M., Fifer, M.A., Thompson, B.T., et al. (2004). Utility of B-type natriuretic peptide for the evaluation of intensive care unit shock. *Critical Care Medicine, 32,* 1643-1647.

USP DI: Drug information for the health care professional (25th ed.). (2005). Greenwood Village, CO: MICROMEDEX Thomson Healthcare.

26

ANTIDYSRHYTHMICS

CHAPTER FOCUS

Although antidysrhythmic drugs are commonly used, the nurse should be aware that these drugs can be as life-threatening as they are lifesaving. An evaluation of the risk-benefit ratio is required with each client. The quality of client care is enhanced by the nurse's knowledge of antidysrhythmic therapy and effectiveness in client teaching.

LEARNING OBJECTIVES

- Identify the medications most commonly used as antidysrhythmic agents.
- Describe the primary electrophysiologic effects and electrocardiographic effects of the major antidysrhythmic agents.
- Relate at least three nursing evaluation strategies for monitoring a client's response to antidysrhythmic therapy.
- Identify the most common adverse effects experienced by older adults receiving specific antidysrhythmic therapy.
- Implement nursing management for the care of individual clients who require the administration of an antidysrhythmic agent.

▲ KEY TERMS

Adams-Stokes syndrome, p. 531
automaticity, p. 524
conductivity, p. 524
dysrhythmia (arrhythmia), p. 523
sinus bradycardia, p. 524
sinus tachycardia, p. 524
Wolff-Parkinson-White syndrome, p. 531

✸ KEY DRUGS

amiodarone, p. 534
lidocaine, p. 531
procainamide, p. 527
propranolol (monograph in Chapter 22, p. 462)

A cardiac **dysrhythmia (arrhythmia)** may be defined as any deviation from the normal rhythm of the heartbeat. Dysrhythmia may be caused by a disorder that modifies the electrophysiologic properties of the cells of the conduction system or cardiac muscle. Chapter 24 reviews the electrophysiologic events of a normal action potential.

Antidysrhythmic drugs are used for the prevention and treatment of cardiac rhythm disorders. Dysrhythmias often develop in individuals approximately 4 to 72 hours after a myocardial infarction ("heart attack"). An abnormal rhythm may also occur in clients recovering from cardiac surgery, in clients with coronary heart disease, and in clients with extracardiac disorders such as pheochromocytoma, electrolyte imbalance, or thyroid disease. Cardiac pathology, such as the idiopathic long QT syndrome, may also be inherited (Goldmuntz, 2004) or drug induced.

☀ What are the common types of disorders in cardiac electrophysiology?

Disorders of cardiac rhythm arise as a result of (1) an abnormality in the spontaneous initiation of an impulse, or **automaticity**, or (2) an abnormality in impulse conduction, or **conductivity**. In some conditions, a combination of both processes may occur.

Abnormality in Automaticity

A disturbance in automaticity may alter the rate, rhythm, or origin of impulse formation in the heart. When the rate of pacemaker activity is affected, a decrease in automaticity of the sinoatrial (SA) node produces **sinus bradycardia** (an abnormal condition in which the myocardium contracts steadily but at a rate less than 60 beats/min); an increase in automaticity of the SA node results in **sinus tachycardia** (an abnormal condition in which the myocardium contracts regularly but at a rate greater than 100 beats/min).

A shift in the origin of impulse formation can generate an abnormal pacemaker or an ectopic focus, resulting in activation of some part of the heart other than the SA node. This is called an ectopic pacemaker, and it may discharge at either a regular or an irregular rhythm. It occurs when the cardiac fibers depolarize more frequently than the SA node.

Abnormal automaticity may develop in cells that usually do not initiate impulses, such as atrial or ventricular cells. Clinical disorders such as hypoxia or ischemia of cardiac tissue can activate sympathetic receptors that in turn become centers to initiate impulses. In addition, ischemic sites can cause impulse disturbances in automaticity and also in conductivity; both manifestations are responsible for ectopic beats. The ectopic beats are classified as escape beats, premature beats or extrasystoles, and ectopic tachydysrhythmia.

Abnormality in Conductivity

Altered conduction of the cardiac impulse probably accounts for more dysrhythmias than a change in automaticity. A disturbance in conductivity is caused by either (1) a delay or block of impulse conduction or (2) the reentry phenomenon.

Delay or Block of Impulse Conduction Normally, the SA node and atrioventricular (AV) junction are poor conductors of impulse transmission. Under abnormal circumstances, the conduction of an atrial impulse to the ventricles may be delayed or blocked either in the AV junction or lower in the conduction pathway. Impaired impulse transmission generally appears in the AV junction and occurs in varying degrees of block. In first-degree AV block, the impulses from the SA node pass through to the ventricles very slowly; this is noted by a prolonged PR interval (>0.20 second) on the electrocardiogram (ECG). In second-degree block, some atrial beats fail to pass into the ventricles through the AV junction and may be referred to as "dropped beats." In third-degree block, or complete heart block, the SA node fires at a normal rate as noted by an adequate number of P waves (60 to 100 per minute), but no impulses are conducted through the AV node to the ventri-

cle. To compensate, the Purkinje fibers initiate their own spontaneous depolarization at a very slow rate (usually 20 to 40 per minute). This results in independent ventricular and atrial rhythms and the slow ventricular response is referred to as ventricular "escape."

Reentry Phenomenon Reentry phenomenon is the mechanism responsible for initiating ectopic beats. A necessary condition for reentry is unidirectional block. A unidirectional block is a barrier that allows an impulse to pass in one direction but not the other (Figure 26-1, B). When an impulse travels down the Purkinje fiber, it normally spreads along two branches; when the impulse enters the connecting branch, it is extinguished at the point of collision in the center (Figure 26-1, A). At the same time, other impulses that begin laterally from the Purkinje fibers activate ventricular muscle tissue. In an abnormal situation, the impulse descending from the central Purkinje fiber travels down the right branch normally but encounters a block in the left branch as a result of ischemia or injury (Figure 26-1, B). This is a unidirectional block. In this left branch, where the impulse is blocked in the forward direction at the site of injury, a retrograde or reverse impulse from the ventricular tissue penetrates or reenters the depressed region from the other direction, provided that the pathway proximal to the block is no longer refractory. When the effective refractory period of the blocked area is over, reentry of the impulse from the ventricular muscle into this site causes the impulse to circulate or recycle repetitively through the loop, resulting in a circular movement that produces dysrhythmia.

Reentry is abolished by certain drug groups, which are explained later in this chapter. Drugs that decrease or slow conduction velocity can convert unidirectional block to a two-way or bidirectional block (see Figure 26-1, C). As the impulses traveling in the antegrade, or forward, direction and those appearing in a retrograde, or reverse, direction are blocked at the injured site, the reentry pathway is interrupted, thereby abolishing the ectopic beats. Some antidysrhythmic agents, including lidocaine, eliminate reentry by stopping unidirectional block (Figure 26-1, D).

☀ How do the antidysrhythmic drugs work and how are they classified?

An increasing number of antidysrhythmic drugs are classified into categories based on their fundamental mode of action on cardiac muscle. Such a grouping of antidysrhythmic mechanisms should be valuable in predicting the therapeutic efficacy of the drug. All drugs belonging to a particular class do not necessarily possess totally identical actions. In some cases, a given agent may have subsidiary properties (extracardiac effects) that alter the basic electrophysiologic actions on the cardiac muscle. The currently available antidysrhythmic drugs are classified into four categories according to their mechanisms of action as developed by Vaughan Williams (1992) (Box 26-1). All of these drugs have one major electrophysiologic property in common: the ability to suppress automaticity.

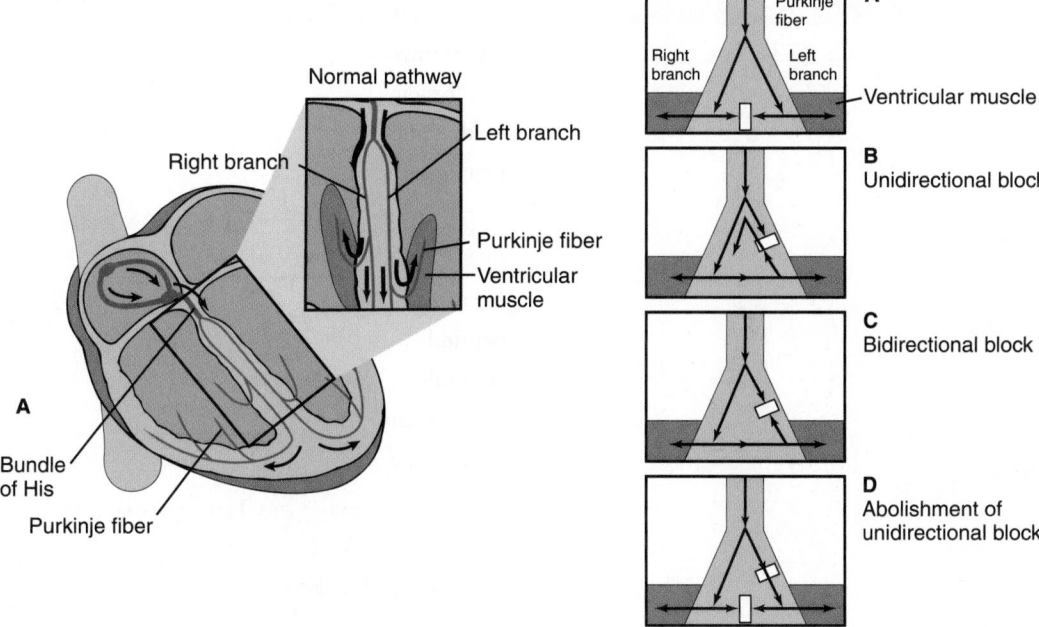

FIGURE 26-1 Reentry phenomenon. Illustration of a branched Purkinje fiber that activates ventricular muscle. **A,** Normal impulse. **B,** Unidirectional block. **C,** Bidirectional block. **D,** Abolishment of unidirectional block.

BOX 26-1 ANTIDYSRHYTHMIC CLASSIFICATIONS

Group I drugs Fast sodium channel blockade in cardiac muscle, resulting in an increased refractory period; subclasses I-A, I-B, and I-C further define the differences between the drugs.

Group II drugs β-Adrenergic-blocking agents that reduce adrenergic stimulation on the heart.

Group III drugs In general, do not affect depolarization but work by prolonging cardiac repolarization.

Group IV drugs Block the slow calcium channel, resulting in the depression of myocardial and smooth muscle contraction, decreased automaticity, and, perhaps, decreased conduction velocity.

Group I compounds are subdivided into groups I-A, I-B, and I-C to reflect the similar electrophysiologic effects of each subgroup. The only exception to the subcategory division is moricizine. Moricizine (Ethmozine) is listed under Group I and has characteristics of all three subgroups (*Drug Facts and Comparisons,* 2005). Group I drugs bind to sodium channels and interfere with sodium influx during phase 0 of the action potential, thus depressing conduction velocity. Group I-A drugs include disopyramide (Norpace), procainamide (Pronestyl), and quinidine. Group I-B drugs are lidocaine, mexiletine (Mexitil), phenytoin (Dilantin), and tocainide (Tonocard). The Group I-B drugs have no effect on conduction velocity, thus they eliminate reentry by stopping unidirectional block entirely. Consequently, normal impulse conduction along the right and left branches of the Purkinje fibers is again restored. Group I-C includes fle-

cainide (Tambocor) and propafenone (Rythmol). Because of their prodysrhythmic effects, Group I-C drugs should be carefully selected and closely monitored when prescribed.

Propranolol (Inderal), acebutolol (Sectral), and esmolol (Brevibloc) are considered Group II drugs because of their β-adrenergic-blocking action.

Group III drugs include bretylium (Bretylol), amiodarone (Cordarone), ibutilide (Corvert), and sotalol (Betapace). The principal action of bretylium is antiadrenergic; it also has a positive inotropic action and prolongs repolarization. Contrary to the typical effects of bretylium, amiodarone increases the refractory period and prolongs the PR interval, QRS complex, and QT interval.

The last category, Group IV drugs, is characterized by a selective calcium antagonistic action. Although there are a number of calcium channel antagonists, only diltiazem (Cardizem) and verapamil (Calan) significantly slow conduction through the AV node. The remaining calcium channel antagonists have minimal activity on cardiac conduction and are not used as antidysrhythmics. Because of its ability to reduce calcium-dependent current in the AV node, adenosine (Adenocard) is often considered a Group IV drug.

Other agents used to treat dysrhythmias include magnesium sulfate, digoxin (see Chapter 25), atropine (see Chapter 21), epinephrine (see Chapter 22), vasopressin (see Chapter 46), and, occasionally, phenytoin (see Chapter 17).

✳ Can drugs cause dysrhythmias?
While myocardial ischemia and infarction are among the most frequent precipitants of dysrhythmias, drugs and electrolyte imbalances also contribute to dysrhythmias. A number of drugs can cause cardiac dysrhythmias, including

BOX 26-2 DRUGS THAT CAN CAUSE CARDIAC DYSRHYTHMIAS

DRUGS THAT PROLONG QT INTERVAL

Cardiac Drugs

amiodarone
disopyramide
dofetilide
ibutilide
procainamide
quinidine
sotalol

Antipsychotics

chlorpromazine
haloperidol
mesoridazine
pimozide
risperidone
thioridazine

Antidepressants

amitriptyline
desipramine
imipramine
maprotiline
nortriptyline

Other Drugs

chloroquine
clarithromycin
domperidone
droperidol

erythromycin
gatifloxacin
methadone
pentamidine

DRUGS REMOVED FROM MARKET OR LIMITED AVAILABILITY

astemizole
bepridil
cisapride
sparfloxacin
terfenadine

DRUGS CAUSING BRADYCARDIA AND/OR AV BLOCK

β-adrenergic blockers
digoxin
diltiazem
verapamil

DRUGS CAUSING TACHYCARDIA

Amphetamines
Antihypertensives (via reflex tachycardia)
β-adrenergic agonists
caffeine
pseudoephedrine
Stimulants
theophylline
Withdrawal of β-adrenergic blockers

---

many of the drugs themselves classified as antidysrhythmic. By altering cardiac conduction, the antidysrhythmics may actually increase risk for dysrhythmias. Of particular concern are the Group I-C agents.

A number of noncardiac drugs can also cause tachycardia or bradycardia, or have the risk of prolonging QT interval on ECG, and are a risk for a life-threatening type of ventricular dysrhythmia known as *torsades de pointes*. Prolongation of the QT interval is a dose-dependent effect of a fair number of drugs. Many times this effect is only observed when very high blood levels are noted, such as when a second interacting drug affects the metabolism of the drug in question. Examples of such drugs include terfenadine (Seldane), cisapride (Propulsid), and thioridazine (Mellaril), all of which have been either removed from the market or largely replaced by safer agents. Box 26-2 lists the more common agents that can cause cardiac dysrhythmias. The implications of pharmacogenetics on the likelihood of

drug-induced dysrhythmias are presented in the Special Considerations for Pharmacogenetics box on p. 527.

✸ What are the key differences among the antidysrhythmics?

Each of the antidysrhythmics differs in pharmacologic effect, adverse effect potential, and indication for use. In 1970, Vaughan Williams proposed a classification of these drugs that subdivides the antidysrhythmics based on their activity on the myocardial action potential. Each of the Vaughan Williams classes is discussed separately. Table 26-1 summarizes the classification and pharmacokinetics of the more commonly used agents.

Group I Drugs

The Vaughan Williams Group I drugs block sodium channels in cardiac muscle, but produce unique physiologic

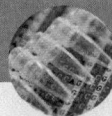 Special Considerations for Pharmacogenetics | ANTIDYSRHYTHMICS

PHARMACODYNAMICS

The effects of genetic variation on β-adrenergic receptors and β blockers were noted in the Special Considerations for Pharmacogenetics box on p. 444 in Chapter 22. Preliminary data in the mouse model suggest a genetic influence on the ability of long-term amiodarone to alter ion channels that affect cardiac rhythms (Le Bouter et al., 2004). Pharmacodynamic changes based on genetics have been established for mexiletine and propafenone (Chang & Altman, 2004).

PHARMACOKINETICS

The variation in cytochrome P450 2D6 that metabolizes encainide, flecainide, propafenone, lidocaine, and a number of β blockers is genetically established. Similarly, cytochrome P450 3A4 activity demonstrates considerable differences in expression across populations and may account for varied levels of dofetilide, disopyramide, lidocaine, diltiazem, verapamil, and quinidine (Wojnowski, 2004; Schaefer, Caracciolo, Frishman, & Charney, 2003b).

ADVERSE EFFECTS

The propensity for drugs, including antidysrhythmic drugs, to produce prolonged QT intervals and the risk for life-threatening ventricular dysrhythmias is believed to be genetically determined (Roden, 2004). Genetic markers have been identified in individuals with prolonged QT intervals and such markers are found nearly twice as often in blacks than in whites (Ackerman et al., 2003). Women also appear to be at higher risk than men for prolonged QT interval syndromes (Schaefer et al., 2003a). The genetic variation in drug-metabolizing enzymes may also play an important role in the prodysrhythmic effects observed with antidysrhythmic agents.

---

properties. These agents are subclassified as Group I-A, I-B, and I-C agents.

Group I-A Agents

The pharmacologic effects of procainamide, quinidine, and disopyramide are similar: they bind to sodium channels and interfere with sodium influx during phase 0 of the action potential. The result is depression of conduction velocity. The ECG effects of these drugs include a widened QRS complex and a prolonged QT interval. Procainamide is the most widely used of these agents and serves as the key drug for this group.

◼⬛ procainamide [proe kane **ah** mide]
(Pronestyl, Procanbid, Procan SR, Apo-Procainamide✤)

Procainamide stabilizes the cell membrane by preventing the ready movement of sodium and potassium across this cellular barrier. This inhibition of cation exchange results in a decrease in the rate of diastolic depolarization from the resting potential during phase 4 and an increase in the threshold potential (the voltage shifts toward 0 mV). Procainamide reduces automaticity, slows electrical conduction and delays repolarization in the atria, ventricles, and Purkinje fibers. Procainamide possesses some negative inotropic activity. Similar properties are seen with its active metabolite, N-acetyl procainamide (NAPA), which accumulates in clients with renal insufficiency.

Indications

Procainamide is indicated for ventricular tachycardia (VT), paroxysmal supraventricular tachydysrhythmia (PSVT), and atrial fibrillation.

Pharmacokinetics/Dosing

Procainamide is fairly well-absorbed orally. It is metabolized via cytochrome P450 2D6 to the active metabolite NAPA. The elimination half-life of procainamide and NAPA for adults with normal renal function is 2.5 to 4.7 hours and 6 to 8 hours, respectively. Half-lives in renal dysfunction are prolonged for both procainamide and NAPA. The typical adult intravenous (IV) dose is 15 to 17 mg/kg slow infusion over 30 minutes, then an infusion of 1 to 4 mg/min. Oral dosing for adults with normal renal function is typically 250 to 500 mg orally every 3 hours or 500 to 1000 mg of extended-release procainamide every 6 hours. Normal therapeutic blood levels for procainamide/NAPA are 4 to 10 mcg/mL and 15 to 25 mcg/mL, respectively, and are usually obtained immediately before the next scheduled dose.

Adverse Effects

Procainamide is associated with hypotension on IV administration, as well as diarrhea, nausea, and vomiting. It may exacerbate heart failure (HF) in clients with preexisting myocardial disease. Procainamide and NAPA have a relatively narrow therapeutic index with the risk for sinus bradycardia and prolonged QT interval observed with levels above the normal range. Long-term use may result in accumulation of antinuclear antibodies in up to 50% of clients and may result in a systemic lupus erythematosus-like state. Bone marrow suppression has also been reported. Procainamide may also cause elevations in liver function tests, including alanine aminotransferase (ALT), aspartate aminotransferase (AST), alkaline phosphatase, lactate dehydrogenase, and bilirubin.

Drug Interactions

Other drugs affecting cytochrome P450 2D6 (e.g., amiodarone, ranitidine, cimetidine, ofloxacin) can result in elevated procainamide levels. Avoid use of procainamide and NAPA in clients with prolonged QT interval or clients receiving other drugs that prolong QT interval (see Box 26-2). Prolonged QT interval significantly increases the risk for torsades de pointes, a stereotypic dysrhythmia with ventricular tachycardia.

quinidine [**kwin** i deen]
(Quinaglute, Apo-Quinidine✤, Quinate✤)
quinidine polygalacturonate
(Cardioquin)
quinidine sulfate
(Quinora)

Quinidine is similar to procainamide with stronger control of abnormal ectopic pacemaker activity and more activity as a cholinergic (muscarinic) antagonist. This atropine-like effect permits the sinus node to accelerate and may often provoke a dangerous sinus tachycardia. Therefore digoxin, verapamil, or a β-blocking agent is usually administered before quinidine to prevent ventricular acceleration

TABLE 26-1 SELECTED ANTIDYSRHYTHMICS: PHARMACOKINETICS

Drug	Time to Peak Level or Effect (hours)	Duration of Action* (hours)	Therapeutic Serum Level† (mcg/mL)
GROUP I-A			
disopyramide	PO: 0.5-3	1.5-8.5	3-6
procainamide	PO: 1-1.5	3	4-10
quinidine	PO: 1-4	6-8	3-6
GROUP I-B			
lidocaine	IV: 1 min	10-20 min	1.5-5
tocainide	PO: 0.5-2	8	4-10
mexiletine	PO: 2-3	—	0.5-2
GROUP I-C			
flecainide	PO: 3	—	0.2-1 (trough)
propafenone	PO: 3.5	—	0.06-1 (trough)
GROUP I (A, B, C)			
moricizine	PO: 0.5-2 level 6-14 effect	10-24	—
GROUP II			
propranolol	PO: 1-1.5	3-5	0.05-0.1
GROUP III			
bretylium	IV: 5-10 min‡ IM: 1‡	6-8 —	0.5-1.5 0.5-2.5
amiodarone	IV: 3-7	Variable	1-2.5§
dofetilide	PO: SS 2-3 days	10	—
sotalol	PO: 2-3	7-18	—
GROUP IV			
diltiazem	IV: <5 min PO: 2-3	Variable	—
verapamil	IV: 1-5 min PO: 2	IV: 10-20 min PO: 6-8	—
adenosine	IV: 10-20 sec	<1-2 min	—

Data from *Drugs Facts and Comparisons*. (2005). St. Louis: Facts and Comparisons; *USP DI: Drug information for the health care professional* (24th ed.). (2005). Greenwood Village, CO: MICROMEDEX Thomson Healthcare; *Physicians' Desk Reference*. (2004). Montvale, NJ: Medical Economics; and White, C.M., Song, J., & Chow, M.S.S. (2005). Cardiac arrhythmias. In M.A. Koda-Kimble, L.Y. Young, W.A. Kradjan, B.J. Guglielmo, B.K. Alldredge, & R.L. Corelli (Eds.), *Applied therapeutics: The clinical use of drugs* (8th ed.). Philadelphia: Lippincott Williams & Wilkins.
IV, Intravenously; *IM*, intramuscularly; *PO*, orally; *SS*, steady state.
*Metabolism/excretion is primarily via the liver/kidneys, with the exception of amiodarone, mexiletine, and moricizine, which are mainly excreted via bile.
†Steady-state plasma level.
‡To treat ventricular fibrillation.
§Steady state following 2 months of drug therapy.

when attempting to convert atrial fibrillation to normal sinus rhythm. The chief noncardiac action of quinidine is peripheral vasodilation, which results from its α-adrenergic blocking effect on vascular smooth muscle.

Indications

Quinidine is indicated for prophylaxis to maintain normal sinus rhythm after cardioversion of atrial fibrillation or atrial flutter, for prevention of PSVT, and for ventricular tachydysrhythmia.

Pharmacokinetics/Dosing

Quinidine salts contain different percentages of the active drug: quinidine gluconate, 62%; quinidine polygalacturonate, 80%; quinidine sulfate, 83%. Consequently, these drugs are not interchangeable without an appropriate dosage adjustment. Quinidine sulfate 200 mg is considered equivalent to 275 mg of quinidine gluconate or quinidine polygalacturonate. The usual adult dosage of quinidine sulfate is 200 to 300 mg orally (PO) three to four times daily. Safety in children has not been established.

Adverse Effects

The adverse effects of quinidine include anorexia, diarrhea, bitter taste, nausea, vomiting, abdominal distress, flushing, rash, tinnitus, confusion, and vision changes. This constellation of effects is often referred to as cinchonism. Severe hypotension and heart failure have been reported. As with procainamide, the potential for prolonged QT interval and torsades de pointes are risks of therapy.

Drug Interactions

Quinidine is metabolized by cytochrome P450 3A4 and inhibits the metabolism of other drugs metabolized by cytochrome P450 2D6 and 3A4. This accounts for a significant number of interactions with other drugs/foods including amiodarone, cimetidine, clarithromycin, diltiazem, erythromycin, grapefruit juice, itraconazole, ketoconazole, ritonavir, and verapamil. Quinidine also increases concurrent digoxin levels and may increase the levels of metoprolol, mexiletine, nifedipine, propafenone, propranolol, and timolol. Concurrent administration with any other drug that prolongs QT interval may increase the risk for torsades de pointes (see Box 26-2).

disopyramide [dye soe **peer** ah mide]
(Norpace, Rythmodan✚)

The effects of disopyramide are similar to those of procainamide and quinidine with the exception that the anticholinergic effects of disopyramide are more prominent. This is the reason why a drug that slows AV conduction is administered with disopyramide for the treatment of atrial flutter or atrial fibrillation. Converting a unidirectional block into a bidirectional block (see Figure 26-1, C) abolishes reentrant dysrhythmias.

Indications

Disopyramide is indicated to treat ventricular dysrhythmia. Because of significant anticholinergic effects, it is often considered a second-line agent.

Pharmacokinetics/Dosing

Disopyramide is reasonably well-absorbed orally and is metabolized to inactive metabolites via cytochrome P450 3A4. See Table 26-1 for the pharmacokinetics of this drug. The dosage of disopyramide is individualized according to response and tolerance. The usual adult loading dose is 300 mg for clients weighing 50 kg or greater; the maintenance dosage is 150 mg every 6 hours. Disopyramide is generally avoided in older adults; if used, older adults require a dosage reduction.

Adverse Effects

The adverse effects of disopyramide are similar to quinidine with exception of tinnitus, visual changes, and rash. In addition, disopyramide may cause dry mouth and throat, difficulty in urination, weight gain, and sexual impotency.

Drug Interactions

Disopyramide interacts with other drugs metabolized by cytochrome P450 3A4 including flecainide, procainamide, quinidine, and propafenone. Concurrent phenytoin, phenobarbital or rifampin will often increase metabolism of disopyramide and result in reduced levels. Additive anticholinergic (antimuscarinic) activity is observed with other muscarinic antagonists (e.g., atropine, antihistamines, tricyclic antidepressants). Disopyramide should be avoided in the presence of prolonged QT interval or with other drugs known to prolong QT interval (see Box 26-2).

✴ **L.S., a 63-year-old woman, presents to the cardiology clinic for a visit following "shortness of breath and palpitations" on the golf course yesterday. She has had hypertension for 20 years and an anterior wall myocardial infarction 5 years ago. Her current medications include atenolol 25 mg PO daily, enalapril 15 mg PO twice daily, digoxin 0.125 mg PO daily, and furosemide 20 mg PO daily. Her physical exam reveals a blood pressure (BP) of 135/85 mm Hg, pulse of 90 beats/min, respiratory rate of 16 breaths/min, and body temperature of 37° C (98.6° F). Her cardiac exam reveals an irregularly irregular pulse without murmurs, rubs, or gallops. She has bibasilar rales and jugular vein distention, but no hepatosplenomegaly. She has 1+ pitting edema bilaterally. L.S.'s ECG shows atrial fibrillation and her chest radiograph is compatible with mild HF. Her lab work is within normal limits and her digoxin serum level is 0.9 ng/mL. Her prescriber adds quinidine gluconate (Quinaglute Dura-Tabs) 324 mg PO every 8 hours and warfarin 5 mg PO at bedtime.**

The goals of L.S.'s therapy are to relieve her symptoms, control her ventricular rate with the Group I-A drug quinidine, and reduce the risk of stroke with the anticoagulant warfarin. Because L.S. has been on her other drugs and warfarin previously (when she had her myocardial infarction), the nurse focuses on the management of her antidysrhythmic therapy with quinidine.

Assessment Careful evaluation is necessary to determine the effect of the dysrhythmia on L.S. The effect on clients may range from benign to life-threatening, depending on the individual's health status and the degree of dysrhythmia. A thorough history, a physical assessment, and an interpretation of the dysrhythmia on the ECG are essential for formulating L.S.'s possible nursing diagnoses. Clients with hepatic or renal function impairment may require decreased dosages to avoid accumulation of the drug and caution is used in clients with a history of thrombocytopenia. Unlike other antidysrhythmic agents, quinidine is unique because if quinidine is administered to clients with myasthenia gravis, it may increase muscle weakness secondary to its weak curare-like action.

In review of L.S.'s concurrent medication regimen, there are a number of drug interactions for which she is at risk. These include inhibition of warfarin metabolism by quinidine, increased digoxin levels with quinidine use, and increased risk for AV block with quinidine, digoxin, and atenolol. Monitor L.S. for signs of additional anticoagulant effects, such as excessive bruising, bleeding gums, black stools, hematuria, and hematemesis. It may be necessary to adjust the anticoagulant dosage both during therapy and after quinidine therapy is discontinued. The concurrent administration of digoxin will possibly increase her serum digoxin concentrations 100%. Monitor digoxin serum levels carefully to prevent toxicity. If quinidine is administered during digoxin intoxication, the effects are additive and may lead to AV block. Question L.S. about her use of antacids, as many clients do not believe over-the-counter drug use is remarkable, but in this case, antacids block the renal excretion of quinidine and may lead to cinchonism. Assess also her intake of grapefruit juice, which inhibits metabolism of cytochrome P450 3A4 hepatic enzymes and may increase quinidine serum concentrations (*USP DI*, 2005).

Obtain a baseline assessment of L.S., including BP, pulse pressure, and any changes caused by postural change; apical pulse rate and rhythm; apical-radial pulse deficit; heart sounds; jugular vein distintion; edema; capillary refill time; urinary output; activity tolerance; the presence of chest discomfort (pain or pressure), shortness of breath, syncope, fatigue, nausea, and perception of heart rate ("skipping beats"); level of consciousness, confusion, and anxiety; serum electrolyte levels (particularly potassium); and ECG.

Nursing Diagnosis Possible nursing diagnoses/collaborative problems that L.S. or other clients may experience while receiving an antidysrhythmic agent include, but are not limited to, the following: impaired comfort (nausea); risk for injury related to hypotension and dizziness; activity intolerance; deficient knowledge; anxiety related to altered heart action; and the potential complications of decreased cardiac output and altered cerebral and peripheral tissue perfusion. In addition to these general nursing diagnoses related to any antidysrhythmic agent, L.S., because of her quinidine therapy, is also at risk for impaired comfort (skin flushing, bitter taste, or abdominal cramping); risk for injury related to cinchonism (blurred vision, dizziness, headache, altered hearing) and anemia (tiredness, weakness); and the potential complications of allergic reaction (fever, rash, wheezing, dyspnea), thrombocytopenia (unusual bruising or bleeding), and further dysrhythmias. Consider these issues in the care and education of clients who are taking antidysrhythmic agents.

Planning While L.S. is on antidysrhythmic drug therapy, she will:
- Experience effective tissue perfusion related to the therapeutic effect of the antidysrhythmic drug.
- Not experience injury related to the adverse effects of antidysrhythmic drug therapy.
- Demonstrate adequate knowledge of the antidysrhythmic drug therapy.
- Effectively manage her therapeutic regimen (e.g., reporting adverse effects appropriately, pulse-taking, maintaining prescriber contact for monitoring and follow up care).

Implementation

Monitoring To determine the effectiveness of L.S.'s antidysrhythmic therapy, continue to assess the indicators of the baseline assessment. Question her about episodes of light-headedness, dizziness, or confusion. Monitor lung sounds and heart rate and rhythm, and monitor her ECG for changes and/or further development of HF. The QT interval is the best indicator of quinidine-induced ventricular dysrhythmia, although serum quinidine serum levels can be monitored as well. Monitor laboratory data as ordered, especially potassium levels. Be alert to premature ventricular contractions (PVCs) not noted before drug administration (appear as ectopic foci by reentry phenomenon), because they may lead to VT or fibrillation, and subsequently to cardiac standstill (asystole). Note that another form of ventricular disorder can cause "quinidine syncope." It produces ventricular tachycardia or fibrillation, causing a decrease in cardiac output, thereby diminishing blood flow to the brain. The symptoms are a feeling of faintness, loss of consciousness, and, ultimately, sudden death.

Intervention Although some clients may require an artificial pacemaker to control their dysrhythmia, most are treated with antidysrhythmic agents some time during the course of their illness. Maintain a quiet environment for L.S.

Education Provide L.S. continuous explanation for the various diagnostic and/or monitoring devices. Instructing her within the clinical setting provides the opportunity for her to self-administer the antidysrhythmic medications safely and accurately. Much anxiety can be allayed through instruction regarding the dysrhythmia and its management. Such instruction is essential because medications may need to be taken for a lifetime. L.S. should be able to take and assess her pulse rate and rhythm accurately, counting for 1 full minute. She should be able to describe the medication regimen, including dosage scheduling, rationale, and the adverse effects of the prescribed medications. L.S. should be able to state signs and symptoms to report to the prescriber, including syncope, chest pain, dizziness, low BP, gastrointestinal (GI) distress, blurred vision, a change in respiratory status or pulse rate or rhythm, swollen feet or ankles, a sudden weight gain, or hypersensitivity (commonly fever with other symptoms 3 to 20 days into therapy). She should be able to state the need for ongoing care and the importance of adhering to the prescribed treatment regimen. Quinidine may be given with food to decrease gastric distress if it occurs. Caution L.S. not to self-medicate without advice from prescriber as some over-the-counter medications, such as antacids and cimetidine, will increase quinidine levels. Teach her to limit coffee, tea, and cola drinks because caffeine can cause an increase in abnormal heart rhythm. She should eat a balanced diet without excesses of alkaline ash foods (e.g., citrus fruit, vegetables, milk) as these will prolong the half-life of quinidine.

Instruct L.S. to make position changes slowly from the recumbent posture if hypotension should occur. Caution her about driving or other hazardous activities, because blurred vision and dizziness may occur. Advise her about the possibility of dry mouth, which can be relieved with sugarless hard candy, gum, or frequent clear-water rinses. Recommend regular dental checkups for the prevention of caries and periodontal disease. In addition, instruct her to avoid alcoholic beverages because of the potential hypotensive effects. Caution L.S. to avoid exertion and hot weather, because heat intolerance and reduced perspiration will occur. Constipation may result from the antimuscarinic effects of the Class I antidysrhythmics. Instruct L.S. about a high-fiber diet, increased fluid intake, moderate exercise, and regular bowel patterning.

Recommend that L.S. carry medical identification. Caution her to alert health care professionals, including dentists, that she is taking quinidine. Instruct her to continue to take the drug, even if feeling well, and to check with her prescriber before discontinuing the medication. Alert L.S. that there are also sources of health information online; see the Technology Link box in Chapter 25, p. 519.

Evaluation The expected outcome of antidysrhythmic therapy is that L.S. will maintain normal cardiac output as evidenced by BP, pulse, and capillary refill within normal limits. She will also increase activity tolerance, as evidenced by less fatigue and less dyspnea; experience less chest pain, palpitations, and associated symptoms; and demonstrate no dysrhythmias on ECG tracings. She will be able to state an understanding of dysrhythmia, the actions to take when experiencing the signs and symptoms of dysrhythmias, and administer her antidysrhythmic therapy safely and accurately. The efficacy of antidysrhythmic medications for L.S. or any client is determined by the achievement of these goals. Modification of the nursing care plan may be necessary for L.S. to achieve the goals for management of the dysrhythmia.

Group I-B Drugs

The Group I-B drugs (e.g., lidocaine [Xylocaine], phenytoin [Dilantin], tocainide [Tonocard], and mexiletine [Mexitil]) differ from Group I-A drugs in that they either increase or have no effect on conduction velocity. Although not approved by the U.S. Food and Drug Administration (FDA), phenytoin is used in the therapy of digoxin-induced dysrhythmias. Lidocaine, tocainide, and mexiletine are related therapeutically and are particularly useful for acute

ventricular dysrhythmia. The high incidence of adverse effects with mexiletine has limited its use. Tocainide can cause the serious adverse effect of agranulocytosis, and therefore it is usually reserved for clients who have not responded to other drug therapies.

lidocaine [lye doe kane]
(Xylocaine, Xylocard✤, Zilactin-L✤)
Lidocaine appears to act primarily on the sodium channel, blocking both the activated and inactivated sodium channels; its greater effect is in depolarized or ischemic tissues. These effects are indicative of the efficacy of lidocaine for suppressing the dysrhythmias associated with depolarization (e.g., ischemia, digoxin-induced toxicity) and of its lack of effectiveness in dysrhythmias that occur in normal polarized tissues (atrial fibrillation, atrial flutter). Lidocaine has few electrophysiologic effects in normal cardiac tissue.

Unlike quinidine and procainamide, lidocaine has no vagolytic properties, nor does it influence cardiac output and arterial pressure. It does not depress myocardial contractility and thereby provides no potential for the development of heart failure. Because lidocaine exerts a limited effect, if any, on the SA node and atrial myocardium, it has no use in the treatment of supraventricular tachycardias. Because electric activities are primarily limited to the ventricular cells, the major use of lidocaine is in abolishing ventricular dysrhythmias (see Figure 26-1, D).

Indications
Lidocaine, an agent used extensively as a local and topical anesthetic agent, is also an antidysrhythmic agent, especially for ventricular dysrhythmias seen after cardiac surgery or an acute myocardial infarction

Pharmacokinetics/Dosing
Lidocaine undergoes very extensive first pass metabolism via cytochrome P450 2D6 and 3A4 hepatic isoenzymes rendering oral administration not practical. Lidocaine is administered IV as an antidysrhythmic (although in an emergency situation, may be administered endotracheally). The adult dosage of lidocaine is by IV bolus, 1 mg/kg at a rate of 25 to 50 mg/min; this may be repeated in 5 minutes if necessary (the maximum dose per hour is 300 mg). Children receive the same 1 mg/kg dose initially, but repeat doses in 5 minutes should not exceed a total of 3 mg/kg. With IV infusion, the dosage is usually 20 to 50 mcg/kg, given at a rate of 1 to 4 mg/min for both adults and children. Topical use of lidocaine is discussed in Chapter 15.

Adverse Effects
Lidocaine is contraindicated in a number of cardiac rhythm disturbances, including Adams-Stokes syndrome (sudden, recurring episodes of loss of consciousness, caused by the transient interruption of cardiac output by incomplete or complete heart block), Wolff-Parkinson-White syndrome (a supraventricular tachycardia), and severe AV block. The adverse effects of lidocaine include dizziness, anorexia, nausea, vomiting, chest pain, and breathing difficulties. Central nervous system toxicity, including seizures, is noted with high levels. Table 26-2 lists the adverse effects of lidocaine as related to serum concentration.

TABLE 26-2 ADVERSE EFFECTS RELATED TO SERUM CONCENTRATIONS OF LIDOCAINE

Serum Concentration	Adverse Effects
1.5-6 mcg/mL	Anxiety, nervousness, drowsiness, dizziness, sensations of cold, heat, or numbness
6-8 mcg/mL	Tremors, twitching, blurred or double vision, nausea, vomiting, tinnitus
>8 mcg/mL	Dyspnea, severe dizziness, fainting, bradycardia, seizures

Drug Interactions
Lidocaine levels may be elevated in clients who receive concurrently administered drugs metabolized by cytochrome P340 2D6 or 3A4, including β-adrenergic blockers. Consult appropriate references for a full listing of interactions. Use of lidocaine with phenytoin or other antidysrhythmic agents may increase the risk for cardiac depression.

tocainide [toe **kay** nide]
(Tonocard)
Tocainide is similar to lidocaine and has been used orally. This agent is not currently available in the United States.

Indications
Tocainide is used for the suppression and prevention of life-threatening ventricular dysrhythmias. Although not FDA approved as an analgesic, it is has been used as an adjunct therapy for neurogenic pain.

Pharmacokinetics/Dosing
Unlike lidocaine, tocainide displays little first-pass metabolism and orally administered doses are well absorbed into systemic circulation. It is metabolized into inactive metabolites. The half-life is 11 to 14 hours in adults, and extends to about 24 hours with concurrent renal or hepatic impairment. The typical oral dose is 400 to 800 mg every 8 hours.

Adverse Effects
Dizziness and nausea are the most common adverse effects of tocainide. Other effects include paresthesias, tremor, ataxia, bone marrow suppression, pulmonary fibrosis, and other dysrhythmias.

mexiletine [mex il **eh** teen]
(Mexitil)
Mexiletine is similar to lidocaine and has been used orally.

Indication
Mexiletine is indicated for the suppression and prevention of life-threatening ventricular dysrhythmias. An unlabeled use is as adjunct therapy for diabetic neuropathic pain.

Pharmacokinetics/Dosing
Similar to tocainide, mexiletine displays little first-pass metabolism. It is metabolized via cytochrome P450 1A2 and 2D6, which explains its interaction potential with other agents. The half-life is 10 to 14 hours in adults and is prolonged in hepatic failure. The oral dose for adults is 200 to 400 mg every 8 hours.

Adverse Effects
Gastrointestinal distress is the most common adverse effect with nausea or abdominal discomfort observed in approximately 40% of clients. Other adverse effects include dizziness, ataxia, tremors, bradycardia, and muscle weakness.

Drug Interactions
Drugs that affect cytochrome P450 1A2 action may result in elevated mexiletine levels. Such drugs include amiodarone, ciprofloxacin, fluvoxamine, ketoconazole, ofloxacin, and rofecoxib. Mexiletine may increase caffeine and theophylline levels. Quinidine may result in increased mexiletine levels. Carbamazepine, phenobarbital, and rifampin may result in reduced mexiletine levels.

✷ **M.M., a 69-year-old man, presents to the emergency department with chest pain. He is diagnosed with an acute myocardial infarction and is treated with a fibrinolytic. He begins to develop PVCs and goes into VT; he is cardioverted successfully, but continues to have PVCs. He is administered a lidocaine 75-mg bolus, followed by another 50 mg in 5 minutes. He is then maintained on a 3 mg/min infusion of lidocaine and his PVCs do not recur.**

✷ **What the nursing management issues of M.M.'s lidocaine therapy?**

Assessment The assessment of M.M.'s relevant preexisting illness includes other cardiac, hepatic, and renal impairment. Do not administer lidocaine in the case of severe heart block or Adams-Stokes syndrome; the administration of lidocaine may worsen the heart block. Use lidocaine with caution in individuals with hypovolemia, shock, incomplete heart block, sinus bradycardia, and Wolff-Parkinson-White syndrome, because these conditions may be aggravated. The risk-benefit ratio should be considered if M.M. has a known history of hypersensitivity to the amide type of local anesthetics. To prevent toxicity in M.M. if he has impaired renal and hepatic function, exercise caution with prolonged use because lidocaine is metabolized mainly in the liver and excreted by the kidney.

Assess M.M.'s concurrent medications for interactions that might contraindicate lidocaine or require careful monitoring. A significant drug interaction may occur when lidocaine is administered with phenytoin (hydantoin antiepileptic drug), as well as other antidysrhythmic agents; it may result in enhanced cardiac depressant effects.

The baseline clinical assessment is the same as for L.S.'s antidysrhythmic regimen in the previous case discussion of quinidine.

Nursing Diagnosis With the administration of lidocaine, assess M.M. for the following selected nursing diagnoses/collaborative problems: impaired comfort related to prolonged IV use (pain at the site of injection); risk for toxicity related to specific serum levels of the drug (see Table 26-1); and the potential complications of allergic reaction (skin rash, urticaria, and dyspnea) and decreased cardiac output related to cardiac conduction disturbances (hypotension, dysrhythmias, heart block, and cardiac arrest).

Planning While M.M. is on antidysrhythmic drug therapy, he will:
- Experience effective tissue perfusion related to the therapeutic effect of the antidysrhythmic drug.
- Not experience injury related to the adverse effects of antidysrhythmic drug therapy.
- Demonstrate adequate knowledge of the antidysrhythmic drug therapy.
- Report any dizziness, chest pain, or shortness of breath to the nursing staff.

Implementation
Monitoring To avoid overdose and toxicity as a result of IV administration, constant ECG monitoring of M.M. is essential. Stop the infusion immediately if excessive cardiac depression occurs, such as prolongation of the PR interval or QRS complex or aggravation of dysrhythmias. Monitor BP and ECG constantly. Assess respiratory status for basilar rales. Monitor M.M.'s neurologic status frequently for drowsiness, dizziness, confusion, changes in perceptual and

visual disturbances, and behavioral changes. Serum electrolyte levels should be determined periodically during prolonged lidocaine infusions to correct imbalances. Observe M.M. for adverse effects of lidocaine (see Table 26-2). Monitor serum lidocaine levels to minimize the chance of toxicity. If the IV administration runs for more than 24 hours, observe for local thrombophlebitis and assess M.M. for the risk of drug accumulation.

Intervention Recheck the drug label; administer only lidocaine hydrochloride without preservatives or epinephrine. The label will specifically read "IV use for cardiac dysrhythmias." Preparations intended for use as an anesthetic contain epinephrine and *should not* be used for treating dysrhythmias. IV infusions of lidocaine are usually prepared as 1 mg/mL solution using 5% dextrose solution; use a precision IV volume control set for continuous infusion. The solution is stable for 24 hours. Do not add to blood transfusions.

M.M's bolus dose was given to rapidly attain therapeutic serum concentrations. Because the loading dose did not provide the desired therapeutic effect within 5 minutes, a second dose was administered (one-half to one-third of the initial dose). Monitor the prescribed IV rate of flow; lidocaine should not exceed 4 mg/min. Terminate the IV infusion as soon as the cardiac rhythm is stable or signs of toxicity develop. Have oxygen, resuscitative equipment and drugs available to treat adverse effects involving the cardiovascular system, respiratory system, and central nervous system.

Note that IV infusions are rarely continued beyond 24 hours. M.M. is then given an oral antidysrhythmic agent for maintenance therapy.

Education Provide M.M. continuous explanation about the monitoring equipment. Instruct him to report any dizziness, chest pain, or shortness of breath.

Evaluation The expected outcome of lidocaine antidysrhythmic therapy is that M.M. will have regular palpable pulses and will experience an absence of or a decrease in ventricular ectopy on the ECG without any adverse effects of the drug.

Group I-C Drugs

The Group I-C drugs include flecainide (Tambocor) and propafenone (Rythmol), which are used to treat and/or prevent life-threatening supraventricular tachydysrhythmia. A landmark trial of flecainide and another I-C agent, encainide, in the late 1980s identified the life-threatening risks of these agents to cause sinus arrest, AV block, and ventricular dysrhythmias (CAST Investigators, 1989). This prodysrhythmic effect is of real concern, especially in clients with poor left-ventricular function or sustained ventricular dysrhythmias. The Group I-C drugs can also aggravate HF. As such, these agents are typically reserved for clients who

are carefully monitored by an electrophysiologic cardiologist who specializes in dysrhythmia suppression.

flecainide [fle kay **nide**]
(Tambocor)
Flecainide is a sodium channel blocking agent with minimal effects on repolarization and has no anticholinergic properties. It suppresses PVCs and in high doses may exacerbate dysrhythmias in clients with a preexisting ventricular tachydysrhythmia or in clients with a previous myocardial infarction.

Indications
Flecainide is indicated for the treatment of ventricular dysrhythmia and as prophylaxis of supraventricular dysrhythmia, such as AV junction reentrant tachycardia.

Pharmacokinetics/Dosing
Flecainide is well-absorbed orally and is hepatically metabolized via cytochrome P450 2D6. The adult dosage of flecainide is 50 to 100 mg PO every 12 hours, titrated every 4 days as necessary.

Adverse Effects
The most serious of adverse effects are the risk for inducing irreversible ventricular dysrhythmias, including ventricular tachycardia (VT) or ventricular fibrillation (VF) which are refractory to treatment and often result in death. Use in clients with hypotension, existing heart failure, electrolyte disturbance or with other agents that affect cardiac conduction (see Box 26-2) may be at particular high risk. Other adverse effects of flecainide include blurred vision, dizziness, headaches, constipation, nausea, weakness, chest pain, irregular heartbeats, and other dysrhythmias.

Drug Interactions
Elevated flecainide levels can increase the risk for irreversible ventricular dysrhythmias. Flecainide levels are increased by concurrently administered cytochrome P450 2D6 inhibitors including amiodarone, amprenavir, cimetidine, digoxin, propranolol, quinidine, and ritonavir. Agents that acidify or alkalinize urine can also affect flecainide levels. Concurrent β-adrenergic blockers or verapamil may increase the risk for heart failure. Extreme caution is exercised when dosing with other drugs known to prolong QT interval (see Box 26-2).

propafenone [proe pa **feen** one]
(Rythmol)
Propafenone is similar to flecainide in its action and therapeutic uses. It also has some β-blocking activity and weak calcium channel blocking activity. It prevents the passage of sodium ions into the fast sodium channels (phase 0), resulting in a decrease in depolarization rate. It also prolongs the refractory period in cardiac tissues.

Indications
It is indicated for the treatment of life-threatening ventricular dysrhythmia.

Pharmacokinetics/Dosing
Propafenone is well absorbed and metabolized by cytochrome P450 2D6. The usual adult dosage is 150 mg PO every 8 hours, with dosage adjustments at 3- to 4-day intervals as necessary. Use in children is not established.

Adverse Effects
The adverse effects of propafenone are similar to flecainide. Propafenone may be more likely to induce heart failure because of negative inotropic effects and should be used with extreme caution in such individuals. Other adverse effects include dizziness, nausea, headaches, constipation, weakness, chest pain, irregular heartbeats, and dysrhythmias.

Drug Interactions
Like flecainide, propafenone is metabolized by cytochrome P450 2D6. Drug interactions with propafenone are similar to those seen with flecainide. Propafenone may also increase the anticoagulant effects of warfarin.

Group IA-IB-IC Drugs

moricizine [mor **i** siz een]
(Ethmozine)
Moricizine (Ethmozine) has the properties of all three classes (A, B, C) and therefore does not belong to one individual classification. It is a fairly potent sodium channel blocking agent that does not prolong the duration of the action potential. It has local anesthetic action and a membrane stabilizing effect; thus it decreases AV junction and His-Purkinje conduction.

Indications
Moricizine is indicated for the treatment of life-threatening ventricular dysrhythmia.

Pharmacokinetics/Dosing
Moricizine has an extensive first pass effect and is metabolized by cytochrome P450 3A4. The adult dosage is 200 to 300 mg PO three times daily every 8 hours; the dosage is titrated as necessary at 3-day intervals. The maximum daily dose is 900 mg.

Adverse Effects
The adverse effects of moricizine include light-headedness, dry mouth, blurred vision, nausea, vomiting, weakness, chest pain, heart failure, and ventricular tachydysrhythmia.

Drug Interactions
Moricizine levels may be increased by other agents metabolized by cytochrome P450 3A4, including cimetidine and diltiazem. Moricizine may result in reduced theophylline levels, although this combination of drugs is not recommended because of the prodysrhythmic nature of theophylline. Caution must be exercised if using other concurrently administered drugs that prolong the QT interval, including digoxin (see Box 26-2).

Group II Drugs

The β-adrenergic blocking drugs have multiple uses including their ability to help control certain cardiac dysrhythmias. These agents are most effective for conditions associated with increased sympathetic discharge and also serve to slow conduction through the AV node (e.g., in the management of atrial fibrillation [Snow et al., 2003]). Subtle differences among the β-adrenergic blockers lead to different indications for use. Sotalol is unique among the β-adrenergic-blocking drugs in that it also blocks potassium channels and is considered a Group III agent (see p. 536). Propranolol, the key drug in the class, can be used to treat dysrhythmias and is presented with other β-adrenergic agents in Chapter 22.

acebutolol [a se **byoo** toe lole]
(Sectral, Monitan✤, Novo-Acebutolol✤, Rhotral✤)
Acebutolol is a β₁-selective adrenergic blocker with modest intrinsic sympathomimetic activity.

Indication
Acebutolol is indicated for ventricular dysrhythmia because of its ability to suppress ectopic ventricular beats. It is also indicated for hypertension and angina.

Pharmacokinetics/Dosing
Like other β-adrenergic blockers, acebutolol has a high first-pass effect on oral administration. For ventricular dysrhythmias, it is dosed at 200 to 600 mg orally twice daily.

Adverse Effects
The adverse effects for acebutolol are similar to other β-adrenergic antagonists and are presented more fully in Chapter 22. Of major concern are the risks for AV block and bradycardia; acebutolol is contraindicated if those states are present before administration. Being cardioselective for β₁ receptors, it has a lower potential for bronchospasm. As a negative inotrope, its use in clients with heart failure (HF) should generally be avoided (see Chapter 25 for a discussion of β-adrenergic blockers in HF).

Drug Interactions
When dosed with other agents that suppress conduction through the AV node, there is an increased risk for AV block (see Box 26-2). β-Adrenergic blockers may mask symptoms of hypoglycemia in clients with diabetes mellitus.

esmolol [ess **moe** lol]
(Brevibloc)
Esmolol is a very short-acting cardioselective β₁-adrenergic-blocking drug. Actions are similar to other β-adrenergic blockers.

Indications
Controlling ventricular rate in atrial fibrillation/atrial flutter, supraventricular tachycardia, and acute management of intraoperative hypertension.

Pharmacokinetics/Dosing
Because esmolol is metabolized by enzymes in red blood cells, its elimination half-life is short at 9 minutes. Adult doses are typically 0.5 to 1 mg/kg bolus with an infusion of 50 to 150 mcg/kg/min infusion.

Adverse Effects
Adverse effects of esmolol are similar to other β-adrenergic antagonists, but are generally short-lived because of its short duration of action. Hypotension, diaphoresis, pain on injection, and nausea are among the most common adverse effects.

Drug Interactions
Drug interactions are similar to those with other β-adrenergic blockers and with acebutolol.

Group III Drugs

The electrophysiologic properties of drugs in this group differ markedly from the drugs previously discussed. Drugs in this group prolong the effective refractory period by prolonging the action potential (delay repolarization). Their action in part is usually related to potassium channel blockade, although other pharmacologic actions exist for most of the agents in this class. Like some of the Class I drugs, these agents can significantly prolong QT interval and pose a risk for ventricular dysrhythmias, including the life-threatening torsades de pointes. Amiodarone is the most frequently used agent in the group and is considered the key drug.

✱🏴 amiodarone [a **mee** oh da rone]
(Cordarone)
Amiodarone is structurally related to thyroid hormone. It increases the refractory period in all cardiac tissues by having a direct effect on the tissues. Amiodarone decreases automaticity, prolongs AV conduction, and decreases the automaticity of fibers in the Purkinje system. It may block potassium, sodium, and calcium channels and β receptors. It has the potential to cause a variety of complex effects on the heart and has serious adverse effects.

Indications
Amiodarone is indicated for life-threatening VF and VT. Unlabeled uses include converting atrial fibrillation to normal sinus rhythm and PSVT. Unlabeled but widely accepted uses (per Advanced Cardiac Life Support [ACLS] guidelines) include cardiac arrest with persistent VT after defibrillation and epinephrine, and control of hemodynamically stable VT, polymorphic VT, or wide-complex tachycardia of uncertain origin.

Pharmacokinetics/Dosing

Oral absorption of amiodarone is variable with an oral bioavailability of approximately 50%. It is extensively metabolized via a number of the cytochrome P450 enzymes including 2C8/9. Amiodarone possesses a very long half-life of 26 to 107 days and its effects can persist for weeks or months after discontinuation of therapy. IV amiodarone is typically administered based on prior use of amiodarone, protocols, and indication. In a life-threatening emergency situation, intravenously administered amiodarone is typically dosed in a "front-loaded" fashion with a bolus IV dose of 150 to 300 mg, followed by a 6-hour infusion of 360 mg, then an 18-hour infusion of 540 mg, and, finally, a continuous rate infusion of 0.5 mg/min. The usual adult oral dosage for ventricular dysrhythmias is 800 mg to 1.6 g PO daily for 1 to 3 weeks until a therapeutic response is noted or adverse effects appear. The dosage is then reduced to 600 to 800 mg daily for 1 month, eventually decreasing to the lowest effective dosage. Amiodarone is generally avoided in women of childbearing age unless life-threatening dysrhythmias not responsive to other therapies are present. (See the Pregnancy Safety box below for FDA pregnancy safety categories.) The pediatric oral dosage is 10 mg/kg/day for 10 days or until a therapeutic response is noted or adverse effects appear. The dosage is then decreased and tapered to lowest effective dosage as outlined in the package insert.

Adverse Effects

The most serious adverse effects of amiodarone are bradycardia, hypotension (frequently observed with IV administration), cardiac dysrhythmias including heart block, heart failure, hepatotoxicity, and pulmonary toxicity. Pulmonary toxicity or hypersensitivity evidenced by cough, fever, and malaise, has been reported in 2% to 17% of clients receiving chronic amiodarone. Hyperthyroidism is noted in approximately 3% of clients on the drug. Amiodarone often is deposited in the cornea and may lead to visual disturbances in approximately 10% of clients on long-term therapy. Other adverse effects of amiodarone include dizziness, bitter taste, headache, flushing, nausea, vomiting, constipation, ataxia, weight loss, tremors, numbness and tingling of the fingers and toes, muscle weakness, photosensitivity, blue-gray skin discoloration, fever, allergic reaction, and blurred vision. For clients on oral dosing, the nausea and vomiting is minimized if amiodarone is taken consistently with meals.

Drug Interactions

Amiodarone is metabolized by a number of the cytochrome P450 enzymes and serves to inhibit the metabolism of a number of other drugs that are metabolized by 1A2, 2A6, 2D6, and 3A4. Among the many drugs interacting with amiodarone is warfarin. Careful monitoring of warfarin dosing and bleeding risk is required with this combination. Because amiodarone can increase the QT interval, other drugs that also prolong QT interval should be avoided (see Box 26-2). Consult with an appropriate reference for potential drug interactions and work with the prescriber and pharmacist to manage them.

PREGNANCY SAFETY
ANTIDYSRHYTHMICS

Category	Drug
B	sotalol, lidocaine, moricizine
C	adenosine, bretylium, disopyramide, dofetilide, flecainide, ibutilide, mexiletine, procainamide, propafenone, quinidine, tocainide
D	amiodarone

Data from *Mosby's drug consult* (15th ed.). (2005). St. Louis: Mosby.

The remaining agents in this group, such as bretylium, dofetilide, ibutilide, and sotalol, are less frequently used.

bretylium tosylate [bre **til** ee um]
(Bretylol, Bretylate✦)

Unlike the other antidysrhythmics, bretylium does not suppress automaticity and has no effect on conduction velocity. The direct electrophysiologic action on the heart appears to be prolongation of the action potential and lengthening of the effective refractory period. This mechanism is believed to help terminate dysrhythmias caused by the reentry phenomenon. Bretylium is also taken up and concentrated in the adrenergic nerve terminals where, after an initial release of norepinephrine, it prevents any further release. This sympatholytic action significantly increases the threshold, producing an antifibrillatory response in the ventricles. Bretylium produces a positive inotropic effect, increasing myocardial contractility. With long-term treatment, the drug shows increased responsiveness to circulating epinephrine and norepinephrine, which may account for the increased myocardial contractility.

Indications

Bretylium is used as second-line therapy to treat VT and VF.

Pharmacokinetics/Dosing

Bretylium is given IV and is primarily eliminated in the urine as unchanged drug. The usual adult dosage for life-threatening VF is 5 mg/kg IV of undiluted solution, followed by 10 mg/kg every 15 to 30 minutes as needed. Refer to a current reference for dosage recommendations for other ventricular dysrhythmias.

Adverse Effects

The adverse effects of bretylium include severe and sudden hypotension and bradycardia. Other undesirable effects include anorexia, headaches, nausea, vomiting, bitter taste, impotency, dizziness, cough, breathing difficulties, fever, paresthesia of the fingers or toes, hand tremors, and weakness.

Drug Interactions

Bretylium prolongs QT interval and, with the exception of use in a life-threatening situation, should be avoided when other agents that prolong QT interval are in use (see Box 26-2).

dofetilide [doe **fet** il ide]
(Tikosyn)

Dofetilide is a class III agent whose action is limited to blockade of the potassium channel. Dofetilide has no action at the sodium channel of adrenergic receptors. It increases the action potential and prolongs the QT interval.

Indication

Dofetilide (Tikosyn) has been approved for the treatment and maintenance of atrial fibrillation and atrial flutter. It is available via a restricted distribution system for prescribers and hospitals that have undergone specific training in proper dosing and drug management.

Pharmacokinetics/Dosing

Dofetilide is well absorbed and partially metabolized via cytochrome P450 3A4. Dosing is dependent on QT interval and renal function.

Adverse Effects

Dofetilide has a narrow therapeutic index. Drug-induced VT and torsades de pointes have been observed in approximately 4% of clients on dofetilide. The risk for torsades de pointes is highest during the first 3 days of treatment, and is higher for clients on high doses and with preexisting heart failure (HF). Other adverse effects include AV block, cardiac arrest, myocardial infraction, bradycardia, cerebrovascular accidents, headache, dizziness, insomnia, hepatic injury, and respiratory difficulty.

Drug Interactions

Dofetilide concentrations are increased when administered concurrently with other drugs that affect the action of cytochrome P450 3A4, including, but not limited to, amiodarone, fluconazole, itraconazole, and grapefruit juice. Drugs that prolong QT interval must also be avoided (see Box 26-2). *Careful management of interactions is a critical component in the safe use of this drug and cannot be underestimated.* Nurses are encouraged to work with the prescriber and the pharmacist to identify potential interacting drugs and appropriately manage such interactions as to avoid interactions that may contribute to ventricular dysrhythmias.

ibutilide [eye **byoo** ti lide]
(Corvert)
Ibutilide prolongs the action potential and increases the atrial and ventricular refractory period. It may produce its effect at the sodium channels by slowing the inward current or by blocking the potassium outward currents. Like other Class III agents, ibutilide prolongs the QT interval.

Indications
Ibutilide is indicated for the conversion of atrial fibrillation or atrial flutter to normal sinus rhythm.

Pharmacokinetics/Dosing
Ibutilide has an extensive first-pass effect and is not used orally. Administered intravenously, ibutilide has an average 6-hour elimination half-life with excretion mainly in the urine. The adult dosage for clients weighing less than 60 kg is 0.01 mg/kg administered over 10 minutes. For clients weighing more than 60 kg, 0.1 mg/kg is administered. If necessary, a second dose of equal strength may be administered 10 minutes after the completion of the first infusion (*Drug Facts and Comparisons*, 2005).

Adverse Effects
The most significant toxicity of ibutilide is torsades de pointes, which may occur in up to 6% of clients receiving therapy. The risk is highest for individuals with preexisting prolonged QT interval. Other adverse effects include headache, nausea, cardiovascular alterations (e.g., AV block, bradycardia, ventricular extrasystoles, and sustained monomorphic ventricular tachycardia), hypotension, and hypertension.

Drug Interactions
Ibutilide should be avoided in the presence of prolonged QT interval or with concurrent administration of other drugs that prolong QT interval (see Box 26-2).

sotalol [soe ta lole]
(Betapace, Betapace AF)
Sotalol is a nonselective β-adrenergic-blocking agent that prolongs the duration of the action potential, increasing the effective refractory period in atrial, ventricular, and AV junction. Unlike other β-adrenergic blockers, sotalol affects potassium channels rendering this drug effective in the treatment of ventricular dysrhythmia.

Indications
Sotalol is indicated for life-threatening ventricular dysrhythmias. One formulation of sotalol (Betapace AF) is indicated for the maintenance of normal sinus rhythm in individuals with atrial fibrillation or atrial flutter and should not be substituted for other formulations.

Pharmacokinetics/Dosing
Sotalol is well-absorbed orally and is eliminated in the urine as unchanged drug. The half-life in adults with normal renal function is 12 hours. Dosing is typically initiated in a hospital setting. Initial adult doses of sotalol are typically 80 mg twice daily with titration to response. Doses up to 640 mg daily in divided doses have been used. Dosage adjustment for renal dysfunction is required.

Adverse Effects
The most significant adverse effect is prolongation of the QT interval and the risk for torsades de pointes. Because sotalol is a β_1- and β_2-adrenergic blocker, it is contraindicated in bronchial asthma, sinus bradycardia, AV block, cardiogenic shock, and heart failure, and in persons who are hypersensitive to sotalol. Other adverse effects include fatigue, dizziness, weakness, dyspnea, confusion, headache, nausea/vomiting, and paresthesias. (See Chapter 22 for additional information regarding the adverse effects of β-adrenergic blockers.)

Drug Interactions
As with other Class III agents, concurrent drugs that prolong QT interval should be avoided (see Box 26-2).

✳ **E.B., a 47-year-old woman, collapses in her real estate office and is unresponsive. When the paramedics arrive, she has no pulse or BP and is in VF. The paramedics institute ACLS protocols for VF. After being defibrillated at 200 J, 300 J, and 360 J, E.B.'s VF continues. She is intubated and an IV line is placed. Epinephrine 1 mg IV push is administered followed by 360-J defibrillation with no change in her VF. Amiodarone (Cordarone) 300 mg IV push is given. She is shocked again and sinus rhythm is established. E.B. is started on a maintenance infusion of amiodarone.**

Epinephrine is recommended for use in cardiopulmonary resuscitation (CPR) with vasopressin as a second-line alternative for CPR. The β-agonist activity of epinephrine enhances automaticity and conduction and increases the force of ventricular contraction in the beating heart; its α-adrenergic activity increases systemic vascular resistance through vasoconstriction. Both properties enhance cerebral and coronary blood flow (White, Song, & Chow, 2005). Recent research, however, demonstrates that if E.B. were in asystole, vasopressin as the CPR agent might improve her chances of hospital admission and hospital discharge (Wenzel, Krismer, Arntz, Sitter, & Stadlbauer, 2004). Because the epinephrine was ineffective in converting E.B.'s VF, an antidysrhythmic agent, amiodarone was administered.

✳ **What are the nursing management issues with amiodarone therapy for E.B.?**

Assessment Because the amiodarone was administered on an emergency basis, an assessment of E.B.'s preexisting health status was not accomplished before initiation of the drug. As soon as laboratory results are available, any electrolyte imbalances must be corrected. As soon as possible, a health history with drug regimen is determined. It would be important to know if E.B. has a history of respiratory, thyroid, or hepatic conditions, or if she were hypertensive. If E.B. were younger, assessment would include determining whether she was pregnant or was planning to become pregnant, or was breastfeeding.

Assess E.B.'s concurrent medication regimen for potential drug interactions. There would be concern if E.B. had been taking anticoagulants, such as warfarin. Because the anticoagulant effect may be increased, the anticoagulant dosage should be reduced by one-third to one-half when adding amiodarone to E.B.'s drug regimen. Prothrombin times or international normalized ratio (INR) should also be closely monitored with concurrent warfarin use. Other antidysrhythmic agents may increase cardiac effects and the risk of inducing tachydysrhythmias. Amiodarone also increases serum levels of quinidine, procainamide, flecainide, and phenytoin. If amiodarone must be given with Group I antidysrhythmic agents, the dosage of the Group I antidysrhythmic drug should be reduced by 30% to 50% several days after starting amiodarone, and the Group I drug gradually withdrawn. If additional treatment with amiodarone is necessary, therapy is usually started at half the usual recommended dosage. Amiodarone may increase the serum level of digoxin resulting in toxicity. Digoxin should be discontinued or the dose reduced to 50% whenever amiodarone is given. Monitor serum levels closely. There may also be additive effects of both drugs on the SA node and AV junction. Amiodarone may also increase serum levels of phenytoin (Dilantin), so phenytoin levels should be monitored for toxicity. Verapamil, diltiazem, and β-adrenergic blocking agents may potentiate sinus bradycardia, sinus arrest, or AV block. Fentanyl and St. John's wort may also cause bradycardia or hypotension. Cimetidine may increase amiodarone levels; cholestyramine may decrease them. Amiodarone increases cyclosporine levels. Ritonavir increases the risk of amiodarone toxicity.

Nursing Diagnosis With the administration of amiodarone, assess E.B. for development of the following nursing diagnoses/collaborative problems: impaired comfort (dizziness, bitter taste, headache, flushing, nausea, and vomiting); constipation; imbalanced nutrition: less than body requirements related to anorexia (severe weight loss); and the potential complications of photosensitivity; pulmonary fibrosis or pneumonitis (cough, dyspnea, fever); hyperthyroidism (weight loss, insomnia, nervousness, sensitivity to heat); hypothyroidism (weight gain, tiredness, sensitivity to cold, dry skin); neurotoxicity (ataxia, numbness in fingers and toes, trembling, weakness of arms or legs); ocular toxicity (blurred vision, corneal deposits); allergic reaction (rash); hepatitis (yellow skin and eyes); and decreased cardiac output related to hypotension, new dysrhythmias, sinus bradycardia, or heart failure (pulmonary edema, edema of feet and lower legs).

Planning While E.B. is on amiodarone therapy, she will:
- Experience effective tissue perfusion related to the therapeutic effect of the antidysrhythmic drug.
- Not experience injury related to the adverse effects of amiodarone therapy.
- Demonstrate adequate knowledge of amiodarone therapy.
- Effectively manage her therapeutic regimen (e.g., reporting adverse effects appropriately, pulse-taking, maintaining prescriber contact for monitoring and follow-up care).

Implementation

Monitoring Monitor ECG, thyroid function studies, liver function studies (ALT, AST, and serum alkaline phosphatase), chest radiography examinations, and pulmonary studies. Also monitor E.B.'s vital signs and fluid balance. Ophthalmologic examinations should be performed if eye symptoms occur. Pulmonary fibrosis may occur in 10% to 30% of clients receiving long-term amiodarone therapy.

This is usually reversible if detected early enough, and thus chest radiography examinations every 3 months are recommended. Thyroid function studies should be performed periodically because of the risk for hyperthyroidism or hypothyroidism.

Intervention Because GI disturbances occur in 25% of clients during loading, care should be taken to minimize these as much as possible. Provide E.B. with a high-fiber diet and increased fluid intake, unless contraindicated, to prevent constipation. Make efforts to stimulate appetite to counteract anorexia.

It is recommended that a central venous catheter with an in-line filter be used for IV administration, with the initial rate not exceeding 30 mg/min. Most clients require 48 to 96 hours of IV amiodarone. If E.B.'s arrhythmia is managed with IV amiodarone, she can be switched to the oral form.

Education If E.B. is maintained on oral amiodarone, instruct her to maintain regular contact with the prescriber to monitor drug use. Alert her to obtain a Cordarone Tablets Medication Guide (see the Medication Safety Alert below). Advise her to carry medical identification at all times and to alert health care professionals unfamiliar with her medication regimen to the amiodarone administration.

Photosensitivity is a potential adverse effect with this drug. Caution E.B. to avoid exposure to the sun and to wear sun-protective clothing and dark glasses. Sunscreen agents are ineffective because they do not block ultraviolet B (UVB) light; barrier sun blocks are needed (e.g., zinc or titanium oxide). In addition, a blue-gray coloration of the skin occurs with long-term use (more than 1 year) and affects sun-exposed parts of the body (e.g., face, neck, and arms) and clients with fair skin.

Alert E.B. to report any of the following signs and symptoms to the prescriber: cough, dyspnea, fever (pulmonary toxicity); ataxia, numbness, tingling, weakness, or spasm of the extremities (neurotoxicity); blurred vision or increased sensitivity of the eyes to light (ocular toxicity); unusual

---

⁂ Medication Safety Alert

FDA Alert Regarding Amiodarone (Cordarone)

The FDA issued an alert relating to amiodarone (Cordarone) in December 2004. It requires pharmacists and other health professionals who dispense medication to distribute Medication Guides directly to each client to whom Cordarone Tablets are dispensed. The Medication Guide developed by Wyeth should not be used as a substitute for talking to clients about the risks relative to the benefits associated with the drug. Clients should be alerted to ask for the Medication Guide each time they refill their prescription as there may be new information about the drug. A copy may be obtained through www.wyeth.com. Click on Products and scroll down to Cordarone, Patient Information.

weight gain or loss, increased sensitivity to heat or cold (thyroid toxicity); pain and swelling of the scrotum if she were male; jaundice (hepatic toxicity); or swelling of the lower limbs (HF).

Evaluation The expected outcome of amiodarone therapy for E.B. is that she will have regular palpable pulses and will demonstrate an absence of or decrease in ventricular ectopy on ECG with minimal adverse effects of the drug.

Group IV Drugs

Agents that interfere with calcium channels in the AV node are among the Group IV drugs. These agents are typically used to slow AV nodal conduction in the treatment of supraventricular dysrhythmia, particularly atrial fibrillation. Diltiazem, verapamil, and the β blockers (Group II agents) are generally preferred over digoxin in the management of ventricular dysrhythmias secondary to atrial fibrillation (Snow et al., 2003). Most prominent are the calcium channel blockers diltiazem (Cardizem) and verapamil (Calan), which are briefly presented here. Chapter 27 has a more complete discussion of calcium channel blockers. Adenosine (Adenocard) has multiple effects, but is often considered a Group IV drug because of its effect on suppressing calcium currents in the AV node.

Diltiazem and verapamil block the flow of calcium into the cell via the slow calcium channels. This results in slowed AV nodal conduction. Other effects include relaxation of coronary vascular smooth muscle, reduction in myocardial contractility, and dilation of the coronary vessels.

diltiazem [dil **tye** a zem]
(Cardizem, Apo-Diltiaz✦, Novo-Diltiazem✦)
Indications
Reducing ventricular response in atrial fibrillation and atrial flutter, paroxysmal supraventricular tachycardia (PSVT). Other indications include hypertension (see Chapter 27), stable angina, and vasospastic angina (see Chapter 28). Calcium channel blockers are also sometimes used in the treatment of diastolic heart failure (see Chapter 25), but are avoided in systolic heart failure because of their negative inotropic effects.
Pharmacokinetics/Dosing
Diltiazem displays significant first-pass effect on oral administration and is metabolized by cytochrome P450 3A4 and other cytochrome P450 isoenzymes. Its half-life is 3 to 4.5 hours with normal renal function. IV dosing for atrial fibrillation, atrial flutter, or PSVT is typically 0.25 mg/kg over 2 minutes IV with a repeat dose if needed. Continuous IV infusions may be used at a rate of 5 to 15 mg/hr. The oral dose for angina or hypertension depends on the formulation and is initially 30 mg four times daily for immediate-release formulations or 120 to 240 mg daily for extended-release formulations.
Adverse Effects
Edema and headache are the most common adverse effects observed with diltiazem. AV block, systolic heart failure, dizziness, GI upset, and muscle weakness have also been reported.
Drug Interactions
Diltiazem interacts with a number of drugs metabolized by cytochrome P450 3A4, including, but not limited to, amiodarone,

cimetidine, digoxin, fluoxetine, ketoconazole, itraconazole, omeprazole, phenytoin, and grapefruit juice. Diltiazem may serve as a negative inotrope and should be used cautiously for clients with preexisting systolic heart failure or on other negative inotropes. Caution should be exercised when using other drugs that prolong QT interval or slow AV nodal conduction (see Box 26-2).

verapamil [ver **ap** a mil]
(Calan, Isoptin, Apo-Verap✦, Novo-Veramil✦)
Indications
Indications for verapamil are similar to those for diltiazem.
Pharmacokinetics/Dosing
Like diltiazem, verapamil displays significant first-pass effect on oral administration and is metabolized by cytochrome P450 3A4 and other cytochrome P450 isoenzymes. Its half-life is 4 to 7 hours with normal renal and hepatic function. Intravenous dosing for atrial fibrillation, atrial flutter, or PSVT is typically 2.5 to 5 mg over 2 minutes IV with a repeat dose of 5 to 10 mg after 15 to 30 minutes if needed. The initial oral dose for angina or hypertension is 40 to 120 mg three times daily for immediate-release formulations.
Adverse Effects
Gingival hyperplasia and constipation are the most common adverse effects observed with verapamil. AV block, hypotension, peripheral edema, reflex tachycardia, dizziness, and GI upset have also been reported.
Drug Interactions
Similar to diltiazem, verapamil interacts with a number of drugs metabolized by cytochrome P450 3A4, as noted above. Similar warnings for drugs with concurrent negative inotropic effects, drugs that prolong the QT interval, or slow AV nodal conduction are appropriate for verapamil as well (see Box 26-2).

adenosine [a **den** oh seen]
(Adenocard)
Adenosine is a natural constituent of muscle tissue. It works via specific G-protein-coupled adenosine receptors to shorten action potential via reduction of calcium current in the AV node.
Indications
Adenosine is indicated for the conversion of PSVT to normal sinus rhythm.
Pharmacokinetics/Dosing
Administered by IV bolus, it is taken up almost immediately by red blood cells and vascular endothelial cells and metabolized to inosine and adenosine monophosphate in the body. The half-life of adenosine is extraordinarily short at less than 10 seconds. Because of this very short half-life, the drug is administered by rapid bolus and immediately followed with 10 mL saline flush to assure the complete administered dose is flushed from the IV line. The usual dose is 6 mg administered rapidly by IV bolus over 1 to 2 seconds. If the dysrhythmia is still present 1 to 2 minutes after the injection, a 12-mg dose may be administered.
Adverse Effects
Adenosine is contraindicated for clients with a recent history of myocardial infarction, AV block, atrial fibrillation, atrial flutter, or cerebral hemorrhage. The adverse effects of adenosine are often dramatic, but thankfully brief. Clients often report significant dyspnea, chest pain, flushing, nausea, headache, dizziness, and tingling in arms, and should be informed before administration that this is a typical response and that it should subside within 1 minute or so. Cardiac effects include pulmonary edema and new dysrhythmias, such as premature ventricular contractions, sinus bradycardia, sinus tachycardia, skipped beats, and chest pain/pressure.
Drug Interactions
Concurrent caffeine or theophylline may reduce the effects of adenosine.

✳ What other types of drugs are used occasionally to treat cardiac dysrhythmias?

Other drugs occasionally used to treat cardiac dysrhythmias include those that augment calcium, potassium, or magnesium levels. Elevated or low levels of potassium contribute to dysrhythmias, and the administration of potassium or enteral potassium-binding resins (e.g., sodium polystyrene sulfonate [Kayexalate]) are used to increase or decrease potassium levels, respectively. Specific to the treatment of ventricular dysrhythmias is the IV administration of magnesium sulfate, which is briefly discussed below.

magnesium sulfate [mag **nee** zee um **sul** fate]

Magnesium is a naturally occurring electrolyte in the body with multiple physiologic properties. Administered IV, magnesium acts to slow the rate of sinoatrial impulses and prolongs conduction time. It also decreases acetylcholine at the motor-nerve junction. Given orally, magnesium acts as an osmotic laxative.

Indications

Treatment of torsades de pointes and other ventricular dysrhythmia. It is also used intravenously for seizure management in preeclampsia or eclampsia of pregnancy and for treatment of hypomagnesemia. As a topical solution, it is used as a soaking aid. Other magnesium salts are used as osmotic laxatives.

Pharmacokinetics/Dosing

For treatment of torsades de pointes, magnesium sulfate 1 to 2 g diluted in 100 mL dextrose 5% in water (D₅W) over 1 to 2 minutes. Magnesium sulfate is very irritating to the vein and must be diluted before use.

Adverse Effects

Hypotension and asystole are the most serious reactions noted with rapid IV administration. Other effects are often dose related and include heart block, respiratory depression, central nervous system depression, depressed muscle reflexes, and irritation to the vein or tissue.

Drug Interactions

Magnesium sulfate is not physically compatible with many other drugs and should be administered via a separate IV site, which is flushed before and after administration.

Summary

Antidysrhythmic agents are used for the treatment and prevention of cardiac rhythm disorders that result from some abnormality in the electrophysiologic properties of the cardiac conduction system cells or cardiac muscle cells. These drugs are classified based on pharmacologic action into four groups according to the Vaughan Williams classification schema.

Group I drugs serve as sodium channel blockers. Although all drugs in this group have the ability to suppress automatic-

ity, they are subdivided into groups I-A, I-B, and I-C to reflect the similar electrophysiologic properties of each subgroup. Group I-A includes disopyramide (Norpace), procainamide (Pronestyl), and quinidine, all of which decrease conduction velocity and prolong the action potential. Group I-B drugs—lidocaine, tocainide (Tonocard), and mexiletine (Mexitil)—either increase or have no effect on conduction velocity. Group I-C drugs—flecainide (Tambocor) and propafenone (Rythmol)—are used to treat or prevent supraventricular tachydysrhythmia; however, they have prodysrhythmic effects that are of concern and require careful monitoring of the client.

Group II drugs, such as propranolol (Inderal), acebutolol (Sectral), and esmolol (Brevibloc), have β-adrenergic-blocking action and are discussed mainly in Chapter 22. The Group III agents—bretylium (Bretylol), amiodarone (Cordarone), ibutilide (Corvert), and sotalol (Betapace)—are antiadrenergic. Group IV consists of the calcium channel blockers, such as diltiazem and verapamil; adenosine is sometimes considered an unclassified agent, although many consider it a Group IV drug based on its action at the AV node. It is indicated for the conversion of paroxysmal supraventricular tachycardia.

Finally, management of potassium, magnesium, and calcium levels are important in preventing and treating cardiac dysrhythmias. The IV administration of magnesium sulfate is considered the drug of choice for treating torsades de pointes ventricular dysrhythmia.

The nursing management of cardiac dysrhythmia with the administration of antidysrhythmic agents should produce the following expected outcomes: the client will maintain cardiac output within normal limits, increase activity tolerance, experience less chest discomfort and associated symptoms, and demonstrate a decrease in or the absence of dysrhythmias on ECG tracings. Client education is focused on developing the client's knowledge of health status and medications, skill at pulse taking, and ability to recognize reportable changes in health status, which enables the client to self-administer antidysrhythmic agents safely and accurately.

✳ Critical Thinking Questions

- How would the differences in the groupings of antidysrhythmic agents affect nursing management of the client's care?

- What concerns do you perceive a client might have if the client is receiving antidysrhythmic therapy?

𝑒-LEARNING SUPPLEMENTS

Student CD-ROM
- Final Exam questions
- NCLEX® Examination review questions
- Pharmacology animations
- Printable chapter summary

Evolve Website (http://evolve.elsevier.com/mckenry)
- Case study on drugs affecting the parasympathetic nervous system

- Content updates, including information on new drugs
- WebLinks corresponding to this chapter
- Answers to the critical thinking questions in this chapter
- *Elsevier ePharmacology Update* newsletter
- *Mosby's Drug Consult* Internet Edition
- Supplemental and reference information

Bibliography

Ackerman, M.J., Tester, D.J., Jones, G.S., Will, M.L., Burrow, C.R., & Curran, M.E. (2003). Ethnic differences in cardiac potassium channel variants: Implications for genetic susceptibility to sudden cardiac death and genetic testing for congenital long QT syndrome. *Mayo Clinic Proceedings, 78*(12), 1479-1487.

Anderson, D.M., Keith, J., & Novak, P.D. (Eds.) (2002). *Mosby's medical, nursing, and allied health dictionary* (6th ed.). St. Louis: Mosby.

Braunwald, E., Zipes, D.P., & Libby, P. (2001). *Heart disease: A textbook of cardiovascular medicine* (6th ed.). Philadelphia: W.B. Saunders.

CAST Investigators. (1989). Preliminary report: Effect of encainide and flecainide on mortality in a randomized trial of arrhythmia suppression after myocardial infarction. *New England Journal of Medicine, 321,* 406-412.

Chang, J.T., & Altman, R.B. (2004). Extracting and characterizing gene-drug relationships from the literature. *Pharmacogenetics, 14*(9), 577-586 and linked supplemental website http://bionlp.stanford.edu/genedrug/gene_drug_predictions.html (as cited December 2, 2004).

DiPiro, J.T., Talbert, R.L., Yee, G.C., Matzke, G.R., Wella, B.G., & Posey, L.M. (Eds.). (2002). *Pharmacotherapy: A pathophysiologic approach* (5th ed.). New York: McGraw-Hill.

Dorian, P., Cass, D., Schwartz, B., Cooper, R., Gelaznikas, R., & Barr, A. (2002). Amiodarone as compared with lidocaine for shock-resistant ventricular fibrillation. *New England Journal of Medicine, 346*(12), 884-890.

Drug facts and comparisons. (2005). St. Louis: Facts and Comparisons.

Goldmuntz, E. (2004). The genetic contribution to congenital heart disease. *Pediatric Clinics of North America, 51*(6), 1721-1737.

Kudenchuk, P.J., Cobb, L.A., Copass, M.K., Cummins, R.O., Doherty, A.M., Fahrenbruch, C.E., et al. (1999). Amiodarone for resuscitation after out-of-hospital cardiac arrest due to ventricular fibrillation. *New England Journal of Medicine, 341*(12), 871-878.

Lacy, C.F., Armstrong, L.L., Goldman, M.P., & Lance, L.L. (2004). *Lexi-Comp's drug information handbook* (12th ed.). Hudson, OH: Lexi-Comp.

Le Bouter, S., El Harchi, A., Marionneau, C., Bellocq, C., Chambellan, A., van Veen, T., et al. (2004). Long-term amiodarone administration remodels expression of ion channel transcripts in the mouse heart. *Circulation, 110*(19), 3028-3035.

Mosby's drug consult (15th ed.). (2005). St. Louis: Mosby.

Roden, D.M. (2001). Antiarrhythmic drugs. In J.G. Hardman & L.E. Limbird (Eds.), *Goodman & Gilman's the pharmacological basis of therapeutics* (10th ed.). New York: McGraw-Hill.

Roden, D.M. (2004). Drug-induced prolongation of the QT interval. *New England Journal of Medicine, 350*(25), 2618-2621.

Schaefer, B., Caracciolo, V., Frishman, W., & Charney, P. (2003a). Gender, ethnicity and genetics in cardiovascular disease. Part 1: Basic principles. *Heart Disease, 5*(2), 129-143.

Schaefer, B., Caracciolo, V., Frishman, W., & Charney, P. (2003b). Gender, ethnicity, and genes in cardiovascular disease. Part 2: Implications for pharmacotherapy. *Heart Disease, 5*(3), 202-214.

Siddoway, L.A. (2003). Amiodarone: Guidelines for use and monitoring. *American Family Physician, 68*(11):2189-2190.

Snow, V., Weiss, K.B., LeFevre, M., McNamara, R., Bass, E., Green, L.A., et al. (2003). Management of newly detected atrial fibrillation: A clinical practice guideline from the American Academy of Family Physicians and the American College of Physicians. *Annals of Internal Medicine, 139,* 1009-1017.

USP DI: Drug information for the health care professional (25th ed.). (2005). Greenwood Village, CO: MICROMEDEX Thomson Healthcare.

Vaughan Williams, E.M. (1992). Classifying antiarrhythmic actions: By facts or speculation. *Journal of Clinical Pharmacology, 32,* 964-977.

Wenzel, W., Krismer, A.C., Arntz, R., Sitter, H., & Stadlbauer, K.H. (2004). A comparison of vasopressin and epinephrine for out-of-hospital cardiopulmonary resuscitation. *New England Journal of Medicine, 350,* 105-113.

White, C.M., Song, J., & Chow, M.S.S. (2005). Cardiac arrhythmias. In M.A. Koda-Kimble, L.Y. Young, W.A. Kradjan, B.J. Guglielmo, B.K. Alldredge, & R.L. Corelli (Eds.), *Applied therapeutics: The clinical use of drugs* (8th ed.). Philadelphia: Lippincott Williams & Wilkins.

Wojnowski, L. (2004). Genetics of the variable expression of CYP3A in humans. *Therapeutic Drug Monitoring, 26*(2), 192-199.

ANTIHYPERTENSIVES

CHAPTER FOCUS

Hypertension (sustained, elevated blood pressure) is a chronic circulatory disease that affects millions around the world. In North America, it has been estimated that between 27% and 30% of adults have systolic and/or diastolic blood pressures higher than 140/90 mm Hg (Kearney, Whelton, Reynolds, Whelton, & He, 2004). Untreated hypertension or subtherapeutic treatment of hypertension increases the risk of stroke, cerebral hemorrhage, heart failure (HF), coronary heart disease (CHD), and renal failure. Risk factors for essential hypertension include family history, race (most common in African Americans), anatomic variation in vasculature, stress, obesity, a high dietary intake of saturated fats or sodium, the use of tobacco or hormonal contraceptives, sedentary lifestyle, and aging. The role of nursing is important not only in the direct care of clients with hypertension but even more so in the prevention and management of the condition through client education.

LEARNING OBJECTIVES

- Describe the physiologic control of blood pressure.
- Define hypertension using criteria established by the Joint National Committee on Detection, Evaluation, and Treatment of High Blood Pressure.
- Describe the stepped-care approach used in drug therapy for hypertension.
- Discuss the special considerations for antihypertensive drug therapy: sexual dysfunction, concerns with children, older adults, pregnant clients, or surgical clients.
- Define the six major categories of antihypertensive drugs: diuretics, adrenergic inhibitors, vasodilators, angiotensin-converting enzyme inhibitors, angiotensin II receptor antagonists, and calcium channel blockers.
- Identify the mechanism of action, pharmacokinetics, adverse effects, interactions, and dosages of commonly used antihypertensive drugs.
- Implement nursing management of clients receiving antihypertensive drug therapy.

▲ KEY TERMS

angiotensin-converting enzyme (ACE) inhibitors, p. 555
angiotensin II receptor blockers (ARBs), p. 557
baroreceptor reflex, p. 543
calcium channel blockers (CCBs), p. 558
diuretics, p. 550
hypertension, p. 542
peripheral vascular resistance, p. 558

★ KEY DRUGS

captopril, p. 556
clonidine, p. 563
hydralazine, p. 569
hydrochlorothiazide, p. 551
losartan, p. 557
nifedipine, p. 559
nitroprusside, p. 571
prazosin, p. 568

Continued

541

✱ What is hypertension?

Hypertension is defined as an elevated systolic blood pressure, diastolic blood pressure, or both. Historically, hypertension has been defined as consistently elevated blood pressure above 140 mm Hg systolic or 90 mm Hg diastolic. The classification for adult hypertension has been refined by the Seventh Report of the Joint National Committee on Prevention, Detection, Evaluation, and Treatment of High Blood Pressure (JNC VII) (2003), U.S. Department of Health and Human Services and is presented in Table 27-1.

The number of persons with the silent killer hypertension is alarming. Although this condition seems relatively harmless, it severely damages major body organs. According to JNC-VII, 30% of individuals with hypertension are unaware of their condition, and only one third of those are adequately controlled (Chobanian, Bakris, & Black, 2003). The need for improving medical care for clients with hypertension is apparent, because cardiovascular disease remains the number one cause of death in North America.

Hypertension can also be classified according to etiology. In approximately 90% of cases, hypertension is considered **primary hypertension** (also referred to idiopathic or essential) because the cause is unknown. **Secondary hypertension** is related to an identifiable cause in which treatment is directed toward correcting the underlying cause. Box 27-1 outlines causes of secondary hypertension.

✱ How is blood pressure maintained?

Blood pressure (BP) is a function of cardiac output and peripheral vascular resistance as outlined below:

Blood pressure (mean arterial pressure) =
    Cardiac output × Peripheral vascular resistance

Cardiac output = Stroke volume × Heart rate

TABLE 27-1 CLASSIFICATION AND MANAGEMENT OF BP FOR ADULTS PER JNC VII*

BP Classification	Systolic Blood Pressure (mm Hg)*	Diastolic Blood Pressure (mm Hg)*	Lifestyle modification	Initial Drug Therapy	
				Without Compelling Indication	**With Compelling Indications**
Normal	<120	and <80	Encourage	No antihypertensive drug indicated.	Drug(s) for compelling indications.†
Prehypertension	120-139	or 80-89	Yes		
Stage 1 Hypertension	140-159	or 90-99	Yes	Thiazide-type diuretics for most. May consider ACEI, ARB, BB, CCB, or combination	Drug(s) for the compelling indications.† Other antihypertensive drugs (diuretics, ACEI, ARB, BB, CCB) as needed.
Stage 2 Hypertension	≥160	or ≥100	Yes	Two-drug combination for most‡ (usually thiazide-type diuretic and ACEI or ARB or BB or CCB).	

Modified from Chobanian, A., Bakris, G.L., Black H.R., et al. and the National High Blood Pressure Education Program Coordinating Committee. (2003). *The Seventh Report of the Joint National Committee on Prevention, Detection, Evaluation, and Treatment of High Blood Pressure: The JNC 7 Report.* Retrieved July 3, 2005, from http://www.nhlbi.nih.gov/guidelines/hypertension/jncintro.htm.
ACEI, angiotensin converting enzyme inhibitor; *ARB,* angiotensin receptor blocker; *BB,* β adrenergic blocker; *CCB,* calcium channel blocker.
*Treatment determined by highest BP category.
†Initial combined therapy should be used cautiously in those at risk for orthostatic hypotension.
‡Treat clients with chronic kidney disease or diabetes to BP goal of <130/80 mm Hg.

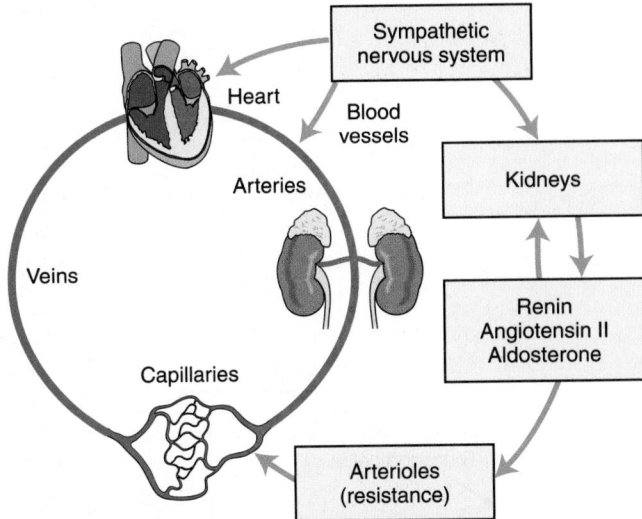

FIGURE 27-1 Blood pressure control mechanisms.

Control of BP involves a complex interaction between the nervous, hormonal, and renal systems; all play a part in regulating arterial BP (Figures 27-1 and 27-2). The body has two primary mechanisms to control BP:

- Adrenergic nervous system or baroreceptor reflex—a rapid-acting system
- Renin-angiotensin-aldosterone (RAA) mechanism—a long-acting system

Adrenergic Nervous System

The adrenergic or sympathetic nervous system uses a reflex mechanism, the **baroreceptor reflex**, to maintain BP. Baroreceptors are nerve endings located in the walls of the internal carotid arteries and the aortic arch. These sensory receptors rapidly respond to changes in BP. Any elevation in pressure stretches the receptors, which causes an impulse to be transmitted along the afferent neuron (vagus nerve) to the vasomotor center in the brainstem. The vasomotor cen-

ter responds to the impulse by causing the following two reactions: (1) a decrease in heart rate and force of myocardial contraction, which lowers cardiac output; and (2) vasodilation of peripheral vessels, which decreases total peripheral resistance. The subsequent reduction in BP is attributed to the reflex activity of the baroreceptor reflex.

When BP is low, this information is projected to the vasomotor center, which then activates sympathetic nerves. Two hormones, norepinephrine (primarily at the effector organ synapse) and epinephrine (primarily in a release from the adrenal medulla), mediate the sympathetic nervous system response. Norepinephrine acts mainly on α-adrenergic receptors (located in the arterioles), whereas epinephrine acts on both α- and β-adrenergic receptors. Stimulation of α receptors produces vasoconstriction, and BP is increased. Stimulation of β_1-adrenergic receptors in the heart increases both the heart rate and the force of myocardial contraction, thereby indirectly elevating BP.

Because it produces dilation of skeletal muscle blood vessels, epinephrine does not cause any increase in peripheral resistance. However, epinephrine does produce a considerable increase in heart rate and force of myocardial contraction; this elevation in cardiac output indirectly raises BP.

The baroreceptor reflex functions as a rapidly acting system for short-term control of low and high BP. It has been demonstrated that the rate of baroreceptor firing diminishes over a prolonged period, even if the BP remains elevated. Therefore it has been speculated that in hypertension these receptors are "reset" to maintain a higher level of BP.

Renin-Angiotensin-Aldosterone Mechanism

The **renin-angiotensin-aldosterone (RAA) mechanism** regulates BP by increasing or decreasing the blood volume through kidney function (Figure 27-3). The initiating factor is renin, an enzyme secreted from the juxtaglomerular cells

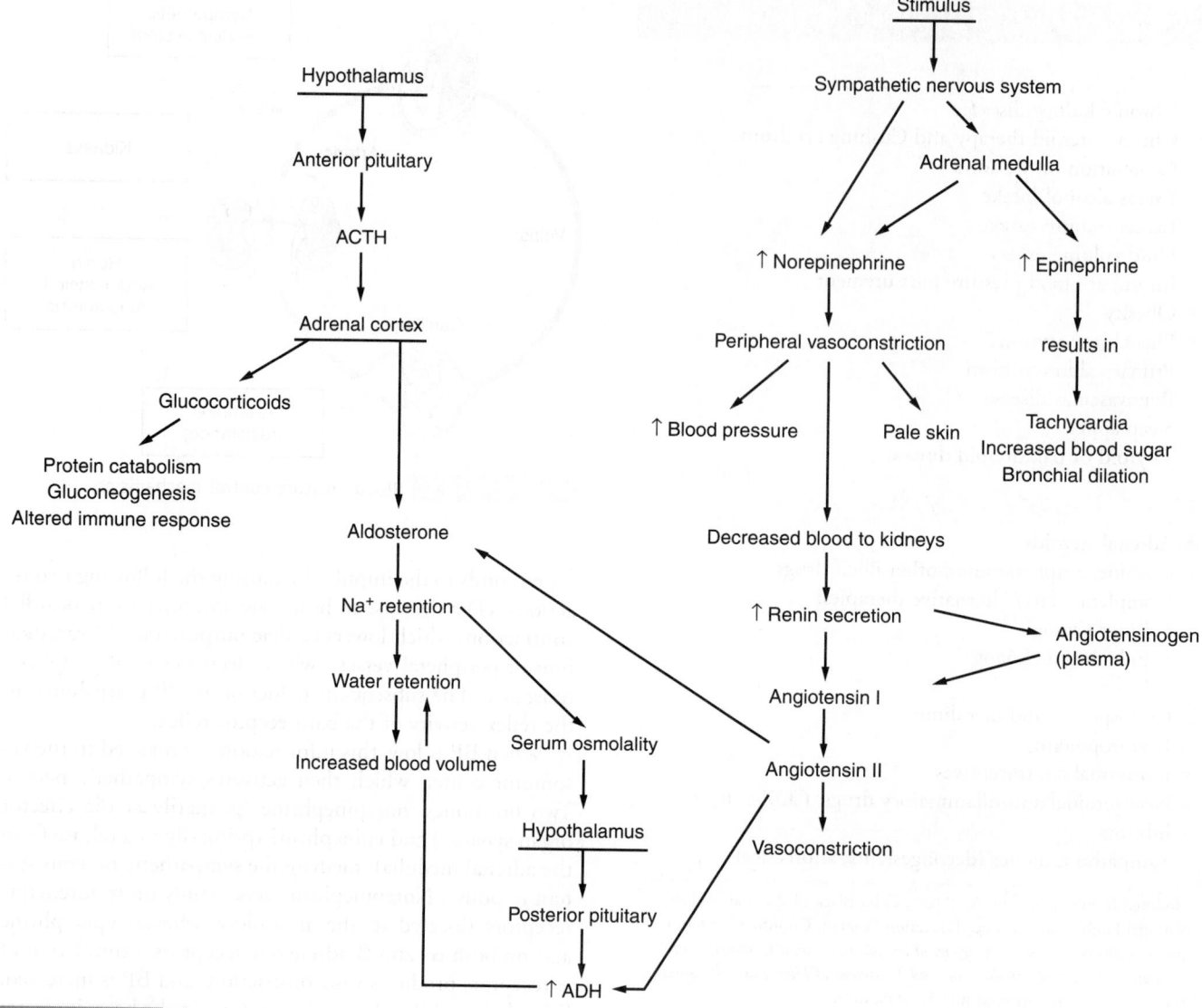

Physiologic control of blood pressure.

located in the afferent arteriolar walls of the nephron. When blood flow through the kidneys is reduced, renal arterial pressure is reduced; this causes the release of renin into the circulation. Renin catalyzes the cleavage of a plasma protein to form angiotensin I, a weak vasoconstrictor. In the small vessels of the lung, angiotensin I is converted by angiotensin-converting enzyme (ACE) to angiotensin II.

Angiotensin II is one of the most potent vasoconstrictors known. It is particularly effective in constricting arterioles, which increases peripheral resistance and raises BP. Additionally, angiotensin II acts on the adrenal cortex to stimulate the secretion of aldosterone, a hormone that promotes sodium reabsorption by the kidneys. The increased sodium elevates the osmotic pressure in the plasma, causing a release of antidiuretic hormone from the posterior pituitary. Angiotensin II acts on the kidney tubules to promote reabsorption of water.

The RAA system involves slow adjustments to changes in fluid volume. Excessive fluid retention is controlled by the negative-feedback mechanism operating within this system so that fluid balance is restored to a normal level. The kidneys are by far the most important organs in the body for long-term regulation of BP. When the operation of the urinary system fails, increased peripheral resistance and retention of fluid volume produces a combination of hypertensive effects, which keep BP constantly elevated.

Knowledge of the normal mechanisms for BP control has led to the development of the pharmacologic agents. For example, β-blocking agents suppress renin release, and ACE inhibitors prevent the conversion of angiotensin I to angiotensin II. The mechanisms of action for the antihypertensive agents are reviewed in this chapter. Figure 27-4 is a diagram of the sites of action of the various antihypertensive drugs in relation to cardiac output and peripheral vascular resistance.

✳ **T.S. is a 5' 8" 195 pound, 48-year-old male in general good health who presents to his health care provider with a BP of 158/105 mm Hg.**

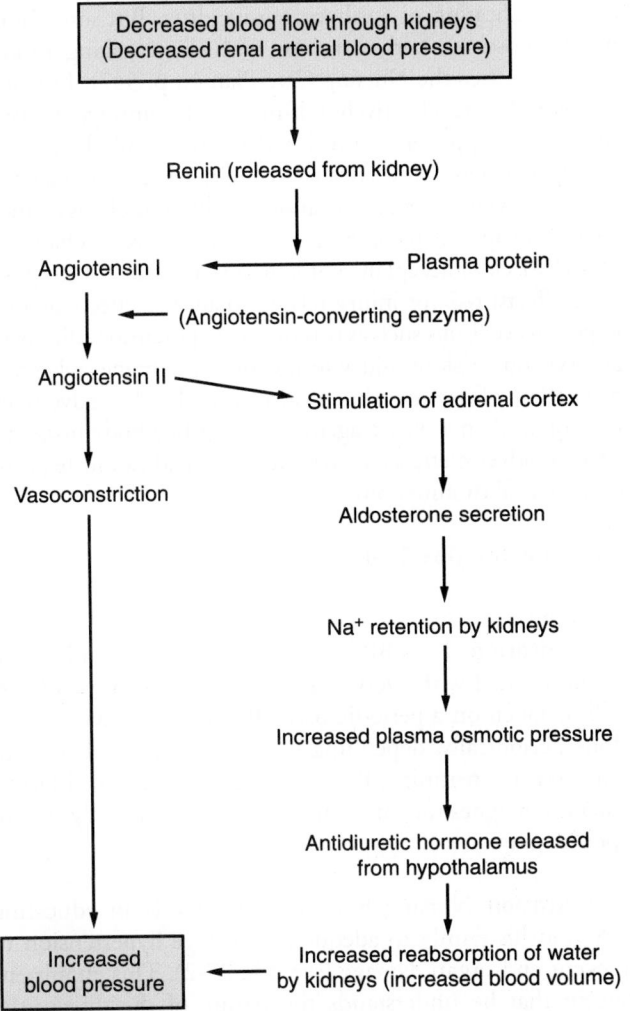

FIGURE 27-3 The renin-angiotensin-aldosterone (RAA) system.

Blood Pressure	=	Cardiac Output	X	Total Peripheral Resistance
		β-Blockers		ACE Inhibitors
				ARBs
				α-Blockers
				α₂-Agonists
		CCBs*		CCBs
		Diuretics		Diuretics
				Sympatholytics
*Non-dihydropyridine CCBs				Vasodilators

FIGURE 27-4 Sites of action of antihypertensive drugs.

BOX 27-2 TARGET ORGAN DAMAGE WITH UNCONTROLLED HYPERTENSION

- Heart
  - Left ventricular (LV) hypertrophy
  - Angina
  - Heart failure
- Brain
  - Stroke or transient ischemic attack
- Chronic kidney disease
- Peripheral arterial disease
- Retinopathy

Modified from Chobanian, A., Bakris, G.L., Black H.R., et al. and the National High Blood Pressure Education Program Coordinating Committee. (2003). *The Seventh Report of the Joint National Committee on Prevention, Detection, Evaluation, and Treatment of High Blood Pressure: The JNC 7 Report*. Retrieved July 3, 2005, from http://www.nhlbi.nih.gov/guidelines/hypertension/jncintro.htm.

What are the risks associated with elevated BP for T.S.?

Uncontrolled hypertension significantly increases risk for multiple organ damage (referred to as target organ damage) including heart disease, renal disease, risk for cerebrovascular accident (CVA) and eye damage (Box 27-2). Individuals with preexisting diabetes mellitus (DM) are at the highest risk for target organ damage with uncontrolled hypertension. Other factors that increase risk for target organ damage include smoking, high blood cholesterol or lipids, and family history of heart disease. Low levels of albumin in the urine often suggest increased risk of hypertension and renal disease in both those with diabetes mellitus and those who do not have diabetes mellitus (Wang et al., 2005) (Box 27-3).

How should T.S.'s blood pressure be assessed and managed?

Assessment Careful assessment of BP is important to establish the diagnosis and identify factors that adversely influence BP. The diagnosis of hypertension is based on obtaining two or more measured BP readings on each of two or more visits. Assessment should be carefully obtained with

---

BOX 27-3 FACTORS THAT INCREASE CARDIOVASCULAR RISK

- Hypertension*
- Cigarette smoking
- Obesity (BMI greater than or equal to 30)*
- Physical inactivity
- Dyslipidemia*
- Diabetes mellitus*
- Microalbuminuria or estimated glomerular filtration rate (GFR) less than 60 mL/min
- Age (greater than 55 years for men, greater than 65 years for women)
- Family history of premature cardiovascular disease (men less than 55 years or women less than 65 years)

Modified from Chobanian, A., Bakris, G.L., Black H.R., et al. and the National High Blood Pressure Education Program Coordinating Committee. (2003). *The Seventh Report of the Joint National Committee on Prevention, Detection, Evaluation, and Treatment of High Blood Pressure: The JNC 7 Report*. Retrieved July 3, 2005, from http://www.nhlbi.nih.gov/guidelines/hypertension/jncintro.htm.
*Components of the metabolic syndrome.

properly calibrated equipment and with the arm at heart level while the client is in the seated position and has been sitting quietly for 5 minutes.

Some clients will experience an elevation in BP in a hospital or office setting, which may not reflect typical BP readings. This is often referred to as "white coat hypertension." If white coat hypertension is suspected, ambulatory or self-monitored BPs may help establish a more accurate baseline BP. (See the Evidence-Based Practice for Nursing box below).

T.S.'s assessment begins with a thorough health history and physical examination. Although T.S. indicates he is in good health, hypertension is known as a "silent killer" because of the lack of client-perceived symptoms. The purpose of the assessment is to determine any underlying causes of hypertension (see Box 27-1), to establish a baseline clinical assessment, and to ensure the safety of the drug regimen. Blood pressure, pulse, heart sounds, breath sounds, respiratory rate and rhythm, and weight are documented and laboratory values that indicate fluid and electrolyte imbalances (serum creatinine, blood urea nitrogen [BUN], potassium, sodium, chloride, calcium, magnesium, and urinalysis with specific gravity), and a lipid profile. Some issues of health status (e.g., pregnancy in a female client or age) or preexisting illness may contraindicate the use of a certain drug or require specific monitoring in the cautious use of a drug.

Nursing Diagnosis Every client's response to medication has the potential to be unique for that client and each medication has expected responses that will be discussed with each classification of antihypertensive drug. But some nursing diagnoses are fairly common with clients taking antihypertensives (see the Nursing Care Plan on p. 547). In working with T.S. to effectively self-manage his antihypertensive therapy, the appropriate nursing diagnoses would be the following: deficient knowledge related to newly prescribed or altered antihypertensive medication and lifestyle changes; ineffective therapeutic regimen management related to change of lifestyle, lack of acceptance of hypertensive state, or drug adverse effects; risk for injury related to adverse effects of antihypertensive drugs such as orthostatic hypotension, dizziness, and syncope; risk of injury to mucous membranes related to drug effect of dry mouth; constipation related to adverse effects of antihypertensive agents; or disturbed body image related to adverse effects of hypertension medication (e.g., fatigue, sexual dysfunction).

Planning See Box 27-4.

Implementation

Monitoring T.S.'s BP, heart and lung sounds, and weight are monitored with every visit. Electrocardiograms (ECGs) will be taken on a periodic basis. Blood studies will also be done periodically, depending on T.S.'s status, and may include serum creatinine, BUN, potassium, sodium, chloride, calcium, magnesium, and a lipid profile; and urinalysis with specific gravity.

Education Nursing has an essential role in educating T.S. and his family to adequately manage hypertension to prevent end-organ damage (see Box 27-2). This entails ensuring that he understands the nature of the disease, its symptoms and treatment, and the importance of complying with the therapies. It may difficult for him to accept that there is no cure for hypertension and that lifestyle changes will need to be life-long and will probably also include drug therapy. Lifestyle adjustments, including diet and exercise are key first steps for all clients, and may serve to reduce systolic BP by up to 20 mm Hg (Table 27-2).

Aggressive control of hypertension is necessary to reduce cardiovascular morbidity and mortality. Box 27-5 lists key points from the JNC-VII report. Although lifestyle changes may improve T.S.'s BP and reduce his risk for cardiovascular morbidity, it is often difficult for clients to adopt these changes long term without significant motivation and support. In most cases, clients will require drug therapy if BP remains above 140/90 mm Hg.

Sources of health information are available online. See the Technology Link box in Chapter 25, p. 519.

✱ **T.S. returns to clinic in 2 weeks and his BP remains elevated at 155/102 mm Hg. He is encouraged to lose weight, exercise, and has an evaluation of his lipid profile to reduce his cardiovascular risk. One week later, he is walking every day, has tried to change his diet, and has lost 2 pounds. His BP is modestly improved at 150/98 mm Hg.**

⁘ Evidence-Based Practice

Home BP monitoring is a useful practice to assist clients to manage their hypertension more effectively.

Cappuccio, Kerry, and Donald (2004) reviewed the literature on home blood pressure monitoring from 1966 to January 2003 on Medline, 1980 to January 2003 on Embase, and other databases for randomized controlled trials of home or self BP monitoring in people with hypertension. Eighteen trials were identified that compared BP control. In total, 1359 people were randomized to home or self BP monitoring and 1355 to a control group of BP monitoring by health professionals in clinical settings. This meta-analysis found that "self" BP monitoring results in better BP control and greater achievement of BP targets than "usual" BP monitoring in the health care system. The difference in BP control between the two methods is small but likely to contribute to an important reduction in vascular complications in the hypertensive population.

Data from Cappuccio, F.P., Kerry, S.M., & Donald, A. (2004). Blood pressure control by home monitoring: meta-analysis of randomized trials. *British Medical Journal*, 329(7464):145.

NURSING CARE PLAN SELECTED NURSING DIAGNOSES RELATED TO ANTIHYPERTENSIVE THERAPY

Nursing Diagnosis	Outcome Criteria	Nursing Interventions
Deficient knowledge related to newly prescribed or altered antihypertensive drug therapy	• Client will describe hypertension; how drug therapy relates to condition; how and when to take medications; common drug interactions, particularly with OTC drugs; safety precautions; common adverse effects and which are reportable; and storage requirements of drugs. • Client will monitor effectiveness of drug therapy with sequential blood pressure readings.	• Assess learning needs and learning readiness. • Plan with client and family for achievement of realistic goals. • Provide information to meet outcome criteria.
Ineffective therapeutic regimen management	• Client will self-administer medications safely and accurately.	• Check refill frequency to determine adherence to the medication regimen. • Explore with client reasons for noncompliance and take appropriate teaching/counseling interventions. • Provide needed drug information concerning rationales for the specific client's hypertensive status. • Emphasize that drug therapy controls but does not cure hypertension, and emphasize the possible need for life-long therapy. • Discuss possibility of rebound hypertension with noncompliance to the medication regimen.
Sexual dysfunction related to antihypertensive drug therapy	• Client will describe the nature of dysfunction, consult with the prescriber for dosage reduction or drug substitution, and resume sexual activity.	• Assess for causative factors. • Encourage client to share concerns. • Provide health teaching and referrals when needed. • Encourage a return to sexual activity.

BOX 27-4 CLIENT GOALS FOR ANTIHYPERTENSIVE DRUG THERAPY

All clients and family/caregivers, within their physical and cognitive abilities should be able to do the following:
• Describe the nature of hypertension, the rationale of drug therapy in relation to the disease, the use of the specific medication, its adverse effects, and appropriate dosing.
• State the adverse effects of the drug and practices interventions to minimize or prevent risk of injury related to those effects.
• Maintain a BP diary and have the requisite knowledge, skills, and equipment to self-monitor health status (access to scale and BP equipment and records periodic BPs,

weights) and any drug adverse effects that may occur (e.g., orthostasis, sexual dysfunction, altered bowel patterns, activity intolerance).
• Effectively maintain the therapeutic regimen (e.g., changes positions slowly, moderate exercise, weight loss if required, DASH diet).
• Meet regularly and collaborate actively with health care personnel to manage his illness and drug regimen.
• Remain adherent and progress satisfactorily toward his expected outcome criteria (see evaluation).

TABLE 27-2 LIFESTYLE MODIFICATIONS FOR THE TREATMENT OF HYPERTENSION*†

Modification	Recommendation	Approximate SBP Reduction (Range)
Weight reduction	Maintain normal body weight (body mass index 18.5-24.9 kg/m^2).	5-20 mm Hg/10 kg weight loss
Adopt DASH eating plan	Consume a diet rich in fruits, vegetables, and low-fat dairy products with a reduced content of saturated and total fat.	8-14 mm Hg
Dietary sodium reduction	Reduce dietary sodium intake to no more than 100 mmol per day (2.4 g sodium or 6 g sodium chloride).	2-8 mm Hg
Physical activity	Engage in regular aerobic physical activity such as brisk walking (at least 30 min per day, most days of the week).	4-9 mm Hg
Moderation of alcohol consumption	Limit consumption to no more than 2 drinks (1 oz or 30 mL ethanol; e.g., 24 oz beer, 10 oz wine, or 3 oz 80-proof whiskey) per day in most men and to no more than 1 drink per day in women and lighter weight persons.	2-4 mm Hg
Stress reduction	Practice of yoga, meditation, and biofeedback on a regular basis	Systolic 1-13 mm Hg Diastolic 6-8 mm Hg

Modified from Chobanian, A., Bakris, G.L., Black H.R., et al. and the National High Blood Pressure Education Program Coordinating Committee. (2003). *The Seventh Report of the Joint National Committee on Prevention, Detection, Evaluation, and Treatment of High Blood Pressure: The JNC 7 Report.* Retrieved July 3, 2005, from http://www.nhlbi.nih.gov/guidelines/hypertension/jncintro.htm. *DASH,* Dietary Approaches to Stop Hypertension.
*For overall cardiac risk reduction, stop smoking.
†The effects of implementing these modifications are dose- and time-dependent, and could be greater for some individuals.

BOX 27-5 KEY POINTS FROM SEVENTH REPORT OF THE JOINT NATIONAL COMMITTEE ON PREVENTION, DETECTION, EVALUATION, AND TREATMENT OF HIGH BLOOD PRESSURE

- For individuals greater than 50 years old, systolic BP greater than 140 mm Hg is significantly greater cardiovascular risk factor than elevated diastolic pressure.
- Each 20 mm Hg rise in systolic BP or 10 mm Hg rise is diastolic BP above 115/75 mm Hg doubles cardiovascular disease risk.
- Individuals who are normotensive at 55 years old have a 90% lifetime risk for developing hypertension.
- Systolic BP of 120 to 139 mm Hg or diastolic BP of 80 to 89 mm Hg is now considered prehypertensive and clients with BP in this range should receive lifestyle modifications to prevent cardiovascular disease.
- BPs above 140/90 mm Hg (or 130/80 mm Hg for those with diabetes or chronic renal disease) require drug therapy.

- Most individuals with hypertension will require two or more drugs to achieve adequate blood pressure control.
- Thiazide diuretics remain the drugs of choice for uncomplicated hypertension with the use of other drug classes dependent on comorbidities or other compelling indications.
- Client motivation is key to successful control of blood pressure.

Modified from Chobanian, A., Bakris, G.L., Black H.R., et al. and the National High Blood Pressure Education Program Coordinating Committee. (2003). *The Seventh Report of the Joint National Committee on Prevention, Detection, Evaluation, and Treatment of High Blood Pressure: The JNC 7 Report.* Retrieved July 3, 2005, from http://www.nhlbi.nih.gov/guidelines/hypertension/jncintro.htm.

✳ What is the role of drug therapy in the treatment of hypertension?

Most clients with hypertension do not achieve goal blood pressures with lifestyle changes alone and often require more than one drug to reach and maintain blood pressures below 140/90 mm Hg (or below 130/80 mm Hg for individuals with DM or chronic renal disease). Antihypertensive drug therapy reduces stroke incidence by 35% to 40%, reduces the

risk for a myocardial infarction by 20% to 25% and lowers the risk of heart failure by over 50% (Chobanian et al., 2003).

JNC VII recommends thiazide diuretics as first line drug therapy for uncomplicated hypertension. Other drugs used in the management of hypertension include the angiotensin converting enzyme (ACE) inhibitors (ACEIs), angiotensin II receptor blockers (ARBs), β-adrenergic blockers, and calcium channel blockers (CCBs). Table 27-3 lists common

TABLE 27-3 COMMONLY USED ORAL DRUGS FOR THE TREATMENT OF HYPERTENSION

Class	Drug (Trade Name)	Usual Oral Adult Dose*
Thiazide diuretics	chlorothiazide (Diuril)	125-500 mg once daily
	chlorthalidone (generic)	12.5-25 mg once daily
	hydrochlorothiazide (Microzide, HydroDIURIL†)	12.5-50 mg once daily
	indapamide (Lozol†)	1.25-2.5 mg once daily
	metolazone (Zaroxolyn)	2.5-5 mg once daily
Loop diuretics	bumetanide (Bumex†)	0.5-2 mg twice daily
	furosemide (Lasix†)	20-80 mg one to two times daily
	torsemide (Demadex†)	2.5-10 mg once daily
Potassium-sparing diuretics	amiloride (Midamor†)	5-10 mg once daily
	triamterene (Dyrenium)	50-100 mg twice daily
Aldosterone receptor blockers	eplerenone (Inspra)	50 mg one to two times daily
	spironolactone (Aldactone†)	25-50 mg one to two times daily
β blockers	atenolol (Tenormin†)	25-100 mg once daily
	betaxolol (Kerlone†)	5-20 mg once daily
	bisoprolol (Zebeta†)	2.5-10 mg once daily
	metoprolol (Lopressor†)	50-100 mg twice daily
	metoprolol extended release (Toprol XL)	50-100 mg once daily
	nadolol (Corgard†)	40-120 mg once daily
	propranolol (Inderal†)	20-160 mg twice daily
	propranolol long-acting (Inderal LA†)	60-180 mg once daily
	timolol (Blocadren†)	10-30 mg twice daily
β blockers with intrinsic sympathomimetic activity	acebutolol (Sectral†)	200-800 mg twice daily
	penbutolol (Levatol)	20-40 mg once daily
	pindolol (generic)	5-30 mg twice daily
Combined α and β blockers	carvedilol (Coreg)	6.25-25 mg twice daily
	labetalol (Normodyne, Trandate†)	100-400 mg twice daily
ACE inhibitors	benazepril (Lotensin†)	10-40 mg one to two times daily
	captopril (Capoten†)	25-100 mg twice daily
	enalapril (Vasotec†)	2.5-20 mg one to two times daily
	fosinopril (Monopril)	10-40 mg once daily
	lisinopril (Prinivil, Zestril†)	10-40 mg once daily
	moexipril (Univasc)	7.5-30 mg once daily
	perindopril (Aceon)	4 mg one to two times daily
	quinapril (Accupril)	10-80 mg once daily
	ramipril (Altace)	2.5-20 mg once daily
	trandolapril (Mavik)	1-4 mg once daily
Angiotensin II receptor blockers (ARBs)	candesartan (Atacand)	8-32 mg once daily
	eprosartan (Tevetan)	400-800 mg daily; may be given in two divided doses
	irbesartan (Avapro)	150-300 mg once daily
	losartan (Cozaar)	25-50 mg daily; maximum dosage 100 mg in one or two divided doses
	olmesartan (Benicar)	20-40 mg once daily
	telmisartan (Micardis)	20-80 mg once daily
	valsartan (Diovan)	80-320 mg once daily

Modified from Chobanian, A., Bakris, G.L., Black H.R., et al. and the National High Blood Pressure Education Program Coordinating Committee. (2003). *The Seventh Report of the Joint National Committee on Prevention, Detection, Evaluation, and Treatment of High Blood Pressure: The JNC 7 Report.* Retrieved July 3, 2005, from http://www.nhlbi.nih.gov/guidelines/hypertension/jncintro.htm.

* These dosages may vary from those listed in the "Physicians' Desk Reference."

† Are now or will soon become available in generic preparations.

‡ A 0.1 mg dose may be given every other day to achieve this dosage.

Continued

TABLE 27-3 COMMONLY USED ORAL DRUGS FOR THE TREATMENT OF HYPERTENSION—CONT'D

Class	Drug (Trade Name)	Usual Oral Adult Dose
Calcium channel blockers—Nondihydropyridines	diltiazem extended release (Cardizem CD, Dilacor XR, Tiazac†)	180-420 mg once daily
	diltiazem extended release (Cardizem LA)	120-540 mg once daily
	verapamil immediate release (Calan, Isoptin†)	80-120 mg three times daily
	verapamil long-acting (Calan SR, Isoptin SR†)	180-240 mg one to two times daily
	verapamil—Coer (Covera HS)	180-480 mg once daily
	verapamil—Coer (Verelan PM)	200-400 mg once daily
CCBs—Dihydropyridines	amlodipine (Norvasc)	2.5-10 mg once daily
	felodipine (Plendil)	2.5-10 mg once daily
	isradipine (DynaCirc CR)	2.5-10 mg twice daily
	nicardipine sustained release (Cardene SR)	30-60 mg twice daily
	nifedipine long-acting (Adalat CC, Procardia XL)	30-60 mg once daily
	nisoldipine (Sular)	10-40 mg once daily
α_1 blockers§	doxazosin (Cardura)	1-16 mg once daily
	prazosin (Minipress†)	1-5 mg two to three times daily
	terazosin (Hytrin)	1-5 mg once daily
Central α_2 agonists and other centrally acting drugs	clonidine (Catapres†)	0.1-0.4 mg twice daily
	clonidine patch (Catapres-TTS)	0.1-0.3 mg/24 hr (one patch per week)
	methyldopa (Aldomet†)	125-500 mg twice daily
	reserpine (generic)	0.05‡-0.25 mg once daily
	guanfacine (generic)	1-3 mg once daily
Direct vasodilators	hydralazine (Apresoline†)	12.5-50 mg twice daily
	minoxidil (Loniten†)	2.5-20 mg one to two times daily

Modified from Chobanian, A., Bakris, G.L., Black H.R., et al. and the National High Blood Pressure Education Program Coordinating Committee. (2003). *The Seventh Report of the Joint National Committee on Prevention, Detection, Evaluation, and Treatment of High Blood Pressure: The JNC 7 Report.* Retrieved July 3, 2005, from http://www.nhlbi.nih.gov/guidelines/hypertension/jncintro.htm.
* These dosages may vary from those listed in the "Physicians' Desk Reference."
† Are now or will soon become available in generic preparations.
‡ A 0.1 mg dose may be given every other day to achieve this dosage.
§Not routinely recommended for the treatment of hypertension (see text).

agents available for oral drug therapy for the treatment of hypertension. Figure 27-5 lists the algorithm for treatment.

✱ **The prescriber for T.S. is considering starting hydrochlorothiazide therapy.**

✱ **What are the key points to consider with thiazide diuretics in the treatment of hypertension?**
Thiazide diuretic drugs play a vital role in lowering BP. The use of **diuretics,** agents that promote the formation and excretion of urine, results in a loss of excess salt and water from the body by renal excretion. The decrease in plasma and extracellular fluid volume subsequently depresses vascular reactivity to sympathetic stimulation. Thus volume depletion, plus the direct thiazide diuretic effect on the arterioles (which produces vasodilation), lowers the BP. This response causes an initial decline in cardiac output followed by a decrease in peripheral resistance and a lowering of BP (Figure 27-6).

When used in maximum therapeutic dosages, the **thiazides** and related sulfonamide diuretics (e.g., chlorthali-

done and hydrochlorothiazide) are effective in decreasing BP. They have also demonstrated efficacy in preventing complications of hypertension and may be more effective than ACE inhibitors and CCBs at preventing heart failure (ALLHAT, 2002). These mild diuretics can be used alone for individuals in the early stages of hypertension. In contrast, many of the other types of antihypertensive agents, when used alone on a long-term basis, cause a gradual retention of sodium and water and expansion of plasma fluid volume. Therefore a low-dose diuretic is often given in combination with vasodilators, or adrenergic inhibitors to prevent fluid retention.

Thiazide diuretics are synthetic agents chemically related to the sulfonamides. They inhibit sodium reabsorption in the early distal tubules in the nephron and work to promote the renal excretion of water, sodium, chloride, and magnesium. Potassium loss is also common with thiazides; this is related to sodium dependent changes in potassium excretion and corresponding effects on diuresis on plasma renin and aldosterone activity. Potassium excretion may be more

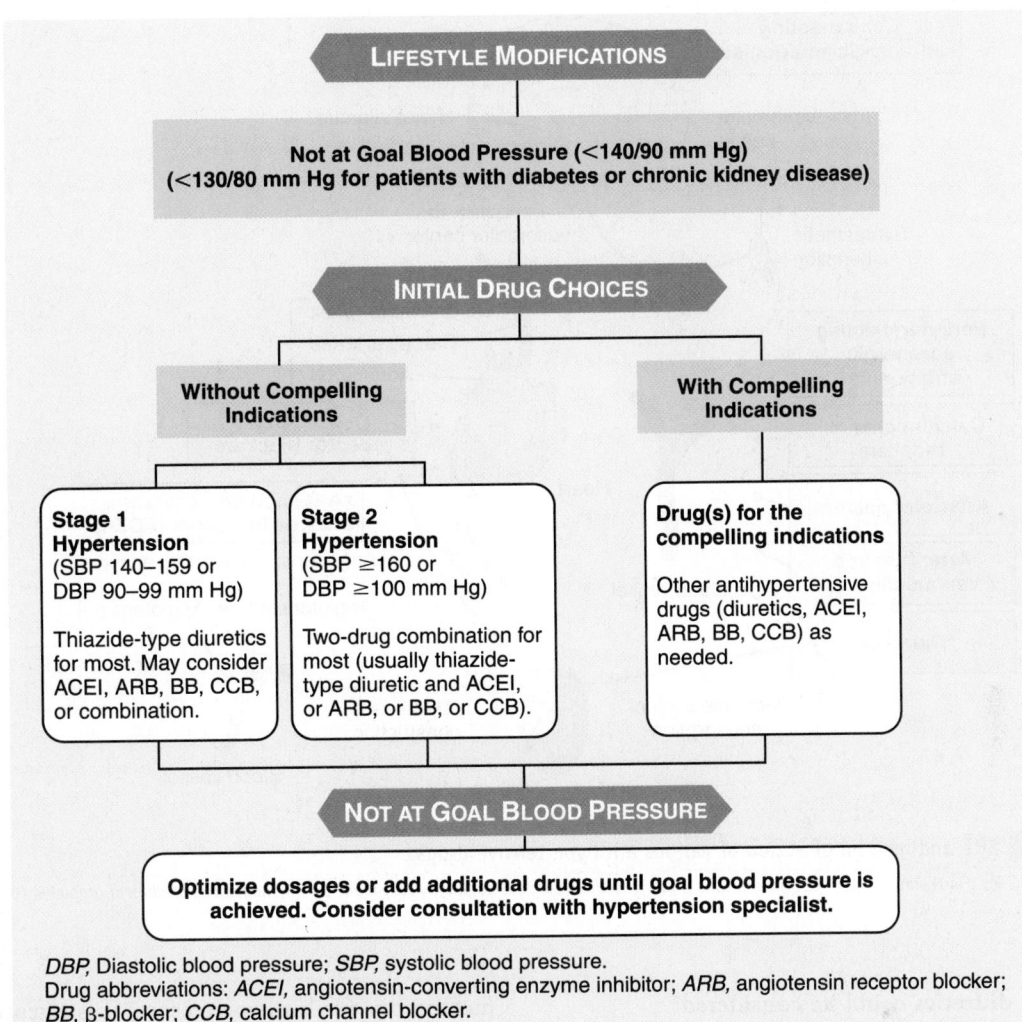

FIGURE 27-5 JNC-VII algorithm for the treatment of hypertension.

From Chobanian, A., Bakris, G.L., Black H.R., et al. and the National High Blood Pressure Education Program Coordinating Committee. (2003). *The Seventh Report of the Joint National Committee on Prevention, Detection, Evaluation, and Treatment of High Blood Pressure: The JNC 7 Report*. Retrieved July 3, 2005, from http://www.nhlbi.nih.gov/guidelines/hypertension/jncintro.htm.

pronounced early in treatment, or with larger doses. Increased serum levels of calcium, glucose, and uric acid are also observed with thiazide diuretics.

The mechanisms of antihypertensive action are believed to be initially because of the reduction in plasma and extracellular fluid volume, which results in a decrease in cardiac output. In time, the cardiac output returns to normal. Thiazide-type diuretics also decrease peripheral resistance by a direct action on the peripheral blood vessels. There are many different thiazide diuretics available including chlorothiazide (Diuril), chlorthalidone (Hygroton), and metolazone (Zaroxolyn). The classic thiazide diuretic is hydrochlorothiazide, which is briefly discussed in the following section.

✷⬛ hydrochlorothiazide [hye dro klor oh **thye** a zide]
(HydroDiuril, Esidrix, Apo-Hydro✚)

Indications
Indications for thiazide-type diuretics include treating hypertension, edema associated with HF, hepatic cirrhosis with ascites, and some types of renal impairment, such as nephrotic syndrome, acute glomerulonephritis, and chronic renal failure.

Pharmacokinetics/Dosing
Hydrochlorothiazide is reasonably well absorbed orally. The onset of diuretic action with hydrochlorothiazide is about 2 hours. It is eliminated in urine as unchanged drug. The typical adult dose for hydrochlorothiazide for hypertension is 12.5 to 25 mg once daily. Although doses as high as 200 mg daily have been used, doses above 50 mg generally do not produce increased response and are more likely to result in disturbances in electrolyte levels. Thiazide diuretics are not effective for individuals with severe renal impairment.

Adverse Effects
As with all diuretics, there is concern for orthostatic hypotension and dehydration, particularly in older adults. Hypokalemia is common and may be problematic with concurrent digoxin therapy. Other adverse effects include GI upset, elevated uric acid levels (potentially aggravating gout), and elevated lipid levels. Rarely, serious hypersensitivity reactions and bone marrow suppression have been observed. Hyperglycemia and impaired glucose tolerance has been reported, but is typically limited to older clients.

Drug Interactions
Thiazide-induced hypokalemia may predispose to digoxin-induced ventricular dysrhythmias. Concurrent administration with lithium may lead to lithium toxicity.

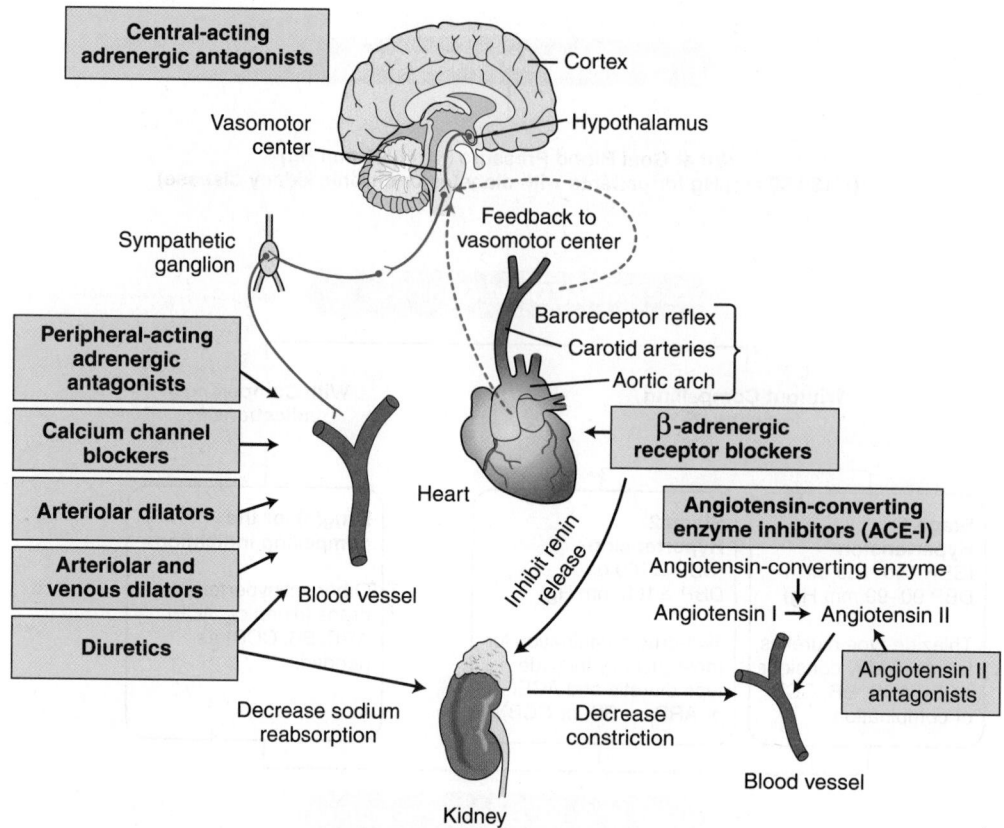

FIGURE 27-6 Site and method of action of various antihypertensive drugs.

Modified from Lewis, S.M., Heitkemper, M.M., & Dirksen, S.R. (2004). *Medical-surgical nursing: Assessment and management of clinical problems* (6th ed.). St. Louis: Mosby.

✳ **What other diuretics could be considered?**

The **potassium-sparing diuretic agents,** such as spironolactone (Aldactone), eplerenone (Inspra), and triamterene (Dyrenium), are useful in counteracting the potassium loss induced by other diuretics. They promote sodium and water loss without an accompanying loss of potassium. These drugs are indicated for the management of hyperaldosteronism and renal vascular hypertension when the client's condition is resistant to other diuretics. For the management of hypertension, they are most often they are used in combination with a thiazide to counteract the hypokalemic effects. Examples of common combinations are hydrochlorothiazide/triamterene (Dyazide, Maxzide) and hydrochlorothiazide/spironolactone (Aldactazide).

The loop diuretics such as furosemide (Lasix) and bumetanide (Bumex) are potent agents commonly used for edema and HF, but do not appear to be as effective in the long-term management of hypertension. See Chapter 33 for a more complete discussion of diuretics.

✳ **T.S. is begun on hydrochlorothiazide 25 mg daily in the morning. What monitoring and education is appropriate before and during therapy?**

Review and reinforcement of the nonpharmacologic interventions (see Table 27-2) would be universal for T.S. and all clients at every contact. Additionally, now that he is taking medications for his hypertension, it is essential for TS (or any client) to accomplish the goals in Box 27-4.

Implementation Implementation of the nursing process in drug therapy, which entails monitoring, interventions, and client education would be specific for each client and each medication.

Monitoring In addition to T.S.'s self-monitoring, review during each visit his BP diary and assess his BP, pulse, weight, respiratory rate, heart and breath sounds, any pedal edema, and his baseline laboratory studies that are repeated periodically. Serum potassium, blood glucose, and uric acid are monitored to detect hydrochlorothiazide-induced hypokalemia, hyperglycemia, and hyperuricemia respectively. Ask specifically for the incidence of medication adverse effects even if not described in his diary. Many clients are hesitant to mention constipation, sexual dysfunction, or other adverse effects as concerns.

Intervention Encourage T.S. to take the single daily dose of hydrochlorothiazide in the morning to minimize the effect of increased frequency of urinary frequency on sleep. T.S. may expect to have a modest diuretic effect within the 2 hours of dosing. Concurrent potassium may be indicated if T.S. is at risk for hypokalemia.

BOX 27-6 KEY POINTS OF INSTRUCTION FOR CLIENTS TAKING ANTIHYPERTENSIVE AGENTS

- Primary hypertension is a life long diagnosis. Lifestyle modifications (see Table 27-2) and/or prescribed medications will always need to be taken. Treatment is necessary to reduce morbidity and mortality; it will control but not cure the disease.
- Clients should be able to verbalize an understanding of their disease and the relationship of their treatment to hypertension. Review the potential long-term consequences of nonadherence to their antihypertensive therapy and uncontrolled BP.
- Taking medication as prescribed is important, not omitting doses or doubling up on doses. Always maintain an adequate supply of medication. Take medication even if feeling better; abrupt discontinuation may result in rebound hypertension; see Box 27-9.
- Self-management of the therapeutic regimen is encouraged as much as possible. Teach clients to self-monitor BP, pulse, and weights and to document these findings to share with their health care provider. See the Evidence-Based Practice box on p. 546.
- Collaboration with the health care provider is essential. Attend scheduled visits to the provider for monitoring. Re-

port any adverse effects to the prescriber. Ask the prescriber for parameters for BP, pulse, and weight above or below and adverse effects that would need to be reported.
- Drug interactions, particularly OTC preparations for colds because of their vasoconstrictive properties that would elevate BP, or other medications that would elevate BP should be avoided. Ask the prescriber which OTC medications may be taken for coughs, colds and headache, or other discomforts.
- Informing all health care providers of his drug therapy and carrying a medical identification card with a list of all current medications (prescribed, OTC, and alternative/complementary medications that are commonly labeled as dietary supplements).
- Antihypertensives are to lower blood pressure. Each additional medication in the antihypertensive regimen increases the risk for orthostatic hypotension. To minimize this adverse effect, change position slowly from lying to sitting or standing, avoid alcohol ingestion, prolonged standing and strenuous exercising, and exercising during hot weather.

Education Providing T.S. with the knowledge, skills, and abilities to self-manage illness and its therapies will help to prevent or minimize any situational powerlessness or disturbance of his self-esteem and promote effective management of his therapeutic regimen. Box 27-6 presents key points for clients taking antihypertensive agents. With hydrochlorothiazide, alert T.S. that reportable symptoms would include the following: fatigue, mood changes, muscle cramps, irregular heartbeat (hypokalemia); confusion, irritability, muscle cramps (hyponatremia); unusual bruising or bleeding (thrombocytopenia); fever or chills, cough, painful urination, or other symptom of infection (agranulocytosis); and joint or lower back pain (gout). Other adverse effects are anorexia, sexual dysfunction, diarrhea or constipation, orthostatic hypotension, and photosensitivity.

T.S. should maintain a high-fiber diet, adequate fluid intake, and moderate exercise to avoid constipation; and avoid sunlight, particularly from 10 AM to 3 PM and tanning beds, and wear sunscreen to minimize the effects of photosensitivity.

Evaluation In evaluating the therapeutic effect of antihypertensive drug therapy for T.S., he should accomplish the evaluation criteria in Box 27-7.

✱ **T.S. returns to clinic every 2 weeks for the next 2 months. His serum potassium is 3.4 mEq/L and fasting blood glucose is at 90 mg/dL. His blood pressures are improved at 145/95 mm Hg, 148/92 mm Hg, 140/90 mm Hg, and 146/96 mm Hg. He uses an ambulatory**

BOX 27-7 EVALUATION CRITERIA FOR ANTIHYPERTENSIVE THERAPY

During antihypertensive therapy, the client should experience:
- An ability to comply with drug regimen and needed lifestyle changes.
- Improvement in BP, less than 140/90 mm Hg, (or 130/80 mm Hg for those with diabetes or chronic renal disease) without adverse effects (e.g., orthostatic hypotension, fatigue, dizziness).
- Absence of any symptoms of target organ disease, such as heart failure, stroke, kidney disease, and retinopathy; see Box 27-2.
- Effective management of therapeutic regimen: monitoring BP; maintaining journals of BP determinations and occurrence of adverse effects; attending follow-up visits; reporting appropriately to prescriber any weight gain (>1 kg/week) or edema; and normal nutritional status (limited sodium intake, diet high in fiber, adequate fluid intake, and avoidance of alcohol).

BP cuff at home twice weekly and obtains similar readings. He is somewhat adherent to diet and exercise and has lost an additional 4 pounds. Is this considered adequate management of hypertension?

T.S. displays a typical response to antihypertensive therapy with a moderate drop in BP. His serum potassium levels are modestly low secondary to the thiazide diuretic, and will be managed with increased dietary potassium sources (e.g., bananas, orange juice); see Box 27-8. His fasting glucose is within normal limits.

Unfortunately, he is not at a consistently adequate goal BP of less than 140/90 mm Hg. Although a higher dose of his current agent could be considered, most individuals do not obtain dramatic improvement in BP control at doses greater than 25 mg daily of hydrochlorothiazide. Like many clients, it appears that T.S. will require two or more drugs to achieve adequate BP control (Chobanian et al., 2003). Additional medications that could be added include β-adrenergic blocking drugs, ACE inhibitors, ARBs, or CCBs.

✱ **The prescriber is considering adding a β-adrenergic blocker to the regimen for T.S.**

✱ **What considerations are appropriate for the use of β-adrenergic blockers in the management of hypertension?**

β blocking agents decrease cardiac output and inhibit renin secretion, which result in a lowering of BP. By competing with epinephrine for available β receptor sites, they inhibit the typical organ or tissue response to β stimulation. Because β-adrenergic blocking agents may have multiple effects, a review of concurrent drugs and conditions is appropriate before initiating β-blocker therapy. Use of a cardioselective agent (e.g., atenolol, metoprolol) over a nonselective agent (e.g., propranolol, nadolol) is likely to be better tolerated.

β blockers, although long considered first line agents for hypertension, may not be best first choices for everyone. Black clients appear less or nonresponsive to the BP lowering effects of these agents (Brewster, van Montfrans, & Kleijnen, 2004). In late 2004, an analysis of earlier studies

comparing atenolol to other antihypertensives noted that atenolol was no more effective at lowering BP, and was associated with higher mortality and stroke rates compared with other antihypertensive therapy (Carlberg, Samuelsson, & Lindholm, 2004). The use of labetalol (Normodyne, Trandate) is usually limited to severe hypertension or hypertensive crisis because it acts as an α_1-, β_1-, and β_2-adrenergic antagonist. A brief review of atenolol is presented here in the context of management of hypertension. Chapter 22 presents a more complete discussion of the β-adrenergic blocking agents.

atenolol [a **ten** oh lole]
(Tenormin, Apo-Atenol✱, Tenolin✱)
Atenolol is a competitive β_1 adrenergic antagonist with little action at β_2 receptors at low to moderate doses. Actions include reduced heart rate, reduced cardiac output, and inhibition of rennin secretion.

Indications
Atenolol is used for the treatment of hypertension and angina, and is an important part of drug management of myocardial infarction (MI). Unlabeled uses include migraine headache prophylaxis.

Pharmacokinetics/Dosing
Atenolol has a high first pass effect, which accounts for difference between oral and parenteral doses. Its half-life in adults with normal renal function is approximately 6 to 8 hours, and it has an antihypertensive effect for up to 24 hours. The typical oral dose for hypertension is 12.5 to 50 mg daily.

Adverse Effects
Like other β-adrenergic blockers, atenolol results in bradycardia, hypotension, and may contribute to dizziness, fatigue, lethargy, and impotence. Caution should be exercised for clients with HF and AV block because these conditions are often aggravated by β-adrenergic blockers. Many clients complain of reduced peripheral circulation. Although less likely than the noncardioselective β blockers, atenolol can result in bronchospasm and wheezing, particularly at high doses.

Drug Interactions
Concurrent dosing with other drugs that slow AV nodal conduction (e.g., digoxin, diltiazem, verapamil) can increase the risk for AV block. β blockers typically mask the symptoms of hypoglycemia (tachycardia, tremors, sweating) for clients on insulin or oral hypoglycemics.

Nursing Management
Alert T.S. to assess his ability to undertake physical exertion because of possible activity intolerance related to atenolol's adverse effects of fatigue and weakness. Teach T.S. to check his pulse before he takes his atenolol; if it is less than 50 bpm to withhold the atenolol and notify his prescriber. He should also alert his prescriber if he experiences any light-headedness, wheezing or shortness of breath, edema, sudden weight gain, or symptoms of depression or sexual dysfunction. See Chapter 22 for more details of nursing management.

✱ **T.S. is started on atenolol 25 mg daily with his hydrochlorothiazide. He checks his BP and pulse every 2 weeks and returns to clinic in 2 months with the following BP and pulse results: 135/82 mm Hg, pulse 60; 138/85 mm Hg, pulse 55; 130/80 mm Hg, pulse 65; 128/78 mm Hg, pulse 60. He has lost an additional 7 pounds and walks daily. His only complaint is that he has a lower libido and some difficulty in obtaining an erection.**

✱ **Is this effect common with atenolol?**

TABLE 27-4 PHARMACOKINETICS OF ACE INHIBITORS

Drug	Duration of Action	Active Metabolite	Usual Adult Dose
benazepril (Lotensin)	24 hours	benazeprilat	10-40 mg PO daily
captopril (Capoten)	6-12 hours		12.5 mg PO twice daily to 50 mg PO three times daily
enalapril (Vasotec)	24 hours	enalaprilat	5 mg PO daily to 20 mg PO twice daily
enalaprilat (Vasotec IV)	6-12 hours		0.625-5 mg IV q6h
fosinopril (Monopril)	24 hours	fosinoprilat	10-40 mg PO daily
lisinopril (Prinivil, Zestril)	24 hours		10-40 mg PO daily
moexipril (Univasc)	24 hours	moexiprilat	7.5 mg PO daily to 15 mg PO twice daily
perindopril (Aceon)	24 hours	peridoprilat	4-8 mg PO daily
quinapril (Accupril)	24 hours	quinaprilat	5 mg PO twice daily to 40 mg PO twice daily
ramipril (Altace)	24 hours	ramiprilat	2.5 mg PO daily to 10 mg PO twice daily
trandolapril (Mavik)	24 hours	trandolaprilat	1-4 mg PO daily

Sexual dysfunction is a common complication of many antihypertensive medications and may be manifested in males as decreased libido, impotence, impaired or retrograde ejaculation, and gynecomastia. In females it may be manifested as decreased libido, decreased vaginal lubrication, and inability to achieve orgasm. Such symptoms may lead to T.S.'s noncompliance with the drug regimen. The nature of the disorder and knowledge of the effects associated with different antihypertensive agents will assist in determining the cause of the symptoms. Agents that have an effect on the autonomic nervous system (e.g., β blockers and the centrally acting adrenergic inhibitors) are most often associated with sexual dysfunction. Only the ACE inhibitors or the ARBs are virtually devoid of this effect. If the sexual dysfunction becomes problematic, clients may become nonadherent to therapy. In such cases, switching to alternate therapy (e.g., ACE inhibitors or ARBs) is often required.

✹ **P.T. is a 63-year-old female who has been newly diagnosed with type 2 DM. At clinic, her BP is 138/85 mm Hg. Her prescriber is considering the addition of antihypertensive therapy. Why is P.T. being treated for hypertension? What therapies are recommended for her?**

Individuals with DM are at two to four times greater risk for cardiovascular events than nondiabetics. Of particular concern is the development of chronic renal failure, which is correlated with hypertension and albumin in the urine for clients with DM. Even mildly elevated blood pressures are correlated with increased risk for negative cardiovascular and renal outcomes (Prisant, 2003).

For individuals with DM, the ACE inhibitors and the ARBs have demonstrated the greatest reduction in target organ damage. They are considered the drugs of choice for individuals with hypertension and DM. ACE inhibitors in diabetes do not have biochemical adverse effects on glucose as other agents may. These agents are also recommended for individuals with concurrent HF and hypertension (see Chapter 25). ACE inhibitors have also been shown to reduce the risk for cerebrovascular events in clients with hypertension (Chobanian et al., 2003).

Angiotensin-converting enzyme (ACE) inhibitors competitively block the angiotensin I converting enzyme necessary for the conversion to angiotensin II. Angiotensin II is a powerful vasoconstrictor that raises BP and also causes the release of aldosterone, resulting in sodium and water retention. Thus the inhibition of ACE has a number of results. First, there is a decrease in vascular tone, thereby directly lowering BP. Second, the release of aldosterone is inhibited, which reduces sodium and water reabsorption. The resultant excretion of fluid is thought to cause only a secondary reduction in BP (a decrease in aldosterone secretion does lead to a slight elevation in serum potassium). Third, there is an increase in plasma renin activity, which is caused by a loss of negative feedback on renin release. (See Figures 27-2 and 27-3 for physiologic BP control and the RAA system.) Captopril (Capoten) is the key or prototype ACE inhibitor. Although the mode of action for each of the ACE inhibitors is similar, they differ in chemical structures. Early data is suggesting that these agents may not all have equal benefit in reducing cardiovascular complications (Pilote, Abrahamowicz, Rodrigues, Eisenberg, & Rahme, 2004), but additional data will be required. Table 27-4 presents a comparison of the pharmacokinetics of ACE inhibitors.

❋┏▪ captopril (**kap** toe pril)

(Capoten, Novo-Captopril✚)

Captopril competitively inhibits ACE, which results in reduced vaso-constriction, inhibition of aldosterone and reduced sodium and wa-ter retention.

Indications

ACE inhibitors are used alone or in combination with thiazide di-uretics or other antihypertensives to treat hypertension. It is also indicated for the treatment of HF, diabetic nephropathy, and left ventricular dysfunction after a myocardial infarction. Blacks appear to be less responsive to the antihypertensive effects of ACE inhibitor therapy (Brewster et al, 2004).

Pharmacokinetics/Dosing

Captopril is fairly well absorbed orally, but oral absorption is signifi-cantly reduced when dosed with food. (Other ACE inhibitors are not as likely to be impacted by concurrent administration with meals). Captopril is metabolized by cytochrome P450 2D6. Its half-life is ap-proximately 2 hours for individuals with normal renal function. Typi-cal dosing for hypertension is 12.5 mg three times daily and in-creased up to 50 mg three times daily as tolerated. Occasionally higher doses have been used.

Adverse Effects

The most serious adverse effects of captopril and other ACE in-hibitors are angioedema and acute renal failure. Angioedema is man-ifested by facial, perioral, epiglottal and/or extremity swelling, in-testinal pain, and/or difficulty breathing and may occur at any time during therapy. Acute renal failure is most likely to occur in clients with preexisting renal insufficiency who are dehydrated or hypona-tremic. Acute renal failure would be unexpected for clients with nor-mal renal function who are adequately hydrated. (Of note, ACE in-hibitor therapy is typically used alone or in combination with an ARB for clients with mild renal impairment to reduce the risk for fur-ther renal insufficiency [Strippoli, Craig, Deeks, Schena, & Craig, 2004; Nakao et al, 2003]. This is achieved by favorably altering ves-sel constriction in the nephron.) Other adverse effects of the ACE inhibitors include hyperkalemia, dry cough, headaches, diarrhea, loss of or altered taste, weakness, nausea, dizziness, hypotension, rash, fever, and joint pain. ACE inhibitors should be avoided in pregnancy; see the Pregnancy Safety box below.

PREGNANCY SAFETY ANTIHYPERTENSIVES	
Category	**Drug**
B	doxazosin, guanadrel, guanfacine, methyldopa
C	clonidine, diazoxide, guanabenz, guanethidine, hydralazine, minoxidil, nitroprusside, prazosin, reserpine, ter-azosin; all ACE inhibitors in the first trimester; eprosartan, irbesartan, losartan, olmesartan, and valsartan in the first trimester
D	trimethaphan; all ACE inhibitors in the second and third trimesters; eprosar-tan, irbesartan, losartan, olmesartan, and valsartan in the second and third trimesters

Modified from *Mosby's drug consult* (15th ed.). (2005). St. Louis: Mosby.

Drug Interactions

Concurrent dosing with potassium salts, potassium sparing diuretics, or ARBs may lead to hyperkalemia. Concurrent dosing with nons-teroidal antiinflammatory drugs (NSAIDs) or cyclooxygenase-2 (COX-2) inhibitors may increase the likelihood of renal insufficiency.

✴ P.T. is started on the ACE inhibitor lisinopril (Prinivil, Zestril) 10 mg daily in the morning. How should her therapy be managed?

Assessment An assessment of P.T.'s health status consid-ers her age and her preexisting medical conditions. There are no significant differences in BP response necessitating lower ACE inhibitor dosages in older adults; however, P.T. may be more sensitive to the positional hypotensive effects of the drug than younger clients. Lisinopril is beneficial in the case of her diabetes because it reduces the risk of stroke and coronary events, and progression of kidney disease, that are often complications of diabetes. Other conditions for which the prescriber would consider the risk-benefit are the following: history of angioedema (increased risk of ACE inhibitor-related angioedema); hyperkalemia; renal artery stenosis or renal transplant (increased risk of renal function impairment; renal function impairment [de-creased elimination of the ACE inhibitor]); and fluid vol-ume deficit, e.g., dialysis or severe dietary sodium restric-tion (increased risk of ACE inhibitor-induced renal failure, especially with HF). Because of her age, pregnancy is not an issue with P.T., however, if it were, ACE inhibitors are Pregnancy Category C in the first trimester and D in the second and third trimesters, and so are discontinued when pregnancy is suspected.

Review P.T.'s current medication regimen for the risk of significant drug interactions. Alcohol, diuretics, and other hypotension-producing medications will cause P.T. to expe-rience added hypotensive effects. Potassium-sparing diuret-ics, low-sodium soups (often high in potassium), low-salt milk (up to 60 mEq of potassium per liter), potassium sup-plements, or potassium-containing medications and salt substitutes may lead to hyperkalemia and necessitate close monitoring of the serum potassium.

Before beginning therapy, a baseline assessment of P.T.'s BP, complete white cell count, proteinuria determination, serum potassium, and hepatic and renal function studies are necessary.

Nursing Diagnosis With the administration of ACE in-hibitors, P.T. may experience the following nursing diag-noses/collaborative problems: risk for injury related to hypotension; imbalanced nutrition: less than body require-ments related to taste impairment (dysgeusia); ineffective protection related to neutropenia and agranulocytosis; im-paired skin integrity (rash); impaired comfort (nausea, headache, dry cough, joint pain, or chest pain); diarrhea; fa-tigue; and the potential complications of anaphylaxis, pan-creatitis, and hyperkalemia (confusion, weakness, cardiac dysrhythmias).

Planning Planning is the same as for other antihypertensive agents; see Box 27-4.

Implementation

Monitoring Obtain white blood cell (WBC) and differential counts every month for the first 3 to 6 months of therapy and periodically thereafter. Instruct the client to report any sign of infection (e.g., sore throat, fever), which indicates possible neutropenia.

Perform urinary protein determinations periodically on P.T.'s first morning urine. If proteinuria is greater than 1 g/day, the drug regimen should be reevaluated. Instruct her to report any edema or weight gain that may occur.

An elevation in potassium level may occur because of depressed aldosterone levels. Monitor the serum potassium and sodium levels.

Monitor BP closely because a precipitous fall can occur in 1 to 3 hours, particularly in clients who have been receiving salt-restricted diets, diuretics, or dialysis. Vomiting, diarrhea, and dehydration can intensify hypotension. P.T. is instructed to discontinue the salt-restricted diet. The hypotensive effect is the same in both the standing and the supine positions. Monitor the pulse rate.

Intervention There are no special considerations for P.T.'s lisinopril in relation to food, however, other ACE inhibitors, such as captopril and moexipril will have reduced absorption if given with meals and so are taken on an empty stomach, 1 hour before meals. Absorption of the other ACE inhibitors is not affected by food (*Drug Facts and Comparisons*, 2005).

Clients with renal disease, particularly those with renal artery stenosis, may experience an increase in BUN and serum creatinine levels. Reduce the dosage of the ACE inhibitor or discontinue diuretic therapy if necessary.

A skin rash may occur during the first 4 weeks of therapy. A dosage reduction or cessation or the administration of an antihistamine usually causes the rash to disappear. Any facial swelling or difficulty breathing could indicate angioedema and requires immediate medical attention.

Education As with other antihypertensive agents, instruct P.T. in nonpharmacologic measures to reduce hypertension (see Table 27-2) and general information on antihypertensive therapy (Box 27-6). Advise P.T. that signs of infection (e.g., sore throat or fever) and easy bruising or bleeding (possible agranulocytosis) should be reported to the prescriber. If taste impairment (dysgeusia) occurs, it generally disappears in 2 or 3 months, but it may cause weight loss. Provide her with nutritional guidance.

Instruct P.T. not to use potassium supplements or substances containing large amounts of potassium (e.g., salt substitutes or low-sodium milk) without prescriber approval. Caution clients with HF to increase their physical activity slowly in response to decreased chest pain.

Evaluation The expected outcome of ACE inhibitor therapy is that the client will maintain a BP within the normal limits without experiencing adverse effects of the drug along with the general outcomes listed in Box 27-7.

⚙ **P.T. seems to be doing well on lisinopril, except that she has developed a persistent dry cough that keeps her up at night. She has no other symptoms of an upper respiratory infection, gastroesophageal reflux or heart failure. Her cough appears to be drug induced. The prescriber starts her on an ARB, losartan 50 mg PO daily and discontinues the lisinopril. P.T.'s cough should resolve over a number of days to 2 weeks after the drug is discontinued.**

The angiotensin II receptor blockers (ARBs) are newer agents. The class includes candesartan cilexetil (Atacand), eprosartan (Teveten HCT), irbesartan (Avapro), losartan potassium (Cozaar), olmesartan (Benicar), telmisartan (Micardis), and valsartan (Diovan). These agents block the receptors for angiotensin II and thus block the vasoconstriction and increase of aldosterone release; however, they have very little effect on serum potassium. Additionally, they do not affect bradykinin and there is no associated cough as with ACEIs. Losartan is considered the key drug in this category.

⚙▀ **losartan potassium** [low **sar** tan]
(Cozaar)
Losartan is an ARB resulting in reduced vasoconstriction and aldosterone release.
Indications
Losartan is indicated for the treatment of hypertension alone or in combination with other antihypertensives, and prevention of diabetic nephropathy in clients with type 2 diabetes mellitus. Although not an official FDA labeled use, ARBs have been used for clients with HF. As with ACE inhibitors, blacks appear less responsive to the antihypertensive action of these agents (Brewster et al, 2004).
Pharmacokinetics/Dosing
Losartan is administered orally and reaches a peak effect in 6 hours. It undergoes substantial first-pass metabolism in the liver and is converted to at least six metabolites via cytochrome P450 2 C9 and 3 A4. One active metabolite (carboxylic acid) is between 10 and 40 times more potent than the parent drug. The half-life of losartan is 2 hours; the half-life of the carboxylic acid metabolite is between 6 and 9 hours. The duration of action is at least 24 hours. Losartan is metabolized in the liver and excreted in the bile (approximately 60%) and kidneys (35%). The initial adult dosage is 50 mg PO daily; the maintenance dosage is 25 to 100 mg daily. The dosage for children has not been established.
Adverse Effects
Like the ACE inhibitors, the ARBs pose the risk for angioedema. The risk for renal failure with concurrent dehydration is also possible. Other adverse effects of losartan include headache, tiredness, back or muscle pain, diarrhea, nasal congestion, dizziness, and upper respiratory infection. A dry cough and insomnia are considered rare effects. ARBs should also be avoided in women who are or potentially become pregnant; see the Pregnancy Safety box on p. 556.

A comparison of the pharmacokinetics of ARBs is presented in Table 27-5.

⚙ **What special monitoring is required now that P.T. is taking an ARB?**

Nursing management, monitoring requirements, contraindications, adverse effects (other than cough), and client

TABLE 27-5 ANGIOTENSIN₂ RECEPTOR BLOCKERS

Drug	Half-life	Usual Adult Dose	Comment
candesartan (Atacand)	9 hours	8 mg PO daily to 16 mg PO twice daily	Has an active metabolite
eprosartan (Teveten)	5-9 hours	400 mg PO daily to 400 mg PO twice daily	
irbesartan (Avapro)	11-15 hours	150-300 mg PO daily	
losartan (Cozaar)	2 hours (6-9 hours for metabolite)	25 mg PO daily to 50 mg PO twice daily	Has an active metabolite
olmesartan (Benicar)	13 hours	20-40 mg PO daily	Lower dose for renal dysfunction
telmisartan (Micardis)	24 hours	20-80 mg PO daily	
valsartan (Diovan)	6 hours	80 mg PO daily to 160 mg PO twice daily	

education are similar for ARBs and ACE inhibitors. Because of the risk of acute renal dysfunction and hyperkalemia secondary to renal insufficiency, serum potassium and creatinine are monitored. ARBs are contraindicated in pregnancy and in clients with volume depletion or renal artery stenosis. Clients with hyponatremia, volume depletion, or heart failure may experience acute hypotension when beginning ARB therapy (Saseen & Carter, 2005).

✳ **S.F. is a 73-year-old black female with a longstanding history of hypertension. For the past 20 years, S.F. has received hydrochlorothiazide 25 mg daily. At her last two clinic visits, her blood pressures have been 161/80 mm Hg and 155/75 mm Hg. Is her hypertension adequately controlled?**
Systolic blood pressure consistently above 140 mm Hg is not considered adequately controlled, even if diastolic pressures remain below 80 mm Hg. S.F.'s treatment regimen needs to be re-evaluated. She evidences isolated systolic hypertension. As noted by the JNC-VII, systolic hypertension in older clients poses a greater risk for target organ damage than does diastolic hypertension. The first line treatment of choice of isolated systolic hypertension is a thiazide diuretic, which S.F. is currently receiving. Further increases above 25 mg are not likely to produce added benefit and would likely increase the risk for hypokalemia.

Calcium channel blockers (CCBs) decrease the force of myocardial contraction by blocking the inward flow of calcium ions through the slow channels of the cell membrane during phase 2 (the plateau phase) of the action potential (see Figure 24-2). The diminished entry of calcium ions into the cells fails to trigger the release of large amounts of calcium from the sarcoplasmic reticulum within the cell. This free calcium is needed for excitation-contraction coupling, an event that activates contraction by allowing crossbridges to form between the actin and myosin filaments of muscle. The force of the contraction of the heart is determined by the number of actin and myosin cross-bridges formed within the sarcomere. Decreasing the amount of

calcium ion released from the sarcoplasmic reticulum results in the formation of fewer actin and myosin crossbridges; this decreases the force of contraction and results in a negative inotropic effect.

In the cardiac conduction system only diltiazem and verapamil significantly decrease automaticity in the SA node and decrease conduction in the AV junction. Their use in the management of supraventricular cardiac dysrhythmias is presented in Chapter 26.

The smooth muscle of the coronary and peripheral vessels has a significant influence on the hemodynamics of circulation. CCBs effectively inhibit calcium ion influx through the slow channels of the membrane of smooth muscle cells. The depressed interaction between actin and myosin results in a decreased force of smooth muscle contraction. As a result, coronary artery dilation occurs, which lowers coronary resistance and improves blood flow through collateral vessels, and oxygen delivery to ischemic areas of the heart. Hence drugs with these actions are useful in the treatment of angina pectoris.

CCBs also inhibit the contraction of smooth muscle of the peripheral arterioles. This results in a widespread reduction in BP and **peripheral vascular resistance** (resistance to blood flow through the body determined by the tone of the vascular musculature and the diameter of the blood vessels). The dihydropyridine CCBs are more active in reducing peripheral vascular resistance and BP. Included in this subgroup are amlodipine (Norvasc), felodipine (Plendil), isradipine (DynaCirc), nicardipine (Cardene), nifedipine (Adalat CC, Procardia, Procardia XL), nimodipine (Nimotop), and nisoldipine (Sular).

Therapeutically, the CCBs have been used to treat a variety of conditions, with each agent having various indications for use. FDA-approved indications include angina pectoris (bepridil, diltiazem, felodipine, mibefradil, nicardipine, nifedipine, verapamil), dysrhythmias (diltiazem, verapamil), hypertension (diltiazem, felodipine, isradipine, mibefradil, nicardipine, nifedipine extended-release tablets, verapamil), subarachnoid hemorrhage (nimodipine), and prophylaxis for vascular headaches (flunarizine [Sibelium🍁]). Some CCBs have also been prescribed for non–FDA-approved indications, such as felodipine, isradipine, nicardipine, and nifedipine for Raynaud's phenomenon, and verapamil for vascular headache prophylaxis and hypertrophic cardiomyopathy. Because these agents differ in specificity and their individual effects on cardiac and peripheral tissues, they may have different indications, such as those discussed in the following paragraphs.

A number of CCBs are also indicated for isolated systolic hypotension. Additionally, data suggest that black clients may achieve better blood pressure control with CCBs and thiazides compared to other agents (Brewster et al, 2004). Treatment of diagnostic hypertension with CCBs in postmenopausal women is not as effective in preventing cardiovascular mortality compared with diuretics, but the role of CCBs for older women with isolated systolic hypertension is less clear (Wassertheil-Smoller et al, 2004). CCBs have multiple effects, including effects on cardiac tissue and vascular smooth muscle.

Bepridil, a structurally unique CCB, is indicated only for chronic stable angina. The potential adverse effects of bepridil, serious ventricular dysrhythmia and agranulocytosis, limit its use. Diltiazem is primarily used for managing ventricular rates for individuals with atrial fibrillation and for reducing coronary artery spasms for individuals with vasospastic angina. Felodipine, nicardipine, and sustained action nifedipine are used to treat hypertension (usually isolated systolic hypertension in older clients) and angina, whereas isradipine is used to treat essential hypertension. Nicardipine is a very potent peripheral vasodilator that does not affect the SA node or AV junction. Because of its pronounced effect on the peripheral vascular bed, nifedipine causes the greatest hypotensive effect. However, it exerts minimal cardiac depressant action.

Nimodipine, which is highly lipophilic, crosses the blood-brain barrier and has a greater effect on the cerebral arteries than on other arteries in the body. It is indicated for the treatment of cerebral arterial spasm after subarachnoid hemorrhage. It also inhibits platelet aggregation. The adult dosage is 60 mg every 4 hours, starting within 96 hours after the subarachnoid hemorrhage and continuing for 3 weeks.

Most of the CCBs are metabolized by the cytochrome P450 enzyme systems, and usually involve cytochrome P450 3 A4. Interactions with other drugs (e.g., azole antifungals, amiodarone) or foods (e.g., grapefruit juice) affecting these systems are possible and caution is advised in managing interactions. Diltiazem and verapamil both suppress AV nodal conduction and should be used cautiously with other drugs with slow conduction through the AV node (see Chapter 26).

Diltiazem and verapamil are available in intravenous (IV) formulations and are more fully discussed in Chapter 26. Clients receiving IV diltiazem or verapamil should be monitored continuously on telemetry with frequent BP measurements. Administer the drug slowly as a direct injection over at least 2 minutes (over at least 3 minutes in older adults). Avoid repeated doses in clients with hepatic or re-nal failure, because an IV dose may prolong the duration of effects. If repeated injections are required, closely monitor BP and the PR interval, and use smaller doses as prescribed. If bolus therapy is successful, the client may be placed on continuous IV administration; use a controlled infusion device for precise dosage. The maximum effects of verapamil occur in 15 to 30 minutes, and therefore adjustments in infusion rates are made at 30-minute intervals. Monitor the client carefully for a return of abnormal ECG readings for several hours after discontinuing the IV verapamil because the drug is excreted over 2 to 5 hours. If the client becomes hypotensive, the infusion rate should be slowed or discontinued. To reduce the hypotensive effects of CCBs, instruct the client to remain in the recumbent position for at least 1 hour following an IV bolus injection.

A comparison of the CCBs is presented in Table 27-6. A brief discussion of the key CCB, nifedipine, will be presented here. The use of diltiazem and verapamil in the management of cardiac dysrhythmias is presented in Chapter 26.

⬦✦🄝 **nifedipine** (nye **fed** i peen)
(Adalat CC, Procardia XL, Adalat FT🍁, Adalat PA🍁, Apo-Nifed🍁)
Nifedipine is a dihydropyridine CCB that blocks calcium from entering the slow channels of vascular smooth muscle and the myocardium. It produces vasodilation and reduces vasospasm for clients with vasospastic angina and isolated systolic hypertension. It, like other dihydropyridines, plays a more secondary role in the management of diastolic hypertension.

Indications
Nifedipine in its sustained action form is indicated for hypertension and angina. Many clinicians reserve its use to black clients or those with isolated systolic hypertension or clients with Prinzmetal's angina (angina secondary to vasospasm).

Pharmacokinetics/Dosing
Its rapid onset of action with immediate release dosing results in a rapid drop in BP that may predispose to myocardial or cerebrovascular ischemia. As such, the immediate release dose forms of this drug are rarely used. Nifedipine is fairly well absorbed orally when administered as a sustained action formulation and is metabolized by cytochrome P450 3 A4 to inactive metabolites. Its elimination half-life is 2 to 4 hours in adults and is prolonged in older adults. Typical doses for hypertension are 30 to 120 mg (sustained release formulation) daily.

Adverse Effects
The rapid decline in BP with immediate release formulations is much less likely to occur with sustained action formulations. Dose related peripheral edema is the most commonly observed adverse effect with the dihydropyridine CCBs. Other effects include reflex tachycardia, excessive hypotension, GI distress, and male sexual dysfunction. CCBs should be avoided for individuals with systolic HF because these agents are negative inotropes.

Drug Interactions
Drugs and foods that inhibit cytochrome P450 3 A4 activity (e.g., azole antifungals, grapefruit juice) should be avoided with most of the dihydropyridine CCBs, including nifedipine. Use of sildenafil (Viagra), tadalafil (Cialis), and vardenafil (Levitra), which are used for male sexual dysfunction, may result in excessive hypotensive episodes.

✱ **S.F. is started on amlodipine (Norvasc) 5 mg daily in addition to her hydrochlorothiazide 25 mg daily.**

TABLE 27-6 COMPARISON OF CALCIUM CHANNEL BLOCKERS

Agent	Contractility	Coronary Artery Tone	Peripheral Vessel Tone	SA Node	AV Node	Indications	Half-Life	Typical Adult Oral Dose
DIHYDROPYRIDINE								
amlodipine (Norvasc)	↑	↓	↓↓↓			Hypertension Angina	34 hours	2.5-10 mg daily
felodipine (Plendil)	↑	↓	↓↓↓			Hypertension HF (cautiously)	10-36 hours	2.5-10 mg daily
isradipine (DynaCirc)	↓	↓↓↓	↓↓↓			Hypertension	8 hours	2.5-10 mg twice daily
nicardipine (Cardene)	↓	↓↓↓	↓↓↓		↓	Chronic stable angina Hypertension	2-4 hours	20-40 mg three times daily Sustained release: 30-60 mg twice daily
nifedipine (Adalat CC, Pro-cardia, Procardia XL)	↓	↓↓↓	↓↓↓		↓	Angina Hypertension Pulmonary hypertension	2-5 hours	Sustained release: 30-60 mg once daily. *Shell of sustained release form may remain in stool.* ***Immediate release forms may result in excessive hypotension***
nimodipine (Nimotop)						Vasospasm following subarachnoid hemorrhage	1-2 hours	60 mg q4h × 21 days
nisoldipine (Sular)						Hypertension	7-12 hours	10-40 mg daily
BENZOTHIAZEPINE								
diltiazem (Cardizem, Dilacor XR)	↓	↓↓↓	↓	↓↓↓	↓↓↓	Hypertension Angina AF/A flutter (IV) PSVT (IV)	4-7 hours	Immediate Release: 30-90 mg q6h Sustained Release: 120-240 mg daily *(depending on indication and formulation)*

TABLE 27-6 COMPARISON OF CALCIUM CHANNEL BLOCKERS—CONT'D

Agent	Contractility	Coronary Artery Tone	Peripheral Vessel Tone	SA Node	AV Node	Indications	Half-Life	Typical Adult Oral Dose
PHENYLALKYLAMINE								
verapamil (Calan, Isoptin)	↓↓	↓↓	↓↓	↓↓↓	↓↓↓	Angina Hypertension AF/A flutter (IV) PSVT (IV) Unlabeled: Migraine, Mania	3-7 hours	Immediate release: 40 mg three times daily to 120 mg four times daily Sustained release: 120-360 mg daily
DIARYLAMINOPROPYLAMINE ETHER								
bepridil (Vascor)	↓	↓↓↓	↓	↓		Chronic stable angina *(for clients not responsive to other therapy because of risk for dysrhythmias)*	24 hours	200-400 mg daily

Modified from Lacy, C.F., Armstrong, L.L., Goldman, M.P., & Lance, L.L. (2004). *Lexi-Comp's Drug Information Handbook* (12th ed.). Hudson, Ohio: Lexi-Comp.
0, No Effect; ↓, slight decrease; ↓↓, moderate decrease; ↓↓↓, significant decrease.

✳ **What nursing management of S.F.'s drug regimen is appropriate?**

Assessment Review S.F.'s health status for conditions that might contraindicate the use of CCBs or indicate the need for special caution with their administration. Do not administer these drugs to clients who have severe hypotension (<90 mm Hg systolic). Administer CCBs with caution to clients with bradycardia, heart failure, cardiogenic shock, acute MI, ventricular dysrhythmias, hypokalemia, and mild to moderate hypotension, because these conditions will be worsened. Clients with renal or hepatic function impairment may have a reduced clearance of CCBs, which results in a prolonged half-life. Intolerance to the prescribed CCBs is also a contraindication. Although not an issue with S.F. because of her age, ask female clients if they are pregnant or plan to become pregnant. Tests on laboratory animals have resulted in teratogenic effects on the fetus (FDA Pregnancy Category C for all CCBs in first trimester, D in second and third trimester).

Older adults, such as S.F., may require more caution in the dosage of CCBs because of age-related renal impairment. The half-life of diltiazem, nimodipine, verapamil, and other CCBs may be increased because of decreased clearance; the half-life of nicardipine has shown no difference in young adults and in clients older than 65 years of age.

Review S.F.'s current medication regimen for the risk of significant drug interactions. Although concurrent administration is beneficial in some clients, the combination of CCBs and β-adrenergic blocking agents, systemic and ophthalmic, should be closely monitored because adverse cardiac effects may occur (bradycardia, hypotension, and heart failure caused by prolonged AV conduction). Rifampin and other hepatic enzyme inducers may reduce serum levels of CCBs. Concurrent administration of 200 mL of grapefruit has been shown to increase CCB serum levels by inhibiting first-pass metabolism.

Additional interactions with CCBs should be considered. Carbamazepine (Tegretol), cyclosporine (Sandimmune), or quinidine concurrent with diltiazem and verapamil may inhibit liver metabolism (cytochrome P450 system), resulting in increased serum levels and toxicity of these drugs. Nifedipine with quinidine may result in reduced serum levels of quinidine. Monitor such combinations closely, because dosage adjustments may be necessary. Increased serum levels of digoxin are reported, especially when administered with verapamil (occurs to a lesser degree with other CCBs); monitor digoxin serum levels closely whenever a CCB is started or discontinued or when the dosage is changed. Monitor for prolonged AV conduction, bradycardia, or AV blocks, especially during the initial week of therapy, because the dosage for digoxin may need to be changed. Do not administer disopyramide (Norpace) within 48 hours before or 24 hours after verapamil because the additive negative inotropic effects may result in serious reactions, including death. Hypokalemia-producing drugs, such as corticosteroids and potassium-depleting diuretics, increase the risk for bepridil-induced dysrhythmias.

S.F.'s baseline assessment should include pulse, BP, heart and breath sounds, respiratory rate and rhythm, weight, and ECG readings. Liver and renal function studies are recommended if long-term therapy is anticipated.

Nursing Diagnosis With amlodipine therapy, S.F. may be at risk for the following nursing diagnoses/collaborative problems: impaired comfort (dry mouth, flushing, dizziness, headache, palpitations, chest pain, and nausea); excess fluid volume related to sodium and water retention as evidenced by swelling of the feet, ankles, and lower legs; and risk for injury related to dizziness, drowsiness, and fainting; activity intolerance related to lethargy and weakness; and the potential complications of allergic reaction (skin rash). With other CCBs, clients may also experience the following: depression, angina, HF, decreased cardiac output related to hypotension, dysrhythmias, or tachycardia; impaired oral mucous membrane (gingival hyperplasia); and constipation or diarrhea.

Planning Planning is the same as for other antihypertensive agents; see Box 27-4.

Implementation

Monitoring Monitor S.F.'s BP and pulse rate. Observe the ECG for a prolonged PR interval, which is caused by the slowing of AV conduction. Heart failure may occasionally occur after the initiation of CCB therapy; assess for peripheral edema, rales, dyspnea, weight gain, and jugular vein distention. Assess intake and output ratios and daily weight. If other antihypertensives are withdrawn before initiating CCB therapy, taper their dosage gradually. Abrupt withdrawal may provoke angina. Hepatic and renal function studies may be required during long-term therapy with CCBs.

Intervention Take S.F.'s pulse before each dose of a CCB; if the pulse rate is 50 beats/min or below, withhold the dose and report to the prescriber. Although amlodipine and other CCBs may be taken without regard to food, nifedipine needs to be taken on an empty stomach. Most CCBs are not to be taken with grapefruit juice.

Education Instruct S.F. in lifestyle changes to support her CCB therapy; see Table 27-2. In particular, she should move from a sitting or lying position to a standing position cautiously to avoid orthostatic hypotension. Advise her of the general instructions for antihypertensive medications, see Box 27-6.

Teach S.F. to take her pulse and report a heart rate of less than 50 beats/min. Instruct her to report headaches, rashes, nausea, and vomiting; additionally, instruct S.F. to report edema and weight gain (more than 1 kg/day), because these two symptoms may indicate HF.

Instruct S.F. to perform meticulous daily dental hygiene and to maintain regular dental examinations and cleaning; this may reduce the incidence or severity of gingivitis and gingival hyperplasia (a rare adverse effect).

Evaluation The expected outcome of CCB therapy is that S.F. will demonstrate a regular sinus rhythm on the ECG and have a BP within the normal limits without adverse effects of the drug; see Box 27-7 for other outcome criteria.

❋ **What other drug choices are available for treating hypertension?**

Although not recommended as first line therapy for hypertension by the JNC-VII, other agents have been used to treat hypertension. The centrally acting adrenergic inhibitors like clonidine (Catapres), methyldopa (Aldomet), guanabenz (Wytensin), and guanfacine (Tenex) have limited use in treating hypertension in treatment-resistant cases or under special circumstances. The peripheral adrenergic inhibitors, guanethidine (Ismelin), guanadrel (Hylorel) and reserpine (Serpalan, Serpasil) are infrequently used because of their adverse effects. The use of α-adrenergic blocking drugs, doxazosin (Cardura), prazosin (Minipress) and terazosin (Hytrin), have been mainly used to treat symptoms of benign prostatic hyperplasia (BPH). Their use for blood pressure control has declined because this class is associated with increased risk for heart failure (ALLHAT, 2002; Stafford et al., 2004). The vasodilating drugs, diazoxide (Hyperstat IV), hydralazine (Apresoline), and minoxidil (Loniten), are occasionally used for severe, drug-resistant hypertension. Drugs used for malignant hypertension (BP >180/110 mm Hg) include nitroprusside (Nipride, Nitropress) and the β blocker labetalol (Normodyne, Trandate).

Centrally Acting Adrenergic Inhibitors

Although thought of as antiadrenergic drugs, centrally acting adrenergic inhibitors are actually central α_2-adrenergic agonists. Central α_2-adrenergic stimulation results in a decreased sympathetic outflow to the heart, kidneys, and peripheral vasculature; this results in decreased heart rate, decreased peripheral vascular resistance and, as a result, decreased systolic and diastolic BP. The centrally acting agents clonidine (Catapres), methyldopa (Aldomet), guanfacine (Tenex), and guanabenz (Wytensin) are effective antihypertensives, especially when combined with a diuretic, but their adverse effect profiles render them agents generally reserved for resistant cases or special circumstances. When given as a single agent, clonidine and methyldopa (and guanfacine and guanabenz to a lesser extent) usually produce sodium and water retention.

✳🎙 clonidine [**kloe** ni deen]

(Catapres, Catapres-TTS, Dixarit✽)

Clonidine is considered the prototype centrally acting adrenergic inhibitor. It reduces systolic and diastolic BP by stimulating central α_2 receptors, which decreases the sympathetic outflow of norepinephrine from the brain to the blood vessels and heart. Decreasing cardiac output, heart rate, and peripheral vascular resistance lowers BP. The depressed cardiac output is the result of a reduction in both heart rate and stroke volume. Consequently, this action can cause bradycardia. Decreased sympathetic outflow to the kidneys reduces renal vascular resistance and thus preserves renal blood flow. Renin activity may be suppressed in some clients. With continued use of clonidine, a diuretic is prescribed to correct fluid retention.

Indications

Clonidine is indicated for management of mild to moderate hypertension. Although not approved indications in the United States, clonidine is also used in the diagnosis of pheochromocytoma, for prophylaxis of migraine or vascular headaches, and for treatment of dysmenorrhea, menopause, attention deficit hyperactive disorder, impulse control disorder, Tourette syndrome, and nicotine and opioid withdrawal. A parenteral formulation (Duraclon) is available for epidural administration as an adjunct to cancer pain management. Perioperative use of clonidine may reduce postoperative mortality (Wallace et al, 2004)

Pharmacokinetics/Dosing

Oral clonidine has an onset of action within 30 to 60 minutes, a peak effect in 2 to 4 hours, duration of action up to 8 hours, and a serum half-life between 12 and 16 hours. It is metabolized in the liver and excreted primarily by the kidneys. Transdermal clonidine is best absorbed from the chest and upper arm. The onset of action and time to peak effect are 2 to 3 days, and the duration of action is approximately 1 week if the drug is in continuous contact with the body (approximately 8 hours if removed from the body). Metabolism and excretion are the same as for oral clonidine. The initial adult dosage for hypertension is 0.1 mg twice daily; this is increased by 0.1 or 0.2 mg every 2 to 4 days as necessary to control BP. For maintenance, the dosage is 0.2 to 0.6 mg daily in divided doses. The dosage for children has not been established.

Catapres-TTS (Clonidine Transdermal System)

Clonidine transdermal is available in various strengths (0.1, 0.2, or 0.3 mg), which are programmed to deliver the specified strength daily for 1 week. The system is composed of four layers: a film that contains a drug reservoir of clonidine, a membrane that controls the rate of drug delivery, an adhesive layer that also contains clonidine to initially saturate the skin site, and a top backing or cover layer. This system was formulated for the drug to flow from a higher concentration to a lower concentration in the body; this is limited by the rate-controlling membrane layer. It takes approximately 2 to 3 days to reach a therapeutic serum level of clonidine on initial application; replacing the system weekly at a new body site will maintain the therapeutic serum level.

Adverse Effects

The adverse effects of clonidine include dry mouth, headaches, constipation, weakness, postural hypotension, impotency or decreased sexual drive, insomnia, anxiety, anorexia, nausea, vomiting, and pruritus. Of significant concern is a withdrawal reaction resulting in significantly elevated BP on abrupt discontinuation. This agent should always be tapered over 1 week when discontinued.

✳ **D.T. is a 47-year-old male CEO of an international corporation with a 5-year history of primary hyperten-**sion. **His current medications are losartan/hydrochlorothiazide 100/25 mg daily and sustained release diltiazem 240 mg daily. His BP is averaging 150/94 mm Hg for the past 3 months. He has been adherent to his drug regimen and lifestyle modifications, but has been unable to stop smoking. His prescriber is going to add to his antihypertensive drug regimen, but D.T. has experienced bothersome side effects from ACE inhibitors, CCBs, and peripherally acting antiadrenergics. So he is started on clonidine (Catapres) 0.1 mg PO twice daily, a central α_2 agonist. The prescriber will increase the dosage 0.1 to 0.2 mg daily every few weeks until the desired BP is reached. She will then switch him to a transdermal patch (Catapres TTS) that is applied every 7 days to make adherence easier given D.T.'s travel schedule. The clonidine may also serve to lessen withdrawal symptoms for D.T. as he attempts smoking cessation again.**

Nursing Management

Assessment Before D.T.'s clonidine therapy begins, his prescriber performs a thorough history and physical exam. She rules out coronary insufficiency, recent MI, or cerebrovascular disease, because the decrease in BP as a result of clonidine may decrease tissue perfusion and increase ischemia. Thromboangiitis, Raynaud's phenomenon, a history of mental depression, and sinus or atrioventricular node dysfunction are also ruled out as clonidine may worsen these conditions. If the transdermal dosage form of clonidine is to be applied, assess the D.T.'s skin for any irritation or abrasion so that these areas can be avoided; absorption may be increased if the drug is applied to such areas. Avoid also any areas of skin involvement with disorders such as systemic lupus erythematosus (SLE) or scleroderma that might decrease drug absorption.

Review D.T.'s current medication regimen for the risk of significant drug interactions, such as β-blocking agents (may lead to a loss of BP control and bradycardia) and tricyclic antidepressants (antihypertensive effectiveness of clonidine may be reduced).

Perform a baseline assessment of D.T.'s BP, health status, and lifestyle before initiating clonidine therapy.

Nursing Diagnosis Although D.T. is receiving clonidine therapy, he has the potential for the following nursing diagnoses/collaborative problems: risk for injury related to orthostatic hypotension, rebound hypertension, or the ineffectiveness of clonidine therapy; impaired skin integrity related to an allergic reaction to the transdermal system (itching, redness of skin); excess fluid volume related to sodium and water retention (edema); constipation; disturbed sleep pattern (drowsiness); impaired oral mucous membrane (dry mouth); fatigue; sexual dysfunction (impotence, loss of libido); impaired comfort (anorexia, nausea, nervousness); disturbed thought processes (confusion); and the potential complications of mental depression and overdose (dyspnea, syncope, pinpoint pupils, bradycardia, fatigue). (See the Nursing Care Plan on p. 547 for other selected nursing diagnoses related to antihypertensive therapy.)

Planning Planning is the same as for other antihypertensive agents; see Box 27-4.

Implementation

Monitoring Monitor D.T.'s BP and pulse closely during initiation of therapy, and continue to observe these parameters until the dosage is properly titrated. Blood pressure should decrease within 30 to 60 minutes of oral administration, and the decrease may persist for 8 hours. Monitor BP and pulse rate regularly on a long-term basis to determine the effectiveness of clonidine.

Observe D.T. for drug tolerance as evidenced by rising BP levels. The prescriber may increase the dosage or, in D.T.'s case, change his diuretic obtain the required antihypertensive response.

Weigh D.T. daily for 3 to 4 days after initiation of therapy; fluid volume excess may occur because of sodium retention and edema. Monitor intake and output ratios, and assess D.T. for dependent edema. If fluid retention exists, a change in the diuretic is needed. Monitor for the anticholinergic effects of dry mouth, constipation, and urine retention.

Intervention When the change in D.T.'s clonidine therapy is made to the transdermal patch, administer his oral clonidine dose the first day because the onset of the initial BP effect to the patch may be delayed for 2 to 3 days when it is first applied. The oral dose is reduced over 2 to 3 days to prevent rebound hypertension until the patch becomes effective. In applying the clonidine transdermal system, select a hairless, intact area of D.T.'s upper arm or torso. Do not trim the patch; doing so will alter the dosage. Reapply a new patch to a different skin site once every 7 days. If the system loosens, cover it with an adhesive overlay from the drug package. The patch should remain in place during bathing or showering. Replace the patch if it falls off or becomes very loose. Discard used patches by folding them in half with the adhesive sides together. If local skin irritation occurs before the patch has been in place for 7 days, it may be removed and a new one applied to a different skin area. A change from transdermal therapy may be required if skin irritation persists.

Prescribed dosage reductions are performed over 2 to 4 days, or preferably longer (1- to 2-week period), to prevent rebound hypertension, a potentially serious adverse syndrome (Box 27-9).

Education Along with the nonpharmacologic interventions (Table 27-2) and antihypertensive drug instruction (Box 27-6), emphasize the importance of periodic follow-up visits so BP can be closely monitored. Be explicit in instructions to D.T. concerning the serious consequences of

---

The abrupt withdrawal or discontinuation of antihypertensive medications may result in rebound hypertension and possibly a hypertensive crisis. In both instances, therapy is instituted to reduce blood pressure as soon as possible (Goldman & Ausiello, 2004).

Rebound hypertension refers to the sudden increase of blood pressure to the pretreatment level or higher. Symptoms of rebound hypertension depend on the elevation of blood pressure. The symptoms usually involve sympathetic system hyperactivity (e.g., sweating, anxiety, tachycardia, insomnia, muscle cramps, chest pain, headache, and nausea).

A hypertensive crisis or hypertensive emergency is a blood pressure greater than 220/140 mm Hg, headaches, confusion, blurred vision, nausea and vomiting, seizures, grade III or IV hypertensive retinopathy, heart failure, and oliguria (Goldman & Ausiello, 2004). In a hypertensive emergency or crisis, the extremely elevated rise in blood pressure may cause target organ damage, such as to the eyes (retina), heart, kidneys, or neurologic system. In such cases, labetalol, a β blocker, is often used as a first-line therapy. IV nitroprusside is used in severe cases or for cases in which labetalol is contraindicated or is not effective. Fenoldopam (Corlopam) is a dopamine and α_2-adrenergic agonist that can also be used intravenously for hypertensive crisis.

---

rebound hypertension caused by missing drug doses or abruptly discontinuing clonidine (Goldman & Ausiello, 2004). If he develops serious adverse effects, D.T. should immediately report the problem to the prescriber so that the dosage may be adjusted or the drug withdrawn gradually over a period of 2 to 4 days. Abrupt withdrawal, including the omission of sequential doses, can result in a hypertensive crisis within 8 to 24 hours. The symptoms of hypertensive crisis are anxiety, sweating, tachycardia, insomnia, salivation, abdominal and muscle cramps, headache, and chest pain. Instruct D.T. on how to apply the transdermal patch and place it at a different site each week.

Alert D.T. that he may have diminished reaction times. If D.T. were older, he might experience impaired cognition and also be more sensitive to the hypotensive effects of clonidine and be at risk for injury related to orthostatic hypotension.

Instruct D.T. to keep an adequate supply of the drug at all times, particularly during travel. Instruct him, while on the oral clonidine to take the last dose before bedtime to ensure continuous BP control during the night and to reduce daytime drowsiness, which occurs in approximately 33% of clients using oral dosage forms. Instruct D.T. to make position changes slowly. Because the risk for orthostatic hypotension is greatly increased with clonidine, D.T. is cautioned to avoid alcohol ingestion, prolonged standing and strenuous exercising, and exercising during hot weather.

Altered comfort related to dry mouth occurs in 40% of the clients using oral dosage forms. Encourage D.T. to use sugarless candy or gum or ice to obtain relief. A saliva substitute such as Salivart or Optimoist may also be used. If dry mouth persists longer than 2 weeks, the prescriber or dentist needs to be consulted because of the increased risk of caries and oral candidiasis.

Altered bowel function occurs as constipation in approximately 10% of clients. Instruct D.T. about maintaining adequate fluid and fiber intake, regular exercise, and establishing a regular bowel pattern to prevent or minimize constipation.

Evaluation The expected outcome of clonidine therapy for hypertension is that D.T.'s BP will remain within normal limits with minimal adverse effects. See Box 27-7 for other outcome criteria.

methyldopa [meth ill **doe** pa]
(Aldomet, Apo-Methyldopa✤, Novomedopa✤)
methyldopate injection [meth ill **doe** payte]
(Parenteral Aldomet)

Although the exact hypotensive mechanism is unknown, the theory is that a metabolite of methyldopa (α-methylnorepinephrine) stimulates the central α_2 receptors, which results in a reduction in norepinephrine (sympathetic) outflow to the heart, kidneys, and peripheral vasculature. It lowers BP in a way that is similar to clonidine.

Indications
Methyldopa is indicated for moderate to severe hypertension. Given its category B rating, it is recommended as a first-line agent in pregnancy when hypertension is first diagnosed during pregnancy (Saseen & Carter, 2005).

Pharmacokinetics/Dosing
In the body, methyldopate is hydrolyzed to methyldopa, which then must undergo the previously described process to produce the hypotensive effect. The antihypertensive effect produced by the parenteral dosage form begins in approximately 4 to 6 hours and therefore should not be used as the primary single drug in a hypertensive emergency.

The peak effect for methyldopa occurs 4 to 6 hours after a single dose or in 48 to 72 hours with multiple dosing. The duration of action is 12 to 24 hours (after oral single dose), 1 to 2 days (after multiple oral doses), or 10 to 16 hours (after IV administration). Methyldopa is metabolized centrally to α-methylnorepinephrine. Excretion is primarily by the kidneys.

The initial adult oral dosage is 250 mg two to three times daily for 2 days, titrated as necessary. The maintenance dosage is 500 to 2000 mg daily, divided into 2 to 4 individual doses; the maximum total daily dosage is 3 g. The initial pediatric dosage is 10 mg/kg PO in 2 to 4 divided doses, increased at 2-day intervals according to the child's response, up to 65 mg/kg or 3 g daily, whichever is less. The parenteral adult dosage is 250 to 500 mg in dextrose 5% injection (100 mL) administered over 30 to 60 minutes every 6 hours as needed. The maximum dosage is 1 g every 6 to 12 hours. The pediatric IV infusion dosage is 20 to 40 mg/kg in dextrose 5% injection over 30 to 60 minutes every 6 hours as needed, up to 65 mg/kg or 3 g daily, whichever is less.

Adverse Effects
The adverse effects include drowsiness, dry mouth, headaches, edema of feet and legs, postural hypotension, impotency, insomnia, depression, anxiety, and nightmares. Hemolytic anemia is a rare but serious adverse effect.

Nursing Management
Assessment
Methyldopa is not used with clients with active hepatic disease (e.g., hepatitis or cirrhosis) or a hypersensitivity to methyldopa. Use with caution in clients with a history of autoimmune hemolytic anemia, pheochromocytoma (interference with catecholamines), or previous liver disease in association with the methyldopa administration. The risk-benefit ratio must be considered in childbearing and lactating women.

Review the client's current medication regimen for the risk of significant drug interactions, such as those that may occur when methyldopa is given concurrently with monoamine oxidase (MAO) inhibitors (hyperexcitability, hallucinations, headache, and hypertension have been reported with this combination) and sympathomimetics, e.g., cocaine, norepinephrine, phenylephrine (a decrease in the antihypertensive effect of methyldopa is reported). If it is necessary to use sympathomimetics, the prescriber should prescribe very small doses of the sympathomimetic agent. Monitor closely.

Complete a baseline assessment of the client's BP, and a complete blood cell count (CBC) and a direct Coombs test.

Nursing Diagnosis
The client receiving methyldopa therapy has the potential for the following nursing diagnoses/collaborative problems: risk for injury related to orthostatic hypotension or the ineffectiveness of methyldopa therapy; ineffective protection related to leukopenia or thrombocytopenia; excess fluid volume related to sodium and water retention (edema); disturbed thought processes (nightmares, vivid dreams); anxiety; diarrhea; disturbed sleep pattern (daytime drowsiness); impaired oral mucous membrane (dry mouth); impaired comfort (headache, nausea, stuffy nose); activity intolerance related to hemolytic anemia; sexual dysfunction (decreased libido, ejaculation failure); and the potential complications of mental depression, drug fever (fever within the first 3 months of therapy), myocarditis (fever, chills, tachycardia), pancreatitis (abdominal pain with nausea and vomiting), SLE–like syndrome (weakness, joint pain, rash), colitis (severe diarrhea, abdominal cramping), or cholestasis or hepatitis (dark urine, pale stools, jaundice).

Planning
Planning is the same as for other antihypertensive agents; see Box 27-4.

Implementation
Monitoring
Take the client's BP and pulse as prescribed during the initiation of therapy, and continue until the drug dosage is properly titrated. To determine the effectiveness of methyldopa, measure the BP at regular intervals, with the client in the lying, sitting, and standing positions.

Observe the client for drug tolerance within the second or third month of therapy as evidenced by rising BP levels. The prescriber may increase the dosage or add a diuretic to obtain the required antihypertensive response. Observe the client for drug-induced depression, and report any symptoms to the prescriber. Observe the client for adverse effects, especially unexplained fever or jaundice, and immediately report any to the prescriber.

If unexplained fever or rash occurs, obtain liver function studies (e.g., AST, bilirubin), especially during the first 2 or 3 months of therapy. If jaundice is present, methyldopa is discontinued to avoid drug-induced hepatitis.

Monitor for fluid volume excess by assessing intake and output ratios, weighing the client daily, and checking for dependent edema; report fluid volume excess to the prescriber. If fluid retention occurs, it may be necessary to add a diuretic to the regimen.

Hemolytic anemia may occur with possible fatal complications. A CBC and direct Coombs test should be performed periodically during treatment. A positive Coombs test may or may not indicate hemolytic anemia. With prolonged use of methyldopa, 10% to 20% of clients develop a positive direct Coombs test; this is not a contraindication to further use of the drug. However, if a positive

Coombs test leads to a diagnosis of hemolytic anemia, the prescriber will discontinue therapy. A positive Coombs test produced by methyldopa therapy may interfere with the crossmatching of blood. If thrombocytopenia or reversible leukopenia occurs, drug therapy should be discontinued.

The refill frequency may be checked to determine the effectiveness of the client's management of the therapeutic regimen.

Intervention
Initiate dosage increases with the evening dose to minimize the effects of sedation.

Intramuscular (IM) or subcutaneous administration of methyldopa is not recommended because of unreliable absorption. Administer an IV infusion slowly over 30 to 60 minutes. When changing a client from the IV to the oral form once the BP has stabilized, the same dosage is used.

Education
Give lifestyle modification (see Table 27-2) and general antihypertensive medication instruction (see Box 27-6). Emphasize the importance of keeping clinical laboratory visits for blood cell counts and hepatic function studies. Methyldopa hepatotoxicity, which is reversible, may occasionally develop 2 to 4 weeks after initiation of therapy. Alert the client to report any flu-like symptoms of chills, fever, headache, anorexia, fatigue, arthralgia, or pruritus. If the results of the liver function tests are positive, therapy will be discontinued. Instruct the client to follow the same precautions as for oral clonidine.

Evaluation
The expected outcome of methyldopa therapy is that the client's BP will be within normal limits without the client experiencing any adverse effects of the drug; see Box 27-7 for other outcome criteria.

guanabenz [**gwahn** a benz]
(Wytensin)
The mechanism of action of guanabenz acetate is believed to be the same as for clonidine; it is a centrally acting α_2 agonist. Cardiac output remains unchanged, and the antihypertensive effect occurs without major changes in peripheral resistance. Peripheral resistance does eventually decrease with continued therapy.

Indications
Guanabenz is indicated for the management of hypertension.

Pharmacokinetics/Dosing
Guanabenz has an onset of action within 1 hour (for a single dose); the peak effect occurs in 2 to 4 hours, and the duration of action is 12 hours. The serum half-life is 6 hours. This drug is metabolized in the liver, and excretion is via the kidneys and feces. The initial adult dosage is 4 mg PO twice daily, increased if necessary every 1 to 2 weeks by increments of 4 to 8 mg daily up to a maximum of 32 mg daily. The dosage for children is not established.

Adverse Effects
The adverse effects of guanabenz include drowsiness, headaches, nausea, and impotency or decreased sexual drive.

Nursing Management
Assessment
Guanabenz is used during pregnancy only if the benefits outweigh the potential risk of adverse effects on the fetus. In animal studies an increase in skeletal abnormalities has been observed, and increased fetal loss and diminished body weight of the neonate. Always inquire whether a female client is pregnant or plans to become pregnant. Do not use guanabenz in clients who are hypersensitive to this substance. It should be used with caution in clients with cerebrovascular or cardiovascular disease or renal or hepatic impairment. Giving guanabenz concurrently with a β-adrenergic blocking agent or other hypotensive agents may result in additive hypotensive effects. Monitor BP closely, because dosage adjustments may be necessary. When discontinuing both drugs in a client (for example, a β-blocking drug and guanabenz), taper the β blocker first to prevent a withdrawal hypertensive reaction. A baseline assessment of the client's BP should be performed.

As with other antihypertensive agents, clients receiving guanabenz therapy might be at risk for the following nursing diagnoses/collaborative problems: risk for injury related to syncope or the ineffectiveness of guanabenz therapy (hypertension); impaired comfort (headache or nausea); impaired oral mucous membrane (dry mouth); fatigue; disturbed sleep pattern (daytime drowsiness); sexual dysfunction; and the potential complications of sympathetic overactivity related to withdrawal (anxiety, chest pain, tachycardia, nausea, insomnia, headache, increased salivation and sweating).

Planning
Planning is the same as for other antihypertensive agents; see Box 27-4.

Implementation
Monitoring
Monitor BP and pulse closely during the initiation of therapy and until the dosage is properly titrated. Closely observe clients with severe hepatic or renal failure, severe coronary insufficiency, recent MI, or cerebrovascular disease; also observe older adults closely, because they are particularly sensitive to the hypotensive effects of the drug. The client's BP should be monitored on a long-term basis.

Intervention
The last dose of each day should be taken at bedtime to ensure overnight control of BP and to reduce daytime drowsiness. Although guanabenz is usually not discontinued before surgery, the anesthetist must be aware that the client is receiving the drug.

Education
Instruct the client in lifestyle modifications (see Table 27-2) and general information regarding antihypertensive medications (see Box 27-6). Emphasize the importance of periodic follow-up visits so that the guanabenz dosage and BP can be monitored. Caution the client against abrupt withdrawal of the drug, even if experiencing unpleasant adverse effects. There is the possibility of withdrawal symptoms, although rebound hypertension does not generally occur. The prescriber should be consulted for recommendations regarding how to proceed.

Evaluation
The expected outcome of guanabenz therapy is that the client will maintain a BP within normal limits without experiencing any adverse effects of the drug. See Box 27-7.

guanfacine [**gwahn** fa seen]
(Tenex)
Guanfacine (Tenex) is a centrally acting α_2-adrenergic agonist antihypertensive similar to clonidine.

Indications
Guanfacine is used to treat hypertension. Other uses not approved by the FDA include management of heroin withdrawal, migraine headache, and attention deficit hyperactive disorder.

Pharmacokinetics/Dosing
Guanfacine is well absorbed orally and has a peak effect in 8 to 12 hours (single dose) or 1 to 3 months (long-term dosing). The onset of action occurs within 7 days of chronic dosing. The duration of effect is 1 day (single dose). This drug is metabolized by the liver and excreted by the kidneys. The adult dosage is 1 mg PO daily at bedtime, increased if needed in 3 to 4 weeks (to 2 mg daily). If necessary, a third increase may be instituted in another 3 to 4 weeks. The pediatric dosage has not been determined.

Adverse Effects
The adverse effects of guanfacine include constipation, dry mouth, sedation, light-headedness, headache, nausea, vomiting, insomnia, impotency, dry or itching eyes, weakness, and depression.

Nursing Management
Except for the precaution regarding the use of guanabenz during pregnancy, the nursing management for guanfacine is the same as for guanabenz. There is also the added concern that the client may experience depression with the use of guanfacine. The client and family/caregiver

should report any symptoms of depression, including appetite disturbance (anorexia or overeating), significant weight gain or loss, sleep disturbance (insomnia or hypersomnia), fatigue, agitation, loss of interest or pleasure in activities, feelings of guilt or worthlessness, difficulty in concentration or decision making, or suicidal thoughts.

Peripheral Adrenergic Inhibitors

The peripherally active adrenergic inhibitors are rarely used older agents and include reserpine (Serpalan, Serpasil), guanethidine (Ismelin), and guanadrel (Hylorel). Reserpine may be used as a second line agent because of its low cost and once daily dosing. Guanadrel and guanethidine have significant adverse effects and should be avoided because of the availability of safer agents.

reserpine [re **ser** peen]
(Serpalan, Serpasil)
Reserpine is a *Rauwolfia* alkaloid obtained from *Rauwolfia serpentina*, a shrub endemic to India and various tropical areas of the world. Reserpine lowers BP by depleting the storage sites of norepinephrine in the peripheral postganglionic adrenergic neuron. Without adequate norepinephrine available for release, discharges of nerve impulses from the peripheral sympathetic neurons, which supply the smooth muscle of arterioles, produce little or no effect on these blood vessels. The resultant vascular relaxation decreases peripheral resistance, thereby reducing BP. These compounds also decrease heart rate and thus lower cardiac output. Reserpine also depletes stores of serotonin.

Indications
Reserpine is indicated for mild to moderate hypertension. Uses beyond the FDA-approved indication include management of tardive dyskinesia and schizophrenia.

Pharmacokinetics/Dosing
Reserpine has an onset of antihypertensive action of days to 3 weeks with multiple dosing, and it has a peak antihypertensive effect within 3 to 6 weeks. The half-life is initially 4.5 hours, but with long-term dosing it is extended to between 45 and 168 hours. Reserpine is metabolized in the liver and excreted primarily in the feces. The adult dosage is 0.1 to 0.25 mg PO daily.

Adverse Effects
The adverse effects of reserpine include nausea, vomiting, anorexia, diarrhea, dizziness, dry mouth, stuffy nose, light-headedness, fluid retention, sexual dysfunction, chest pain, bradycardia, and bronchospasm. Clinical depression has also been noted with reserpine therapy.

Nursing Management
Assessment
Determine if the client has a history of mental depression, in which case reserpine is used cautiously. Reserpine therapy is discontinued at the first sign of despondency; otherwise continued therapy could result in suicide. Use reserpine cautiously in clients with a history of gallstones (to prevent biliary colic) or a history of renal insufficiency (to avoid the decreased renal tissue perfusion that may result from lower BP levels). Use cautiously in clients who are receiving electroconvulsive therapy or in clients with epilepsy, cardiac dysrhythmias, respiratory problems, parkinsonism, or pheochromocytoma. Clients with ulcerative colitis or acute peptic ulcer disease may experience increased GI motility; use reserpine with caution in such cases. Do not use reserpine with clients who are hypersensitive to *Rauwolfia* derivatives.

Review the client's current medication regimen for the risk of significant drug interactions, such as CNS depressants and/or alcohol enhanced CNS depressant effects) or MAO inhibitors (may result in hyperpyrexia and hypertension (moderate, severe, or even crisis level). Concurrent administration is not recommended. Clients receiving MAO inhibitors should be taken off this medication for at least 2 weeks before beginning administration of a *Rauwolfia* alkaloid.

Perform a baseline assessment of the client's BP, mental status, and renal function.

Nursing Diagnosis
With the administration of reserpine, the client may experience the following nursing diagnoses/collaborative problems: impaired tissue perfusion related to the client's underlying condition; risk for injury related to cardiovascular and CNS effects (light-headedness, dizziness, orthostatic hypotension); anxiety; disturbed thought processes (inability to concentrate); sexual dysfunction (impotence or decreased sexual interest); diarrhea; impaired oral mucous membrane (dry mouth, stuffy nose); disturbed sleep pattern (nightmares, early morning insomnia); ineffective protection (thrombocytopenia); impaired comfort (abdominal cramps, headache, chest pain); anxiety; and the potential complications related to GI effects (tarry stools, hematemesis, peptic ulcer), mental depression, or dysrhythmias.

Planning
Planning is the same as for other antihypertensive agents; see Box 27-4.

Implementation
Monitoring
Monitor the client's BP and pulse rate frequently and compare with baseline readings, particularly before parenteral administration. A decrease in BP may be a result of bradycardia. Weigh the client daily. Excessive weight gain indicates fluid retention, which should be reported to the prescriber.

Intervention
Administer the oral medication with meals or with milk or other food to minimize gastric irritation, because the drug increases gastric secretions.

Note that the *Rauwolfia* derivatives have a slow onset of action and a long duration of action; therefore therapeutic benefits may take approximately 2 weeks to develop. This means that dosage adjustments should be made no more frequently than every 7 to 14 days so that the full effect of the previous dosage can be evaluated. Action may persist for approximately 1 month after discontinuation of therapy. Reserpine no longer needs to be withdrawn if a client requires a general anesthetic, including for dental surgery; however, the anesthetist must be aware of the therapy. It is recommended that reserpine be withdrawn 2 weeks before electroconvulsive therapy is instituted.

Education
Review with the client lifestyle modifications that accompany antihypertensive therapy (Table 27-2), and standard information related to antihypertensive drugs (Box 27-6).

Although orthostatic hypotension does not usually occur with reserpine, advise the client to make position changes slowly to avoid potential dizziness and fainting. Alert the client that the drug may cause drowsiness and to take precautions about driving and other hazardous activities until the CNS effects are known. Advise the client not to take alcohol or other CNS depressants, which will increase the sedative effects of reserpine.

Instruct the client or caregiver about the possible adverse effects that may occur and those that should be reported to the prescriber, such as nightmares, weight gain, nasal stuffiness, or a significant change in BP. Mental depression (anorexia, self-deprecation, detached attitude, and powerlessness) may lead to suicide. This usually occurs in clients who receive high dosages. Clients should report despondency, early morning insomnia, anorexia, impotence, and feelings of low self-esteem.

If nasal stuffiness occurs, nasal decongestants or other over-the-counter (OTC) preparations containing sympathomimetics should not be used without first consulting the prescriber. A dry mouth may be relieved with warm water rinses, OTC saliva substitutes, sugarless gum, or sour hard candy.

Evaluation
The expected outcome of reserpine therapy is that the client will maintain a BP within normal limits without experiencing any adverse effects of the drug; see Box 27-7 for other outcome criteria.

The α-Adrenergic Blocking Agents

The α-adrenergic blocking agents used in the management of hypertension include phenoxybenzamine (Dibenzyline), phentolamine (Regitine), doxazosin (Cardura), prazosin (Minipress), terazosin (Hytrin), and tamsulosin (Flomax). Phenoxybenzamine and phentolamine are relatively nonselective alpha blockers; they antagonize responses mediated by both α_1 and α_2 receptors. Hence, they lower BP by preventing norepinephrine from activating α_1 receptors on vascular smooth muscle to produce vasoconstriction; see Chapter 22. Doxazosin, prazosin, and terazosin are more selective in activity and are classed as α_1-adrenergic blocking agents. Although these agents are effective at lowering BP, they are not as effective as thiazides in blood pressure control and are associated with increased risk for heart failure (ALLHAT, 2002; Davis, Furberg, Wright, Cutler, & Whelton, 2004). Doxazosin, prazosin, terazosin, and tamsulosin all act to improve urinary flow in clients with BPH, which accounts for their use for this indication. Tamsulosin has less activity on vascular smooth muscle and is less inclined to lower BP. A brief review of prazosin is presented as representative of this class.

Prazosin is a selective α_1-adrenergic blocking agent that dilates both arterioles and veins. This action results in decreased peripheral vascular resistance and lowered BP. Modest reflex tachycardia is associated with doxazosin use.

⭐🔲 **prazosin [pra** zoe sin]
(Minipress)

Indications
Prazosin is used in the treatment of hypertension and managing symptoms of BPH.

Pharmacokinetics/Dosing
The onset of action for prazosin is about 2 hours; the duration of action is about 10 to 24 hours. Prazosin is metabolized in the liver and is excreted primarily in the urine. The initial adult dosage of prazosin is 1 mg PO daily at bedtime for the first dose, then 1 mg two or three times daily. Dosages may be titrated up to a maximum daily dose of 20 mg. On rare occasions, doses as high as 40 mg daily have been used.

Adverse Effects
The adverse effects of the α-adrenergic blocking drugs include weakness, nausea, vomiting, stuffy nose, orthostatic hypotension, angina, edema of the lower extremities, headaches, syncope, and shortness of breath. First dose orthostatic hypotension is often dramatic and occurs within 90 minutes of the first dose. As such, the client should be instructed to take the first dose immediately before bed and not arise for a few hours.

Nursing Management

Assessment
Do not administer α_1 blockers if a client has a sensitivity to the drug. Clients with impaired renal and hepatic function may have a prolonged hypotensive effect and require lower dosages. Older adults may be more sensitive to the effects of α-adrenergic blocking agents. The concurrent use of NSAIDs (cause sodium and fluid retention), other hypotensive agents (may have an additive effect), and sympathomimetics (reduce antihypertensive effects) should be avoided. Document a baseline BP.

Nursing Diagnosis
The nursing diagnoses/collaborative problems to be considered with α_1 blockers include the following: risk for injury related to the cardiovascular and CNS effects (drowsiness, dizziness, and orthostatic hypotension); excess fluid volume (dependent edema, shortness of breath, and weight gain); fatigue; impaired oral mucous membrane (dry mouth); impaired comfort (nasal stuffiness, headache, chest pain, joint pain, nausea, and vomiting); decreased cardiac output (tachycardia, palpitations); and the potential complication of "first-dose orthostatic hypotensive reaction" and priapism.

Planning
Planning is the same as for other antihypertensive agents; see Box 27-4.

Implementation

Monitoring
Monitor the client's BP 2 to 6 hours postdose with the first dose and each dosage increase because orthostasis is most likely to occur at this time. Dosage increases are based on standing blood pressures taken at 2 to 6 hours and 24 hours post dose. Assess heart sounds for dysrhythmias and tachycardia and for symptoms of HF, e.g., peripheral edema, adventitious lung sounds, dyspnea.

Intervention
"First-dose hypotensive reaction," a syncope along with dizziness, light-headedness, or a sudden loss of consciousness, may occur, generally 30 to 120 minutes after an initial dose or a rapid dosage increase. These symptoms may also appear when other antihypertensive agents are added to the regimen. Occasionally the syncopal episode is preceded by severe tachycardia (heart rate of 120 to 160 beats/min). To minimize this reaction, the initial dose of α_1 blockers is limited to 1 mg and then increased slowly. When a diuretic or other antihypertensive agent is added, the dose is reduced to 1 or 2 mg and then increased as needed. It is recommended that the initial dose be administered at bedtime to minimize the "first-dose hypotensive reaction."

Education
Inform the client of "first-dose hypotensive reaction." Instruct the client to avoid rapid postural changes, particularly from recumbent to upright positions. Teach the client to lie down if dizziness occurs. Reassure the client that this effect tends to disappear with continued use of the drug or dosage reduction. Instruct the client not to drive or operate hazardous machinery during the early period of adjustment to drug therapy. Note that the full effect of the drug may not be achieved for 4 to 6 weeks.

Teach the client to weigh daily and to report any significant increase (over 1 kg per day) to the prescriber. Because these agents tend to increase fluid retention, instruct the client to minimize sodium intake.

Emphasize the importance of complying with the drug regimen and in keeping appointments with the prescriber. Ineffectiveness usually occurs within several months if tolerance develops, and the prescriber will need to alter the drug regimen. As with other antihypertensive agents, instruct the client in nonpharmacologic measures to reduce hypertension (see Table 27-2) and general instructions regarding antihypertensive medications (see Box 27-6).

Evaluation
The expected outcome of α-adrenergic blocking therapy is that the client will maintain a BP within normal limits and not experience any untoward effects of the drug. See Box 27-7 for other criteria for the evaluation of antihypertensive therapy. If the α-adrenergic drug is administered to improve the symptoms of benign prostatic hyperplasia, the client with have increased ease of starting his urinary stream, more complete bladder emptying, and less dribbling of urine.

Vasodilating Drugs

Vasodilators exhibit a direct action on the smooth muscle walls of the arterioles and veins, thereby lowering peripheral resistance and BP. Although various theories have been proposed, the mechanism of action, at least in part, involves the direct relaxation of vascular smooth muscle by stimulation of the calcium-binding process. The drop in BP stimulates the sympathetic nervous system and activates the baroreceptor reflexes, increasing heart rate and cardiac output. This also increases the release of renin. Therefore combined therapy is recommended. To inhibit sympathetic reflex response, the use of a β-adrenergic blocker such as propranolol (Inderal) has been advocated along with a diuretic to alleviate the sodium and water retention that occurs during vasodilator therapy.

There are two types of vasodilators: (1) arteriolar dilators (e.g., hydralazine [Apresoline], and minoxidil [Loniten]), which exert a selective effect on arterioles; and (2) arteriolar and venous dilators (e.g., sodium nitroprusside [Nipride, Nitropress]), which lower BP by acting on both arteriolar resistance vessels and venous capacitance vessels.

Labetalol (Normodyne) is an α_1-, β_1-, and β_2-adrenergic blocker with significant vasodilatory properties. Although its effects on vasculature are primary on arterioles, it may also have some effect on venous capacitance. Like nitroprusside, it is used intravenously for hypertensive emergencies and thus is presented here. A further discussion of adrenergic antagonists is presented in Chapter 22.

Arteriolar Dilator Drugs

✱◪ hydralazine [hye **dral** a zeen]
(Apresoline, Novo-Hylazin✺)
Hydralazine is believed to produce its hypotensive effects by direct relaxation of vascular smooth muscle (particularly the arterioles) with little effect on the veins; this results in a reduction in peripheral resistance. Consequently, renal blood flow is increased, which provides an advantage to clients with renal failure. Hydralazine also maintains cerebral blood flow and produces sodium and water retention. However, the resultant hypotension is thought to stimulate the baroreceptor reflex, causing an increase in heart rate and cardiac output. Although this response offsets the antihypertensive effects of the drug, it proves beneficial in the reduction of afterload, explaining its use in the treatment of heart failure. Its combination with nitrates has proven beneficial for black clients with heart failure (Taylor et al, 2004).

Tolerance to the antihypertensive action of hydralazine may be offset by the addition of a diuretic to the drug regimen. The diuretic enhances the antihypertensive effect and reduces the potential for increased cardiac output and fluid retention. Hydralazine decreases diastolic pressure more than systolic pressure. It also increases plasma renin activity.

Indications
Hydralazine is indicated for the management of moderate to severe hypertension and as adjunct therapy in the management of HF.

Pharmacokinetics/Dosing
The onset of action of hydralazine is 45 minutes for an oral dose or within 10 to 20 minutes for an IV dose. Its peak effect is within 1 hour (oral dose) or 15 to 30 minutes (IV dose). The half-life for both the oral and IV dosage forms is between 3 and 7 hours, and the duration of action is 3 to 8 hours. Hydralazine is metabolized in the liver and excreted by the kidneys. The adult oral dosage is 40 mg daily PO for 2 to 4 days, then 100 mg daily in divided doses for the remainder of the first week. The maintenance dosage is 50 mg four times daily or the lowest effective dosage. Children receive 0.75 mg/kg divided into 2 to 4 doses, increased slowly over 1 to 4 weeks as necessary to a maximum of 7.5 mg/kg. For parenteral administra-

tion for hypertension, the adult dosage is 10 to 40 mg IM or IV; repeat if necessary. The parenteral pediatric dosage is 1.7 to 3.5 mg/kg divided into 4 to 6 daily doses.

Adverse Effects
The adverse effects of hydralazine include diarrhea, nausea, vomiting, tachycardia, anorexia, headache, facial flushing, stuffy nose, edema, angina, rash peripheral neuritis, and SLE–like syndrome. The SLE-like syndrome may include myalgia, arthralgia, arthritis, weakness, fever, and skin changes.

Nursing Management

Assessment
Hydralazine hydrochloride is contraindicated in clients with coronary artery disease (CAD) (anginal attacks may be intensified); rheumatic mitral valvular disease (may increase pulmonary artery pressure and precipitate HF); and hypersensitivity to hydralazine. Acute aortic dissection may worsen if hydralazine is administered. Clients with cerebrovascular disease may be at risk for increased cerebral ischemia, and those with impaired renal function may need lower dosages of hydralazine. The concurrent use of NSAIDs (cause sodium and fluid retention), other hypotensive agents (may have an additive effect), and sympathomimetics (reduce antihypertensive effects) should be avoided. Before the initiation of hydralazine therapy, obtain a baseline BP. ANA titer determinations are documented for comparison if the client develops a drug-induced SLE. CBC is determined as periodic monitoring for blood dyscrasias will be done throughout therapy. A baseline assessment includes ECG, heart and lung sounds, and BP.

Nursing Diagnosis
With the administration of hydralazine, the client may experience the following nursing diagnoses/collaborative problems: risk for injury related to hypotension (dizziness, light-headedness); excess fluid volume related to sodium and water retention (swelling of feet or lower legs); impaired comfort (headache, nasal congestion, watery eyes, flushing of face, skin rash, anorexia, nausea, and vomiting); diarrhea; constipation; and the potential complications of SLE-like syndrome (malaise, sore throat, fever, arthralgia), angina (chest pain), blood dyscrasias (agranulocytosis, leukopenia, purpura), peripheral neuritis (tingling, numbness, and weakness in hands or feet), lymphadenopathy, and an allergic response.

Planning
Planning is the same as for other antihypertensive agents; see Box 27-4.

Implementation

Monitoring
Check the BP and pulse of clients receiving parenteral hydralazine every 5 minutes until stabilized; continue to check frequently (approximately every 10 to 15 minutes) during parenteral therapy. Monitor intake and output ratios during parenteral therapy; output may be increased with improved renal blood flow. Monitor BP periodically if oral hydralazine is used.

Weigh the client daily to check for fluid retention. Report to the prescriber any weight gain. Advise the client to reduce salt intake.

Observe the mental status of the client. Report to the prescriber any signs of anxiety or mental depression; this condition may indicate cerebral ischemia.

CBC, SLE cell preparation, and antinuclear antibody (ANA) titer tests are indicated if the client develops fever, sore throat, arthralgia, chest pain, and chronic malaise. Repeat these tests periodically if the client is receiving prolonged therapy. SLE-like syndrome may occur in clients receiving higher dosages (more than 200 mg daily), in slow acetylators, and in clients with renal impairment. Discontinue the drug if tests are positive.

Intervention
Administer the parenteral form of hydralazine immediately after opening the ampule. The drug may change color when added to infusion fluids. Hydralazine is usually administered with a diuretic and a sympatholytic to prevent fluid retention and excessive sympathetic stimulation of the heart. Most clients can be changed to oral dosage forms after 24 to 48 hours of parenteral therapy. Administer oral hy-

dralazine with meals or food; this minimizes the first-pass metabolism of the drug in the intestinal wall, thereby enhancing bioavailability. The drug should be administered consistently in relation to food. The oral solution may be mixed with a small amount of fruit juice or applesauce just before administering it.

Education

Review with the client lifestyle modifications that accompany antihypertensive therapy (see Table 27-2), and standard information related to antihypertensive drugs (see Box 27-6). Teach the client the importance of taking the medication at the same time each day and to take it exactly as prescribed, even when feeling well. Inform the client that the drug should not be discontinued even if adverse effects occur; instead, the prescriber should be contacted. This agent should be discontinued gradually; abrupt withdrawal will precipitate a sudden rise in BP and heart failure. After long-term administration of hydralazine, drug tolerance may develop, which necessitates adjustment of the drug regimen.

Inform the client that palpitations and headache may occur during the early stages of oral administration, but these symptoms usually subside with continued therapy. A β blocker such as propranolol is usually prescribed to prevent reflex tachycardia.

Instruct the client to report any signs of peripheral neuritis (numbness, tingling, and paresthesias) so that pyridoxine (vitamin B_6) may be prescribed to combat the antipyridoxine response of hydralazine.

Evaluation

The expected outcome of hydralazine therapy is that the client will maintain a BP within normal limits and not experience any adverse effects of the drug; see Box 27-7 for other outcome criteria.

minoxidil [mih **nox** i dill]
(Loniten)

Minoxidil (Loniten) is an orally effective, direct-acting peripheral vasodilator. It reduces BP by decreasing peripheral vascular resistance in the arteriolar vessels with little effect on veins. It does not cause orthostatic hypotension. It is a potent vasodilator but also causes a reflex increase in cardiac output, induces sodium retention, promotes the development of edema, and increases plasma renin activity.

Indications

Minoxidil is reserved for severe hypertension unresponsive to traditional agents (e.g., severe hypertension associated with chronic renal failure). Concomitant administration of a β-adrenergic blocking agent such as propranolol (Inderal) is necessary to prevent severe reflex tachycardia. Administration of a diuretic agent is also essential to counteract sodium and water retention. Topical minoxidil is used to promote hair growth.

Pharmacokinetics/Dosing

Minoxidil has an onset of action in 30 minutes and a peak effect in 2 to 3 hours (after a single dose). The half-life of this drug and its metabolites is 4.2 hours. Its duration of effect is between 1 and 2 days. It is metabolized in the liver and excreted mostly by the kidneys. The dosage for adults and children 12 years and older is 5 mg PO daily, increased in 100% increments as necessary (e.g., to 10 mg, 20 mg, 40 mg). It is usually recommended that dosage increases be on a minimum 3-day schedule, but in certain cases increases can be made every 6 hours with close monitoring of the client. For children up to 12 years of age, the dosage is 0.2 mg/kg/day.

Adverse Effects

The adverse effects of minoxidil include nausea; vomiting; tachycardia; edema; anorexia; headaches; excessive hair growth (hypertrichosis), usually on the face, arms, and back; red flushing of the skin; angina; and pericarditis.

Nursing Management
Assessment

Inquire if the client is pregnant or has plans for pregnancy, because studies about the risk to the fetus are inconclusive. Hypertrichosis has been reported in newborns following maternal therapy with minoxidil. Do not use in clients with pheochromocytoma, because minoxidil may stimulate catecholamine secretion from the tumor. Use minoxidil cautiously in clients with MI, pericardial effusion, coronary insufficiency, and HF, because this drug may further limit blood flow to the myocardium. Clients with renal function impairment may require lower dosages.

Review the client's current medication regimen for the risk of significant drug interactions, such as guanethidine, nitrates or potent parenteral antihypertensives, e.g., nitroprusside (Nitropress). This combination may result in severe hypotensive reaction. The concurrent use of NSAIDs (cause sodium and fluid retention), other hypotensive agents (may have an additive effect), and sympathomimetics (reduce antihypertensive effects) should be avoided.

A baseline assessment of the client should include BP, pulse, weight, respiratory rate, heart and breath sounds, assessment for pedal edema, and laboratory studies for serum electrolytes.

Nursing Diagnosis

With the administration of minoxidil, the client may experience the following nursing diagnoses/collaborative problems: excess fluid volume related to sodium and water retention (dependent edema, rapid weight gain); disturbed body image related to hypertrichosis; impaired comfort (rash, itching, paresthesia, and chest pain); and the potential complications of allergic reaction, angina, cardiac effusion, Stevens-Johnson syndrome, and reflex sympathetic activation (tachycardia, flushing of skin).

Planning

Planning is the same as for other antihypertensive agents; see Box 27-4.

Implementation
Monitoring

When minoxidil is first administered, clients are monitored in a controlled setting to prevent too rapid a decrease in BP. Take BP and pulse rate before administering minoxidil, and use these parameters as a guideline to determine progress. Monitor BP and pulse rate regularly during therapy. Report to the prescriber any sharp drop in BP, which can precipitate a stroke or MI.

Monitor weight gain, intake and output ratios, and the presence of edema. Inform the prescriber of an increase in weight (kg/day) so that fluid retention can be corrected.

Monitor electrolyte balance, especially potassium levels if the client is receiving a diuretic that may produce hypokalemia. Potassium replacement therapy should be prescribed. Watch for pericardial effusion with or without tamponade; this reaction may occur in approximately 3% of clients not receiving dialysis. This requires more vigorous diuretic therapy; if pericardiocentesis does not alleviate the condition, discontinuation of minoxidil is necessary.

Observe for anginal symptoms or tachycardia, which can be relieved by concomitant administration of a β-adrenergic blocker.

Intervention

Closely monitor clients with renal failure or those receiving dialysis to prevent exacerbation of renal failure or precipitation of cardiac failure. Lower dosages of minoxidil are indicated for these clients. It is recommended that a 3-day interval occur between dosage adjustments. In an acute care setting, more rapid dosage changes may occur with careful monitoring of the BP.

Education

Instruct the client to count the radial pulse rate for 1 minute before taking minoxidil and to report to the prescriber an increase of at least 20 beats/min above baseline. Advise the client receiving combination therapy to take each medication at the proper time. A diuretic is given to reduce salt and fluid retention, and a β blocker is given to control reflex tachycardia. Combined therapy is indicated to increase the effectiveness of the drug and to minimize adverse effects by lowering the dosage of minoxidil. Advise the client to weigh daily and to report any sharp 2 kg increase in weight to the prescriber.

Inform the client that a missed dose may be taken a few hours later. A missed dose should not be made up the next day; instead, the regular dosing schedule should be resumed. Consult the prescriber if there is any question.

Emphasize the importance of drug compliance despite uncomfortable adverse effects. Inform the client that minoxidil is a powerful drug for reducing BP and that by relaxing small blood vessels, more blood flow protects vital organs (heart, kidney, and brain).

Inform the client that hypertrichosis will likely occur (incidence is 80%) 3 to 6 weeks after starting therapy. This involves elongation, thickening, and increased pigmentation of fine body hair over the temples, eyebrows, sideburns, malar area, shoulders, back, legs, and forearms. This adverse effect is particularly troublesome to women. Advise the client that this condition is reversible within 2 to 6 months following discontinuation of therapy. No endocrine abnormalities have been found to account for this distressing effect. Hair remover (depilatory creams) or shaving may be effective in removing unwanted hair.

Instruct the client that minoxidil may be taken with or without food. Advise the client against increasing salt intake, and request that a dietitian provide information regarding appropriate dietary choices. Inform the client to notify the prescriber if difficulty in breathing occurs, especially when lying down, because this may indicate impending HF. As with other antihypertensive medications, teach the client about nonpharmacologic therapies to reduce BP (see Table 27-2) and general information about antihypertensive drug therapy.

Evaluation

The expected outcome of minoxidil therapy is that the client will maintain a BP within normal limits and not experience any adverse effects of minoxidil; see Box 27-7 for general outcome criteria for antihypertensives.

Arterial and Venous Dilator Drugs

✱▪ nitroprusside [nye troe **prus** ide]

(Nipride, Nitropress)

Nitroprusside is a potent and fast direct-acting vasodilator agent that greatly reduces arterial BP. It relaxes both arterial and venous smooth muscles but is more active on veins. Therefore nitroprusside reduces cardiac load; that is, the decrease in systemic resistance results in a reduction in preload and afterload, which improves cardiac output in the client with HF.

Indications

Nitroprusside is indicated for rapid reduction of BP in hypertensive emergencies, adjunct therapy in MI and valvular regurgitation, and also as an antidote for ergot alkaloid toxicity.

Pharmacokinetics/Dosing

Sodium nitroprusside has an almost immediate onset of action and peak effect (within minutes) after administration by IV infusion. The half-life of nitroprusside is 2 minutes; the half-life of thiocyanate, a possible toxic metabolite, is 3 days. The duration of effect is between 1 and 10 minutes after discontinuance of the infusion. It is metabolized by erythrocytes (to cyanide) and the liver (cyanide to thiocyanate), and it is excreted by the kidneys. For the adult and pediatric dosage, mix the contents of the vial in dextrose 5% injection only, and administer by IV infusion. The initial dosage is 0.3 mcg/kg/min, which is slowly increased in increments of 0.3 mcg according to client response. The usual dosage is 0.003 mg (3 mcg)/kg/min.

Adverse Effects

The adverse effects of nitroprusside include dizziness, excessive sweating, headaches, anxiety, abdominal cramps, tachycardia, hypothyroidism, flushing, rash, and muscle twitching. If the client has thiocyanate toxicity, ataxia, blurred vision, headache, nausea, vomiting, tinnitus, shortness of breath, delirium, and unconsciousness may occur. Hypotension, metabolic acidosis, pink coloration, very shallow breathing pattern, decreased reflexes, coma, and widely dilated pupils may be observed in clients with cyanide toxicity.

Nursing Management

Assessment

Do not use the drug in clients with inadequate cerebral or coronary artery circulation because there is a reduced tolerance for hypotension. Sodium nitroprusside should be used cautiously in clients with renal or hepatic function impairment, Leber hereditary optic atrophy, vitamin B_{12} deficiency, or tobacco amblyopia, because these conditions influence the metabolism and excretion of the drug. Clients with encephalopathy and other conditions in which they are at risk for increased intracranial pressure may experience pressure increases. If the client is also taking dobutamine, a higher cardiac output and lower pulmonary wedge pressure may result. Concurrent use of other antihypertensive agents is an indication for closer monitoring of the BP, because there may be an additive effect. A baseline BP should be obtained.

Nursing Diagnosis

With the administration of sodium nitroprusside, the client may experience the following nursing diagnoses/collaborative problems: risk for injury related to rebound hypertension with abrupt withdrawal of the drug or related to hypotension (dizziness, restlessness, tachycardia); impaired tissue integrity (pain at infusion site); impaired comfort (headache, abdominal cramping); and the potential complications of thiocyanate toxicity (ataxia, blurred vision, delirium, dizziness, nausea and vomiting, ringing of the ears) and cyanide toxicity (decreased consciousness progressing to coma).

Planning

Planning is the same as for other antihypertensive agents; see Box 27-4.

Implementation

Monitoring

To prevent rapid hypotension, monitor the BP every 30 seconds when the infusion is first started. Later, check it every 5 minutes. Facilities and personnel must be adequate for this purpose; intensive care facilities are recommended. Observe the client for any precipitous drop in BP, which may occur if large doses are given. Do not allow the infusion rate to exceed 10 mcg/kg/min. If an adequate reduction in BP does not occur in 10 minutes, the drug is discontinued.

Monitor intake and output ratios. Monitor the client for thiocyanate toxicity (tinnitus, blurred vision, and delirium). Because sodium nitroprusside is converted to thiocyanate, monitor the blood thiocyanate level when infusion is continued for more than 72 hours, especially in clients with renal dysfunction.

Intervention

After starting an IV solution of sodium nitroprusside, promptly wrap the container in the supplied opaque sleeve or aluminum foil or other opaque material to protect the drug from light. Use fresh solution, and do not keep it longer than 24 hours. Freshly prepared solution has a faint brown tinge; discard it if it is highly colored (e.g., blue, green, or dark red).

Administer the infusion using a volumetric infusion pump; these devices allow precise measurement of the prescribed flow rate. Do not add other drugs to the nitroprusside infusion. Avoid extravasation, because it results in tissue damage.

If the blood thiocyanate level exceeds 10 mg/dL, the infusion should be discontinued or decreased to prevent toxicity. A potential for cyanide intoxication exists with prolonged treatment and overdose. (Note that nitroprusside is metabolized first to cyanide, then to thiocyanate.) Discontinue nitroprusside in the event of cyanide toxicity (coma, dilated pupils, pink color, shallow respirations, imperceptible pulse rate, distant heart sounds, hypotension, and absent reflexes). Continue to observe the client for several hours to prevent the recurrence of signs of overdose. (See the Management of Drug Overdose box on p. 572.)

Be aware that the client's therapy will be changed to oral antihypertensive agents as soon as a response occurs. As oral therapy is instituted, the client will require lower doses of nitroprusside.

Education

Keep the client advised about the care that is taking place.

Evaluation

The expected outcome of sodium nitroprusside therapy is that the BP will return to normal parameters without the client experiencing any adverse effects of the drug.

labetalol [la **bet** a lole]
(Normodyne, Trandate)
Indications

Labetalol is used orally to treat moderate to severe hypertension and is used intravenously to treat hypertensive emergencies.

⚙ Management of Drug Overdose

Nitroprusside

- The structure of nitroprusside contains five cyanide groups which, when the drug is administered IV, splits off to free cyanide and nitric oxide, the active substance. Nitric oxide then activates the enzyme guanylate cyclase to produce cyclic GMP and vasodilation. The free cyanide is converted to hydrogen cyanide (prussic acid), which is metabolized in the liver by rhodanase and a sulfur donor (such as thiosulfate) to convert it to thiosulfate, which is then excreted by the kidneys.

- When the amount of sulfur donors are limited or overwhelmed by high-dose nitroprusside therapy, hydrogen cyanide may accumulate in the body and cause toxicity. Some investigators report that if thiosulfate is mixed in the nitroprusside infusion at a 5 to 10:1 ratio (such as 250 mg to 500 mg thiosulfate to 50 mg nitroprusside) during administration of the nitroprusside, the less toxic thiocyanate will be formed and excreted. This method reduces the potential for cyanide accumulation and toxicity (*USP DI*, 2005).

- Thiocyanate toxicity may occur in clients with chronic therapy and renal impairment. The half-life of nitroprusside in normal renal function is 2.7 days; in renal failure it is 9 days. Therefore, depending on the amount of drug administered to the client, this toxicity is usually more apt to occur than the cyanide toxicity.

- For severe hypotension, slow or discontinue the infusion. Placing the client supine with the legs elevated on pillows will maximize venous return.

- For cyanide toxicity, discontinue nitroprusside and administer sodium nitrite (3% solution) in dose of 4 to 6 mg/kg IV over 2 to 4 minutes. Amyl nitrite inhalation should be used if IV sodium nitrite is not immediately available. Nitrites buffer the cyanide by converting approximately 10% of the client's hemoglobin to methemoglobin. After administering sodium nitrite, administer sodium thiosulfate (150 to 200 mg/kg) to convert the cyanide to thiocyanate. Thiocyanate is less toxic and rarely a problem; use hemodialysis if thiocyanate toxicity occurs. Be aware however, that hemodialysis does not remove cyanide. If necessary, this regimen (nitrite and thiocyanate) may be repeated after 2 hours, in one-half the original dose.

Pharmacokinetics/Dosing

Administered intravenously, labetalol has an onset of action within 2 to 5 minutes, a peak effect in 5 to 15 minutes, and a duration of action of 2 to 4 hours. Orally administered labetalol has an onset of 20 minutes to 2 hours and a duration of effect between 8 and 24 hours depending on dose. As with other β blockers, labetalol undergoes extensive first-pass metabolism and is metabolized primarily via cytochrome P450 2D6. It is lipid soluble and distributes to many tissues, including the CNS and across the placenta, which may account for fatigue and fetal bradycardia, respectively. The oral adult dose for hypertension is 100 mg twice daily initially, with doses increased by 100-mg increments daily every 2 to 3 days until an adequate dose response is obtained. Typical doses are 200 to 400 mg orally twice daily, but doses as high as 1200 mg orally twice daily have been used. In the treatment of hypertensive emergencies, an IV dose of 20 mg is typically administered initially over 2 minutes, then doses of 40 to 80 mg IV every 10 minutes (or an IV infusion of 2 mg/min) are used up to a maximum total IV dose of 300 mg. When blood pressure is controlled with IV labetalol, dosing is often converted to 200 mg orally for one dose, then 200 to 400 mg orally every 6 to 12 hours.

Adverse Effects

The most common adverse effect with labetalol is significant hypertension, particularly with the IV formulation. Dosing of IV labetalol requires careful monitoring. Other adverse effects of labetalol are similar to other nonselective β blockers (see Chapter 22) and include bradycardia, bronchospasm, sexual dysfunction, mental depression, and delayed conduction through the AV node. It is considered a category C agent by the manufacturer, but many consider it a category D agent during the second and third trimester because of its ability to cross the placenta and affect fetal heart rate and blood flow.

Drug Interactions

Labetalol has the potential to interact with a number of other drugs, including drugs that interfere with cytochrome P450 2D6 activity. Such drugs include quinidine, propoxyphene, and propafenone. Other vasodilatory or antihypertensive agents may result in excessive hypotension. A more complete discussion of β blockers, their interactions, and nursing management is presented in Chapter 22.

✳ Are there special considerations in the choice of antihypertensives?

Matching the most appropriate therapy to the client is important to assure optimal BP control and reduced target organ damage, adherence to therapy and minimal adverse effects. Considerations include age of client, culture/genetics, pregnancy status, comorbidities and surgical status.

Age Age differences affect BP. Elevated systolic BP, elevated diastolic BP, or both, occurs in a significant proportion of persons older than 65 years of age and increases their risk of cardiovascular morbidity and mortality. Antihypertensive drugs should be started at smaller than usual doses, increased by smaller than usual amounts, and scheduled at less frequent intervals with older adults, because they are more sensitive to volume depletion and sympathetic inhibition than are younger clients. They commonly have impaired cardiovascular reflexes, which makes them more susceptible to hypotension.

In older adults with isolated systolic hypertension who are treated with antihypertensive drugs, the systolic pressure should be cautiously decreased to 140 to 160 mm Hg. Consideration should be given to further lowering the systolic value only if this medication level is tolerated without serious adverse effects. The response of older adults to both nonpharmacologic and pharmacologic therapies should be monitored closely.

The goal of therapy for children and adolescents with hypertension is to reduce BP without producing adverse effects that limit compliance or interfere with normal growth and development. The causative factors, the presence of complications, and the degree of hypertension will determine the type of intervention. Nonpharmacologic measures (weight control, reduction of dietary sodium, exercise, avoidance of smoking and alcohol, and reduction of saturated fat) are strongly recommended. Pharmacologic therapy should be considered if children do not respond to nonpharmacologic measures or if their blood pressures place them at risk for organ damage.

Pharmacologic interventions for children also follow the stepped approach. Continued assessment of the child and family is necessary to ensure satisfactory BP control and compliance with the pharmacologic or nonpharmacologic therapeutic program.

Culture/Genetics African Americans generally respond better to diuretics and calcium antagonists than to ACE inhibitors or β-blocking agents. (See the Special Considerations for Pharmacogenetics box below for additional clinical responses to antihypertensive agents among different racial and ethnic groups.) Gender differences in response to antihypertensive agents have not been identified. Hypertension is reported to be two to three times more common in women who have used hormonal contraceptive agents for 5 years or longer as compared with those not taking any hormonal contraceptives. This risk increases with age, smoking, and higher doses of estrogen and progesterone. If hypertension occurs, the usual treatment is to discontinue the hormonal contraceptive; BP usually normalizes in 3 to 6 months. If BP does not return to normal, lifestyle modifications and antihypertensive drugs should be instituted.

Pregnancy Hypertension during pregnancy is a serious condition that requires early detection and treatment. The following are two major diagnostic categories and treatment:

- *Chronic hypertension.* Hypertension is present before pregnancy or is diagnosed before the twentieth week of gestation. Diuretics, methyldopa (Aldomet), or other antihypertensive medications may be used. ACE inhibitors and ARBs are to be avoided; serious neonatal problems, including renal failure and death, have been reported with their use. (For more information, see the Pregnancy Safety box on p. 556.)
- *Preeclampsia-eclampsia.* This condition is a pregnancy-induced hypertension and is a primary factor in maternal and fetal morbidity and mortality. It has been estimated to occur in 3% to 7% of nulliparas and 0.8% to 5% of multiparas, mostly in teenagers or in primigravida women over 35 years of age (Sibai et al., 2000).

The signs and symptoms of preeclampsia may range from mild to severe; the severe form may include systolic BP greater than or equal to 160 mm Hg, diastolic BP greater than or equal to 110 mm Hg, proteinuria, elevated serum

---

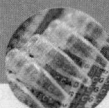 **Special Considerations for Pharmacogenetics | ANTIHYPERTENSIVES**

PHARMACODYNAMICS

Blacks are considerably less likely to respond to the antihypertensive effects of β-adrenergic blockers, ACE inhibitors, and ARBs compared with whites, although they appear to respond well to diuretics and CCBs (Brewster et al, 2004). Similarly, blacks respond well to the combination of hydralazine and nitrates in the treatment of heart failure (Taylor, 2004). The basis for these findings likely lies in genetic variation in pharmacodynamic response. The effects of genetic variation on β adrenergic receptors and β blockers were noted in the Special Considerations for Pharmacogenetics box on p. 506 in Chapter 25. There also appears to be a correlation between genetic markers and the likelihood of β blockers or ARBs to prevent left ventricular hypertrophy in hypertension independent of blood pressure reduction (Liljedahl et al, 2004). Similar data exists for drugs which bind to angiotensin II receptors (Jones et al, 2004). These findings may have future importance in drug selection based on genetics to determine which candidates would best respond to therapies that reduce long-term risks of hypertension.

PHARMACOKINETICS

The variation across populations in the activity of P450 2D6 (affecting metabolism of many β blockers), and 3 A4 (impacting metabolism of CCBs and quinidine) appears to be genetically determined (Wojnowski, 2004; Schaefer, Caracciolo, Frishman, & Charney, 2003).

ADVERSE EFFECTS

Up to 7% of the Chinese population may display genetic markers for low P450 2 C19, which metabolizes propranolol (Si et al, 2004). This may explain the observation that many Chinese are more sensitive to the effects of propranolol. The risk for angioedema, a potentially life-threatening hypersensitivity reaction to ACE inhibitors is related to a gene that codes for altered degradation of bradykinin (an inflammatory mediator) (Dykewicz, 2004). It remains to be seen whether future genetic testing could help predict individuals who might be at risk for adverse events to antihypertensives.

creatinine, headache, visual disturbances, gastric pain, retinal damage (e.g., hemorrhage, exudate), pulmonary edema, decreased platelet count (less than $100,000/mm^3$), and/or eclampsia or seizures in a woman with preeclampsia.

Therapy includes bed rest, hospitalization (controversial today) and, if the fetus is mature, a timely delivery. The use of antihypertensive agents is based on maternal safety, with most clinicians initiating treatment when the diastolic BP is greater than or equal to 100 mm Hg. If delivery is not planned for within 24 hours, an oral agent such as methyldopa (Aldomet) is the drug of choice, although labetalol (Normodyne), magnesium sulfate, parenteral hydralazine, calcium blocking agents, and various beta-adrenergic agents have also been used. Low-dose aspirin (60 mg) is sometimes used to prevent preeclampsia in high-risk clients. Aspirin reverses the imbalance between prostacyclin and thromboxane that may be responsible for preeclampsia. As mentioned previously, the ACEIs and ARBs are not recommended for use during pregnancy (Sibai et al., 2000).

Women receiving continuous antihypertensive therapy should be advised not to breastfeed, because most of the agents are transferred to breast milk.

Comorbid States Persons with concurrent disease/illness may respond best or, in some instances, adversely to certain medications. For example, β-blocking agents and CCBs are the preferred agents for hypertensive clients who also have angina or atrial tachycardia and fibrillation. In type 2 DM, ACE inhibitors or ARBs are recommended unless there is a significant contraindication to their use (Tan, Kuppuswamy, Whaley-Connell, Kurukulasuriya, & Sowers, 2004). β-blocking agents are usually preferred with preoperative hypertension but should be avoided with asthma, heart block, depression, or dyslipidemia.

Surgical Clients To prevent rebound hypertension, clients scheduled for elective surgery should receive their antihypertensive medications up to the time of surgery and as soon afterward as possible. Parenteral diuretics, adrenergic inhibitors, and vasodilators, plus sublingual nifedipine or transdermal clonidine, are available for clients who are unable to take oral medications. Clients taking an adrenergic inhibitor before surgery are more at risk for rebound hypertension (see Box 27-9).

The client's electrolyte status should be carefully checked before surgery. If hypokalemia is detected, it should be corrected before the scheduled operation. The anesthetist should always be completely informed about the client's medication regimen; this is vital information that may alter the medications or the monitoring methods used.

✳ **How can the nurse support adherence to antihypertensive therapy?**
Client adherence to hypertensive therapy is often difficult because hypertension is usually asymptomatic yet the drugs are often associated with troublesome adverse effects. Ways to help improve adherence to therapy include education about hypertension and its risks and the role of med-

ications. Creating an environment in which the client can openly ask questions or raise concerns about therapy or adverse effects is also important to identify obstacles to optimal therapy. Ask open-ended questions about the client's perception of the effectiveness of the therapeutic regimen. Provide encouragement for achieving goals. With the client's approval, involve clients' families and/or caregivers in the antihypertensive therapy. Provide oral and written instructions and information on the drug regimens and the goals of therapy. Provide assistance for clients having difficulty with compliance (e.g., drug doses written on a calendar; compartmentalized pill boxes; more frequent follow up appointments; mail, email and/or telephone refill reminders).

Advise the client that there are multiple agents for the treatment of hypertension and alternative medications may be prescribed to decrease adverse effects, minimize expense and/or increase the opportunity for compliance. Drugs can be prescribed with an adverse effect profile tolerable to the client, lower doses, and use of combination products that reduce "pill burden" may be helpful to increase compliance. Multiple combinations of thiazide diuretics with β blockers or ACE inhibitors are available and may be useful once the client has tolerated each agent. Collaborate with other health care professionals (e.g., nurses, pharmacists, physicians, nurse practitioners, therapists) and the client and family and/or caregivers to increase the effectiveness of the client's therapeutic regimen (Chobanian et al., 2003).

Summary

Hypertension is the most common cardiovascular health problem and affects more than 30 million Americans. Ninety percent of such cases are considered to be essential, idiopathic, or primary hypertension—that is, the specific cause of the hypertension is not known. Because individuals with hypertension are at higher risk for cardiovascular injury, they are treated nonpharmacologically and/or pharmacologically to reduce their BP and therefore reduce their risk of premature death or disability.

Nonpharmacologically, clients are encouraged to modify their lifestyles to include weight reduction, sodium restriction, elimination or limited consumption of alcohol and tobacco, reduction of dietary saturated fats, regular exercise, and behavior modification to promote relaxation.

Pharmacologically, a stepped-care approach is recommended by the Joint National Committee on the Detection, Evaluation, and Treatment of High Blood Pressure. This plan is a progressive approach that begins with the administration of a single drug, increases the dosage of that drug and then, in sequential order, gradually adds more potent agents as the need for more intensive therapy is indicated.

The antihypertensive drugs currently used to reduce BP are classified into five major categories: diuretics, adrenergic inhibitors (central and peripheral), ACE inhibitors and ARBS, CCBs, and vasodilators. The use of diuretics or the β-blocking agents in hypertension have resulted in a reduction in morbidity and mortality.

Diuretic drugs play an important role in the management of hypertension. Their administration results in the loss of excess salt and water from the body by renal excretion. This volume depletion, and a direct effect on the arterioles to produce vasodilation, result in a decrease in BP. Diuretic drugs are discussed primarily in Chapter 33.

Captopril, enalapril, and doxazosin are angiotensin II antagonists that inhibit vasoconstriction and the action of the RAA system, a disturbance of which may cause hypertension. ARBs, the newest class of antihypertensives, also inhibit vasoconstriction and the release of renin; they do this by blocking angiotensin II receptors. These agents are drugs of choice in treating hypertension in individuals with DM or HF.

Adrenergic-inhibiting agents were discussed in Chapter 22. β-adrenergic blockers are frequently used to treat hypertension, especially to manage reflex tachycardia associated with vasodilators. The centrally acting drugs clonidine, methyldopa, guanabenz, and guanfacine are sometimes used for resistant hypertension, particularly when combined with a diuretic. The peripheral adrenergic inhibitors (guanethidine, guanadrel, and *Rauwolfia* derivatives) are rarely used antihypertensives because of risks of therapy. Adrenergic-blocking agents such as doxazosin, prazosin, and terazosin lower BP by preventing norepinephrine from activating α_1 receptors on vascular smooth muscle to produce vasoconstriction, but their use is primarily in the management of benign prostatic hyperplasia because no reduction in morbidity or mortality has been demonstrated with these drugs.

Vasodilators act on the smooth muscle walls of the arterioles and veins, lowering peripheral resistance and BP. The arteriolar dilator agents administered for hypertension are diazoxide, hydralazine, and minoxidil. Sodium nitroprusside is a direct-acting vasodilator that relaxes both arteriolar and venous smooth muscle, which greatly reduces arterial BP, but cyanide accumulation limits its long-term use.

Nurses have a major role in the administration of antihypertensive agents when involved in the direct care of the client. By far the greatest contribution of nursing is client education to sustain adherence to the accurate and safe self-administration of antihypertensive agents. This guidance will assist the client in changing his or her lifestyle to incorporate the modifications to promote a decrease in hypertension and thus a healthier life.

Critical Thinking Questions

- Tim Rogers, 46 years old, has mild primary hypertension for which his health care provider has prescribed reserpine, 0.1 mg PO daily. About which past medical conditions would the nurse specifically ask during the drug history, which needs to be obtained before Mr. Rogers begins his reserpine therapy?

- Stella Parr, 52 years old, expresses her relief now that her prescriber has placed her on a diuretic as part of her antihypertensive medications. She states, "Now I won't have to struggle with all that tasteless food without salt. If I get water retention, the diuretic will take care of it." How should the nurse respond? What other lifestyle issues need to be explored with Ms. Parr?

Bibliography

The ALLHAT Officers and Coordinators for the ALLHAT Collaborative Research Group. (2002). Major outcomes in high-risk hypertensive patients randomized to angiotensin-converting enzyme inhibitor or calcium channel blocker vs diuretic: The Antihypertensive and Lipid-Lowering treatment to prevent Heart Attack Trial (ALLHAT). *Journal of the American Medical Association*, 288:2981-2997.

Anderson, D.M., Keith, J., & Novak, P.D. (Eds.) (2002). *Mosby's medical, nursing, and allied health dictionary* (6th ed.). St. Louis: Mosby.

Brewster, L.M., van Montfrans, G.A., Kleijnen, J. (2004). Systematic review: Antihypertensive drug therapy in black patients. *Annals of Internal Medicine*, 141(8):614-627.

Cappuccio, F.P., Kerry, S.M., & Donald, A. (2004). Blood pressure control by home monitoring: meta-analysis of randomized trials. *British Medical Journal*, 329(7464):145.

Carlberg, B., Samuelsson, O., Lindholm, L.H. (2004). Atenolol in hypertension: Is it a wise choice? *Lancet*, 364:1684-1689.

Carter, B.L., & Saseen, J.J. (2002). Hypertension. In J.T. DiPiro, R.L. Talbert, G.C. Yee, G.R. Matzke, B.G. Wells, & L.M. Posey (Eds.), *Pharmacotherapy: A pathophysiological* approach (3rd ed.). Norwalk, CT: Appleton & Lange.

e-LEARNING SUPPLEMENTS

Student CD-ROM
- Final Review questions
- NCLEX® Examination review questions
- Pharmacology animations
- Printable chapter summary

Evolve Website (http://evolve.elsevier.com/mckenry)
- Case study on drugs affecting the parasympathetic nervous system

- Content updates, including information on new drugs
- WebLinks corresponding to this chapter
- Answers to the critical thinking questions in this chapter
- *Elsevier ePharmacology Update* newsletter
- *Mosby's Drug Consult* Internet Edition
- Supplemental and reference information

Chobanian, A., & Hill, M. (2000). National Heart, Lung and Blood Institute Workshop on Sodium and Blood Pressure: A critical review of current scientific evidence. *Hypertension, 35*:858-863.

Chobanian, A., Bakris, G.L., Black H.R., et al. and the National High Blood Pressure Education Program Coordinating Committee. (2003). *The Seventh Report of the Joint National Committee on Prevention, Detection, Evaluation, and Treatment of High Blood Pressure: The JNC 7 Report.* Retrieved July 3, 2005, from http://www.nhlbi.nih.gov/guidelines/hypertension/jncintro.htm.

Davis, B.R., Furberg, C.D., Wright, J.T., Cutler, J.A., Whelton, P., and the ALLHAT Collaborative Research Group. (2004). ALLHAT: Setting the Record Straight. *Annals of Internal Medicine, 141*(1):39-46.

DiPiro, J.T., Talbert, R.L., Yee, G.C., Matzke, G.R., Wella, B.G., & Posey, L.M. (Eds.). (2002). *Pharmacotherapy: A pathophysiologic approach* (5th ed.). New York: McGraw-Hill.

Drug facts and comparisons (58th ed.). (2005). St. Louis: Facts and Comparisons.

Dykewicz, M.S. (2004) Cough and angioedema from angiotensin-converting enzyme inhibitors: new insights into mechanisms and management. *Current Opinion in Allergy & Clinical Immunology, 4*(4):267-270.

Goldman, L., & Ausiello, D. (Eds.) (2004). *Cecil's Textbook of Medicine* (22nd ed.). Philadelphia: W.B. Saunders.

He, J., Whelton, P.K., Appel, L.J., Charlston, J., & Klag, M.J. (2000). Long-term effects of weight loss and dietary sodium on incidence of hypertension, *Hypertension, 35*:544-549.

Jones, A., Dhamrait, S., Payne, J.R., et al. (2003). Genetic variants of angiotensin II receptors and cardiovascular risk in hypertension. *Hypertension, 42*(4):500-506.

Kearney, P., Whelton, M., Reynolds, K., Whelton, P., & He, J. (2004). Worldwide prevalence of hypertension: a systematic review. *Journal of Hypertension, 22*(1):11-19.

Lacy, C.F., Armstrong, L.L., Goldman, M.P., & Lance, L.L. (2004). *Lexi-Comp's Drug Information Handbook* (12th ed.). Hudson, Ohio: Lexi-Comp.

Liljedahl, U., Kahan, T., Malmqvist, K., et al. (2004). Single nucleotide polymorphisms predict the change in left ventricular mass in response to antihypertensive treatment. *Journal of Hypertension, 22*(12):2321-2328.

McCraty, R., Atkinson, M., & Tomasino, D. (2003). Impact of a workplace stress reduction program on blood pressure and emotional health in hypertensive employees. *Journal of alternative and Complementary Medicine, 9*(3):355-369.

Mosby's drug consult (15th ed.). (2005). St. Louis: Mosby.

Nakao, N., Yoshimura, A., Morita, H., Takada, M., Kayano, T., Ideura, T. (2003). Combination treatment of angiotensin-II receptor blocker and angiotensin-converting-enzyme inhibitor in non-diabetic renal disease (COOPERATE): A randomised controlled trial. *Lancet, 361*:117-24.

Pilote, L., Abrahamowicz, M., Rodrigues, E., Eisenberg, M.J., Rahme, E. (2004). Mortality rates in elderly patients who take different angiotensin-converting enzyme inhibitors after acute myocardial infarction: A class effect? Annals of Internal Medicine, 141:102-112.

Prisant, L.M. (2003). Diabetes mellitus and hypertension: A mandate for intense treatment according to new guidelines. *American Journal of Therapeutics, 10*(5):363-369.

Sacks, F.M., Svetsky, L.P., Vollmer, W.M., Appel L.J., Bray, G.A., Harsha, D., et al. (2001). Effects on blood pressure of reduced dietary sodium and the Dietary Approaches to Stop Hypertension

(DASH) diet. DASH-Sodium Collaborative Research Group. *New England Journal of Medicine, 344*:3-10.

Saseen, J.J., & Carter, B.L. (2005). Essential hypertension. In M.A. Koda-Kimble, L.Y. Young, W.A. Kradian, B.J. Guglielmo, B.K. Alldredge, & R.L. Corelli. (Eds.), *Applied therapeutics: The clinical use of drugs* (8th ed.). Philadelphia: Lippincott, Williams & Wilkins.

Schaefer, B., Caracciolo, V., Frishman, W., Charney, P. (2003). Gender, Ethnicity, and Genes in Cardiovascular Disease. Part 2: Implications for Pharmacotherapy. *Heart Disease, 5*(3):202-214.

Si, D., Guo, Y., Zhang, Y., Yang, L., Zhou, H., Zhong, D. (2004). Identification of a novel variant CYP2 C9 allele in Chinese. *Pharmacogenetics, 14*(7):465-469.

Sibai, B.M., Hauth, J., Caritis, S., Lindheimer, M.D., MacPherson, C., & Klebanoff, M. for the Network of Maternal-Fetal Medicine Units of the National Institute of Child Health and Human Development. (2000). Hypertensive disorders in twin versus singleton pregnancies. *American Journal of Obstetrics & Gynecology, 182*:938.

Stafford, R.S., Furberg, C.D., Finkelstein, S.N., Cockburn, I.M., Alehegn, T., Ma, J. (2004). Impact of Clinical Trial Results on National Trends in α-Blocker Prescribing, 1996-2002. Journal of the American Medical Association, 291(1):54-62.

Strippoli, G.F., Craig, M., Deeks, J.J., Schena, F.P., Craig, J.C. (2004). Effects of angiotensin converting enzyme inhibitors and angiotensin II receptor antagonists on mortality and renal outcomes in diabetic nephropathy: Systematic review. British Medical Journal, 329:828-831.

Tan, A.S., Kuppuswamy, S., Whaley-Connell, A.T., Kurukulasuriya, L.R., Sowers, J.R. (2004). Recommendations for special populations: The Treatment of hypertension in diabetes mellitus. *Endocrinologist, 14*(6):368-381.

Taylor, A.L., Ziesche, S., Yancy, C., et al., and the African-American Heart Failure Trial Investigators. (2004). Combination of isosorbide dinitrate and hydralazine in blacks with heart failure. New England Journal of Medicine, 351:2049-2057.

USP DI: Drug information for the health care professional (25th ed.). (2005). Greenwood Village, CO: MICROMEDEX Thomson Healthcare.

Wallace, A.W., Galindez, D., Salahieh, A., et al. (2004). Effect of clonidine on cardiovascular morbidity and mortality after noncardiac surgery. *Anesthesiology, 101*:284-293.

Wang, T.J., Evans, J.C., Meigs, J.B., Rifai, N., Fox, C.S., D'Agostino, R.B., et al. (2005). Low-grade albuminuria and the risks of hypertension and blood pressure progression. *Circulation 2005, 111*, 1370-1376.

Wassertheil-Smoller, S., Psaty, B., Greenland, P., Oberman, A., Kotchen, T., Mouton, C., et al. (2004). Association between cardiovascular outcomes and antihypertensive drug treatment in older women, *Journal of the American Medical Association, 292*, 2849-2859.

Whelton, S.P., Chin, A., Xin, X., & He, J. (2002). Effect of aerobic exercise on blood pressure: A meta-analysis of randomized, controlled trials. *Annals of Internal Medicine, 136*:493-503.

Wojnowski, L. (2004). Genetics of the Variable Expression of CYP3 A in Humans. *Therapeutic Drug Monitoring, 26*(2):192-199.

Xin, X., He, J., Frontini, M.G., Ogden, L.G., Motsamai, O.I., & Whelton, P.K. (2001). Effects of alcohol reduction on blood pressure: A meta-analysis of randomized controlled trials, *Hypertension, 38*:1112-1117.

VASODILATORS AND BLOOD VISCOSITY–REDUCING AGENTS

CHAPTER FOCUS

Nitrates have been prescribed for more than 100 years to treat ischemic heart disease. Because of their vasodilatory properties, they are also used to reduce preload and afterload in heart failure (HF). The blood viscosity–reducing agents have a more limited use in improving microcirculatory flow for clients with intermittent claudication.

LEARNING OBJECTIVES

- Identify three therapeutic objectives for the use of antianginal agents.
- Compare the effects of nitrates, β blockers, and calcium channel blockers on the heart.
- Describe the mechanism of action, adverse effects, significant drug interactions, and dosages for nitrates.
- Instruct a client in the self-management of a transdermal system for the administration of nitroglycerin.
- Implement nursing management of a client receiving vasodilators.
- Define the science of hemorrheology.
- Implement nursing management of a client receiving pentoxifylline.

▲ **KEY TERMS**

angina pectoris, p. 578
hemorrheology, p. 585
ischemic, p. 578
myocardial infarction, p. 578
nitrates, p. 579
silent ischemia, p. 578
stable angina, p. 578
unstable angina, p. 578
vasospastic angina, p. 578

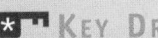 **KEY DRUGS**

nitroglycerin, p. 580
pentoxifylline, p. 586

Vasodilators are used to treat vascular disorders, including peripheral vascular conditions. These agents produce peripheral vasodilation by relaxing smooth muscle in blood vessel walls. Some drugs act primarily on veins or arterioles, and others dilate both types of blood vessels.

Chapter 27 reviews the vasodilators used to treat hypertension. This chapter addresses the use of vasodilators for angina and peripheral occlusive arterial disease and the use of blood viscosity–reducing agents in treating peripheral vascular disease. The blood viscosity–reducing agents improve microcirculatory blood flow to ischemic tissues (tissues with a decreased oxygenated blood supply).

✳ What are the important pathologic considerations of angina?

The term angina pectoris refers to a temporary interference with the flow of blood, oxygen, and nutrients to heart muscle, or intermittent myocardial ischemia. Angina is a manifestation of coronary artery disease and associated atherosclerosis. Angina is often characterized by pain behind the sternum. Differentiation of the type of myocardial ischemia is important before treatment is instituted. Stable angina refers to chest pain that occurs with exercise or stress and is relieved by rest. This type of angina is often predictable with increased oxygen demand. It can often be minimized with the use of coronary vasodilators. Vasospastic angina occurs when spasms of the coronary arteries reduce blood flow and may predispose to cardiac dysrhythmias. Unstable angina reflects chest pain that occurs independent of exercise or stress and reflects reversible myocardial ischemia. Unstable angina is potentially life-threatening. Unstable angina often is caused by an atherosclerotic lesion in a coronary vessel that triggers the clotting cascade. Emergency treatment of unstable angina with antiplatelets, anticoagulants and/or fibrinolytics (see Chapter 30), and/or cardiac catheterization is important to prevent a myocardial infarction (MI), an irreversible ischemic event with injury to myocardial tissue (Box 28-1).

Angina pectoris occurs when the workload on the heart is too great and/or oxygen delivery is inadequate. Coronary flow is very responsive to the oxygen requirements of the heart. Inadequate oxygenation of the heart results from coronary blood flow less than the amount needed. When coronary blood flow is inadequate (such as with coronary atherosclerosis or vasomotor spasm), hypoxia causes an accumulation of pain-producing substances, such as lactic acid (anaerobic metabolite), and other chemical irritants, such as potassium ions, kinins, and prostaglandins. These products stimulate the cardiac sensory nerve endings, which transmit impulses to the central nervous system (CNS) to produce the typical anginal pain response.

Other causes of anginal pain may be pulmonary hypertension and valvular heart disease. Individuals with severe anemia, even with minimal coronary artery disease, may suffer from anginal attacks because of inadequate oxygen supply. The presence of carbon monoxide hemoglobin (carboxyhemoglobin) in smokers, who have reduced amounts of available blood oxygen, is another factor in causing angina pectoris.

Myocardial ischemia can usually be detected on the electrocardiogram as ST segment depression. Myocardial infarction usually presents on electrocardiogram (ECG) as ST segment elevation. Significantly reduced blood flow to the heart and ST segment changes on ECG can occur in the absence of symptoms. This asymptomatic ischemia is termed silent ischemia.

✳ S.P. is a 63-year-old male who reports to his physician with a new complaint of substernal chest

pain when walking up two flights of stairs. He describes the pain as a sensation of a weight on his chest, feeling of tightness, and some pain in his jaw. He rates the pain as 7 on a 0 to 10 scale. The pain lasts for about 5 minutes and is relieved with rest. His blood pressure is 148/95 mm Hg and his pulse is 90 beats/min. He has a history of hypertension, which is moderately well controlled with hydrochlorothiazide 25 mg daily. He takes a multivitamin and calcium supplement daily.

✳ What are the goals of therapy in treating angina?

Drug therapy for angina pectoris is aimed at increasing myocardial oxygen supply, reducing myocardial oxygen demand, and minimizing or removing the occlusion.

Box 28-1 Types of Angina Pectoris

Stable Angina

(also referred to as classic angina, exercise-induced angina, effort angina)

This type of pain is usually associated with coronary arteriosclerosis. The attack can be precipitated by exertion or stress (e.g., cold, fear, and emotion) and by eating. The pain lasts up to 15 minutes and disappears with rest or nitrates.

Vasospastic Angina

(also referred to as variant angina or Prinzmetal's angina)

This type of pain may be associated with spasms of the coronary arteries, and it usually occurs in the presence of coronary stenosis. The pain often occurs during rest and without any cause. Its occurrence follows a regular pattern (e.g., it appears at the same time during the night). Dysrhythmias often accompany the attack. Calcium channel blockers are considered the drugs of choice for this type of angina.

Unstable Angina

(also referred to as crescendo angina or preinfarction angina)

This is a progressive form of angina in which pain occurs more frequently and becomes more severe in time. The attack may appear during rest and may last longer with less relief provided by antianginal drugs. Individuals with unstable angina eventually show signs and symptoms of impending myocardial infarction or coronary failure.

Silent Ischemia

This asymptomatic condition presents as ST segment changes of the electrocardiogram consistent with myocardial ischemia. It is most common in individuals with pre-existing coronary artery disease and is associated with an increased risk for myocardial events. Silent ischemia may coexist with other forms of angina.

Agents that serve to increase myocardial oxygen supply include the coronary vasodilators (e.g., nitrates and calcium channel blockers). Calcium channel blockers are particularly useful when reduced oxygen supply is related to spasm of the coronary artery (vasospastic or Prinzmetal's angina). Calcium channel blockers are discussed more fully in Chapters 26 and 27.

Drugs that reduce myocardial oxygen demand serve to reduce heart rate. The β-adrenergic blockers are key drugs that serve this purpose. They are used both acutely during an impending MI and prophylactically to prevent angina. They are discussed in Chapter 22 and briefly in Chapters 26 and 27. Table 28-1 compares the pharmacologic effects of nitrates, β blockers, and calcium channel blockers.

In unstable angina or a myocardial infarction, acute treatment targeting platelets, fibrin, and/or the clotting factors is used. Acute treatment includes the antiplatelets (e.g., aspirin), the anticoagulants (e.g., heparin), and the fibrinolytics (e.g., alteplase). These agents are reviewed in Chapter 30. Drugs that help prevent future occlusions are the antiplatelets (e.g., aspirin, clopidogrel [Plavix]) and the antihyperlipidemic drugs (e.g., atorvastatin [Lipitor], which is discussed in Chapter 31). Occasionally an anticoagulant (e.g., warfarin) is used to prevent future vessel occlusion as well. Nondrug interventions, including diet and exercise, are also important to prevent coronary artery disease.

✱ S.P. is not in acute distress and is evaluated by the cardiologist for angina. An ECG and exercise tolerance test are consistent with stable angina. He is started on a β blocker, atenolol, 25 mg daily for angina and hypertension and nitroglycerin 0.4 mg sublingually (SL) as needed (p.r.n.) for chest pain.

✱ What is the role of β blockers in the management of angina?
Although not a vasodilator, the β blockers help prevent future angina attacks by decreasing heart rate, thereby decreasing myocardial oxygen demand. They are also ideal for clients with other comorbidities that benefit from β-adrenergic blockers (e.g., hypertension). A more complete discussion of β-adrenergic blockers is found in Chapters 22, 26, and 27.

✱ How do the nitrates work?
The **nitrates**, including nitroglycerin, are effective in treating stable angina pectoris because of their dilating effect on the veins and arteries. The pooling of blood in the veins (capacitance blood vessels) decreases the amount of blood returned to the heart (preload), which reduces left ventricular end-diastolic volume. This decrease in blood return may help to reduce the demand for myocardial oxygen.

Not all clients with coronary artery disease obtain relief from nitroglycerin, however. Similarly, not all responders to nitroglycerin have demonstrated coronary artery disease. (Henrikson et al., 2003).

Nitroglycerin (NTG) is the key drug in the nitrate category. It is available as sublingual tablets (Nitrostat), extended-release buccal tablets (Nitrogard SR), lingual aerosols (Nitrolingual), extended-release capsules (Nitroglyn E-R), parenteral injections (Nitro-Bid, Nitrol), ointments (Nitro-Bid, Nitrostat), and transdermal topical systems (Nitro-Dur). The other drugs in the nitrate drug category include amyl nitrite inhalant and isosorbide mononitrate (Imdur, ISMO, Monoket) and isosorbide dinitrate (Isordil, Sorbitrate).

Nitrates dilate venous capacitance and arterial resistance vessels, which results in reduced myocardial oxygen demand and a more efficient distribution of blood in the myocardium. The antihypertensive effect of nitrates is also a result of peripheral vasodilation. Figure 28-1 illustrates the biochemical steps for nitrates.

Amyl nitrite has been used to treat acute angina attacks, but the other, safer nitrate dosage forms have replaced it. Although not approved by U.S. Food and Drug Administration labeling in the United States, amyl nitrite has been used as an antidote for cyanide poisoning and in cardiac function tests to assess reserve cardiac function. This prod-

TABLE 28-1 COMPARISON OF EFFECTS OF NITRATES, β BLOCKERS, AND CALCIUM CHANNEL BLOCKERS

	Nitrates	β Blockers	Calcium Channel Blockers
Systolic blood pressure	↓	↓	↓
Ventricular volume	↓	↑	↓, ↑, or (0)
Heart rate	↑	↓	↓, ↑, or (0)
Myocardial contractility	(0)	↓	↓
Coronary blood flow	↑	↑ or (0)	↑
Coronary vessel resistance	↓	↑ or (0)	↓
Coronary spasms	↓	↑ or (0)	↓
Collateral flow	↑	(0)	↓

↓, Decreased; ↑, increased; (0), no change.

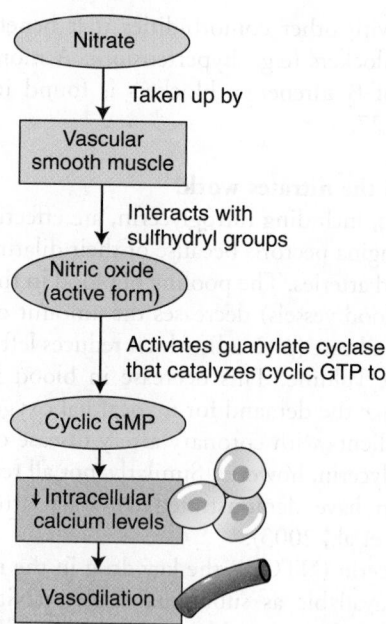

Figure 28-1 Pharmacologic action of nitrates.

uct has also been abused and used as a sexual stimulant or euphoric agent, but such applications are extremely dangerous and should be avoided.

Nitroglycerin is the key drug in this class and is discussed in greater depth in the following monograph.

nitroglycerin [nye troe glih ser in]
(Minitran, Nitrostat, Nitrogard SR, Nitrolingual, Nitrocap, Nitro-Bid, Nitrol, Nitro-Dur, Nitrong)

Indications
NTG and the other nitrates are used to reduce or prevent the pain of angina, to treat heart failure (HF), and on rare occasions, to treat hypertension (nitroglycerin injection).

Pharmacokinetics/Dosing
Nitroglycerin has a large first-pass effect on oral administration. This is avoided by administering nitroglycerin sublingually or topically. Nitroglycerin has a short half-life of 1 to 4 minutes and is eliminated in the urine primarily as unchanged drug. A number of dosage formulations are available, including sublingual tablets and sprays, sustained-release oral tablets, and topical delivery systems. Table 28-2 compares nitrate formulations and kinetics; Box 28-2 discusses transdermal delivery systems.

Adverse Effects
The most common adverse effect of nitrates is headache, which is related to vasodilation of cerebral vessels. Other undesirable effects include dizziness, nausea or vomiting, agitation, facial flushing, increased pulse rate, dry mouth, rash, prolonged headaches, and blurred vision. Tolerance to the vasodilatory effects of nitroglycerin is noted within 24 to 48 hours of continuous administration. This may be related to volume expansion or to cellular depletion of sulfhydryl groups (Kerins, Robertson, & Roberson, 2001). Tolerance is avoided by institution of an 8- to 12-hour nitrate-free period each day.

Drug Interactions
Nitrates interact with other vasodilators. Of greatest concern is the concurrent use of sildenafil (Viagra), tadalafil (Cialis), and vardenafil (Levitra), which can result in significant drops in blood pressure if dosed within the same 24-hour period. Concurrent ethanol can also contribute to excessive hypotension.

✱ What nursing care is provided to S.P. regarding the use of sublingual nitroglycerin?

Assessment S.P.'s health history and physical exam would focus on preexisting illnesses that require the cautious use of nitrates such as recent MI (the resultant hypotension and tachycardia may aggravate ischemia); glaucoma (may increase intraocular pressure); recent head trauma or cerebral hemorrhage (may increase cerebrospinal fluid pressure); severe anemia; or hyperthyroidism. If S.P. has hypotension evidenced by low systolic pressure, he may experience further hypotension with paradoxical bradycardia and increased angina pectoris. Although it is rare, clients who are intolerant of one nitrate may show intolerance to other nitrates.

S.P.'s current medication regimen is reviewed for significant drug interactions, such as with other vasodilators, because concurrent use may exaggerate the orthostatic hypotensive effects of the drugs; dosage adjustments may be necessary. The concurrent use of any drug with hypotensive effects such as alcohol, opioid analgesics, or antihypertensive agents should be used cautiously, if at all, for the same reasons. If it is not possible for S.P. to avoid concurrent administration, monitor closely because dosage reductions may be necessary. Question S.P. carefully about the possible use of anti-impotence agents such as sildenafil (Viagra), tadalafil (Cialis), and vardenafil (Levitra), as they potentiate the hypotensive effects of nitrates and deaths have been reported.

A baseline clinical assessment for S.P. includes the ECG and exercise tolerance test already performed, respiratory pattern and rate, blood pressure (BP) (lying, sitting, and standing), and pulse rate. A description of S.P.'s anginal attacks, including characteristics of chest pain (precipitating factors, intensity, character, area of radiation, what resolves it), dizziness, and syncope, will aid in evaluating drug effectiveness.

Nursing Diagnosis With the administration of nitrates, S.P. may experience the following nursing diagnoses: deficient knowledge related to first-time use of nitrates for angina; acute pain related to cardiac tissue ischemia and ineffectiveness of the nitrate; impaired comfort related to dry mouth, flushing, headache, rash, dizziness, and nausea and vomiting; and risk for injury related to orthostatic hypotension or blurred vision.

Planning While S.P. is on nitrates, he will:
- Experience fewer episodes of chest pain with less severity.
- Evidence greater activity tolerance.
- State the adverse effects of nitrates and interventions to minimize or prevent risk of injury related to those effects.
- Effectively maintain the therapeutic regimen (e.g., keep a journal of angina symptoms, know what action to take when chest pain is unrelieved, weight loss if required, report symptoms of adverse effects appropriately).

TABLE 28-2 PHARMACOKINETICS OF NITRATES

Drug	Formulation	Onset	Duration	Typical Adult Dose
nitroglycerin	Sublingual tablet (Nitroquick, Nitrostat)	1-3 min	30-60 min	0.2-0.6 mg SL every 5 min for a maximum of 3 doses. If no relief after 3 doses, go to hospital immediately. Do not chew or swallow tablet.
	Sublingual aerosol (Nitrolingual)	2-4 min		
	Extended-release buccal tablet (Nitrogard)	3 min	5 hr	1 mg q3-5h while awake
	Extended-release oral capsule (Nitro-Time)		8-12 hr	2.5-9 mg two to three times daily
	Ointment (Nitro-Bid, Nitrol)	30 min	4-8 hr	2% ointment: ½ inch on arising in the morning, and repeated 6 hr later; dose may be increased up to 2 inches as tolerated.
	Transdermal patch* (Minitran, Nitro-Dur)	30 min	8-24 hr	0.2-0.4 mg/hr titrated up to 0.8 mg/hr if needed; typically patch is applied for 12-14 hr/day and removed for 10-12 hr/day
	Intravenous (Nitro-Bid IV, Tridil)	Immediate	Several minutes	5 mcg/min increased by 5 mcg/min every 3-5 min with titration up to 200 mcg/min as tolerated; must prepare in glass, use special administration set for nitroglycerin, and administer via infusion pump or controller
isosorbide mononitrate	Regular Tablet (Ismo, Monoket)	30-50 min	7-8 hr	5-20 mg twice daily (on arising, then 7 hr later)
	Extended-release tablet (Imdur)	30-50 min	12-16 hr	30-60 mg once daily on arising; may titrate up to 240 mg if tolerated
isosorbide dinitrate	Sublingual tablet (Isordil)	2-5 min	1-2 hr	2.5-10 mg q4-6h
	Oral tablet (Isordil)	15-40 min	4-6 hr	5-40 mg three to four times daily
	Chewable tablet (Isordil)	2-5 min	1-2 hr	5-10 mg q2-3h
	Sustained-release capsule (Isordil)	30 min	12 hr	40 mg twice daily

*To prevent nitrate tolerance, it is recommended that the patch be left on only 12-14 hours per day, with the next daily patch applied 10-12 hours later.

BOX 28-2 TRANSDERMAL NITRATE SYSTEMS

Because transdermal nitroglycerin delivery systems are quite popular, the nurse should be familiar with several issues and concerns associated with these products. Three systems are currently available; the actual amount of nitroglycerin delivered by each system varies depending on the system and the individual client's skin absorption of the nitroglycerin. The mechanism of drug delivery may vary. For example, Nitro-Dur contains a gel-like matrix surrounded by fluid. Nitroglycerin moves from the matrix to the fluid to the skin.

Drug absorption in all systems is by passive diffusion and is based on processes relating to heat transfer (or Fick's first law of diffusion).

Transdermal systems are not interchangeable because patch size, nitroglycerin content, and the average amount of nitroglycerin delivered in 24 hours can differ. Although many individuals reportedly control their conditions with or have responded to this dosage form, other clients do not achieve adequate therapeutic blood levels or a clinically significant therapeutic response. Maintaining stable nitroglycerin serum levels over 24 hours is not always desirable because this leads to drug tolerance and the need to increase dosage. The intermittent use of transdermal products (e.g., application for 12 to 16 hours followed by removal for the night) results in prolonged clinical results without the development of significant drug tolerance.

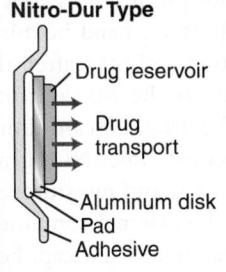

Nitro-Dur Type

Drug reservoir

Drug transport

Aluminum disk
Pad
Adhesive

- Meet regularly and collaborate actively with health care personnel to manage his illness and drug regimen.

Implementation

Monitoring To determine effectiveness, assess S.P.'s chest pain on a scale of 1 to 10 before administration and 5 minutes after administration of the sublingual dose. Monitor pulse and blood pressure before and after administration. With S.P. in a resting position, an appropriate dosage produces a fall in blood pressure of 10 mm Hg or a rise in heart rate of 10 beats/min.

Intervention Doses may be repeated every 5 minutes for 15 minutes for a total of three doses if necessary. If there is no relief after three doses, emergency personnel should be called. For a hospitalized individual, a specific number of tablets (approximately 25) may be prescribed for placement at the bedside in an appropriate container and properly labeled for the client's use. Monitor and document the client's self-administration of nitroglycerin in this setting.

Education Instruct S.P. to sit or lie down and to take the medication at the first indication of an oncoming anginal attack. This position prevents postural hypotension. The signs and symptoms of postural hypertension include dizziness, syncope, and weakness. Instruct him to keep a record of the frequency of anginal attacks, the precipitating factors, the number of tablets used, and the occurrence of adverse effects. The buccal, lingual, sublingual, and chewable oral dosage forms of nitrates are used to prevent angina. Instruct S.P. to take his SL tablet 5 to 10 minutes before the occurrence of the anticipated stressor.

Warn S.P. of transient headaches, which usually last 5 to 20 minutes after the sublingual administration of nitroglycerin. He should notify the prescriber if the headache persists. Headaches may disappear within several days to weeks and may be relieved by aspirin, acetaminophen, or a temporary dosage reduction. Dizziness, light-headedness, and a slight headache may occur with the administration of nitrates. Instruct S.P. to report to the prescriber if blurred vision, dry mouth, or severe headaches occur; these are signs of overdose and require immediate attention.

Explain to S.P. that a sublingual tablet should be placed under the tongue or in the buccal pouch and allowed to dissolve; it is not to be swallowed. Avoid eating, drinking, or smoking while the drug dissolves. The potency of the drug is usually indicated by a burning or stinging sensation under the tongue. However, some of the newer, more stable preparations may not produce this effect.

Keep a fresh supply on hand because the drug loses its potency about 3 to 6 months after the bottle has been opened, depending on the manufacturer; read the insert that accompanies the drug. Discard unused tablets after the manufacturer's specified time. Nitroglycerin is inactivated by exposure to air, heat, and moisture. Store the stock supply of the drug in the original container, which should be tightly closed with a metal screw cap. Federal regulation requires that the sublingual form of nitroglycerin be dispensed in the original, unopened manufacturer's container. Do not leave the cotton or package insert in the container after opening; these articles may absorb some of the drug, which reduces potency. A supplementary stainless steel container has been approved for carrying small amounts of nitroglycerin. The pendant-like container may be worn on a chain around the neck to provide a convenient supply of the drug when it is needed. Be sure the hands are dry if handling nitroglycerin, because moisture hastens its deterioration. Cold and heat affect nitroglycerin. Do not store it in the refrigerator or in the bathroom medicine or kitchen cabinets.

Instruct the client not to change the dosage or medication without consulting the prescriber and to report regularly for cardiac function monitoring.

Inform P.S. about the importance of learning to identify stressful situations that precipitate anginal attacks. These include emotional stress, overeating, smoking, temperature extremes, and a sudden increase in physical activity. Explain the need to pace activities and to plan for rest periods. He should receive support to modify behaviors that precipitate anginal attacks.

Sources of health information are available online. See the Technology Link box in Chapter 25, p. 519.

Evaluation The expected outcome of nitrate therapy is that S.P. will report a decrease in the frequency and severity of angina attacks along with increased activity tolerance with minimal adverse effects, such as hypotension, headache, tachycardia, fainting, and flushing of the face. He will verbalize those symptoms to report to the physician (syncope, severe headache, or chest pain) and what actions to take when the chest pain is unrelieved.

Other forms of nitrates for treatment of acute attacks of angina might have been prescribed for S.P., such as chewable tablets and aerosol lingual. These differ in their manner of delivery of the nitroglycerin. The chewable tablet is chewed thoroughly and held in the mouth for 2 minutes before swallowing. With the aerosol lingual dose, spray 1 to 2 metered doses onto or under the tongue by holding the can vertically. Do not inhale the spray or swallow it immediately and do not shake the can beforehand. No more than 3 metered doses are recommended within 15 minutes. If the chest pain persists, seek medical attention. The spray may also be used prophylactically 5 to 10 minutes before engaging in activities that usually precipitate an attack.

Intravenous forms may be used for acute attacks if the client is hospitalized. Hypovolemia must be corrected before the use of intravenous (IV) nitroglycerin because of the risk of producing severe hypotension and shock. Clients with low pulmonary capillary wedge pressure may also be sensitive to its hypotensive effects. There are special nitroglycerin infusion sets made of non-polyvinylchloride (PVC) plastic to prevent the adsorption of nitroglycerin into PVC containers and tubing; 40% to 80% of dosage is adsorbed into the tubing in a standard IV set. When non-PVC sets are used, dosage instructions should be followed with care because in changing from the regular (PVC) set to the non-PVC set may result in excessive NTG dosage. Expect dosage differences to be made if there is a change in delivery system.

✸ What other interventions are appropriate for S.P.?

S.P. should be counseled and evaluated for coronary artery disease. Lifestyle changes including diet and moderate exercise should be encouraged as tolerated. Consideration of antiplatelet therapy (e.g., low-dose aspirin or clopidogrel [Plavix]; see Chapter 30), evaluation of lipid levels with consideration of antihyperlipidemic medication (see Chapter 31), management of his hypertension (see Chapter 27), and assessment for other conditions that increase risk (e.g., screening for diabetes mellitus, which increases cardiovascular risk; see Chapter 49) are all appropriate for S.P.

✸ L.S. is a 68-year-old female with HF. She is maintained on enalapril (Vasotec) 10 mg daily and furosemide (Lasix) 40 mg daily. Her cardiologist is recommending the addition of transdermal nitroglycerin to her regimen.

✸ How can nitrates help HF?

Nitrates decrease preload and, to a modest extent, afterload. These actions improve stroke volume and cardiac output in many clients with HF. (Chapter 24 discusses the concepts of preload, afterload, stroke volume, and cardiac output; Chapter 25 reviews the principles of management of HF.) Before the widespread use of angiotensin-converting enzyme (ACE) inhibitors or angiotensin II receptor blockers (ARBs), nitrates were commonly used to help manage the symptoms of HF. In combination with hydralazine, nitrates are quite effective in the treatment of heart failure, particularly in black clients who may be less responsive to ACE inhibitors or ARBs (Taylor et al., 2004). Refer to the Special Considerations for Pharmacogenetics box in Chapter 27, p. 573.

✸ What nursing care is appropriate for L.S. when she uses transdermal nitroglycerin?

Assessment L.S.'s assessment would be the same as S.P.'s above with angina, but with the addition of the following indicators of HF: BP; apical pulse rate; breath and heart sounds; weight; laboratory values such as potassium, sodium, magnesium, and calcium; ECG; renal function laboratory studies (e.g., blood urea nitrogen, serum creatinine); and liver function studies (aspartate aminotransferase, alanine aminotransferase, creatine phosphokinase, lactate dehydrogenase, and alkaline phosphatase).

Nursing Diagnosis Although the nursing diagnoses for the use of nitrates would generally be the same as S.P. in the last case, differences would relate to the use of nitrates for HF rather than angina or the form of the drug. Thus, relevant nursing diagnoses include deficient knowledge related to first-time use of nitrates for HF, risk of injury related to

hypotension and the signs and symptoms of HF (decreased urinary output; increased weight; increased edema; shortness of breath, dyspnea, and rales; fatigue; and decreased peripheral pulses) and ineffectiveness of the nitrate, as well as impaired skin integrity (erythema) related to the application of topical dosage form.

Planning While L.S. is on transdermal nitroglycerin, she will:

- Exhibit decreased signs and symptoms of heart failure.
- Experience greater activity tolerance.
- State the adverse effects of nitrates and interventions to minimize or prevent risk of injury related to those effects.
- Effectively maintain the therapeutic regimen (e.g., daily weights, application of patches, compliance with medications, weight loss if required, Dietary Approaches to Stop Hypertension [DASH] diet, reporting symptoms of adverse effects appropriately).
- Meet regularly and collaborate actively with health care personnel to manage her illness and drug regimen.

Implementation

Monitoring Over the course of long-acting nitrate therapy for the treatment of HF, L.S. is monitored for the nursing diagnoses above, particularly the status of her HF (see the symptoms mentioned previously), as well as hypotension. Measure BP and pulse rate after L.S. has been at rest 10 minutes; take her BP in both arms and in the sitting and standing position. Follow up on other indicators in the baseline clinical assessment.

Intervention Remove the old transdermal patch and apply the new one at the same time each day. To prevent nitrate tolerance, a drug-free interval of 6 to 8 hours is typically prescribed. Work with L.S. and the prescriber to identify optimal times to remove and reapply the patch. The system should be applied to a clean, dry, and hairless skin area of the chest, shoulder, or inside of the upper arm. Avoid skin folds, areas distal to the knee or elbow, and irritated or excessively scarred areas. Rotate application sites to prevent irritation. Apply a new system if the current one becomes loosened. Do not trim the units, because doing so will alter the dosage (see Box 28-2). Alert the client to use caution near microwave ovens when wearing a transdermal system that has a metallic backing, because leaking radiation may heat the backing and cause a burn.

Education Rotate sites. Wash the skin when the patch is removed. Remove the patch for 10 to 12 hours every day to prevent tolerance. Patches with aluminum backings should be removed before defibrillation, because the electric current may cause it to burn the skin.

Instruct L.S. to avoid alcoholic beverages while taking nitrates because a shock-like syndrome (flushing, weakness, pallor, hypotension, and syncope) can occur.

The used patch should be folded with adhesive sides together and disposed of in such a way that children and small animals will be unable to access the drug.

Evaluation If nitrates are administered for HF, the client will demonstrate a clearing of peripheral edema and the lung fields, a urinary output of more than 30 mL/hr, and a blood pressure, pulmonary artery pressure, and pulmonary wedge pressure within normal limits.

Other forms of nitrates for the treatment of HF or chronic angina may be prescribed.

Ointment Squeeze the prescribed dose of nitroglycerin onto the specially designed dose-measuring applicator supplied with the package; 1 inch (25 mm) contains 15 mg of NTG. The dosage will start with ½ to 1 inch and then increase each dose by a ½ inch until the individualized dose produces the desired clinical result without symptomatic hypotension. *Avoid using the fingers* to spread the ointment. Apply a thin, uniform layer to a premarked, 6-square-inch applicator and then place on the skin surface (a clean, dry, hairless skin area of chest or back) covering at least a 2¼- × 3½-inch area. Rotate sites to prevent inflammation. Do not massage or rub in the ointment, because rapid absorption will interfere with the sustained action of the drug. Cover the area with an occlusive dressing, if ordered, and secure it with tape. The ointment is usually applied every 8 hours during the day and at bedtime. If the client experiences breakthrough angina, the dose may be prescribed for application every 4 to 6 hours. Continuous use beyond 48 hours may result in tolerance; therefore a daily nitrate-free interval is instituted. Instruct the client to apply the ointment as described previously; cleanse the area before applying a new dose. Instruct the caregiver not to get ointment on his or her hands, because the medication may precipitate a headache. Tell the client to store nitroglycerin ointment in a cool place and in the original container with the tube tightly capped.

Transmucosal Controlled Extended-Release Tablets Instruct the client to place the tablet between the upper lip and gum (buccal area) to dissolve, or above the incisors if food or drink is to be taken within the 3 to 5 hours it takes to dissolve. Caution the client against using these tablets at bedtime, because aspiration is a risk. The tablet may be replaced if swallowed.

Oral Sustained-Release Tablets or Capsules Administer these tablets on an empty stomach (1 hour before or 2 hours after meals) with a full glass of water; instruct the client to swallow the medication whole. Alert the client to notify the prescriber if undigested tablets are found in stools. Tolerance may also develop; consider using a daily or twice daily dosing rather than three or four times daily. For isosorbide dinitrate, three times daily dosing with a 12-hour drug-free interval is often used (e.g., 7 AM, 1 PM, 7 PM). For isosorbide mononitrate, the drug is dosed based on the manufacturer's recommendation of once or twice daily, timed to allow for a 12-hour drug-free interval.

Other Nitrates

Isosorbide dinitrate (Isordil) and its longer acting active metabolite isosorbide mononitrate (Ismo, Monoket, Imdur) are orally available nitrates. Isosorbide dinitrate is also available as a sublingual formulation. These nitrates are sometimes used long term for the management of angina of HF and share similar pharmacology to nitroglycerin.

isosorbide dinitrate [eye soe **sor** bide dye **nye** trate]
(Isordil)
Indications
Isosorbide dinitrate is used to prevent and treat angina, to treat HF, and occasionally to treat esophageal spasms associated with gastroesophageal reflux.
Pharmacokinetics/Dosing
Isosorbide dinitrate exhibits an onset of action typically within 45 minutes after ingestion of the oral tablet. Response to the sublingual tablet and chewable tablet is 2 to 3 minutes and 3 minutes, respectively. Duration of action is longest (at 4 to 6 hours) with the oral tablet and is under 2 hours with the chewable and sublingual formulations. Isosorbide dinitrate is metabolized to two different active metabolites: isosorbide 2-mononitrate and isosorbide 5-mononitrate, which are marketed as isosorbide mononitrate (see the next monograph). Oral isosorbide dinitrate is dosed at 5 to 40 mg three to four times daily. As with nitroglycerin, a nitrate-free interval is recommended with chronic use.
Adverse Effects
The adverse effects of isosorbide dinitrate are similar to nitroglycerin. As with nitroglycerin, tolerance to the vasodilatory effects may be noted if drug-free intervals are not instituted each day.
Drug Interactions
See nitroglycerin.

isosorbide mononitrate [eye soe **sor** bide mon oh **nye** trate]
(Imdur, Ismo, Monoket)
Indications
Isosorbide mononitrate is used to prevent and treat angina and to treat HF.
Pharmacokinetics/Dosing
Isosorbide mononitrate has an onset of action within 50 minuets of oral dosing and varies in duration of action depending on formulation. Ismo and Monoket have durations of 7 to 8 hours, whereas Imdur has effects for up to 16 hours. Dosing is reflective of these durations. Ismo and Monoket are dosed at 5 to 10 mg twice daily (on arising and 7 hours later), whereas Imdur is dosed at 30 to 60 mg (up to 240 mg) once daily on arising.
Adverse Effects
Similar to isosorbide dinitrate and nitroglycerin.
Drug Interactions
See nitroglycerin.

✳ **What other vasodilators are available?**
A number of other agents with vasodilatory properties are available. Many of these agents—including the thiazide diuretics, ACE inhibitors, ARBs, adrenergic-inhibiting drugs, diazoxide (Hyperstat IV), hydralazine (Apresoline), minoxidil (Loniten), and nitroprusside (Nipride)—are discussed

in Chapter 27. Their use in treating angina is limited. Dipyridamole (Persantine) is a vasodilator with antiplatelet activity (see Chapter 30) that was originally developed as a coronary artery vasodilator; however, it is no longer indicated for that use.

Papaverine (Pavabid) and isoxsuprine (Vasodilan) are vasodilators with questionable efficacy (Kerins et al., 2001). Both agents have historically been used to promote cerebral vascular flow associated with dementia and other neurologic and psychiatric conditions. Isoxsuprine has also been historically used, with variable effect, to relieve symptoms of Raynaud's phenomenon and other peripheral vascular conditions. Given the lack of strong evidence of their effectiveness, these agents are rarely used today.

Occasionally, IV vasodilators are used in the long-term management of pulmonary hypertension. Epoprostenol (Flolan) directly dilates the pulmonary and systemic arteries and also inhibits platelet aggregation. It is administered via continuous injection through a central venous catheter. It is used for long-term treatment of pulmonary hypertension that has not responded to other therapies or for pulmonary hypertension associated with scleroderma. Reconstitute epoprostenol according to the manufacturer's instructions and do not mix with other parenteral solutions. In addition to the nursing care associated with an indwelling venous catheter to prevent sepsis and local infection, monitor the client for dizziness, flushing, headache, jaw pain, tachycardia, anxiety, diarrhea, and thrombocytopenia. Epoprostenol therapy should not be discontinued abruptly.

⚹ **T.M. is a 63-year-old male who complains of bilateral leg pain while walking. His health care provider diagnoses intermittent claudication and prescribes pentoxifylline (Trental) 400 mg three times daily.**

⚹ **What is intermittent claudication?**

Intermittent claudication is a syndrome that results from an insufficient supply of blood to the skeletal muscles in the legs. Reduced microcirculatory blood flow causes ischemia and pain. This syndrome is a common complication of atherosclerosis and is characteristic of Buerger's disease. While walking, affected individuals first experience pain in the muscles, which is followed by cramps and weakness.

Hemorrheology is a science that deals with the deformation and flow properties of blood under physiologic and pathophysiologic conditions. Because arteriosclerosis reduces blood flow to tissues distal to the obstruction, blood viscosity is elevated; this further diminishes the flow of blood. In addition, impaired blood flow at the microcirculatory level affects the normal capacity of the red blood cells (RBCs) to flex as they enter the narrowed capillary lumen, which has a mean diameter smaller than the erythrocytes.

A major function of RBCs is to transport the hemoglobin that carries oxygen that is converted to energy for muscle movement such as walking during the metabolic process. The decreased flexibility of the RBCs and the elevated blood viscosity are responsible for diminishing tissue oxygenation. Hence during exercise, the demand for an increase in blood flow and tissue oxygenation may result in claudication, thereby limiting the distance a person can walk.

Drug therapy for the treatment of intermittent claudication is limited. Ginkgo biloba, a complementary/alternative therapy, is reasonably effective for the treatment of intermittent claudication (see Chapter 12). Horse chestnut has some efficacy in treating symptoms of chronic venous insufficiency (see the Complementary and Alternative Considerations box below). Pentoxifylline is the most common allopathic medicine used in the treatment of intermittent claudication.

⚹ **How does pentoxifylline work?**

Pentoxifylline represents an important development in the therapy for peripheral vascular disorders, because the ability of vasodilators to improve blood flow by the dilation of rigid, arteriosclerotic blood vessels is somewhat limited. Furthermore, capillary walls lack smooth muscle, and therefore dilation by this group of drugs is often unlikely to occur.

⁘ Complementary and Alternative Considerations

Horse Chestnut

Horse chestnut is used in seed extract, leaf, branch bark, and flower form. Its proposed uses are for the treatment of varicose veins, hemorrhoids, phlebitis, diarrhea, soft-tissue swelling, fever, and enlarged prostate. Although there is insufficient reliable information available about the effectiveness of horse chestnut for its other uses, clinical studies do show that horse chestnut seed extract is effective in chronic venous insufficiency. Pittler and Ernst (2003) evaluated horse chestnut seed extract for chronic venous insufficiency. In this study, the evidence from randomized clinical trials was reviewed to assess the efficacy and safety of oral horse chestnut seed extract (HCSE) versus placebo, or reference therapy for the treatment of chronic venous insufficiency. Placebo-controlled trials suggest that horse chestnut results in an improvement in chronic venous insufficiency–related signs and symptoms. Six trials addressing leg pain reported a significant reduction of leg pain in the HCSE groups compared with the placebo groups. A meta-analysis of four trials (N = 239) reporting adequate data suggests a significant reduction in pain using HCSE compared with placebo. Adverse effects are usually mild and infrequent. The evidence suggests that HCSE is effective and safe in short-term treatment for chronic venous insufficiency; however, more randomized controlled trials are required to assess the long-term efficacy of this treatment option.

Data from Pittler, M.H., & Ernst, E. (2003). Horse chestnut seed extract for chronic venous insufficiency. Cochrane Peripheral Vascular Diseases Group. *Cochrane Database Systematic Review, 2003, 3.*

Pentoxifylline is considered a blood viscosity–reducing agent that increases microcirculatory blood flow and oxygenation of tissues. Pentoxifylline improves microcirculation, which involves the flow of blood through the fine vessels (arterioles, capillaries, and venules). Although the mechanism of action of pentoxifylline is not completely understood, current evidence shows that it possesses several properties to improve microcirculatory blood flow to ischemic tissues, including the following:

- It restores RBC flexibility, probably by its inhibition of phosphodiesterase, which results in an increase in cyclic adenosine monophosphate (cAMP) in RBCs.
- It lowers blood viscosity by decreasing fibrinogen concentrations and inhibiting the aggregation of RBCs and platelets.

✳ ⬛ **pentoxifylline** [pen tox ih **fi** leen]
(Trental)

Indications
Pentoxifylline is indicated as an adjunct to surgery for the treatment of intermittent claudication caused by occlusive arterial disease of the limbs.

Pharmacokinetics/Dosing
Pentoxifylline is administered orally and, on absorption, binds to erythrocyte membranes. It has a half-life of 0.4 to 0.8 hours for the primary drug and 1 to 1.6 hours for the metabolites. Peak concentration in the blood occurs in 2 to 4 hours, and the onset of action with chronic dosing is between 2 and 4 weeks. It is metabolized by RBCs and in the liver and is excreted primarily by the kidneys. The adult dosage is 400 mg orally three times daily with meals. If undesirable adverse effects occur, such as gastrointestinal (GI) upset or CNS disturbances, the dosage should be decreased to 400 mg twice daily.

Adverse Effects
The most common adverse effect of pentoxifylline is GI upset with abdominal distress, nausea and vomiting. Other adverse effects of pentoxifylline include dizziness and headaches. Rare adverse effects are chest pain and an irregular heart rate. With an overdose the client experiences increased sedation, flushing of the skin, a feeling of faintness, increased excitability, or seizures.

⚙ **What nursing care is provided to T.M. regarding the use of pentoxifylline?**

Assessment Because pentoxifylline is a xanthine derivative, do not administer it to T.M. if he has an intolerance to other xanthine derivatives (e.g., caffeine, theophylline, or theobromine), because excessive CNS stimulation may result. Pentoxifylline should also be used with caution in clients with impaired hepatic and renal function; it may accumulate and dosages may need to be lowered. Because pentoxifylline enhances microcirculation, careful monitoring is required for any client at risk for bleeding, particularly a cerebral or retinal hemorrhage.

Nursing Diagnosis With the administration of pentoxifylline, T.M. may be at risk for impaired comfort related to GI effects (e.g., nausea, vomiting, and abdominal cramping) and the CNS effects (dizziness, drowsiness, and headache). The potential complications may be angina and dysrhythmias.

Planning While T.M. is taking pentoxifylline, he will:
- Walk greater distances with less discomfort.
- State the adverse effects of pentoxifylline and interventions to minimize or prevent risk of injury related to those effects.
- Effectively maintain the therapeutic regimen (e.g., keep a journal of symptoms, report symptoms of adverse effects appropriately).
- Meet regularly and collaborate actively with health care personnel to manage his illness and drug regimen.

Implementation
Monitoring Monitor blood pressure periodically in clients receiving concurrent antihypertensive therapy. Small decreases in blood pressure have been noted in clients receiving pentoxifylline alone, and a reduction of the hypotensive agent might be indicated. Monitor the client with peripheral vascular disease for an improvement in walking distance and duration. Monitor pulses, color, and temperature of the affected extremities.

Intervention Administer pentoxifylline with food, milk, or antacids to decrease GI distress. If GI adverse effects persist, notify the prescriber to consider a reduction in the dosage. *The tablets should not be crushed.*

Education Instruct T.M. to swallow extended-release tablets whole without crushing or chewing them. Instruct the client that an improvement in clinical status may not occur before 8 weeks of therapy and that it is essential for the medication to be taken as prescribed until discontinued by the prescriber. Advise the client to quit smoking, because nicotine constricts the blood vessels and defeats the purpose of the medication. The client should receive support in smoking cessation through group or individual counseling.

Evaluation The expected outcome of pentoxifylline therapy is that the client will experience an improvement in pulse volume and in skin color and temperature, report decreased pain, and demonstrate increased activity tolerance.

Summary

Both vasodilators and blood viscosity–reducing (antihemorrheologic) agents are used in the treatment of vascular disorders. Vasodilators produce vasodilation by relaxing smooth muscle in the blood vessel walls, whereas blood viscosity–reducing agents improve microcirculatory blood flow to ischemic tissues by lowering blood viscosity as well as increasing cAMP in the RBCs. Vasodilators are more effective in treating angina and intermittent myocardial ischemia than they are for peripheral vascular disease.

The goals of therapy with nitrates, the classic antianginal agents, are to decrease the duration and intensity of pain during an attack, decrease the frequency of attacks, and improve work capacity even though angina may occur. Nursing management of the client taking nitrates is to assist in determining the appropriate dosages for the client; this is accomplished through medication administration and evaluation and is based on symptom control. The nurse also prepares the client for the safe and accurate self-administration of nitrates.

Chronic occlusive arterial disease is less successfully treated with vasodilating agents. The blood viscosity–reducing agent pentoxifylline increases microcirculatory blood flow, thereby increasing oxygenation of the tissues. It is a valuable adjunct treatment for occlusive arterial diseases of the limbs such as Buerger's disease.

✳ Critical Thinking Questions

- Mr. Scott has been taking sublingual nitroglycerin for years. He has now been prescribed a transdermal patch. How will Mr. Scott need to modify his therapeutic regimen?

- In obtaining a drug history from Mr. Slattery, who is about to begin pentoxifylline therapy, you determine that he has an intolerance to milk and coffee, and smokes a pack of cigarettes a day. What action would you take?

Bibliography

Anderson, D.M., Keith, J., & Novak, P.D. (Eds.). (2002). *Mosby's medical, nursing, and allied health dictionary* (6th ed.). St. Louis: Mosby.

Drug facts and comparisons (58th ed.). (2005). St. Louis: Facts and Comparisons.

Henrikson, C.A., Howell, E.E., Bush, D.E., Miles, J.S., Meininger, G.R., Friedlander, T., et al. (2003). Chest pain relief by nitroglycerin does not predict active coronary artery disease. *Annals of Internal Medicine, 139*, 979-986.

Kerins, D.M., Robertson, R.M., & Roberson, D. (2001). Drugs used for the treatment of myocardial ischemia. In J.G. Hardman & L.E. Limbird (Eds.), *Goodman & Gilman's the pharmacological basis of therapeutics* (10th ed.). New York: McGraw-Hill.

Lacy, C.F., Armstrong, L.L., Goldman, M.P., & Lance, L.L. (2004). *Lexi-Comp's drug information handbook* (12th ed.). Hudson, OH: Lexi-Comp.

Mosby's drug consult (15th ed.). (2005). St. Louis: Mosby.

Talbert, R.L. (2002). Ischemic heart disease. In J.T. DiPiro, R.L. Talbert, G.C. Yee, G.R. Matzke, B.G. Wella, & L.M. Posey (Eds.), *Pharmacotherapy: A pathophysiologic approach* (5th ed.). New York: McGraw-Hill.

Taylor, A.L., Ziesche, S., Yancy, C., Carson, P., D'Agostino, R. Jr., Ferdinand, K., et al. (2004). Combination of isosorbide dinitrate and hydralazine in blacks with heart failure. *New England Journal of Medicine, 351*, 2049-2057.

Trujillo, T.C., & Nolan, P.E. (2005). Ischemic heart disease: Anginal. In M.A. Koda-Kimble, L.Y. Young, W.A. Kradian, B.J. Guglielmo, B.K. Alldredge, & R.L. Corelli (Eds.), *Applied therapeutics: The clinical use of drugs* (8th ed.). Philadelphia: Lippincott Williams & Wilkins.

USP DI: Drug information for the health care professional (25th ed.). (2005). Greenwood Village, CO: MICROMEDEX Thomson Healthcare.

 ## *e*-LEARNING SUPPLEMENTS

Student CD-ROM
- Final Exam questions
- NCLEX® Examination review questions
- Pharmacology animations
- Printable chapter summary

Evolve Website (http://evolve.elsevier.com/mckenry)
- Case study on vasodilators and blood viscosity–reducing (antihemorrheologic) agents

- Content updates, including information on new drugs
- WebLinks corresponding to this chapter
- Answers to the critical thinking questions in this chapter
- *Elsevier ePharmacology Update* newsletter
- *Mosby's Drug Consult* Internet Edition
- Supplemental and reference information

OVERVIEW OF THE BLOOD

CHAPTER FOCUS

Because cells in the body are metabolically active, the blood plays an important role in maintaining homeostasis by providing constant nutrition and waste removal. Because the blood affects every other body system, it is a consideration in the assessment and care of most clients. Many drugs have adverse effects that cause disorders of the blood such as thrombocytopenia or agranulocytosis. The nurse therefore needs to be knowledgeable about hematology—the study of blood and blood-forming tissues.

LEARNING OBJECTIVES

- Describe the functions of the blood.
- Identify the three types of blood cells and their functions.
- Compare and contrast the five types of white blood cells.
- Describe the role of platelets in blood clotting.
- Identify the three major blood proteins and their functions.
- Describe the major blood types.
- Describe the significance of Rh factor.

▲ KEY TERMS

albumin, p. 592
anemia, p. 589
erythrocytes, p. 589
erythropoietin, p. 589
fibrinogen, p. 592
globulins, p. 592
hematocrit, p. 589
hemoglobin, p. 589
hemostasis, p. 592
leukocytes, p. 589
leukocytosis, p. 589
leukopenia, p. 589
phagocytosis, p. 589
plasma, p. 588
platelets, p. 589
thrombocytes, p. 589
thrombocytopenia, p. 591

✱ What are the functions of blood in the body?

Blood is the major transport system in the body. It is also vitally important for proper functioning and regulation of the human body. Pumped by the heart, blood carries nutrients and oxygen from the digestive and respiratory systems to cells throughout the entire body. Additionally, it picks up waste products from body cells and delivers them to the proper system for excretion, usually the liver, kidneys, and lungs. Hormones, enzymes, buffers, and many other bio-chemical substances are transported by the blood from one site in the body to the receptors or target cells. Blood also helps to regulate body heat by absorbing and transporting heat from the body core to where it can be more easily dispersed.

✱ What is the composition of blood?

Blood is composed of billions of cells and **plasma,** a fluid portion in which the cells are suspended. Although blood volume can vary from person to person, the average blood volume in a normal adult is approximately 5000 mL (5 L). Of this volume, 3000 mL is usually plasma; the remainder is primarily red blood cells (RBCs). **Hematocrit** is the packed cell volume of the RBCs expressed as a percentage of the total blood volume, or the blood viscosity. Hematocrit is measured by a laboratory test performed on a blood sample. The higher the hematocrit, the greater the blood viscosity. For example, persons with polycythemia may have a hematocrit of 60 or 70 because of an excessive number of red blood corpuscles. Increased blood viscosity can retard the flow of blood through blood vessels, resulting in headaches, fatigue, weakness, dyspnea, and perhaps an enlarged spleen and increased basal metabolism.

Blood is composed of the following three types of blood cells: (1) **erythrocytes**, or RBCs, that transport oxygen and carbon dioxide; (2) **leukocytes,** or white blood cells (WBCs), that defend the body against bacteria and infections; and (3) **platelets,** or **thrombocytes,** that are necessary for blood coagulation. Proteins such as serum albumin, globulins, and fibrinogen are also present in the blood.

Plasma may contain thousands of other substances, such as glucose, electrolytes, vitamins, hormones, and waste products. The discussion in this chapter is limited to blood cells, blood proteins, and blood groups (or types).

Erythrocytes RBCs (erythrocytes) are small and disk shaped. They are the cells present in the largest quantities in the bloodstream, and they have a life span of approximately 120 days. The major function of the RBCs is to carry **hemoglobin,** a complex protein-iron compound in the blood. Each hemoglobin molecule contains four iron atoms; these four iron atoms combine with four oxygen molecules to transport oxygen from the lungs to the tissues. Hemoglobin can also combine with carbon dioxide and carry it from the cells to the lungs for excretion. It also serves as an acid-base buffering system in whole blood.

After birth, RBCs are produced by the bone marrow. In early life most bones manufacture RBCs, but after 20 years of age most RBCs are produced in the bone marrow of the vertebrae, sternum, ribs, and ilia.

Males have more hemoglobin in their blood than do females. In general, most men have between 14 and 16 g/dL, whereas women have a range of 12 to 14 g/dL. A person with a hemoglobin count below 10 g/dL is usually diagnosed as having **anemia.** Anemias are classified according to both the size and the number of functional RBCs in the blood.

RBCs are rapidly formed and destroyed in the body. It has been estimated that more than 100 million RBCs are produced every minute during adulthood. The normal healthy adult has between 4.5 and 5.5 million cells/mm³ of blood. The body balances the production versus the destruction of these cells to maintain a relatively constant level of RBCs. The exact mechanism for this is unknown.

It is known that the rate of RBC production can increase if a considerable decrease in RBCs occurs or if tissue hypoxia develops. In such cases the kidneys are stimulated to increase secretion of **erythropoietin,** a hormone that acts to stimulate the production of RBCs by bone marrow. With maximum bone marrow stimulation, RBC production can be increased to nearly seven times over normal.

To make new RBCs, the bone marrow needs adequate supplies of vitamin B_{12}, iron, and other substances. A deficiency in the absorption of vitamin B_{12} from the gastrointestinal (GI) tract, which is caused by a lack of intrinsic factor (see Chapter 67), can lead to pernicious anemia.

Anemia can also be induced by increased red cell destruction that can occur with infections or cancer, or from bone marrow suppression caused by radiation therapy and many cancer chemotherapeutic agents and other drugs (Box 29-1).

Leukocytes There are five types of leukocytes, which are classified according to the presence or absence of granules in the cell cytoplasm. The granular leukocytes are neutrophils, eosinophils, and basophils; the nongranular leukocytes are lymphocytes and monocytes. The granular leukocytes have two or more nuclear lobes and are therefore referred to as polymorphonuclear leukocytes or "polys."

Under normal circumstances, blood contains between 5000 and 9000 leukocytes per cubic milliliter (Table 29-1). A differential count may be ordered by the health care provider to aid in diagnosis. In acute appendicitis, for example, the percentage of neutrophils increases, as does the total leukocyte count. A shift to the left in the differential count, or a predominance of immature leukocytes, is usually indicative of an infection or inflammation. This term derives from a graph of blood components in which immature cell frequencies appear on the left side of the graph. A shift to the right indicates a preponderance of "polys," which indicates a relative lack of blood-forming activity, such as in severe liver disease and advanced pernicious anemia.

Leukocytes are produced primarily in the bone marrow. However, lymphocytes are produced mainly in lymph tissues and organs (e.g., the spleen, thymus, tonsils) and in various other lymphoid tissue in the bone marrow, GI tract, and elsewhere. Several terms are important to understand. **Leukopenia** refers to an abnormal decrease in the number of leukocytes to fewer than 5000/mm³; **leukocytosis** refers to an abnormal increase in the number of leukocytes.

Neutrophils, monocytes, lymphocytes, and basophils are very mobile. They can leave the capillaries and migrate to organisms or foreign particles that have entered the body. Neutrophils and monocytes ingest and destroy the invaders in a process known as **phagocytosis.** The absolute neutrophils count is used to determine the status of the immune system, particularly in response to chemotherapy, bone marrow transplantation, or radiation (Box 29-2). Lymphocytes defend the body against bacteria, fungi, and viruses by forming B lymphocytes or T lymphocytes. (Chapter 61 provides an overview of the immune system.)

Eosinophils are considered weak phagocytes and have limited mobility. An increased level of eosinophils is usually

BOX 29-1 DRUGS THAT CAUSE BONE MARROW DEPRESSION

amphotericin B, systemic (Fungizone)

antithyroid medications

aspariginase (Elspar)

azathioprine (Imuran)

busulfan (Myleran)

carmustine (Bicnu)

chlorambucil (Leukeran)

chloramphenicol (Chloromycetin)

cisplatin (Platinol-AQ)

clozapine (Clozaril)

colchicine

cyclophosphamide (Cytoxan, Procytox)

cytarabine (Cytosar-U, Cytosar)

dacarbazine (DTIC, DTIC-Dome)

dactinomycin (Cosmegen)

daunorubicin (Cerubidine)

doxorubicin (Adriamycin)

etoposide (Etopophos, Toposar, VePesid)

floxuridine (FUDR)

flucytosine (Ancobon, Ancotil)

fluorouracil, systemic (5-FU, Adrucil)

gold salts

hydroxyurea (Hydrea)

interferon (Roferon-A, Intron-A)

linezolid (Zyvox)

lomustine (CeeNU)

mechlorethamine, systemic (Mustargen)

melphalan (Alkeran IV)

mercaptopurine (Purinethol)

methotrexate (Mexate)

mitomycin (Mutamycin)

pentamidine (Pentam)

phenytoin (Dilantin)

plicamycin (Mithracin)

procarbazine (Matulane, Natulan)

sodium iodide ^{131}I (Iodotope)

sodium phosphate P_{32}

sulfamethoxazole/trimethoprim (Bactrim, Septra)

streptozocin (Zanosar)

thioguanine

thiotepa (Thioplex)

uracil mustard

vinblastine (Velban, Velbe)

vincristine (Oncovin)

zidovudine (Retrovir)

TABLE 29-1 NORMAL ADULT WHITE BLOOD CELL COUNT WITH DIFFERENTIAL

The normal range for total white blood cell count in adults is 4500 to 11,000/mm³

White Blood Cells	% of Total
Neutrophils (polymorphonuclear)	40%-78%
Segs (mature neutrophils)	35%-66%
Bands (almost mature neutrophils)	5%-11%
Eosinophils (polymorphonuclear)	0%-3%
Basophils (polymorphonuclear)	0%-1%
Monocytes	3%-6%
Lymphocytes	24%-44%
Atypical lymphocytes	0%-8%

Data from Lacy, C.F., Armstrong, L.L., Goldman, M.P., Lance, L.L. (2004). *Lexi-Comp's drug information handbook* (12th ed.). Hudson, OH: Lexi-Comp.

Box 29-2 Absolute Neutrophil Count (ANC)

The Absolute Neutrophil Count (ANC) reflects the number of white blood cells (WBCs) the client has available to fight infection. These WBCs include both mature segmented neutrophils (sometimes referred to as "Segs") and immature but functional neutrophils ("Bands"). The ANC is calculated from the differential WBC (see Table 29-1) using the following formula:

ANC (per mm³ = Total WBCs ×
          (% Neutrophils/100 + % Band cells/100)

An example a calculated ANC:
- Total WBC count: 5000 cells/mm³:
- Neutrophils (segmented or mature neutrophils): 20%
- Bands (immature neutrophils): 5%

ANC = 5000 cells/mm³ × (20/100 + 5/100)

ANC = 5000 cells/mm³ × (25/100)

ANC = 5000 cells/mm³ × 0.25

ANC = 1250 cells/mm³ (Sometimes presented as an ANC of 1.25)

Calculation and interpretation of the ANC is important in assessing and monitoring clients who are at risk for infection and/or who receive drugs that may cause bone marrow suppression (e.g., antineoplastic therapy, clozapine) or suppress immune function (immunosuppressants used in transplant medicine and autoimmune diseases). The following table highlights how ANC is often interpreted in clinical settings.

ANC Value	Interpretation	Comments
1800-8000 cells/mm³ (1.8-8)	Normal	No added risk for infection
1000-1800 cells/mm³ (1-1.8)	Mild neutropenia	Low risk for infection
500-1000 cells/mm³ (0.5-1)	Moderate neutropenia	Moderate risk for infection
Less than 500 cells/mm³ (0-0.49)	Severe neutropenia	High risk for infection

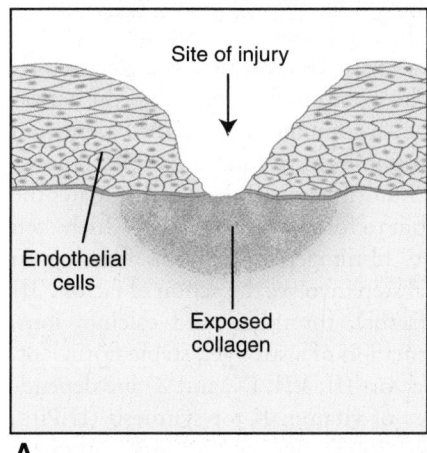
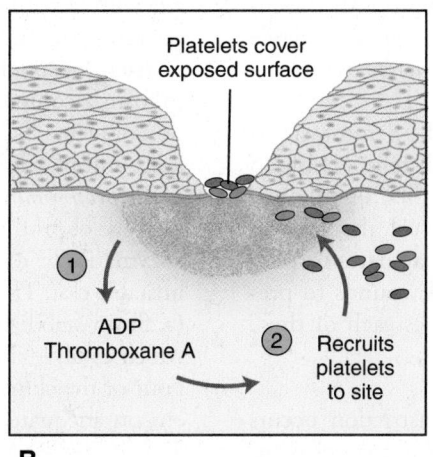
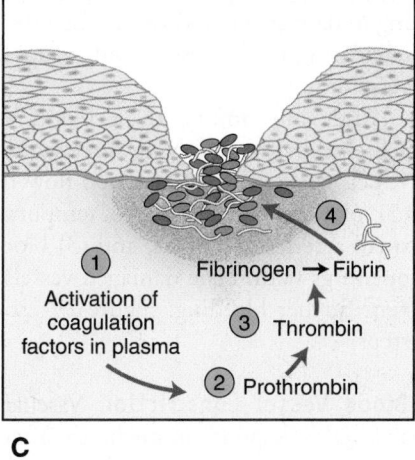

FIGURE 29-1 Formation of a hemostatic plug. **A,** Exposed collagen triggering the formation of a platelet plug. **B,** ADP and thromboxane A release (1) promotes recruitment of more platelets to the site and completes the initial platelet plug (2). **C,** The activation of coagulation factors (1) leads eventually to the formation of fibrin strands being intermeshed with the platelet plug forming a clot (2, 3, 4).

seen with allergic reactions or a cell injury caused by parasites (e.g., hookworm).

The life span of granular leukocytes (granulocytes) is estimated to be 4 to 8 hours in the bloodstream and 3 to 5 days in body tissues. If involved in the ingestion of invading organisms, this life span can be reduced to only a few hours, because during this process they are also destroyed. Monocytes also have a short life span in blood, but they can live for months or even years in the body tissues if not destroyed by phagocytosis. Monocytes in the tissues often increase in size to become tissue macrophages, and in this way they often provide a first line of defense against tissue infections.

Platelets Platelets, or thrombocytes, are small, round, or oval colorless cells produced by the bone marrow. They have a life span of 5 to 8 days. A normal platelet level in the blood is between 150,000 and 350,000/mm³.

Platelets are key substances for blood clotting in the body. If a blood vessel is injured and blood is escaping, platelets quickly congregate at the site and clump together to form a plug and stop the bleeding. If the wound is large, platelets set off a series of chemical reactions within the body to form a clot and seal the injury (Figure 29-1).

Persons with **thrombocytopenia** have a low quantity of platelets. Such persons tend to bleed, and their skin usually displays small purple spots—hence the name thrombocytopenia purpura. Bleeding problems usually do not occur until the platelets decrease to levels below 50,000/mm³. Thrombocytopenia is often induced by irradiation injury to the bone marrow or from aplasia of the bone marrow induced by specific drugs.

Blood Proteins The blood contains three major proteins: albumin, globulins, and fibrinogen. **Albumin** is responsible for the osmotic pressure gradient produced at the capillary membrane. This prevents plasma fluid from leaving the capillaries to enter the interstitial spaces.

Globulins are divided into alpha, beta, and gamma globulins. Gamma globulin and perhaps, to a lesser extent, beta globulin help to protect the body against infections. Gamma globulin is involved with humoral immunity. Alpha and beta globulins are also believed to perform other functions, such as transporting certain substances in the blood by reversibly combining with them. They may also be a substrate to form other substances.

Fibrinogen, a plasma protein that is converted to fibrin by thrombin in the presence of calcium ions, is necessary for coagulation.

✳ What mechanisms exist to arrest bleeding?

Hemostasis is a process that spontaneously stops the bleeding in damaged blood vessels. Blood is normally fluid while circulating in the vessels, but it rapidly clots at the site of vessel injury.

After any injury to a blood vessel, hemostasis is achieved by the following three sequential steps: (1) blood vessels constrict to slow blood flow from the injured area, (2) platelet plugs form to temporarily seal the leaking small arteries and veins, and (3) blood coagulates to plug openings within the damaged vessels and wounds to prevent further bleeding. Figure 29-1 outlines each of these steps.

Blood Vessel Constriction Vascular constriction occurs as a reflex response immediately after a blood vessel is injured. This response instantly slows the flow of blood from the ruptured vessel.

Platelet Plug Formation When a blood vessel is injured, the interruption of the continuity of its endothelial lining exposes the collagen (a fibrous protein) in the underlying connective tissue. Platelets immediately adhere to this exposed collagen to form a dense aggregate in a process known as platelet adhesion. This attachment triggers the release of adenosine diphosphate (ADP), which causes the outer surface of the platelets to become extremely sticky so that other adjacent platelets adhere to one another at the damaged site. Thromboxane A2 (TXA2) is a prostaglandin that promotes vasoconstriction and further release of ADP. This process eventually forms the platelet plug. This plug is relatively unstable; it can stop bleeding quickly as long as the damage to the vessel is small. For long-term effectiveness the platelet plug must be reinforced with fibrin. This involves a chemical mechanism called blood coagulation.

Coagulation Blood coagulation is the final stage of a complex series of events in hemostasis. This process ultimately results in the formation of a stable fibrin clot, which is composed of a meshwork of fibrin threads that entraps platelets, blood cells, and plasma. The physical formation of a blood clot or thrombus plays a key role in hemostasis by permanently closing the hole in the injured vessel to prevent further bleeding.

The chemical events in the blood coagulation mechanism involve two distinct pathways: the intrinsic pathway and the extrinsic pathway.

Intrinsic Pathway Because all the chemical substances involved in coagulation are normally found in the circulating blood, this pathway is referred to as the *intrinsic system of coagulation*. In this pathway the activation of specific blood coagulation factors is initiated by injury to the endothelial lining of the blood vessel wall. When blood contacts the exposed underlying collagen, the Hageman factor (factor XII) is activated by enzymatically converting it to the active form (factor XIIa). The simultaneous damage of platelets also causes the release of platelet phospholipid (platelet factor 3), which is required later in the coagulation process. Factor XIIa then activates factor XI to XIa. The reaction of factor XIa with factor IX requires calcium ions for the formation of activated factor IXa. In the presence of calcium ions and platelet phospholipids, factor IXa interacts with factor VIII to form a complex. This combination speeds up the activation of factor X. Factor Xa combines with factor Va, calcium ions, and platelet phospholipids to form a complex known as the *prothrombin* activator (factor II). Factor II initiates the cleavage of prothrombin to form thrombin (IIa), which then enzymatically converts fibrinogen into fibrin, forming an unstable clot. The final step involves the action of factor XIII (a fibrin-stabilizing factor), thrombin, and calcium ions, which catalyze the formation of a stronger, stable fibrin clot. Four of the clotting factors (II, VII, IX, and X) are dependent on adequate stores of vitamin K for synthesis (DiPiro, Talbert, Yee, & Matzke, 2002). (Figure 29-2 lists a summary of the main events of the intrinsic pathway.)

Extrinsic Pathway The extrinsic pathway is activated by trauma to the vascular wall or to the tissues outside the blood vessels. In this pathway, clotting occurs when products of tissue damage gain access to the blood. The tissue factor thromboplastin is released and becomes part of a complex with factor VII and calcium ions. This combination of components activates factor X, which is the step at which the extrinsic pathway converges with the intrinsic pathway; coagulation then continues through a common route with the resultant formation of a final stable clot. (Figure 29-2 shows the extrinsic pathway.)

The final pathway, which is common to both the intrinsic and the extrinsic coagulation systems, begins with the activation of factor X and ends with the formation of fibrin. Both systems function simultaneously in the body. The lack of a normal factor in either system will usually result in a blood disorder.

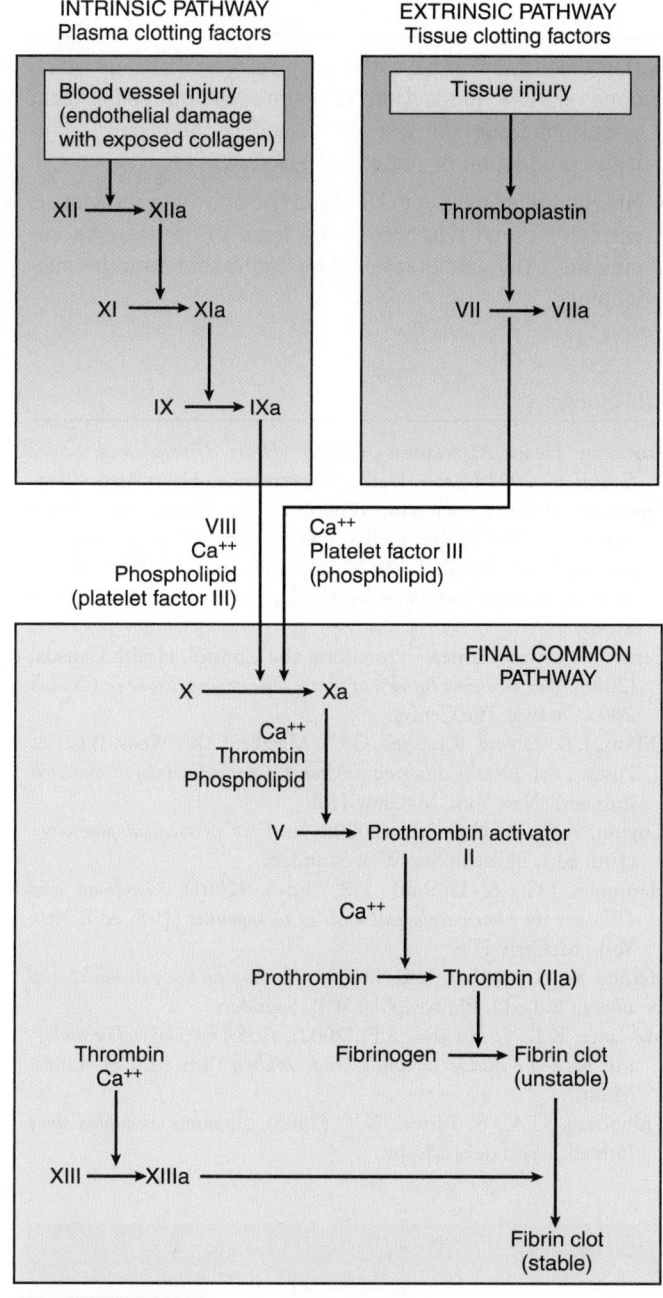

INTRINSIC PATHWAY
Plasma clotting factors

Blood vessel injury
(endothelial damage
with exposed collagen)

XII ——→ XIIa

XI ——→ XIa

IX ——→ IXa

VIII
Ca⁺⁺
Phospholipid
(platelet factor III)

EXTRINSIC PATHWAY
Tissue clotting factors

Tissue injury

Thromboplastin

VII ——→ VIIa

Ca⁺⁺
Platelet factor III
(phospholipid)

FINAL COMMON
PATHWAY

X ——→ Xa

Ca⁺⁺
Thrombin
Phospholipid

V ——→ Prothrombin activator
II

Ca⁺⁺

Prothrombin ——→ Thrombin (IIa)

Fibrinogen ——→ Fibrin clot
(unstable)

Thrombin
Ca⁺⁺

XIII ——→ XIIIa ————————————————→

Fibrin clot
(stable)

FIGURE 29-2 The coagulation system.

What abnormalities of blood coagulation are observed in clinical practice?

Diseases associated with abnormally clotting vessels cause many deaths. Venous thromboembolism occurs for the first time in about 100 people per 100,000 each year in the United States. About one third of these are pulmonary embolism (PE), and about two thirds have deep vein thrombosis (DVT) alone. DVT is when a blood clot occurs in the legs. PE occurs when that clot travels through the bloodstream, and obstructs a vessel in the lungs. There are more than 200,000 new cases of venous thromboembolism annually. Of these people, 30% die within 3 days. PE causes death in one fifth of these cases suddenly and within a month of diagnosis in 12% of cases (American Heart Association, 2004).

Diseases caused by intravascular clotting include some of the major causes of death from cardiovascular sources—coronary occlusion and cerebrovascular accidents. Cardiovascular disease was the primary or contributing factor to 400,000 death certificates in 2002, of which 53% were because of coronary heart disease (CHD) and 18% because of stroke (American Heart Association, 2005). Over 80% of the Canadian population has at least one risk factor for cardiovascular events (Centre for Chronic Disease Prevention and Control, Health Canada, 2003). Therefore, knowledge of drugs that inhibit clotting is important to a nurse's practice.

Local trauma, vascular stasis, and systemic alterations in the coagulability of blood are considered the main factors in the initiation of thrombosis. Basically, coagulation mechanisms are responsible for forming two types of thrombi: arterial thrombi and venous thrombi. Arterial thrombi are most commonly associated with atherosclerotic plaques, high blood pressure, and turbulent blood flow that damage the endothelial lining of the blood vessel and cause platelets to stick and aggregate in the arterial system. Arterial thrombi are mostly platelets, and their formation is associated with the intrinsic pathway of the coagulation mechanism.

Venous thrombi occur most often in areas in which blood flow is reduced or static. This appears to initiate clotting and produces a thrombus in the venous system. The formation of thrombi involves the extrinsic pathway of the coagulation mechanism. Current anticoagulants are more effective in preventing venous thrombi.

What are the major blood types and their significance?

Blood type refers to the type of antigen located on RBC membranes. Although many antigens have been identified, antigens A, B, and Rh are the most important ones involved with blood transfusions and newborn survival. Every person belongs to one of the four blood groups and is also Rh positive or Rh negative. The ABO blood groups are as follows:

- Type A: A antigen on RBCs (the plasma has antibody B)
- Type B: B antigen on RBCs (the plasma has antibody A)
- Type AB: A antigen and B antigen on RBCs (the plasma contains no antibodies)
- Type O: neither A nor B antigens on RBCs (the plasma contains A and B antibodies)

Persons with type A blood can safely receive blood from type A and type O donors. Persons with type B blood can safely receive blood from type B and type O donors. People with AB blood are known as the universal recipients because their blood is compatible with types AB, A, B, and O. However, crossmatching of the blood is necessary before transfusion, because other agglutinins may be present. Type O persons can receive only type O blood; they are called universal donors because they can donate blood to anyone. (Chapter 30 discusses additional information on blood transfusion.)

A person who is Rh-positive carries the Rh antigen on the RBCs. A person who is Rh-negative does not have any Rh antigens on the RBCs. Approximately 85% of the population is Rh-positive. Rh factor is particularly important when an Rh-negative woman is impregnated by an Rh-positive man. The mother may have antibodies against the Rh antigen, which can cross the placenta and attack the fetus should its blood be Rh-positive. If this occurs, the infant may develop jaundice or be stillborn.

An Rh-negative woman could acquire Rh antibodies via blood transfusions. It is also possible for her to develop them if fetal blood enters her bloodstream during childbirth or miscarriage. Regardless, the first pregnancy usually has less risk associated with it than subsequent pregnancies because there is less of a chance that the woman has Rh antibodies.

Prescribers can reduce this danger by administering an anti-Rh antibody (Gamulin Rh, RhoGAM, or HypRho-D) to Rh-negative women after each pregnancy. These drugs prevent their systems from making antibodies to Rh-positive blood. Rh-negative women who have a spontaneous or induced abortion or a termination of an ectopic pregnancy of up to and including 12 weeks' gestation are given a microdose of immune globulin (MICRhoGAM or Mini-Gamulin Rh) if the father is Rh-positive.

Summary

The role of blood is to transport cellular requirements and products from one part of the body to another. The continuous exchange between the interstitial fluid and the blood serves to maintain a cellular environment that fluctuates only within narrow limits. An appreciation of the role of blood in maintaining homeostasis in the body is essential.

⊛ Critical Thinking Questions

- Many medications have the adverse effect of depressing bone marrow production of various blood cells. What symptoms would you expect to see if a client had diminished production of platelets? RBCs? WBCs?
- Mrs. Chandler has type AB blood. At one time individuals with this blood type were considered to be universal recipients. Why was that so? Why might that term be misleading?

Bibliography

American Heart Association. (2004). *Heart Disease and Stroke Statistics – 2004 Update.* Dallas, TX: American Heart Association.

American Heart Association. (2005). *Heart Disease and Stroke Statistics – 2005 Update.* Dallas, TX: American Heart Association.

Anderson, D.M., Keith, J., & Novak, P.D. (Eds.) (2002). *Mosby's medical, nursing, and allied health dictionary* (6th ed.). St. Louis: Mosby.

Centre for Chronic Disease Prevention and Control, Health Canada. (2003). *The Growing Burden of Heart Disease and Stroke in Canada 2003* Ottawa: The Centre.

DiPiro, J.T., Talbert, R.L., Yee, G.C., Matzke, G.R., Wells, B.G., & Posey, L.M. (2002). *Pharmacotherapy: A pathophysiologic approach* (5th ed.). New York: McGraw-Hill.

Guyton, A.C., & Hall, J.E. (2000). *Textbook of medical physiology* (10th ed.). Philadelphia: W.B. Saunders.

Hardman, J.G., & Limbird, L.E. (Eds.). (2001). *Goodman and Gilman's the pharmacological basis of therapeutics* (10th ed.). New York: McGraw-Hill.

Herlihy, B., & Maebius, N.K. (2003). *The human body in health and illness* (2nd ed.). Philadelphia: W.B. Saunders.

McCance, K.L., & Huether, S.E. (2002). *Pathophysiology: The biological basis for disease in adults and children* (4th ed.). St. Louis: Mosby.

Thibodeau, G.A., & Patton, K.T. (2003). *Anatomy and physiology* (5th ed.). St. Louis: Mosby.

e-LEARNING SUPPLEMENTS

Student CD-ROM
- Final Exam questions
- NCLEX® Examination review questions
- Pharmacology animations
- Printable chapter summary

Evolve Website (http://evolve.elsevier.com/mckenry)
- Content updates, including information on new drugs
- WebLinks corresponding to this chapter
- Answers to the critical thinking questions in this chapter
- *Elsevier ePharmacology Update* newsletter
- *Mosby's Drug Consult* Internet Edition
- Supplemental and reference information

ANTIPLATELETS, ANTICOAGULANTS, FIBRINOLYTICS, AND BLOOD COMPONENTS

CHAPTER FOCUS

Blood affects every body system because it transports gases, nutrients, metabolic wastes, blood cells, immune cells, and hormones throughout the body. The nurse must manage the client's therapeutic regimen for antiplatelets, anticoagulants, fibrinolytics, and blood components effectively to ensure the most positive outcome possible for clients with a wide variety of illnesses and injuries.

LEARNING OBJECTIVES

- Identify the disease processes that require the administration of drugs to inhibit clotting.
- Describe the advantages and disadvantages of antiplatelet therapy.
- Differentiate between the mechanisms of action of parenteral and oral anticoagulant agents.
- Implement the nursing management of a client receiving anticoagulant therapy.
- Describe the use of protamine sulfate and vitamin K as anticoagulant antagonists.
- Differentiate between the actions of fibrinolytics and anticoagulant drugs on blood clots.
- Describe drugs that may be successfully used in treating hemophilia.
- Implement the nursing management of a client receiving blood component therapy.

▲ KEY TERMS

anticoagulants, p. 596
antiplatelet drugs, p. 596
embolus, p. 595
fibrinolytics, p. 596
hemophilia, p. 619
thrombus, p. 595

KEY DRUGS

abciximab, p. 601
alteplase, p. 617
aspirin (Monograph in Chapter 14, p. 268)
clopidogrel, p. 598
enoxaparin, p. 606
heparin, p. 606
protamine sulfate, p. 615
warfarin, p. 607

This chapter reviews the drugs and substances that affect hemostasis or blood clotting, preformed thrombi, and blood administration. Normal blood clotting is a defense mechanism constantly available for protection against excessive hemorrhage. However, the development of a throm-

bus in a blood vessel can obstruct blood flow and cause an infarction with resultant tissue necrosis. A **thrombus** is an aggregation of platelets, fibrin, clotting factors, and the cellular elements of the blood that becomes attached to the inner wall of a blood vessel—a blood clot. An **embolus,** a mass of undissolved matter that breaks off from the thrombus, can travel in the blood vessel and lodge in areas of the body; this can cause death. By contrast, a defect in the blood clotting mechanism may lead to excessive bleeding or hemorrhage, even after a minor injury. Both thrombotic and hemorrhagic disorders can be treated with drugs. The following discussion describes the rationale for the use of various groups of therapeutic agents.

✳ What drugs are available to prevent or treat a thrombus or embolus?

Drugs that interfere with clot formation or accelerate clot degradation fall into one of three broad categories: antiplatelets, anticoagulants, and fibrinolytics.

Antiplatelet drugs inhibit platelet aggregation. Classic examples include the orally administered drugs, aspirin and clopidogrel (Plavix). These agents are commonly used to prevent or treat a number of conditions, including myocardial infarction (MI) and thromboembolic cerebrovascular accident (CVA). Parenterally administered antiplatelets include the IIb/IIIa inhibitors abciximab (ReoPro), eptifibatide (Integrilin), and tirofiban (Aggrastat). Their use is limited to the hospital setting in the treatment of unstable angina and as adjunct therapy for interventional cardiac catheterization procedures.

The anticoagulants interfere with one or more of the clotting factors in the clotting cascade and include the parenterally administered heparins and the orally administered warfarin (Coumadin). Anticoagulants are used to prevent and/or treat deep vein thrombosis (DVT) and pulmonary embolism (PE). Although they are used to treat thrombosis, they do not dissolve clots, but prevent the extension of existing clots. A number of other anticoagulants are either in use or under investigation for their clinical utility.

Finally, the fibrinolytics (formerly known as the thrombolytics) include derivatives of alteplase (tPa) and streptokinase. These agents degrade fibrin strands and are used to help dissolve an existing clot. Their use includes the treatment of MI and thromboembolic CVA. In lower doses, they are also instilled locally by specialists in vascular medicine to help break up other thrombi or emboli.

✳ What are the risks of using antiplatelets, anticoagulants, and fibrinolytics?

As expected, agents that interfere with hemostasis pose significant risks. The primary risk for each of these agents is bleeding. Bleeding may be manifested by impaired ability to clot after a cut, or internal bleeding from numerous sites (e.g., gastrointestinal (GI), retroperitoneal, cerebrovascular). Agents and classes vary in the likelihood for a bleeding event and the careful evaluation of risk and benefit of these treatments must be made before therapy is initiated. Many conditions being prevented or treated with these drugs have a significant risk for morbidity or mortality if untreated, and as such, drug therapy is instituted.

Other risks for these drugs include hypersensitivity reactions, or changes related to bleeding events. These will be discussed with individual agents.

✳ **B.K. is a 58-year-old female with a recent history of stable angina and hypertension. She is stabilized on metoprolol (Lopressor) 50 mg every 12 hours and her health care provider is considering antiplatelet therapy to help prevent an MI.**

✳ What oral antiplatelets are used to prevent or treat a thromboembolic event?

The composition of arterial thrombi is primarily platelet aggregates; venous thrombi are usually composed of fibrin and red blood cells (RBCs). Therefore the anticoagulant drugs are used to reduce the risks or complications of venous thrombi, whereas the antiplatelet agents are used for arterial thrombi.

The most commonly used antiplatelet drugs in North America are aspirin and clopidogrel (Plavix). Other oral antiplatelet drugs, or drugs that inhibit platelet aggregation, include anagrelide (Agrylin), cilostazol (Pletal), dipyridamole (Persantine), and ticlopidine (Ticlid). The intravenously administered antiplatelet glycoprotein IIb/IIIa inhibitors include abciximab (ReoPro), eptifibatide (Integrilin), and tirofiban (Aggrastat).

Oral Antiplatelets

Aspirin, also known as acetylsalicylic acid (ASA), has numerous properties related to its ability to inhibit prostaglandin synthesis. At doses of 80 to 325 mg daily, aspirin inhibits cyclooxygenase, an enzyme necessary for the synthesis of thromboxane A_2 (TXA_2). TXA_2 promotes platelet aggregation and vasoconstriction, and aspirin suppresses these actions (see Chapter 29). Higher doses of aspirin result in antiinflammatory, analgesic and antipyretic properties. The inhibition of prostaglandins observed with aspirin also poses a risk for GI irritation or bleeding and is one of the concerns with its use. Additional concerns with aspirin use are the potential to trigger bronchoconstriction in a client with asthma, and renal insufficiency for clients with preexisting renal impairment. More information on aspirin is presented in Chapter 14.

✳ **B.K.'s health care provider has determined that she has no history of GI bleeding or renal insufficiency, and she is started on enteric-coated aspirin 325 mg daily to help prevent an MI.**

✳ How should B.K.'s drug regimen be managed by nursing?

Assessment Because aspirin and other antiplatelet drugs prolong bleeding time, they are contraindicated for clients with bleeding ulcers or erosive gastritis, other active bleeding states (intracerebral or intraocular hemorrhage), and hemophilia or other bleeding problems (coagulation or platelet disorders). In clients with nasal polyps or a history of asthma, aspirin should be avoided as it may precipitate a severe episode of bronchospasm.

Aspirin should be held 5 days before major surgery (Cahill et al., 2005).

Review B.K.'s current medication regimen for significant drug interactions. With aspirin and the other antiplatelet agents, the concomitant use of anticoagulants and antiplatelet and fibrinolytic agents would result in additive bleeding effects. In addition, the risk for acute MI (AMI) may be increased for up to 1 month after stopping nonaspirin NSAIDs (Fischer, Schlienger, Matter, Jick, & Meier, 2004). Other drugs that may cause hypoprothrombinemia (e.g., cefamandole [Mandol], cefoperazone [Cefobid], or cefotetan [Cefotan], will also increase the risk of bleeding. See Box 30-1 for other medications with platelet aggregation-inhibiting activity. Giving aspirin with drugs that have the potential for ototoxicity, such as vancomycin, increases the risk of hearing loss. Aspirin is not recommended for concurrent administration with medications used to treat hyperuricemia (probenecid, sulfinpyrazone) because it decreases their effects. It may also increase the risk of methotrexate toxicity if given concurrently.

A baseline assessment of B.K. includes a cardiovascular assessment in relation to her angina, and a complete blood count (CBC) (hematocrit, platelet count) and prothrombin time (PT) or international normalized ratio (INR) for comparison during her aspirin therapy.

Nursing Diagnosis The client receiving aspirin as platelet therapy may be at risk for the following nursing diagnoses/collaborative problems: impaired comfort (dyspepsia, heartburn, nausea); ineffective airway clearance related to bronchospasm (shortness of breath, dyspnea, wheezing); risk for injury related to dizziness; activity intolerance related to anemia; disturbed sensory perception related to tinnitus and hearing loss; ineffective tissue perfusion related to thrombus formation and the ineffectiveness of the aspirin; and the potential complications of hemorrhage related to altered clotting factors, hepatotoxicity and allergic reaction.

Planning The goals for B.K.'s aspirin therapy are that she will:

- Not experience a thrombotic episode, such as CVA or MI.
- Remain free of injury from the adverse effects of the aspirin.
- Be compliant with the medication regimen.
- Demonstrate adequate knowledge regarding the aspirin therapy and its potential adverse effects.
- Effectively manage the aspirin regimen, including lifestyle changes and collaboration with health care providers for monitoring and treatment.

Implementation

Monitoring All platelet aggregate inhibitor therapy should be discontinued if the platelet count is less than 80,000 cells/mm³. Monitor B.K. for bleeding—epistaxis, bleeding gums, hematuria, conjunctival hemorrhage, GI bleeding, or excessive bruising. If she experiences invasive

---

BOX 30-1 SELECTED MEDICATIONS WITH PLATELET AGGREGATION-INHIBITING ACTIVITY

ANTIPLATELET AGENTS

abciximab (ReoPro)

anagrelide (Agrylin)

aspirin

clopidogrel (Plavix)

dipyridamole (Persantine)

eptifibatide (Integrilin)

ticlopidine (Ticlid)

tirofiban (Aggrastat)

THROMBIN INHIBITORS

argatroban (Acova)

bivalirudin (Angiomax)

OTHER AGENTS

alprostadil, systemic (Edex), prostaglandin

antiinflammatory drugs, nonsteroidal (NSAIDs), analgesics

calcium channel blockers (CCBs)

contrast agents, radiopaque (intravascular administration)

dextran (Dextran 70), blood former and coagulant

divalproex (Depakote), antiepileptic drug

epoprostenol (Flolan), vasodilator

garlic, complementary/alternative therapy

gingko, complementary/alternative therapy

mezlocillin (Mezlin), antibiotic

pentoxifylline (Trental), blood-viscosity reducer

piperacillin (Pipracil), antiinfective

plicamycin (Mithracin), antineoplastic

sulfinpyrazone (Antazone), antigout agent

ticarcillin (Ticar), antiinfective

valproic acid (Depakene), antiepileptic drug

---

procedures, monitor catheter insertion sites, arterial and venous puncture sites, cutdown sites, and needle puncture sites. Coagulation studies should also be performed.

Intervention The extended-release tablet may give incomplete absorption. If B.K. uses the delayed release tablet, it must be swallowed whole.

Education If B.K. had been instructed to take the nonenteric-coated aspirin form, she should take it after meals or with food to minimize stomach irritation. Take any of the oral dosage forms with a full glass of water and do not lie down for 15 to 30 minutes after taking. Discard aspirin if it has a strong vinegar-like odor. See also Box 30-2.

- Monitor for and report signs of bleeding (e.g., bleeding gums, skin bruises, tarry stools, hematuria, epistaxis).
- Inform physicians, dentists, and other health care providers of antiplatelet and anticoagulant therapy before invasive procedures.
- Certain medications can inhibit or potentiate antiplatelet and anticoagulant effect. Consult with your pharmacist or prescriber before taking any new medications, including OTCs and herbal products. Ask your prescriber for a list of OTCs that may be taken for colds, headache, and other common health alterations.
- Do not discontinue your medication without consulting your prescriber. Discontinuing your medication will place you at higher risk for thrombotic episodes, e.g., MI, CVA, or DVT.
- If on warfarin therapy, be consistent in your dietary intake of foods high in vitamin K as vitamin K decreases anticoagulant action. These foods include turnip greens, asparagus, broccoli, cabbage, lettuce, watercress, beef liver, and green tea. Your medication dosage is regulated on the basis of blood coagulation studies. By changing vitamin K intake, the effect of the anticoagulant may be altered. Have a normal, balanced diet and do not to change dietary patterns radically or take vitamins or dietary supplements without consulting the prescriber.
- Apply direct pressure on cuts and abrasions, they may bleed longer than usual. Menstrual flow may also be heavier, but is not usually problematic. Report excessive bleeding in either case at once.
- Avoid alcohol because the risk for bleeding may be increased.
- Avoid participating in activities with a substantial risk of injury and contact prescriber immediately if injury occurs.
- Take nonpharmacologic interventions to support anticoagulant therapy. Avoid wearing constrictive clothing, crossing legs at the knees, sitting or standing for long periods of time, or putting pressure on ischemic areas. If you smoke, ask for assistance with smoking cessation.
- Wear Medic Alert identification, especially if receiving chronic anticoagulant therapy.
- Follow-up care with your prescriber is essential to effectively regulate the dosage of your medication.

Modified from Carpenito-Moyet, L.J. (2004). *Nursing diagnosis: Application to clinical Practice.* (10th ed.). Philadelphia: J.B. Lippincott.

Alert B.K. that clients usually notice bleeding problems when their gums bleed during brushing their teeth, as the initial sign of increased bleeding tendency, but she might notice persistent heartburn, pink urine (hematuria), dark stools, excessive bruising, or activity intolerance. These symptoms should be reported to the prescriber.

Evaluation The expected outcome of B.K.'s antiplatelet therapy with aspirin is that she:
- Will not experience any thrombotic episodes, such as CVA or MI.
- Is free of bruising, bleeding problems, or other adverse effects of the aspirin.
- States the adverse effects, how to monitor for the adverse effects of aspirin therapy, the importance of follow-up appointments with her prescriber, and when to contact the prescriber for bothersome adverse effects or hemorrhage.

✳ **B.K. was compliant with her ASA 325 mg for 6 months. However, her constant bruising was bothersome to her and her dose was decreased to 81 mg daily. She has been taking this dosage for about 6 months. Last week she was hospitalized for rapidly worsening angina. She is discharged with a prescription for clopidogrel (Plavix) 75 mg PO daily along with her ASA therapy.**

✳ **What is the role of clopidogrel therapy? Is it appropriate to take two antiplatelet drugs concurrently?**
Clopidogrel is an antithrombotic and inhibitor of platelet aggregation. It inhibits ADP binding to platelet receptors, thus interfering with the ADP activation of a glycoprotein complex. This results in the inhibition of platelet aggregation. The combination of aspirin and clopidogrel is appropriate to significantly reduce the occurrence of death from cardiovascular causes, nonfatal MI or CVA (The Clopidogrel in Unstable Angina to Prevent Recurrent Events Trial Investigators, 2001) and may be added to fibrinolytic therapy in treating AMI (Sabatine et al., 2005)

✳◼ **clopidogrel** [kloe **pid** oh grel]
(Plavix)
Indications
Clopidogrel is indicated for the prophylaxis of MI, thromboembolic stroke, and vascular death. It is slightly more effective than aspirin in the treatment of coronary heart disease (CHD) and secondary prevention of MI, but not significantly so. It is often used for clients who have a contraindication to aspirin therapy (Frishman, Lerner, Klein, & Roganovic, 2003). It may also be used in combination with aspirin in high-risk clients.
Pharmacokinetics/Dosing
Administered orally, clopidogrel is biotransformed in the liver to an active metabolite by P450 3 A4. The active metabolite produces approximately 85% of its effects. It has an onset of action in 2 hours after a single dose and reaches peak serum levels in 1 hour and peak effects with repeated dosing between day 3 and day 7. It is excreted by the kidneys (50%) and in the feces (approximately 46%). The usual adult dosage of clopidogrel is 75 mg PO daily.
Adverse Effects
The adverse effects of clopidogrel include GI distress, arthralgia, back pain, headache, dizziness, anxiety, weakness, constipation, cough, diarrhea, hypoesthesia or paresthesia, insomnia, pruritus, nausea, leg cramps, depression, vomiting, and rash. Additionally, chest pain, purpura, upper respiratory infection, dysrhythmias, bronchitis, dyspnea, edema, GI hemorrhage, hypertension, urinary tract infection (UTI), and syncope are possible. Clopidogrel alone causes

significantly greater rates of recurrent ulcer bleeding than aspirin with esomeprazole, a proton pump inhibitor to prevent aspirin-induced GI bleeding (Chan et al., 2005).

Drug Interactions

It is unclear if other concurrently administered drugs metabolized by P450 3 A4 (e.g., many "statin" drugs like atorvastatin [Lipitor]) could interfere with the conversion of clopidogrel to its active form (Lau et al., 2003), but this is probably not clinically important (Saw et al, 2003). Concurrent use of clopidogrel with other antiplatelets, with anticoagulants or fibrinolytics, or with some herbals (garlic, gingko) may increase bleeding risk. Use of NSAIDs may increase risk for GI bleeding.

✱ What is the nursing management of B.K.'s clopidogrel therapy?

The nursing management of clopidogrel therapy is similar to aspirin. The major concern with B.K. taking two antiplatelet medications is the increased risk of bleeding because there is an additive effect. This risk should be closely monitored, along with adverse effects more unique to clopidogrel that occur in over 5% of cases: headache, flu-like symptoms, dyspepsia, dizziness, back pain, arthralgia, and stomach pain. It is recommended that clopidogrel be discontinued 7 days prior to elective surgery.

In addition to reinforcing the client instructions in Box 30-2, inform B.K. that clopidogrel may be taken with or without food.

✱ Are there other antiplatelet drugs that might have been considered for B.K.?

Not really. Ticlopidine is associated with bone marrow suppression, and less data are available to document the benefit of dipyridamole in preventing MI. The other antiplatelet drugs are indicated primarily for thrombocythemia.

anagrelide [an **ah** greh lide]

(Agrylin)

The antiplatelet effect of anagrelide is unknown, but studies indicate that it decreases megakaryocyte hypermaturation, inhibits cyclic adenosine monophosphate (cAMP) phosphodiesterase and adenosine diphosphate (ADP), and inhibits collagen-related platelet aggregation.

Indications

Anagrelide is indicated for the treatment of essential thrombocythemia.

Pharmacokinetics/Dosing

The initial adult dosage is 1 mg twice daily (or 0.5 mg four times daily) for 1 week; the dosage is then adjusted to the lowest effective dose that maintains a platelet count <600,000/mcL. The dosage may be increased by 0.5 mg/day weekly, up to a maximum dose of 2.5 mg four times daily.

Adverse Effects

The adverse effects of anagrelide include stomach pain, tachycardia, edema, diarrhea, and headaches. Adverse effects may include heart failure (HF), cardiomyopathy, heart block, atrial fibrillation, pulmonary hypertension, and seizures.

Drug Interactions

Sucralfate may reduce absorption. Other drugs which affect platelets or coagulation could also increase bleeding risk; see Box 30-1.

Nursing Management

Assessment

Review the client's history for preexisting illness (e.g., cardiac disease, hepatic function impairment, renal function impairment) in which the

risk-benefit of anagrelide should be considered. Cardiac disease is a concern because anagrelide has positive inotropic effects and cardiac adverse effects. Close monitoring is important with impairment of hepatic and renal function because of its hepatotoxic and renal toxic effects.

Assess the client's concurrent medication regimen for drug combinations that might be contraindicated or might require more careful monitoring. See drug interactions above.

A baseline assessment of the client includes a cardiovascular examination and platelet count.

Nursing Diagnosis

The client receiving anagrelide therapy is at risk for the nursing diagnoses of risk for injury related to dizziness (hypotension) and weakness; altered comfort related to headache, nausea, dyspepsia, or flatulence; diarrhea; impaired gas exchange related to pulmonary fibrosis or pulmonary infiltrates; pain related to pancreatitis or peptic ulcer; and the potential complications of cardiotoxicity (HF, complete heart block) and asthma, bronchitis, or pneumonia.

Planning

The goals for anagrelide therapy are that the client:

- Remains free from injury from either the thrombocythemia or the adverse effects of anagrelide.
- Is compliant with anagrelide therapy.
- Demonstrates adequate knowledge regarding the drug regimen and its potential adverse effects.
- Collaborates with health care professionals for monitoring and follow up care.

Implementation

Monitoring

Clients on anagrelide therapy are monitored closely for cardiovascular effects (tachycardia, signs and symptoms of HF [dyspnea, adventitious lung sounds, pedal edema, weight gain]). Standing BPs are monitored for orthostatic hypotension. Platelet counts are monitored every 2 days for the first week of therapy and weekly thereafter until maintenance doses are established without causing thrombocytopenia.

Intervention

Anagrelide requires close medical supervision. If thrombocytopenia (<100,000 per mcL) occurs, the dosage of anagrelide is reduced or withdrawn; platelet counts usually promptly recover.

Education

Emphasize the need for close supervision by the physician. Advise the client to report any symptoms of chest pain, palpitations, or edema to the prescriber. Instruct the client to seek emergency assistance immediately if signs and symptoms of a heart attack occur.

Evaluation

The client on anagrelide therapy will have the following outcomes:

- Maintains platelet counts within normal limits, 150 to 450 × 10^3/mm^3
- Is free of the adverse effects of anagrelide.
- States the rationale for anagrelide therapy, the adverse effects, the importance for follow-up visits, and adverse effects to report to the prescriber.

cilostazol [sil **os** tah zol]

(Pletal)

Cilostazol and several of its metabolites are inhibitors of cAMP phosphodiesterase III, which results in an increase in cAMP levels, vasodilation, and the inhibition of platelet aggregation. The antiplatelet effects of this drug may also be induced by a variety of other mechanisms.

Indications

Cilostazol is indicated for intermittent claudication. Intermittent claudication and its treatment are also discussed in Chapter 28.

Pharmacokinetics/Dosing

The adult dosage is 100 mg twice daily administered 30 minutes before or 2 hours after the morning and evening meals (see Drug Interactions).

Adverse Effects

The adverse effects of cilostazol include headache, pharyngitis, fever, diarrhea, nausea, and peripheral edema. Adverse effects include tachycardia, HF, cerebral ischemia, atrial fibrillation, and atrial flutter.

Drug Interactions

If the client is taking ketoconazole, itraconazole, erythromycin, or diltiazem (CYP3 A4 inhibitors) or omeprazole (CYP2 C19 inhibitor), the adult dosage is 50 mg twice daily. Clients should avoid the consumption of grapefruit juice because it is associated with CYP3 A4 inhibition. Bleeding risk may be increased when other antiplatelet agents are used.

Nursing Management

Although cilostazol does not exhibit the cardiotoxicity of anagrelide, the precautions about administration to clients with HF exist. Monitor the client for improvement in intermittent claudication; decreased pain on walking and walking for longer distances. Cilostazol is taken at least 30 minutes before meals or 2 hours after breakfast and dinner. Instruct the client to avoid consuming grapefruit juice. Assist the client to contact a smoking cessation program if the client is still smoking. Instruct the client on the drug interactions and reportable adverse effects listed above. The client will experience relief from the intermittent claudication without adverse effects of the drug and be able to effectively self-manage the therapeutic regimen.

dipyridamole [dye peer **id** a mole]

(Persantine, Apo-Dipyridamole✣, Apo-Dipyridamole FC✣)

Dipyridamole, originally developed as a coronary artery vasodilator, has more commonly been used for its antiplatelet action. Multiple mechanisms of platelet inhibition for dipyridamole have been postulated, including the following:

- Thromboxane A_2 formation, a potent platelet activator
- Phosphodiesterase, which results in an increase in cyclic-3′ 5′ monophosphate in the platelets
- RBC uptake of adenosine, a platelet aggregation inhibitor

Indications

Dipyridamole is used in combination with oral anticoagulants for the prevention of postsurgical thromboembolic complications after cardiac valve replacement. It is used intravenously (IV) as a diagnostic aid in the evaluation of coronary artery disease (CAD).

Pharmacokinetics/Dosing

After an oral dose, dipyridamole reaches peak serum levels in approximately 75 minutes. This drug is highly protein bound, metabolized in the liver, and excreted in bile. The usual adult dosage is 75 to 100 mg PO four times daily.

Adverse Effects

The adverse effects of dipyridamole include hypotension, headache, tachycardia, dizziness, abdominal upset, and rash.

Drug Interactions

Concurrent use of antiplatelets or anticoagulants may increase bleeding risk (see Box 30-1). Adenosine effects may be more pronounced with concurrent dipyridamole therapy. Theophylline therapy should be held for 48 hours before the IV use of dipyridamole for diagnostic evaluation because theophylline reduces the coronary artery vasodilation effects of dipyridamole.

Nursing Management

The nursing management for oral dipyridamole is as for clopidogrel therapy, except there is no prohibition on grapefruit juice.

ticlopidine [tye **kloe** pih deen]

(Ticlid, Apo-Ticlopidine✣)

Ticlopidine is believed to produce an irreversible, ADP-induced inhibition of platelet-fibrinogen binding. Its use has waned given safer alternatives available.

Indications

It is indicated to decrease the risk of stroke for clients who have had warning of a thrombotic stroke or for those who have had a thrombotic stroke. *Because of the risk for potentially life-threatening bone marrow suppression, ticlopidine use should be limited to clients who have not responded to or tolerated other antiplatelet therapy.*

Pharmacokinetics/Dosing

Administered orally, ticlopidine reaches peak serum levels in approximately 2 hours and a peak effect with repeated dosing in 8 to 11 days. It is metabolized by the liver and excreted by the kidneys. The recommended adult dosage is 250 mg twice daily with food.

Adverse Effects

The most serious adverse effects of ticlopidine are bone marrow suppression including neutropenia, agranulocytosis, thrombocytopenia, and purpura. Other adverse effects of ticlopidine include nausea, stomach cramps, bloating or gas, dizziness, skin rash, diarrhea, tinnitus, bleeding, and pruritus.

Drug Interactions

Ticlopidine is metabolized by P450 3 A4 and inhibits the metabolism of drugs metabolized by P450 2 C19. Cimetidine is known to increase ticlopidine levels. Ticlopidine may increase phenytoin and theophylline levels. Concurrent use of antiplatelet or anticoagulant therapy and NSAIDs, will increase the potential for bleeding.

Nursing Management

Assessment

Assess the client for preexisting illness for which ticlopidine may be contraindicated, such as any hemostatic disorders (bleeding or hemophilia) or severe hepatic function impairment, because of the risk of increased bleeding. Hematopoietic disorders such as neutropenia or thrombocytopenia may be exacerbated. Clients with a history of thrombocytopenic purpura are also excluded from ticlopidine therapy because of the risk of recurrence. Greater caution is used with the care of any condition that places the client at risk for bleeding such as trauma, surgery, or peptic ulcer. Renal impairment will increase drug concentrations.

Concurrent medications that interact to increase the risk of hemorrhage would be anticoagulants, fibrinolytics, aspirin, NSAIDs, and other platelet inhibitors (see Box 30-1). Question the prescribing of these drugs concurrently. Assess what over-the-counter drugs (OTCs) the client uses for minor pain, such as headache or backache, to determine usage of aspirin and/or other NSAIDs. Because ticlopidine increases phenytoin concentrations resulting in sleepiness and lethargy, plan for more careful observation of the client's alertness if the drugs are used concurrently.

A baseline assessment for the use of ticlopidine for thromboembolic CVA prophylaxis includes a mental status and neurologic examination, and a CBC with platelet count, RBC morphology, and white blood cell (WBC) differentials.

Nursing Diagnosis

The client on ticlopidine therapy is at risk for the following nursing diagnoses: altered comfort (nausea, indigestion); diarrhea; impaired skin integrity (rash); and potential complications of hemorrhage, neutropenia, thrombocytopenia, hepatitis, and severe skin rash (erythema multiforme, Stevens-Johnson syndrome, thrombotic thrombocytopenic purpura [TTP]).

Planning

The client receiving ticlopidine will:

- Remain free from CVA and side/adverse effects (bruising, bleeding or other effects) of ticlopidine.
- Be compliant with ticlopidine therapy.
- Demonstrate adequate knowledge of therapy and its adverse effects to effectively manage the therapeutic regimen.

Implementation

Monitoring

With ticlopidine, monitor the CBC every 2 weeks until the third month of therapy. Monitor more frequently if the neutrophil count is declining or is 30% less than the baseline count. After the third month, obtain a CBC only if the client has signs and symptoms of an infection. Any unexplained reduction in hemoglobin or platelets prompts further investigation for TTP.

Intervention

Ticlopidine is taken with meals to enhance absorption and decrease GI irritation. The drug may be discontinued temporarily if the client is injured with increased risk for bleeding. It is recommended that ticlopidine be discontinued 10 to 14 days before elective surgery, including tooth extraction.

Education

In addition to the client instruction in Box 30-2, inform the client of the adverse effects and how to manage them. Alert the client that the risk of bleeding may continue for 1 to 2 weeks after ticlopidine is discontinued.

Evaluation

The expected outcome of ticlopidine therapy is that the client:

- Will not experience a CVA.
- Is free of bruising, bleeding problems, or other adverse effects of ticlopidine.
- States the adverse effects, how to monitor for the adverse effects of ticlopidine therapy, the importance for follow-up appointments with prescriber, and when to contact the prescriber for bothersome adverse effects or hemorrhage.

Glycoprotein IIb/IIIa Inhibitors

The glycoprotein IIb/IIIa receptors are targets for fibrinogen and von Willebrand factor that allows platelets to adhere to each other and to foreign surfaces. By occupying these receptors, the glycoprotein IIb/IIIa inhibitors hinder platelet aggregation. These IV agents are strong antiplatelet agents reserved for acute coronary events in part because of their higher risk for bleeding, and also because of their expense and need for careful IV administration. Abciximab (ReoPro) is a monoclonal antibody fragment that strongly binds to the platelet receptors. Abciximab, a monoclonal antibody fragment, inhibits platelet aggregation by binding or blocking the glycoprotein (GP) IIb/IIIa receptor involved in the pathway for platelet aggregation. Eptifibatide (Integrilin) and tirofiban (Aggrastat) reversibly bind to platelet receptors and each has a relatively short duration of action.

★ abciximab [ab **six** ih mab]
(ReoPro)

Indications

It is indicated as adjunct therapy (to aspirin and heparin) for prevention of acute cardiac vessel ischemic complications in clients undergoing percutaneous transluminal coronary angioplasty or atherectomy (PTCA). It is also indicated for the management of unstable angina. The use of abciximab is contraindicated in clients with active bleeding or a high risk for bleeding.

Pharmacokinetics/Dosing

After IV administration, abciximab binds to platelets and produces its antiplatelet action. Unbound abciximab has an elimination half-life of approximately 30 minutes, but the duration of action of abciximab may continue for 24 hours or more beyond discontinuation of the infusion. The recommended adult dosage is 0.25 mg/kg administered 10 to 60 minutes before the procedure. The maintenance dosage by IV infusion is 0.125 mcg/kg/min up to a maximum dose of 10 mcg/min. The dose for refractory unstable angina is 0.25 mg/kg IV over 10 to 60 minutes, then 10 mcg/min IV over 18 to 24 hours.

Adverse Effects

The adverse effects of abciximab include major bleeding episodes and hypotension. Nausea, vomiting, and back pain have also been frequently reported. As with all antibody therapy, there is a potential for hypersensitivity reactions, including anaphylaxis.

Drug Interactions

Increased risk for bleeding is noted when abciximab is administered with other antiplatelets, anticoagulants or fibrinolytics. Although many protocols for its use recommend concurrent anticoagulant and/or oral antiplatelet therapy, monitoring for bleeding is required.

eptifibatide [ep ti **fib** a tide]
(Integrilin)

Indications

Eptifibatide is indicated for the treatment of acute coronary syndrome (unstable angina or non-Q wave MI) and as adjunct therapy for those undergoing percutaneous coronary interventions (PCIs).

Pharmacokinetics/Dosing

Eptifibatide reversibly binds to the platelet with platelet activity returning to normal within 4 hours of discontinuation of the infusion. The adult dosage of eptifibatide for acute coronary syndrome (ACS) is an initial IV bolus of 180 mcg/kg. This is followed by an IV infusion of 2 mcg/kg/min until hospital discharge or until coronary artery bypass graft (CABG) surgery is initiated, which is usually up to 72 hours. Refer to a current package insert or reference for additional dosing parameters and monitoring guidelines.

Adverse Effects

The most common adverse effect is bleeding, which can range from minor bleeding to intracranial (stroke) and retroperitoneal bleeding. Thus close monitoring of platelet counts, hemoglobin, and other laboratory tests are necessary before treatment and at regular intervals (at least daily if not more often) during treatment. Other adverse effects include bradycardia, edema, hypersensitivity (including the potential for anaphylaxis) and leg pain.

Drug Interactions

Similar to abciximab.

tirofiban [ter **ro** fi ban]
(Aggrastat)

Indications

Similar to eptifibatide.

Pharmacokinetics/Dosing

Tirofiban also reversibly binds to platelets and has a half-life of approximately 2 hours. Tirofiban is administered in combination with heparin for ACS. Most clients receive an initial IV dose of 0.4 mcg/kg/min for 30 minutes, followed by 0.1 mcg/kg/min for 48 to 108 hours or 12 to 24 hours after coronary intervention.

Adverse Effects

See eptifibatide.

Drug Interactions

Similar to abciximab.

Nursing Management of Glycoprotein IIb/IIIa Inhibitor Therapy

Assessment Assess the client for conditions that would be contraindications for glycoprotein (GP) IIb/IIIa therapy and increase the client's risk for bleeding: intracranial aneurysm, arteriovenous malformation or neoplasm; active bleeding; GI or genitourinary (GU) bleeding, major surgery or trauma within the last 6 weeks; bleeding diathesis, CVA with significant residual neurologic deficit or within the last 2 years; uncontrolled severe hypertension; thrombocytopenia ($<$100,000/mcL or history of vasculitis. Consider also the risk-benefit if the client is older than 65 years of age; weighs less than 75 kg; has a history of GI disease, or failed or prolonged PTCA or one within 12 hours of the onset of acute MI.

Review the client's concurrent drug regimen for other drugs that would increase the risk for bleeding such as oral anticoagulants, platelet aggregation inhibitors, dextran, dipyridamole, ticlopidine, and fibrinolytic agents.

The baseline assessment includes: an examination of potential bleeding sites and laboratory determinants of clinical significance, such as the activated clotting time (ACT), activated partial thromboplastin time (aPTT), PT/INR, and platelet counts.

Nursing Diagnosis The client on GP IIb/IIIa therapy is at risk for the following nursing diagnoses of decreased cardiac output related to bradycardia (peripheral edema, dyspnea, fatigue, hypotension) and potential complications of hemorrhage, thrombocytopenia, leukocytosis, and pleural effusion or pleurisy.

Planning The client receiving GP IIb/IIIa therapy will:
- Remain free from PTCA thrombosis and adverse effects (bleeding, thrombocytopenia or other effects) of GP IIb/IIIa therapy. With eptifibatide and tirofiban, client remains free of ACS-related thrombosis.
- Be compliant with ticlopidine therapy.
- Demonstrate adequate knowledge regarding therapy and its adverse effects to effectively collaborate with the therapeutic regimen.

Implementation

Monitoring Pay careful attention to all potential bleeding sites; catheter insertion sites, arterial and venous puncture sites, needle puncture sites, and GI and GU sites. Coagulation studies are monitored frequently; ACT, aPTT, PT/INR, and platelet counts.

Intervention Minimize the use of invasive procedures, such as intramuscular (IM) injections, urinary catheters, nasogastric tubes and automatic BP cuffs. Noncompressible sites, such as subclavian or jugular veins, are not to be used for IV access. For specific parameters for dosing, see the package insert. If the client begins to bleed, stop the infusion immediately and institute supportive therapy. Eptifibatide is administered as a bolus or continuous IV infusion. See package insert for IV incompatibilities.

Education Keep the client apprised of the progress of therapy. Instruct the client to report any nausea, vomiting, confusion, or bleeding immediately.

Evaluation The client will undergo a successful PTCA without any evidence of bleeding or thrombocytopenia, or allergic response. With eptifibatide and tirofiban, the client will remain free of ACS-related thrombosis without adverse effects.

✱ **R.P. is a 68-year-old man of 60 kg with long-standing osteoarthritis of the knee and has just com-** pleted a 12-hour airplane trip with his family in South America. He presents to the emergency room with calf tenderness and swelling. His prescriber diagnoses a DVT brought on by immobility and is concerned for the risk of developing a PE. The prescriber initiates the anticoagulant enoxaparin (Lovenox) 60 mg subcutaneously twice daily with warfarin (Coumadin) therapy 5 mg orally one time 6 hours after start of enoxaparin.

✱ **How are anticoagulants used clinically?**
Anticoagulant therapy is directed toward preventing intravascular thrombosis by decreasing blood coagulability. This therapy has no direct effect on a blood clot that has already formed or on ischemic tissue injured by an inadequate blood supply because of the clot. Anticoagulant drug therapy is primarily prophylactic because these agents act by preventing (1) fibrin deposits, (2) extension of a thrombus, and (3) thromboembolic complications. Although long-term anticoagulant therapy remains controversial, there is evidence that such therapy reduces the incidence of thrombosis and therefore prolongs life in clients at high risk for thromboembolic events. Clients at high risk for short-term thromboembolic events include postsurgical clients (particularly with procedures that limit lower extremity movement, such as hip and knee surgery). Clients with atrial fibrillation, pregnancy, cardiac valve replacement, and a history of hypercoagulability (e.g., observed with some cancers) or thrombotic events are also at higher risk for developing thrombosis and/or thromboembolic events. Clients with existing thrombosis, such as a DVT, pose a grave risk for life-threatening embolic events (e.g., PE) and are also typically treated with higher doses of anticoagulants. Clients with unstable angina, MI, or thromboembolic CVA are also candidates for higher dose anticoagulant therapy.

✱ **How are the anticoagulants differentiated?**
The two main groups of anticoagulant drugs are (1) parenteral anticoagulant drugs, and (2) oral anticoagulant drugs.

The parenteral anticoagulants include heparin and the low molecular weight (LMW) heparins. These agents consist of long chains of monosaccharides and proteins and have a large molecular weight. The LMW agents are isolated from standard heparin and possess shorter monosaccharide/protein chains. These LMW heparins (dalteparin, enoxaparin, tinzaparin) have longer durations of action and are typically dosed once or twice daily via (subcutaneous) injection. All heparins (including the LMW agents) are derived primarily from the mucosal lining of pig intestine (porcine source) but occasionally obtained from bovine lung (beef source). The heparins potentiate antithrombin III action leading to decreased fibrin formation. Heparin effect is measured with the activated partial thromboplastin time (aPTT) (Box 30-3). The LMW heparins have more specific antifactor Xa activity and the aPTT is not helpful in evaluating effect. The antidote for heparin is protamine sulfate. Table 30-1 lists heparin and LMW heparins, which are discussed in greater depth in the following sections.

Box 30-3 Laboratory Monitoring of Anticoagulants

Anticoagulants must be carefully dosed to achieve adequate anticoagulation with minimal risk for bleeding. To assure safe and effective anticoagulation, frequent monitoring of blood is usually required when using these agents. An overview of each of these tests and their role is presented here.

Partial Thromboplastin Time (PTT)/Activated Partial Thromboplastin Time: (aPTT)

The PTT detects defects in the intrinsic thromboplastin system. The aPTT is a more sensitive version of the PTT and largely replaces it.

- *Use:* The activated PTT is used to identify deficiencies in the intrinsic coagulation system and to monitor heparin therapy.
- *Normal values for a PTT:* 21 to 35 seconds (subtle variation from lab to lab)
- *Goal ranges with anticoagulation:* 1.5 to 2.5 times the normal lab value (some references suggest 2 to 2.5 times normal lab value).

Prothrombin Time (PT)/International Normalized Ratio (INR)

Prothrombin is a vitamin K–dependent protein produced by the liver involved in coagulation. Prothrombin is also known as Clotting Factor II. PTs vary with each lab based on the laboratory reagents (thromboplastin) used in the testing process. The sensitivity of thromboplastin used by each laboratory is considered with the reported PT result and calculated as the INR. This calculated value is standard across different laboratories at different times and has become the routine reported parameter to utilize when evaluating oral warfarin dosing.

- *Use:* The PT is used to evaluate the activity of the clotting cascade and sometimes used as an indicator of liver function (because prothrombin is manufactured by the liver). The INR is the routine test to evaluate the degree of anticoagulation with warfarin.

- *Normal values:* PT: 11 to 13 seconds (varies significantly with different laboratories) INR: 1
- *Goal ranges with anticoagulation:* Depending on indication: Target INR for prevention and treatment of most thromboembolic events is 2.5 (range 2 to 3). For individuals with recurrent systemic emboli or mechanical heart valves, goal INR may be as high as 3 (range 2.5 to 3.5), and occasionally higher. INR result reflects warfarin dose administered 36 to 72 hours prior to testing.

Activated Coagulation Time (ACT)

The ACT evaluates coagulation status and responds to a broader range of heparin levels than does the aPTT. Its lack of standardization makes this test less commonly used outside of cardiac surgery.

- *Use:* Bedside procedure to evaluate efficacy of anticoagulants, including argatroban, bivalirudin and high dose heparin (e.g., as used during cardiac surgery)
- *Normal values:* 150 to 180 seconds.
- *Goal ranges with anticoagulation:* 175 to greater than 500 seconds (varies with indication and laboratory).

Antithrombin III (AT-III)

AT-III inhibits a number of activated clotting factors, including factors II, IX, X, XI, and XII. Deficiency of AT-III may predispose to recurrent thromboembolism.

- *Use:* Identify AT-III deficiency
- *Normal values:* 17 to 30 mg/dL
- *Goal ranges with anticoagulation:* Obtain normal levels for clients with AT-III deficiency

Antifactor Xa Assay

Antifactor Xa measures the activity of Factor Xa.

- *Use:* Measuring the degree of anticoagulation with LMW heparins, danaparoid, and fondaparinux
- *Normal values:* 0 units/mL
- *Goal ranges with anticoagulation:* 0.4 to 1.1 units/mL depending on agent used and indication.

Other parenteral anticoagulants include antithrombin III (ATnativ, Thrombate III), argatroban, bivalirudin (Angiomax), fondaparinux (Arixtra), lepirudin (Refludan) and danaparoid (Orgaran). Antithrombin III binds covalently to thrombin and its use is limited to clients with documented antithrombin III deficiencies. Argatroban is a thrombin inhibitor used to treat thromboembolic events in clients with heparin-induced thrombocytopenia. Bivalirudin, also known as Hirulog, is a reversible polypeptide thrombin inhibitor indicated for use with aspirin for clients with unstable angina undergoing cardiac catheter procedures. Fondaparinux is a synthetic pentasaccharide that selectively inhibits factor Xa. It was released on the market in 2002, and its role in the prevention and treatment of thromboembolic events is evolving. Lepirudin is derived

from the medicinal leech and is used for clients who cannot tolerate heparin (typically because of heparin-induced thrombocytopenia). Effect of lepirudin is monitored with the aPTT. Danaparoid is a heparin-like derivative from porcine intestinal mucosa and has a low cross-reactivity with heparin. Danaparoid, like the LMW heparins, is more specific for factor Xa. Table 30-2 lists these agents.

The oral anticoagulant most commonly used is warfarin (Coumadin). Warfarin interferes with the production of vitamin K–dependent clotting factors. Other similar agents include dicumarol and anisindione (Miradon), but are infrequently used. The safety and efficacy of warfarin is evaluated with the PT and the INR (see Box 30-3). The lag time between warfarin administration and decay of the vitamin K–dependent clotting factors is typically 36 to 72

TABLE 30-1 COMPARISON OF HEPARIN ANTICOAGULANTS

Agent	Indication	Typical Adult Dose†	Lab Monitor	Adverse Effect	Comment
HEPARIN					
heparin (Hep-lock, Liquiprin)	Line flush	100 units/mL	Dosing: none Toxicity: platelets/CBC, occult blood	Risk of heparin-induced thrombocytopenia (HIT)	Frequency based on line, institutional protocols
	Prophylaxis for DVT	5000 units subcutaneously q8-12h		Risk of HIT, bleeding	Typically known as "low-dose" or "mini-dose" heparin
	Treatment of: DVT/PE Acute coronary syndromes (unstable angina*/MI)	60-80 units/kg IV push, then 12-18 units/kg/hr with adjustment for 1.5-2.5 × normal aPTT per institutional protocol†	Dosing: aPTT (often q6h per institutional protocol) Toxicity: platelets/CBC, occult blood	Risk of HIT, bleeding, hypotension	IV infusion must be administered via pump or line controller‡ Typically lower dose range if concurrent fibrinolytic therapy or treating unstable angina; higher range for DVT/PE
LOW-MOLECULAR-WEIGHT HEPARIN					
dalteparin (Fragmin)	Prophylaxis for lower risk DVT	2500 units subcutaneously 1-2 hr presurgery then daily × 5-10 days)	Dosing: usually none; occasionally antifactor Xa Toxicity: platelets/CBC, occult blood	Risk of HIT (lower than heparin), bleeding (see comments)	*Avoid if recent or anticipated spinal/epidural anesthesia or lumbar puncture because of risk of spinal or epidural hematoma*
	Prophylaxis for higher risk DVT	2500-5000 units subcutaneously prior to surgery, then 5000 units subcutaneously daily × 5-14 days‡			
	Treatment of DVT*	100 units/kg twice daily or 200 units/kg daily			
	Acute coronary syndromes (unstable angina/MI)	120 units/kg (max 10,000 units) subcutaneously q12h × 5-8 days with aspirin			
enoxaparin (Lovenox)	Prophylaxis for DVT (First dose: 12-24 hr after surgery)	30 mg subcutaneously twice daily or 40 mg subcutaneously once daily × 7-14 days‡			
	Treatment of DVT/PE	1 mg/kg q12h or 1.5 mg/kg/day‡			
	Acute coronary syndromes (unstable angina/MI)	1 mg/kg q12h × 2-8 days			
tinzaparin (Innohep)	Treatment DVT/PE	175 anti-Xa international units/kg/day			

CBC, complete blood count; *DVT*, deep vein thrombosis; *PE*, pulmonary embolism; *MI*, myocardial infarction.
*Not FDA approved use.
† These doses are given in USP Heparin Units. The strengths of heparin preparations available in the United States are labeled in USP Heparin Units per mL. The strengths of heparin preparations available in Canada may be labeled in USP units or in international units (IU) per mL. USP Heparin Units are not identical to IU. Consult the prescriber's order and the package insert for appropriate dosing.
‡ See package insert or other reference for more complete dosing information.

Table 30-2 Comparison of Other Parenteral Anticoagulants

Agent	Indication	Typical Adult Dose†	Lab Monitor	Adverse Effect	Comment
Thrombin Inhibitor					
antithrombin III (ATnativ, Thrombate III)	Prophylaxis or treatment of thromboembolic events in clients with antithrombin III deficiency	50-100 international units/min IV‡	Dosing: Antithrombin III activity levels Toxicity: CBC, occult blood	Bleeding	Use limited to clients with documented antithrombin III deficiency.
argatroban (Acova)	Prophylaxis or treatment of thromboembolic events in clients with HIT	Dose widely variable†‡	Dosing: aPTT, ACT Toxicity: CBC, occult blood	Bleeding	Dose depending on indication.†
bivalirudin [also known as Hirulog] (Angiomax)	Adjunct to PTCA in clients with unstable angina	1 mg/kg IV × 1 then 2.5 mg/kg/hr × 4 hr; dosed with 325 mg oral aspirin‡	Dosing: ACT Toxicity: CBC, occult blood	Bleeding, hypotension	Dosage adjustment required for clients with renal insufficiency.
lepirudin [also known as recombinant hirudin] (Refludan)	Prophylaxis or treatment of thromboembolic events in clients with HIT	Dose widely variable‡	Dosing: aPTT Toxicity: CBC, occult blood	Bleeding	Dose dependent on indication, renal function.
Heparinoid					
danaparoid (Orgaran)	Prophylaxis for DVT	750 anti-Xa units subcutaneously twice daily × 7-10 days	Dosing: Usually none. Occasionally antifactor Xa Toxicity: Platelets/CBC, occult blood	HIT, bleeding	Dose based on weight of client and if new event or event occurred >5 days prior.
	Treatment of DVT/PE*	1250-3750 anti-Xa units IV × 1 then 150-500 units/hr IV or varying doses subcutaneously‡			
Selective Factor Xa Inhibitor					
fondaparinux (Arixtra)	Prophylaxis for DVT	2.5 mg subcutaneously daily × 5-28 days‡	Dosing: Usually none. Occasionally Factor Xa activity Toxicity: CBC, occult blood	Bleeding (see comments)	Avoid in clients >75 yr, <50 kg, or with renal dysfunction because of risk of bleeding.

CBC, complete blood count; *DVT*, deep vein thrombosis; *PE*, pulmonary embolism; *MI*, myocardial infarction; *PTCA*, percutaneous transluminal coronary angioplasty; *HIT*, heparin-induced thrombocytopenia
*Not FDA approved use.
†These doses are given in USP Heparin Units. The strengths of heparin preparations available in the United States are labeled in USP Heparin Units per mL. The strengths of heparin preparations available in Canada may be labeled in USP units or in international units (IU) per mL. USP Heparin Units are not identical to IU. Consult the prescriber's order and the package insert for appropriate dosing.
‡See package insert or other reference for more complete dosing information.

hours, making warfarin dosing more complicated than heparin. Interactions with other drugs and foods also confound therapy. The antidotes for warfarin include vitamin K and fresh frozen plasma. Warfarin is often used when longer term anticoagulation is required.

For effective anticoagulation, the manner of use for both parenteral and oral anticoagulants is important. They have been used to complement each other, and often the administration of both a rapidly acting parenteral anticoagulant (heparin) and one of the oral anticoagulants is started shortly thereafter. Heparin is usually discontinued as soon as the PT/INR has been sufficiently increased and the oral compound is producing a full therapeutic effect.

Parenteral Anticoagulants Heparin is a rapidly acting, injectable anticoagulant. Heparin produces its anticoagulant effect by combining with antithrombin III (heparin cofactor), a naturally occurring anticlotting factor in the plasma. This compound is unrelated to factor III (tissue thromboplastin), a factor in the process of blood coagulation. The binding of heparin with antithrombin III forms a complex that acts at multiple sites in the normal coagulation system, inactivating factors IXa, Xa, XIa, and XIIa. Inactivation of factor Xa of the intrinsic and extrinsic pathways prevents the conversion of prothrombin to thrombin, thereby inhibiting the formation of fibrin from fibrinogen. Furthermore, by preventing the activation of factor XIII (fibrin stabilizing factor), heparin also prevents the formation of a stable fibrin clot. Because fibrin is associated with venous thrombi, heparin is useful in preventing venous thrombosis. Heparin does not have fibrinolytic activity. It will not dissolve existing clots but can prevent the extension of existing clots.

The normal function of antithrombin III is to maintain intravascular fluidity of the blood. Thromboembolism commonly occurs in individuals with acquired or congenital deficiency of this plasma protein. In the absence of antithrombin III, heparin is unable to exert its anticoagulant effect.

⬛🔳 **heparin [hep a rin]**
(Liquiprin, Hepalean✦, Heparin Leo✦)
Indications
Heparin is used to prevent and treat all types of thromboses and emboli. It is used prophylactically to prevent blood clotting in surgery of the heart or blood vessels, during blood transfusion, in clients with disseminated intravascular coagulation (DIC), and in the hemodialysis process. It is considered the drug of choice for sudden arterial occlusion, because its action is immediate and can be readily reversed if surgery is necessary.

Heparin is superior to the coumarin drugs in preventing pulmonary complications in cases of thrombophlebitis. It is also the preferred treatment of thrombophlebitis during pregnancy, because it does not cross the placental barrier and is not excreted in breast milk. When rapid anticoagulation is necessary, it is used before the oral anticoagulants (see Table 30-1).

Pharmacokinetics/Dosing
Heparin is administered via the parenteral route of administration because its large molecular size and polarity prevent any GI absorption. The onset of action of the IV injection is immediate. A subcutaneous injection usually results in an onset of action within 20 to 60 minutes. The half-life is dose dependent but averages 1.5 hours (range: 1 to 6 hours). This drug is highly protein bound, metabolized in the liver, and excreted by the kidneys.

The dosage of heparin is expressed in USP Heparin Units/mL in the United States. In Canada, the dosage is expressed in USP units or in international units. USP Heparin Units are not equivalent to international units. Because the potency may vary between USP and international units, the student should review the current package insert for dosage instructions whenever packages are labeled in international units. The recommended dosages in the following paragraphs are given in USP Heparin Units. The adult dosage for heparin sodium is dependent on indication; see Table 30-1.

The dosage of heparin is closely monitored with coagulation tests (usually the aPTT). For consistency, it is recommended that a single laboratory be used to monitor a client undergoing heparin therapy.
Adverse Effects
As with other anticoagulants, the major adverse effect of heparin is bleeding. Bleeding risk is particularly prominent when the aPTT is markedly elevated above goal ranges. Other risks include easy bruising, GI complaints, and hypersensitivity reactions. Chronic use is associated with reduced bone density and osteoporosis.

A serious reaction known as heparin-induced thrombocytopenia (HIT) has been reported in 1% to 2% of clients receiving heparin therapy. Heparin-induced thrombocytopenia is an immune-based reaction where platelet counts drop by 50% or more after the initiation or reinstitution of heparin therapy. It is a potentially life-threatening condition that can result in further thromboembolic events including gangrene to the extremities. It is treated by stopping all heparin products and instituting a non–heparin-derived anticoagulant (often lepirudin).
Drug Interactions
Increased risk for hemorrhage is noted when heparin is used concurrently with other anticoagulants, antiplatelets, or fibrinolytics. These combinations, however, are often used for clients with life-threatening thromboembolic events. The NSAIDs (e.g., ibuprofen, indomethacin, aspirin) may also increase bleeding risk, particularly GI bleeding.
Antidote
Protamine sulfate is the antidote for heparin overdose. (See monograph on p. 615).

Enoxaparin (Lovenox, Klexane) was the first LMW heparin (LMWH) released in the United States for the prevention of postsurgical DVT after hip- and knee-replacement surgery. The LMWHs appear to have the advantage of having slightly fewer hemorrhagic complications than standard heparin (Bick, Frenkel, Walenga, Fareed, & Hoppensteadt, 2005). Other LMWHs available in the United States include dalteparin (Fragmin) and tinzaparin (Innohep). Each product differs in its pharmacologic profile and so they are not interchangeable (Bick et al., 2005).

LMWHs are made by chemically processing regular heparin into fragments based on molecular weight. These LMWHs have a mean molecular weight between 4000 and 6000 daltons, whereas the mean molecular weight of unfractionated heparin ranges between 12,000 and 15,000 daltons. This difference in molecular weight produces an anticoagulant with considerably different properties than heparin. Both types of heparin can inactivate factor Xa, but inactivating factor IIa (thrombin) requires the larger molecular weight heparin. See Table 30-3 for a comparison of heparin and LMWHs.

⬛🔳 **enoxaparin [ee nox ah pa rin]**
(Lovenox, Klexane✦)
Indications
The indications for enoxaparin include prophylaxis of DVT, treatment of DVT and/or PE, and as part of management for ACSs (e.g., unstable angina, MI). Indications for other LMWHs vary based on agent and are presented in Table 30-1.

TABLE 30-3 COMPARISON OF REGULAR HEPARIN AND LOW-MOLECULAR-WEIGHT HEPARIN

Properties	Regular Heparin	LMW Heparin
Molecular weight range	3000-30,000	1000-10,000
Mean molecular weight	12,000-15,000	4000-6000
Mechanism of action	Inactivates factor Xa and IIa (thrombin)	Inactivates factor Xa
APTT monitoring required	Yes	No
Inhibits platelet function	++++ (high)	++ (medium)
Route of administration	IV, subcutaneous	Subcutaneous only
Protein binding	++++ (high)	+ (low)
Vascular permeability increased	Yes	No
Treatment of drug overdose	Protamine	Protamine

From Salerno, E. (1999). *Pharmacology for health professionals.* St. Louis: Mosby.

Pharmacokinetics/Dosing

The LMWHs are administered subcutaneously and have a very low protein-binding ratio, therefore their anticoagulant effect is more predictable. Peak serum levels are reached in 3 to 5 hours with enoxaparin. The elimination half-life is 3 to 6 hours. All LMWHs are primarily excreted by the kidneys. Their efficacy may be reduced in obese clients, and they may increase the risk for bleeding in those with renal failure (Kucher et al., 2005). Factor Xa levels are sometimes used to guide dosing, particularly for clients in renal failure or who are obese. Dosing is presented in Table 30-1 but may need to be reduced in renal failure (Thorevska et al, 2004).

Adverse Effects

The adverse effects of the enoxaparin and the other LMWHs include local irritation effects such as erythema, hematomas, urticaria, and pain at injection sites. Thrombocytopenia and bleeding episodes may occur less frequently. Use is generally avoided for clients who have recently had, or are expected to have lumbar punctures or epidural or spinal anesthesia because of the risk of spinal or epidural hematoma. As with unfractionated heparin, long-term use can contribute to osteoporosis.

Drug Interactions

Similar to heparin.

Oral Anticoagulants

✶🔲 warfarin [war far in]
(Coumadin, Warfilone✤)

Warfarin is an orally administered anticoagulant that requires a few days of therapy to become effective. Warfarin interferes with liver synthesis of the vitamin K–dependent clotting factors X, IX, VII, and II (prothrombin). Factor VII is depleted quickly; the sequential depletion of factors IX, X, and II follows. Like other anticoagulants, warfarin does not affect established clots but instead prevents further extension of formed clots. This reduces the potential for secondary thromboembolic complications.

Indications

Warfarin is used for the prophylaxis and treatment of DVT and pulmonary thromboembolism. It is also used for the prophylaxis of thromboembolism associated with chronic atrial fibrillation or MI.

Pharmacokinetics/Dosing

The major advantage of warfarin is that it is available as a once a day oral medication. The disadvantages of warfarin are the lag time between initial dosing and effect, as well as the great number of drug and food interactions. Warfarin is absorbed well from the GI tract, is highly protein bound (99%), metabolized in the liver, and excreted by the kidneys.

Dosing of warfarin can be tricky and is based on indications, potential interacting drugs and foods, client age, and risk for bleeding. Most clinicians use standard protocols to assist dosing and base dosing on the degree of rise or fall of the INR (see Box 30-3). Typical adult doses of warfarin range between 1 mg and 5 mg orally daily. Older clients are often more sensitive to warfarin. This may in part relate to a greater likelihood for a vitamin K–deficient state.

It is important to remember that warfarin reduces the production of vitamin K clotting factors, so a full therapeutic effect is typically observed about 3 days after dosing. Clinicians must cautiously interpret the INR keeping in mind that today's result reflects the dose administered 2 to 3 days ago. It is important to consider what dose of warfarin and what interacting foods or drugs have been administered in the prior 3 days. Such consideration can help predict whether the INR is rising or falling.

Adverse Effects

Bleeding is the major risk with warfarin therapy. The risk for intercranial hemorrhage is increased for those with an INR above 3.5 and for all clients over 85 years of age (Fang et al., 2004). Other adverse effects include alopecia, anorexia, abdominal cramps or distress, leukopenia, nausea, vomiting, diarrhea, purple toes syndrome (rare), and kidney damage (rare). Fetal abnormalities and facial anomalies of newborns have been reported following use of the drug during pregnancy. If an anticoagulant is necessary during pregnancy, LMWHs are the drugs of choice.

Rarely, an increased risk for thrombosis can be seen early in therapy. This may be due to the inhibition of protein C and protein S, which serve as naturally occurring anticoagulants. This risk can be reduced by initially anticoagulating with heparin or LMWH for clients with inherited protein C or protein S deficiency.

Drug Interactions

Warfarin interacts with many drugs and foods. It is metabolized by cytochrome P450 2 C8/9 and other enzymes. Changes in Vitamin K intake can also alter warfarin action. See Box 30-4 for warfarin interactions.

Antidote

Vitamin K is the antidote for warfarin overdose. Vitamin K administration will reverse the effects of warfarin over 24 to 48 hours. Many clinicians recommend low-dose oral vitamin K for clients with moderately elevated INRs (e.g., >5) and absence of bleeding. Excessive use of vitamin K may make future anticoagulation with warfarin impossi-

---

BOX 30-4 SIGNIFICANT INTERACTIONS WITH WARFARIN

The oral anticoagulants have a great potential for causing drug interactions; therefore clients must be cautioned against taking any drug and/or making significant dietary changes without prior consultation with their prescriber. A list of some of the many drugs interacting with warfarin is presented below.

Agents that may increase the anticoagulant effect, often necessitating a dosage reduction

allopurinol	clofibrate	grapefruit juice	piperacillin
amiodarone	danazol	indomethacin	plicamycin
anabolic steroids	dextran	itraconazole	propylthiouracil
androgens	dextrothyroxine	levofloxacin	quinidine
aspirin	diflunisal	mefenamic acid	salicylates
azlocillin	dipyridamole†	meperidine	streptokinase
carbenicillin (parenteral)	disulfiram	methimazole	sulfinpyrazone
cefamandole	erythromycins	metronidazole	sulfonamides
cefoperazone	fenoprofen	mezlocillin	sulindac
chloral hydrate*	fluconazole	mifepristone	thyroid hormone
chloramphenicol	gemfibrozil	nalidixic acid	ticarcillin
cimetidine	ginkgo	ofloxacin	urokinase
ciprofloxacin	ginseng	phenytoin‡	

Agents that may decrease the anticoagulant effect, often necessitating an increase in anticoagulant dosage

oral antidiabetic agents§	colestipol	estrogens¶	primidone
barbiturates	contraceptives, hormonal¶	ethchlorvynol	rifampin
carbamazepine	estramustine	griseofulvin	Vitamin K
cholestyramine			

*Usually occurs during first 2 weeks of therapy. With chronic concurrent therapy, the anticoagulant effect may return to normal or be decreased.
†With doses of dipyridamole over 400 mg daily.
‡Increased anticoagulant effect occurs initially. With chronic concurrent therapy decreased activity may occur. May also see a decrease in metabolism of phenytoin, possibly leading to increased serum levels and toxicity.
§May initially increase anticoagulant effects, but with long-term concurrent therapy, such effects may decrease. Also, the decrease in metabolism of the antidiabetic agent may increase serum levels and cause prolonged half-life, hypoglycemia, and toxicity.
¶Estrogens and hormonal contraceptives may increase risk for thromboembolic events and are generally avoided in clients with conditions necessitating anticoagulants.

---

ble for the next 7 to 14 days. If acute bleeding is present, administration of fresh frozen plasma (with active clotting factors) is indicated.

✳ **R.P. is hospitalized until his condition is stabilized.**

✳ **What is the role of nursing in R.P.'s anticoagulant therapy?**

Nursing Management of Anticoagulant Therapy

The role of the nurse with the client receiving anticoagulant therapy is primarily one of monitoring R.P. for the increased risk of bleeding and educating him for the safe and accurate self-administration of the particular anticoagulant agent.

Assessment Before initiating anticoagulation therapy, assess R.P. for any preexisting health conditions that would contraindicate anticoagulation or would indicate the need for caution in the use of anticoagulant therapy. Anticoagula-

tion is contraindicated in instances in which bleeding would be imminently life-threatening, such as threatened or incomplete abortion, cerebral or aortic aneurysm, cerebrovascular hemorrhage, active bleeding, severe hypertension, hemorrhagic blood dyscrasias (hemophilia, thrombocytopenia), other hemorrhagic tendencies (leukemia, polycythemia vera), eclampsia or preeclampsia, pericarditis, and recent or contemplated neurosurgery or ophthalmic surgery.

Caution is required if R.P. has any of the following conditions in which an increased risk of hemorrhage is present: acute bacterial endocarditis; severe renal function impairment; severe trauma, especially to the central nervous system (CNS); severe vasculitis; wounds; active ulcers or lesions of the GI, GU, or respiratory tract, or recent childbirth, if R.P. were a female client.

Be concerned if R.P. has any condition that might increase the response to anticoagulant therapy, such as visceral carcinoma, severe hepatic impairment, and vitamin C or K deficiency; or if the client is to undergo a procedure that presents the risk of bleeding and a risk for injury, such as regional or lumbar block anesthesia or spinal puncture. (See the Pregnancy Safety box on p. 609 for Food and Drug Administration [FDA] classifications of the various anticoagulant agents.)

Category	Drug
B	aprotinin, clopidogrel, dalteparin, dipyridamole, enoxaparin, ticlopidine, tranexamic acid, urokinase
C	abciximab, alteplase, aminocaproic acid, anistreplase, antiinhibitor coagulant complex, antithrombin III, factor IX, heparin, protamine, reteplase, streptokinase, tenecteplase
D	aspirin
X	anisindione, warfarin

Data from *Mosby's drug consult* (15th ed.). (2005). St. Louis: Mosby.

R.P.'s current medication regimen is reviewed for significant drug interactions. In addition to the specific drug interactions listed within the discussion of heparin and the oral anticoagulants, consider that the risk of hemorrhage may be increased by the concurrent use of any medication that inhibits platelet aggregation or causes hypoprothrombinemia, thrombocytopenia, or GI ulcers (see Boxes 30-1 and 30-4).

The appropriate laboratory tests to determine coagulation times (PT or INR), and a hematocrit and CBC, including platelets, are performed before the initiation of anticoagulant therapy.

Nursing Diagnosis While receiving anticoagulant therapy, R.P. is at risk for ineffective tissue perfusion (cardiopulmonary, cerebral, GI, peripheral, renal) related to an underlying condition, and the potential complication of hemorrhage and excessive bruising related to the anticoagulant effect of the drugs.

Planning Although R.P. is receiving anticoagulants, he will:
- Exhibit increased tissue perfusion as the result of anticoagulant therapy.
- Experience increased comfort and/or does not experience a new thrombosis.
- Remain free from injury related the anticoagulant.
- Manage effectively his therapeutic regimen, including medication and supportive lifestyle changes.
- Demonstrate knowledge regarding anticoagulant therapy and its potential adverse effects.

Implementation
Monitoring Remain vigilant to the early signs of bleeding with R.P. while he is receiving anticoagulant therapy. Assess him for signs of overdose, such as ecchymosis, petechiae, hematomas, nosebleeds, and unusual bleeding from gums, cuts, wounds, and tube insertion sites. Internal

bleeding will reveal itself as abdominal pain or swelling, backache, bloody or black tarry stools, dizziness, headache, hematemesis, hematuria, hemoptysis, or joint pain. Check R.P.'s urine and stool periodically for occult blood.

Monitor laboratory values before the drug is administered to ensure that R.P.'s coagulation times are in the therapeutic, not the dangerous, range. See Box 30-3 for coagulation tests used with these drugs.

Intervention The dosage of anticoagulants is individualized for R.P. and adjusted according to the appropriate laboratory test.

Education See Box 30-2.

Evaluation
The expected outcomes of R.P.'s anticoagulant therapy are that he will:
- Remain in the therapeutic range of his appropriate coagulation study determinations.
- Experience a decrease in the symptoms such as pain and swelling with increased tissue perfusion.
- Remain free of bruising and other symptoms of increased bleeding tendencies, or any other adverse effect of the anticoagulant.
- State the rationale for the use of the anticoagulant in relation to health status.
- State the adverse effects and how to manage them, indicate reportable ones, and state the importance of collaborating with the health care team in monitoring the effects of anticoagulant therapy.

In addition to the previous general discussion concerning anticoagulants, information needs to be reviewed specific to parenteral and oral anticoagulants. The goal is to begin R.P. on a rapid-acting parenteral drug and add warfarin, which is an oral drug that takes longer to become therapeutic, but one with which R.P. will be discharged. He will need sufficient teaching to be able to self-manage his therapy.

Nursing Management of Parenteral Anticoagulant Drugs, Heparin (UFH), and Low-Molecular-Weight Heparin (LMWH) Therapy

Assessment Assess R.P. to determine that heparin is not contraindicated by preexisting conditions, such as those listed in the discussion of the nursing management of anticoagulant therapy. Caution is used in administering heparin if R.P. were to have any condition in which hemorrhage is possible. Because he is older than 60 years of age, he is more susceptible to the hemorrhagic effects of heparin. Women are even more susceptible to these effects. As an aside to R.P.'s case, heparin is the anticoagulant of choice for use during pregnancy because it does not cross the placenta and affect clotting mechanisms in the fetus. Because of the risk of maternal bleeding, it is used with caution only in the last trimester of pregnancy and during the postpartum period.

A baseline assessment should consist of an aPTT, a platelet count, and a hematocrit evaluation, and an assessment of R.P.'s underlying problem, DVT, for which the heparin is being administered.

A review of R.P.'s current medication regimen for the risk of significant drug interactions includes the ones detailed in Box 30-4. However, UFH may be administered before or after fibrinolytics, such as alteplase, anistreplase, streptokinase, or urokinase for an additive anticoagulant effect in conjunction with percutaneous transluminal coronary angioplasty (PTCA) or other invasive procedures.

Nursing Diagnosis With the administration of heparin, R.P. is at risk for the following nursing diagnoses/collaborative problems: ineffective tissue perfusion related to the underlying condition and ineffectiveness of the heparin; risk for injury related to increased bleeding tendencies; impaired comfort such as irritation, pain, or redness at the injection site related to parenteral administration; disturbed body image related to unusual hair loss (long-term therapy); and the potential complications of allergic reaction, thrombocytopenia, and osteoporosis with long-term therapy. The Nursing Care Plan below lists other se-

NURSING CARE PLAN SELECTED NURSING DIAGNOSES FOR CLIENTS RECEIVING ANTICOAGULANT THERAPY

Nursing Diagnosis	Outcome Criteria	Nursing Interventions
Ineffective tissue perfusion: reduced blood flow (prevention and treatment of thromboembolic disorders)	• Clotting studies are maintained within therapeutic range; aPTT is prolonged to 1.5-2.5 times the control (heparin). • PT is prolonged to 1.5-2.5 times the control (warfarin) (INR 2.0-3.0) • Extension of the thrombus or embolization of thrombi does not occur.	• Monitor clotting studies as ordered. • Administer anticoagulant therapy and assess effectiveness. • Monitor vital signs, including blood pressure every 4 hours. Report immediately any adverse change in vital signs. • Auscultate breath sounds every 4 hours. • Report the development of crackles. • Assess for signs of developing pulmonary emboli, such as dyspnea, cough, or hemoptysis. • Apply antiembolism stockings or sequential compression devices as ordered. • Measure calf circumference bilaterally; compare and record every 8 hours.
Risk for injury: hemorrhage	• No signs of hemorrhage occur.	• Administer subcutaneous heparin rather than IM heparin to prevent hematoma formation. Inject into lower abdomen using a small-gauge needle (25-27); do not massage injection sites. Rotate sites. • Alert all personnel that the client is receiving anticoagulant therapy. • Keep venipunctures and injections to a minimum and apply pressure to prevent bleeding when performed. • Observe the client for excessive bruising, bleeding gums, nosebleed, blood in urine, feces, and/or secretions and report any findings.
Deficient knowledge related to medication regimen	• Client will describe the underlying condition, how the drug relates to the condition, how and when to take the medication, common drug interactions, safety precautions, common side effects, and which adverse effects warrant reporting. • Client will self-administer warfarin safely and accurately.	• Assess learning needs and learning readiness. Plan with the client for the achievement of realistic goals. • Provide information to meet outcome criteria. • Caution the client to use a soft toothbrush and an electric razor. • Recommend to the client that all health care personnel be informed of anticoagulant therapy before treatment. • Advise the client on the importance of having blood studies performed as ordered. • Instruct the client on the need to report any signs of bleeding.

lected nursing diagnoses for clients receiving anticoagulant therapy.

Implementation

Monitoring R.P.'s dose of enoxaparin will be administered as prescribed with coagulation studies being done daily and then with decreasing frequency as his coagulation times are stabilized within the therapeutic range. Remember these results are not "normal" or "within normal limits"; extended coagulation times from normal values demonstrate that R.P. is therapeutically anticoagulated. If R.P. were switched to UFH, anticipate that each dose of UFH will be individualized after the prescriber has evaluated the coagulation effect or provided a sliding scale or protocol by which specific doses will be administered based on the laboratory values. Check to be sure that these tests are performed as ordered (before each IV or subcutaneous injection or daily depending on dose and indication) and that the results are reported promptly. If no dosage adjustments have been required for 2 weeks, further monitoring need not be as frequent. The exception is pregnant women, who need to be monitored throughout therapy because heparin requirements increase as the client's blood volume increases with the progression of pregnancy.

In the treatment of an active thromboemoblic event, the dosage of UFH is adjusted to maintain the aPTT between 1.5 and 2.5 times normal control level. Occasionally, LMWH is dosed based on factor Xa activity (goal varies with agent and laboratory used, often 0.4 to 1.1 units/mL). Report any value under or over these ranges to the prescriber immediately. In all cases, R.P. should be observed to assure he remains free of signs of thromboembolism or

hemorrhage as discussed in the section on the nursing management of anticoagulant therapy.

Test stools and urine for occult blood daily to determine hidden bleeding. Monitor the platelet count for any possible thrombocytopenia. Hematocrit tests are performed at frequent intervals.

There is the possibility of genetic "heparin resistance" usually associated with conditions such as infection, thrombophlebitis, fever, pleurisy, cancer, MI, and extensive surgery in which the client requires much higher doses of heparin. (See the Special Considerations for Pharmacogenetics box below.) Additionally, be aware that the abrupt withdrawal of R.P.'s heparin may precipitate an increase in coagulability. R.P. is having a full dose of heparin followed by oral anticoagulants for prophylaxis. There generally is an overlap of both drugs for 3 to 5 days while the heparin is being tapered off and the INR is approaching the goal range with warfarin.

Intervention UFH and LMWH differ in their administration. Where with UFH, the dose is based on the previous result of a blood coagulation study, LMWHs are administered subcutaneously every 12 to 24 hours on at fixed doses. The LMWHs, enoxaparin (Lovenox), dalteparin (Fragmin), and tinzaparin (Innohep) have replaced the use of UFH in many clinical settings. Be alert to safety issues with the administration of heparin; see the Medication Safety Alert box on p. 612.

For subcutaneous administration, use the smallest gauge (25 to 27) $\frac{3}{8}$- to $\frac{5}{8}$-inch needle to prevent hematoma at the injection site. Use a "bunching" technique (pull the fatty layer away from the underlying tissue). Inject the heparin

---

Special Considerations for Pharmacogenetics | ANTIPLATELETS, ANTICOAGULANTS, FIBRINOLYTICS

PHARMACODYNAMICS

Response to the effects of the antiplatelet clopidogrel is correlated with genetic markers (Angiolillo et al, 2004a) and may have an impact on dosing of clopidogrel for clients undergoing coronary procedures (Angiolillo et al, 2004b). Similar findings may be true for the antiplatelet activity of aspirin as well (Schafer, 2003).

PHARMACOKINETICS

A wide variation in the dose requirements and time to stabilization of warfarin dosing is correlated with genetic markers which code for the cytochrome P450 isoenzyme 2 C9 (King, Khan, Aithal, Kamali, & Daly, 2004; Kirchheiner et al, 2004). Variation in markers for this isoenzyme has been noted in various populations, including Chinese clients (Si et al, 2004). This variation could explain, in part, why some clients respond to low doses of warfarin and others require higher doses and longer titration periods (Leung et al, 2002). Although many

factors, including diet and drug interactions can affect warfarin dosing, genotyping may assist clinicians in the future with initial dosing recommendations for warfarin (Hillman et al, 2004). The metabolism of the antiplatelet ticlopidine is also believed to be genetically determined (Chang et al, 2004).

ADVERSE EFFECTS

Use of pharmacogenomics may assist clinicians in the future in avoiding excessive anticoagulation and bleeding events for clients on warfarin (Visser et al, 2004). Presence of an enzyme that may be genetically determined is correlated with risk for hemorrhagic complications associated with the administration of alteplase (Montaner et al, 2003), but the clinical utility of this finding is unclear. Women appear to have a higher risk than men for severe thromboembolic complications with heparin induced thrombocytopenia (HIT), but clear genetic markers for this risk have yet to be identified (Carlsson et al, 2003).

Medication Safety Alert

UFH and LMWH

UFH and LMWH come in many concentrations: carefully check the vial and the prescriber's order. Errors have been known to occur between the vials of 1000 USP units/mL and 10,000 USP units/mL, and between the vials of 2000 USP units/mL and 20,000 USP units/mL; watch the decimal points. Be alert, too, that the heparin-lock flush solution maintains the patency of the indwelling venipuncture unit and that the flush solution is not used for systemic anticoagulation. The nurse working with premature neonates should be aware that some heparin sodium injections contain benzyl alcohol as a preservative; these preparations should not be administered to these infants. Clients with a history of allergies or asthma should receive a test dose of 1000 USP units of heparin before treatment is initiated, because heparin is derived from animal tissue.

deep into the fatty tissue above the iliac crest or into the abdominal fat layer. Avoid the umbilical veins by avoiding a 2-inch radius around the umbilicus. This distance should also be maintained from scars and lesions. Do not aspirate, and *do not massage the injection site.* Hold the needle in place for 10 seconds after administration, and withdraw it gently to minimize bruising. Apply direct pressure for 1 to 2 minutes if needed. Rotate sites to prevent the formation of hematomas.

Document the location of injection sites graphically. IM administration is not recommended because it causes hematomas, irritation, and pain at the injection site and causes erratic absorption.

With IV administration, full-dose therapeutic UFH requires a loading dose (usually preceding a continuous infusion), or heparin may be administered intermittently via a heparin lock. This IV dose may be given undiluted over at least 1 minute. Many clinicians prefer continuous IV infusions for the administration of heparin because it provides a more constant blood level of the drug and because the risk for bleeding complications is decreased. For continuous IV infusion of heparin, use an infusion pump or a volume control unit; check the system frequently to prevent overdose or underdose. Never add other drugs to the heparin infusion or piggyback other drugs into an IV line containing heparin, because many other drugs inactivate heparin.

For clients receiving intermittent doses of UFH—either subcutaneously or by heparin lock—ensure that the blood samples for the aPTT are drawn 30 minutes before each dose to avoid a falsely high aPTT. This false reading can also be avoided for the client with a continuous heparin infusion by drawing the sample from the arm opposite the infusion site.

Although controversy exists in clinical practice regarding whether normal saline or diluted heparin solutions (10 to 100 units of heparin sodium/mL) should be used to irrigate

and maintain patency of an indwelling venipuncture device, be aware that the purpose of the device is to maintain an open IV line so that intermittent bolus doses of drugs, IV solutions, or both may be administered through this line. Obtain information within each clinical practice setting about the accepted protocol concerning the solution to be used and how often the device should be flushed if not in frequent use; then closely monitor the unit for patency.

If a heparin solution is being used to maintain the patency of an indwelling peripheral venipuncture device, 1 mL of a heparin-lock flush solution is usually effective for 4 to 8 hours. If the device is being used to administer a drug that is incompatible with heparin, it should be flushed with 0.9% sodium chloride for injection before and after the drug is administered. Inject the heparin-lock flush solution after the second flush. If the device is being used to obtain blood samples for laboratory analysis and heparin might alter the results of the test, the heparin solution should be cleared from the device by aspirating and discarding 1 mL of solution before the blood sample is taken. After the blood sample is drawn, the device is again filled with 1 mL of heparin-lock flush solution. Heparin is also used for irrigation for patency of central lines according to health organization policy. See the Evidence-Based Practice box on p. 613.

Heparin is to be stopped immediately if the client complains of chills, low back pain (a sign of abdominal bleeding), or spontaneous bleeding. Notify the prescriber, and have protamine sulfate on hand. In some cases it may be necessary to administer whole blood or plasma.

Alert other staff members that the client is receiving heparin (e.g., place a sign over the client's bed). Apply pressure to venipuncture and injection sites to minimize bruising. These invasive procedures should be avoided if at all possible. Consult the prescriber regarding a change from the IM administration of other drugs to other routes of administration while the client is receiving anticoagulants.

Education In addition to the client education information discussed in Nursing Management of Anticoagulant Therapy (p. 608), inform R.F. of the potential for diuresis beginning 36 to 48 hours after the initial dose of heparin and lasting 36 to 48 hours after the termination of therapy.

Advise any client on long-term heparin therapy that alopecia may occur several months after the initiation of the drug and that the condition is reversible when the drug is discontinued. Irreversible osteoporosis may also occur with long-term therapy.

Evaluation For expected outcomes of R.P.'s LMWH therapy, see the evaluation statement within the general management of anticoagulant therapy. Additionally, R.P.'s blood counts, including platelet counts, hematocrit or hemoglobin, and urinalysis are within normal limits; occult blood stool tests are negative.

The expected outcome of UFH therapy is that the client's aPTT will show values 1.5 to 2.5 times the control value in seconds or ACT values 2 to 3 times the control

Irrigation of Central Venous Lines with Heparin to Ensure Patency of the Line for IV Access to the Client

Rabe and associates (2002) examined the practice of sealing intermittently used central venous catheters with vitamin C solution, heparin solution or saline solution between use to avoid occlusion. The prospective randomized study performed on a nine-bed medical intensive care unit (ICU) and on medical wards of an academic tertiary care center. Ninety-nine central venous line placements were prospectively included in the study and randomized into three treatment groups: sodium chloride 0.9%, vitamin C (200 mg/mL) and heparin (5000 international units/mL) sealing solutions. Catheters were filled with the respective sealing solution and patency was tested once every 2 days using a standardized routine. Catheter patency was compared among the three groups. There was a significant difference in catheter patency between the three groups (p <0.03, log-rank test). A comparison of catheter survival between the catheters filled with heparin and those filled with sodium chloride, but not between those filled with vitamin C solution and with sodium chloride solution, exhibited significant differences in catheter patency (p <0.04, log-rank test). Local anticoagulation of intermittently used central venous catheters prolongs catheter patency. High-dose (5000 international units/mL) heparin solution is a useful anticoagulant for this purpose, whereas vitamin C solution does not prolong catheter patency.

Modified from Rabe, C., Gramann, T., Sons, X., Berna, M., Gonzalez-Carmona, M.A., Klehr, H.U., et al. (2002). Keeping central venous lines open: a prospective comparison of heparin, vitamin C and sodium chloride sealing solutions in medical patients. *Intensive Care Medicine*, 28(8), 1172-1176.

value in seconds. Additionally, the client will not show evidence of any signs or symptoms of bleeding or thrombus formation.

Other parenteral anticoagulants include antithrombin III (ATnativ, Thrombate III), argatroban, bivalirudin (Angiomax), fondaparinux (Arixtra), lepirudin (Refludan) and danaparoid (Orgaran). The nursing management of the miscellaneous antithrombin agents is the same as for the nursing management of LMWHs.

Nursing Management of Oral Anticoagulant Drugs

Oral anticoagulation is the most common anticoagulation modality outside of institutional settings, so there is a higher expectation for clients to be able to effectively manage their drug therapy. R.P. is started on warfarin

(Coumadin) while hospitalized and will be discharged on warfarin therapy for his DVT. This discussion of oral anticoagulants assumes the foundation of the general discussion of the nursing management of anticoagulant therapy, p. 608.

Assessment As with the parenteral anticoagulants, assess R.P. for health conditions for which oral anticoagulant therapy is contraindicated or for which R.P. may be at risk for adverse effects. (Review the assessment content within the discussion of the nursing management of anticoagulant therapy.) If R.P. were a woman, it would be important to ascertain if she is pregnant and inform her of the potential risk of congenital malformations before beginning therapy; warfarin is Pregnancy Category X. The Special Considerations for Older Adults box on p. 614 discusses the issues involved in oral anticoagulant therapy with older adults.

Review R.P.'s current medication for significant drug interactions. Although all interactions between the oral anticoagulants and the other medications have not been identified, a listing of the medications known to cause interactions is found in Box 30-4.

A baseline assessment should consist of an INR determination, a platelet count, a hematocrit evaluation, and an examination of the status of his DVT. Anticipate that the dosage of these drugs will be individualized after the prescriber has evaluated R.P.'s INR.

Nursing Diagnosis With the administration of oral anticoagulant therapy, R.P. is at risk for the following nursing diagnoses/collaborative problems in addition to the ones cited above: impaired skin integrity related to allergic dermatitis (necrosis of skin); impaired comfort (bloated stomach or gas); diarrhea related to GI effects; and the potential complications of acute adrenal insufficiency (diarrhea, nausea with or without vomiting, abdominal cramps) and hepatotoxicity (dark urine, yellow sclera, and skin).

Planning Same as for parenteral anticoagulants.

Implementation

Monitoring Anticipate that the dosage is based on the PT or INR. Check to be sure that one of these tests is performed as ordered, and report the results to the prescriber immediately. The therapeutic aim for clients undergoing anticoagulant therapy with warfarin is to prolong the INR from usually 2 to 3. If the client is at higher risk for thrombus, then a prolongation of the INR from 3 to 4 is the therapeutic level sought. Once the maintenance dosage has been determined, further monitoring need not be as frequent. (Review client monitoring within the discussion of the nursing management for anticoagulant therapy.)

Intervention Be aware that the onset of action of the oral anticoagulants is slow; therefore LMWH is usually given during the first few days of treatment. The duration of warfarin therapy for the treatment of DVT is often 3 to

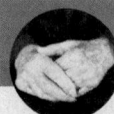

Special Considerations for Older Adults | ANTICOAGULANTS

- Older adults may be more susceptible to the effects of anticoagulants including warfarin (Coumadin). A lower maintenance dose is usually recommended for the older client along with very close supervision and monitoring. This is particularly true for clients who receive warfarin and may be vitamin K deficient because of low intake of green leafy vegetables.
- The primary adverse effects of excessive drug usage are prolonged bleeding from gums when brushing teeth or from small shaving cuts, excessive or easy skin bruising, blood in urine or stools, and unexplained nosebleeds. These may be early signs of overdose that indicate the need for medical intervention.
- Caution clients to carry an identification card indicating the use of an anticoagulant. Also, remind client to always consult the prescriber before starting any new drug, including OTC medications and vitamins, or if changing a medication dose or when any drug product is discontinued. Many medications can change the effects of an anticoagulant in the body.
- Be aware that administration of concurrent drug therapy that may induce gastric irritation increases the risk for

GI bleeding. Drugs such as the nonsteroidal antiinflammatory agents (NSAIDs such as ibuprofen, indomethacin) that are commonly prescribed for the older adult client often cause GI effects.
- Alcohol consumption can alter the effect of this medication in the body. Clients should be instructed to avoid alcohol or at the least limit their daily alcohol intake to one alcoholic drink a day. Alcohol may cause liver damage and cause minor GI bleeding, both of which increase the individual's sensitivity to anticoagulants (*USP DI*, 2005).
- The nurse should be aware that diet can interfere with the anticoagulant effect. In a previously stabilized person, vitamin C deficiency, chronic malnutrition, diarrhea, or other illnesses may result in an increased anticoagulant effect, although increased intake of green leafy vegetables (such as broccoli, cabbage, collard greens, lettuce, spinach, and others) or the consumption of a nutritional supplement or multiple vitamin containing vitamin K can result in decreased anticoagulant effectiveness.

---

6 months. For other indications, such as preventing thromboembolic events for clients with atrial fibrillation or prosthetic heart valves, therapy may be lifelong. When discontinuing oral anticoagulant therapy, it is usually terminated gradually over a 3- or 4-week period to prevent rebound thromboembolic complications. Vitamin K_1 (phytonadione) should be readily accessible if bleeding occurs.

Education In addition to the points discussed in Nursing Management of Anticoagulant Therapy (p. 608), stress with R.P. the importance of adhering to the schedule of laboratory procedures and prescriber's appointments once maintenance therapy is established. The INR should be performed at intervals of 1 to 4 weeks, depending on dosage. Periodic urinalysis, blood counts, stool guaiac, and liver function tests are also performed. Ensure that the client is aware of different dosage tablets, because the prescriber may vary the dosage by phone on the basis of the INR. Instruct R.P. to take the medication at the same time every day to limit excessive fluctuations in drug response. He should never "double up" on a missed dose unless instructed to do so by the prescriber.

Evaluation In addition to the previously mentioned general expected outcomes for anticoagulant therapy, the expected outcome of oral anticoagulant therapy is that R.P.'s INR will show values 2 to 3, or 3 to 4 if he is considered at higher risk for thrombus.

✴ **R.P. received his second dose of enoxaparin subcutaneously and his first dose of warfarin 5 mg PO last evening at 6:00 PM. His INR is reported from the laboratory this morning at 1.3.**
Given that R.P. has an existing DVT, he would be considered at a higher risk for thrombosis at this time so the preference would be to have his INR in the 2 to 3 range. However, the onset of warfarin effect is 2 to 3 days. As a consequence, the prescriber will maintain the heparin therapy until R.P.'s INR is in the therapeutic range.

✴ **R.P. is maintained on enoxaparin for the first 4 days of warfarin therapy and receives warfarin 5 mg PO each day. On day four of warfarin therapy, the INR is at 2.7 (goal range 2 to 3) and enoxaparin is discontinued. Warfarin therapy is continued daily at 5 mg PO daily. On day 10 of warfarin therapy, the lab reports the INR for R.P. is elevated at 8. R.P. is brought into the prescriber's office and evaluated. R.P. indicates that he misunderstood instructions and thought he was supposed to take warfarin 5 mg twice daily. He has no overt signs of bleeding, his vital signs are stable (normal blood pressure and pulse).**

✴ **How is excessive intake of an anticoagulant managed?**
Management of excessive anticoagulation is dependent on the presence and/or risk of bleeding, the degree of antico-

agulation, and the anticoagulant used. In mild cases where bleeding is not present and anticoagulant levels are only moderately elevated, the drug is often held until the lab test used (e.g., aPTT, INR or Factor Xa) returns to the goal range. In such circumstances, clients are carefully monitored for the presence of bleeding and bleeding risk. An evaluation of why the client presented with an exaggerated response to anticoagulation is important before reinstitution of anticoagulation. Factors that may predispose to increased response include dosing errors, drug interactions, and food interactions.

With excessive UFH or LMWH levels resulting in bleeding, the antidote protamine is often used, and effect is observed almost immediately. In the event of severe bleeding, support with blood, blood products (specifically fresh frozen plasma [FFP] with clotting factors present), and fluid replacement may be utilized.

★▆▀ protamine sulfate [**proe** ta meen]
(heparin antidote)

Protamine sulfate, a protein-like substance derived from the sperm and mature testes of salmon and other fish, is an antidote for a heparin overdose. Protamine is a very weak anticoagulant alone. When it is given in conjunction with heparin, however, a combination is formed that dissociates the heparin–antithrombin III complex, thus reducing the anticoagulant action of heparin.

Indications
Protamine is indicated for the treatment of a severe heparin overdose that has resulted in hemorrhaging. Blood transfusions may be necessary. Protamine is also used to neutralize the effects of heparin administered during dialysis or cardiac or arterial surgery.

Pharmacokinetics/Dosing
When administered intravenously, protamine has an onset of action within 30 to 60 seconds, with duration of effect of usually 2 hours. Protamine is administered by slow IV injection at a rate of 1 mg/min. One milligram of protamine is necessary to neutralize approximately 100 USP units of heparin. It is recommended that not more than 50 mg of protamine be given in any 10-minute period and that no more than 100 mg be administered over a 2-hour period. Close monitoring with blood coagulation tests is required.

Adverse Effects
When protamine is administered too rapidly, respiratory difficulties, bradycardia, and a sudden hypotensive effect may result. Less frequently reported symptoms are bleeding (caused by protamine overdose or a rebound of heparin activity), hypertension, anaphylaxis, back pain, a feeling of warmth and/or tiredness, flushing, nausea, or vomiting. Coughing spells, facial edema, or rash also occur and should be reported to the prescriber immediately.

Nursing Management
Assessment
Protamine is used as an antidote to severe heparin overdose (including the LMWHs) as evidenced by frank hemorrhaging or abnormally high values on the aPTT or ACT. If a large amount of bleeding has occurred, administration of packed RBCs may be necessary as well. Protamine is not used in instances of minor heparin overdose, which can be treated by withholding the doses of heparin. Ascertain that the client has not had a previous allergic reaction to protamine. Obtain a hemoglobin and hematocrit, and aPTT for baseline.

Planning
The goals of therapy are to stop the hemorrhage, stabilize the client, and then return the client to normal or therapeutic aPTT or ACT ranges.

Nursing Diagnosis
The client receiving protamine sulfate is at risk for the following nursing diagnoses/collaborative problems: ineffective tissue perfusion and deficient fluid volume related to the underlying hemorrhage; impaired comfort (back pain, feelings of warmth and flushing, and nausea or vomiting); and the potential complications of cardiovascular collapse related to too rapid administration, anaphylaxis, bleeding related to protamine overdose or rebound heparin activity, and pulmonary edema.

Implementation
Monitoring
Frequent assessment of the client's vital signs and some estimation of blood loss are essential. An ACT, aPTT, or thrombin time (TT) should be performed 5 to 15 minutes after the initial administration of protamine as an antidote for heparin and repeated as needed. The aPTT and TT may not be useful in monitoring protamine therapy after the administration of enoxaparin, because it does not alter the results of these tests in therapeutic doses. Observe the client for spontaneous bleeding or heparin "rebound" (the effects of heparin last longer than the effects of protamine) after procedures involving extracorporeal circulation such as cardiac or arterial surgery or dialysis. This may occur as long as 18 hours after the initial neutralization of the heparin.

Intervention
Discontinue the heparin immediately. Protamine sulfate should be administered by a physician. It should be administered IV slowly—over 1 to 3 minutes—not more than 50 mg in any 10-minute period. Too rapid administration may cause injury, dyspnea, and shock. Emergency equipment should be available. Reversal of heparin's anticoagulant activity takes place in as few as 5 minutes. For UFH, usually 1 mg can reverse the effects of 100 units of UFH, with LMWH, the ratio is 1 mg of protamine to 1 mg of LMWH.

Education
Keep the client apprised of situation and explain each of the interventions taken in this urgent situation.

Evaluation
The expected outcome of protamine sulfate therapy is that the client will not evidence bleeding, the hemoglobin and hematocrit will stabilize within normal limits, males: 13.6 to 17.5 g/dL, females 12 to 15.5 g/dL and males: 39% to 49%, females: 35% to 45% respectively, and the aPTT or ACT will be within normal or therapeutic limits (see Box 30-3).

In the case of excess warfarin intake, vitamin K may be utilized, but its activity is not fully realized for at least 24 to 48 hours. In severe cases, fresh frozen plasma is utilized with vitamin K to arrest bleeding immediately. Recombinant human factor VIIa concentrate has also been used (Deveras & Kessler, 2002). Administration of blood or blood products may also be required if severe bleeding is noted. Vitamin K is essential to the hepatic synthesis of prothrombin (factor II) and factors VII, IX, and X. It contributes to the activation of an enzyme necessary to the formation of prothrombin. A deficiency of vitamin K leads to hypoprothrombinemia and hemorrhage. Vitamin K is available in several forms, including menadiol sodium diphosphate (Synkayvite) and phytonadione (Mephyton, AquaMEPHYTON).

Vitamin K is used to prevent and treat hypoprothrombinemia. A prothrombin deficiency may occur because of inadequate absorption of vitamin K from the intestine (usually caused by biliary disease, in which bile fails to enter the intestine) or because of the destruction of intestinal organisms, which may occur with antibiotic therapy. It is also seen in the newborn, in which case it is probably caused by the fact that the intestinal organisms have not yet become established. It may result from therapy with certain medications, such as salicylates, sulfonamides, quinine, quinidine, or broad-spectrum antibiotics.

Vitamin K is useful only in conditions in which the prolonged bleeding time is caused by a low concentration of prothrombin in the blood and not by damaged liver cells. Vitamin K is routinely administered to newborns to help prevent hemorrhage. Although prothrombin levels may be normal at birth, they decline until about the sixth to the eighth day, when the liver is able to form prothrombin. Phytonadione is usually the preferred agent. It is important to measure the prothrombin activity of the blood frequently when the client is receiving a preparation of vitamin K.

phytonadione [fye toe na **dye** one]
(Mephyton, AquaMEPHYTON)
Indications

Phytonadione is used to prevent or treat hypoprothrombinemia related to drug-induced vitamin K deficiency—specifically as an antidote for warfarin. It is also used to treat hemorrhagic disease of the newborn and is administered to clients with deficient prothrombin, particularly those with obstructive jaundice.

Pharmacokinetics/Dosing

Parenteral preparations should be administered if intestinal absorption is impaired. Natural vitamin K is normally synthesized by the intestinal flora. When synthetic forms of vitamin K are administered, the absorption is good, but phytonadione requires the presence of bile salts. The onset of action for oral phytonadione it is 6 to 12 hours, and for the injectable form it is 1 to 2 hours. Vitamin K is metabolized in the liver and excreted by the kidneys and in the bile. As an antidote for drug-induced hypoprothrombinemia, the oral dosage is between 1 and 10 mg daily. Many clinicians use vitamin K sparingly in clients on warfarin with elevated INRs and no bleeding, because aggressive doses make future anticoagulation problematic.

Adverse Effects

The most serious adverse effects are hypersensitivity, particularly on parenteral administration. Other adverse effects include facial flushing, taste alterations, and redness or pain at the injection site.

Nursing Management
Assessment

Vitamin K is used as an antidote to severe warfarin overdose as evidenced by frank hemorrhaging or abnormally high values on the INR. Assess the client for preexisting conditions in which vitamin K therapy would entail some risk, such as hepatic function impairment (large doses of vitamin K might increase the impairment), or glucose-6-phosphate dehydrogenase (G6PD) deficiency (menadiol might induce erythrocyte hemolysis).

Ascertain the amount of hemorrhage or the risk of bleeding from the INR as a baseline assessment. Obtain a hemoglobin and hematocrit and INR.

Nursing Diagnosis

The administration of vitamin K may place the client at risk for impaired comfort (facial flushing, unusual taste, and discomfort and redness at the injection site) and the potential complications of hemolytic anemia or a rare hypersensitivity-like reaction.

Planning

The goals of therapy are to stop or prevent hemorrhage, stabilize the client and then return the client normal or therapeutic INR.

Implementation
Monitoring

Monitor INR as a baseline measurement and throughout vitamin K therapy to evaluate the client's response. During IV infusion, ob-

serve for signs of adverse effects such as flushing, weakness, and hypotension, and report them to the prescriber.

Intervention

Discontinue warfarin. Because vitamin K has a delayed onset of 36 to 42 hours to reverse warfarin's effects, the administration of plasma or fresh whole blood may be necessary with severe bleeding. The dose and route of administration of vitamin K will depend on the acuity of the client's condition. IV administration is not generally recommended because of the risk of hypersensitivity reactions; if IV administration is necessary, administer the drug by slow IV infusion over 2 to 3 hours, and protect the infusion container from light by wrapping it in aluminum foil. High doses of vitamin K (10 to 15 mg) given IV can reverse the anticoagulation within 6 hours. However, with such a dose vitamin K will maintain its reversal effect for a week. This will make it difficult to reinstitute warfarin therapy when it must be restarted. Lower doses help to minimize this effect. AquaMEPHYTON, a parenteral solution, contains benzyl alcohol, which may cause a toxic fatal syndrome in neonates; avoid using this solution with infants.

Education

Advise the client of the goals of therapy. If the client evidences a high INR and has not experienced frank bleeding, advise the client to avoid hazardous activities until the INR is in the therapeutic range again.

Evaluation

The expected outcome of vitamin K therapy is that the client's INR is 2 to 3 and the client will not show evidence of bleeding.

✳ **K.P. is a 62-year-old semi-retired construction worker (80 kg) who abruptly develops facial drooping and slurred speech on the worksite. He is rushed to the hospital and is evaluated for a cerebral vascular accident. The neurologist conducts a complete examination and immediately orders a computed tomography (CT) of the head. K.P. is diagnosed with a thromboembolic CVA and 7 mg of the fibrinolytic alteplase (t-PA, Activase) is given as an IV bolus over 1 minute, then 65 mg are administered via IV infusion over 60 minutes.**

✳ **What is the role of fibrinolytic drug therapy?**
Fibrinolytic (also referred to as thrombolytic) drugs are used to treat acute thromboembolic disorders. Unlike anticoagulants, they dissolve clots and are used in a hospital setting only by health care providers who are experienced in the management of diseases caused by thrombosis. These agents alter the hemostatic capability of the client more profoundly than does anticoagulant therapy. Consequently, when bleeding occurs, it is more severe and very difficult to control.

These agents are indicated for life-threatening conditions such as MI, thromboembolic CVA, and PE. In lower doses these drugs can be used locally to clear thrombosed catheters and by the interventional radiologist or other specialist to dissolve thrombus or emboli from other localized sites.

Fibrinolytic drugs dissolve clots via the endogenous fibrinolytic system. All six drugs have similar biochemical mechanisms of action on the fibrinolytic system—converting plasminogen in the blood to plasmin. Plasmin, an enzyme with fibrinolytic activity, digests or dissolves fibrin clots wherever they exist and wherever they can be reached by plasmin. A number of fibrinolytics are available for use and include alteplase (Activase), anistreplase (Eminase), reteplase (Retavase), streptokinase (Streptase), and tenecteplase (TNKase) and urokinase (Abbokinase). Indications and dosing vary by agent. Although streptokinase was the first fibrinolytic agent released, many consider alteplase to be more representative of the class.

⚹ ◠ alteplase [**al** ti plase]
(Activase)

Indications

Alteplase is indicated for the treatment of acute pulmonary thromboembolism and for the treatment of acute ischemic stroke when initiated within 3 hours of the onset of symptoms. (*USP DI*, 2005). It can also be used to treat acute coronary arterial thrombosis associated with an AMI. Their use for AMI has declined over the past decade because of advances in interventional cardiology techniques, availability of the glycoprotein II b/III a inhibitors, and increased availability of cardiac catheterization laboratories in acute care settings. Active bleeding or a high risk for bleeding is a contraindication for use (see the nursing assessment in a later section).

Pharmacokinetics/Dosing

Alteplase is administered IV and/or intra-arterially. It has an elimination half-life of 35 minutes with a duration of the fibrinolytic effect of approximately 4 hours. In an acute coronary artery thrombosis that evolves into a transmural MI, fibrinolytic therapy is most effective when started within 3 to 4 hours after the onset of symptoms. For AMI, a 15 mg IV bolus is followed by 0.75 mg/kg (maximum dose 50 mg) over 30 minutes, then 0.5 mg/kg (maximum dose 35 mg) over 60 minutes. It is typically dosed with heparin. For acute ischemic stroke, therapy must be initiated within 3 hours of the onset of symptoms and is dosed at 0.9 mg/kg (maximum dose 90 mg) over 60 minutes, with 10% of that dose given as an IV bolus over 1 minute. The adult dose for PE is 100 mg IV over 2 hours. Refer to the package insert for more specific information.

Adverse Effects

Bleeding is a major and real complication of fibrinolytic therapy. Hemorrhage from any site is possible. Risk of bleeding is highest with high dose therapy and for older clients (especially >75 years of age). Anaphylaxis is possible with any agent in the class.

⚙ **K.P. tolerates the infusion of alteplase.**

⚙ **What monitoring is appropriate during and after administration of alteplase to K.P.?**
The nursing management of fibrinolytic therapy usually occurs in emergency or critical care settings.

Assessment Note that fibrinolytic therapy would be contraindicated for K.P. if there were the risk of uncontrollable bleeding because of preexisting conditions such as aneurysm or arteriovenous malformation, active bleeding, brain tumor, CVA, intracranial or intraspinal surgery within the last 2 months, recent thoracic surgery, or CNS trauma. Such therapy is also contraindicated for severe uncontrolled hypertension (>200 mm Hg systolic and/or >120 mm Hg diastolic) because of the risk of cerebral hemorrhage. Alteplase therapy for acute ischemic stroke is initiated only after the exclusion of intracranial hemorrhage by a cranial computed axial tomography (CAT) scan

or other diagnostic imaging method. Use fibrinolytics with caution for any condition in which the risk of bleeding is present or would be difficult to control because of its location. In addition to those already listed are childbirth, organ biopsy, puncture of noncompressible blood vessel, or major surgery within past 10 days; uncontrolled coagulation defects; subacute bacterial endocarditis; neurosurgical procedures within the prior 2 months; recent severe trauma; and mitral stenosis with atrial fibrillation or other indicators of potential left heart thrombus. If K.P. has been treated previously with anistreplase or streptokinase, the formation of antibodies to the drug may cause either a resistance to the therapeutic effects of the drug or a severe allergic reaction.

Review K.P.'s current medication regimen for the risk of significant drug interactions, such as those that may occur when fibrinolytic agents are given concurrently with anticoagulants because of the increased risk of bleeding and hemorrhage. However, heparin has been administered with fibrinolytic agents to treat an acute coronary arterial occlusion; monitor closely when concurrent therapy is prescribed. Other drugs of concern for significant interaction are: antifibrinolytic drugs (may inhibit the effectiveness of fibrinolytic agents); NSAIDs or platelet aggregation inhibitors, especially sulfinpyrazone and ticlopidine (may inhibit platelet aggregation and increase the potential for GI ulceration and bleeding); cefamandole, cefoperazone, cefotetan, plicamycin, or valproic acid (may cause hypoprothrombinemia, inhibit platelet aggregation, and increase risk of hemorrhage).

Before fibrinolytic therapy, coagulation tests such as TT, aPTT, PT, fibrin/fibrinogen degradation product (FDP/fdp) titer, and fibrinogen concentration are be performed; however, therapy for acute coronary arterial occlusion must not be delayed until the test results are available. Additionally, an electrocardiogram (ECG) and hematocrit, hemoglobin, and platelet counts are needed.

Nursing Diagnosis With the administration of fibrinolytic agents, K.P. is at risk for the following nursing diagnoses: risk for injury related to increased bleeding tendencies; acute pain related to cardiac ischemia; ineffective tissue perfusion related to cardiac dysrhythmias; hyperthermia; and the potential complication of hypotension (not related to hemorrhage), stroke (hemorrhagic or thromboembolic). Additionally, the client is at risk for the complication of an allergic reaction with the use of anistreplase, streptokinase, and urokinase.

Planning While receiving antifibrinolytic therapy, K.P. will:
- Experience increased comfort and relief of pain.
- Evidence increased tissue perfusion.
- Remain free of injury from either the original disease process or the fibrinolytic therapy.
- Demonstrate adequate knowledge regarding fibrinolytic therapy and the potential risks of bleeding and other adverse effects.

Implementation

Monitoring During the early phase of therapy, observe K.P. carefully for allergic reactions. With urokinase, relatively mild reactions (e.g., bronchospasm, skin rash) are reported. Alteplase is not antigenic and does not cause antibody formation; this allows for a second course of the drug if reocclusion occurs without fear of anaphylaxis. However, other fibrinolytics, such as anistreplase and streptokinase may produce more serious reactions, and possibly anaphylaxis. If allergic manifestations occur, discontinue the infusion and treat appropriately (if anaphylaxis, with epinephrine, antihistamines, and corticosteroids). Fever should be treated symptomatically with acetaminophen.

Monitor vital signs frequently (i.e., pulse rate, temperature, respiratory rate, and BP), at least every 4 hours. To avoid possible dislodgement of deep vein thrombi, do not take BP in the lower extremities. Monitor client carefully for bleeding: every 15 minutes for the first hour, every 30 minutes for the next 8 hours, and every 4 hours until therapy is discontinued. Notify the prescriber immediately if bleeding occurs. Therapy should be discontinued if bleeding occurs that is not controlled by local pressure. In addition to observing for overt bleeding, observe K.P. for internal bleeding—bloody sputum, hematuria, hematemesis, dark stools (e.g., guaiac positive), flank and abdominal pain, and neurologic and mental status changes (intracranial bleeding). For uncontrollable bleeding, stop treatment and be ready to administer whole blood (fresh blood if available), packed red cells, cryoprecipitate or fresh-frozen plasma, and aminocaproic acid (an antifibrinolytic).

Observe the extremities and palpate the pulses of the affected extremities every hour. The prescriber should be notified immediately if there are signs of circulatory impairment. Observe K.P. carefully for dysrhythmias during and after intracoronary infusion of the fibrinolytic. Rapid lysis of coronary thrombi has caused atrial and ventricular dysrhythmias. ECG monitoring is recommended for all clients receiving fibrinolytic therapy.

Continue to observe K.P. for bleeding during and after treatment. Coagulation tests such as aPTT, INR, and TT are used to assess fibrinolytic activity. Because the fibrinolytic effects of the drug last for several hours, the sites of invasive devices are common areas for hematoma formation.

After therapy, monitor fibrinogen levels—which are decreased by fibrinolytic agents—until they return to normal.

Intervention Fibrinolytic therapy is administered as soon as possible following the onset of symptoms because the resistance to lysis increases with the age of the thrombus. It is beneficial if fibrinolytic therapy is initiated for AMI, within 6 to 12 hours; thromboembolic CVA, within 3 hours; PE, 5 to 7 days; DVT, 3 to 4 days; and noncoronary thromboembolism or arterial thrombosis, 3 days. Fibrinolytic therapy is administered only by personnel who are experienced in the management of thrombotic diseases and only where skilled personnel and laboratory resources are available. Typed and crossmatched whole blood and packed red cells should be available in case of hemorrhage. Follow the manufacturer's instructions when reconstituting and diluting the drugs to minimize the formation of fibrin:

- Have equipment and drugs for treating anaphylaxis available in the immediate environment. In the case of streptokinase, a glucocorticoid and/or antihistamine may be given before administration to reduce the risk of adverse reactions, such as hypersensitivity and fever. However, the prophylactic effectiveness of these interventions has not been proven.
- Do not add any other medication to the container of alteplase, anistreplase, streptokinase, or urokinase solution or administer other medications through the same IV line. Do not administer by IM injection because of the danger of hematoma. Use venipuncture sites for other purposes as seldom as possible (use a 23-gauge or smaller needle), and perform this procedure with care. Maintain pressure dressings at the site for at least 30 minutes, and check frequently for bleeding.
- Therapy is discontinued immediately if bleeding occurs that is not controlled by local pressure. To prevent bruising during therapy, avoid unnecessary handling of the client. Keep K.P. on bed rest, and pad the side rails of his bed. Place pressure dressings on recently invaded sites. Avoid invasive procedures such as IM injections and biopsies. Only essential procedures and diagnostic tests are performed.
- After the completion of fibrinolytic therapy, begin continuous IV infusion of heparin (without a loading dose) when TT has decreased to less than twice the normal control value (usually within 2 hours after completion of the infusion). Use an infusion pump for heparin. Later the client may receive oral anticoagulant therapy, a procedure that prevents the recurrence of thrombosis.

Evaluation The expected outcome of alteplase therapy for acute ischemic stroke is that K.P.'s symptoms of stroke will resolve and he will not experience intracranial hemorrhage or other adverse effects of the drug.

When fibrinolytic therapy is used for the emergency treatment of coronary artery thrombosis, the expected outcome is that the client will experience a cessation of chest pain, improved ECG values, and the absence of coronary occlusion with cardiac catheterization. When fibrinolytic therapy is administered for the treatment of venous thrombosis, pulmonary embolism, and arterial thrombosis and embolism, the client will demonstrate increased tissue perfusion as evidenced by the absence of ischemic pain, a return of normal peripheral pulses, and good capillary refill. When administered for pulmonary embolus, the client will demonstrate normal blood gases and a normal lung scan.

What role does pharmacotherapy have in the treatment of hemophilia?

Hemophilia is a hereditary disorder caused by a deficiency of one or more plasma protein clotting factors. This condition usually leads to persistent and uncontrollable hemorrhage after even a minor injury. Symptoms include excessive bleeding from wounds and hemorrhage into joints, the urinary tract, and on occasion, the CNS. There are two types of hemophilia: (1) hemophilia A, the classic type, in which factor VIII activity is deficient; and (2) hemophilia B, or Christmas disease, in which factor IX complex activity is deficient. In recent years a correct diagnosis of the coagulation disorder has led to specific factor replacement therapy; this medical advance has resulted in effective management of the client at home.

Individuals treated for hemophilia before 1986 may be seropositive for human immunodeficiency virus (HIV) infection transmitted via the various antihemophilic factors. Standard treatment of hemophilia A is based on infusion of factor VIII concentrates, now heat treated to reduce the likelihood of transmission of HIV. Recombinant factor VIII appears safe and effective, although expensive, and should impose no risk of transmitting HIV or other viruses. Since 1986, there has been no transmission of HIV through factor concentrates to clients with hemophilia in the United States. Factor VIII products other than the recombinant form have been implicated in cases of hepatitis A and C (Dunn & Abshire, 2004). Desmopressin acetate or DDAVP, a form of vasopressin, may be used for minor bleeding episodes in hemophilia A; see Chapter 46. A new agent, recombinant factor VIIa is thought to be hemostatically active only at the site of tissue injury so the risk of systemic thrombotic events is minimal. Factor VII may also be effective for clients with intracerebral hemorrhage, but its expense (in excess of $20,000 in the United States) would limit its use (Mayer et al., 2005). Because it is not a plasma-derived product, viral transmission is unlikely. Its drawback is its short half-life that necessitates dosing every 2 hours.

Factor VIII, or the antihemophilic factor (AHF), is a glycoprotein necessary for hemostasis and blood clotting. In the intrinsic pathway of the coagulation mechanism, AHF is required for the transformation of prothrombin to thrombin.

Two recombinant DNA-derived factor VIII preparations (Recombinate and Kogenate) were marketed in 1993. Before these products, concentrates were prepared from donor plasma pools; some concentrates have been the source of transmission of various viruses, such as hepatitis, HIV, and others. The recombinant products are essentially free of viruses because they are prepared by genetic engineering in a controlled laboratory setting. They appear to be as effective as the plasma source concentrates, although presently they are much more expensive than the other products (*USP DI*, 2005).

factor VIII
(Koate-HP, Recombinate, Kogenate-FS)
Indications
In the treatment or prevention of hemophilia A, factor VIII administration is based on replacing the missing plasma clotting factor to control and prevent bleeding.

Pharmacokinetics/Dosing
When administered IV, factor VIII has a distribution half-life of 2.4 to 8 hours and an elimination half-life of 8.4 to 19.3 hours. The time to peak effect is between 1 and 2 hours after IV administration.

The dosage of factor VIII must be individualized according to the client's weight, severity of the deficiency, and the amount of blood loss. During hemorrhage, the dosage is adjusted so that a level of 25% of normal levels of factor VIII can produce hemostasis. Clients who develop inhibitors to factor VIII may not respond to factor VIII therapy. After careful evaluation of the client, the administration of antiinhibitor coagulant complex, which reduces factor VIII inhibitors, may be indicated to correct this condition.

Adverse Effects
Mild to severe allergic reactions have been reported, such as bronchospasm, elevated temperature, chills, or rash. Other adverse effects that may be related to the rate of infusion include headache, increased heart rate, tingling of fingers, fainting, lethargy, sedation, hypotension, back pain, nausea or vomiting, visual disturbances, and chest constriction. No significant drug interactions are reported with factor VIII.

antiinhibitor coagulant complex
(Autoplex, Feiba VH)
Antiinhibitor coagulant complex is made from pooled human plasma. It contains variable quantities of clotting factors and kinin system factors and has been standardized to help correct clotting time in factor VIII–deficient individuals or to treat factor VIII–deficient individuals who have plasma-containing inhibitors to factor VIII.

Indications
Antiinhibitor coagulant complex is indicated for clients with factor VIII inhibitors who are bleeding or are being prepared for surgery. Approximately 10% of factor VIII–deficient individuals have inhibitors to factor VIII. Clients with factor VIII inhibitor levels greater than 10 Bethesda Units (BU) are usually treated with this product.

Pharmacokinetics/Dosing
Antiinhibitor coagulant complex is administered only by IV infusion. The recommended dosage varies from 25 to 100 units/kg depending on the site and severity of the hemorrhage. Check the current package insert or *USP DI* for specific recommendations.

Adverse Effects
Allergic reactions and hypersensitivity reactions (fever, chills, rash, hypotension) have been reported with the use of antiinhibitor coagulant complex. If antiinhibitor coagulant complex is administered too rapidly, the recipient may experience flushing, headache, and changes in BP and heart rate. These are indications to slow the rate of flow or to stop the infusion until the symptoms disappear. Concurrent administration with epsilon-aminocaproic acid or tranexamic acid is not recommended.

Nursing Management
Weigh the benefits of the antiinhibitor complex against the risk of hepatitis associated with its administration. (See Nursing Management of Antihemophilic Factors on p. 620.) The client is also at risk for the potential complications of thrombotic complications such as DIC, MI, and DVT. Because this complex is prepared from human plasma, the risk of transmitting hepatitis, HIV, and other viral diseases exists.

factor IX complex
(Mononine, Proplex T)
Factor IX complex is a purified plasma fraction prepared from pooled units of plasma. It contains factors II, VII, IX, and X, which are known as the vitamin K coagulation factors.

Indications
Factor IX complex is used for therapy during hemorrhage or before surgery in individuals with a deficiency of these factors. It is also indicated for hemophilia B in which factor IX (Christmas disease) is deficient. Factor IX complex is used to prevent or control bleeding in individuals with factor IX deficiency. It is also used to treat clients with

bleeding problems that have inhibitors to factor VIII and will reverse the hemorrhage induced by coumarin anticoagulants.

Pharmacokinetics/Dosing

Factor IX has an elimination half-life of 18 to 32 hours; the time to peak effect after IV administration is 10 to 30 minutes. Factor IX should be administered slowly by IV injection or IV infusion. The dosage is individualized according to the client's coagulation assay, which is performed before treatment. Check current references for specific dosing recommendations.

Adverse Effects

The adverse effects of factor IX include chills and fever, especially when large doses are given. Thrombosis and disseminated intravascular coagulation (DIC) have occurred as a result of the administration of factor IX. MI, PE, and anaphylaxis have also been reported.

Nursing Management of Antihemophilic Factors

Assessment It must be determined that the client has hemophilia A as it is the only indication for factor VIII or AHF, the treatment or prophylaxis of bleeding in these clients. If the client has developed antibodies to AHF to the level of 5 to 10 BU/mL, which about 15% those having received AHF do, then alternative therapies would be factor IX complex concentrates, or porcine AHF (Linker, 2003). Collaboration with the client and/or family is necessary. Although almost all of the plasma-derived AHF products currently available are purified, they are made from pooled sources and no procedure has been shown to be totally effective in removing the risk of viral infections. The alternatives to factor VIII, such as factor IX may still transmit hepatitis A and other viruses. Hemophilia B requires a deficiency of factor IX to be replaced.

There are no drugs that would contraindicate the use of these factors, but concurrent administration of aminocaproic acid or tranexamic acid is not recommended because such a combination would increase the risk of thrombotic complications.

A baseline clinical assessment includes an assessment of the client's bleeding or risk of bleeding before dental/surgical procedures, factor VIII or IX determinations, and coagulations studies; aPTT, plasma fibrinogen, and platelet counts.

Nursing Diagnosis The client is at risk for altered comfort (headache, increased heart rate, tingling of fingers, fainting, lethargy, sedation, hypotension, back pain, nausea, or vomiting) and the potential complications of allergic response and thrombotic complications such as DIC, MI, and DVT. Depending on the preparation of these factors, the risk of transmitting hepatitis and other viral diseases exists.

Planning The client receiving antihemophilic factor therapy will:

- Experience decreased risk or severity of hemorrhage.
- Remain free from injury related to the factor therapy.
- Be adherent to necessary lifestyle changes and factor therapy.

- Demonstrate adequate knowledge regarding the risks associated with factor therapy and its potential adverse effects.

Implementation

Monitoring Observe for adverse effects during IV therapy (flushing, hypotension, symptoms of allergic response). Monitor the client's vital signs over the course of administration. Adverse effects are related to the rate of administration. Slow the rate of flow or stop the infusion until the symptoms of flushing, headache, and alterations of blood pressure and pulse disappear. Review laboratory results as available; antibody determinations will determine that adequate concentrations have been achieved for the client. Periodic determinations of factor VIII antibodies will help to predict the client's ability to respond to AHF therapy (<10 BU/mL may receive increased amounts of AHF, >10 BU/mL not likely to respond to AHF). Also monitor hematocrit and platelet counts.

Intervention Refrigerate the factor concentrate until ready for use, but do not freeze it. Do not refrigerate after reconstitution, because the active ingredient may precipitate. Warm the concentrate and diluent to room temperature before reconstitution. Gently rotate (do not shake) the vial containing the concentrate and diluent until it is completely dissolved. This may take as long as 5 to 10 minutes. Because the factor concentrate is filtered before administration, the active components will be filtered out if it is not fully dissolved. Although factor concentrate remains stable for 12 to 24 hours at room temperature after reconstitution, it should be used within 3 hours. Do not mix it with other medications. Factor concentrate is for IV infusion only.

If factor therapy is administered too rapidly, the recipient may experience flushing, headache, and changes in blood pressure and heart rate. These are indications to slow the rate of flow or to stop the infusion until the symptoms disappear.

Education Instruct the client to wear a Medic Alert bracelet to alert medical personnel in an emergency situation that factor therapy may be required. Encourage clients with newly diagnosed hemophilia to be vaccinated for hepatitis A and B.

It is common for families to learn to manage factor concentrate therapy at home. Parents may learn to infuse factor for younger children, and older children and adult clients may learn self-administration. This requires extensive client education in home IV therapy beyond the scope of this text; see a home health care text for detail.

Evaluation The expected outcome of factor concentrate therapy is that the client's appropriate plasma factor levels will be adequate and the client will not experience any abnormal bleeding. The client will state the rationale for the use of factor concentrate therapy, adverse effects, how to monitor for the occurrence of adverse effects, and the importance of collaboration with the health team for follow-up appointments and appropriate laboratory studies.

✳ **What drugs are available to help reduce bleeding risk?**
Hemostatic agents are compounds used to hasten clot formation to reduce bleeding. The purpose of these agents is to control the rapid loss of blood. They are divided into IV agents for a systemic effect and topically administered agents for a local effect. Specific agents that affect gastric acidity or offer protection to the gastric mucosa to reduce upper GI bleeding are discussed in Chapter 40.

Systemic Hemostatics

Agents used systemically to hasten clot formation are often used to help manage care for clients at high risk for bleeding, including post surgical interventions where bleeding risk may be high. Available systemic hemostatic agents include aminocaproic acid (Amicar), tranexamic acid (Cyklokapron) and aprotinin (Trasylol).

aminocaproic acid [a mee noe ka **proe** ik]
(Amicar)
Aminocaproic acid is a synthetic compound that inhibits fibrinolysis when excessive bleeding occurs. This drug acts as a competitive antagonist of plasminogen, therefore reducing the conversion of plasminogen to plasmin or fibrinolysin. To a lesser degree, it directly inhibits plasmin (fibrinolysin) by noncompetitive mechanisms.

Indications
Aminocaproic acid is used in the treatment of hyperfibrinolysis-induced hemorrhage such as fibrinolytic bleeding after heart surgery, prostatectomy, nephrectomy, and for hematologic disorders such as aplastic anemia, hepatic cirrhosis, and neoplastic disease states. Although not an approved indication, it has also been used as a specific antidote for an overdose of fibrinolytic drugs.

Pharmacokinetics/Dosing
Aminocaproic acid is absorbed orally and reaches a peak concentration within 2 hours. The therapeutic serum concentration is 130 mcg/mL to inhibit systemic hyperfibrinolysis or 150 to 300 mcg/mL to prevent recurrent subarachnoid hemorrhage. It is excreted mainly by the kidneys. The recommended adult dosage of aminocaproic acid is 5 g PO or parenterally (IV infusion) initially, followed by 1 g/hr for up to 8 hours or until the desired response is achieved. The maximum dosage is 30 g/24 hr. The pediatric dosage (oral or parenteral) is 100 mg/kg body weight the first hour followed by 33.3 mg/kg/hr up to 18 g/m²/24 hr.

Adverse Effects
The adverse effects of aminocaproic acid include nausea; diarrhea; menstrual difficulties; increased weakness; severe muscle pain; a decrease in urination; edema of the face, feet, or lower legs; unusual weight gain; slow or irregular heart rate; abdominal pain; rash; stuffy nose; tinnitus; bloodshot eyes; and thrombosis.

Drug Interactions
Concurrent use of estrogens or hormonal contraception may increase the risk for thromboembolic events when aminocaproic acid is used.

Nursing Management
Assessment
Aminocaproic acid is contraindicated for use in clients with active intravascular clotting because of the risk of serious thrombus formation. It is used cautiously in individuals with a history or predisposition to thrombosis or in those with cardiac disease (may cause hypotension and bradycardia), hepatic disease (may make diagnosing the cause of bleeding more difficult), renal disease (may accumulate) or sensitivity to the drug.

Assess the female client's current drug regimen for estrogen or estrogen-containing contraceptives, because they will increase the risk for thrombus formation if administered concurrently with aminocaproic acid. Avoid concurrent use. Antifibrinolytic agents are

mutually antagonistic. Use of aminocaproic acid with factor IX complex and antiinhibitor coagulant complex may increase the risk of thrombotic complications.

Assess baseline vital signs and coagulation studies initially and periodically during administration.

Nursing Diagnosis
With the administration of aminocaproic acid, the client is at risk for development of the following nursing diagnoses/collaborative problems: impaired comfort (headache, myopathy, tinnitus, stuffy nose, rash, nausea, abdominal cramping, or unusual menstrual cramping); diarrhea; impaired urinary elimination related to bladder obstruction caused by blood clot formation; fatigue; sexual dysfunction (dry ejaculation); risk for injury related to hypotension; and the potential complications of renal failure (sudden decrease in urinary output, edema) or thromboembolism (sudden headache; pains in chest, groin, or legs; sudden shortness of breath; slurred speech; vision changes; or weakness of arm or leg).

Planning
The client receiving aminocaproic acid will:
- Experience reduction in bleeding tendencies without a thrombotic episode.
- Demonstrate adequate knowledge of aminocaproic acid therapy and its potential adverse effects.

Implementation
Monitoring
Observe the client for signs of thromboembolic complications such as thrombophlebitis, pulmonary embolus, MI, and CVA. Monitor for the signs and symptoms of the previously listed nursing diagnoses. Aminocaproic acid therapy is usually discontinued when bleeding stops or when laboratory values of fibrinolysis indicate that the drug is no longer necessary.
Intervention
Dilute before administering IV. Administer slowly; an infusion that is too rapid may result in hypotension or bradycardia. Take care with insertion and positioning of the infusion needle to minimize thrombophlebitis. The syrup form of the drug may be used as an oral rinse to prevent bleeding during dental and oral surgery in clients with hemophilia.
Education
Inform the client of the purpose of the medication and subjective symptoms to report, such as headache, dizziness, tinnitus, and abdominal cramping.

Evaluation
The expected outcome of aminocaproic acid therapy is that the client's laboratory values for fibrinolysis will be within normal limits and that the client will have no signs of bleeding. The client states the rationale for the use of aminocaproic acid and its adverse effects.

tranexamic acid [tran ex am **ik**]
(Cyklokapron)
Tranexamic acid is a competitive inhibitor of plasminogen activation; at high doses, it is a noncompetitive inhibitor of plasmin. Its effects are similar to aminocaproic acid, but it is approximately 5 to 10 times more potent in vitro.

Indications
Tranexamic acid is used after dental surgery in clients with hemophilia to reduce or prevent bleeding episodes.

Pharmacokinetics/Dosing
Peak plasma levels are reached 3 hours after oral administration; the peak plasma level is 8 mcg/mL after a 1-g dose. The duration of action in serum is 7 to 8 hours, and excretion is by the kidneys. The dosage before dental surgery for adolescents and adults with hemophilia is 25 mg/kg PO three or four times daily, starting 1 day before the planned dental procedure. Clotting factors VIII or IX should also be given before surgery. Postsurgically, the dosage is 25 mg/kg PO three or four times daily for 2 to 8 days. Availability of the oral formulation of tranexamic acid is limited and is no longer marketed in the United States. The parenteral postsurgical dose is

usually reserved for persons who are unable to use the oral product. By injection, the dosage is 10 mg/kg IV before surgery and 10 mg/kg IV postsurgically three or four times daily for 2 to 8 days.

Adverse Effects

The adverse effects of tranexamic acid include nausea, vomiting, and diarrhea. Visual disturbance, thrombosis, and menstrual discomfort have been infrequently reported.

Drug Interactions

Similar to aminocaproic acid.

Nursing Management

In addition to the previous discussion of the nursing management of aminocaproic acid therapy, tranexamic acid places the client at risk for visual disturbances. For this reason ophthalmologic examinations (visual acuity, color vision, eye grounds, and visual fields) are suggested before and periodically during therapy. It is recommended that administration of the drug be discontinued if visual changes occur or if thromboembolic complications occur. Tranexamic acid, as an IV medication, should not be mixed with blood or added to any solution containing penicillin.

aprotinin [a **pro** ti nin]

(Trasylol)

Aprotinin is a proteinase inhibitor obtained from bovine lung that directly prevents fibrinolysis by inhibiting plasmin and kallikrein, an enzyme of the renal cortex.

Indications

Aprotinin is used in cardiopulmonary bypass surgery to reduce blood loss and the need for blood transfusions.

Pharmacokinetics/Dosing

Aprotinin is administered IV and is rapidly distributed in the extracellular space with a terminal half-life between 5 and 10 hours. It is slowly metabolized by lysosomes in the kidneys and excreted primarily in the urine. The recommended adult dosage is 10,000 Kallikrein inhibitor units (KIU) (1 mL) as a test IV dose first, administered at least 10 minutes before the loading dose. If no allergic-type reaction occurs, all other dosages should be administered via a central venous line, and no medications should be given in this line. See the current *USP DI* or the package insert for dosing recommendations.

Adverse Effects

Adverse effects are rare but include allergic-type reactions (skin rash), and anaphylaxis (respiratory difficulties, nausea, tachycardia, hypotension, bronchospasm).

Drug Interactions

Similar to aminocaproic acid. Additionally, aprotinin may interfere with the activated coagulation time (ACT), which is sometimes used during cardiac surgery to assess the degree of anticoagulation of heparin. Aprotinin blocks the fibrinolytic action of alteplase and other fibrinolytics. The antihypertensive effects of ACE inhibitor therapy (e.g., captopril) may be blunted by concurrent aprotinin.

Nursing Management

Assessment

Determine if the client is allergic to aprotinin by obtaining a history and administering a test dose. Ensure that the client receives a test dose (1 mL) IV at least 10 minutes before a loading dose is administered. There is an increased risk of allergic reactions with reexposure to the drug.

Review the client's current medication profile to determine drug-drug interactions, such as fibrinolytic agents that will increase the risk for hemorrhage.

Assess the client's pulse, blood pressure, respirations, breath sounds, and skin for color, temperature, and other indicators of peripheral perfusion. A baseline ECG and renal and hepatic function studies should be performed.

Nursing Diagnosis

The client receiving aprotinin is at risk for the potential complication of anaphylaxis.

Planning

The client receiving aprotinin will:
- Experience reduction in bleeding tendencies without a thrombotic episode.
- Demonstrate adequate knowledge of aprotinin therapy and its potential adverse effects.

Implementation

Monitoring

Continue to monitor the client by the indicators in the baseline assessment and ACT and activated partial prothrombin time (aPTT). Monitor closely for anaphylaxis that may occur even with a negative test dose.

Intervention

For clients with reexposure to aprotinin, a prophylactic dose of an H_1 histamine antagonist is recommended before the loading dose of aprotinin, even after a successful response to a test dose. After a loading dose over 20 to 30 minutes, a continuous infusion of 50 mL/hr is used. All IV doses are to be administered through a central venous line, and no other medication should be administered through the same line.

Education

Inform the client of the purpose of aprotinin and any subjective symptoms that should be reported, such as palpitations and beginning dyspnea.

Evaluation

The expected outcome of aprotinin therapy is that the client will show no evidence of blood loss or anaphylaxis, and the pulse, blood pressure, and ECG will remain within normal limits. The client states the rationale for the use of aprotinin and its adverse effects.

Topical Hemostatics

Topical hemostatic agents are often used during surgical procedures to help limit excessive blood loss. Various agents and delivery systems are available.

absorbable gelatin sponge

(Gelfoam)

Absorbable gelatin sponge is a specially prepared, nonantigenic gelatin capable of holding many times its weight in whole blood. It is used in thin strips to control capillary bleeding and may be left in place in a surgical wound because it is completely absorbed in 4 to 6 weeks. It should be well moistened with isotonic saline solution or thrombin solution before being applied to a bleeding surface. Its presence does not induce excessive scar formation. Sterile technique must be used to avoid infection.

When inserted into cavities or tissue spaces, the gelatin sponge reduces bleeding by acting as a tampon. Contact with the sponge damages platelets, liberating the thromboplastin needed for clot formation. This product completely dissolves within 2 to 5 days when applied to bleeding areas on the skin or in the nose, rectum, or vagina.

An absorbable gelatin sponge is indicated in surgical procedures as an adjunct to hemostasis when bleeding is not controlled by ligature or when such methods are impractical. It is also used by dentists to aid in hemostasis.

Insertion of the gelatin sponge in the prostatic cavity promotes hemostasis in open prostatic surgery. The gelatin sponge may provide a site for infection. Monitor the surgical incision and implantation site closely for redness, swelling, or discomfort, and for signs of recurrent bleeding.

No significant drug interactions have been reported. This product is available in different sizes and diameters. Application instructions and size depend on the area to be treated.

absorbable gelatin powder

(Gelfoam)

A sterile absorbable gelatin powder (Gelfoam) is also available to promote hemostasis. This powder can be made into a paste to control bleeding from bone areas when standard procedures such as ligatures are ineffective or impractical. It is also used to treat chronic leg ulcers and decubitus ulcers.

oxidized cellulose
(Oxycel, Surgicel)

Oxidized cellulose is a specially treated form of surgical gauze or cotton that exerts a hemostatic effect but is absorbable when buried in the tissues. The hemostatic action is caused by the formation of an artificial clot by cellulosic acid. Absorption of oxidized cellulose occurs between the second and the seventh days following implantation, although the absorption of large amounts of blood-soaked material may take 6 weeks or longer. Oxidized cellulose is valuable in controlling bleeding during surgery that involves organs such as the liver, pancreas, spleen, kidney, thyroid, and prostate. Its hemostatic action is not increased by the addition of other hemostatic agents. It should not be used as a surface dressing except for the control of bleeding, because cellulosic acid inhibits the growth of epithelial tissue. It also interferes with bone regeneration and therefore should not be implanted in fractures.

No significant drug interactions are reported. Do not moisten the oxidized cellulose, and use sterile technique when applying or inserting it. Serious adverse reactions are related to the site of application, the amount used, and the pressure applied to a blood vessel or specific area. Careful application and monitoring are necessary to reduce complications such as obstruction, necrosis, and stenosis. A burning sensation has been reported when used after nasal polyp removal or hemorrhoidectomy. Headache, stinging, and sneezing may also occur.

microfibrillar collagen hemostat
(Avitene)

Microfibrillar collagen hemostat is an absorbable topical hemostatic substance that will attract platelets and platelet aggregation in the area when placed on a bleeding surface, forming thrombi. It is used as an adjunct to hemostasis during surgery when ligature or standard procedures are ineffective or impractical.

Adhesions, allergic or foreign body reactions, hematomas, or infections such as abscesses may occur. Monitor the client closely, because these conditions may cause serious problems. No significant drug interactions have been reported.

In general, microfibrillar collagen hemostat is applied directly on the source of bleeding in a dry form. Do not moisten or wet this substance, and do not resterilize it. Apply pressure over the area with a dry sponge for a minute or more. Use dry forceps to handle it because it will adhere to wet gloves or instruments. Do not use gloved fingers to apply the necessary pressure.

thrombin
(Thrombostat)

Thrombin is a hemostatic agent prepared as a sterile powder; it is obtained from bovine prothrombin that has been treated with thromboplastin in the presence of calcium. Thrombin catalyzes the conversion of fibrinogen to fibrin. It has several additional mechanisms, which may include stimulating the release, reaction, and aggregation of platelets. It is used topically to treat capillary bleeding. It has also been used during various surgeries with absorbable gelatin sponge for hemostasis.

Febrile and allergic-type reactions have been reported when thrombin is used for epistaxis. No significant drug interactions are reported.

Thrombin may be applied topically as a powder or solution. Concentration of the preparation varies with its use (see the package insert).

Nursing Management of Topical Hemostatics

Assessment Ascertain whether or not the client is sensitive to bovine products.

Nursing Diagnosis The client undergoing topical hemostatic therapy may be at risk for infection and the potential complications of an allergic reaction and bleeding related to the ineffectiveness of the therapy.

Planning The client receiving topical hemostatics will:
- Experience reduction in bleeding.
- Not experience adverse effects of the topical hemostatic such as infection and an allergic reaction.

Implementation
Monitoring Monitor the client for recurrent bleeding, infection, and allergic reaction.

Intervention Sponge—do not wipe—all blood from the recipient surface before applying the topical hemostatic. If applied as a powder, thrombin may need to be pulverized with a sterile instrument before use. To avoid disturbing the clotting, do not sponge once the hemostatic agent is applied. Some agents can be combined; thrombin may be used in association with an absorbable gelatin foam. In this case the saturated sponge is applied to the bleeding area for 10 to 15 seconds to promote hemostasis. Use thrombin solution within a few hours of reconstitution, or freeze it and use within 48 hours. Do not inject thrombin into large blood vessels, because extensive intravascular clotting and even death may result.

Evaluation The expected outcome of thrombin therapy is that the client's bleeding will diminish and eventually cease without experiencing the adverse effects of infection and/or allergy. The client will state the rationale for the hemostatic therapy and follow-up that is prescribed.

Blood and Blood Components

The bloodstream is the main mode of transport and distribution in the body. As such, it functions to deliver vital nutrients, water, and oxygen from the digestive and respiratory systems to all body parts. Wastes are retrieved for excretion by the bloodstream. In the kidneys, the bloodstream provides the hydrostatic pressure necessary to create urine as an excretory vehicle for those waste products. It conveys hormones from endocrine glands and enzymes, vitamins, buffers, and other biochemical substances to target areas. The bloodstream buffers and regulates the body's heat exchange processes by absorbing and transferring core body heat to the surface for dissipation, and it buffers the body's acid-base balance. The bloodstream also carries components such as platelets, blood cells, and antibodies to sites where a sudden need for these exists, such as in hemorrhage, inflammation, or infection.

The bloodstream creates oncotic or colloid osmotic pressure to regulate the volume of interstitial fluids. It also transports therapeutic additives such as medications, fluids, electrolytes, and nutrients to their respective sites of action.

Abnormal States of Blood Components

Normally, a thrifty bodily balance is maintained between the production and loss, attrition, or excretion of all components that comprise the bloodstream. Pathologic conditions result from a disturbance in production or an excessive loss or excretion of one or more components. Hemorrhage results in a generally impoverished bloodstream and may significantly alter many body functions. Impaired production or the increased destruction of any one component may impinge on one or more functions. All this is a matter of degree. If the impairment is minor or is detected early, correction of the cause and replenishment by natural or therapeutic means may restore functioning.

Naturally harmful or foreign substances may build up in the bloodstream when excretory systems fail (e.g., renal failure) or when metabolizing capabilities fail (e.g., liver failure). Some examples of abnormal states of blood components follow.

Depending on the individual's size and preexisting blood integrity, an acute whole blood loss of more than 500 mL is manifested by signs of anemia. Chronic, gradual, and unnoticed blood loss from GI tract malignancy, ulcers, or hemorrhoids may be compensated for naturally, or iron deficiency anemia may develop. Signs of anemia usually reflect the true importance of RBC loss. Deficiencies in intake or in the functioning of certain essential nutritional elements may result in iron deficiency anemia or one of the megaloblastic anemias, which usually are caused by deficiencies in vitamin B_{12} or folic acid. A pathologic overabundance of erythrocytes can be compensation for longstanding hypoxia from pulmonary or cardiac disease, certain tumors, or polycythemia vera. Delayed or disordered production of erythrocytes (aplastic anemia) may result from disorders of the reticuloendothelial system, primarily the bone marrow, which is responsible for their systematic production. The bone marrow is particularly vulnerable to certain drugs, poisons, and antineoplastic agents. On the other hand, too-rapid destruction of erythrocytes can lead to hemolytic anemia.

Leukocytes also are lost in hemorrhage, but reductions in their numbers most often are associated with certain specific conditions. Each of the five types of WBCs—neutrophils, eosinophils, basophils, lymphocytes, and monocytes—is associated with different disorders. For example, abnormally low neutrophil counts are associated with certain aplastic diseases, and with acute reactions to drugs such as sulfonamides, propylthiouracil, and chloramphenicol. Excessively high neutrophil counts are found primarily with bacterial infections, and with some inflammatory disorders, leukemia, and hyperplastic disorders.

Thrombocytes may be present in inadequate numbers because of their rapid destruction, typically caused by idiopathic thrombocytopenia purpura. Conversely, excessive platelet counts are associated most often with hyperplastic disorders, iron deficiency anemia, splenectomy, and chronic inflammatory conditions such as tuberculosis. Other factors crucial to the clotting process may be absent in hemophilia and similar disorders.

Losses of the liquid portion of the blood can create dehydration problems, impede metabolic processes that function only through the use of hydrogen or oxygen molecules, or subvert hydrodynamic and hydraulic processes.

In addition to hemorrhage, plasma proteins may be lost through burn wounds or wound drainage or may be insufficient because of a lack of adequate available substrates such as amino acids. The results vary depending on the type of plasma protein and may include deficiencies in immune status, blood viscosity, or colloid osmotic pressure (oncotic pressure).

Replacement Therapies

Therapy to replace all or certain components of the bloodstream is a common practice in most health facilities. Because blood is considered a tissue, transfusions are technically tissue transplants. The usual treatment of choice is replacement of the blood component that is deficient rather than whole blood, because the body is better able to replace intravascular fluids than formed elements of the blood. Transfusing only the depleted blood fraction serves two other purposes: (1) it prevents fluid overload in high-risk individuals such as older adults and those with cardiovascular or renal disease, and (2) it more efficiently uses the remaining blood fractions for other clients' needs. Table 30-4 outlines the indications for this therapy. When a client is to receive blood, the nurse is largely responsible for its safe administration.

Nursing Management of Blood and Blood Component Replacement Therapies

Assessment Obtain the client history regarding previous transfusions and the client's response to them. Report any history of an adverse effect to the prescriber and the blood bank. Assess the client for adequacy of venous access. Gather baseline data about the client's blood studies and vital signs before administration, and observe the general appearance and demeanor of the client.

Nursing Diagnosis The client is at risk for injury related to a hemolytic or allergic reaction (anaphylactic shock), excess fluid volume (pulmonary congestion, circulatory overload), a response to aged blood (hyperkalemia), transfusion-related lung injury (TRALI), or infection.

Planning The client receiving blood products will:
- Experience relief from symptoms that necessitated the administration of the blood product.
- Remain free from injury from the administration of the blood product.
- Demonstrate adequate knowledge of the blood product to be administered and its potential adverse effects that are reportable to the health care provider.

TABLE 30-4 INDICATIONS FOR COMMON BLOOD COMPONENT THERAPIES

Component	Indications
Whole blood	Hemorrhage, hypovolemic shock
Fresh whole blood	Multiple transfusions, exchange transfusions; priming agent for hemodialysis machines (normal saline may also be used)
Packed red blood cells	Transfused when whole blood could result in circulatory overload
Deglycerolized or washed red cells	Transfused when hypersensitivity reactions are likely, as in immunosuppressed clients and those with a history of reactions or extreme hypersensitivity
Fresh-frozen plasma (FFP)	Clotting deficiencies, especially factors V and VII; blood volume expansion in burns, shock, or protein deficiencies (believed to be overused for these deficiencies); warfarin overdose
Plasma exchange (plasmapheresis): blood drawn off, cleansed, and components returned	Immune-related disorders: multiple myeloma, glomerulonephritis, systemic lupus erythematosus, rheumatoid arthritis, myasthenia gravis
Plasma expanders (Dextran—large polysaccharide polymer)	Temporary volume expansion in hemorrhagic shock states (sole use for Dextran 70 or 75); not a substitute for blood or plasma
Granulocytes	Granulocyte counts below 500/mm^3
Platelets	Platelet counts at or below 20,000/mm^3
Cryoprecipitate (fresh-frozen plasma precipitate; contains factors I and VIII)	Hemophilia, fibrinogen deficiency, von Willebrand's disease
Antihemophilic factor concentrate	Treatment of hemophilia; preferred over fresh-frozen plasma
Factor VIIa	Treatment of hemophilia A and B in clients who have developed inhibitor antibodies to factor VIII
Factor IX complex	Hemophilia B; deficiencies of clotting factors II, VII, X; warfarin overdose
Plasma protein fraction (PPF)	Hypovolemic shock, protein replacement, burns, adult respiratory distress syndrome, dehydration, and hypoalbuminemia; as an additive to complement packed cells when necessary
Fibrinogen	When fibrinogen levels are insufficient for adequate control of bleeding
Albumin	Blood volume expansion by oncotic pressure; prevention and treatment of cerebral edema
Gamma globulins	Exposure to hepatitis; to prevent complications of mumps

Implementation

Monitoring As administration begins, remain with the client and observe the client closely for reactions for 15 minutes or more while the flow rate is kept at a keep-open rate, because transfusion reactions are more likely to occur within this timeframe. Assess and record vital signs before starting the transfusion and several times during the first 15 minutes. If a reaction occurs, stop the transfusion and administer the prescribed corrective measures. Observe the client for the development of the following:

1. Immune-mediated transfusion reactions
   - Allergic transfusion reactions (cutaneous): local erythema, urticaria, pruritus caused by hypersensitivity to donor protein. Antihistamines are used as therapy

or prophylactically, it may or may not be necessary to stop the transfusion
- Anaphylactic transfusion reaction caused by hypersensitivity to donor proteins; apprehension; restlessness; flushed skin; increased pulse and respiratory rates; burning sensations, fever, chills, dyspnea, urticaria, swellings of the skin, face, or throat, pruritus, shock, profound hypotension, cardiac arrest. Discontinue the transfusion immediately, administer 0.3 to 0.5 mL of subcutaneous epinephrine (1:1000); provide hemodynamic and respiratory support.
- Immune-mediated hemolytic transfusion reactions: hemolytic event from the administration of incompatible blood evidenced by fever accompanied by chills, tachypnea, cyanosis, pain at infusion site,

chest, back or flank, abdominal pain; symptoms will depend on the amount of blood transfused. Discontinue the transfusion immediately, rapid administration of fluids may avoid progression to renal failure. May require hemodialysis and red cell or plasma exchange. Analgesics, diuretics, and pressor agents may be used.

- Febrile nonhemolytic reaction: It is the most common transfusion reaction, 43% to 75% of all reactions (Blecher, 2003). It is a reaction between preformed recipient WBC antibodies directed against transfused WBC in the product or cytokines that accumulate in the blood bag during storage. The symptoms are fever 1° C above baseline, with or without chills, and no other causes of fever, headache, or flushing. Antipyretic premedication will prevent this reaction.

- Cardio-respiratory events: Transfusion-related acute lung injury (TRALI) is thought to be sequestration of WBCs in pulmonary microvasculature that leads to vascular permeability and pulmonary edema (Kuriyan & Carson, 2004). It is evidenced by dyspnea, cyanosis, hypotension, fever, and chill with bilateral pulmonary edema occurring within 1 to 2 hours of transfusion and needs to be differentiated from volume overload and acute respiratory distress syndrome (ARDS). Because the disease is self-limiting, ventilatory assistance and circulatory support are needed and diuretics are contraindicated. Circulatory overload on the other hand is evidenced by dyspnea, cough, hypertension, tachycardia, and headache, requires treatment with diuretics, oxygen, and perhaps phlebotomy.

2. Nonimmune-mediated transfusion reactions
- Noninfectious, nonimmune transfusion reaction: It is caused by the hemolyzation of RBCs related to unacceptable flow rates and pressures, inadequate catheter size, too much heat or cold, or being mixed with hypo- or hypertonic solutions in a common venous access. Potassium imbalance, acid-based imbalance, hypothermia, or circulatory overload may occur. Administer blood only with 0.9% saline.

- Acute infectious (bacterial), nonimmune transfusion reaction: Bacterial contamination of the transfusion may result from donor infections, faulty aseptic technique during donor arm preparation, blood product storage, and transportation issues, or when the transfusion exceeds 4 hours. Signs and symptoms are high fever, shock, pain anywhere, and hemoglobinuria. Inspect blood products for clots, discoloration, and gas formation. Treatment is with antibiotics and supportive treatment of symptoms.

3. Delayed hemolytic transfusion reactions. These are immune-mediated events occurring about 1 week after transfusion with unexpected anemia, fever, chills, jaundice, asymptomatic falling hematocrit, or rising bilirubin. These effects may be prevented by the use of compatible RBCs.

4. Delayed nonhemolytic reactions: These reactions are varied.
- Platelet alloimmunization, very common in clients with hematologic disorders or cancers, occurs because of immunoglobulin (Ig) G directed against human leukocyte antigen (HLA), WBC, or platelet-specific antigens (Blecher, 2003). Fever and chills occur with shortened platelet survival. Affected clients are treated with antipyretics and crossmatch or HLA-matched platelets.

- Posttransfusion purpura: This severe thrombocytopenia is associated with life-threatening hemorrhages and occurs within 5 to 10 days of transfusion, usually of RBCs (Blecher, 2003). This complication occurs more commonly in women with a history of recent surgery associated with transfusions (Kuriyan & Carson, 2004). Spontaneous recovery typically occurs within 7 to 48 days. Treatment includes use of IgG or plasma exchanges and corticosteroids.

- Transfusion-associated graft-versus-host disease: This acute, and if severe, fatal complication occurs 2 to 30 days after transfusion and involves whole-body erythroderma, desquamation, nausea, vomiting, profuse diarrhea, liver dysfunction, and bone marrow failure. It is caused by transplantation of sufficient numbers of immunocompetent lymphocytes to immunocompromised clients. No effective therapy exists, but corticosteroids and cyclosporine are frequently tried. It can be prevented by gamma irradiation of blood products for susceptible clients.

- Transfusion-associated immunomodulation: WBCs produce cytokines during blood storage that may interfere with immune function that may increase the risk of recurrent cancer and bacterial infection (Claridge, Sawyer, Schulman, McLemore, & Young, 2002; Engoren et al., 2002; Taylor et al., 2002). However, the clinical significance regarding cancer recurrence and risk of bacterial infection awaits further data.

- Transfusional hemosiderosis: Hemosiderosis, or iron overload, is a risk for clients with thalassemias, other hemoglobinopathies, and bone marrow failure (Blecher, 2003). Iron overload may result in impairment of the liver, pancreas, and other endocrine glands, or cardiac involvement because each unit of RBCs contains 225 mg of iron. This can be prevented by chelation therapy of susceptible clients receiving many units of blood.

5. Transfusion-transmitted diseases, viral infections: Treatment is for the specific disease.
- HIV: There has been almost complete eradication of transfusion transmission of HIV with stringent donor eligibility and more sensitive testing for antibodies, antigens, and nucleic acid amplification (NAT) testing. The transmission rate is one per 2 million transfusions (Centers for Disease Control and Prevention, 2002).

- Hepatitis: Hepatitis A virus (HVA) infection is rarely transmitted through blood transfusion, which can only be prevented by widespread control of the disease. HAV is typically spread through fecally contaminated food and water and is more prevalent elsewhere, including Mexico and parts of the Caribbean. Hepatitis B (HBV) is uncommon because of routine testing of blood and donor screening. However, it is transmitted more commonly than HIV. The disease is expected to become less common with routine HBV vaccination of health care workers and children. However, the tests used to screen blood for the virus may be negative in HBV carriers, so a small number of recipients may still develop hepatitis B. Hepatitis C virus (HCV) leads to relatively mild acute disease. With NAT testing, the risk of receiving HCV from a unit of blood is reduced to about 1 in 2 million transfusions (Kuriyan & Carson, 2004).

- Cytomegalovirus (CMV): CMV is a virus belonging to the herpes family that may be transmitted by transfusion. Although such infection is usually mild, it could be serious or fatal in immunocompromised clients. Clients at high risk should only receive blood that tests negative for CMV.

6. Transfusion-transmitted diseases, parasitic and emerging infections: Because of global population shifts or travel, Chagas' disease and malaria are possible complications of blood transfusion. Screening for prevention prohibits donors who have had Chagas' disease and from people who have visited malarial areas in the past year or have emigrated from a malarial area in the last 3 years. A number of new infections that might be transmitted by blood transfusion are being investigated including Creutzfeldt-Jakob disease (CJD), West Nile virus, Ehrlichiosis, the human herpes virus family (Epstein-Barr virus, herpes virus 8) and parvovirus B19. Bioterrorism has also raised the possibility of transmission of anthrax from blood transfusion. Treatment is for the specific disease.

Frequent assessment of the needle insertion site is essential because the absorption of infiltrated blood is very slow. If no symptoms of reactions appear after the first 15 minutes, the flow rate may be calculated and set so that therapy is concluded in 30 to 120 minutes (volumes are usually between 250 and 500 mL). Continue to monitor vital signs and observe for symptoms throughout administration. The importance of the early detection of a transfusion reaction, particularly in a critically ill client, cannot be overemphasized.

Intervention Administer blood components promptly to ensure that the transfused product is fresh, uncoagulated, and without toxic breakdown products. Before administration, the product should remain out of the blood bank's refrigerator and untransfused for no longer than 30 minutes. Refrigeration in the standard hospital units or home refrigerator will not prevent deterioration. Blood and blood components must not lie unused at the nursing station but must be returned to the blood bank refrigerator if administration

has not started within 30 minutes. A unit of whole blood or packed RBCs cannot be returned to a blood bank if it has been out of a monitored environment (1° C to 6° C) for more than 30 minutes. Once the infusion has started, whole blood or packed RBCs should be transfused within 2 hours, 4 hours at the most.

Because incompatibility is a possibility, especially after multiple doses of these products, take precautions such as scrupulously comparing the product ordered with the label on the product before administration. The worst adverse reactions to blood transfusions often result from misidentification of the blood or the client. Although the procedures of various institutions vary, at least two persons (often two registered nurses) must verify the identification of blood product and client. This will vary with the administration of blood products in the home (see the Community and Home Health Considerations box below). Client identifica-

---

✸✸ Community and Home Health Considerations

Blood Component Administration

It is becoming increasingly common for whole blood, blood components, or expanders to be administered in the home setting. The administration of these substances allows for the restoration of blood volume or the replacement of serum, plasma, RBCs, platelets, or albumin in a more cost effective and comfortable environment for the client.

The client and caregiver(s) need to understand the purpose of the blood administration. Ask them if they understand the procedure and why it is being done. Assess the client's allergy history and ascertain any previous reactions to blood products.

Make the client comfortable in bed or in a reclining chair. Have the client void before the procedure begins. Check the blood bag information with the client identification with at least one other person. Check the bag for leaks. Select an appropriate site and perform the venipuncture using aseptic technique. See the discussion of nursing management for infusion techniques. Determine the drip rate per minute and time for blood completion. Administer the blood slowly for the first 15 minutes and monitor the client and vital signs carefully during this time. Monitor vital signs every hour while the blood is infusing; check the drip rate every 15 minutes. Assess the infusion site for infiltration. Assess the client for symptoms of transfusion reaction as discussed in the text. Change the blood tubing and filter if more than one unit is to be administered. Remove the IV needle or cannula after transfusion and ensure that it is intact. Document the procedure as described in the text.

If the client experiences any untoward symptoms, stop the transfusion and transfuse normal saline. Follow the health care agency protocols for emergency action. Stay with the client until the situation is resolved.

tion must match, and the prescriber's name, the blood type, the Rh factor, and the unit number. Note the Venereal Disease Research Laboratories' (VDRL) information and expiration date. Compare the client's identification bracelet or tag with the label on the container. A blood bank identification bracelet is also used as an additional means of correctly identifying the client, and to ensure that the client receives the correct blood product. (See the Medication Safety Alert box below.)

Nurses should be aware of transfusion hazards in certain blood-type combinations. Careful typing and cross-matching help to prevent serious complications. The incidence of transfusion reactions following transfusion with whole blood is approximately 2.5 times greater than the incidence of reactions following transfusion with packed RBCs. Additionally, whole blood contains antigenic leukocytes and serum proteins, which may produce allergic reactions (a risk of 1%). The donor and the recipient should be ABO- and Rh-compatible. About 85% of individuals possess the D antigen and are classified as Rh(D) positive; the remaining 15%, who lack the D antigen, are classified as Rh(D) negative. ABO antigen-

antibody reactions result from the following and must be avoided:

RECIPIENT'S BLOOD TYPE	SHOULD NOT RECEIVE
A	Type B or AB
B	Type A or AB
0	Any type except type 0

RECIPIENT'S BLOOD TYPE	REACTIONS WITH MULTIPLE TRANSFUSIONS
A	Type 0
B	Type 0
AB	Type A, B, or 0

Immediately report to the blood bank any discrepancies between the information on the compatibility tag, the unit of blood, and the prescriber's order on the clinical record; blood that is past its expiration date; or any signs of contamination.

Hypersensitivity is also common, because most of these products are essentially foreign proteins. Exceptions include autologous transfusions collected previously from the client's own blood or transfusions of inert, synthetic products. Diphenhydramine (Benadryl) 25 mg, taken orally or injected into blood transfusion tubing before the transfusion, is recommended to prevent mild allergic reactions.

Return the product to the blood bank or laboratory if the contents appear unusual because of discoloration, gas bubbles, or an overly full (gaseous) appearance. Mix the contents by gently upending the container once or twice; take care not to bruise or damage blood cells or other fragile components by squeezing or agitating the bag carelessly. Note that many of these agents require the concomitant use of a 170-mcg filter incorporated into the transfusion tubing to remove the debris and tiny clots found in the blood. Check the filter often to ensure that it is not clogged and slowing the transfusion. If the rate of transfusion is too slow, it may be necessary to use a filter with a larger surface area. This may also be necessary when administering packed RBCs because of the viscosity of the product. Access to the vein should be provided by fresh tubing and a needle no smaller than 19 gauge. However, a 22- or 23-gauge needle is recommended for adults with small veins and for children.

A normal saline solution should be hung in tandem with the blood product using a Y-set multiple lead tubing. Use the saline solution to prime the tubing before connecting it to the insertion site. Using straight tubing limits the possibility of stopping the transfusion while keeping the vein open if the client has an untoward response to the blood. Piggybacking on an established IV line is not recommended; there may be compatibility issues and it increases the risk of contamination, especially with the administration of multiple units of blood. Change the filter and administration set at least every 4 hours; do not transfuse more than 2 units per administration set.

Infuse approximately 60 mL of saline through the tubing before and after the transfusion. Do not use dextrose and other solutions with RBC products, because they may react with the product in the tubing to clump cells and cause hemolysis. When inserting the spike of the administration set

---

✦ Medication Safety Alert

Transfusion Errors

Despite the discussion of the complications of transfusions, the most common cause of adverse reactions from blood transfusions results from human errors (Callum et al., 2001; Linden, Wagner, Voytovich, & Sheehan, 2000). The major transfusion errors result from giving the wrong unit of blood, which may lead to a hemolytic reaction. Other events from human error include air embolism and circulatory overload. In pediatric populations, massive or excess transfusion results in metabolic derangement because of errors in judgment of size. And clients may be undertransfused by the overly cautious.

Hemolytic transfusion reactions resulting from administration of the wrong unit of blood may be prevented by strict adherence to factors affecting safety such as client identification, specimen collection, confirmation of sample identity and testing, issue from blood bank, blood administration and client monitoring, and handling of the transfusion reaction (Blecher, 2003). New York state reports erroneous transfusion of blood in 1 of 19,000 units. More than half are bedside errors, of which 13% were in collection of the wrong blood sample for crossmatching and 38% the administration of the right blood to the wrong client. Of these, 15% involve multiple errors (Linden et al., 2000).

New information technology systems are being developed to design error out of the transfusion process. One of these is a unique barcode on each client's wrist to identify the client's crossmatch blood samples and each unit of blood prepared for that client. Nurses then electronically match each unit of blood with the client's wrist identification before administering blood.

into the port of the blood bag, guide it straight into the container to avoid puncturing the side of the bag. Note that infusion pumps intended specifically for maintaining transfusion rates are safe and reliable when used with the appropriate tubing and filters. Raising the height of the container or applying a pressure sleeve to the bag (at pressures up to 300 mm Hg) is also useful to maintain transfusion flows at prescribed rates. Higher pressures may burst the bag. If use of a pressure bag is necessary, use the lowest effective pressure possible to avoid damaging blood components.

To maintain the prescribed infusion rate, agitate the blood by inverting the bag frequently during administration. A blood-warming device (up to 37° C [98.6° F]) is necessary if a rapid transfusion is to be made through a central venous catheter line. Do not administer any medications through the same tubing while any blood products are being infused.

Documentation should include the client's baseline vital signs before the transfusion was started; the signatures of the two persons who identified the client and the blood product; the blood product administered; the time the transfusion was started and completed; the total volume of fluid transfused, listing the starter solution separately; the client's response to

the transfusion; and any nursing interventions taken in response to an adverse reaction to the blood.

Be aware that the risks of nursing personnel contracting diseases such as hepatitis when accidentally injected with pooled blood, especially repeatedly, are not entirely known. Therefore use standard precautions when manipulating these products and their equipment.

If the client experiences any of the untoward symptoms previously discussed, stop the transfusion and infuse normal saline. Notify the prescriber. Continue to monitor vital signs, monitor intake and output, observe the client, and follow the health care organization's emergency measures. Obtain a blood sample and the first voided urine specimen after the reaction. Many agencies have a form that must be completed as part of agency policy when a reaction occurs.

Education Explain the transfusion procedure to the client, especially the reason why it has been ordered. Many older adults associate a blood transfusion with being critically ill and may be upset about the need for the transfusion. Ensure that a consent form for the procedure has been signed (Box 30-5).

BOX 30-5 LEGAL IMPLICATIONS: CONSENT FOR TRANSFUSION

Before any transfusion is given, informed consent should be obtained from the client or guardian. If a client is damaged by a transfusion administered without a valid consent, damages may be recovered even though the defendant did everything properly. The law is clear that ordinarily a physician has the sole and exclusive right to obtain a client's informed consent to surgery. However, who bears the responsibility to obtain the client's informed consent to a blood transfusion? Whose duty is it to apprise the client of all of the risks attendant to the transfusion of donated blood? Must the client be informed that there are several options, including donations from "anonymous" sources, direct donations (usually from family or friends), or an autologous donation (in which the client donates blood before surgery) for use during surgery? The informed consent process involves a discussion of transfusion-associated risks (including risks related to not receiving a transfusion), benefits, and alternatives.

In *Jones v. Philadelphia Coll. of Osteo. Med.* (813 F. Supp. 1125-PA [1993]) informed consent was at issue. On October 6, 1986, J. Jones was admitted to the hospital by his primary treating physician to undergo a lumbar myelogram to diagnose the cause of his severe low back pain. Following this examination his physician recommended surgery to alleviate his condition. During surgery Mr. Jones lost blood and received nine units of packed cells and two units of fresh frozen plasma. One of the units of fresh frozen plasma came from an "anonymous" donor who was infected with the HIV virus. Before his transfusion Mr. Jones was never advised by the physicians or the hospital of the potential risk of contracting acquired immune deficiency syndrome (AIDS) as a result of the use of contaminated blood products. He brought suit against the hospital and physicians involved in the surgery, alleging that he received HIV-contaminated blood

during the surgery. Although the risk of HIV is now negligible, risks for other viral infections are possible as discussed above.

The United States District Court for the Eastern District of Pennsylvania held that informed consent was necessary for blood transfusions. The law of Pennsylvania is that consent is valid only if the individual grants it after being fully apprised of such important matters as the nature of the therapy, the seriousness of the situation, the disease and organs involved, and the potential results of the treatment. In determining whether a client's consent was "informed," the standard is whether the physician disclosed all the facts, risks, and alternatives that a reasonable person in the situation would deem significant. In this state the doctrine of informed consent is limited to cases involving surgery or operative procedures. However, the Court held that a physician cannot inform a client of all of the risks of a surgical procedure without also informing him or her of the risks associated with blood transfusion when transfusion is a potential part of the procedure.

Although the Court held that only the primary treating physician could be held liable for failure to obtain informed consent, there was also a basis for liability on the part of the hospital. Because the hospital was bound by FDA regulations requiring it to obtain informed consent and because the hospital could also be held liable for battery (lack of informed consent) because it intended that the client come in contact with a foreign substance as a part of a planned procedure, the hospital had Mr. Jones sign two documents for informed consent for transfusion. In doing so the hospital "gratuitously undertook an obligation to obtain informed consent." Because of this the Court concluded that Mr. Jones may indeed have a valid claim against the hospital and the physician.

How would this knowledge of informed consent influence your nursing practice in relation to clients receiving blood transfusion?

Instruct the client to report any symptoms of an adverse reaction, such as nausea, chills, burning sensations, or headache.

Evaluation The client will experience increased hemoglobin and hematocrit levels without any adverse effects of the transfusion. One unit of whole blood typically raises the average adult's hemoglobin level by 1 to 1.5 g/dL and the hematocrit by 2% to 3%. The client states the rationale for the administration of the blood product and reportable adverse reactions.

Summary

This chapter reviewed substances that concern antiplatelet, anticoagulant, and fibrinolytic therapy, hemostatic agents, and blood component administration. Antiplatelet drugs are used for the treatment and prevention of ischemic events. The oral agents, including aspirin and clopidogrel, are used for both acute and chronic management although the II b/III a inhibitors are used for ACSs.

Anticoagulant therapy is primarily prophylactic; it acts to prevent fibrin deposits, thrombus extension, and thromboembolic complications by decreasing blood coagulability. Anticoagulants may be administered parenterally or orally. Administered parenterally, heparins act almost immediately but have a short duration of action (less than 4 hours). Warfarin is administered orally; the onset of action is slow (24 to 48 hours) and the duration is long (2 to 5 days). This allows heparin and warfarin to be used in a complementary fashion. They are often started on the same day; heparin is used when an immediate anticoagulant effect is needed, and its dosage is tapered off as the oral agent produces its full therapeutic effect. In the administration of both types of anticoagulants, the client has the potential for injury related to increased bleeding tendencies; nursing care focuses on the observation, protection, and education of the client to prevent injury. There are specific antidotes for both parenteral and oral anticoagulants: protamine sulfate is the antidote for heparin, and vitamin K is the antidote for the oral anticoagulants.

Whereas anticoagulants are used prophylactically, fibrinolytic agents are used to dissolve clots in the treatment of acute thromboembolic disorders. Fibrinolytic enzyme therapy with streptokinase, urokinase, alteplase, or anistreplase alters the hemostatic capability of the client to a greater extent than anticoagulant therapy; therefore when bleeding does occur, it is more severe and more difficult to control.

Hemostatic agents are compounds used to hasten clot formation to reduce bleeding and therefore control rapid blood loss. Both systemic and topical therapies are available. Aminocaproic acid, a hemostatic agent, has been used as an antidote for the fibrinolytic agents, but this use is not approved.

The antihemophilic agents are specific factors within the clotting process that can be used in replacement therapy for clients who have hemophilia, a deficiency of one or more plasma protein clotting factors. With accurate diagnosis of the specific missing factor, this replacement therapy has allowed for the successful management of these clients at home.

Blood transfusion is an important intervention for many critically ill clients, but it is not without adverse effects. The nurse's knowledge of the type of symptoms associated with these reactions, and the awareness that any symptom that occurs in the client during a transfusion is suspect until proven otherwise, is essential for client safety. Assessment of appropriate blood use criteria and strict adherence to standard policies and procedures for the client, sample, and product identification will minimize risks and make blood transfusions the beneficial therapy they were meant to be.

✳ Critical Thinking Questions

- Mary Brickland, 58 years old, is admitted to a general medical unit for the treatment of acute thrombophlebitis in her right calf. Orders include strict bed rest and heparin 5000 units by IV bolus followed by 1000 units/hr. Why would heparin be the anticoagulant of choice? How would you best monitor the effectiveness of the heparin therapy? In preparation for discharge, the prescriber adds warfarin to Ms. Brickland's medication regimen. How will this affect her response to the heparin therapy?

- George Thomas, 45 years old, has been admitted to the emergency department (ED) with an AMI. In the brief medical history that was obtained, it was determined that Mr. Thomas was seeing his primary care physician for an active peptic ulcer for which he was taking antacids and cimetidine. The emergency physician decides to administer alteplase IV. What will be of major concern for the client's safety? What assessments are required to monitor Mr. Thomas' condition?

- What is the informed consent policy for the transfusion of blood products within your practice setting? What part do you play in this policy as a nursing student? What will your role be as a registered nurse?

Bibliography

Anderson, D.M., Keith, J., & Novak, P.D. (Eds.) (2002). *Mosby's medical, nursing, and allied health dictionary* (6th ed.). St. Louis: Mosby.

Angiolillo, D., Fernandez-Ortiz, A., Bernardo, E., Ramirez, C., Escaned, J., Moreno, R., et al. (2004a). 807 C/T Polymorphism of the glycoprotein Ia gene and pharmacogenetic modulation of platelet response to dual antiplatelet treatment. *Blood Coagulation & Fibrinolysis*, 15(5):427-433.

Angiolillo, D., Fernandez-Ortiz, A., Bernardo, E., Alfonso, F., Sabate, M., Fernandez, C., et al. (2004b). PlA polymorphism and platelet reactivity following clopidogrel loading dose in patients undergoing coronary stent implantation. *Blood Coagulation & Fibrinolysis*, 15(1):89-93.

Bick, R.L., Frenkel, E.P., Walenga, J., Fareed, J., & Hoppensteadt, D.A. (2005). Unfractionated heparin, LMW heparins and pentasaccharide: Basic mechanisms of action, pharmacology, and clinical use. *Hematology and Oncology Clinics of North America,* 19(1):1-51.

Blecher, M.E. (Ed.) (2003). *Technical Manual.* Bethesda: American Association of Blood Banks.

Bockert, B. & Kwiatkowski, J.L. (2002). Coagulation disorders. In J.T. DiPiro, R.L. Talbert, G.C. Yee, G.R. Matzke, B.G. Wells, & L.M. Posey (Eds.), *Pharmacotherapy: A pathophysiological approach* (3rd ed.). Norwalk, CT: Appleton & Lange.

Bosker, G. (Ed.). (2004). *Primary and acute care medicine: Practice, protocols, pathways,* (2nd ed.). Atlanta: Thomson American Health Consultants.

Cahill, R.A., McGreal, G.T., Crowe, B.H., Ryan, D.A., Manning, B.J., Cahill, M.R., et al. (2005). Duration of increased bleeding tendency after cessation of aspirin therapy. *Journal of the American College of Surgeons, 200,* 564-573.

Callum, J.L., Kaplan, H.S., Merkley, L.L., Pinkerton, P.H., Rabin, F.B. Romans, R.A. (2001). Reporting of near-miss events for transfusion medicine: improving transfusion safety. *Transfusion,* 41(10):1204-1211.

Carlsson, L., Lubenow, N., Blumentritt, C., Kempf, R., Papenberg, S., Schroder, W., et al. (2003). Platelet receptor and clotting factor polymorphisms as genetic risk factors for thromboembolic complications in heparin-induced thrombocytopenia. *Pharmacogenetics,* 13(5):253-258.

Centers for Disease Control and Prevention. (2002). Summary of notifiable diseases, United States, 2000. *MMWR Morbidity & Mortality Weekly Report,* 49(53):i-xxii, 1-100.

Chan, F.K., Ching, J.Y., Hung, L.C., Wong, V.W., Leung, V.K., Kung, N.N., et al. (2005). Clopidogrel versus aspirin and esomeprazole to prevent recurrent ulcer bleeding, *New England Journal of Medicine,* 352;238-244.

Chang, J.T., Altman, R.B. (2004). Extracting and characterizing gene-drug relationships from the literature. *Pharmacogenetics,* 14(9):577-586. Retrieved December 2, 2004, from http://bionlp.stanford.edu/genedrug/gene_drug_predictions.html

Claridge, J.A., Sawyer, R.G., Schulman, A.M., McLemore, E.C., & Young, J.S. (2002). Blood transfusions correlate with infections in trauma patients in a dose-dependent manner. *American Surgeon,* 68(7):566-572.

The Clopidogrel in Unstable Angina to Prevent Recurrent Events Trial Investigators. (2001). Effects of clopidogrel in addition to aspirin in patients with acute coronary syndromes without ST-segment elevation. *New England Journal of Medicine,* 345: 494-502.

Deveras, R.A.E., & Kessler, C.M. (2002). Reversal of warfarin-induced excessive anticoagulation with recombinant human factor VIIa concentrate. *Annals of Internal Medicine,* 137:884-888.

Drug facts and comparisons. (58th ed.). (2005). St. Louis: Facts and Comparisons.

Dunn, A.L., & Abshire, T.C. (2004). Recent advances in the management of the child who has hemophilia. *Hematology and Oncology Clinics of North America,* 18(6):1249-1276.

Engoren, M.C., Habib, R.H., Zacharias, A., Schwann, T.A., Riordan, C.J. & Durham, S.J. (2002). Effect of blood transfusion on long-term survival after cardiac operation, *Annals of Thoracic Surgery,* 74(4):1180-1186.

Fang, M.C., Chang, Y., Hylek, E.M., Rosand, J., Greenberg, S.M., Go, A.S., et al. (2004). Advanced age, anticoagulation intensity, and risk for intracranial hemorrhage among patients taking warfarin for atrial fibrillation. *Annals of Internal Medicine, 141,* 745-752.

Fischer, L.M., Schlienger, R.G., Matter, C.M., Jick, H., & Meier, C.R. (2004). Discontinuation of nonsteroidal anti-inflammatory drug therapy and risk of acute myocardial infarction. *Archives of Internal Medicine, 164,* 2472-2476.

Frishman, W.H., Lerner, R.G., Klein, M.D., & Roganovic M. (2003). Antiplatelet and antithrombotic drugs. In W.H. Frishman, E.H. Sonnenblick, & D.A. Sica. (Eds.), *Cardiovascular Pharmacotherapeutics* (2nd ed.). New York: McGraw-Hill.

Hardman, J.G., & Limbird, L.E. (Eds.). (2001). *Goodman & Gilman's the pharmacological basis of therapeutics* (10th ed.). New York: McGraw-Hill.

Hillman, M.A., Wilke, R.A., Caldwell, M.D., Berg, R.L., Glurich, I., Burmester, J.K. (2004). Relative impact of covariates in prescribing warfarin according to CYP2 C9 genotype. *Pharmacogenetics,* 14(8):539-547.

King, B.P., Khan, T.I., Aithal, G.P., Kamali, F., Daly, A.K. (2004). Upstream and coding region CYP2 C9 polymorphisms: correlation with warfarin dose and metabolism. *Pharmacogenetics,* 14(12):813-822.

Kirchheiner, J., Ufer, M., Walter, E.C., Kammerer, B., Kahlich, R., Meisel, C., et al. (2004). Effects of CYP2 C9 polymorphisms on the pharmacokinetics of R- and S-phenprocoumon in healthy volunteers. *Pharmacogenetics,* 14(1):19-26.

Kucher, N., Leizorovicz, A., Vaitkus, P.T., Cohen, A.T., Turpie, A.G., Olsson, C.G., et al. (2005). Efficacy and safety of fixed low-dose dalteparin in preventing venous thromboembolism among obese or elderly hospitalized patients: A subgroup analysis of the PREVENT trial. *Archives of Internal Medicine, 165,* 341-345.

Kuriyan, M., & Carson, J.L. (2004). Blood transfusion risks in the intensive care unit. *Critical Care Clinics,* 20(2):255-268.

Lacy, C.F., Armstrong, L.L., Goldman, M.P., & Lance, L.L. (2004). *Lexi-Comp's Drug Information Handbook* (12th ed.). Hudson, Ohio: Lexi-Comp.

Lau, W.C., Waskell, L.A., Watkins, P.B., Neer, C.J., Horowitz, K., Hopp, A.S., et al. (2003). Atorvastatin reduces the ability of clopi-

e-LEARNING SUPPLEMENTS

Student CD-ROM
- Final Exam questions
- NCLEX® Examination review questions
- Pharmacology animations
- Printable chapter summary

Evolve Website (http://evolve.elsevier.com/mckenry)
- Case study on antiplatelets, anticoagulants, fibrinolytics, and blood components

- Content updates, including information on new drugs
- WebLinks corresponding to this chapter
- Answers to the critical thinking questions in this chapter
- *Elsevier ePharmacology Update* newsletter
- *Mosby's Drug Consult* Internet Edition
- Supplemental and reference information

dogrel to inhibit platelet aggregation: a new drug–drug interaction. *Circulation*, 107:32–37.

Leung, A.Y., Chow, H.C., Kwong, Y.L., Lie, A.K., Fung, A.T., Chow, W.H., et al. (2001). Genetic polymorphism in exon 4 of cytochrome P450 CYP2 C9 may be associated with warfarin sensitivity in Chinese patients. *Blood*, 98:2584–2587.

Linden, J.V., Wagner, K., Voytovich, A.E., & Sheehan, J. (2000). Transfusion errors in New York State: An analysis of 10 years' experience. *Transfusion*, 4(10):1207-1213.

Linker, C.A. (2003). Blood. In L.M. Tierney, Jr., S.J. McPhee, & Papadakis, M.A (eds.), *Current medical diagnosis & treatment.* New York: Lange Medical Books/McGraw-Hill.

Mayer, S.A., Brun, N.C., Begtrup, K., Broderick, J., Davis, S., Diringer, M.N., et al. (2005). Recombinant activated factor VII for acute intracerebral hemorrhage. *New England Journal of Medicine, 352,* 777-785.

Montaner, J., Fernandez-Cadenas, I., Molina, C., Monasterio, J., Arenillas, J., Ribo, M., et al. (2003). Safety profile of tissue plasminogen activator treatment among stroke patients carrying a common polymorphism (C-1562 T) in the promoter region of the matrix metalloproteinase-9 gene. *Stroke*, 34(12):2851-2855.

Mosby's drug consult (15th ed.). (2005). St. Louis: Mosby.

Sabatine, M.S., Cannon, C.P., Gibson, C.M., Lopez-Sendon, J.L., Montalescot, G., Theroux, P., et al. (2005). Addition of clopidogrel to aspirin and fibrinolytic therapy for myocardial infarction with ST-segment elevation. *New England Journal of Medicine, 352,* 1179-1189.

Saw, J., Steinhubl, S.R., Berger, P.B., Kereiakes, D.J., Serebruany, V.L., Brennan, D., et al, and the Clopidogrel for the Reduction of Events During Observation Investigators. (2003). Lack of adverse clopidogrel-atorvastatin clinical interaction from secondary analysis of a randomized, placebo-controlled clopidogrel trial. *Circulation*, 108:921-924.

Schafer, A.I. (2003). Genetic and Acquired Determinants of Individual Variability of Response to Antiplatelet Drugs. *Circulation*, 108(8):910-911.

Si, D., Guo, Y., Zhang, Y., Yang, L., Zhou, H., Zhong, D. (2004). Identification of a novel variant CYP2 C9 allele in Chinese. *Pharmacogenetics*, 14(7):465-469.

Taylor, R.W., Manganaro, L., O'Brien, J., Trottier, S.J., Parkar, N., & Veremakis, C. (2002). Impact of allopathic packed red blood cell transfusion on nosocomial infection rates in the critically ill patient. *Critical Care Medicine,* 30(10):2249-2254.

Thorevska, N., Amoateng-Adjepong, Y., Sabahi, R., Schiopescu, I., Salloum, A., Muralidharan, V., et al. (2004). Anticoagulation in hospitalized patients with renal insufficiency: A comparison of bleeding rates with unfractionated heparin vs enoxaparin. *Chest*, 125:856-863.

USP DI: Drug information for the health care professional (25th ed.). (2005). Greenwood Village, CO: MICROMEDEX Thomson Healthcare.

Visser, L.E., van Vliet, M., van Schaik, R.H.N., Kasbergen, A.A.H., De Smet, P.A., Vulto, A.G., et al. (2004). The risk of overanticoagulation in patients with cytochrome P450 CYP2 C9*2 or CYP2 C9*3 alleles on acenocoumarol or phenprocoumon. *Pharmacogenetics*, 14(1):27-33.

Wittkowsky, A.K. (2005). Thrombosis. In M.A. Koda-Kimble, L.Y. Young, W.A. Kradjan, B.J. Guglielmo, B.K. Alldredge, & R.L. Corelli (Eds.), *Applied therapeutics: The clinical use of drugs* (8th ed.). Philadelphia: Lippincott Williams & Wilkins.

31

ANTIHYPERLIPIDEMIC DRUGS

CHAPTER FOCUS

A strong link exists between coronary heart disease (CHD) and elevated plasma lipoprotein concentrations. These elevated lipids, or hyperlipidemia, may develop as the result of high dietary fat intake, systemic disease, or genetic factors. The nurse needs to be knowledgeable about drugs that lower serum lipids, and factors that increase lipid levels, to provide appropriate information to clients to prevent the coronary artery disease (CAD) that might result from hyperlipidemia.

LEARNING OBJECTIVES

- Define hyperlipidemia and describe the pathophysiology of this condition.
- Identify the four types of lipoprotein and differentiate them according to their lipid content.
- Discuss the importance of combining dietary modifications with drug therapy to treat hyperlipidemia.
- Implement nursing management of clients receiving antihyperlipidemic agents.

▲ KEY TERMS

apolipoproteins, p. 635
atherosclerosis, p. 633
chylomicrons, p. 635
high-density lipoproteins (HDLs), p. 635
hyperlipidemia, p. 633
lipoprotein, p. 634
low-density lipoproteins (LDLs), p. 635
very low-density lipoproteins (VLDLs), p. 634

KEY DRUGS

cholestyramine, p. 642
gemfibrozil, p. 644
lovastatin, p. 638
niacin, p. 641

Hyperlipidemia is a metabolic disorder characterized by increased concentrations of cholesterol and triglycerides, two of the major serum lipids in the body. Antihyperlipidemic or antilipemic drugs are used along with dietary modifications to treat hyperlipidemia. Clinical and experimental studies offer evidence that an important relationship exists between atherosclerosis and high levels of circulating triglycerides and cholesterol. **Atherosclerosis** is a disorder characterized by inflammatory lipoprotein lipid deposits in the lining of large- and medium-sized arteries, which eventually produces degenerative changes and obstructs blood flow.

Atherosclerosis is a causative factor in CHD, which may result in angina, heart failure (HF), myocardial infarction (MI), cerebral arterial disease that results in senility or cerebrovascular accidents (CVAs), peripheral arterial occlusive disease (which may cause gangrene and loss of limb), and renal arterial insufficiency. It is also a factor in hypertension. Intensive research is being conducted to better understand the pathogenesis of atherosclerosis and develop more effective and safer antihyperlipidemic drugs.

❋ **What are the key factors in the pathogenesis of atherosclerosis?**

The accumulation of lipoproteins and other inflammatory mediators is an important element in the progression of atherosclerosis. Various protein-carbohydrate complexes are found in arterial walls and contribute to arterial wall integrity and are synthesized in part by macrophages. The incorporation of fatty acid in the synthesis of these complexes by macrophages in the presence of low-density lipoproteins may be an important step in the generation of an atherosclerotic plaque (Khalil, Wagner, & Goldberg, 2004). Macrophages in the arterial wall, in the presence of oxidative stress and large amounts of cholesterol, are transformed into foam cells, which are primary players in development of inflammatory processes leading to atherosclerosis. The ability of macrophages to effectively scavenge and regulate lipid balance is controlled by intracellular transcription factors. These transcription factors regulate lipid uptake, genesis, metabolism, and movement in the macrophage (Ricote, Valledor, & Glass, 2004).

Atherosclerotic lesions may not develop at the same rate at all vascular sites, but instead may be influenced by hemodynamic factors in localized arteries. The inflammatory process of atherosclerosis appears greatest in large and medium sized arteries, is affected by blood flow patterns in the vessel and is probably genetically determined (Vander-Laan, Reardon, & Getz, 2004). Sustained high blood pressure (BP) is known to be a risk factor for the development of atherosclerosis. Angiotensin II, inducing vasoconstriction, has also been implicated in contributing to inflammation in the arterial wall, facilitating the conversion of vessel macrophages into foam cells, and increasing oxidative stress by promoting the formation of superoxide radicals (Ferrario et al., 2004). Infection with human immunodeficiency virus (HIV) is also a risk factor for development of atherosclerosis, and may be related to inflammation by the virus itself, and/or concurrent drug therapy (e.g., protease inhibitors) (Hsue et al., 2004). Markers for inflammation, including C-reactive protein, interleukin-6, myeloperoxidase, cell adhesion molecules, and fibrinogen are associated with CHD and are sometimes used to help predict risk (Rackley, 2004).

Each of these variables—blood and tissue lipids, oxidative stress, macrophage activity, inflammation, genetic determinants for macrophage transcription factors and vessel

susceptibility, and hypertension—are likely targets for drug and nondrug therapies to prevent and treat atherosclerosis. The effective prevention and treatment of atherosclerosis involves identifying and adjusting controllable risk factors for its development. Although clients can do little to control inherited risks, lifestyle changes including a diet high in fiber and low in saturated fat and sodium, moderate exercise, and smoking cessation can all reduce risk. Other controllable factors include BP control (see Chapter 27) and control of elevated lipid levels. Although the first step to improved lipid levels involves lifestyle changes, many clients require drug therapy to adequately reduce risk.

✱ How are lipids classified?

Lipid compounds do not circulate freely in the bloodstream but are bound to plasma proteins (albumin, globulin), that act as carriers. These complexes are called lipoproteins. A **lipoprotein** has a protein shell and an interior composed of a core lipid (cholesterol, triglycerides) (Table 31-1). Hyperlipoproteinemia is always associated with an increased concentration of one or more lipoproteins, particularly cholesterol.

Lipoprotein complexes are classified according to their densities and electrophoretic mobilities. The three primary lipoproteins found in the blood of fasting individuals are very low-density lipoproteins, low-density lipoproteins, and high-density lipoproteins.

The **very low-density lipoproteins (VLDLs)** contain a large amount of triglycerides (50% to 65%) and 20% to 30% cholesterol. VLDLs are formed in the liver from endogenous fat sources and contain 15% to 20% of the total blood cholesterol and most of the triglycerides found in the body (McKenney, 2005). Because these particles are quite large, they are not believed to be involved in atherosclerosis.

After secretion from the liver, the VLDL particles will in time become smaller particles as the triglyceride content is removed. Two enzymes, lipoprotein lipase and hepatic lipase, are involved with triglyceride removal. Medications that increase the action of lipoprotein lipase will lower triglyceride levels. Triglyceride-depleted lipoprotein is smaller and contains a higher quantity of cholesterol. VLDL is eventually broken down into intermediate-density lipoprotein (IDL), which contains 50% each of cholesterol and triglyc-

TABLE 31-1 LIPOPROTEINS: CORE LIPIDS AND TRANSPORT/FUNCTION

Lipoproteins	Core Lipid	Transport/Function
Chylomicrons	Dietary triglycerides	Dietary triglycerides
Chylomicron remnants	Dietary cholesterol	Dietary cholesterol
Very-low-density lipoproteins (VLDLs)	Endogenous cholesterol	Endogenous triglycerides
Intermediate-density lipoprotein (IDL)	Endogenous cholesterol and triglycerides	Endogenous cholesterol
Low-density lipoprotein (LDL)	Endogenous cholesterol	Endogenous cholesterol
High-density lipoproteins (HDL)	Endogenous cholesterol	Removes cholesterol

erides. Approximately 50% of this substance is converted to the cholesterol-rich lipoprotein, or low-density lipoprotein. These smaller remnant VLDL particles include VLDL, intermediate-density lipoprotein (IDL), and low-density proteins. These lipoproteins can now be involved in the development of atherosclerosis.

The **low-density lipoproteins (LDLs)** contain the major portion of cholesterol in the blood and are considered to be the most harmful. They carry 60% to 70% of total blood cholesterol. Elevated LDL levels suggest that an individual has a greater potential for developing atherosclerosis.

The **high-density lipoproteins (HDLs)** are the smallest and most dense lipoproteins. Their function is to transport cholesterol from peripheral cells to the liver, where it is metabolized and excreted. This transport mechanism prevents the accumulation of lipids in the arterial walls, thereby providing protection against the development of CHD. Thus high levels of HDL are considered beneficial. The higher the HDL levels, the lower the potential risk for developing cardiovascular disease.

Chylomicrons are large particles that transport cholesterol and fatty acids from the diet and/or the gastrointestinal (GI) tract to the liver. This is known as the *exogenous* system of transport. The lipoproteins transporting cholesterol from the liver to peripheral cells are part of the *endogenous* system. Chylomicrons consist mainly of triglycerides (85% to 95%). Normally they are produced in the small intestine during absorption of a fatty meal and are cleared from the bloodstream by lipoprotein lipase after 12 to 14 hours. A deficiency of this enzyme is rare and results in increased levels of chylomicrons, causing a disease called *exogenous* hyperlipoproteinemia. This condition is usually found in children but may also be induced by alcoholism. Therapy is aimed at keeping the diet low in fat.

Lipoproteins contain proteins on their surface called **apolipoproteins**. These proteins have a number of functions, including helping the lipoprotein bind with cell receptors, activating the enzyme system, and providing structure for the lipoprotein. An increased risk of atherosclerosis exists if the metabolism of apolipoproteins is impaired. Therefore blood levels of apolipoproteins are important in evaluating lipid disorders. The clinically important apolipoproteins are A-I, A-II, B-100, C-II, and E. A deficiency of the C-II apolipoprotein in VLDL particles results in impaired triglyceride metabolism and hypertriglyceridemia. The quantity of apolipoprotein B present is used to determine the number of VLDL and LDL substances in circulation. High levels of apolipoprotein A-I in HDL correlate more closely with a lower incidence of CHD than do HDL particles that have both A-I and A-II (McKenney, 2005).

Figure 31-1 reviews the normal lipid transport system. Dietary fats and cholesterol are orally consumed and transported into the system by bile acids (Figure 31-1, *A*); in the endogenous transport system, the liver converts excess calories from carbohydrates and fatty acids into triglycerides. The liver ultimately produces both HDL and LDL (Figure 31-1, *B*). The function of HDL is to carry approximately 25% of blood cholesterol to the liver, where it is processed into bile acids (Figure 31-1, *C*). Because the cholesterol carried by HDL is for ultimate excretion, HDL is known as "good cholesterol." LDL carries more than 50% of the total blood cholesterol, and this LDL-cholesterol combination can penetrate arterial walls, resulting in atherosclerotic plaques; thus in excess, this combination is referred to as "bad" cholesterol (Figure 31-1, *D*).

Plasma lipoproteins are usually in a state of dynamic equilibrium because the LDL needed to transport fats such as fatty acids and cholesterol is located throughout the body. When cells outside the liver need cholesterol, they produce LDL receptors on their surfaces (see Figure 31-1, *D*). These receptors are necessary for LDL to enter the cells, where it is broken down into amino acids and free cholesterol. When the cellular need for cholesterol is met, the production of LDL receptors stops, and the excess cholesterol is discarded into the plasma. LDL receptors are also located in the liver, where they function to monitor plasma levels of LDL. When the appropriate level of LDL is present in the plasma, the liver will suppress its production. This is essentially a feedback system that functions like a thermostat in the home; it maintains adequate plasma levels of LDL to provide cholesterol to body cells on demand.

✱ **B.T. is a 48-year-old male with a sedentary lifestyle who presents to his health care provider for an employment physical exam. He has not seen a health care provider for the past 7 years, and describes himself in general good health. He does not smoke. He has no family history of CHD. His blood pressure is 142/88 mm Hg in the office. He is 5'8" and weighs 94 kg. His lipid profile is as follows: total cholesterol, 225 mg/dL; LDL, 180 mg/dL; HDL, 38 mg/dL; and triglycerides, 185 mg/dL.**

✱ **What are the goals for lipid profiles?**
The National Cholesterol Education Program (NCEP) Expert Panel on Detection, Evaluation, and Treatment of High Blood Cholesterol in Adults in the United States, in conjunction the National Heart, Lung and Blood Institute, American College of Cardiology Foundation and the American Heart Association have revised recommended goals for Low Density Lipoproteins–Cholesterol (LDL-C) based on a risk stratification (Grundy et al., 2004). These are based on the strong correlation of elevated LDL-C and CHD and the cardiovascular benefits associated with lowering LDL-C levels. For clients with elevated triglycerides (≥ 200 mg/dL), levels of non-high density lipoproteins (non-HDL-C) that are the sum values of VLDL and low density lipoproteins (LDL-C) are also evaluated. There is some correlation with elevated high density lipoproteins (HDL-C) and reduced cardiovascular risk, but the revised NCEP 2004 guidelines have not specified treatment goals for HDL-C, although levels above 60 mg/dL are desirable.

Lipid profiles should be obtained in the fasting state at least every 5 years for all individuals over the age of 20 years. Included in the profile should be a total cholesterol, HDL-C, LDL-C, and triglyceride level.

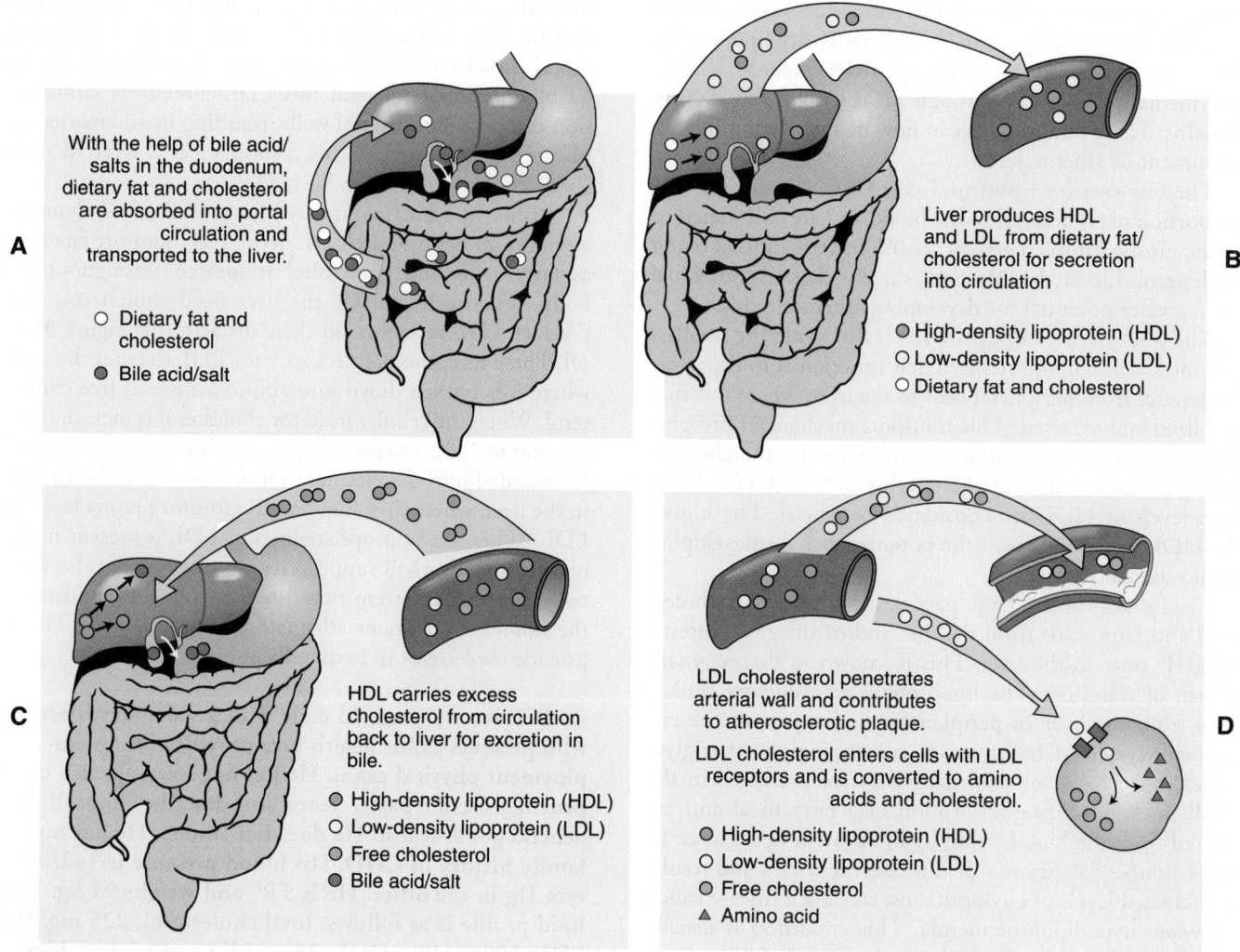

FIGURE 31-1 Dietary carbohydrates, fatty acids, and cholesterol: conversion sites and processes. The absorption of dietary fats and cholesterol **(A)**, production of HDL and LDL **(B)**, function of HDL **(C)**, and actions of LDL **(D)** are depicted.

The highest risk individuals for future cardiovascular events include those clients with existing CHD, which includes clients with a history of MI, angina, myocardial ischemia, or clients who have undergone coronary artery procedures. Considered at similar risk are individuals with diabetes and two or more other risk factors (Table 31-2), clients with noncoronary forms of atherosclerotic disease (including transient ischemic attacks or cerebrovascular accident). Such clients are considered to have a greater than 20% likelihood of a CHD event over the next 10 years.

At moderate risk are those clients without existing CHD with two or more risk factors (Box 31-1). These clients are considered to have between a 10% and 20% risk for developing CHD over the next 10 years, although a subset of these individuals are at lower risk, primarily based on age. Individuals with one or fewer risk factors are considered at low risk for developing CHD over the next 10 years. To more accurately quantify risk, the National Institutes of Health (NIH) has made available a 10-year risk calculator to assist clinicians and clients. The calculator is available online at http://www.nhlbi.nih.gov/guidelines/cholesterol/ as are the latest updated guidelines.

Goal LDL-C levels are stratified by risk. With each risk group, NCEP has recommended when to initiate therapeutic lifestyle changes (diet/exercise) and drug therapy. These recommendations are presented in Table 31-2. For high risk individuals, goal LDL-C levels are set at less than 100 mg/dL with an optimal goal set at less than 70 mg/dL for very high-risk clients. Goals of less than 130 mg/dL and less than 160 mg/dL are recommended for moderate- and low-risk individuals respectively. Institution of therapeutic lifestyle changes is considered for all clients whose LDL-C is above the goal, particularly for clients with obesity, physical inactivity, elevated triglycerides, or low HDL-C levels. For high-risk and moderately high-risk individuals, drugs are also recommended if LDL-C is not in goal range. For moderate and low risk individuals, drugs are usually not initially recommended unless LDL-C is considerably above goal range (see Table 31-2).

✲ **B.T. is considered at moderately high risk for CHD. Although he does not have a family history of CHD and doesn't smoke, he is obese, hypertensive, and has a LDL of 180 mg/dL. Using the web-based NIH**

TABLE 31-2 NCEP ADULT TREATMENT PANEL III 2004 GOALS FOR LDL-C

Risk Category	Goal LDL-C	Cut Off for Initiating Therapeutic Lifestyle Changes	Cutoff for Considering Drug Therapy†
High Risk (CHD, diabetes with 2+ risk factors,* existing atherosclerotic disease)	<100 mg/dL (Optimal <70 mg/dL)	≥100 mg/dL	≥100 mg/dL
Moderately High Risk (2+ risk factors,* 10-year risk 10-20%)	<130 mg/dL	≥130 mg/dL	≥130 mg/dL
Moderate Risk (2+ risk factors,* 10-year risk <10%)	<130 mg/dL	≥130 mg/dL	≥160 mg/dL
Lower Risk (0-1 risk factors)*	<160 mg/dL	≥160 mg/dL	≥190 mg/dL

Modified from Grundy, S.M., Cleeman, J.I., Merz, C.N., Brewer, H.B., Clark, L.T., Hunninghake, D.B., et al.; National Heart, Lung, and Blood Institute; American College of Cardiology foundation; American Heart Association. (2004). Implications of recent clinical trials for the National Cholesterol Education Program Adult Treatment Panel III guidelines. *Circulation, 110*(6), 763.
*Risk factors are presented in Box 31-1.
†May consider drug therapy below these levels based on evidence, other client factors.

BOX 31-1 RISK FACTORS FOR CORONARY HEART DISEASE

Based on NCEP guidelines, each of the following are risk factors for CHD:
- Cigarette smoking
- Hypertension (BP = 140/90 mm Hg or on antihypertensive therapy)
- Low HDL-C (<40mg/dL)
- Male first-degree relative with CHD under 55 years of age or female first-degree relative with CHD under 65 years of age
- Age (men ≥45 years of age, women ≥55 years of age)

10-year risk calculator, B.T. is considered at an 18% risk of developing CHD over the next 10 years, and is a candidate for lifestyle changes and drug therapy.

✱ What therapeutic lifestyle changes are recommended by NCEP?

Therapeutic lifestyle changes for B.T. include diet and moderate exercise, and if he smoked, it would include smoking cessation. The Healthy Heart Diet guidelines recommend limiting saturated fat to 8% to 10% of total calories, that no more than 30% of total calories be obtained from fat, and limiting cholesterol intake to less than 300 mg daily. Sodium intake should be limited to 2400 mg daily as well. Caloric restriction is also recommended to achieve or maintain a healthy weight. Adoption of a Mediterranean-style diet (high vegetable, nut, fish, and monounsaturated fats intake) combined with smoking cessation, modest alcohol consumption, and physical activity are associated with significantly lower risks for CHD (Knoops et al., 2004) and

lower levels of C-reactive protein and interleukins (Esposito et al., 2004).

✱ What drug treatment options are available for achieving lipid goals?

Treatment recommendations are based on the client's cholesterol level and the presence of CHD, age, and other risk factors as discussed previously. Most drug studies in the treatment of hyperlipidemia have focused on drug response in middle age men to reduce CHD. Mortality is significantly reduced for clients with CHD when statins are combined with aspirin and β blockers or angiotensin-converting enzyme (ACE) inhibitor therapy (Hippisley-Cox & Coupland, 2005). Drug therapy may also reduce risk for thromboembolic CVAs as well (Collins, Armitage, Parish, Sleight, & Peto, 2004). For women, drug therapy is indicated with existing CHD to reduce future cardiac disease. Its role in women without existing cardiac disease, however, is debated (Walsh & Pignone, 2004). Benefit is seen with moderate lipid lowering in older adults (Shepherd et al., 2002), although very low cholesterol levels may be correlated with increased mortality risk (Brescianini et al., 2003). For children (8 through 18 years of age), a 2-year trial of statins appeared safe and effective in controlling familial hyperlipidemias (Wiegman et al., 2004). Benefit is also observed when lipid lowering agents are used to treat even modestly elevated cholesterol levels for individuals with diabetes mellitus (DM) (Collins, Armitage, Parish, Sleigh, & Peto, 2003). Modest reductions in cardiac morbidity are observed when drugs are used to treat individuals with hypertension and only normal or only modestly elevated cholesterol levels, but it is not clear if this benefit is worth the risk and costs of therapy (Sever, 2003). Genetics also influences drug response (see the Special Considerations for Pharmacogenetics box on p. 638).

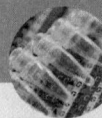

Special Considerations for Pharmacogenetics | ANTIHYPERLIPIDEMICS

PHARMACODYNAMICS

The pathology of atherosclerosis is highly influenced by genetics. Known factors for its risk and risk of CHD, including HDL, LDL, hypertension, and DM, are largely hereditary. The synthesis of a major protein component of HDL, apolipoprotein A-I, is genetically based (Dudley-Brown, 2004). Variation in another gene, CETP, is correlated with variations in lipid levels and CHD risk (Boekholdt et al., 2003). Variation in 5-lipoxygenase genotypes is also correlated with atherosclerosis risk (Dwyer et al., 2004). Identification of multiple genes which are known to increase risk for CHD or related factors, known as multilocus gene testing, is a potential future avenue to identify candidates and individualize treatments in the future (Lusis, Fogelman, Fonarow, & Gregg, 2004). Response to drugs, including statins (e.g., pravastatin, simvastatin) and fibric acid derivatives (e.g., fenofibrate, gemfibrozil), have been correlated with genetic markers (Caslake &

Packard, 2004; Chang & Altman, 2004; Chasman et al., 2004; Foucher et al., 2004). It is not yet practical, however, to use gene typing for drug selection (Zineh, 2004).

PHARMACOKINETICS

The statins are extensively metabolized by the cytochrome P450 enzymes. A correlation in the genetic variation in P450 3A4/5 and simvastatin, atorvastatin, and lovastatin response has been reported (Kivisto et al., 2004). Differences in metabolism of fluvastatin via 2C19 and 2C9 is also noted to have a genetic basis (Chang & Altman, 2004).

ADVERSE EFFECTS

Variation in the metabolism of simvastatin by P450 2D6 may predispose to the risk for rhabdomyolysis (Vermes & Vermes, 2004). Genetic markers have also been correlated with variable pravastatin levels (Niemi et al., 2004) and could lead to toxicity.

Drug classes used in the management of lipid disorders include the HMG-Co-A reductase inhibitors ("statins"), niacin, fibric acid derivatives, bile acid sequestering agents, and a newer class, the azetidinones. Complementary and alterative therapies include garlic, green tea and red yeast rice (see Chapter 12). The relative efficacy of each class on LDL-C, HDL-C and triglycerides is presented in Table 31-3. Each class will be discussed briefly.

HMG-Co-A Reductase Inhibitors ("Statins")

The inhibitors of 3-hydroxy-3-methylgluraryl coenzyme A (HMG-CoA) have become a mainstay of drug therapy for hyperlipidemia. They are highly effective in lowering LDL-C by 20% to 50%. They also modestly raise HDL-C and lower triglyceride levels. They are competitive inhibitors of HMG-CoA reductase, an enzyme necessary for cholesterol biosynthesis. The decrease in cholesterol production in the liver leads to an increase in the synthesis of cholesterol and also stimulates hepatocytes to produce more LDL receptors. The result is that more LDL cholesterol is removed from the blood. The ability of statins to lower C-reactive protein level, a marker for atherosclerotic inflammation, may be important as well (Ridker et al., 2005; Nissen et al., 2005). Long-term use of statins may also reduce the risk for colon cancer, a cancer that is associated with elevated HMG-CoA reductase expression (Poynter et al., 2005). Agents in this class include atorvastatin (Lipitor), fluvastatin (Lescol), lovastatin (Mevacor), pravastatin (Pravachol), rosuvastatin (Crestor), and simvastatin (Zocor). These agents are generally considered safe, but rates of muscle injury vary with the

agent, prompting the removal of cerivastatin (Baycol) from the market in 2001 (Graham et al., 2004; Psaty, Furberg, Ray, & Weiss, 2004). A U.S. Food and Drug Administration (FDA) public health advisory notes an increased risk for myopathy and rhabdomyolysis with rosuvastatin (FDA, March 2005). Lovastatin was the first available agent in the class and is considered the prototype HMG-CoA reductase inhibitor.

★▄▀ lovastatin [**loe** vah sta tin]
(Mevacor)
Indications
Lovastatin and other HMG-CoA reductase inhibitors are indicated as adjuncts for the treatment of primary hypercholesterolemia caused by an elevated LDL cholesterol level not controlled by diet or other treatment measures.

Pharmacokinetics/Dosing
On absorption, lovastatin has an extensive first-pass hepatic extraction and is highly protein bound. Peak serum levels are reached in 2 to 4 hours. Lovastatin is converted by the liver via cytochrome P450 enzymes to several active metabolites. The initial response is seen within 1 to 2 weeks, with the maximum therapeutic response occurring within 4 to 6 weeks of chronic drug administration. Excretion is primarily fecal. The adult dosage of lovastatin is 20 mg daily with the evening meal, increased monthly as necessary according to the client's response to therapy, up to a maximum of 80 mg daily.

Adverse Effects
One of the most important adverse effects with this class of drugs is myopathy, which is manifested by myalgias, myositis, and the risk for rhabdomyolysis (necrosis of skeletal muscle with the release of myoglobulin, which may result in myopathy and acute renal failure). This risk may be highest for rosuvastatin (Crestor) (FDA, June 2004). This reaction is noted with higher HMG-CoA reductase inhibitor levels, which can be seen with high doses or with concurrent administration of interacting foods or drugs. Other adverse effects of the HMG-CoA reductase inhibitors include gas, stomach cramps or pain, rash, constipation or diarrhea, nausea, headaches, and, rarely, impo-

TABLE 31-3 COMPARATIVE EFFICACY OF ANTIHYPERLIPIDEMIC THERAPIES

Class	Effect on			Common Adverse Effects
	LDL-C	HDL-C	Triglycerides	
HMG-CoA reductase inhibitors ("statins")	↓ 18%-55%	↑ 5%-15%	↓ 7%-30%	Myopathy ↑ Liver function test values
Niacin/nicotinic acid	↓ 5%-25%	↑ 15%-35%	↓ 20%-50%	Flushing Hyperglycemia Hyperuricemia/Gout Upper GI upset Hepatotoxicity
Fibric acids	↓ 5%-20%	↑ 10%-20%	↓ 20%-50%	Dyspepsia Gallstones Myopathy Unexplained non-CHD deaths in WHO study
Bile acid sequestrants	↓ 15%-30%	↑ 3%-5%	No change	Gastrointestinal distress Constipation Decreased absorption of other drugs
Azetidinones (usually used as add on therapy; limited data on efficacy as monotherapy)	↓ 16%-20%	↑ 1%-4%	↓ 5%-6%	Gastrointestinal distress Headache Joint pain

Modified from the Third Report of the National Cholesterol Education Program (NCEP) Expert Panel on Detection, Evaluation, and Treatment of High Blood Cholesterol in Adults (Adult Treatment Panel III) Executive Summary, NIH publication No. 01-3670. (2001). Retrieved July 15, 2004, from http://www.nhlbi.nih.gov/guidelines/cholesterol/atp3xsum.pdf; Lacy, C.F., Armstrong, L.L., Goldman, M.P., & Lance, L.L. (2004). *Lexi-Comp's Drug Information Handbook* (12th ed.). Hudson, Ohio: Lexi-Comp; Goldberg, A.C., Sapre, A., Liu, J., Capece, R., Mitchel, Y.B., for the Ezetimibe Study Group. (2004). Efficacy and safety of ezetimibe coadministered with simvastatin in patients with primary hypercholesterolemia: A randomized, double-blind, placebo-controlled trial. *Mayo Clinic Proceedings, 79*(5), 620-629.

tency and insomnia. Liver toxicity is possible but is not common. Obtaining baseline liver function tests is appropriate before initiating treatment, but long-term monitoring is probably essential only for those clients with interacting drugs or significant comorbidities (Charles, Olson, Sandhoff, McClure, & Merenich, 2005). All drugs in this class are category X drugs and should not be used in pregnant women or women who could become pregnant while on therapy. They also enter breast milk and are contraindicated for women who are breast feeding.

Drug Interactions
Drugs that interact with the HMG-CoA reductase inhibitors increase the risk for rhabdomyolysis (as noted above). Most of the HMG-CoA reductase inhibitors are metabolized by cytochrome P450 3A4 and interact with a number of drugs and foods, including cyclosporine (Neoral, Sandimmune), grapefruit juice, and azole antifungals. Table 31-4 outlines the P450 isoenzyme that primarily metabolizes each drug and Box 31-2 identifies other commonly used drugs which could result in elevated levels of statins which are metabolized by P450 3A4. Risk for rhabdomyolysis is also possible with concurrent gemfibrozil (Lopid) or niacin therapy, however these combinations are sometimes used in very high-risk clients.

✱ **B.T. is encouraged to initiate dietary and exercise modification and is started on atorvastatin (Lipitor) 10 mg daily. He is also being evaluated for hypertension.**

✱ **What nursing management of B.T.'s drug therapy is appropriate?**

Assessment B.T. is tested for liver function impairment because active hepatic disease is a contraindication for HMG-CoA reductase inhibitors. These drugs are used with caution in clients with organ transplant and immunosuppressant therapy because of the increased risk of rhabdomyolysis and renal failure. B.T.'s history and physical exam also rule out conditions in which there is increased risk of secondary renal failure if rhabdomyolysis occurs, such as hypotension, severe infection, uncontrolled seizures, major surgery, trauma, and severe metabolic, endocrine, or electrolyte disorders.

B.T.'s concurrent medication regimen is reviewed to prevent interactions with such drugs as cyclosporine, niacin, gemfibrozil, and other fibrates (increased risk of rhabdomyolysis and acute renal failure); antacids (decrease atorvastatin levels 35%); and digoxin (increases serum digoxin levels). He is questioned about his use of grapefruit juice because 200 mL of grapefruit juice increases atorvastatin levels and increases the risk of myopathy. If B.T. were a female client, hormonal contraceptive use would be discussed as atorvastatin increases estrogen and ethinyl estradiol serum concentrations. As indicated earlier, all drugs in this class are Pregnancy Category X and are contraindicated for pregnant women, women who could become pregnant, and breastfeeding women.

TABLE 31-4 HMG-CoA REDUCTASE INHIBITORS (STATINS)

Agent	Adult Dose Range	Drug Interaction Potential	Cytochrome P450 Isoenzymes Responsible for Metabolism*	Comments
atorvastatin (Lipitor)	10-80 mg daily	Moderate-High	**3A4**	Dose any time of day
fluvastatin (Lescol)	20-80 mg daily	Moderate	2C8/9, 2D6, 3A4	Dose in evening with or without meals
lovastatin (Mevacor)	20-80 mg daily	High	**3A4**	Dose with evening meal
pravastatin (Pravachol)	10-80 mg daily	Moderate	3A4	Dose any time of day
rosuvastatin (Crestor)	10-40 mg daily	Moderate	2C9, 3A4	Dose any time of day *May have higher risk for rhabdomyolysis, particularly at higher doses*
simvastatin (Zocor)	5-80 mg daily	High	**3A4**	Dose in evening with or without meals

Modified from Lacy, C.F., Armstrong, L.L., Goldman, M.P., & Lance, L.L. (2004). *Lexi-Comp's Drug Information Handbook* (12th ed.). Hudson, Ohio: Lexi-Comp.
Bold indicates major metabolic pathway and greater likelihood for interactions with inhibitors of this enzyme (See Box 31-2 for inhibitors of P450 3A4).

BOX 31-2 EXAMPLES OF POTENT INHIBITORS OF P450 3A4

amiodarone	itraconazole
amprenavir	ketoconazole
atazanavir	miconazole
cimetidine	nefazodone
clarithromycin	nelfinavir
diltiazem	nicardipine
erythromycin	norfloxacin
fluconazole	quinidine
fosamprenavir	ritonavir
grapefruit juice	saquinavir
imatinib	verapamil
indinavir	voriconazole
isoniazid	

Data from Lacy, C.F., Armstrong, L.L., Goldman, M.P., & Lance, L.L. (2004). *Lexi-Comp's Drug Information Handbook* (12th ed.). Hudson, Ohio: Lexi-Comp.

A baseline assessment includes a serum cholesterol and liver function studies, including serum transaminase. Weight and a dietary profile will be helpful to determine any lifestyle changes that may be required.

Nursing Diagnosis B.T. is at risk for the following nursing diagnoses: deficient knowledge about hyperlipidemia and its complications; ineffective management of therapeutic regimen related to need for lifestyle changes, dietary requirements, and unfamiliar medication regimen; impaired comfort (headache, heartburn, gas, and nausea); risk for injury related to dizziness; constipation; diarrhea; impaired skin integrity (rash) and the potential complications of myalgia, myositis or rhabdomyolysis (fever, muscle aches, weakness).

Planning Box 31-3 lists the goals for B.T. when receiving antilipidemics.

Implementation

Monitoring Liver function studies should be performed periodically, because reductase inhibitors may elevate transaminase levels and serum creatine concentrations. Serum creatine kinase (CK) levels should be determined if B.T. develops muscular tenderness. Serum cholesterol levels determine the efficacy of treatment. Review with B.T. his progress on dietary changes, weight, and exercise.

Intervention Atorvastatin may be taken without regard to meals and at any time so long as it is consistent. Discontinue reductase inhibitor therapy if serum transaminase concentrations increase to three times the upper limit of normal, if creatine kinase (CK) concentrations markedly increase, or if myositis occurs.

Education As with other antihyperlipidemic medications, an appropriate diet, exercise, and weight reduction program for obese clients should be instituted along with drug therapy. Work with B.T. to find a substitute if grapefruit juice is a regular part of his diet, because it greatly increases the bioavailability of atorvastatin and simvastatin (Lilja, Kivisto, & Neuvonen, 1999).

Evaluation Box 31-3 outlines the expected outcomes of B.T.'s antilipidemic therapy.

✴ **How do nicotinic acid derivatives help to lower serum lipid levels?**

Nicotinic Acid Derivatives

✴◼ niacin [**nye** a sin]
(nicotinic acid, Nicobid)

Niacin (vitamin B_3) is a water-soluble vitamin that can lower total cholesterol and triglyceride levels by inhibiting VLDL-C synthesis and can also increase HDL cholesterol levels. Niacin has long been used to treat hyperlipidemia, but its association with significant vasodilation and flushing on initial dosing has limited its use. There is renewed interest in niacin and its efficacy (McKenney, 2004). Because nicotinic acid inhibits lipolysis in adipose tissue, it lowers the plasma concentration of free fatty acids, which usually is the main source of triglyceride synthesis in the liver.

Indications
Niacin is used as sole or adjunctive therapy in the treatment of both hypertriglyceridemia and hypercholesterolemia (Expert Panel on Detection, Evaluation and Treatment of High Blood Cholesterol in Adults, 2001). It is also used to prevent and treat niacin (vitamin B_3) deficiency.

Pharmacokinetics/Dosing
Niacin is well absorbed orally and has a half-life of approximately 45 minutes. It reduces cholesterol levels several days after initiating therapy; a reduction in triglyceride levels occurs within several hours of taking an oral dose. Niacin is metabolized in the liver and excreted by the kidneys. The adult dosage of niacin for an antihyperlipidemic effect is 1 g PO three times daily. The dosage may be increased to 500 mg daily every 2 to 4 weeks as necessary. The maximum dosage is 6 g daily.

Adverse Effects
The most obvious adverse effect of niacin is an increased feeling of warmth, flushing, or red skin on the face and neck. This flushing is common and can be minimized by initiating with very low doses of niacin and slowly increasing doses over the first few weeks or months of therapy, dosing niacin with aspirin, and using a formulation associated with reduced flushing (e.g., with inositol, or an extended release formulation of niacin). Long-acting formulations of niacin (designated as LA niacin) have been associated with increasing hepatic enzyme levels compared to immediate release or extended-release formulations (designated as ER niacin). LA niacin should therefore be avoided (McKenney, 2004). Hyperuricemia, elevated blood glucose levels, and myalgia have been reported. Other rare adverse effects include dysrhythmias, dry skin or eyes, dizziness, diarrhea, and aggravation of peptic ulcers; these are more likely with high dosages.

Drug Interactions
Concurrent use of vasodilators may increase the likelihood of flushing and postural hypotension. The effect of oral hypoglycemic agents may be reduced with niacin use. Bile acid sequestrants (e.g., cholestyramine) reduce the absorption of niacin. Use of niacin with statin drugs may increase the risk for rhabdomyolysis or hepatotoxicity, but this combination is sometimes required for high-risk clients.

✴ **What nursing management is needed for a client receiving a nicotinic acid derivative?**

Assessment Assess the client for preexisting conditions that would contraindicate the use of niacin, such as peptic ulcers, asthma, or allergy to niacin or niacinamide, because niacin should be used cautiously in these clients. Nicotinic acid causes a release of histamine and stimulates the secretion of hydrochloric acid. Niacin also should be used cautiously in individuals with arterial bleeding and hypotension (the vasodilating effects of the drug may worsen these conditions), hepatic dysfunction (may cause hepatic damage), glaucoma (may worsen the condition), diabetes mellitus (may impair glucose tolerance), and gout (may cause hyperuricemia).

Assess the client's concurrent medication regimen for medications that might contraindicate the use of niacin or require careful monitoring if they are taken at the same time; see drug interactions above.

A baseline assessment includes a serum cholesterol, glucose, and uric acid, and liver function studies, including serum transaminase. An eye exam for the presence of glaucoma and a baseline BP will provide comparative data during the course of therapy. Weight and a dietary profile will be helpful to determine any lifestyle changes that may be required.

Nursing Diagnosis With the administration of niacin, the client may experience the following nursing diagnoses/collaborative problems: impaired comfort (flushing of the skin of the head and neck, headaches, dizziness, nausea, and vomiting); diarrhea; impaired skin integrity (pruritus); and the potential complications of peptic ulcer (stomach pain), hyperglycemia (frequent urination, unusual thirst), hyperuricemia (joint pain, flank pain), hepatotoxicity (anorexia, abdominal discomfort, dark urine, light-colored stools, jaundice), dysrhythmias, or myalgia (fever, muscle aches, or cramping).

Planning See Box 31-3.

Implementation

Monitoring Monitor the results of periodically drawn serum cholesterol levels to evaluate the effectiveness of drug therapy; also monitor results of blood glucose, uric acid, and hepatic function studies to determine adverse effects. Monitor for orthostatic hypotension, especially if the client is also taking antihypertensive agents. Prolonged treatment with niacin has resulted in hepatic disease.

Intervention Give the drug with meals or with antacids, which may reduce the incidence and severity of gastric distress. If facial flushing is problematic, products containing inositol may be preferred because of its lack of vasodilating effect.

Education Instruct the client to swallow the extended-release form whole, without chewing or crushing. The powder within the capsule may be mixed with jam or applesauce for ease of administration. Encourage the client to adhere to the dietary regimen—low cholesterol and low saturated fats. Instruct the client to maintain clinical appointments so that serum cholesterol and triglycerides may be monitored on a periodic basis. Emphasize the importance of not taking more or less of the medication; or discontinuing the drug (blood lipids may increase significantly).

Alert the client that numerous and often disagreeable adverse effects may occur from niacin. Common adverse effects include severe GI upset, flushing, pruritus, nervousness, and urticaria. Although tolerance to the flushing, pruritus, and GI effects usually occurs within 2 weeks, these effects may be minimized by starting the client's therapy with a low dosage and increasing it slowly. If flushing continues to be a discomfort for the client, 300 mg of aspirin may be taken 30 minutes before each dose of niacin.

Evaluation See Box 31-3. If used for niacin deficiency, the client will experience a decrease or absence in the symptoms of pellagra, such as dermatitis, dementia, and diarrhea.

✱ **What are bile acid sequestering agents and how do they help to lower serum lipid levels?**

Bile Acid Sequestering Agents

These agents are nonabsorbable anion-exchange resins that are also called bile acid sequestrants. These drugs are used for their cholesterol-lowering effects. Cholesterol is the major precursor of bile acids that are normally secreted from the gallbladder and liver into the small intestine. Here the bile acids perform two functions: (1) they emulsify the fat

present in food to facilitate chemical digestion, and (2) they are required for the absorption of lipids (including fat-soluble vitamins A, D, E, and K). After their physiologic performance, the major portion of the bile acids is returned to the liver.

The anion-exchange resins bind bile acids in the intestine, thus preventing their absorption and producing an insoluble complex that is excreted in the feces. To compensate for the loss of bile acids removed by the drugs, the liver increases the rate of oxidation of cholesterol by converting more cholesterol to bile acids. Subsequently, the long-term fecal loss of bile acids causes a reduction of serum cholesterol levels and LDL cholesterol. These agents are less commonly used because of frequent GI distress and drug interactions. They are also less effective than other agents (see Table 31-3). Available agents include cholestyramine (Questran), colesevelam (Welchol) and colestipol (Colestid). Cholestyramine is considered the prototype agent.

✱◼▔▔ **cholestyramine** [koe less **tear** a meen]
(Questran)
Indications
Cholestyramine is used in the treatment of hyperlipidemia of primary hypercholesterolemia. Although not FDA-approved indications, it is also used to treat the pruritus induced by bile acid deposits in dermal tissues (from partial biliary obstruction), as an antidiarrheal agent for diarrhea caused by bile acids (not for common diarrhea) and as an antidote for negatively charged drugs and other medications by binding them in the gut before systemic absorption (e.g., digoxin, oral penicillin, tetracyclines, and thyroid medication).
Pharmacokinetics/Dosing
Plasma cholesterol levels usually decrease 1 to 2 weeks after the initiation of therapy, and plasma cholesterol levels may continue to fall for up to 1 year. After the initial decrease, plasma cholesterol levels may increase to previous levels in some individuals or even exceed these levels with continued therapy. Close monitoring for effectiveness is necessary. Plasma cholesterol levels increase approximately 2 to 4 weeks after the withdrawal of cholestyramine. If used to treat pruritus, pruritus often returns within 1 to 2 weeks. Cholestyramine is available as Questran and Questran Light (sugar free) powders for oral suspension. The adult dosage of cholestyramine is 4 g once or twice daily before meals; the maintenance dosage is 8 to 24 g daily in 2 to 6 divided doses as necessary. The pediatric dosage is 4 g daily in 2 divided doses initially, then 8 to 24 g in 2 or more divided doses as necessary.
Adverse Effects
The adverse effects of the bile acid sequestering agents include constipation, indigestion, abdominal pain, nausea and vomiting, abdominal pain, gas, dizziness, headache, and, rarely, gallstones, pancreatitis, bleeding ulcers, and malabsorption syndrome.
Drug Interactions
The bile acid sequestrants may reduce systemic absorption of a number of orally administered drugs, including digoxin, HMG Co-A reductase inhibitors, corticosteroids, and warfarin. This interaction can be minimized by consistently dosing the bile acid sequestrants apart from other drugs.

✱ **What nursing management is needed for a client receiving a bile acid sequestrant?**

Assessment Ascertain whether the client has a preexisting condition for which the drug would be used with great caution or contraindicated. The risk of cholestyramine and colestipol therapy should be considered in clients with constipation because it may induce fecal impaction. Because of its tendency to enhance constipation, this therapy should be used with caution in clients with medical conditions that could be aggravated by severe constipation, such as hemorrhoids or CHD. It should also be used with caution in older adults and in clients with peptic ulcer, gallstones, malabsorption states, bleeding disorders, and impaired renal function. Clients with complete biliary obstruction or complete atresia will have no bile acids in the GI tract to bind with cholestyramine and colestipol. Clients with phenylketonuria will be sensitive to the phenylalanine in aspartame in the sugar-free preparation of cholestyramine. Colestipol is contraindicated in clients with primary biliary cirrhosis because it may further increase concentrations of serum cholesterol. These drugs are contraindicated for use in clients who have an allergy to bile acid sequestrants.

The safety of these drugs for use by pregnant women and lactating mothers is Pregnancy Category C (see the Pregnancy Safety box below for FDA pregnancy safety classifications). However, because the drugs are almost totally unabsorbed after ingestion, there is a risk for impaired maternal absorption of vitamins and other nutrients.

Review the client's current medication regimen for the risk of significant drug interactions, such as those that may occur when cholestyramine, colesevelam, or colestipol are given concurrently with the following drugs. Bile acid sequestrants significantly decrease the absorption of warfarin and vitamin K; thus the anticoagulant effect may be increased or decreased. Oral anticoagulants should be given 6 hours before cholestyramine, colesevelam, or colestipol; monitor INRs closely, because dosage adjustments of warfarin may be necessary. Because the half-life of digoxin, and GI absorption, may be reduced, bile acid sequestrants should be administered at least 8 hours after digoxin to reduce the potential for interactions. If these bile acid sequestrants are discontinued in a client who is also taking digoxin, monitor the client closely for digoxin toxicity. Oral dosages of thiazide diuretics, propranolol, penicillin G, or

tetracyclines may have decreased absorption, and the therapeutic effect of orally administered vancomycin in the treatment of *Clostridium difficile* colitis may be impaired; administer such medications several hours before or after the sequestrants. Finally, because decreased absorption of thyroid hormone products has been reported, administer thyroid first on the medication administration schedule, then administer bile acid sequestrants several hours later.

Before beginning bile acid sequestrants, the client should undergo a lipid profile, including serum cholesterol and triglyceride concentration determinations to provide a baseline by which to evaluate therapy. A baseline dietary and exercise record is helpful in charting client progress with lifestyle changes.

Nursing Diagnosis Clients receiving bile acid sequestrants are at risk for the following nursing diagnoses/collaborative problems: constipation in approximately 10% of clients (mild to severe) and possible fecal impaction; impaired comfort (headache, belching, bloating, heartburn, nausea or vomiting, and abdominal discomfort); and the potential complications of gallstones or pancreatitis (severe stomach pain with nausea and vomiting), GI bleeding or peptic ulcer (black, tarry stools), steatorrhea or malabsorption syndrome (sudden loss of weight), or myalgia (with colesevelam).

Planning See Box 31-3.

Implementation

Monitoring Continue to monitor serum cholesterol and triglyceride levels in relation to baseline periodically and at regular intervals. (Table 31-3 compares the antilipemic effects of these drugs.) Additionally, INR values should be monitored, because a vitamin K deficiency may occur with the chronic use of cholestyramine and colestipol that could put the client at risk for increased bleeding tendencies. With the chronic use of cholestyramine, monitor serum calcium concentrations because of decreased calcium absorption.

Monitor digoxin levels in clients who are receiving digoxin and a bile sequestering agent simultaneously. To avoid toxicity, the dosage of the digoxin should be adjusted before discontinuing the anion-exchange resin.

Monitor progress on adequate fluid intake to prevent constipation as a side effect of these drugs and moderate exercise and limitation on dietary fat intake to evaluate progress of lifestyle changes.

Intervention Administer cholestyramine and colestipol before meals, and colesevelam with meals. To increase the palatability of cholestyramine and colestipol granules, sprinkle the powder on the surface of 2 ounces of a preferred liquid or semiliquid, such as cold beverages, hot cereals, thin soups (tomato, chicken noodle), or pulpy fruit (fruit cocktail, pears, peaches, or pineapple). Allow the drug to sit on the surface of the liquid for 1 to 2 minutes before stirring vigorously to prevent lumpiness. Add an additional

PREGNANCY SAFETY	
ANTIHYPERLIPIDEMIC DRUGS	
Category	**Drug**
C	cholestyramine, colestipol, clofibrate, ezetimibe, gemfibrozil, niacin (doses used for hyperlipidemia)
X	atorvastatin, cerivastatin, fluvastatin, lovastatin, pravastatin, simvastatin

Data from *Mosby's drug consult* (15th ed.). (2005). St. Louis: Mosby.

2 to 4 ounces of diluent, and shake vigorously again. Be sure the drug is thoroughly mixed, because it does not dissolve. Incomplete mixing of the dry form may result in mucosal irritation and esophageal impaction, or it may be accidentally inhaled. Rinse the glass or cup with a small amount of liquid, and have the client drink it to ensure that the complete dose is taken. Colesevelam may be taken in combination with a HMG-CoA reductase inhibitor.

Concurrent administration of a laxative or stool softener may help to prevent constipation. The client should also increase fluid intake to 2500 mL daily if not contraindicated.

Because resins interfere with the absorption of other drugs when taken concurrently, administer other drugs 1 hour before or 4 to 6 hours after cholestyramine or colestipol.

Education Instruct the client in the preparation of the medication for administration as discussed previously. Warn the client that the sudden withdrawal of resins could lead to uninhibited absorption of other drugs taken concomitantly, resulting in overdose or toxicity.

Supplemental parenteral or water-soluble vitamins A, D, E, and K, and folic acid, are prescribed to prevent vitamin deficiencies in clients receiving long-term therapy. Instruct the client to report early symptoms of bleeding immediately: petechiae, ecchymoses, bleeding from mucous membranes of gums or nose, or tarry stools (which indicate hypoprothrombinemia). The administration of vitamin K_1 (parenteral) and vitamin K_2 (oral) may be necessary.

Encourage the client to maintain regular bowel elimination patterns and to adhere to a high-fiber diet (e.g., grains, fruits, raw vegetables) and an increased fluid intake as an adjunct therapy to the drug. If constipation occurs, the dosage may be lowered to prevent fecal impaction, or a stool softener or laxative may be prescribed. Instruct the client to report GI symptoms to the prescriber: gastric distress, nausea and vomiting (pancreatitis), and unusual weight loss (steatorrhea).

Evaluation The expected outcome of bile acid sequestering agent therapy is that the client's serum cholesterol and LDL levels will decrease to within normal range. The drug is usually withdrawn if the response is unsatisfactory after 3 months of therapy. See also Box 31-3.

✷ **What are fibric acid derivatives and how do they help to lower serum lipid levels?**

Fibric Acid Derivatives

The fibric acid derivatives include gemfibrozil and fenofibrate. Clofibrate, also a fibric acid derivative, is associated with significant adverse effects and is no longer marketed. These agents appear to inhibit peripheral lipolysis and a decrease the hepatic extraction of free fatty acids, which result in a reduction of triglyceride production. Additionally, they may accelerate the turnover and removal of cholesterol from the liver, which is ultimately excreted in the feces. Like niacin, these agents are highly effective at lowering triglyceride levels and are considered drugs of choice for hypertriglyceridemia. Unlike gemfibrozil, fenofibrate has not demonstrated reductions in cardiovascular risks and is associated with increased toxicity and therefore is less frequently used.

✷🔲 **gemfibrozil** [jem **fye** broe zil]
(Lopid, Apo-Gemfibrozil✤, Novo-Gemfibrozil✤)
Gemfibrozil is an agent that primarily decreases the serum triglycerides found in VLDL-C and increases HDL-C.

Indications
Gemfibrozil is indicated for the treatment of hyperlipidemia, particularly when triglyceride levels are elevated.

Pharmacokinetics/Dosing
Oral gemfibrozil is well absorbed from the GI tract and reaches peak levels in 1 to 2 hours. The onset of action in reducing serum VLDL-C levels is within 2 to 5 days, and the peak effect is seen in 4 weeks. It is metabolized in the liver and excreted by the kidneys and in the feces. The adult dosage is 1.2 g daily in 2 divided doses, preferably before breakfast and dinner. Pediatric dosages have not been established.

Adverse Effects
The adverse effects of gemfibrozil include muscle aches and cramps, nausea, vomiting, rash, diarrhea, gas, and abdominal distress.

Drug Interactions
An increased anticoagulant effect is reported when gemfibrozil is given with warfarin. Monitor PTs/INRs closely because the anticoagulant dosage may need to be decreased significantly. If administered with an HMG-CoA reductase inhibitor (e.g., lovastatin), an increased risk of rhabdomyolysis and myoglobinuria may result in acute renal failure. This has been reported after 3 weeks to several months of combined drug therapy. Clients should be monitored for muscle pain or change in urinary patterns.

fenofibrate [fen oh **fi** brate]
(Tricor, Apo-Fenofibrate✤)
Fenofibrate is similar to clofibrate and gemfibrozil. Although its exact mechanism of action is unknown, the active metabolite fenofibric acid is believed to lower triglyceride levels by inhibiting triglyceride synthesis and stimulating the breakdown of triglyceride-rich lipoproteins (VLDL-C).

Indications
It is indicated as an adjunct to diet for the treatment of very high plasma levels of triglycerides (types IV and V hyperlipidemia) in adults who have not responded to diet alone or in persons who are at risk for pancreatitis.

Pharmacokinetics/Dosing
Fenofibrate reaches peak levels in 6 to 8 hours, is highly protein bound (99%), and has a half-life of 20 hours. It is metabolized in the liver and excreted primarily by the kidneys. The usual adult dosage is based on tablet formulation and ranges between 48 and 145 mg orally once daily.

Adverse Effects
The adverse effects of fenofibrate therapy include constipation, GI distress, eye irritation, decreased libido, skin photosensitivity or rash, dizziness, flu-like syndrome, infections, and pruritus.

✷ **What nursing management is needed for a client receiving a fibric acid derivative?**

Assessment Obtain a complete health assessment to ensure that the client does not have a preexisting condition for which the administration of fibric acid derivatives would be contraindicated or entail risk. The presence of primary biliary cirrhosis precludes the use of fibric acid derivatives because the drug may further raise serum cholesterol levels. Hepatic and renal dysfunction may require a reduced dosage to avoid an increased incidence of adverse effects, especially myopathy. There is an increased risk of biliary complications in the presence of gallstones with these agents.

Obtain a family health history; because of the genetic tendency of the disease, children and other family members should be screened for abnormal lipid levels. As a baseline assessment, a complete blood count (CBC), liver function tests, and serum cholesterol and triglyceride levels are determined.

Review the client's medication regimen to detect significant drug interactions. An increased anticoagulant effect is reported when these drugs are given with oral anticoagulants. Monitor INRs closely because the anticoagulant dosage may need to be decreased significantly. With fenofibrate, cyclosporine may increase renal dysfunction and HMG-CoA reductase inhibitors increase the risk of myopathy and rhabdomyolysis.

Nursing Diagnosis Clients undergoing fibric acid derivative therapy are at risk for developing the following nursing diagnoses/collaborative problems: impaired comfort (nausea, vomiting, flu-like syndrome, headache, heartburn, and abdominal discomfort); diarrhea; impaired oral mucous membrane (stomatitis); sexual dysfunction (decreased sexual ability); and the potential complications of myopathy (muscle aches, cramps or weakness), angina (chest pain, shortness of breath), cardiac dysrhythmias, anemia or leukopenia (abnormal blood counts and signs of infection—fever or chills, cough, painful urination), pancreatitis or gallstones (severe stomach pain with nausea and vomiting), and renal toxicity (blood in urine, decreased urinary output, pedal edema).

Planning See Box 31-3.

Implementation

   Monitoring In addition to clinically monitoring the client for signs and symptoms of adverse effects, monitor CBCs for signs of anemia or leukopenia, monitor hepatic function studies for abnormalities, and monitor serum cholesterol and triglyceride levels for the effectiveness of the drug. These drugs may increase the risk of biliary diseases such as cholelithiasis and cholecystitis; the appropriate diagnostic tests should be performed if signs and symptoms of biliary disease occur. Consult with the prescriber to withdraw the drug if any of the test results are abnormal.

   Intervention Administer clofibrate and fenofibrate with meals to prevent gastric distress whereas gemfibrozil is to be taken in two divided doses 30 minutes before the morning and evening meals.

   Education Advise the client to adhere to the recommended diet. The diet is usually low in fats, cholesterol,

and/or sugars. Encourage weight reduction and physical exercise.

A decrease in serum lipid levels during the first and second months of therapy indicates a therapeutic response. Warn the client that a paradoxical rise in levels may occur in 2 or 3 months, but afterward a further decrease is customary.

Instruct the client to keep clinical appointments for laboratory studies and reevaluation by the prescriber. If serum cholesterol and triglyceride levels are not lowered within 3 months, drug therapy is usually discontinued.

Advise the client to report any flu-like symptoms (muscular aching, soreness, cramping). This condition may be remedied by a dosage reduction. Instruct the individual to check with the prescriber about alcohol intake, because alcohol may be restricted to prevent hypertriglyceridemia.

The client should be aware that there is no substantial evidence that the drug reduces the incidence of CHD or fatal MI. Increased incidences of cardiac dysrhythmias, thromboembolism, intermittent claudication, and angina have been reported in clients treated with clofibrate.

Evaluation The client undergoing fibric acid derivative therapy will experience a reduction in serum lipid levels to within normal limits. See also Box 31-3.

✱ What other agents are used to manage hyperlipidemia?

Other agents used to treat hyperlipidemias include the azetidinones, ezetimibe (Zetia) and probucol (Lorelco), which are discussed in the following section. A number of complementary and alternative therapies are used by many clients to improve lipid profiles and include garlic, red yeast rice, and omega-3 fatty acids. Because it is so commonly used, garlic is discussed in the Complementary and Alternative Considerations box on p. 646. Red yeast rice is also discussed in Chapter 12.

Azetidinones

ezetimibe [e **zet** ih mibe]
(Zetia, Ezetrol ✤)
Ezetimibe is classified as a 2-azetidinone. It inhibits cholesterol absorption at the brush border of the small intestine. By interfering with enterohepatic circulation of cholesterol, reduced LDL-C and triglyceride levels are achieved as is a modest increase in HDL-C levels.

Indications
Ezetimibe is indicated for treating hyperlipidemia as monotherapy or in combination with an HMG Co-A reductase inhibitor (e.g., ezetimibe/simvastatin [Vytorin]). It is less effective at lowering cholesterol than are the statins, but in combination with statins, results in improved cholesterol lowering compared to statins alone (Goldberg, Sapre, Liu, Capece, & Mitchel, 2004; Pearson et al., 2005). Its role in lipid management is evolving.

Pharmacokinetics/Dosing
Ezetimibe displays variable absorption and is metabolized to an active metabolite. The majority of ezetimibe and its metabolite un-

Complementary and Alternative Considerations

Garlic

Garlic is widely used for flavoring in foods and beverages. Medicinally, it is used to reduce blood pressure, prevent age-related vascular changes, decrease LDLs and VLDLs, increase HDLs, and reduce blood clotting (antiplatelet effect). The lipid-lowering effects of garlic are attributed to its inactivation of the enzymes involved in lipid synthesis through an interaction with enzyme thiol groups. It is considered to be effective for lowering blood pressure and reducing serum cholesterol, LDLs, and triglycerides when taken orally as fresh garlic. Some controversy exists about the particular garlic supplements used in some studies. In general, data suggest that in addition to its lipid-lowering abilities, garlic has demonstrated antihypertensive, antithrombotic, and hypoglycemic activity. Garlic ingestion in the amounts commonly found in foods is considered safe unless the person has a sensitivity to garlic. It is possibly safe in larger amounts, but it may be contraindicated in clients with bleeding disorders, GI infection, or inflammation. Close monitoring is required for all clients with diabetes (because of garlic's hypoglycemic effects) and for clients taking anticoagulants (because additive effects may increase bleeding tendencies). The dose-related effects of garlic are breath odor, oral and GI burning or irritation, nausea, vomiting, flatulence, and diarrhea. Large amounts of garlic are contraindicated in children and in women who are pregnant or lactating. Garlic enhances the effects of warfarin as measured by the INR. Theoretically, it may also increase the effects of other anticoagulant drugs, antiplatelet drugs, and hypoglycemic drugs. Monitor more carefully clients with diabetes who are taking larger amounts of garlic, because the control of diabetes may be affected by the garlic. Although larger doses are taken to obtain the cholesterol-lowering and antihypertensive effects of garlic, the usual dosage is 1 clove of fresh garlic daily. Garlic is also available in various over-the-counter (OTC) preparations. Aged garlic extract can reduce total and LDL-C by 5% to 10% in hypercholesterolemic clients. Most studies of garlic preparations have been poorly controlled, short in duration, and without standardization of the type of garlic preparation, making evaluation of efficacy difficult. Until larger random controlled trials of longer duration, which correct the existing methodological flaws, are designed and carried out, it is best not to recommend garlic be used to treat mild to moderate hyperlipidemia. (For further information, see Chapter 12.) Green tea and red yeast rice have also been used for hyperlipidemia; see Chapter 12.

From Borek, C. (2001). Antioxidant health effects of aged garlic extract. *Journal of Nutrition, 131*(3s), 1010S–1015S. Alder, R., Lookinland, S., Berry, J.A., & Williams, M. (2003). A systematic review of the effectiveness of garlic as an antilipidemic agent. *Journal of the American Academy of Nurse Practitioners,* 13(3)120-129; and Jellin, J.M., Batz, F., & Hitchens, K. (2004). *Pharmacist's letter/prescriber's letter natural medicines comprehensive database.* Stockton, CA: Therapeutic Research Faculty.

dergo enterohepatic circulation and the majority of the drug is eliminated in the feces. The typical adult dose is 10 mg daily and is typically dosed concurrent with an HMG Co-A reductase inhibitor.

Adverse Effects

Ezetimibe is well tolerated with headache and GI upset among the most frequently reported adverse effects. Hypersensitivity reactions, sinusitis and pharyngitis, have been reported.

Drug Interactions

Use of cyclosporine, gemfibrozil, clofibrate, or fenofibrate may increase levels of ezetimibe, but it is not clear if this is clinically important. Dosing with bile acid sequestrants (e.g., cholestyramine) reduces absorption.

Nursing Management

As for the fibric acid derivatives above, except that clients on ezetimibe therapy are more at risk for an upper respiratory infection.

probucol [**proe** byoo kole]
(Lorelco)

Probucol is an antihyperlipidemic agent; it lowers levels of both LDL cholesterol and the desired HDL cholesterol, which limits the usefulness of this product. It is available in Canada, but not in the United States.

Indications

Probucol is used for persons with primary hypercholesterolemia who have not responded to other measures. In addition to lowering cholesterol levels, probucol induces the regression of xanthomas in persons with homozygous familial hypercholesterolemia and inhibits atherosclerosis as result of its antioxidant properties.

Pharmacokinetics/Dosing

Probucol is administered orally and has a variable absorption pattern. It tends to accumulate in fatty tissues with chronic therapy. Peak serum levels increase slowly and reach a steady state after 3 or 4 months of treatment; the peak effect usually occurs in 20 to 50 days after initiation of the drug. The half-life ranges from 12 to 500 hours. Probucol is excreted as bile in the feces. The adult dosage is 500 mg PO twice daily with breakfast and dinner. A pediatric dosage has not been established.

Adverse Effects

The adverse effects of probucol include gas, diarrhea, nausea, vomiting, abdominal distress, ventricular dysrhythmias and, rarely, anemia, angioneurotic edema, and thrombocytopenia.

Drug Interactions

It has no reported significant drug interactions.

Nursing Management

Assessment

Probucol is usually administered to individuals who do not respond adequately to dietary management and weight reduction. Do not give probucol to clients with primary biliary cirrhosis because it may further raise cholesterol levels, and do not give to clients with QT interval prolongation because the risk of additive QT interval may increase the risk of ventricular tachycardia. If there is evidence of myocardial damage and unresponsive heart failure (HF), the drug should be used with caution and only with electrocardiogram (ECG) monitoring, because these conditions may be exacerbated. A baseline assessment should include serum cholesterol and serum triglycerides.

Nursing Diagnosis

With the administration of probucol, the client may experience the following nursing diagnoses/collaborative problems: impaired comfort related to GI irritation (bloating, nausea, vomiting, abdominal discomfort), dizziness, headache, and tingling of the fingers and toes; and potential complications that include eosinophilia, anemia, thrombocytopenia, QT interval prolongation, and ventricular dysrhythmias.

Planning

See Box 31-3.

Implementation

Monitoring

Serum cholesterol and triglyceride levels should be obtained periodically during therapy to determine the efficacy of treatment. A baseline and periodic ECG readings should be monitored, especially for QT prolongation. Observe for syncope and pulse irregularities.

Intervention

If syncope occurs, probucol should be discontinued and the client monitored with an ECG. Probucol is usually discontinued if the client's response is not adequate after 4 months of therapy. When the drug is discontinued, continue to monitor serum lipids because serum cholesterol levels may rise up to or above the original base.

Education

If medication is given, adherence to a low-cholesterol, low-fat diet and physical exercise should continue. Instruct the individual to take the drug with food to minimize gastric irritation.

Evaluation

The client will show evidence of serum lipid concentrations that are within normal limits. See also Box 31-3.

Summary

Along with lifestyle modifications, antihyperlipidemic agents are used to treat hyperlipidemia, a metabolic disorder characterized by increased serum concentrations of cholesterol and triglycerides. High levels of these serum lipids have been associated with atherosclerosis, in which lipids are deposited in the linings of medium- and large-sized arteries.

Atherosclerosis is a causative factor in hypertension, CHD, cerebral artery disease, peripheral artery occlusive disease, and renal arterial insufficiency. Although atherosclerosis has many causes, such as dietary saturated fats, faulty fat metabolism, genetic influences, and others, some clinicians believe that the progression of atherosclerosis can be controlled if serum lipid levels can also be controlled.

The nurse is a key player in helping the client understand and achieve internationally accepted guidelines for lipid management. Management consists of encouraging the client to adopt positive therapeutic lifestyle changes including diet, exercise, and smoking cessation. Drug therapy is now considered an essential component for many clients to achieve goal lipid levels and reduce CHD risk.

As HMG CoA reductase inhibitors, atorvastatin, fluvastatin, lovastatin, pravastatin, rosuvastatin and simvastatin inhibit the synthesis of cholesterol in the liver and are effective for clients with primary hypercholesterolemia. Niacin, although associated with flushing, is highly effec-

tive in lowering both LDL-C and triglycerides. The bile acid sequestering agents, cholestyramine, colesevelam, and colestipol hydrochloride, combine with bile acids in the intestine to prevent their absorption and promote their loss from the body in feces. To compensate for their loss, the liver increases its rate of oxidation of cholesterol to replace the bile acids, which causes a reduction of serum cholesterol levels. The fibric acid derivatives, including gemfibrozil, are more effective in lowering serum triglyceride levels than cholesterol. Ezetimibe, a newer agent classified as an azetidinone, interferes with cholesterol absorption at the brush border of the small intestine. Each agent varies in effectiveness and adverse effects.

✳ Critical Thinking Questions

- Mr. Clark has been taking atorvastatin for 6 months. During this office visit he indicates that he has been experiencing muscle aches more frequently. What might be happening?
- How would the nurse counteract the common belief of clients that drug therapy replaces dietary restrictions in the management of hyperlipidemia?

Bibliography

Anderson, D.M., Keith, J., & Novak, P.D. (Eds.) (2002). *Mosby's medical, nursing, and allied health dictionary* (6th ed.). St. Louis: Mosby.

Boekholdt, S.M., Kuivenhoven, J.A., Hovingh, G.K., Jukema, J.W., Kastelein, J., van Tol, A. (2003). CETP gene variation: relation to lipid parameters and cardiovascular risk. *Current Opinion in Lipidology, 15*(4), 393-398.

Bosker, G. (Ed.). (2004). *Primary and acute care medicine: Practice, protocols, pathways,* (2nd ed.). Atlanta: Thomson American Health Consultants.

Brescianini, S., Maggi, S., Farchi, G., Mariotti, S., Di Carlo, A., Baldereschi, M., et al., and the ILSA Group. (2003). Low total cholesterol and increased risk of dying: Are low levels clinical warning signs in the elderly? Results from the Italian Longitudinal Study on Aging. Journal of the American Geriatric Society, *51,* 991-996.

Caslake, M., Packard, C.J. (2004). Phenotypes, genotypes and response to statin therapy. *Current Opinion in Lipidology, 15*(4), 387-392.

𝓮-LEARNING SUPPLEMENTS

Student CD-ROM
- Final Exam questions
- NCLEX® Examination review questions
- Pharmacology animations
- Printable chapter summary

Evolve Website (http://evolve.elsevier.com/mckenry)
- Case study on antihyperlipidemic drugs
- Content updates, including information on new drugs

- WebLinks corresponding to this chapter
- Answers to the critical thinking questions in this chapter
- *Elsevier ePharmacology Update* newsletter
- *Mosby's Drug Consult* Internet Edition
- Supplemental and reference information

Chang, J.T., Altman, R.B. (2004). Extracting and characterizing gene-drug relationships from the literature. *Pharmacogenetics, 14*(9), 577-586. Retrieved December 2, 2004, from http://bionlp.stanford.edu/genedrug/gene_drug_predictions.html.

Charles, E.C., Olson, K.L., Sandhoff, B.G., McClure, D.L., & Merenich, J.A. (2005). Evaluation of cases of severe statin-related transaminitis within a large health maintenance organization. *American Journal of Medicine, 118,* 618-624.

Chasman, D.I., Posada, D., Subrahmanyan, L., Cook, N.R., Stanton, V.P. Jr, Ridker, P.M. (2004). Pharmacogenetic study of statin therapy and cholesterol reduction. Journal of the American Medical Association, *291,* 2821-2827.

Collins, R., Armitage, J., Parish, S., Sleigh, P., Peto, R. and the Heart Protection Study Collaborative Group. (2003). MRC/BHF Heart Protection Study of cholesterol-lowering with simvastatin in 5963 people with diabetes: A randomised placebo-controlled trial. *Lancet, 361,* 2005-2016.

Collins, R., Armitage, J., Parish, S., Sleigh, P., Peto, R. and the Heart Protection Study Collaborative Group. (2004). Effects of cholesterol-lowering with simvastatin on stroke and other major vascular events in 20 536 people with cerebrovascular disease or other high-risk conditions. *Lancet, 363,* 757-767.

Drug facts and comparisons (58th ed.). (2005). St. Louis: Facts and Comparisons.

Dudley-Brown, S. (2004). A shot of good cholesterol: Synthetic HDL, a new intervention for atherosclerosis. *Journal of Cardiovascular Nursing, 19*(6), 421-424.

Dwyer, J.H., Allayee, H., Dwyer, K.M., Fan, J., Wu, H., Mar, R., et al. (2004). Arachidonate 5-Lipoxygenase Promoter Genotype, Dietary Arachidonic Acid, and Atherosclerosis. *New England Journal of Medicine, 350*(1), 29-37.

Esposito, K., Marfella, R., Ciotola, M., Di Palo, C., Giugliano, F., Giugliano, G., et al. (2004). Effect of a Mediterranean-style diet on endothelial dysfunction and markers of vascular inflammation in the metabolic syndrome: A randomized trial. *Journal of the American Medical Association, 292,* 1440-1446.

Expert Panel on Detection, Evaluation and Treatment of High Blood Cholesterol in Adults (2001). Executive Summary of the third report of the National Cholesterol Education Program (NCEP) expert panel on detection, evaluation, and treatment of high blood cholesterol in adults (Adult Treatment Panel III). *Journal of the American Medical Association, 285,* 2486-2497.

Ferrario, C.M., Richmond, R.S., Smith, R., Levy, P., Strawn, W., Kivlighn, S. (2004). Renin-angiotensin system as a therapeutic target in managing atherosclerosis. *American Journal of Therapeutics, 11*(1), 44-53.

Foucher, C., Rattier, S., Flavell, D.M., Talmud, P.J., Humphries, S., Kastelein, J., et al., for the DAIS investigators. (2004). Response to micronized fenofibrate treatment is associated with the peroxisome-proliferator-activated receptors alpha G/C intron7 polymorphism in subjects with type 2 diabetes. *Pharmacogenetics, 14*(12), 823-829.

Goldberg, A.C., Sapre, A., Liu, J., Capece, R., & Mitchel, Y.B. for the Ezetimibe Study Group. (2004): Efficacy and safety of ezetimibe coadministered with simvastatin in patients with primary hypercholesterolemia: A randomized, double-blind, placebo-controlled trial. *Mayo Clinic Proceedings, 79*(5), 620-629.

Graham, D.J., Staffa, J.A., Shatin, D., Andrade, S.E., Schech, S.D., LaGrenade, L., et al. (2004). Incidence of hospitalized rhabdomyolysis in patients treated with lipid-lowering drugs. *Journal of the American Medical Association, 292,* 2585-2590.

Grundy, S.M., Cleeman, J.I., Merz, C., Noel, B., Brewer, H., et al., for the Coordinating Committee of the National Cholesterol Education Program. (2004). Implications of recent clinical trials for the National Cholesterol Education Program Adult Treatment Panel III Guidelines. *Circulation, 110*(2), 227-239.

Hardman, J.G., & Limbird, L.E. (Eds.). (2001). *Goodman & Gilman's the pharmacological basis of therapeutics* (10th ed.). New York: McGraw-Hill.

Hippisley-Cox, J., & Coupland, C. (2005). Effect of combinations of drugs on all cause mortality in patients with ischaemic heart disease: Nested case-control study. *British Medical Journal, 330,* 1059-1063.

Hsue, P.Y., Lo, J.C., Franklin, A, Bolger, A.F., Martin, J.N., Deeks, S.G., et al. (2004). Progression of atherosclerosis as assessed by carotid intima-media thickness in patients with HIV infection. *Circulation, 109,* 1603-1608.

Khalil, M.F., Wagner, W.D., Goldberg, I.J. (2004). Molecular interactions leading to lipoprotein retention and the initiation of atherosclerosis. *Arteriosclerosis, Thrombosis & Vascular Biology, 24*(12), 2211-2218.

Kivisto, K.T., Niemi, M., Schaeffeler, E., Pitkala, K., Tilvis, R., Fromm, M.F., et al. (2004). Lipid-lowering response to statins is affected by CYP3A5 polymorphism. *Pharmacogenetics. 14*(8), 523-525.

Knoops, K.T., de Groot, L.C., Kromhout, D., Perrin, A.E., Moreiras-Varela, O., Menotti, A., et al. (2004). Mediterranean diet, lifestyle factors, and 10-year mortality in elderly European men and women: The HALE Project. *Journal of the American Medical Association, 292,* 1433-1439.

Lacy, C.F., Armstrong, L.L., Goldman, M.P., & Lance, L.L. (2004). *Lexi-Comp's Drug Information Handbook* (12th ed.). Hudson, Ohio: Lexi-Comp.

Lilja, J.J., Kivisto, K.T., & Neuvonen, P.J. (1999). Grapefruit juice increases serum concentrations of atorvastatin and has no effect on pravastatin. *Clinical Pharmacology & Therapeutics, 66*(2), 118-127.

Linker, C.A. (2003). Blood. In L.M. Tierney, Jr., S.J. McPhee, & Papadakis, M.A. (Eds.), *Current Medical Diagnosis & Treatment.* New York: Lange Medical Books/McGraw-Hill.

Lusis, A.J., Fogelman, A.M., Fonarow, Gregg C. (2004). Genetic basis of atherosclerosis: Part II: Clinical implications. *Circulation, 110*(14), 2066-2071.

McKenney, J.M. (2005). Dyslipidemias, atherosclerosis, and coronary heart disease. In M.A. Koda-Kimble, L.Y. Young, W.A. Kradjan, B.J. Guglielmo, B.K. Alldredge, & R.L. Corelli (Eds.), *Applied therapeutics: The clinical use of drugs* (8th ed.). Philadelphia: Lippincott, Williams & Wilkins.

McKenney, J. (2004). New perspectives on the use of niacin in the treatment of lipid disorders. *Archives of Internal Medicine, 164*(7), 697-705.

Mosby's drug consult (15th ed.). (2005). St. Louis: Mosby.

Niemi, M., Schaeffeler, E., Lang, T., Fromm, M.F., Neuvonen, M., Kyrklund, C., et al. (2004) High plasma pravastatin concentrations are associated with single nucleotide polymorphisms and haplotypes of organic anion transporting polypeptide-C (OATP-C, SLCO1B1). *Pharmacogenetics, 14*(7), 429-440.

Nissen, S.E., Tuzcu, E.M., Schoenhagen, P., Crowe, T., Sasiela, W.J., Tsai, J., et al. (2005). Reversal of Atherosclerosis with Aggressive Lipid Lowering (REVERSAL) Investigators: Statin therapy, LDL cholesterol, C-reactive protein, and coronary artery disease. *New England Journal of Medicine, 352,* 29-38.

Pearson, T.A., Denke, M.A., McBride, P.E., Battisti, W.P., Brady, W.E., & Palmisano, J. (2005) A community-based, randomized trial of ezetimibe added to statin therapy to attain NCEP ATP III goals for LDL cholesterol in hypercholesterolemic patients: The Ezetimibe Add-On to Statin for Effectiveness (EASE) trial. *Mayo Clinic Proceedings, 80,* 587-595.

Poynter, J.N., Grubner, S.B., Higgins, P.D., Almog, R., Bonner, J.D., Rennert, H.S et al. (2005). Statins and the risk of colorectal cancer. *New England Journal of Medicine, 352,* 2184-2192.

Psaty, B.M., Furberg, C.D., Ray, W.A., & Weiss, N.S. (2004). Potential for conflict of interest in the evaluation of suspected adverse drug reactions: Use of cerivastatin and risk of rhabdomyolysis. *Journal of the American Medical Association, 292,* 2622-2631.

Rackley, C.E. (2004). New clinical markers predictive of cardiovascular disease: The role of inflammatory mediators. *Cardiology in Review, 12*(3), 151-157.

Ricote, M., Valledor, A.F., Glass, C.K. (2004). Decoding transcriptional programs regulated by PPARs and LXRs in the macrophage: Effects on lipid homeostasis, inflammation, and atherosclerosis. *Arteriosclerosis, Thrombosis & Vascular Biology, 24*(2), 230-239.

Ridker, P.M., Cannon, C.P., Morrow, D., Rifai, N., Rose, L.M., McCabe, C.H., et al. (2005). Pravastatin or atorvastatin evaluation and infection therapy: Thrombolysis in myocardial infarction. *New England Journal of Medicine, 352,* 20-28.

Sever, P.S., Dahlof, B., Poulter, N.R., Wedel, H., Beevers, G., Caulfield, M., et al., the ASCOT investigators. (2003). Prevention of coronary and stroke events with atorvastatin in hypertensive patients who have average or lower-than-average cholesterol concentrations, in the Anglo-Scandinavian Cardiac Outcomes Trial — Lipid Lowering Arm (ASCOT-LLA): A multicentre randomised controlled trial. *Lancet, 361,* 1149-1158.

Shepherd, J., Blauw, G.J., Murphy, M.B., Bollen, E.L., Buckley, B.M., Cobbe, S.M., and the Prospective Study of Pravastatin in the Elderly at Risk (PROSPER) study group. (2002). Pravastatin in elderly individuals at risk of vascular disease (PROSPER): A randomised controlled trial. *Lancet, 360,* 1623-1630.

Talbert, R.L. (2002). Hyperlipidemia. In J.T. DiPiro, R.L. Talbert, G.C. Yee, G.R. Matzke, B.G. Wells, & L.M. Posey (Eds.), *Pharmacotherapy: A pathophysiological* approach (3rd ed.). Norwalk, CT: Appleton & Lange.

Third Report of the National Cholesterol Education Program (NCEP) Expert Panel on Detection, Evaluation, and Treatment of High Blood Cholesterol in Adults (Adult Treatment Panel III) Executive Summary. (2001). NIH publication No. 01-3670. Retrieved July 15, 2004, from http://www.5nhlbi.nih.gov/guidelines/cholesterol/atp3xsum.pdf.

U.S. Food and Drug Administration. (2004). FDA Public Health Advisory for Crestor (rosuvastatin). Retrieved December 30, 2004, from http://www.fda.gov/cder/drug/advisory/crestor.htm.

U.S. Food and Drug Administration. (2005). FDA Public Health Advisory on Crestor (rosuvastatin). Retrieved July 8, 2005, from http://www.fda.gov/cder/drug/advisory/crestor_3_2005.htm.

USP DI: Drug information for the health care professional (25th ed.). (2005). Greenwood Village, CO: MICROMEDEX Thomson Healthcare.

VanderLaan, P.A., Reardon, C.A., Getz, G.S. (2004). Site specificity of atherosclerosis: Site-selective responses to atherosclerotic modulators. *Arteriosclerosis, Thrombosis & Vascular Biology, 24*(1), 12-22.

Vermes, A., Vermes, I. (2004). Genetic polymorphisms in cytochrome P450 enzymes: Effect on efficacy and tolerability of HMG-CoA reductase inhibitors. *American Journal of Cardiovascular Drugs, 4*(4), 247-255.

Walsh, J., Pignone, M. (2004). Drug treatment of hyperlipidemia in women. *Journal of the American Medical Association, 291*(18), 2243-2252.

Wiegman, A., Hutten, B.A., de Groot, E., Rodenburg, J., Bakker, H.D., Buller, H.R., et al. (2004). Efficacy and safety of statin therapy in children with familial hypercholesterolemia: A randomized controlled trial. *Journal of the American Medical Association, 292,* 331-337.

Zineh, I. (2004). Genetic polymorphisms and statin therapy. *Journal of the American Medical Association, 292*(11), 1302-1303.

32

OVERVIEW OF THE URINARY SYSTEM

CHAPTER FOCUS

The urinary system functions with other organs to regulate the volume and composition of fluid within the body, retaining essential materials and excreting waste. Because of this function, the urinary system affects other body systems and the client's general health. Many pharmacologic effects are diminished or enhanced by the activity of the urinary system, and therefore the nurse must be knowledgeable about its anatomy and physiology.

LEARNING OBJECTIVES

- Describe the anatomy and physiology of the urinary system.
- Identify the functions of the various segments of the nephron.
- Describe the major functions of the kidneys.
- Describe the sites of action and primary effects of antidiuretic hormone, vasopressin, and aldosterone on the nephrons.

▲ **KEY TERMS**

aldosterone, p. 653
antidiuretic hormone (vasopressin) , p. 653
electromagnetic gradient, p. 652
glomerular filtration, p. 651
glomerulus, p. 651
hypertonic, p. 653

hypotonic, p. 653
osmotic gradient, p. 652
threshold concentration, p. 652
tubular reabsorption, p. 652
tubular secretion, p. 652
tubular transport maximum, p. 652

The urinary system is composed of organs that manufacture and excrete urine from the body: two kidneys, two ureters, the bladder, and the urethra (Figure 32-1). Urine formed in the kidneys flows through the ureters to the bladder, in which it is stored. When approximately 250 mL of urine is collected, bladder expansion results in a feeling of distention and a desire to void. The urine flows from the bladder into the urethra to be expelled from the body.

In males the urethra is surrounded by the prostate gland; it then passes through fibrous tissue connected to the pubic bones and terminates at the urinary meatus, or tip of the penis (Figure 32-2). The male urethra serves a dual purpose—elimination of urine from the body and the transport of semen. In females the urethra is the final vehicle for urination (Figure 32-3).

The kidneys regulate homeostasis in the body; they are responsible for the maintenance of body fluids, electrolytes, and acid-base balance and the elimination of body waste, urea, and urine. The primary focus of this chapter is the kidneys.

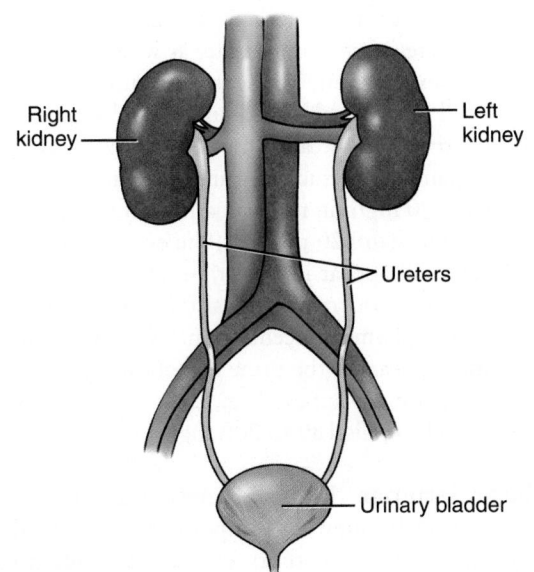

FIGURE 32-1 Urinary system.

✳ **What are the key physiologic features of the kidney?**
The kidney is composed of millions of individual units
called nephrons. Each nephron consists of a glomerulus and
a tubular system (Figure 32-4). The volume and composition of urine as a result of concentration and dilution depend on three major processes in the kidney: glomerular filtration, tubular reabsorption, and tubular secretion.

Glomerular Filtration Glomerular filtration occurs as
a result of plasma flowing across a cluster of capillary blood
vessels and into the urinary space of the Bowman capsule.
This capillary cluster is enveloped within a thin wall,
branching into uriniferous tubules; it is called the **glomerulus.** The heart works to create pressure in the blood vessels,
which in turn provides the force necessary to accomplish
glomerular filtration. Blood flow to the kidney occurs at a
rate of 1200 mL/min, which is 20% to 25% of cardiac output. The blood pressure (BP) within the glomerular capillaries is approximately 60% of arterial pressure. Systemic

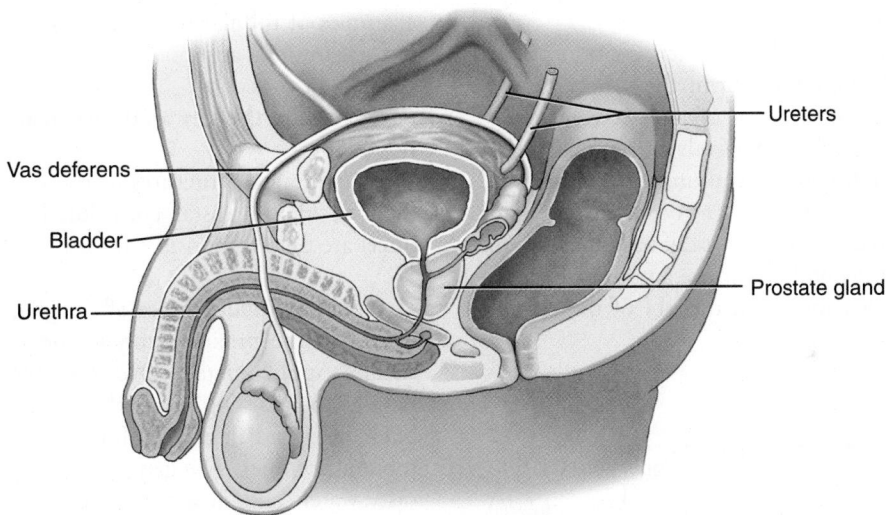

FIGURE 32-2 Sagittal section of the male pelvis.

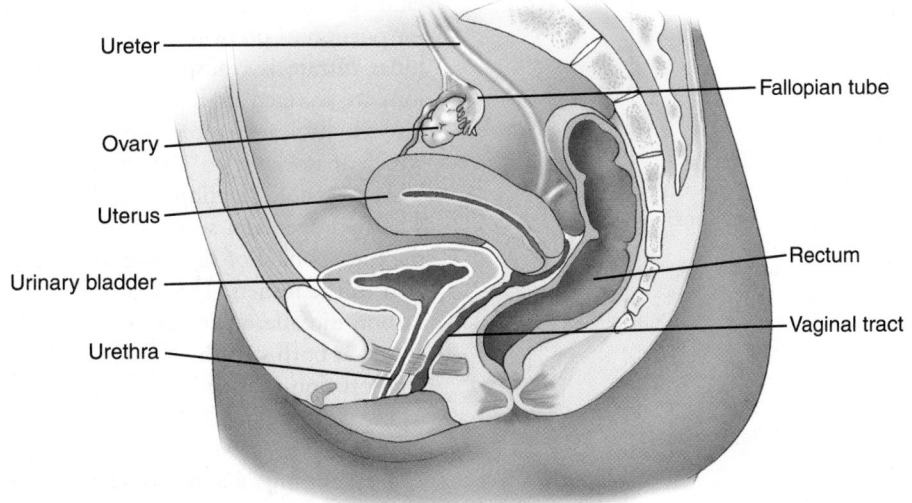

FIGURE 32-3 Sagittal section of the female pelvis.

BP must be significantly reduced before glomerular filtration is greatly altered. Usually some degree of filtration exists if the mean BP remains above 50 mm Hg. Maintenance of glomerular hydrostatic pressure is aided by the ability of the afferent and efferent arterioles to alter vessel resistance effectively.

In the absence of disease, the glomerular membrane does not filter plasma proteins greater than 100 angstroms in diameter (e.g., hemoglobin and albumin and the small amount of protein-bound substances). Otherwise the glomerular filtrate is almost identical to plasma. The rate of filtration in an average adult is approximately 125 mL/min; 99% of this tubular filtrate is ultimately reabsorbed throughout the tubule.

Tubular Reabsorption Tubular reabsorption involves both active and passive transport of substances into the tubular epithelial cell and into the extracellular fluid compartment. Passive transport, or diffusion, through the tubular membrane occurs because of a difference in particle concentration (**osmotic gradient**) or electrical charge (**electromagnetic gradient**).

In the proximal tubule, sodium is *actively* transported across the tubular cell membrane from the tubule filtrate. Chloride follows passively because of an electromagnetic gradient. Water in turn follows passively in response to an osmotic gradient established by sodium chloride solute. Then diffusion of 60% of urea content occurs to maintain a chemical gradient. Weak acids and weak bases may be reabsorbed by diffusion depending on the amount of a drug in ionized or nonionized form and the pH of the tubular fluid.

For almost every substance actively transported across the membrane, there is a maximum rate at which the transport mechanism can function; above this maximum, the excess substance will not be reabsorbed and the substance will appear in the urine. This is called the **tubular transport maximum.** For example, the tubular transport maximum for glucose averages 320 mg/min for most adults. If the tubular load becomes greater than 320 mg/min, the excess will not be reabsorbed and will appear in the urine. Every substance that has a tubular transport maximum also has a **threshold concentration,** the plasma concentration below which none of the substance appears in the urine and above which progressively larger quantities appear (e.g., the approximate plasma threshold for glucose is 180 to 200 mg/dL).

Tubular Secretion Tubular secretion affects the composition of urine by allowing compounds such as penicillin, histamine, probenecid, methotrexate, and thiazides to enter into tubular fluid from peritubular or interstitial capillaries. This is accomplished via specific transport mechanisms for the secretion of organic compounds. Other very important examples of tubular secretion include that of the hydrogen ions, ammonia, and potassium ions.

✳ What are the key anatomic features of the nephron?

The anatomical structures of the tubule (proximal tubule, loop of Henle, distal convoluted tubule, and collecting duct) are each responsible for unique functions.

Proximal Tubule Most of the glomerular filtrate is reabsorbed in the proximal tubule and returned to the bloodstream. Approximately 70% of salt and water is reabsorbed rapidly, maintaining nearly the same osmolality between tubular fluid and interstitial fluid at the end of the proximal tubule (isotonic). The general mechanism for sodium, chloride, water, and urea reabsorption is tubular reabsorption with respect to gradient transport. There are no dilutional or concentration changes of these ions in the proximal tubule.

Other substances reabsorbed in the proximal tubule include glucose, amino acids, phosphate, uric acid, and a major portion of potassium. Nearly 90% of bicarbonate in tubular filtrate is reabsorbed as carbon dioxide if hydrogen ions are secreted in the tubular lumen. Plasma carbon dioxide is hydrolyzed in the tubular cell to form carbonic acid, which dissociates to give bicarbonate and hydrogen ion. This reversible reaction is catalyzed by carbonic anhydrase. The hydrogen ion secreted into the lumen combines with the bicarbonate of the glomerular filtrate to form carbonic acid in the lumen. This again dissociates to give water and carbon dioxide, which are reabsorbed. This reaction is catalyzed at both steps by carbonic anhydrase. Proximal tubule reabsorption is usually constant despite moderate changes in the glomerular filtration rate.

Descending Loop of Henle This portion of the nephron is permeable to water; water is passively taken up to equilibrate medullary interstitial osmolality. This pro-

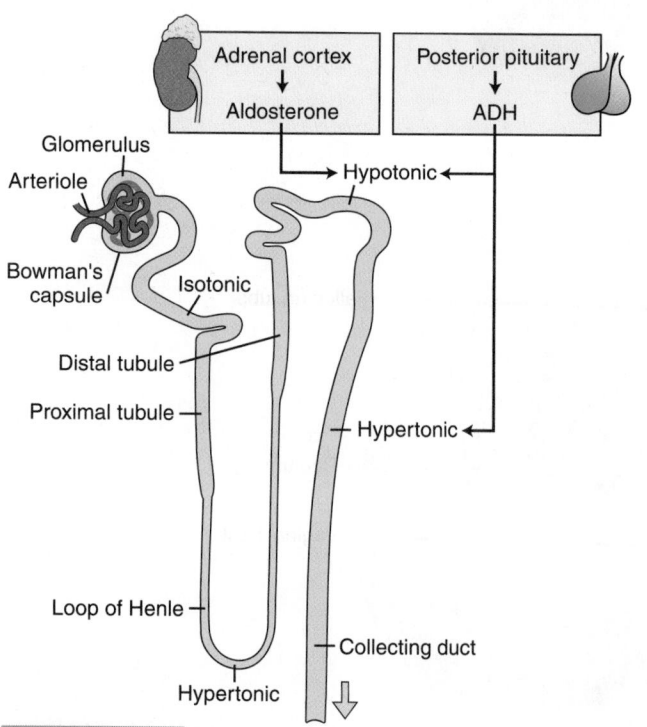

FIGURE 32-4 Components of the nephron.

duces a hypertonic (more concentrated) filtrate at the tip of the loop of Henle, the papilla. There is very low sodium and urea permeability in this segment.

Ascending Loop of Henle Water permeability is almost nil in the ascending limb of the loop of Henle, whereas sodium and chloride permeability is high. Approximately 20% to 25% of sodium load in glomerular filtrate is reabsorbed, and chloride follows passively. As a result, two very important situations occur. The concentration of tubular filtrates becomes very dilute, or hypotonic; this is often termed "free water production." Meanwhile, the medullary interstitium becomes hypertonic, which is necessary to the concentration capacity of the countercurrent multiplier. The concentration gradient established across the tubular epithelium becomes multiplied in a longitudinal direction, resulting in a large osmotic gradient between the isosmotic renal cortex and the hyperosmotic medulla and papilla. Unlike other segments, the ascending limb of the loop of Henle is not responsive to any hormones.

Distal Convoluted Tubule Between 5% and 10% of sodium reabsorption actively occurs in the distal tubule. This uptake is largely determined by the presence of aldosterone. When the extracellular fluid volume is decreased, the renin-angiotensin system becomes involved and stimulates the release of aldosterone. Increased levels of aldosterone act to increase the active reabsorption of sodium. Although an increase in potassium secretion is seen, a simple sodium-potassium exchange pump is no longer recognized.

Collecting Duct The hypotonic fluid entering the collecting duct may be altered in the medullary portion by the presence of antidiuretic hormone (ADH), or vasopressin. The released ADH acts at the distal tubule and collecting duct to reabsorb water to increase plasma volume, thus lowering plasma osmolality. Thus the collecting duct is responsible for urine concentration.

✱ **What metabolic processes are regulated by the kidney?**

The kidneys excrete metabolic byproducts of the body, especially nitrogenous-type substances such as urea. They maintain electrolyte homeostasis (e.g., sodium, potassium, chloride) and body fluids. Sodium is actively reabsorbed in the proximal tubules (approximately 65%) and ascending loop of Henle (27%). Approximately 8% of sodium reaches the distal tubules; the rate of reabsorption in the distal tubules depends on the presence of aldosterone. If large quantities of aldosterone are present, sodium is reabsorbed. A lack of aldosterone leads to elimination of sodium in the urine. In general, healthy kidneys excrete the daily sodium intake. Potassium is reabsorbed from the proximal tubules and loop of Henle in percentages equivalent to sodium. Thus approximately 8% of the filtered potassium reaches the distal tubules. Aldosterone controls potassium secretion; in its presence, sodium is reabsorbed and potassium is secreted in the distal tubules. The daily potassium intake is generally excreted daily in the kidneys. Table 32-1 summarizes nephron functions.

ADH is a water-conserving hormone synthesized in the hypothalamus and stored in the posterior pituitary gland. When plasma osmolarity increases as a result of dehydration or water deprivation, osmoreceptors in the supraoptic area of the hypothalamus stimulate the release of ADH. The released ADH acts at the distal tubule and collecting duct to reabsorb water to increase plasma volume, thus lowering plasma osmolality. Urine output is decreased, and the urine is more concentrated.

Acid-base balance is partially controlled in the kidneys. The kidneys are one of three pH control mechanisms in the body; the others are blood buffering and the respiratory adjustment mechanism. As the blood pH becomes more acidic, the kidneys respond by increasing the renal tubule excretion of hydrogen and ammonia, which results in an increase in blood bicarbonate and an increase in pH (toward normal). This is an effective method of adjusting hydrogen ions within the system.

The hormone erythropoietin is synthesized in the kidneys. A decrease in red blood cells (RBCs) below normal, or tissue hypoxia, stimulates an increased release of erythropoietin from the kidneys. The increased serum concentra-

TABLE 32-1 NEPHRON FUNCTIONS	
Site	**Major Functions**
Glomerulus	Filtration
Proximal tubule	Reabsorption of glucose, potassium, sodium, amino acids, water, and nutrients; remaining fluid isotonic.
Loop of Henle	Sodium and chloride reabsorbed in ascending loop. Countercurrent mechanism produces decrease in osmolality of filtrate in ascending loop of Henle (e.g., sodium chloride but not water is transported into the body). Filtrate leaves loop of Henle as hypotonic urine.
Distal tubule	Sodium and bicarbonate are reabsorbed. Potassium, hydrogen, and ammonia may be secreted. ADH is necessary to reabsorb water at this site. Filtrate leaves the distal tubule as hypotonic urine.
Collecting duct	ADH, if present, will reabsorb water at this site. Urine may be hypertonic. If ADH is unavailable or not functioning, dilute urine (hypotonic) may be excreted.

tion of erythropoietin stimulates the bone marrow to increase its production of RBCs so that the RBC average is restored to normal.

Some basic functional studies to assess overall renal function are important for the nurse to monitor:

- Creatinine clearance (Cl_{Cr}): This is a widely used test of urine to determine glomerular filtration (GFR). It is theoretically reliable, but is commonly compromised because of the difficulty of getting a complete 24 hour specimen. Normal adult values are 90 to 130 mL/min/1.73 m² BSA.
- Serum creatinine (Cr): This is a readily available, inexpensive measure of GFR. Endogenous creatinine is a product of metabolism in muscle and so its production is directly dependent on muscle mass. Creatinine is excreted through the kidney by glomerular filtration and so as GFR declines, the serum creatinine concentration increases. It is not sensitive to early changes in renal mass or single-kidney and may overestimate GFR in some conditions (e.g., cirrhosis, clients with reduced muscle mass, older adults). Normal adult values are about 0.6 to 1.2 mg/dL or 50 to 100 μmol/L. The use of serum creatinine in estimating renal function is discussed in Chapter 35.
- Blood urea nitrogen (BUN): Urea, an end product of protein metabolism is excreted by the kidney. It is directly related to protein intake and nitrogen metabolism. Urea concentration in glomerular filtrate is the same as in plasma, but its tubular reabsorption is inversely related to the rate of urine production or the client's hydration. Therefore, in general, creatinine determinations have largely replaced urea and urea nitrogens in the evaluation of renal function. Normal adult values are about 8 to 20 mg/dL or 2.9 to 7.1 mmol/L.
- Urinalysis (UA): The urinalysis, particularly by dipstick, is readily available method for assessing a number of results. The results may be nonspecific and influenced by a number of diseases, but it is a useful screening tool. A single dipstick may measure specific gravity, pH, protein, glucose, ketone, bilirubin, blood, nitrite, and leucocytes in the urine. The dipstick will be color-coded for specific values for each substance. Other substances can be identified in urine assisting with diagnosis (e.g., drug testing) or monitoring the management of conditions.

- Urine cultures (C&S): Culture of urine can assist the identification of the causative microorganism in a number of conditions, such as cystitis, pyelonephritis, prostatitis, and other genitourinary (GU) infections. The sensitivity component of the C&S determines which antiinfectives the identified organism is sensitive or resistant to, thereby enhancing the selection of the appropriate drug.
- Computed tomographic (CT) scans, nuclear imaging, angiography, and magnetic resonance imaging (MRI) are additional procedures available for the evaluation of GFR, renal masses, unexplained hematuria, or obstruction. Finally, for client with suspected primary glomerular disease or unexplained renal failure, a renal biopsy may be indicated after all other available means of establishing a diagnosis have been exhausted.

The role of the nurse may be to prepare the client for these examinations, both physiologically and psychologically, but to also monitor the results and intervene with appropriate nursing care based on the data.

Summary

The kidneys as part of the urinary system participate with other body organs to regulate the volume and composition of interstitial fluid within a narrow range of values. They remove waste products from the blood and are important in controlling blood volume, the concentration of ions in the blood, and the pH of the blood. The kidneys also function in the control of RBC production. As the major excretory organs in the body, the kidneys are essential in maintaining a normal environment for the body cells.

> ### ✱ Critical Thinking Questions
>
> - Sally Bownes has eaten a large box of salty pretzels. What effect will this have on her urine concentration and volume? Why?
> - Mr. Smith has had a course of acyclovir for a week at the high level of the dosage range and needs continued encouragement to drink fluids. Knowing that a potential complication of this drug is renal toxicity, what laboratory values would you be monitoring? How would you expect them to change if Mr. Smith began to develop toxicity and why?

ℓ-LEARNING SUPPLEMENTS

Student CD-ROM
- Final Exam questions
- NCLEX® Examination review questions
- Pharmacology animations
- Printable chapter summary

Evolve Website (http://evolve.elsevier.com/mckenry)
- Content updates, including information on new drugs
- WebLinks corresponding to this chapter
- Answers to the critical thinking questions in this chapter
- *Elsevier ePharmacology Update* newsletter
- *Mosby's Drug Consult* Internet Edition
- Supplemental and reference information

Bibliography

Anderson, D.M., Keith, J., & Novak, P.D. (Eds.) (2002). *Mosby's medical, nursing, and allied health dictionary* (6th ed.). St. Louis: Mosby.

Guyton, A.C., & Hall, J.E. (2000). *Textbook of medical physiology* (10th ed.). Philadelphia: W.B. Saunders.

Hardman, J.G., & Limbird, L.E. (Eds.). (2001). *Goodman and Gilman's the pharmacological basis of therapeutics* (10th ed.). New York: McGraw-Hill.

Herlihy, B., & Maebius, N.K. (2003). *The human body in health and illness* (2nd ed.). Philadelphia: W.B. Saunders.

McCance, K.L., & Huether, S.E. (2002). *Pathophysiology: The biological basis for disease in adults and children* (4th ed.). St. Louis: Mosby.

Nicoll, D., Chou, T.M., & Detmer, W.M. (2004). *Pocket Guide to Diagnostic Tests* (4th ed.) New York: McGraw-Hill.

Thibodeau, G.A., & Patton, K.T. (2003). *Anatomy and physiology* (5th ed.). St. Louis: Mosby.

33

DIURETICS

CHAPTER FOCUS

Diuretics play a leading role in many therapies, including heart failure (HF) and hypertension. Although diuretics can be beneficial, they may also result in many adverse effects and drug interactions. With the appropriate nursing assessment and intervention, diuretic therapy can have positive effects in the treatment of hypertension and edema with a minimum of adverse effects.

<table>
<tr><td>

LEARNING OBJECTIVES

</td><td>

- Compare and contrast the five classifications of diuretics.
- Identify the most common agents within the five classifications of diuretics, and the site within the nephron where the action of each classification occurs.
- Identify the signs and symptoms of fluid and electrolyte imbalances associated with diuretic therapy.
- Explain the nursing care and client education required for clients receiving potassium-depleting diuretics and those receiving potassium-sparing diuretics.
- Implement the nursing management of a client receiving diuretic therapy.

</td></tr>
</table>

▲ **KEY TERMS**

diuretics, p. 656
loop diuretics, p. 656
osmotic diuretics, p. 657
potassium-sparing diuretics, p. 657
proximal tubule diuretics, p. 657
thiazide-type diuretics, p. 656

KEY DRUGS

acetazolamide, p. 667
furosemide, p. 658
hydrochlorothiazide (see the monograph in Chapter 27, p. 551)
mannitol, p. 668
spironolactone, p. 665

Diuretics modify renal function to induce diuresis, or the loss of body water by urination. In addition to water, diuretics increase the excretion of electrolytes, primarily sodium chloride. Understanding their action requires knowledge of the events that take place along each of the tubular segments (see Chapter 32). Diuretics are among the most commonly used medications. Thiazide diuretics represent the mainstay in the treatment of hypertension (see also Chapter 27) and are an integral part of drug therapies in edematous conditions such as cirrhosis, nephrotic syndrome, chronic renal failure, and acute and chronic HF.

Chapters 21 and 53 discuss the drugs that affect bladder function.

✴ **How are diuretics classified?**

Therapeutically, drug selection is best understood if each diuretic is presented according to its major site of action. This approach does not preclude the drug's effect at other sites in the nephron.

Clinically, among the most frequently used diuretics are those that act in the loop of Henle (referred to as "loop diuretics," and include furosemide (Lasix). These **loop diuretics** are highly effective for diuresis and are used to manage fluid overload conditions such as HF (see Chapter 25). The **thiazide type diuretics** (including hydrochlorothiazide) act in the diluting segment of the distal tubule and these are moderately effective at diuresis. They are sometimes used for fluid overload states such as HF, but are more commonly used to treat hypertension because of their effects in also reducing blood pressure (see Chapter 27). **Potassium-sparing diuretics** work in the distal tubule and are weak diuretics. They have specific action and are sometimes used in combination with other diuretics for synergistic effect and to offset the potassium wasting seen with the loop or thiazide diuretics. The carbonic anhydrase inhibitors like acetazolamide (Diamox) act as **proximal tubule diuretics** and have very specific roles in the management of glaucoma and short term management of certain seizure types. Osmotic diuretics like mannitol act as diuretics by drawing fluid into the lumen of the tubule. **Osmotic diuretics** are used to reduce cerebral edema in neurologic states and intraocular pressure in glaucoma. Fluid and electrolyte balance is affected by the use of diuretics. Figure 33-1 shows the various sites of action of diuretic drug groups by means of water and electrolyte transport system in a kidney nephron. Box 33-1 outlines signs and symptoms of fluid and electrolyte imbalance associated with diuretic therapy.

✳ **T.L. is a 67-year-old female admitted to the emergency department (ED) in respiratory distress with bilateral lung crackles. She has a history of heart failure and is diagnosed with pulmonary edema (PE). The ED physician orders the loop diuretic, furosemide (Lasix) 80 mg intravenously (IV) × 1 dose.**

✳ **What physiologic effects do the loop diuretics possess?**
The loop diuretics are so called because they inhibit the reabsorption of sodium and water in the ascending loop of Henle. Agents that work here at the Na^+-K^+-$2\ Cl^-$ co-

---

BOX 33-1 SIGNS AND SYMPTOMS OF FLUID AND ELECTROLYTE IMBALANCES ASSOCIATED WITH DIURETIC THERAPY

Hypovolemia: hypotension, weak pulse, tachycardia, clammy skin, rapid respirations, and reduced urinary output

Hyponatremia: low serum sodium levels (normal range 135 to 145 mEq/L [mmol/L]), lethargy, disorientation, muscle tenseness, seizures, and coma

Hypokalemia: low serum potassium levels (normal range 3.5 to 5.0 mEq/L [mmol/L]), weakness, abnormal ECG, postural hypotension, and flaccid paralysis

Hypocalcemia: low serum calcium levels (normal range 8.4 to 10.2 mg/dL or 2.1 to 2.6 mmol/L), irritability, vomiting, diarrhea, twitching, hyperactive reflexes, cardiac dysrhythmias, tetany, and seizures

Hypochloremia: low serum chloride levels (normal range 95 to 105 mEq/L [mmol/L])

Hypomagnesemia: low serum magnesium levels (normal range 1.6 to 2.4 mEq/L, 1.8 to 3.0 mg/dL, or 0.8 to 1.20 mmol/L), nausea and vomiting, lethargy, muscle weakness, tremors, and tetany

With potassium-sparing diuretics, be alert for the following:

Hyperkalemia: above-normal values for potassium serum levels, nausea, diarrhea, muscle weakness, postural hypotension, and ECG changes

---

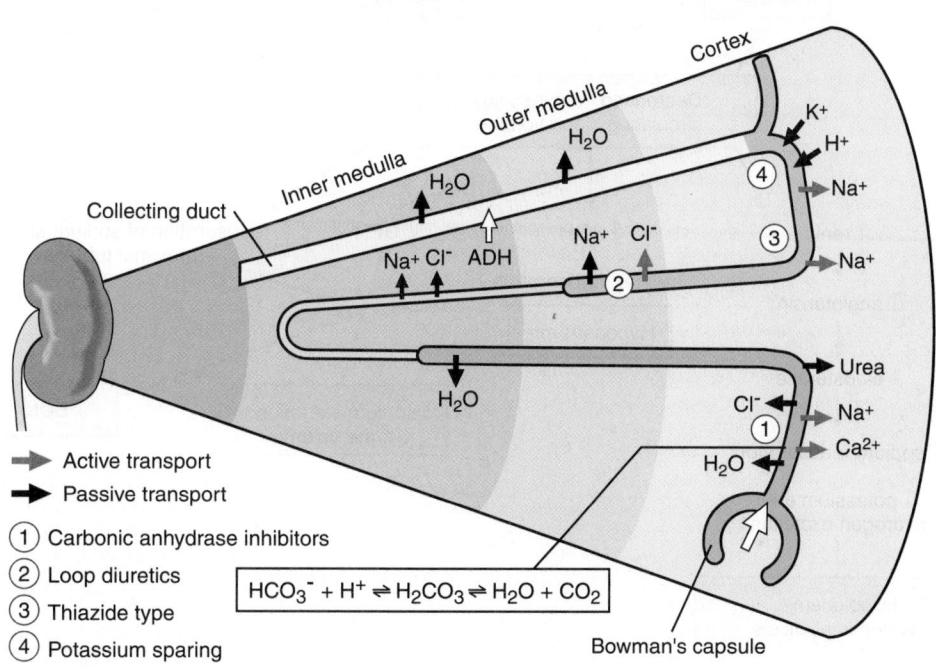

Active transport
Passive transport
① Carbonic anhydrase inhibitors
② Loop diuretics
③ Thiazide type
④ Potassium sparing

$$HCO_3^- + H^+ \rightleftharpoons H_2CO_3 \rightleftharpoons H_2O + CO_2$$

FIGURE 33-1 Site of action of diuretics.

transport (or carrier transfer site) in the ascending limb are most effective because the diuretic effect is greater than that reported with the other diuretic sites (Jackson, 2001).

Included among the loop diuretics are furosemide (Lasix), bumetanide (Bumex, Burinex♣), and torsemide (Demadex). Ethacrynic acid (Edecrin) is also classified as a loop diuretic, but is rarely used because of a risk for serious ototoxicity. These agents inhibit sodium reabsorption in the ascending limb of the loop of Henle, as shown by the marked reduction of free-water clearance during hydration and tubular free-water reabsorption during dehydration. The reabsorption of chloride in the ascending loop is also blocked by loop diuretics, which may have an additional action in the proximal tubule.

With the loop diuretics (and the thiazides discussed later and in Chapter 27 for hypertension therapy), an increased sodium load is presented to the distal tubule. This prompts a corresponding increase in potassium secretion. Additionally, plasma renin activity and aldosterone levels increase as extracellular fluid volume decreases, with a resulting potassium loss (Figure 33-2). This loss is dose-related, occurring early in treatment (first month) and in individuals with a high sodium intake. However, in many cases the loss is intermittent and neither harmful nor clinically observable. Hypokalemia may predispose the client with cirrhosis to hepatic encephalopathy and coma. Health care providers often recommend increased intake of dietary potassium with diuretics to offset this potassium loss. Clients who have renal insufficiency, a history of hyperkalemia, or who are on angiotensin-converting enzyme (ACE) inhibitors, angiotensin receptor blockers (ARBs), potassium sparing diuretics, or potassium supplements should not routinely be encouraged to increase dietary potassium intake because they may be predisposed to hyperkalemia.

furosemide [fur **oh** se myde]

(Lasix, Furoside, Apo-Furosemide♣)

Furosemide was the first loop diuretic, most frequently used, and is considered the prototype for the class.

Indications

The indications for the loop diuretics include the treatment of edema associated with HF, cirrhosis, or renal disease. They are also used as adjunct therapy in clients with acute pulmonary edema and in clients who are refractory to the other diuretics. Furosemide is also used to treat hypertension, although thiazide diuretics are generally preferred. Use of furosemide does not alter outcomes for clients in acute renal failure (Cantarovich, Rangoonwala, Lorenz, Verho, & Esnault, 2004).

Pharmacokinetics/Dosing

Furosemide is fairly well absorbed orally, is highly protein bound, metabolized in the liver, and excreted by the kidneys and in bile. Table 33-1 lists the pharmacokinetics and dosage information for the loop diuretics.

Adverse Effects

The most prominent adverse effects of the loop diuretics are dehydration and hypokalemia. Dehydration is particularly pronounced when higher doses are used in older adults. Dehydration may be manifested by postural hypotension, confusion, or difficulty in ambulation. Furosemide also increases the excretion of magnesium and calcium, which may result in hypomagnesemia and hypocalcemia. Furosemide (like bumetanide and torsemide), can produce reversible toxicity to the ear (manifested by ringing in the ears) when administered by rapid IV push. (This differs from the ototoxicity of ethacrynic acid, which results in irreversible ototoxicity.) As such, IV doses should be administered slowly over a few minutes. Hyperglycemia, hyperuricemia, increases in low-density lipoprotein (LDL) cholesterol and triglycerides, and a decrease in high-density lipoprotein (HDL) cholesterol plasma levels are reported with furosemide, but furosemide and other loop diuretics are not considered con-

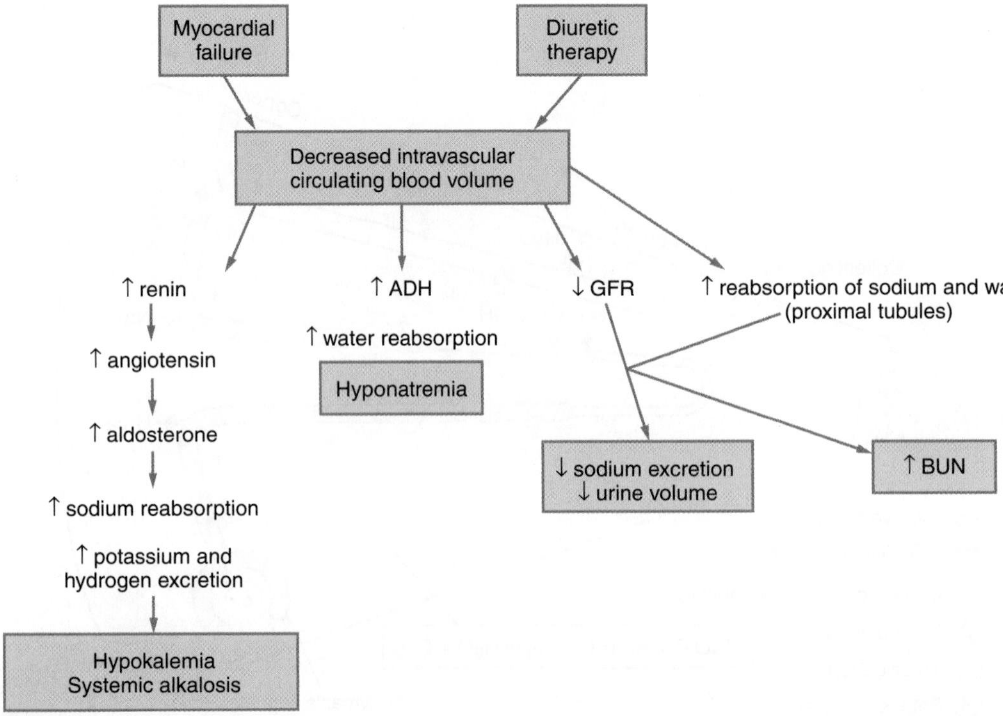

FIGURE 33-2 Body adaptation to extracellular volume depletion.

TABLE 33-1 SELECTED DIURETICS: PHARMACOKINETICS AND DOSAGES*

Category/Generic (Trade Name)	Onset of Action (hours)	Peak Effect (hours)	Duration of Action (hours)	Initial Dosage Adults	Initial Dosage Children
THIAZIDE DIURETICS					
chlorothiazide (Diuril)	PO: 2	4	6-12	125-250 mg one to two times daily	6 months and older: 10-20 mg/kg/day
chlorthalidone (Hygroton)	PO: 2	2	48-72	12.5-25 mg daily	2 mg/kg/day
hydrochlorothiazide (Esidrix)	PO: 2	4	6-12	12.5-25 mg daily	1-2 mg/kg/day
metolazone (Zaroxolyn)	PO: 1	2	12-24	2.5-5 mg daily (2.5 mg daily if used with loop diuretic)	Not established
LOOP DIURETICS					
bumetanide (Bumex)	PO: 0.5-1 IV: minutes	1-2 0.25-0.5	4-6 3.5-4	0.5-2 mg daily	Not established
ethacrynic acid (Edecrin)	PO: 0.5 IV: within 5 minutes	2 0.25-0.5	6-8 2	25-100 mg daily 50 mg; repeat in 2-4 hr if needed	25 mg daily 1 mg/kg
furosemide (Lasix)	PO: ⅓-1 IV: within 5 minutes	1-2 0.5	6-8 2	20-80 mg daily, then adjust as necessary q6-8h 20-40 mg IM or IV	2 mg/kg/day 1 mg/kg IM or IV
torsemide (Demadex)	PO: 0.5-1 IV: within 10 minutes	1-2 0.5-1	6-8 6-8	5-20 mg daily	Not established
POTASSIUM-SPARING DIURETICS					
amiloride (Midamor)	PO: 1-2	6-10	24	5-10 mg daily	Not established
eplerenone (Inspra)	PO: N/A	N/A	N/A	25-50 mg daily	Not established
spironolactone (Aldactone)	PO: 24-48	48-72	48-72	50-100 mg daily or in divided doses	1-3 mg/kg/day
triamterene (Dyrenium)	PO: 2-4	24-72	7-9	50-100 mg twice daily	2-4 mg/kg/day
OSMOTIC DIURETICS					
glycerin (Osmoglyn)	PO: 20 minutes	1	5	1-1.5 g/kg initially, then 0.5 g q6h	Same initial dose; may repeat in 4-8 hr
isosorbide	PO: N/A	1-1.5	5-6	1.5 g/kg two to four times daily	Not established
mannitol (Osmitrol)	IV Diuresis: 1-3 Lowering intraocular pressure: 0.25	0.5-1	6-8	Varies with indication 50-100 g as 5%-25% IV infusion	0.25-2 g/kg as 15%-20% IV infusion
urea (Ureaphil)	IV: 10 minutes	1-2	3-10	0.5-1.5 g/kg as 30% IV infusion	2 years and older: see adult dosage

Data from *Drug facts and comparisons* (58th ed.). (2005). St. Louis: Facts and Comparisons; and *USP DI: Drug information for the health care professional* (25th ed.). (2005). Greenwood Village, CO: MICROMEDEX Thomson Healthcare.

*Dosages are titrated as needed and tolerated.

traindicated for clients with diabetes mellitus, gout, or hyperlipidemia. Other adverse effects of furosemide and the other loop diuretics include blurred vision, headaches, abdominal distress, diarrhea, anorexia, and anxiety. Photosensitivity has been reported with furosemide. Hepatotoxicity, bone marrow suppression, and rash are also infrequently observed with furosemide use.

Drug Interactions

Potassium wasting associated with the loop diuretics can predispose to digoxin toxicity when used concurrently. Potassium wasting can be pronounced when used with the antifungal, amphotericin B. Excessive diuresis can predispose to renal failure, particularly with concurrent ACE inhibitors, ARBs, or nonsteroidal antiinflammatory agents (NSAIDs). Lithium toxicity is more probable for clients on lithium who are sodium depleted, as may be observed with the use of loop diuretics.

✱ What nursing implications for loop diuretics are present for T.L.?

Assessment Assess T.L. for any preexisting health condition that would contraindicate the use of furosemide. The use of a loop diuretic such as furosemide is not recommended in the presence of anuria or severe renal impairment because of decreased effectiveness. If it is used, the reduced clearance with renal function impairment may require higher doses but at more prolonged dosing intervals to reduce accumulation and the resultant risk of ototoxicity. The use of loop diuretics with liver dysfunction increases the risk of dehydration and electrolyte imbalance. Check the results of screenings done for diabetes and hyperuricemia because loop diuretics may increase blood glucose and uric acid concentrations. If T.L. were younger, the Pregnancy Category of furosemide would need to be considered (see the Pregnancy Safety box below).

Review T.L.'s current medication regimen for the risk of significant drug interactions, such as those that may occur when loop diuretics are given concurrently with the following drugs. Parenteral amphotericin B increases the risk for ototoxicity, nephrotoxicity, and electrolyte imbalance (especially hypokalemia). Anticoagulant therapy effects may be decreased with concurrent furosemide therapy. There is an increased risk of hypokalemia when loop diuretics are administered concurrently with other drugs that also cause

hypokalemia. Monitor serum potassium levels and electrocardiograms (ECGs) carefully; potassium supplements may be required. There is an increased risk of lithium toxicity because of reduced renal clearance; lithium and furosemide are not taken concurrently unless the client can be closely monitored. Other nephrotoxic or ototoxic medications increase the risk for these adverse effects, especially in clients with renal impairment.

Obtain a baseline assessment of T.L.'s HF (e.g., weight, BP, pulse, heart and lung sounds, extent and severity of fluid volume excess [edema]) and hearing. Blood chemistries will be monitored for abnormalities in electrolyte, blood urea nitrogen (BUN), carbon dioxide, glucose, and uric acid concentrations. Hepatic and renal function studies are part of the baseline assessment.

Nursing Diagnosis Because T.L. is receiving furosemide therapy, assess her for the development of the following nursing diagnoses/collaborative problems: risk for injury related to orthostatic hypotension (most common adverse effect); excess or deficient fluid volume; impaired comfort related to headache, local irritation at the site of injection, and abdominal cramping; impaired urinary elimination (frequency and amount); diarrhea; constipation; and disturbed sensory perception (visual: blurred vision); and the potential complications of allergic reaction (rash), increased skin sensitivity on exposure to sunlight; ototoxicity as evidenced by tinnitus (deafness), gout (joint pain, back pain), hepatotoxicity (yellow eyes or skin), pancreatitis (severe abdominal pain with nausea and vomiting), thrombocytopenia (unusual bleeding or bruising, black stools, hematuria, petechiae), and agranulocytosis or leukopenia (fever, chills, cough, dysuria).

Planning Client goals related to diuretic therapy are listed in Box 33-2.

Implementation

Monitoring Weigh T.L. at the initiation of therapy and periodically thereafter to monitor fluid loss. During the acute phase of her HF, it is necessary to weigh her daily to monitor for decreases in excess fluid volume. For the most accurate readings, weigh T.L. at the same time each day, preferably before breakfast, in similar clothing, and on the same scale. Weight loss and a reduction in the extent of the edema indicate effectiveness of the drug. Monitor also fluid intake and output ratios while T.L. is hospitalized. Monitor

PREGNANCY SAFETY DIURETICS	
Category	**Drug**
B	amiloride, chlorothiazide, chlorthalidone, ethacrynic acid, hydrochlorothiazide, metolazone, torsemide, triamterene
C	acetazolamide, bumetanide, furosemide, isosorbide, mannitol, urea

Data from *Mosby's drug consult* (15th ed.). (2005). St. Louis: Mosby.

BOX 33-2 CLIENT GOALS RELATED TO DIURETIC THERAPY

While receiving diuretic therapy, the client will:
- Regain fluid and electrolyte balance.
- Remain free of injury related to the effects of diuretic therapy.
- Effectively manage the diuretic therapy regimen.

blood pressure (BP) periodically; a reduction in BP to values within normal limits is also sought. Observe T.L. closely, because of her age, for the following: extreme blood pressure changes; postural hypotension; dehydration (e.g., weight loss of more than 2 pounds per day); allergic reactions (rashes); constipation, nausea, vomiting, and diarrhea; ototoxicity (tinnitus, hearing loss); and serum potassium deficiency.

Check reports of serum electrolytes, uric acid, blood and urine glucose tests, BUN and creatinine levels, and hepatic function studies for abnormalities. Excessive doses or too frequent administration can lead to prolonged water loss, electrolyte depletion, dehydration, blood volume reduction, and circulatory collapse, with possible vascular thrombosis and embolism, especially in older adults. Be aware that hyperuricemia may occur. A reversible elevation of BUN and creatinine levels may occur, especially in association with dehydration and particularly in clients with renal insufficiency.

Be aware that T.L. may develop hypokalemia. Monitor serum potassium levels periodically; potassium supplements or potassium-sparing diuretics may be necessary. Periodic determinations of other electrolytes are advised when high dosages are taken for prolonged periods, particularly in clients on low-salt diets. If T.L. were also experiencing potassium loss through causes other than the diuretic (e.g., vomiting, diarrhea, diaphoresis, gastrointestinal [GI] drainage, or paracentesis), she would be at higher risk for hypokalemia. Determine her blood sugar periodically, as T.L. may develop hyperglycemia.

Intervention Use of the intramuscular (IM) route can produce temporary pain at the site; therefore oral or IV routes are preferable. Administer diuretics so that the onset and peak of action coincides with access to toilet facilities. Administer the IV injection of furosemide to T.L. slowly over at least 4 minutes, which is equal to 20 mg/min. When high doses are ordered IV, a reduced injection rate of 4 mg/min will reduce the risk of ototoxicity.

When T.L. is stabilized, her furosemide will be given orally, usually with a potassium supplement. Liquid potassium for oral use, although unpleasant tasting, may be disguised in cold juices and taken with food. Regular tomato juice is not recommended for this purpose because its sodium content is high; low-sodium juices do well to disguise the taste of potassium. The use of enteric-coated potassium tablets or extended-release tablets should be carefully monitored because they have been implicated in ulcerations of the GI tract lining. Administer with food if GI upset occurs with oral forms. When administering oral solutions, use the calibrated dropper provided by the manufacturer for accurate dosages.

If loop diuretics are added to the medication regimen of hypertensive clients, expect that the medications will be adjusted to minimize the potential for orthostatic hypotension.

Education A comprehensive educational program is provided over the course of T.L.'s hospitalization. A dietitian is available for menu planning, but nurses support that teaching by assisting T.L. with her menu choices on the unit. T.L.'s expectation is that she will be back in her garden soon. It is important to alert her that photosensitivity is a problem for some clients taking furosemide; caution her to avoid prolonged exposure to the sun (or to sunlamps); encourage her to use sun-blocking lotions and to cover skin areas with protective clothing. Other instructions common to all diuretics are found in Box 33-3.

Evaluation The expected outcome of loop diuretic therapy is that T.L. will experience diuresis and an absence of lung crackles and pedal edema. Additionally, her BP, central venous pressure (CVP), and pulmonary artery pressure (PAP) will be within normal limits without T.L. experiencing any adverse effects of the drug. See Box 33-4 for general health outcomes of diuretic therapy.

✱ **C.T. is a 68-year-old male with mild heart failure and moderate isolated systolic hypertension (150/80**

BOX 33-3 CLIENT EDUCATION FOR DIURETIC THERAPY

- Move carefully from a sitting or lying position to an upright position because of positional (orthostatic) hypotension.
- Alcohol ingestion, hot weather, and standing or lying for long periods also increases the risk of orthostatic hypotension.
- Weigh daily on arising on the same scale in similar clothing. Report any overnight 2-pound increase to the prescriber. Take your pulse and BP as often as directed by your prescriber. Maintain a record to take for office visits.
- Maintain follow up visits to your prescriber for laboratory tests and monitoring of your condition.
- Electrolyte imbalances may occur on diuretic therapy particularly hypokalemia (loop diuretics, thiazide and thiazide-like diuretics) or hyperkalemia (potassium-sparing diuretics). For symptoms of the various electrolyte imbalances, see Box 33-1.
- Dietary changes may be required to support a high potassium (except for potassium-sparing diuretics) and low sodium diet. See Table 33-2 and Box 25-6, Tips for Low-Sodium Dining on p. 518.
- Dryness of the mouth may occur. If troublesome, use sugarless candies or small sips of water or ice chip for relief (unless on fluid restriction). Maintain regular dental checkups to monitor the development of caries and gum disease, which may occur as the result of xerostomia.
- Constipation may be prevented by a high-fiber diet, adequate amounts of fluids (unless restricted), moderate exercise, and establishing a routine. If it becomes problematic, ask your prescriber for a recommendation for a stool softener or laxative.

mm Hg). His heart failure is manifested by 1+ pitting ankle edema, shortness of breath on exertion, and mild inspiratory rales and rhonchi bilaterally. His prescriber initiates hydrochlorothiazide 25 mg daily.

✱ **What are the key actions of the thiazide diuretics?**

Thiazide diuretics are active in the diluting segments of the kidney. They are synthetic drugs that are chemically related to the sulfonamides. Hydrochlorothiazide is one of the most commonly used thiazides. Because these agents are similar, all the diluting segment diuretics will be described collectively as the thiazide-type diuretics.

A great number of thiazide and thiazide type diuretics are available and are listed below, and include:

- **bendroflumethiazide** [ben droe floo meth **eye** a zide] (Naturetin)
- **benzthiazide** [benz **thye** a zide] (Exna, Hydrex)
- **chlorothiazide** [klor oh **thye** a zide] (Diuril)
- **chlorthalidone** [klor **thal** i doan] (Hygroton)
- **cyclothiazide** [sye kloe **thye** a zide] (Anhydron)

- **hydrochlorothiazide** [hye droe klor oh **thye** a zide] (HydroDIURIL, Esidrix)
- **hydroflumethiazide** [hye droe floo meth **eye** a zide] (Diucardin, Saluron)
- **indapamide** [in **dap** a mide] (Lozol)
- **methyclothiazide** [meth ee kloe **thye** a zide] (Enduron)
- **metolazone** [me **tole** a zone] (Zaroxolyn)
- **polythiazide** [pol i **thye** a zide] (Renese)
- **quinethazone** [kwin **eth** a zone] (Hydromox)
- **trichlormethiazide** [trye klor meth **eye** a zide] (Metahydrin, Naqua)

The primary action and site of action of the thiazide and thiazide-type drugs appear to be inhibition of sodium reabsorption in the early distal tubules in the nephron, the cortical diluting segment. These drugs are less potent than the loop diuretics, because the maximum portion of the sodium load they can affect at the distal tubule is less than 10% of the glomerular filtrate. Therefore the thiazide-type diuretics primarily promote the renal excretion of water, sodium, chloride, potassium, and magnesium. They also may increase serum levels of calcium, glucose, and uric acid. The reduction in calcium elimination may explain the modest reduction in fracture risks associated with individuals receiving thiazide diuretics (Schlienger, Kraenzlin, Jick, & Meier, 2004). Thiazides are not particularly effective for clients with moderate to severe renal impairment (e.g., creatinine clearance less than 30 mL/min). Their role in reducing cardiovascular risks may be related to genetic variability in promoting sodium excretion (see the Special Considerations for Pharmacogenetics box below).

An especially important feature of thiazide-type diuretics is their ability to impair free water clearance with no effect on concentration ability. The initial natriuretic effect lasts for approximately 1 week and then resets at a lower level. This diuretic tolerance occurs because of increased aldosterone levels and a decreased sodium load at the distal tubule. The mechanisms of antihypertensive action are believed to be initially because of the reduction in plasma and

---

BOX 33-4 EXPECTED OUTCOMES FOR DIURETIC THERAPY

While receiving diuretic therapy, the client will:

- Return to normal electrolyte values.
- Demonstrate normal cardiac output as evidenced by vital signs (BP 120/80 mm Hg, pulse rate greater than 60 and less than 100, respiratory rate 12-20 breaths/min), and appropriate fluid balance ratios.
- Demonstrate an absence of adventitious lung sounds and dependent edema.
- Not experience any adverse effects of diuretic therapy.
- Effectively manage the therapeutic regimen including medication compliance, daily weights, monitoring vital signs, low sodium diet, changing positions slowly, reporting adverse effects appropriately, and maintaining prescriber visits for monitoring and follow up care.

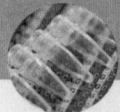 Special Considerations for Pharmacogenetics | DIURETICS

PHARMACODYNAMICS

Sodium reabsorption in the kidney is correlated with a genetic marker (α-adducin variant). For individuals with this variant, diuretics appear to be significantly more effective at lowering the risk for myocardial infarction and stroke (Psaty et al., 2002). Another genetic marker, C825 T, is also noted to correlate with response to thiazide diuretics and may explain in part why African Americans appear to be more responsive to thiazide diuretics than other populations (Terra & Johnson, 2002). Genetic variability in aldosterone synthesis has also been noted and may influence response to spironolactone (Bleumink et al., 2004).

PHARMACOKINETICS

Variation in P450 2 C8/9 activity, which is genetically determined, is noted for torsemide and may explain altered levels and response in different population (Chang & Altman, 2004). The metabolism of other diuretics are probably not significantly affected by genetic influence.

ADVERSE EFFECTS

The effect of pharmacogenetic influences on the potential for adverse effects of diuretics has not been well studied.

extracellular fluid volume that result in a decrease in cardiac output. In time, the cardiac output returns to normal. Thiazide-type diuretics also decrease peripheral resistance by a direct action on the peripheral blood vessels.

Like loop diuretics, thiazides can result in hypokalemia, and other electrolyte disturbances. Thiazides may result in elevated uric acid levels and contribute to the development of gout. They are also associated with modestly elevated LDL and triglyceride levels, but the benefit of lowering BP continues to render these agents advantageous in reducing target organ damage associated with hypertension. Similarly, modest elevations in blood glucose levels associated with thiazides usually are not problematic for most clients with diabetes mellitus (DM).

Hydrochlorothiazide is considered the prototype thiazide diuretic and is widely used to treat hypertension. It is also used to treat edema. Chapter 27 presents the monograph for hydrochlorothiazide.

✷ What is the nurse's role in the management of thiazide diuretics for C.T.?

Assessment Assess C.T. for preexisting conditions that would contraindicate the use of thiazide diuretics. Thiazide-type diuretics are given with caution to clients with severe renal impairment (may be ineffective or precipitate azotemia), hepatic impairment (may precipitate hepatic coma), DM (the dosages of hypoglycemic agents may need to be altered), gout (may elevate uric acid levels), or electrolyte imbalances (may be exacerbated). Check C.T.'s creatinine clearance because of his age to ensure adequate renal function before administering thiazide-type diuretics.

Review C.T.'s current medication regimen for the risk of significant drug interactions, such as those that may occur when thiazide or thiazide-type diuretics are given concurrently with the following drugs. Bile acid sequestrants (cholestyramine [Questran] or colestipol [Colestid]) may reduce the GI absorption of thiazide-type diuretics. Schedule the administration of diuretics 1 hour before or 4 hours after the administration of these drugs. If C.T. is on digoxin for HF there is an increased risk of digoxin toxicity in the presence of hypokalemia that is a possibility with these diuretics. Concurrent use of lithium is not recommended. An increased risk of lithium toxicity is possible because of decreased lithium excretion; there is also the potential for nephrotoxic adverse effects.

A baseline assessment of C.T.'s underlying conditions should be obtained, including the BP for his hypertension, the extent and severity of pedal edema, and adventitious lung sounds with HF. Baseline blood chemistries for glucose, electrolytes, BUN, serum uric acid, lipid profile and serum creatinine are recommended before diuretic therapy is begun.

Nursing Diagnosis During thiazide diuretic therapy, C.T. is at risk for the following nursing diagnoses/collaborative problems: impaired comfort (nausea); impaired urinary elimination (frequency and amount); diarrhea; constipation; risk for injury related to orthostatic hypotension; and the potential complications of electrolyte imbalances (hypokalemia [irregular heart-beat, mental changes, weakness, weak pulse], hyponatremia [confusion, fatigue, irritability, muscle cramps], and hypochloremic alkalosis), allergic reaction, agranulocytosis (fever, low back pain, dysuria), gout, hepatotoxicity, thrombocytopenia (unusual bleeding and bruising, petechiae, and blood in the urine or stools), and photosensitivity.

Planning See Box 33-2.

Implementation

Monitoring Take C.T.'s BP before administering the diuretic to ensure that he is not hypotensive. Obtain a daily weight and monitor intake and output ratios to assist in determining the progress of diuretic therapy. Because electrolyte imbalances are possible, monitor laboratory reports, particularly serum potassium and sodium levels. Monitoring is particularly important when digoxin is part of C.T.'s regimen, because hypokalemia potentiates the toxic cardiac effects of digoxin (e.g., bradycardia or ventricular irritability). Latent diabetes or gout may occasionally occur; monitor laboratory reports for hyperglycemia or hyperuricemia. Observe C.T. for signs and symptoms of fluid and electrolyte imbalances: hypovolemia, hyponatremia, hypokalemia, hypocalcemia, hypochloremia, or hypomagnesemia (see Box 33-1). Monitoring serum cholesterol and triglycerides is recommended after 6 months of therapy and then as part of C.T.'s annual physical examination.

Intervention Although potassium loss is usually not significant enough to require potassium supplementation, add potassium-rich foods to the diet to help prevent hypokalemia. See Table 33-2 for the potassium content of selected foods. Discontinue thiazide-type diuretics before performing parathyroid function tests, because they may alter serum calcium concentrations. As with other diuretics, plan dosing schedules to minimize the inconvenience of diuresis for C.T.

Education Alert C.T. that thiazide-type diuretics may make him feel unusually tired. Advise C.T. that diuretic drugs prescribed for a chronic condition need to be taken as an integral part of his lifestyle. For general teaching related to diuretics, see Box 33-3.

Evaluation See Box 33-4.

✷ **C.T. returns to clinic after 2 months of hydrochlorothiazide 25 mg daily. Symptoms of his HF are improved (reduced ankle swelling, clear lungs), and blood pressure is at 135/80 mm Hg. His potassium, however, is low at 3.2 mEq/L despite eating a banana and drinking a glass of orange juice each day. His prescriber discontinues the hydrochlorothiazide tablet and starts hydrochlorothiazide 25 mg/spironolactone 25 mg (Aldactazide 25/25) once daily.**

TABLE 33-2 FOODS RICH IN POTASSIUM

Food	Amount	Potassium (mg)
FRUIT		
Apple, raw, with skin	1 medium	159
Banana, medium	1	451
Cantaloupe	1 cup, pieces	494
Dates, dried	10	541
Figs, dried	10	1332
Orange, navel	1 medium	250
Prunes, dried	10	626
Raisins, seedless	⅔ cup	751
VEGETABLES		
Artichoke, boiled	1 medium	316
Asparagus, boiled	½ cup (6 spears)	279
Avocado, raw	1 medium	1097
Broccoli, raw	½ cup, chopped	143
Brussels sprouts, boiled	½ cup (4 sprouts)	247
Carrots, raw	1 medium	233
Corn, yellow, boiled	½ cup	204
Mushrooms, boiled	½ cup, pieces	277
Potato, baked with skin	1 medium	844
Spinach, boiled	½ cup	419
Sweet potato, baked	1 medium	397
Tomato, raw	1 medium	254
MEAT, POULTRY, AND FISH		
Beef, top round, lean, broiled	3.5 oz.	442
Chicken, dark meat, roasted, without skin	3.5 oz.	240
Chicken, light meat, roasted, without skin	3.5 oz.	247
Halibut, baked	3 oz.	490
Salmon, baked	3 oz.	319
Trout, rainbow, baked	3 oz.	539
DRINKS		
Milk, whole	8 fl. oz.	368
Milk, skim	8 fl. oz.	406
Orange juice, fresh	8 fl. oz.	486

Modified from Nix, S. (2005). *Williams' basic nutrition and diet therapy* (12th ed.). St. Louis: Mosby.

✱ How are the potassium-sparing agents utilized?

The potassium-sparing diuretics are similar in action to other diuretics and are generally considered to be weak diuretics that act at the distal renal tubules. They block sodium reabsorption in the distal tubule, thus increasing sodium and water excretion; at the same time, they conserve potassium so generally that they are primarily considered useful when combined with other potassium-wasting diuretics.

Amiloride (Midamor) and triamterene (Dyrenium) directly inhibit the reabsorption of sodium and water, whereas spironolactone is an aldosterone antagonist. Any of the three agents may be used when it is necessary to restore or preserve the normal serum potassium level, if other concurrent diuretic therapy causes hypokalemia, and when potassium supplementation by medication or diet is inappropriate. These agents are highly effective for this purpose. If prescribed singly, however, their efficacy may actually result in an undesirable and rapidly developing hyperkalemia.

Spironolactone, a synthetic steroidal compound, antagonizes the effect of aldosterone by binding competitively to the protein that permits potassium secretion at the distal tubule. This response is directly related to the amount of circulating aldosterone in the serum. Spironolactone produces a very mild diuresis of sodium and water at the distal tubule by means of this mechanism. It does not interfere with the renal tubule transport of sodium and chloride and does not inhibit carbonic anhydrase. Triamterene directly depresses the renal tubular transport of sodium in the distal tubule independent of the presence of aldosterone. In 1999, spironolactone (Aldactone) was discovered to be beneficial for HF. When compared with other therapies for severe heart failure, the addition of spironolactone reduced the risk of death and hospitalization by 30%. The combination of spironolactone with an ACE inhibitor provides an additive blockade on aldosterone (i.e., the ACE inhibitor lowers the synthesis of aldosterone), whereas spironolactone blocks the aldosterone receptors. Therefore the addition of spironolactone protects the heart from too much aldosterone, which can reduce the capability of the heart to pump (Sligl, McAlister, Ezekowitz, & Armstrong, 2004).

Spironolactone is considered the prototype potassium potassium-sparing diuretic and is presented here.

✱ ⯀ spironolactone [speer oh no **lak** tone]
(Aldactone, Novospiroton✤)
Indications
All of the potassium-sparing diuretics, including spironolactone, are indicated for prevention and treatment of hypokalemia and as adjunct therapy in treating edema and hypertension. Spironolactone is used in the diagnosis and treatment of primary hyperaldosteronism and hyperaldosteronism secondary to ascites. Spironolactone is also indicated for HF alone or in combination with other diuretics and/or ACE inhibitors. Combinations of these agents with other diuretics are presented in Table 33-3.

Pharmacokinetics/Dosing
Spironolactone is well absorbed orally, metabolized by the liver, and excreted by the kidney. See Table 33-1 for the pharmacokinetics and dosages of these potassium-sparing diuretics.
Adverse Effects
Of greatest concern with these agents is the risk for hyperkalemia. Other adverse effects of the potassium-sparing diuretics include abdominal cramps, diarrhea, nausea, vomiting, gynecomastia, hirsutism, sexual dysfunction, dry mouth, and sedation. Photosensitivity and rash may also be possible
Drug Interactions
Caution must be exercised when these agents are used in combination with other agents that can elevate serum potassium, including the ACE inhibitors, ARBs, and potassium supplements. As with other diuretics, these agents may result in lithium toxicity for clients on lithium therapy.

✱ What are the important nursing implications of adding spironolactone to C.T.'s regimen?

The potassium-sparing diuretic, spironolactone, was prescribed in combination with the thiazide diuretic to manage C.T.'s thiazide-induced hypokalemia and for the beneficial effects of spironolactone in HF. Most potassium loss secondary to thiazide diuretics can by replaced by dietary sources of potassium. When this is not the case, a combination product that includes a potassium-wasting and a potassium-sparing diuretic is frequently prescribed. Potassium-sparing diuretics have modest antihypertensive effects compared to thiazide diuretics. The discussion of nursing management that follows relates more to monotherapy with potassium-sparing diuretics, but the issues should be kept in mind with combination products also.

Assessment Before administering these compounds, ascertain that C.T. has no related drug history of allergy or hyperkalemia (potassium-sparing diuretics may further increase serum potassium levels). Greater caution is required in administering these diuretics to clients who are at risk for developing hyperkalemia because of preexisting conditions (e.g., impaired renal or hepatic function or DM), to severely ill clients, and to clients with decreased urine volumes, which might aggravate electrolyte imbalances.

Review C.T.'s current medication regimen for the risk of significant drug interactions, such as those that may occur when distal tubule/potassium-sparing diuretics are given concurrently with the following drugs. Increased potassium levels leading to hyperkalemia can result from use of blood from the blood bank (up to 30 mEq of potassium per liter of plasma or up to 65 mEq of potassium per liter of whole blood when stored more than 10 days), ACE inhibitors, ARBs, cyclosporine (Sandimmune), other potassium-sparing diuretics, low-sodium milk, potassium-containing medications, salt substitutes, or potassium supplements. Monitor serum electrolytes closely. Concurrent use of lithium increases the risk of lithium toxicity by reducing renal clearance. In addition to these general drug interactions with potassium-sparing diuretics, spironolactone alone increases the half-life of digoxin. Dosage reductions of digoxin may

TABLE 33-3 EXAMPLES OF FIXED DOSE DIURETIC COMBINATIONS

Trade Name	Contents
Accuretic 10/12.5, 20/12.5, 20/25	quinapril 10 or 20 mg, hydrochlorothiazide 12.5 or 25 mg
Aldactazide 25/25, 50/50	spironolactone 25 or 50 mg; hydrochlorothiazide 25 or 50 mg
Apresazide 25/25, 50/50, 50/100	hydralazine 25 or 50 mg; hydrochlorothiazide 25, 50, or 100 mg
Atacand HCT 16/12.5, 32/12.5	candesartan 16 or 32 mg; hydrochlorothiazide 12.5 mg
Avalide 150/12.5, 300/12.5	irbesartan 150 or 300 mg; hydrochlorothiazide 12.5 mg
Benicar HCT 20/12.5, 40/12.5, 40/25	olmesartan 20 or 40 mg; hydrochlorothiazide 12.5 or 25 mg
Capozide 25/15, 25/25, 50/15, 50/25	captopril 25 or 50 mg; hydrochlorothiazide 15 or 25 mg
Combipres 0.1/15, 0.2/15, 0.3/15	clonidine 0.1, 0.2, or 0.3 mg; hydrochlorothiazide 15 mg
Diovan HCT 80/12.5, 160/12.5, 160/25	valsartan 80 or 160 mg; hydrochlorothiazide 12.5 or 25 mg
Dyazide 37.5/25, 50/25	triamterene 37.5 mg; hydrochlorothiazide 25 mg
Hyzaar 50/12.5, 100/25	losartan 50 or 100 mg; hydrochlorothiazide 12.5 or 25 mg
Inderide LA 40/25, 80/25	propranolol 40 or 80 mg; hydrochlorothiazide 25 mg
Lotensin HCT 5/6.25, 10/12.5, 20/12.5, 20/25	benazepril 5, 10 or 20 mg; hydrochlorothiazide 6.25, 12.5, or 25 mg
Lopressor HCT 50/25, 100/25, or 100/50	metoprolol 50 or 100 mg; hydrochlorothiazide 25 or 50 mg
Maxzide 37.5/25, 75/50	triamterene 37.5 or 75 mg; hydrochlorothiazide 25 or 50 mg
Micardis HCT 40/12.5, 80/12.5, 80/25	telmisartan 40 or 80 mg; hydrochlorothiazide 12.5 mg
Minizide 1/0.5, 2/0.5, 3/0.5	prazosin 1, 2 or 5 mg; polythiazide 0.5 mg
Moduretic 5/50	amiloride 5 mg, hydrochlorothiazide 50 mg
Monopril HCT 10/12.5, 20/12.5	fosinopril 10 or 20 mg; hydrochlorothiazide 12.5 mg
Prinzide 10/12.5, 20/12.5, 20/25	lisinopril 10 or 20 mg; hydrochlorothiazide 12.5 or 25 mg
Teveten HCT 600/12.5, 600/25	eprosartan 600 mg; hydrochlorothiazide 12.5 or 25 mg
Ureteric 7.5/12.5, 15/12.5, 15/25	moexipril 7.5 or 15 mg; hydrochlorothiazide 12.5 or 25 mg
Vaseretic 5/12.5, 10/25	enalapril 5 or 10 mg; hydrochlorothiazide 12.5 or 25 mg
Zestoretic 10/12.5, 20/12.5, 20/25	lisinopril 10 or 20 mg; hydrochlorothiazide 12.5 or 25 mg
Ziac 2.5/6.25, 5/6.25, 10/6.25	bisoprolol fumarate 2.5, 5, or 10 mg; hydrochlorothiazide 6.25 mg

be required by either reducing the dose or the frequency of dosing. Monitor serum digoxin levels carefully.

In addition to assessing the underlying condition for which the diuretic was prescribed, a baseline health assessment should include blood pressure, serum electrolyte concentrations (especially potassium, sodium, and uric acid), and BUN and/or serum creatinine levels.

Nursing Diagnosis With the administration of spironolactone (and other distal tubule/potassium-sparing diuretics), C.T. should be assessed for the following nursing diagnoses/collaborative problems: impaired comfort related to muscle cramps, headache, dizziness, and GI effects (nausea,

vomiting, and abdominal cramping); constipation; diarrhea; disturbed body image related to decreased libido, gynecomastia in males, and hirsutism in females secondary to the antiandrogenic effects of the drug (rare); and the potential complications of hyperkalemia (confusion, dysrhythmias, paresthesia, fatigue) and allergic reactions (shortness of breath, rash).

Planning See Box 33-2.

Implementation

Monitoring Monitor daily weights, blood pressure, weight loss, and fluid balance to evaluate the effectiveness of the diuretic. Evaluate C.T.'s compliance at frequent intervals. Although C.T. is at low risk for adverse effects of his potassium-sparing diuretic, be alert to an irregular heartbeat (often the first clinical sign of hyperkalemia) or peaked T waves on the ECG. Other warning signs of hyperkalemia are confusion, tingling in the extremities, breathing difficulties, unexplained anxiety, fatigue, and physical weakness. Serum electrolyte determinations and an ECG are probably indicated if these occur.

Check laboratory reports closely, especially if C.T. is taking other similar drugs or potassium-rich foods. Rapidly increased serum potassium levels may occur. Act immediately to reverse hyperkalemia if the serum potassium level exceeds 6 to 6.5 mEq/L, and anticipate treatment with sodium bicarbonate, glucose and regular insulin preparations, or other therapy. Hyponatremia may occur as evidenced by fatigue, drowsiness, increased thirst, and dry mouth.

Remain sensitive to cues that C.T. may be concerned about body image changes if he has any antiandrogenic effects (breast enlargement, inability to have or keep an erection) from the spironolactone that may threaten his sexual identity.

Intervention Administering potassium-sparing diuretics with food or milk may prevent some GI symptoms and possibly enhance bioavailability.

Education Counsel C.T. to avoid excessively stringent low-salt diets and relatively concentrated potassium intake in the form of citrus juices, cola beverages, low-sodium milk, some salt substitutes, and other potassium supplements. See Box 33-3 for additional client education for diuretic therapy.

Evaluation The expected outcome of C.T.'s potassium-sparing diuretic therapy is that he will experience diuresis and an absence of rales and edema; blood pressure and serum potassium values will be within normal limits. See the general outcomes for diuretic therapy in Box 33-4.

✸ **T.R. is a 58-year-old female who is newly diagnosed by her ophthalmologist with open-angle glaucoma. She is started on a carbonic anhydrase inhibitor, acetazolamide (Diamox) 500 mg sustained release tablet twice daily.**

✸ **What are the key pharmacologic considerations of carbonic anhydrase inhibitors?**
Acetazolamide, a sulfonamide, is the prototype of the proximal tubule diuretics, which act primarily to reduce the volume of sequestered fluids, especially of the aqueous humor. It inhibits the action of the enzyme carbonic anhydrase, which in turn prevents the reabsorption of bicarbonate ions from the proximal tubules. These bicarbonate ions then act to increase tubular osmotic pressure, causing osmotic diuresis. With long-term use, however, the diuretic effect of these drugs is lost.

✸◖◗ **acetazolamide** [a set a **zole** a mide]
(Diamox, Acetazolam, Apo-Acetazolamide✤)
Acetazolamide is widely used as an antiglaucoma agent because it lowers intraocular pressure by decreasing the production of aqueous humor by more than 50% (see Chapter 42 for further discussion).
Indications
Acetazolamide is used to treat open-angle glaucoma and is also used as adjunct treatment with antiepileptic drugs to manage absence seizures (petit mal), generalized tonic-clonic seizures (grand mal), mixed seizure patterns, and myoclonic seizures. It has been found especially useful for women who experience an increase in seizures during their menstrual periods. It has also been found to decrease the incidence and severity of symptoms of altitude sickness in mountain climbers when taken orally. Additionally, acetazolamide produces alkaline urine, which may help to increase the excretion of weakly acidic drugs in cases of drug overdose. It is also used to reverse metabolic alkalosis.
Pharmacokinetics/Dosing
Acetazolamide is well absorbed orally. It reaches a peak level in 2 to 4 hours after a 500 mg dose or in 8 to 12 hours after a 500 mg extended-release capsule. Its half-life is 10 to 15 hours, and excretion is mainly by the kidneys. The adult dosage for glaucoma is 250 mg PO one to four times daily. The antiepileptic drug dosage is 8 to 30 mg/kg PO divided into four doses per day. For acute mountain sickness, the dosage is 500 to 1000 mg daily in divided doses or sustained-release capsules. The safety and effectiveness of acetazolamide in children has not been established. Acetazolamide is also available as a parenteral injection for IV or IM use. Refer to the current package insert for dosing instructions.
Adverse Effects
The adverse effects of acetazolamide therapy include headaches, increased nervousness, anorexia, nausea, vomiting, depression, tremors, rash, alopecia, ataxia, and chest, groin, or leg pain.
Drug Interactions
Acetazolamide may increase cyclosporine levels, and may result in decreased lithium levels. By alkalinizing the urine, serum levels of amphetamines and salicylates may be affected.

✸ **How should T.R.'s drug therapy be managed for the safe and effective use of acetazolamide?**

Assessment Ascertain whether T.R. has diabetes or a familial history of diabetes, because acetazolamide has caused elevations of serum blood glucose and glycosuria in such individuals. Do not give acetazolamide to T.R. if she is allergic to sulfonamides. Assess for preexisting health conditions that might increase the risk for exacerbation of electrolyte imbalances, such as adrenocortical insufficiency, renal or respiratory acidosis, or hepatic impairment. If she has had a history of calcium-containing renal stones, she may experience a recurrence of calculi.

Review T.R.'s current medication regimen for the risk of significant drug interactions, such as those that may occur when acetazolamide is given concurrently with the following drugs. Because of the alkalinization of urine, the excretion of amphetamines, mecamylamine (Inversine), or quinidine is decreased; increased serum levels and toxicity may be seen. Acetazolamide results in alkaline urine that will reduce the effectiveness of methenamine (Mandelamine).

Determine T.R.'s baseline intraocular pressure to assess her glaucoma. If acetazolamide is administered for other conditions, an assessment of the underlying condition is obtained, such as the neurologic status of the client with seizures, and neurologic and respiratory status with altitude (acute mountain) sickness.

Nursing Diagnosis With the administration of acetazolamide, T.R. is at risk for the following nursing diagnoses/collaborative problems: impaired comfort (headache, bitter taste, nausea, vomiting, and numbness or tingling of the fingers, toes, lips, or tongue); impaired urinary elimination with an increase and frequency of urination; diarrhea; constipation; fatigue; imbalanced nutrition: less than body requirements related to anorexia (weight loss); and the potential complications of decreased cardiac output (ventricular dysrhythmias secondary to hypokalemia), mental depression, electrolyte imbalance such as hypokalemia (dry mouth, increased thirst, irregular heartbeats, muscle cramps, fatigue), and renal calculi or nephrotoxicity (hematuria, lower back pain, burning on urination).

Planning While on acetazolamide therapy, T.R. will:
- Remain free of the signs and symptoms of glaucoma.
- Be compliant with therapy.
- Remain free from adverse effects of acetazolamide.
- Effectively manage her therapeutic regimen, including appropriately reporting adverse effects of the drug and maintaining visits with her prescriber for monitoring and follow up care.

Implementation

Monitoring Observe T.R. for signs of allergic reaction (fever, hives, itching, rash). Monitor electrolytes, especially serum potassium levels and blood glucose levels, and intraocular pressure periodically.

Intervention Administer the oral forms of acetazolamide with meals or with antacids to decrease GI distress. For clients who are unable to tolerate tablets for oral administration, crush acetazolamide tablets and mix with a flavored syrup such as chocolate or cherry. Although up to 500 mg may be prepared in 5 mL syrup, it is more palatable if only 250 mg/5 mL is used. Refrigeration also increases the palatability but not the stability of the preparation; use within a week of preparation. Mixing the drug with solutions containing alcohol or glycerin is not as satisfactory.

Plan a high fluid intake to prevent hypercalciuria (excessive calcium in the urine), which is necessary because of the risk of renal calculi. Establish dosing schedules that minimize the inconvenience of diuresis that results from altered urinary elimination patterns. When acetazolamide is used in diuretic therapy, provide a high-potassium diet.

When acetazolamide is used to prevent or minimize high-altitude sickness, it is not a substitute for rapid descent if the climber manifests signs of pulmonary or cerebral edema.

Education A high fluid intake, 2500 to 3000 mL daily, is necessary to reduce the risk of renal calculi. Caution T.R. that the ability to accomplish tasks requiring mental alertness or physical coordination may be impaired. Although the sensation of "not feeling well" is common with the use of acetazolamide, malaise should be reported to the prescriber so that monitoring for acidosis, blood dyscrasias, or hypokalemia may be done. Advise the client to notify the prescriber if paresthesias (numbness, tingling, or burning) of the mouth, fingers, or toes occur. See also Box 33-3.

Evaluation The expected outcome for T.R. receiving acetazolamide therapy for glaucoma is a reduction of intraocular pressure readings to within the normal limits when measured with a tonometer. If the drug is administered to prevent seizures, the client will be free of seizures. If taken for altitude illness, the client will not evidence signs of an attack, such as shortness of breath, headache, or syncope.

✸ What is the role of osmotic diuretics?

Osmotic diuretics include both parenteral agents (mannitol and urea) and oral agents (glycerin and isosorbide). The two parenteral agents cause diuresis by adding to the solutes already present in the tubular fluid; they are particularly effective in increasing osmotic pressure because they are not reabsorbed by the tubules. Thus more water is pulled into tubular fluid, and the kidneys reabsorb less sodium, chloride, and water in an effort to equalize the higher solute content. These excesses are then excreted in the urine. The oral agents are primarily used to reduce intraocular pressure before and after intraocular surgery and to interrupt an acute attack of glaucoma. The parenteral agents (mannitol and urea) are used to treat cerebral edema and secondary glaucoma when other methods have been unsuccessful.

✸◾ mannitol [**man** i tole]
(Osmitrol)
Indications
Mannitol is used to treat cerebral edema, to reduce intraocular pressure, to increase the urinary excretion of toxic substances (salicylates, barbiturates, lithium, bromides), as an irrigating preparation to prevent hemolysis and hemoglobin accumulation during transurethral prostatic resection, and as an adjunct to other therapies in the treatment of edema in acute renal failure.
Pharmacokinetics/Dosing
Very little if any mannitol is metabolized in the liver. See Table 33-1 for the pharmacokinetics and dosages of the osmotic diuretics.
Adverse Effects
The adverse effects of mannitol include nausea, vomiting, dry mouth, headache, increased urination, and weakness. Mannitol may also cause visual disturbances, dizziness, and rash.

✸ What are the key nursing issues regarding the use of the osmotic diuretics?

Assessment Ascertain that the client does not have preexisting severe dehydration, anuria, or severe pulmonary congestion; osmotic diuretics are contraindicated for these conditions. Intracranial bleeding, except during craniotomy, would negate the use of mannitol and urea. Use caution in administering osmotic diuretics to clients with significant renal dysfunction or severe cardiopulmonary impairment, because the sudden increase in extracellular fluid might lead to circulatory overload and HF. The risk-benefit of urea administration is considered in severe hepatic dysfunction because it may lead to elevated levels of blood ammonia. The concurrent use of osmotic diuretics with digoxin may increase the risk of digoxin toxicity associated with hypokalemia.

Recommend baseline serum electrolyte and renal function determinations if they have not already been performed, and monitor the results.

Nursing Diagnosis Clients receiving osmotic diuretics are at risk for the following nursing diagnoses/collaborative problems: impaired comfort (dry mouth, nausea, vomiting, headache, dizziness, rash); hyperthermia; impaired urinary elimination (frequency and amount); and the potential complications of electrolyte imbalance, blurred vision, chest pain, pulmonary congestion, and thrombophlebitis.

Implementation

Monitoring Because these are potent osmotic drugs, it is essential to be alert to rapidly changing client conditions; assess urinary output and vital signs at frequent intervals for changing intravascular volume, pulmonary edema, or hemoconcentration. Monitor fluid and electrolyte balance, particularly serum and urine potassium and sodium levels. When urea is administered, measure BUN before and frequently during IV administration. If the BUN exceeds 75 mg/dL or if there is no diuresis within 6 to 12 hours, slow or stop the infusion and have the client reevaluated. If the osmotic diuretics are administered to reduce intraocular pressure, monitor the pressure determinations closely.

Intervention If the adequacy of renal function is suspect before the administration of mannitol, a test dose is usually prescribed and is given as an IV infusion over 3 to 5 minutes. Urine flow should increase to at least 30 to 50 mL/hr for 2 to 3 hours after this or a second test dose. If it does not, mannitol should be withheld and the client reevaluated.

Infuse mannitol and urea separately from other drugs and blood. Crystallization in solution is common; it may be countered by warming the solution until the crystals are invisible and by inserting a filter in the line whenever this drug is infused. Avoid the extravasation of urea and mannitol; observe the IV site periodically for tissue inflammation, irritation, and necrosis. Electrolyte-free mannitol should not be administered concurrently with blood, because pseudoagglutination may occur. If concurrent administration is necessary, at least 20 mEq of sodium chloride should be added to each liter of mannitol to minimize this effect.

Infuse urea into large veins. For both urea and mannitol, avoid using lower extremity IV sites because phlebitis and thrombosis may occur, particularly in older adults. Do not infuse urea more rapidly than 4 mL/min, because hemolysis and cerebral vasomotor symptoms may occur.

To assist in the prevention and relief of headache caused by cerebral dehydration, have the client lie down during and after the administration of these parenteral drugs.

Use an indwelling catheter with comatose clients to ensure urinary drainage. The use of a urometer that allows for precise measurement of output is important because the therapy is based on the accurate evaluation of intake and output. For clients who are alert, provide for their elimination needs keeping in mind their convenience, comfort, and privacy.

When osmotic diuretics are administered preoperatively, the dosing schedule should be as follows: glycerin, isosorbide, and mannitol, 30 minutes to 60 minutes before surgery; urea, 1 hour before surgery if administered for the reduction of intraocular pressure or at the time of scalp incision during intracranial surgery.

To increase palatability, isosorbide comes in a vanilla-mint–flavored syrup that may be iced, and glycerin may be mixed with iced, unsweetened fruit juice; sip through a straw. With repeated doses of these drugs, maintain adequate fluid and electrolyte balance.

Education Prepare the client for the diuresis that will occur with these drugs.

Advise the client to visit the physician regularly for intraocular pressure monitoring if taking glycerin and isosorbide for the reduction of intraocular pressure.

Evaluation If osmotic diuretics are administered for increased intracranial pressure, the expected outcome is that the client will have an intracranial pressure value within an acceptable range. If the indication for the drugs is increased intraocular pressure, the client will demonstrate a reduced intraocular pressure value with tonometer measurement. If these drugs are being given for acute renal failure, the client will experience diuresis and an improvement in BUN and serum creatinine values.

Summary

Diuretics are valuable assets in the therapeutic regimen for the treatment of hypertension and other conditions in which fluid volume excess is an issue, such as HF, cirrhosis, and nephrotic syndrome. These drugs act on the tubular function of the kidneys and inhibit solute reabsorption; water reabsorption is affected because water diffuses passively across the tubular membrane when sodium transport occurs. In general, diuretics are grouped by their major site of action along the tubule: proximal tubule diuretics, diluting segment diuretics, loop diuretics, and distal tubule diuretics. Osmotic diuretics act by adding to the solutes already present in tubular fluid; because they are not reabsorbed, more water is pulled into tubular fluid and less sodium, chloride, and water are reabsorbed by the kidneys in an effort to equalize the higher solute volume that is excreted in the urine. Combinations of diuretic agents are used for clients with stabilized conditions.

Nursing management focuses on the education of the client for the safe and accurate self-administration of diuretics, particularly in the early recognition of adverse effects. Hypokalemia is common except in clients taking potassium-sparing diuretics; clients should understand the importance of including potassium-rich foods in their diet if a potassium supplement has not been prescribed. An evaluation of the effectiveness of the therapeutic regimen through accurate measurement of the client's blood pressure, fluid balance, and weight is essential.

✱ Critical Thinking Questions

- What conditions place clients receiving loop diuretics at higher risk for hypokalemia? What observations by the nurse are particularly important for these clients?

- What conditions place clients receiving distal tubule and potassium-sparing diuretics at higher risk for hyperkalemia? What observations by the nurse are particularly important for these clients?

- Mrs. Williams, an 82-year-old woman, lives alone in substandard urban housing. Although she has hypertension and chronic HF, she maintains her independence with the assistance of members of her church, who shop for her, bring her meals occasionally, and take her for visits to her doctor. Her current medication regimen is as follows: digoxin, 0.25 mg PO daily; furosemide, 20 mg PO two times daily; K-Dur 20, one tablet PO daily; verapamil SR, 240 mg PO daily; and isosorbide dinitrate, 10 mg PO four times daily. For what nursing diagnoses/collaborative problems is Mrs. Williams at risk? Why? As her home health care nurse, what will be your plan of care?

Bibliography

Anderson, D.M., Keith, J., & Novak, P.D. (Eds.) (2002). *Mosby's medical, nursing, and allied health dictionary* (6th ed.). St. Louis: Mosby.

Bleumink, G., Schut, A.F., Sturkenboom, M.C., Deckers, J.W., van Duijn, C.M., & Stricker, B.H. (2004). Genetic polymorphisms and heart failure. *Genetics in Medicine*, 6(6), 465-474.

Bosker, G. (Ed.). (2004). *Primary and acute care medicine: Practice, protocols, pathways*, (2nd ed.). Atlanta: Thomson American Health Consultants.

Cantarovich, F., Rangoonwala, B., Lorenz, H., Verho, M., Esnault, V.L. (2004). High-dose furosemide for established ARF: A prospective, randomized, double-blind, placebo-controlled, multicenter trial. *Am J Kidney Dis.* 44, 402-409.

Chang, J.T., & Altman, R.B. (2004). Extracting and characterizing gene-drug relationships from the literature. Pharmacogenetics. 14(9):577-586 Retrieved December 2, 2004, from http://bionlp.stanford.edu/genedrug/gene_drug_predictions.html

Drug facts and comparisons. (58th ed.). (2005). St. Louis: Facts and Comparisons.

Jackson, E.K. (2001). Diuretics. In J.G. Hardman & L.E. Limbird (Eds.), *Goodman & Gilman's The pharmacological basis of therapeutics* (10th ed.). New York: McGraw-Hill.

Lacy, C.F., Armstrong, L.L., Goldman, M.P., & Lance, L.L. (2004). *Lexi-Comp's Drug Information Handbook* (12th ed.). Hudson, Ohio: Lexi-Comp.

Lau, A.H. (2005). Fluid and electrolyte disorders. In M.A. Koda-Kimble, , L.Y. Young, W.A. Kradjan, B.J. Guglielmo, B.K. Alldredge, & R.L. Corelli (Eds.), *Applied therapeutics: The clinical use of drugs* (8th ed.). Philadelphia: Lippincott, Williams & Wilkins.

Massie, B.M., & Amidon, T.M. (2003). Heart. In L.M. Tierney, Jr., S.J. McPhee, & Papadakis, M.A. (Eds.), *Current Medical Diagnosis & Treatment.* New York: Lange Medical Books/McGraw-Hill.

Mosby's drug consult (15th ed.). (2005). St. Louis: Mosby.

Psaty, B.M., et al. (2002). Diuretic Therapy, the α-Adducin gene variant, and the risk of myocardial infarction or stroke in persons with treated hypertension. *Journal of the American Medical Association*, 287(13), 1680-1689.

Saseen, J.J., & Carter, B.L. (2005). Essential hypertension. In M.A. Koda-Kimble, , L.Y. Young, W.A. Kradjan, B.J. Guglielmo, B.K. Alldredge, & R.L. Corelli (Eds.), *Applied therapeutics: The clinical use of drugs* (8th ed.). Philadelphia: Lippincott, Williams & Wilkins.

Schlienger, R.G., Kraenzlin, M.E., Jick, S.S., Meier, C.R.. (2004). Use of ß-blockers and risk of fractures. *Journal of the American Medical Association*, 292, 1326-1332.

Sligl, W., McAlister, F.A., Ezekowitz, J., & Armstrong, P.W. (2004). Usefulness of spironolactone in a specialized clinic. *American Journal of Cardiology*, 94(4), 443-447.

Terra, S.G., & Johnson, J.A. (2002), Pharmacogenetics, pharmacogenomics, and cardiovascular therapeutics: The way forward. *American Journal of Cardiovascular Drugs*, 2(5), 287-296.

USP DI: Drug information for the health care professional (25th ed.). (2005). Greenwood Village, CO: MICROMEDEX Thomson Healthcare.

ℓ-LEARNING SUPPLEMENTS

Student CD-ROM
- Final Exam questions
- NCLEX® Examination review questions
- Pharmacology animations
- Printable chapter summary

Evolve Website (http://evolve.elsevier.com/mckenry)
- Case study on diuretics
- Content updates, including information on new drugs

- WebLinks corresponding to this chapter
- Answers to the critical thinking questions in this chapter
- *Elsevier ePharmacology Update* newsletter
- *Mosby's Drug Consult* Internet Edition
- Supplemental and reference information

34

URICOSURIC DRUGS

CHAPTER FOCUS

Gout, a disorder of uric acid metabolism in the body, affects nearly half a million Americans. Although it can affect both males and females, nearly all of the cases affect men; fewer than 5% of diagnosed cases involve postmenopausal women, probably because estrogen promotes the excretion of uric acid. The nurse manages care during the acute episodes but primarily provides teaching and counseling for clients to self-manage the therapeutic regimen to prevent the painful attacks of gout.

LEARNING OBJECTIVES

- Explain the process of the production of uric acid in the body.
- Describe the classic symptoms of gout and the objectives for treatment of gout.
- Identify other diseases in which a secondary hyperuricemia may occur and common drugs that may increase or decrease a client's uric acid level.
- List the common adverse effects and the significant drug interactions for uricosuric drugs.
- Implement the nursing management of drug therapy for a client receiving a uricosuric drug.

▲ KEY TERMS
gout, p. 671
hyperuricemia, p. 671
urate nephropathy, p. 674

＊◖ KEY DRUGS
allopurinol, p. 675
colchicine, p. 672

Hyperuricemia and gout occur in persons with an abnormality in uric acid production and/or excretion. Risk factors for gout include obesity, hypertension, alcohol consumption, and lead exposure. Recurrent gouty arthritis is painful and can cause crystal deposits throughout the body, which results in an inflammatory response and, in some instances, kidney stones.

✹ **L.B., a 54-year-old male who started taking hydrochlorothiazide last month for hypertension, presents to the emergency department (ED) with toe and foot pain he rates at 8 of 10 on a pain scale. On observation his great right toe is swollen and erythematous.**

His serum uric acid level is 10.1 mg/L. He is diagnosed with gout.

✹ **What is gout?**

Gout is a disease associated with an inborn error of uric acid metabolism that increases the production or inhibits the excretion of uric acid. The hallmark of gout is **hyperuricemia,** or high levels of uric acid in the blood.

Gout is characterized by defective purine metabolism and manifests itself by attacks of acute pain, swelling, and tenderness of joints, such as those of the big toe, ankle, instep, knee, and elbow. The amount of uric acid in the blood becomes elevated, and tophi, which are deposits of uric acid or urates, form in the cartilage of various parts of the body. These deposits tend to increase in size and are seen most often along the edge of the ear. Chronic arthritis, nephritis, and premature sclerosis of the blood vessels may develop if gout is uncontrolled.

✱ **L.B. is diagnosed with gout and is told that he will need treatment for this acute attack.**

✱ **How is gout treated?**

The goals of treatment for gout are to (1) end the acute gouty attack as soon as possible, (2) prevent a recurrence of acute gouty arthritis, (3) prevent the formation of uric acid stones in the kidneys, and (4) reduce or prevent disease complications that result from sodium urate deposits in the joints and kidneys.

The drugs used to treat an acute attack of gout include colchicine, nonsteroidal antiinflammatory drugs (NSAIDs), and corticosteroids. The NSAIDs are primarily used to treat the acute inflammation and have no effect on the underlying metabolic problem; they are often prescribed to relieve an acute gout attack. Colchicine should be reserved for persons who do not respond to or cannot tolerate these agents (*USP DI*, 2005). Chapter 14 reviews NSAIDs. Colchicine is used specifically to treat gout and is reviewed in this chapter. Allopurinol, probenecid, sulfinpyrazone, and salicylates have also been used to treat chronic gouty arthritis or to prevent gout attacks. Salicylates require very high daily dosages, such as 4 to 6 g daily. Because few individuals can tolerate such high dosages on a long-term basis, they are not commonly prescribed for gout.

The nurse should be aware that low dosages of aspirin can interfere with the excretion of uric acid, resulting in an exacerbation of gout, and that a secondary hyperuricemia may occur from neoplastic diseases, cancer, psoriasis, Paget's disease, and other common and rare disease states. Many drugs have also been reported to increase or decrease levels of uric acid (Box 34-1).

It is preferable for the prescriber to identify the cause of the hyperuricemia and then decide whether or not to treat it. Asymptomatic hyperuricemia in an older adult may or may not be drug induced and often is not treated by the prescriber because of the potential adverse drug effects and the cost of the medications (Figure 34-1). However, specific treatments are indicated if symptoms are present or a treatable disease state is identified.

✱▀▀ **colchicine** [**koal** cheh seen]

The mechanism of action of colchicine for the treatment of gout is unknown but is reported to have antiinflammatory effects in gout. It also decreases phagocytosis, leukocyte motility, lactic acid production, and the release of a glycoprotein produced during urate crystal phagocytosis. These effects result in a decrease in urate deposits and inflammation even though the drug does not affect levels of uric acid in the circulatory system.

Indications

Colchicine is used in the treatment and prophylaxis of acute gouty arthritis and in the treatment of chronic gouty arthritis.

BOX 34-1 MEDICATIONS AFFECTING SERUM URIC ACID LEVELS

INCREASE LEVELS OF SERUM URIC ACID

ACE inhibitors (lisinopril, ramipril, trandolapril)

alcohol

aminoglycosides

cancer chemotherapeutic agents

diuretics (thiazides, furosemide)

ethambutol

levodopa

methyldopa

pancrelipase

salicylates (less than 2 g daily)

DECREASE LEVELS OF SERUM URIC ACID

acetohexamide

adrenocorticotropic hormone

allopurinol

chloramphenicol

probenecid

radiopaque dyes

salicylates (more than 3 g daily)

streptomycin

tetracycline (outdated)

Data from *USP DI: Drug information for the health care professional* (25th ed.). (2005). Greenwood Village, CO: MICROMEDEX Thomson Healthcare; and Russell T.M., & Young, L.Y. (2005). Gout and hyperuricemia. In M.A. Koda-Kimble, L.Y. Young, W.A. Kradjan, B.J. Guglielmo, B.K. Alldredge, & R.L. Corelli (Eds.), *Applied therapeutics: The clinical use of drugs* (8th ed.). Philadelphia: Lippincott, Williams & Wilkins.

Pharmacokinetics/Dosing

In acute gouty arthritis, colchicine has an onset of action within 12 hours after oral administration and intravenous (IV) injection. The peak effect for relief of pain and inflammation is reached in 1 to 2 days, but the reduction of swelling may require 3 days or more. Colchicine is metabolized in the liver and excreted mainly in bile. The adult dosage for gout prophylaxis is 0.5 to 0.6 mg PO daily, increased if necessary to twice daily. The dosage for acute gouty attacks is 0.5 to 1.2 mg (one to two tablets) initially, followed by one tablet every 1 to 2 hours until pain is relieved; until the adverse effects of nausea, vomiting, or diarrhea occur; or until the maximum dose of 6 mg has been reached. Parenteral colchicine is generally avoided due to greater toxicity observed when given IV. For use in acute gouty attacks when oral therapy is not possible, the dosage is 2 mg IV initially followed by 0.5 mg every 6 to 12 hours until the desired effect is achieved. Pediatric dosages have not been established.

Adverse Effects

The adverse effects with the oral administration of colchicine include diarrhea, nausea, vomiting, abdominal pain, anorexia and, with chronic therapy, alopecia. Colchicine administered IV can be very irritating to the vein, and extravasation can cause tissue injury.

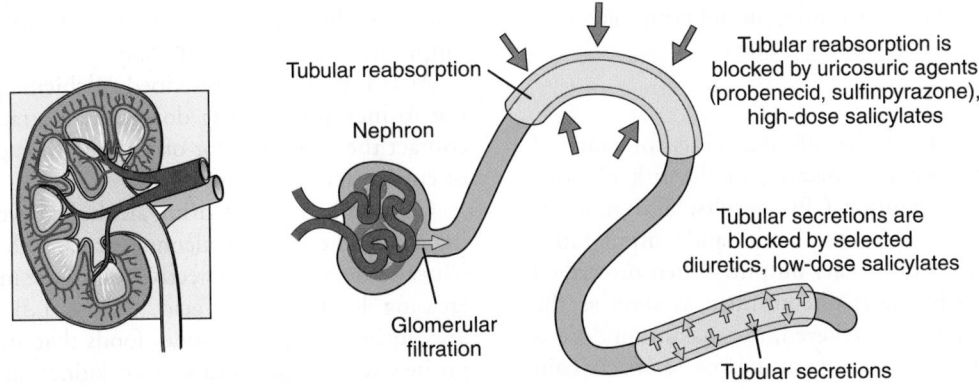

FIGURE 34-1 Drug effects on uric acid excretion in the kidney.

PREGNANCY SAFETY URICOSURIC DRUGS	
Category	**Drug**
B	probenecid,
C	allopurinol, sulfinpyrazone
D	colchicine

Data from *Mosby's drug consult* (15th ed.). (2005). St. Louis: Mosby.

Colchicine-induced toxicity depends on the total dose given over time, and the amount of single doses, especially IV doses. (See the Pregnancy Safety box above).

Drug Interactions
Colchicine is metabolized by P450 3 A4 and the drug may accumulate with known inhibitors of P450 3 A4, including grapefruit juice, azole antifungals, and protease inhibitors. Inducers of 3 A4, including rifampin, carbamazepine, phenytoin, and phenobarbital may result in reduced levels of colchicine. The clinical significance of these interactions is not clear.

✳ **L.B. is started on colchicine two tablets immediately, then one tablet every hour until pain is gone or he exhibits gastrointestinal (GI) upset. He is also asked to follow up with his primary health care provider to re-evaluate the hydrochlorothiazide therapy, which may have precipitated the gout.**

✳ **What care should the nurse provide regarding the safe and effective use of colchicine for L.B.?**

Assessment Although L.B. is only 54 years old, use caution when giving colchicine to older adults, because they often have diminished renal function and are more likely to experience cumulative toxicity, as are those with cardiac, re-nal, or hepatic disease. Assess him also for a GI disorder as colchicine may cause additional injury to GI tissues in clients with GI disorders or in those taking medications, such as NSAIDs, that may increase GI ulceration. Assess also any sensitivity to colchicine. The risk of inducing bone marrow depression or other serious, toxic, hematologic effects may be increased when colchicine is given concurrently with radiation therapy or drugs that induce blood dyscrasia or bone marrow depression (e.g., chloramphenicol [Chloromycetin], phenylbutazone, antineoplastics).

Before initiating therapy, obtain a baseline assessment of L.B.'s general health status, uric acid levels, complete blood count (CBC), frequency and severity of gout symptoms, and current joint pain and stiffness.

Nursing Diagnosis L.B. is at risk for the following selected nursing diagnoses/collaborative problems: diarrhea (up to 80% of clients experience diarrhea with oral doses); acute pain related to gout/ineffectiveness of the medication; impaired comfort related to rash, stomach pain, anorexia, nausea, and vomiting; hyperthermia; disturbed thought processes related to mood and mental changes; disturbed body image related to hair loss secondary to long-term use of drug; and the potential complications of thrombocytopenia (increased tendency to bleed), agranulocytosis (ineffective protection), aplastic anemia, hypersensitivity, myopathy (muscle weakness), and peripheral neuritis (numbness and tingling of the hands and feet). IV administration, although not relevant for L.B., increases the risk for cardiac dysrhythmias (administration too rapid) and localized reactions (thrombophlebitis, neuritis in injected arm).

Planning While taking colchicine, L.B. will be able to:
- Describe the use of the drug as it relates to the relief of his gout symptoms.
- Experience pain relief and relief of his other gout symptoms so that he may return to his usual activities of daily living (ADL).
- Effectively manage his therapeutic regimen (e.g., adherence with medication as prescribed, reporting ad-

verse effects to prescriber, using nonpharmacologic interventions to enhance drug therapy).

Implementation

Monitoring Monitor L.B.'s affected joints for range of motion, pain, and swelling. Because of the risk of bone marrow depression, monitor CBC results; also monitor serum uric acid levels. Monitor intake and output ratios to assess the adequacy of urinary output. When prescribed for acute gout, colchicine is discontinued as soon as the pain of the acute episode is relieved, the maximum dose is reached, or diarrhea, nausea, vomiting, or stomach pain occur.

Intervention To be effective, colchicine must be given properly at the first indication of an oncoming attack, and the dosage must be adequate. Once the dosage that will cause diarrhea has been determined, it is often possible to reduce subsequent doses to prevent diarrhea and still achieve satisfactory pain relief. Record the total amount of the drug taken before the occurrence of GI symptoms, so that in subsequent attacks treatment may be discontinued before this cumulative dose is reached. To avoid the toxic effects of accumulation, additional colchicine should not be administered for at least 3 days after a course of oral therapy or for at least 7 days (up to 21 days for older adults) after a course of IV treatment for an acute episode.

Oral colchicine may be administered with food to prevent GI distress. Oral administration is preferred for prophylaxis. However, IV administration is preferable for clients who are alcohol-dependent because they are more susceptible to GI toxicity, which is more likely to occur with oral administration.

Colchicine cannot be given subcutaneously or intramuscularly (IM) because it is highly irritating and will cause tissue necrosis. Extravasation must be avoided when colchicine is given IV. It is recommended that colchicine injection *not* be diluted with or injected into IV tubing containing 5% dextrose solution, solutions containing a bacteriostatic agent, or any solution that would change the pH of the colchicine solution; it will precipitate if mixed with or injected into these substances. To dilute colchicine, use 0.9% sodium chloride injection or sterile water for injection. Change the needle before administration. Administer the IV injection over a period of 2 to 5 minutes.

Education Alert L.B. to start the medication at the earliest sign of an attack but to discontinue it when the pain is relieved, when the maximum dose is reached, or at the first sign of diarrhea, nausea, vomiting, or stomach pain. The course of therapy should not be repeated for at least 3 days unless otherwise instructed by the prescriber. Because colchicine has such a narrow margin of safety, alert L.B. to report to the prescriber as soon as possible any signs of nausea, vomiting, diarrhea, sore throat, unusual bleeding or bruising, or unusual tiredness. Advise him to visit the health care provider regularly so that progress can be monitored.

Encourage him to increase fluid intake to ensure a urinary output of at least 2000 mL daily.

Alert L.B., if he is prescribed colchicine prophylactically, not to increase the drug dosage if an attack occurs but to contact the prescriber for other drug therapy (e.g., NSAID or corticosteroid therapy).

Caution L.B. not to drink alcoholic beverages while taking colchicine, because alcohol increases the risk of GI toxicity and decreases the effectiveness of the medication by increasing levels of uric acid. Advise L.B. to maintain a low-purine diet that excludes foods that are rich sources of purines (e.g., organ meats, liver, kidney, and sweetbreads), as well as red meats, poultry, and fish. Milk, eggs, cheese, and some vegetable sources of protein may be used as replacements. Instruct him to inform other health care providers that he is taking colchicine before any surgical or dental procedures are performed.

Evaluation The expected outcomes of colchicine therapy are that L.B. will experience pain relief associated with the gout attack or will not experience an acute episode of gout. His serum uric acid levels will remain 2.4 to 7.4 mg/dL. L.B. identifies factors that aggravate his gout and nonpharmacologic measures to use to promote comfort and increase ADLs. He states the adverse effects of the drug (e.g., GI upset, nausea and vomiting, anorexia) and identifies those to be reported to the prescriber (e.g., epigastric distress, diarrhea, abnormal bleeding, unusual bleeding or sore throat). L.B. maintains follow-up visits with his prescriber for monitoring.

✱ **L.B. uses colchicine to resolve his acute attack and follows up with his primary care provider over the following week. His prescriber discontinues the thiazide diuretic and replaces it with atenolol (Tenormin) 25 mg daily for his hypertension. He also starts allopurinol (Zyloprim) 300 mg daily.**

✱ **How does allopurinol affect uric acid levels?**
Allopurinol decreases the production of uric acid by inhibiting xanthine oxidase, the enzyme necessary to convert hypoxanthine to xanthine and xanthine to uric acid (Figure 34-2). It also increases the reutilization of both hypoxanthine and xanthine for nucleic acid synthesis, thus resulting in a feedback inhibition of purine synthesis. The result is a decrease of uric acid in both the serum and in the urine. This decrease of uric acid will prevent or decrease urate deposits, thus preventing or reducing both gouty arthritis and urate nephropathy. The reduction in urinary urate levels prevents **urate nephropathy,** the formation of uric acid or calcium oxalate calculi in the kidneys.

The client should be advised that allopurinol helps to prevent, but does not relieve, acute episodes of gout. Allopurinol use may initially induce an acute attack of gout in predisposed individuals. Concurrent colchicine may reduce this risk (Borstad et al., 2004).

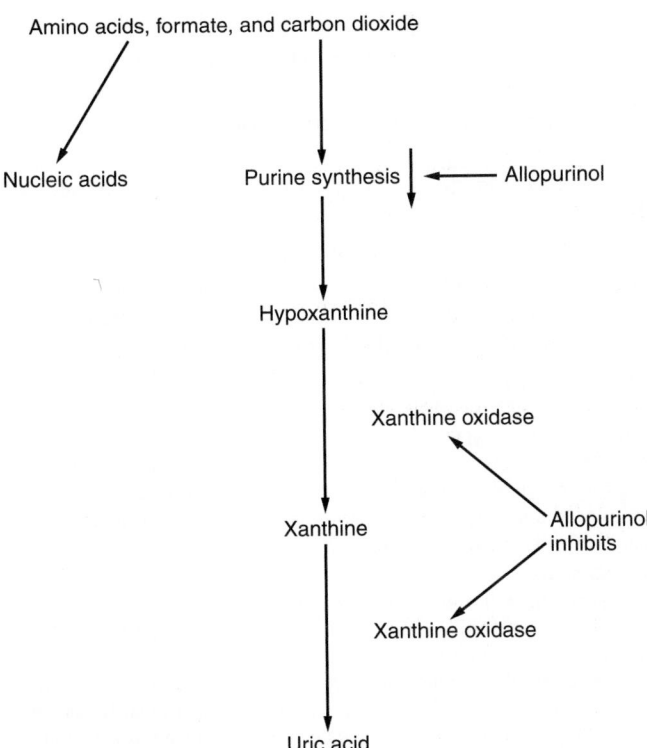

Amino acids, formate, and carbon dioxide

Nucleic acids

Purine synthesis ← Allopurinol

Hypoxanthine

Xanthine oxidase

Xanthine ← Allopurinol inhibits

Xanthine oxidase

Uric acid

FIGURE 34-2 The effects of allopurinol on uric acid production.

allopurinol [al low **pure** ih nawl]
(Zyloprim, Purinol)

Indications

Allopurinol is indicated for the treatment of chronic gouty arthritis and for the prophylaxis and treatment of hyperuricemia, urate nephropathy, and renal calculi associated with gout, tumor lysis after antineoplastic therapy, and other conditions.

Pharmacokinetics/Dosing

Allopurinol is well absorbed orally; the onset of action in reducing serum uric acid is 2 to 3 days. Approximately 70% of a dose is metabolized in the liver to an active metabolite, oxypurinol. The reduction of uric acid to a normal range occurs in 1 to 3 weeks, whereas a decrease in the frequency of acute gout attacks may require several months of drug therapy. Excretion is via the kidneys. The adult antihyperuricemic dosage is 100 mg PO daily initially, increased by 100 mg daily at 7-day intervals if necessary. The maximum daily dosage should not exceed 800 mg. The maintenance dosage is 100 to 200 mg PO two to three times daily or 300 mg once daily. For the treatment of hyperuricemia (from antineoplastic therapy), initially administer 600 to 800 mg PO daily, beginning 2 to 3 days before chemotherapy or radiation therapy. For maintenance therapy, adjust the dosage according to serum uric acid levels, which are analyzed approximately 2 days after the initiation of allopurinol and periodically thereafter. Discontinue allopurinol during the period of tumor regression.

To treat uric acid calculi, the dosage is 100 to 200 mg PO one to four times daily or 300 mg daily as a single dose. For the pediatric dosage as an antihyperuricemic agent in antineoplastic therapy, refer to a current package insert or the *USP DI*.

Adverse Effects

The adverse effects of allopurinol include pruritus, allergic reaction, rash, hives, diarrhea, abdominal distress, nausea, vomiting, alopecia, dermatitis and, rarely, bone marrow depression, liver toxicity, hypersensitivity reaction, peripheral neuritis, renal failure, and nosebleeds. (See the Pregnancy Safety box on p. 673.)

Drug Interactions

Allopurinol has the potential to accentuate the bone marrow suppression effects of other drugs, including agents used in the treatment of cancer. Other interactions with cancer chemotherapy are possible, including increased effects with azathioprine or mercaptopurine. The potential for kidney stones may be higher when allopurinol is administered with large doses of ascorbic acid (vitamin C). Metabolism of warfarin may be impaired. Hypersensitivity reactions may be more common when clients also receive other drugs known to induce hypersensitivity (e.g., ACE inhibitors, amoxicillin, thiazide diuretics).

✹ What are the nursing management issues associated with the use of allopurinol for L.B.?

Assessment Monitor renal function to detect the need for a dosage reduction. Allopurinol may accumulate and increase the risk of allergic reactions or other adverse effects if L.B. has impaired renal function, or any illness that may predispose him to a change in renal function (e.g., diabetes mellitus, hypertension). Assess also L.B.'s sensitivity to allopurinol.

Review L.B.'s concurrent medication regimen for the risk of significant drug interactions. Allopurinol may inhibit the metabolism of the oral anticoagulant warfarin, resulting in an increase in serum levels, activity, and perhaps toxicity. Monitor prothrombin levels closely, because a dosage adjustment may be necessary. When allopurinol is administered with azathioprine (Imuran), an immunosuppressant, or mercaptopurine (Purinethol), an antineoplastic, the effect of allopurinol in inhibiting xanthine oxidase may result in a decreased metabolism of these medications, leading to an increased potential for therapeutic and/or toxic effects (especially bone marrow depression). Monitor closely, because interventions or dosage adjustments may be necessary.

A baseline assessment of L.B. includes serum uric acid levels, CBC, hepatic and renal function determinations, and assessments of joint stiffness and pain.

Nursing Diagnosis While receiving allopurinol, L.B. is at risk for the following nursing diagnoses/collaborative problems: impaired comfort (headache, indigestion, anorexia, nausea, and vomiting); diarrhea; disturbed body image related to hair loss; and the potential complications of hypersensitivity, peripheral neuritis (numbness and tingling of the hands and feet), allergic dermatitis (rash, hives, itching), hepatotoxicity, bone marrow suppression (thrombocytopenia [increased tendency to bleed], anemia [fatigue], agranulocytosis [fever, mouth ulcers, sore throat]), exfoliative dermatitis, erythema multiforme (chills, fever, sores in mouth, skin rash), Stevens-Johnson syndrome, or toxic epidermal necrolysis (chills, fever, muscle ache, skin peeling).

Planning While taking allopurinol, L.B. will be able to:
• Describe the use of the drug as it relates to the prevention of his gout symptoms.

- Experience an absence of pain and his other gout symptoms so that he maintains his usual ADL.
- Effectively manage his therapeutic regimen (e.g., adherence with medication as prescribed, reporting adverse effects to prescriber, using nonpharmacologic interventions to enhance drug therapy).

Implementation

Monitoring For proper dosing, monitor results of serum uric acid levels. CBCs and renal and hepatic function studies are recommended at periodic intervals during therapy, particularly during the first few months. Monitor L.B.'s intake to ensure an adequate fluid intake. Observe his pain level and the mobility status of his affected joints.

Intervention Administer allopurinol with food to minimize GI distress. A high fluid intake (80 to 96 ounces daily to produce 2 L of urine) and alkalinization of the urine are necessary to lessen the risk of stone formation and sludging of the tubules with urates.

A single dose of allopurinol should not exceed 300 mg; it may be given in divided doses.

Education Encourage L.B. to comply with the medication regimen. Advise him that allopurinol helps to prevent, but does not relieve, acute episodes of gout.

Caution L.B. not to drink alcoholic beverages, because alcohol increases concentrations of uric acid. Alert him that drowsiness may occur and that hazardous activities requiring mental alertness, such as driving, need to be avoided until his response to the medication has been determined. Stress the importance of a large amount (2.5 to 3 L daily) of fluid intake to ensure the adequacy of fluid output.

Elevated uric acid levels increase the risk for nephrolithiasis. Obesity increases this risk (Taylor, Stampfer, & Curhan, 2005). To minimize the formation of calcium oxalate stones, teach L.B. to maintain a diet that enhances the alkalinity of the urine. This diet includes milk, fruits (except plums, prunes, and cranberries), carbonated beverages, vegetables (except corn and lentils), molasses, and baking soda and baking powder. He should avoid aspirin and large doses of vitamin C. Advise L.B. to maintain a low-purine diet.

Advise L.B. to report to his prescriber immediately any signs of a skin rash or other adverse effects. A skin rash usually precedes severe hypersensitivity reactions. Regular visits to the prescriber are necessary to monitor progress through periodic blood testing and the assessment for adverse effects. Contact the prescriber if an acute attack of gout occurs while undergoing prophylaxis therapy; additional drug therapy with NSAIDs or corticosteroids may be prescribed.

Evaluation The expected outcome of allopurinol therapy is that L.B. will experience fewer or an absence of acute attacks of gout. His serum uric acid levels will remain 2.4 to 7.4 mg/dL. L.B. identifies factors that aggravate his gout (alcohol ingestion, inappropriate diet) or increase the risk of drug adverse effects (inadequate fluid intake, acidic urine). He states the adverse effects of the drug (e.g., GI upset, nausea and vomiting, anorexia) and identifies those to be reported to the prescriber (e.g., chills, fever, muscular aches and pains, nausea or vomiting, skin rash). L.B. maintains follow-up visits with his prescriber for monitoring.

✱ What other drugs are used to lower uric acid serum levels?

Probenecid (Benemid) and sulfinpyrazone (Anturane) both inhibit the reabsorption of urate in the proximal renal tubule and are indicated for hyperuricemia and gout. Each are briefly described in the following sections.

probenecid [proe **ben** ah sid]
(Benemid, Benuryl✤)

Probenecid lowers serum levels of uric acid by competitively inhibiting the reabsorption of urate at the proximal renal tubule, thus increasing the urinary excretion of uric acid. It has no antiinflammatory action or analgesic effects.

Indications

Probenecid is indicated for the treatment of hyperuricemia and chronic gouty arthritis and as an adjunct to antibiotic therapy. As an adjunct to antibiotic therapy, probenecid competitively inhibits the secretion of weak organic acids, such as penicillin and some of the cephalosporins, at both the proximal and distal renal tubules in the kidneys. The result is an increase in blood concentrations and the duration of action of these antibiotics. This combination is sometimes used to treat sexually transmitted diseases (e.g., gonorrhea, acute pelvic inflammatory disease [PID], and neurosyphilis).

Pharmacokinetics/Dosing

Probenecid is well absorbed orally and is highly bound to plasma proteins, especially to albumin. The therapeutic serum level for uricosuric effect is 100 to 200 mcg/mL, and 40 to 60 mcg/mL for the suppression of penicillin excretion. The peak uricosuric effect is reached within 30 minutes, whereas the peak suppression of penicillin excretion is noted in 2 hours and lasts nearly 8 hours. Probenecid is metabolized in the liver and excreted by the kidneys. The adult dosage is 250 mg twice daily for 7 days, and then increased to 500 mg twice daily. As an adjunct to penicillin/cephalosporin drug therapy, the dosage is 500 mg four times daily. The pediatric dosage as an antihyperuricemic agent has not been established. As an antibiotic adjunct, check a current drug reference for recommended dosing schedules.

Adverse Effects

The adverse effects of probenecid include headaches, anorexia, mild nausea or vomiting, sore gums, pain and/or blood on urination, and lower back pain.

Drug Interactions

Probenecid can result in reduced renal elimination and increased serum levels of methotrexate, fluoroquinolone antimicrobials (e.g., ciprofloxacin), penicillins, cephalosporins, acyclovir, NSAIDs, zidovudine, and benzodiazepines. See Figure 34-2.

✱ What are the key nursing issues with the use of probenecid?

Assessment Probenecid is well tolerated by most clients. However, probenecid is contraindicated for clients who are at increased risk of uric acid renal calculi formation or urate nephropathy, such as clients undergoing cancer chemotherapy or radiation therapy or those with moderate to severe renal function impairment. Its use is carefully considered in clients with blood dyscrasias, a history of uric acid kidney stones, or mild renal function impairment, because these conditions may be exacerbated. Assess the client carefully for allergy to probenecid.

Review the client's drug history for the risk of significant drug interactions, such as those that may occur when probenecid is given concurrently with antineoplastic cytolytic drugs because this combination increases the potential toxicity of uric acid nephropathy. Additionally, the rapidly acting antineoplastic drugs may increase plasma levels of uric acid and interfere with any control of the previous hyperuricemia and gout. Avoid concurrent use or a potentially serious drug interaction may occur. The concurrent use of aspirin or salicylates is not recommended; salicylates in moderate to high doses given chronically will inhibit the effectiveness of probenecid. Additionally, if high doses of salicylates are being given for their uricosuric effects, probenecid may lower the excretion of salicylates, which may result in elevated serum salicylate levels and toxicity. Probenecid decreases the renal tubular secretion of penicillin and selected cephalosporins, which may result in an increased serum level and a prolonged duration of action of the antibiotic. Cephalosporins not affected by probenecid include cefoperazone (Cefobid), ceforanide (Precef), ceftazidime (Fortaz), and ceftriaxone (Rocephin). The anticoagulant effects of heparin may be enhanced and prolonged increasing the client's risk of bleeding. If given concurrently with indomethacin (Indocin), ketoprofen (Orudis), and other NSAIDs, probenecid decreases renal excretion of these drugs, leading to an increase in NSAID serum levels and possibly toxicity. Monitor closely because the prescriber may need to lower the daily dose of NSAID if adverse effects are reported. Probenecid may decrease the renal excretion of methotrexate (Folex, Mexate), which may increase the risk of serious toxicity with methotrexate. Probenecid may decrease the renal tubular secretion of nitrofurantoin (Macrodantin), resulting in an increase in serum levels and possibly toxicity. This may reduce the urinary levels and so the effectiveness of nitrofurantoin in the treatment of urinary tract infections. Concurrent drug administration of zidovudine (AZT) may lead to an inhibition of zidovudine metabolism and secretion, resulting in elevated serum levels and an increased risk of zidovudine toxicity. The administration of probenecid may permit a reduced daily dose schedule for zidovudine.

A baseline assessment of the client should include serum uric acid determinations, acid-base balance determination, and an assessment of the frequency and severity of acute episodes of gout.

Nursing Diagnosis While taking probenecid, clients are at risk for the following selected nursing diagnoses/collaborative problems: acute pain related to underlying gout and ineffectiveness of medication; impaired comfort (headache, stomach pain, anorexia, nausea, and vomiting); hyperthermia; disturbed body image related to hair loss; and the potential complications of allergic dermatitis, uric acid renal calculi (low back pain), thrombocytopenia (increased tendency to bleed), or anemia.

Planning The goals for probenecid therapy are the same as for allopurinol.

Implementation

Monitoring Monitor the client's involved joints for range of motion, pain, and swelling during the course of medication, and serum uric acid levels and CBCs and, if urinary alkalizers are used, acid-base balance values.

Intervention Probenecid may be administered with an antacid or food to minimize GI distress. A high fluid intake (2.5 to 3 L of water daily) to produce copious volumes of urine is recommended to minimize the formation of uric acid stones and the occurrence of renal colic and hematuria.

Alkalinization of the urine may be required to minimize the formation of kidney stones. Sodium bicarbonate, potassium citrate, and acetazolamide are agents recommended for the alkalinization of urine. As with allopurinol therapy, diet therapy is recommended with probenecid.

Education Encourage the client to comply with the medication regimen. Variations in the dosage may precipitate an acute episode of gout. It is important for the client to understand that probenecid helps to prevent attacks but does not relieve acute episodes of gout. Regular visits to the prescriber are necessary to monitor progress. If an acute attack of gout occurs, contact the prescriber for additional medication (e.g., NSAIDs or colchicine).

Stress the importance of maintaining adequate fluid intake. Caution the client not to drink alcohol, because doing so increases uric acid levels. The client should also avoid use of aspirin and other salicylates because they decrease the effectiveness of probenecid and may precipitate a gout attack. Advise the client to read the labels of over-the-counter (OTC) medications carefully because aspirin and other salicylates are common ingredients of OTC medications for cold and flu-like symptoms.

Caution the client to report to the prescriber any symptoms of hypersensitivity (skin rash), renal stones (hematuria, dysuria, low back pain), or blood dyscrasias (sore throat, fever, unusual bleeding or bruising, or unusual fatigue).

Evaluation The expected outcome of probenecid therapy is that the client will not experience attacks of gout, or the attacks will be diminished in frequency and severity. Serum uric acid levels will remain 2.4 to 7.4 mg/dL. The client identifies factors that aggravate gout (alcohol ingestion, inappropriate diet) or increase the risk of adverse effects (inadequate fluid intake, acidic urine). The client states adverse effects (e.g., GI upset, nausea and vomiting, anorexia), identifies those to be reported to the prescriber (e.g., chills, fever, sore gums, lower back pain, blood in urine), and maintains follow-up visits with his prescriber for monitoring.

sulfinpyrazone [sul fin **peer** a zone]
(Anturane)

The mechanism of action of sulfinpyrazone is similar to probenecid; it inhibits the reabsorption of urate at the proximal renal tubule, thus increasing the excretion of uric acid in the urine.

Indications

Sulfinpyrazone is indicated for the treatment of chronic gouty arthritis and hyperuricemia.

Pharmacokinetics/Dosing

Sulfinpyrazone is well absorbed orally and is highly bound to plasma proteins. It is metabolized in the liver into four active metabolites via P450 2 C8/9; the p-hydroxy-sulfinpyrazone metabolite contributes between 33% and 50% of the uricosuric effect of sulfinpyrazone. The duration of the uricosuric effect is usually 4 to 6 hours. Sulfinpyrazone is excreted by the kidneys. The adult antigout dosage is 100 to 200 mg PO twice daily initially, increased gradually at 2-day intervals if necessary until it is sufficient to control the elevated serum uric acid levels (usually 400 to 800 mg daily). The maintenance dosage is 200 to 400 mg daily. The pediatric dosage has not been established.

Adverse Effects

The adverse effects of sulfinpyrazone include nausea, vomiting, abdominal pain, and a rash or allergic reaction.

Drug Interactions

Sulfinpyrazone may increase serum levels and effects of oral hypoglycemics, anticoagulants, and acetaminophen. Concurrent enzyme inducing agents such as rifampin, phenobarbital, phenytoin, and carbamazepine may result in reduced sulfinpyrazone serum levels and response.

Nursing Management

The nursing management of sulfinpyrazone is as for probenecid, except for its drug interactions. When sulfinpyrazone is administered concurrently with the following drugs the potential for bleeding is increased: alprostadil (Prostin VR), anagrelide, aspirin, dextran, carbenicillin (parenteral), cefotetan (Cefotan), cefoperazone (Cefobid), dipyridamole (Persantine), divalproex (Depakote), NSAIDs, plicamycin (Mithramycin), ticarcillin (Ticar), ticlopidine (Ticlid), valproic acid (Depakene), anticoagulants or thrombolytics. Monitor closely for early signs of bleeding. With rapidly cytolytic antineoplastic agents, an increased risk of inducing uric acid nephropathy or losing control of uric acid serum levels (preexisting levels) and gout is possible. When aspirin and other salicylates are given long term in moderate to high doses, the uricosuric effect of sulfinpyrazone may be inhibited (see comments about probenecid). Sulfinpyrazone may decrease kidney excretion of nitrofurantoin (Macrodantin), which may increase the risk of nitrofurantoin toxicity and reduce the effectiveness of nitrofurantoin as a urinary tract antiinfective agent.

Summary

Gout is a metabolic disorder characterized by hyperuricemia. The aims of therapy for gout are to end the acute attack quickly, prevent a recurrence, prevent uric acid renal calculi, and prevent or minimize the complications of sodium urate deposits in the joints. Agents used for these purposes are colchicine, allopurinol, probenecid, and sulfinpyrazone.

✳ Critical Thinking Questions

- Mr. Stevens, 56 years old, comes to the clinic with a red, swollen great toe on his left foot. He is accompanied by his wife. He indicates that he has had pain, redness, and swelling for approximately 1 week, and it has been unrelieved by aspirin. For what risk factors of gout will you assess Mr. Stevens? How will his medical diagnosis be confirmed? Given what Mr. Stevens has already said, what health teaching does the client and family require?

- Why is a diet that enhances alkalinity of the urine recommended for clients with gout? What should be included in such a diet? What dietary limitations are prescribed for these clients?

Bibliography

Anderson, D.M., Keith, J., & Novak, P.D. (Eds.) (2002). *Mosby's medical, nursing, and allied health dictionary* (6th ed.). St. Louis: Mosby.

Borstad, G.C., Bryant, L.R., Abel, M.P., Scroggie, D.A., Harris, M.D., & Alloway, J.A. (2004). Colchicine for prophylaxis of acute flares when initiating allopurinol for chronic gouty arthritis. *Journal of Rheumatology, 31,* 2429-2432.

Bosker, G. (Ed.). (2004). *Primary and acute care medicine: Practice, protocols, pathways,* (2nd ed.). Atlanta: Thomson American Health Consultants.

Drug facts and comparisons. (58th ed.). (2005). St. Louis: Facts and Comparisons.

e-LEARNING SUPPLEMENTS

Student CD-ROM
- Final Exam questions
- NCLEX® Examination review questions
- Pharmacology animations
- Printable chapter summary

Evolve Website (http://evolve.elsevier.com/mckenry)
- Case study on uricosuric drugs

- Content updates, including information on new drugs
- WebLinks corresponding to this chapter
- Answers to the critical thinking questions in this chapter
- *Elsevier ePharmacology Update* newsletter
- Mosby's Drug Consult Internet Edition
- Supplemental and reference information

Hawkins, D.W., & Rahn, D.W. (2002). Gout and hyperuricemia. In J.T. DiPiro, R.L. Talbert, G.C. Yee, G.R. Matzke, B.G. Wells, & L.M. Posey (Eds.), *Pharmacotherapy: A pathophysiological* approach (5th ed.). New York: McGraw-Hill.

Hellman, D.B., & Stone, J.H. (2003). Arthritis and musculoskeletal disorders.. In L.M. Tierney, Jr., S.J. McPhee, & Papadakis, M.A. (Eds.), *Current Medical Diagnosis & Treatment.* New York: Lange Medical Books/McGraw-Hill.

Lacy, C.F., Armstrong, L.L., Goldman, M.P., & Lance, L.L. (2004). *Lexi-Comp's Drug Information Handbook* (12th ed.). Hudson, Ohio: Lexi-Comp.

Mosby's drug consult (15th ed.). (2005). St. Louis: Mosby.

Roberts, L.J., & Morrow, J.D. (2001). Analgesic-antipyretic and antiinflammatory agents and drugs employed in the treatment of gout. In Hardman, J.G. & Limbird, L.E. (Eds.), *Goodman & Gilman's The pharmacological basis of therapeutics* (10th ed.). New York: McGraw-Hill.

Russell, T.M., & Young, L.Y. (2005). Gout and hyperuricemia. In M.A. Koda-Kimble, L.Y. Young, W.A. Kradjan, B.J. Guglielmo, B.K. Alldredge, & R.L. Corelli (Eds.), *Applied therapeutics: The clinical use of drugs* (8th ed.). Philadelphia: Lippincott Williams & Wilkins.

Schnell, Z.B., Van Leeuwen, A.M., & Kranpitz, T.R. (2003). *Davis's comprehensive laboratory and diagnostic test handbook – with nursing implications.* Philadelphia: F.A. Davis.

Taylor, E.N., Stampfer, M.J., & Curhan, G.C. (2005). Obesity, weight gain, and the risk of kidney stone. *Journal of the American Medical Association, 293,* 455-462.

USP DI: Drug information for the health care professional (25th ed.). (2005). Greenwood Village, CO: MICROMEDEX Thomson Healthcare.

DRUG THERAPY FOR RENAL SYSTEM DYSFUNCTION

CHAPTER FOCUS

Renal dysfunction can alter the bioavailability, distribution, and protein binding of drugs by modifying systemic pH, altering the configuration and amount of albumin, and altering body hydration and renal excretion. Even with drugs that are not excreted renally, renal dysfunction may cause toxic metabolites to accumulate. Drug-induced nephrotoxicity may also occur. The nurse needs to be acutely aware of the effects of renal system dysfunction on drug therapy and vice versa.

LEARNING OBJECTIVES

- Differentiate between acute renal failure and chronic renal insufficiency.
- Identify two laboratory tests used to evaluate renal impairment.
- Explain why dietary protein, fluid intake, potassium, magnesium, and phosphorus are restricted in chronic renal insufficiency.
- Describe the differences between the drug dosage reduction method and the interval extension method of treatment, and describe the advantages of each.
- Implement the nursing management of drug therapy for the client with renal system dysfunction.

▲ **KEY TERMS**

acute renal failure, p. 680
azotemic, p. 682
chronic renal insufficiency, p. 681

end-stage renal disease (ESRD), p. 681
hemodialysis, p. 682
peritoneal dialysis, p. 682

Monitoring renal function is an important aspect of providing care for clients. A number of drugs are toxic to the kidney and must be used carefully to avoid renal damage. Other drugs accumulate in clients with renal insufficiency and require dosage adjustment for their safe use. Finally, clients in end-stage renal disease have specific physiologic needs that are partially met with drug therapy.

✴ How does acute renal failure differ from chronic renal insufficiency?

Acute renal failure, a condition characterized by oliguria, rapid accumulation of nitrogenous wastes in the blood, and

a rapid decline in renal function, occurs in 2% to 5% of all hospitalized individuals and in up to 1% of hospital admissions from the community (Brophy, 2005). Primary causes include trauma, pregnancy, and renal ischemia as a result of surgery, severe hemorrhage, severe volume depletion, and shock.

There are a number of mechanisms of drug induced acute renal failure (Table 35-1). In some instances, nephrotoxic agents such as heavy metals, radiopaque contrast dyes and aminoglycoside antibiotics (tobramycin, gentamicin) are toxic to the renal tubule (known as acute tubular necrosis or ATN) (Figure 35-1). Acute renal damage can be a re-

TABLE 35-1 DRUGS ASSOCIATED WITH RENAL TOXICITY OR DYSFUNCTION

Mechanism of Renal Insufficiency	Drugs
Acute tubular necrosis	Aminoglycosides (e.g., gentamicin, tobramycin) amphotericin B Radiographic contrast media
Interstitial nephritis	allopurinol NSAIDs penicillins sulfonamides
Glomerular damage	gold salts heroin lithium
Nephrolithiasis	acyclovir (high dose) indinavir topiramate
Renal ischemia	ACE inhibitors/angiotensin receptor blockers (ARBs) Excessive antihypertensive therapy (especially in older adults) Excessive diuretic use with hypotension NSAIDs Vasopressors (e.g., norepinephrine, IV dopamine)

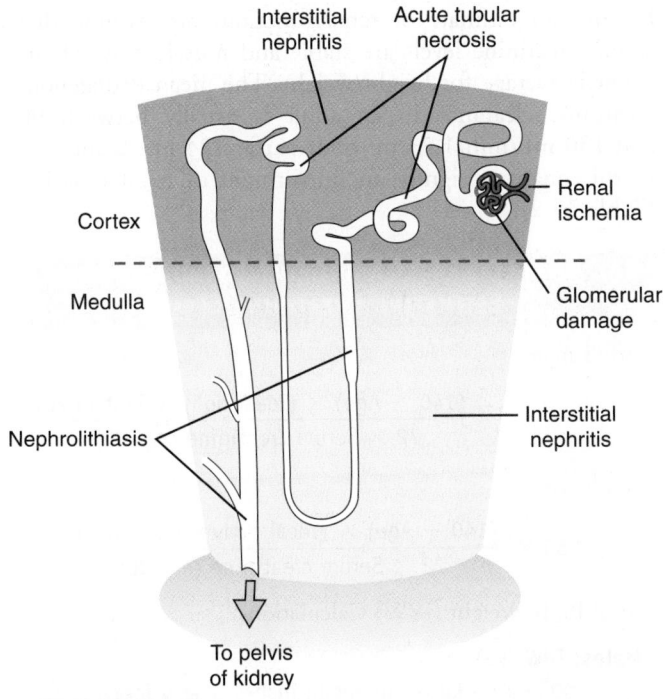

FIGURE 35-1 Sites of drug-induced nephrotoxicity.

sult of inflammation of the interstitial tissue (interstitial nephritis) as may be observed with some penicillins. A third way renal damage is noted acutely with drugs is via damage to the glomerulus as is seen with lithium or gold salts. Ad-

ditional considerations are drugs that may form crystals in the urine and lead to obstruction. Drugs like the antiviral acyclovir, the human immunodeficiency virus (HIV) drug indinavir, and the antiepileptic topiramate, can predispose to nephrolithiasis and lead to obstructive acute renal failure. Finally, acute renal failure is sometimes observed when blood flow to the kidney is temporarily impaired, as is seen in shock, dehydration, or with a number of drugs that impair renal blood flow, including vasoconstrictors, angiotensin-converting enzyme (ACE) inhibitors and nonsteroidal antiinflammatory drugs (NSAIDs). If recognized early and treated promptly, acute renal failure may be reversed before acute tubular necrosis or permanent damage occurs.

Chronic renal insufficiency is a progressive disease usually caused by an irreversible kidney injury that results in the permanent loss of nephrons or renal mass. The most common causes are glomerulonephritis, diabetes mellitus (DM), hypertension, polycystic kidney disease, and other diseases that may lead to the destruction or impaired functioning of the kidneys. Long term use of drugs like lithium (Lepkifker, Sverdlik, Iancu, Ziv, Segev, & Kotler, 2004) and acetaminophen (Curhan, Knight, Rosner, Hankinson, & Stampfer, 2004) are sometimes associated with declining renal function as well. Initially, individuals with chronic renal insufficiency may be treated conservatively, but in **end-stage renal disease (ESRD)** the kidney is so severely damaged or scarred that hemodialysis or organ transplantation may be necessary for survival.

Chronic renal insufficiency and ESRD are major health concerns in North America. In the United States, nearly 300,000 people are on long-term dialysis and more than 20,000 have a functioning transplanted kidney. The most common cause of ESRD in the United States is diabetes. ESRD almost always follows chronic kidney failure, which may exist for 10 to 20 years or more before progression to ESRD. The incident rate for ESRD caused by diabetes has begun to stabilize, and that for ESRD caused by glomerulonephritis has begun to decline. These findings indicate that efforts to address the progression of chronic kidney disease to ESRD, including the use of ACE inhibitors, angiotensin receptor blockers (ARBs), and antihypertensive medications, may be paying off (United States Renal Data System, 2004) In Canada, the rates of ESRD were 79.8 per million population and expected to increase by 5.8% annually through 2005 (Schaubel, Morrison, Desmeules, Parsons, & Fenton, 1999). Treatments for chronic renal insufficiency and ESRD are hemodialysis, peritoneal dialysis, and transplantation of kidneys. **Hemodialysis** is a procedure in which impurities or wastes are removed from the blood; the blood is shunted from the body through a machine for diffusion and ultrafiltration and then returned to the client's circulation. **Peritoneal dialysis** is another form of dialysis but one in which the peritoneum is used as the diffusible membrane. A solution known as dialysate is placed into the peritoneal cavity via a catheter and retained for a specified time; osmosis, diffusion, and filtration pass needed electrolytes into the bloodstream and remove wastes into the dialysate, which is then drained by gravity from the abdominal cavity.

✱ What are the signs and symptoms of renal failure or renal insufficiency?

One of the more common signs of acute renal failure is a marked alteration in expected urine output, usually a significant reduction (less than 400 mL daily). This is referred to as the oliguric phase. Phase two is the diuretic phase; in this phase the individual experiences an increase in urine volume for a few days but remains **azotemic,** retaining excessive amounts of nitrogenous compounds (blood urea nitrogen [BUN] and creatinine) in the blood. Phase three is considered the recovery phase as azotemia decreases and renal function is recovering. The recovery phase may occur over weeks to months, depending on the damage caused by the original insult to the kidneys (Hudson & Johnson, 2005). Signs of acute renal failure in the presence of reduced urine production are usually the result of fluid overload: edema, weight gain, weakness, hypertension, and tachycardia.

The most common complaints with chronic renal insufficiency are increasing weakness, fatigue, and lethargy. Gastrointestinal (GI) signs include anorexia, GI distress, nausea, vomiting, thirst, and weight loss. Paresthesias, pruritus, peripheral neuropathy, seizures, and neuromuscular irritability may also occur. On examination, the client may appear pale and dehydrated and have an increased respiratory rate and uremic breath. Hypertension with retinopathy, cardiac hypertrophy, pulmonary edema, or pericarditis may often be present.

A detailed client history, thorough physical examination, urinalysis, and blood chemistry levels are important for the assessment, diagnosis, and determination of an appropriate treatment plan. The degree of renal impairment is usually estimated by reviewing the levels of serum creatinine and BUN. Concurrent elevated levels of creatinine and BUN indicate a decrease in renal clearance, which predisposes the individual to drug toxicity.

✱ How is renal function measured?

Many formulas and nomograms are available to determine the client's approximate creatinine clearance and the drug dosage adjustment necessary to minimize the risk of toxicity. Creatinine, a byproduct of muscle, is often used as a predictor of renal function because it is only eliminated by the body via glomerular filtration. Normal values may vary from laboratory to laboratory, but in general the range of serum creatinine, which varies with age (approximately 10% increase with each decade after 40 years of age), is usually between 0.5 and 1.2 mg/dL and a normal BUN ranges between 5 and 20 mg/dL.

One of the most reliable tests is to physically measure creatinine clearance. Because it is difficult to obtain an accurate collection of all urine excreted for a 24-hour period, many clinicians use a formula to estimate creatinine clearance; others may prefer to use a nomogram. The formulas most commonly used are noted in Box 35-1. These formulas give an estimate of renal function, but assume that serum creatinine levels are stable and muscle mass of the client is average for height/weight. The mean endogenous creatinine clearance in an adult is usually between 90 and 130 mL/min/1.73 m² body surface/24 hr. Reductions in this quantity signify an impairment of renal function (Table 35-2).

BOX 35-1 COCKROFT AND GAULT FORMULAS FOR ESTIMATING CREATININE CLEARANCE

Adult male

$$= \frac{(140 - \text{Age}) \times (\text{Ideal body weight in kg})}{72 \times \text{Serum creatinine (mg/dL)}}$$

Adult female

$$= 0.85 \times \frac{(140 - \text{Age}) \times (\text{Ideal body weight in kg})}{72 \times \text{Serum creatinine (mg/dL)}}$$

Ideal Body Weight (IBW) Calculations

Males: IBW (kg) =
50 + (2.3 kg × Height in inches over 5 feet)

Females: IBW (kg) =
45.5 + (2.3 kg × Height in inches over 5 feet)

Data from Cockroft, D.W., & Gault, M.H. (1976). Prediction of creatinine clearance from serum creatinine. *Nephron, 16,* 31-41.

Another important factor in evaluating serum levels of drugs in clients with renal failure or renal impairment is an assessment of serum albumin and total protein. Serum protein is decreased in individuals with renal insufficiency. Blood urea nitrogen is also elevated in clients with renal insufficiency and can displace highly plasma protein–binding drugs from their binding sites. These factors can alter the interpretation of serum levels of drugs that are protein bound (90% or more) in persons with normal renal function. Individuals with a lower albumin and/or elevated BUN may have elevated free levels of phenytoin, valproate, warfarin, or other highly plasma protein–bound drugs and be at risk for drug toxicity with standard doses.

What drugs require dosage adjustment with renal insufficiency?

Drugs that are eliminated from the body primarily as unchanged drug or as pharmacologically active metabolites in the urine typically require dosage adjustment for clients with reduced renal function. This is particularly true for drugs with a low therapeutic index like lithium, digoxin, and gentamicin.

In individuals with significant renal insufficiency or impairment, the drug dose may be decreased (dosage reduction method) with the usual dosage interval maintained; if the dose remains the same, the interval between doses is lengthened (interval extension method). Usually the dosage reduction method is preferred for drugs that require a constant therapeutic level in the blood. For most clients receiving a loading dose, the dose is similar to the dose given to a client without renal impairment. This permits a therapeutically desirable blood level that is then maintained by either the dosage reduction method or the interval extension method. Table 35-3 gives typical dosing recommendations for selected medications along with a list of drugs that may or may not be removed by hemodialysis or peritoneal dialysis. Refer to the current package inserts or renal failure dosing guides for specific data.

Can renal failure be prevented?

Acute renal failure is often a potentially preventable event, and its risk can be avoided by careful use and/or avoidance of drugs which are prone to induce acute renal failure (examples in Table 35-1). Reduced renal perfusion and acute

TABLE 35-2 TYPICAL GRADING OF RENAL IMPAIRMENT USING CREATININE CLEARANCE

Degree of Renal Failure	Creatinine Clearance
Normal	Men: 90-139 mL/min Women: 80-125 mL/min
Mild impairment	50-79 mL/min
Moderate impairment	30-49 mL/min
Severe impairment	10-29 mL/min
End-stage renal disease	Less than 10 mL/min

TABLE 35-3 EXAMPLES OF MEDICATION DOSING FOR ADULTS WITH RENAL INSUFFICIENCY

Medication	Normal Function to Mild Renal Insufficiency	Moderate Renal Insufficiency	Renal Failure	Half-Life Normal	Half-Life Anuric
acyclovir (Zovirax)	5 mg/kg IV q8h	5 mg/kg IV q12-24h	2.5 mg/kg IV q24h	2.5 hr	20 hr
ampicillin (Omnipen-N)	1-2 g IV q4-6h	1-1.5 g IV q6h	1 g IV q8-12h	0.8-1.5 hr	20 hr
cefazolin (Ancef)	1-2 g IV q8h	500-1500 mg IV q12h	500-1000 mg IV q24h	1.8-2.6 hr	12-40 hr
ciprofloxacin (Cipro)	250-750 mg PO q12h	250-500 mg PO q12h	250-750 mg PO q24h	4 hr	8.5 hr
fluconazole (Diflucan)	Varies with indication 100-200 mg IV/PO q24h	Varies with indication 50-100 mg IV/PO q24h	Varies with indication 50-100 mg IV/PO q24h	20-50 hr	98 hr
meperidine (Demerol)	50-100 mg IV/subcutaneous q3-4h (Based on response)	25-100 mg IV/subcutaneous q6h (Based on response)	Avoid	3-7 hr	Prolonged and accumulation of active metabolite (normeperidine)

Data from Quan, D.J., & Aweeka, F.T. (2005). Dosing of drugs in renal failure. In M.A. Koda-Kimble, L.Y. Young, W.A. Kradjan, B.J. Guglielmo, B.K. Alldredge, & R.L. Corelli (Eds.), *Applied therapeutics: The clinical use of drugs* (8th ed.). Philadelphia: Lippincott, Williams & Wilkins; *USP DI: Drug information for the health care professional* (25th ed.). (2005). Greenwood Village, CO: MICROMEDEX Thomson Healthcare; *Mosby's GenRx* (2004). St. Louis: Mosby.

renal failure secondary to dehydration is a commonly observed complication of aggressive diuretic use in the older adult. More appropriate dosing and use of diuretics or antihypertensives could prevent such events. For some drugs that are known to be nephrotoxic, adequate hydration before administration can often prevent renal injury. Examples of drugs in which hydration before therapy reduces risk include the antifungal, amphotericin, and the cancer drug, cisplatin. Sometimes the osmotic diuretic mannitol is used in combination with hydration to help reduce toxic drug levels in the kidney and thereby prevent injury. For other drugs, (e.g., the aminoglycoside antibacterials, such as gentamicin), careful monitoring of dose, schedule, and levels can reduce risk for kidney damage. Use of less hyperosmotic contrast dyes (Aspelin et al., 2003), the use of acetylcysteine (Birck et al., 2003; Kay et al., 2003). or sodium bicarbonate (Merten et al., 2004) with contrast dyes can help prevent contrast dye-induced acute tubular necrosis

Chronic renal insufficiency is often secondary to other conditions like hypertension, diabetes mellitus. Use of antihypertensives (e.g., ACE inhibitors, ARBs) and controlling hyperglycemia with insulin or oral therapies for individuals with diabetes mellitus (DM) can all help reduce the risk or slow the development of chronic renal insufficiency for many individuals. See Chapters 27 and 49 for a further discussion.

✴ What are the nursing implications for pharmacologic therapies in renal insufficiency?

Assessment The initial assessment includes a history of recent weight changes, edema, malaise, decreased activity tolerance, pruritus, tremor, increasing irritability or mental changes, polyuria and nocturia (caused by reduced ability to concentrate urine), headache, dizziness, GI disturbances, and hypertension—all symptoms of uremia.

Because other body systems may be affected by renal dysfunction, conduct a thorough multisystem assessment. A baseline assessment of the client's laboratory values includes BUN, serum creatinine, serum electrolytes, CBC, and urinalysis. For clients receiving drugs that are highly bound to plasma proteins, assessment of serum albumin levels may also be helpful. Review the client's current drug regimen to determine the risk for drug toxicities related to drug accumulation. If the client is receiving medications with significant toxicities, the appropriate serum drug levels are carefully monitored to help prevent overdosing the client. Table 35-1 lists the medications most commonly associated with inducing renal dysfunction.

Nursing Diagnosis The client undergoing pharmacologic therapy for renal system dysfunction is at risk for the following selected nursing diagnoses/collaborative problems: excess fluid volume related to an inability to adequately excrete fluids and electrolytes and/or an excessive fluid intake during periods of decreased renal function; ineffective breathing pattern related to circulatory volume overload and/or metabolic acidosis leading to hyperventilation; imbalanced nutrition: less than body requirements related to anorexia, nausea, and vomiting; fatigue secondary to anemia and uremia; risk for infection related to a debilitated state and the use of indwelling catheters and other invasive procedures; and the potential complications of dysrhythmias related to renal failure, anemia related to bone marrow suppression and increased hemolysis and bleeding tendencies, and altered levels of consciousness related to electrolyte imbalances, the accumulation of waste products in the blood, and hypoxia.

Planning The client with renal insufficiency receiving pharmacologic therapy will:
- Maintain normal fluid volume and electrolyte levels.
- Participate in activities of daily living (ADLs) as tolerated.
- State rationale for treatment and adverse effects of various prescribed agents, including those to report to the physician.
- Effectively self-manage the therapeutic regimen as much as possible.
- Collaborate with health team for monitoring and evaluation of the therapeutic regimen.

Implementation

Monitoring Weigh the client at the same time each day, with the same amount of clothing, and with the same scale. The client at home may be better able to establish a routine by weighing first thing in the morning after the first voiding and before dressing or eating. The daily weight is evaluated in light of the 24-hour intake and output ratio for determining fluid volume excess or deficit.

Accurately record the fluid intake and output of the client on a 24-hour basis. Calculate the 24-hour balance by subtracting the output from the intake. In monitoring fluid balance, it is helpful to remember that 500 mL of fluid equates to about 1 pound of body weight. Monitor BUN and serum creatinine levels to ascertain the client's degree of ESRD and to anticipate the clinical signs and symptoms of physiologic injury that require nursing intervention and client education.

Serum potassium levels are monitored daily. Cardiovascular monitoring becomes more intense when the level exceeds 6 mEq/L. In addition to measuring blood pressure and apical heart rate, assessment by cardiac monitor is required. Serum levels of calcium and phosphate should be monitored every 3 to 4 days, and the client is clinically assessed for hypocalcemia and hyperphosphatemia as evidenced by irritability, muscular twitching, and tetany.

In acute circumstances, the client's arterial blood gases may also be monitored. Clinically, observe the client for increased respiratory rate and depth and changes in mental status that would indicate impending metabolic acidosis. CBCs are performed periodically; assess the client for signs and symptoms of anemia that might necessitate interventions such as iron supplements and anabolic steroids or, in the extreme, the transfusion of packed or frozen red blood cells (RBCs).

Intervention Fluid intake may be restricted. If so, plan fluid allotments with the client regarding the types of fluids and time of intake to enhance the client's acceptance of the regimen and to maintain the client's feeling of control. Dietary sodium is usually restricted, and dietary limitations are planned with the client based on the degree of restriction. Drug therapy is based on each client's particular form of dysfunction and its cause. Many body systems are affected by renal dysfunction, and therefore several medications may be used. The more common agents are diuretics to control fluid balance, edema, and hypertension and antibiotics to treat infection. In ESRD, treatments to control calcium/phosphate balance and to manage anemia are routinely used and are discussed later in this chapter. Because altered renal function also alters the pharmacokinetics of many drugs, dosages and dose intervals are adjusted based on the drug and degree of renal system dysfunction.

Education As with any condition, particularly those with multisystem consequences, deficient knowledge is likely. Instruct the client in the purpose of the medications, such as antihypertensives, diuretics, calcium supplements, vitamin D, and phosphate binders. Additionally, inform the client of the adverse effects, because with increasing renal insufficiency the margin of safety with any medication is diminished. Multiple drug therapy increases the chance of a drug interaction. The stressors placed on the client with increasing renal insufficiency are multiple. Changes in lifestyle and body image, and the impact of the disease on the client, require the nurse to exercise skill in supporting and educating the client and family to minimize the potential for ineffective coping.

Evaluation The expected outcome of pharmacologic therapy for renal system dysfunction is that the client will adhere to the prescribed fluid restrictions and will be normovolemic as evidenced by stable weight, normal breath sounds, an absence of edema, and a blood pressure and pulse within the client's normal range. Additionally, the client will verbalize orientation to person, place, and time; will experience a decrease in fatigue; and will increase participation in activities. The client will be free of infection, as evidenced by normothermia, a white blood cell count (WBC) within normal limits, clear urine, normal breath sounds, and an absence of drainage at catheter sites.

✱ **L.J. is a 63-year-old male with a 20-year history of poorly controlled DM. He is newly diagnosed with ESRD and presents to the nephrology clinic to begin hemodialysis three times per week. He complains of lethargy, nausea, and anorexia. His lab values are significant for elevated creatinine (7.8 mg/dL [normal range 0.5 to 1.4 mg/dL]), elevated phosphate levels (7.5 mg/dL [normal range 2.8 to 4.2 mg/dL]), normal**

calcium 9 mg/dL [normal range 8.6 to 10.3 mg/dL] and anemia (hematocrit 26% [normal range 41% to 50%]).

✱ **What are the special needs of clients with end stage renal failure?**
Clients with chronic renal insufficiency have a number of needs, including symptom management, control of diet and fluids, monitoring of electrolytes, and management of anemia. Many clients with ESRD have depression and anxiety as components of their disease.

Diets may be restricted in fluid intake, protein, phosphate, and sodium. In general, dietary protein is usually restricted to 0.5 to 1 g/kg of lean body weight daily. This limitation will reduce the incidence of azotemia, hyperkalemia, and acidosis. Fluid intake is based on daily losses and metabolic needs. Dietary sodium is restricted to approximately 2 g or 90 mEq daily. Potassium, magnesium, and phosphorus are also restricted. While fluid overload and hyperkalemia are commonly observed in these clients, diuretics do not improve outcomes for clients with ESRD (Cantarovich, Rangoonwala, Lorenz, Verho, & Esnault, 2004). The reduced excretion of phosphates, magnesium, and potassium from the kidneys in chronic renal insufficiency can lead to elevated serum levels or hypermagnesemia, hyperkalemia, and hyperphosphatemia, which in turn lead to hypocalcemia and osteodystrophy. Calcium supplements and vitamin D are often prescribed for these clients to reduce or prevent hyperparathyroidism and bone disease. Magnesium levels are kept somewhat in check if the client avoids magnesium-containing antacids and laxatives.

To control calcium and phosphate balance, most clients require active vitamin D replacement and usually require additional calcium supplementation. Since vitamin D is metabolized to its physiologically active form (1,25 dihydroxy-ergocalciferol) by the kidney, clients with renal insufficiency do not benefit from standard vitamin D, but must receive active vitamin D (1, 25 dihydroxy-ergocalciferol) either orally (calcitriol, dihydrotachysterol/DHT) or parenterally (calcitriol [Calcijex], paricalcitol [Zemplar]). See also Chapter 68.

Restriction of dietary phosphate is difficult and as such calcium salts (e.g., calcium acetate) are dosed *with meals* to help impair dietary phosphate absorption. Alternatives to calcium are considered when both calcium and phosphate levels are high. Under such circumstances, calcium supplementation may precipitate calcium phosphate crystals in tissues and alternative oral therapies dosed with meals to reduce phosphate absorption (e.g., sevelamer [Renagel]). Historically, aluminum salts were used as dietary phosphate binders, but the accumulation of aluminum in clients with renal insufficiency can lead to altered mental status. For a further discussion of calcium/phosphate balance, see Chapter 47.

✱ **Because reduction of serum phosphorus is difficult for L.J. to achieve with dietary restriction alone, a phosphorus-binding agent, calcium acetate (PhosLo)**

667 mg, 2 tablets three times daily with meals is included in his drug regimen.

calcium acetate [**kal** see um **ass** e tate]
(PhosLo)
Calcium acetate binds to dietary phosphate in the gut to form calcium phosphate, which is not absorbed and instead is eliminated in the stool.

Indications
Calcium acetate is indicated for the control of hyperphosphatemia in ESRD. It should be avoided, however, if very high phosphate levels are observed as this may result in calcium phosphate deposits in tissue.

Pharmacokinetics/Dosing
Unlike other forms of calcium (e.g., carbonate, citrate), the acetate form of calcium is not well absorbed, even in the presence of vitamin D. It is available as a 667 mg tablet (providing 169 mg of elemental calcium) and is typically dosed at two to four tablets with each meal. Dosing with meals is important to bind adequate phosphate in the gut.

Adverse Effects
The most common adverse effect of calcium acetate is constipation. Severe hypercalcemia (levels greater than 12 mg/dL) can manifest with mental status changes and coma.

Drug Interactions
Excessive calcium intake with thiazide diuretics could result in hypercalcemia. Calcium may decrease the absorption of orally administered tetracyclines, fluoroquinolone antimicrobials (e.g., ciprofloxacin) or alendronate (Fosamax) if dosed together. Calcium salts may increase the potential for digoxin toxicity, and reduce the efficacy of calcium channel blockers.

✴ **What are the nursing issues for L.J. with calcium acetate?**
In addition to the nursing care described above for clients with renal insufficiency, nursing management of calcium acetate therapy for L.J. includes the following.

Assessment Hypercalcemia is a contraindication for calcium supplements in renal insufficiency, however, L.J.'s serum calcium is 9.4 mg/dL, within the normal range of 8.6 to 10.3 mg/dL. Assess L.J.'s concurrent drug regimen for other calcium-containing preparations, including dietary supplement and antacids.

Nursing Diagnosis With the administration of calcium acetate L.J. is at risk for nursing diagnoses related to the potential complication of hypercalcemia: altered comfort (nausea, vomiting, pruritus); constipation; and sensory-perceptual alteration evidenced by confusion.

Planning The goal is to maintain L.J.'s serum phosphate concentrations below 6 mg/dL without precipitating severe hypercalcemia. Additionally, see nursing care described previously for clients with renal insufficiency.

Implementation
Monitoring Review results of serum calcium and serum phosphate concentrations drawn twice a week. Serum cal-

cium levels greater than 10.5 mg/dL are considered mild hypercalcemia and greater than 12 mg/dL indicate severe hypercalcemia and the dosage of calcium acetate is reduced or discontinued depending on the severity.

Intervention As an antihyperphosphatemic, calcium acetate is administered three times a day with meals. The dosage is increased gradually to keep serum phosphate levels below 6 mg/dL.

Education Inform L.J. about avoiding other calcium-containing preparations, such as dietary supplements and antacids. It may be necessary to estimate daily dietary calcium intake and modify if needed. L.J. should report constipation, anorexia, nausea, or vomiting to the prescriber, as these are early symptoms of hypercalcemia. The importance of follow up for blood tests is stressed.

Evaluation L.J. will maintain serum calcium concentrations within 8.6 to 10.3 mg/dL and a serum phosphorus level less than 6 mg/dL without experiencing adverse effects of calcium acetate. He will state symptoms reportable to the prescriber and maintain follow up visits with his provider. L.J. will remain compliant with his medication and increase his participation in ADLs as much as possible.

✴ **L.J. develops severe hypercalcemia over a period of time, 11 mg/dL with elevated phosphate levels (8 mg/dL [normal range 2.8 to 4.2 mg/dL]). He is switched to a noncalcium-based phosphate binder, sevelamer (Renagel) 1600 mg three times daily with meals.**

sevelamer [se **vel** a mer]
(Renagel)
Sevelamer is a polymer that binds phosphate in the GI tract. It results in decreased absorption of dietary phosphate. Sevelamer is recommended for clients with elevated calcium and phosphate levels. In such circumstances, its use avoids hypercalcemia associated with calcium salts and reduces the potential for calcium phosphate deposits in tissue, which can be seen if the calcium phosphate product (calcium level × phosphate level) exceeds 70.

Indications
Sevelamer is indicated for managing hyperphosphatemia in clients with ESRD

Pharmacokinetics/Dosing
Sevelamer is not absorbed orally, but instead binds phosphate in the GI lumen. It is typically dosed based on phosphate levels. For phosphate levels between 6 and 7.5 mg/dL, the usual adult dose is 800 mg three times daily. For phosphate levels between 7.5 and 9 mg/dL, 1200 to 1600 mg is given three times daily. For phosphate levels above 9 mg/dL, 1600 mg is given three times daily.

Adverse Effects
Sevelamer is generally well tolerated, but may be associated with diarrhea or other GI complaints.

Drug Interactions
Sevelamer may bind to other orally administered drugs in the gut and reduce their absorption, but the significance of this potential interaction is not clear.

What are the nursing management issues associated with the administration of sevelamer to L.J.?

In addition to the general nursing management related to pharmacologic therapy in the client with renal insufficiency, L.J.'s sevelamer therapy also includes the following.

Assessment Sevelamer is contraindicated in clients with hypophosphatemia, bowel obstruction, or hypersensitivity to sevelamer. As L.J. has hyperphosphatemia (8 mg/dL [normal range 2.8 to 4.2 mg/dL]), an absence of GI symptoms, and no history of hypersensitivity to the drug, sevelamer therapy is initiated. Assess his concurrent drug therapy because as a binding drug, sevelamer may have effect on other drugs. If this interaction is clinically significant, administer the drug 1 hour before or 3 hours after sevelamer and the prescriber should consider monitoring blood levels of the affected drug.

Nursing Diagnosis See general discussion for client with renal insufficiency.

Planning In addition to general goals for nursing management discussed above, the goal is to maintain serum phosphate concentrations below 6 mg/dL without precipitating diarrhea or other GI complaints.

Implementation
Monitoring The dosage of sevelamer is titrated on the basis of serum phosphorus levels. See dosing schedule above.

Intervention Sevelamer is always administered with meals.

Education Reinforce the importance of monitoring serum levels and the maintenance of regular follow-up visits to the prescriber.

Evaluation L.J. will maintain a serum phosphorus level less than 6 mg/dL without experiencing adverse effects of sevelamer. He will state that he report any GI symptoms to the prescriber and maintain follow-up visits with his provider. L.J. will remain compliant with his medication and increase his participation in ADLs as much as possible.

How does chronic renal insufficiency lead to anemia and how is this managed?

Decreased production of RBCs (erythropoiesis) in chronic renal insufficiency leads to anemia, weakness, and fatigue. Iron therapy may be prescribed for clients with iron-deficiency anemia resulting from chronic blood loss; folic acid, vitamin C, and soluble B-complex vitamins are often given to replace the substances usually lost during dialysis. Epoetin is used specifically to stimulate erythropoiesis in chronic renal insufficiency. It is also used with other anemias associated with a deficiency of erythropoietin, including that observed postcancer chemotherapy with other drugs known to induce anemia responsive to epoetin (e.g.,

zidovudine in the treatment of advanced human immunodeficiency virus (HIV) disease).

Epoetin is a glycoprotein chemically identical to human erythropoietin. It is produced by recombinant DNA technology that contains the same 165 amino acids in the same sequence as human erythropoietin. Epoetin stimulates bone marrow erythropoiesis and also induces the release of reticulocytes from the marrow so they can mature into erythrocytes. Human erythropoietin is produced mainly in the kidneys.

Because endogenous erythropoietin is manufactured mainly in the kidneys, the anemia resulting from chronic renal insufficiency is caused by an inadequate production of the hormone. With the use of epoetin, an initial increase in reticulocytes is seen within 7 to 10 days; an increase in red cell count, hematocrit, and hemoglobin occurs within 2 to 6 weeks. Clients on epoetin typically require aggressive iron supplementation and close monitoring of iron stores (e.g., ferritin levels).

epoetin [eh **poe** e tin]
(Epogen, Procrit, Eprex ✹)
Indications
Epoetin is indicated for anemia of chronic renal insufficiency, anemias related to cancer chemotherapy for nonmyeloid malignancies, and anemia related to zidovudine therapy. It is also used prior to surgery for clients undergoing certain elective procedures.
Pharmacokinetics/Dosing
Epoetin reaches a peak serum level within 15 minutes of IV administration and within 5 to 24 hours of an subcutaneous dose. The half-life is between 4 and 13 hours after IV or subcutaneous administration. When therapy is discontinued, the hematocrit decreases over approximately 2 weeks (duration of action). The initial adult dosage is 50 to 100 units/kg IV or subcutaneously three times weekly. Dosage increments of 25 units/kg may be instituted if the hematocrit has not increased after 2 months of therapy by at least 5 to 6 points and the client is still below the desired range of 30% to 33%. For maintenance, decrease the dosage gradually 25 units/kg monthly until the lowest dosage that maintains the hematocrit at the desired level is reached. The dosage has not been determined for children below 12 years of age. Pregnancy safety has been established by the Food and Drug Administration (FDA) as Category C.
Adverse Effects
Hypertension is one of the most common adverse effects of epoetin. Other adverse effects of epoetin include arthralgias or bone pain, asthenia (severe muscle weakness), nausea and vomiting, weakness, diarrhea, chest pain, edema of the extremities or face, weight gain, tachycardia, headache, clotting of the arteriovenous (AV) shunt and/or dialyzer, polycythemia, and seizures. Reports of thromboembolic events and increased mortality prompted the manufacturer to revise labeling to avoid use of erythropoietin when hemoglobin levels rise above 12 g/dL in clients treated for anemias secondary to cancer (Ortho Biotech, August 13, 2004). No significant drug interactions have been reported.

L.J. is slated to begin hemodialysis three times per week and will receive injectable calcitriol and epoetin with each dialysis treatment. L.J. is initiating a dose of sevelamer 1200 mg with each meal and will be followed up in one week to determine if ongoing sevelamer is indicated. Once phosphate levels are below

6 mg/dL, sevelamer will be discontinued, and he will start of calcium acetate (PhosLo) 667 mg, two tablets with each meal. L.J. will also start iron supplementation with epoetin.

✳ **What are the key nursing management issues of epoetin therapy for L.J.?**

Assessment Monitor L.J.'s blood pressure (BP) for hypertension because the resultant increase in hematocrit from epoetin increases blood viscosity and peripheral vascular resistance, leading to a rise in blood pressure.

Clients with poorly controlled hypertension should delay undergoing epoetin therapy until the hypertension is controlled. Even then, the BP of the hypertensive client (and the previously normotensive client) should be monitored closely because of the increased risk of hypertension, which may lead to hypertensive encephalopathy. Antihypertensive drugs may be required or the dosages of a current regimen may need to be increased. The drug should not be used if L.J. is hypersensitive to human albumin or to products derived from mammalian cells, such as beef and pork insulin.

Nursing Diagnosis With the administration of epoetin, L.J. may be at risk for the following selected nursing diagnoses/collaborative problems: impaired comfort related to arthralgias, headache, dizziness, chest pain, nausea, vomiting, and flu-like syndrome for 1 to 12 hours after IV administration; fatigue; excess fluid volume (weight gain, swelling of the face, fingers, feet, and ankles); hyperthermia; impaired skin integrity (skin reaction at administration site; diarrhea; and the potential complications of polycythemia (increased clotting tendency), severe muscle weakness, seizures, and increased BP.

Planning In addition to general goals for the client with renal insufficiency, the hematocrit should stabilize in the 30% to 36% range.

Implementation

Monitoring As mentioned, monitor L.J.'s blood pressure. Assess the results of complete blood counts (CBC), as ordered by the prescriber, for change. Hematocrit values are particularly important, with baseline and twice-weekly frequencies recommended as a guide for dosage and efficacy. However, at least 4 weeks' time should elapse between dosage adjustments because the response to a change in dosage may require 2 to 6 weeks. A rise in the hematocrit of more than 4 points in a 2-week period or a value over 36%, which is considered the safety limit for the prevention of adverse reactions, should be brought to the prescriber's attention. An increase in L.J.'s heparin dosage may be required; because increases in RBC volume as a result of epoetin may lead to increased blood clotting in the dialyzer or arteriovenous shunt for vascular access

It is recommended that the status of L.J.'s iron stores be monitored to determine the need and the amount of iron supplementation for the client. Because iron is incorporated into hemoglobin as a result of the effectiveness of the drug, his iron stores may be depleted, causing a decrease in the efficacy of epoetin.

Perform neurologic assessments periodically for premonitory signs of the risk of seizures, particularly during the first 90 days of therapy and at times when the hematocrit rises rapidly. Monitor also the results of renal function studies (BUN, serum creatinine, serum phosphorus, serum potassium, serum sodium, and serum uric acid), because the need to increase dialysis may occur with the administration of epoetin. Weight L.J. daily, and monitor the fluid balance ratio.

Intervention Epoetin is administered IV or subcutaneously. With L.J. it will be given IV because there is IV access with his hemodialysis. Each single-dose vial of epoetin should be used to administer one dose only because the injection contains no preservative. Discard any unused portion of the drug. Do not shake the vial; shaking may denature the substance and render it biologically inactive. Do not mix epoetin with other medications. The multidose vial contains benzyl alcohol, which is not recommended for neonates.

Education Alert L.J. to avoid activities that may be hazardous if seizures would occur, especially during the first 90 days of therapy. Instruct him about dietary sources of iron, folic acid, and B_{12} as adjuncts to iron and other vitamin supplementation. Review with L.J. dietary restrictions associated with the antihypertensive regimen and restrictions pertinent to clients with chronic renal insufficiency. The correction of anemia may result in an increased appetite, making it more difficult for him to maintain compliance with the required dietary restrictions. Encourage him to keep prescriber and dialysis appointments.

If epoetin is prescribed for L.J. to self-administer, ensure that he knows the proper injection technique.

Evaluation In addition to the general outcomes for clients with renal insufficiency, the expected outcome of epoetin therapy is that a clinically significant increase in the red cell count, hematocrit, and hemoglobin should be seen in 2 to 6 weeks of the initiation of therapy. The hematocrit should stabilize in the 30% to 36% range. With correction of L.J.'s anemia, he will demonstrate an improved activity tolerance, decreased fatigue, and an improved appetite, sleep pattern, cognitive function, and sense of well-being without adverse effects of epoetin.

Summary

Renal system dysfunction may be a source of tremendous stress for the client and family, and it also presents a challenge for the nurse. Therapy is complicated by the need to use multiple drugs and the need to be aware of altered pharmacokinetics. Drug interactions or adverse effects may appear at any time, and therefore it is essential that the nurse monitor closely the client's renal function and the effects of the drug. Additional areas for nursing intervention include nondrug therapy (e.g., diet modification and fluid restriction, psychosocial support) and the involvement of other body systems.

Bibliography

Anderson, D.M., Keith, J., & Novak, P.D. (Eds.) (2002). *Mosby's medical, nursing, and allied health dictionary* (6th ed.). St. Louis: Mosby.

Aspelin, P., Aubry, P., Fransson, S.G., Strasser, R., Willenbrock, R., Berg, K.J. and the Nephrotoxicity In High-risk patients study of iso-osmolar and low-osmolar non-ionic contrast media study investigators. (2003). Nephrotoxic effects in high-risk patients undergoing angiography. *New England Journal of Medicine, 348*, 491-499.

Birck, R., Krzossok, S., Markowetz, F., Schnulle, P., van der Woude, F.J., & Braun, C. (2003). Acetylcysteine for prevention of contrast nephropathy: Meta-analysis. *Lancet, 362*, 598-603.

Bosker, G. (Ed.). (2004). *Primary and acute care medicine: Practice, protocols, pathways*, (2nd ed.). Atlanta: Thomson American Health Consultants.

Brophy, D.F. (2005). Acute renal failure. In M.A. Koda-Kimble, L.Y. Young, W.A. Kradjan, B.J. Guglielmo, B.K. Alldredge, & R.L. Corelli (Eds.), *Applied therapeutics: The clinical use of drugs* (8th ed.). Philadelphia: Lippincott, Williams & Wilkins.

Cantarovich, F., Rangoonwala, B., Lorenz, H., Verho, M., Esnault, V.L. (2004). High-dose furosemide for established ARF: A prospective, randomized, double-blind, placebo-controlled, multicenter trial. *American Journal of Kidney Disease, 44*, 402-409.

Cockroft, D.W., & Gault, M.H. (1976). Prediction of creatinine clearance from serum creatinine. *Nephron, 16*, 31-41.

Curhan, G.C., Knight, E.L., Rosner, B., Hankinson, S.E., & Stampfer, M.J. (2004). Lifetime nonnarcotic analgesic use and decline in renal function in women. *Arch Intern Med, 164*, 1519-1524.

Drug facts and comparisons. (58th ed.). (2005). St. Louis: Facts and Comparisons.

Hudson, J.Q., & Johnson, C.A. (2005). Chronic renal failure. In M.A. Koda-Kimble, L.Y. Young, W.A. Kradjan, B.J. Guglielmo, B.K. Alldredge, & R.L. Corelli (Eds.), *Applied therapeutics: The clinical use of drugs* (8th ed.). Philadelphia: Lippincott Williams & Wilkins.

Kay, J., et al. (2003). Acetylcysteine for prevention of acute deterioration of renal function following elective coronary angiography and intervention: A randomized controlled trial. *Journal of the American Medical Association, 289*, 553-558.

Lacy, C.F., Armstrong, L.L., Goldman, M.P., & Lance, L.L. (2004). *Lexi-Comp's Drug Information Handbook* (12th ed.). Hudson, Ohio: Lexi-Comp.

Lepkifker, E., Sverdlik, A., Iancu, I., Ziv, R., Segev, S., & Kotler, M. (2004). Renal insufficiency in long-term lithium treatment. *Journal of Clinical Psychiatry, 65*(6), 850-856.

Massie, B.M., & Amidon, T.M. (2003). Heart. In L.M. Tierney, Jr., S.J. McPhee, & Papadakis, M.A. (Eds.), *Current Medical Diagnosis & Treatment.* New York: Lange Medical Books/McGraw-Hill.

Merten, G.J., et al. (2004). Prevention of contrast-induced nephropathy with sodium bicarbonate: A randomized controlled trial. *Journal of the American Medical Association, 291*, 2328-2334.

Mosby's drug consult. (15th ed.). (2005). St. Louis: Mosby.

Mueller, B.A. (2002). Acute renal failure. In J.T. DiPiro, R.L. Talbert, G.C. Yee, G.R. Matzke, B.G. Wells, & L.M. Posey (Eds.), *Pharmacotherapy: A pathophysiological* approach (3rd ed.). Norwalk, CT: Appleton & Lange.

Ortho Biotech Correspondence: "Dear Health Care Professional," August 13, 2004. Retrieved January 2, 2005, from http://www.fda.gov/medwatch/SAFETY/2004/Procrit_dearhcp.pdf

Quan, D.J., & Aweeka, F.T. (2005). Dosing of drugs in renal failure. In M.A. Koda-Kimble, L.Y. Young, W.A. Kradjan, B.J. Guglielmo, B.K. Alldredge, & R.L. Corelli (Eds.), *Applied thera-*

✴ Critical Thinking Questions

- Mrs. Defrees, a 54-year-old female client, has been admitted to your unit for HF. She is 5 feet, 3 inches tall, and she weighs 175 pounds. She has been prescribed digoxin, 0.25 mg daily for her condition. She indicates a history of renal failure, and you are concerned about the level of her renal function with the administration of digoxin. You are aware that a creatinine clearance is the best indicator of renal function, but it is a 24-hour test. The laboratory has just called to the unit with her serum creatinine value of 3.2 mg/dL. Estimate her creatinine clearance to determine the severity of her renal impairment. What action would you take on the basis of your findings?

- Two commonly used tests of renal impairment determination are the BUN and the serum creatinine. Which test is considered to be the most sensitive of renal function and why?

---

e-LEARNING SUPPLEMENTS

Student CD-ROM
- Final exam questions
- NCLEX® Examination review questions
- Pharmacology animations
- Printable chapter summary

Evolve Website (http://evolve.elsevier.com/mckenry)
- Case study on drug therapy for renal system dysfunction

- Content updates, including information on new drugs
- WebLinks corresponding to this chapter
- Answers to the critical thinking questions in this chapter
- *Elsevier ePharmacology Update* newsletter
- *Mosby's Drug Consult* Internet Edition
- Supplemental and reference information

peutics: The clinical use of drugs (8th ed.). Philadelphia: Lippincott Williams & Wilkins.

Reikes, S.T. (2000). Trends in end-stage renal disease: Epidemiology, morbidity, and mortality, *Postgraduate Medicine, 108*(1), 124-142.

St. Peter, W.L., Lewis, M.J., & Collins, A. (2002). End-stage renal disease. In J.T. DiPiro, R.L. Talbert, G.C. Yee, G.R. Matzke, B.G. Wells, & L.M. Posey (Eds.), *Pharmacotherapy: A pathophysiological* approach (3rd ed.). Norwalk, CT: Appleton & Lange.

Schaubel, D.E., Morrison, H.I., Desmeules, M., Parsons, D.A. & Fenton, S. (1999). End-stage renal disease in Canada: prevalence projections to 2005. *Canadian Medical Association Journal, 160*, 1557-1563.

Schnell, Z.B., Van Leeuwen, A.M., & Kranpitz, T.R. (2003). *Davis's comprehensive laboratory and diagnostic test handbook—with nursing implications.* Philadelphia: F.A. Davis.

USP DI: Drug information for the health care professional (25th ed.). (2005). Greenwood Village, CO: MICROMEDEX Thomson Healthcare.

United States Renal Data System. (2004). Retrieved July 3, 2005, from http:www.usrds.org/adr.htm

36

OVERVIEW OF THE RESPIRATORY SYSTEM

CHAPTER FOCUS

The respiratory system functions to maintain the exchange of oxygen and carbon dioxide in the lungs and cells and to regulate the pH of body fluids; therefore a change within this system affects other body systems. The reverse is also true—disorders of other body systems may increase the body's need for oxygen, such as with fever, and therefore increase the work of respiration. Many respiratory problems require direct nursing care and education of the client and caregivers for effective management of the therapeutic regimen at home. This chapter provides a review of anatomy and physiology as a background for understanding the drugs affecting the respiratory system.

LEARNING OBJECTIVES

- Explain the three interrelated processes of respiration.
- Identify the two sources of respiratory secretions.
- Describe the β_2 receptor theory of bronchodilation.
- Describe the effect of the parasympathetic nervous system on the respiratory system.
- Describe the central and peripheral control of respiration.

▲ KEY TERMS

bronchial glands, p. 692
bronchoconstriction, p. 693
bronchodilation, p. 693

cellular respiration, p. 691
gas transport, p. 691
goblet cells, p. 692
mucokinesis, p. 692
pulmonary ventilation, p. 691

✳ **What are the key features of the respiratory system?**
The respiratory system includes all structures involved in the exchange of oxygen and carbon dioxide, such as the airway passages, lungs, nasal cavities, pharynx, larynx, trachea, bronchi, bronchioles, pulmonary lobules with their alveoli, the diaphragm, and all muscles concerned with respiration itself.

The most urgent and critical need for maintaining life is a continued, uninterrupted supply of oxygen. Oxygen is supplied to the body through the process of respiration. The term *respiration* is loosely used to describe three distinct but interrelated processes:

- **Pulmonary ventilation,** which involves the movement of air into and out of the lungs
- **Gas transport,** which involves the exchange of gases between the air in the lungs, the blood, and the cell
- **Cellular respiration,** which involves the use of oxygen in the catabolism of energy-yielding substances for the production of energy

Respiration, one of the body's regulating systems, helps to maintain physiologic dynamic equilibrium. It also compensates for rapid adjustment to changes in metabolic states.

The air passages permit air to flow from the external environment to pulmonary blood, and they modify the air taken in by warming it, moistening it, and removing noxious substances. Airway efficiency is determined by the following factors:

- Shape and size of each portion of the respiratory tract (nasal cavity, pharynx, larynx, trachea, bronchi, bronchioles, alveolar sacs)
- Presence of a ciliated, mucus-secreting, epithelial lining throughout most of the respiratory tract
- Character and thickness of respiratory tract secretions
- Compliance of the cartilaginous and bony supports
- Pressure gradients
- Traction on airway walls
- Absence of foreign substances in the lumen of the respiratory tract

An alteration of any of these factors will affect the ease with which air flows through the air passages, or effective airway clearance. Congenital anomalies, injuries, allergies, or disease will cause airflow resistance if these factors are abnormally affected. For example, resistance occurs if there is stenosis or narrowing of any portion of the respiratory tract, a loss of the cilia that ordinarily sweep out foreign substances, any thick or tenacious secretions, a loss of elasticity, or the presence of foreign objects.

✹ How do respiratory secretions interplay with normal physiology and pathologic states?

The tracheobronchial tree is made up of repeated branching tubes. It is a tubular airway that serves as a conduit for the passage of air from the external environment to the alveolar-capillary exchange unit (Figure 36-1, *A*). The inner surface of the tracheobronchial tree is lined with ciliated columnar epithelium interspersed with goblet cells (see Figure 36-1, *B*). The gelatinous mucus (gel layer) produced by **goblet cells** is normally discharged into the tubular lumen. In some obstructive pulmonary diseases, mucus secretion is greatly increased, making it difficult for the cilia to transport secretions along the airway.

The **bronchial glands,** which are located in the submucosa of the tracheobronchial tree, secrete a relatively watery fluid (sol layer) through ducts leading to the surface of the

ciliated epithelium (see Figure 36-1, *B*). Under vagal (parasympathetic) control, the bronchial glands can be stimulated by irritant agents or aerosol drugs to release their contents into the lumen of the airway.

The products of the goblet cells and bronchial glands form the sol-gel film that makes up the mucociliary blanket. This protective blanket of fluid bathes the ciliated epithelium of the tracheobronchial tree. Additionally, the cilia continuously propel the sol-gel film up toward the larynx along the respiratory tree. The normal adult produces approximately 100 mL of respiratory secretions per day and swallows this material without being aware of it. The process of moving mucus along the tracheobronchial tree is called **mucokinesis.** The mucociliary blanket is a basic concern in most chronic obstructive pulmonary disease (COPD). The cilia must sustain appropriate function; a dry atmosphere causes the respiratory secretions to become thick and tenacious, which tends to interfere with ciliary movements. Thus adequate humidity should be maintained to prevent a change in the normal consistency of the respiratory secretions.

✹ What are the key features of bronchial smooth muscle?

Smooth Muscle Arrangement An important structure of the tracheobronchial tree is the smooth muscle. The mass of muscle fibers along the bronchi progressively increases as it extends down toward the distal bronchioles. Isolated muscle fibers may be found as far down as the alveolar ducts. The smooth muscle fibers are arranged along the length of the tubular tree in a double helical or spiral pattern, and this formation profoundly influences the diameter or the lumen of the airways. Because of this structural feature, the effect of muscle contraction reduces both the diameter and the length of the bronchus (see Figure 37-1, *B*).

Nerve Supply The airway or tracheobronchial tree is innervated by the autonomic nervous system. The balance

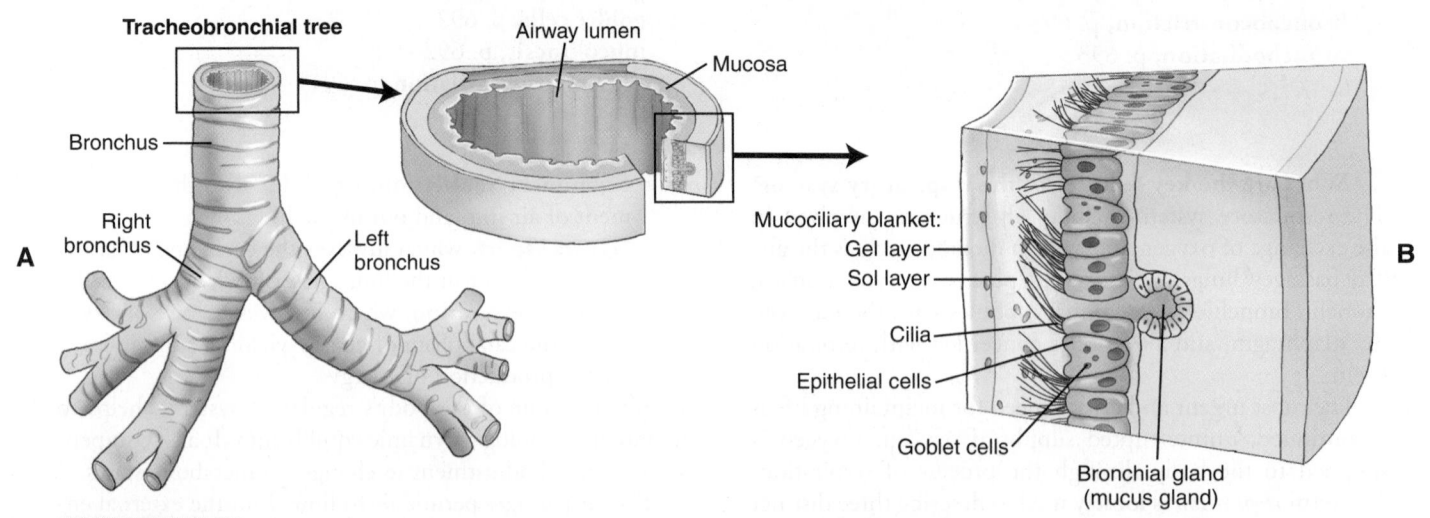

FIGURE 36-1 Tracheobronchial tree **(A)** and cross-section of tracheobronchial tissue **(B)**.

maintained between parasympathetic and sympathetic stimuli during rest influences the tone of the bronchial smooth muscle. Activation of the parasympathetic fiber (vagus nerve) releases acetylcholine, which results in **bronchoconstriction,** a narrowing of the lumen of the bronchial airway. By contrast, stimulation of the sympathetic fiber and the sympathoadrenal system releases epinephrine and norepinephrine from the adrenal medulla into the circulation. Their action on the β_2 receptor sites in the bronchial smooth muscle produces **bronchodilation** by means of smooth muscle relaxation, which improves ventilation to the lungs.

Receptors Several types of receptors are found along the bronchial airway. The release of acetylcholine activates muscarinic receptors during stimulation of the parasympathetic system, whereas the sympathetic system affects adrenergic receptors. Most of the adrenergic receptors present in the bronchial smooth muscle are β_2 receptors that are stimulated mainly by epinephrine released from the adrenal medulla. β_1 receptors are also found, although the ratio of β_2 to β_1 receptors is approximately 3:1. Thus bronchial smooth muscle is supplied primarily by β_2 receptors. The sympathomimetic drugs used principally as bronchodilators stimulate the β_2 receptors. Because many of these agents are not purely selective in their pharmacologic effect, they also stimulate the β_1 receptors in the heart, and α receptors in the lungs and peripheral arterioles. The adverse effects on the heart are increased cardiac output, tachycardia, and dysrhythmia. The presence of α receptors on the bronchial smooth muscle is relatively scarce, and their stimulation results in only mild bronchoconstriction.

Bronchodilation The β_2-adrenergic receptors mediate bronchodilation. Presumably this mechanism is initiated by epinephrine released from the adrenal medulla and norepinephrine released from the peripheral sympathetic nerves. Also located in the cell membrane is an enzyme system known as adenyl cyclase. In the presence of magnesium ions, adenyl cyclase catalyzes the action of adenosine triphosphate (ATP) in the cytoplasm of the cell to produce cyclic 3'5' adenosine monophosphate (cyclic 3'5' AMP). Cyclic 3'5' AMP then performs its important function—inducing the relaxation of bronchial smooth muscle, or bronchodilation. The hormone epinephrine is designated as the "first messenger"; cyclic 3'5' AMP is designated as the "second messenger." As a final action, cyclic 3'5' AMP is inactivated by an enzyme, phosphodiesterase, which catalyzes it to the inactive 5' AMP. This results in a fall in the cyclic 3'5' AMP level. A xanthine drug such as theophylline may inhibit the action of phosphodiesterase (Undem & Lichtenstein, 2001). As a consequence, the cyclic 3'5' AMP level remains elevated, thereby affecting smooth muscle dilation (see Figure 37-3).

Circulating catecholamines can exert their effects on β_1, β_2, and α receptors. Clients with asthma may have a normal reaction to both α and β stimulation through a reduced cyclic AMP response, by an abnormally sensitive response to α stimulation, and by an exaggerated response to the muscarinic agonists via the vagal pathways. This exaggerated bronchoconstrictive airway response may result from the effects of a decrease in cyclic AMP, histamine effects on smooth muscle, the vagal reflex pathway, an increase in cyclic guanylic acid secondary to calcium influx, and/or a histamine-induced release of the contents of mast cells. Bronchodilation is induced by circulating catecholamines or the administration of a sympathomimetic agent.

Circulating catecholamines reach the lung via the circulation and interact with the β_2-adrenergic receptors in the cell membrane of the bronchial smooth muscle cell.

Bronchoconstriction The bronchial smooth muscle is innervated by the parasympathetic fibers from the vagus nerve. Acetylcholine released from the terminal interacts with the muscarinic receptors on the membrane of the cell. Stimulation of the muscarinic receptor increases the activity of the enzyme guanylate cyclase in the membrane, thereby promoting the rate of formation of cyclic 3'5' guanosine monophosphate (cyclic 3'5' GMP) from guanosine triphosphate (GTP) (see Figure 37-3). The cyclic 3'5' GMP level affects the bronchial muscle by producing bronchoconstriction. α receptors found on the bronchial smooth muscle have a similar involvement with this mechanism. On activation, the α receptors also increase the level of cyclic GMP. Furthermore, cyclic 3'5' GMP stimulates the release of chemical mediators from the mast cell during an asthmatic attack, and these mediators are responsible for causing bronchoconstriction.

✷ How is respiration controlled?

Central Control The basic rhythm for respiration is initiated and maintained in the medullary rhythmicity area, which is located beneath the lower part of the floor of the fourth ventricle in the medial half of the medulla. Neurons that control inspiration and expiration intermingle and discharge or fire impulses alternately. Signals from the spinal cord, the cerebral cortex and midbrain, the apneustic area of the pons, and the pneumotaxic area of the upper pons can enter the medullary rhythmicity area, modify the rhythm of respiration, and contribute to the normal pattern of respiration.

Normally, the human organism is unaware of the respiratory process. However, voluntary influence and control of breathing are possible. This is important when a client must learn to voluntarily control breathing patterns.

Peripheral Control The medullary rhythmicity area is also influenced by various sensory and peripheral stimuli, the vasomotor center, reflex mechanisms (e.g., the Hering-Breuer reflex), the chemoreceptors in the carotid and aortic bodies, and the baroreceptors in the carotid sinus and aortic arch. Fear, pain, stress, blood pressure, body temperature, and blood levels of oxygen and carbon dioxide can all modify the activity of the respiratory centers.

The humoral regulation of respiration is achieved primarily through changes in the concentrations of oxygen, carbon dioxide, or hydrogen ions in body fluids. In a healthy individual, carbon dioxide is the chief respiratory stimulant. An increase in the carbon dioxide tension of the blood directly stimulates the inspiratory and expiratory centers, which increases both the rate and the depth of breathing. This results in a blowing off of carbon dioxide to keep the carbon dioxide tension of the blood constant. The pH of the blood is determined by the ratio of bicarbonate ion (HCO_3) to carbon dioxide. When the carbon dioxide content of the blood is increased, there is a subsequent increase in the formation of carbonic acid in the blood. This alters the bicarbonate/carbonic acid ratio from the normal value of 20:1 and results in acidosis. Conversely, a decrease in the carbon dioxide content of the blood results in alkalosis. Therefore respiration is important for regulating the pH of the blood by controlling the carbon dioxide tension of the blood.

Changes in arterial oxygen concentration have little, if any, direct effect on the respiratory center. However, if the arterial oxygen concentration falls below normal, the chemoreceptors in the carotid and aortic bodies are stimulated and in turn stimulate the respiratory center to increase alveolar ventilation. This mechanism operates primarily under abnormal conditions such as COPD.

Summary

The highest priority for the survival of the human organism is an adequate, uninterrupted supply of oxygen. Oxygen is supplied to the various body tissues by the processes of pulmonary ventilation, gas transport, and cellular respiration. Although it is possible to influence and control the respiratory pattern voluntarily, the rhythm and depth of pulmonary ventilation are generally initiated and maintained centrally in the medulla and influenced peripherally by reflex mechanisms, chemoreceptors, and baroreceptors.

✴ Critical Thinking Questions

- You are caring for Tommy, a 3-year-old, who threatens to hold his breath. What effect will holding his breath have on his blood pH? What would happen to his blood pH if he hyperventilated?

- It is known that smoking decreases the number of cilia in the respiratory airway. What is likely to occur as the result of this change?

Bibliography

Anderson, D.M., Keith, J., & Novak, P.D. (Eds.). (2002). *Mosby's medical, nursing, and allied health dictionary* (6th ed.). St. Louis: Mosby.

Guyton, A.C., & Hall, J.E. (2000). *Textbook of medical physiology* (10th ed.). Philadelphia: W.B. Saunders.

Herlihy, B., & Maebius, N.K. (2003). *The human body in health and illness* (2nd ed.). Philadelphia: W.B. Saunders.

McCance, K.L., & Huether, S.E. (2002). *Pathophysiology: The biological basis for disease in adults and children* (4th ed.). St. Louis: Mosby.

Thibodeau, G.A., & Patton, K.T. (2003). *Anatomy and physiology* (5th ed.). St. Louis: Mosby.

Undem, B.J., & Lichtenstein, L.M. (2001). Drugs used in the treatment of asthma. In J.G. Hardman & L.E. Limbird (Eds.), *Goodman and Gilman's The pharmacological basis of therapeutics* (10th ed.). New York: McGraw-Hill.

e-LEARNING SUPPLEMENTS

Student CD-ROM
- Final Exam questions
- NCLEX® Examination review questions
- Pharmacology animations
- Printable chapter summary

Evolve Website (http://evolve.elsevier.com/mckenry)
- Content updates, including information on new drugs

- WebLinks corresponding to this chapter
- Answers to the critical thinking questions in this chapter
- *Elsevier ePharmacology Update* newsletter
- Mosby's Drug Consult Internet Edition
- Supplemental and reference information and reference information

37

BRONCHODILATOR, ANTIASTHMATIC, AND MUCOLYTIC DRUGS

CHAPTER FOCUS

Clients using bronchodilator, respiratory antiinflammatory and mucokinetic drugs may have ineffective breathing patterns, ineffective airway clearance, or impaired gas exchange. Nurses involved in caring for clients with these nursing diagnoses use a variety of technologies with which they must be knowledgeable. These agents are used with clients who have respiratory disorders and with clients who have respiratory problems caused by nonrespiratory disorder.

LEARNING OBJECTIVES

- Describe effective aerosol therapy, including the number and size of droplets, adverse effects, and expected outcomes for client respiratory status.
- Compare the advantages and disadvantages of water and saline as diluents.
- Identify the therapeutic goals of mucolytic and bronchodilator drugs.
- Compare and contrast the sympathomimetic bronchodilator drugs.
- Identify drugs and beverages in the xanthine group.
- Explain the use of cromolyn and nedocromil, sympathetic agonists, ipratropium, leukotriene antagonists, xanthine derivatives, and corticosteroid drugs in the treatment of asthma.
- Implement the nursing management of clients receiving mucokinetic and bronchodilator drug therapy.

▲ KEY TERMS

aerosol therapy, p. 715
expectorant, p. 716
mucokinetic agents, p. 716
mucolytic agents, p. 716
mucus, p. 716
nebulizer, p. 716
sputum, p. 716
xanthine derivatives, p. 697

★ KEY DRUGS

albuterol, p. 702
cromolyn, p. 713
ipratropium, p. 704
montelukast, p. 713
theophylline, p. 704

✳ What drugs are available to treat respiratory conditions?

The three broad categories of respiratory drugs are bronchodilators, antiinflammatory agents and mucokinetic drugs. They are aimed at reversing bronchoconstriction, reducing respiratory inflammation and/or promoting elimination of excessive respiratory secretions respectively. Although they can be used alone, they are often used together to help promote improved airway clearance for a number of conditions, including asthma and chronic obstructive pulmonary disease (COPD). Asthma affects an estimated 17 million Americans or 6.4% of the U.S. population. Children account for 4.8 million of the nation's asthma sufferers. Each year, nearly 500,000 Americans are hospitalized and more than 5000 die from asthma (National Institute of Allergy and Infectious Disease, 2001). Ten percent of adolescents and young adults, and 5% of adults, are affected with asthma in Canada (Chen, Daks, Tang, & Krewski, 2002).

✳ T.F. is a 7-year-old boy who is admitted to the emergency department (ED) with a first episode of wheezing and agitation. He is monitored with pulse oximetry, which reveals a reading of 86% (normal ≥95%). His medical history is noncontributory, but his mother notes they just purchased a new kitten. He is diagnosed with asthma and is administered a dose of the bronchodilator albuterol by updraft.

✳ How is asthma categorized?

Asthma (also referred to as bronchial asthma) may involve bronchial smooth muscle contraction, mucosal edema or inflammation, and mucus hypersecretion (Figure 37-1). The National Institutes of Health (NIH) defines asthma as a lung disease with reversible airway obstruction, airway inflammation, and increased airway sensitivity to stimuli (Self, 2005). In the past asthma was classified on the basis of the stimuli that induce the attack, such as intrinsic asthma caused by emotional factors or exercise and extrinsic asthma caused by pollens, molds, dust, or animal hair. Because many asthmatics have a combination-type asthma, this type of classification is not considered useful. The National Asthma Education and Prevention Program (NAEPP) Expert Panel of the U.S. Department of Health and Human Services identifies a step approach for categorizing and treating asthma. Consistent implementation of these national guidelines is associated with reduced hospitalizations and improved client outcomes (Cloutier, Hall, Wakefield, & Bailit, 2005). Categories of asthma are ranked by severity and include mild intermittent, mild persistent, moderate persistent, and severe persistent asthma as follows.

Clients are classified according to the frequency and severity of their asthma attacks (mild, moderate, or severe); this information is the most useful when considering pharmacologic interventions:

- *Mild intermittent.* Intermittent attacks occur less than two times weekly or nocturnal asthma symptoms occur less than two times monthly. Peak expiratory flow

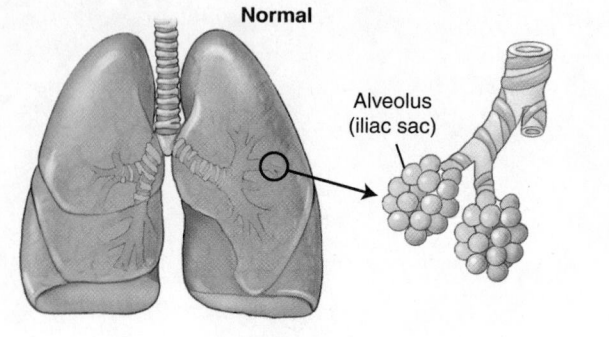

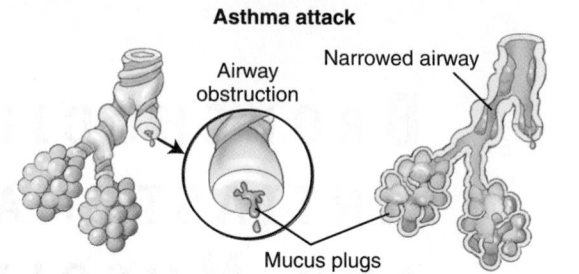

FIGURE 37-1 Bronchiole in normal state (**A**) and during an asthma attack (**B**). An asthmatic attack is illustrated by bronchial muscle spasms, inflammation, and excessive mucus, resulting in mucus plugs, edema, and trapped air in the air sacs (alveoli); this causes airway obstruction. Total amount of air inhaled and exhaled is decreased because of air trapped in the lungs after expiration.

(PEF) is greater than 80% and is normal after bronchodilator use; PEF variability is less than 20%.

- *Mild persistent.* Attacks occur more than two times weekly but not daily, or nocturnal asthma symptoms occur more than twice a month. A β-agonist inhaler is used almost daily. PEF is routinely remains 80% and is normal after bronchodilator use; PEF variability is 20% to 30%.

- *Moderate persistent.* Attacks occur daily more than two times weekly, or nocturnal asthma symptoms occur more than once a week. Exacerbations affect activity and may last days. A β-agonist inhaler is used almost daily. PEF is 60% to 80% and is normal after bronchodilator use; PEF variability is usually greater than 30%.

- *Severe persistent.* Asthmatic symptoms are frequent and continuous (including nocturnal asthma) with PEF less than 60% and variability greater than 30%. Limited physical activity occurs with frequent exacerbations. Often these clients have been hospitalized for asthma in the previous year.

See Figure 37-2 for an overview of the effects of various antiasthmatic medications.

Treatments are based on the severity of asthma and often include use of antiinflammatory agents in addition to the use of bronchodilators like albuterol (Tables 37-1 and 37-2).

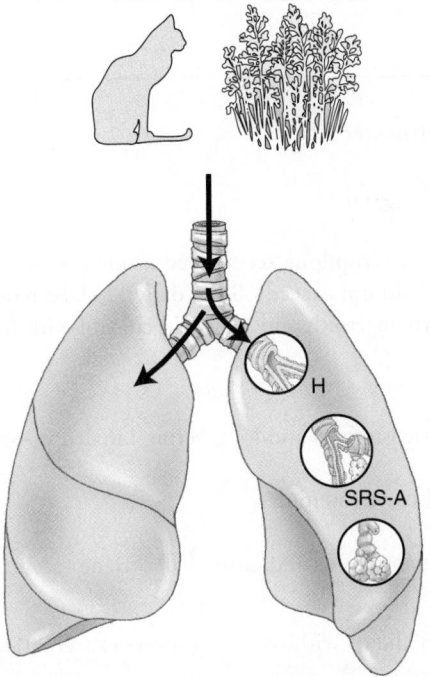

ALLERGENS such as dust, wool blankets, feather pillows, pollen, etc., in hypersensitive persons with IgE antibodies stimulate mast cells in lungs to release histamine (H) and slow-reacting substance of anaphylaxis (SRS-A).

HISTAMINE stimulates larger bronchi to cause smooth muscle spasms, inflammation, and edema.

SRS-A stimulates small bronchi to cause smooth muscle swelling.

Result is spasms of smooth bronchial muscle, increased mucus secretions, swollen mucosa, hyperinflation of alveoli eventually leading to loss of elasticity and collapsed alveoli.

LEUKOTRIENE ANTAGONISTS block the release of leukotrienes in the lungs. Inflammation causes an increase in leukotrienes, substances that constitute the slow-reacting substance of anaphylaxis (SRS-A).

THEOPHYLLINE increases cyclic AMP to inhibit breakdown of sensitized mast cells that stimulate the release of histamine, serotonin, and SRS-A.

MAST CELL STABILIZERS inhibit the release of histamine from mast cells to reduce allergic effects.

SYMPATHETIC AGONISTS stimulate sympathetic systems to decrease mucus secretions and relax bronchial muscle spasms.

CORTICOSTEROIDS produce an antiinflammatory effect and reduce mucus secretions and tissue histamine.

FIGURE 37-2 Overview of the effects of various antiasthmatic medications.

❋ **T.F. would be considered as having mild intermittent asthma at this point. It appears that an allergic component to asthma is likely with T.F., which may be triggered by animal dander. As needed inhaled β₂ agonists (bronchodilators) are appropriate for his management at this time.**

• • •

❋ **B.T. is a 13-year-old boy with a long history of asthma. He has been maintained on salmeterol inhaled twice daily (Serevent Diskus) and albuterol metered dose inhaler PRN acute attacks (both β₂-agonist bronchodilators).**

❋ **What is the role of bronchodilators in the management of asthma and COPD?**

Bronchodilators are a mainstay in the treatment of asthma. They are used on an as needed basis in milder forms of asthma, and on a regular basis for more severe asthma.

Bronchodilators are also used in chronic bronchitis to manage airways. They are primarily composed of agents that stimulate the sympathetic nervous system (SNS) or serve as antagonists in the parasympathetic nervous system (see Chapters 21 and 22).

The most commonly used bronchodilators are administered via inhalation and include the β₂ selective agents albuterol (Proventil, Ventolin) and salmeterol (Serevent), and the antimuscarinics including ipratropium (Atrovent). Older sympathomimetics such as epinephrine and isoproterenol (Isuprel) have fallen out of use because of their cardiac effects with excessive stimulation of β₁ receptors. The **xanthine derivatives** (theophylline, caffeine, theobromine) have central nervous system (CNS) stimulatory properties, produce diuresis and relax smooth muscle. Of these, theophylline is still utilized for clients with moderate persistent asthma. Understandably, drugs that serve as antagonists to the β₂ receptor (e.g., β blockers like propranolol [Inderal]) or muscarinic agonists (e.g., bethanechol [Duvoid]) can worsen respiratory status by inducing bronchoconstriction. Bronchodilators are presented in Table 37-3.

Text continued on p. 702

TABLE 37-1 STEPWISE APPROACH FOR MANAGING INFANTS AND YOUNG CHILDREN (5 YEARS OF AGE AND YOUNGER) WITH ACUTE OR CHRONIC ASTHMA

Classify Severity: Clinical Features Before Treatment or Adequate Control		Medications Required to Maintain Long-Term Control
	Symptoms (Day, Night)	Daily Medications
Step 4 Severe Persistent	Day: Continual Night: Frequent	Preferred Treatment: • High-dose inhaled corticosteroids AND • Long-acting inhaled β_2-agonists AND, if needed, • Corticosteroid tablets or syrup long-term (prednisone/prednisolone 2 mg/kg/day, generally do not exceed 60 mg daily). (Make repeat attempts to reduce systemic corticosteroids and maintain control with high-dose inhaled corticosteroids.)
Step 3 Moderate Persistent	Day: Daily Night: Greater than 1 night/week	Preferred treatments: • Low-dose inhaled corticosteroids and long-acting inhaled β_2-agonists OR • Medium-dose inhaled corticosteroids. Alternative treatment: • Low-dose inhaled corticosteroids and either leukotriene receptor antagonist or theophylline. If needed (particularly in clients with recurring severe exacerbations): Preferred treatment: • Medium-dose inhaled corticosteroids and long-acting β_2-agonists. Alternative treatment: • Medium-dose inhaled corticosteroids and either leukotriene receptor antagonist or theophylline.
Step 2 Mild Persistent	Day: Greater than 2/week but not daily Night: Greater than 2 nights/month	Preferred treatment: • Low-dose inhaled corticosteroid (with nebulizer or MDI with holding chamber with or without face mask or DPI). Alternative treatment (listed alphabetically): • Mast cell stabilizer (nebulizer is preferred or MDI with holding chamber) OR leukotriene receptor antagonist.
Step 1 Mild Intermittent	Day: Less than 2 days/week Night: Less than 2 nights/month	No daily medication needed.
Quick Relief All Clients	Bronchodilator as needed for symptoms. Intensity of treatment will depend on severity of exacerbation. • Preferred treatment: Short-acting inhaled β_2-agonists by nebulizer or face mask and space/holding chamber • Alternative treatment: Oral β_2-agonist With viral respiratory infection • Bronchodilator q4-6h up to 24 hours (longer with physician consult); in general, repeat no more than once every 6 weeks • Consider systemic corticosteroid if exacerbation is severe or client has history of previous severe exacerbations Use of short-acting β_2-agonists greater than 2 times a week in intermittent asthma (daily, or increasing use in persistent asthma) may indicate the need to initiate (increase) long-term control therapy.	

Step down: Review treatment every 1 to 6 months; a gradual stepwise reduction in treatment may be possible.
Step up: If control is not maintained, consider step up. First, review client medication technique, adherence, and environmental control.

From National Asthma Education and Prevention Program. (2002). Guidelines for the diagnosis and management of asthma. Retrieved July 12, 2005, from http://www.nhlbi.nih.gov/guidelines/asthma/asthgdln.pdf.

GOALS OF THERAPY: ASTHMA CONTROL

- Minimal or no chronic symptoms day or night
- Minimal or no exacerbations
- No limitations on activities; no school/parent's work missed
- Minimal use of short-acting inhaled β_2-agonist
- Minimal or no adverse effects from medications

NOTE

- The stepwise approach is intended to assist, not replace, the clinical decision making required to meet individual client needs.
- Classify severity: assign client to most severe step in which any feature occurs.
- There are very few studies on asthma therapy for infants.
- Gain control as quickly as possible (a course of short systemic corticosteroids may be required); then step down to the least medication necessary to maintain control.
- Minimize use of short-acting inhaled β_2-agonists. Overreliance on short-acting inhaled β_2-agonists (e.g., use of approximately one canister a month even if not using it every day) indicates inadequate control of asthma and the need to initiate or intensify long-term control therapy.
- Provide parent education on asthma management and controlling environmental factors that make asthma worse (e.g., allergies and irritants).
- Consultation with an asthma specialist is recommended for clients with moderate or severe persistent asthma. Consider consultation for clients with mild persistent asthma.

TABLE 37-2 STEPWISE APPROACH FOR MANAGING ASTHMA IN ADULTS AND CHILDREN OLDER THAN 5 YEARS OF AGE: TREATMENT

	Classify Severity: Clinical Features Before Treatment or Adequate Control		Medications Required to Maintain Long-Term Control
	Symptoms (Day, Night)	PEF or FEV$_1$ PEF Variability	Daily Medications
Step 4 Severe Persistent	Day: Continual Night: Frequent	Day: Less than 60% predicted Night: More than 30%	Preferred treatment: • High-dose inhaled corticosteroids AND • Long-acting inhaled β_2-agonists AND, if needed, • Corticosteroid tablets or syrup long term (prednisone 2 mg/kg/day, generally do not exceed 60 mg daily). (Make repeat attempts to reduce systemic corticosteroids and maintain control with high-dose inhaled corticosteroids.)
Step 3 Moderate Persistent	Day: Daily Night: More than 1 night/week	Day: 60% to 80% predicted Night: More than 30%	Preferred treatment: • Low-to-medium-dose inhaled corticosteroids and long-acting inhaled β_2-agonists Alternative treatment (listed alphabetically): • Increase inhaled corticosteroids within medium-dose range OR • Low-to-medium-dose inhaled corticosteroids and either leukotriene receptor antagonist or theophylline. If needed (particularly in clients with recurring severe exacerbations): Preferred treatment: • Increase inhaled corticosteroids within medium-dose range and add long-acting inhaled β_2-agonists Alternative treatment (listed alphabetically): • Increase inhaled corticosteroids within medium-dose range and add either leukotriene receptor antagonist or theophylline.

Continued

TABLE 37-2 STEPWISE APPROACH FOR MANAGING ASTHMA IN ADULTS AND CHILDREN OLDER THAN 5 YEARS OF AGE: TREATMENT—cont'd

Classify Severity: Clinical Features Before Treatment or Adequate Control		Medications Required to Maintain Long-Term Control
Symptoms (Day, Night)	**PEF or FEV$_1$ PEF Variability**	**Daily Medications**
Step 2 Mild Persistent	Day: More than 2 times/week but not daily Night: More than 2 nights/month	Day: More than 80% predicted Night: 20%-30%	Preferred treatment: Low-dose inhaled corticosteroids. Alternative treatment: leukotriene receptor antagonist and/or mast cell stabilizer OR sustained-release theophylline to serum concentration of 5-15 mcg/mL.
Step 1 Mild Intermittent	Day: Less than 2 times/week Night: Less than 2 nights/month	Day: More than 80% predicted Night: Less than 20%	No daily medication needed. Severe exacerbations may occur, separated by long periods of normal lung function and no symptoms. Severe exacerbation may require systemic corticosteroids.

Quick Relief All Clients
- Short-acting bronchodilator: 2-4 puffs short-acting inhaled β$_2$-agonists as needed for symptoms.
- Intensity of treatment will depend on severity of exacerbation; up to 3 treatments at 20-minute intervals or a single nebulizer treatment as needed. Course of systemic corticosteroids may be needed.

Use of short-acting β$_2$-agonists greater than 2 times a week in intermittent asthma (daily, or increasing use in persistent asthma) may indicate the need to initiate (increase) long-term control therapy.

Step down: Review treatment every 1 to 6 months; a gradual stepwise reduction in treatment may be possible.

Step up: If control is not maintained, consider step up. First, review client medication technique, adherence, and environmental control.

GOALS OF THERAPY: ASTHMA CONTROL

- Minimal or no chronic symptoms day or night
- Minimal or no exacerbations
- No limitations on activities; no school/work missed
- Maintain (near) normal pulmonary function
- Minimal use of short-acting inhaled β$_2$-agonist
- Minimal or no adverse effects from medications

NOTE

- The stepwise approach is intended to assist, not replace, the clinical decision making required to meet individual client needs.
- Classify severity: assign client to most severe step in which any feature occurs (PEF is % of personal best; FEV$_1$ is predicted).
- Gain control as quickly as possible (consider a short course of systemic corticosteroids); then step down to the least medication necessary to maintain control.
- Minimize use of short-acting inhaled β$_2$-agonists. Overreliance on short-acting inhaled β$_2$-agonists (e.g., use of approximately one canister a month even if not using it every day) indicates inadequate control of asthma and the need to initiate or intensify long-term control therapy.
- Provide education on self-management and controlling environmental factors that make asthma worse (e.g., allergies and irritants).
- Refer to an asthma specialist if there are difficulties controlling asthma or if step 4 care is required. Referral may be considered if step 3 care is required.

From National Asthma Education and Prevention Program. (2002). Guidelines for the diagnosis and management of asthma. Retrieved July 12, 2005, from http://www.nhlbi.nih.gov/guidelines/asthma/asthgdln.pdf.

TABLE 37-3 COMPARISON OF BRONCHODILATORS

Drug	Typical Adult Dose	Onset*	Duration*
SHORT-ACTING β₂-AGONISTS			
albuterol (Proventil, Ventolin)	1.25-5 mg via inhalation q4-8h	<5 min	3-8 hr
isoetharine	0.2-0.5 mL of 1% solution diluted in nebulizer q4h	<5 min	1-3 hr
levalbuterol (Xopenex)	0.65-1.25 mg via nebulizer three times daily	10-15 min	5-6 hr
metaproterenol (Alupent)	0.65 mg per inhalation puff: 2-3 puffs q3-4h	5-30 min	2-6 hr
pirbuterol (Maxair)	0.2 mg per inhalation puff: 2 puffs q4-6h	<5 min	5 hr
terbutaline (Brethine, Bricanyl)	2.5-5 mg PO three times daily	~1 hr (oral)	3-6 hr
LONG-ACTING β₂-AGONISTS			
formoterol (Foradil)	12 mcg by inhalation q12h	3-5 min	12 hr
salmeterol (Serevent Diskus)	50 mcg by inhalation q12h	5-15 min	12 hr
β₁- AND β₂-AGONIST			
isoproterenol (Isuprel)	80 mcg per inhalation puff: 1 puff q4h PRN	2-5 min	30 min to 2 hr
α,- β₁,- AND β₂-AGONIST			
epinephrine (Primatene Mist)	160-250 mcg per inhalation puff: 1-3 puffs four to six times daily	1-5 min	1-3 hr
ANTIMUSCARINIC AGENTS			
ipratropium (Atrovent)	18 mcg per inhalation puff: 2-3 puffs three to four times daily	1-5 min	3-6 hr
tiotropium (Spiriva HandiHaler)	18 mcg per inhalation capsule: one capsule via HandiHaler q24h	<30 min	24 hr
XANTHINE AGENTS			
aminophylline	5 mg/kg IV loading dose over 30 min, then 0.4-0.7 mg/kg/hr IV	<30 min IV	Varies
theophylline (Uniphyl, others)	5-13 mg/kg/24 hr (maximum 900 mg/24 hr) in divided dose depending on formulation titrated to levels	Varies with formulation	Varies with formulation
COMBINATION THERAPY			
ipratropium/albuterol (Combivent)	Ipratropium: 18 mcg/puff; albuterol: 90 mcg/puff: two inhalations four times daily	5 min	3-8 hr

Modified from Lacy, C.F., Armstrong, L.L., Goldman, M.P., & Lance, L.L. (2004). *Lexi-Comp's Drug Information Handbook* (12th ed.). Hudson, Ohio: Lexi-Comp.
*Onset and duration assume inhalation unless otherwise specified.

Short-Acting β₂ Agonists

Of the short-acting β₂ agonists, albuterol is by far the most commonly used agent in North America and is considered the prototype. Albuterol, a sympathomimetic bronchodilator, possesses a relatively selective specificity for β₂-adrenergic receptors in the lungs and therefore is less likely to cause unwanted cardiovascular effects. Its interaction with the β₂ receptor in the cell membrane of the bronchial smooth muscle stimulates the enzyme adenyl cyclase to produce cyclic 3'5' AMP, which results in relaxation of the smooth muscle of the bronchi (Figure 37-3), thus relieving bronchospasm and decreasing airway resistance. Additionally, this mechanism causes relaxation of the smooth muscle of the uterus and the blood vessels of skeletal muscle. Although most clients achieve therapeutic effects with β-agonists, there appears to be some genetically based variation in response to these agents. See the Special Considerations for Pharmacogenetics box below. Albuterol is not helpful in the management of viral bronchiolitis in infants and children (Patel et al., 2003); inhaled epinephrine may be preferred for viral bronchiolitis (Hartling, Wiebe, Russell, Patel, & Klassen, 2003), although conflicting data exist to suggest no adrenergic agonist is helpful (Mull et al., 2004). Higher doses are usually required to inhibit uterine contractions to delay premature labor (see the Pregnancy Safety box above).

An R-isomer of racemic albuterol, levalbuterol (Xopenex), is also available as a nebulized solution to prevent and treat bronchospasm in clients at least 6 years of age (*USP DI*, 2005). However, further study is needed to determine whether this higher potency drug offers any clinically significant advantage over racemic albuterol to justify its higher cost.

albuterol [al **byoo** ter ole]
(Proventil, Ventolin, Novosalmol✦)
Indications
Albuterol is indicated for reversible airway obstruction in asthma and COPD, and is used to prevent exercise induced bronchoconstriction.
Pharmacokinetics/Dosing
Albuterol is primarily administered by inhalation. Inhaled albuterol has an onset of action between 5 and 15 minutes, a peak effect in 30 to 90 minutes after two inhalations, and a duration of action of 3 to 6 hours. Orally, its onset of action is between 15 and 30 minutes, its peak effect is in 2 to 3 hours, and its duration of action is 8 hours or more (12 hours for the sustained-release dosage form). This drug is metabolized in the liver and excreted by the kidneys and in the feces. The adult bronchodilator dosage for inhalation is 200 to 400 mcg every 4 to 6 hours. The oral dosage is 2 to 4 mg three or four times daily. This dose may be increased to a maximum of 8 mg four times daily if necessary. Extended-release tablets are administered 4 or 8 mg PO every 12 hours. Refer to the package insert for the pediatric dosage schedule.

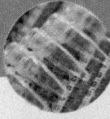

Special Considerations for Pharmacogenetics | PULMONARY AGENTS

PHARMACODYNAMICS

A strong correlation exists between genes that code for leukotriene receptors and the presence of asthma in Japanese individuals (Fukai et al., 2004). Similar findings have been identified in North American and European populations (Pillai et al., 2004). Presence or absence of the genetic markers for enzymes involved in leukotriene synthesis strongly predicts drug response to leukotriene antagonists (Wechsler & Israel, 2002). Variation in β₂ receptor affinity has been linked to genetic markers and resistance to β₂-agonists (Dishy et al., 2004; Israel et al., 2001). Some variation in response to inhaled corticosteroids and antimuscarinics may be explained by genetics (Joos & Sandford, 2002), but their correlations of response to genetic markers are less strong than that observed with β-agonists and leukotriene antagonists. These findings help explain why some clients are resistant to asthma drug therapy and may have future implications in predicting who is responsive to leukotriene antagonists and β-agonists (Holgate, 2004).

PHARMACOKINETICS

Wide variation in the pharmacokinetics of salmeterol elimination suggests a genetic explanation, but to date, the role of genetics in the elimination of salmeterol is unclear (McKenzie, 2004). The wide variation in theophylline metabolism may have a genetic basis (Chang et al., 2004; Miller, Slusher, & Vesell, 1985).

ADVERSE EFFECTS

Although not directly attributed to genetic influence, increased asthma-related deaths with salmeterol were reported in 2003 by the FDA in African Americans (FDA, January 23, 2003). Genetic variation in β-adrenergic receptor sensitivity may predict which individuals would be at highest risk for cardiovascular and other complications associated with β-agonist use (Evans & McLeod, 2003). Theophylline toxicity is closely correlated with metabolic clearance, and may be genetically influenced.

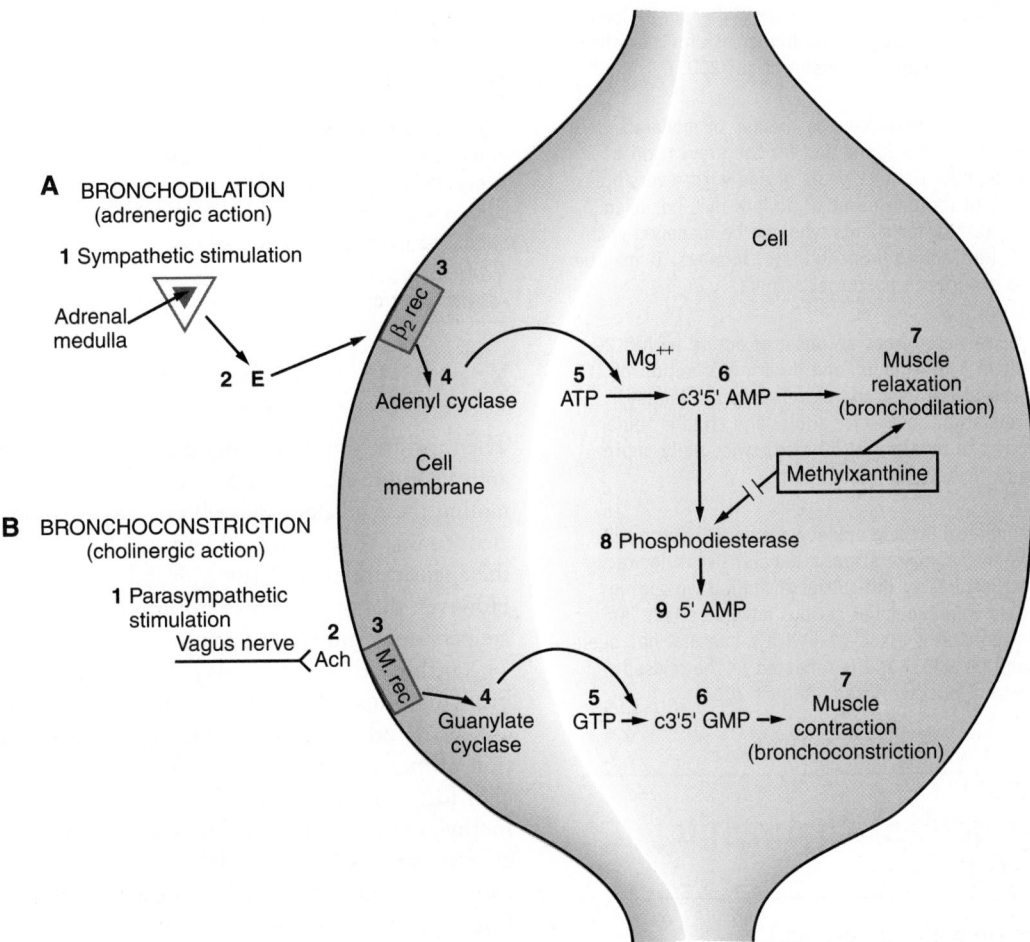

A BRONCHODILATION
(adrenergic action)

1 Sympathetic stimulation

Adrenal medulla

2 E

3 β₂ rec

4 Adenyl cyclase

Cell membrane

5 ATP

Mg⁺⁺

6 c3'5' AMP

7 Muscle relaxation (bronchodilation)

Methylxanthine

8 Phosphodiesterase

9 5' AMP

Cell

B BRONCHOCONSTRICTION
(cholinergic action)

1 Parasympathetic stimulation
Vagus nerve
2 Ach

3 M. rec

4 Guanylate cyclase

5 GTP

6 c3'5' GMP

7 Muscle contraction (bronchoconstriction)

FIGURE 37-3 Mechanisms of bronchial smooth muscle action. **A,** Bronchodilation pathway. **B,** Bronchoconstriction pathway. *E,* Epinephrine; *Ach,* acetylcholine, *β₂ rec,* β₂ receptor; *M. rec,* muscarinic receptor.

Adverse Effects
The adverse effects of albuterol include nausea, increased anxiety, palpitations, tremors, tachycardia, sedation, hypokalemia, difficulty in urination, dizziness, headaches, heartburn, muscle cramping, insomnia, increased sweating, vomiting, increased weakness, hypotension or hypertension, and an unusual taste in the mouth.

Drug Interactions
Inhaled albuterol has few clinically important drug interactions. Concurrent use of drugs with cardiac stimulant properties (e.g., sympathomimetics, monoamine oxidase [MAO] inhibitors, tricyclic antidepressants) may increase the potential for tachycardia or dysrhythmias. β-adrenergic blockers (e.g., propranolol) will blunt the effect of albuterol.

terbutaline [tur **byoo** ta leen]
(Brethine, Bricanyl)
Like albuterol, terbutaline serves as an agonist to β₂-adrenergic receptors in the bronchioles. It is only available in the United States as an oral or injectable formulation. Its use to help prevent premature labor is explained by its agonist activity at β₂ receptors in the uterus.

Indications
Terbutaline is used as a bronchodilator for asthma and COPD. It is also used as a tocolytic in clients with premature labor because of its activity to suppress uterine contractions.

Pharmacokinetics/Dosing
Orally, its onset of action is within 1 to 2 hours, with a peak effect in 2 to 3 hours and duration of action of 4 to 8 hours. Parenterally, its onset of action is within 15 minutes, with a peak effect in 30 to

60 minutes and duration of action of 1.5 to 4 hours. It is metabolized in the liver and excreted by the kidneys. For oral administration, a 2.5 to 5 mg tablet three times daily (every 6 hours during waking hours) is recommended. For children 12 to 15 years of age, the dosage is 2.5 mg PO three times daily. Parenterally, the dosage is 250 mcg subcutaneously, which may be repeated in 15 to 30 minutes. A total dose of 500 mcg is the maximum in a 4-hour period.

Adverse Effects
The adverse effects of terbutaline include tremors, increased anxiety, restlessness, dizziness, sedation, headaches, hypertension, muscle cramps, nausea, vomiting, palpitations, insomnia, sweating, tachycardia, weakness, dry mouth or throat, and an unusual taste in the mouth. Rare adverse effects include chest pain and an increase in respiratory difficulties.

Drug Interactions
Similar to albuterol.

Long Acting β₂-Agonists

salmeterol [sal **met** er ole]
(Serevent, Serevent Diskus)
Salmeterol is utilized to prevent asthma attacks. The mechanism of action of salmeterol is the same as for albuterol, but it has a slower onset and longer duration of action. Its long onset of action renders this drug not useful for treating acute asthmatic attacks. An FDA Talk paper in January 2003 identified a potential increased rate of asthma episodes and asthma-related deaths associated with salmeterol use

(FDA, January 23, 2003). Risk, if present, may be higher for African Americans. More recent analysis suggests no higher risk for mortality with long-acting β-agonist therapy (Anderson et al., 2005).

Indications

Salmeterol is indicated for the maintenance therapy of moderate persistent and severe persistent asthma and for the prevention of bronchospasm in clients older than 12 years of age with reversible airway disease. Because of its long onset of action, it is not used for acute asthmatic attacks or for clients who can be managed with the occasional use of short-acting bronchodilator inhalers. It may be used with clients who experience nocturnal asthma.

Pharmacokinetics/Dosing

The inhalation form of salmeterol has an onset of action within 20 minutes, a peak effect in 3 to 4 hours, and duration of action of 12 hours. It is metabolized in the liver and excreted by the kidneys. The bronchodilator inhalation dosage for adults and children older than 12 years of age is one inhalation (50 mcg) twice daily, morning and evening, approximately 12 hours apart.

Adverse Effects

Adverse effects of salmeterol include anxiety, insomnia, dizziness, headaches, nausea, vomiting, palpitations, tremors, sweating, tachycardia, and weakness. Respiratory difficulties including worsening asthma episodes, are an infrequent but serious adverse effect. An increased asthma-related deaths associated with salmeterol has been reported (FDA, January 23, 2003) and is reflected in the revised package insert (Salmeterol package insert, August 2003).

Drug Interactions

Similar to albuterol.

Antimuscarinic (Anticholinergic) Bronchodilators

★➤ ipratropium [ih prah **troe** pee um]
(Atrovent)

Ipratropium is an anticholinergic drug with affinity for muscarinic receptors that produces a local bronchodilation after inhalation. Its chemical structure is highly ionized and therefore is not well absorbed orally. As such, it is not associated with significant systemic antimuscarinic properties.

Indications

Ipratropium is indicated for maintenance therapy (not for acute episodes) in clients with COPD (chronic bronchitis or emphysema). Although not an FDA-approved use, it is commonly used as an adjunct bronchodilator inhaler with other therapies for asthma.

Pharmacokinetics/Dosing

After administration, the onset of action is between 5 and 15 minutes, with a peak effect in 1 to 2 hours and duration of action of 3 to 6 hours. The usual adolescent or adult dosage is two to three inhalations three or four times daily, administered every 4 hours. Shake the unit well before using.

Adverse Effects

The adverse effects of ipratropium include dry mouth or throat, coughing, headache, anxiety, gastrointestinal (GI) distress and, rarely, eye pain, blurred vision, tremors, tachycardia, bronchospasm, glaucoma, hives, skin rash, or stomatitis.

Drug Interactions

Significant drug interactions with ipratropium are infrequent. Additive anticholinergic effects (e.g., dry mouth, urinary retention, constipation) might be expected when used with other antimuscarinic agents (e.g., atropine, benztropine, tolterodine, trihexyphenidyl).

tiotropium [tee oh **troe** pee um]
(Spiriva)

Tiotropium is a long-acting antimuscarinic for inhalation similar to ipratropium but with a longer duration of action.

Indications

Similar to ipratropium.

Pharmacokinetics/Dosing

Tiotropium is available as a dry powder capsule for inhalation utilizing a handheld device specific for this formulation. Like ipratropium, minimal drug is systemically absorbed on inhalation. The usual dose is one 18-mcg capsule by inhalation daily.

Adverse Effects

Similar to ipratropium.

Drug Interactions

As with ipratropium.

Xanthine Derivatives

The xanthine group of drugs includes caffeine, theophylline, and theobromine. Beverages from the extracts of plants containing these alkaloids have been used by humans since ancient times. They are less widely used because of their narrow therapeutic index and the availability of safer alternatives. However, theophylline is still utilized for clients with moderate persistent and severe persistent asthma.

Xanthine derivatives relax smooth muscle (particularly bronchial muscle), stimulate cardiac muscle and the CNS, and also produce diuresis, probably through a combined action of increased renal perfusion and increased sodium and chloride ion excretion. The drugs in this category are methylated forms of xanthines or methylxanthines. Their effectiveness as bronchodilators depends on their conversion to theophylline, which is the active constituent. Therefore, with the exception of dyphylline, the action of xanthine depends on the content of theophylline. Xanthines inhibit mast cell degranulation and the release of histamine and other mediators that are responsible for bronchoconstriction. Methylxanthines also inhibit phosphodiesterase (see Figure 37-3), but it is unclear how much this property contributes to therapeutic benefit.

★➤ theophylline [thee **off** ih lin]
(Bronkodyl, Elixophyllin, Slo-Phyllin)

Theophylline is the prototype and most frequently used of the xanthine derivatives. It competitively inhibits the action of phosphodiesterase (the enzyme that degrades cyclic 3'5' AMP), resulting in bronchodilation. Aminophylline and oxtriphylline (Choledyl) are infrequently used salts of theophylline. The dose of aminophylline and oxtriphylline differ from theophylline. Aminophylline is available for intravenous (IV) and oral administration.

Indications

Theophylline is used for the prevention and treatment of bronchial asthma and for the treatment of bronchitis, pulmonary emphysema, and COPD.

Pharmacokinetics/Dosing

Oral liquids and uncoated tablets of theophylline are rapidly absorbed, whereas enteric-coated tablets have a delayed and, at times, an unreliable pattern of absorption. The extended-release dosage forms are slowly absorbed and sometimes unreliable. Slow-release theophylline products can vary in their rate of absorption and therapeutic effects, even if they have the same strength and active ingredient. It has been recommended that pharmacists not substitute for these drugs if the new product does not have proven bioequivalence (USP DI, 2005). Some states do not permit generic substitution for theophylline slow-release products. Peak levels of theophylline are reached in 1 to 2 hours with the oral solution, immediate-release capsules, or tablets; in approximately 4 hours with delayed-release tablets; and in 4 to 13 hours with extended-release products.

Theophylline is metabolized by the liver to caffeine by P450 1 A2, 2 E1, 3 A4, and other isoenzymes. Caffeine concentrations may average approximately 30% of the theophylline concentration in adults, but in neonates it may be much more. Caffeine does not accumulate in adults. The half-life of theophylline varies by age and with concurrent illness. For example, with premature newborns, the half-life is approximately 30 hours during the first 15 days of life; for children 1 to 4 years of age, it is 3.4 hours; for adult nonsmokers with uncomplicated asthma, 8.2 hours; and for older adults, nearly 10 hours. In clients with acute hepatitis, the half-life is 19 hours; for cirrhosis, 32 hours; and for hyperthyroidism, 4.5 hours (*USP DI*, 2005). The half-life of theophylline in an adult smoker is only 3 to 4 hours (Metz, Gregersen, & Malhotra, 2004).

The therapeutic serum levels for bronchodilator effects with theophylline are usually between 10 and 20 mg/L. Some studies have indicated that a therapeutic response may be seen with serum levels of 5 to 15 mg/L; however, some clients have minimal gain at this level, and others experience toxicity at levels of 15 to 20 mg/L (Kelly & Sorkness, 2002). Therefore it is necessary to provide close supervision with dosage adjustments according to client's therapeutic response or the presence of toxic effects. As a respiratory stimulant, serum levels of theophylline are between 5 and 10 mg/L. The rapid IV administration of theophylline and its derivatives has caused severe and even fatal acute circulatory failure; therefore the drug should be administered slowly, over 20 to 30 minutes. Because theophylline has a low therapeutic index, it is essential to use caution when determining the dosage. When administering theophylline by "piggyback," turn off the other IV solution already in place or start another IV line, because theophylline will need to be titrated according to the client's response. For IV administration, monitoring theophylline serum concentrations and the client's response is essential to prevent toxicity. Box 37-1 lists factors that affect the therapeutic effects of theophylline.

Adverse Effects

The adverse effects of theophylline preparations include nausea, increased anxiety, restlessness, gastric upset, vomiting, gastroesophageal reflux, headache, increased urination, insomnia, trembling, increased nervousness, tachycardia and, with aminophylline, dermatitis. Toxic levels are associated with seizures and cardiac dysrhythmias (see the Management of Overdose box above). Inhaled corticosteroids are often preferred in pregnancy over theophylline (Dombrowski et al., 2004).

Drug Interactions

Theophylline is a narrow therapeutic index drug that is metabolized by cytochrome P450 1 A2/3 and 3 A4. As such, a number of other

---

 Management of Drug Overdose

Theophylline (Xanthine)

- Treatment is supportive and symptomatic because there is no known specific antidote.
- To decrease drug absorption, administer an activated charcoal preparation orally or via a nasogastric tube. Charcoal should be premixed with sorbitol or a single dose of sorbitol should follow the charcoal dose. Sorbitol is considered to be more effective than magnesium-containing laxatives.
- Gastric lavage if instituted early (within an hour of ingestion) or whole bowel irrigation with a polyethylene glycol and electrolyte solution are useful for very large overdoses of theophylline.
- If the client has seizures, establish an airway and administer oxygen. Diazepam or phenobarbital IV may be administered to control the seizures.
- Charcoal hemoperfusion may be necessary when theophylline serum concentration is very high (greater than 40 mcg/mL in chronic overdose or if other risk factors are present, such as an older adult client, concurrent illnesses, etc.). Hemodialysis and peritoneal dialysis are less or ineffective, respectively, for theophylline toxicity (*USP DI*, 2005).
- Monitor vital signs and provide supportive care as required.

---

drugs and food can affect the elimination of theophylline, including the macrolide antibacterials (e.g., erythromycin, azithromycin) and fluoroquinolone antibacterials (e.g., ciprofloxacin, gatifloxacin, levofloxacin) and antiepileptic drugs (carbamazepine, phenytoin, phenobarbital). Many other drugs also affect theophylline clearance. Smokers are more rapid metabolizers of theophylline than nonsmokers, and intake of broiled or charred foods also results in increased metabolism (see Box 37-1). Health care team members should review drug regimens for potential interactions, particularly when drugs are added or discontinued.

BOX 37-1 FACTORS AFFECTING THE THERAPEUTIC EFFECTS OF THEOPHYLLINE

MAY BE INCREASED BY

- Age: older adult and newborn
- Drugs: Many, including erythromycin, cimetidine, ciprofloxacin
- Disease states: cirrhosis, pulmonary edema, heart failure, and severe COPD
- Diet: high carbohydrate

MAY BE DECREASED BY

- Substances: tobacco, marijuana
- Drugs: phenobarbital, phenytoin, carbamazepine
- Diet: high protein
- Age: adolescence

❋ **What nursing management is appropriate for B.T. regarding the use of the bronchodilators salmeterol and albuterol?**

Assessment Assess B.T. for a previous intolerance to adrenergic bronchodilators because this may indicate intolerance to albuterol and salmeterol. Take a history to exclude cardiac insufficiency; potentially, but rarely, inhaled adrenergic bronchodilators may worsen cardiac disorders.

In the assessment of his concurrent drug therapies, it is determined that B.T. is not using any other medications known to induce bronchospasm. Therapies that can produce bronchospasm include β-adrenergic blockers (e.g., propranolol), parasympathomimetics (e.g., bethanechol), or other drugs that might trigger an allergic response.

Include in a baseline assessment a description of B.T.'s respiratory status—respiratory rate and effort, the use of accessory muscles, nasal flaring or lip pursing, breath sounds per auscultation, circumoral pallor or cyanosis, the presence of cough and/or sputum, activity intolerance, peak expiratory flow (PEF) readings, blood pressure (BP), pulse oximetry, and signs of impaired gas exchange (e.g., anxiety, confusion, and irritability). A detailed allergy history is essential. Additionally, the following diagnostic tests may be performed: chest x-ray examination, sputum culture, complete blood count (CBC), pulmonary function studies, and electrocardiogram (ECG).

Nursing Diagnosis Because respiratory disorders interfere with the basic human need for air, expect B.T. to exhibit anxiety, not only during acute episodes but also in anticipation of them. Ineffective airway clearance, ineffective breathing pattern, impaired gas exchange, and activity intolerance are nursing diagnoses common to clients receiving bronchodilator therapy. Additionally, these adrenergic bronchodilators increase B.T.'s risk for impaired comfort (dryness of the mouth and throat, taste changes, coughing,

flushing of the face, increased sweating, nausea and vomiting, heartburn, headache, restlessness, nervousness, trembling, palpitations, and chest pain); anxiety; disturbed sleep pattern (drowsiness or insomnia); and the potential complications of paradoxical bronchospasm (increase in dyspnea and wheezing), hypertension, and tachycardia. (See the Nursing Care Plan below for other selected nursing diagnoses.)

Planning While on bronchodilator therapy, B.T. will:
- Experience minimal exacerbations of asthma symptoms (e.g., coughing or breathlessness during the night or after exertion).
- Maintain (near) "normal" pulmonary function while compliant with his drug therapy.
- Effectively manage his therapeutic regimen, including compliance with medications and supportive non-pharmacologic interventions.
- Collaborate with health care providers for monitoring and ongoing care.

NURSING CARE PLAN SELECTED NURSING DIAGNOSES RELATED TO BRONCHODILATORS

Nursing Diagnosis	Outcome Criteria	Nursing Interventions
Ineffective airway clearance related to reversible airway obstruction	• Coughs effectively and expectorates sputum • Absence of abnormal breath sounds • Absence of sputum production • Maintains fluid intake of at least 3000 mL/24 hr unless contraindicated	• Assess respiratory status every 4 hours • Assist client to turn, cough, and deep breathe as necessary • Provide adequate humidification as ordered • Monitor characteristics of sputum every 8 hours and record • Encourage fluids to at least 3000 mL daily
Activity intolerance related to reversible airway obstruction	• Increases level of activity • Pulse, respiration, and blood pressure remain within acceptable limits during activity	• Plan with client for increasing levels of activity including activities that have priority for client • Identify and limit the factors that decrease the client's tolerance for activity • Monitor pulse rate, respiration, and blood pressure (BP) while increasing the level of activity
Deficient knowledge related to medication regimen	• Describes underlying condition and how the drug relates to the condition, how and when to take the medication, common drug interactions, safety precautions, common adverse effects and which of those warrant reporting • Self-administers medication safely and accurately	• Administer oral forms with food to minimize gastrointestinal (GI) distress • Emphasize the need for drug to be taken as prescribed around the clock • Caution the client not to self-administer any over-the-counter (OTC) drugs without prescriber consultation • Advise the client to notify the prescriber if the usual dose fails to be therapeutic or if condition worsens after treatment • Instruct the client to minimize ingestion of foods and beverages containing xanthine (coffee, chocolate, colas) • Emphasize the need for ongoing contact with the prescriber for serum levels and evaluation

Implementation

Monitoring Determine B.T.'s respiratory status on an ongoing basis to evaluate the drug's effectiveness using indicators from the baseline assessment. Monitor for adverse effects of bronchodilators, including tachycardia and dysrhythmias.

Intervention Although B.T.'s inhalers are prescribed for prophylaxis (salmeterol) and rescue (albuterol), albuterol and other adrenergic bronchodilators are also used in more severe asthma attacks with either a metered dose inhaler or a nebulizer to deliver the drug. (See Figure 37-4 for a metered-dose inhaler and nebulizer.) Short-acting aerosolized β_2 agonists are the agents of choice for hospital management of asthma (National Asthma Education and Prevention Program, 2002). A spacing device is typically used to improve the delivery of drugs via metered dose inhaler. A mouthpiece or a face mask may be used to administer the inhalation solution through a nebulizer. The nebulizer may be used with compressed air or oxygen, 6 to 10 L/min. A treatment lasts about 10 minutes. Children younger than 5 years old and infants as young as 2 months old appear to respond as well to the use of metered-dose inhalers with a spacer compared to nebulizer-delivered therapy, with less cost, greater ease, and lower rates of hospitalization (Castro-Rodriguez & Rodrigo, 2004; Delgado, Chou, Silver, & Crain, 2003).

In the acute setting, provide supportive nursing care with oxygen and fluid replacement to bring respirations within the normal range for rate, depth, and effort during acute episodes. Nebulized bronchodilator solutions are available as both nonsterile and sterile-filled products. Nonsterile products contain additives (e.g., sulfites, benzalkonium chloride, or chlorobutanol) to prevent bacterial growth. These additives are capable of inducing bronchospasm in a concentration-dependent manner that diminishes the bronchodilator effects of the drug for some clients. For hourly or continuous nebulization of bronchodilator drugs, use only additive-free solutions.

Education An important aspect of nursing management is to provide B.T. with information that enables him to maintain some measure of control over what is happening to him and thus decrease his anxiety. Education for B.T. is an integral part of his care and includes instruction on factors that tend to precipitate an acute episode.

Encourage B.T. to use a diary to record the administration of as-needed (PRN) medications and his response. A health care provider should routinely review the diary to monitor for continued beneficial effects or the presence of adverse effects and early treatment failures. This information may provide the first warning of the incorrect use of the medication or failure to take early preventive measures, or it may indicate the need for a change in dosage, a change in medication, or additional medication.

Assess B.T.'s ability to hold and manipulate a metered-dose inhaler. Provide instructions on inhaler use and cleansing. Written instructions are provided in addition to verbal discussion. Ensure that he is able to use the inhaler; see Box 37-2.

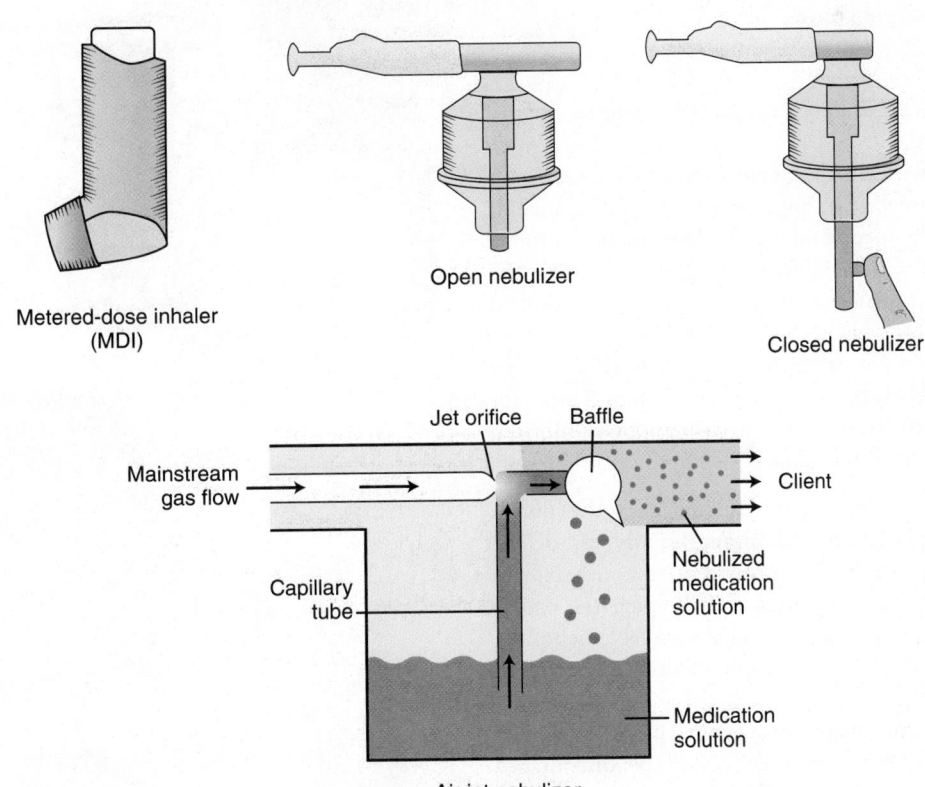

Metered-dose inhaler (MDI)

Open nebulizer

Closed nebulizer

Air jet nebulizer

Jet orifice   Baffle

Mainstream gas flow

Client

Capillary tube

Nebulized medication solution

Medication solution

FIGURE 37-4 Example of a metered-dose inhaler, open nebulizer, closed nebulizer, and air jet nebulizer.

BOX 37-2 CLIENT EDUCATION: USING A METERED-DOSE INHALER (MDI)

It is important that the client be instructed in the correct use of a MDI before it is needed to relieve an asthma attack. The prescriber will indicate whether a spacer or the open-mouth technique is to be used. The spacer is a small tube that fits into the MDI mouthpiece and goes into the client's mouth, to enhance the delivery of aerosolized agent to the bronchioles. If the open-mouth technique is used incorrectly, the dose may be dispersed into the air or sprayed onto the surface of the pharynx. Because only 10% of an inhaled dose reaches the lungs under the best of conditions, the ability to use the MDI appropriately is essential for the client. A placebo inhaler should be used for demonstration. This will enable the client to repeat the demonstration a number of times until the inhaler can be easily and correctly used.

THE SPACER TECHNIQUE (FIGURE A)

1. Attach the spacer to the mouthpiece.
2. Shake the MDI for 2 to 5 seconds (not required for dry powder inhalers).
3. Hold the MDI so the mouthpiece is at the bottom (with the drug container upside down).
4. Place the spacer mouthpiece in the mouth, closing lips tightly around it.
5. Exhale steadily and completely through nose.
6. Inhale slowly and deeply, and at the same time press the container down on the mouthpiece.
7. Hold breath for as long as possible before exhaling and remove mouthpiece from your mouth.
8. Wait 15 seconds.
9. Repeat steps 1 through 6 above.
10. If no relief is achieved after 5 minutes and condition worsens, contact prescriber.

THE OPEN-MOUTH TECHNIQUE (FIGURE B)

1. Shake the MDI for 2 to 5 seconds (not required for dry powder inhalers).
2. Hold the MDI with the drug container upside down.
3. Hold the mouthpiece two finger widths (about 1½ inches) in front of widely opened mouth. Hold container upright.
4. Exhale deeply, then inhale slowly through mouth and at the same time press down firmly on the container. Continue to breathe deeply.
5. Hold breath for a few seconds, then exhale slowly. After taking a few normal breaths, then repeat steps 3 to 5 for second inhalation. (Keep eyes closed—temporary blurring of vision may occur if the aerosol is sprayed into the eyes.)

Advise client that rinsing the mouth after using the inhaler reduces systemic absorption and minimizes dryness of the mouth. The mouthpiece should be rinsed at least once daily to avoid clogging. Stress the importance of keeping the equipment clean to prevent infection. If using a refillable nebulizer, do not place more than a day's supply of drug in nebulizer. Change solution daily.

Clients with asthma benefit greatly from the use of sympathomimetic inhalers; however, they should be discouraged from using over-the-counter (OTC) inhalers because of the nonselective ß-agonist drug effect of the epinephrine base. The nurse needs to recognize the possibility of misuse and the consequences of abuse in order to successfully help the client with inhalant drug therapy.

CLEANING

1. Once a day clean the spacer and mouthpiece by rinsing it in warm running water. Let it dry before you use it again. Have another spacer and mouthpiece to use while it is drying.
2. Twice a week, wash the plastic mouthpiece and spacer with mild dishwashing soap and warm water. Rinse and dry well before putting it back.

KNOWING WHEN TO REFILL YOUR MDI

1. Start with a brand new MDI.
2. Divide the number of puffs in the canister—the canister will usually have this number printed on it—by the number of puffs you take each day. The number you get will be the number of days the canister should last. (For example, if you take four puffs each day from a 200-puff canister, you will need to have a new canister every 50 days.)
3. Using a calendar, count forward that many days to see when your medicine will run out. So you won't run out of the medicine that you use every day, choose a day 1 or 2 days before this date to have your prescription refilled.
4. Write the refill date on the canister using a permanent marker.

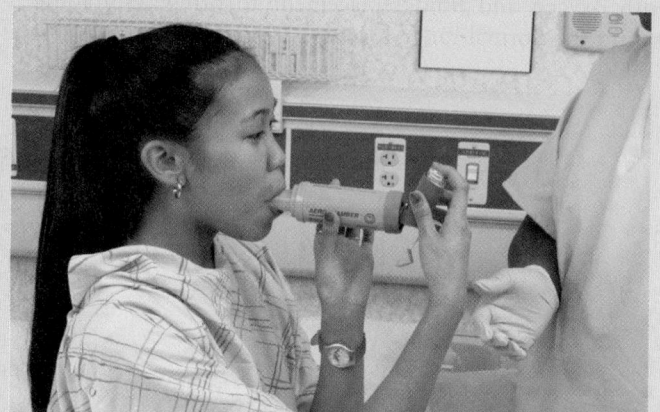

A

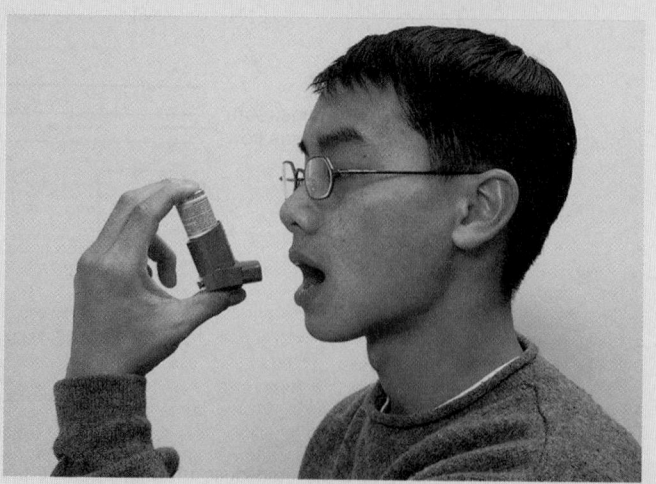

B

Stress the importance of not changing the dosage or frequency of albuterol without consulting the prescriber. Advise him against floating the metered-dose inhaler in water to estimate the amount of drug remaining in the canister; instead, B.T. should keep a record of the number of inhalations for accuracy (see the Evidence-Based Practice box below).

Instruct B.T. in ways to control known risk factors whenever possible to support the treatment plan and help to prevent recurrences (Box 37-3), measures to take during an attack and the signs and symptoms to report to the health care provider (chest pain, extreme dizziness and light-headedness, severe headache, palpitations, continuing tachycardia, dysrhythmias, or hypertensive episodes).

⁘ Evidence-Based Practice

Instruct the client to properly administer a MDI and to count the number of MDI doses administered as the only accurate method to determine when a canister should be discarded

Rubin and Durotoye (2004) evaluated how fifty consecutive clients attending the Brenner Children's Asthma Center determined that MDI canisters were empty. If clients do not recognize when a MDI is empty, they will not replace it and may continue to use the device without receiving required medication. Of the 50 children and parents questioned, 74% did not know how many doses were in their canisters, and all used the MDI until they could no longer "hear" the medication during inhalation. Only half shook the canister before actuating. Shaking the canister before using increased the number of actuations per canister for chlorofluorocarbon (CFC) canisters but not hydrofluoroalkane (HFA) canisters. Storing the MDI stem-down reduced the total dose delivered in the first actuation by 25% despite shaking the MDI before use (Everard et al., 1995). Canister flotation was ineffective in determining when a MDI was depleted. Not only are flotation characteristics product-specific, but water obstructs the valve opening and reduces the medication output (Brock et al., 2002; Cain & Oppenheimer, 2001).

BOX 37-3 ENVIRONMENTAL ALLERGENS

Although some allergens may be impossible to avoid, many occupational or environmental allergens may be reduced or eliminated. For example, smoke is an irritant to many asthmatics, especially children. Asthmatic attacks may be precipitated or aggravated by dust, dust mites, cat or dog hair, hairspray, perfumes, temperature changes, and physical exertion. Air pollution is also correlated with asthma frequency and severity (Gent et al., 2003). Whenever possible, changes that can reduce or eliminate the irritants should be attempted, such as keeping the house as dust free as possible and avoiding shag carpeting, heavy draperies, dust on silk flower arrangements, use of perfumed soap and products, and smokers or smoke-contaminated areas.

Monitoring PEF, initially in the morning and in the evening, is a method of objectively measuring lung function at home. After establishing a personal best PEF or "green zone," B.T. will probably be able to verify his optimal therapy once daily in the early morning on a peak flow meter. (See Figure 37-5 for an illustration of a peak flow meter.)

Green, yellow, and red zones are similar to those on a traffic light and are used as a guide for clients and clinicians. The "green" zone refers to a PEF that is 80% to 100% of "personal best" and generally indicates that therapy is in good control. Until B.T.'s "personal best" can be determined, a predicted PEF rate (L/min) is estimated using age and height. His prescriber uses green, yellow, and red tape directly on the PEF meter. The "yellow" zone indicates a PEF that 50% to 79% of personal best. B.T. is instructed to call his prescriber for adjustment in his preventative medication if his PEF stays in the "yellow" zone after using two puffs of his albuterol inhaler. The "red" zone indicates a PEF that is less than 50% of personal best. B.T. should call his health care provider immediately if his albuterol inhaler does not bring him into the yellow or green zone. He should initiate an emergency plan provided by his prescriber or go to an ED.

Evaluation The expected outcome of bronchodilator therapy for B.T. is that he will have an adequate respiratory status as evidenced by the absence of adventitious breath sounds, PEF readings in the "green" range, and a normal ar-

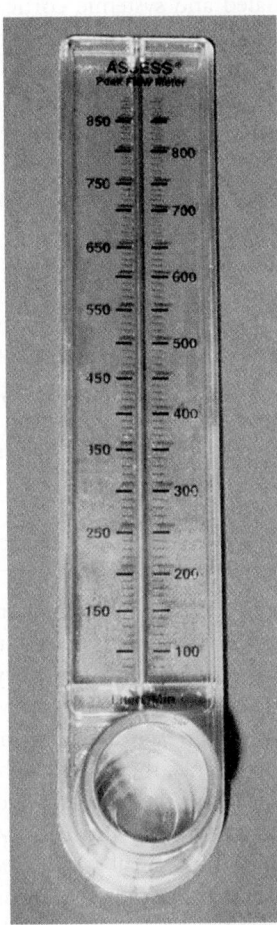

FIGURE 37-5 Peak flow meter.

terial blood oxygen saturation of 95% or more. If B.T. had been in acute distress, ABGs would be obtained, and they would be within normal limits (PaO$_2$ greater than 80 mm Hg, PaCO$_2$ 35 to 45 mm Hg), pH 7.35 to 7.45. Respirations are unlabored and within the normal limits for age. He describes the disease process and his precipitating factors, maintains his asthma "diary," describes the importance of taking his various medications, appropriately contacts his prescriber if he experiences a "yellow" or "red" reading on his PEF meter, and collaborates with his health care providers for monitoring and treatment of his asthma by keeping scheduled appointments.

✳ **B.T. experiences daily asthma attacks. His peak flow readings are about 70% of his predicted best. His attacks appear to be triggered by animal dander and pollen. His prescriber initiates inhaled corticosteroid therapy with fluticasone (Flovent Rotadisk) one inhalation 100 mcg twice daily and starts B.T. on the leukotriene antagonist montelukast (Singulair) 10 mg daily in the evening. The prescriber is also considering the addition of nedocromil inhalation two puffs four times daily if B.T.'s attacks persist.**

✳ **What is the role of agents that target inflammation in the treatment of asthma?**
Inflammation is an important component of persistent asthma. Antiinflammatory agents that affect leukotrienes, including the inhaled and systemic corticosteroids such as prednisone and the leukotriene antagonists, are important modalities to prevent future attacks, and, to some degree, limit inflammatory progression of an existing attack. Antiinflammatory agents that target cyclooxygenase (e.g., the cyclooxygenase (COX)-1 and 2 and the COX-2 inhibitors like ibuprofen and celecoxib respectively) do not help asthma management, and may in fact trigger attacks. Agents that stabilize the mast cell membrane from degranulation (e.g., cromolyn [Intal]) are also useful modalities prophylactically for individuals in whom there is an allergic component to their asthma. Omalizumab (Xolair), a monoclonal antibody with affinity to immunoglobulin (Ig)E on mast cells, is also available for parenteral use in cases of moderate to severe persistent allergic asthma.

Corticosteroids

Corticosteroid drugs are used in chronic asthma to decrease airway obstruction. Corticosteroids are also used in the management of other pulmonary inflammatory states, such as that observed with exposure to pulmonary toxins (see the Pharmacologic Issues in an Age of Terrorism box on p. 711). As antiinflammatory agents, they stabilize the membranes of lysosomes, thus preventing the release of hydrolytic enzymes that produce the inflammatory process in the tissues. The exact mechanism in asthma is still poorly understood but involves the suppression of antibody formation that is responsible for provoking the asthmatic attack. Additionally, corticosteroids inhibit the synthesis of leukotriene, thus reducing bronchoconstriction and mucus secretion.

Daily administration of systemic (e.g., oral, parenteral) corticosteroid therapy provides great therapeutic benefits, but the high incidence of adverse effects has led to the use of short-term or alternate-day schedule of treatment when possible. These agents are most often reserved for severe persistent asthma, and usually dosed for very short courses (e.g., 5 to 10 days) in tapering doses ("burst" or "pulse" dosing) to prevent suppression of the body's normal release of cortisol from the adrenal gland. Alternate-day regimens provide the best risk-benefit ratio for prolonged therapy because they minimize the likelihood of unwanted adverse effects. The corticosteroids generally used have an intermediate-acting duration of action. Chapter 48 discusses corticosteroids, including prednisone, prednisolone, and methylprednisolone.

Chronic use of the inhaled steroid aerosols has resulted in a decrease in bronchial hyperreactivity and respiratory symptoms. Inhaled corticosteroids are the most important therapeutic agents for the pharmacologic control of pulmonary inflammation in clients with moderate persistent asthma. For clients with mild persistent asthma, inhaled corticosteroids offer less benefit but are still recommended in national guidelines (Boushey et al., 2005). Inhaled corticosteroids also result in improved outcomes when added to β-agonist therapy in COPD (Calverley et al., 2003). Inhaled corticosteroid therapy offers the possibility of limiting action at the site of application and thereby avoiding the systemic effects of the oral agents. By chemically modifying the structural arrangement of the steroid molecule, compounds have been developed to diminish systemic absorption from the respiratory tract. The products available for inhaled therapy of asthma are beclomethasone (Vanceril, Beclovent), budesonide (Pulmicort), flunisolide (AeroBid), and triamcinolone (Azmacort).

Inhaled corticosteroids offer the advantage of producing few systemic adverse effects, including that of limited or no adrenal suppression and a lower risk for developing osteoporosis (Elmstahl, 2003), and appear well tolerated during pregnancy (Dombrowski et al., 2004). The aerosols are rapidly absorbed from the pulmonary tissues with limited GI absorption. The maximum improvement in pulmonary function may take 1 to 4 weeks. The adverse effects of the corticosteroid drugs include abdominal distress, anorexia, cough without infection, dizziness, headache, unpleasant taste in the mouth, and oral fungal infection or candidiasis. Table 37-4 compares the inhaled corticosteroids.

Leukotriene Antagonists

Zafirlukast (Accolate), zileuton (Zyflo), and montelukast (Singulair) are inhibitors of the leukotriene receptors and block lipoxygenase. By doing so, these drugs interfere with the formation of substances that cause mucus plugs and constrict bronchial airways. Clinically, they reduce the inflammation, mucus secretion, and bronchoconstriction associated with asthma. As with β-agonists, most (but not all) clients fully respond to these agents. See the Special Considerations for Pharmacogenetics box on p. 702. The leukotriene antagonists are not quite as effective as the corticosteroids in preventing future asthma attacks (Ducharme, 2003), but they are often used in mild to moderate persistent asthma to improve management. All three agents are available on the North American market. Montelukast, however, allows for once daily dosing and has fewer potential drug interactions than the other two agents. Table 37-4 compares these three agents.

⁂ Pharmacologic Issues in an Age of Terrorism

Pulmonary Toxins

It is important for the nurse to recognize the types of agents that could be used in a terrorist attack. A number of aerosolized agents can pose a risk if released into the environment. Chapter 21 discusses those gases that are systemically absorbed and affect parasympathetic nervous system (nerve gases) (Pharmacologic Issues in an Age of Terrorism box, pp. 432 and 433). Chapters 58, 59, and 62 discuss aerosolized or airborne infectious agents (e.g., anthrax, smallpox). Chapter 65 discusses those agents that are toxic to skin and mucous membranes, and are referred to as vesicants (Pharmacologic Issues in an Age of Terrorism box, p. 1166). Chapter 72 discusses other toxins, including cyanide (Pharmacologic Issues in an Age of Terrorism box, p. 1289). This box discusses agents that are aerosolized and are directly toxic to bronchopulmonary tissue.

Among the lung irritants are chlorine, phosgene, and perfluoroisobutylene. Sulfur mustard (mustard gas) is considered a vesicant that is damaging to mucous membranes, bronchioles, and dermal tissue. It is discussed more fully in Chapter 65 (Pharmacologic Issues in an Age of Terrorism box, p. 1166). Chlorine, phosgene and mustard gas were used as part of chemical warfare during World War I. Their use alarmed many and prompted much debate about the use of such agents during war. The effects of these lung irritants include direct damage to the respiratory tract, significant hypersensitivity reactions or, possibly, asphyxiation.

Chlorine

Chlorine has a distinct bleach-like odor and is heavier than air. The odor threshold is typically 0.2 to 0.4 parts per million (ppm). Irritation to the eyes and nose is noted at about 1 ppm, and it may be considered a significant health risk at levels above 10 ppm.

Presentation

Mild exposure to chlorine can result in a choking/suffocation sensation, bronchospasm, chest tightness, cough, and irritation to the eyes and nose. Higher exposures also result in hoarseness and pulmonary edema within a few hours. Very high exposures also produce severe dyspnea, pulmonary edema within 30 to 60 minutes, and increased airway secretions. Such very high exposures can induce laryngospasm and be lethal.

Management

The principles of management include limiting or preventing further exposure, controlling the airway, and reducing exertion on the part of the victim. Corticosteroids (e.g., prednisone) have helped reduce inflammation and pulmonary edema related to these toxins.

Phosgene

Phosgene, like chlorine, is heavier than air. The odor threshold is 1.5 ppm, but it may produce injury before odor is recognized. At higher levels, its odor is similar to freshly mown hay or green corn.

Presentation

With low exposures, cough and dyspnea may be the only presenting signs. Moderate exposures result in irritation to the eyes with tearing. High levels produce severe cough, dyspnea, and pulmonary edema typically within 2 to 6 hours, although the onset of symptoms may be delayed 24 hours or more in some cases. Laryngospasm is also possible and increases the risk for fatality.

Management

Management is similar to chlorine. Strict bed rest should be maintained. Any exertion has the potential to precipitate a sudden onset and often fatal pulmonary edema.

Perfluoroisobutylene (PFIBs)

Perfluoroisobutylene is an organofluoride polymer used in many commercial applications as a sealant or protectant (e.g., Teflon). Aerosolized exposure is highest when these polymers are ignited and release toxic fumes.

Presentation

Typically clients will have been exposed to smoke inhalation of toxic polymer fumes. In moderate to severe cases, pulmonary edema, high fever (as high as 104° F), and flu-like cough, chills, sore throat, and chest tightness are observed.

Management

Management is similar to chlorine and phosgene. Bed rest should be encouraged.

Data from Evison, D., Hinsley, D., Rice, P. (2002). Chemical weapons. British Medical Journal. 2002;324(72333), 332–335; Emergency Preparedness and Response: Center for Disease Control. Accessed February 22, 2003, at http://www.bt.cdc.gov; Maynard, R.M., & Tetley, T.D., (2004). Bioterrorism: the lung under attack. *Thorax, 59*(3), 188-189; Reilly, C.M., & Deason, D. (2003). How would you respond to a chemical release? *Nursing,33*(1), 36-43; and Stokes, E., Gilbert-Palmer, D., Skorga, P., Young, C., & Persell, D. (2004). Chemical agents of terrorism: Preparing nurse practitioners. *Nurse Practitioner, 29*(5), 30-39.

TABLE 37-4 COMPARISON OF ASTHMA ANTIINFLAMMATORY AGENTS

Drug	Dose Form*	Typical Adult Dose	Comment
INHALED CORTICOSTEROIDS			
beclomethasone dipropionate (Beclovent, Vanceril)	MDI: 42 mcg/puff and 84 mcg/puff	1-4 puffs two to four times daily	Typically administered after bronchodilator therapy to improve lung penetration. Recommend client rinse mouth after use to reduce risk of oral/pharyngeal candidiasis
beclomethasone dipropionate HFA (QVAR)	MDI: 40 mcg/puff and 80 mcg/puff	1-2 puffs two to four times daily	
budesonide (Pulmicort)	DPI: 200 mcg/inhalation	1-4 inhalations twice daily	
flunisolide (AeroBid, AeroBid-M)	MDI: 250 mcg/puff	2-6 puffs twice daily	
fluticasone propionate (Flovent)	MDI: 44, 110, 220 mcg/puff	1-4 puffs twice daily	
triamcinolone acetonide (Azmacort)	DPI: 50, 100, or 250 mcg/inhalation MDI 100 mcg/puff	1-5 puffs three to four times daily	
COMBINATION INHALER			
fluticasone propionate/ salmeterol	salmeterol/fluticasone: 50 mcg/50 mcg per inhalation 50 mcg/100 mcg per inhalation 50 mcg/250 mcg per inhalation	1 puff twice daily	
ORAL CORTICOSTEROID			
prednisone (Deltasone)	Oral tablet, liquid	Varies: Typical "Burst/Pulse" Dosing: Day 1: 60 mg Day 5: 20 mg Day 2: 50 mg Day 6: 10 mg Day 3: 40 mg Day 7: 0 mg Day 4: 30 mg	See Chapter 48 for use of systemic corticosteroids
LEUKOTRIENE ANTAGONISTS			
montelukast (Singulair)	Oral tablet, granules	10 mg daily in the evening	See text
zafirlukast (Accolate)	Oral tablet	20 mg twice daily	
zileuton (Zyflo)	Oral tablet	600 mg four times daily	
MAST CELL STABILIZERS			
cromolyn (Intal)	MDI: 800 mcg/puff NEB: 20 mg/2 mL	2 puffs four times daily or 20 mg NEB four times daily	Not for PRN use Dose may ↓ to twice daily if stable
nedocromil (Tilade)	MDI: 1.75 mg/puff	2 puffs four times daily	
ANTI IgE MONOCLONAL ANTIBODY			
omalizumab (Xolair)	Injection	150-375 mg subcutaneously every 2-4 weeks Dose dependent on age and IgE levels	See prescribing information for further details

Modified from Lacy, C.F., Armstrong, L.L., Goldman, M.P., Lance, L.L. (2004). *Lexi-Comp's Drug Information Handbook* (12th ed.). Hudson, Ohio: Lexi-Comp.
*MDI, Metered Dose Inhaler; *DPI*, Dry Powder Inhaler; *NEB*, Nebulizer solution.

✴☐ montelukast [mon **tee** loo cast]

(Singulair)

Indications

Montelukast is indicated for the prophylaxis and chronic treatment of asthma in adults and children older than 1 year old. It is also indicated for the treatment of seasonal allergic rhinitis in adults and children older than 2 years.

Pharmacokinetics/Dosing

Montelukast is rapidly absorbed and bound to plasma proteins (mainly albumin). The onset of action occurs after the first dose, and peak levels are reached in 3 to 4 hours; the duration of action of montelukast is 24 hours. It is metabolized in the liver and excreted primarily in feces. The adult and adolescent dosage of montelukast, it is 10 mg PO in the evening.

Daily dose for those younger than 5 years old is 4 mg daily whereas those aged 6 to 14 years old are treated with 5 mg daily.

Adverse Effects

The adverse effects of montelukast include headache, GI distress, weakness, cough, dental pain, fever, nasal congestion, and rash.

Drug Interactions

Montelukast in metabolized by P450 2 C8/9 and 3 A4, but clinically important interactions have not been identified.

Mast Cell Stabilizers

Cromolyn (Intal) and nedocromil (Tilade) are antiinflammatory agents that inhibit the release of histamine, leukotrienes, and other mediators of inflammation from mast cells, macrophages, and other cells associated with asthma. Neither drug has any bronchodilator effect, nor do they have any effect on inflammatory mediators already released in the body. While not officially a mast cell stabilizer, the monoclonal antibody omalizumab (Xolair) binds to IgE on mast cells and is used subcutaneously every 2 to 4 weeks for clients with more severe persistent allergic asthma.

✴☐ cromolyn [**kroe** moe lin]

(Intal, Apo-Cromolyn✤)

Indications

Cromolyn is indicated for the prevention of bronchospasm and bronchial asthmatic attacks. It has no benefit for treating asthma acutely, and inconsistent or "PRN" intake results in little or no benefit.

Pharmacokinetics/Dosing

Administered by oral inhalation, cromolyn has approximately 8% to 10% absorption in the lungs; it has an onset of action within 4 weeks and is excreted in the kidneys and bile. The dosage of cromolyn for adults and children (5 years of age and older) to prevent bronchial asthma is two oral inhalations (1.6 or 2 mg) four times daily at 4- or 6-hour intervals. A dosage has not been established for children younger than 5 years old.

Adverse Effects

The adverse effects of cromolyn and other mast cell stabilizers include cough, hoarseness, dry mouth or throat, nasal congestion, sneezing, diarrhea, myalgia, difficulty sleeping, stomach pain, rash, sneezing, bronchospasm, and a bad taste in the mouth after use of the inhaler.

omalizumab [oh mah **liz** uh mab]

(Xolair)

Omalizumab is an IgG antibody derived from recombinant genetic technology that binds to IgE receptor sites on the mast cell. Its use requires regular subcutaneous injections every 2 to 4 weeks based on IgE levels and is not effective in managing acute attacks.

Indications

Omalizumab is indicated for moderate to severe persistent asthma know to be allergic in nature. Its use in generally limited to clients who have had inadequate control with high-dose inhaled corticosteroids and other modalities.

Pharmacokinetics/Dosing

It is slowly absorbed following subcutaneous injection and reaches its peak action about 7 days after administration. It is available as an injection in 150-mg increments and doses range from 150 mg every 4 weeks up to 375 mg every 2 weeks depending on client weight and baseline IgE serum levels. The maximum dose per injection site is 150 mg.

Adverse Effects

Local injection site irritation is the most common reaction noted. Other reactions include an increased rate of viral or respiratory tract infections, headache, joint pain, and fatigue.

✳ How should B.T.'s antiinflammatory regimen be managed?

Because inflammation is a major component of B.T.'s asthma, inhalation corticosteroid therapy (fluticasone) and montelukast (Singulair) are added to the therapeutic regimen. The assessment of his respiratory status is continued as described earlier in the case for bronchodilating drugs as is the planning and evaluation process.

Assessment Before initiating corticosteroid therapy, assess B.T. for preexisting health conditions that might contraindicate the use of inhalation corticosteroids, such as ocular herpes simplex or an untreated systemic infection that might be worsened by the use of the drug. Tuberculosis may be reactivated with long-term corticosteroid inhalation therapy; so if B.T. has a positive Mantoux test, he would require careful monitoring. B.T.'s age is of concern because significant systemic absorption of inhaled corticosteroids as the result of high dosages over an extended period has been reported to cause growth inhibition in children and adolescents related to hypothalamic-pituitary-adrenal (HPA) axis suppression. Obtain his height and weight as part of the baseline assessment. With adults, glaucoma and cataracts may result. With the use of properly administered doses of inhalation corticosteroid, systemic adverse effects do not often occur unless the client has bronchitis or is taking systemic corticosteroid drugs; in such cases, all concerns related to systemic corticosteroids may occur (see Chapter 48). Sensitivity to montelukast is the only contraindication for Singulair.

A baseline assessment of B.T.'s respiratory status should be completed (see the assessment within the nursing management of bronchodilator drug therapy, p. 705). Drug interactions are unlikely to occur with the usual dosages of inhalation corticosteroids.

Nursing Diagnosis With the administration of corticosteroids by inhalation, B.T. is at risk for the following nursing diagnoses/collaborative problems: impaired comfort (unpleasant taste, dry/irritated mouth and throat, and cough and hoarseness without signs of infection, headache, nausea); and the potential complications of oral candidiasis (creamy, white patches within the mouth), monilial esophagitis (difficulty in swallowing), upper respiratory tract infection, bronchospasm, and allergic reaction. Psychologic changes (nervousness, restlessness, depression) have been reported with fluticasone. For montelukast, there may be altered comfort (headache) and the potential complication of elevated hepatic enzymes.

Planning Therapeutic goals for B.T. are the same as for bronchodilator drugs. The emphasis for these inhalers is prevention of asthmatic episodes.

Implementation

Monitoring Monitor B.T.'s respiratory status on an ongoing basis to evaluate the effectiveness of the drug. Monitor for adverse effects of corticosteroid therapy and symptoms of overdosage, cushingoid syndrome (fullness of face, neck and trunk, elevated BP, muscle wasting, weakness, growth velocity retardation, emotional change). Record his height and weight at each visit to determine his growth pattern. Check B.T.'s proper use of the inhaler at periodic intervals.

Intervention When B.T. uses a separate bronchodilator inhaler, it should be used 15 minutes before the corticosteroid inhalation. This opens the respiratory passages to allow for greater penetration of the fluticasone. If B.T.'s response to the corticosteroid begins to diminish, the prescriber should be notified so the dosage can be adjusted. Box 37-4 reviews the inhalants used for the treatment of asthma. The use of a spacer greatly decreases the occurrence of candidiasis and hoarseness. Montelukast is available in regular tablets or chewable tablets for use in children 6 to 15 years of age. Taper montelukast dosage when the drug is being discontinued.

Education Stress the importance of self-management as previously described. Alert B.T. that oral fungal infections may occur with inhaled corticosteroids. Instruct him to examine his mouth daily for redness and/or white patches indicative of candidiasis. He can prevent infection by rinsing his mouth after each treatment and washing and drying the inhaler thoroughly after each use.

Stress the importance of compliance with the daily regimen with montelukast for the prevention of asthmatic episodes even if symptom free. This drug may allow for a decrease in the corticosteroid dosage. Although its use is not for the management of acute asthma, it is not to be discontinued during these episodes. Alert B.T. that he should always have rescue medications available even though he takes his corticosteroid inhaler and the montelukast daily.

Evaluation The expected outcome of B.T.'s corticosteroid inhalation therapy is as described for bronchodilating drugs. Additionally, he will not experience the adverse effects of corticosteroid therapy.

✳ **If B.T.'s prescriber determines that he also requires the addition of nedocromil to his existing regimen of bronchodilators and/or inhaled corticosteroid for**

BOX 37-4 NURSING REVIEW: INHALANTS FOR ASTHMA TREATMENT

With the wide variety of medications that may be used concurrently for the treatment of asthma, the nurse should be aware of the following:

- For prophylactic use, the antiinflammatory inhalation drugs cromolyn (Intal) or nedocromil (Tilade) are recommended to decrease airway hyperactivity. These drugs have no bronchodilator effects, and so, no role in the treatment of acute asthmatic attacks.
- Corticosteroid inhalers such as beclomethasone (Beclovent, Vanceril), flunisolide (AeroBid), etc., are for preventive use only, and they may cause localized fungal infections in the mouth and pharynx. Advise client to rinse mouth with water or mouthwash after each use and also to thoroughly rinse and dry the inhaler tip after each use. This will help reduce the incidence of dry, sore throat and oropharyngeal candidiasis.
- β_2-agonist inhalers have no antiinflammatory effects but are considered the most effective drugs for treatment of acute bronchospasm and asthma. Subcutaneous injection of β-agonists has not been found to be more effective than inhalation, and it has been reported to cause more systemic adverse effects.
- Multiple inhalers and/or inhaler combinations of a β agonist, anticholinergic, and/or corticosteroid are often used to optimize bronchodilation and reduce inflammation.

WHAT INSTRUCTIONS WOULD YOU OFFER THE CLIENT WITH ASTHMA?

Instruct the client in the proper technique for use of a metered-dose inhaler (MDI) and other inhaling devises as ordered. Spacer units are often suggested for young children and at times, other clients with coordination difficulties also may benefit from their use. Home use of peak flow meters and the documentation of the results are often recommended for clients with moderate to severe asthma. Peak flow meters objectively measures peak expiratory flow (PEF) rate and daily variability determinations before and after use of medications, especially bronchodilators. With proper use, this device may help in the early detection of airflow obstruction, which allows for timely intervention.

Inhalers with combinations of corticosteroids and bronchodilators may improve adherence, but their use is limited to chronic management of stable asthma. If the prescriber has not given specific dosing instructions for individuals inhalers, generally the order of administration to obtain optimal drug effects is as follows:

1. The β-agonist is used first to open the airways.
2. The anticholinergic agent is administered.
3. The corticosteroid is administered.

Instruct client to wait approximately 5 minutes between each medication and to rinse mouth thoroughly without swallowing the rinse, after the corticosteroid dose.

bronchospasm prophylaxis, what additional nursing management is required?

If nedocromil is added to B.T.'s antiinflammatory therapy, a reduction in dosage of the corticosteroid or bronchodilator may be achieved. Even without the addition of mast cell stabilizers, nearly half of clients with moderate to severe asthma can tolerate a reduction in inhaled corticosteroid therapy once stable (Hawkins et al., 2003). However, the dosage reduction will be gradual and under close supervision of his prescriber to avoid an exacerbation of asthma. A decrease in the severity of his symptoms or in the need for his concomitant therapy will usually be evident in the first 2 to 4 weeks of nedocromil.

If B.T. requires a mast cell stabilizer, the nursing management of his drug therapy would be as listed in the following sections.

Assessment During the initial assessment, determine that B.T. does not have a sensitivity to nedocromil. Documentation, as described previously, of a baseline history of his frequency and severity of asthma episodes will help with the evaluation of drug therapy.

Nursing Diagnosis With the administration of nedocromil, B.T. has the potential for impaired comfort (unpleasant taste, headache, throat irritation, nausea), impaired airway clearance (rhinitis, cough) or the potential complications of arthritis, neutropenia, leukopenia, or increased bronchospasm because of sensitivity to the drug or fluorocarbon propellants.

Planning Therapeutic goals for B.T. are the same as for previously discussed drugs. The emphasis is on prevention of asthmatic episodes.

Implementation

Monitoring Monitor B.T. for the frequency and intensity of asthma attacks or other symptoms of allergy.

Intervention Nedocromil helps to prevent but does not relieve asthma or bronchospasm attacks. It may be continued during an attack unless B.T. becomes intolerant to the use of inhaled drugs. If B.T. is also using a bronchodilator inhaler, he should use it 15 minutes before the nedocromil inhalation.

Education Ensure B.T. can administer the drug correctly. Caution B.T. to avoid getting the medication in his eyes if using the aerosol form. Teach B.T. to rinse the mouth and gargle after an inhalation treatment to relieve dryness of the mouth and throat and the unpleasant aftertaste. Advise B.T. to prime his nedocromil inhaler with three sprays into the air before using it the first time or if it has not been used in more than 7 days. Instruct B.T. not to float the canister to test fullness but to keep a record of sprays.

Advise B.T. and his parents that it may be as long as 4 weeks before the drug is fully beneficial. Compliance with the regimen is necessary to achieve these results. With the use of these prophylactic agents it may be possible to lower the dosages of other antiasthmatic medications. However, alert B.T. that it is important to maintain any concurrent therapies, such as adrenocorticoids, until modified or discontinued by the prescriber. The prescriber should be notified if his condition does not improve or worsens.

Evaluation The expected outcome of nedocromil therapy for B.T. is a reduction in the number of attacks, reduced cough, decreased sputum production, and/or a decreased need for other antiasthma drugs within 4 weeks of initiating therapy. Some clients show improvement in pulmonary function. Only if B.T. demonstrates improvement in 4 weeks should he continue to receive nedocromil.

✷ How are inhaled drugs administered?

Inhaled drugs can be administered primarily by one of three modalities—aerosol by metered-dose inhaler, aerosol by nebulizer, or aerosol by dry powder inhaler. **Aerosol therapy** is a form of inhaled, topical pulmonary treatment. An aerosol is a suspension of fine liquid or solid particles dispersed in a gas or in a solution that is deposited in the respiratory tract. Liquid or solid particles range in size from approximately 0.005 to 50 μm in diameter. Nebulizers are devices that disperse a solution into a maximum number of particles of a desired size for inhalation. The terms *aerosol therapy* and *nebulization therapy* are often used interchangeably. Aerosol therapy promotes the following:

- Bronchodilation and pulmonary decongestion
- Loosening of secretions
- Topical application of corticosteroids and other drugs
- Moistening, cooling, or heating of inspired air

The effectiveness of nebulization therapy depends on the number of droplets that can be suspended in an inhaled aerosol. This number is directly related to the size of the droplets, with smaller droplets suspended in greater numbers than large droplets. Small droplets (approximately 2 to 4 μm in diameter) are more likely to reach the periphery of the lungs—the alveolar ducts and sacs. Small droplets are more effective for the absorption of bronchodilators. Larger droplets (8 to 15 μm in diameter) are deposited primarily in the bronchioles and bronchi. Droplets of more than 40 μm in diameter are deposited primarily in the upper airway (mouth, pharynx, trachea, and main bronchi).

The rate and depth of breathing are other factors that determine the effectiveness of nebulization therapy. Rapid or shallow breathing decreases the number, and the retention, of droplets that reach the periphery of the lungs. Rapid breathing permits significant amounts of fine droplets to escape during expirations; few droplets will escape if the breath is held long enough after deep inspiration to permit droplet deposit in the lung periphery.

Almost all large droplets are retained somewhere in the larger air passages. Large droplets are used for keeping large airways (nose, trachea) moist and for loosening secretions. Slow and deep breathing is required for proper lung aeration and penetration of the mist into peripheral lung areas. The breath should be held for a few seconds after a full inspiration.

✿ Medication Safety Alert

Drug Reconcentration with Jet and Ultrasonic Nebulizers

Drug reconcentration can occur with both jet and ultrasonic nebulizers if a humidity deficit occurs. The evaporation of water molecules causes a gradual increase in drug concentration in the droplets, thus increasing the risk of drug toxicity. Controlling temperature and humidity can prevent this toxicity.

It is important to remember that the lung is an absorptive organ and is therefore a route of access for drugs to enter the systemic circulation. When used as a method of administering drugs, aerosol therapy is supposed to minimize systemic absorption and adverse effects. Certain bronchodilator aerosols produce cardiovascular effects simply because the drug may possess a property that adversely influences cardiac action after absorption into the bloodstream.

Droplet size can be controlled by the amount of pressure used to force oxygen or room air through the solution to produce a mist. The nebulizer tubing diameter, its length, and its number of bends affect turbulent flow and mist temperature. With most nebulizers the maximum density of the inhaled mist is achieved by making the flow of mist as smooth and direct as possible. Nebulizers commonly used in hospitals produce similar mists. See also the Medication Safety Alert box above.

When combination inhalation aerosols are prescribed for a client without specific instructions for the sequence of administration, the nurse should be aware of the proper recommendations for drug administration. The most efficacious of the client's bronchodilators is administered first. For example, if corticosteroids (Beclovent, Vanceril) or cromolyn (Intal) or nedocromil (Tilade) are prescribed to be administered with ipratropium (Atrovent), the ipratropium should be administered 5 minutes before either of the other drugs to promote bronchodilation. Whenever a β-agonist (Alupent, Proventil) is prescribed with ipratropium (Atrovent), the β-agonist is always administered first, with a 5-minute wait before administration of the second drug. Combined albuterol and ipratropium solution is now common for nebulizers to help prevent confusion and promote compliance. Do not administer separate aerosols in rapid sequence, because there is the possibility of inducing fluorocarbon toxicity; such rapid administration also decreases the effectiveness of the drug. Advair contains fluticasone and salmeterol in fixed dosage and is administered by a combined inhaler device. Combivent contains ipratropium and albuterol combined in an aerosol container. It is indicated for bronchospasm in clients with COPD.

✿ What drugs improve the clearance of respiratory tract secretions?

Drugs that improve clearance of respiratory tract secretions can be categorized as either mucokinetic agents (expectorants), mucolytic agents, or agents that suppress bronchial secretions. **Mucokinetic agents** promote the removal of abnormal or excessive respiratory tract secretions by thinning hyperviscous mucus, which allows for a more effective ciliary action. **Mucolytic agents** actually serve to breakdown mucus. The term **expectorant** is often used to describe an agent that has mucokinetic and/or mucolytic properties. Drugs with antimuscarinic properties suppress bronchial secretions, but may serve to thicken existing secretions. The antimuscarinics (e.g., ipratropium [Atrovent]) are primarily used for their bronchodilator effects. Chapters 14 and 21 discuss the antimuscarinic scopolamine transdermal sometimes used in palliative care to reduce respiratory secretions.

Sputum (or phlegm) may be defined as an abnormal, viscous secretion that is an excretory production of the lower respiratory tree. It consists mainly of **mucus,** a proteinaceous material that has a mucopolysaccharide as its major component. Additionally, sputum contains deoxyribonucleic acid (DNA) molecules, which are derived from the breakdown of mucosal cells, leukocytes, and bacteria. These products are responsible for the characteristic heavy quality and yellow color of the sputum. The terms *sputum* and *mucus* should not be used interchangeably. Sputum is an abnormal secretion originating in the lower respiratory tract, whereas mucus is a normal secretion produced by the surface cells in the mucous membrane.

Individuals with respiratory disorders such as chronic bronchitis develop disturbances of the mucociliary blanket, resulting in a significant impairment of the process of mucus clearance (see Figure 37-1). Mucus plugging and the pathogenic colonization of microorganisms occur in the lower respiratory tract. These changes lead to an overproduction of thick, tenacious sputum. The advantage provided by the adequate hydration is that they alter the consistency of the sputum, thereby promoting the eventual expectoration, or expulsion, of these secretions.

Water and hydration is probably the most effective mucokinetic agent. Maintaining adequate hydration and administering water by nebulizer can help prevent sputum retention, which may result from abnormal ciliary activity, defects in airflow, or a modification in cough effectiveness. Guaifenesin is the only expectorant listed by the Food and Drug Administration (FDA) in Category I (safe and effective); Chapter 11 reviews its usage.

Diluents

Water

The most commonly used agent to dilute respiratory secretions is water. Persons with COPD often suffer from dehydration; thus respiratory secretions are retained. These secretions become highly viscous in consistency and lead to widespread plug formation in the respiratory tree. Water may be administered by ultrasonic **nebulizer,** a device for producing a fine spray. Small amounts of water deposited on the gel layer of the respiratory tree appear to reduce the adhesive characteristics and general viscosity of the gelatinous substances found in this layer. Care is needed with clients receiving restricted fluid intake, because water can be absorbed through the inhalation route. If fluid intake is being measured, water added to the nebulizer and absorbed through the inhalation route must be added to the client's intake record. If a client's fluid intake is not restricted, large amounts of water are usually encouraged to liquefy the respiratory secretions.

Saline Solutions

Normal saline (0.9% sodium chloride) is a physiologic (isotonic) salt solution that exerts the same osmotic pressure as plasma fluids. Therapy by nebulization is well tolerated, resulting in the hydration of respiratory secretions. A hypotonic solution (0.45% sodium chloride) is thought to provide deeper penetration into the more distal airways or into the alveoli via the inhalation route, whereas inhalation of a hypertonic solution (1.8% sodium chloride) stimulates a productive cough because the particles deposited on the respiratory mucosa are irritating. A hypertonic solution osmotically attracts fluid out of the mucosa and into the respiratory secretions, thereby promoting their excretion.

Mucolytics

Mucolytics exert a disintegrating effect on mucus and promote coughing or spitting and thereby the removal of mucus or other exudates from the lung, bronchi, or trachea. Examples of mucolytics are acetylcysteine and dornase alfa.

acetylcysteine [ah see tyl **sis** teen]
(Mucomyst, Acetadote, Parvolex✚)
Acetylcysteine reduces the thickness and stickiness of purulent and nonpurulent pulmonary secretions by decreasing the viscosity of the respiratory mucoprotein molecules into smaller, more soluble and less viscous strands. It also effects similar changes in the DNA molecule and cellular debris. This decrease in the viscosity of bronchial secretions aids their removal by coughing, postural drainage, or suctioning.

When administered systemically, acetylcysteine is a specific antidote for an acetaminophen overdose; it reduces the extent of liver injury by altering hepatic metabolism, and it maintains or restores concentrations of glutathione. Glutathione is necessary for inactivation of an intermediate metabolite of acetaminophen, which is believed to be hepatotoxic on accumulation.

Indications
Acetylcysteine is indicated as an adjunct treatment for thick or abnormal mucus in bronchopulmonary disease, cystic fibrosis, or atelectasis caused by a mucus obstruction. It is also used as a diagnostic aid in a variety of bronchial studies, such as bronchospirometry and bronchograms. The benefit of acetylcysteine in COPD appears limited (Decramer et al., 2005). Acetylcysteine is also the antidote for acetaminophen (Tylenol) overdose and Chapter 14 discusses its usage.

Pharmacokinetics/Dosing
With inhalation therapy, some acetylcysteine is absorbed from the pulmonary epithelium, although its primary effects are local on the mucus in the lungs. It produces an effect within 1 minute when inhaled; direct instillation via an intratracheal catheter produces an immediate effect. The peak response from inhalation occurs within 5 to 10 minutes. Acetylcysteine is metabolized in the liver. The usual dosage for adults and children by nebulization using a face mask,

mouthpiece, or tracheostomy is 3 to 5 mL of a 20% solution or 6 to 10 mL of a 10% solution inhaled three or four times daily. To treat an acetaminophen overdose, acetylcysteine is administered orally in a dose of 140 mg/kg initially, then 70 mg/kg every 4 hours for an additional 17 doses.

Adverse Effects
The adverse effects of acetylcysteine include fever, nausea, vomiting, runny nose, throat or lung irritation, unpleasant odor during drug administration, clammy skin, sore mouth, stomatitis, hemoptysis, rash, and respiratory difficulties. No significant drug interactions have been reported with acetylcysteine when administered by inhalation.

Nursing Management
Assessment
Use acetylcysteine with caution in older adults, in debilitated clients, and in clients with asthma or severe respiratory insufficiency. This drug may increase airway obstruction with respiratory secretions, and/or bronchospasm may occur in susceptible clients. Determine the client's sensitivity to acetylcysteine.

Nursing Diagnosis
With the administration of acetylcysteine, the client is at risk for the following nursing diagnoses/collaborative problems: impaired comfort related to the unpleasant odor of the drug during administration, facial stickiness after nebulization by face mask, nausea or vomiting, and throat irritation; impaired oral mucous membrane (stomatitis); ineffective airway clearance related to increased amounts of sputum; and the potential complications of allergic dermatitis and bronchospastic allergic reaction.

Planning
The client receiving acetylcysteine therapy will:
• Develop a productive cough
• Be able to expectorate mucus effectively
• Have clear or improved breath sounds
• Effectively manage the acetylcysteine therapy

Implementation
Monitoring
Observe and document the frequency of the client's cough, its character, and the character and quantity of expectorated material. Percuss and auscultate the chest on a periodic basis.
Intervention
Ultrasonic nebulizers are recommended for administration of acetylcysteine. Hand nebulizers are discouraged because the output is too small and the fluid particles too large. The prescriber may order the administration of a bronchodilator before acetylcysteine therapy. The nebulized drug may be inhaled either directly or by the use of a plastic face mask, mouthpiece, tracheostomy, or croupette. The nebulizer may be used with an intermittent positive pressure breathing (IPPB) apparatus. An IPPB apparatus is a ventilator that assists or controls respiration by delivering compressed gas under positive pressure into a person's airways until a preset pressure is reached. Passive exhalation is allowed through a valve, and the cycle begins again as the flow of gas is triggered by inhalation. When the drug is nebulized using a drying gas, the drug may become concentrated because of evaporation of the solution. The last remaining quarter of the drug can be diluted with an equal part of sterile water for injection to continue nebulization so the client is ensured of receiving the appropriate dosage.

After nebulization, encourage the client to wash the face with water to remove the sticky coating left by the drug. Clean the equipment immediately after use to prevent blockage of the fine parts and corrosion of the metal ones. In many health care agencies, respiratory therapists administer these treatments, but nurses are responsible for evaluating the effectiveness of treatments, and they may be responsible for administering them at night and with the client in the home.

Some clients may develop nausea and vomiting; this may result from the disagreeable odor of the nebulized drug and quantity of respiratory secretions eliminated. With the aid of these agents and postural drainage, most individuals can expectorate pulmonary secretions without further assistance; however, suctioning may be indicated for older adults or debilitated clients. Provide mouth care after inhalation treatment to minimize nausea and vomiting.

Because of the release of hydrogen sulfide, solutions of acetylcysteine will harden rubber and become discolored on contact with certain metals. Acetylcysteine solutions should be used with equipment made of glass, plastic, or stainless steel. If the vacuum seal has been broken on the bottle, the solution should be refrigerated to slow oxidation and used within 48 hours.

Education

Alert the client to the disagreeable odor of the drug and the expected result of increased expectoration. Teach the client to clear the airway by coughing before the drug is administered by aerosol. Provide instructions on the correct use of the nebulizer.

Evaluation

The expected outcome of acetylcysteine mucolytic therapy is that the client will experience increased sputum production and expectoration and a decrease or absence of adventitious breath sounds. The client will effectively manage the acetylcysteine therapy, including medication compliance, correct use of the nebulizer, and collaboration with the health care providers for monitoring and follow-up care.

Antidotal Use

When acetylcysteine is administered as an antidote for acetaminophen toxicity, it is most beneficial when started within 10 hours of the overdose, but it is still beneficial if started within the first 24 hours (*USP DI,* 2005). The oral solution is tolerated better if it is well chilled (over ice), diluted in soft drinks or citrus juices, and sipped with a straw from a covered container. The diluted solution should be used within the hour. Depending on the nature of the acetaminophen ingestion, the client should be supported through gastric lavage or induced emesis, the administration of activated charcoal, and other appropriate therapies. The greatest risk of acetaminophen overdose is hepatotoxicity. The potential for hepatotoxicity can be assessed from plasma acetaminophen concentrations; monitoring these concentrations and liver function studies is essential. Liver function studies should be performed every 24 hours for at least 96 hours after the ingestion of the overdose. Monitor fluid and electrolyte balances, renal function, and cardiac function. Nursing care is provided for the client with risk for poisoning or a high risk for self-harm.

The expected outcome of acetylcysteine as an antidote for acetaminophen toxicity is that the client's liver function studies will be within normal limits and that the underlying issue, risk for poisoning or high risk for self-harm, will be resolved.

dornase alfa
(Pulmozyme)

Recombinant human DNase or dornase alfa (Pulmozyme) is used to increase expectoration in cystic fibrosis. Cystic fibrosis (CF) is a respiratory disease associated with thick secretions caused by an accumulation of DNA from degenerating neutrophils and inflammation. Dornase alfa is an enzyme that digests extracellular DNA, thus improving pulmonary function and reducing the risk for the respiratory tract infections common with CF. The use of this product has resulted in a decrease in respiratory infections, hospitalizations, and medical costs.

Indications

Management of respiratory status in clients with CF.

Pharmacokinetics/Dosing

A significant improvement in pulmonary function is seen within 3 to 7 days, and a decrease in respiratory infections is seen within weeks to several months. The usual dosage for adults and children 5 years and older is 2.5 mg daily (up to 2.5 mg twice daily) inhaled via nebulization.

Adverse Effects

The adverse effects of dornase alfa include chest pain, sore throat, laryngitis, skin rash, conjunctivitis, hoarseness, upset stomach, dyspnea, fever, and rhinitis.

Nursing Management
Assessment

Determine that the client does not have a sensitivity to dornase alfa. Although drug interactions have not been studied with dornase alfa, it has been administered safely with other medications commonly taken by clients with CF (e.g., bronchodilators, antibiotics, corticosteroids, enzymes, vitamins, and analgesics). Establish a baseline assessment of the client's respiratory status.

Nursing Diagnosis

The client receiving dornase alfa has the potential for the following nursing diagnoses: impaired comfort (chest pain, dyspepsia, sore throat, hoarseness, conjunctivitis); impaired skin integrity (rash); and the potential complication of decreased forced vital capacity.

Planning

The goals for dornase alfa therapy include that the client will:
- Maintain a patent airway and an effective respiratory pattern without adverse drug effects.
- Effectively manage the dornase alfa therapy.

Implementation
Monitoring

Monitor the client's respiratory status carefully for cough, breath sounds, sputum, forced expiratory volume, vital capacity, and tidal volume.

Intervention

Dornase alfa is administered via a nebulizer. Refer to the package literature for recommended devices. Wash hands thoroughly before assembling the nebulizer and mouthpiece. Do not mix or dilute dornase alfa with other agents. It should be administered every day; a decrease in pulmonary function occurs within 48 hours after therapy is stopped.

Education

Instruct the client on the appropriate nebulizer and ensure its correct use with dornase alfa. Advise the client not to use a face mask but only a mouthpiece. Do not use the medication if it is cloudy or discolored. Advise the client to administer the treatment at the same time each day and that compliance is essential. Although some improvement may be seen a week after therapy starts, it may require weeks or months for the full benefits to be experienced.

Evaluation

The expected outcome of dornase alfa therapy is that the client's airway is patent, the breathing pattern is effective without fatigue or dyspnea, and the breath sounds are clear. The client will effectively manage the dornase alfa therapy, including compliance with the medication and collaboration with the health care providers for monitoring and follow-up care.

Summary

In clients with ineffective airway clearance, nursing interventions along with bronchodilator and antiinflammatory drugs are used to control the client's condition. Bronchodilators diminish airway obstruction by bronchial smooth muscle relaxation. β_2-adrenergic agonists and antimuscarinics are the most commonly used bronchodilators, although theophylline is utilized in some clients.

Antiinflammatory drugs are critical in the management of asthma to improve outcomes. Inhaled corticosteroids are the primary antiinflammatory agent used in asthma, with systemic corticosteroids reserved for severe persistent asthma. Other antiinflammatory agents are used to prevent future attacks and include the leukotriene antagonists and mast cell stabilizers. Mucokinetic and mucolytic agents have a more limited role and help promote the removal of abnormal or excessive respiratory tract secretions.

Nursing management of the care of the client receiving these agents is focused on the client experiencing increased ease of respiration, decreased wheezing, and a decrease in medication use. The nurse should stress the need for responsible self-management of the therapeutic medication regimen. The nurse can play a crucial role in reducing the morbidity and mortality of asthma by keeping current on the guidelines and treatment of asthma and by taking an active role in applying the clinical skills of assessment, intervention, client education, and evaluation.

✴ Critical Thinking Questions

- John Holt, 62 years old, was admitted to the hospital with the symptoms of fatigue, weakness, dyspnea, malaise, and a persistent, nonproductive cough. He was diagnosed as having a viral upper respiratory tract infection. Would a mucolytic drug be appropriate for this client? Why or why not?

- What nursing interventions would be considered appropriate to the nursing management of a client receiving either a mucolytic or bronchodilating drug?

- Stanley Myers, 22 years old, a college student with a history of asthma, has come to the clinic for a regularly scheduled visit. In reviewing his inhalant therapy, he indicates that he takes the medications in any order "just to get it over with." What would be the most appropriate response by the nurse?

Bibliography

Anderson, D.M., Keith, J., & Novak, P.D. (Eds.) (2002). *Mosby's medical, nursing, and allied health dictionary* (6th ed.). St. Louis: Mosby.

Anderson, H.R., Ayres, J.G., Sturdy, P.M., Bland, J.M., Butland, B.K., Peckitt, C., et al. (2005). Bronchodilator treatment and deaths from asthma: Case-control study. *British Medical Journal, 330,* 117-120.

Bosker, G. (Ed.). (2004). *Primary and acute care medicine: Practice, protocols, pathways* (2nd ed.). Atlanta: Thomson American Health Consultants.

Boushey, H.A., Sorkness, C.A., King, T.S., Sullivan, S.D., Fahy, J.V., Lazarus, S.C., et al. (2005). Daily versus as-needed corticosteroids

for mild persistent asthma. *New England Journal of Medicine, 352,* 1519-1528.

Brock, T.P., Wessell, A.M., Williams, D.M., et al. (2002). Accuracy of float testing for metered-dose inhaler canisters. *Journal of American Pharmaceutical Association, 42,* 582-586.

Cain, W.T., & Oppenheimer, J.J. (2001). The misconception of using floating patterns as an accurate means of measuring the contents of metered-dose inhaler devices. *Annals of Allergy Asthma & Immunology, 87,* 417-419.

Calverley, P., et al., and the Trial of Inhaled Steroids and Long-Acting Beta2 Agonists Study Group. (2003). Combined salmeterol and fluticasone in the treatment of chronic obstructive pulmonary disease: A randomised controlled trial. *Lancet, 361,* 449-456.

Castro-Rodriguez, J.A., & Rodrigo, G.J. (2004). β-agonists through metered-dose inhaler with valved holding chamber versus nebulizer for acute exacerbation of wheezing or asthma in children under 5 years of age: A systematic review with meta-analysis. *Journal of Pediatrics, 145,*172-177.

Chang, J.T., Altman, R.B. (2004). Extracting and characterizing gene-drug relationships from the literature. Pharmacogenetics, 14(9), 577-586. Retrieved December 2, 2004, from http://bionlp.stanford.edu/genedrug/gene_drug_predictions.html

Chen, Y., Daks, R., Tang, M., & Krewski, D. (2002). Association between income adequacy and asthma in Canadians. *Proceedings of Statistics Canadian Symposium.* Ottawa: Modelling Survey Data for Social and Economic Research.

Chesnutt, M.S., & Prendergast, T.J. (2003). Lung. In L.M. Tierney, Jr., S.J. McPhee, & Papadakis, M.A. (Eds.), *Current Medical Diagnosis & Treatment.* New York: Lange Medical Books/McGraw-Hill.

Cloutier, M.M., Hall, C.B., Wakefield, D.B., & Bailit, H. (2005). Use of asthma guidelines by primary care providers to reduce hospitalizations and emergency department visits in poor, minority, urban children. *Journal of Pediatrics, 146,* 591-597.

Decramer, M., Rutten-van Molken, M., Dekhuijzen, P.N., Troosters, T., van Herwaarden, C., Pellegrino, R., et al. (2005). Effects of N-acetylcysteine on outcomes in chronic obstructive pulmonary disease (Bronchitis Randomized on NAC Cost-Utility Study, BRONCUS): A randomised placebo-controlled trial. *Lancet, 365,* 1552-1560.

Delgado, A., Chou, K.J., Silver, E.J., & Crain, E.F. (2003). Nebulizers vs metered-dose inhalers with spacers for bronchodilator therapy to treat wheezing in children aged 2 to 24 months in a pediatric emergency department. *Archives of Pediatric & Adolescent Medicine, 157,* 76-80.

Dishy, V., et al. (2004). β₂-adrenoceptor Thr164 Ile polymorphism is associated with markedly decreased vasodilator and increased vasoconstrictor sensitivity in vivo. *Pharmacogenetics, 14*(8), 517-522.

𝑒-LEARNING SUPPLEMENTS

Student CD-ROM
- Final Exam questions
- NCLEX® Examination review questions
- Pharmacology animations
- Printable chapter summary

Evolve Website (http://evolve.elsevier.com/mckenry)
- Case study on bronchodilator, antiasthmatic and mucolytic drugs
- Interactive concept map on asthma

- Content updates, including information on new drugs
- WebLinks corresponding to this chapter
- Answers to the critical thinking questions in this chapter
- *Elsevier ePharmacology Update* newsletter
- Mosby's Drug Consult Internet Edition
- Supplemental and reference information

Dombrowski, M.P., et al., and the National Institute of Child Health and Human Development Maternal-Fetal Medicine Units Network; National Heart, Lung, and Blood Institute. (2004). Randomized trial of inhaled beclomethasone dipropionate versus theophylline for moderate asthma during pregnancy. *American Journal of Obstetrics and Gynecology, 190*,737-744.

Drug facts and comparisons (58th ed.). (2005). St. Louis: Facts and Comparisons.

Ducharme, F.M. (2003). Inhaled glucocorticoids versus leukotriene receptor antagonists as single agent asthma treatment: Systematic review of current evidence. *British Medical Journal, 326,* 621-623.

Elmstahl, S., et al. (2003). Is there an association between inhaled corticosteroids and bone density in postmenopausal women? *The Journal of Allergy and Clinical Immunology, 111,* 91-96.

Evans, W.E., McLeod, H.L. (2003). Drug therapy: Pharmacogenomics—drug disposition, drug targets, and side effects. *New England Journal of Medicine, 348*(6), 538-549.

Everard, M.L., et al. (1995). Factors affecting total and "respirable" dose delivered by a salbutamol metered dose inhaler. *Thorax, 50,* 746-749.

FDA Talk Paper T03-06 (January 23, 2003) Study of Asthma-Drug Halted. Washington DC: Food and Drug Administration. Retrieved January 3, 2005, from http://www.fda.gov/bbs/topics/ANSWERS/2003/ANS01192.html

Fukai, H., et al. (2004). Association between a polymorphism in cysteinyl leukotriene receptor 2 on chromosome 13 q14 and atopic asthma. *Pharmacogenetics, 14*(10), 683-690.

Gent, J.F., et al. (2003). Association of low-level ozone and fine particles with respiratory symptoms in children with asthma. *Journal of the American Medical Association, 290,* 1859-1867.

Hartling, L., Wiebe, N., Russell, K., Patel, H., Klassen, T.P. (2003). A meta-analysis of randomized controlled trials evaluating the efficacy of epinephrine for the treatment of acute viral bronchiolitis. *Archives of Pediatric & Adolescent Medicine, 157,* 957-964.

Hawkins, G., McMahon, A.D., Twaddle, S., Wood, S.F., Ford, I., Thomson, N.C. (2003). Stepping down inhaled corticosteroids in asthma: Randomised controlled trial. British Medical Journal, 326, 1115-1118.

Holgate, S.T. (2004). Pharmacogenetics: the new science of personalizing treatment. *Current Opinion in Allergy & Clinical Immunology, 4*(1), 37-38.

Israel, E., et al., and the National Heart, Lung, and Blood Institute's Asthma Clinical Research Network. (2001). Effect of polymorphism of the beta(2)-adrenergic receptor on response to regular use of albuterol in asthma. *International Archives of Allergy & Immunology, 124*(1-3), 183-186.

Joos, L., & Sandford, A.J. (2002). Genotype predictors of response to asthma medications. *Current Opinion in Pulmonary Medicine, 8*(1), 9-15.

Kelly, H.W., & Sorkness, C.A. (2002). Asthma. In J.T. DiPiro, R.L. Talbert, G.C. Yee, G.R. Matzke, B.G. Wells, & L.M. Posey (Eds.), *Pharmacotherapy: A pathophysiological approach* (5th ed.). New York: McGraw-Hill.

Konzem, S.L., & Stratton, M.A. (2002). Chronic obstructive lung disease. In J.T. DiPiro, R.L. Talbert, G.C. Yee, G.R. Matzke, B.G.

Wells, & L.M. Posey (Eds.), *Pharmacotherapy: A pathophysiological approach* (5th ed.). New York: McGraw-Hill.

Lacy, C.F., Armstrong, L.L., Goldman, M.P., & Lance, L.L. (2004). *Lexi-Comp's Drug Information Handbook* (12th ed.). Hudson, Ohio: Lexi-Comp.

McKenzie, D.C. (2004). Salbutamol and the competitive athlete. *Clinical Journal of Sport Medicine, 14*(5), 316.

Metz, C.N., Gregersen, P.K., & Malhotra, A.K. (2004). Metabolism and biochemical effects of nicotine for primary care providers. *Medical Clinics of North America 88*(6), 1399-1413.

Miller, C.A., Slusher, L.B., & Vesell, E.S. (1985). Polymorphism of theophylline metabolism in man. *Journal of Clinical Investigation, 75,* 1415–1425.

Mosby's drug consult (15th ed.). (2005). St. Louis: Mosby.

Mull, C.C., et al. (2004). A randomized trial of nebulized epinephrine vs albuterol in the emergency department treatment of bronchiolitis. *Archives of Pediatric & Adolescent Medicine, 158,* 113-118.

National Asthma Education and Prevention Program. (2002). Guidelines for the diagnosis and management of asthma. Retrieved July 12, 2005, from http://www.nhlbi.nih.gov/guidelines/asthma/asthgdln.pdf.

National Institute of Allergy and Infectious Disease (NIAID). (2001). *Asthma: A concern for minority populations.* NIAID Fact Sheet.

Patel, H., et al. (2003). Randomized, double-blind, placebo-controlled trial of oral albuterol in infants with mild-to-moderate acute viral bronchiolitis. *Journal of Pediatrics, 142,* 509-514.

Pillai, S.G., et al., and the investigators of the GAIN Network. (2004). A coding polymorphism in the CYSLT2 receptor with reduced affinity to LTD4 is associated with asthma. *Pharmacogenetics, 14*(9), 627-633.

Rubin, B.K., & Durotoye, L. (2004). How do patients determine that their metered-dose inhaler is empty? *Chest, 126,* 1134-1137.

Salmeterol Package Insert. Research Triangle Park, NC: Galaxo-SmithKline. August 2003. Retrieved January 3, 2005, from http://www.fda.gov/medwatch/SAFETY/2003/serevent_PI.pdf

Self, T.H. (2005). Asthma. In M.A. Koda-Kimble, L.Y. Young, W.A. Kradian, B.J. Guglielmo, B.K. Alldredge, & R.L. Corelli (Eds.), *Applied therapeutics: The clinical use of drugs* (8th ed.). Philadelphia: Lippincott Williams & Wilkins.

Undem, B.J., Lichtenstein, L.M. (2001). Drugs Used in the Treatment of Asthma. In Hardman, J.G. & L.E. Limbird (Eds.), (2001). *Goodman & Gilman's The pharmacological basis of therapeutics* (10th ed.). New York: McGraw-Hill.

USP DI: Drug information for the health care professional (25th ed.). (2005). Greenwood Village, CO: MICROMEDEX Thomson Healthcare.

Wechsler, M.E., & Israel, E. (2002) Pharmacogenetics of treatment with leukotriene modifiers. *Current Opinion in Allergy & Clinical Immunology, 2*(5), 395-401.

Williams, D.M., & Kradjan, W.A. (2005). Chronic obstructive pulmonary disease. In M.A. Koda-Kimble, L.Y. Young, W.A. Kradian, B.J. Guglielmo, B.K. Alldredge, & R.L. Corelli (Eds.), *Applied therapeutics: The clinical use of drugs* (8th ed.). Philadelphia: Lippincott Williams & Wilkins.

38

OXYGEN AND MISCELLANEOUS RESPIRATORY AGENTS

CHAPTER FOCUS

An understanding of oxygen therapy and other associated therapies is essential to the delivery of effective respiratory care. Clients with different types of respiratory conditions may require varied treatment modalities and respiratory agents. Assessment and management of the client with altered respiratory function is more efficacious when the approach is multidisciplinary and collaborative.

LEARNING OBJECTIVES

- Describe how the body uses oxygen and the result of oxygen deprivation.
- Implement the nursing interventions applicable to each of the various methods of oxygen administration.
- Identify the effects of carbon dioxide.
- Implement nursing management of clients receiving respiratory stimulants and depressants.
- Describe antitussive agents and the proper method of administration.
- Explain the three actions of histamine in the body.
- Implement nursing management of clients receiving antihistamine therapy.

▲ KEY TERMS

analeptics, p. 727
hypercapnia, p. 724
hypoxemia, p. 722
hypoxia, p. 722
pulse oximetry, p. 725

✳▄ KEY DRUGS

diphenhydramine, p. 733
oxygen, p. 721

✳ What is the role of oxygen in respiratory care?

✳▄ Oxygen—a gas that is essential for life—is colorless, odorless, and tasteless. It is not flammable, but it supports combustion much more vigorously than does air. Inspired air normally contains 20.9% oxygen that, at an atmospheric pressure of 760 mm Hg, exerts a partial pressure (P_{O_2}) or tension of 159 mm Hg. As oxygen passes through the bronchial airway, the inspired air becomes saturated with water vapor, which reduces the P_{O_2} in the alveoli to approximately 100 mm Hg. Finally, the oxygen appears in dissolved form in the arterial blood. The P_{O_2} of arterial blood is normally above 80 mm Hg.

Oxygen must be continuously supplied to tissue cells; no fiber or cell can survive very long without oxygen. The adult human brain consumes from 40 to 50 mL of oxygen per minute. The cortex consumes more than the centers in the medulla or spinal cord. Cerebral oxygen consumption proceeds without pausing, and the replenishment of oxygen by the blood must be maintained continuously. Whenever any circulatory stress exists, cerebral blood flow tends to be preserved at the expense of other, less vital organs. Of all the tissues affected by hypoxia (inadequate cellular oxygen), the brain is most susceptible to disruption of normal function and irreversible damage. An acute reduction of the PO_2 to 50 mm Hg decreases mental functioning, emotional stability, and finer muscular coordination. Further reduction of the PO_2 to 40 mm Hg produces impaired judgment, decreased pain perception, and impairment of muscular coordination. When the PO_2 is reduced to 32 mm Hg or less, unconsciousness and a progressive, descending depression of the central nervous system (CNS) ensue.

The kidneys are vital organs in which there must be considerable constancy of blood flow and oxygen supply. Oxygen consumption is greater in the renal cortex; renal medullary tissue has an oxygen consumption that is 15% less than that of the renal cortex. This difference is related to the variation in pressure gradient and to the fact that cortical flow is rapid whereas the medullary flow is slower. The renal cortex is highly dependent on oxygen, whereas the renal medulla can function relatively independently of the oxygen supply.

The rate of oxygen consumption by the kidneys is approximately 0.06 mL/g/min, more than most other tissues. For each 100 mL of blood entering the kidney, 1.4 mL of oxygen is consumed. The oxygen consumed by the kidneys is primarily used for sodium reabsorption.

Renal vasoconstriction occurs when the renal arterial content falls to less than 55% of normal. This response is believed to be mediated by chemoreceptors that stimulate the vasomotor center to produce renal vasoconstriction. Renal vasoconstriction also occurs as a result of the action of ether, barbiturates, and other anesthetics. Renal blood flow is also decreased during periods of exercise. It is important to note that autoregulation of renal perfusion does occur.

In the skeletal muscles, oxygen consumption is related to blood flow. Oxygen consumption and blood flow are decreased when the muscle is at rest and significantly increased during exercise.

Some investigators regard the reduction of oxygen supply to the intestinal tract as a key factor for inadequate splanchnic vasoconstriction during hypotension.

An inadequate oxygen supply impairs myocardial metabolism and function. Severe hypoxia may produce changes in the ST segment and T wave of the electrocardiogram (ECG), dysrhythmias, ectopic beats, and myocardial infarction (MI).

When used alone, arterial blood pressure (BP) determinations are unreliable indicators of the adequacy of tissue perfusion. Arterial blood gas determinations are obtained, because these results provide a more accurate and reliable indication of the shifts in the partial pressures of oxygen and carbon dioxide.

Oxygen is used chiefly to treat hypoxia and hypoxemia (diminished oxygen tension in the blood). Basically, there are four types of hypoxia:

- Hypoxemic hypoxia: decreased oxygen level in the blood, resulting in decreased oxygen diffusion into the tissues

- Ischemic hypoxia: inadequate blood flow to an organ or tissue in the presence of a normal PO_2 and hemoglobin content
- Anemic hypoxia: inadequate hemoglobin to carry oxygen in the presence of a normal PO_2
- Histotoxic hypoxia: adequate PO_2 and hemoglobin but an inability of the tissues to use the delivered oxygen because of a toxic agent

Clinically, hypoxemic hypoxia is the most common form of hypoxia. A variety of pathologic conditions result in hypoxemic hypoxia and necessitate the use of oxygen treatment. These conditions include hypoventilation, increased airway resistance, pneumothorax, respiratory center depression, abnormal ventilation-perfusion ratio, congenital cyanotic heart disease, decreased pulmonary compliance, and breathing oxygen-poor air. The use of oxygen is also indicated in heart failure (HF) or decompensation and coronary occlusion, and anesthesia administration (to increase the safety of general anesthesia).

Exposure to 100% oxygen for a period of 6 hours causes an inflammatory response with subsequent destruction of the alveolocapillary membrane of the respiratory tract and the development of pulmonary edema that is not cardiac in origin. Toxicity is often difficult to recognize, but the most common symptoms are substernal distress (ache or burning sensation behind the sternum), an increase in respiratory distress, fatigue, nausea, vomiting, restlessness, tremors, twitching, paresthesias, and seizures.

❋ How is oxygen administered?

Oxygen is administered by inhalation. Various methods are used, and each method has its advantages and disadvantages (Figure 38-1).

A *nasal catheter* is made of soft plastic. When used, it should be lubricated with water-soluble K-Y Jelly and passed through the nose until the tip is just above the epiglottis. This distance is usually the same as the distance from an individual's external nares to the tragus of the ear, minus 1 cm. The catheter should not be inserted so far that the client swallows oxygen, because this will cause stomach distention and abdominal discomfort. The catheter is fastened with tape to the forehead and/or nose. The flow rate varies according to individual need, but 4 to 8 L/min of a 25% to 40% concentration of oxygen is commonly used. This form of therapy is very drying to the mucous membrane, and therefore the oxygen should be humidified. Additionally, nasal and oral hygiene are important to maintain cleanliness and an intact mucous membrane and to prevent infection and discomfort. Most clients receiving oxygen therapy are mouth breathers, and frequent mouth care is required to prevent alteration of the mucous membranes. Nasal catheters become obstructed with encrusted secretions and must be removed and cleaned or replaced several times a day.

A *nasal cannula* is much more comfortable for the client than is a catheter. Cannulas have either single or double, short prongs that are inserted into the lower part of the nos-

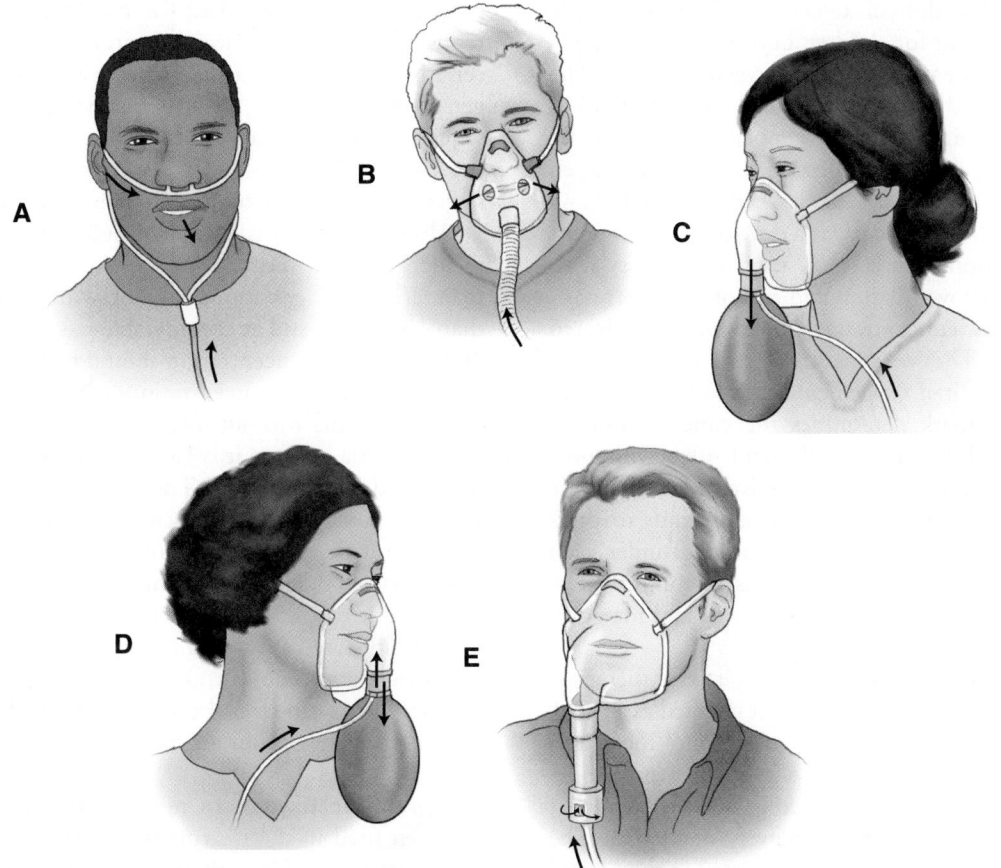

FIGURE 38-1 Various oxygen delivery systems. **A,** Nasal cannula. **B,** Simple face mask. **C,** Partial rebreathing mask. **D,** Nonrebreathing mask. **E,** Venturi mask.

trils. Cannulas are less likely to become obstructed with secretions. The nasal and oral mucosa still require frequent attention. A flow of 1 to 6 L/min of a 23% to 42% concentration of oxygen is adequate for many clients.

An *oxygen mask* is the most effective means of delivering needed oxygen. Oxygen concentrations up to 100% can be administered by mask. To be effective, the mask must fit well over the nose and mouth; to some extent, high flow rates can compensate for a poor fit. Masks are better tolerated when used intermittently or when disposable plastic masks are used. Only absolutely clean and uncontaminated rubber masks should be used, because they can be a source of nosocomial infection. There are two main types of oxygen masks: those that deliver low concentrations of oxygen and those that deliver high concentrations of oxygen.

A *simple face mask,* which is lightweight and disposable, is useful for short-term oxygen administration, such as in the early postoperative period or when intermittent oxygen therapy is required. The flow rate is only 6 to 8 L/min at a low-oxygen concentration of 40% to 60%. Because the mask is loose fitting and can leak, simple face masks are suitable for individuals with carbon dioxide retention. They are also indicated for clients who cannot use a nasal cannula, such as those who have a nasal obstruction.

A *partial rebreathing* mask is a disposable, lightweight plastic face mask that consists of a reservoir bag and a partial rebreathing valve. It is commonly used by individuals who require oxygen. On expiration, only a portion of the exhaled air enters the reservoir bag; it conserves roughly one third of the client's exhaled air. Because this air comes from the trachea and bronchi and does not participate in gas exchange in the lungs, it is rich in oxygen. To prevent the rebreathing of carbon dioxide, the reservoir bag should deflate only slightly on inhalation. By this method, a concentration of 50% to 75% oxygen can be delivered at a flow rate of 8 to 11 L/min.

A *nonrebreathing mask* is designed to fit tightly over the face and is usually made of rubber with a reservoir bag and a nonrebreathing valve. On inhalation, oxygen flows into the bag and mask, and the one-way valve prevents exhaled air from flowing back into the bag. The expired air instead escapes through the one-way flap valve in the mask. The concentration of oxygen is 80% to 100%, and the flow is adjusted to keep the reservoir bag fully inflated. This type of mask is used for short-term therapy, such as counteracting smoke inhalation. The rubber can become hot and sticky; prolonged use can cause discomfort.

An *oxygen tent* is of limited value, particularly when it is necessary to open the canopy for monitoring vital signs and administering care to the client. The rate of flow is 20 L/min at an oxygen concentration of 60%. Obviously, the oxygen concentration falls each time the tent is opened, which makes the flow difficult to control. Oxygen tents are now used rarely, except for children beyond early infancy.

Plastic hoods may be used to deliver oxygen to infants. The clear plastic head hood allows low and high concentrations of oxygen to be maintained without hampering most nursing care. A rate of 4 to 5 L/min is needed to maintain oxygen concentrations and remove the exhaled carbon dioxide.

The *Ventimask (Mix-O-Mask)* is a development originating from the Venturi mask. It is used for clients with chronic alveolar hypoventilation and carbon dioxide retention. Exact low-flow concentrations of oxygen are delivered to the individual. The Ventimask provides an air-oxygen mixture with the desired oxygen concentration. The size of the orifice to the mask determines the concentration of oxygen—24% or 28%, 31%, 35%, and 40% with flow rates of 4, 6, 8, and 10 L/min, respectively. A thin elastic band holds the Ventimask in position and tends to press into the skin behind the ears. Gauze padding under each side of the elastic band will alleviate this discomfort. The device must be removed when the client eats and may give the client a feeling of being smothered.

Most of the oxygen administered in hospitals for therapy is provided from a central source in which it is stored as a gas or as liquid oxygen. The gas is piped into a client's room at a standard pressure of 50 pounds per square inch (psi) at the gauge. Compressed oxygen is marketed in steel cylinders that are fitted with reducing valves for delivery of the gas. The cylinders are usually color-coded; green is used in the United States. Because the gas is under considerable pressure, the tanks must be handled carefully to prevent falling or jarring.

The effectiveness of oxygen administration depends on the carbon dioxide content of the blood. Individuals with chronic obstructive pulmonary disease (COPD) have difficulty with carbon dioxide and oxygen exchange and are subject to **hypercapnia** (high carbon dioxide content in the blood). Because of chronic hypercapnia, the medullary center of these individuals is relatively insensitive to stimulation with carbon dioxide; rather, a low PaO_2 serves as a stimulant to respiration. Therefore oxygen flow rates are kept low (1 to 2 L/min) for clients with COPD. Administration of high rates of oxygen to clients with chronic hypercapnia may result in respiratory arrest. Nursing care should prevent a greater accumulation of carbon dioxide by encouraging the improvement of gas exchange. This involves having the client turn, deep breathe, and use pursed lip breathing periodically. Toxic carbon dioxide levels may result in further depression of respiration and respiratory acidosis. The nurse should be alert to neurologic symptoms that indicate an accumulation of carbon dioxide, including drowsiness, mental confusion, paresthesias, and visual disturbances. The occurrence of carbon dioxide narcosis may be prevented by gradually increasing the concentration of oxygen administered.

✲ **What special circumstances impact on how oxygen is administered?**

Oxygen Administration in the Premature Infant Nurses caring for premature infants in incubators must be constantly aware of the danger of retrolental fibroplasia (retinopathy of prematurity). This is a vascular proliferative disease of the retina that occurs in some premature infants who have received high concentrations of oxygen at birth. Excessive oxygen constricts the developing retinal vessels of the eye. Consequently, normal vascularization is suppressed, but because the endothelial cells become disorganized, they cause destruction of the immature retina. The result is blindness.

Although there has been a considerable reduction in the incidence and severity of this condition, infants younger than 28 weeks' gestational age or with birth weights less than 1000 g are still at considerable risk (Ibarra & Capone, 2004). Oxygen concentration should be kept between 30% and 40%. Higher concentrations can be administered to cyanotic infants without increasing the danger of retrolental fibroplasia because it is PaO_2, not inspired PO_2, which is implicated in this disease. Therefore careful monitoring of arterial blood gases is essential. Some incubators are equipped with a safety valve that automatically releases any excess oxygen outside the chamber. When orders for an infant include oxygen PRN, the nurse must make certain that it is administered at low concentrations and only as needed rather than continuously. Often the removal of a very small plug of mucus can clear the airway and enable the infant to breathe oxygen without assistance.

Hyperbaric Oxygen In recent years hyperbaric oxygen has been used in the treatment of various conditions. The intermittent use of hyperbaric oxygen is controversial in the treatment of infections caused by *Clostridium perfringens, C. septicum,* or *C. histolyticum*—anaerobic bacilli that produce gas gangrene. It is believed that increased oxygen pressure in the tissue may exert an inhibitory effect on the enzyme systems of these bacteria. This same inhibitory effect may be implicated in the use of hyperbaric oxygen on other anaerobic microorganisms.

Hyperbaric oxygen has also been used in certain circulatory disturbances, such as air or gas embolism, decompression sickness, carbon monoxide, and cyanide poisoning, and exceptional blood loss. It has also been used in certain local circulatory disturbances such as necrotizing soft-tissue infections; acute traumatic ischemia, crush injury, and compartment syndrome; compromised (ischemic) grafts and flaps; radiation necrosis; refractory osteomyelitis; and enhancement of healing in selected problem wounds.

Helium-Oxygen Mixtures Helium-oxygen mixtures have been used to treat obstructive types of dyspnea. Helium is an inert gas and so light that a mixture of 80% helium and 20% oxygen is only one third as heavy as air. Helium is only slightly soluble in body fluids and has a high rate of diffusion. Because of its low specific gravity, mixtures of this gas with oxygen can be breathed with less effort than either oxygen or air alone when air passages are obstructed. These mixtures are recommended for individuals with status asthmaticus, bronchiectasis, and emphysema, and during anesthesia induction for clients with respiratory tract obstruction.

✲ **What considerations are important for the nurse regarding oxygen use?**

BOX 38-1 PULSE OXIMETRY

Pulse oximetry works by passing light of differing wavelengths through living tissue and analyzing the differences in absorption. Oxygenated hemoglobin absorbs light differently, and these variations in absorption serve as the basis of calculations that determine the presence and amount of oxygenated hemoglobin compared to nonoxygenated hemoglobin. This provides a continuous reading of arterial blood oxygen saturation. A saturation of 95% or greater is desired for clients. (This correlates with a PaO_2 of 60.)

Pulse oximeters work with a small probe (light source and detector) that may be placed on a client's ear, finger, toe, bridge of the nose, nasal septum, or temple. Pulse oximetry monitors are relatively inexpensive, noninvasive, safe, extremely accurate, require no calibration, and provide almost instantaneous results. Although initially used with clients during anesthesia, recovery, and critical care, the use of pulse oximetry is an immediate and safe method of determining tissue oxygenation in any client having respiratory difficulties in any health care setting.

BOX 38-2 NORMAL VALUES FOR ARTERIAL BLOOD GASES

pH: 7.35-7.45

$PaCO_2$: 35-45 mm Hg

PaO_2: 80-95 mm Hg

O_2 saturation: 95% or above

HCO_3: 18-23 mEq/L

Assessment Dyspnea or an increased respiratory rate may indicate the need for oxygen therapy. The best means of gauging the need for oxygen or the effectiveness of oxygen therapy is via arterial blood gas evaluations or pulse oximetry before and during therapy (Box 38-1). Additionally, document the client's BP and pulse, level of consciousness, and respiratory status, including respiratory rate, effort, adventitious breath sounds, cyanosis, and activity intolerance.

It is important to know normal blood gas values and be able to recognize deviations (Box 38-2). The goal of oxygen therapy is to return the arterial oxygen pressure to normal (80 to 95 mm Hg) or the client's normal baseline often 60 mm Hg or above with respiratory disease, or oxygen saturation greater than 95% by pulse oximetry.

In chronic carbon dioxide retention, the PaO_2 may decrease to as low as 55 to 60 mm Hg. An arterial blood gas analysis is required 30 minutes after the oxygen dosage is changed unless the oxygen saturation is being monitored.

Oxygen should be given with extreme caution to some clients. In clients with chronic hypoxemia and/or hypercapnia, the central chemoreceptors no longer act as the primary stimulus for breathing. In such cases respiratory drive is maintained by peripheral chemoreceptors that are sensitive to changes in PaO_2. If oxygen therapy causes PaO_2 to ex-

ceed 60 mm Hg, the stimulus to breathe is lost, and apnea results. Low-flow oxygen is administered to these clients, and pulse oximetry values are checked frequently.

Nursing Diagnosis The client receiving oxygen therapy may experience ineffective airway clearance, ineffective breathing pattern, and impaired gas exchange. Additionally, oxygen therapy places the client at risk for the following nursing diagnoses/collaborative problems: impaired skin integrity of the face related to the mask; infection related to contamination of the oxygen equipment; risk for injury related to the combustibility of oxygen; impaired oral mucous membrane related to the drying effects of oxygen; and the potential complications of oxygen toxicity and, for infants, retrolental fibroplasia.

Planning The client receiving oxygen therapy will:
- Experience minimal exacerbations of respiratory symptoms (e.g., coughing or breathlessness during the night or after exertion).
- Maintain (near) "normal" pulmonary function while compliant with his drug therapy.
- Effectively manage his therapeutic regimen with oxygen.
- Collaborate with health care providers for monitoring and ongoing care.

Implementation

Monitoring Monitor the client's vital signs—pulse rate, BP, and respiratory rate and pattern. Also observe level of consciousness, skin temperature, and color. Report any abnormal findings to the prescriber. Examine the client and the equipment frequently to see that the skin and mucous membranes in contact with the equipment are intact and without irritation; the equipment is patent, without leaks, and properly positioned; the flow rate is at the prescribed level; the humidifier contains solution; and, if an oxygen cylinder is being used, that it is stabilized and contains enough oxygen. Pulse oximetry, and blood gases, may be required periodically. If high concentrations of oxygen are used, positive end-expiratory pressure (PEEP) or continuous positive airway pressure (CPAP) values are used to determine the best oxygenation without hemodynamic compromise and thereby prevent oxygen toxicity.

Intervention To prevent dryness of the nose and throat and respiratory complications, add sterile, distilled water to the humidifying device, and administer oxygen concentration and liter flow as prescribed. Because oxygen is a dry gas, adequate humidification is essential to the client and must be monitored frequently.

Oxygen supports combustion, and combustible materials (linens, wooden furniture, plastic articles) burn with greater ease and intensity in the presence of oxygen. Therefore smoking, or use of matches, woolen blankets, clothing, or electric equipment (radios, electric razors, hair dryers) that may cause sparks are strictly forbidden in rooms in which oxygen is being administered. "No smoking" signs are also posted within the home environment. In some health agencies, these signs are posted on the individual's door and above the bed, even though smoking is not permitted within the agency.

Because oxygen therapy is often administered to debilitated clients, take special care to avoid contamination of the equipment; this will help to prevent a nosocomial infection. Nasal cannulas, Ventimasks, other masks, tubing, nebulizers, and other equipment exposed to moisture need to be changed daily. Nasal catheters should be changed every 8 to 12 hours. If the client's condition permits, remove the oxygen mask periodically to dry, powder, and massage the skin around the mask.

Education Show the equipment for oxygen administration to the client and family. Explain the procedure and the benefits of oxygen therapy. Explain to the client and visitors the importance of not lighting candles or smoking in the client's room. (Because oxygen supports combustion, the possibility of fire always exists.) Prepare the client and caregivers for oxygen use in the home (see the Community and Home Health Considerations box below).

Evaluation The expected outcome of oxygen therapy is that the client will have adequate gas exchange as evidenced by a respiratory rate of 12 to 20 breaths/min or a rate in keeping with the client's baseline; the following blood gas values: PaO_2 greater than 60 mm Hg, $PaCO_2$ 35 to 45 mm Hg, and pH 7.35 to 7.45; and/or pulse oximetry of 95% or

greater. The client describes the disease process and its precipitating factors, manages the oxygen equipment safely and effectively, and collaborates with the health care providers for monitoring and treatment by keeping scheduled appointments.

How is carbon dioxide used clinically?

Carbon dioxide is a colorless, odorless gas that is heavier than air. Carbon dioxide used as a pharmacologic agent affects respiration, circulation, and the CNS. Inhaling carbon dioxide for a short time increases both the rate and the depth of respiration unless the respiratory center is depressed by opioids or disease. However, mechanical assistance in respiration and oxygen administration is the usual treatment in cases of respiratory depression.

Carbon dioxide stimulates the cells of the sympathetic nervous system (SNS), respiratory center, and peripheral chemoreceptors. It depresses the cerebral cortex, myocardium, and smooth muscle of the peripheral blood vessels. Carbon dioxide may also interfere with nerve conduction and transmission. When carbon dioxide increases the rate and force of respiration, venous return to the heart is usually enhanced because of decreased peripheral resistance; the rate and force of myocardial contraction improves, and there is less likelihood of myocardial irritability and dysrhythmias.

Although the use of carbon dioxide has been suggested for many commonly encountered clinical situations, other therapies are usually more effective and have fewer disad-

---

Community and Home Health Considerations

Home Management of Oxygen Therapy

For home use of oxygen, the client and family must understand how the system works, how to determine that the system is not functioning, and how to "troubleshoot" the system, how to contact the supplier, and what to do in an emergency. Essentially there are three methods of delivery for home oxygen systems. (1) The liquid oxygen system in which liquid oxygen is provided in large reservoir canisters with smaller portable units that can be refilled by the client. It has the advantage of delivering 100% oxygen on all flow rates so higher liter flow is achievable. The disadvantages are that the stationary unit must be refilled periodically (a small amount evaporates), and it may be the most costly method. (2) The oxygen concentrator system, that extracts oxygen from ambient air, is inexpensive and convenient, but the main unit is not portable so the client also needs a portable oxygen unit. It is heavy and the client must have a backup system in case of power failure. (3) Compressed oxygen tanks deliver 100% oxygen on all flow rates so a higher liter flow is achievable. But it is heavy and unsightly, a safety hazard if not stored properly, and it must be replaced by periodic delivery. The Centers for Medicare and Medicaid Services (CMS) uses a "modality neutral" method, which applies a fixed reimbursement regardless of the mode of delivery (Bailey, 2004).

Whatever the system, the client or caregiver should check it daily. The assessment should include proper function of the

equipment, prescribed flow rates, remaining liquid or compressed gas content, and backup supply to meet the client's needs. The supplier's name and phone number need to be in a handy place for reordering or in case of emergency. Fire hazards can be prevented by instructing the client and family not to smoke or use an open flame in the room when the oxygen is on. Electrical appliances, such as razors and electric blankets, should not be used in the vicinity of the administration of the oxygen. No oil (Vaseline, hair oils, body oils), wool blankets, or flammable liquids (alcohol) should be used in the area. "No smoking" signs should be posted as reminders. The local fire department should be alerted to the presence of oxygen tanks in the house.

A respiratory care practitioner or nurse should visit at least monthly to clinically assess the client and to reinforce appropriate practices and performance by the client and caregivers and assure that the equipment is being maintained in accordance with the manufacturer's recommendations.

To ensure consistent quality of care and to maximize the client's financial reimbursement, the physician's order for oxygen therapy needs to include the disorder for which the oxygen is required, the amount of oxygen flow and the conditions for its use, i.e., continuous, PRN, or nighttime only.

vantages. Too much carbon dioxide has a depressant effect and results in acidosis and unresponsiveness of the respiratory center to the gas. Therefore it is important that carbon dioxide be administered with caution.

carbon dioxide

Indications

Carbon dioxide is occasionally used by anesthesiologists to manage respiratory and anesthesia status, as a respiratory stimulant, and for postoperative management of hiccups. Carbon dioxide initially speeds up anesthesia by increasing pulmonary ventilation. By lessening the sense of asphyxiation, it reduces struggling. In the postanesthesia period, it hastens the elimination of many anesthetics. Inhalation of 5% to 7% carbon dioxide increases cerebral blood flow by approximately 75%, primarily by dilation of the cerebral vessels.

The use of carbon dioxide as a respiratory stimulant in the presence of depressed respiration is limited, and requires close monitoring of pulse oximetry and Pa_{O_2}. Relief from hiccups is apparently accomplished by stimulating the respiratory center; this causes large excursions of the diaphragm that suppress spasmodic contractions of that muscle, thereby promoting regular contractions.

Pharmacokinetics/Dosing/Administration

Carbon dioxide is kept in metal cylinders and vaporizes as it is delivered from the cylinder. It is administered in combination with oxygen when used for medical purposes. A 5% to 10% concentration of carbon dioxide delivered through a tight-fitting face mask is inhaled by the client until the depth of respiration is definitely increased, which usually occurs within 3 minutes. For postoperative clients, the procedure is repeated every hour or two for the first 48 hours and then several times a day for several days.

Another way of administering carbon dioxide is to allow the client to hyperventilate with a paper bag held over the face. Reinhaling expired air causes the carbon dioxide content to be continually increased.

Adverse Effects

Signs of carbon dioxide overdose are dyspnea, breath holding, markedly increased chest and abdominal movements, nausea, and increased systolic BP. Administration of the gas should be discontinued when these symptoms appear. The administration of 5% carbon dioxide may produce severe mental depression if given over an hour; a 10% concentration can lead to a loss of consciousness within 10 minutes. The administration should be stopped as soon as the desired effects on the client's respiration have been obtained.

❊ What other agents affect respiratory drive?

Rate and depth of respirations can be affected by respiratory stimulants or respiratory depressants. Direct respiratory stimulants come under a broader classification of CNS stimulants and are often referred to as **analeptics** (see Chapter 18). These drugs act directly on the medullary center to increase respiratory rate and tidal exchange. Although these drugs are available for stimulating the depth and rate of respiration, airway management and ventilation support are more effective in the treatment of respiratory depression. The mechanical support of ventilation is often superior to the use of drugs, because respiratory stimulants in large doses can cause seizures.

In the past, respiratory stimulants (analeptics) have been advocated in the treatment of drug-induced respiratory depression. However, these drugs are not specific antagonists to sedatives or opioids, and thus their use in drug-induced respiratory depression is now considered obsolete. Indeed, repeated doses of an analeptic may potentiate the depressant effects of CNS depressants. See Chapter 18 for information on the direct respiratory stimulant doxapram.

An aromatic ammonia spirit is given by inhalation for its action as a reflex respiratory stimulant. In cases of fainting, it is administered by inhaling the vapor. Reflex stimulation of the medullary center occurs through peripheral irritation of sensory nerve receptors in the pharynx, esophagus, and stomach. The rate and depth of respiration are then increased through afferent messages to the respiratory control centers. Reflex stimulation of the vasomotor center results in a rise in BP.

The most important respiratory depressants are barbiturates and opium and its derivatives. These agents depress the respiratory center, thereby making breathing slower and more shallow and lessening the irritability of the respiratory center. Respiratory depression is seldom desirable or necessary, but it is sometimes unavoidable. It is an adverse effect of otherwise very useful drugs.

Low doses of morphine decrease the sense of breathlessness and improve sleep patterns for clients with severe dyspnea related to end stage respiratory conditions like COPD (Abernethy et al., 2003). However, such therapy is not without risk. Monitoring respiratory status is important when opioids are used for clients with underlying respiratory conditions. Refer to Chapter 14 for a more complete discussion of opioids.

❊ What agents suppress the cough reflex?

A number of agents are used to stop a dry hacking cough, which is uncomfortable for the client and interferes with sleep. Treatment of the cough is secondary to treatment of the underlying disorder; that is, the therapeutic objective is to decrease the intensity and frequency of the cough yet permit adequate elimination of tracheobronchial secretions and exudates.

Chapter 11 reviews the most commonly used cough suppressant, dextromethorphan, an over-the-counter (OTC) agent. Deaths associated with the abuse of dextromethorphan have been reported with adolescents (U.S. Food and Drug Administration [FDA], 2005). Diphenhydramine (Bena-dryl) is an antihistamine with some cough suppressant activity and is presented later in this chapter. Prescription cough suppressants are usually reserved for a nonproductive cough that is inadequately controlled by or nonresponsive to OTC medications. Prescription agents include those structurally related to morphine (opioids) and the nonopioid cough suppressants.

Opioids such as morphine and hydromorphone are potent suppressants of the cough reflex, but their clinical usefulness is limited by their adverse effects. They inhibit the ciliary activity of the respiratory mucous membrane, depress respiration, and may cause bronchial constriction in clients with allergies or asthma. Additionally, they can cause drug dependence. Co-deine and hydrocodone are widely used; they exhibit fewer pronounced antitussive effects but have fewer adverse effects. (See Chapter 14 for information on opioid agents.)

The nonnarcotic, nonopioid antitussive drugs produce fewer gastrointestinal (GI) adverse effects than do codeine and the related compounds. Benzonatate is the most common of the prescription nonopioid cough suppressants.

benzonatate [ben **zow** nah tate]
(Tessalon Perles, Tessalon)
Benzonatate is chemically related to the local anesthetic tetracaine. Benzonatate relieves coughing by peripherally anesthetizing the stretch or cough receptors in the lungs and respiratory passages, and it may also have a central effect on the cough reflex.

Indications
Benzonatate is indicated for the symptomatic treatment of a nonproductive cough.

Pharmacokinetics/Dosing
The onset of action is within 15 to 20 minutes after oral administration, with duration of action of up to 8 hours. The dosage for adults and children older than 10 years is 100 mg three times daily. The maximum daily dose is 600 mg.

Adverse Effects
Adverse effects include drowsiness, headache, dizziness, tightness or numbness in chest, nausea, constipation, abdominal upset, skin eruptions, nasal congestion, and a vague sensation of chill.

✱ **A.R., a 54-year-old female, has been prescribed a variety of antihypertensive agents trying to bring her BP under control without experiencing what she describes as unacceptable side effects: dizziness, lightheadedness, and sexual dysfunction. Her recently prescribed drug regimen includes valsartan (Diovan), an angiotensin receptor blocker (ARB) to which she attributes a dry cough. Although ARBs have lower rates of dry cough compared to ACE inhibitors, it has been reported rarely. She wishes to stay on the medication because her present drug regimen brings her BP into an acceptable range without "major" side effects; she believes this will enhance her compliance with her antihypertensive therapy. Her primary care provider has ruled out any other etiology for her cough and agrees to prescribe a cough suppressant, benzonatate (Tessalon) 100 mg three times daily PRN that she may take when the cough is bothersome.**

✱ **What are the nursing management issues involved in using cough suppressants for A.R.?**

Assessment The cause of A.R.'s cough has been determined, which is important because a cough suppressant such as benzonatate would be contraindicated if heart failure or other disease was the cause of the cough. Benzonatate is contraindicated for a productive cough because secretions are retained if the cough is suppressed. No significant drug interactions have been reported with this drug, although there is an increased risk of drowsiness if benzonatate is taken with CNS depressants. Obtain a baseline assessment of A.R.'s respiratory status and cough. Assess from her history that she has no known hypersensitivity to benzonatate or related compounds (local anesthetics).

Nursing Diagnosis With the administration of benzonatate, A.R. is at risk for the following nursing diagnoses/collaborative problems: impaired comfort related to GI effects (nausea, heartburn), nasal congestion, and continued cough; constipation; impaired skin integrity related to the occurrence of rash; risk for injury related to CNS effects (confusion if concurrently taking CNS depressants); and the potential complications of allergic reaction, or bronchospasm or laryngospasm related to local anesthesia secondary to chewing or sucking the capsule rather than swallowing it whole.

Planning While taking drug therapy for cough suppression, A.R. will:
- Experience an absence of or acceptable decrease in her dry cough.
- Effectively manage her benzonatate and antihypertensive regimen.
- Collaborate with health care providers for monitoring and ongoing care.

Implementation
Monitoring Observe A.R. for drowsiness and dizziness, nausea, GI distress, constipation, and rash. Assess her cough to determine if it remains nonproductive. Report symptoms of other pulmonary conditions to the prescriber (e.g., productive cough, chest pain, crackles, or rhonchi).

Intervention Activities by A.R. that would be supportive of antitussives are deep-breathing exercises, frequent changes of position, limitation or cessation of smoking, maintenance of adequate humidity in the environment, and adequate hydration. If a specific stimulus that adds to A.R.'s cough can be identified (e.g., dust, smoking, or pollen), attempts should be made to minimize exposure to these substances.

Education Teach A.R. that the capsule should be swallowed whole. Temporary local anesthesia of the oral mucosa results if it is chewed or dissolved in the mouth. Caution A.R. about operating a car or other machinery until she assesses its effects, because the drug may cause drowsiness or dizziness. Advise her to report a cough that becomes productive or worsens.

Evaluation The expected outcome of benzonatate therapy is that A.R. will experience a decrease in the intensity and frequency of coughing without adverse drug effects. A.R. describes the cough and its precipitating factors, manages her therapeutic regimen effectively (including medication compliance and stating reportable adverse effects), and collaborates with the health care providers for monitoring and treatment by keeping scheduled appointments.

✱ **What is the role of histamine in the body?**
Histamine is a chemical mediator that occurs naturally in almost all body tissues. It is present in highest concentration in the skin, lung, and GI tract. These structures are often exposed to environmental assaults and require protection against damage. When liberated from its cells, the free form of histamine plays an early transient role in the inflammatory process that defends the exposed tissues against injury.

In many tissues the chief site of production and storage of histamine occurs in the cytoplasmic granules of the mast cell or, in the case of blood, the basophil (which closely resembles the mast cell in function). The mast cells are small, ovoid structures widely distributed in the loose connective tissue. They are especially abundant along small blood vessels and along the bronchial smooth muscle cell, which appears to have the highest concentration of mast cells of any organ in the body. Both the mast cells and basophils make up the mast-cell histamine pool.

A second major site of histamine production is known as the nonmast pool, in which the amine is stored in the cells of the epidermis, GI mucosa, and the CNS. Although histamine is present in various foods and is synthesized by intestinal flora, the amount absorbed does not contribute to the body's stores of this amine.

The reactions mediated by histamine are attributed to receptor activity, which involves two distinct populations of receptors: H_1 and H_2. The principal actions of histamine are summarized in Table 38-1 and are outlined in the following sections.

Vascular Effects In the microcirculatory component of the cardiovascular system (arterioles, capillaries, venules), the liberation of histamine has been shown to involve both H_1 and H_2 receptors. Stimulation of these receptors dilates the capillaries and venules, producing an increased localized blood flow, increased capillary permeability, erythema, and edema. By activating the H_1 and H_2 receptors on the smooth muscles of the arterioles, histamine is also capable of eliciting a systemic response (vasodilation of the arterioles), which can result in a profound fall in BP.

Smooth Muscle Effects Although histamine exerts a powerful relaxing effect on the smooth muscle of the arterioles, it produces a contractile action on the smooth muscles of many nonvascular organs, such as the bronchi and GI tract. In sensitized individuals, activation of the H_1 receptors of the lungs can cause marked bronchial muscle contraction that often progresses to dyspnea and airway obstruction.

Exocrine Glandular Effects Histamine stimulates the gastric, salivary, pancreatic, and lacrimal glands, with the main effect seen in the gastric glands. Stimulation of H_2 receptors in the exocrine glands of the stomach increases the production of gastric acid secretions. The high concentration of hydrochloric acid in the stomach is attributed to the activity of the parietal cells and is implicated in the development of peptic ulcers.

Central Nervous System Effects Histamine is also known to be present throughout the tissues of the brain. Its effects seem to involve both H_1 and H_2 receptor mediation. The activation of H_1 receptors of the semicircular canals is associated with motion sickness.

✳ What are the pathologic effects of histamine?

Histamine as a chemical mediator is implicated in many pathologic disorders. Conditions for which drugs are used to counteract this compound are concerned with the hypersensitivity response known as the allergic reaction. There are four different types of hypersensitivity responses to immunologic injury; the type I anaphylactic reaction is associated with the disorders caused by histamine release.

Individuals with type I–mediated hypersensitivity develop allergies as a result of sensitization to a foreign agent that may be ingested, inhaled, or injected. An incalculable number of these agents act as antigens. They vary widely— seasonal exposure to pollens, grasses, and weeds, or nonseasonal exposure to agents such as house dust, feathers, molds, and other similar substances can produce different forms of allergic reactivity.

Hypersensitivity to a variety of foods such as shellfish or strawberries requires ingestion of the antigen. Insects such as bees or wasps and even drugs, particularly penicillin, also possess allergic properties that may induce a severe response in hypersensitive individuals.

TABLE 38-1 HISTAMINE: PRINCIPAL ACTIONS

Structure	Histamine Receptors	Pharmacologic Effects
Vascular system		
Capillary (microcirculation)	H_1 and H_2	Dilation, increased permeability
Arteriole (smooth muscle)	H_1 and H_2	Dilation
Smooth muscle		
Bronchial, bronchiolar	H_1	Contraction
Gastrointestinal	H_1	Contraction
Exocrine glands		
Gastric	H_2	Gastric acid secretion (HCl)
Epidermis	H_1	Triple response (flush, flare, wheal)
Adrenal medulla	—	Epinephrine and norepinephrine release
Central nervous system	H_1	Motion sickness

Thus type I anaphylactic hypersensitivity accounts for a substantial number of allergic disorders, and it involves a complex series of anomalies that range from mild urticaria to anaphylactic shock. The mechanism of type I anaphylactic reaction involves the attachment of an antigen (Ag) to an antibody (Ab), specifically immunoglobulin E (IgE); this complex becomes fixed to the mast cell. The pathologic manifestations of an Ag-IgE interaction are caused by mast cell degranulation, which results in the release of histamine and other mediators responsible for producing the allergic symptoms. The type I anaphylactic reaction is responsible for various disorders, such as urticaria, atopy (allergic rhinitis, hay fever), food allergies, bronchial asthma, and systemic anaphylaxis.

Urticaria Urticaria is a vascular reaction of the skin; it is characterized by immediate formation of a wheal and flare and is accompanied by severe itching. Contact with an external irritant, such as drugs or foods, produces the Ag-IgE–mediated response with the resultant release of histamine from the mast cell into the skin. The local vasodilation produces the red flare, and the increased permeability of the capillaries leads to tissue swelling. These swellings are called "hives"; giant hives are known as angioneurotic edema. Antihistaminic drugs administered before exposure to the antigen will prevent this response.

Atopy Atopy occurs in genetically susceptible individuals and is usually caused by seasonal pollen. This condition is manifested as an upper respiratory tract disorder known as allergic rhinitis (hay fever) and may be confused with the common cold or influenza by clients (Table 38-2). (See Chapter 11 for additional information.) After the interaction of the Ag-IgE complex on the surface of the bronchial mast cells, histamine is released, producing local vascular dilation and increased capillary permeability. This change produces a rapid leakage of fluid into the tissues of the nose, which results in swelling of the nasal linings. Antihistaminic therapy can prevent the edematous reaction in certain individuals if the drug is administered before antigenic exposure.

Food Allergies Food allergies involve the interaction of the Ag-IgE complex and mast cells in the intestine; this occurs when antigens are ingested. If the upper GI tract is affected, vomiting results; if the lower GI tract is invaded, cramps and diarrhea occur. The ingestion of a large amount of antigen has also been known to produce systemic anaphylaxis.

Asthma When the inhaled antigen combines with the IgE antibody, stimulation of the mast cells triggers the release of mediators in the lower respiratory tract, usually in the bronchi and bronchioles. Histamine plays a minor role in this response because the slow-reacting substance of anaphylaxis (SRS-A) is a more potent mediator, causing long-term contraction of the bronchiolar smooth muscle. The difficulty in breathing may be relieved by a bronchodilator such as epinephrine. Because more potent chemical mediators than histamine are responsible for causing the reaction, the administration of antihistaminic drugs actually has no value in relieving this condition.

Systemic Anaphylaxis Systemic anaphylaxis is a generalized reaction manifested as a life-threatening systemic condition. The Ag-IgE mediator response involves the basophils of the blood and the mast cells in the connective tissue. The most common precipitating causes of this response are drugs (particularly penicillin), insect stings (wasps and bees), and occasionally certain foods. The release of massive amounts of histamine into the circulation causes widespread vasodilation, resulting in a profound fall in BP. The excessive dilation also allows plasma to leave the capillaries, and a loss of circulatory volume ensues. When the reaction is fatal, death is usually caused not only by shock but also by laryngeal edema. The symptoms of the latter condition include smooth muscle contraction of the bronchi and pharyngeal edema, which usually leads to asphyxiation. Because the mediator SRS-A is also released from the cells, the resulting spasm of the smooth muscle of the bronchioles elicits the asthma-like attack. See Chapter 22 for the use of epinephrine in the management of anaphylaxis.

TABLE 38-2 COLDS, ALLERGIC RHINITIS, AND INFLUENZA: SIGNS OR SYMPTOMS

Signs or Symptoms	Common Cold	Allergic Rhinitis	Influenza
Fever	Rare	Absent	Common—sudden onset, may range 102°-104° F
Aches and pains	Slight	Absent	May be severe
Sneezing	Usual	Common	Infrequent
Pruritus	Absent or rare	Common	Absent
Cough	Mild-moderate	Uncommon	Common
Headaches	Rare	Can occur	Prominent
Causative	Usually viruses	Usually allergens	Usually viruses
Occurrence	Anytime	Usually seasonal	Anytime
Complications	Sinus congestion, earache	Uncommon	Bronchitis, pneumonia

Antihistaminic drugs are less effective against systemic anaphylaxis because these agents do not antagonize the SRS-A mediator that causes the severe bronchoconstriction. Accordingly, a drug such as epinephrine, a bronchodilator, is indicated for this life-threatening situation. The relief produced by this drug results from the β_2-receptor action that relaxes the bronchial smooth muscles.

Drug allergies often develop in susceptible individuals who show no adverse reactions after the first dose of drug administration. However, a second or subsequent reexposure to even an extremely small amount of this same antigen may elicit an exaggerated local or systemic IgE response. Individuals who exhibit such reactions are said to be allergic to the drug. The IgE-mediated response, particularly with penicillin, may occur either in the skin, producing severe urticaria, and/or in the respiratory tract, causing bronchial asthma.

In certain sensitized individuals, even limited contact can produce a fatal systemic anaphylaxis. Some of the drugs that elicit an allergic response include penicillin, chloramphenicol, streptomycin, sulfonamides, aspirin, and phenacetin. Allergic reactions to penicillin account for nearly 100 deaths per year in the United States. Therefore even the mildest sign of an allergic response or rash, particularly one with a rapid onset, should be reported immediately to the prescriber. In all probability the drug will be discontinued to avoid the possibility of an exaggerated type I hypersensitivity reaction.

✺ Is histamine administered as a pharmacologic or therapeutic agent?

Histamine is not used therapeutically. Instead, it has limited use as a diagnostic agent in testing for gastric acid secretory functions. If achlorhydria is the response to histamine, the client may have pernicious anemia, gastric polyps, gastric carcinoma, or atrophic gastritis. If hypersecretion of gastric acid occurs after the histamine, a duodenal ulcer or Zollinger-Ellison syndrome may be the problem.

Histamine testing of gastric function is contraindicated in clients who have a history of hypersensitivity to the drug, bronchial asthma, vasomotor instability, urticaria, or severe cardiac, pulmonary, or renal disease. Histamine should be used cautiously in clients with pheochromocytoma. Histamine H_2-receptor antagonists, such as cimetidine and ranitidine, are not to be administered for 24 hours before the test because they will antagonize the effects of the histamine. Antacids and anticholinergics are also withheld before the examination. The procedure and any anticipated effects of the histamine test should be explained to the client.

The client should fast for a minimum of 12 hours and be at rest under basal conditions. Use a nasogastric tube to empty the stomach contents before the examination and to obtain specimens during the examination. A baseline or basal acid output is obtained by obtaining four samples of aspirant 15 minutes apart; clamp the nasogastric tube between samples. The histamine dose of 0.01 mg/kg (equal to histamine phosphate 0.0275 mg/kg) is administered subcutaneously. Epinephrine or ephedrine may be administered if the adverse effects of flushing, headache, nasal stuffiness, dizziness, faintness, and nausea become too severe. Epinephrine and ephedrine antagonize the effects of histamine (except the effects of gastric secretion).

Monitor the client's pulse rate and BP closely. Prevent the client from swallowing saliva, because its alkalinity may interfere with test results. Obtain four samples for volume and acidity of gastric contents, 15 minutes apart for analysis. The maximal acid output is determined by adding the total milliequivalent of all samples collected after the injection of the gastric acid stimulant. The maximal acid output should be 1.5 to 3 times the baseline acid output. The maximum effect from the histamine is usually seen in approximately 30 minutes. *This test should be performed by or under the direction of a physician.*

Pentagastrin (Peptavlon) is another drug used to induce gastric secretion. It is a useful test for achlorhydria and is helpful in diagnosing pernicious anemia, atrophic gastritis, and gastric carcinoma. It is as effective as histamine and produces significantly fewer side effects and less severe adverse reactions.

✺ What agents counteract the effects of histamine?

Antihistamines are drugs that compete with histamine for its receptor sites. With the discovery of two histamine receptors (H_1 and H_2), the antihistamines are divided into the H_1-receptor antagonists and the H_2-receptor antagonists. Chapter 11 discusses agents that block H_1 receptors and are used to diminish symptoms of allergic rhinitis and seasonal allergies (see the following section). Chapters 11 and 40 discuss the H_2-receptor blocking agents, which include cimetidine (Tagamet), ranitidine (Zantac), famotidine (Pepcid), and nizatidine (Axid) that inhibit gastric acid secretion in the stomach. Although not direct histamine receptor antagonists, corticosteroids administered nasally are also indicated for control of allergic rhinitis and seasonal allergy symptoms. They are well tolerated and may be more effective than the H_1 antagonists at controlling symptoms. Chapter 37 discusses inhibitors of mast cell degranulation (e.g., cromolyn, nedocromil) and antibodies directed against IgE on the mast cell (omalizumab) that prevent histamine release. Chapter 37 discusses leukotriene antagonists (e.g., montelukast) that are also used in the treatment of allergic rhinitis.

✺ What is the role of H_1 antagonists?

Antihistamines prevent the physiologic action of histamine by preventing it from reaching its site of action; thus the H_1 antihistamines have the greatest therapeutic effect on nasal allergies. They do not inhibit histamine already attached to receptors; therefore these drugs are more effective if administered before histamine is released. They relieve symptoms better at the beginning of the pollen season than during its height, but they fail to relieve the asthma that often accompanies allergic rhinitis. These preparations are palliative and do not immunize the individual or protect over time against allergic reactions.

Antihistamines do not have much impact on the bronchioles or blood vessels directly and do not replace standard sympathomimetic treatments for anaphylaxis (e.g., epinephrine) or asthma (e.g., β_2-agonists). Dozens of antihistamine drugs are available and generally differ from each other by potency, duration of action, and incidence of adverse effects, particularly sedation. The newer antihistamines including desloratadine (Clarinex), fexofenadine (Allegra), and loratadine (Alavert, Claritin) are usually less sedating because of reduced distribution to the CNS (Bender, Berning, Dudden, Milgrom, & Tran, 2003). Many of the antihistamines currently on the market are now over-the-counter (OTC) and Chapter 11 discusses their use. Table 38-3 compares antihistamines, pharmacokinetics, and dosing.

TABLE 38-3 HISTAMINE₁ ANTAGONISTS

Agent	Prescription/ OTC	Typical Oral Adult Dose	Typical Oral Children's Dose	Comment
NONSEDATING				
desloratadine (Clarinex, Aerius❦)	Prescription	5 mg daily	6-11 mo: 1 mg daily 12 mo-5 yr: 1.25 mg daily 6-11 yr: 2.5 mg daily ≧12 yr: 5 mg daily	Metabolite of loratadine
fexofenadine (Allegra)	Prescription	60 mg twice daily (allergic rhinitis: 180 mg once daily)	6-12 yr: 30 mg twice daily	
loratadine (Alavert, Claritin)	OTC	10 mg daily	2-6 yr: 5 mg daily >6 yr: 10 mg daily	
SEDATING				
azatadine (Optimine)	Prescription	1-2 mg PO twice daily	Not recommended	
brompheniramine (Dimetane)	OTC	4 mg q4-6h	<6 yr: 0.125 mg/kg q6h 6-12 yr: 2-4 mg q6-8h	
cetirizine (Zyrtec)	Prescription	5-10 mg daily	6-12 mo: 2.5 mg daily 12-24 mo: 2.5 mg daily to twice daily 2-6 yr: 2.5-5 mg daily >6 yr: adult dose	Metabolite of hydroxyzine Probably less sedating than other agents in this group
chlorpheniramine (Chlor-Trimeton)	OTC	4 mg q4-6h	2-6 yr: 1 mg q4-6h 6-12 yr: 2 mg q4-6h	
clemastine fumarate (Tavist)	OTC	1.34-2.68 mg two to three times daily	6-12 yr: 0.67-1.34 mg twice daily	
cyproheptadine (Periactin)	Prescription	2-8 mg three to four times daily	2-6 yr: 2 mg q8-12h 7-14 yr: 4 mg q8-12h	Used for cluster headaches Also used as appetite stimulant at higher end of dose range
diphenhydramine (Benadryl, Benylin)	Prescription/ OTC depending on dose	25-50 mg q4-6h	2-6 yr: 6.25 mg PO q4-6h 6-12 yr: 12.5-25 mg PO q4-6h	
hydroxyzine (Atarax, Vistaril)	Prescription	25-100 mg q6h	<6 yr: 0.5 mg/kg q6-8h 6-12 yr: 12.5-25 mg q6-8h	Also used for anxiety, nausea, insomnia

Modified from Lacy, C.F., Armstrong, L.L., Goldman, M.P., & Lance, L.L. (2004). *Lexi-Comp's Drug Information Handbook* (12th ed.) Hudson, Ohio: Lexi-Comp.
*As base drug.

✳️⁀ diphenhydramine [dye fen **high** dra meen]

(Allerdryl✤, Benadryl)

Diphenhydramine is a H_1 antagonist and is available both OTC and by prescription. Unlike other antihistamines, it also depresses the cough center in the medulla of the brain.

Indications

Diphenhydramine is indicated for the symptomatic relief of allergic rhinitis, allergic dermatosis, and other histamine-based allergic reactions. Unique among the H_1 antagonists, diphenhydramine is also used as a cough suppressant, for treatment of nausea and vomiting, and to treat acute dystonic reactions associated with the dopamine-blocking antipsychotics. As a sedating antihistamine, it is also used as an OTC treatment for insomnia.

Pharmacokinetics/Dosing

The adult dosage for an antitussive effect is 25 mg PO (syrup) every 4 to 6 hours; for an antihistamine effect, the dosage is 25 to 50 mg PO every 4 to 6 hours when necessary; and as a sedative-hypnotic, the dosage is 50 mg given 20 to 30 minutes before bedtime. The dosage for antidyskinetic or antiparkinson effects is 50 to 150 mg PO daily in divided doses. For antiemetic or antivertigo effects, the dosage is 25 to 50 mg PO 30 minutes before traveling and before each meal as necessary. Older adults may be more sensitive to the effects of this drug; lower adult dosages should be prescribed, with close monitoring for any adverse effects. The maximum recommended daily dose is 300 mg in divided doses. The antihistamine dosage for children is 1.25 mg/kg PO every 4 to 6 hours up to 300 mg daily. Do not use diphenhydramine in premature or full-term neonates.

The adult dosage of diphenhydramine injection for antihistamine or antidyskinetic effects is 10 to 50 mg intramuscularly (IM) or IV every 2 to 3 hours. For antiemetic or antivertigo effects, the initial dosage is 10 mg IM or IV, which may be increased to 20 to 50 mg every 2 or 3 hours. In children the parenteral dosage for antihistamine or antidyskinetic effects is 1.25 mg/kg IM four times daily. Do not use in premature or full-term neonates.

Adverse Effects

The most common adverse effects with diphenhydramine include sedation and antimuscarinic effects, including dry mouth, urinary retention, and constipation. Urinary retention may be particularly problematic in older men with benign prostatic hyperplasia (BPH). Other effects include increased appetite, diarrhea, blurred vision, and thickened bronchial secretions.

Drug Interactions

The sedative effects of diphenhydramine can produce excessive sedation when used with other CNS sedatives or drugs with sedating properties. Similarly, additive antimuscarinic effects are observed when diphenhydramine is used with other antimuscarinic agents. Diphenhydramine may also interfere with the gastric absorption of levodopa.

✱ How are nasal steroids used in the management of allergic rhinitis?

The nasally administered corticosteroids are effective in the management of allergic rhinitis symptoms and offer an alternative to antihistamines. There is some evidence that they are more effective in controlling symptoms than the antihistamines, and that the addition of antihistamines to nasal corticosteroid therapy offers no additional benefit. Nasal corticosteroids may result in some burning on administration, but are not associated with adrenal suppression or osteoporosis (Suissa, Baltzan, Kremer, & Ernst, 2004) as is seen with parenteral corticosteroid use. Nasal administration of these agents has no effect on control of lower respiratory inflammatory states (e.g., asthma) and these formulations should not be confused with the inhaled corticosteroids for asthma. Table 38-4 compares available nasal corticosteroids. Chapter 48 presents a more complete discussion of corticosteroids.

✱ E.F. is a 51-year-old librarian with allergic rhinitis to mold spores. Her symptoms include itchy watery eyes and a runny nose, and they appear worse on days she has to work in the "old book" section. She has just seen her allergist who gave her a prescription for fexofenadine (Allegra) 60 mg PO twice daily and fluticasone nasal (Flonase) two sprays each nostril daily. Instructions from the allergist were to decide which one of the two therapies she preferred, and have only one of the prescriptions filled. She seeks counsel from her brother who is a nursing student.

✱ What nursing considerations are recommended for E.F. with the use of antihistamines and nasal corticosteroids?

Assessment Assess E.F. for renal function impairment because the increased half-life with fexofenadine would necessitate one daily dosing. With the nasal fluticasone, determine that E.F. does not have any systemic infection, ocular herpes simplex, or tuberculosis of the respiratory tract for which the nasal corticosteroid may mask or exacerbate the infection. If E.F. has had any recent nasal ulcers, trauma or surgery, the drug would inhibit wound healing. Review E.F.'s health history to determine if there is a previous intolerance to corticosteroids or antihistamines. If E.F. were of childbearing age, the pregnancy safety category of her medications would need to be considered (see the Pregnancy Safety box on p. 734).

TABLE 38-4 COMPARATIVE NASAL CORTICOSTEROIDS FOR ALLERGIC RHINITIS

Agent	Adult Nasal Dose
beclomethasone (Beconase AQ)	1-2 sprays each nostril twice daily
budesonide (Rhinocort Aqua)	1-4 sprays each nostril daily
fluticasone (Flonase)	2 sprays each nostril daily
flunisolide (Nasarel)	2 sprays each nostril two to three times daily
mometasone (Nasonex)	2 sprays each nostril daily
triamcinolone (Nasacort AQ, Nasacort HFA)	1-2 sprays each nostril daily

Category	Drug
B	azatadine, brompheniramine, cetirizine, clemastine, cyproheptadine, dexchlorpheniramine, dimenhydrinate, diphenhydramine, loratadine
C	benzonatate, chlorpheniramine, codeine, desloratadine, dextromethorphan, fexofenadine, hydroxyzine

Data from *Mosby's drug consult* (15th ed.). (2005). St. Louis: Mosby.

In reviewing E.F.'s current medication regimen, she indicates that she takes no other medications except for antacids on occasion for heartburn. Advise her to take the fexofenadine either 1 hour before or 2 hours after the antacid when she takes it. Obtain a baseline assessment of E.F.'s allergic rhinitis symptoms.

Nursing Diagnosis With the administration of fexofenadine as with other antihistamines, E.F. is at risk for the following nursing diagnoses/collaborative problems: impaired comfort related to dryness of the mouth and throat, rash, and/or tinnitus; risk for injury related to dizziness or drowsiness; ineffective airway clearance related to thickened mucus; and fatigue. If she elects to use the fluticasone nasal spray, the nursing diagnosis/collaborative problems may be: altered comfort (headache, sore throat) and risk for injury (crusting inside nose, epistaxis, irritation or ulceration of the nasal mucosa).

Planning In the discussion with E.F. and a review of the route of administration, adverse effects, cost, and other compliance issues, she indicates that although she would prefer to take a pill rather than a nasal spray, she feels her compliance would be greater with a once a day medication. Additionally, the fluticasone would be less expensive on a monthly basis. For these reasons, she elects to manage her allergic rhinitis with a nasal spray. Either medication will meet the goals for her drug therapy for allergic rhinitis that include:
- Decreased symptoms of allergic rhinitis with altered nasal mucosa.
- Effective management of her therapeutic drug regimen.
- Collaboration with health care providers for monitoring and ongoing care.

Implementation

Monitoring Monitor for resolution of symptoms of allergic rhinitis, including rhinorrhea and eye irritation (pruritus, erythema, excessive tearing). Fluticasone nasal spray is not continued for more than 3 weeks unless there is improvement in symptoms of allergy.

Intervention Regular use is required to obtain optimal therapeutic effect. Shake container well before using the spray.

Education Instruct E.F. in the proper administration technique. Have her blow her nose before delivering the spray and aim spray away from nasal septum (aim for inner corner of the eye). If she experiences blocked nasal passages, she may use a topical decongestant just prior to her nasal corticosteroid; however, because of congestive rebound, nasal decongestants should be used only for 3 to 5 days. Stress the importance of not using more medication than prescribed because of enhanced absorption and increased adverse effects. It may be 3 weeks before E.F. experiences optimal benefits. Unless approved by her physician, she should avoid immunizations while taking nasal corticosteroids because of a lack of immunologic response or possible neurologic hazard (*USP DI,* 2005). Advise E.F. to check with her prescriber before using any other nasal medication; if she experiences signs of infection of the nose, throat, or sinuses occur; if she experiences no improvement in her symptoms in 3 weeks; or if her condition worsens.

Evaluation E.F. will demonstrate relief from itching, sneezing, and nasal secretions without nasal irritation of ulceration, manage her therapeutic regimen effectively, and collaborate with the health care providers for monitoring and treatment by keeping scheduled appointments.

✳ **T.F. is a newborn of 26 weeks' gestation who, immediately after delivery, is administered the surfactant beractant (Survanta) to help prevent respiratory distress syndrome (RDS).**

✳ **What is the role of surfactants in preventing and treating RDS of the premature newborn?**
Naturally occurring surfactant is produced in the fetus by 24 weeks gestation but secretion into fetal airways may lag an additional 2 to 6 weeks. Surfactant is an important lipid-protein mixture that reduces surface tension in the lung and prevents alveolar collapse or atelectasis. Inadequate surfactant can lead to the development of RDS in the premature newborn.

Administration of lung surfactant intratracheally to the premature newborn reduces the severity of RDS. Three surfactants are available for administration. Beractant (Survanta) and calfactant (Infasurf) are a bovine source surfactant, whereas colfosceril (Exosurf Neonatal) is synthetically derived. Each is used to prevent or treat RDS in low-birth-weight (LBW) neonates or those who have evidence of surfactant deficiency. Refer to product information for specific issues regarding dosing and administration of these products.

Summary

The drugs discussed in this chapter cover a wide range of therapeutic effects on the respiratory system. Oxygen, a therapeutic gas, is essential to sustain life, and its administration is required for many clients. Although most acute care facilities have a respiratory therapy department, the nurse is responsible for evaluating the client's response to oxygen and, in some circumstances, initiating oxygen therapy.

In general, cough suppressants are used for nonproductive coughs in which prolonged coughing is annoying, exhausting, and painful. (Chapter 14 discusses opioid antitussive drugs.) Nonnarcotic (nonopioid) antitussive drugs may be effective and produce fewer GI adverse effects.

Histamine is a chemical mediator that occurs naturally in most body tissues and has been implicated in a number of pathologic conditions, such as urticaria, atopy, food allergies, bronchial asthma, and systemic anaphylaxis. This makes antihistamines, which compete with histamines at receptor sites to prevent their physiologic actions, invaluable as medications. Antihistamines are contained in numerous antitussive preparations, cough and cold products, OTC sleeping compounds, and oral analgesic products. The nasal corticosteroids are also highly effective in the treatment of allergic rhinitis.

Surfactant therapy is generally limited to premature neonates to prevent or treat respiratory distress syndrome of the newborn. Its use requires specialized administration procedures and monitoring typically observed in the neonatal intensive care unit.

✴ Critical Thinking Questions

- Mr. Hodges, a 72-year-old with COPD, has been receiving low-flow oxygen therapy at 2 L/min per nasal cannula. When you check the flow meter, you discover it is set at 6 L/min. What assessment do you need to make of Mr. Hodges immediately? Why?

- You are preparing Mr. Hodges and his wife for his return home, where he will be continuing his oxygen therapy. Although Mr. Hodges has given up smoking since he became so ill, you have noticed that both his wife and his son, with whom he lives, smoke. What action will you take?

Bibliography

Abernethy, A.P., Currow, D.C., Frith, P., Fazekas, B.S., McHugh, A., & Bui, C. (2003). Randomised, double blind, placebo controlled crossover trial of sustained release morphine for the management of refractory dyspnoea. *British Medical Journal, 327*, 523-526.

Anderson, D.M., Keith, J., & Novak, P.D. (Eds.) (2002). *Mosby's medical, nursing, and allied health dictionary* (6th ed.). St. Louis: Mosby.

Andy, C., & Thering, A. (2002). How effective are nasal steroids combined with nonsedating antihistamines for seasonal allergic rhinitis? *Journal of Family Practice, 51*(7), 616.

Bailey, R.E. (2004). Home oxygen therapy for the treatment of patients with chronic obstructive pulmonary disease, *American Family Physician, 70*(5), 864-865.

Bender, B.G., Berning, S., Dudden, R., Milgrom, H., & Tran, Z.V. (2003). Sedation and performance impairment of diphenhydramine and second-generation antihistamines: A meta-analysis. *The Journal of Allergy & Clinical Immunology, 111*, 770-776.

Bosker, G. (Ed.). (2004). *Primary and acute care medicine: Practice, protocols, pathways*, (2nd ed.). Atlanta: Thomson American Health Consultants.

Brown, N.J., Roberts, L.J. (2001). Histamine, bradykinin, and their antagonists. In: Hardman, J.G., & Limbird, L.E. (Eds.). (2001). *Goodman & Gilman's The pharmacological basis of therapeutics* (10th ed.). New York: McGraw-Hill.

Chesnutt, M.S., & Prendergast, T.J. (2003). Lung. In L.M. Tierney, Jr., S.J. McPhee, & Papadakis, M.A. (Eds.), *Current Medical Diagnosis & Treatment*. New York: Lange Medical Books/McGraw-Hill.

Drug facts and comparisons (58th ed.). (2005). St. Louis: Facts and Comparisons.

Ibarra, M.S., & Capone, Jr., A. (2004). Retinopathy of prematurity and anterior segment complications, *Ophthalmology Clinics of North America, 17*(4), 577-582.

Kelly, H.W., & Sorkness, C.A. (2002). Asthma. In J.T. DiPiro, R.L. Talbert, G.C. Yee, G.R. Matzke, B.G. Wells, & L.M. Posey (Eds.), *Pharmacotherapy: A Pathophysiological Approach* (5th ed.). New York: McGraw-Hill.

Konzem, S.L., & Stratton, M.A. (2002). Chronic obstructive lung disease. In J.T. DiPiro, R.L. Talbert, G.C. Yee, G.R. Matzke, B.G. Wells, & L.M. Posey (Eds.), *Pharmacotherapy: A Pathophysiological Approach* (5th ed.). New York: McGraw-Hill.

Lacy, C.F., Armstrong, L.L., Goldman, M.P., & Lance, L.L. (2004). *Lexi-Comp's Drug Information Handbook* (12th ed.). Hudson, Ohio: Lexi-Comp.

Laffey, J.G. (2003). Carbon dioxide attenuates pulmonary impairment resulting from hyperventilation. *Critical Care Medicine, 31*(11), 2634-2640.

Mosby's drug consult (15th ed.). (2005). St. Louis: Mosby.

Schnell, Z.B., Van Leeuwen, A.M., & Kranpitz, T.R.. (2003). *Davis's Comprehensive handbook of laboratory and diagnostic tests and nursing implications*. Philadelphia: F.A. Davis.

e-LEARNING SUPPLEMENTS

Student CD-ROM
- Final Exam questions
- NCLEX® Examination review questions
- Pharmacology animations
- Printable chapter summary

Evolve Website (http://evolve.elsevier.com/mckenry)
- Case study on oxygen and miscellaneous respiratory agents
- Content updates, including information on new drugs

- WebLinks corresponding to this chapter
- Answers to the critical thinking questions in this chapter
- *Elsevier ePharmacology Update* newsletter
- Mosby's Drug Consult Internet Edition
- Supplemental and reference information

Self, T.H. (2005). Asthma. In M.A. Koda-Kimble, L.Y. Young, W.A. Kradian, B.J. Guglielmo, B.K. Alldredge, & R.L. Corelli (Eds.), *Applied therapeutics: The clinical use of drugs* (8th ed.). Philadelphia: Lippincott Williams & Wilkins.

Suissa, S., Baltzan, M., Kremer, R., Ernst, P. (2004). Inhaled and nasal corticosteroid use and the risk of fracture. *American Journal of Respiratory and Critical Care Medicine, 169,* 83-88.

U.S. Food and Drug Administration. (May 2005). FDA warns against abuse of dextromethorphan (DXM). Retrieved July 10, 2005, from http://www.fda.gov/bbs/topics/ANSWERS/2005/ANS01360.html.

USP DI: Drug information for the health care professional (25th ed.). (2005). Greenwood Village, CO: MICROMEDEX Thomson Healthcare.

Williams, D.M., & Kradjan, W.A. (2005). Chronic obstructive pulmonary disease. In M.A. Koda-Kimble, L.Y. Young, W.A. Kradian, B.J. Guglielmo, B.K. Alldredge, & R.L. Corelli (Eds.), *Applied therapeutics: The clinical use of drugs* (8th ed.). Philadelphia: Lippincott Williams & Wilkins.

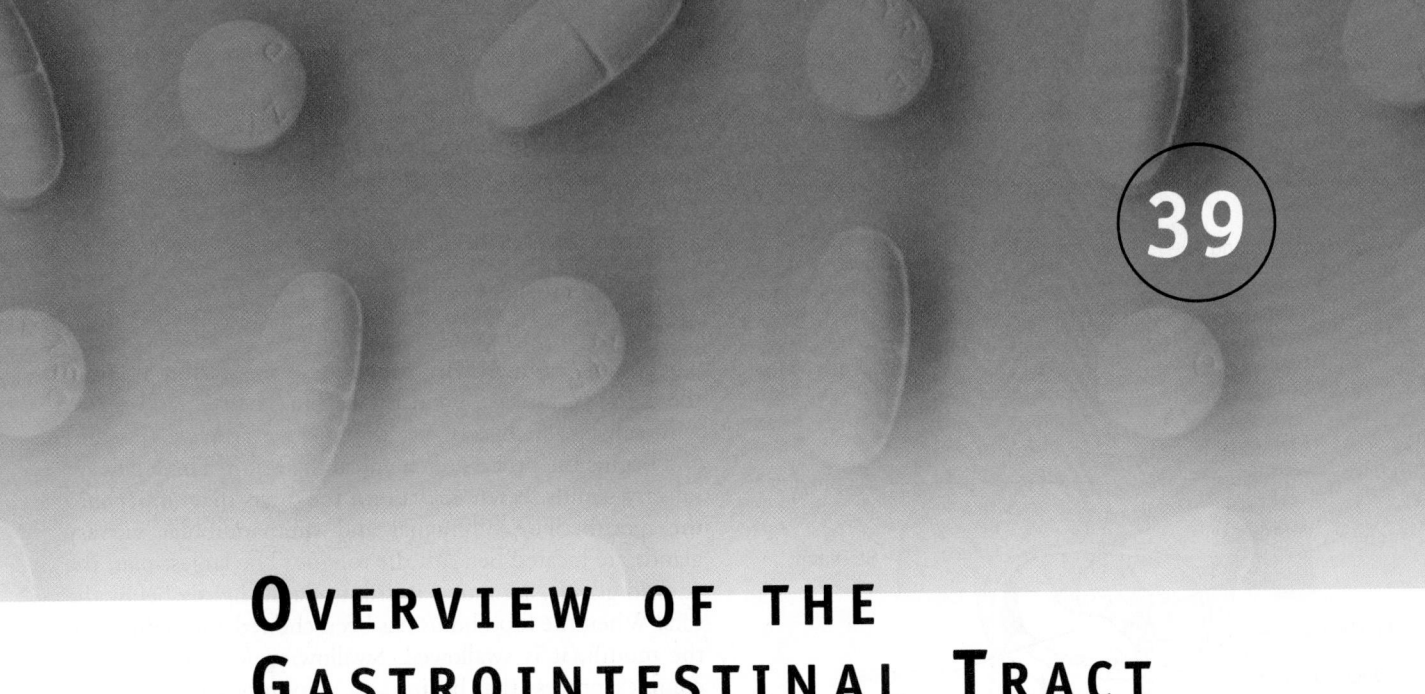

Overview of the Gastrointestinal Tract

Chapter Focus

The gastrointestinal (GI) system is responsible for the digestive processes of the body and for supplying nutrients to fuel the body. This function contributes to a client's wellness by influencing overall health. The nurse should assess every client's nutritional-metabolic need. This assessment requires a thorough knowledge of the anatomy and physiology of the GI system and provides the background for the nurse to plan for and deliver appropriate care to clients with GI disorders. This chapter provides a review of GI anatomy and physiology.

Learning Objectives

- Identify the major parts of the GI tract.
- Describe the functions of individual components of the GI tract.
- List the effects of parasympathetic and sympathetic innervation on the GI tract.
- Describe common disorders affecting the GI tract.

▲ Key Terms

Disorders of the gastrointestinal (GI) tract such as indigestion, gastroesophageal reflux disease (GERD), constipation, diarrhea, and peptic ulcers are very common problems reported by large numbers of the population. Because the cause of many GI diseases remains unclear, pharmacologic management is often directed at relieving symptoms rather than at control or cure. In this chapter the anatomy and functions of the GI tract are reviewed.

✳ **What are the key structures and functions of the gastrointestinal tract?**

The GI system is made up of the alimentary canal (or digestive tract), the biliary system, and the pancreas (Figure 39-1). The alimentary canal extends from the mouth to the anus. Food substances entering the canal undergo mechanical and chemical changes called **digestion.** These changes permit nutrients to be absorbed and indigestible materials to be excreted by the body. Absorbed nutrients may be used as an energy source or stored (as glycogen for glucose or as fat for carbohydrates). **Peristalsis** is the movement of the smooth muscle fibers surrounding the canal that (1) mixes the contents by seg-

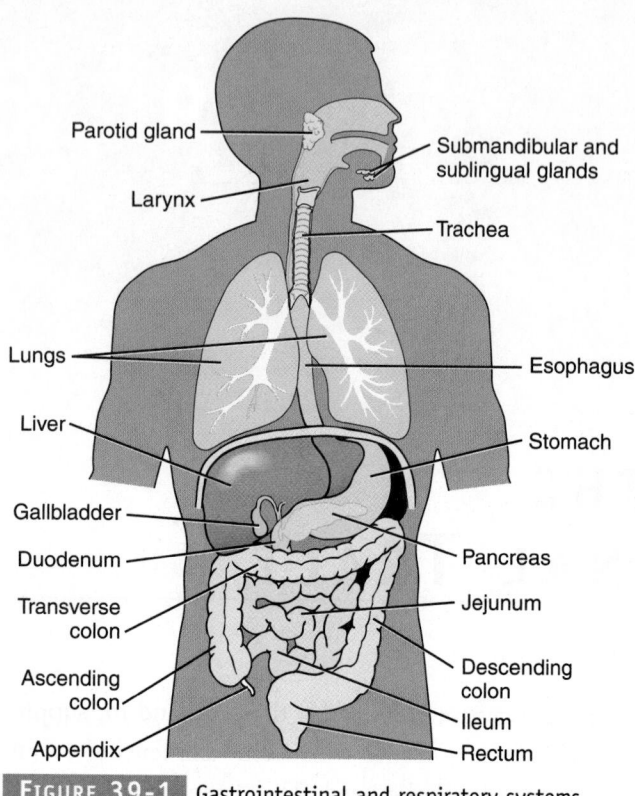

FIGURE 39-1 Gastrointestinal and respiratory systems.

Labels on figure: Parotid gland · Submandibular and sublingual glands · Larynx · Trachea · Lungs · Esophagus · Liver · Stomach · Gallbladder · Duodenum · Pancreas · Transverse colon · Jejunum · Ascending colon · Descending colon · Appendix · Ileum · Rectum

mental contractions and (2) moves the mass through the tract by peristalsis.

The secretory and muscular activities of the GI system are regulated by neural mechanisms. An interconnecting network of neurons is located in the smooth muscle and secretory cells. This system is self-regulating; it is capable of controlling exocrine gland secretions and muscular contractions without any external influence.

By contrast, the external innervation of the GI system is supplied by the divisions of the autonomic nervous system. Their major function is to correlate activities between different regions of the GI system and also between this system and other parts of the body. The influence of the parasympathetic division is mediated by two branches of the vagus nerve and exerts an excitatory action, which increases digestive secretions and muscular activity. In contrast, the splanchnic nerves of the sympathetic division are primarily inhibitory, depressing digestive secretions and muscular activity. Under normal conditions, the two divisions of the autonomic nervous system maintain a delicate balance of control of functions.

✸ By what mechanisms do drugs act in the GI tract?

Drugs affecting the GI tract exert their action mainly on muscular and glandular tissues. The action may be directly on the smooth muscle and gland cells or indirectly on the autonomic nervous system. Drugs may also increase or decrease function, tone, emptying time, or peristaltic action of the stomach or bowel. Additionally, they may be used to relieve enzyme deficiency, to counteract excess acidity or gas formation, to produce or prevent vomiting, or to aid with diagnosis.

✸ What are the normal and pathological states for the mouth, pharynx and esophagus?

Each of these areas provides unique functions in digestion and is associated with unique pathology.

Mouth (Oral Cavity)

The mouth, or oral cavity, functions as the starting point of the digestive process. Food is taken in, chewed, and mixed with saliva, which contains the enzyme amylase (ptyalin) and begins the process of chemical digestion. Three pairs of salivary glands secrete saliva into the ducts that empty into the mouth. The sublingual and submandibular salivary glands are located beneath the tongue. The largest pair, the parotid glands, are found in front of and slightly below the ears. When the food bolus has been chewed and reduced in the mouth, it is swallowed. Swallowing (deglutition) is a complex process that begins as a voluntary movement but continues as an involuntary muscular reflex as the food is propelled through the GI tract.

Disorders Affecting the Mouth Systemic diseases, nutritional deficiencies, and mechanical trauma can cause irritation or inflammation of the buccal structures. Dental disorders (e.g., caries, gingivitis, and pyorrhea) and bacterial, viral, or fungal infections (e.g., candidiasis or herpes simplex) can affect the structures of the oral cavity, causing symptoms such as mouth blistering or other lesions, swelling, pain, and inflammation. Drug therapy such as cancer chemotherapy is can also result in irritation to these tissues. Chapter 40 discusses agents acting on the oral cavity.

Pharynx

The pharynx (throat), a tube-like passageway connecting the mouth and the esophagus, is important in swallowing. Food and fluid pass through the pharynx into the esophagus. During this passage the trachea is closed to prevent aspiration into the lungs.

Disorders Affecting the Pharynx Like the mouth, various systemic diseases can affect the pharynx. It can become irritated and inflamed (e.g., from sinusitis or the "common cold") and treated symptomatically with an antiinflammatory agent. It can also become a locus of infection (e.g., strep throat), which requires systemic antibiotic therapy.

Esophagus

The esophagus is a pliable muscular structure approximately 25 cm long that extends from the pharynx to the cardiac end of the stomach. It extends through the diaphragm as it drops from the thoracic cavity into the abdominal cavity. The esophagus is considered the beginning of the digestive system proper; the rest of the organs of the GI tract function only in digestion and/or excretion. The esophagus continues the process of swallowing and begins the peristaltic process, or the squeezing of the food bolus down the GI tract by band contraction. The peristaltic band wave stimulates the lower esophageal sphincter, which closes to prevent gastroesophageal reflux and then returns the esophagus to its normal resting state.

Disorders Affecting the Esophagus Esophageal disorders are characterized by retrosternal pain (heartburn) and difficulty in swallowing (dysphagia). The sources of pain are numerous; potential causes include diffuse esophageal spasm, achalasia, pyloric or duodenal ulcers, scleroderma, postural changes (bending forward), excessive alcohol ingestion, and nonspecific dysmotility.

Heartburn commonly results from **gastroesophageal reflux disease (GERD)**, in which the incompetent lower esophageal sphincter permits gastric contents to flow back into the esophagus; or from hiatal hernia, in which a part of the stomach protrudes into the diaphragm. GERD is quite common and affects an estimated 20% to 40% of North American adults (Locke, 1997). One type of hiatal hernia, paraesophageal hernia, may be associated with esophageal obstruction and strangulation. Difficulty in swallowing can be a symptom of esophageal obstruction, mechanical interference with or paralysis of the muscles of deglutition, neuromuscular incoordination, achalasia, carcinoma of the esophagus, anxiety states, hysteria, or schizophrenic hallucinations.

Inflammation of the esophagus can have many causes: reflux esophagitis associated with hiatal hernia, irritant ingestion, infection, peptic ulceration, prolonged gastric intubation, and uremia.

✳ What are the key anatomic and physiologic features of the stomach?

The stomach, a pouch-like structure lying below the diaphragm, has three divisions: the fundus, the body, and the pylorus. Two sphincter muscles—the cardiac sphincter and the pyloric sphincter—regulate the stomach opening. Gastric glands secrete mucus and gastric juice composed of enzymes and hydrochloric acid. They also produce intrinsic factor, a protein essential for the absorption of vitamin B_{12}, which is needed for erythropoiesis (red blood cell [RBC] formation).

The stomach functions as a temporary storage site for food as it is being digested. It also manufactures gastrin, a hormone that regulates enzyme production to facilitate digestion. The stomachs of males and females differ both in storage capacity and in size; females have smaller and more slender stomachs. The stomach is capable of holding 1500 to 2000 mL. It distends after eating and gradually collapses as the food bolus moves into the small intestine. Its churning action further breaks down the food bolus and mixes it with gastric juice to continue chemical digestion. A limited amount of nutrient and drug absorption takes place in the stomach.

The time required for digestion in the stomach depends on the amount of food eaten. Normal emptying time is 2 to 6 hours. However, gastric emptying time may be affected by drug administration, physical activity of the individual, and body position during digestion. Gastric emptying time is a factor to consider in the timing of drug administration, because the presence of food may block the absorption of some drugs.

✳ What pathologic states affect the stomach?

Acute gastritis is an inflammatory response of the stomach lining to the ingestion of irritants, such as ethanol or nonsteroidal antiinflammatory agents, including aspirin. Symptoms include epigastric discomfort, nausea, abdominal tenderness, and GI hemorrhage. Treatment consists of lifestyle modifications and drugs such as antacids, antiemetic agents, anticholinergics, and antihistamines (see Chapter 40).

Chronic gastritis is a long-term inflammation of the stomach lining, generally with degeneration of the gastric mucosa; its causes are not well established. It is more common in women, and the incidence increases with age, excessive smoking, and ethanol use. Symptoms are nonspecific but may include flatulence, epigastric fullness after meals, diarrhea, and bleeding. Iron deficiency anemia and pernicious anemia may result from chronic gastritis. Treatment is the same as for acute gastritis. The usual therapeutic regimen involves treatment of symptoms with antacids, anticholinergics, and sedatives (and vitamin B_{12} if pernicious anemia is present), and the elimination of possible causative or aggravating factors (e.g., aspirin use).

Peptic ulcer disease is a broad term encompassing both gastric and duodenal ulcers. Although both types of ulcers produce a "break" in the gastric mucosa, the causes differ. With gastric ulcers the ability of the gastric mucosa to protect and repair itself seems to be defective; with duodenal ulcers the hypersecretion of gastric acid is responsible for the erosion of the gastric mucosa. Gastric colonization with *Helicobacter pylori*, a gram-negative bacillus, has been identified as a causative agent in clients with peptic ulcer disease not caused by nonsteroidal antiinflammatory drugs. Treatment with various antibacterial combinations has resulted in healing and a low recurrence rate. *H. pylori* has been identified in nearly all persons with duodenal ulcers and in nearly 75% of persons with gastric ulcers.

Duodenal ulcers are more common than gastric ulcers; they account for nearly 80% of all peptic ulcers. Duodenal ulcers usually occur more often in younger persons. Overall, the reported incidence of peptic ulcers is much lower in females. In addition to antibacterial combination therapies, pharmacologic treatment of peptic ulcer disease may include the use of proton pump inhibitors, antacids, H_2-receptor antagonists, and sucralfate (Hoogerwerf & Pasricha, 2001). Nondrug treatment (diet and lifestyle modification) is equally important (see Chapter 40). Hereditary factors, the use of some drugs (e.g., aspirin and corticosteroids), psychological factors, stress, and diet have been implicated in the development of peptic ulcer disease.

✳ What features of liver structure and function are essential?

Immediately under the diaphragm and above the stomach is the liver, the largest gland in the body. It weighs approximately 1.5 kg and is an extremely active and important organ that performs more than 100 different functions.

The liver consists of two lobes, which are composed of multitudes of lobules that function to remove toxins from the bloodstream, store nutrients such as iron and some vitamins, and secrete bile. Bile is transported via the hepatic ducts to the gallbladder for storage. In the intestine, bile aids in the digestion, emulsification, and absorption of fat. Because it is normally alkaline, bile also functions to neutralize gastric acid in the duodenum. The liver also is responsible for the manufacture of key substances, including albumin and clotting factors.

Venous blood goes directly to the liver from the intestinal tract; nutrients and absorbed drugs pass through the liver before reaching the systemic circulation. Thus the liver plays an active role in absorbing and metabolizing fats, carbohydrates, and proteins. It also stores iron and vitamins A, B_{12}, and D. Some drugs are taken up by the liver, released into the bile, and excreted in the feces. Other drugs move from the bile into the small intestine, where they are reabsorbed and recirculated. Still other drugs are transformed by the liver and excreted in the urine. In all of these cases the liver metabolizes the drug to make it more water soluble. This biotransformation changes the parent compound to a metabolite that may have greater, lesser, or equal activity; cytochrome P450 in the liver is responsible for biotransformation. There are also drugs that pass through the body and are excreted unchanged in the urine. See Chapter 3 for more detail.

Disorders Affecting the Liver Viral hepatitis, Laënnec cirrhosis, postnecrotic cirrhosis, carcinoma, and chronic alcoholism cause liver damage and liver cell dysfunction. Complications of advanced liver disease include coagulopathies, portal hypertension, ascites, esophageal varices, and hepatic encephalopathy. Because pathology of the liver impedes drug biotransformation, pharmacologic therapy for those with liver disease is very carefully monitored. Drugs may be given in smaller doses or at less frequent intervals, and drugs that are particularly toxic to the liver may be avoided altogether.

What are the important issues to consider in gallbladder and pancreatic function?

Gallbladder

Lying on the undersurface of the liver is the gallbladder, a pear-shaped organ 7 to 10 cm long and 2.5 to 3.5 cm wide. The gallbladder can hold 30 to 50 mL of bile. It concentrates the bile and stores it until it is needed for digestion in the stomach and small intestine.

Disorders Affecting the Gallbladder Cholecystitis, inflammation of the gallbladder, is often associated with the presence of gallstones (cholelithiasis). The stones lodge in the ducts or neck of the gallbladder, causing congestion and edema as bile builds up. This condition may be acute or

chronic. Treatment of cholecystitis and cholelithiasis includes the administration of analgesics, antispasmodics, and chenodeoxycholic acid. Malignant tumors of the gallbladder are uncommon.

Pancreas

The pancreas is a gland that is approximately 15 to 20 cm long and 5 cm wide, and it weighs approximately 75 g. The gland has three major segments: the head (found in the curve of the duodenum), the body, and the tail (which touches or nearly touches the spleen). The role of the pancreas is twofold: the exocrine cells secrete the digestive enzymes found in pancreatic juice, and the endocrine cells help to control the metabolism of carbohydrates by producing glucagon and insulin.

Disorders Affecting the Pancreas With the exception of diabetes mellitus (DM), many pancreatic diseases have symptoms that are not readily diagnosed. Inflammation of the pancreas, referred to as pancreatitis, may be acute or chronic. Among the many causes are blockage of the pancreatic ducts, trauma to the pancreas, alcohol consumption, drug use, tumors, cysts, or abscesses. Symptoms are nonspecific but ultimately include severe pain. Carcinoma of the pancreas is as difficult to diagnose as other pancreatic disorders.

What are the structure and function of the small and large intestines?

Small Intestine

The small intestine is a coiled tube approximately 21 feet long. It consists of the duodenum, jejunum, and ileum. Within the small intestine the food bolus is thoroughly mixed with the digestive juices to complete the "breakdown" process. The intestinal mucosa then absorbs nutrients and drugs, which are filtered through the liver before entering the circulatory and lymphatic systems.

Disorders Affecting the Small Intestine Diarrhea and constipation are two disorders that affect the entire lower GI tract. Chapters 11 and 40 discuss these disorders along with the drugs used in their treatment. Diarrhea (frequent, profuse, and/or loose stools) may be due to drugs, foods, infections, or other conditions. Constipation, which involves reduced stool frequency or difficulty in passing stool, may be related to diet, dehydration, lack of exercise, or drugs.

Other disorders affecting the small intestine include obstruction, malabsorption syndrome, and blind loop syndrome. Symptomatic treatment is customary while the underlying causative factors are investigated.

Large Intestine

The cecum, colon, and rectum make up the large intestine. The distal 2.5 cm of the rectum is known as the anal canal. The large intestine is approximately 5 feet long and completes the digestive and absorptive processes. The large intestine is involved mainly with water absorption (from 1800 to 3000 mL/day) and synthesis of vitamin K. The lining of the large intestine secretes mucus to coat the undigested residue and protect the bowel lining. The indigestible residue is expelled through the reflex action known as defecation.

Disorders Affecting the Large Intestine Diarrhea and constipation, discussed in Chapters 11 and 40, also affect the large intestine. Other disorders include diverticular disease, which has no specific pharmacologic therapy; ulcerative colitis, which is treated with lifestyle modifications, antidiarrheals, and steroids; carcinoma; Crohn's disease; and irritable bowel syndrome (IBS). Hemorrhoids (varicosities of the external or internal hemorrhoidal veins) are common.

Summary

Food sustains life and determines nutritional status, which contributes to an individual's state of health, levels of achievement, and resistance to and ability to handle disease. The primary function of the GI tract is to provide the body cells with nutrients, electrolytes, and water through the processes of ingestion, digestion, and absorption of food and fluid and the elimination of waste products and residue. Drugs affect the GI tract by acting primarily on muscular and glandular tissue. Although some drugs are prescribed primarily for their effect on the GI tract, the nurse needs to be aware that most drugs prescribed for other reasons also produce GI adverse effects.

✳ Critical Thinking Questions

- Imagine being a bolus of food progressing through the GI tract; describe what the journey would be like.
- Patty Smith has been diagnosed as having achlorhydria, a condition in which the stomach stops producing hydrochloric acid. What effect will this have on her digestion? On her RBC count?

Bibliography

Anderson, D.M., Keith, J., & Novak, P.D. (Eds.) (2002). *Mosby's medical, nursing, and allied health dictionary* (6th ed.). St. Louis: Mosby.

Guyton, A.C., & Hall, J.E. (2000). *Textbook of medical physiology* (10th ed.). Philadelphia: W.B. Saunders.

Hardman, J.G., & Limbird, L.E. (Eds.). (2001). *Goodman and Gilman's The pharmacological basis of therapeutics* (10th ed.). New York: McGraw-Hill.

Herlihy, B., & Maebius, N.K. (2003). *The human body in health and illness* (2nd ed.). Philadelphia: W.B. Saunders.

Hoogerwerf, W.A., & Pasricha, P.J. (2001). Agents used for control of gastric acidity and treatment of peptic ulcers. In: Hardman, J.G. & Limbird, L.E. (Eds.), *Goodman and Gilman's The pharmacological basis of therapeutics* (10th ed.). New York: McGraw-Hill.

Locke, G.R., Talley, N.J., Fett, S.L., Zinsmeister, A.R., & Melton, L.J. (1997). Prevalence and clinical spectrum of gastroesophageal reflux: A population-based study in Olmsted County, Minnesota. *Gastroenterology, 112,* 1448-1456.

McCance, K.L., & Huether, S.E. (2002). *Pathophysiology: The biological basis for disease in adults and children* (4th ed.). St. Louis: Mosby.

Thibodeau, G.A., & Patton, K.T. (2003). *Anatomy and physiology* (5th ed.). St. Louis: Mosby.

e-LEARNING SUPPLEMENTS

Student CD-ROM
- Final Exam questions
- NCLEX® Examination review questions
- Pharmacology animations
- Printable chapter summary

Evolve Website (http://evolve.elsevier.com/mckenry)
- Content updates, including information on new drugs

- WebLinks corresponding to this chapter
- Answers to the critical thinking questions in this chapter
- *Elsevier ePharmacology Update* newsletter
- Mosby's Drug Consult Internet Edition
- Supplemental and reference information

DRUGS AFFECTING THE GASTROINTESTINAL TRACT

CHAPTER FOCUS

The gastrointestinal (GI) tract affects the overall health of the individual because it has the essential task of supplying necessary nutrients to fuel the physiologic processes of other vital organs (brain, lungs, and heart) and of eliminating the body's wastes. Many GI disorders present with pain, nausea, constipation, and diarrhea, which negatively affect the client's quality of life. To assist clients toward self-management and optimal health, the nurse needs to be knowledgeable and skillful in the management of the pharmacologic therapeutic regimen related to the GI tract.

LEARNING OBJECTIVES

- Describe the use and side effects of antacids.
- List four drugs administered to promote digestion.
- Differentiate the five classes of antiemetic medications and their sites of action.
- Explain the effect of proton pump inhibitors and H_2 receptor antagonists on gastric acid secretion.
- Explain the use of mesalamine, olsalazine, sulfasalazine, and infliximab in the treatment of inflammatory and ulcerative bowel disease.
- Differentiate between various types of laxatives, their mechanisms of action, and the best indication for each type.
- Implement nursing management of clients receiving agents that affect the GI tract.

▲ KEY TERMS

antiemetics, p. 758
chemoreceptor trigger zone (CTZ), p. 758
constipation, p. 771
diarrhea, p. 753
emetic center, p. 758
laxatives, p. 771

✱▀ KEY DRUGS

cimetidine, p. 750
mesalamine, p. 768
metoclopramide, p. 760
omeprazole, p. 748
ondansetron, p. 762

✱ What drugs affect the upper GI tract?

A number of modalities impact on prevention or treatment of disease, or on client comfort related to perioral and stomach ailments. These include oral rinses, dental products, antiinfectives, and saliva substitutes in the treatment of oral conditions, and a number of drugs affecting acidity, ulcers/erosions, and nausea/vomiting treat conditions of the lower esophagus and stomach.

✱ T.M. is an 8-year-old boy who has recently started prednisone (Deltasone) therapy orally for asthma. He also is finishing up a 10-day course of antibiotics for bronchitis. He presents to the school nurse with white lesions on his tongue. The nurse suspects oral candidiasis and arranges a visit with the nurse practitioner.

✱ How does oral candidiasis present?

Oral candidiasis (or "thrush"), caused by *Candida albicans*, can present as cream-colored or bluish white patches of exudate on the tongue, mouth, or pharynx that reveal bloody engorgement when scraped. A culture of the fungus may be obtained before initiating antifungal therapy. Clients who have acquired immunodeficiency syndrome (AIDS) or are taking antineoplastic or immunosuppressive drugs (e.g., corticosteroids) are particularly at risk for oral candidiasis. Concurrent antibacterial therapy may also predispose to candidiasis.

✱ How is oral candidiasis treated?

Treatment of oral candidiasis includes both topical treatments (nystatin oral rinse, clotrimazole troches or lozenges) and systemically administered antifungals (e.g., fluconazole [Diflucan]). Chapter 59 discusses systemically administered agents whereas topical treatments for perioral candidiasis will be discussed here.

Clotrimazole and nystatin inhibit the synthesis of sterols in the fungal wall; this increases the permeability of the fungal cell membrane, which results in the loss of important cellular contents. Clotrimazole also inhibits oxidative enzyme activity, which may increase intracellular hydrogen peroxide to toxic levels and thus contribute to the destruction of the fungal cells and their contents. Additionally, they inhibit fungal synthesis of triglycerides and phospholipids. Clotrimazole and nystatin are indicated for the oral-local treatment of candidiasis or fungal infections caused by *Candida* species.

clotrimazole [kloe **trye** ma zole]
(Mycelex troches)
Indications
The clotrimazole troche (or lozenge) is indicated for the treatment of superficial oropharyngeal candidiasis. Other formulations of topical clotrimazole are available, including vaginal preparations and topical creams for fungal or candidal infections in other body areas (see Chapter 65).
Pharmacokinetics/Dosing
Troches are to be slowly dissolved in the mouth and drug levels remain in saliva for 3 hours or more. Typical dose for children over 3 years of age or adults is one 10 mg troche dissolved three times daily during risk times (prophylaxis with cancer chemotherapy or corticosteroid use) or five times daily × 14 days for treatment of active candidiasis.
Adverse Effects
Nausea and vomiting have been reported, as have elevated liver function tests when the troche is used.
Drug Interactions
Serious drug interactions with the use of clotrimazole troches are unlikely. Clotrimazole is a moderate inhibitor of P450 3 A4 and may result in moderate elevations in levels of drugs metabolized by this system.

nystatin [nye **stat** in]
(Mycostatin, Nilstat)
Indications
Nystatin solution or troches is indicated for the treatment of candidal infections of the perioral area.
Pharmacokinetics/Dosing
Nystatin is poorly absorbed systemically from topical perioral use. The dosage of nystatin for adults and children (over 5 years of age) is 400,000 to 600,000 units of oral suspension, four times daily (one half of the dose in each side of mouth, retaining the drug as long as possible before swallowing—this application procedure is often referred to as "swish and swallow"). The troche or lozenge is an alternative, which is dosed at 200,000 to 400,000 units of troches, four to five times daily.
Adverse Effects
Stomach upset, nausea, and vomiting have been reported on occasion.
Drug Interactions
Serious interactions are not observed with nystatin use.

✱ The nurse practitioner decides to treat T.M.'s candidiasis with either clotrimazole lozenges or nystatin suspension. Given that the side effect profile of both drugs is similar, she discusses the different forms of medication and dosing with T.M. and his parents. There is agreement that the probability of compliance would be higher for the nystatin oral suspension as "swishing the solution around in his mouth and gargling seems a lot more fun" than remembering to not chew or swallow a clotrimazole lozenge for 15 to 30 minutes.

✱ What are the nursing management issues for T.M. in the use of topically applied antifungals for perioral use?

Assessment Inspect T.M.'s oropharynx using a tongue depressor and a flashlight. Although T.M. at 8 years old almost surely does not have dentures, clients should be asked to remove any partial or complete dentures for the examination of the oral cavity. Poorly fitting dentures also can be a source of inflammation. T.M. is at risk for candidiasis because of his corticosteroid and antibacterial therapies. Also at particular risk are clients who have AIDS or who are taking antineoplastic, broad spectrum or long-term antimicrobial, or immunosuppressive drugs. The normal mucosa is pink, although dark-skinned clients may have bluish or patch-type pigmented mucosa. Candidiasis presents as cream-colored or bluish white patches of exudate on the tongue, mouth, or pharynx that reveal bloody engorgement when scraped. A culture of the fungus may be obtained before initiating antifungal therapy, but usually with the presence of the characteristic lesions and documented risk exposure as in T.M.'s case, therapy is begun without a culture. Ascertain that T.M. is not allergic to nystatin.

Nursing Diagnosis T.M. may experience the following nursing diagnoses with his oral suspension antifungal therapy: impaired oral mucous membrane related to the underlying condition and the ineffectiveness of or sensitivity to the oral antifungal drug; or impaired comfort related to the GI effects of the drug as evidenced by nausea or vomiting, diarrhea, and perhaps abdominal cramping.

Planning Goals for T.M. and his parents include the following:
- T.M. experiences relief from his symptoms of candidiasis with minimal or no adverse effects from his therapy.
- T.M.'s parents effectively manage his nystatin therapy.

Implementation

Monitoring Using a tongue blade and flashlight, inspect and document the size and condition of the affected areas of the mouth. If T.M. were hospitalized, this would be done on a daily basis.

Intervention Have T.M. brush his teeth and cleanse the area carefully before he takes each dose. For infants and dependent clients, gently swab nystatin on the oral mucosa. Clients with full or partial dentures need to soak them nightly in an oral suspension of nystatin to eliminate the fungus. To minimize the amount of nystatin solution to be used, place the dentures in a small self-sealing plastic bag with a small amount of the solution and express the air from the bag to ensure coverage of the dentures with the solution.

When administering the oral suspension, shake it well to ensure consistency in dosing. When preparing the oral suspension from powder, shake it well and use it immediately, because it contains no preservatives.

Education Instruct T.M. in good oral hygiene techniques. Inform his parents that a dental examination every 6 months is recommended.

When using the oral suspension forms of nystatin, instruct T.M. to swish the medication around in his mouth and maintain contact with the mucosa as long as possible before swallowing, then gargle and swallow the solution. If T.M. were using the troche form of nystatin or of clotrimazole, provide a careful explanation that the troche is to be dissolved slowly in the mouth (15 to 30 minutes). It is not to be chewed or swallowed whole. The saliva is swallowed. The troche may be cut in half to facilitate administration. Avoid the use of troches with children younger than 5 years of age, because they may be unable to safely manage that form of the medication and present a choking hazard.

Instruct T.M. and his parents to have him continue taking the medicine for the full duration prescribed and to report to the nurse practitioner if symptoms persist.

Evaluation The expected outcome of antifungal therapy to prevent and/or treat altered oral mucous membranes is that T.M. will experience normal-colored, intact oropharyngeal mucous membranes without adverse effects of the drug. His parents effectively manage his nystatin therapy, including medication compliance for the full prescription, stating of the common adverse effects of the drug and which are reportable to the prescriber, and collaboration with the health care provider for monitoring and follow-up care.

✱ **T.L. is a 64-year-old woman who is receiving the antimuscarinic tolterodine (Detrol) 2 mg twice daily for the treatment of overactive bladder. She is complaining of very dry mouth (xerostomia) and irritated dentures, and asks the nurse what she can do to be more comfortable.**

✱ **What alternatives are available to treat xerostomia?**
Xerostomia, or dry mouth, can be caused by a number of conditions, but is often a complication of antimuscarinic (anticholinergic) therapy. Drugs with antimuscarinic properties include those used to treat overactive bladder (e.g., tolterodine [Detrol]), antihistamines (e.g., diphenhydramine [Benadryl]), and the tricyclic antidepressants (e.g., imipramine [Tofranil]). Xerostomia can affect the comfort of dentures for older clients who wear them. Treatment can include the frequent use of ice chips or small sips of water, or sugar-free hard candy to promote salivation, or the addition of a saliva substitute.

Saliva substitutes (Orex, Xero-Lube, Moi-Stir, Salivart) are used to relieve dry mouth and throat when simpler modalities are not effective. They are available as solutions in squirt bottles and as pump or aerosol sprays. They contain electrolytes (potassium phosphate, magnesium chloride, potassium chloride, calcium, and sodium), sodium fluoride, sorbitol, and carboxymethylcellulose as the base. Muscarinic agonists (e.g., pilocarpine [Salagen] and cevimeline [Evoxac]) are sometimes used orally for severe xerostomia but would be contraindicated for antimuscarinic-induced dry mouth.

✱ **F.G. is a 43-year-old woman with breast cancer undergoing cancer chemotherapy. Five days after completing her second cycle of cancer chemotherapy, she develops oral lesions with blisters, irritation, tissue sloughing, and pain. The oncology team diagnoses stomatitis and recommends initiation of "magic mouthwash" and systemic antiviral therapy.**

✱ **What treatments are available for stomatitis?**
A number of acute and chronic diseases contribute to mouth blistering and erosions. Determining the etiology of stomatitis or mouth irritation is important before treatment is initiated. Stomatitis can be caused by herpes-type viruses, or aggravated by drugs like cancer chemotherapy. Acute viral diseases such as herpes simplex, herpes zoster, and varicella are commonly implicated and are treated with antiviral therapy. Acyclovir (Zovirax), an antiviral agent, is effective against herpes simplex virus and varicella zoster virus, the viruses associated with skin manifestations. It acts

to reduce viral shedding, time to crusting, duration of local pain, and severity of symptoms. Acyclovir is available in topical, oral, and parenteral dosage forms. Chapter 59 discusses acyclovir and other antivirals.

To improve comfort for clients with stomatitis, a number of treatments are available, including topically anesthetics (e.g., lidocaine), antihistamines (e.g., diphenhydramine) and antacids (e.g., magnesium/aluminum hydroxide). Often health care settings have their own formula for combinations of these ingredients and often refer to the solution or suspension as "Magic Mouthwash." Use of such products is often helpful, but the addition of antimicrobials or corticosteroids to these solutions may complicate therapy and lead to increased risk for candidiasis or viral infection.

For prevention of severe antineoplastic-induced mucositis in clients undergoing stem cell transplantation, palifermin (Kepivance), a recombinant human keratinocyte growth factor, is sometimes given intravenously for 3 days before, during, and for 3 days after chemotherapy. Severe hypersensitivity reactions and tumor growth are the most serious reported adverse effects. Refer to package labeling for more information.

✱ What other drugs are used for perioral care?

In general, medications have little effect on the mouth. Good oral hygiene, which includes brushing properly after meals and at bedtime, flossing, and stimulating the gums, has more influence on the tissues of the mouth than most medicines. Many mouth and throat preparations are available with corticosteroids, anesthetics, and antiseptics for various disorders of the oral cavity, including chapped lips, sun and fever blisters, inflammatory lesions, ulcerative lesions secondary to trauma, gingival lesions, teething pain, toothache, irritation caused by orthodontic appliances or dentures, and abrasions of the oral cavity. Most agents that affect the mouth may be purchased over-the-counter (OTC).

Mouthwashes and Gargles

Mouthwashes and gargles are dilute aromatic solutions that contain a sweetener and an artificial coloring agent. They may also contain an antiseptic (e.g., alcohol, cetylpyridinium chloride, phenol), anesthetic (eugenol, clove oil), astringent (zinc chloride), or anticaries agent (sodium fluoride). Mouthwashes with high alcohol content may be problematic for certain populations (see the Medication Safety Alert box above).

Several products claim to contain ingredients that reduce plaque formation. Clinical trials have demonstrated some success with volatile oils and cetylpyridinium chloride alone or in combination with domiphen bromide. Commercial products that contain at least one of these active ingredients include Cepacol (cetylpyridinium chloride), Listerine (volatile oils), and Scope (cetylpyridinium chloride and domiphen bromide). A detergent-type product to lessen plaque (Plax) is also available on the market. The client should be informed that these products do not replace good oral hygiene but instead are recommended as an adjunct to proper brushing and flossing of the teeth.

✸ Medication Safety Alert

Warnings for Mouthwashes with High Alcohol Content

Pediatric Alert

The leading mouthwashes usually contain from 14% to 27% alcohol. Parents of young children should be cautioned to store these products in a safe area, preferably a locked cabinet. The use of mouthwash in young children is not recommended because children often swallow the mouthwash rather than expectorate it.

Alcohol Abuse

Clients with alcoholism may substitute alcohol-containing products such as mouthwashes and cough-cold preparations when beverage alcohol is not readily available. The health care professional should be alert for ingestion abuse of alcohol-containing products in persons with a history of alcohol abuse.

Oropharyngeal Cancer

As an ingredient in ingestible products, there has been concern that the use of alcohol-containing mouthwash may increase the risk of developing oropharyngeal cancer. A study by Cole, Rodu, & Mathisen (2003) reviewed all nine English-language epidemiologic studies of oropharyngeal cancer that made reference to mouthwash and determined that it is unlikely that the use of alcohol-containing mouthwashes increase the risk of developing oropharyngeal cancer (Cole et al., 2003).

Mouthwashes are often used for halitosis, or "bad breath," or as gargles to treat colds or sore throats. In general, they are not considered effective for such problems. Mouthwashes may improve mouth odor briefly; however, if such a problem persists, the underlying cause needs to be identified and treated (e.g., poor dental hygiene, various gum diseases, and many other potential causes).

Sore throats are usually caused by infection, most often viral rather than bacterial. Gargling cannot reach the site of infection, which is usually deep in the throat tissues. Sodium chloride solution (one half teaspoon of salt to an 8-ounce glass of warm water) has been recommended for use as a gargle and mouthwash. Although recommended by a number of sources (e.g., Mayo Clinic, Discovery Health website, numerous university health centers, *American Family Physician*), there is no evidence that it is efficacious, other than as a comfort measure.

Oxygen-Releasing Agents Hydrogen peroxide is a weak antibacterial agent used to clean topical and oral wounds. The antibacterial effect depends on the liberation of oxygen, which occurs when the peroxide comes in contact with the tissue enzyme catalase. The resulting effervescence (bubbling action) loosens pus and tissue debris, which helps to reduce bacterial content. Hydrogen peroxide is usually used in a 1.5% to 3% solution for cleaning wounds or as a mouthwash. As a gargle, the 3% solution should be diluted with an equal amount of water before use.

A number of other oxygen-releasing products are commercially available. Perimax Perio Rinse (hydrogen peroxide) is used for the treatment of canker sores, denture irritation, and irritation following orthodontic intervention. The solution is expectorated. Hydrogen peroxide gel (Peroxyl) is also available for minor mouth irritation and is applied and expectorated after use.

Fluoridated Mouthwashes A number of fluoride-containing preparations, including mouthwash (Fluorigard), toothpaste, tablets, and solutions are available for use as anticaries agents. Fluoride prevents decay through three specific mechanisms, it: (1) reduces the solubility of enamel in acid by converting hydroxyapatite into less soluble fluorapatite; (2) exerts an influence directly on dental plaque by reducing the ability of plaque organisms to produce acid; and (3) promotes the remineralization or repair of tooth enamel in areas that have been demineralized by acids. The remineralization effect of fluoride is of prime importance. Fluoride ions in and at the enamel surface result in fortified enamel that is not only more resistant to decay, but enamel that can repair or remineralize early dental decay caused by acids from decay-causing bacteria (American Dental Association, 2005).

Supported by more than half a century of research, the benefits of fluoride toothpastes are firmly established. Taken together, the trials are of relatively high quality, and provide clear evidence that fluoride toothpastes are efficacious in preventing caries (Marinho, Higgins, Logan, & Sheiham, 2003).

Fluoridated mouthwashes are generally used once a day (rinsed for a minute and expectorated), preferably after brushing and flossing. The client should be taught to avoid taking anything by mouth for approximately 30 minutes after use. See Box 40-1 for information regarding fluoride toxicity.

Antiseptic Mouthwashes Phenol penetrates plaque and is a local anesthetic and antimicrobial agent. Chloraseptic mouthwash contains phenol and sodium phenolate. Preparations that provide temporary relief of sore gums caused by teething often contain phenol or benzocaine. Phenol or phenol-type compounds are also present in several OTC lozenges, liquids, and sprays for the treatment of sore throat. The liquid is diluted with equal parts of water or may be sprayed full strength.

Dentifrices

A dentifrice is a substance used to aid in cleaning the teeth. An ordinary dentifrice contains one or more mild abrasives, a foaming agent, and flavoring materials made into a powder or paste (toothpaste) to aid in the mechanical cleansing of accessible parts of the teeth. Fluoride dentifrices are effective anticaries agents. These products carry the American Dental Association ADA) Seal of Acceptance as an important symbol of a dental product's safety and effectiveness.

Dentifrices are also available for the treatment of hypersensitive teeth, which usually occur from exposed root areas at the cement-enamel junction. The exposed area allows pain stimuli access to the nerve fibers in the pulp area. Dentists often suggest desensitizing dentifrices that contain 5% potassium nitrate, such as Promise, Mint Sensodyne, or Denquel.

✳ **P.G. is a 32-year-old advertising executive who eats "on the run," drinks 5 to 6 cups of coffee daily and eats poorly. He has gained 35 pounds over the past year, and complains of frequent epigastric pain and burning. His symptoms include a burning sensation behind his sternum and he often notes an acid taste in his mouth. To relieve discomfort and alter this bad taste, he uses peppermint candy, but notes that symptoms have worsened since starting to use mint. He visits his health care provider who diagnoses gastroesophageal reflux disease (GERD).**

✳ **What are the key issues regarding GERD?**
GERD is a common ailment manifested by retrosternal burning or stinging, acid regurgitation, and occasionally difficulty swallowing (dysphagia). Other symptoms include abdominal pain, cough, hoarseness, belching or bloating, or wheezing. Substernal chest pain may be confused with symptoms of angina or a myocardial infarction (MI). The wheezing and cough are often confused with asthma, particularly in children. Dental erosions can be a complication of acid reflux as well.

A decrease in lower esophageal tone combined with high gastric acid levels account for the pathology of GERD. A

BOX 40-1 FLUORIDE TOXICITY

Community water fluoridation remains the safest, most cost-effective and most equitable method of reducing tooth decay in a community in the developed world. A controlled study conducted in 1990 demonstrated that average tooth decay experience among schoolchildren who were lifelong residents of communities having low fluoride levels in drinking water was 61% to 100% higher as compared with tooth decay experience among schoolchildren who were lifelong residents of a community with an optimal level of fluoride in the drinking water (Selwitz, Nowjack-Raymer, Kingman, & Driscoll, 1998). However, fluoride is capable of producing an acute toxic reaction that may be fatal if not treated promptly. A chronic toxic state resulting in mottling or discoloration of the tooth enamel and possible osteosclerosis has been reported. This effect may occur when excessive fluoride is consumed during childhood. In severe cases, the teeth appear as brown- to black-stained corroded areas. Fluoridated water supplies usually contain 1 ppm (part per million) of fluoride, which is accepted as a safe level that is effective in reducing the incidence of caries in permanent teeth. Health care professionals, particularly in primary health care settings, need to be aware of the amount of fluoride in their water supplies and to recommend and/or closely supervise the use of additional fluoride products by their clients. Fluoride supplements are recommended when community drinking water contains less than 0.7 ppm of fluoride (USP DI, 2005).

number of drugs or foods decrease lower esophageal sphincter (LES) tone. Additionally, any factor that increases pressure on the abdomen is likely to increase pressure on the stomach and LES and predispose to acid backwash in the esophagus. Weight gain, tight fitting clothing, or bending/stooping can induce GERD symptoms. Estrogen use in women is also cor-

related with worsening GERD symptoms (Nilsson, Johnsen, Ye, Hveem, Lagergren, 2003). These contributing factors are listed in Box 40-2.

How is GERD treated?

Nondrug treatments include avoiding foods and drugs that aggravate GERD, weight loss, avoiding tight fitting clothing, and elevating the head of the bed with wooden blocks to reduce nocturnal symptoms. Smoking cessation should also be strongly encouraged.

Drug treatments include the use of proton pump inhibitors (e.g., omeprazole [Prilosec]), histamine$_2$ (H$_2$) receptor antagonists (e.g., cimetidine [Tagamet]), antacids (e.g., magnesium and aluminum hydroxide [Maalox, Mylanta], each of which increase gastric pH. Chapter 11 discusses many of these agents, which are also available OTC. The promotility agents (e.g., metoclopramide [Reglan]) are reserved for clients who do not respond to other modalities and will be discussed with the treatments for nausea and vomiting later in this chapter. Other drugs for gastric conditions, including sucralfate (Carafate) and misoprostol (Cytotec) have not demonstrated improvement in GERD, but will be discussed later in the chapter. See the Special Considerations for Older Adults box below.

How do proton pump inhibitors decrease gastric acidity?

Proton pump inhibitors (PPIs) suppress gastric acid secretion by inhibiting the hydrogen/potassium adenosine triphosphatase (ATPase) enzyme system at the secretory surface of the gastric parietal cells. Therefore they block the final step of acid production, inhibiting both basal and stimulated gastric acid secretion. They are indicated for the treatment of GERD, peptic ulcer disease, and hypersecretory conditions with excessive gastric acid such as Zollinger-Ellison syn-

---

BOX 40-2 CONTRIBUTING FACTORS TO GASTROESOPHAGEAL REFLUX DISEASE (GERD)

A number of drugs and foods decrease the tone of the lower esophageal sphincter (LES) and are associated with aggravation of GERD. Other conditions also worsen GERD symptoms. These are listed below:

FOODS THAT ↓ LES TONE OR WORSEN GERD

Caffeine	Mint
Chocolate	Spicy foods
Fatty foods	Alcoholic beverages

DRUGS THAT ↓ LES TONE OR WORSEN GERD

Caffeine	Nitrates
Calcium channel blockers	Theophylline
Inhaled sympathomimetics	

CONDITIONS THAT WORSEN GERD

Bending or stooping	Pregnancy
Eating late in day	Tight fitting waistbands
Increased abdominal girth	Tobacco/smoking

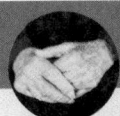

Special Considerations for Older Adults | ANTIULCER THERAPIES

Gastrointestinal symptoms are very common in older adult clients. Every symptom should be properly evaluated before instituting drug therapy.

The use of aluminum-containing antacids should be avoided with older adult clients. They are more apt to have age-related impaired renal function, which may lead to aluminum retention. Chronic use of aluminum-containing antacids may aggravate metabolic bone disease through the actions of phosphorus depletion, hypercalciuria, and inhibition of the absorption of intestinal fluoride (*USP DI*, 2005). Although the neurotoxicity of aluminum is well established, at present, aluminum exposure is not thought to be a major risk factor for Alzheimer's disease (Goetz, 2003; Rondeau, 2000).

With the routine administration of H$_2$ blockers, confusion and dizziness are more commonly reported by older adults than in younger adults (*USP DI*, 2005). With cimetidine, famotidine, and ranitidine, mental status changes have been

reported, especially in older adult persons that have impaired liver or renal function or are severely ill. Acute mental changes in older adult may indicate the need for lowering the drug dose or discontinuing the medication.

In older adult using PPIs, elimination rates of the drugs are decreased and bioavailability is increased. However, these differences in pharmacokinetics do not necessitate dosage adjustments.

Many older adults take NSAIDs for the discomfort of osteoarthritis and are at risk for NSAID-induced gastric ulcers as the result of NSAID inhibition of prostaglandin synthesis. PPIs are often used with NSAIDs to reduce this risk for upper GI bleeding. Misoprostol, a synthetic prostaglandin E1 analog, has mucosal protective properties and is an alternative to PPIs. However, serum levels of misoprostol are increased in the older adult so monitor clients carefully to see if the usual dose is not tolerated (*Drug Facts and Comparisons*, 2005).

TABLE 40-1 COMPARISON OF AGENTS THAT INCREASE GASTRIC pH

Drug	Typical Adult Dose	Comments
PROTON PUMP INHIBITOR		
esomeprazole (Nexium)	Erosive esophagitis/GERD: 20-80 mg PO daily *H. pylori*: 40 mg PO daily × 10 days (with amoxicillin and clarithromycin)	Active metabolite of omeprazole
omeprazole (Prilosec)	Erosive esophagitis/GERD: 20-80 mg PO daily *H. pylori**: 20 mg PO twice daily × 10 days/40 mg PO daily × 14 days Hypersecretion: 60 mg PO daily to 120 mg PO three times daily Peptic ulcer: 20-40 mg PO daily Ulcer prophylaxis with NSAIDs*: 20-40 mg PO daily	Available OTC
lansoprazole (Prevacid)	Erosive esophagitis/GERD: 15-30 mg PO daily to twice daily *H. pylori*: 30 mg PO two to three times daily × 14 days Peptic ulcer: 15-30 mg PO daily to twice daily	
pantoprazole (Protonix)	Erosive esophagitis: 40 mg IV daily or 40 mg PO daily to twice daily Hypersecretion: 40-120 mg PO twice daily Peptic ulcer*: 80 mg IV × 1 then 8 mg/hr continuous IV	Available as IV formulation *Glass vial breakage is possible with use of spiked IV adaptors (Kentrup, August 2004)*
rabeprazole (Aciphex)	Erosive esophagitis/GERD: 20 mg PO daily to twice daily Hypersecretion: 60-120 mg PO daily *H pylori*: 20 mg PO twice daily × 7 days Peptic ulcer: 20 mg PO daily	
HISTAMINE-2 RECEPTOR BLOCKERS		
cimetidine (Tagamet)	Peptic ulcer: 300 mg PO four times daily or 600 mg PO twice daily; 300 mg q6-8h by IM, IV, or IV infusion	May have greater potential for interactions than other H₂ blockers
famotidine (Pepcid)	Peptic ulcer: 20-40 mg PO once daily at bedtime or 20 mg PO twice daily; 20 mg IV q12h	

*Not an FDA-approved indication.

drome. PPIs are also indicated in combination with antimicrobials (most often amoxicillin and clarithromycin) in a number of peptic ulcer disease treatment protocols to eradicate *H. pylori*. In addition, PPIs are used to prevent and treat NSAID-induced upper GI ulcers (Hawley et al., 2005) but may not protect against NSAID-induced lesions in the jejunum or ileum (Maiden, Thjodleifsson, Theodors, Gonzalez, & Bjarnason, 2005). Oral PPI therapy appears to be as effective as parenteral therapy in managing active upper GI bleeding (Leontiadis, Sharma, & Howden, 2005). The first proton pump inhibitor, omeprazole (Prilosec), will be discussed in depth, but the other agents are very similar and are compared in Table 40-1.

★ ⚏ omeprazole [oh **mep** ra zole]
(Prilosec)
Indications
Omeprazole (and other PPIs) are indicated for the treatment of severe erosive esophagitis that occurs with gastroesophageal reflux, for the treatment of duodenal ulcer, and for the long-term treatment of hypersecretory gastric conditions (Freston, 2004; Poe & Kallay, 2003; Vanderghoff & Tahboub, 2002). The PPIs are also used in combination with antimicrobials to treat *H. pylori*-related peptic ulcer disease.

Pharmacokinetics/Dosing
Administered orally, the onset of action for omeprazole is within 1 hour, and the peak effect is in 2 hours. Complete acid suppression, however, may not be observed until 24 to 48 hours after the initial dose. The duration of action is 3 to 4 days (the time needed for production of new enzyme). It is metabolized in the liver by P450 2 C19 and 3 A4 and excreted by the kidneys. Variation in metabolism among different populations is noted (see the Special Considerations for Pharmacogenetics box on p. 750). The adult dosage of omeprazole for gastroesophageal reflux is 20 mg PO (delayed-release capsule) daily for 1 to 2 months. For gastric hypersecretory conditions, the dosage is 60 mg PO daily, with dosage adjustments as necessary. For older adults the dosage should not exceed 20 mg daily. While not officially indicated in children, GERD doses of 10 mg PO daily for children less than 20 kg, and 20 mg daily for children greater than 20 kg are recommended.

Adverse Effects
PPIs are very well tolerated. The adverse effects of omeprazole include stomach colic or pain and infrequently, abdominal distress, increased weakness, muscle aches, dizziness, headache, sedation, chest pain, heartburn, constipation or diarrhea, gas, nausea, vomiting, or skin rash. Rare adverse effects include anemia, neutropenia, pancytopenia, thrombocytopenia, and urinary tract infections (UTIs).

Drug Interactions
By altering gastric acid secretion, PPIs may result in decreased oral absorption of some of the azole antifungals (itraconazole, ketoconazole) and some protease inhibitors (atazanavir, indinavir). As an in-

TABLE 40-1 COMPARISON OF AGENTS THAT INCREASE GASTRIC pH—*cont'd*

Drug	Typical Adult Dose	Comments
HISTAMINE-2 RECEPTOR BLOCKERS—*cont'd*		
nizatidine (Axid)	Peptic ulcer: 150-300 mg PO once daily at bedtime or 150 mg PO twice daily	Not available parenterally
ranitidine (Zantac)	Peptic ulcer: 150 mg PO twice daily or 300 mg PO once daily at bedtime; 50 mg IM/IV q6-8h or continuous infusion at 6.25 mg/hr	
ANTACIDS		
aluminum hydroxide (Amphojel, Alternagel)	Gastritis: Varies, typically 5-15 mL PO three times daily and half-strength PRN	More likely to cause constipation Avoid in renal insufficiency
calcium carbonate (Tums)	Gastritis: Varies, typically 250-500 mg PO three times daily and half-strength PRN	May cause constipation See Chapters 11, 35, 47, and 69
magnesium hydroxide (MOM)	Gastritis: Varies, typically 5-15 mL PO up to four times daily PRN	Causes diarrhea Often used as a laxative Avoid in renal insufficiency
sodium bicarbonate	Gastritis: 325 mg to 2 grams PO up to four times daily PRN	Not recommended because of high sodium load
aluminum and magnesium hydroxides (Maalox, Mylanta)	Gastritis: Varies and may range from 10-50 mL PO three times daily and PRN	Combination offsets constipation/diarrhea

*Not an FDA-approved indication.

hibitor of P450 2 C19, omeprazole may result in elevated warfarin effect and international normalized ratio (INR) for clients receiving this oral anticoagulant. Serum levels of benzodiazepines, phenytoin, and other drugs may also be increased with omeprazole therapy.

✳ What is the role of histamine 2 (H₂) receptor antagonists?

The H_2 blockers are somewhat less effective in acid suppression when compared to the PPIs. As such, their use is more often limited to clients who have less severe conditions, and for the management of intermittent gastritis.

Histamine is found in the mucosal cells of the GI tract; this substance activates H_2 receptors to increase gastric acid secretion. The major components of gastric secretion include hydrochloric acid (HCl) and intrinsic factor (IF), both of which are produced by the parietal (acid-forming) cells; pepsinogen, which is synthesized by the chief cells, and mucus. The principal function of mucus is to protect the epithelial cells of the GI tract from an attack by pepsin and irritation by the HCl secreted by the stomach. Pepsinogen, an enzyme, is the precursor of pepsin; HCl catalyzes the cleavage of pepsinogen to active pepsin by providing a

low pH environment in which pepsin can initiate the digestion of proteins.

Gastric secretion is regulated by a neural mechanism (parasympathetic [vagus] fibers) and a hormonal mechanism (gastrin). Activation of the vagus nerve causes the secretion of vast quantities of pepsinogen and HCl. The hormonal mechanism involves the actual presence of food, which distends the stomach and stimulates the antral mucosa to release gastrin. This hormone is then absorbed into the blood and carried to the parietal cells and chief cells, which secrete HCl and pepsinogen, respectively. It is believed that histamine activates the gastric mucosa much the same as gastrin does. Additionally, caffeine and alcohol are potent stimuli for gastrin release. When the acidity of the gastric juice is increased to a pH of 2, a negative feedback mechanism helps to block gastric secretion from the parietal and chief cells. Thus the inhibition of gastric gland secretion plays an essential role in protecting the stomach against excessively acidic secretions, which are responsible for causing peptic ulcerations. Clinical evidence has shown that histamine released by severe injuries, particularly burns, may also lead to the formation of peptic ulcers.

Special Considerations for Pharmacogenetics | GASTROINTESTINAL AGENTS

PHARMACODYNAMICS

Significant genetic differences in serotonin subtype receptors are observed (DePonti, 2004). While about 30% of clients receiving 5-HT$_3$ receptor antagonists for nausea and vomiting (e.g., ondansetron) do not respond adequately, a specific genetic variant explaining this finding remains elusive (Kaiser et al., 2004; Tremblay et al., 2003). Differences in genetic markers for α_2 receptors and serotonin transporter function are correlated with irritable bowel syndrome (IBS) (Kim et al., 2004). It is unclear whether this finding is related to the efficacy of tegaserod in IBS in women but not men.

Significant subtypes of IBS have been identified with strong genetic influences (Ahmad, Marshall, & Jewell, 2003). Biomarkers for disease subtypes, that are genetically influenced, may help predict responders to therapy for inflammatory bowel disease (Beaven & Abreu, 2004). About one third of clients who receive infliximab do not respond significantly to therapy (Gwo-Tzer, Lees, & Satsangi, 2004), but a genetic link has not yet been recognized. To date drugs specifically targeted for genetic variation affecting pathogenesis of Crohn's disease have not been identified (Gasche & Grundtner, 2005).

PHARMACOKINETICS

Approximately 2% to 5% of Caucasian and 11% to 23% of Asians are considered poor metabolizers of drugs metabolized by P450 2 C19, including omeprazole (Tassaneeyakul et al., 2002). Variation in the metabolism of omeprazole by Chinese subjects is attributed to significantly altered omeprazole pharmacokinetics when dosed with other inducing or inhibiting agents, including the complementary and alternative therapy Ginkgo biloba (Yin, Tomlinson, Waye, Chow, & Chow, 2004).

ADVERSE EFFECTS

Metabolism of 6-mercaptopurine, used as treatment for advanced inflammatory bowel disease, is highly influenced by genetics (Derijks et al., 2004). Toxicity and efficacy of azathioprine and 6-mercaptopurine is correlated with thiopurine methyltransferase (TPMT) gene activity (Gwo-Tzer et al., 2004). Until the use of genetic markers becomes more standardized, therapeutic drug monitoring of 6-mercaptopurine levels is recommended to avoid toxicity.

The H$_2$ receptor blockers include cimetidine (Tagamet), ranitidine (Zantac), famotidine (Pepcid), and nizatidine (Axid). They act to prevent histamine from stimulating the H$_2$ receptors on the gastric parietal cells, thus reducing the volume of gastric acid secretion (from stimuli such as food, pentagastrin, histamine, caffeine, and insulin) and the concentration (acid content) of these secretions. All four drugs are presently considered to be equally effective, but the pharmacokinetics, adverse effects, and drug interactions may differ. Table 40-1 compares these drugs and cimetidine, the first drug available in this class, is discussed below.

cimetidine [sye **me** ti deen]
(Tagamet, Apo-Cimetidine✦, Novocimetine✦, Peptol✦)
Indications
Cimetidine and other H$_2$ blockers are used to treat and prevent duodenal ulcers and to treat gastritis, gastric ulcers, gastroesophageal reflux, and hypersecretory gastric states.
Pharmacokinetics/Dosing
Cimetidine is fairly well absorbed orally, has an onset of action in about 1 hour and duration of action for 6 hours. It is metabolized by the cytochrome P450 enzyme systems, particularly 1A2, 2C19, 2D6, and 3A4, but most of the drug is eliminated unchanged in the urine. Adult doses of 300 mg four times daily orally or 300 mg intravenously (IV) every 6 hours are recommended for treatment of active ulcers. Doses of 600 mg twice daily or 800 mg once daily at bedtime have also been used. Dosage adjustment for renal insufficiency is recommended to avoid a change in mental status and confusion.
Adverse Effects
Cimetidine is associated with stronger antimuscarinic properties than the other H$_2$ blockers. Properties include constipation, confusion, and dry mouth, which are more problematic in older clients

with renal insufficiency. Other adverse effects of H$_2$ receptor blockers include diarrhea, headache, stomach cramps or pain, dizziness, and rash. Breast swelling or pain in males and females has been reported. Less common and rare adverse effects include neutropenia, bradycardia, tachycardia, and agranulocytosis.
Drug Interactions
Cimetidine may interfere with the metabolism of a number of drugs metabolized by the cytochrome P450 enzyme systems and result in increased levels or effect of those drugs. Drugs with a potential for elevated response with concurrent use include warfarin, amiodarone, benzodiazepines, calcium channel blockers, carbamazepine, citalopram, tricyclic antidepressants and theophylline.

❋ How are the antacids utilized?
Antacids are chemical compounds that buffer or neutralize HC1 in the stomach and thereby increase gastric pH. The major ingredients in antacids include aluminum salts, calcium carbonate, magnesium salts, and sodium bicarbonate, alone or in combination. Most antacids may be purchased as OTC preparations.

Traditionally, the antacids have been classified as nonsystemic or systemic. The term *nonsystemic* indicates that an almost negligible amount of drug is absorbed into the circulation; activity occurs only locally within the GI tract. The nonsystemic metal ion is absorbed to some degree; however, the aluminum ion is absorbed the most and magnesium the least, and calcium is absorbed slightly more than magnesium.

Antacids are indicated for the relief of symptoms associated with the hyperacidity related to peptic ulcer, gastritis, gastric esophageal reflux disease (GERD), gastric hyperacidity, heartburn, or hiatal hernia. In general, antacids have a rapid onset of action. The antacid effect lasts from 20 to 40 minutes when administered in a fasting state. If administered 1 hour after meals, the effects may be extended for up to 3 hours. A small amount of absorbable antacid is absorbed (15% to 30%), with the remainder broken down via the digestive process and excreted in the feces. Accumulation of magnesium or aluminum can be problematic in clients with renal failure, however, and these agents are typically avoided in such clients. Table 40-1 compares the elemental antacids. See Table 11-2 for adverse effects of antacids.

✴ What types of interactions occur between antacids and other drugs?

Many drugs are either weak acids or weak bases, and the pH of the stomach is an important factor in their absorption. Changes in pH modify drug solubility and stability, which also affects absorption. Therefore antacids affect the absorption of most drugs to some degree. Drugs that are weak acids are nonionized in the acidic environment of the stomach, are lipid soluble, and are absorbed by simple diffusion across the gastric mucosal cells. The administration of an antacid either with a weak acidic drug or shortly before or after its administration will raise the pH of the stomach contents; as a result, a more ionized drug is formed and is not absorbed to the degree to which the nonionized, lipid-soluble form was absorbed. A weakly basic drug is absorbed in a more alkaline medium.

Drugs that are weak bases include morphine sulfate, quinine, pseudoephedrine, antihistamines, amphetamines, theophylline, tricyclic antidepressants, and quinidine. Examples of weak acids are isoniazid, barbiturates, nalidixic acid, nonsteroidal antiinflammatory drugs, sulfonamides, salicylates, nitrofurantoin, and warfarin.

Antacids have been reported to reduce the absorption of many drugs. Most significantly affected are the quinolone antibiotics (e.g., ciprofloxacin), the tetracyclines, ketoconazole, and digoxin. Additionally, dosing of antacids with sucralfate reduces the efficacy of sucralfate action locally in the upper GI tract. Therefore carefully schedule the majority of medications 1 hour before or 2 hours after the administration time for an antacid. Close monitoring for both therapeutic response and possible adverse effects is also recommended.

✴ P.G. is encouraged to lose weight, exercise, and avoid mints, coffee, and foods that worsen GERD. He is prescribed omeprazole 40 mg PO daily.

✴ What are the nursing considerations for PPI therapy for P.G?

Assessment It is determined that P.G. does not have a sensitivity to omeprazole or a history of or current chronic hepatic disease that would require a reduced dosage (hepatic dysfunction increases the half-life). Review P.G.'s concurrent medications because PPIs increase gastric pH and have the potential to affect the bioavailability of medications that depend on pH for absorption. Omeprazole may interact

and cause an inhibition of the hepatic P450 enzyme system, thus decreasing the metabolism of warfarin, diazepam, and phenytoin. Serum levels of these agents may rise resulting in toxicity. Because sucralfate requires an acid medium to create a matrix in the GI tract, its use is avoided with PPIs. A baseline assessment of P.G.'s GERD includes: severity of heartburn and factors that increase its intensity, reflux of sour or bitter gastric contents into the mouth, and "atypical" symptoms of asthma, chronic cough, chronic laryngitis, sore throat, and chest pain.

Nursing Diagnosis With PPI therapy, P.G. is at risk for the following nursing diagnoses: impaired comfort (heartburn, flatulence, abdominal pain or colic, pruritus, headache); risk for injury related to dizziness or drowsiness; fatigue; diarrhea; constipation; and risk for injury related to central nervous system (CNS) disturbance (dizziness or drowsiness); and the potential complications of blood dyscrasias (thrombocytopenia, eosinopenia, leukocytosis, anemia), UTI, and generalized skin reactions (toxic epidermal necrolysis, erythema multiforme, or Stevens-Johnson syndrome).

Planning See Box 40-3.

Implementation

Monitoring Monitor P.G. for decreased GI reflux or heartburn and signs of generalized skin reactions (blisters; chills; fever; redness, tenderness, itching, burning, or peeling of skin). Record the frequency, character, and color of stools. Monitor hepatic function studies, complete blood counts (CBCs) for blood dyscrasias, and urinalysis (UA) for hematuria or proteinuria (UTI). Monitor concurrent therapy closely.

Intervention Therapy for the healing of ulcers should continue for at least 4 to 6 weeks but rarely beyond 8 weeks. Maintenance therapy for ulcer prophylaxis or hypersecretory gastric conditions may be long-term. Administer immediately before meals, preferably in the morning. Antacids may be taken concurrently with omeprazole to minimize gastric discomfort.

Education Assist P.G. to identify foods that would aggravate his hyperacidity and acceptable substitutes for them. Discuss various weight control programs with him and pro-

---

BOX 40-3 GOALS FOR CLIENTS ON ACID-REDUCING DRUGS

Clients on acid-reducing drug therapy will:
- Experience minimal or no epigastric pain or burning during and following therapy.
- Experience minimal or no adverse effects during therapy.
- Effectively self-manage therapeutic regimen including medication compliance, supportive lifestyle changes, and collaboration with health care providers for treatment and monitoring.

vide him with a written list of such programs and contacts in his area. Instruct P.G. to swallow the capsule whole; it is not to be crushed or chewed. With lansoprazole, another PPI, if the client has difficulty swallowing, the capsule may be opened and the intact granules sprinkled on a tablespoon of applesauce and swallowed immediately. For clients with a nasogastric tube, the intact granules of the lansoprazole capsule may be mixed in 45 mL of apple juice and placed in the tube; flush the tube with additional apple juice to clear it.

Evaluation The expected outcome of PPI therapy is that P.G.'s hyperacidity is alleviated without producing adverse effects of the drug. He will experience increased comfort, be compliant with his drug therapy and supportive lifestyle changes, and maintain his visits to the prescriber for follow-up care.

✱ **T.P. is a 31-year-old chef with a recent history of mid-epigastric pain relieved by food. The discomfort often awakens him at night. He smokes one pack of cigarettes per day. He is evaluated by his health care provider, is tested for *H. pylori* and is found positive on breath test. He is started on a combination of lansoprazole 30 mg/amoxicillin 500 mg/clarithromycin 500 mg (Prevpac) twice daily for 2 weeks.**

✱ **What is the pathology of peptic ulcer disease and how is it treated?**
Normally the mucosal surface of the stomach and upper duodenum is protected from the irritation of gastric acid by a layer of mucus and bicarbonate. Factors that decrease this defense system can lead to mucosal damage. Aggravating factors include agents that interfere with prostaglandin synthesis in the stomach, which produces mucus (e.g., COX-1 inhibitors like aspirin, ibuprofen). If a circumscribed area of the mucosal surface is damaged and fails to repair rapidly, it may become eroded, forming an ulcer at one of these sites. When gastric acid comes in contact with this inflamed region, pain may result. Additionally, clinical studies have suggested that esophageal, gastric, and duodenal ulcers (peptic ulcers) are associated with the excessive production of gastric acid. Infection with *H. pylori* is also a major cause of gastric and duodenal ulcers, gastric adenocarcinoma and lymphoma (Marshall & Windor, 2005). Smoking increases the risk for mucosal damage as well.

H. pylori bacteria have been found in persons with gastritis and gastric and duodenal peptic ulcers. It has been reported that persons who have a colony of *H. pylori* in the stomach are more prone to gastritis and gastric and duodenal ulcers. It has been recommended that all persons with a non–drug-induced peptic ulcer be treated with a combination of antibacterials and proton pump inhibitors to eradicate *H. pylori* (Marshall & Windor, 2005). Controlling or eradicating these bacteria vastly improves the chances that the ulcer will not recur. Unfortunately, resistance to commonly used antibacterials has emerged (McMahon et al., 2003) and may require alternate choices for antimicrobial therapy in the future.

✱ **What nursing management of T.P.'s drug regimen is appropriate?**
In general, the nursing management of T.P.'s drug therapy would be the same as P.G.'s because each dose of his Prevpac contains lansoprazole 30 mg, a PPI, to reduce gastric acidity. Each Prevpac dose also has two antimicrobials, amoxicillin 2 × 500 mg and clarithromycin 500 mg, for the eradication of *H. pylori*. So in addition to the care provided above, perform the following.

Assessment Do not use a Prevpac in clients with a creatinine clearance of less than 30 mL/min because the doses provided assume normal renal function (see Chapter 35). Because there may be cross-sensitivity between the cephalosporins and penicillins, ensure T.P. is not sensitive to penicillin, cephalosporins and clarithromycin, erythromycins, or other macrolide antibiotics. Both amoxicillin and clarithromycin interact with a variety of drugs; see Chapter 58. A baseline of T.P.'s symptoms includes: severity of epigastric pain and factors that precipitate it or relieve it, nausea and vomiting, fecal occult blood testing, and hemoglobin and hematocrit (H&H). Upper endoscopy is the procedure of choice for determining the location and size of the ulcer or a barium upper GI series may be done.

Nursing Diagnosis See previous discussion for PPIs and Chapter 58 for the antimicrobials.

Planning See Box 40-3.

Implementation
Monitoring Observe T.P. for an allergic response to the drug; anaphylaxis, rash or serum-sickness-like reaction. Monitor for signs of a superinfection (e.g., candidiasis, *C. difficile* colitis). Perform fecal occult blood testing and monitor results of H&H as required.

Education Instruct T.P. that the Prevpac is a package of the doses for the day; divide the tablets so that he takes the combination of one lansoprazole tablet, two amoxicillin tablets, and one clarithromycin tablet, twice a day (morning and evening). If T.P. has difficulty in affording the Prevpac as packaged, the drugs may be obtained individually at a reduced cost but may require additional education and support to ensure adherence. Inform him of the harm of smoking with peptic ulcers and provide him with information about smoking cessation.

Evaluation The expected outcome of PPI therapy is that T.P.'s upper endoscopy or barium upper GI series is negative for an ulcer. His H&H is within normal limits and his fecal occult blood remains negative. T.P.'s epigastric pain is alleviated without producing adverse effects to the drug. He will experience increased comfort, be compliant with his drug therapy and supportive life style changes, and maintain his visits to the prescriber for follow-up care.

✱ **O.W. is a 27-year-old police officer who reports occasional heartburn and asks her neighbor, who is a** nurse, whether she should take famotidine (Pepcid) or calcium carbonate (Tums) for her heartburn.

What are the important implications for the use and monitoring of H₂ blockers and antacids with O.W.?

The nurse discusses what is related to the contraindications, drug interactions, and effective management of each of the classifications of these drugs. O.W. decides that she will keep both drugs on hand, preferring calcium carbonate for her occasional mild heartburn because it will add to her calcium intake, but will resort to the famotidine if she gets "a heavy duty" episode.

What is the nursing management of antacid therapy for O.W.?

Although antacids are considered to be OTC preparations (and are therefore discussed in Chapter 11), these medications are commonly administered by nurses in a variety of health care settings. Additionally, the nurse is ideally placed within the health care delivery system to offer clients instruction, such as with O.W., on the safe use of antacids as OTC medications.

Assessment A baseline assessment of O.W.'s heartburn includes the severity and frequency of her discomfort and the aggravating and mitigating factors in her condition. Determine her sensitivity to medications containing calcium because O.W. would be taking calcium carbonate (Tums), or if she were considering another antacid, sensitivity to aluminum, magnesium, simethicone, or sodium bicarbonate.

Antacids would be carefully considered if it were determined that O.W. has a history of renal function impairment. Clients who have renal failure and are receiving magnesium-containing antacids are particularly at risk for hypermagnesemia. If such antacids are given to clients with renal dysfunction, low dosages (50 mEq magnesium daily) should be administered under close monitoring by a health care provider. Antacids that contain magnesium may also cause diarrhea, the frequent passage of loose, watery stools; caution should be used in clients with an ostomy or any condition that might be worsened by diarrhea, such as hemorrhoids, ulcerative colitis, or diverticulitis.

On the other hand, aluminum- and calcium-containing antacids tend to be constipating and would be taken by O.W. with caution if she has a history of constipation or hemorrhoids that might be aggravated. Clients with hypercalcemia or hypoparathyroidism should not receive calcium-containing antacids. Antacids should be used cautiously in clients with symptoms of appendicitis, undiagnosed GI bleeding, and intestinal obstruction, because the laxative or constipating effects may worsen the condition. Aluminum-containing antacids are avoided in clients with renal failure and may exacerbate Alzheimer's disease. Calcium-containing antacids may affect hypothyroidism and sarcoidosis. Consult with the prescriber about low-sodium antacids for clients with sodium restrictions.

Review O.W.'s current medication regimen, keeping in mind that antacids have an effect on most oral forms of drugs necessitating a scheduling of doses of other medications either 1 before or 2 hours after an antacid.

Nursing Diagnosis With the administration of antacids, O.W. may experience pain related to the underlying condition and the ineffectiveness of the antacid. Other concerns for clients are related to the type of antacid administered. With aluminum- or calcium-containing antacids, constipation may result from an alteration of bowel function, whereas diarrhea may result from magnesium-containing antacids. Excessive use of calcium- and sodium bicarbonate–containing antacids may place the client at risk for the potential complication of metabolic alkalosis (mood/mental changes, muscle twitching, decreased respiratory rate, unpleasant taste, fatigue). With the long-term use of aluminum- and sodium bicarbonate–containing antacids, hypercalcemia associated with milk-alkali syndrome (headache, urinary frequency, anorexia, nausea/vomiting, fatigue) and osteomalacia/osteoporosis caused by phosphate depletion (bone pain, wrist or ankle joint swelling) may occur. Clients with renal impairment may experience neurotoxicity (mood swings, mental changes) with the chronic use of aluminum-containing antacids, or hypermagnesemia (fatigue, dizziness) with the chronic use of magnesium-containing antacids.

Planning See Box 40-3.

Implementation

Monitoring O.W.'s subjective response to antacid therapy and the nurse's objective observations (e.g., frequency with which the client takes the antacid) can help determine the effectiveness of therapy. Assess epigastric discomfort at the time of each dose. If O.W.'s epigastric pain continues to be bothersome, she should see her primary care provider for treatment.

Note the frequency and consistency of stools. If O.W. develops constipation, a magnesium hydroxide antacid or an increase in the intake of bran and other fiber in the diet may be instituted. If diarrhea occurs, it may be advantageous to change to another antacid, such as magnesium hydroxide with magnesium trisilicate or aluminum hydroxide.

Monitor clients undergoing long-term aluminum antacid therapy regularly for serum phosphate levels, because phosphate depletion may result in osteoporosis; monitor serum calcium levels for milk-alkali syndrome (headache, anorexia, nausea and vomiting, weakness, fatigue).

Intervention The dosing schedule of antacid therapy is important. Antacids given immediately after meals will delay gastric emptying and the buffering effect. When given at 1 and 3 hours after meals and at bedtime, the gastric pH remains at approximately 3 throughout the day. Because of their ability to interact with numerous medications, scheduling in relation to other medications is considered. Administer antacids 1 hour before or 2 hours after other drugs, such as digoxin, tetracyclines, phenothiazines, and all enteric-coated medications. Antacids combined with ibuprofen, indomethacin, phenylbutazone, potassium chloride supplements, reserpine, sulindac, and tolmetin can help to reduce the gastric distress associated with these drugs.

O.W. is taking Tums tablets rather than a liquid antacid for the convenience of being able to carry them with her easily. If she were taking liquid preparations of antacids, they would need to be shaken vigorously before administration to achieve a uniform suspension. Refrigerate liquid antacids to make them more palatable, but do not freeze them. When administering antacids via a nasogastric tube, assess the placement and patency of the tube before giving the medication, and follow the dose with sufficient water to clear the tube.

Do not administer calcium carbonate antacids with milk, milk products, or other foods or vitamin supplements high in vitamin D, because milk-alkali syndrome may occur.

Education Discuss with O.W. the sodium content and side effects of various antacids (see Table 11-2 for the adverse effects of antacids). Inform clients that antacids vary in their sodium content, which can be significant for clients who are on low-sodium diets or who take antihypertensive drugs or diuretics. Instruct clients with hypertensive, cardiac, or renal disease to avoid antacids containing sodium, particularly if antacids are used frequently.

Inform O.W. that liquid antacids have superior neutralizing properties compared with tablets. Instruct O.W. that chewing the antacid tablets thoroughly and drinking a full glass of water will facilitate the action of the antacid tablets.

Caution O.W. about adverse effects, and instruct her to consult her prescriber if these occur. Alert her to check the expiration dates of the antacids, because the effectiveness of antacids decreases with age. Alert her to check the name carefully when purchasing OTC antacids. Names may be similar (Mylanta vs. Mylanta II), but dosage requirements differ. Advise O.W. to seek medical care if she is self-medicating with antacids for recurring GI symptoms, because she is treating the symptoms rather than the cause of the problem. Because antacids are OTC drugs and there is no medically supervised restriction, clients may abuse or misuse antacids.

Assist O.W. to identify sources of gastric discomfort, such as overeating, smoking, tension, anxiety, or other emotional stress; this may teach her to avoid the causes of discomfort and help to eliminate the need for antacid therapy.

Evaluation The expected outcome of antacid therapy is that the O.W. will experience decreased discomfort or an absence of pain without adverse effects (e.g., constipation or diarrhea). She will effectively and safely use occasional antacids, but consult her primary care provider if her dyspepsia continues.

✳ What is the nursing management of H₂ receptor antagonist therapy for O.W.?

Assessment Determine O.W.'s sensitivity to H₂ receptor blockers. Note that clients with impaired renal function may require a dosage reduction for cimetidine, famotidine, ranitidine, or nizatidine because of delayed excretion and

the risk for increased adverse effects, particularly CNS effects. A further reduction in dosage may be necessary in clients with impaired liver function. Alert O.W. that H₂ receptor blockers are Pregnancy Category B.

If O.W. were going to take H₂ receptor antagonists for more than occasional use, her current medication regimen would need to be reviewed for the risk of significant drug interactions, such as itraconazole, ketoconazole, and antacids. Antacids may be indicated for the relief of pain but should not be administered within 1 hour of administration of the H₂ blocker as its absorption may be decreased. An increase in GI pH induced by the H₂ blocker (any of the four agents) may result in a reduced absorption of itraconazole and ketoconazole. Advise clients to talk with their health care provider about this combination. Assess the underlying condition. If O.W.'s dyspepsia persists, she needs to seek medical attention. Assess her smoking history, precipitating factors for her dyspepsia, and dietary patterns.

A baseline assessment of O.W.'s GI pain is obtained. If her discomfort is persistent, a CBC and a stool guaiac for occult blood is obtained. Upper GI barium series or upper endoscopy may be necessary to rule out more serious etiology.

Nursing Diagnosis With the administration of H₂ blocker, O.W. is at risk for the following nursing diagnoses/collaborative problems: impaired comfort (headache, breast tenderness, muscle ache, anorexia, nausea or vomiting, rash, and dizziness); sexual dysfunction (decreased sexual ability); constipation; diarrhea; disturbed sleep pattern (drowsiness); disturbed thought processes (confusion); hyperthermia; and the potential complications of allergic reaction, blood dyscrasias, bradycardia or tachycardia, and bronchospasm. O.W.'s intention of occasional use of famotidine places her at low risk for any of these conditions.

Planning See Box 40-3.

Implementation

Monitoring Assess O.W. regularly for GI pain. A periodic evaluation of blood counts is required during a course of prescribed therapy. Be aware that mild bilateral gynecomastia in males and galactorrhea in females have been observed in some clients after long-term treatment with H₂ blockers (1 month or more).

Intervention Administer H₂ blockers with meals, because the maximum therapeutic effect occurs when the stomach is protected by the buffering effect of food. A bedtime dose protects the stomach from the nocturnal hypersecretion of gastric acid. Ulcer healing rates may be greatest with a bedtime only regimen. Although the symptoms of duodenal ulcers may diminish in a week or two, therapy should be continued for 4 to 6 weeks (rarely beyond 8 weeks).

Note that the parenteral form of the drug is stable for 48 hours at room temperature. Cimetidine, ranitidine, and famotidine are compatible for dilution with IV solutions of 0.9% sodium chloride and dextrose 5%. Rapid IV bolus administration (less than 2 minutes) may result in cardiac dysrhythmias and hypotension.

Education If O.W. smokes, encourage her to discontinue smoking altogether or at least after the last dose of the day. Smoking diminishes the effectiveness of H_2 receptor antagonists in inhibiting nocturnal gastric acid secretions. Instruct her to keep clinical and laboratory appointments as scheduled.

Evaluation The expected outcome of H_2 blocker therapy is that the client will report diminished pain or an absence of pain and demonstrate healing or an absence of ulceration by endoscopic or radiograph examination. O.W. will effectively and safely use occasional H_2 blockers, but consult her primary care provider if her dyspepsia continues.

✳ **What other drugs are available to prevent or treat gastric mucosal injury?**
Two other modalities are available to treat prevent and treat gastric mucosa damage, but are less frequently utilized. Sucralfate (Carafate) is an orally administered tablet or suspension composed of an aluminum salt. It binds to the ulcer site in the presence of acid to form a protective barrier. Misoprostol (Cytotec) is a prostaglandin used to help prevent nonsteroidal antiinflammatory drug (NSAID)-induced peptic ulcer disease. These drugs have little or no effect on gastric acidity. Both agents require four times a day dosing and are discussed briefly in the following monographs.

sucralfate [soo **kral** fate]
(Carafate, Novo-Sucralate✤, Sulcrate✤)
Sucralfate is a local topical agent composed of sulfated sucrose and aluminum hydroxide; in the presence of acid, albumin and fibrinogen, this substance forms a protective, acid-resistant shield in the ulcer crater. This barrier hastens the healing of the peptic ulcer by protecting the mucosa for up to 6 hours.
Indications
This drug is indicated for short-term treatment of a duodenal ulcer (up to 8 weeks).
Pharmacokinetics/Dosing
Sucralfate is administered orally, and there is minimal systemic absorption (up to 5%). Excretion is primarily in the feces. The adult dosage for the treatment of a duodenal ulcer is 1 g four times daily, 1 hour before each meal and at bedtime. The dosage for the prophylaxis of recurrence of duodenal ulcer is 1 g twice daily on an empty stomach.
Adverse Effects
The side effects of sucralfate are minimal; the most common one reported is constipation. Other possible effects include diarrhea, nausea, gastric discomfort, dry mouth, dizziness, drowsiness, back pain, rash, and itching.
Drug Interactions
Sucralfate may decrease the absorption of other orally administered drugs, including the quinolone antibacterials (e.g., ciprofloxacin), tetracyclines, warfarin, theophylline, phenytoin, and digoxin. Sucralfate requires an acid medium to adequately form a protective coating on gastric mucosa. Concurrent use of antacids, H_2 blockers or PPIs reduces the efficacy of sucralfate.
Nursing Management
Assessment
A baseline assessment should include the client's underlying condition, sensitivity to sucralfate, and renal status. Obtain a serum aluminum level in clients with renal failure. Sucralfate is used with caution in

clients with renal failure because the absorption of the aluminum in the drug may cause aluminum toxicity, especially with long-term use.

Review the client's current medication regimen for the risk of significant drug interactions, such as those that may occur when sucralfate is given concurrently with the following drugs: antacids (concurrent use may interfere with sucralfate binding, thus reducing its effect; administer antacids either 30 minutes before or 1 hour after the administration of sucralfate); ciprofloxacin (Cipro), norfloxacin (Noroxin), or ofloxacin (Floxin), (sucralfate is reported to decrease the absorption and serum levels of these antibiotics; advise clients to take antibiotics 2 to 3 hours before sucralfate); digoxin (Lanoxin) or theophylline (Elixophyllin) (sucralfate interferes with the absorption of these drugs; advise clients to take digoxin or theophylline 2 hours before or after sucralfate); and phenytoin (Dilantin) (concurrent administration with sucralfate may decrease serum levels of phenytoin, resulting in a loss of seizure control; advise clients not to take sucralfate within 2 hours of phenytoin administration).
Nursing Diagnosis
The client receiving sucralfate is at risk for the following nursing diagnoses: constipation; diarrhea; disturbed sleep pattern (drowsiness); impaired oral mucous membrane (dry mouth); and impaired comfort (nausea, itching, indigestion, dizziness, backache).
Planning
Although sucralfate is not an acid-reducing drug, the goals for therapy would be the same as in Box 40-3.
Implementation
Monitoring
Monitor the client's bowel elimination for constipation or diarrhea. The ulcer will be monitored by radiographic or endoscopic examination.
Intervention
Administer sucralfate with water to the client 1 hour before meals and at bedtime; sucralfate is taken on an empty stomach. If the client's regimen also includes antacids, they may be administered 30 minutes before or 1 hour after the sucralfate. The use of sucralfate via a nasogastric tube has resulted in the formation of bezoar as a result of the protein-binding properties of the drug.
Education
Instruct the client not to chew the tablet. An oral suspension is available for clients who are unable to swallow tablets. Encourage compliance with the regimen for at least 4 to 8 weeks, until healing has been documented by radiograph or endoscopic examination. Sucralfate therapy is not recommended for longer than 8 weeks.
Evaluation
The expected outcome of sucralfate therapy is that the client's duodenal ulcer will heal within 8 weeks as evidenced by radiographic or endoscopic examination. The client's epigastric pain is alleviated without producing adverse effects to the drug. The client will experience increased comfort, be compliant with drug therapy and supportive lifestyle changes, and maintain visits to the prescriber for follow-up care.

Prostaglandins normally protect the stomach by decreasing gastric acid secretion and increasing gastric cytoprotective mucus and bicarbonate. NSAIDs inhibit prostaglandin synthesis, which reduces the protective mechanisms and may result in gastric ulcers.

misoprostol [mye soe **prost** ole]
(Cytotec)
Misoprostol, a synthetic prostaglandin E_1 analogue, suppresses gastric acid secretion and thus helps to heal gastric ulcers. Its use in treating gastric ulcers has waned over the past decade due to a risk for teratogenicity (Category X) and adverse effects (especially diarrhea).
Indications
Misoprostol, a gastric mucosa–protecting agent, is indicated for the prevention of gastric ulcers associated with the use of NSAIDs, especially in persons at increased risk for developing complications from

gastric ulcers (Saad & Scheiman, 2004; Shiotoni & Graham, 2002). Other uses (not approved by the U.S. Food and Drug Administration [FDA]) include chronic constipation, cervical ripening, and early pregnancy termination.

Pharmacokinetics/Dosing

Misoprostol is rapidly absorbed orally; it reaches a peak serum level in approximately 15 minutes and has a duration of action of 3 to 6 hours. It is metabolized to an active metabolite that is later metabolized to inactive metabolites in various tissues. It is excreted primarily by the kidneys. The adult dosage is 0.2 mg PO four times daily after meals and at bedtime, or 0.4 mg PO twice daily, with the last dose at bedtime. A pediatric dosage has not been established.

Adverse Effects

The most common adverse effects associated with misoprostol are stomach distress and diarrhea, which are dose-related. Less common adverse effects include constipation, gas, headache, nausea, or vomiting. At the present time, no significant drug interactions have been noted with misoprostol. Misoprostol can induce uterine contractions via its prostaglandin activity and exposure to it must be avoided for individuals who may be pregnant. Misoprostol is a Pregnancy Safety Category X drug; see the Pregnancy Safety box below.

Nursing Management

Assessment

Determine if the client is sensitive to other prostaglandins or prostaglandin analogues, because there may be cross-sensitivity. Use misoprostol with caution in clients with cerebrovascular or coronary artery disease; although it has not been reported with this drug, prostaglandins can cause hypotension, which would worsen these conditions. Use this drug cautiously in clients with epilepsy; prostaglandins administered by routes other than the oral route have been reported to cause seizures, although this effect has not been reported with misoprostol itself.

It should be determined if the client is pregnant, because this drug increases the frequency and intensity of uterine contractions and may cause miscarriages. It is used as a non-FDA approved indication as an abortifacient (*Mosby's Drug Consult*, 2005; Feldman, Borgida, Rodis, Leo, & Campbell, 2003). The drug carries a FDA "black box" warning (highest warning) that misoprostol should not be used for reducing the risk of NSAID-induced ulcers in women of childbearing potential unless the client is at high risk of complications from gastric ulcers associated with use of the NSAID, or is at high risk of developing gastric ulceration. In such clients, misoprostol may be prescribed if the client:

- Has had a negative serum pregnancy test within 2 weeks prior to beginning therapy.
- Is capable of complying with effective contraceptive measures.
- Has received both oral and written warnings of the hazards of misoprostol, the risk of possible contraception failure, and the danger to other women of childbearing potential should the drug be taken by mistake.
- Will begin misoprostol only on the second or third day of the next normal menstrual period.

Nursing Diagnosis

The client receiving misoprostol is at risk for the following nursing diagnoses/collaborative problems: diarrhea; constipation; impaired comfort (mild abdominal pain, flatulence, headache, nausea and vomiting); and the potential complications of uterine stimulation and vaginal bleeding.

Planning

Although misoprostol is indicated for the prevention of gastric ulcers, the goals in Box 40-3 are appropriate.

Implementation

Monitoring

Monitor for GI distress and discomfort and the stools for type, amount, color, and guaiac determinations. Diarrhea associated with misoprostol is dose-related; it occurs early in the course of therapy and is self-limiting, usually in the first 8 days of therapy.

Intervention

Administer misoprostol with or after meals. Start the course of therapy at the same time as the NSAIDs. Taking it with food or milk will decrease the diarrhea and abdominal cramping associated with the drug. Misoprostol may be administered with antacids, but magnesium-containing antacids are not recommended because they may aggravate misoprostol-induced diarrhea. Therapy should continue for 4 weeks unless healing has been documented by endoscopic examination.

Education

Alert the client to report to the prescriber any episode of diarrhea that lasts more than 1 week. Misoprostol is not to be taken for longer than 4 weeks unless otherwise prescribed, and then only for another 4 weeks if necessary. Instruct the client not to give the drug to any other person. Misoprostol has an expiration date of 18 months after its manufacture.

Evaluation

The expected outcome of misoprostol therapy is that the client will remain ulcer-free as evidenced by endoscopic examination and will not experience any adverse effects of misoprostol. The client will experience increased comfort, be compliant with drug therapy and supportive lifestyle changes, and maintain visits to the prescriber for follow-up care.

PREGNANCY SAFETY	
AGENTS AFFECTING THE GASTROINTESTINAL SYSTEM	
Category	**Drug**
B	aprepitant, balsalazide, cimetidine, diphenhydramine, dimenhydrinate, dolasetron, dronabinol, esomeprazole, famotidine, granisetron, lactulose, lansoprazole, meclizine, mesalamine, metoclopramide, nizatidine, ondansetron, palonosetron, pantoprazole, paregoric, rabeprazole, ranitidine, sucralfate, sulfasalazine, tegaserod, ursodiol
C	calcium carbonate, chlorpromazine, clotrimazole, dexamethasone, difenoxin and atropine, diphenoxylate and atropine, droperidol, haloperidol, infliximab, nystatin, olsalazine, omeprazole, pancreatin, pancrelipase, polyethylene glycol, prochlorperazine, promethazine, scopolamine, sodium bicarbonate
D	lorazepam
X	misoprostol, thiethylperazine

Data from *Mosby's drug consult* (15th ed.). (2005). St. Louis: Mosby.

✴ **T.C. is a 5-year-old male who was recently diagnosed with cystic fibrosis (CF) and is started on pancreatic enzymes with meals. His pediatrician orders pancrelipase (lipase 5000 units/protease 1875 units/amylase 16,600 units [Creon 5]) one capsule with each meal.**

✴ **What is the role of pancreatic enzymes?**

Pancreatic enzymes are considered digestants or drugs that promote the process of digestion in the GI tract. Problems with digestion may be caused by a deficiency of HC1, digestive substances, enzymes, or bile salts; organic disease states (stomach cancer, pernicious anemia, cholecystectomy); or, possibly, a reaction to emotional situations or stress. Digestive enzymes secreted by the mouth, stomach, small intestine, pancreas, and liver are necessary for the digestion of food. Pepsin is the stomach enzyme that reduces protein to smaller particles. It can be given alone or in combination with a HC1 source in clients with hypochlorhydria or achlorhydria.

HC1 keeps the gastric pH level below 4 and protects the proteolytic activity of pepsin. A pH level of 1.5 to 2.5 is usually the optimal range. Pepsin is not considered a critical enzyme because proteolytic enzymes released from the pancreas and intestine cause the same effects.

In clinical practice, pancreatic enzymes are the most commonly utilized digestants for treatment. Pancrelipase is a combination of lipase, protease, and amylase, which help in the digestion of fats, proteins and carbohydrates respectively. The pancreas normally releases these digestive enzymes and bicarbonate into the duodenum. Bicarbonate neutralizes acid and thus helps to protect the enzymes from both acid and pepsin. When acid chyme enters the duodenum, vagal stimulation regulates pancreatic secretion; therefore enzyme replacement therapy may be necessary for clients who have had their vagal fibers surgically severed or have undergone surgical procedures that cause food to bypass the duodenum. Replacement therapy is usually necessary in cases of exocrine pancreatic enzyme deficiency states, chronic pancreatitis, CF, pancreatic tumors, pancreatic obstruction, and pancreatectomy.

pancrelipase [pan kre li pase]
(Creon, Pancrease, Pancrease MT, Ultrase)
Pancrelipase contains the enzymes amylase, trypsin, and lipase, but pancrelipase has greater enzyme activity in the neutral or alkaline media of the GI tract. It has approximately 12 times the lipolytic and 4 times the proteolytic and amylolytic activities of pancreatin. These agents are not interchangeable because they are not bioequivalent.

Indications
Pancrelipase is indicated for clients with pancreatic insufficiency such as that observed with CF and chronic pancreatitis.

Pharmacokinetics
Pancrelipase is available in enteric-coated capsules to avoid destruction in the stomach. The enteric-coated microsphere formulation resists gastric inactivation, so enzymes reach the duodenum to hydrolyze fats into glycerol and fatty acids, proteins into proteases, and starch into dextrins and sugars. The adult dosage for pancrelipase is 1 to 3 capsules or tablets or 1 or 2 packets before or with meals or snacks. The dosage should be adjusted as necessary. With extreme deficiency, the dosage interval may be changed to hourly if no nausea or diarrhea develops.

Adverse Effects
The adverse effects of pancreatin and pancrelipase include nausea, abdominal cramps, hyperuricemia, intestinal obstruction, allergic reaction, and loose stool.

✱ How should T.C.'s drug regimen be managed?

Assessment A baseline assessment should include T.C.'s discomfort levels associated with eating, and bowel status and serum and urine uric acid levels. Treatment with pancrelipase is contraindicated if T.C. has acute pancreatitis or sensitivity to pork protein, pancrelipase, or pancreatin. Consideration should be given to clients whose religious beliefs prohibit the use of pork products.

Review T.C.'s medications for drug interactions. The most significant drug interaction occurs when calcium and magnesium antacids negate the action of the enzyme pancrelipase. Absorption of iron supplements is decreased by pancreatic extracts.

Nursing Diagnosis While T.C. is receiving digestant therapy, he is at risk for the following nursing diagnoses/collaborative problems: impaired comfort (nausea and abdominal cramps); impaired oral mucous membrane related to the enzymatic digestion of mucous membranes when the tablet is held in the mouth; diarrhea; and potential complications related to an allergic reaction (rash), or sensitization induced by inadvertent inhalation of the powder dosage form (dyspnea, nasal congestion, wheezing).

Planning While receiving digestant therapy, T.C. will:
- Maintain normal digestion and nutritional status without adverse effects of pancrelipase.
- Effectively self-manage therapeutic regimen including medication compliance, supportive lifestyle changes, and collaboration with health care providers for treatment and monitoring.

Implementation
Monitoring Monitor for discomfort associated with eating, diarrhea, irritated mouth, respiratory status, and elevated serum and urine levels of uric acid. Fatty stools would indicate a deficiency of lipase. A weight below ideal for growth and development suggests inadequate absorption of nutrients. Both would be indications for increased doses of pancreatic enzymes.

Intervention Pancreatin is inactivated by gastric pepsin and acid pH; therefore cimetidine or antacids (except for those containing calcium and magnesium) may be prescribed to be taken concurrently. For children or adults who cannot swallow the capsules, sprinkle the powdered form or the powder from the opened capsule on soft food (e.g., applesauce, gelatin) that have a pH less than 5.5 and that do not require chewing. The soft food is to be swallowed immediately and followed with a glass of water or juice. Avoid the inhalation of capsule contents.

Education Instruct T.C.'s parents to give pancrelipase and pancreatin before or with meals for the greatest effectiveness. If he is switched to enteric-coated tablets, instruct him to swallow the tablets whole; do not crush them or allow them to be chewed, because irritation of the mouth may occur. Instruct T.C. and his family on the rationale for taking the pancreatic enzyme preparations, and not to discontinue the medication without prescriber approval. Urge them to have T.C. adhere to the prescribed diet (usually a high-calorie diet that is high in protein and low in fat), because the dosage for pancrelipase is individualized and determined by his indigestion and malabsorption and the fat content of the diet.

If capsules need to be opened for administration, advise the client to be careful not to inhale the contents or spill them on the hands; the contents are very irritating to the nasal membranes, respiratory tract, and skin. If the capsules contain enteric-coated spheres, they should be taken with liquids or small amounts of foods that do not need chewing. Tablet forms should be followed with one or two mouthfuls of food to decrease the risk of esophageal irritation, particularly in clients in a recumbent position. Instruct the client to contact the prescriber if adverse effects such as nausea, abdominal cramping, and diarrhea occur. Consult with the prescriber before changing brands.

Evaluation The expected outcome of digestant therapy is that T.C. will experience normal digestion without fatty stools and will maintain a normal growth pattern for his age. The client and family will manage the digestant therapy effectively without T.C. experiencing any adverse effects, and they will collaborate with health care providers for monitoring and follow-up care.

✸ What mechanisms are involved in vomiting?

The vomiting or **emetic center,** which is located in the medulla oblongata, may be stimulated by smells, strong emotion, severe pain, increased intracranial pressure, labyrinthine disturbances (motion sickness), endocrine disturbances, toxic reactions to drugs, GI disease, radiation treatments, and chemotherapy (Figure 40-1). The stimuli may involve neurotransmitters and vagal and/or sympathetic afferent nerve transmission.

The **chemoreceptor trigger zone (CTZ)** is an area of sensory nerve cells; this area is activated by chemical stimuli and relays messages to the emetic center. It has various receptors (serotonin, dopamine, opioid) that detect irritat-

ing drugs or toxins in the blood to stimulate or mediate emesis. The CTZ itself is not able to induce vomiting. Because the CTZ is located close to the respiratory center in the brain, it is difficult to completely control vomiting initiated from this site without affecting respiration. If the emetic center is activated by stimuli, it sends impulses (via the efferent nerves) to the diaphragm, stomach muscles, esophagus, and salivary glands, resulting in vomiting.

The cerebral cortex is involved in anticipatory nausea and vomiting, a conditioned response caused by a stimulus connected with a previous unpleasant experience. For example, a client who vomited after receiving cancer chemotherapy might vomit at the sight of the hospital, doctor, or nurse, even before treatment is given (Lindley, 2005). See also Chapter 56.

The primary pathways for the vomiting reflex are as follows:

1. Higher central nervous system or cerebral cortex stimulation
   a. Emotional or anticipatory vomiting
2. Peripheral or central nerve transmission secondary to body tissue or organ alterations
   a. Irritation of GI tract
   b. Increased intracranial pressure
   c. Vestibular stimulation
3. Stimulation from the CTZ
   a. Toxins circulating in blood

✸ What agents are utilized to prevent or treat nausea and vomiting?

Antiemetics are drugs given to prevent or relieve nausea and vomiting. Control of vomiting is important and at times may be difficult. Numerous preparations have been used, but effective treatment usually depends on treating the cause.

Antiemetics vary widely in their chemical class, receptor site affinity and sites of action. They may exert their effects on the vomiting center, the cerebral cortex, the CTZ, or the vestibular apparatus and bind to a number of different receptors. The neurotransmitters involved in controlling or preventing nausea and vomiting include dopamine (D_2) receptors located in the GI tract and CTZ, acetylcholine (ACh) receptors in the vestibular and vomiting center impacting on motion sickness, histamine (H_1) receptors in the vestibular and vomiting centers and serotonin (5-HT_3) receptors in the GI tract, CTZ, and vomiting centers (Table 40-2). Ginger, a complementary/alternative therapy for nausea and vomiting, (see the Complementary and Alternative Considerations box on p. 760) is discussed more fully in Chapter 12.

Vomiting as a result of cancer chemotherapy can be serious enough to limit the dosages of chemotherapeutic agents given to a client. Because antiemetics are usually more effective in preventing vomiting than they are in treating it, they should be administered prophylactically before chemotherapy administration. The effective treatment of chemotherapy-induced vomiting may require several antiemetic agents with different sites of action—for example, metoclopramide (Reglan) and lorazepam (Ativan), metoclopramide and dexamethasone

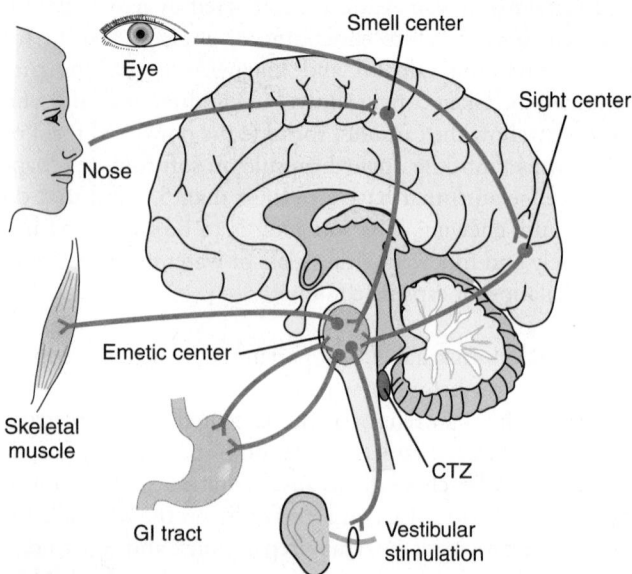

FIGURE 40-1 CTZ and other sites that activate the emetic center.

TABLE 40-2 CLASSIFICATIONS OF ANTIEMETICS

Drug	Class	Mechanism of Action	Anatomic Sites of Action	Comments
chlorpromazine (Thorazine)	Phenothiazine	Dopamine$_2$ (D$_2$) blockade	CTZ Peripheral	Extrapyramidal effects and tardive dyskinesia possible (See Chapter 19) Prolonged QT on ECG with droperidol, haloperidol
prochlorperazine (Compazine)				
promethazine (Phenergan)				
thiethylperazine (Torecan)				
droperidol (Inapsine)	Butyrophenone			
haloperidol (Haldol)				
metoclopramide (Reglan)	Prokinetic GI agent	D$_2$ blockade, 5-HT$_3$ antagonist		
scopolamine (Transderm-Scop)	Anticholinergic	Muscarinic receptor blockade	Emetic center Vestibular Cerebral cortex Peripheral	Antimuscarinic effects
diphenhydramine (Benadryl)	Antihistamine	H$_1$ blockade (partial muscarinic receptor blockade)	Vestibular Emetic center	Antimuscarinic effects
dimenhydrinate (Dramamine)				
meclizine (Antivert)				
dolasetron (Anzemet)	Selective serotonin receptor antagonist	5-HT$_3$ receptor antagonists	CTZ Emetic center Peripheral	Use primarily limited to chemotherapy induced and postoperative nausea and vomiting
granisetron (Kytril)				
ondansetron (Zofran)				
palonosetron (Aloxi)				
lorazepam (Ativan)	Benzodiazepine	Benzodiazepine receptor	Cerebral cortex	See Chapter 16
dexamethasone (Decadron)	Glucocorticoid	Glucocorticoid receptors	Unknown	See Chapter 48
dronabinol (Marinol)	Cannabinoid	? CB1 receptor	Emetic center Cerebral Cortex	Schedule II substance
aprepitant (Emend)	Substance P/ neurokinin 1 receptor antagonist	Sub P/NK1 receptor antagonist	NK1 receptors in brain	Use limited to preventing vomiting for highly emetic chemotherapy

CTZ, Chemoreceptor trigger zone; *ECG*, electrocardiogram; *GI*, gastrointestinal.

(Decadron), or ondansetron (Zofran) and dexamethasone. A number of clients respond well to the serotonin receptor antagonists alone if properly scheduled according to the manufacturer's recommendations. Representative agents are outlined in the following sections.

Phenothiazines/Butyrophenones

The phenothiazines and butyrophenones are potent D$_2$ blockers with significant antiemetic properties. Among the more commonly used agents for nausea and vomiting are prochlorperazine (Compazine) and promethazine (Phener-

Ginger

Ginger is an herbal remedy that has been used throughout the world to flavor foods as well to aid digestion, relieve nausea, and treat motion sickness. Ginger (*Zingiber officinale*) is often advocated as beneficial for nausea and vomiting. Whether the herb is truly efficacious for this condition is, however, still a matter of debate. Ernest & Pittler (2000) performed a systematic review of the evidence from randomized controlled trials for or against the efficacy of ginger for nausea and vomiting. Six studies met all inclusion criteria and were reviewed. Three on postoperative nausea and vomiting were identified and two of these suggested that ginger was superior to placebo and equally effective as metoclopramide. The pooled absolute risk reduction for the incidence of postoperative nausea, however, indicated a nonsignificant difference between the ginger and placebo groups for ginger 1 g taken before operation. One study was found for each of the following conditions: seasickness, morning sickness and chemotherapy-induced nausea. These studies collectively favored ginger over placebo. Ginger is considered safe in pregnancy and lactation when used in food amounts; however, greater amounts are contraindicated in pregnancy because of ginger's abortifacient (abortion-inducing) activity. (See Chapter 12 for more information.)

gan), which are available in oral, rectal and injectable formulations. Haloperidol (Haldol) and droperidol (Inapsine) are effective antiemetics, but prolonged QT intervals following their use have resulted in reduced use over the past decade. Chapter 19 discusses these agents more fully.

Benzamides

metoclopramide [met oh **kloe** pra mide]
(Reglan, Maxeran, Apo-Metoclop✚)

Metoclopramide is classified as a benzamide and has both a central and peripheral action in preventing or relieving nausea and emesis. Centrally, it blocks dopamine receptors in the CTZ; peripherally, it increases motility of the upper GI tract, increases peristalsis, and overcomes the immobility, dilation, and reverse motility that occurs with the vomiting reflex.

Indications
Metoclopramide is used for diabetic gastroparesis (Hasler, 2003), gastroesophageal reflux, and parenterally for the prevention of nausea and vomiting secondary to emetogenic cancer chemotherapeutic agents, radiation, and opioid medications. It is also used as an adjunct for GI radiologic examinations because it hastens the transit of barium through the upper GI tract by stimulating gastric emptying and accelerating intestinal transit.

Pharmacokinetics/Dosing
Parenteral metoclopramide may be used to facilitate intestinal intubation. The onset of action of metoclopramide is 30 minutes to 1 hour after oral administration, 10 to 15 minutes after an intramuscular (IM) dose, and within 3 minutes after an IV dose. The duration of action is 1 to 2 hours, and the half-life is 4 to 6 hours. It is metabolized by the liver and excreted by the kidneys. To treat diabetic gas-

troparesis or gastroesophageal reflux in an adult, the oral dosage of metoclopramide is 10 mg 30 minutes before each meal and at bedtime (up to four times daily). Check the package insert for further instructions. The IV dosage is 10 mg as a single dose. The antiemetic adult dosage (for chemotherapy-induced emesis) is 1-2 mg/kg by IV infusion 30 minutes before chemotherapy; the dose may be repeated every 2 to 3 hours as necessary. The oral pediatric dosage of metoclopramide is 0.1 to 0.2 mg/kg 30 minutes before meals and at bedtime to increase peristalsis in delayed GI emptying. Refer to current drug references for additional dosing recommendations.

Adverse Effects
Most common adverse effects of metoclopramide include diarrhea, sleepiness, restlessness, increased weakness and, rarely, extrapyramidal (parkinsonian) effects, hypotension, hypertension, tachycardia, and agranulocytosis. Long term use has been associated with tardive dyskinesia. See Chapter 19 and Box 19-4 for further discussion of extrapyramidal effects and tardive dyskinesia.

Drug Interactions
Concurrent use of typical antipsychotic drugs increases the potential for extrapyramidal effects and possibly the development of tardive dyskinesia. Use of metoclopramide may increase the rate (but usually not the extent) of other orally administered drugs.

⚙ **M.S. is a 54-year-old woman receiving chemotherapy for breast cancer with cyclophosphamide and doxorubicin. Despite prophylaxis for acute chemotherapy-induced emesis with ondansetron and dexamethasone before therapy and a prescription for oral ondansetron (8 mg twice daily) and oral dexamethasone (8 mg twice daily) for delayed emesis, she experiences refractory emesis. The oncologist prescribes high dose metoclopramide (2 mg/kg IV bolus, followed by 5 to 7.5 mg IV every 2 hours for 6 to 8 hours.**

⚙ **How will the addition of the metoclopramide alter M.S.'s drug therapy?**

Assessment Assess M.S. for preexisting conditions that might cause concern with the addition of metoclopramide to her drug therapy. The drug is often avoided in clients with epilepsy (isolated seizures have been reported) or to those in whom stimulation of GI motility is hazardous (e.g., those with GI hemorrhage, perforation, or mechanical obstruction); these conditions may be aggravated by metoclopramide. Clients with liver or renal dysfunction may experience decreased clearance of these agents. Extrapyramidal effects may be increased if metoclopramide is administered to clients with chronic renal failure. With metoclopramide, clients with pheochromocytoma are at risk for a hypertensive crisis. Assess M.S. for sensitivity to metoclopramide. Clients with intolerance to procaine and procainamide may experience a cross-sensitivity to metoclopramide.

Review M.S.'s medication regimen for the risk of significant drug interactions, such as those that may occur when metoclopramide is given concurrently with alcohol and CNS depressants (concurrent administration may increase the CNS depressant effects of either or both drug). Consider that the increased GI motility and decreased gastric emptying time caused by metoclopramide may decrease the absorption of oral medications from the stomach, whereas absorption from the small intestine may be enhanced. Obtain a baseline assessment of blood pressure, mental status, and underlying nausea and vomiting.

Nursing Diagnosis With the administration of metoclopramide, M.S. may be at risk for the following nursing diagnoses/collaborative problems: disturbed sleep pattern (drowsiness); impaired comfort (headache, dryness of the mouth, breast tenderness and swelling, and dizziness); disturbed thought processes (confusion, agitation, restlessness, depression); fatigue; ineffective protection related to agranulocytosis (chills, fever, sore throat, fatigue); risk for injury related to postural hypotension; diarrhea; and the potential complications of parkinsonian extrapyramidal effects, tardive dyskinesia, and altered cardiac output related to tachycardia and hypertension.

Planning See Box 40-4.

Implementation

Monitoring Monitor M.S.'s CBC, blood pressure (BP), mental status, and bowel status; also monitor for the presence of extrapyramidal effects and tardive dyskinesia and the incidence of nausea and vomiting. Be aware that extrapyramidal adverse effects may be seen with therapeutic dosages of metoclopramide and are more likely to occur in children and young adults.

Intervention Administer oral preparations of metoclopramide 30 minutes before meals and at bedtime. Administer IV injections of metoclopramide slowly over 1 to 2 minutes; a more rapid administration will produce a brief episode of anxiety and restlessness followed by drowsiness. For an IV infusion, dilute in 50 mL of the appropriate IV solution and infuse for a period of time (not less than 15 minutes). Solutions of parenteral metoclopramide may be kept for 48 hours after dilution if protected from light; if solutions are not protected from light, discard unused portions after 24 hours. Metoclopramide injection has a number of incompatibilities; see package insert for full listing.

Education Because metoclopramide can cause drowsiness, caution M.S. against operating any potentially haz-

---

BOX 40-4 GOALS FOR CLIENTS RECEIVING ANTIEMETIC DRUGS

The client receiving antiemetic drugs will:
* Remain free of nausea, vomiting, and adverse effects of antiemetic drug regimen, regaining normal fluid volume status.
* Effectively manage the therapeutic regimen, including medication compliance, supportive measures to reduce nausea and vomiting, and reporting adverse drug effects appropriately.
* Collaborate with health care providers for monitoring and follow-up care.

---

ardous equipment. Caution her against using alcohol or other CNS depressants. Metoclopramide may cause an increased rate of alcohol absorption from the small intestine leading to a CNS depressant effect. Instruct M.S. on symptoms to report to the prescriber; fainting, dizziness, irregular heartbeat, or any other unusual symptoms.

Evaluation The expected outcome of metoclopramide is that M.S. will report relief from nausea without experiencing any adverse effects or vomiting episodes. She will remain compliant with therapies, maintain supportive measures, and continue supervision with her provider for monitoring and follow-up care.

Antimuscarinics/Anticholinergics/ Antihistamines

Antimuscarinics appear effective in preventing vestibular induced nausea and vomiting. Scopolamine is the classic antimuscarinic used for this purpose, but trimethobenzamide (Tigan) is also included here. The antihistamines, which have strong antimuscarinic properties, are also used for motion-induced nausea and vomiting. Chapter 38 discusses these antihistamines. Antimuscarinics are also discussed in Chapter 21.

scopolamine transdermal [skoe **pol** a meen]
(Transderm-Scop, Transderm-V✤)
Scopolamine is an antimuscarinic agent used to prevent motion-induced nausea and vomiting by depressing conduction in the labyrinth of the inner ear. Overstimulation in this area is responsible for the nausea and vomiting of motion sickness. Scopolamine is metabolized in the liver and excreted by the kidneys.
Indications
Scopolamine transdermal is indicated for motion sickness prevention. It is also used in palliative care to reduce respiratory tract secretions.
Pharmacokinetics/Dosing
Scopolamine transdermal is recommended for use in adults only. In the United States, the product is a four-layered film that releases 0.5 mg of scopolamine over a 3-day period. It is applied on the skin behind the ear, usually 4 hours before the antiemetic effect is desired. In Canada, it is formulated to release 1 mg of scopolamine over a 3-day period, and it should be applied 12 hours before the antiemetic effect is desired.
Adverse Effects
The adverse effects of scopolamine are related to its anticholinergic effects: decreased sweating, sleepiness, dry mouth, nose, throat, or skin. Impaired memory and insomnia (paradoxical reaction) have been reported in older adults.
Drug Interactions
Use of other antimuscarinics or drugs with antimuscarinic properties may result in additive effects.

✱ **N.M. is a 30-year-old woman who has no significant medical history except motion sickness associated with air travel. She has self-treated with dimenhydrinate (Dramamine) before flights with moderate success; however, she did experience drowsiness as a result of the medication. She is engaged to be married and she and her future husband are planning a Mediterranean cruise for their honeymoon. She is concerned**

about having motion sickness for 7 days or sleeping her honeymoon away with the dimenhydrinate. Her primary care provider gives her a prescription for scopolamine patches.

✱ What is the nursing management of the antivertigo therapy for N.M.?

Motion sickness occurs when perceptions of motion by different proprioceptors (e.g., visual, vestibular, sensory) provide conflicting information. Antihistamines are the agents of choice for mild to moderate motion sickness. The scopolamine patch is as efficacious as, or more efficacious than, dimenhydrinate and has the advantage of providing continuous systemic concentrations of scopolamine for 72 hours at a time.

Assessment Because antihistamines have anticholinergic effects, assess N.M. for asthma, narrow-angle glaucoma, pyloric or intestinal obstruction, urinary tract obstruction, and also diminished renal or hepatic function. Assess whether N.M. is pregnant as scopolamine is used cautiously, if at all, in women who are pregnant or breastfeeding. Other cautions for use of this drug are: older adults are more susceptible to the effects of scopolamine and it is not used with children because of adverse effects. Although N.M. is not currently on other medications, alert her that the effects of anticholinergic/antimuscarinic drugs or CNS depressants, which would include alcohol, may be potentiated when used concurrently with scopolamine.

Nursing Diagnosis Using a scopolamine transdermal patch, N.M. is at risk for the following nursing diagnoses: disturbed sleep pattern (drowsiness); impaired comfort (headache, nasal congestion, dry mouth); constipation; impaired urinary elimination (urinary hesitancy and retention); and risk for injury related to blurred vision.

Planning While taking scopolamine transdermal, N.M. will:

- Remain free of nausea, vomiting and any adverse effects of the scopolamine.
- Effectively manage the therapeutic regimen, including medication compliance and supportive measures to prevent nausea and vomiting.

Implementation

Monitoring N.M. may have a dilated pupil on the side that the patch is worn that may persist for 2 weeks after the patch is worn. Be aware that clients can develop tolerance to the drug after prolonged use.

Intervention Depending on the type of patch, apply the system at least 4 hours or 12 hours before the antiemetic effect is desired. Wash and dry the hands thoroughly before and after applying the system. Apply it to intact skin in the hairless area behind the ear.

Education Warn N.M. it would be best to have her husband drive on any shore breaks because it would be hazardous for her to do so because of potential drowsiness, disorientation, confusion, and blurred vision.

Evaluation The expected outcome of scopolamine transdermal therapy is that N.M. will not experience motion sickness, nausea, and vomiting or any adverse effects of the drug.

trimethobenzamide [trye meth oh **ben** za mide]
(Tigan)

Although not a classic antimuscarinic, trimethobenzamide possesses antimuscarinic activity. It may depress the CTZ in the medulla rather than the vomiting center directly. As an antiemetic, it is not as effective as metoclopramide.

Indications

Trimethobenzamide is indicated for the control of nausea and vomiting.

Pharmacokinetics/Dosing

Trimethobenzamide is metabolized in the liver and excreted in the urine. The adult oral dosage of trimethobenzamide is 250 mg three or four times daily. For rectal or IM administration, 200 mg is given three or four times daily. With children over 13.6 kg, the dosage is 15 mg/kg PO daily, divided into 3 or 4 doses. Its use is not recommended for children weighing less than 13.6 kg. Refer to a current drug reference for additional recommendations.

Adverse Effects

The reported adverse effects include sleepiness, blurred vision, diarrhea, dizziness, headache, muscle cramps and, rarely, allergic reactions, seizures, blood dyscrasias, impaired liver function, tremors, Reye syndrome, and depression (USP DI, 2005).

5-HT$_3$ Receptor Antagonists

Ondansetron was the first of a new class of serotonin receptor (5-HT$_3$) antagonists approved by the Food and Drug Administration (FDA) for the prevention of nausea and vomiting associated with the use of antineoplastic agents. Granisetron (Kytril), dolasetron (Anzemet), and palonosetron (Aloxi) are also selective serotonin antagonists. Serotonin (5-HT$_3$) receptors are located peripherally on the vagus nerve terminal and centrally in the CTZ. It is believed that antineoplastics cause the release of stored serotonin from the enterochromaffin cells of the GI tract (*USP DI,* 2005). Serotonin stimulates serotonin receptors in the vagus nerve in the GI tract, which then stimulates serotonin receptors in the CTZ, inducing vomiting. When ondansetron or granisetron are administered before antineoplastic therapy, they block serotonin receptors in the brainstem and GI tract. As a result, serotonin released in response to the administration of antineoplastic agents cannot bind with the serotonin receptors, and vomiting is prevented. Ondansetron and dolasetron are also effective for postoperative nausea and vomiting.

✱🔳 ondansetron hydrochloride [on **dan** se tron]
(Zofran)

Indications

Ondansetron is indicated for the prevention of chemotherapy-induced and radiation-induced nausea and vomiting and for prevention of postoperative nausea and vomiting.

Pharmacokinetics/Dosing

Ondansetron peaks in 1 to 2 hours when administered orally; the elimination half-life is 3 to 4 hours, and it is metabolized in the liver by P450 3 A4 and other isoenzymes and excreted primarily by the kidneys.

The parenteral dosage for ondansetron to prevent cancer chemotherapy-induced nausea and vomiting in adults and children 4 to 18 years of age is 0.15 mg/kg IV infused over 15 minutes beginning 30 minutes before chemotherapy, followed by 0.15 mg/kg 4 and 8 hours after the first dose of ondansetron. The oral adult dosage is 8 mg 30 minutes before cancer chemotherapy, then 8 mg at 8 hours after the first dose, followed by 8 mg every 12 hours for several days. The oral dosage for children is 4 mg in the same schedule as for adults.

Adverse Effects
The adverse effects of ondansetron include fever, headache, constipation, diarrhea and, rarely, anaphylaxis, chest pain, and bronchospasm. Prolongation of QT interval, which increases risk for life-threatening cardiac dysrhythmias, has been reported with other drugs in this class (dolasetron, palonosetron).

Drug Interactions
Concurrent use of enzyme inducing agents (e.g., rifampin, carbamazepine, barbiturates, phenytoin) may reduce the efficacy of ondansetron or necessitate higher doses to achieve desired effects.

✳ **A.U. is a 6-year-old girl who is admitted to the ambulatory center for placement of tympanostomy tubes. Balanced anesthesia consisting of propofol, fentanyl, and isoflurane is administered for the operative procedure. To prevent postoperative nausea and vomiting, A.U. is administered ondansetron 4 mg IV intraoperatively.**

✳ **What nursing management of antiemetic therapy is required for A.U.?**

Assessment For all antiemetic therapy, a baseline assessment includes an allergy history in relation to the antiemetic, fluid balance ratio data, the degree of nausea reported by A.U., and the frequency of vomiting. For A.U., the antiemetic is given to prevent postoperative nausea and vomiting, but as a rule, do not give antiemetics until the underlying cause of nausea has been established. For example, a drug overdose or increased intracranial pressure may cause nausea. Additionally, ondansetron may increase hepatic enzymes (ALT/AST) and therefore is contraindicated at its standard dosage and schedule for clients with hepatic impairment.

Nursing Diagnosis With the administration of antiemetic therapy, A.U. may experience the following nursing diagnoses: impaired comfort (nausea) related to the underlying postoperative status and/or ineffectiveness of the antiemetic agent; deficient fluid volume or imbalanced nutrition: less than body requirements related to vomiting; or disturbed sleep pattern (drowsiness). In addition with ondansetron therapy, she is at risk for impaired comfort (headache, abdominal cramping, dry mouth, rash); fatigue; diarrhea; and constipation; and the potential complication of bronchospasm.

Planning For goals of antiemetic therapy for A.U., see Box 40-4.

Implementation

Monitoring For all antiemetics, monitor for nausea and vomiting, a general sense of well-being, and fluid balance ratio. Additionally, for ondansetron, monitor A.U.'s bowel status for diarrhea or constipation.

Intervention As in A.U.'s case, the antiemetic is given prophylactically for best results. To support the administration of antiemetics, provide a quiet environment, make A.U. comfortable, and give ice chips or small sips of ginger ale, if allowed. If it is decided to give another dose, ondansetron may be administered by oral solution, tablet, disintegrating tablet or IV solution. The disintegrating tablet dissolves when placed on the tongue and does not require water. If given IV, dilute the IV injection in 50 mL of 5% dextrose or 0.9% sodium chloride solution before administering; infuse over 15 minutes. This dose may be repeated twice at 4-hour intervals. Ondansetron sometimes precipitates in the vial at the stopper/vial interface in vials stored upright; shake the vial vigorously to restabilize it.

Education Instruct A.U. and her parents to report any symptoms of hypersensitivity or continued vomiting. Most antiemetics cause drowsiness as a side effect. If an antiemetic is prescribed on discharge, caution A.U. against performing hazardous tasks (e.g., bicycle riding) until the effects of the drug have subsided. Caution her parents against combining her antiemetic with alcohol (e.g., some cough and cold medication contain alcohol) or any CNS depressants. The CNS depressant effects of the drug can be potentiated when these drugs are combined.

Evaluation The expected outcome of antiemetic therapy is that A.U. experience the absence of or diminished nausea and vomiting and maintain an adequate fluid balance. She and her parents will report symptoms of nausea and vomiting and/or adverse effects of the drug to the health care team.

✳ **D.D. is a 64-year-old man with newly diagnosed adenocarcinoma. He scheduled to receive his first course of chemotherapy with cisplatin 100 mg/m² on day 1 and fluorouracil 1 g/m² daily for 5 days by continuous infusion. One of his expressed concerns is about the nausea and vomiting associated with the chemotherapy. "I had a friend who told me the nausea and vomiting with this stuff is terrible."**

Nausea and vomiting are common complications of chemotherapy. However, D.D. should be reassured that medications are available to minimize these symptoms.

One study reported that nausea was present in 50% and vomiting in 27% of an outpatient population receiving a variety of chemotherapy regimens (Lindley, 2005). Although nausea and vomiting are most common in the first 24 hours following chemotherapy, they may persist for up to 5 days in a significant number of clients. The emetogenic potential of the most emetogenic chemotherapy agent administered as part of the combination therapy has the greatest influence on acute nausea and vomiting after antineoplastic chemotherapy. See Chapter 56 for the emetogenic potential of specific antineoplastic agents. Combination antineoplastic chemotherapy is at least as emetogenic as the most emetogenic agent in the combination. Regimens that are moderate or moderately high to high risk for chemotherapy-induced emesis require prophylactic antiemetic therapy with the maximally effective dose of 5-HT$_3$ antagonist, dexamethasone, or prochlorperazine (Lindley, 2005).

✱ What is the nursing management of 5-HT$_3$ antagonist therapy for D.D.?

Assessment A sensitivity to granisetron, dolasetron, ondansetron, or palonosetron would contraindicate 5-HT$_3$ antagonist therapy for D.D. Drug clearance and half-life alterations of the 5-HT$_3$ antagonists may occur with drugs that induce hepatic enzymes or ones that inhibit hepatic enzymes as the 5-HT$_3$ antagonists are metabolized by hepatic cytochrome P450 enzymes. D.D.'s baseline assessment includes a description of his previous experience with antiemetic therapy, nutritional status, bowel status, serum electrolytes, and respiratory status. An ECG may be warranted for clients with cardiovascular risk, especially with the use of dolasetron or palonosetron, which can prolong QT intervals.

Nursing Diagnosis With 5-HT$_3$ antagonist therapy, D.D. is at risk for the following nursing diagnoses: impaired comfort (headache, abdominal cramping, dry mouth, rash); fatigue; disturbed sleep pattern (drowsiness); diarrhea; and constipation. He is also at risk for the following potential complications: with ondansetron, bronchospasm; with granisetron, weakness; and with dolasetron and palonosetron, cardiac dysrhythmias.

Planning See Box 40-4.

Implementation

Monitoring Observe D.D.'s vital signs, nausea, vomiting, and comfort status. Monitor his fluid and electrolytes, bowel status, and activity tolerance.

Intervention The time of administration of the prophylactic antiemetic agent will depend on the chemotherapeutic regimen prescribed. To support the administration of antiemetics, provide a quiet environment, make D.D. comfortable, and give ice chips, small sips of ginger ale or, if allowed, hot tea to drink. Vomiting as the result of cancer chemotherapy can cause serious electrolyte imbalance and a nutritional deficit. These drugs have a number of incompatibilities; check package insert for specific drugs.

Dolasetron is to be administered before chemotherapy; 1 hour before with oral doses and 30 minutes before with IV doses. The IV injection preparation of dolasetron is not to be mixed with other medications, and the IV infusion line should be flushed before and after administration.

Dilute granisetron with 5% dextrose or 0.9% sodium chloride injection to a total volume of 20 to 50 mL; infuse over 5 minutes about 30 minutes before the administration of cancer chemotherapy.

With ondansetron, dilute the IV injection in 50 mL of 5% dextrose or 0.9% sodium chloride solution before administering; infuse over 15 minutes. This dose may be repeated twice at 4-hour intervals.

The injection solution of dolasetron may be mixed in apple juice or grape juice for oral administration to children.

Education Alert D.D. that headache may occur; this can be relieved by an analgesic. Instruct the client to eat small frequent meals or small nutritional snacks between meals.

Evaluation The expected outcome of 5-HT$_3$ antagonist therapy is that the client will not experience postoperative or antineoplastic drug–induced nausea and vomiting or any adverse effects of the drug. The client will maintain normal fluid balance. The client will collaborate with the health care providers by reporting adverse effects, maintaining medication compliance, and participating in nonpharmacologic interventions to reduce nausea and vomiting.

Benzodiazepines

Benzodiazepines like lorazepam (Ativan) are frequently used as part of combination therapy to prevent chemotherapy induced nausea and vomiting. Their anxiolytic and amnesic actions reduce negative associations with the chemotherapy treatment process and thereby may reduce future anticipatory nausea and vomiting (Pasricha, 2001). Chapter 16 discusses benzodiazepines more fully.

Glucocorticoids

Corticosteroids have been reported to be effective for chemotherapy-induced nausea and vomiting alone or when used in combination with other antiemetics (Lindley, 2005). The mechanism of action is unknown, but it has been proposed that these drugs may inhibit the synthesis of prostaglandins, which may be involved in chemotherapy-induced vomiting. Some prostaglandins (especially the PGE series) can induce nausea and vomiting.

Many studies with corticosteroids have involved the use of dexamethasone and methylprednisolone, but corticotropin and hydrocortisone may also be used. Their effectiveness as antiemetics was a serendipitous discovery—clients receiving various chemotherapeutic regimens experienced less nausea and vomiting when prednisone was one of the agents administered. Thus the corticosteroids (usually dexamethasone) are used as antiemetics in cancer chemotherapy, especially in clients who are not responsive to other drug therapies. See Chapter 48 for a discussion related to corticosteroids.

Cannabinoids

Marijuana and its derivatives have been controversial treatments to reduce nausea and stimulate appetite. Dronabinol is the most frequently used cannabinoid in clinical practice for these purposes.

dronabinol [droe **nah** bih nol]
(Marinol)
Dronabinol is the synthetic derivative of THC (delta-9-tetrahydrocannabinol) and a Schedule III substance by the U.S. Drug Enforcement Agency (DEA).

Indications

Dronabinol is indicated as a second-line agent to prevent the nausea and vomiting associated with chemotherapy when other antiemetics are ineffective. It is also used as an appetite stimulant to treat anorexia and weight loss in persons with AIDS.

Pharmacokinetics/Dosing

Dronabinol reaches peak serum levels in 2 to 4 hours; the duration of action is 4 to 6 hours for psychologic effects and 1 day or longer for appetite-stimulating effects. It is metabolized in the liver and excreted mainly in the feces. The oral dosage for adults is 5 mg/m² of body surface 1 to 3 hours before chemotherapy, then every 2 to 4 hours afterward (4 to 6 doses daily). If the initial dose is ineffective, it may be increased in increments of 2.5 mg/m² (the maximum dose is 15 mg/m² per dose). The dosage for appetite stimulation is 2.5 mg twice daily before lunch and supper, which may be increased if necessary up to a maximum of 20 mg daily. The pediatric dosage is similar to the adult dosage.

Adverse Effects

The adverse effects of dronabinol include ataxia, light-headedness, nausea, vomiting, blurred vision, dry mouth, restlessness, weakness, drowsiness, tachycardia or bradycardia, and CNS adverse effects such as confusion, delusions, hallucinations, depression, mood alterations, restlessness, and anxiety. Older adults are particularly prone to the adverse effects in the CNS.

✸ What is the nursing management of cannabinoid therapy?

Assessment Sensitivity to dronabinol or sesame oil may preclude the use of cannabinoids. These agents should be used with caution in clients with cardiac disorders, because dysrhythmias may occur with an increase in sympatho-mimetic activity. Clients with mental disorders such as manic, depressive, and schizophrenic states may have increased symptoms. Clients with a history of substance abuse may tend to abuse these agents. The concurrent use of dronabinol with alcohol and other CNS depressants may potentiate the effects of the CNS depressants. Assess the client's weight and nutritional status, symptoms of nausea and vomiting, fluid volume status, cardiac status, and mental status before therapy.

Nursing Diagnosis The client receiving dronabinol therapy is at risk for the following nursing diagnoses/collaborative problems: disturbed sleep pattern (drowsiness); disturbed thought processes as a result of the psychotomimetic effects of the drug (mood swings, confusion, inability to think, anxiety, hallucinations); impaired oral mucous membrane (dry mouth); risk for injury related to blurred vision, orthostatic hypotension, and light-headedness; and the potential complications of mental depression and altered cardiac output (tachycardia).

Planning

See Box 40-4.

Implementation

Monitoring Document the client's weight, fluid volume status, and frequency of nausea and vomiting. Monitor the client's vital signs and mental status. Some clients report feelings of well-being and euphoria; others have transient psychoses characterized by hallucinations and depersonalization.

Intervention Dronabinol is administered while the client is being supervised. It is administered 1 to 3 hours before chemotherapy. The amount dispensed should be limited to that necessary to accompany a single cycle of chemotherapy. Clients may experience withdrawal (irritability, insomnia, restlessness, diarrhea, sweating, anorexia) when the drugs are abruptly discontinued after 12 to 16 days of therapy; to prevent this, clients should be weaned gradually from the drug.

Education Alert the client to make position changes slowly, particularly from the recumbent to upright position to prevent the dizziness and fainting of orthostatic hypotension. Caution the client to avoid ingesting alcoholic beverages and other CNS depressants while taking dronabinol because of the additive CNS depressing effects. Alert the client to use caution when driving or performing other activities that require alertness. Inform the client that dronabinol may be habit-forming.

Evaluation The expected outcome of dronabinol therapy is that the client will not experience nausea and vomiting or any adverse effects of the drug. The client will effectively manage the drug regimen, including compliance with medication, notifying the prescriber of reportable adverse effects, and maintaining scheduled visits with health care providers for monitoring and follow-up care.

Substance P/NK1 Receptor Antagonists

A newer approach to reduce chemotherapy induced nausea and vomiting is to target an antagonist for the NK1 subtype of the substance P receptor in central afferent fibers. The first of this group is aprepitant (Emend).

aprepitant [ah **preh** pih tant]
(Emend)

Indications

Aprepitant is indicated for the prevention of acute and delayed nausea and vomiting secondary to highly emetogenic chemotherapy.

Pharmacokinetics/Dosing

Aprepitant is moderately well absorbed orally and is metabolized extensively by cytochrome P450 3 A4. Its levels and effect peaks 4 hours after dosing and the half-life is between 9 and 13 hours. It is typically dosed at 125 mg orally on the first day of chemotherapy 1 hour before chemotherapy begins, followed by 80 mg on days 2 and 3. It is administered in combination with dexamethasone and a 5-HT₃ antagonist (e.g., ondansetron).

Adverse Effects

The most common adverse effects are dizziness, weakness, hiccups, dizziness, and diarrhea. Other GI complaints have also been reported.

Drug Interactions

Aprepitant may affect the metabolism of other drugs metabolized by cytochrome P450 systems and current references should be consulted before use.

Nursing Management

Assessment

Aprepitant is contraindicated for lactating clients and clients younger than 18 years of age. Determine the presence of any underlying cardiovascular disease or hypersensitivity to aprepitant. Review the client's concurrent medications for any drug that is also metabolized by the CYP3 A4 isoenzyme, because aprepitant is an inhibitor of this isoenzyme and elevated plasma concentrations of these drugs may occur (e.g., ketoconazole, itraconazole, nefazodone, troleandomycin, clarithromycin). As an inducer of CYP 2 C9, concurrent use may result in lower plasma concentrations, and so efficacy, of some drugs (e.g., hormonal contraceptives, warfarin, tolbutamide, phenytoin). Obtain a baseline of the client's health status preparatory to initiating aprepitant therapy, including serum electrolytes, UA, and CBC, and a PT/INR if the client is on warfarin.

Nursing Diagnosis

While receiving aprepitant, the client is at risk for the following nursing diagnoses: fatigue, diarrhea, impaired comfort (GI distress, anorexia, nausea, hiccups, myalgia); disturbed sensory perception (tinnitus), confusion; and the potential complications of anemia, neutropenia, hypokalemia, and deep vein thrombosis.

Planning

See Box 40-4.

Implementation

Monitoring

Monitor PT/INR 7 to 10 days after a 3-day regimen of aprepitant if the client is taking warfarin concurrently. Monitor phenytoin serum levels if the client is taking the drug concurrently. Monitor serum electrolytes, UA, and CBC.

Intervention

Give aprepitant 1 hour before chemotherapy is to begin. Ensure that the capsule is swallowed whole with a full glass of water. Do not crush or open the capsule.

Education

Report to the prescriber any shortness of breath, changes in BP, heart rate, dizziness, confusion, any sudden severe or sharp pain in the legs or stomach. Use barrier contraception in addition to hormonal contraceptives while taking aprepitant. Do not add any medications, prescription, OTC or herbal, without consulting the prescriber of aprepitant therapy.

Evaluation

The expected outcome of aprepitant therapy is that the client will not experience nausea and vomiting or any adverse effects of the drug. The client will effectively manage the drug regimen, including compliance with medication, notifying the prescriber of reportable adverse effects, and maintaining scheduled visits with health care providers for monitoring and follow-up care.

✳ What drugs are used to induce vomiting?

Emetic drugs, such as ipecac syrup, exert their effects on the same centers as antiemetic drugs but have the opposite effect. They have historically been used to induce vomiting as part of the treatment for certain drug overdoses and poisonings. Because their use can complicate the management of poisonings, their use has been largely abandoned. Refer to Chapter 72 for a review of the role of emetics in poison management.

✳ What drugs affect the gallbladder?

The major pathology associated with the gallbladder includes obstruction and reduced biliary flow. A number of drugs can adversely affect the gallbladder by forming crystals or stones in bile, or by inducing spasms of the musculature. Commonly used drugs causing such issues include estrogens and hormonal contraceptives, opioids, and the cephalosporin antibiotic ceftriaxone. Most pathology of the gallbladder, however, is not correlated with drug use. Gallstone development is one of the most common pathologies.

ursodiol [er so dye all]
(Actigall)

Drugs have a limited role in treating gallstones. The most frequently used drug to treat gallstones is ursodiol. Ursodiol, an analog of chenodiol, is an oral product used to dissolve cholesterol gallstones in clients with uncomplicated gallstone disease. It is more effective against small, floatable stones and is not indicated for the treatment of calcified cholesterol stones, radiopaque (calcium-containing) stones, or radiolucent bile pigment–type stones or when surgery is clearly necessary.

Although its exact mechanism of action is unknown, ursodiol inhibits the intestinal absorption of cholesterol and also decreases cholesterol synthesis and secretion in the liver. A decrease in cholesterol saturation allows for the gradual dissolution of cholesterol from the gallstones. Ursodiol also increases the flow of bile in the body. However, 6 to 24 months of oral therapy may be necessary for gallstone dissolution depending on the composition and size of the stone. Therapy is monitored by performing ultrasonograms at 6-month intervals during the first year. If partial effectiveness is not recorded after 1 year of treatment, ursodiol is usually determined to be ineffective and drug therapy is discontinued. If therapy is successful, ursodiol is recommended for at least 3 months after complete dissolution of the stones to ensure the removal of small particles that are not visible with the ultrasonogram. Complete dissolution does not occur in all clients and recurrence of stones within 5 years has been observed in 50% of clients who do dissolve their stones on bile acid therapy (*Drug Facts and Comparisons,* 2005).

Indications

Ursodiol is indicated for the client with radiolucent stones who has a well-opacified, functioning gallbladder but who is at increased risk with elective surgery because of systemic disease, age, or cardiovascular, renal, or respiratory disease.

Pharmacokinetics/Dosing

When administered orally, ursodiol is absorbed from the small intestine, reaches a peak concentration in 1 to 3 hours, and is metabolized by the liver to taurine and glycine conjugates that are secreted in bile. Excretion is mainly in the feces. The oral dosage for adults is 8 to 10 mg/kg daily, divided into 2 or 3 doses taken with meals. A pediatric dosage has not been established.

Adverse Effects

An uncommon adverse effect reported with ursodiol is diarrhea. Ursodiol may cause hepatotoxicity, but liver injuries have not been reported to date.

Nursing Management

Assessment

Although ursodiol is indicated for the dissolution of cholesterol gallstones, administer it with caution if the client's health status is further compromised with bile duct abnormalities, complications of gallstones such as cholecystitis or pancreatitis, or chronically impaired hepatic function. The client will usually undergo ultrasonogram and/or hepatic function studies to determine if these conditions exist before beginning a regimen of ursodiol. Hepatic function studies are performed to rule out preexisting liver disease. No significant drug interactions have been reported with ursodiol, but keep in mind that antacids (containing aluminum), cholestyramine, or colestipol may decrease the absorption and effectiveness of ursodiol when administered concurrently. A nursing baseline assessment includes ursodiol sensitivity, pain status, and bowel status.

Nursing Diagnosis

During the course of ursodiol therapy the client may experience altered comfort (nausea, dyspepsia, headache, metallic taste, biliary pain, flatulence), fatigue, and diarrhea as an adverse effect of the drug.

Planning

The client receiving ursodiol will:
- Remain free of biliary colic and other abdominal discomfort without experiencing adverse effects of the drug.

- Effectively manage the therapeutic regimen, including medication compliance, supportive measures to reduce nausea and vomiting, and reporting adverse drug effects appropriately.
- Collaborate with health care providers for monitoring and follow-up care.

Implementation

Monitoring

Ultrasonograms, cholecystograms, and/or hepatic function studies are usually performed periodically over the course of drug therapy to determine the dissolution of gallstones and the development of hepatotoxicity. Have the client monitor bowel elimination for the frequency and character of stools.

Intervention

Administer ursodiol with meals, but administer antacids and bile-sequestering agents at least 2 hours apart from ursodiol. If partial dissolution has not occurred after 6 to 12 months of therapy, the drug is considered ineffective and is discontinued.

Education

Instruct the client to take ursodiol with meals because it dissolves more rapidly when bile and pancreatic enzymes are present. Encourage compliance and caution the client to be patient, because gallstone dissolution may take 6 months to 2 years depending on the size and number of stones.

Evaluation

If ursodiol therapy is successful, the client's gallstones should diminish in size and number as demonstrated by the ultrasonogram, and the client will not experience any adverse effects of the drug. The client will effectively manage the drug regimen, including compliance with medication, notifying the prescriber of reportable adverse effects, and maintaining scheduled visits with health care providers for monitoring and follow-up care.

❋ What treatments are used to manage complications of end-stage liver disease?

End-stage liver disease, a consequence of chronic liver inflammation because of infectious or toxin etiologies, is often complicated by portal hypertension, coagulopathies, ascites, hepatic encephalopathy, and/or esophageal variceal bleeding.

Portal hypertension is often managed with β-adrenergic blockers and/or nitrates (Merkel et al., 2004), although endoscopic banding may be more effective than drugs in preventing bleeding from esophageal varices (Jutabha et al., 2005; Sarin, Wadhawan, Agarwal, Tyagi, & Sharma, 2005). (See Chapters 22, 27 and 28.) Coagulopathies, a result of reduced production of clotting factors, may benefit in part from vitamin K supplementation (see Chapter 30), although this is only helpful for clients who are nutritionally deficient. Ascites is often managed with diuretics—specifically spironolactone (refer to Chapter 33). Lactulose is sometimes used to help trap ammonia retained in the colon for clients with encephalopathy (see p. 771), although this practice has been questioned (Als-Nielsen, Gluud, & Gluud, 2004). Esophageal variceal bleeding risk can be reduced by managing portal hypertension and coagulopathies, and is treated acutely with octreotide or vasopressin (see Chapter 46). Milk thistle is also known to stimulate bile flow and have protective effects on the liver. See Complementary and Alternative Considerations box above.

❋ P.F. is a 43-year-old woman with a five year history of Crohn's disease who is receiving sulfasalazine (Azul-

❋ Complementary and Alternative Considerations

Milk Thistle

The above-ground parts of milk thistle, and its fruit and seed, have been used for thousands of years for treating dysfunction of the gallbladder and liver and other dyspeptic disorders. Milk thistle contains silymarin, which is a mixture of chemicals (flavonoids) that help protect the liver not only by reducing inflammation, but by promoting regeneration of the liver cells and helping them become more efficient at detoxifying the blood. The dose is based on the percent of silymarin. Clinically, silymarin has been found to reduce liver transaminase levels and result in improvement of both acute and chronic viral hepatitis. It has also been found to prolong survival in clients with cirrhosis. The client should take 300 mg three times daily (210 mg silymarin three times daily). The standard dose of milk thistle is based on the silymarin content, which is 70% of the bulk herb; therefore, 300 mg of milk thistle is equal to 210 mg of silymarin (Rakel, 2003). For further information, see Chapter 12.

fidine) 1 g orally q6h. While her symptoms were in reasonable control over the past few years, she now is demonstrating significant cramping and diarrhea (5 to 6 times daily) and mucus in the stool.

❋ How are inflammatory bowel diseases differentiated?

The two most common types of inflammatory bowel diseases are ulcerative colitis and Crohn's disease. Other similar conditions include irritable bowel disease and diverticulitis. Irritable bowel disease is associated with similar symptoms ulcerative colitis and Crohn's disease. Diverticulitis involves inflammation of the diverticuli of the colon and may be treated with antimicrobials. Genetic variation among the different inflammatory bowel diseases is noted, and may account for variations in response to treatment (see the Special Considerations for Pharmacogenetics box on p. 750).

Ulcerative colitis is more common than Crohn's disease. Ulcerative colitis presents with abdominal pain, cramping, and frequent diarrhea. Rectal bleeding is a common finding, as is weight loss and fever. Inflammation is restricted to the rectum and colon, and is typically limited to the local mucosa and is usually contiguous.

Unlike ulcerative colitis, the lesions of Crohn's disease penetrate through the entire gut wall and may be observed throughout the GI tract from the mouth to the anus. Like ulcerative colitis, diarrhea is common, but it is less likely to contain blood.

Irritable bowel syndrome (IBS) is not an inflammatory state, but instead functional state involving cramps, diarrhea or constipation, and bloating. Episodes may be triggered by stress or diet, but pathologically, no inflammatory lesions are present. Many clients find symptomatic relief with complementary/alternative therapies, such as pepper-

Peppermint Oil

Peppermint oil is a common flavoring agent in foods and beverages. When taken orally, peppermint oil is used for nausea and vomiting, colds, cough, inflammation of the mouth and pharynx, liver and gallbladder complaints, dyspepsia, and as an antiflatulent. Topically, peppermint oil is used for headache, neuralgias, toothaches, mucosal inflammation, and pruritus. When used for relief of irritable bowel syndrome (IBS), it is considered to be possibly effective. There is some evidence (Pittler & Ernest, 1998) that peppermint oil can reduce abdominal pain, distention, flatulence, and bowel movements in clients with IBS. It relaxes GI smooth muscle by reduction of calcium influx (Hasler, 2003). It is considered an effective antispasmodic agent (Somers & Lembo, 2003). Its spasmolytic effect was demonstrated in a randomized, double-blind, double dummy controlled trial (Hiki et al., 2003).

Peppermint oil is associated with reduced lower esophageal sphincter tone and can worsen the symptoms of GERD. Although there may be some burning and ulceration of the mouth in clients with contact sensitivity, enteric-coated capsules may reduce the incidence of these symptoms and heartburn. The usual dose of peppermint oil for irritable bowel syndrome is 0.2 to 0.4 mL three times daily in enteric-coated capsules.

mint oil. See the Complementary and Alternative Considerations box above.

✪ What drugs are used to treat inflammatory bowel disease?

A number of drugs are used to treat inflammatory bowel disease and are classified as aminosalicylates, immunomodulators, corticosteroids, and biologic response modifiers. Antimicrobials are also used in the treatment of inflammatory bowel diseases. Tegaserod (Zelnorm) is a 5-HT$_4$ antagonist in the colon indicated for irritable bowel disease in women and for chronic constipation refractory to other treatments.

The aminosalicylates have long been used to treat ulcerative colitis and Crohn's disease. These include mesalamine or 5-aminosalicylic acid (Asacol, Pentasa, Rowasa), balsalazide (Colazal), olsalazine (Dipentum), and sulfasalazine (Azulfidine). These agents are used to treat both acute conditions and help maintain remission in clients with relatively good control of symptoms.

The immunomodulators used to treat inflammatory bowel disease include azathioprine (Azasan, Imuran), methotrexate, mercaptopurine (Purinethol) and occasionally cyclosporine (Sandimmune). These drugs suppress the immune system and are reserved for more advanced cases. These are reviewed in Chapter 63.

Corticosteroids like prednisone are used topically as rectal formulations and systemically to reduce inflammation during flare ups. These agents are discussed more fully in Chapter 48.

The biologic response modifiers are monoclonal antibodies directed against tumor necrosis factor alpha (TNF-α). Infliximab (Remicade) is used for the treatment of Crohn's disease. Infliximab and other similar agents are used for the other serious inflammatory conditions such as progressive rheumatoid arthritis. Infliximab is reserved for advanced cases of Crohn's disease. Like the immunomodulators and corticosteroids, they also suppress immune function and increase risk for infections.

✦◼ mesalamine [me **sal** a meen]
(Asacol, Pentasa, Rowasa, Mesasal✦, Salofalk✦)
Although the exact mechanism of action of mesalamine is unknown, it appears to decrease inflammation by inhibiting cyclooxygenase and lipoxygenase, which results in a decrease in the production of prostaglandin and leukotriene.

Indications
Mesalamine is indicated for the treatment of mild to moderate ulcerative colitis. It is also used in mild cases of Crohn's disease in which lesions are limited to the distal colon. Mesalamine is also indicated to maintaining remission of such cases.

Pharmacokinetics/Dosing
Mesalamine is available in extended-release capsules and tablets (Pentasa), delayed-release tablets (Asacol) and rectal suppositories and rectal suspensions (Rowasa). The nurse should be aware that there is a difference between the extended-release and delayed-release preparations; therefore one product should not be substituted for the other.

The absorption of oral mesalamine is 20% to 30%. Asacol has a coating (acrylic-based resin) that delays dissolution until the tablet is at a pH of 7 or more; therefore it is released in the distal ileum and colon. Pentasa contains cellulose-coated granules, which permits the continuous release of mesalamine in the small and large intestine, independent of pH. The half-life of mesalamine from Asacol is 3 hours; the half-life of Pentasa cannot be determined because of the continuous release of the product. A peak serum level occurs in 4 to 12 hours for Asacol and in 3 hours for Pentasa. Excretion of the unchanged drug is primarily in the feces for Asacol (80%) but reduced for Pentasa (13%). The absorbed mesalamine is excreted renally as the metabolite (N-acetyl-5-aminosalicylic acid [Ac-5-ASA]).

Adverse Effects
The adverse effects of mesalamine include stomach cramps or pain, diarrhea, headache, nausea, vomiting, weakness, rhinitis and, infrequently or rarely, acne, alopecia, loss of appetite, back pain, indigestion, hepatitis, pancreatitis, or pericarditis.

Drug Interactions
Mesalamine may decrease the absorption of digoxin. Bone marrow suppression may be more likely with other immunosuppressant therapies.

olsalazine [ole **sal** a zeen]
(Dipentum)
Olsalazine is a salicylate compound that is converted in the colon by bacteria to mesalamine, so the active ingredient is mesalamine.

Indications
Similar to mesalamine.

Pharmacokinetics/Dosing
Olsalazine remains primarily unabsorbed until it reaches the colon, where it is converted to mesalamine by colonic bacteria. Mesalamine is absorbed slowly, which results in a high local concentration of mesalamine in the colon. The excretion of mesalamine occurs in the feces (80%); the absorbed portion is excreted by the kidneys as the metabolite (Ac-5-ASA). The adult dosage of olsalazine is 500 mg twice daily.

Adverse Effects

The adverse effects of olsalazine include GI adverse effects similar to mesalamine; infrequent or rare effects include rash, joint and muscle pain, mood alterations, sedation, headache, insomnia, exacerbation of ulcerative colitis, hepatitis, and pancreatitis.

Drug Interactions

Similar to mesalamine. Olsalazine may also increase the anticoagulant effect of warfarin.

sulfasalazine [sul fa **sal** a zeen]
(Azulfidine, Salazopyrin✽, SAS-500✽)

Indications
See mesalamine.

Pharmacokinetics/Dosing
Sulfasalazine is poorly absorbed orally (20%); the remaining dose is converted by bacteria in the colon to sulfapyridine and mesalamine. Most of the sulfapyridine (60% to 80%), and approximately 25% of the mesalamine, is absorbed in the colon. The half-life of sulfapyridine is 6 to 14 hours; for mesalamine it is 0.6 to 1.4 hours. The peak serum level is between 1.5 and 6 hours for sulfasalazine (oral suspension and tablets) and between 9 and 24 hours for sulfapyridine. Enteric-coated tablets take longer to peak—between 3 and 12 hours for sulfasalazine and between 12 and 24 hours for sulfapyridine. Excretion is primarily by the kidneys for sulfasalazine and sulfapyridine, whereas it is mainly fecal for mesalamine. The adult dosage of sulfasalazine is 1 g every 6 to 8 hours initially, which is reduced to 500 mg every 6 hours for maintenance dosing.

Adverse Effects
For sulfasalazine, the adverse effects include GI effects similar to mesalamine, continuous headache, allergic reaction, photosensitivity; infrequent or rare effects include blood dyscrasias, hepatitis, Stevens-Johnson syndrome, systemic lupus erythematosus–like syndrome, and exacerbation of colitis.

Drug Interactions
Similar to mesalamine. Additionally, sulfasalazine use may result in elevated phenytoin and methotrexate levels, and may increase the effect of oral hypoglycemics and warfarin.

infliximab [in **flix** i mab]
(Remicade)
Infliximab is a monoclonal antibody that binds and neutralizes the TNF-a, which is a primary cytokine that is believed to activate the inflammatory response in clients with Crohn's disease.

Indications
Infliximab therapy is reserved for clients with moderate to severe Crohn's disease who do not adequately respond to other therapy. It is also indicated for the treatment of moderate to severe rheumatoid arthritis not responsive to other modalities.

Pharmacokinetics/Dosing
Infliximab is administered by IV infusion and has a prolonged half-life; a single infusion of 5 mg/kg has a half-life of approximately 9.5 days. The adult dosage of infliximab for moderate to severe cases of Crohn's disease is 5 mg/kg by a single dose (IV infusion). Fistulizing Crohn's disease may require additional doses 2 and 6 weeks after the first dose, then every 8 weeks if needed.

Adverse Effects
The most serious adverse effects of infliximab are immunosuppression, increased malignancy risk and liver injury. Immunosuppression with the risk for serious or life-threatening infection (particularly tuberculosis, fungal infections, and other opportunistic infections) is a real concern with this and other immunomodulator therapies. Tuberculosis should be ruled out before initiating therapy. Infliximab use is also associated with increased risk for lymphomas and other malignancies (Everitt, 2004).

Serious hepatic injury, including liver failure, jaundice, cholestasis, and hepatitis, has been reported for clients receiving infliximab therapy (Everitt, 2004). A few cases resulted in death or required liver transplant. Infusion-related reactions are common (e.g., dyspnea, flushing, headache, rash), occurring during or 1 to 2 hours after the infusion. Other undesirable effects include nausea, stomach pain, weakness, fever, vomiting, pharyngitis and, infrequently, hypotension, hypertension, tachycardia, acne, alopecia, and other skin disorders, constipation, gas, intestinal obstruction, and urinary tract infection (*Drug Facts and Comparisons*, 2005).

tegaserod [teg a **ser** od/the **gah** she rod]*
(Zelnorm)
Tegaserod is a 5-HT₄ (serotonin 4) antagonist in the colon. It affects colonic motility predominantly. Efficacy in the treatment of irritable bowel syndrome have identified benefit limited to women in which symptoms were primarily constipation. It is also used for the treatment of severe chronic constipation with limited effect (Kamm et al., 2005). It has no role in the treatment of Crohn's disease or ulcerative colitis.

Indications
Tegaserod is indicated for short-term management of constipation-predominant irritable bowel syndrome (IBS) in women. It is also indicated for chronic idiopathic constipation in adults under 65 years of age for whom other interventions are ineffective.

Pharmacokinetics/Dosing
Tegaserod is poorly absorbed orally and is metabolized predominantly by gut enzymes. It is dosed at 6 mg twice daily before meals for 4 weeks, then if adequate response is achieved, an additional 4 to 6 weeks of therapy may be considered. It should not be used in clients with severe renal or hepatic dysfunction. For chronic constipation, the dose is 6 mg twice daily for up to 12 weeks.

Adverse Effects
The FDA recommended revised labeling secondary to adverse effects of tegaserod (FDA Talk Paper, 2004). This was prompted because of reports of diarrhea with hypovolemia and dehydration requiring hospitalization associated with tegaserod therapy. Intestinal ischemia with rectal bleeding or worsening abdominal pain or cramping and potential for gangrene has also been reported. Clients should inform their health care provider of any significant change in upper or lower GI symptoms while on this agent. Other adverse effects include headache, nausea, flatulence, back pain. On rare occasions, its use has been associated with angina, altered liver function tests, and syncope.

✺ **P.F. is evaluated by the gastroenterologist. She continues with sulfasalazine, and is started on prednisone 60 mg orally once daily. She also receives one dose of infliximab at 5 mg/kg intravenously in the clinic with two additional doses scheduled at 2 and 6 weeks.**

✺ **What is the nursing management of the drugs used in inflammatory bowel disease?**

Sulfasalazine is widely used for treating clients with mild to moderately symptomatic Crohn's disease. In general, clients with mild active disease are started on a 5-ASA agent (e.g., sulfasalazine, olsalazine, mesalamine, balsalazide), although more severe disease is often treated with corticosteroids. See Chapter 48 for a discussion of the role of corticosteroids in inflammation. Once P.F. is in remission, the prednisone will be tapered by 5% to 10% per week, taking several weeks or months to complete. Infliximab has been prescribed for inducing and maintaining a remission of P.F.'s Crohn's disease because she stopped responding to her usual therapy.

---

*Tegaserod was voluntarily removed from the market in March 2007.

Assessment Determine if P.F. has a sensitivity to mesalamine, olsalazine, infliximab, or salicylates and her response to prior sulfasalazine therapy. Be aware that with sulfasal-azine, that there are related drugs that have cross-sensitivity, including sulfonamides, furosemide, thiazide diuretics, sulfonylureas, and carbonic anhydrase inhibitors. Concern for renal function impairment exists with all of these agents, but the use of sulfasalazine is contraindicated in clients with intestinal or urinary obstruction. Some clients with severe allergies or asthma risk developing an increasing hypersensitivity to sulfasalazine. Because of the risk for immunosuppression and infection is so significant, ensure that P.F. does not have an active infection before beginning therapy. Clients with blood dyscrasias, a deficiency of glucose-6-phosphate dehydrogenase (G6PD), and porphyria may develop more symptomatic conditions. Sulfonamides are metabolized in the liver and may cause hepatitis in clients with a preexisting hepatic impairment.

Review P.F.'s concurrent medication regimen for the risk of significant drug interactions. Of the 5-ASA drugs, sulfasalazine has the most drug-drug interactions. In addition to those listed with olsalazine, sulfasalazine interacts with anticoagulants, but also with antiepileptic drugs (hydantoins), oral antidiabetic sulfonylureas, and methotrexate (Folex). Sulfasalazine may displace these drugs from protein-binding sites and/or inhibit their metabolism, resulting in a prolonged effect or toxicity. Dosage adjustments may be necessary during and after sulfonamide therapy. Sulfasalazine also increases the potential for hemolysis with methyldopa (Aldomet), nitrofurantoin (Furadantin), and quinidine (Quinaglute). This requires careful monitoring of CBCs. With other hepatotoxic drugs, such as alcohol, angiotensin-converting enzyme (ACE) inhibitors, NSAIDs, isoniazid, valproic acid (Depakene), zidovudine (Retrovir), and others, sulfasalazine increases the risk of hepatotoxicity, especially in clients with a history of liver disease. Monitor P.F.'s hepatic function studies carefully.

A baseline assessment of P.F.'s health status should include weight, dietary patterns, bowel status, CBCs, blood urea nitrogen (BUN), serum creatinine, UA, liver function studies, and proctoscopy and sigmoidoscopy determinations.

Nursing Diagnosis While P.F. is undergoing 5-ASA therapy, she is at risk for the following nursing diagnoses/collaborative problems: impaired comfort (headache, anorexia, heartburn, abdominal cramping, flatulence, nausea or vomiting); fatigue; diarrhea; and the potential complications of hypersensitivity reaction (fever, skin rash, itching, aching joints), hepatitis (jaundice, right upper abdominal quadrant tenderness), blood dyscrasias (agranulocytosis, neutropenia, aplastic anemia, thrombocytopenia), exacerbation of the client's ulcerative colitis, Stevens-Johnson syndrome (aching of joints, peeling of skin, fatigue), or systemic lupus erythematosus–like syndrome (skin rash or blisters, general feeling of illness).

Planning While receiving drug therapy for her Crohn's disease, P.F. will:
- Remain free of diarrhea and abdominal cramping, and fever, and will have an improved sense of well-being, gain weight, and maintain a good nutritional status without experiencing adverse effects of her drug therapy.
- Effectively manage the therapeutic regimen, including medication compliance, supportive measures to reduce symptoms of Crohn's disease, and reporting adverse drug effects appropriately.
- Collaborate with health care providers for monitoring and follow-up care.

Implementation

Monitoring Check the results of CBCs and renal and hepatic function studies that are performed periodically. P.F.'s progress is monitored by proctoscopy and sigmoidoscopy. Her comfort, weight, diet, bowel status, and general health are also to be monitored. Because the risk for immunosuppression and infection with infliximab is so significant, monitor P.F. for body temperature, WBC, and signs and symptoms of infection (e.g., night sweats, fever, fatigue, involuntary weight loss, headache, cough, presence of sputum). Serum sulfapyridine levels may be useful, because concentrations greater than 50 mcg/mL seem to result in a higher incidence of adverse effects in clients receiving sulfasalazine.

Intervention Sulfasalazine (and olsalazine) are administered with food. P.F. may be placed on maintenance doses when improvement is demonstrated by endoscopy. Mesalamine should be administered before meals and at bedtime with a full glass of water. In addition to sulfasalazine, P.F. will be coming to the clinical setting for her IV infusion of infliximab, non-5-ASA drug that has been added to her regimen reduce her symptoms in this acute attack. The infusion is given over 2 hours with additional doses in 2 and 6 weeks. Stop the infusion if severe reactions occur (chest pain, dyspnea, hypertension, hypotension, syncope)

Education Advise a well-balanced diet and a fluid intake of at least 1500 mL daily to minimize the risk of tissue dehydration and urinary tract infection associated with low urinary output. Instruct P.F. to avoid trauma (e.g., breaks in the skin) and to seek medical treatment for wounds that do not heal quickly. Encourage meticulous oral hygiene, including the cautious use of toothbrushes, dental floss, and toothpicks, as well as regular dental care to minimize gingival inflammation and for early detection of altered oral mucous membranes. The ingestion of alcohol and aspirin should be avoided to minimize the risk of GI bleeding. Instruct P.F. to report any signs or symptoms of infection. Advise her to consult her prescriber before taking any OTC or complementary/alternative medications or receiving any immunizations. Reinforce the importance of keeping appointments with the health care team for monitoring and follow-up care. See Chapter 63 for further details of caring for the immunosuppressed client.

Stress the importance of adherence to the full course of therapy, consulting with the prescriber on a regular basis to check progress, and not switching brands of medications without checking with the prescriber. Sulfasalazine (and olsalazine) are taken in evenly divided doses throughout the day. If P.F. were taking mesalamine, she would swallow mesalamine tablets whole and not to chew, crush, or break them; the empty tablet may be seen in the stool after the medication has been absorbed.

With sulfasalazine, maintain a fluid intake of 1200 to 1500 mL/daily. Alert P.F. about sun precautions to protect against photosensitivity effects: avoid sun exposure between 10 AM and 3 PM, apply sunscreen lotion with at least a 15 SPF to sun-exposed body parts, and wear sunglasses, long sleeves, pants, and a hat when outside during the day. She may experience an orange-yellow discoloration of the urine and skin from the sulfasalazine. This coloration is clinically insignificant but may be alarming to the unsuspecting client.

Evaluation The expected outcome for inflammatory bowel disease drug therapy is that P.F.'s underlying condition will improve as evidenced by an absence of abdominal cramping, fever, and diarrhea, a weight gain to a normal weight for height, and an improved sense of well-being. She will not experience any adverse effects of the immunosuppressing effects of infliximab (e.g., signs and symptoms of infection, bleeding). P.F. will effectively manage the drug regimen, including compliance with medication, notifying the prescriber of reportable adverse effects, and maintaining scheduled visits with health care providers for monitoring and follow-up care.

✱ **G.N. is a 78-year-old male who was recently admitted to Shady Pines Nursing Home. His last bowel movement was 3 days ago and was described as hard. He has vague abdominal complaints and asks the nurse for something to move his bowels.**

✱ **How is constipation manifested?**
Bowel elimination is often a major concern of clients, particularly constipation in the older client. Clients admitted to various health care agencies for short stays in acute care institutions or for extended stays in long-term care facilities often experience constipation or diarrhea.

Constipation is defined as difficult fecal evacuation as a result of degree of hardness and perhaps infrequent movements. Regular bowel movements may range from three per day to three per week. A subjective aspect of constipation is the individual's feeling or attitude of dissatisfaction regarding bowel function, pattern of elimination, or perceived constipation. Chronic constipation is sometimes caused by organic disease (e.g., tumors); bowel obstruction; megacolon; metabolic abnormalities (e.g., diabetes mellitus or hypercalcemia); rectal disorders; diseases of the liver, gall-

bladder, or muscles; neurologic abnormalities (e.g., multiple sclerosis and Parkinson's disease); and pregnancy. Persons who suffer from disorders of the GI tract often complain of constipation. On the other hand, many persons complain of constipation when no organic disease or lesion can be found.

When it is not a result of organic factors, constipation is generally attributable to faulty eating habits, a failure to respond to defecation impulses, insufficient fluid intake or exercise, or being hospitalized (off the usual routine, and in a strange place). For example, a diet that provides inadequate fiber will contribute to the development of constipation. The GI tract should function normally if fluids and fiber are supplied in sufficient quantities to keep the stool formed but soft.

Another common cause of constipation is a failure to respond to the normal defecation impulses and insufficient time to permit the bowel to produce an evacuation. Sedentary habits and insufficient exercise may be factors. Clients with impaired physical mobility may be constipated because of inactivity or an unnatural position for defecation, such as using a bedpan.

Another causative factor is the effect of drugs. The use of antacids, diuretics, morphine, tricyclic antidepressants, codeine, aluminum hydroxide, and anticholinergics often leads to constipation as an adverse effect. Constipation can also be a symptom of both functional and organic disorders, such as febrile states, psychosomatic disorders, anemias, and tension headaches. A less common cause of constipation may be atonic and hypotonic conditions of the musculature of the colon. These conditions may result from habitual use of cathartics—substances that produce a liquid or fluid evacuation of the bowel.

✱ **What treatments are available for the prevention and treatment of constipation?**
Laxatives are drugs given to induce defecation. Laxatives may be classified according to their source, site of action, degree of action, or mechanism of action (see Chapter 11). Box 40-5 summarizes the types of laxatives. Most of these agents are available as OTC drugs and discussed more fully in Chapter 11. The prescription laxatives lactulose and polyethylene glycol (PEG)/electrolytes are discussed here.

lactulose [lak tyoo lose]
(Chronulac, Duphalac✥, Laxilose✥)
Lactulose is composed of galactose, fructose, and other sugars; in the GI tract, the normal colonic bacteria (*Lactobacillus, Bacteroides, Escherichia coli,* and *Streptococcus faecalis*) metabolize lactulose syrup to organic acids, primarily lactic, acetic, and formic acids. These acids produce an osmotic effect, with an increase in fluid accumulation, distention, peristalsis, and bowel movements within 24 to 72 hours. Lactulose is also used to decrease serum levels of ammonia in persons with hepatic encephalopathy secondary to chronic liver disease.

Indications
Lactulose is indicated for the treatment of chronic constipation. In higher doses, it is used to prevent or treat portal-systemic en-

Saline laxatives retain and increase water content of feces by virtue of osmotic qualities

Stimulant laxatives increase peristalsis in the colon by irritating intramural sensory nerve plexuses in the mucosa

Bulk laxatives absorb water and increase the volume, bulk, and moisture of nonabsorbable intestinal contents, thereby distending the bowel and initiating reflex bowel activity

Intestinal lubricants mechanically lubricate feces to facilitate defecation

Emollients, or fecal softening agents act as dispersing wetting agents, facilitating mixture of water and fatty substances within the fecal mass; when a homogeneous mixture is produced, the feces become soft

Hyperosmotic agents increase the intraluminal osmotic pressure in the bowel; because they are not absorbed, they draw water into the intestine, resulting in an increased volume that stimulates peristalsis

cephalopathy by trapping ammonia in the colon, although its efficacy for this indication has been questioned (Als-Nielsen et al., 2004).

Pharmacokinetics/Dosing
The absorption of lactulose is minimal after oral administration, and it is excreted by the kidneys. For constipation, the adult dosage is 1 to 2 tablespoons (15 to 30 mL) daily after breakfast, which is increased in 5 and 10 mL increments to 60 mL daily after breakfast. Oral doses as high as 30 to 45 mL three to four times daily have been used for the management of hepatic encephalopathy, with doses titrated until the client has 2 to 3 soft stools per day. Alternatively, a 300-mL retention enema may be considered every 4 to 6 hours.

Adverse Effects
Dose-related flatulence and intestinal cramps, gas, and belching are reported. Excessive doses may produce some diarrhea (hypokalemic) and nausea (caused by the sweet taste).

Drug Interactions
The effectiveness of lactulose may be reduced if it is used concomitantly with an antibiotic that destroys the normal colonic bacteria. A nonabsorbed antibiotic such as neomycin destroys enough luminal colonic bacteria to interfere with lactulose. Most systemic, highly absorbable antibiotics do not affect the colonic bacteria in the lumen.

polyethylene glycol (PEG) and electrolytes (pol ee **eth** ih leen **gleye** kohl and ee **lek** troe lites)
(GoLYTELY, Klean-Prep✤, Peglyte✤, Pro-Lax✤)
A mixture of polyethylene glycol (nonabsorbable osmotic substance) with sodium salts (sulfate, bicarbonate, and chloride) and potassium chloride is isotonic with body fluids and is used when bowel cleansing is required before diagnostic examinations. Because it is isotonic, fluids and electrolytes are neither absorbed nor secreted in the GI tract; thus it can be used in clients who are dehydrated or have renal impairment or cardiac disease. The drug acts as an osmotic agent.

Indications
GoLYTELY is used for bowel cleansing before colonoscopy and before the administration of a barium enema for radiologic examination.

Pharmacokinetics/Dosing
Minimal systemic absorption of polyethylene glycol occurs. Dosage is based on indication, with lower amounts used for constipation management and higher doses utilized for bowel evacuation. With higher

dosing, the onset of effect is observed within 1 to 2 hours. Its use in children, although not FDA indicated, appears safe (Pashankar, Loening-Baucke, & Bishop, 2003).

Adverse Effects
There is a low incidence of nausea, vomiting, bloating, cramps, and abdominal fullness.

✪ **G.N. indicates he has not had a bowel movement in 5 days and is evaluated by the nurse for constipation. Based on protocol orders, the nurse administers 30 mL of milk of magnesia and starts docusate (Colace) 100 mg orally twice daily.**

✪ **What are the nursing implications of laxative use with G.N.?**

Assessment Determine G.N.'s bowel status by careful assessment. The occurrence of the last bowel movement, the quality of bowel sounds, defecation habits, dietary patterns, fluid intake, level of daily activity, and the use of laxatives are important components of the nurse's assessment. Ensure that the client does not have intestinal obstruction, paralytic ileus, perforated bowel, or toxic bowel; laxatives are contraindicated for these conditions. Review G.N.'s medical history for causative factors. Before initiating laxative therapy, assess his current medication regimen for drugs that might contribute to the constipation or produce significant drug interactions when laxatives are administered. These include the following:

- High-fiber and bulk-forming laxatives may decrease the effects of tetracycline, anticoagulants, digoxin, or salicylates by binding with the drug or delaying its absorption. Separate the administration of these substances by at least 2 hours.
- Magnesium salts may interact with quinolone antibacterials (e.g., ciprofloxacin) or tetracyclines, forming a nonabsorbable complex when administered within 1 to 2 hours of the antimicrobial. The diarrhea produced by these drugs may interfere with absorption as well.
- Stimulant/contact/irritant laxatives such as bisacodyl oral tablets, that contain an enteric coating, will be prematurely released in the stomach when administered with antacids or proton pump inhibitors, producing severe cramping in the stomach and duodenum.
- Lubricant/emollient laxatives such as mineral oil may interfere with the absorption of antibiotics, anticoagulants, hormonal contraceptives, digoxin, and fat-soluble vitamins when concurrently administered; this reduces their therapeutic effectiveness. Mineral oil is not recommended for children under the age of 6 years or for bedridden older adults because they are more at risk for aspirating the droplets coating the pharynx; this may result in lipid pneumonia. Do not give mineral oil routinely to pregnant women; it decreases vitamin K availability to the fetus, resulting in hypoprothrombinemia and hemorrhagic disease. The chronic use of mineral oil in any client may decrease vitamin K absorption and lead to an increased poten-

tial for bleeding. Additionally, clients may experience anal leakage of the oil with long-term use.

- Stool softener/surfactant or wetting agent laxatives may increase the absorption of mineral oil if administered together. Granuloma formation or tumor-like deposits in tissues are also reported.
- The use of lactulose during pregnancy has not been evaluated. Lactulose use in clients with diabetes may cause elevations in blood glucose levels; therefore another type of laxative without galactose or lactose may be preferred. Older adults and debilitated clients receiving lactulose for 6 months or more should undergo periodic evaluations of serum electrolytes (potassium, chloride, and carbon dioxide). Lactulose contains galactose (less than 2.2 g/15 mL) and is therefore contraindicated in low-galactose diets.
- Other oral medications given within an hour of administration of a PEG-electrolyte solution may be expelled from the GI tract without absorption.

Do not use laxatives when an emergency surgical condition in the abdomen might be suspected, such as appendicitis, bowel obstruction, hemorrhage, or intussusception.

Nursing Diagnosis When G.N. takes a laxative, he is at risk for the following nursing diagnoses/collaborative problems: constipation related to ineffectiveness of the laxative or to intestinal obstruction (bulk laxatives); diarrhea related to the misuse of laxatives; impaired comfort (abdominal cramping, flatulence, nausea); and the potential complications of allergic reaction or electrolyte imbalance (weakness, muscle cramping, confusion).

Planning G.N. will report bowel movements at least every 2 to 3 days without experiencing any side effects of laxative therapy. He will effectively manage the laxative regimen, including using the laxative appropriately, notifying his primary care provider if his constipation persists, and implementing supportive measures to prevent constipation.

Implementation
Monitoring Have G.N. report the frequency, consistency, and color of his stools and his comfort during defecation.

Intervention Encourage nonpharmacologic interventions to relieve constipation. Depending on G.N.'s health assessment, encourage measures to relieve constipation including adding fresh fruits, vegetables, and whole grains to increase fiber in the diet; allowing for a calm, adequate, and routine time for defecation; ensuring a daily fluid intake of eight to ten glasses of water for adequate hydration; and increasing the amount of daily exercise. When laxatives are indicated, use the mildest laxative necessary. See Chapter 11 for further discussion of laxatives.

Lactulose Mix lactulose in water, juice, or milk to make it more palatable. Results may occur 24 to 36 hours after administration. The solution may darken on exposure to high temperature, but this does not change its therapeutic effect. Freezing does not alter the therapeutic effect.

Polyethylene Glycol and Electrolytes (GoLYTELY) GoLYTELY is given orally, 4 L at a rate of 240 mL every 10 minutes (rapidly swallowed). Fasting 3 to 4 hours before use is necessary. In general, a midmorning examination permits 3 hours for consumption followed by a 1-hour period for bowel movement. Less stool is retained after its use, but the water or electrolyte balance does not change. Only clear liquids are permitted after its administration and before examination. After reconstitution of the powder, refrigerating the solution improves palatability. The reconstituted solution must be used within 48 hours.

Bulk-Forming Laxative (psyllium and others) Because there is a possibility of impaction or obstruction if fluid intake is not substantial, avoid the use of bulk-forming laxatives in clients with stenosis, adhesions, or dysphagia. Administer these laxatives with a full glass of liquid (240 mL) plus additional liquid every day to prevent intestinal impaction. Some preparations contain sugar and sodium and may not be used with clients for whom these substances are restricted.

Bisacodyl (Dulcolax) Because bisacodyl tablets are enteric coated, instruct clients not to chew them or ingest them when they are chipped. Instruct clients to swallow bisacodyl tablets whole no sooner than 1 hour before or after the ingestion of dairy products or antacids. (Milk or antacids can break down the enteric coating, which can lead to gastric irritation, cramping, and vomiting.) See Chapter 11 for additional information on bisacodyl.

Calcium Polycarbophil (Mitrolan) Instruct the client with constipation to follow each dose of calcium polycarbophil with at least 8 ounces of water or other liquid. If this drug is being used to treat diarrhea, administer less fluid with each dose. Instruct the client to chew polycarbophil tablets thoroughly before swallowing.

Castor Oil Castor oil is rarely used today due to its adverse effect profile. It may be unpleasant and nauseating. This effect may be overcome by disguising the taste of the oil. To do this, emulsify it in a blender or mix it with cold orange juice or other fruit juices, and have the client drink the mixture immediately. Neoloid is a preemulsified preparation. Castor oil is contraindicated in pregnancy. Its administration often results in engorgement of the pelvic area, which may reflexively stimulate the gravid uterus.

Education Based on the original assessment of G.N.'s health behaviors, review the preventative techniques discussed in the "Intervention" section.

Encourage G.N. to avoid the habitual use of laxatives. Inform him that misuse or overuse may result in a dependence on laxatives for routine bowel function. Instruct him not to take laxatives unnecessarily. For example, some individuals believe that laxatives are to be taken to "clean out" the system, as a tonic, in the case of colds, or at the change of seasons.

Caution G.N. to forbid children free access to laxative preparations that are in a candy-like form, chewing gum, or mint. Children are likely to regard these substances as ordinary candy or gum and take an overdose of the drug. Deaths have been reported from such accidents.

Evaluation The expected outcome of laxative therapy is that G.N. reports bowel movements of soft stool without straining or pain. If the drug was administered for bowel cleansing before a colonoscopy or barium enema, there will be an absence of stool in the colon. G.N. will effectively manage the drug regimen, including compliance with medication, notifying the prescriber of reportable adverse effects, and maintaining scheduled visits with health care providers for monitoring and follow-up care.

✳ **B.D. is a 32-year-old school teacher who complains of passing three unformed stools without blood and experiencing abdominal cramping over the past 8 hours. She calls her health care provider for advice.**

✳ **What are the causes and complications of diarrhea?**
Clients with diarrhea present with frequent watery stools. Diarrhea can be classified as acute or chronic. Acute diarrhea is often subclassified as infectious or noninfectious.

Acute diarrhea is typically of sudden onset. Infectious etiologies include viral (accounting for almost one third of infectious diarrhea cases) or bacterial. Bacterial pathogens include strains of *Campylobacter jejuni, Salmonella, Shigella,* or *E. coli* and are often acquired from food. *Clostridium difficile* toxin diarrhea may be noted in clients with recent broad spectrum antimicrobial use and requires aggressive and immediate treatment with metronidazole (Flagyl) or vancomycin. Travelers may be predisposed to other pathogens, including the *Giardia,* or *Cryptosporidium.* Individuals with immunocompromised status are also at risk for infectious diarrhea from multiple pathogens.

Non-infectious acute diarrhea may be related to diet, stress, drugs, or other etiologies. Drug-induced diarrhea may be noted with a great number of agents, including antimicrobials that change gut flora, β-adrenergic blockers, cholinergic agonists (e.g., treatments for Alzheimer's disease), misoprostol (Cytotec), colchicine, cancer chemotherapy, magnesium-containing products, and laxatives.

Chronic diarrhea may be related to a number of chronic conditions, including ulcerative colitis, Crohn's disease and irritable bowel syndrome as noted above.

Complications of diarrhea are primarily related to hydration and electrolyte status. Elevated temperatures, profuse or bloody diarrhea, or changes in hemodynamics requires immediate medical attention. This is particularly true for infants, young children, and older adults.

✳ **How is diarrhea treated?**
The first step in the treatment of diarrhea is to assess the client both in terms of complications (e.g., fluid and elec-

trolyte status) and for possible etiologies based on presenting symptoms. Removal of the cause, or treating infectious diarrhea with the appropriate antimicrobial therapy, is an essential management strategy. Rehydration is a critical component of diarrhea management, especially in infants, children, and older adults. Oral rehydration is usually preferred over IV rehydration for noncritical cases when tolerated (Fonseca, Holdgate, & Craig, 2004). Once the cause is addressed and fluid and electrolyte status is maintained, symptomatic treatment of diarrhea with antidiarrheals is often utilized.

A number of agents to treat diarrhea are available over the counter and include loperamide (Imodium) and bismuth subsalicylate (Pepto-Bismol), which are discussed in Chapter 11. Prescription antidiarrheals include opioids and opioid/ antimuscarinic combinations. Cholestyramine (Questran) is sometimes also used to bind toxins that cause diarrhea in the GI tract. Cholestyramine is discussed in Chapter 31.

The opioids (codeine and paregoric—DEA Class III) act by virtue of their constipating and sedative action. They lower the propulsive motility of the bowel, reduce pain, and relieve tenesmus (rectal spasms). The delay in transit time of food permits intestinal contact time with the absorptive surface of the bowel; this increases the reabsorption of water and electrolytes and reduces stool frequency and net volume.

The anticholinergics and opium derivatives decrease bowel motility. They should not be used when the cause of diarrhea is an invading organism (e.g., toxigenic bacteria or pseudomembranous enterocolitis), because these drugs decrease intestinal motility and subsequently lower the excretion of the organisms and their toxins, resulting in epithelial penetration and multiplication of the organisms.

Codeine and paregoric cause depression and sedation. Because of the additive effects, this factor must be considered if the client is taking other CNS depressant drugs. The opioids are short acting; frequent administration (4- to 6-hour intervals) is needed to control the function of smooth muscle in the GI tract. Chapter 14 discusses opioids in greater detail.

Opioids

opium tincture, deodorized (DTO)
Tincture of opium, a hydroalcoholic (19% alcohol) solution, contains 10% opium.
Indications
DTO is indicated for the treatment of diarrhea or relief of pain.
Pharmacokinetics/Dosing
Absorption is variable and duration of action is 4 to 5 hours. The average dosage is 0.6 mL four times daily. This substance is a class II prescription under the Controlled Substances Act.
Adverse Effects
Refer to Chapter 14 for the adverse effects of opioids.

paregoric (camphorated tincture of opium)
[par e **gor** ik]
Paregoric (camphorated opium tincture, although camphor is no longer required in this formulation in the United States) requires a prescription. It is a class III drug that is equivalent to 2 mg of morphine/5 mL. It is important that the nurse not confuse deodorized opium tincture (10 mg morphine equivalent/1 mL), and camphorated opium tincture (0.4 mg morphine equivalent/1 mL); deodorized opium tincture has 25 times more morphine equivalent than

camphorated opium tincture. Addiction liability has been reported with these preparations. Paregoric becomes a class V product when combined with another drug if the combination contains no more than 100 mg of opium or 25 mL of paregoric/100 mL of the mixture.

Indications
Paregoric is indicated for the treatment of diarrhea and for pain relief. It is also used as part of neonatal opioid withdrawal protocols.

Pharmacokinetics/Dosing
The pharmacokinetics are similar to deodorized opium tincture. The adult antidiarrheal dosage is 5 to 10 mL one to four times daily. The pediatric dosage is 0.25 to 0.5 mL/kg one to four times daily.

Adverse Effects
See Chapter 14.

Synthetic Opioids/Antimuscarinics

diphenoxylate and atropine [dye fen ox i late/a troe peen]
(Lomotil)
Diphenoxylate, a controlled substance in the United States (Class V), inhibits intestinal propulsive motility by acting directly on intestinal smooth muscles to decrease transit time. It is typically combined with the antimuscarinic, atropine.

Indications
Diphenoxylate/atropine is indicated as an adjunct to fluid and electrolyte replacement for the treatment of acute and chronic diarrhea in adults. It is not recommended for use in children.

Pharmacokinetics/Dosing
The onset of action for diphenoxylate is between 45 to 60 minutes; the half-life is 2.5 hours, and the duration of action is 3 to 4 hours. It is metabolized in the liver and excreted primarily by the kidneys. For adults and children 12 years of age and older, the dosage is 1 to 2 tablets PO three or four times daily.

Adverse Effects
The adverse effects of diphenoxylate/atropine include drowsiness, dizziness, confusion, tachycardia, dry mouth, hyperthermia, abdominal distress, rash, urinary retention, and agitation.

difenoxin/atropine [dye fen ox in/a troe peen]
(Motofen)
A second product in the synthetic opioid category is difenoxin with atropine (Motofen). Difenoxin is the active metabolite derived from diphenoxylate; therefore it is effective at one-fifth the dose of diphenoxylate.

Indications
It is indicated for the treatment of acute nonspecific diarrhea and acute exacerbations of chronic diarrhea.

Pharmacokinetics/Dosing
Peak serum levels of difenoxin are reached between 40 and 60 minutes. It is metabolized in the liver and excreted primarily by the kidneys and in the feces. The adult oral dosage is 2 tablets initially, then 1 tablet after each loose stool or 1 tablet every 3 to 4 hours as needed. The maximum daily dose is 8 tablets.

Adverse Effects
See diphenoxylate/atropine sulfate.

✱ **Although B.D. has had abdominal cramping and three unformed stools over the past 8 hours, there has been no blood or pus in the stools and she has had no nausea or vomiting or fever.**

✱ **What are the nursing issues involved in the use of antidiarrheals for B.D.?**

This section focuses on prescription drugs that have a direct pharmacologic effect on the GI tract. Although many antidiarrheal preparations may be purchased as over the counter (as discussed in Chapter 11), the nurse may also administer these same preparations within a health agency setting.

Assessment The objectives of treatment of B.D. is to replenish fluid and electrolyte loss; ascertain, if possible, the cause or causes of diarrhea; and treat the underlying cause or causes. Reducing the frequency of evacuation may be contraindicated if the diarrhea is infectious and self-limiting. It is important to determine the cause of the diarrhea through careful evaluation of client data. Ask questions about the following to aid in discovering the cause or causes of the diarrhea:
- Age of the client
- Occupation
- Duration of diarrhea (precipitating factors tantamount to onset)
- Stool description (frequency of evacuation, rectal bleeding or black stool appearance, foul odor, light color, or greasy consistency)
- Medication profile (prescribed and self-administered OTC and complementary/alternative drugs)
- Presence or absence of anorexia, weight reduction (involuntary), fever, abdominal tenderness, dehydration
- Ingestion of foods, toxic substances, milk, alcohol
- Travel outside the United States or Canada or camping in primitive areas
- Symptom description (location)
- Relief obtained, if any, and treatment modality
- Chronic diseases, the presence of acute or concurrent illness, emotional or behavioral problems

Nursing Diagnosis If B.D. is placed on antidiarrheal therapy, she is at risk for the following nursing diagnoses/collaborative problems: diarrhea related to the underlying cause and ineffectiveness of the antidiarrheal agent; impaired comfort related to abdominal cramping; and the potential complications of hypovolemia and electrolyte imbalances.

Planning During antidiarrheal therapy, B.D. will:
- Remain free of fluid and electrolyte disturbances related to changes in bowel patterns.
- Maintain normal bowel pattern without experiencing any adverse effects of the drug therapy.
- Effectively manage the drug regimen, including compliance with medication, notifying the prescriber of reportable adverse effects, and maintaining scheduled visits with health care providers for monitoring and follow-up care.

Implementation
Monitoring Fluid and electrolyte loss may cause tachycardia, postural hypotension, elevated hematocrit or blood urea nitrogen, and poor skin turgor. The stool specimen

may reveal occult blood (GI bleeding), fecal leukocytes, parasites, or fat.

Intervention Nonspecific measures are directed at treating stool frequency, which burdens daily lifestyle; alleviating abdominal cramps; preventing dehydration and metabolic acidosis from fluid and electrolyte loss; and minimizing weight loss and nutritional deficits resulting from malabsorption. Specific treatment is directed at the cause or condition creating the diarrhea, as demonstrated by the Nursing Care Plan below.

Hospitalization is needed for dehydration that would compromise a client with heart failure or chronic renal disease; these conditions complicate fluid replacement efforts. If a child or infant is unable to consume oral replacement fluids, hospitalization is needed to replace fluids and maintain urine flow. Bed rest alone may reduce stool frequency. Children, infants, older adults with a poor medical history, clients with chronic illness (heart disease, asthma), and pregnant women are at risk from acute or chronic diarrhea.

Maintaining fluid and electrolyte balance is the most important goal of supportive therapy in acute diarrhea. If left untreated, a loss of anions (bicarbonate, organic anions as short-chain fatty acids) will create a gain of hydrogen ions, resulting in metabolic acidosis. This gain will be exacerbated by the (often) concomitant ketoacidosis of starvation and the acidosis of prerenal azotemia. As volume increases in diarrhea, a rise in sodium and chloride develops with a decrease in potassium concentration. The decreased contact time of the luminal contents with the mucosal surface decreases the passive secretion of potassium. The electrolyte composition of stool water is then close to that of plasma. The electrolyte replacement of sodium, potassium, chloride, and bicarbonate is the basis of therapy.

It is recommended that clear liquids (noncarbonated soft drinks, fruit juice, diluted and flavored gelatin, and apple juice) and a bland diet be continued for 1 to 2 days. According to the cause of the diarrhea, several different medications can be given along with bed rest. Such medications include activated charcoal, absorbents, anticholinergic drugs, and many other drug products.

OTC antidiarrheals may contain the following ingredients: limited amounts of opiates; adsorbents such as bismuth salts, aluminum salts, attapulgite, kaolin, pectin, activated charcoal, and belladonna alkaloids (hyoscyamine, hyoscine, scopolamine, atropine); and calcium salts. Inactive ingredients vary, but the nurse should be aware of the variation in alcohol content (1.5% to 18%).

Antidiarrheal products have a warning stating that they are not to be used for longer than 2 days, not to be used if a fever is present, and not to be used in infants or children under 3 years of age. The prescriber may modify these instructions.

Intractable diarrhea of infancy is traditionally treated with clear liquids and a gradual reintroduction of milk or formula, with the addition of oral elemental diets or total parenteral nutrition. The infant syndrome is described as loose stools that result in dehydration and a failure to

NURSING CARE PLAN SELECTED NURSING DIAGNOSES: ANTIDIARRHEAL MEDICATION ADMINISTRATION

Nursing Diagnosis	Outcome Criteria	Nursing Interventions
Diarrhea	• Decrease in number of stools to less than three per day • Formed stools	• Record frequency, number, consistency of stools • Encourage bland diet and liquids • Administer antidiarrheal agents as prescribed
Potential complications: hypovolemia and electrolyte imbalance	The client will: • Maintain electrolytes within normal limits • Maintain normal fluid balance • Experience fewer episodes of diarrhea • Maintain normal body weight	• Monitor client's intake and output ratios • Monitor bowel movements, recording diarrhea as output • Weigh client daily • Administer antidiarrheal agents as prescribed • Assess client for signs of dehydration and hypokalemia • Encourage high fluid intake • Monitor serum electrolyte determinations
Risk for impaired comfort related to abdominal cramping and diarrhea	The client will: • Verbalize comfort or pain relief • Maintain ADL without disruption because of discomfort	• Assess comfort status of client • Instruct client in appropriate diet to minimize intestinal cramping • Provide suggestions for nondrug pain management (positioning, activities, distraction) • Administer antidiarrheal medications as prescribed • Consult prescriber if additional pain relief is needed

ADL, Activities of daily living.

thrive. Because a newborn's total body weight is usually 75% water, a 10% or greater weight loss may occur with severe diarrhea. If an infant has eight to ten bowel movements in a 24-hour period, the fluid loss may cause circulatory collapse and renal impairment. Diarrhea in infants should be considered serious enough to warrant immediate referral of the client to a prescriber for evaluation.

Persistent diarrhea in older adults can result in fluid and electrolyte loss, dehydration, and perhaps more serious medical complications. Such clients should be referred to a prescriber without delay.

Education Explain the effects of diarrhea on hydration and electrolytes. Instruct the client on interventions to prevent future episodes. Instruct caregivers in appropriate solutions and technique for oral rehydration of children (see the Evidence-Based Practice box below).

Evaluation The expected outcome of antidiarrheal drug therapy is that the client will experience a decrease in the number, frequency, and fluidity of stools.

✱ **B.D. is willing to replace her fluids and electrolytes by taking small sips of a sport rehydration drink. However, she is flying to Houston on business tomorrow and would feel more confident taking an antidiarrheal. The physician prescribes diphenoxylate and atropine (Lomotil).**

Assessment Assess B.D.'s health status for conditions for which diphenoxylate therapy would be contraindicated or would indicate risk. For example, it should not be used with pseudomembranous colitis (*Clostridium difficile* toxin) sec-

ondary to broad-spectrum antibiotic therapy. With infectious diarrhea, slowing peristalsis would inhibit the evacuation of toxins from the bowel and thereby worsen the client's diarrhea. The risk associated with the use of diphenoxylate for dehydration, particularly in children, requires caution because it may predispose clients to delayed diphenoxylate intoxication. Antidiarrheal agents (e.g., diphenoxylate, loperamide, or opioids are carefully considered in instances of acute diarrhea or traveler's diarrhea caused by bacteria (enterotoxin-producing strains of *E. coli, Campylobacter jejuni, Salmonella,* or *Shigella*), parasites *(Giardia lamblia),* and viruses (parvovirus or rotavirus); these organisms penetrate the intestinal wall if retained in the intestine and therefore must be eliminated in the feces. The cautious use of antidiarrheals is also true of diarrhea that is caused by poisoning until the toxic materials have been eliminated from the GI tract.

Assess B.D. for any preexisting condition that would contraindicate her drug therapy. Diphenoxylate may precipitate a hepatic coma in clients with impaired hepatic function. Children and older adults are more susceptible to the respiratory depressant effects of diphenoxylate. Toxic megacolon may develop as the result of inhibition of intestinal motility in clients with acute ulcerative colitis. B.D.'s current drug regimen is reviewed for significant drug interactions, which include the following: The CNS depressant effects are potentiated by alcohol and other CNS depressant drugs. Concurrent use with monoamine oxidase (MAO) inhibitors may precipitate a hypertensive crisis because of the chemical similarity to meperidine. Additive effects are seen with drugs that have anticholinergic/antimuscarinic effects because of the atropine present. The administration of naltrexone will block the therapeutic effects of diphenoxylate and will precipitate withdrawal symptoms if the client is physically dependent on diphenoxylate.

Obtain a baseline assessment of B.D.'s bowel disorder, including vital signs, GI status, and the frequency of diarrhea.

Nursing Diagnosis While undergoing diphenoxylate therapy, B.D. is at risk for the following nursing diagnoses/collaborative problems: diarrhea related to ineffectiveness of the drug regimen; constipation related to the adverse effects of the drug; ineffective breathing pattern related to the effect of the drug on respiratory depression; disturbed thought processes related to the CNS effects of drug (confusion); urinary retention related to the anticholinergic effects of the drug; impaired comfort (blurred vision, dry mouth, flushing of skin, dizziness) related to the anticholinergic effects of the drug; and the potential complications of paralytic ileus (nausea, vomiting, constipation, severe abdominal pain), mental depression, or withdrawal symptoms.

Planning Same as described in previous section.

Implementation

Monitoring Monitor hepatic function if B.D. were receiving long-term therapy. Dehydration in clients may cause variability in the response to diphenoxylate. B.D. can

---

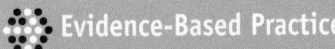
Evidence-Based Practice

Enteral Rehydration Is an Effective Way to Rehydrate Children with Gastroenteritis

Enteral rehydration is effective based on a meta-analysis of data from 16 randomized trials involving 1545 children with gastroenteritis who were younger than 15 years of age (Fonseca, Holdgate, & Craig, 2004). Compared with children who received IV rehydration, children who received enteral rehydration had significantly briefer hospital stays (mean, 21 hours). Enteral rehydration included nasogastric and oral approaches. Duration of diarrhea and weight gain at discharge were similar for enteral- and IV-treated children. Serious major adverse effects occurred significantly more often in the IV-treated group. Given the lack of evidence to support IV rehydration as a first line therapy for children, why is it that it is assumed that more intensive care or technology-based therapy is better than simpler approaches? Perhaps the current culture of health care focuses too often on the technical. In the case of rehydration of children with gastroenteritis, the simpler enteral approach often is better (Taylor, 2004).

have a delayed toxic response; observe for bloating, constipation, abdominal pain, and diminished bowel sounds indicative of paralytic ileus or toxic megacolon. Discontinue the drug if abdominal distention occurs. Electrolytes must be monitored and dehydration corrected in hospitalized clients. As B.D. is not hospitalized, fluid intake should be increased to prevent dehydration. Until diarrhea is controlled, have B.D. weigh daily to monitor fluid loss. Monitor B.D.'s fluid balance ratio.

Monitor carefully the frequency and character of stools to observe for constipation (a potential adverse effect) or to see if diarrhea is diminishing, which indicates the efficacy of therapy.

Intervention Have B.D. modify her diet to support hydration and help control diarrhea. Instruct her to provide good skin care to the perianal area.

Education Caution B.D. about taking alcohol and CNS depressants with diphenoxylate. Instruct about its habit-forming potential. Because dizziness and drowsiness are common adverse effects, caution B.D. regarding tasks that involve alertness. Refer her to her prescriber if diarrhea increases or fever develops.

Evaluation The expected outcome of diphenoxylate therapy is that B.D. will experience a decrease in or an absence of diarrhea without experiencing adverse effects of the drug. B.D. will effectively manage the drug regimen, including compliance with medication, notifying the prescriber of reportable adverse effects, and maintaining scheduled visits with health care providers for monitoring and follow-up care.

Summary

Drugs and agents that affect the mouth are usually used for the provision of good oral hygiene. Dentifrices are helpful as mechanical aids for brushing teeth. Clotrimazole and nystatin are specific agents for the treatment of oral candidiasis.

Drugs that affect the stomach are classified as antacids, antiflatulents, digestants, antiemetics, emetics, and those used in the treatment of peptic ulcer and GERD. Antacids are used to neutralize HCl in the stomach and may be composed of aluminum salts, calcium carbonate, magnesium salts, or sodium bicarbonate (alone or in combination). Digestants are administered to promote the process of digestion when there is a deficiency of some substance essential to that process. Antiemetics are given for the relief of nausea and vomiting; it is essential to determine the cause of the gastric distress, because these drugs may mask the symptoms of more serious illnesses. Emetics, administered to induce vomiting, are rarely used today as a part of drug overdoses or poisonings. Drugs used in the treatment of peptic ulcer are cytoprotective agents, which act locally to promote healing; H_2-receptor antagonists, which prevent

histamine from stimulating the H_2 receptor; and PPIs, which block acid production and so increase the pH of the stomach. Sucralfate and misoprostol are also occasionally used for cytoprotection.

Ursodiol, which affects the gallbladder, is administered to dissolve radiolucent cholesterol gallstones in clients who may be surgical risks because of preexisting conditions.

Drugs affecting the lower GI tract include treatments for inflammatory or irritable bowel, laxatives or antidiarrheal agents. Mesalamine and its derivatives, antimicrobials, corticosteroids, immunosuppressants and the biologic modifying drug infliximab, are used for the treatment of Crohn's disease and other inflammatory bowel diseases. Tegaserod is a serotonergic agent used for short-term treatment of irritable bowel syndrome in women.

Laxatives are given to relieve or prevent constipation, to expel parasites or poisonous substances, to obtain a specimen, or to cleanse the bowel for diagnostic examination. They are usually classified by their mechanism of action: saline, stimulant, bulk-forming, emollient, lubricant laxatives, or bowel evacuants. The goal is to return the client to a normal, adequate bowel pattern.

Antidiarrheals are administered to reduce the frequency of evacuations. This is only part of a treatment plan that should also include replenishment of fluid and electrolyte loss, diagnosis and treatment of the underlying cause, and restoration of the intestinal flora. Again, the goal of treatment is to return the client to a normal, adequate bowel pattern.

⊛ Critical Thinking Questions

- Given the questionable efficacy of mouthwashes and gargles, why is advertising money spent for these products?

- Why is it important to establish the underlying cause of vomiting before administering any antiemetic?

- What lifestyle teaching would be important in supporting the treatment of GERD?

- What would be the laxative of choice for Mr. Preston, a 56-year-old client, 3 days after his myocardial infarction? For Jimmy Tyrone, 7 years old, whose last bowel movement was 4 days ago? For Mrs. White, a 42-year-old client being prepared for a colonoscopy? Why would it be the drug of choice, and what disadvantages are involved in its use?

- Alice Reagan, a 27-year-old teacher, has just returned from a week's vacation in Mexico with severe diarrhea of 3 days' duration. What criteria should be considered in the selection of an antidiarrheal agent?

Bibliography

Ahmad, T., Marshall, S., & Jewell, D., (2003). Genotype-based phenotyping heralds a new taxonomy for inflammatory bowel disease. *Current Opinion in Gastroenterology, 19*(4), 327-335.

Als-Nielsen, B., Gluud, L.L., & Gluud, C. (2004). Non-absorbable disaccharides for hepatic encephalopathy: Systematic review of randomised trials. *British Medical Journal, 328*, 1046-1050.

American Dental Association. (2005). Fluoridation facts. Retrieved July 14, 2005, from http:www.ada.org

Anderson, D.M., Keith, J., & Novak, P.D. (Eds.) (2002). *Mosby's medical, nursing, and allied health dictionary* (6th ed.). St. Louis: Mosby.

Beaven, S.W., & Abreu, M.T. (2004). Biomarkers in inflammatory bowel disease. *Current Opinion in Gastroenterology, 20*(4), 318-327.

Berardi, R.R. (2002). Peptic ulcer disease. In J.T. DiPiro, R.L. Talbert, G.C. Yee, G.R. Matzke, B.G. Wells, & L.M. Posey (Eds.), *Pharmacotherapy: A pathophysiological approach* (5th ed.). New York: McGraw-Hill.

Bosker, G. (Ed.). (2004). *Primary and acute care medicine: Practice, protocols, pathways,* (2nd ed.). Atlanta: Thomson American Health Consultants.

Carpenito-Moyet, L.J. (2004). *Nursing diagnosis: Application to clinical practice* (10th ed.). Philadelphia: Lippincott, Williams & Wilkins.

Cole, P., Rodu, B., & Mathisen, A. (2003). Alcohol-containing mouthwash and oropharyngeal cancer: a review of the epidemiology. *Journal of the American Dental Association, 134*(8), 1079-1087.

Committee on Injury, Violence and Poison Prevention, American Academy of Pediatrics Policy Statement. (2003). Poison treatment in the home. *Pediatrics, 112*, 1182.

De Ponti, F. (2004), Pharmacology of serotonin: what a clinician should know. *Gut, 53*(10), 1520-1535.

Derijks, L.J., et al. (2004). Pharmacokinetics of 6-mercaptopurine in patients with inflammatory bowel disease: Implications for therapy. *Therapeutic Drug Monitoring, 26*(3), 311-318.

Drug facts and comparisons (58th ed.). (2005). St. Louis: Facts and Comparisons.

Ernest, E., & Pittler, M.H. (2000). Efficacy of ginger for nausea and vomiting: a systematic review of randomized clinical trials. *British Journal of Anaesthesia, 84*(3), 367-371.

Everitt, D.E. (2004). Important Drug Warning. Malvern, PA: Centocor, Inc. Retrieved January 4, 2005, from http://www.fda.gov/medwatch/SAFETY/2004/remicade_dearhcp.pdf

FDA Talk Paper T04-10 (April 28, 2004). FDA Updates Zelnorm Labeling with New Risk Information Washington DC: Food and Drug Administration. Retrieved January 5, 2005, from http://www.fda.gov/bbs/topics/ANSWERS/2004/ANS01285.html

Feldman, D.M., Borgida, A.F., Rodis, J.F., Leo, M,V., & Campbell, W.A. (2003). A randomized comparison of two regimens of misoprostol for second-trimester pregnancy termination. *American Journal of Obstetrics and Gynecology, 189*(3), 710-713.

Flu and colds: Information from your family doctor. (2004). *American Family Physician, 70*(1), 1341-1342.

Fonseca, B.K., Holdgate, A., & Craig, J.C. (2004). Enteral vs. intravenous rehydration therapy for children with gastroenteritis: A meta-analysis of randomized controlled trials. *Archives of Pediatric and Adolescent Medicine, 158*, 483-490.

Freston, J.W. (2004). Therapeutic choices in reflux disease: defining the criteria for selecting a proton pump inhibitor. *American Journal of Medicine, 117*(Suppl 5A), 14 S-22 S.

Gasche, C., & Grundtner, P. (2005). Genotypes and phenotypes in Crohn's disease: do they help in clinical management? *Gut, 54*(1), 162-167.

Goetz, C.G. (2003). *Textbook of Clinical Neurology* (2nd ed.). Philadelphia: W.B. Saunders.

Gwo-Tzer, M., Lees, C., & Satsangi, J. (2004). Pharmacogenetics and inflammatory bowel disease: Progress and prospects. *Inflammatory Bowel Diseases, 10*(2), 148-158.

Hasler, W.L. (2003). Pharmacotherapy for intestinal motor and sensory disorders. *Gastroenterology Clinics of North America, 32*(2), 707-732.

Hawkey, C., Talley, N.J., Yeomans, N.D., Jones, R., Sung, J.J., Langstrom, G., et al.; NASA1 SPACE1 Study Group. (2005). Improvements with esomeprazole in patients with upper gastrointestinal symptoms taking non-steroidal antiinflammatory drugs, including selective COX-2 inhibitors. *American Journal of Gastroenterology, 100*, 1028-1036.

Hiki, N., et al. (2003). Peppermint oil reduces gastric spasm during upper endoscopy: a randomized, double blind, double dummy, controlled trial. *Gastrointestinal Endoscopy, 57*(4), 475-482.

Jutabha, R., Jensen, D.M., Martin, P., Savides, T., Han, S.H., & Gornbein, J. (2005). Randomized study comparing banding and propranolol to prevent initial variceal hemorrhage in cirrhotics with high-risk esophageal varices. *Gastroenterology, 128*, 870-881.

Kaiser, R., Tremblay, P.B., Sezer, O., Possinger, K., Roots, I., & Brockmoller, J. (2004). Investigation of the association between 5-HT3 A receptor gene polymorphisms and efficiency of antiemetic treatment with 5-HT3 receptor antagonists. *Pharmacogenetics, 14*(5), 271-278.

Kamm, M.A., Muller-Lissner, S., Talley, N.J., Tack, J., Boeckxstaens, G., Minushkin, O.N., et al. (2005). Tegaserod for the treatment of chronic constipation: A randomized, double-blind, placebo-controlled multinational study. *American Journal of Gastroenterology, 100*, 362-372.

Kentrup, W.A. (August, 2004). Dear Health Care Professional. Collegeville, PA: Wyeth Pharmaceuticals. Retrieved January 4, 2005, from http://www.fda.gov/medwatch/SAFETY/2004/PROTONIX%20 IV_Dear%20 HCP_2004-08-27.pdf.

Kim, H.J., et al. (2004). Association of distinct α_2 adrenoceptor and serotonin transporter polymorphisms with constipation and somatic symptoms in functional gastrointestinal disorders. *Gut, 53*(6), 829-837.

Lacy, C.F., Armstrong, L.L., Goldman, M.P., & Lance, L.L. (2004). *Lexi-Comp's Drug Information Handbook* (12th ed.). Hudson, Ohio: Lexi-Comp.

Leontiadis, G.I., Sharma, V.K., & Howden, C.W. (2005). Systematic review and meta-analysis of proton pump inhibitor therapy in peptic ulcer bleeding. *British Medical Journal, 330*, 568-575.

e-LEARNING SUPPLEMENTS

Student CD-ROM
- Final Exam questions
- NCLEX® Examination review questions
- Pharmacology animations
- Printable chapter summary

Evolve Website (http://evolve.elsevier.com/mckenry)
- Case study on drugs affecting the GI tract
- Interactive concept map on gastroesophageal reflux

- Content updates, including information on new drugs
- WebLinks corresponding to this chapter
- Answers to the critical thinking questions in this chapter
- *Elsevier ePharmacology Update* newsletter
- Mosby's Drug Consult Internet Edition
- Supplemental and reference information

Lindley, C. (2005). Nausea and vomiting. In M.A. Koda-Kimble, L.Y. Young, W.A. Kradian, B.J. Guglielmo, B.K. Alldredge, & R.L. Corelli (Eds.), *Applied therapeutics: The clinical use of drugs* (8th ed.). Philadelphia: Lippincott Williams & Wilkins.

Maiden, L., Thjodleifsson, B., Theodors, A., Gonzalez, J., & Bjarnason, I. (2005). A quantitative analysis of NSAID-induced small bowel pathology by capsule enteroscopy. *Gastroenterology, 128,* 1172-1178.

Marinho, V.C.C., Higgins, J.P.T., Logan, S., & Sheiham, A. (2003). Fluoride toothpastes for preventing dental caries in children and adolescents. *The Cochrane Database of Systematic Reviews, 1*(3), 679-684.

Marshall, B.J., & Windor, H.M. (2005). The relation of H. pylori to gastric adenocarcinoma and lymphoma: pathophysiology, epidemiology, screening, clinical presentation, treatment, and prevention. *Medical Clinics of North America, 89*(2), 313-344.

McMahon, B.J., et al. (2003). The relationship among previous antimicrobial use, antimicrobial resistance, and treatment outcomes for Helicobacter pylori infections. *Annals of Internal Medicine, 139,* 463-469.

McQuaid, K.R. (2003). Alimentary tract. In Tierney, L.M. Jr., McPhee, S.J., & Papadakis, M.A. (Eds.), *Current Medical Diagnosis & Treatment.* New York: Lange Medical Books/McGraw-Hill.

Merkel, C., et al., and the Gruppo Triveneto per l'Ipertensione Portale. (2004). A placebo-controlled clinical trial of nadolol in the prophylaxis of growth of small esophageal varices in cirrhosis. *Gastroenterology, 127,* 476-484.

Mosby's drug consult.(15th ed.). (2005). St. Louis: Mosby.

Nilsson, M., Johnsen, R., Ye, W., Hveem, K., & Lagergren, J. (2003). Obesity and estrogen as risk factors for gastroesophageal reflux symptoms. *Journal of the American Medical Association, 290,* 66-72.

Pashankar, D.S., Loening-Baucke, V., & Bishop, W.P. (2003). Safety of polyethylene glycol 3350 for the treatment of chronic constipation in children. *Archives of Pediatric and Adolescent Medicine, 157,* 661-664.

Pasricha, P.J. (2001). Prokinetic agents, antiemetics, and agents used in irritable bowel syndrome. In Hardman, J.G., & Limbird, L.E. (Eds.), *Goodman & Gilman's The pharmacological basis of therapeutics* (10th ed.). New York: McGraw-Hill.

Pittler, M.H., & Ernst, T. (1998). Peppermint for irritable bowel syndrome: A critical review and meta analysis. *American Journal of Gastroenterology, 93*(7), 1131-1135.

Poe. R.H., & Kalley, M.C. (2003). Chronic cough and gastroesophageal reflux: experience with specific therapy for diagnosis and treatment. *Chest, 123*(3), 679-684.

Rakel, D. (2003). *Integrative Medicine.* Philadelphia: W.B. Saunders.

Rondeau, V. (2000). A review of epidemiologic studies on aluminum and silica in relation to Alzheimer's disease and associated disorders. *Review of Environmental Health, 17*(2), 107-121.

Saad, R.J., & Schieman, J.M. (2004). Diagnosis and management of peptic ulcer disease. *Clinics in Family Practice, 6*(3), 569-587.

Sarin, S.K., Wadhawan, M., Agarwal, S.R., Tyagi, P., & Sharma, B.C. (2005). Endoscopic variceal ligation plus propranolol versus endoscopic variceal ligation alone in primary prophylaxis of variceal bleeding. *American Journal of Gastroenterology, 100,* 797-804.

Selwitz, R.H., Nowjack-Raymer, R.E., Kingman, A., & Driscoll, W.S. (1998). Dental caries and dental fluorosis among schoolchildren who were lifelong residents of communities having either low or optimal levels of fluoride in drinking water. *Journal of Public Health Dentistry, 58*(1), 28-35.

Shiotani, A., & Graham, D.Y. (2002). Pathogenesis and therapy of gastric and duodenal ulcer disease. *Medical Clinics of North America, 86*(6), 1447-1466.

Siepler, J. Smith-Scott, C. (2005). Upper gastrointestinal disorders. In M.A. Koda-Kimble, L.Y. Young, W.A. Kradian, B.J. Guglielmo, B.K. Alldredge, & R.L. Corelli (Eds.), *Applied therapeutics: The clinical use of drugs* (8th ed.). Philadelphia: Lippincott Williams & Wilkins.

Somers, S.C., & Lembo, A. (2003). Irritable bowel syndrome: evaluation and treatment. *Gastroenterology Clinics of North America, 32*(2), 507-529.

Tassaneeyakul, W., et al. (2002). Analysis of the CYP2 C19 polymorphism in a North-eastern Thai population. *Pharmacogenetics, 12*(3), 221-225.

Taylor, J.A. (2004). Oral rehydration: In pediatrics, less is often better. *Archives of Pediatric and Adolescent Medicine, 158,* 420-421.

Tremblay, P.B., et al. (2003). Variations in the 5-Hydroxytryptamine type 3 B receptor gene as predictors of the efficacy of antiemetic treatment in cancer patients. *Journal of Clinical Oncology, 21*(11), 2147-2155.

USP DI: Drug information for the health care professional (25th ed.). (2005). Greenwood Village, CO: MICROMEDEX Thomson Healthcare.

Vanderghoff, B.T., & Tahboub, R.M. (2002). Proton pump inhibitors: an update. *American Family Physician, 67*(6), 1189-1190.

Wall, G. (2005). Lower gastrointestinal disorders. In M.A. Koda-Kimble, L.Y. Young, W.A. Kradian, B.J. Guglielmo, B.K. Alldredge, & R.L. Corelli (Eds.), *Applied therapeutics: The clinical use of drugs* (8th ed.). Philadelphia: Lippincott Williams & Wilkins.

Williams, D.B. (2002). Gastroesophageal reflux disease. In DiPiro J.T., Talbert R.L., Yee G.C., Matzke, G.R., Wells B.G., & Posey, L.M. (Eds.), *Pharmacotherapy: A Pathophysiological Approach* (5th ed.). New York: McGraw-Hill.

Williams, D.M., & Kradjan, W.A. (2005). Chronic obstructive pulmonary disease. In M.A. Koda-Kimble, L.Y. Young, W.A. Kradian, B.J. Guglielmo, B.K. Alldredge, & R.L. Corelli (Eds.), *Applied therapeutics: The clinical use of drugs* (8th ed.). Philadelphia: Lippincott Williams & Wilkins.

Yin, O., Tomlinson, B., Waye, M., Chow, A., & Chow, M. (2004). Pharmacogenetics and herb-drug interactions: experience with Ginkgo biloba and omeprazole. *Pharmacogenetics, 14*(12), 841-850.

OVERVIEW OF THE EYE

CHAPTER FOCUS

Approximately 70% of all sensory information is perceived through the eyes. Visual impairment, which often accompanies ophthalmic disorders, affects the client's ability to function independently and diminishes his or her perception of the environment. Disorders of the eye are becoming increasingly common as the population ages. To appropriately assess and care for clients with ophthalmic problems, the nurse needs to have a thorough understanding of the anatomy and physiology of the eye.

LEARNING OBJECTIVES

- Describe the anatomy and physiology of the eye.
- Identify the muscles involved with miosis and mydriasis, and explain their functions.
- Define accommodation and cycloplegia.
- Name four protective mechanisms associated with the eye.

▲ KEY TERMS

accommodation, p. 782
cataract, p. 782
cornea, p. 781
cycloplegia, p. 782
miosis, p. 782
mydriasis, p. 782

✳ **What are the key issues in anatomy, physiology, and pathophysiology of the eye?**

The eye is the receptor organ for one of the most delicate and valuable senses—vision. Figure 41-1 shows the parts of the eye. The eyeball has three layers or coats: the protective external layer (cornea and sclera), the middle layer (which contains the choroid, iris, and ciliary body), and the light-sensitive retina.

The eyeball is protected in a deep depression of the skull called the orbit. It is moved in the orbit by six small extraocular muscles.

The anterior covering of the eye is the **cornea.** The cornea is normally transparent and allows light to enter the eye. It has no blood vessels and receives its nutrition from the aqueous humor and its oxygen supply by diffusion from the air and surrounding structures. The corneal surface consists of a thin layer of epithelial cells that are quite resistant to infection. An abraded cornea, however, is very susceptible to infection. The cornea is also supplied with 60 to 80 sensory fibers that elicit pain whenever the corneal epithelium is damaged. Seriously injured corneal tissue is replaced by scar tissue, which is usually not transparent. Increased intraocular pressure also results in a loss of transparency.

The sclera, which is continuous with the cornea, is non-transparent; it is the white fibrous envelope of the eye. The conjunctiva is the mucous membrane that lines the anterior part of the sclera and the inner surfaces of each eyelid.

The iris gives the eye its brown, blue, gray, green, or hazel color. It surrounds the pupil, whose size is altered by the sphincter and dilator muscles in the iris. The sphincter mus-

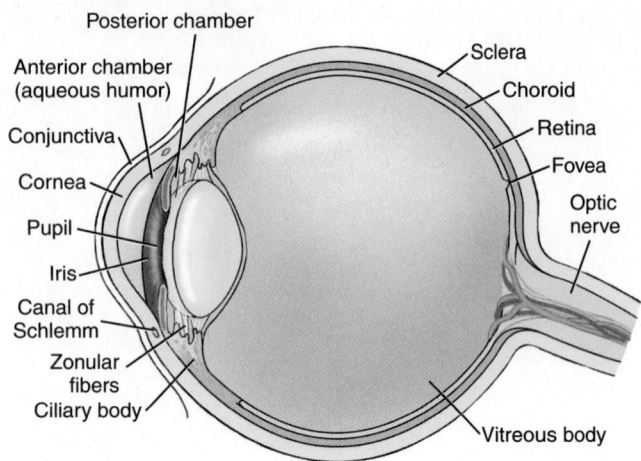

FIGURE 41-1 Parts of the eye.

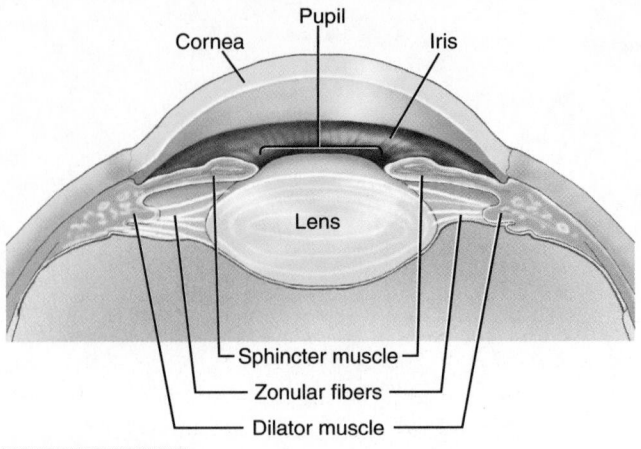

FIGURE 41-2 Accommodation and pupillary alterations.

cle, which encircles the pupil, is parasympathetically innervated; the dilator muscle, which runs radially from the pupil to the periphery of the iris, is sympathetically innervated. Contraction of the sphincter muscle, either alone or with relaxation of the dilator muscle, causes constriction of the pupil, or **miosis.** Contraction of the dilator muscle and relaxation of the sphincter muscle causes dilation of the pupil, or **mydriasis** (Figure 41-2). Drugs producing miosis (miotics) act by (1) interfering with cholinesterase activity or (2) acting like acetylcholine at receptor sites in the sphincter muscle. Drugs producing mydriasis (mydriatics) act by (1) interfering with the action of acetylcholine or (2) stimulating sympathetic or adrenergic receptors (Moroi & Lichter, 2001). Pupil constriction normally occurs in bright light or when the eye is focusing on nearby objects. Pupil dilation normally occurs in dim light or when the eye is focusing on distant objects.

The lens is situated behind the iris. It is a transparent mass of uniformly arranged fibers encased in a thin elastic capsule. Its protein concentration is higher than that of any other tissue of the body. The function of the lens is to ensure that the image on the retina remains in sharp focus. The lens does this by changing shape (**accommodation**) to adjust to variations in distance. This occurs readily in young persons, but the lens becomes more rigid with age. The ability to focus on close objects is then lost, and the near point (the closest point that can be seen clearly) recedes.

With age the lens may also lose its transparency and become opaque; this is known as a **cataract.** Blindness can occur unless the cataract can be treated or removed surgically. Vision is not compromised if the opaque (cataract) portion is located peripherally in the lens.

The lens has suspensory ligaments called zonular fibers around its edge. These fibers connect with the ciliary body, and their tension helps to change the shape of the lens. In the unaccommodated eye the ciliary muscle is relaxed and the zonular fibers are taut. When zonular fibers contract, the pupil dilates; this results in sharp distant vision and blurred near vision (unaccommodated eye). Parasympathetic stimulation accommodates the eye for near vision; the pupil constricts in response to contraction of the sphincter muscle, and the zonular fibers are relaxed.

Accommodation depends on the following two factors: (1) ciliary muscle contraction and (2) the ability of the lens to assume a more biconvex shape when tension on the ligaments is relaxed. The ciliary muscle is innervated by parasympathetic fibers. Paralysis of the ciliary muscle is termed **cycloplegia.**

Aqueous humor is formed by the ciliary body. It bathes and feeds the lens, iris, and posterior surface of the cornea. After it is formed, it flows forward between the lens and the iris into the anterior chamber. It drains out of the eye through drainage channels located near the junction of the cornea and sclera. A trabecular meshwork called the canals of Schlemm drains the aqueous humor into the venous system of the eye (see Figure 42-1).

The retina contains nerve endings plus the rods and cones that function as visual sensory receptors. It is connected to the brain by the optic nerve, which leaves the orbit through a bony canal in the posterior wall.

Eyelashes, eyelids, blinking, and tears serve to protect the eye. Each eye has approximately 200 eyelashes. A blink reflex occurs whenever a foreign body touches the eyelashes. The lids close quickly to prevent the foreign substance from entering the eye. Blinking, which is bilateral, occurs every few seconds during the waking hours. This process keeps the corneal surface free of mucus and spreads the lacrimal fluid evenly over the cornea. Tears are secreted by the lacrimal glands and contain lysozyme, a mucolytic enzyme with bactericidal action. Tears provide lubrication for lid movements, and they wash away noxious agents. By forming a thin film over the cornea, tears provide a good optical surface. Tear fluid is lost by evaporation and by draining into two small ducts (the lacrimal canaliculi) at the inner corners of the upper and lower eyelids.

Summary

The eyes provide much of the information of the world around us. These delicate structures are protected from direct sunlight, damaging particles, and dryness of the environment by accessory structures such as eyelids, eye muscles, and tear glands.

Critical Thinking Questions

- Mrs. B. has telephoned to make an appointment to have her eyes examined. During the examination her pupils will be dilated. As a preexamination instruction, you tell her she will be unable to drive home and should have someone drive her to the appointment. Why?

- One of your classmates cannot see the whiteboard during class and moves to the front row, but still gets headaches. What do you think is happening, and what causes this?

Bibliography

Anderson, D.M., Keith, J., & Novak, P.D. (Eds.) (2002). *Mosby's medical, nursing, and allied health dictionary* (6th ed.). St. Louis: Mosby.

Guyton, A.C., & Hall, J.E. (2000). *Textbook of medical physiology* (10th ed.). Philadelphia: W.B. Saunders.

Hardman, J.G., & Limbird, L.E. (Eds.). (2001). *Goodman and Gilman's The pharmacological basis of therapeutics* (10th ed.). New York: McGraw-Hill.

Herlihy, B., & Maebius, N.K. (2003). *The human body in health and illness* (2nd ed.). Philadelphia: Saunders.

McCance, K.L., & Huether, S.E. (2002). *Pathophysiology: The biological basis for disease in adults and children* (4th ed.). St. Louis: Mosby.

Moroi, S.E., Lichter, P.R. (2001). Ocular Pharmacology. In: Hardman, J.G. & Limbird, L.E. (Eds.), *Goodman and Gilman's The pharmacological basis of therapeutics* (10th ed.). New York: McGraw-Hill.

Thibodeau, G.A., & Patton, K.T. (2003). *Anatomy and physiology* (5th ed.). St. Louis: Mosby.

e-LEARNING SUPPLEMENTS

Student CD-ROM
- Final Exam questions
- NCLEX® Examination review questions
- Pharmacology animations
- Printable chapter summary

Evolve Website (http://evolve.elsevier.com/mckenry)
- Content updates, including information on new drugs

- WebLinks corresponding to this chapter
- Answers to the critical thinking questions in this chapter
- *Elsevier ePharmacology Update* newsletter
- Mosby's Drug Consult Internet Edition
- Supplemental and reference information

42

OPHTHALMIC DRUGS

CHAPTER FOCUS

Eye disorders and the sensory-perceptual alterations that occur can cause varying degrees of disability. The early detection and treatment of eye disorders can minimize limitations of vision. Ophthalmic drugs make a significant contribution to the treatment of eye disorders and the preservation of vision.

LEARNING OBJECTIVES

- Describe the nursing management of ophthalmic drug administration.
- Compare and contrast the antiglaucoma agents.
- Identify the systemic effects of ophthalmic drugs.
- List antiinfective and antiinflammatory ophthalmic agents.
- Implement the nursing management of clients receiving ophthalmic agents.

▲ **KEY TERMS**
glaucoma, p. 793
miotics, p. 796
mydriasis, p. 799

◼▀ **KEY DRUGS**
levocabastine, p. 802
latanoprost, p. 795
pilocarpine, p. 797

✳ **What drugs are available to treat ophthalmologic conditions?**

Drugs used to treat eye disorders can be divided into three major groups: the antiinfectives/antiinflammatory agents, the antiglaucoma agents, and the mydriatics and cycloplegics. Many eye preparations are available, including ophthalmic diagnostic products, enzymes, irrigating solutions, eyewashes, and hyperosmolar preparations.

✳ **What are the nursing management issues with using drugs that affect the eye?**

Assessment Ask the client if he wears glasses or contact lenses or has a history of glaucoma, cataracts, vision loss, or retinitis. Determine if the client is taking any medications; some drugs may cause visual disturbances. For example, digoxin causes the client to see yellow halos around bright lights (Abdollahi, Shafiee, Bathaiee, Sharifzadeh, & Nikfar,

2004). Assess the pregnancy safety of female clients of childbearing age (see the Pregnancy Safety box on p. 785). Assess the eyes for redness, swelling, tearing, discharge, a decrease in visual acuity, and pain. Check the pupils for size, equality, reactivity, light reaction, and accommodation. In the case of glaucoma, tonometry will indicate increased intraocular pressure (IOP). Assess fine motor skills of the client and/or caregiver that enable self-management of ophthalmic drops or ointment.

Nursing Diagnosis With a course of therapy with ophthalmic preparations, the client is at risk for the following nursing diagnoses/collaborative problems: deficient knowledge related to self-administration of the medication and the condition for which it is administered; risk for injury related to blurred vision as the result of the instillation of drops or ointment into the eye; risk for infection related to contaminated eye drops or ointment; and the potential

PREGNANCY SAFETY
OPHTHALMIC DRUGS

Category	Drug
B	atropine, brimonidine, cromolyn, diclofenac, dipivefrin, emedastine, erythromycin, flurbiprofen, lodoxamide, nedocromil, polymyxin B, prednisolone, tobramycin
C	acetazolamide, apraclonidine, azelastine, bacitracin, betamethasone, betaxolol, bimatoprost, brinzolamide, carbachol, carteolol, chloramphenicol, ciprofloxacin, cyclopentolate, cyclosporine, dexamethasone, dichlorphenamide, dorzolamide, echothiophate, epinastine, epinephrine, fluorescein, fluorometholone, gentamicin, homatropine, hydrocortisone, hydroxyamphetamine, idoxuridine, ketorolac, ketotifen, latanoprost, levocabastine, levobunolol, medrysone, methazolamide, metipranolol, naphazoline, natamycin, norfloxacin, ofloxacin, olopatadine, pemirolast, phenylephrine, pilocarpine, proparacaine, scopolamine, sulfacetamide, suprofen, tetracaine, tetrahydrozoline, timolol, travoprost, trifluridine, unoprostone, vidarabine
D	neomycin
X	demecarium
Unclassified	chymotrypsin

Data from *Mosby's drug consult* (15th ed.). (2005). St. Louis: Mosby.

complications of hypersensitivity, superinfections, and systemic effects of the drug. The Nursing Care Plan on p. 786 provides other selected nursing diagnoses to consider for clients who are receiving ophthalmic conditions.

Planning The goals of ophthalmic medications are that the client will:
- Remain free of signs and symptoms of infection of the eye or pain related to eye disorder.
- Return to normal vision or preinfection or predisorder status.
- Effectively manage drug regimen, including correct administration technique, compliance with medications and use of supportive measures (compresses, analgesics).
- Collaborate with health care providers, reporting adverse effects appropriately and maintaining scheduled appointment with health care providers for monitoring and treatment.

Implementation

Monitoring Monitor the affected eye(s) on a daily basis for improvement of the condition for which the medication was prescribed. Assess for redness, itching, swelling, and a burning sensation that was not present before therapy started; such reactions might indicate hypersensitivity. Systemic absorption may occur with eyedrops and cause adverse systemic reactions (Table 42-1).

Intervention In addition to developing a working knowledge of the available ophthalmic agents, be especially aware of the special considerations in administering these drugs. Ocular drugs are administered by topical application of a solution or ointment (Box 42-1). Ocular solutions are sterile and easily administered and usually do not interfere with vision. Their main disadvantage is that the drug is in contact with the eye for only a short time. Ocular ointments have the advantages of being quite comfortable on instillation and staying in longer contact with the eye for more prolonged effects. However, ointments form a film or haze over the eye that interferes with vision, and they have a higher incidence of contact dermatitis than do solutions. Additionally, most ointments are not sterile.

Packs may also be used to apply drugs to the eye. Packs are cotton pledgets that are saturated with an ophthalmic solution and inserted into the inferior or superior cul-de-sac. Ocular drugs may also be physician-administered by iontophoresis, subconjunctival (sub-Tenon's) injection, retrobulbar injection, or injection directly into the vitreous or anterior chamber of the eye.

Ocular gel formulations and Ocusert (an elliptical unit that is placed in the cul-de-sac of the eye to provide continuous drug release) provide delivery systems for pilocarpine and other medications. These systems were developed to overcome some of the problems with conventional eye drops or ointments. Their longer duration of action improves client management of the therapeutic regimen and avoids the peak-and-valley response associated with previous solutions and ointments. A steady release or range of pilocarpine should reduce drug-induced adverse effects and improve treatment outcome.

Education Instruct the client and/or home caregiver in the proper administration of eye medications (see Box 42-1). Caution the client to always check the bottle label for correct medication and concentration, such as 0.1% or 1%. Checking labels is increasingly important because many beauty aids and home products (glues) are packaged in similar containers. Discard ophthalmic solutions that have darkened or become cloudy.

Contact lenses are not to be worn during eye infections. Check with the prescriber regarding when it would be safe to use them again or if they may be worn during drug regimens with other ophthalmic conditions.

Store medications as directed on the label; some may need refrigeration. Once opened, most medications have a limited life (3 months or the end of the current illness). If stored longer, the medication is more likely to become con-

NURSING CARE PLAN SELECTED DIAGNOSES RELATED TO OPHTHALMIC DRUGS

Nursing Diagnosis	Outcome Criteria	Interventions

Deficient knowledge related to new ophthalmic drug regimen	The client will:
	• Express understanding of purpose, function, adverse effects
	• Demonstrate proper handling and administration
	• Discuss possible drug interactions
		• Assess client's level of understanding.
		• Determine the educational needs of the client.
		• Instruct client in the following:
		  • Purpose and function of medicine
		  • Adverse effects that may occur, and the appropriate response
		  • Proper storage and handling
		  • Correct method of administration
		  • Systemic reactions that may occur with topically applied eye preparations

Anxiety related to possible decrease in or loss of vision	The client will: • Verbalize fears and concerns	• Assess client for perceptions and fears related to the eye disorder. • Encourage open communication about fears. • Provide emotional support. • Provide information related to the effectiveness of drug therapy. • Allay unwarranted fears.
Impaired comfort related to ophthalmic disorder	The client will: • Express a decrease in discomfort • Provide rest and limiting of eye activity (e.g., reading)	• Closely assess the client's symptoms and level of comfort. • Provide rest and limiting of eye activity (e.g., reading). • Provide emotional support and encouragement.
Risk for injury related to impaired vision	The client will: • Maintain activity appropriate for level of vision without injury • Discuss necessary lifestyle adjustments	• Assess level of vision impairment. • Provide safety measures as needed. • Encourage client to adjust activities in accordance with client's level of vision.

taminated and lead to an infection of the eye. To avoid such contamination from the outset, the sterility of the preparation and/or dropper must be maintained. Do not allow the tube tip or dropper to touch anything, including the skin. Hold the dropper with the tip down. Never allow medication to flow into the bulb of the dropper. Keep the container closed when not in use. If two or more family members are using eye medications, each should have a separate vial to prevent cross-contamination.

Inform the client of the signs of adverse effects of the medication, and signs of progress. Advise the client when to contact or return to the prescriber for assessment.

Evaluation The expected outcome is that the client experiences a decrease in or absence of the symptoms for which the agent was prescribed. The client states signs and symptoms of eye pain, redness, drainage and when to report them to the prescriber. The client/care giver demonstrates the correct method for instilling eye medication. Client shows improvement in visual acuity to normal vision or preinfection or predisorder status.

✱ **P.M. is a 19-year-old male college student who presents to the college infirmary with itchy, inflamed conjunctiva with yellow discharge of 2 days duration.**

✱ **What are the common types of eye infections?**
Among the most common ocular infections are conjunctivitis, hordeolum, and blepharitis. Also common are keratitis and uveitis. These and other types of eye infections are presented in Box 42-2.

✱ **How are eye infections treated?**
To treat ocular infections, the drug of choice and the required dosage should ideally be determined by laboratory isolation of the offending organism. The initial culture from the infected area is obtained before any ophthalmic agent is applied. However, treatment is not withheld if the time required to make these determinations may cause increased severity of infection and if the type of infection (e.g., most cases of conjunctivitis, which tend to be self-limiting) does not warrant the expense of laboratory analysis.

TABLE 42-1 OPHTHALMIC DRUGS: ADVERSE SYSTEMIC EFFECTS

Ophthalmic Drug	Reported Adverse Effect
ANTIMICROBIAL AGENTS	
chloramphenicol eyedrops	Aplastic anemia
sulfacetamide eyedrops	Stevens-Johnson syndrome, systemic lupus erythematosus
ANTICHOLINERGIC AGENTS	
atropine eyedrops	Tachycardia, elevated temperature, fever, delirium
cyclopentolate	Seizures, hallucinations
scopolamine eyedrops	Acute psychosis
ANTIGLAUCOMA AGENTS	
β-blocking agents (timolol)	Bradycardia, syncope, low blood pressure, asthmatic attack, heart failure, hallucinations, loss of appetite, headaches, nausea, weakness, depression
anticholinesterase (echothiophate)	Asthmatic attack, systemic cholinergic effects
parasympathomimetic (pilocarpine)	Nausea, stomach pain, increased sweating, salivation, tremors, bradycardia, lightheadedness
ADRENERGIC AGENTS	
phenylephrine (10%)	Severe hypertension, cerebral hemorrhage, dysrhythmias, myocardial infarction
epinephrine eyedrops	Tremors, increased sweating, headaches, hypertension
dipivefrin	
CARBONIC ANHYDRASE INHIBITORS	
brinzolamide	Bitter taste, headache
dorzolamide	

BOX 42-1 GUIDELINES FOR THE INSTILLATION OF EYEDROPS AND OPHTHALMIC OINTMENTS

INSTILLATION OF EYEDROPS

- Wash your hands and put on gloves if necessary.
- Gently cleanse exudates from the eye if necessary.
- Ask the client to tilt the head toward the side of the affected eye.
- Gently pull the lower eyelid down and ask the client to look up.
- Instill the correct number of drops in the sac formed by the lower eyelid.
- Take care not to touch the dropper to the eye or eyelashes.
- Gently apply pressure for 30 seconds to 1 minute over the inner canthus next to the nose to prevent absorption through the tear duct and premature drainage of the medication away from the eye.
- Ask the client to close the eye gently, which distributes the solution. Warn against squeezing the eye tightly, which forces out the medication.
- Wipe away any excess medication.
- If both eyes are to be medicated, do the second instillation quickly before the client begins to blink and tear as a reaction to the burning sensation occurring in the first eye.

INSTILLATION OF EYE OINTMENT

- The procedure is the same except that the ointment is expressed directly into the exposed conjunctival sac from the inner to outer canthus with a small individual tube.
- Have the client close his or her eye; gently massage the eye to distribute the medication.

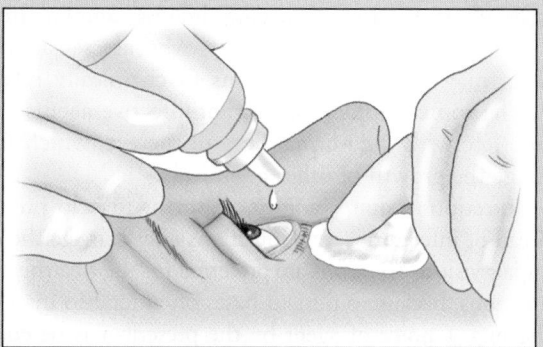

- *Conjunctivitis:* An acute inflammation of the conjunctiva resulting from a bacterial invasion or viral infection. It is a common sign in severe colds. "Pink eye" is the acute contagious epidemic form of conjunctivitis usually caused by *Haemophilus* organisms. Symptoms include redness and burning of the eye, lacrimation, itching, and at times photophobia. Conjunctivitis is usually self-limiting. The eye should be protected from light.
- *Hordeolum (sty):* An acute localized infection of the eyelash follicles and the glands of the anterior lid margin, which results in the formation of a small abscess or cyst.
- *Chalazion:* Infection of the meibomian (sebaceous) glands of the eyelids. A hard cyst may form from blockage of the ducts.
- *Blepharitis:* Inflammation of the margins of the eyelid resulting from bacterial infection or allergy. Symptoms are crusting, irritation of the eye, and red and edematous lid margins.
- *Keratitis:* Corneal inflammation caused by bacterial infection; herpes simplex keratitis is caused by a viral infection.
- *Uveitis:* Infection of the uveal tract or the vascular layer of the eye, which includes the iris, ciliary body, and choroid.
- *Endophthalmitis:* Inflammation of the inner eye structure caused by bacteria.

In general, the prophylactic use of antiinfective/antiinflammatory agents is useless, wasteful, and potentially dangerous because a large proportion of ophthalmic inflammatory diseases are caused by viruses or other agents that are not susceptible to currently available antiinfective agents. Systemic medications that can induce ocular adverse effects need to be considered before an antiinfective or antiinflammatory agent is introduced. See Table 42-2 for drugs that induce adverse effects involving the eye.

Most antiinfective agents do not readily penetrate the eye when applied. Some drugs do penetrate the inflamed eye when the blood-aqueous barrier is decreased by injury or inflammation. Topically applied antiinfective agents can cause sensitivity reactions (stinging, itching, angioneurotic edema, urticaria, dermatitis). Clients who are sensitive to one drug may show cross-reactions to chemically related drugs. The topical application of antiinfective agents may also interfere with the normal flora of the eye, which may encourage the growth of other organisms.

Eye infections require prompt treatment to help prevent the spread of infection; severe infections may damage the eye and impair vision. Solutions are preferred for the treatment of eye infections, because ointment bases often tend to interfere with healing. Choice of agent by the prescriber is based on whether the infection is bacterial, viral, or fungal.

To avoid possible sensitization to systemic antiinfective drugs and to discourage the development of resistant strains of offending organisms, the antibiotic of choice is not given systemically. Instead these agents are administered topically, subconjunctivally, or intrauveally. The selection of an antibiotic for ocular infection is based on (1) clinical experience, (2) the nature and sensitivity of the organisms most commonly causing the condition, (3) the disease itself, (4) the sensitivity and response of the client, and (5) laboratory results. Unfortunately, antibiotic resistance by pathogenic ophthalmic microorganisms is emerging (Abel & Sorensen, 2005).

✳ **P.M. is diagnosed with bacterial conjunctivitis and is prescribed erythromycin ophthalmic ointment to be used four times daily.**

✳ **What topical agents are available to treat bacterial eye infections?**
Antibiotic ophthalmic preparations include bacitracin, chloramphenicol, ciprofloxacin, erythromycin, gentamicin, norfloxacin, ofloxacin, polymyxin B, and tobramycin. Combination preparations usually contain various combinations of these ingredients and/or neomycin, gramicidin, oxytetracycline, or trimethoprim. Some combinations also contain a corticosteroid to reduce inflammation, but the addition of a corticosteroid increases the risk for viral and/or fungal growth. Selected antibiotic ophthalmic products are discussed in the following sections.

erythromycin [eh rith roe **my** sin]
(Ilotycin)
Erythromycin ophthalmic ointment is a bacteriostatic agent, but it may be bactericidal in high concentrations against very susceptible organisms. It is a commonly used agent with good coverage of common pathogens and has a low likelihood of adverse effects.
Indications
Ophthalmic erythromycin is indicated for the treatment of neonatal conjunctivitis caused by *Chlamydia trachomatis* and for the prevention of ophthalmia neonatorum (against *Neisseria gonorrhoeae* or *C. trachomatis*) and other ocular infections caused by susceptible organisms.
Dosing
For adults and children with ocular infections, a thin ointment strip is applied into the conjunctival sac daily, or more often (up to 8 times daily) if necessary. To prevent ophthalmia neonatorum, the ointment should not be flushed from the eye.
Adverse Effects
Eye irritation not present before therapy is rarely reported with this drug.

✳ **What are the nursing considerations for P.M.'s antimicrobial ophthalmic drug therapy?**

Assessment Antibiotic eye medications are contraindicated if P.M. has had a previous allergic reaction to the drug. A baseline assessment of the ocular infection is required. A specimen for culture and sensitivity may be obtained before therapy is initiated.

Nursing Diagnosis While taking antimicrobial ophthalmic drug therapy, P.M. is at risk for the following nursing diagnosis/collaborative problem: risk for injury related to the ineffectiveness of the drug; and the potential complication of

TABLE 42-2 OCULAR ADVERSE EFFECTS INDUCED BY SYSTEMIC MEDICATIONS

Drug	Possible Ocular Adverse Effect Induced	Drug	Possible Ocular Adverse Effect Induced
allopurinol	Retinal hemorrhage, exudative lesions	hydralazine	Lacrimation, blurred vision
amiodarone	Reduced lacrimation, altered pigmentation, corneal and conjunctival deposits, cataracts	ibuprofen	Altered color vision, blurred vision, allergic conjunctivitis
anticholinergics/ tricyclic antidepressants/ antihistamines	Reduced lacrimation, altered vision, altered accommodation, mydriasis	indomethacin	Mydriasis, retinopathy
		isoniazid	Optic neuritis
		lithium carbonate	Exophthalmos, oculogyric crisis
antineoplastics	Toxic conjunctivitis	nifedipine	Periorbital edema
antipsychotics, typical	Corneal and conjunctival deposits, cataracts, retinopathy, oculogyric crisis	nitroglycerin	Transient elevation in IOP
		opioids	Miosis, nystagmus
		phenytoin	Nystagmus
aspirin	Allergic dermatitis including keratitis and conjunctivitis	quinine, chloroquine	Blurring of vision, optic neuritis, blindness (reversible), conjunctivitis, corneal deposits, photoallergic reactions
barbiturates	Nystagmus		
β-adrenergic blockers	Reduced lacrimation		
busulfan	Cataracts	rifampin, rifabutin	Staining of tears, lens
cannabis, marijuana	Nystagmus, conjunctivitis, double vision	sildenafil (Viagra)	Optic neuropathy with risk for vision loss*
carbamazepine	Nystagmus	statins (HMG Co-A reductase inhibitors)	Cataracts
chloral hydrate	Eyelid edema, conjunctivitis, miosis	sulfonamides	Stevens-Johnson syndrome with severe dry eye syndrome
chloroquine	Lenticular and corneal opacity, retinopathy	tadalafil (Cialis)	Optic neuropathy with risk for vision loss*
clarithromycin	Corneal opacity	tetracycline	Swelling of optic disc, conjunctival deposits
clomiphene citrate	Blurred vision, light flashes	thiazide diuretics	Acute transient myopia, yellow coloring of vision
clonidine	Miosis		
corticosteroids	Cataracts, increased IOP, papilledema, exophthalmos	vardenafil (Levitra)	Optic neuropathy with risk for vision loss*
diazoxide	Oculogyric crisis	vincristine	Ptosis, paresis of extraocular muscles
digoxin	Scotomas, optic neuritis	vitamin A overdose or toxicity	Papilledema, increased IOP
ethambutol	Optic nerve damage		
ethyl alcohol	Nystagmus	vitamin D toxicity	Calcium deposits in cornea
guanethidine	Miosis, ptosis, blurred vision		

Data from Abdollahi, M., Shafiee, A., Bathaiee, F.S., Sharifzadeh, M., & Nikfar, S. (2004). Drug-induced toxic reactions in the eye: An overview. *Journal of Infusion Nursing, 27*(6):386-398; Challa, P. (2004). Glaucoma genetics: Advancing new understandings of glaucoma pathogenesis. *International Ophthalmology Clinics, 44*(2):167-185; and U.S. Food and Drug Administration. (July 2005). FDA Alert: Cialis (tadalafil). Retrieved July 10, 2005, from http://www.fda.gov/cder/drug/infopage/cialis/default.htm.
IOP, Intraocular pressure.
*Ocular hemorrhage, pain, photophobia, and other adverse ocular effects have also been reported.

a hypersensitivity response (burning, itching, redness, and swelling not present before therapy).

Planning While receiving an antimicrobial ophthalmic drug, P.M. will:

- Remain free of signs and symptoms of infection of the eye.
- Return to normal vision or preinfection status.
- Effectively manage drug regimen, including correct administration technique, compliance with medications and use of supportive measures (compresses, analgesics).
- Collaborate with health care providers, reporting adverse effects appropriately and maintaining scheduled appointments with health care providers for monitoring and treatment.

Implementation

Monitoring The status of the infected eye(s) should be monitored regarding pain, redness, swelling, and drainage.

Intervention The presence of exudate interferes with the effectiveness of the medication. It is removed before the medication is applied with a separate warm damp cotton ball for each eye. A thin strip (approximately 1 cm) of ointment is placed into the conjunctival sac. Be careful not to touch the tip of the tube to the surface of the eye.

Education Instruct P.M. and his roommate in the application of the ointment. Alert them to symptoms of hypersensitivity that need to be reported to the prescriber. Maintain all personal grooming items and bath linens separate. Do not share eye ointment with others. Continue the medication for the full course of therapy.

Evaluation The expected outcome is P.M.'s ocular infection will be resolved as evidenced by the absence of pain, redness, swelling, and drainage. P.M. demonstrates medication compliance, demonstrates the correct method for instilling eye medication, demonstrates correct cleansing of the eye and the use of compresses, and states when to contact his prescriber if the infection does not improve or if the area becomes more reddened with the application of the ointment.

•   •   •

The sulfonamide agents are effective against a wide variety of bacteria, but have a higher likelihood for localized allergic reactions than erythromycin. The action of sulfonamides is reduced by the presence of para-aminobenzoic acid (PABA) or its derivatives, procaine and tetracaine, and also by the presence of purulent drainage or exudate (purulent matter contains PABA). Therefore lid exudate should be removed before the drugs are instilled.

sulfacetamide [sul fah **see** tah mide]
(Bleph-10, Sulamyd, Cetamide✤, Diosulf✤)
Indications
Sulfacetamide ophthalmic is used in the treatment of conjunctivitis due to sensitive pathogens.

Pharmacokinetics/Dosing
Absorption is possible with ophthalmic use. Before administration, the client should check to see that the solution has not darkened in color; if so, it is to be discarded. Solutions are instilled at a rate of 1 drop every 1 to 3 hours during the day, with increased time intervals during the night. Instillation of the drops may cause some mild pain and discomfort.
Adverse Effects
Allergic reactions, burning on instillation, and conjunctivitis are the most common adverse effects. A small risk for Stevens-Johnson syndrome is possible, particularly in clients who are immunocompromised.
Drug Interactions
Because the activity of sulfacetamide may be inhibited by the concurrent administration of ophthalmic anesthetics, such drugs are applied 30 to 60 minutes apart. Sulfonamides are physically incompatible with thimerosal (an ingredient in some contact lens cleaning solutions) and silver preparations.

triple antibiotic ophthalmic ointment (neomycin, polymyxin B sulfate, and bacitracin ophthalmic ointment) [nee oh **my** sin, polly **mix** in, bass i **tray** sin]
(Mycitracin, Neosporin)
Triple antibiotic ophthalmic ointment (neomycin, polymyxin B, and bacitracin) has been widely used historically in dermal and ophthalmic preparations. This combination, however, has fallen out of favor because of the highly sensitizing nature of neomycin. Bacitracin is rarely used systemically because of its nephrotoxic effects but is particularly useful in treating surface superficial infections caused by gram-positive bacteria (inhibiting protein synthesis). Bacitracin does penetrate the conjunctiva or the cornea slightly, is nonirritating to the eye, is excreted in the nasolacrimal system, and produces no systemic effects.

A broader spectrum of antimicrobial activity is produced when bacitracin is used in combination with other antibiotics than when used alone. The combination dosage form provides a bactericidal effect against many gram-positive and gram-negative organisms.
Indications
Neomycin, polymyxin, and bacitracin ophthalmic ointment is indicated for the treatment of superficial ocular infections caused by susceptible organisms.
Dosing
A small amount (1 cm) of ointment is usually applied into the conjunctival sac every 3 to 4 hours.
Adverse Effects
The greatest concern is the risk for hypersensitivity reactions with neomycin. Localized erythema, conjunctivitis, and systemic reactions are all possible.

chloramphenicol [klor am **fen** ih kole]
(Chloroptic)
Chloramphenicol is a bacteriostatic that prevents peptide bond formation and protein synthesis in a wide variety of gram-positive and gram-negative organisms. Thus it is a useful drug for superficial intraocular infections.
Indications
Ophthalmic preparations of chloramphenicol are used to treat superficial intraocular infections to sensitive pathogens.
Dosing
For adults, a thin strip of ophthalmic ointment is applied into the conjunctival sac every 3 hours (more often if necessary). The adult dosage of the solution is 1 drop into the conjunctival sac every 3 hours.
Adverse Effects
Serious adverse effects to the ophthalmic formulation are usually rare. Burning and stinging on instillation have been reported. Irreversible aplastic anemia has been reported with the systemic formulations of chloramphenicol, but not with the ophthalmic form. Nev-

ertheless, it would be prudent to monitor for blood dyscrasias with prolonged use.

Nursing Management

With prolonged (more than 3 days) or frequent use, monitor complete blood counts (CBCs). Monitor the client for pallor, sore throat and fever, unusual bleeding or bruising, and unusual tiredness, which may indicate irreversible bone marrow depression associated with aplastic anemia. See Table 42-1 for the systemic effects of a variety of ophthalmic agents.

•   •   •

Gentamicin and tobramycin are aminoglycoside antimicrobials effective against a wide variety of gram-negative pathogens including *Pseudomonas*, *Proteus*, and *Klebsiella* organisms and *Escherichia coli*. As a topical agent in high doses. Aminoglycosides may be active against some strains of staphylococci and streptococci that have developed a resistance to other antibiotics.

gentamicin [jen tah **my** sin]
(Garamycin, Genoptic)

Indications

Gentamicin is indicated for ophthalmic infections due to sensitive pathogens.

Pharmacokinetics/Dosing

Gentamicin is very water-soluble and systemic absorption is low with standard dosing. It is applied as an ointment two or three times daily; with the solution, 1 drop is applied every 4 hours.

Adverse Effects

Adverse effects include ocular toxicity and hypersensitivity, including lid itching, swelling, and conjunctival erythema. Systemic toxicity from absorption may occur from excessive use; to minimize these risks, applying pressure to the inner aspect of the eye for 1 minute during and after administration is recommended.

tobramycin [toe bra **my** sin]
(Tobrex)

Indications

As with gentamicin.

Pharmacokinetics/Dosing

See gentamicin.

Adverse Effects

Minimal and similar to gentamicin.

✷ What agents are available to treat fungal eye infections topically?

natamycin [na ta **my** sin]
(Natacyn)

Natamycin ophthalmic suspension is used to treat fungal blepharitis, conjunctivitis, and keratitis. It produces altered membrane permeability by binding to steroids in the cell membrane of the fungus; this causes a loss of the cellular constituents. Overwhelming fungal infections of the eye in a client who is immunocompromised will likely require systemic antifungal therapy.

Indications

Natamycin is indicated for the treatment of conjunctivitis, blepharitis, and keratitis caused by susceptible fungi.

Pharmacokinetics/Dosing

Because natamycin is retained mainly in the conjunctival area, significant drug levels in the ocular fluids are not achieved. It is not systemically absorbed. For fungal keratitis, 1 drop of the 5% solu-

tion is instilled into the conjunctival sac at 1- to 2-hour intervals initially for 3 or 4 days, after which the solution is instilled 6 to 8 times daily. For fungal blepharitis and conjunctivitis, 1 drop 4 to 6 times daily is usually adequate.

Adverse Effects

Natamycin may cause irritation of the eye.

✷ What treatments exist for viral eye infections?

The topical antiviral preparations for eye infections include idoxuridine, trifluridine, and vidarabine. Because these infections can be serious, and the antiviral agents have a short duration of action, frequent dosing is required. The nursing management is as for the antimicrobial ophthalmic medications, except some of these solutions may need to be refrigerated. Trifluridine is a similar agent with identical indications for use.

idoxuridine [eye dox **yoor** i deen]
(Stoxil, Herplex)

Idoxuridine resembles thymidine, a substance necessary for viral deoxyribonucleic acid (DNA); thus idoxuridine replaces thymidine and inhibits the replication of viral DNA.

Indications

Idoxuridine is indicated for the treatment of herpes simplex virus keratitis.

Dosing

The adult dosage of the idoxuridine solution for the treatment of herpes simplex virus keratitis is 1 drop hourly during the waking hours and every 2 hours during the night. With the ointment, apply a thin strip every 4 hours (five times daily) during the waking hours.

Adverse Effects

Less common adverse effects include hypersensitivity (eye redness, pruritus, irritation), visual disturbance, and photosensitivity not present before therapy.

trifluridine [try **flure** i deen]
(Viroptic)

Indications

Trifluridine is also used to treat herpes simplex virus keratoconjunctivitis.

Dosing

The usual adult dosage is 1 drop (1% solution) into the conjunctival sac every 2 hours during the waking hours. The maximum daily dose is 9 drops. Therapy is continued until the cornea has recovered; the dosage is then reduced to 1 drop every 4 hours during the waking hours (minimum of 5 drops per day) for 1 week.

Adverse Effects

A commonly reported side effect is burning or stinging on application. Rare adverse effects include increased IOP, blurred vision, and hypersensitivity reaction as evidenced by redness, swelling, or eye irritation not present before therapy.

vidarabine [vye **dare** a been]
(Vira-A)

Vidarabine is also used to treat herpes simplex viral (HSV) infections. The antiviral mechanism of action is due to the conversion of vidarabine to intracellular substances that inhibit viral DNA polymerase or other enzymes specific to virus DNA.

Indications

Vidarabine is indicated for the treatment of HSV keratitis and keratoconjunctivitis.

Pharmacokinetics/Dosing

Systemic absorption is not expected after ocular administration. The usual adult dosage is a thin strip of ointment applied into the conjunctival sac every 3 hours five times daily. Therapy is continued until the cornea is completely reepithelialized; the dosage is then decreased to twice daily for 7 to 10 days.

Adverse Effects
The adverse effects of vidarabine include increased tear flow and a sensation that something is in the eye. The prescriber should be contacted if there is an occurrence of photosensitivity, redness, eye swelling, or increased eye irritation not present before treatment.

What is the role of antiseptics in treating eye infections?

Many antiseptics that were used to treat surface infections of the eye before the advent of antibiotics are now obsolete. Inorganic mercuric salts such as yellow mercuric oxide ophthalmic ointment (1% to 2%), thimerosal (Merthiolate), and ammoniated mercury formerly served as bacteriostatic agents. They are seldom used today because they do not completely sterilize, spores are resistant to them, and they are irritating to the eye. Silver nitrate is still occasionally used as a topical antiseptic, but its role in preventing neonatal conjunctivitis has been abandoned because it does not protect against chlamydial infection and it can be irritating.

When are corticosteroids used topically in the eye?

The use of corticosteroids in the eye is usually under the direction of an ophthalmologist. They are indicated for the treatment of allergic and inflammatory ophthalmic disorders of the conjunctiva, cornea, and anterior segment of the eye. Although these drugs will reduce inflammation, they can also increase the risk for infection.

Many corticosteroids are available as topical solutions, suspensions, or ointments for ophthalmic use. These include betamethasone (Betnesol), dexamethasone (Maxidex, Decadron), fluorometholone (FML S.O.P., FML), hydrocortisone (Cortamed), medrysone (HMS Liquifilm) and prednisolone (Pred-Forte, Predair-A). These drugs are available in varying strengths and in combination with various antibiotics or mydriatics. They are indicated for the treatment of allergic and inflammatory ophthalmic disorders of the conjunctiva, cornea, and anterior segment of the eye.

Rare adverse effects include burning or lacrimation. Blurred vision or visual disturbances, eye pain, headaches, ptosis, or enlarged pupils should be reported to the prescriber. For dosage and administration, refer to the current *USP DI* or to current package inserts.

What are the nursing management issues with using ophthalmic corticosteroid therapy?

Assessment Ophthalmic corticosteroid therapy is not used for pyogenic (pus-producing) inflammations of the eye because corticosteroids decrease defense mechanisms and reduce resistance to pathogenic organisms. Corticosteroid therapy is not recommended for minor corneal abrasions. Steroids may actually increase ocular susceptibility to fungal, viral, or tuberculosis infection. Cataracts and chronic open-angle glaucoma may be worsened. When steroids are used for various eye conditions, they should be used for a limited time only, and the eye should be checked for increased IOP. Corticosteroids may diminish the resistance to infection and may also mask the allergic reactions or hypersensitivity reactions to other drugs. A baseline assessment of the client's ocular inflammation and vision should be noted.

Nursing Diagnosis The client using ophthalmic corticosteroids is at risk for the following nursing diagnoses/collaborative problems: risk for injury related to ineffectiveness of the drug; impaired comfort (burning, stinging, or watering of the eyes); and the potential complications of hypersensitivity and the long-term effects of the drug (open-end glaucoma, optic nerve damage, infection, cataracts, defects in vision).

Planning The client receiving corticosteroid ophthalmic medications will:
* Remain free of signs and symptoms of inflammation of the eye.
* Return to normal vision or preinfection or predisorder status.
* Effectively manage drug regimen, including correct administration technique, compliance with medications and use of supportive measures (compresses, analgesics).
* Collaborate with health care providers, reporting adverse effects appropriately and maintaining scheduled appointment with health care providers for monitoring and treatment.

Implementation
Monitoring Periodic tonometry and slit-lamp examinations is performed to monitor client progress. Assess the eye for infection at periodic intervals; report any infection to the prescriber.

Intervention The glucocorticoids used in ophthalmology may be applied topically, injected into the conjunctiva by the ophthalmologist, or given systemically to diminish leukocyte infiltration where inflammation exists.

Education Alert the client that temporary stinging may occur after application. For adequate dispersion of the active ingredients, instruct the client to shake the ophthalmic suspensions well before use. Contact lenses should not be used during and for some time after corticosteroid therapy because of the risk of infection. Caution the client not to stop taking the medication without consulting the prescriber. The return of inflammation secondary to the abrupt cessation of ophthalmic steroid administration may be overcome by using dose-frequency reduction (from every 3 hours, to every 6 hours, to 3 times daily, to twice daily, to once daily, and to every other day) or by decreasing the percentage strengths and using the dose-frequency reduction schedule. This is typically done under the supervision of an ophthalmologist.

Evaluation The expected outcome of ophthalmic corticosteroid therapy is that the client's inflammation will be resolved (e.g., decreased pain, swelling, redness) without the occurrence of infection (e.g., purulent exudate). The client states signs and symptoms of infection of the eye and when to report them to the prescriber. The client/care giver demonstrates the correct method for instilling eye medication, medication compliance, and the use of supportive measures (e.g., use of compresses, proper eye cleansing, use of analgesics). Client shows improvement in visual acuity to normal vision or preinfection or predisorder status. Client maintains appointments with health care providers for monitoring and follow-up care.

❂ A.S. is a 63-year-old semi-retired construction worker who is diagnosed with glaucoma in his right eye on routine ophthalmologic examination.

❂ What is the pathology of glaucoma?

Glaucoma is an eye disease characterized chiefly by an abnormally elevated IOP, which may result from the excessive production of aqueous humor or diminished ocular fluid outflow. Increased pressure, if sufficiently high and persistent, may lead to irreversible blindness. Although glaucoma is primarily a disease of middle age—occurring in approximately 2% of all persons 40 years and older—it has also been diagnosed in younger adults and children. There are three major types of glaucoma: primary, secondary, and congenital.

Primary glaucoma includes angle-closure (acute congestive) glaucoma and open-angle (chronic simple) glaucoma (Figure 42-1). Persons with angle-closure glaucoma have closure of the angle of the anterior chamber, possibly because of a physiologic or anatomic predisposition. Drugs are needed to control the acute attack associated with angle-closure glaucoma; this is usually followed by surgery, such as iridectomy or laser surgery. Open- or wide-angle glaucoma is more common, occurring in approximately 90% of individuals with primary glaucoma. The increased IOP is secondary to an increased production of aqueous humor or a decreased outflow caused by degenerative changes in the outflow system. It has a gradual insidious onset, and its control depends on drug therapy or perhaps a peripheral iridectomy. Secondary glaucoma may result from previous eye disease or may follow cataract extraction (Abel & Sorensen, 2005). Therapy for secondary glaucoma usually involves drug therapy, whereas congenital glaucoma requires surgical treatment.

❂ A.S. is prescribed betaxolol (Betoptic) one drop to the right eye twice daily.

❂ What drugs are used to treat glaucoma?

Primary medications used to treat glaucoma include β-adrenergic blocking agents, prostaglandins, sympathomimetics, carbonic anhydrase inhibitors and cholinergics. The selection of a particular drug is determined largely by the requirements and individual response of the client. Preference is also given to agents that can be dosed more easily or less frequently to improve adherence. In severe cases, osmotic agents are given intravenously or orally to reduce IOP. In general, these agents do not cross the blood aqueous barrier into the anterior chamber of the eye and are rarely found in the ocular humor. (See Chapter 33 for a discussion of the osmotic agents.) Table 42-3 lists topical agents used to reduce IOP.

β-Adrenergic Blocking Agents

The β-adrenergic blocking agents administered topically in the eye include betaxolol (Betoptic), carteolol (Ocupress), levobunolol (Betagen), metipranolol (OptiPranolol), and timolol (Istalol, Timoptic). The systemic effects of β blockers are presented in Chapter 22. Betaxolol is a cardioselective (β_1) blocking agent, whereas all the other β blockers are noncardioselective and block both β_1- and β_2-adrenergic receptors. Timolol is also used to treat selected cases of secondary glaucoma. Betaxolol is indicated for the treatment of open-angle glaucoma and ocular hypertension and may be a drug of choice for clients with pulmonary disease because of its selective β_1-blocking effects; the nurse should still monitor for respiratory difficulties. Systemic effects can be minimized by applying pressure for 30 seconds to one minute over the inner canthus next to the nose. This prevents systemic absorption through the tear duct. These agents work alone or in combination with other drugs to

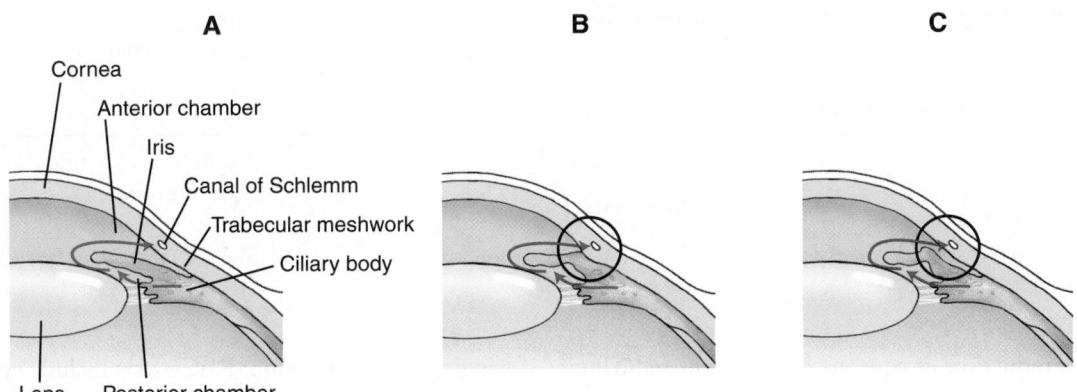

FIGURE 42-1 Main structures of the eye and enlargement of the canal of Schlemm showing aqueous flow in normal (**A**), angle-closure (**B**), and open-angle glaucoma (**C**).

TABLE 42-3 TOPICAL TREATMENTS FOR GLAUCOMA

Agent	Typical Adult Dose to Affected eye(s)	Comments
β-ADRENERGIC BLOCKERS		
betaxolol (Betoptic, Betoptic S)	0.25% or 0.5% twice daily	Apply pressure to inner canthus to reduce systemic absorption. Monitor for systemic effects including bradycardia and respiratory distress.
carteolol (Ocupress)	1% twice daily	
levobetaxolol (Betaxon)	0.5% twice daily	
levobunolol (Betagan)	0.25% or 0.5% daily or twice daily	
metipranolol (OptiPranolol)	0.3% twice daily	
timolol (Betimol, Istalol, Timoptic, Timoptic XE)	0.25% or 0.5% daily or twice daily	
PROSTAGLANDIN AGONISTS		
bimatoprost (Lumigan)	0.03% daily in PM	May cause pigmentation.
latanoprost (Xalatan)	0.005% daily in PM	
travoprost (Travatan)	0.004% daily in PM	
unoprostone (Rescula)	0.15% twice daily	
SYMPATHOMIMETICS		
apraclonidine (Iopidine)	0.5% or 1% two to three times daily	Apply pressure to inner canthus to reduce systemic absorption. Monitor for systemic effects including tachycardia.
brimonidine (Alphagan P)	0.15% three times daily	
dipivefrin (Propine)	0.1% twice daily	
epinephrine (Epifrin)	0.5%, 1% or 2% daily or twice daily	
phenylephrine (Neo-Synephrine)	10% three or four times daily 2.5% for ocular congestion	
DIRECT-ACTING CHOLINERGICS		
carbachol (Carbastat, Isopto Carbachol)	0.75%, 1.5%, 2.25% or 3% daily up to three times daily	Apply pressure to inner canthus to reduce systemic absorption. Monitor for systemic effects including wheezing, GI upset, dysrhythmias.
pilocarpine (Pilocar, others)	0.5%, 1%, 2%, 3%, 4%, 5%, 6%, 8% Drops: Three times daily up to six times daily Ointment: Once daily	
CHOLINESTERASE INHIBITOR		
echothiophate (Phospholine Iodide)	0.03%-0.25% daily or twice daily	Apply pressure to inner canthus to reduce systemic absorption.
CARBONIC ANHYDRASE INHIBITORS		
brinzolamide (Azopt)	1% three times daily	Monitor for allergic reactions, bitter taste.
dorzolamide (Trusopt)	2% three times daily	

Modified in part from Lacy, C.F., Armstrong, L.L., Goldman, M.P., & Lance, L.L. (2004). *Lexi-Comp's Drug Information Handbook*, (12th ed.). Hudson, Ohio: Lexi-Comp.

decrease the production of aqueous humor, thus reducing IOP in open-angle glaucoma. However, the exact mechanism of action for these agents is unknown.

The adverse effects of the β-adrenergic blocking ophthalmic agents are primarily local reactions, such as burning, stinging, or eye irritation. Rare effects include eye inflammation, visual disturbance, pruritus, or allergic reaction. These agents can be systemically absorbed to cause bradycardia or tachycardia, confusion, insomnia, weakness, wheezing, respiratory difficulties, depression, ataxia, edema of the lower ex-

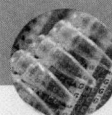 Special Considerations for Pharmacogenetics | OPHTHALMIC AGENTS

PHARMACODYNAMICS

Glaucoma is believed to have a genetic basis with genes correlated with glaucoma development (Challa, 2004). Further identification of the genetic basis for glaucoma might lead to earlier and more tailored therapy.

PHARMACOKINETICS

The metabolism of timolol eye drops and associated risk for systemic effects is related to the genetic potential for P450 2D6 metabolism (Lutz et al., 2002). It is unclear if this finding also impacts response to non–β-adrenergic blocker ophthalmic agents.

ADVERSE EFFECTS

Impaired or blurred vision is noted with a number of drugs, including proton pump inhibitors, but a genetic basis for this response has remained elusive (Lutz et al., 2002). Individuals who are slow acetylators and metabolize drugs more slowly are at higher risk for developing cataracts (Meyer et al., 2003). Identification of further methodologies may help predict who is more likely to develop cataracts with phenothiazine antipsychotics and corticosteroids.

---

tremities, nausea, and vomiting. Hallucinations have been reported with timolol only.

Betaxolol and timolol are among the most frequently used ophthalmic β-adrenergic blocking drugs.

betaxolol [beh **tax** oh lol]
(Betoptic)
Indications
The ophthalmic preparation of this product is indicated for chronic open-angle glaucoma and ocular hypertension.

Pharmacokinetics/Dosing
Onset of action of topical betaxolol is approximately 30 minutes with a duration of over 12 hours. Systemic absorption is possible with ophthalmic preparations and can be limited by applying pressure to the inner aspects of the eye during and after administration. Typical dose is one drop to affected eye(s) twice daily.

Adverse Effects
Redness, stinging, and eye pain are the more common adverse effects of betaxolol. If systemically absorbed, respiratory wheezing is possible, but less likely with this β_1-selective agent.

timolol [**tye** moe lole]
(Istalol, Timoptic, Apo-Timol✿, Apo-Timop✿, Gen-Timolol✿)
Indications
Ophthalmic administration of timolol is indicated elevated IOP or ocular hypertension.

Pharmacokinetics/Dosing
Similar to betaxolol. Systemic absorption is possible and can be limited with pressure to the inner canthus. Usual dose is one drop to affected eye(s) once or twice daily. Pharmacogenetic variation in response has been noted (see the Special Considerations for Pharmacogenetics box above).

Adverse Effects
As with betaxolol, but higher risk for bronchospasm if systemically absorbed because of β_2-adrenergic blocking actions.

✱ **A.S. follows up with the ophthalmologist over the next 2 months and IOP determinations in the right eye remain elevated. The ophthalmologist adds the prostaglandin latanoprost (Xalatan) one drop to the right eye daily in the evening.**

✱ **How are prostaglandins agonists used in treating glaucoma?**
Latanoprost (Xalatan) was the first prostaglandin agonist approved to treat open-angle glaucoma and ocular hypertension. It reduces IOP by increasing aqueous humor outflow. Other similar agents are bimatoprost (Lumigan), travoprost (Travatan) and unoprostone (Rescula). These agents are well tolerated, have a long duration of action, and are frequently chosen as first-line agents for clients who do not adequately respond to or cannot tolerate β-adrenergic blocking agents. Continuous use may result in developing a brown pigment in the eye.

latanoprost [la **tan** oh prost]
(Xalatan)
Indications
Latanoprost is indicated for reducing IOP in clients with glaucoma or ocular hypertension.

Pharmacokinetics/Dosing
Latanoprost's duration of action is in excess of 24 hours. Typical dosing is one drop to affected eye(s) once daily in the evening.

Adverse Effects
The adverse effects of latanoprost include blurred vision, burning and stinging, itching, photophobia, and conjunctival hyperemia. Clients should be informed that this drug may cause an increase in iris pigmentation (brown).

✱ **A.S. follows up with the ophthalmologist over the next six months and IOP determinations in the right eye remain elevated despite betaxolol and latanoprost. The ophthalmologist is considering addition of the sympathomimetic dipivefrin (Propine) or a topical carbonic anhydrase inhibitor, brinzolamide (Azopt).**

✱ **What is the role of sympathomimetics in glaucoma?**
The primary sympathomimetic agents are dipivefrin (Propine), which is converted to epinephrine by enzyme hydrolysis in the eye, and epinephrine, a direct-acting sympathomimetic agent. The chemical modification of dipivefrin

results in a more lipophilic compound that facilitates absorption and penetration through the cornea into the anterior chamber of the eye. The penetration and absorption of dipivefrin is greater than that of epinephrine.

Other ophthalmic sympathomimetics include apraclonidine (Iopidine), brimonidine (Alphagan), epinephrine (Epifrin) and phenylephrine (Neo-Synephrine). The mechanism of action of the sympathomimetic agents is unknown, but it appears that they lower IOP via action at α-adrenergic receptors by increasing aqueous humor outflow. This is in contrast to β-adrenergic blockers, which reduce the production of aqueous humor. Sympathomimetics are indicated for the treatment of open-angle glaucoma. Like the prostaglandin agents, the sympathomimetics are well tolerated and considered for clients who are not responsive to or cannot tolerate β-adrenergic blockers.

dipivefrin [dye pih **veh** frin]
(Propine)
Indications
Reducing IOP in ocular hypertension and open glaucoma.
Pharmacokinetics/Dosing
Onset of action of dipivefrin is approximately 30 minutes. The duration of action is approximately 12 hours. Systemic absorption is possible. The pediatric and adult dosage is 1 drop (0.1%) topically every 12 hours.
Adverse Effects
The adverse effects of the sympathomimetic ophthalmic agents are rarely troublesome; they include burning, stinging or eye irritation, headache, brow pain, and watering eyes. The signs and symptoms of systemic absorption include tachycardia, palpitations, hypertension, increased sweating, tremors, and light-headedness.

✳ What is the role of carbonic anhydrase inhibitors in treating glaucoma?
The carbonic anhydrase inhibitors are less well tolerated. The oral carbonic anhydrase inhibitors include the more widely used acetazolamide (Diamox) and dichlorphenamide (Daranide), and methazolamide (Neptazane). The carbonic anhydrase inhibitors are sulfonamides (nonbacteriostatic) with an undetermined mechanism of action, but they appear to lower IOP by decreasing the aqueous production to approximately one-half its baseline measurement.

The topical applied brinzolamide (Azopt) and dorzolamide (Trusopt) are carbonic anhydrase inhibitors that are systemically absorbed. Although not as effective as the oral agents in reducing IOPs, but do not have the same level of adverse effects as do the oral agents.

The oral drugs are used for the treatment of open-angle, secondary, and angle-closure glaucoma, whereas eyedrops are indicated for open-angle glaucoma and ocular hypertension. Adverse effects with the oral carbonic anhydrase inhibitor agents include diarrhea, discomfort, diuresis, anorexia, metallic taste in mouth, nausea, vomiting, weight loss, and tingling or numbness (paresthesia) of the fingers, hands, and toes. Prescriber intervention is necessary if the client has the signs and symptoms of acidosis, blood dyscrasias, or hypokalemia. The adverse effects of the eyedrops include a topical allergic reaction of the eye, a bitter

taste in the mouth, photosensitivity, and superficial punctate keratitis. Chapter 33 discusses acetazolamide in greater depth.

brinzolamide [brin **zoe** lah mide]
(Azopt)
Indications
Brinzolamide is indicated as second-line therapy for clients with elevated IOP or open-angle glaucoma.
Pharmacokinetics/Dosing
Systemic absorption contributes to its adverse effect profile. Although brinzolamide has a relatively long duration of action, it requires frequent dosing. It is typically dosed as a 1% suspension up to three times daily. The suspension should be shaken prior to administration.
Adverse Effects
Topical allergic reactions are among the most common adverse effects; also observed are photosensitivity, keratitis, and bitter taste.

dorzolamide [dor **zole** a mide]
(Trusopt)
Indications
As with brinzolamide.
Pharmacokinetics/Dosing
Dorzolamide, like brinzolamide, is systemically absorbed. Dosage is 2% solution to affected eye three times daily.
Adverse Effects
As with brinzolamide.

✳ What cholinergic drugs are available to treat elevated IOP?
The cholinergic agents have long been used for treating glaucoma, but their adverse effects render them second line therapy. Cholinergic medications or **miotics,** so called because they cause pupillary constriction, are topically applied agents useful in treating open-angle and angle-closure glaucoma. Cholinergic miotics (direct acting) are chemically related to acetylcholine, the neurotransmitter that mediates nerve impulse transmission at all cholinergic or parasympathetic nerve sites. When applied topically to the eye, cholinergic drugs cause contraction of the sphincter muscle of the iris. This action results in pupil constriction (miosis) and contraction of the ciliary muscle attached to the trabecular meshwork, thus opening the spaces in the meshwork and increasing the outflow of aqueous humor. The contracted ciliary muscle leaves the eye in accommodation of near vision.

Cholinergic miotics (direct-acting) drugs include carbachol (Carboptic) and pilocarpine (Isopto Carpine). Anticholinesterase drugs inhibit the enzymatic destruction of acetylcholine by activating cholinesterase. This action permits acetylcholine to act on the iris sphincter and ciliary muscles, producing pupil constriction (miosis) and ciliary muscle contraction (accommodation). The irreversible anticholinesterase drugs (echothiophate [Phospholine Iodide] and isoflurophate [Floropryl]) form stable complexes with cholinesterase and thus irreversibly impair the destructive function of the enzyme. The destruction of acetylcholine then depends on the synthesis of new enzymes. Demecarium (Humorsol) is more toxic than the other agents in this category and therefore is not as commonly used. Although it is a reversible inhibitor, its prolonged action has results similar to the irreversible inhibitors. The cholinesterase inhibitors are usually reserved for clients who respond inadequately to the first-line agents, such as β blockers, prostaglandins, cholinergics (pilocarpine), and sympathomimetics (dipivefrin).

The adverse effects of the cholinergic agents include visual blurring, irritation, myopia, ciliary spasm, brow pain, and headache resulting from the stimulation of accommodative ancillary muscles. Miosis also makes it difficult to adjust quickly to changes in illumination. This may be serious in older adults, because their light adaptation and visual acuity are often reduced. Nighttime is particularly hazardous for these individuals.

Cysts of the iris, synechiae (adhesions of the iris to the cornea or lens of the eye), retinal detachments, obstruction of tear drainage, and even cataracts may develop with prolonged use of cholinergic agents, especially with the long-acting anticholinesterases. In general, adverse effects caused by direct-acting cholinergic agents are less severe and occur less often than those caused by anticholinesterase agents. Systemic adverse effects include salivation, nausea, vomiting, diarrhea, precipitation of asthmatic attack, decrease in blood pressure, and other symptoms of parasympathetic stimulation.

Direct-Acting Cholinergic Agents

carbachol [**kar** ba kole]
(Carbastat)
Indications
Carbachol is indicated for the treatment of glaucoma. It is also effective for inducing miosis during surgery.
Pharmacokinetics/Dosing
The onset of action of carbachol is approximately 15 minutes and has a duration of up to 24 hours. Typical dose is one or two drops of the 0.75%, 1.5% or 3% solution to affected eye up to three times daily.
Adverse Effects
In addition to local irritation, systemic effects such as increased salivation, wheezing, or nausea and vomiting may occur if absorbed.

⭐◼◻ pilocarpine [pye loe **kar** peen]
(Isopto Carbine, Pilocar, Salagen)
Indications
Pilocarpine is used in the treatment of open-angle and closed-angle glaucoma. An oral formulation is available for treating severe xerostomia (dry mouth).
Pharmacokinetics/Dosing
Pilocarpine's onset of action for miosis is 10 to 30 minutes and about 1 hour for decreasing IOP. Duration of IOP reduction is 4 to 12 hours. Typical dose is one to two drops to affected eye up to six times daily for the 0.5%, 1%, 2%, or 4% solution.
Adverse Effects
As with carbachol.

Cholinesterase Inhibitors

echothiophate iodide [eck oh **thye** oh fate **eye** oh dide]
(Phospholine Iodide)
Indications
Echothiophate iodide is indicated for the treatment of open-angle and isolated cases of closed-angle glaucoma.

Pharmacokinetics/Dosing
Echothiophate produced miosis within 1 hour of administration and reduced IOP is observed within 4 hours. The cholinesterase inhibitors have a fairly long duration of action, typically 24 to 48 hours based on inhibition of acetylcholinesterase.
Adverse Effects
Adverse effects are as with carbachol but may be more pronounced. Application of pressure to the inner aspects of the eye for 1 minute during and after administration is encouraged to limit systemic absorption.

✴ What are the nursing implications of using these cholinergic agents to treat A.S.'s glaucoma?

Assessment Determine A.S.'s history of sensitivity to sulfites or the drug being used. Obtain baseline assessments of A.S.'s vision status, IOP, pupil size, and vital signs.

Betaxolol and Other β-Adrenergic Blocking Agents
Use caution when administering β-adrenergic blocking agents to A.S. if he has a positive history for bronchial asthma, severe chronic obstructive pulmonary disease, sinus bradycardia or greater than first-degree heart block, cardiogenic shock, or overt heart failure. There is sufficient absorption from the conjunctiva and nasopharynx to produce systemic nonselective β-adrenergic (β₁ and β₂) effects such as cardiopulmonary complications, exacerbation of asthma, and hypotension. Symptoms of hypoglycemia may be masked if these agents are used for clients with diabetes mellitus. These agents may mask symptoms of hyperthyroidism and precipitate a thyroid storm if suddenly discontinued. Because A.S.'s β blocking agent may be absorbed systemically, review his current medication regimen for drug interactions, such as those listed for systemic β-adrenergic blocking agents in Chapter 22.

Latanoprost and Other Prostaglandin Agonists Assess A.S. for aphakia (the absence of a crystalline lens), preexisting or a history of macular edema, or pseudophakia because latanoprost may contribute to macular edema.

Dipivefrin and Other Sympathomimetic Agents Sympathomimetic ophthalmic agents are contraindicated if A.S. has narrow-angle glaucoma or a predisposition to it, because pupil dilation may aggravate the condition. Dipivefrin or epinephrine may cause macular edema in clients with aphakia. Ophthalmic epinephrine should be administered with caution if A.S. has hypertension or other cardiovascular disease, hyperthyroidism, parkinsonism, asthma, or diabetes mellitus. A.S.'s drug history is reviewed to determine the risk for drug interactions. Epinephrine may be absorbed systemically to interact with ophthalmic β-blockers, digoxin, or monoamine oxidase (MAO) inhibitors.

Brinzolamide and Other Carbonic Anhydrase Inhibitors If the prescriber decides to add a topical carbonic anhydrase inhibitor, assess A.S.'s health status would be assessed for conditions that might indicate that carbonic anhydrase inhibitors are to be administered cautiously, such as if A.S. had adrenocortical insufficiency and would be more at risk for electrolyte imbalances. Reactions to sulfonamide agents (thiazide diuretic, oral sulfonylureas) raise suspicion for cross-sensitivity and hypersensitivity. Contraindications include clients with decreased sodium/potassium serum levels or other electrolyte imbalances, or hepatic or renal dysfunction (potential for renal calculi formation). For potential drug interaction, see Chapter 33. In addition to the previous baseline assessment of the client's vision, IOP, ocular pain, vital signs, include an urinalysis (UA), CBC, platelet count, and serum electrolytes.

Nursing Diagnosis While taking any antiglaucoma medication, A.S. is at risk for altered comfort (stinging of eye or other eye irritation on administration of the medication and increased sensitivity of eye to light), risk for infection related to improper administration of ophthalmic medication, and risk for injury related to transient blurred vision and decreased night vision.

With β-adrenergic blocking ophthalmic agents, A.S. is at risk for the potential complication of decreased cardiac output (hypotension, decreased heart rate) and other symptoms related to systemic absorption of the drug. With latanoprost, he may experience the potential complication of increased pigmentation of the iris, eyelashes, and periorbital tissue.

While receiving sympathomimetic ophthalmic solution, A.S. is at risk, if the agent is absorbed systemically, for the potential complication of altered cardiac output (tachycardia, hypertension).

With carbonic anhydrase inhibitors, A.S. is at risk for impaired comfort in a variety of ways, including metallic taste, dry eye, and rhinitis.

Planning The client receiving antiglaucoma ophthalmic medications will:

- Remain free of signs and symptoms of glaucoma without adverse effects of the drug.
- Return to normal vision or preglaucoma status.
- Effectively manage drug regimen, including correct administration technique and compliance with medications.
- Collaborate with health care providers, reporting adverse effects appropriately and maintaining scheduled appointment with health care providers for monitoring and treatment.

Implementation

Monitoring To ensure the effectiveness of therapy, the prescriber evaluates A.S.'s condition at periodic intervals throughout therapy with fundus and IOP examinations. Assess for decreased visual acuity and ocular discomfort. Monitor the eye for inflammation; although these agents are usually well tolerated, occasional signs of mild ocular irritation may occur. Local hypersensitivity (rash) occurs rarely. Obtain periodic pulse and blood pressure determinations to assess for systemic effects such as tachycardia and elevated blood pressure with sympathomimetics, or hypotension, bradycardia, or wheezing with the β-adrenergic blocking agents.

Any eye medication is discontinued if signs of hypersensitivity or other serious reactions occur.

Intervention Wait 10 minutes between using two different ophthalmic preparation to avoid "washing out" one with the other. Shake ophthalmic suspensions well before administering.

Review A.S.'s regimen carefully if the prescriber decides to add the sympathomimetic dipivefrin with other antiglaucoma ophthalmic solutions. Although the dipivefrin is not replacing epinephrine in A.S.'s case, but if it were, the epinephrine is discontinued when the dipivefrin is started. If dipivefrin were to replace something other than epinephrine, that agent is discontinued on the second day of dipivefrin administration. If administered in addition to other antiglaucoma agents, dipivefrin is given at the usual adult dosage.

To minimize systemic absorption, maintain pressure on the lacrimal sac during and for 1 to 2 minutes after instillation of these drugs.

Education Review with A.S. the safe and accurate techniques for the self-administration of ophthalmic agents. Stress the importance of compliance with antiglaucoma drugs. Advise him to wear sunglasses and avoid bright light. A.S. should ask his prescriber about the use of contact lenses during therapy. Instruct him about which symptoms to report to the prescriber. Instruct A.S. to alert health practitioners to his drug therapy if surgery is considered; some prescribers recommend that these agents be gradually withdrawn 48 hours before surgery. Encourage regular consultation with the prescriber to check IOP.

If he has diabetes, alert him that symptoms of hypoglycemia may be masked, such as tachycardia and trembling with β-adrenergic blocking agents. Alert A.S. that his eyelashes may become longer, thicker, and darker, and the iris and skin around the eye may also become darker. This hyperpigmentation may be reason to discontinue latanoprost.

Evaluation The expected outcome of these antiglaucoma drugs is that A.S. will experience a therapeutic reduction in IOP without experiencing clinically significant, systemic responses. The expected outcome of latanoprost therapy is it contributes to decreased IOP without significant hyperpigmentation of the iris and periorbital tissue. A.S. states significant adverse signs and symptoms of eye pain, redness, drainage and when to report them to the prescriber. He demonstrates the correct method for instilling eye medication. A.S. shows improvement in visual acuity to normal vision or preglaucoma status. He effectively manages his medication regimen, maintaining medication compliance and collaborating with health care providers for monitoring and follow-up care.

❋ What drugs are used during ophthalmic evaluations?

Both anticholinergics (antimuscarinics) and adrenergic agonists are used to produce pupil dilation (mydriasis), and cycloplegic agents paralyze ciliary muscle, impairing accommodation. These agents are used primarily for the diagnosis of ophthalmic disorders. The effects of these agents depend on the client's age, race, and color of iris. For example, mydriatic agents evoke less of a response in persons with heavily pigmented (dark) irides than in those with lighter pigmented (blue) irides. Topical anesthetics are also used during ophthalmic evaluations.

Anticholinergics

Anticholinergic agents are indicated for the treatment of inflammations such as uveitis and keratitis; they relieve ocular pain by relaxing inflamed intraocular muscles. They are also used for the relaxation of ciliary muscle to allow accurate measurement of refractive errors (which permits proper lens determination for eyeglasses) and for preoperative and postoperative use in intraocular surgery. Contraction of the iris sphincter by anticholinergics leads to relaxation and a possible increase in IOP and should be avoided in clients with glaucoma. Atropine, the classic anticholinergic, is not used clinically because of its long-lasting effects.

Local adverse effects that are reported with the use of anticholinergic ophthalmic agents include stinging or an increase in IOP. Allergic lid reactions, red eye, and various eye irritation injuries may be induced with chronic use. Systemic absorption of these agents may result in mild to serious adverse effects such as dryness of the mouth, inhibition of sweating, flushing, tachycardia, ataxia, hallucinations, psychiatric and behavioral problems, fever, delirium, seizures, respiratory depression, and coma. Deaths have been recorded in children after systemic absorption. Pupillary dilation from either local or systemic administration can precipitate acute glaucoma in persons with a predisposition to this condition. Blindness can result if this condition is left unrecognized or untreated.

Adrenergic Agonists

Topical adrenergic agents mimic (direct acting) or potentiate (indirect acting) the action of epinephrine on the dilator muscle of the iris; this results in mydriasis and decreased congestion of the conjunctival blood vessels. The adrenergic drugs used in ophthalmology include the agents used primarily for glaucoma (discussed above—epinephrine [Epifrin], dipivefrin [Propine], phenylephrine [Ak-Nefrin, Prefrin, Neo-Synephrine]), and those used primarily for their vasoconstrictive properties to improve conjunctival erythema (naphazoline [Allerest, VasoClear, Vasocon], and tetrahydrozoline [Murine Plus, Visine]).

Adrenergic drugs applied topically to the eye elicit the following sympathetic responses: vasoconstriction, pupil dilation, an increase in the outflow of aqueous humor, a decrease in aqueous humor formation, and relaxation of the ciliary muscle. Exactly how these effects are produced remains un-

certain, but there is some evidence that α-adrenergic receptors are present in the outflow mechanism of the eye. When stimulated, they increase outflow of aqueous humor. It has also been shown experimentally that vasoconstriction decreases the rate of aqueous humor formation (Abel, 2005).

Adrenergic drugs are used to treat wide-angle glaucoma and glaucoma secondary to uveitis, to produce mydriasis for ocular examination, and to relieve congestion and hyperemia. Adrenergic drugs are contraindicated in the treatment of narrow-angle glaucoma or abraded cornea because dilation of the pupil will further restrict ocular fluid outflow, which may cause an acute attack of glaucoma.

Serious systemic adverse effects are unusual; typical undesired effects include local pain and brow ache. Systemic absorption may be a concern for clients with cardiovascular disease, because tachycardia and elevated blood pressure can occur with these agents. Sweating, tremors, and confusion may also occur. As with other ophthalmic drugs, the potential for systemic drug interactions exists if significant absorption occurs.

Combinations of anticholinergic and adrenergic agonist eyedrops include Cyclomydril and Murocoll-2. These agents in combination produce a greater mydriasis than either drug alone. Table 42-4 presents anticholinergics, adrenergic agonists, and combination drugs.

Topical Anesthetics

Local anesthetics stabilize neuronal membranes so they become less permeable to ions; this prevents the initiation and transmission of nerve impulses. It is theorized that sodium ion permeability is limited by these agents. Local anesthetics are used to prevent pain during surgical procedures (removal of sutures and foreign bodies) and tonometry examinations. The local anesthetics have a rapid onset (within 20 seconds) and last for 15 to 20 minutes. Classic agents include tetracaine and proparacaine.

tetracaine [**tet** ra kane]
(Pontocaine)
Indications
Tetracaine is a widely used anesthetic used topically for rapid, brief, superficial anesthesia.
Pharmacokinetics/Dosing
One to two drops of a 0.5% solution will produce anesthesia within 30 seconds; the client may feel a burning or stinging sensation. The anesthetic effect lasts for 10 to 15 minutes.
Adverse Effects
Tetracaine can cause epithelial damage and systemic toxicity and therefore is not recommended for prolonged home use by clients.
Drug Interactions
Tetracaine is physically incompatible with the mercury or silver salts often found in ophthalmic products.

proparacaine [proe **par** a kane]
(Ophthaine, Ophthetic)
Indications
Indications for proparacaine are similar to tetracaine.

TABLE 42-4 MYDRIATIC AND CYCLOPLEGIC AGENTS

ANTICHOLINERGICS FOR MYDRIASIS OR CYCLOPLEGIA

Agent	Typical Adult Dose	Onset Mydriasis	Recovery Mydriasis	Onset Cycloplegia	Recovery Cycloplegia
atropine (Isopto Atropine)	1% × 1 drop	30-40 min	7-10 days	60-180 min	6-12 days
cyclopentolate (Cyclogyl)	0.5%-2% × 1 drop	30-60 min	1 day	25-75 min	6-24 hr
homatropine (Isopto Homatropine)	2%-5% × 1 drop	40-60 min	1-3 days	30-60 min	1-3 days
scopolamine (Isopto Hyoscine)	0.25% × 1 drop	20-130 min	3-7 days	30-60 min	3-7 days
tropicamide (Mydriacil)	0.5%-1% × 1 drop	20-40 min	6 hr	30 min	6 hr

ADRENERGICS

Agent	Typical Adult Dose	Indications
epinephrine (Epifrin)	0.5%, 1%, or 2% daily or twice daily	Glaucoma, increased IOP
naphazoline (Vasocon)	0.012%, 0.03%, or 0.1% up to four times daily	Ocular congestion
phenylephrine (Neo-Synephrine)	Glaucoma: 10% three to four times daily Mydriasis/Cycloplegia: 2.5%-10% × 1 drop Uveitis: 10% three to four times daily Ocular congestion: 2.5% q3-4h PRN	IOP Mydriasis/Cycloplegia Anterior uveitis Ocular congestion
tetrahydrozoline (Visine)	0.05% four times daily PRN	Ocular congestion

COMBINATION ANTICHOLINERGICS/ADRENERGICS

Agent	Typical Adult Dose	Indications
cyclopentolate 0.2% phenylephrine 1% (Cyclomydril)	0.2%/1%: one drop q5-10min up to three times daily	Mydriasis
phenylephrine 10% scopolamine hydrobromide 0.3% (Murocoll-2)	10%/0.3%: one drop × 1, may repeat in 5 min × 1	Mydriasis, cycloplegia, iritis

IOP, Intraocular pressure.

Pharmacokinetics/Dosing

A 0.5% solution is administered by topical instillation. Anesthesia is produced within 20 seconds and lasts for 15 minutes.

Adverse Effects

Proparacaine is relatively free from the burning and discomfort of other anesthetics, but it is highly toxic if it enters the systemic circulation. Adverse effects include allergic contact dermatitis, softening and erosion of the corneal epithelium, pupillary dilation, cycloplegia, conjunctival congestion and hemorrhage, stromal edema, and delayed corneal healing after photorefractive keratectomy.

✳ What are the nursing implications of drugs used during ophthalmic evaluations?

Assessment Anticholinergic and adrenergic agonist therapy are used with caution in clients with primary glaucoma or a predisposition to angle-closure glaucoma. Dilation of the pupil causes a narrowing of the iridocorneal angle in which the canal of Schlemm is located. This restricts the drainage of intraocular fluids and because secretion continues, the IOP rises. This may precipitate an attack of acute glaucoma.

Obtain a baseline assessment of the client's vision status and IOP.

Nursing Diagnosis The client receiving anticholinergics or adrenergic agonists for ophthalmic examination is at risk for the following nursing diagnoses: disturbed sensory perception related to blurred vision and increased sensitivity of the eyes to light; impaired tissue integrity related to eye irritation not present before therapy and swelling of the eyelids; and risk for injury related to systemic absorption (confusion, dizziness, dryness of skin, fever, slurred speech, tachycardia, drowsiness, dryness of the mouth).

With topical anesthetics of the eye, the client is at risk for injury due to loss of sensation of the eye.

Planning The client receiving ophthalmic medications during an eye examination will:

- Experience pupil dilation during the ophthalmic examination and/or anesthesia.
- Take precautions to prevent injury until the medications wear off.
- Collaborate with health care providers, report adverse effects appropriately and maintain scheduled appointments with health care providers for monitoring and treatment of ophthalmic disorders and/or routine eye exams.

Implementation

Monitoring The client's IOP and vision is monitored during the ophthalmic examination. The potential for systemic adverse effects of anticholinergics is more pronounced in infants, young children, children with blond hair or blue eyes, clients with Down syndrome, children with brain damage, and older adults. Monitor these clients for a fast, irregular pulse, skin dryness, confusion, slurred speech, dry mouth, fever, and unusual drowsiness or weakness.

Intervention If the ointment form is to be used for refraction, apply it several hours before the vision examination to minimize any impairment of corneal transparency.

Although 2 drops are the recommended dosage by some manufacturers, the conjunctival sac will usually hold only 1 drop. To minimize systemic absorption, the lacrimal duct should be compressed during administration of the drops and for 2 to 3 minutes after administration.

The practice of repeatedly applying a topical anesthetic agent to the eye will delay wound healing and produce sensitivity, permanent corneal opacification, vision loss, or perforation of the cornea. Patching the anesthetized eye is prudent because the blink reflex is lost, and the cornea needs to be protected from debris and irritants.

Education Alert the client that he or she may be unable to focus on nearby objects during therapy (blurred vision) and will be unusually sensitive to light. Dark glasses are worn to decrease the photophobia. The eye will be accommodated for distant vision.

To prevent damage to the eye during use of a topical anesthetic agent, instruct the client not to touch or rub the eye until the anesthetic agent has worn off.

Evaluation The expected outcome of anticholinergic ophthalmic therapy is that the client will experience cycloplegia. If administered for uveitis, the condition will be alleviated as evidenced by a lack of discomfort, redness, and drainage from the eye.

The expected outcome of topical ophthalmic anesthetic agent therapy is that the client will experience no discomfort and experience no adverse effects or injuries.

⚹ **What other ophthalmic preparations are available?**

A myriad of other ophthalmic agents are available to lubricate the eye, prevent or treat allergies, reduce inflammation, facilitate diagnostics, and irrigate the eye. Representative agents are listed in the following sections.

Artificial Tear Solutions and Lubricants

Lubricants or artificial tears are used to provide moisture and lubrication for diseases in which tear production is deficient, to lubricate artificial eyes and moisten contact lenses, to remove debris, and to protect the cornea during procedures on the eye. These agents are also incorporated into ophthalmic preparations to prolong the contact time of topically applied drugs.

These products have a balanced salt solution (equivalent to 0.9% sodium chloride), buffers to adjust pH, highly viscous agents (methylcellulose, propylene glycol, and others) to extend contact time with the eye, and preservatives to maintain sterility. These products are usually administered three or four times daily.

An artificial tear insert (Lacrisert) was devised to extend the effect of this preparation. It is usually inserted daily or at most twice daily for selected clients.

Ointment preparations are also used as ocular lubricants. They help to protect the eye, such as during and after eye surgery, and to lubricate the eye. They are particularly valuable for clients who have an impaired blink reflex (e.g., sedated clients in surgery or critical care) and for nighttime use. Examples include Lacri-Lube, Duratears, and Hypo Tears.

Antiallergic Agents

Antiallergic ophthalmic agents available include ophthalmic antihistamine and mast cell stabilizers. The histamine 1 (H_1) blockers available in ophthalmic formulations include azelastine (Optivar), epinastine (Elestat), emedastine (Emadine), levocabastine (Livostin) olopatadine (Patanol). Like the oral products, they serve as antagonists at the H_1 receptor and reduce symptoms of erythema and tearing. The mast cell stabilizers include cromolyn (Crolom, Opticrom), lodoxamide (Alomide), nedocromil (Alocril), and pemirolast (Alamast). Cromolyn sodium inhibits the degranulation of sensitized mast cells that occurs after exposure to a specific antigen. This inhibition of mast cell release prevents the mediators of inflammation (histamine and slow-releasing substance of anaphylaxis) from producing their characteristic effects. To be effective, they must be used regularly (not on an as needed basis) to prevent degranulation of the mast cell. Ketotifen (Zaditor) possesses both H_1 antagonist and mast cell stabilizing properties. Chapter 37 discusses H_1 antagonists and mast cell stabilizers in greater depth. A few representative agents are presented here. Lodoxamide ophthalmic is another antiallergic and mast cell stabilizer used for allergic ophthalmic reactions.

✱🔲 levocabastine [lee voe **kab** as teen]
(Livostin)

Indications
Levocabastine is a topical antihistamine indicated for allergic conjunctivitis.

Dosing
The usual adult dosage is 1 drop in the eyes four times daily.

Adverse Effects
The adverse effects are mild and consist of burning, stinging, visual alterations, eye pain, red eyes, and headaches.

cromolyn sodium [**kroe** moe lin]
(Crolom, Opticrom, Apo-Cromolyn✦)

Indications
Cromolyn sodium ophthalmic is used for allergic eye disorders (vernal and allergic keratoconjunctivitis, papillary conjunctivitis, keratitis) that have symptoms of itching, tearing, redness, and discharge.

Dosing
In adults and children over 4 years of age, instill 1 drop of 4% solution in each affected eye four to six times daily at regular intervals.

Adverse Effects
The adverse effects of cromolyn sodium include a stinging and burning sensation in the eyes. Concomitant corticosteroids may be necessary, but are usually avoided if infection is present.

lodoxamide [loe **dox** a myde]
(Alomide)

Indications
Lodoxamide is used for the treatment of vernal conjunctivitis, vernal keratitis, and several other eye disorders. Lodoxamide inhibits Type I immediate hypersensitivity reactions by interfering with histamine release, and it inhibits the release of SRS-A and eosinophil chemotaxis.

Dosing
The usual dosage for adults and children 2 years and older is 1 drop of 0.1% solution in each affected eye four times daily for up to 3 months (*Drug Facts and Comparisons*, 2005).

Adverse Effects
The adverse effects of lodoxamide include a transient burning of the eye. Less commonly reported effects are blurred vision, pruritus of the eye, tearing, or eye irritation.

ketotifen fumarate [kee toe **tih** fen]
(Zaditor)

Indications
Ketotifen is a histamine antagonist with mast cell–stabilizing properties. It is used to treat allergic conjunctivitis.

Dosing
The usual adult dosage is 1 drop in the affected eye(s) every 8 to 12 hours.

✳ What are the nursing implications for ophthalmic antiallergy agents?

Assess the client for itching, tearing, redness, and discharge from the eyes. Determine the client's sensitivity to the drug. The client receiving antiallergy agents should be assessed for the following nursing diagnoses/collaborative problems: risk for injury related to the ineffectiveness of the drug; impaired comfort (burning, stinging, sensation of foreign body); and the potential complications of hypersensitivity or chemosis (severe swelling of the conjunctiva). Note that the signs and symptoms of relief will appear within days but that treatment may be required at regular intervals for as long as 6 weeks. Refrigerate cromolyn, keep it out of direct sunlight, and dis-

card any unused portion after 4 weeks. Although manufacturers recommend not wearing soft contact lenses while using antiallergy solution, medical experts believe this precaution is unnecessary in most instances. Have the client check with the prescriber about contact lens use before using the drug. The expected outcome of antiallergy agents is that client's eyes will not evidence an allergic reaction; itching, tearing, redness, and discharge will not be present.

Ophthalmic Diagnostic Aids

fluorescein [fluh **ress** ee in]
(Fluorescite, Fluor-I-Strip)

Fluorescein is a nontoxic, water-soluble dye that is used as a diagnostic aid. When applied to the cornea, corneal lesions or ulcers are stained a bright green, and foreign bodies appear to be surrounded by a green ring. These effects permit the location of foreign bodies and corneal epithelial defects caused by injury or infection. Fluorescein dye is also used in fitting hard contact lenses. Areas that lack fluorescein-stained tears will appear black under ultraviolet light, indicating that the contact lens is touching the cornea at those areas. Fluorescein is used in retinal photography to determine retinal vascular status and to identify defects in the retinal pigment epithelium. Additionally, it may be used to test the patency of the lacrimal apparatus; if the dye appears in the nasal secretions after being instilled into the eye, the nasolacrimal drainage system is open. A fluorescein injection is used in ophthalmic angiography to examine the fundus, vasculature of the iris, and aqueous flow; to make a differential diagnosis of cancerous and noncancerous tumors; and to determine the time for circulation in the eye.

Indications
Fluorescein is an ophthalmic dye used in diagnostics.

Dosing
If a topical solution is being used to detect foreign bodies and corneal abrasions, instill 1 or 2 drops of the 2% solution. Check a current drug reference for instructions regarding strip application and injection.

Adverse Effects
Topical application is well tolerated. Reactions after injection include nausea, headache, abdominal distress, vomiting, hypotension, hypersensitivity reactions, and anaphylaxis.

Enzyme Preparations

chymotrypsin [kye moe **trip** sin]
(Catarase)

Chymotrypsin, a proteolytic enzyme, is used in selected cases to facilitate cataract extraction. It is injected by an ophthalmologist behind the iris and into the posterior chamber to dissolve the filaments or zonules that hold the lens; this facilitates intracapsular lens extraction.

Indications
Chymotrypsin is used to facilitate lens extraction during cataract surgery

Pharmacokinetics/Dosing
Desired effect is usually obtained in 5 to 15 minutes, with total lysis of the entire zonular membrane reported within 30 minutes.

Adverse Effects
Adverse effects include a transient postoperative glaucoma that lasts approximately 1 week; this effect can be relieved by the use of pilocarpine.

Hyperosmolar Preparation

sodium chloride
(ointment: Muro-128, solution: Adsorbonac)
Highly osmotic saline is sometimes used topically to reduce local edema.

Indications

The 5% ointment and 2% or 5% solution of sodium chloride are used to reduce the corneal edema that occurs in certain corneal dystrophies and after cataract extraction.

Dosing

The dosage is 1 to 2 drops of solution in the affected eye(s) every 3 to 4 hours as directed. A small amount of the 5% ointment is administered to the affected eye once daily or as needed.

Ophthalmic Nonsteroidal Antiinflammatory Agents

Flurbiprofen, suprofen, diclofenac, and ketorolac tromethamine are available topically for ophthalmic use. These agents are nonsteroidal antiinflammatory drugs (NSAIDs) with various antiinflammatory indications. Flurbiprofen (Acular) and suprofen (Profenal) are used to inhibit intraoperative miosis, diclofenac (Voltaren, Diclotec❋, Novo-Difenac❋) is used to treat postoperative inflammation after cataract extraction whereas ketorolac is used to treat conjunctivitis and seasonal allergic ophthalmic pruritus. Flurbiprofen is presented here as an example.

flurbiprofen [flure **bi** proe fin]
(Ocufen, Froben❋)
Indications
Flurbiprofen is used to inhibit intraoperative miosis.
Dosing
Flurbiprofen is typically dosed one drop to affected eye every 30 minutes for 2 hours prior to surgery for a total of four drops.
Adverse Effects
These agents may produce a systemic effect if absorbed. Because they have the potential to cause increased bleeding, monitor their use closely in clients who are known to have bleeding tendencies. The most commonly reported adverse effect is transient burning or stinging on application. Other minor symptoms of ocular irritation have also been reported, such as itching, redness, discomfort, allergic reaction.
Nursing Management
For the nursing management of NSAIDs, see the nursing management of drugs affecting the eye, p. 784. Additionally, it should be determined if the client has a sensitivity to aspirin, phenylacetic acid derivatives, such as diclofenac, or other ophthalmic or systemic NSAIDs.

Agents for Severe Inflammation-Associated Ocular Dryness

Cyclosporine, an immunomodulator used to prevent organ transplant rejection and sometimes used in autoimmune diseases like rheumatoid arthritis and severe psoriasis (see Chapter 63), is available as an ophthalmic agent in the treatment of keratoconjunctivitis sicca. It is not recommended for use for mild to moderate cases of dry eye. Cyclosporine 0.05% ophthalmic suspension (Restasis) is typically dosed in adults as a single drop to each eye every 12 hours. The adverse effects of cyclosporine administered systemically is associated with significant interactions and potential for adverse effects. The most common adverse effect of the ophthalmic preparation is burning or eye irritation. Serious reactions or interactions have yet to be noted with ophthalmic use, but an increased risk for ophthalmic infection may be possible given its immunosuppressive action.

Irrigating Solutions

Sterile isotonic external irrigating solutions are used in tonometry, fluorescein procedures, and the removal of foreign material. They are also used to cleanse and soothe the eyes of clients who wear hard contact lenses. These external products do not require a prescription and are available as drops, irrigations, and eyewashes. Examples of irrigating solutions include Blinx, Dacriose, Eye Stream, and Eye Wash.

Summary

Although there are a myriad of ophthalmic preparations, the drugs used to treat eye disorders can be divided into three major groups: the antiinfective/antiinflammatory, antiglaucoma agents, and the mydriatics and cycloplegics. Antiinfective/antiinflammatory agents used in the treatment of ocular infections may be antibacterial agents, antifungal agents, or antiviral agents, antiallergics, corticosteroids, and NSAIDs.

Antiglaucoma agents may be miotics. These cause pupillary constriction either by (1) direct action (cholinergic) to minimize the effects of acetylcholine at autonomic synapses or the neuroeffector junction of the parasympathetic nervous system, or (2) indirect action (anticholinesterase), inactivating the enzyme cholinesterase by preventing hydrolysis of acetylcholine. Antiglaucoma drugs may be α-adrenergic agents that increase the outflow of aqueous humor or β-adrenergic blockers that reduce aqueous humor production. Carbonic anhydrase inhibitor agents and osmotic agents are also used in the treatment of glaucoma.

Mydriatic and cycloplegic agents used for ophthalmic disorders are topically applied autonomic drugs that cause dilation of the pupils (mydriasis) and paralysis of accommodation (cycloplegia). In addition to being used for the specific treatment of ophthalmic disorders, they are also used during eye examinations and in preparation of the client for intraocular surgery.

The role of the nurse in the clinical management of the client receiving ophthalmic drugs focuses on safe administration and the preparation of the client for the self-administration of these drugs.

✳ Critical Thinking Questions
- How would the teaching plan for the self-administration of ophthalmic agents vary among antiglaucoma agents, antiinfective agents, and corticosteroids?
- Steve Cameron has had his ophthalmic medication changed from an optic solution to an optic ointment. What instruction will you provide Mr. Cameron to prepare him for safe self-administration of the new form of medication?

Bibliography

Abdollahi, M., Shafiee, A., Bathaiee, F.S., Sharifzadeh, M., & Nikfar, S. (2004). Drug-induced toxic reactions in the eye: An overview. *Journal of Infusion Nursing, 27*(6):386-398.

Abel, S.R., & Sorensen, S.J. (2005). Eye disorders. In M.A. Koda-Kimble, L.Y. Young, W.A. Kradian, B.J. Guglielmo, B.K. Alldredge, & R.L. Corelli. (Eds.), *Applied therapeutics: The clinical use of drugs* (8th ed.). Philadelphia: Lippincott Williams & Wilkins.

Anderson, D.M., Keith, J., & Novak, P.D. (Eds.) (2002). *Mosby's medical, nursing, and allied health dictionary* (6th ed.). St. Louis: Mosby.

Bosker, G. (Ed.). (2004). *Primary and acute care medicine: Practice, protocols, pathways,* (2nd ed.). Atlanta: Thomson American Health Consultants.

Challa P. (2004) Glaucoma genetics: Advancing new understandings of glaucoma pathogenesis. *International Ophthalmology Clinics, 44*(2):167-185.

Drug facts and comparisons (58th ed.). (2005). St. Louis: Facts and Comparisons.

Edeki, T.I., He, H., & Wood, A.J. (1995). Pharmacogenetic explanation for excessive beta-blockade following timolol eye drops: Potential for oral-ophthalmic drug interaction. *Journal of the American Medical Association, 274*(20):1611-1613.

Hardman, J.G., & Limbird, L.E. (Eds.). (2001). *Goodman & Gilman's The pharmacological basis of therapeutics* (10th ed.). New York: McGraw-Hill.

Lacy, C.F., Armstrong, L.L., Goldman, M.P., & Lance, L.L. (2004). *Lexi-Comp's Drug Information Handbook* (12th ed.). Hudson, Ohio: Lexi-Comp.

Lesar, T.S. (2002). Glaucoma. In DiPiro, J.T., Talbert, R.L., Yee, G.C., Matzke, G.R., Wells, B.G., & Posey, L.M. (Eds.), *Pharmacotherapy: A Pathophysiological Approach* (5th ed.). New York: McGraw-Hill.

Lutz, M., et al. (2002) Visual disorders associated with omeprazole and their relation to CYP2C19 polymorphism. *Pharmacogenetics, 12*(1):73-75.

Meyer, D., et al. (2003). NAT2 slow acetylator function as a risk indicator for age-related cataract formation. *Pharmacogenetics, 13*(5):285-289.

Mosby's drug consult (15th ed.). (2005). St. Louis: Mosby.

Riordan-Eva, P. (2003). Eye. In Tierney, L.M. Jr., McPhee, S.J., & Papadakis, M.A. (Eds.), *Current Medical Diagnosis & Treatment.* New York: Lange Medical Books/McGraw-Hill.

USP DI: Drug information for the health care professional (25th ed.). (2005). Greenwood Village, CO: MICROMEDEX Thomson Healthcare.

e-LEARNING SUPPLEMENTS

Student CD-ROM
- Final Exam questions
- NCLEX® Examination review questions
- Pharmacology animations
- Printable chapter summary

Evolve Website (http://evolve.elsevier.com/mckenry)
- Case study on ophthalmic drugs
- Content updates, including information on new drugs

- WebLinks corresponding to this chapter
- Answers to the critical thinking questions in this chapter
- *Elsevier ePharmacology Update* newsletter
- Mosby's Drug Consult Internet Edition
- Supplemental and reference information

43

OVERVIEW OF THE EAR

CHAPTER FOCUS

Disorders of the ear can be painful and impair the client's ability to hear and maintain balance. Pharmacologic interventions for the ear are somewhat limited. However, many systemic drugs have ototoxic effects. To appropriately assess and care for clients with ear disorders, the nurse needs to have a thorough understanding of the anatomy and physiology of the ear.

LEARNING OBJECTIVES

- Differentiate between the external, middle, and inner ear with respect to structure and function.
- Identify the three bones of the inner ear.
- Describe the function of the eustachian tube.
- List disorders that commonly affect the ear.

▲ KEY TERMS

auditory ossicles, p. 805
cochlea, p. 806
eustachian tube, p. 805
external ear, p. 805

inner ear, p. 806
middle ear, p. 805
otitis media, p. 806
tympanic membrane, p. 805

✳ **What are the key anatomic and physiologic features of the ear?**

The ear consists of three sections or parts: external ear, middle ear, and inner ear (Figure 43-1). The **external ear** has two divisions, the outer ear (or pinna) and the external auditory canal. The external auditory canal leads to the eardrum (or **tympanic membrane**), which is a thin, transparent partition of tissue between the auditory canal and the middle ear. The function of the external ear is to receive and transmit auditory sounds to the eardrum. The tympanic membrane protects the middle ear from foreign substances and transmits sound to the bones of the middle ear.

The **middle ear** is an air-filled cavity in the temporal bone that contains three small bones called the **auditory ossicles.** The auditory ossicles consist of the malleus (ham-

mer), incus (anvil), and stapes (stirrup). The tip of the malleus is attached to the surface of the tympanic membrane. Its head is attached to the incus, which in turn is attached to the stapes. The ossicles amplify and transmit sound waves to the inner ear.

The middle ear is also directly connected to the nasopharynx by the eustachian (auditory) tube. The **eustachian tube** is usually collapsed except during swallowing, chewing, yawning, or jaw movements. This tube joins the nasopharynx and the tympanic cavity, which allows for the equalization of air pressure in the inner ear with atmospheric pressure to prevent the tympanic membrane from rupturing. Pressure changes on airline flights are relieved by the action of the eustachian tube when the individual chews gum, yawns, or deliberately swallows.

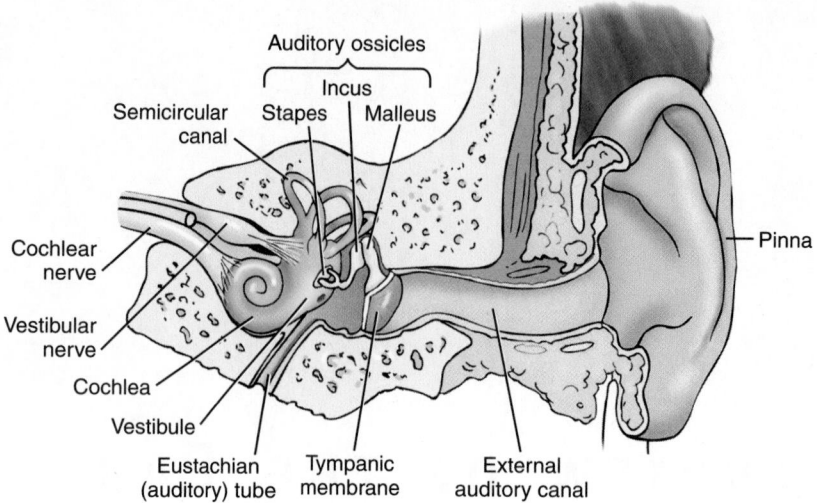

Auditory ossicles
Incus
Semicircular canal · Stapes · Malleus

Cochlear nerve

Vestibular nerve

Cochlea

Vestibule

Eustachian (auditory) tube

Tympanic membrane

External auditory canal

Pinna

FIGURE 43-1 Anatomy of the ear.

The **inner ear** is the complex structure of the ear that communicates directly with the acoustic nerve, which transmits sound vibrations from the middle ear. The inner ear, also referred to as the labyrinth because of its series of canals, has two main divisions: the bony labyrinth and the membranous labyrinth. The bony labyrinth consists of the vestibule, cochlea, and semicircular canals, and the membranous labyrinth consists of a series of sacs and tubes within the bony labyrinth. The **cochlea** is the primary organ of hearing; fibers of the cochlear division of the acoustic nerve pass through this organ. The vestibular apparatus is necessary for maintaining equilibrium and balance (see Figure 43-1).

What are the common ear disorders observed in clinical practice?

The most common ear disorders include infections of the ear (bacterial or fungal), earwax accumulation, and various other painful or distressing conditions. Many ear disorders are minor and are easily treated or self-limiting. Persistent pain or ear problems should be professionally evaluated, because some untreated disorders can lead to hearing loss.

External ear disorders usually include trauma, such as lacerations or scrapes to the skin. These conditions are often minor and heal with time. If the injury results in bleeding and perhaps a hematoma, a referral to a primary health care provider is necessary. Localized infections of the hair follicles may result in boils. Clients with recurring boils and small boils that do not respond to good hygiene and topical compresses should be referred to a provider for evaluation and possible treatment with systemic antibiotics.

Dermatitis of the ear, itching, local redness, weeping, or drainage are also reported. Such conditions must be individually evaluated, because the causes can vary from inflammation induced by seborrhea, psoriasis, or contact dermatitis to head trauma that produces ear discharge. Self-medication should be discouraged when infection is suspected, when there are known injuries to the ear, or whenever drainage, pain, and dizziness are present.

Middle ear disorders are not to be treated with over-the-counter medications. The most commonly reported problem is middle ear inflammation, or **otitis media**. This condition occurs most often in children, but chronic otitis media may be caused in adults by a nasopharyngeal tumor. Pain, fever, malaise, pressure, a sensation of fullness in the ear, and hearing loss are common symptoms. Clients with such conditions should be treated promptly by a prescriber. Acute tympanic membrane perforation from foreign objects or from water sports (e.g., diving or water skiing) will result in a multitude of symptoms if left untreated. Pain at the time of injury that subsides, diminished hearing acuity, tinnitus, nausea, vertigo, and otitis media or mastoiditis may be noted. An examination by a physician is vital when a perforated tympanic membrane is suspected.

Loss of hearing, especially a unilateral hearing loss, may result from a viral infection of the inner ear. Genetic diseases or slowly progressive diseases such as otosclerosis or Ménière's disease may cause hearing deficits. Untreated external and middle ear infections may also affect hearing and the functioning of the inner ear.

The nurse also needs to be aware of drugs that include ototoxicity as an adverse effect, which can result in impaired hearing for the client (see Chapter 44).

Summary

Pharmacologic interventions for the ear are limited. To appropriately assess and care for clients receiving otic agents, the nurse needs to have a thorough understanding of the anatomy and physiology of the ear.

✱ Critical Thinking Questions

- It is not uncommon to hear infants begin to cry when airplanes begin their descent and cabin pressure changes. Why does this occur, and what action would you recommend to caregivers to minimize this response?

- Mr. Jones worked with heavy equipment at construction sites for a number of years before regulations of the Occupational Safety and Health Administration required ear protection. He admits to having difficulty hearing. Why do you think this has happened?

- Mrs. Harris, 84 years old, has come to the emergency department with a broken arm from a fall in her home. She states having increasing problems maintaining her balance. Why might this be so?

Bibliography

Anderson, D.M., Keith, J., & Novak, P.D. (Eds.) (2002). *Mosby's medical, nursing, and allied health dictionary* (6th ed.). St. Louis: Mosby.

Guyton, A.C., & Hall, J.E. (2000). *Textbook of medical physiology* (10th ed.). Philadelphia: W.B. Saunders.

Hardman, J.G., & Limbird, L.E. (Eds.). (2001). *Goodman and Gilman's The pharmacological basis of therapeutics* (10th ed.). New York: McGraw-Hill.

Herlihy, B., & Maebius, N.K. (2003). *The human body in health and illness* (2nd ed.). Philadelphia: W.B. Saunders.

McCance, K.L., & Huether, S.E. (2002). *Pathophysiology: The biological basis for disease in adults and children* (4th ed.). St. Louis: Mosby.

Thibodeau, G.A., & Patton, K.T. (2003). *Anatomy and physiology* (5th ed.). St. Louis: Mosby.

e-LEARNING SUPPLEMENTS

Student CD-ROM
- Final Exam questions
- NCLEX® Examination review questions
- Pharmacology animations
- Printable chapter summary

Evolve Website (http://evolve.elsevier.com/mckenry)
- Content updates, including information on new drugs

- WebLinks corresponding to this chapter
- Answers to the critical thinking questions in this chapter
- Elsevier ePharmacology Update newsletter
- Mosby's Drug Consult Internet Edition
- Supplemental and reference information

Drugs Affecting the Ear

44

Chapter Focus

Persons with ear disorders may experience impaired communication related to hearing loss, or they may experience difficulty with balance and vertigo. Otic drugs may be prescribed for ear disorders; however, systemic drugs prescribed for a variety of diagnoses may result in ototoxicity, causing a loss of both hearing and balance. The nurse needs to be concerned about the client's comfort, auditory perception, and risk of injury related to vestibular dysfunction; the nurse also needs to be knowledgeable about drugs that affect the ear to provide client instruction for effective self-management of the therapeutic drug regimen.

Learning Objectives
- List the drugs commonly used to treat ear infections.
- Describe the various preparations used to treat ear ailments.
- Identify five drugs reported to cause ototoxicity.
- Implement the nursing management of the client receiving drugs that affect the ear.

▲ Key Terms
cerumen, p. 809
ototoxicity, p. 810
tinnitus, p. 811
vertigo, p. 811

Disorders and infections of the external ear canal are treated with antibiotic solutions, corticosteroids, and miscellaneous preparations such as wax emulsifiers, antibacterials, antifungals, local anesthetics, antiinflammatory agents, and local analgesic–type preparations. The potent systemic medications that may adversely affect the client's hearing and/or balance are also reviewed in this chapter.

✳ **T.S. is a 9-year-old boy who repeatedly reports ear pain and drainage during the summer months after swimming in the local swimming hole. He is diagnosed as having otitis externa ("swimmer's ear") and on advice of his pediatrician, he is started on ciprofloxacin/hydrocortisone to each ear twice daily × 7 days. When** his ciprofloxacin/hydrocortisone regimen is completed, he is to use aluminum and acetic acid solution (Domeboro Otic) in each ear after swimming.

✳ **What antimicrobial agents are used topically in the ear?**
Antibiotic ear preparations are used as topical agents to treat infections of the external auditory canal surface (otitis externa). Clients often refer to this condition as "swimmer's ear." Choice of agent depends on likely pathogens, client age and history, and presenting symptoms. For bacterial otitis externa, ciprofloxacin or ofloxacin otic preparations are sometimes used. Often these preparations are combined with hydrocortisone to reduce inflammation. The antimi-

crobial ophthalmic preparations, although less viscous than otic preparations, are also safe to use in the ear if the tympanic membrane is intact. As discussed in Chapter 42, topical preparations containing neomycin are often avoided because of their sensitizing potential.

Agents that alter environmental pH such as dilute aluminum acetate and acetic acid solution (Otic Domeboro) are also sometimes used to treat or prevent superficial otitis externa. Other similar agents used alone or in combination for their antibacterial or antifungal effects include acetic acid, boric acid, benzalkonium chloride, benzethonium, and aluminum acetate (Burow's solution). These agents are somewhat effective in treating and preventing "swimmer's ear" when used as prophylaxis after bathing or swimming.

ciprofloxacin/hydrocortisone otic suspension
[sip roe **floks** a sin + hye droe **kor** ti sone]
(Cipro HC Otic)
Ciprofloxacin is a fluoroquinolone antibacterial effective against gram-negative and some gram-positive pathogens. Hydrocortisone is a corticosteroid antiinflammatory agent. A similar product combination of ciprofloxacin/dexamethasone (Ciprodex) is also available.

Indications
Ciprofloxacin/hydrocortisone is indicated for the treatment of acute otitis externa.

Dosing
Ciprofloxacin 0.2%/hydrocortisone 1% suspension for otic use is administered to children older than 1 year and adults as three drops to fill the ear canal twice daily for 7 days.

Adverse Effects
This product is well tolerated. It is contraindicated if the tympanic membrane is not intact. Secondary fungal, viral, or resistant bacterial infection is the most common adverse effect reported.

What corticosteroids are used in the ear?
Corticosteroid otic solutions include betamethasone, hydrocortisone (Betnesol and Cortamed), and dexamethasone (Decadron). Hydrocortisone combinations with antibacterials (see Cipro HC, Ciprodex above), acetic acid (VoSol HC, Acetasol HC), with alcohol (EarSol-HC), or with acetic acid and benzethonium (AA-HC Otic) are also available. Hydrocortisone is included for its antiinflammatory, antipruritic, and antiallergic effects (*USP DI,* 2005). The combination of topical corticosteroid to acetic acid is associated with improved response in otitis externa compared to acetic acid alone (van Balen, Smit, Zuithoff, Verheij, 2003).

Corticosteroids may be combined with the antibiotics neomycin and polymyxin B to treat infections in the external ear canal or mastoid cavity. Many such products are available that may also include other ingredients, such as those included in over-the-counter (OTC) otic preparations. These are prescription otic solutions such as AK-Spore HC, Cort-Biotic, Cortisporin, and Cortomycin (*USP DI*, 2005).

What other products are available?
Glycerin, mineral oil, and olive oil (sweet oil) are used as emollients to help relieve itching and burning in the ear, whereas propylene glycol enhances the antibacterial effect and acidity of acetic acid. Carbamide peroxide (urea hydrogen peroxide) is an antibacterial agent that releases oxygen to help remove accumulations of cerumen (earwax). Thus combinations of these ingredients are often included in OTC otic solutions.

A wide variety of both single and combination products is used to treat impacted cerumen, inflammation, bacterial or fungal infections, ear pain, and other minor or superficial problems associated primarily with the external ear canal. To prevent complications, a health care provider's thorough evaluation and intervention is required for more serious problems such as an earache secondary to an upper respiratory tract infection, ear discharge or drainage, persistent or recurrent otitis, or ear pain caused by recent injury or head trauma. Systemic medications with or without ear preparations are usually necessary in such cases.

Although most OTC otic preparations are considered safe and effective, clients should be advised to see a provider if symptoms do not improve within several days of using these preparations or if an adverse effect occurs. Table 44-1 lists selected examples of OTC otic solutions.

What are the nursing management issues for T.S.'s drug therapy and other otic drugs?

Assessment Before initiating therapy, assess T.S.'s hearing and the extent of symptoms (earache, pain, erythema, vertigo, drainage, and others) that may be present. Before instilling the eardrops, assess that the ear canal is clear and not impacted with cerumen and that the tympanic membrane is intact.

To identify areas for education, assess the client for improper hygiene or health practices that may contribute to

TABLE 44-1 SELECTED EXAMPLES OF OVER-THE-COUNTER (OTC) OTIC PREPARATIONS

Ingredients (Trade Names)	Indications
carbamide peroxide (Auro Ear Drops, Debrox)	Ear wax
boric acid and isopropyl alcohol (Auro-Dri Ear Drops)	Swimmer's ear
isopropyl alcohol in glycerin (Swim-Ear Drops)	Swimmer's ear
carbamide peroxide and glycerin (E.R.O. Ear Drops, Murine Ear Drops)	Ear wax
hydrocortisone, propylene glycol, alcohol, benzyl benzoate (Earsol-HC Drops)	Inflammation, itching

Data from *Drug facts and comparisons* (58th ed.) (2005). St. Louis: Facts and Comparisons.

the development of infections, such as cleaning the ear canal with a cotton swab, or in T.S.'s case, not drying the ears after swimming.

Nursing Diagnosis T.S. is at risk for the following nursing diagnoses/collaborative problems: impaired verbal communication related to hearing loss, acute pain related to infection of the outer ear, and risk for infection related to poor hygiene after swimming; and the potential complication of spread of current infection.

Planning While receiving otic medications, T.S. will:
- Remain free of signs and symptoms of ear infection or pain related to ear disorder.
- With his parents, effectively manage drug regimen, including correct administration technique, compliance with medications, and use of supportive measures (drying ears after swimming).
- Collaborate with health care providers, reporting adverse effects appropriately and maintaining scheduled appointment with health care providers for monitoring and treatment.

Implementation

Monitoring Monitor T.S.'s affected ear(s) for improvement of the condition for which the eardrops are being administered. Monitor for possible hypersensitivity to the eardrops as evidenced by burning, redness, and swelling that was not present when the medication was started. If hypersensitivity occurs, discontinue the drops and notify the prescriber. Monitor T.S.'s level of comfort, ear drainage, hearing, and temperature at periodic intervals.

Intervention Eardrops are more comfortably tolerated if they are warmed (if not contraindicated) before instillation. This can be achieved by running warm water over the bottle (on the side without the label) or by immersing the bottle in warm water in a medicine cup. Even simply carrying the bottle in a pocket for half an hour or so will help to warm the drops.

Assist T.S. to a comfortable position before attempting to administer eardrops. To prepare for the instillation of eardrops, cleanse any drainage from the ear and position him so that the ear to be medicated is facing upward.

The instillation of eardrops requires knowledge of anatomic structure across the life span; the shape of the auditory canal of a young child is different from that of an adult. To instill eardrops in children 3 years of age or younger, gently pull the pinna of the ear slightly down and back. In older children and adults, hold the pinna up and back. Gently massaging the area immediately anterior to the ear will facilitate the entry of the drops into the ear canal (Figure 44-1).

Education Instruct T.S. to remain on his side for 5 minutes after instillation. A small cotton pledget may be gently inserted into the ear canal if desired. Alert T.S. to the hazard of impaired hearing related to the eardrops, the cotton

pledget, or the ear ailment itself. Instruct T.S. and his parents about how to appropriately instill eardrops according to the client's age.

Evaluation The expected outcome of otic drug therapy is that T.S. will show no clinical signs of infection (fever, pain, redness, heat, odor, drainage) or hearing loss and will have a normal white cell count (WBC). Cultures of the ear canal will be negative for pathogenic growth. T.S. and his parents state the signs and symptoms of otitis externa and when to report them to the prescriber and the prevention of further infections. His caregivers demonstrate the correct method for instilling ear medications and follow up with health care providers for monitoring and treatment.

⭐ **Which systemic drugs produce ototoxicity?**
Many medications have reportedly caused **ototoxicity** in humans. This condition may affect hearing (auditory or

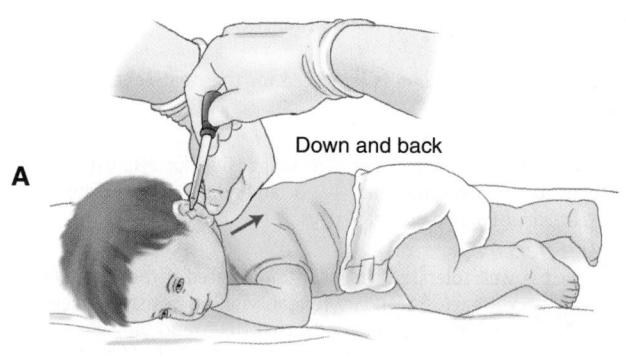

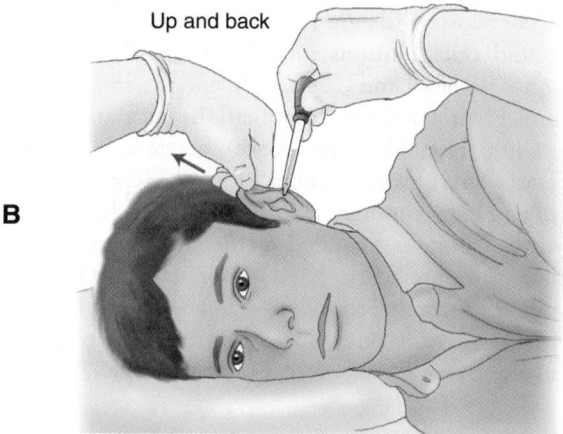

FIGURE 44-1 Administration of eardrops. The infant or child is positioned on the side of the unaffected ear. **A,** To administer eardrops to infants and children less than 3 years, the nurse pulls the pinna down and back. **B,** To administer eardrops to children older than 3 years (and to adults), the nurse gently pulls the pinna up and back. The nurse should stabilize his or her hand on the client's head for safety and instill the prescribed number of drops. The drops are directed toward the ear canal to avoid hitting the tympanic membrane, which can cause pain. The client should remain in position for 5 to 10 minutes. To prevent nausea or vertigo, otic drugs should be warmed before being instilled.

cochlear function), balance (vestibular function), or both. The most common symptom reported is **tinnitus,** a ringing or buzzing sound in the ears.

Cochlear ototoxicity causes a progressive or continuing hearing loss. High-pitched tinnitus or a loss of the highest tones occurs first and then progresses to affect the lowest tones. Because of this slow progression, most clients are not aware that it is occurring. Vestibular toxicity may start with a severe headache of 1 to 2 days' duration, followed by nau-sea, vomiting, dizziness, ataxia, and difficulty with equilibrium. The client may feel as if the room is in motion (**vertigo).** Ototoxicity is usually bilateral and may be reversible, but it can become irreversible if not recognized early enough to stop the offending medications. Most drug-induced ototoxicity is associated with the use of aminoglycosides, such as streptomycin, gentamicin, tobramycin, and others. Table 44-2 lists selected drugs reported to induce ototoxicity. Whether antiinflammatory or antioxidant therapy can help

TABLE 44-2 SELECTED DRUGS REPORTED TO CAUSE OTOTOXICITY

Drug	Comments
ANALGESICS	
aspirin and NSAIDs	Salicylates, especially in high doses, can cause tinnitus, vertigo, and hearing loss. It is generally reversible if drug is reduced or discontinued, although some cases of irreversible hearing loss are documented. With NSAIDs, hearing disturbances and loss are reported.
ANTIMICROBIALS	
aminoglycosides	Incidence of ototoxicity is 1%-5% and may be irreversible. The toxicity may be vestibular, auditory, or both.
clarithromycin	Hearing loss reported (usually reversible). Occurs more often in older adult women.
erythromycin	Reversible hearing loss has been reported in persons with liver and/or kidney impairment, in persons 50 years and older and in individuals that received high doses (>4 g daily) IV erythromycin has resulted in irreversible ototoxicity.
vancomycin	Hearing loss reported, especially in persons with kidney impairment or those receiving another ototoxic medication concurrently.
ANTINEOPLASTIC AGENTS	
cisplatin	Ototoxicity with tinnitus, hearing loss, and possible deafness has been reported. This effect is especially severe in children (younger than 12 years old). This effect is cumulative, particularly with doses over 400 mg/m². Audiometric testing is recommended.
mechlorethamine	Tinnitus and, less frequently, hearing loss reported.
LOOP DIURETICS	
bumetanide, ethacrynic acid, furosemide	Reversible (bumetanide, furosemide) and irreversible (ethacrynic acid) hearing loss reported, usually with too rapid IV injection, high diuretic dosages, concurrent use with other ototoxic medications, and in renal impairment.
OTHER DRUGS	
quinidine	Dose-related tinnitus and headache seen as part of cinchonism symptom complex.
quinine	Tinnitus and hearing loss have been noted with high doses.
valproate	Tinnitus and hearing loss have been reported.

Modified from Bertolini, P., Lassalle, M., Mercier, G., Raquin, M.A., Izzi, G., Corradini, N., et al. (2004) Platinum compound–related ototoxicity in children: Long-term follow-up reveals continuous worsening of hearing loss. *Journal of Pediatric Hematology/Oncology.* 26(10), 649-655; Black, F.O., Pesznecker, S., Stallings, V. (2004). Permanent gentamicin vestibulotoxicity. Otology & Neurotology. 25(4), 559-569; *Drug facts and comparisons.* (57th ed.). (2004). St. Louis: Facts and Comparisons; Folmer, R.L., Martin, W.H., Shi, Y., (2004). Tinnitus: Questions to reveal the cause, answers to provide relief. *Journal of Family Practice.* 53(7), 532-540.
IV, intravenous; *NSAIDs,* nonsteroidal antiinflammatory drugs.

reduce ototoxicity risk remains to be evaluated more completely (Kalkanis, Whitworth, & Rybak, 2004; Park, Choi, Russell, John, & Jung, 2004; Rybak & Kelly, 2003).

✳ **L.S., an 82-year-old woman, has been on quinidine sulfate extended-release tablets (Quinidex Extentabs) 300 mg twice daily for some years for atrial fibrillation. Recently she has developed dyspepsia for which she has been taking large amounts of antacids. Two days ago, she developed a buzzing in her ears. Today she sees her primary care provider for impaired hearing.**

✳ **What are the nursing management issues with ototoxicity?**

Assessment Assess L.S.'s hearing status. Her ototoxicity is a result of increased quinidine serum levels (Roden, 2001), because the antacids modified the pH of L.S.'s urine, causing quinidine to be reabsorbed into the body. If she were being prescribed a more potential ototoxic drug, her hearing would be tested before starting therapy. Concurrent administration of more than one ototoxic drug may increase the potential for hearing loss. Use caution when administering ototoxic drugs to clients who have any condition that may increase their risk of having an adverse effect. One such condition is renal failure, which alters the elimination of aminoglycosides and may result in ototoxic serum levels.

Obtain a thorough drug history, particularly with a client who is experiencing tinnitus or a sudden hearing loss. Aspirin is the most widely used drug that causes tinnitus, but also keep in mind others such as nonsteroidal antiinflammatory drugs, aminoglycosides, quinine and its synthetic substitutes, diuretics, and antineoplastics (see Table 44-2).

Nursing Diagnosis L.S., who is taking a drug that could cause ototoxicity, is at risk for the following nursing diagnoses/collaborative problems: disturbed sensory perception related to ototoxicity (auditory deficit, tinnitus); impaired verbal communication related to hearing loss; risk for injury related to vestibular dysfunction (ataxia, dizziness); and the potential complication of deafness.

Planning While receiving ototoxic medications, L.S. will:
- Remain free of tinnitus, ataxia, dizziness, impaired hearing, and other signs and symptoms of ototoxicity.
- Effectively manage drug regimen, including compliance with medications and checking with prescriber before adding medications to her regimen.
- Collaborate with health care providers, report adverse effects appropriately, and maintain scheduled appointment with health care providers for monitoring and treatment.

Implementation
Monitoring The serum levels of some drugs may be monitored to help detect the development of dangerously high blood levels. Monitor and have L.S.'s family monitor her ability to hear by observing for cues that indicate increasing hearing loss (inappropriate responses to the conversation of others, speaking loudly, moving closer to others when they speak) and by noting any comments by her regarding an inability to hear or understand what others are saying. Report increased hearing loss to the prescriber. For clients who are at higher risk for permanent ototoxicity (e.g., those receiving repeat or long-term aminoglycosides), close monitoring of drug serum levels and evaluation by an audiologist may be indicated.

Intervention Although not the etiology of L.S.'s impaired hearing, the administration of ototoxic drugs increases the risk when given intravenously. Administer such drugs (e.g., aminoglycosides, furosemide) at the rate suggested by the manufacturer to avoid high peak levels.

Education Instruct L.S. to report tinnitus or any other hearing impairment immediately. Auditory damage is usually reversible if the causative drug is discontinued early.

Evaluation The expected outcome of therapy with drugs that induce ototoxicity is that the client will not experience tinnitus or deafness, will be able to understand others, and will express satisfaction with sensory input. The client states signs and symptoms of tinnitus, ataxia, and impaired hearing and when to report them to the prescriber.

✳ **L.S.'s quinidine dosage was withheld for 2 days and her hearing returned. She is undergoing tests to determine the cause of her dyspepsia.**

Summary

Drugs that affect the ear may relate to the treatment of inflammation, excess cerumen, bacterial or fungal infection, or ear discomfort, or they may cause ototoxicity as an adverse effect when administered for some other condition. In both instances the nurse needs to be concerned about the client's comfort and auditory perception and the risk for injury as a result of adverse effects of the drugs or an extension of the client's symptoms.

✳ **Critical Thinking Questions**

- Joan Stevens is a 10-month-old infant who is brought to the clinic by her mother because of irritability, tugging at her ear, and a fever of 101°F. What would the nurse consider to be essential in her assessment of Joan?
- What clients are particularly at risk for drug-related ototoxicity and why?

Bibliography

Anderson, D.M., Keith, J., & Novak, P.D. (Eds.) (2002). *Mosby's medical, nursing, and allied health dictionary* (6th ed.). St. Louis: Mosby.

Bertolini, P., Lassalle, M., Mercier, G., Raquin, M.A., Izzi, G., Corradini, N., et al. (2004). Platinum compound-related ototoxicity in children: long-term follow-up reveals continuous worsening of hearing loss. *Journal of Pediatric Hematology/Oncology, 26*(10), 649-655.

Black, F.O., Pesznecker, S., & Stallings, V. (2004). Permanent gentamicin vestibulotoxicity. *Otology & Neurotology, 25*(4), 559-569.

Bosker, G. (Ed.). (2004). *Primary and acute care medicine: Practice, protocols, pathways,* (2nd ed.). Atlanta: Thomson American Health Consultants.

Drug facts and comparisons. (58th ed.). (2005). St. Louis: Facts and Comparisons.

Folmer, R.L., Martin, W.H., & Shi, Y. (2004). Tinnitus: Questions to reveal the cause, answers to provide relief. *Journal of Family Practice, 53*(7), 532-540.

Jackler, R.K., & Kaplan, M.J. (2003). Ear, nose & throat. In L.M. Tierney, Jr., S.J. McPhee & Papadakis, M.A. (Eds.), *Current Medical Diagnosis & Treatment.* New York: Lange Medical Books/McGraw-Hill.

Kalkanis, J.G., Whitworth, C., & Rybak, L.P. (2004). Vitamin E reduces cisplatin ototoxicity. *Laryngoscope, 114*(3),538-542.

Lacy, C.F., Armstrong, L.L., Goldman, M.P., & Lance, L.L. (2004). *Lexi-Comp's Drug Information Handbook* (12th ed.). Hudson, Ohio: Lexi-Comp.

Mosby's drug consult. (15th ed.). (2005). St. Louis: Mosby.

Park, S.K., Choi, D., Russell, P., John, E.O., & Jung, T. (2004). Protective effect of corticosteroid against the cytotoxicity of aminoglycoside otic drops on isolated cochlear outer hair cells. *Laryngoscope, 114*(4), 768-771.

Roden, D.M. (2001). Antiarrhythmic drugs. In: Hardman, J.G. & Limbird, L.E. (Eds.), *Goodman & Gilman's The pharmacological basis of therapeutics* (10th ed.). New York: McGraw-Hill.

Rybak, L.P., Kelly, T. (2003). Ototoxicity: bioprotective mechanisms. *Current Opinion in Otolaryngology & Head & Neck Surgery, 11*(5), 328-333.

USP DI: Drug information for the health care professional (25th ed.). (2005). Greenwood Village, CO: MICROMEDEX Thomson Healthcare.

van Balen, F.A., Smit, W.M., Zuithoff, N.P., & Verheij, T.J. (2003). Clinical efficacy of three common treatments in acute otitis externa in primary care: Randomised controlled trial. *British Medical Journal, 327,* 1201-1203.

 e-LEARNING SUPPLEMENTS

Student CD-ROM
- Final Exam questions
- NCLEX® Examination review questions
- Pharmacology animations
- Printable chapter summary

Evolve Website (http://evolve.elsevier.com/mckenry)
- Content updates, including information on new drugs

- WebLinks corresponding to this chapter
- Answers to the critical thinking questions in this chapter
- *Elsevier ePharmacology Update* newsletter
- Mosby's Drug Consult Internet Edition
- Supplemental and reference information

45

OVERVIEW OF THE ENDOCRINE SYSTEM

CHAPTER FOCUS

The endocrine and nervous systems serve as the communication system of the body. The endocrine glands respond to signals from the internal and external environment by synthesizing and releasing hormones into the circulation. To provide care to clients with disorders of the endocrine system, it is essential that the nurse be knowledgeable about the anatomy and physiology of this complex system.

✳ **What are the functions of hormones?**

Hormones are active, natural chemical substances secreted into the bloodstream from the endocrine glands. These substances initiate or regulate the activity of an organ or group of cells in another part of the body. They also have specific, well-defined physiologic effects on metabolism. The list of major hormones includes the secretions from the anterior and posterior pituitary glands, the thyroid hormones,

parathyroid hormone, pancreatic insulin and glucagon, epinephrine and norepinephrine from the adrenal medulla, several potent steroids from the adrenal cortex, and the gonadal hormones of both genders (Figure 45-1).

The major types of hormones are the steroid hormones and the hormones derived from amino acids. Steroid hormones are secreted by the adrenal gland and the sex glands. They transport proteins in the plasma; their physiologic ef-

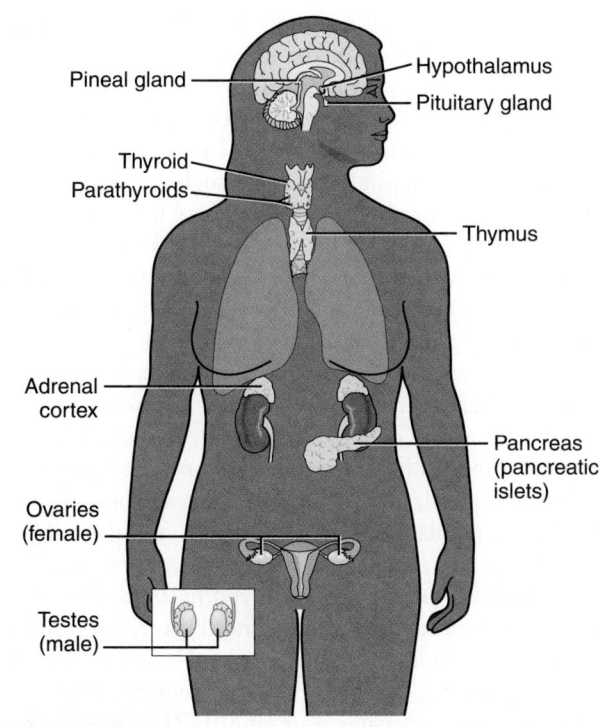

FIGURE 45-1 Locations of the major endocrine glands.

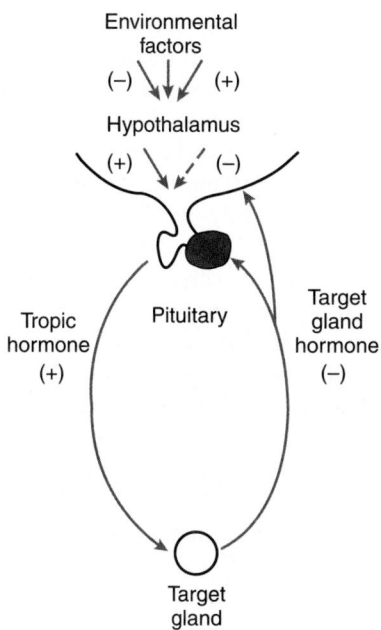

FIGURE 45-2 Various internal and external factors may inhibit or stimulate the hypothalamus to secrete inhibitory (−) or releasing (+) factors to control the output of hormones from the anterior pituitary and ultimate hormone release from the target glands.

fect begins when the steroid enters the cell, with subsequent binding to the specific cytosol or nuclear protein receptor.

Hormones from the various endocrine glands work together to regulate vital processes, including the following:

- Secretory and motor activities of the digestive tract
- Energy production
- Composition and volume of extracellular fluid
- Adaptation, such as acclimatization and immunity
- Growth and development
- Reproduction and lactation

Hormones may exert their effects by controlling the formation or destruction of an intracellular regulator (cyclic adenosine monophosphate [cAMP]), controlling protein synthesis, or controlling membrane permeability and the movement of ions and other substances. The effect of a hormone depends on its interaction with a receptor and is determined by the level of the circulating active hormone.

To maintain the internal environment, hormone secretion must be controlled. This is achieved by a self-regulating series of events known as **negative feedback,** in which a hormone produces a physiologic effect that, when strong enough, inhibits further secretion of that hormone, thereby inhibiting the physiologic effect. Increased hormonal secretions may be evoked in response to stimuli from the external environment; the cessation of the external stimuli ends the internal secretion response (Figure 45-2).

Hormones are not "used up" in exerting their physiologic effects; they must be inactivated or excreted if the internal environment is to remain stable. Inactivation occurs enzymatically in the blood or intercellular spaces, in the liver or kidney, or in the target tissues. The excretion of hormones is primarily via the urine and, to a lesser extent, the bile.

The wide range in the onset and duration of hormonal activity contributes to the flexibility of the endocrine system. Most hormones are destroyed rapidly, with a half-life of 10 to 30 minutes in blood. Some hormones (e.g., catecholamines) have a half-life of seconds, and thyroid hormones have a half-life measured in days. Some hormones exert their physiologic effects immediately, whereas others require minutes or hours before their effects occur. Some effects end immediately when the hormone disappears from the circulation; other responses may persist for hours after hormone concentrations have returned to basal levels. The exposure of a tissue to an active hormone is also controlled by that hormone's pathway for metabolism, including molecular alterations, consumption at the site of action, and hepatorenal excretion.

A major development in biology and medicine has been the recognition, isolation, purification, and chemical and cellular understanding of most known hormones. Duplicating hormones by chemical synthesis becomes theoretically possible once their chemical structure is known. This has been accomplished for some but not all hormones.

✳ How are hormones used in clinical practice?

In medicine, hormones generally are used in three ways: (1) for replacement therapy, as exemplified by the use of insulin in diabetes or of adrenal steroids in Addison disease; (2) for pharmacologic effects beyond replacement, as in the use of larger-than-endogenous doses of adrenal steroids for their antiinflammatory effects; and (3) for endocrine diagnostic testing.

Research in endocrinology has advanced the concept of specific receptors within or on the surface of cells. This has led to knowledge of hormone specificity and the essential cellular mechanisms involved in the hormone-receptor complex. The recognition and activation properties found in the hormone-receptor complex come from different receptor molecular sites. Only specific receptor material binds a hormone and begins its activity; the hormone has no effect on tissues that do not carry specific receptors.

Alterations in either hormone secretion or hormone receptor responses may culminate in endocrine disease states. Certain cell surface receptors may become antigenic and develop antibodies that accelerate receptor destruction, block receptor function, or mimic the action of the target tissue. Among the receptor-like disorders, which are referred to as antireceptor autoimmune diseases, are myasthenia gravis, Graves' disease, insulin-resistant diabetes mellitus (DM), and bronchial asthma.

Pituitary Gland

✷ What are the functions of the pituitary gland?

The hormones of the pituitary gland exert an important effect in regulating the secretion of other hormones. The pituitary body is approximately the size of a pea and occupies a niche in the sella turcica of the sphenoid bone. It consists of an anterior lobe (adenohypophysis), a posterior lobe (neurohypophysis), and a smaller pars intermedia composed of secreting cells. The anterior lobe is particularly important in sustaining life. The function of the pars intermedia is not well understood. Figure 45-3 shows the major pituitary hormones and their principal target organs.

✷ How is anterior pituitary function regulated?

The pituitary and target glands have a negative feedback relationship. A trophic hormone from the pituitary stimulates the target gland to secrete a hormone that inhibits further secretion of the trophic hormone by the pituitary. When the serum concentration of the target gland hormone falls below a certain level, the pituitary again secretes the trophic hormone until the target gland produces enough hormone to inhibit the pituitary secretion. However, the negative feedback concept alone is not enough to account for changes in the serum levels of target gland hormones, especially those caused by changes in the external environment. The central nervous system (CNS) plays a decisive role in regulating pituitary function to meet environmental demands through activity of the hypothalamus.

Some neurons in the hypothalamus have endocrine functions. Their axons secrete releasing hormones into the blood that stimulate the anterior pituitary to release its own hormones responsible for growth and hormone secretion by sex glands, thyroid, and the adrenal cortex. The hormones from the hypothalamus may stimulate or inhibit functions of the body (e.g., prolactin-releasing hormone and prolactin-inhibiting hormone). The hypothalamus adjusts the secretion of the anterior pituitary and the anterior pituitary adjusts the secretions of its target glands. Among the important hormones secreted by the hypothalamus are: growth hormone-releasing hormone (GRH), growth hormone-inhibiting hormone (GIH), corticotropin-releasing hormone (CRH), thyrotropin-releasing hormone (TRH), gonadotropin-releasing hormone (GnRH), prolactin-releasing hormone (PRH), and prolactin-inhibiting hormone (PIH).

✷ What are the anterior lobe pituitary hormones and their functions?

The number of hormones secreted by the anterior pituitary gland is unknown. However, at least seven relatively pure extracts have been prepared, and these have definite specific action:

1. A growth factor influences the development of the body and promotes skeletal, visceral, and general growth. Acromegaly, gigantism, and dwarfism are

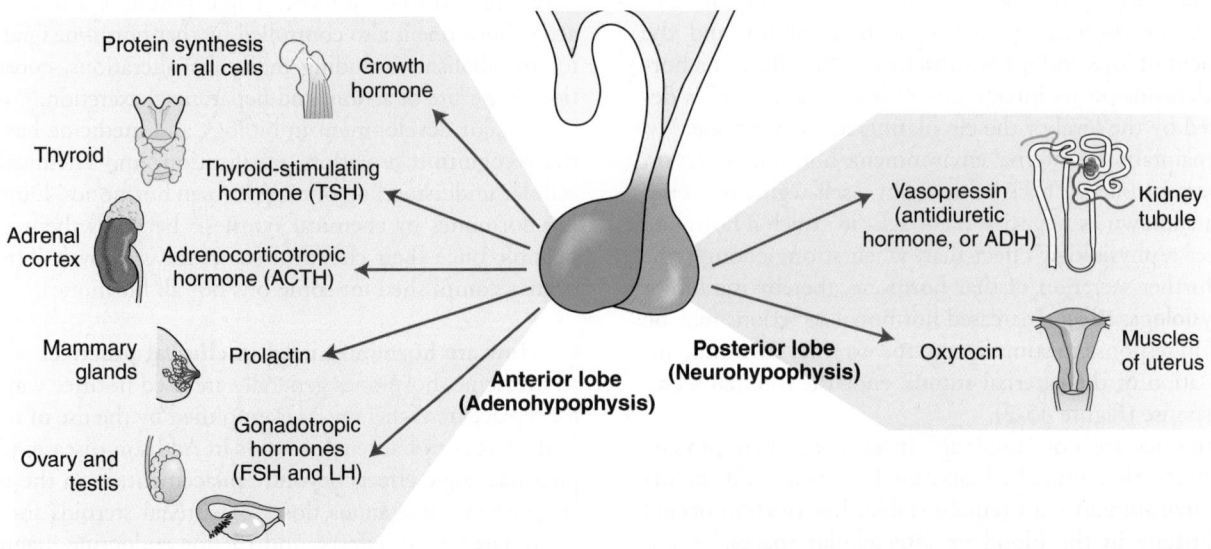

FIGURE 45-3 Pituitary hormones. Some of the major hormones of the adenohypophysis and neurohypophysis and their principal target organs.

associated with pathologic conditions of the anterior lobe of the pituitary gland. Growth hormone (GH) (somatotropin, somatropin, somatotropic hormone [STH]) has been obtained as a small crystalline protein but currently has no established place in medicine, except in documented clinical and laboratory evidence of growth hormone deficiency, especially that associated with chronic renal insufficiency *(Drug Facts and Comparisons,* 2005). Its use in various clinical conditions is largely experimental. (See Chapter 46 for further discussion on growth hormone.)

2. Follicle-stimulating hormone (FSH) stimulates the growth and maturation of the ovarian follicle, which in turn brings on the characteristic changes of estrus (menstruation in women). This hormone also stimulates spermatogenesis in men. FSH appears to be a protein or associated with a protein, but this human pituitary gonadotropin has not yet been obtained in a highly purified form.

3. Luteinizing hormone (LH), also known as the interstitial cell–stimulating hormone (ICSH), together with FSH (Pergonal) causes maturation of the graafian follicles, ovulation, and the secretion of estrogen in females. It causes spermatogenesis, androgen formation, and the growth of interstitial tissue in males. LH also promotes the formation of the corpus luteum in females.

4. Thyroid-stimulating hormone (TSH, thyrotropic hormone, thyrotropin) is necessary for the normal development and function of the thyroid gland. If too much is present, it produces hyperthyroidism and increases the size of the gland in laboratory animals.

5. A lactogenic factor (prolactin or mammotropin) plays a part in the proliferation and secretion of the mammary glands of mammals. This may be identical to the hormone responsible for the development of the corpus luteum. In its absence the corpus luteum fails to produce progesterone.

6. Adrenocorticotropic hormone (corticotropin or ACTH) stimulates the cortex of the adrenal gland.

7. Melanocyte-stimulating hormone (intermedin or MSH) is probably produced in the intermediate lobe. Its physiologic role is unknown, but it darkens the skin when injected into human beings.

The hormones produced by the anterior lobe of the pituitary gland are important physiologically, and purified preparations have become available, at least for clinical study; such preparations are both expensive and limited in supply. They may become useful in combating certain disorders in the future as chemically defined preparations become available.

✱ What are the functions of the posterior lobe pituitary hormones?

Two hormones obtained from the posterior lobe of the pituitary gland have been identified and chemically analyzed. These compounds, **oxytocin** (a hormone that stimulates the smooth muscle of the uterus to contract) and **vaso**pressin (the **antidiuretic hormone**), are both peptides; each contains eight amino acids. It has proved possible to synthesize them chemically. The availability of these hormones in pure form has clarified their mechanism of action and has allowed better control of their therapeutic use. A certain overlap of pharmacologic action exists even in the pure preparation; pure oxytocin, for example, has some vasopressor activity. The antidiuretic potency of vasopressin is much greater than its pressor potency.

A deficiency of antidiuretic hormone leads to **diabetes insipidus,** a condition with dilute urine, polydipsia (increased thirst), and polyuria (increased urine volume). Diabetes insipidus, not to be confused with diabetes mellitus, can be secondary to drugs (e.g., lithium) or other conditions.

The syndrome of inappropriate antidiuretic hormone (SIADH) is due to increased ADH secretion and can result in significant dilutional hyponatremia. SIADH may also be drug induced (e.g., carbamazepine). Diabetes insipidus and SIADH are discussed in greater depth in Chapter 46.

Although vasopressin is available in a natural state, synthetic formulations (e.g., lypressin and desmopressin) have been developed, and they act primarily as antidiuretic hormone. These formulations have very little, if any, pressor or oxytocic activity. Chapter 52 discusses oxytocin.

Thyroid Gland

✱ What is the function of the thyroid gland?

The thyroid gland, one of the most richly vascularized tissues of the body, secretes three hormones essential for the proper regulation of metabolism: thyroxine (T_4) and triiodothyronine (T_3) from follicular cells, and calcitonin from parafollicular cells. Because of its role in calcium metabolism, calcitonin is discussed in greater detail in the section on parathyroid gland hormones (see Chapter 47).

The large amount of iodine in thyroid hormones and the availability of radioactive iodine have led to detailed knowledge about the physiology of the thyroid gland and its role in metabolism. Iodine is essential for the synthesis of thyroid hormone. Approximately 1 mg of iodine is required per week, most of which is ingested in food, water, and iodized table salt. Approximately two thirds of this iodine is reduced in the gastrointestinal (GI) tract, enters the circulation as iodide, and is excreted into the urine. The remaining third is taken up by the thyroid gland for hormone synthesis. This process is aided by the "iodide pump," which takes up the iodide from the extracellular fluid, traps it, and concentrates it to many times that found in plasma. The ratio of iodide in the thyroid gland to that in the serum is expressed as the T/S ratio; normally this ratio is 20:1. In hypoactivity the ratio may be 10:1; in hyperactivity it may be as great as 250:1.

Thyroglobulin is synthesized first. It contains tyrosine, an amino acid that reacts with iodine to form thyroid hormones. The thyroglobulin–thyroid hormone complex is stored in the follicles of the thyroid gland and is called "colloid." Approximately 30% of the thyroid mass is stored thyroglobulin, which contains enough thyroid hormone to meet normal requirements for 2 to 3 months without any further synthesis.

Normally thyroglobulin is not released into the circulation but undergoes proteolytic digestion (a coupling reaction), which releases the active thyroid hormones T_3 and T_4. Hormone synthesis—iodine trapping, iodination and proteolysis of thyroglobulin, and hormone release—is controlled by the thyroid-stimulating hormone (thyrotropin, TSH) from the beta cells of the anterior pituitary gland. Thyroid secretion is maintained by this TSH secretion. Decreased serum levels of T_3 and T_4 stimulate thyrotropin-releasing hormone (TRH) from the hypothalamus, which stimulates the pituitary gland to secrete TSH; this in turn stimulates release of thyroxin from thyroglobulin.

TSH secretion is negatively regulated by T_3 and T_4, which directly inhibit the thyrotropic cells of the pituitary gland. An increase in free, unbound thyroid hormone causes a decrease in TSH secretion and inhibits TRH production; a decrease in the free unbound hormone stimulates TRH production and causes an increase in TSH secretion—a negative feedback mechanism.

✳ What effects are observed with thyroid hormones?

The precise physiologic role of the thyroid hormones is not yet known, but several hormonal actions have been identified and studied. The three following generalizations can be made about thyroid hormones:

1. They have a diffuse effect and do not seem to have any specific target organ effect; no special cells or tissues appear to be particularly affected by the thyroid hormones.
2. Their long delay in onset of action and their prolonged duration of action rule them out as minute-to-minute regulators of physiologic function. Instead, their role is more likely to be that of establishing and maintaining long-term functions such as growth, maturation, and adaptation.
3. They are not necessary for survival, although reduced levels can affect quality of life.

Triiodothyronine (T_3) and thyroxine (T_4) appear to have the same physiologic actions, but T_3 is far more potent than T_4.

Effects on Growth and Maturation A normal, functioning thyroid is essential for normal growth. Thyroid hormones stimulate the production of messenger ribonucleic acid (RNA) molecules, which are involved in the synthesis of various proteins; this facilitates growth and development. The hormones must be present in the right amounts if growth is to occur at the normal rate. The growth rate is slowed in children with hypothyroidism; this may lead to shortness of stature. Conversely, children with hyperthyroidism may have excessive skeletal growth and become taller than they otherwise would. However, if there is premature closing of the epiphyses because of accelerated bone maturation, stunting of growth results. In the adult, excess thyroid hormone causes increased bone demineralization and an increased loss of calcium and phosphate.

Calcitonin is produced by cells in the interstitial tissue between the follicles of the thyroid gland; the effect of this hormone is to reduce the concentration of calcium ions in the blood—the exact opposite effect of parathyroid hormone. Calcitonin is essential for bone formation in children because it promotes the deposition of calcium. Calcitonin has a very weak effect on plasma concentration in adults because the absorption and deposition of calcium are slow in the adult and because the effects of calcitonin are rapidly overridden by parathyroid hormone.

Effects on the Central Nervous System From the time of birth through the first year of life, thyroid hormone must be present for normal cerebral development; irreversible mental retardation occurs if the hormone is not present. In the adult, hypothyroidism causes listlessness, a general dulling of mental capacity, decreased sensory capacity, slow speech, impaired memory, and somnolence. Hyperthyroidism in the adult results in hyperexcitability, irritability, restlessness, exaggerated responses to environmental stimuli, and emotional instability. Psychosis can occur in either hypothyroidism or hyperthyroidism.

Effects on Basal Metabolic Rate Thyroid hormones increase oxygen consumption in most cells of the body; the lungs, spleen, gastric smooth muscle, gonads, and accessory sex organs are not affected. The basal metabolic rate is subnormal with hypothyroidism; it may be 40% to 60% above normal with hyperthyroidism.

Effects on Carbohydrate and Lipid Metabolism Thyroid hormones accelerate glucose catabolism, increase cholesterol synthesis, and enhance the ability of the liver to excrete cholesterol in the bile. Because the effect on cholesterol excretion is greater than that on cholesterol synthesis, the result is a decrease in plasma cholesterol level. The hormones also stimulate the mobilization of fatty acids from adipose tissue. Individuals with hypothyroidism have an elevated serum cholesterol level and increased blood levels of phospholipids and triglycerides.

Effects on Protein Metabolism Thyroid hormones are essential for the development of protein mass. In hypothyroidism both the synthesis and the breakdown of protein are diminished, but the effect on protein synthesis is more profound. The deposition of mucoproteins occurs in subcutaneous spaces, which osmotically attract water, causing "puffiness." Increased catabolism of protein, or the breakdown of muscle mass, and increased nitrogen excretion occur with hyperthyroidism.

Effects on Gastrointestinal Function Thyroid hormones increase GI motility, the absorption of food, and the secretion of digestive juices. Hypothyroidism decreases both intestinal absorption and the secretion of pancreatic enzymes. Constipation may also occur with hypothyroidism.

Effects on Water and Electrolyte Balance Water and electrolytes accumulate in subcutaneous spaces when thyroid hormone is deficient. The result of administering thyroid hormone is diuresis and a loss of fluid and electrolytes from the subcutaneous spaces.

Effects on Cardiovascular Function Because the thyroid hormones increase metabolism, the tissues have an increased need for oxygen and nutrients; this in turn demands increased blood flow. In hyperthyroidism these effects cause increased cardiac output, increased pulse pressure, and tachycardia. If these effects are prolonged, cardiac hypertrophy and even high-output heart failure may occur (see Chapter 24). The opposite effects occur in hypothyroidism.

Effects on Muscle Function Moderate increases in thyroid hormone make muscles react with vigor; large increases result in muscle weakness because of excess protein catabolism. A characteristic sign of hyperthyroidism is a fine muscle tremor. Hypothyroidism causes the muscles to be sluggish.

Effects on Temperature Regulation Thyroid hormones must be present for an increase in heat production or a decrease in heat loss to occur. Although the hormones do not initiate the physiologic response to cold, they appear to magnify the body's response to catecholamine effects, which innervate the sympathetic system during exposure to cold. Hypothyroidism causes decreased tolerance to cold.

Effects on Lactation Thyroid hormone is necessary for normal milk production; without thyroid hormone, the fat content of milk and total milk production are greatly reduced.

Effects on Reproduction Thyroid hormone is required for normal rhythmicity in the reproductive cycle.

✳ What are the common disorders of the thyroid gland?

The three most frequently observed thyroid disorders in clinical practice are goiter, which results in an enlarged thyroid gland, hypothyroidism with reduced thyroid hormone release, and hyperthyroidism/thyrotoxicosis with risks for cardiovascular pathology.

Goiter The synthesis of the thyroid hormones and their maintenance in the blood in adequate amounts depend largely on an adequate intake of iodine. Iodine ingested through food or water is changed into iodide and is stored in the thyroid gland before reaching the circulation. Prolonged iodine deficiency in the diet results in enlargement of the thyroid gland, known as a simple goiter. When thyroid hormones fail to be synthesized because of a lack of iodine, the anterior lobe of the pituitary is stimulated to increase the secretion of thyrotropic hormone, which in turn causes hypertrophy and hyperplasia of the gland. The enlarged thyroid then removes residual traces of iodine from the blood. Providing an adequate supply of iodine for young persons can prevent this type of goiter (simple or nontoxic). Iodine is not abundant in most foods except fish and seafood; iodized salt is often the primary source of iodine in areas where seafood is expensive or not readily available.

Hypothyroidism Clients with primary hypothyroidism have decreased T_3 and T_4 levels and an elevated TSH level. Those with pituitary (secondary) hypothyroidism and hypothalamic (tertiary) hypothyroidism, much less frequently observed, have decreased levels of T_3, T_4, and TSH.

The TSH test, the most sensitive index of hypothyroidism, is elevated in primary hypothyroidism and depressed in secondary hypothyroidism. The free thyroxine index is depressed in clients with both primary and secondary hypothyroidism but elevated in clients with hyperthyroidism. The T_3 resin uptake (RT_3U) is depressed in pregnancy and in clients with primary and secondary hypothyroidism but is elevated in clients with hyperthyroidism. The serum T_3 level is depressed in both secondary and primary hypothyroidism but elevated in hyperthyroid states and T_3 thyrotoxicosis. The total T_4 is elevated in pregnancy and hyperthyroidism but depressed in both primary and secondary hypothyroidism. The free T_4 (unbound) is depressed in both primary and secondary hypothyroid states but is elevated in hyperthyroid states.

Hypothyroidism in the young child is known as cretinism. It is characterized by the cessation of physical and mental development, which leads to dwarfism and mental retardation. Clients with cretinism usually have thick, coarse skin; a thick tongue; a gaping mouth; a protruding abdomen; thick, short legs; poorly developed hands and feet; and weak musculature. This condition may result from faulty development or atrophy of the thyroid gland during fetal development. Failure of the gland to develop may be caused by a lack of iodine in the mother.

In children, normal skeletal growth is evidence of adequate therapy; an increase in serum alkaline phosphatase indicates that growth will occur. In cases of cretinism, thyroid hormone levels equal to or above those required for the adult must be established immediately after birth to prevent permanent mental and physical retardation. If cretinism is not treated until a later time, treatment will not reverse the mental retardation that has already occurred. Clients with hypothyroidism need to be informed of their lifelong need for replacement therapy.

Severe hypothyroidism in an adult is called myxedema. When it is the last stage of a long-standing, inadequately treated, or untreated hypothyroidism, coma sets in and is accompanied by hypotension, hypoventilation, hypothermia, bradycardia, hyponatremia, and hypoglycemia. The development of myxedema is usually insidious and causes gradual slowing of physical and mental functions. There is gradual infiltration of the skin and a loss of facial lines and facial expression, which results in a puffy, expressionless face. The formation of subcutaneous connective tissue causes the hands and face to appear puffy and swollen. The basal metabolic rate becomes subnormal, the skin is cold and dry, the hair becomes scant and coarse, movements become sluggish, cardiac output is reduced, and the client becomes hypersensitive to cold.

Hyperthyroidism Excessive formation of the thyroid hormones and their escape into the circulation result in a toxic state called thyrotoxicosis. This occurs with diffuse toxic goiter, exophthalmic goiter (Graves' disease), thyroid cancer, and in some forms of adenomatous goiters.

Primary hyperthyroidism is characterized by elevated levels of T₃ and T₄ and decreased levels of TSH. T_3, T_4, and TSH levels increase with pituitary (secondary) hyperthyroidism. Hyperthyroidism leads to symptoms quite different from those seen in myxedema. The metabolic rate is increased, sometimes as much as 60% or more. The body temperature is often above normal, the pulse rate is fast, and the client complains of feeling too warm. Other symptoms include restlessness, anxiety, emotional instability, muscle tremor and weakness, sweating, and exophthalmos. The increased thyroxine levels may cause cardiomegaly, tachycardia, atrial fibrillation, heart failure, hepatic alterations (necrosis, dysfunction, fatty changes), lymphoid hyperplasia, osteoporosis, pretibial myxedema, and neurologic irritability. In thyroid storm, elevated thyroxine levels cause a sudden onset of hyperthyroid symptoms, especially those affecting the nervous and cardiovascular systems.

Before the advent of antithyroid drugs, treatment was limited to a subtotal resection of the hyperactive gland. Propylthiouracil is the most commonly used antithyroid medication. However, antithyroid drugs provide less rapid control of hyperthyroidism than do surgical measures. Radioactive therapy is used primarily in treatment of middle-aged clients and older adults.

Parathyroid Glands

✲ What are the functions of the parathyroid glands and parathyroid hormones?

Lying just above and behind the thyroid gland are bean-shaped glands known as the parathyroids. Humans have two pairs of these glands. The adult glands consist of encapsulated masses of cells, between which are abundant adipocytes and vascular channels. The primary function of the parathyroids is to maintain adequate levels of calcium in the extracellular fluid. Parathyroid hormone has multiple effects, ultimately culminating in the mobilization of calcium from bone. It also reduces the concentration of phosphate, which permits more calcium to be mobilized.

Parathyroid hormone (PTH) is a polypeptide. The active component has a half-life of 30 minutes, and the inactive component has a half-life of 7 to 10 days. PTH circulates in elevated concentrations in clients with hyperplastic parathyroid glands as a result of diminished calcium levels; this condition occurs in persons with impaired renal function or intestinal malabsorption. Elevated PTH levels may cause metabolic bone disease, including osteoporosis and osteomalacia.

The mechanism of action of PTH in the bone or kidney is not completely understood. Some researchers suggest that PTH receptor binding and adenylate cyclase activity are coupled events that are subject to down regulation of the receptors. Clients with hyperparathyroidism may be resistant to PTH action in the kidney and bone. The decreased number of these receptors, not their altered affinity, produces a reduction in PTH-stimulated adenylate cyclase activity.

Cholesterol-derived provitamin D is converted to vitamin D₃ by the action of sunlight on the skin. The vitamin is also present as a milk additive. Along with PTH, vitamin D₃ is converted to its active form in the kidney. It is involved in the metabolism of calcium, phosphate, and magnesium in the bone and GI tract.

✲ What are the disorders of parathyroid function?

Primary hyperparathyroidism is caused by adenomas, chief cell hyperplasia, or hypertrophy. PTH elevations alter the function of renal tubular cells, bone cells, and GI tract mucosa. Elevated levels of calcium and increased bone resorption with the development of renal calculi generally occur in hyperparathyroidism. In secondary hyperparathyroidism, an overactive parathyroid gland causes increased calcium excretion and possibly kidney stones, but serum calcium levels generally remain stable because of an effective feedback mechanism.

Hypoparathyroidism leads to manifestations of hypocalcemia and tetany, the symptoms of which include muscle spasms, seizures, gradual paralysis with dyspnea, and death from exhaustion. GI hemorrhages and hematemesis commonly occur before death. At death the intestinal mucosa is congested, and the calcium content of the heart, kidney, and other tissues is increased.

Symptoms of tetany are relieved by administration of calcium salts. Large doses of vitamin D also help to relieve tetany and to restore the normal calcium level in the blood. The client is hospitalized because frequent assessment of blood calcium and phosphate levels is essential.

Adrenal Glands

✲ What is the role of the adrenal glands?

The adrenal glands are located just above the kidneys. They consist of two parts: the inner medulla and the outer cortex. The adrenal cortex synthesizes three important classes of hormones: the **glucocorticoids** (cortisol), **mineralocorticoids** (primarily aldosterone), and **androgens** (primarily dehydroepiandrosterone). The adrenal medulla is responsible for catecholamine production (e.g., epinephrine).

✲ How are the glucocorticoids, mineralocorticoids, and androgens differentiated?

Glucocorticoids The glucocorticoids—adrenocortical steroid hormones that increase glyconeogenesis, exert an antiinflammatory effect, and influence many body functions—are synthesized primarily in the zona fasciculata and are under the control of ACTH from the pituitary gland. The basal production rate averages 30 mg every 24 hours; under stressful conditions (trauma, major surgery, infection), there is a reserve capacity production of up to 300 mg daily. Increases in glucocorticoid production may be related to proportional increases in the release of ACTH by the pituitary. Chapter 48 discusses the uses and effects of glucocorticoids.

Mineralocorticoids The mineralocorticoids are synthesized specifically in the zona glomerulosa of the adrenal cortex. Production is primarily under the control of both the renin-angiotensin axis system (discussed later in this chapter) and the blood potassium level. The production of **aldosterone,** the primary mineralocorticoid, is stimulated by salt depletion and causes sodium retention in the kidney at the distal convoluted tubule to preserve extracellular fluid volume. Mineralocorticoids also increase the urinary excretion of potassium and hydrogen ions and maintain normal blood volume.

Aldosterone is the primary mineralocorticoid to regulate the balance of sodium and potassium in the blood. It is synthesized in the adrenal zona glomerulosa, which is the outer edge of the adrenocortical tissue below the adrenal capsule. The production of aldosterone is maintained primarily by the renin-angiotensin system and the concentration of circulating serum potassium. A drop in the circulating arterial volume stimulates volume receptors in the juxtaglomerular apparatus. As a result, renin (a proteolytic enzyme) is produced and acts on angiotensinogen, which is synthesized by the liver to form angiotensin I. When angiotensin I passes through the pulmonary circulation, two amino acids are cleared from it to form angiotensin II. Angiotensin II stimulates the adrenal zona glomerulosa to produce aldosterone. Aldosterone promotes sodium reabsorption in the kidney at the distal convoluted tubule to preserve extracellular fluid volume. Aldosterone secretion is normally stimulated by a decrease in circulating volume (e.g., loss of blood, excessive diuresis, low salt intake) and increased potassium levels. Aldosterone secretion is suppressed by an elevation of sodium levels in the blood (e.g., by excessive dietary salt intake). It restricts the loss of sodium and its accompanying anions, chloride and bicarbonate, and thereby helps to maintain extracellular fluid volume. It also maintains acid-base and potassium balance.

Androgens The androgens are synthesized in the zona fasciculata and the zona reticularis and essentially enhance male characteristics and control the growth of hair follicles in the skin.

✱ How does adrenal function change in response to stress?

A reaction to serious stress normally causes a prompt and noticeable increase in the production of cortisol and aldosterone; these hormones operate together to maintain the cardiovascular tone essential for survival. A client under stress who has impaired ability to produce these hormones incurs the risk of developing an acute adrenal crisis. The production of cortisol is under the control of a continuous feedback mechanism involving the pituitary and ACTH production, which in turn is inhibited by the circulating cortisol levels. Stress is a stimulus that overrides this inhibition and initiates the secretion of corticotropin-releasing factor; this culminates in the release of ACTH and activation of the adrenal cortex, which leads to an increased production of cortisol.

✱ What are the pathologic states involving adrenal function?

The two most common disorders or adrenal function are adrenal insufficiency (Addison's disease or hypoaldosteronism) and adrenal hyperfunction (adrenal virilism, hyperaldosteronism, Cushing's disease and pheochromocytoma).

Adrenal Insufficiency States In adrenal insufficiency or Addison's disease, there is a deficit of aldosterone, cortisol or both. One of the most common etiologies of adrenal insufficiency is abrupt withdrawal of chronically administered corticosteroids (e.g., prednisone) or inadequate corticosteroid dose during times of stress for clients maintained on chronically administered corticosteroids. Aldosterone deficit is manifest by inhibition of sodium reabsorption and decreased potassium excretion. Hyperkalemia and mild acidosis occur. Cortisol deficit results in altered carbohydrate, protein, and fat metabolism and altered insulin sensitivity.

In early adrenal insufficiency, weakness, fatigue, and orthostatic hypotension are often noted. In severe cases, adrenal insufficiency is manifested by abdominal pain, nausea, vomiting, diarrhea, shock, vascular collapse, and cardiac dysrhythmias. This may lead to death unless a mineralocorticoid, salt, and water are administered immediately.

Adrenal Hyperfunction Syndromes of adrenal hyperfunction depend on which zones and which hormones are elevated. If androgens are elevated, adrenal virilism with hirsutism, baldness, acne, and deeper voice are noted. Elevations in aldosterone can produce weakness, tetany, and hypertension with elevated serum sodium and chloride levels and hypervolemia. Pheochromocytoma is most often secondary to tumor growth and results in elevated catecholamine levels (e.g., epinephrine, norepinephrine) and intermittent but significant hypertensive episodes (often with tachycardia and sweating). Cushing's disease is manifested by body fat redistribution, poor wound healing, muscle wasting, and weakness. Fat deposits on the face (moonface) or back ("buffalo hump") with slender arms, legs, and fingers are a common presentation. Cushing's disease is related to overactivity of cortisol, and is most often secondary to chronic corticosteroid (e.g., prednisone) therapy.

Pancreas

✱ What are the endocrine functions of the pancreas?

The pancreas is a gland that lies transversely across the posterior wall of the abdomen. It secretes a limpid, colorless fluid that digests proteins, fats, and carbohydrates. It also produces internal secretions—insulin and glucagon—that affect blood sugar levels.

Insulin is a hormone secreted by the beta cells of the islets of Langerhans in the pancreas in response to increased levels of glucose in the blood. On hydrolysis, this hormone yields several amino acids. In its crystalline state it appears to be chemically linked with certain metals (zinc, nickel, cadmium, or cobalt). Normal pancreatic tissue is rich in zinc, which may be significant to the natural storage of the hormone. Insulin consists of two polypeptide chains and contains 51 amino acids, the exact sequence of which is known. Insulin is stored in the beta cells as a larger protein known as proinsulin. Because relatively small amounts of insulin are necessary in the body tissues, it is thought that insulin acts as a catalyst in cellular metabolism.

Carbohydrate metabolism is controlled by a finely balanced interaction of several endocrine factors (adrenal, anterior pituitary, thyroid, insulin), but the particular phase of carbohydrate metabolism that is affected by insulin is not entirely known. An subcutaneous injection of insulin produces a rapid lowering of blood sugar in both diabetic and nondiabetic persons. Moderate amounts of insulin in diabetic animals promote the storage of carbohydrate in the liver and also in the muscle cells, particularly after the ingestion of carbohydrate. The deposit of muscle glycogen also increases in the nondiabetic animal, but apparently the level of liver glycogen does not. In both diabetic and nondiabetic persons, the oxygen consumption increases and the respiratory quotient rises.

Glucagon, like insulin, is a pancreatic extract and is thought to oppose the action of insulin. Glucagon is a product of the alpha cells of the islets of Langerhans. Glucagon acts primarily by mobilizing hepatic glycogen and converting it to glucose, which produces an elevation in the concentration of glucose in the blood.

✴ What are the diseases of the pancreas?

Pathology of the pancreas can be related to altered exocrine or altered endocrine functions. Chapters 39 and 40 discuss altered exocrine functions, including states resulting in changes in amylase, lipase, and protease. The endocrine-based pathologic state most commonly associated with the pancreas is diabetes mellitus.

Diabetes mellitus (DM) is a heterogenous complex disorder of carbohydrate, fat, and protein metabolism that is primarily a result of a relative or complete lack of insulin or defects of the insulin receptors. Type 1 DM results in lack of insulin production and is usually presents as a childhood onset. Type 2 DM involves altered insulin sensitivity at the tissue level and is typically observed in older, obese individuals. Obesity, certain drugs, viruses, autoimmune phenomena, genetic predisposition, and age may have roles in its development. The blood glucose becomes elevated, and when it exceeds a certain amount, the excess is secreted by the kidney (glycosuria). Symptoms include increased appetite (polyphagia), thirst (polydipsia), weight loss, increased urine output (polyuria), weakness (fatigue), and itching (e.g., pruritus vulvae).

In DM, glycogen fails to store in the liver, although the conversion of glycogen back to glucose or the formation of glucose from fatty acids and proteins (**gluconeogenesis**) is not necessarily impaired. As a result, the level of blood glucose rapidly rises. For clients with type 1 disease, this derangement of carbohydrate metabolism results in an abnormally high metabolism of proteins and fats. The ketone bodies, which result from the oxidation of fatty acids, accumulate faster than the muscle cells can oxidize them, resulting in ketosis and acidosis.

The course of untreated DM is progressive. The symptoms of diabetic coma and acidosis are directly or indirectly the result of the accumulation of acetone, β-hydroxybutyric acid, and diacetic acid. Unless treatment is started promptly, respirations become rapid and deep, the breath has an odor of acetone, the blood glucose is elevated, the client becomes dehydrated, and stupor and coma develop.

The long-term complications of DM can lead to an increase in morbidity and mortality. Some of the most commonly associated problems are peripheral atherosclerosis, which may result in coronary artery disease (CAD), infections, gangrene, or stroke; and diabetic retinopathy, which can include vitreal hemorrhage, retinal detachment, and blindness. Renal disease, peripheral sensory neuropathy, and cardiomyopathy leading to heart failure are also frequent complications of uncontrolled DM.

DM is usually treated with diet, exercise, and when necessary, medication. Those with type 1 DM require exogenous insulin. Clients with type 2 diabetes are treated often with drugs that enhance insulin action, but exogenous insulin can be used in more advanced cases. Glucose and insulin promote the formation and retention of glycogen in the liver, and the oxidation of fat in the liver is arrested. Therefore the rate of formation of acetone bodies is slowed and the acidosis is checked. Other supportive measures, such as restoring the fluid and electrolyte balance of the body, are very important in treatment.

Advances in diabetic therapy include the following: (1) the synthesis insulin analogs and human insulin by bacteria genetically altered by recombinant DNA technology, (2) islet cell and/or pancreas transplantation, (3) external and implanted continuous insulin infusion pumps, and, (4) an increasing array of oral agents to treat type 2 disease. Stem cell research appears promising and may ultimately lead to better management of DM.

Summary

The endocrine system carries out integrative and regulatory functions within the body through the actions of hormones. Hormones regulate mechanisms that allow the body to meet its needs. The endocrine system consists of specialized glands and their hormones, which act on specific target cells and stimulate various responses. The overproduction or underproduction of hormones results in pathologic conditions. Hormonal replacement therapy is the major concern in the underproduction of hormones by the endocrine system.

Critical Thinking Questions

- Given that the hospital laboratory has the ability to determine blood levels of TSH, T$_3$, and T$_4$, create a protocol for determining whether hyperthyroidism is the result of a pituitary abnormality or the production of a nonpituitary thyroid-stimulating substance.

- A client is admitted to the emergency department with polydipsia (thirst), polyuria (excess urine production), and urine with low specific gravity. The prescriber wants to reverse these symptoms. Which of the following substances will he or she ask you to administer: insulin, glucagon, antidiuretic hormone, or aldosterone? Explain why.

- A client arrives at the emergency department. He is unconscious, and his MedicAlert bracelet indicates that he has diabetes. The client may be in diabetic coma or insulin shock. How do you distinguish between these two conditions, and what treatment would you recommend for each condition?

Bibliography

Anderson, D.M., Keith, J., & Novak, P.D. (Eds.) (2002). *Mosby's medical, nursing, and allied health dictionary* (6th ed.). St. Louis: Mosby.

Drug facts and comparisons (58th ed.). (2005). St. Louis: Facts and Comparisons.

Guyton, A.C., & Hall, J.E. (2000). *Textbook of medical physiology* (10th ed.). Philadelphia: W.B. Saunders.

Herlihy, B., & Maebius, N.K. (2003). *The human body in health and illness* (2nd ed.). Philadelphia: W.B. Saunders.

McCance, K.L., & Huether, S.E. (2002). *Pathophysiology: The biological basis for disease in adults and children* (4th ed.). St. Louis: Mosby.

Merck Manual Online. (2005). Retrieved July 21, 2005, from http://www.merck.com/mrkshared/mmanual/section2/chapter9/9 a.jsp

Parker, K.L., & Schimmer, B.P. (2001). Pituitary hormones and their hypothalamic releasing factors. In: Hardman, J.G. & Limbird, L.E. (Eds.), *Goodman and Gilman's The pharmacological basis of therapeutics* (10th ed.). New York: McGraw-Hill.

Thibodeau, G.A., & Patton, K.T. (2003). *Anatomy and physiology* (5th ed.). St. Louis: Mosby.

e-LEARNING SUPPLEMENTS

Student CD-ROM
- Final Exam questions
- NCLEX® Examination review questions
- Pharmacology animations
- Printable chapter summary

Evolve Website (http://evolve.elsevier.com/mckenry)
- Content updates, including information on new drugs

- WebLinks corresponding to this chapter
- Answers to the critical thinking questions in this chapter
- *Elsevier ePharmacology Update* newsletter
- Mosby's Drug Consult Internet Edition
- Supplemental and reference information

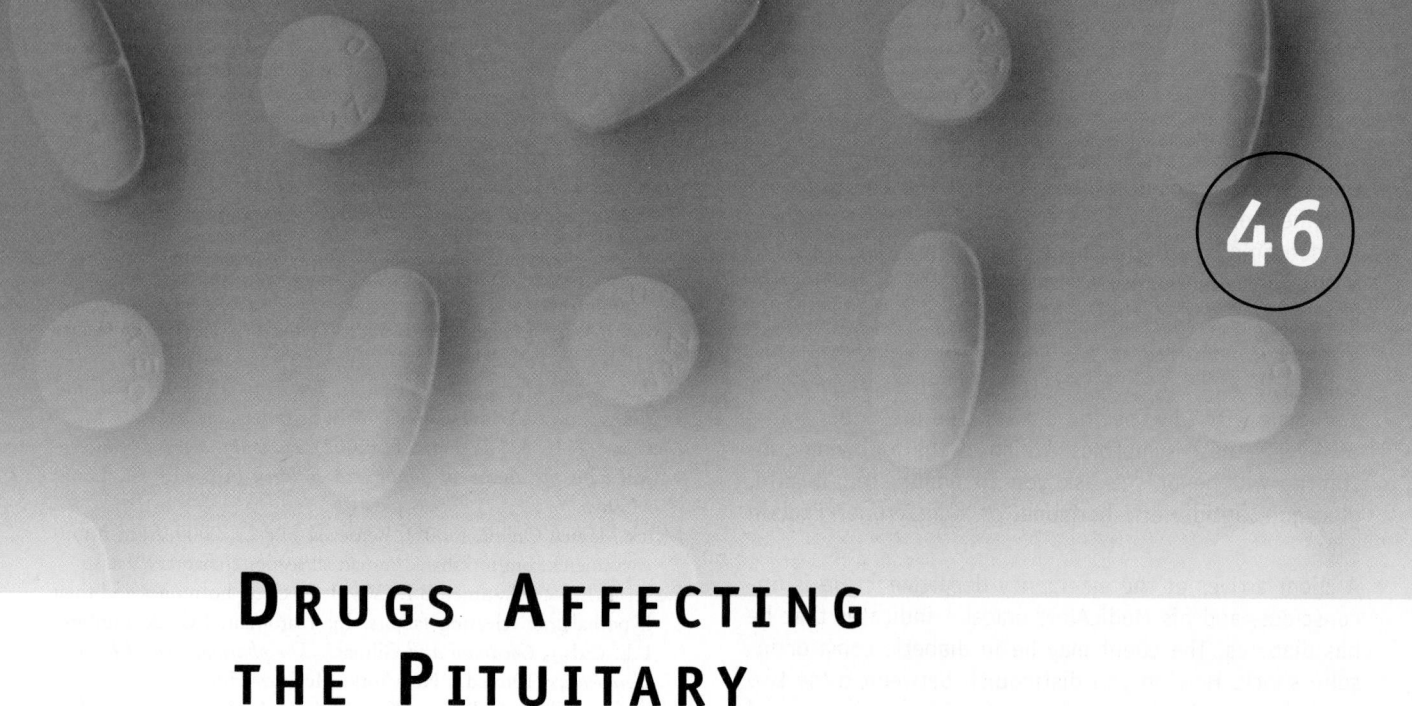

46

DRUGS AFFECTING THE PITUITARY

CHAPTER FOCUS

Although the pituitary secretes numerous hormones, this chapter discusses only the growth hormones (GHs) and the antidiuretic hormone, vasopressin. Other hormones are discussed in chapters more directly related to the endocrine glands they affect. Although disorders involving these two hormones are not common, the nurse is expected to appropriately assess and care for clients with pituitary dysfunction.

LEARNING OBJECTIVES	• Describe the primary functions of the anterior and posterior pituitary hormones. • Describe the effects of somatrem, somatropin, and octreotide. • List the effects of vasopressin. • Implement the nursing management of the client receiving drugs affecting the pituitary.

▲ **KEY TERMS**
dwarfism, p. 825
gigantism, p. 825
growth hormone–inhibiting hormone (somatostatin), p. 825
growth hormone–releasing hormone, p. 825

KEY DRUGS
somatrem, p. 825
vasopressin, p. 828

 What is the role of the pituitary-related hormones?
The variety of available preparations that affect the pituitary gland are sometimes used as replacement therapy for hormone deficiency, as drug therapy for specific disorders to produce a therapeutic hormonal response, and as diagnostic aids to determine hypofunctional or hyperfunctional hormone states.

A number of hormones have been identified, and many have been synthesized, including the following: GH-releasing hormone (GH-RH), GH-inhibiting hormone (somatostatin), thyrotropin-releasing hormone (TRH), corticotropin-releasing hormone (CRH), gonadotropin-releasing hormone (GnRH), and prolactin-inhibiting hormone (PIH or dopamine). Six anterior pituitary hormones and two posterior pituitary hor-

mones have also been identified and are reviewed in Chapter 45. The anterior pituitary hormones include GH, thyrotropin (thyroid-stimulating hormone [TSH]), adrenocorticotropin (ACTH), follicle-stimulating hormone (FSH), luteinizing hormone (LH), and prolactin. The posterior pituitary hormones are vasopressin and oxytocin. This chapter covers specific agents that affect the pituitary.

Chapter 51 discusses gonadotropin-releasing hormone; Chapters 47 and 48 discuss thyrotropin-releasing hormone and corticotropin-releasing hormone, respectively. Although a true hormone with prolactin-inhibiting effects has not been identified, dopamine does inhibit prolactin to some degree. Chapters 23 and 52 review bromocriptine, a drug with dopamine-agonist properties.

❊ **S.P. is an 8-year-old diagnosed with growth failure by his pediatrician. He is being considered for GH therapy.**

❊ **What hormones are administered to affect growth?**
The anterior pituitary is responsible for secreting hormones that affect growth. Of these substances, human growth hormone (hGH) is used to treat growth failure in children and for the treatment of GH-deficient states in both children and adults. Somatrem and somatropin are synthetic derivatives of hGH. In addition to treating growth failure or GH-deficient states, these substances are also used to treat Prader-Willi syndrome, Turner's syndrome, and muscle wasting observed in acquired immune deficiency syndrome (AIDS).

Growth hormone–releasing hormone has been identified in vivo but is still under investigation. This substance has been found to stimulate the release of GH after intranasal application, but its optimal dosage, route, and frequency of administration have not been determined (Larsen, 2003).

At one time the **growth hormone–inhibiting hormone** (**somatostatin**—not to be confused with the similar sounding somatrem and somatropin) was obtained from human cadaver pituitaries, but its distribution in the United States was stopped in 1985. Creutzfeldt-Jakob disease (a neurotropic virus), which is very rare in young people, was diagnosed in some clients and resulted in the death of several persons 5 to 7 years after receiving this product. Several biosynthetic hormones grown through recombinant deoxyribonucleic acid (DNA) technology are available in the United States. The most widely used analog of somatostatin is octreotide, which is used to inhibit the release of GH and for specific actions in the gastrointestinal (GI) tract. Pegvisomant (Somavert) is an antagonist of GH used on a restricted basis to treat acromegaly.

Growth Hormone Agonists

❊▣ somatrem [**soe** ma trem] (also known as human growth hormone)
(Protropin)
Somatrem contains the identical sequence of the pituitary-derived hGH plus one additional amino acid, methionine. In tests it has been demonstrated to be therapeutically equivalent to somatropin, the pituitary hGH.

The anabolic effects of somatrem result from the indirect effect of other hormones known as somatomedin-C or insulin-like growth factors (IGF-1) (Heck, Yanovski, & Calis, 2002). IGF-1 is directly responsible for the growth of skeletal and soft tissue, and it increases the number of cells in the body rather than cell size. Therefore a major pharmacologic consequence of the use of somatrem is an increase in longitudinal growth; a deficiency in GH usually results in **dwarfism,** an abnormal underdevelopment of the body.

Somatrem also has metabolic effects. It decreases insulin sensitivity and may also affect glucose transport. It also increases lipolysis; promotes cellular growth by retaining phosphorus, sodium, and potassium; and enhances protein synthesis by increasing the retention of nitrogen.

Indications
Somatrem is indicated for the treatment of growth failure in children as a result of a deficiency in pituitary GH. It is also used for the treatment of short stature in children who are 2.5 standard deviations below the mean in height. It is sometimes abused by athletes seeking increased size and strength (Box 46-1).

Pharmacokinetics/Dosing
Although the half-life of parenteral (IV) somatrem is 20 to 30 minutes (3 to 5 hours for intramuscular [IM] and subcutaneous forms), the duration of action for IV, IM, and subcutaneous preparations is 12 to 48 hours. Somatrem is metabolized in the liver and excreted by the kidneys. With children, the dosage and administration of somatrem for injection (Protropin) is up to 0.1 mg/kg IM or subcutaneous (preferred) three times weekly. The growth rate response is monitored in 3 to 6 months to determine if a dosage adjustment is necessary. Therapy is usually continued until epiphyseal closure occurs or there is no further response. If therapy is unsuccessful (less than 2 cm per year), treatment should be discontinued and the child reevaluated (*Drug Facts and Comparisons,* 2005; *USP DI,* 2005).

Adverse Effects
Antibodies to somatrem have been reported in 30% to 40% of treated clients during the first 3 to 6 months of therapy, but only 5% of the clients develop neutralizing antibodies. It is rare that a client does not respond to therapy. However, pain and edema have been reported at the site of injection; an allergic-type reaction (rash, itching) is rare. Excessive doses may produce **gigantism** in

---

BOX 46-1 GROWTH HORMONE ABUSE

Some athletes use GH to either increase their size and strength or their ultimate height, depending on the age of the user. The anabolic effects of short-term usage in sports are difficult to predict and may not truly offer athletic advantage (Godfrey, Whyte, & Head, 2004; Rennie, 2003). Users are at risk for the adverse effects of the drug—acromegalic syndrome, with symptoms such as increased size of facial bones, thickened hands and fingers, osteoporosis, long-term heart failure, diabetes, impotence, and amenorrhea. Additionally, because the drug is injectable, there are the added risks of hepatitis and AIDS as the result of shared needles and syringes.

Under an amendment to the Food, Drug, and Cosmetic Act, "whoever knowingly distributes, or possesses, hGH for any use in humans other than the treatment of disease or other recognized medical condition, or such use as has been authorized by the Secretary of Health and Human Services under Section 505 and pursuant to the order of a physician, is guilty of an offense punishable by not more than 5 years in prison, such fines as are authorized by Title 18, United States Code, or both." This legislation clearly defines GH distribution as a serious federal offense, and federal authorities are authorized to investigate these practices.

Fortunately, its cost and the fact that anabolic steroids are simply more enticing to the athlete limit the abuse of GH. However, there are adverse effects with which many athletes are unfamiliar and education of the potential consequences of GH excess is important in counseling athletes considering its use.

Modified from Godfrey, R., Whyte, G., Head, T. (2004). Acute Human Growth Hormone Response in Elite Rowers After 12 weeks of Training. Medicine & Science in Sports & Exercise, 36(5) Supplement, S303; Rennie, M.J. (2003). Claims for the anabolic effects of growth hormone: a case of the emperor's new clothes? *British Journal of Sports Medicine, 37,* 100-105.

children, an abnormal condition characterized by excessive size and stature. Therefore growth failure must be carefully documented before the drug is used, and dosages and individual responses must be closely monitored. Hypothyroidism is rarely reported.

Long-term risks for use include inhibition of pituitary function, and may pose increased risk for adrenal insufficiency and hypoglycemia. An analysis of over 6000 recipients of earlier forms of GH from 1963 to 1985 identified a fourfold increase in mortality with its use (Mills et al., 2004). Mortality rates were lowest for those who had idiopathic GH deficiency.

Drug Interactions

The growth response effects of somatrem may be impaired when given concurrently with adrenocorticoids, glucocorticoids, or corticotropin (ACTH). ACTH should not be given concurrently; if it is necessary to treat with an adrenocorticoid agent, the daily doses should be limited. For example, the total daily dose per square meter of body area should not be greater than the following: cortisone (12.5 to 18.8 mg), hydrocortisone (10 to 15 mg), methylprednisolone (2 to 3 mg), prednisone or prednisolone (2.5 to 3.75 mg), betamethasone (300 to 450 mcg), and dexamethasone (250 to 500 mcg).

somatropin, biosynthetic [soe mah **troe** pin]
(Humatrope)

Somatropin is a DNA recombinant product that is identical to the amino acid sequence of hGH. It is used to stimulate linear growth in clients who lack sufficient endogenous GH; this stimulation results in increased skeletal growth (an increased length of the epiphyseal plates of long bones is reported). The number and size of muscle cells, organs, and red cell mass are also increased. An increase in cellular protein synthesis and lipid mobilization resulting in a decrease in body fat stores is also reported.

Indications
Similar to somatrem.

Pharmacokinetics/Dosing
The recommended dosage is individualized—the maximal replacement weekly dosage is 0.3 mg/kg subcutaneous or IM divided into equal doses given either on 3 alternate days, 6 times a week, or daily for growth hormone–deficient pediatric clients (*Mosby's Drug Consult,* 2005).

Adverse Effects
Similar to somatrem.

Growth Hormone Antagonist

pegvisomant [peg **vi** soe mant]
(Somavert)

Pegvisomant is similar in chemical structure to GH. It displays affinity for GH receptors and competitively blocks the binding of endogenous GH to GH receptors. Reduced levels of IGF-1 are observed and often used as a measure of response. The drug consists of a protein affixed to polyethylene glycol (PEG) polymers, which extend its duration of action.

Indications
Pegvisomant is used to treat acromegaly resistant to other interventions. In the United States, its availability is limited through the pharmaceutical manufacturer.

Pharmacokinetics
After subcutaneous injection, it achieves a peak level in the blood at 33 to 77 hours (Lacy, Armstrong, Goldman, & Lance, 2004). The elimination half-life is approximately 6 days. Dosage is typically 40 mg subcutaneous as an initial loading dose, then 10 mg subcutaneous daily with dosage adjustments every 4 to 6 weeks based on IGF-I levels and response.

Adverse Effects
A number of adverse effects are attributed to pegvisomant, including infections, flu-like syndrome, hypertension, peripheral edema, pain on injection, diarrhea, and back pain. Development of antibodies to GH is observed in many clients, but the clinical significance of this finding is not clear.

✷ **S.P. (20 kg) is started on somatropin recombinant (Humatrope) at 0.025 mg/kg (0.5 mg) subcutaneously three times weekly on Mondays, Wednesdays, and Fridays.**

✷ **What are the nursing management issues with hGH?**

Assessment A baseline assessment includes a family history, a history of the child's growth patterns and previous health status, physical examination, psychosocial evaluation, radiographic surveys, and endocrine studies. It is ascertained that S.P. does not have a malignancy, especially an intracranial tumor. GH is also contraindicated in clients with closed epiphyses or in those with a known sensitivity to benzyl alcohol, such as neonates. It is ascertained that S.P. does not have untreated hypothyroidism, because the response to the GH would be adversely affected.

Review S.P.'s current medication regimen to ensure he is not receiving adrenocorticoids, glucocorticoid, or corticotropin, which inhibit the growth response to somatrem. Hydrocortisone and cortisone are allowed for brief administration of stress dosages during acute febrile illness or other acute stress.

Nursing Diagnosis While receiving somatrem therapy, S.P. is at risk for the following nursing diagnoses/collaborative problems: delayed growth and development related to an underlying lack of endogenous GH secretion and an ineffective response to the drug; fatigue; impaired tissue integrity (pain and swelling at the injection site); and the potential complications of allergic reaction (rash), slipped capital femoral epiphysis (limp, pain in hip or knee), and hypothyroidism.

Planning While receiving GH, S.P. will:
- Demonstrate an acceleration of growth velocity until achievement of height appropriate to family height.
- With his parents, effectively manage his drug regimen, including correct administration technique and compliance with medications
- Collaborate with health care providers, reporting adverse effects appropriately and maintaining scheduled appointment with health care providers for monitoring and treatment.

Implementation

Monitoring Monitor bone age determinations, thyroid function studies, blood glucose determinations (hGH can cause insulin resistance) and anti–GH antibodies periodically during therapy. If the growth rate does not exceed the pretreatment rate by 2 cm per year, S.P. should be monitored for noncompliance or other factors such as antibody formation, hypothyroidism (lethargy, intolerance to cold, weight gain, constipation, dry skin, and brittle, lackluster hair), or malnutrition. Antibodies to somatrem may form in some clients after several months of therapy, but these rarely reduce the response to therapy. Ineffectiveness to therapy is more a function of the binding capacity of antibodies rather than the antibody titer.

Observe the injection site; pain and swelling can occur at the site of injection.

Intervention A HumatroPen has a cartridge that allows a specific dose to be administered by dialing in increments of 0.048 mL per click of the dosage knob (e.g., the 6-mg cartridge contains a 0.1-mg dose per click of the dosage knob). A sterile disposable needle should be used for each administration of Humatrope. Other manufacturers also have a cartridge system for drug administration.

Optimal dosing is often achieved when the drug is administered at bedtime. Physiologic release is more normally simulated as a result of pituitary release of GH during the first 45 to 90 minutes after the onset of sleep.

Decision to discontinue drug is made jointly by client, family, and health care team. Radiologic evidence of epiphyseal closure is a criterion for ending therapy.

Education Instruct S.P. in self-administration techniques. This is particularly important to increase S.P.'s self-esteem as it is not uncommon for people to juvenilize children who are short in stature.

Advise S.P. and his parents of the importance of regular visits to the pediatric endocrinologist for the monitoring of blood and urine studies, thyroid function studies, and growth rate and bone age determinations.

Evaluation The expected outcome of somatrem therapy is that the client will experience an increase in the growth pattern at a minimum of 2 cm per year. Therapy is usually continued as long as the client is responsive and until a mature adult stature is reached or S.P.'s epiphyses close. S.P. and his parents state the signs and symptoms of adverse effects to the GH and when to report them to the prescriber. S.P. and his parents demonstrate the correct method for subcutaneous injections of the GH.

What other agents affect growth?

octreotide [ok **tree** oh tide]
(Sandostatin)
Octreotide is a long-acting agent with an effect similar to somatostatin, the GH-inhibiting hormone; however, octreotide is a more potent inhibitor of GH, glucagon, and insulin (*Drug Facts and Comparisons*, 2005). It demonstrates other effects as well, including GI effects, rendering it effective for a number of GI ailments.
Indications
Octreotide is indicated to lower blood levels of GH and IGF-1 to normal in persons with acromegaly who have not responded to other therapies, such as surgery, radiation, and bromocriptine. It is also used to treat symptoms associated with carcinoid tumors, such as flushing and severe diarrhea. It also has many unapproved uses, including the treatment of diarrhea associated with AIDS. It is used acutely to control bleeding of esophageal varices.
Pharmacokinetics/Dosing
Octreotide is rapidly absorbed after subcutaneous injection and reaches a peak serum concentration in approximately 25 minutes; the half-life is 1.7 hours. Its duration of action is variable but can be up to 12 hours depending on the tumor. The IV and subcutaneous dosages are considered equivalent in effect. The dosage for the treatment of acromegaly is 50 mcg subcutaneously or IV three times daily; the dosage is adjusted according to the client's response and the presence of adverse effects. Dosing for controlling

esophageal variceal bleeding is typically 25 to 50 mcg IV × 1, then 25-50 mcg/hr by continuous IV infusion. Dosage for other indications vary. Refer to package insert for more information.
Adverse Effects
The adverse effects of octreotide include pain, swelling, and pruritus at the injection site; sinus bradycardia; diarrhea and stomach distress (30% to 58% in clients with acromegaly, and only 5% to 10% in clients with other disorders); headache, dysrhythmias, and cold-like symptoms. Hyperglycemia, hypoglycemia, and hypothyroidism are also reported primarily in clients with acromegaly. Refer to a current reference for a list of other potential adverse effects.

What nursing issues are involved in the use of octreotide?

Assessment Determine that the client does not have active gallbladder disease or gallstones or a history of these conditions; there is an increased risk of cholelithiasis because of decreased gallbladder motility and the alteration of fat absorption with the administration of octreotide. If the client has diabetes mellitus, hypoglycemic medications may have to be adjusted. A baseline and periodic ultrasonograms may be necessary to assess for the presence of gallstones. Thyroid function studies and serum GH levels are needed for baseline determinations.

Review the client's current medication regimen for oral antidiabetic agents, insulin, glucagon, or GH; the use of these medications in combination with octreotide may result in hypoglycemia or hyperglycemia. A baseline determination of blood glucose concentrations is recommended.

Record a detailed assessment of the condition for which the octreotide is administered before initiating therapy. Determine also the client's sensitivity to octreotide.

Nursing Diagnosis The client receiving octreotide is at risk for the following nursing diagnoses/collaborative problems: impaired comfort (abdominal cramping, headache, flushing of the face, nausea and vomiting); impaired tissue integrity (pain and redness at the injection site); diarrhea; fatigue; and the potential complications of altered cardiac output (dysrhythmias, bradycardia), acute pancreatitis, and hypoglycemia or hyperglycemia.

Planning The client receiving octreotide will:
- If administered for acromegaly, demonstrate a significant decrease in GH concentration and an improvement in clinical symptoms. If administered for GI tumors, experience fewer episodes of severe diarrhea and facial flushing.
- Effectively manage his drug regimen, including correct administration technique and compliance with medications
- Collaborate with health care providers, reporting adverse effects appropriately and maintaining scheduled appointment with health care providers for monitoring and treatment.

Implementation
Monitoring Monitor GH levels at periods appropriate to the selected administration schedule. Monitor blood glu-

cose determinations, particularly during dosage changes in the medication regimen. Observe the client for hypoglycemia (anxiety, cool/pale skin, headache, hunger, nausea, difficulty concentrating, nervousness, shakiness, weakness, unconsciousness) and hyperglycemia (drowsiness, red/dry skin, anorexia, acetone-like breath, thirst, nausea and vomiting, rapid weight loss, lethargy, unconsciousness). Urinary 5-hydroxyindoleacetic acid (5-HIAA) determinations are recommended periodically during therapy for clients with carcinoid tumors. Periodic ultrasonograms are done to assess the presence of gallstones.

Intervention Octreotide comes in two formulations. To initiate therapy, the octreotide acetate injection is administered two or three times a day for at least 2 weeks. When responsiveness to octreotide is determined, the client is switched to the injectable suspension with injections monthly.

Octreotide is administered subcutaneously, with the hip, thigh, and abdomen being the preferred sites. Administration into the deltoid causes severe discomfort. Administer octreotide slowly at room temperature, and rotate injection sites to prevent tissue irritation. Administer between meals and at bedtime to minimize the GI symptoms of octreotide.

Education Counsel the client about the importance of close monitoring by the prescriber. Instruct the client regarding proper injection technique, to rotate and select injection sites and to report any signs of irritation at the injection sites or any symptoms of hyperglycemia, hypoglycemia, or cholelithiasis.

Evaluation The expected outcome of octreotide therapy administered for a pituitary tumor is that, there will be a reduction in the secretion of GH as evidenced by suppressed tumor growth and a decrease in the client's symptoms of acromegaly. If administered as an antidiarrheal for GI tumors or AIDS, the outcome is that the client will experience fewer, firmer stools or a bowel elimination pattern that is normal for that client. The client will effectively manage the drug regimen by remaining medication compliant and correctly administering his or her own injections. The client will report symptoms of hypoglycemia or hyperglycemia and other adverse effects to the prescriber and will maintain scheduled appointments for monitoring and ongoing treatment.

✪ **W.S. is a 7-year-old boy with nocturnal enuresis. His pediatrician is discussing the use of desmopressin (DDAVP) nasal solution with T.C. and his father.**

✪ **What are the clinically used posterior pituitary gland hormones?**
The hormones secreted by the posterior pituitary gland are oxytocin and vasopressin (antidiuretic hormone [ADH]). Chapter 52 discusses oxytocin with the drugs related to labor and delivery.

Vasopressin is obtained from natural sources; lypressin and desmopressin are synthetic derivatives of vasopressin. Desmopressin has a longer duration of activity than the other agents.

The ADH effect of these agents is the result of increasing water reabsorption in the collecting ducts of the nephron. This leads to a decreased urine volume with a higher osmolarity. At higher than physiologic dosages, vasopressin stimulates peristalsis through a direct effect on GI motility; increases the secretion of corticotropin, GH, and follicle-stimulating hormone; and may increase blood pressure secondary to a vasoconstrictive effect. The synthetic formulations (desmopressin [DDAVP] and lypressin [Diapid]) act as ADH with little vasopressor activity.

These agents are used to treat diabetes insipidus, a metabolic disorder characterized by extreme polyuria and polydipsia and caused by the deficient production or secretion of ADH centrally. Desmopressin is available as an intranasal solution and is also frequently used for the treatment of nocturnal enuresis. Vasopressin, desmopressin, and lypressin are not effective for polyuria induced by renal impairment, nephrogenic diabetes insipidus, psychogenic diabetes insipidus, hypokalemia, hypercalcemia, or drug-induced diabetes insipidus (lithium).

⭐▀ **vasopressin** [vay soe **press** in]
(Pitressin, Pressyn✱)
Indications
Vasopressin (Pitressin) is used to treat diabetes insipidus and for treatment of GI hemorrhage, including bleeding esophageal varices. It is also used as part of cardiac resuscitation protocols for cardiac asystole, and may be slightly more effective for this indication compared with epinephrine (Wenzel et al., 2004).
Pharmacokinetics/Dosing
Vasopressin administered IM or subcutaneously has a half-life of 10 to 20 minutes; the duration of effect is 2 to 8 hours. It is metabolized in the liver and kidneys and excreted by the kidneys. The adult dosage of aqueous vasopressin injection (Pitressin) is 5 to 10 units IM or subcutaneously two or three times daily when needed to treat central diabetes insipidus. In children the dosage for the treatment of central diabetes insipidus is 2.5 to 10 units three or four times daily.
Adverse Effects
See Table 46-1.

desmopressin [des moe **press** in]
(DDAVP, Stimate, Octostim✱)
Indications
Desmopressin intranasal is used for primary nocturnal enuresis and nocturnal polyuria in men. The oral, intranasal, and parenteral dosage forms are used to treat central diabetes insipidus, whereas only the parenteral dosage form of desmopressin is used for homeostasis in clients with hemophilia A and von Willebrand's disease.
Pharmacokinetics/Dosing
Desmopressin nasal has a half-life of approximately 3.5 hours, and peak serum concentration is reached in 40 to 45 minutes; oral and intranasal dosage forms reach a peak serum level in 30 to 90 minutes. The onset of antidiuretic effects with desmopressin tablets is within 1 hour, with the maximum effect reached between 4 and 7 hours. For primary nocturnal enuresis, the dosage of desmopressin intranasal for adults and children 6 years and older is 20 mcg at bedtime, adjusted as necessary. The adult intranasal dosage for central diabetes insipidus is 10 to 40 mcg daily as a single dose or in divided doses. The parenteral dosage is 1 to 2 mcg subcutaneously or IV twice daily. The oral adult dosage starts with 50 mcg twice daily and is adjusted according to response.
Adverse Effects
See Table 46-1.

TABLE 46-1 POSTERIOR PITUITARY HORMONES: ADVERSE EFFECTS

Drug	Minor/Moderate Adverse Effects*	Serious Adverse Effects†
desmopressin (DDAVP, Stimate)	Less frequent: headache, nausea, mild stomach cramps, vulvar pain. Injection: local redness, burning or swelling, facial flush, slight increase or decrease in blood pressure.	Rare: severe allergic reaction including anaphylaxis with parenteral administration.
lypressin (Diapid)	Less frequent: abdominal distress, headache, heartburn, eye pain, nasal irritation or itching, runny nose, increase in bowel movements.	Rare: continuous coughing, chest pain, shortness of breath, difficulty breathing.
vasopressin (Pitressin)	Less frequent: abdominal distress, gas, sweating, nausea, vomiting, tremors, increased pressure for bowel evacuation, headache.	Rare: chest pain due to angina or myocardial infarction; allergic reaction; increased or continuing headaches, confusion, coma, seizures, weight gain, drowsiness, urinary difficulties (usually the result of water retention or intoxication).

*If minor/moderate adverse effects continue, increase, or disturb the client, inform the prescriber.
†If serious adverse effects occur, contact the prescriber because medical intervention may be necessary.

lypressin [lye **press** in]
(Diapid)
Indications
Lypressin is used to treat clients with diabetes insipidus who are either nonresponsive to or cannot tolerate other interventions. This product prevents or controls the polydipsia, polyuria, and dehydration caused by insufficient ADH.
Pharmacokinetics/Dosing
Lypressin nasal spray has an immediate onset of antidiuretic activity, peaks in 30 to 90 minutes, and has a duration of action between 3 and 8 hours. The adult dosage for lypressin nasal spray is 1 or 2 sprays to one or both nostrils when urinary frequency increases or when a significant thirst sensation occurs. The usual pediatric and adult dosage is 1 or 2 sprays in each nostril four times daily.
Adverse Effects
See Table 46-1.

⬟ **W.S. is started on desmopressin (DDAVP) nasal solution 100 mcg/mL dosed at 20 mcg at bedtime.**

⬟ **What are the nursing implications for the use of antidiuretic hormone therapy for W.S.?**

Assessment After discussion of the various treatments for nocturnal enuresis with W.S. and his father, desmopressin is selected because it reduces the number of nights of primary nocturnal enuresis by at least 1 per week, and increases the likelihood of a "cure" (defined as 14 consecutive dry nights) while treatment is continued (Glazener, Evans, & Petro, 2003).

Of the antidiuretic hormones, desmopressin and lypressin and have fewer pressor effects than vasopressin; therefore cardiovascular precautions are not as great for these two drugs. However, if W.S. has allergic rhinitis, nasal congestion, or an upper respiratory infection, he may experience less efficacy because of a decrease in absorption with the nasal form of these drugs.

A baseline assessment determines that W.S. is without cardiovascular problems and that his fluid and electrolyte balance is within normal limits before beginning desmopressin therapy.

Although vasopressin is not a consideration for use with W.S., it is used for treatment of diabetes insipidus. Use vasopressin with caution in clients with inadequate coronary circulation (the drug may precipitate anginal pain and myocardial infarction) and in clients with hypertension (the drug may increase blood pressure). Use with caution in older adults because of the risk of water intoxication and hyponatremia. Its use is avoided if at all possible in clients who have chronic nephritis with nitrogen retention.

Nursing Diagnosis While receiving antidiuretic agents, W.S. has the potential for the following nursing diagnoses: excess fluid volume related to water intoxication (confusion, drowsiness, increasing headache, weight gain, seizures, hyponatremia); ineffective airway clearance with nasal dosage forms (runny or stuffy nose); impaired comfort (abdominal cramping, belching, nausea); diarrhea; and the potential complications of altered cardiac output related to increased fluid volume and the vasopressor effect of the drug. With vasopressin, there is the potential complication of angina and myocardial infarction (MI) (chest pain, shortness of breath).

Planning While receiving desmopressin therapy, W.S. will:
- Demonstrate a significant decrease in enuresis.
- With his family, effectively manage his drug regimen, including correct administration technique, adoption of supportive measures, and compliance with medications
- Collaborate with health care providers, reporting adverse effects appropriately and maintaining scheduled appointment with health care providers for monitoring and treatment.

Implementation

Monitoring Obtain fluid and electrolyte determinations periodically during therapy. To evaluate the effectiveness of the drug, monitor the number of dry nights. Monitor his weight, urine specific gravity, and blood pressure because of the possible fluid retention, or in the case of nonresponse to the drug, hypotension. Factor VIII coagulant concentrations and other bleeding factors should be monitored if desmopressin is used for clients with hemophilia A or von Willebrand disease.

Be alert for early signs of water toxicity/dilutional hyponatremia—such as confusion, headache, drowsiness, and weight gain—which progress to seizures. Withdraw the drug and restrict fluid intake until the specific gravity of urine is at least 1.015 and polyuria occurs. Notify the prescriber immediately.

Intervention For W.S., desmopressin is administered as a nasal spray, although it may be administered in a parenteral form for IV or subcutaneous use, or through a flexible catheter known as a rhinyle for nasal dosages less than 10 mcg. W.S. should be reassured, encouraged to limit fluids and void before bedtime, take responsibility for changing his bedding, and praised for dry nights. Behavioral modification with alarms or bladder-stretching exercises may also help.

Other ADH medications: Lypressin is administered intranasally; it is not to be inhaled. If lypressin is not effective with 3 sprays, it is recommended to increase the frequency of administration rather than the number of sprays per dose.

Vasopressin may be administered IM, subcutaneously, IV, or intraarterially. To allow for a precise IV or intraarterial flow rate, administer the vasopressin aqueous injection by an infusion pump. Avoid extravasation, because it is a vasopressor and tissue necrosis and gangrene may result.

Education Alert W.S. and his father that it is important to take the medication as prescribed and to maintain supervision by the prescriber. Instruct them to hold the medication and report symptoms of water intoxication (e.g., weight gain, headache, confusion, and drowsiness). Fluid intake may need to be adjusted to decrease the risk for water intoxication, particularly in children and older adults. The dosage of desmopressin is adjusted to control nocturia.

Evaluation The expected outcome for W.S.'s desmopressin therapy is that his nocturnal enuresis will diminished and become nonexistent. W.S. and his father state the signs and symptoms of adverse effects of desmopressin (e.g., headache, confusion, drowsiness, weight gain) and when to report them to the prescriber. W.S. remains compliant with his medication and demonstrates the correct method for nasal administration of desmopressin. His parents maintain scheduled appointments for monitoring and follow-up care for W.S.

For other antidiuretic agents administered for diabetes insipidus is that the client will experience a decreased urinary output, and the client's urinalysis will indicate an increased osmolality and specific gravity.

Summary

Drugs affecting the pituitary gland are generally used as replacement therapy for hormone deficiency, as drug therapy for a specific disorder, or as diagnostic aids to diagnose hypofunctional or hyperfunctional hormone states. Somatrem is therapeutically equivalent to somatropin (the hGH from the anterior pituitary); it is used for the treatment of growth failure in children caused by a deficiency of that hormone. Octreotide is used as a GH–inhibiting agent and to treat bleeding esophageal varices.

The two posterior pituitary hormones are oxytocin and vasopressin. Chapter 52 discusses oxytocin. Vasopressin and the other antidiuretic agents (lypressin and desmopressin) are used for the treatment of diabetes insipidus, which results from a deficiency of ADH. Desmopressin is also used in the management of nocturnal enuresis. The pituitary gland serves a major role in the regulation of the endocrine system.

⊛ Critical Thinking Questions

- Timmy Johnson, age 14, is receiving somatrem to enhance his growth process. In the last 6 months he has grown 3 cm. Would you consider the drug to be effective? A current radiograph examination indicates epiphyseal closure. How does this impact his therapy?

- Your client, Polly Jones, has been receiving vasopressin for her diabetes insipidus. Now she is disoriented, irritable, and short of breath. Her vital signs are stable on assessment: blood pressure, 124/70 mm Hg; pulse, 82 beats/min; respirations, 24 breaths/min; and temperature, 96.8°F (36°C). Her laboratory results are as follows:

Client	Normal Values
BLOOD	
Sodium, 116 mEq/L	135-145 mEq/L
Chloride, 86 mEq/L	100-108 mEq/L
Potassium, 3.6 mEq/L	3.5-5 mEq/L
Blood urea nitrogen, 10 mg/dL	8-20 mg/dL
Serum creatinine, 1 mg/dL	0.5-1.1 mg/dL for women
Serum osmolality, 243 mOsm/kg H$_2$O	275-295 mOsm/kg H$_2$O
URINE	
Urine osmolality 1.541 mOsm/kg H$_2$O	300-1000 mOsm/kg H$_2$O
Urine sodium, 320 mEq/24 hr	130-280 mEq/24 hr
Urine specific gravity, 1.04	1.025-1.032

What is happening to Ms. Jones? How should the nurse intervene?

Bibliography

Anderson, D.M., Keith, J., & Novak, P.D. (Eds.) (2002). *Mosby's medical, nursing, and allied health dictionary* (6th ed.). St. Louis: Mosby.

Bosker, G. (Ed.). (2004). *Primary and acute care medicine: Practice, protocols, pathways,* (2nd ed.). Atlanta: Thomson American Health Consultants.

Drug facts and comparisons (58th ed.). (2005). St. Louis: Facts and Comparisons.

Fitzgerald, P.A. (2003). Endocrinology. In Tierney, L.M., Jr., McPhee, S.J., & Papadakis, M.A. (Eds.), *Current Medical Diagnosis & Treatment.* New York: Lange Medical Books/McGraw-Hill.

Glazener, C.M., Evans, J.H., & Petro, R.E. (2003). Desmopressin for nocturnal enuresis in children. *Cochrane Database Systematic Review 3,* CD002112.

Godfrey, R., Whyte, G., & Head, T. (2004). Acute Human Growth Hormone Response in Elite Rowers After 12 Weeks of Training. Medicine & Science in Sports & Exercise, 36(5) Supplement, S303.

Heck, A.M., Yanovski, J.A., & Calis, K.A. (2002). Pituitary gland disorders. In DiPiro, J.T., Talbert, R.L., Yee, G.C., Matzke, G.R., Wells, B.G., & Posey, L.M. (Eds.), *Pharmacotherapy: A Pathophysiological Approach* (5th ed.). New York: McGraw-Hill.

Lacy, C.F., Armstrong, L.L., Goldman, M.P., & Lance, L.L. (2004). *Lexi-Comp's Drug Information Handbook* (12th ed.). Hudson, Ohio: Lexi-Comp.

Larsen, P.R., Kronenberg, H.M., Melmed, S., & Polonsky, K.S. (2003). *Williams textbook of endocrinology* (10th ed.). St. Louis: Mosby.

Lau, A.H. (2005). Fluid and electrolyte disorders. In M.A. Koda-Kimble, L.Y. Young, W.A. Kradian, B.J. Guglielmo, B.K. Alldredge, & R.L. Corelli (Eds.). *Applied therapeutics: The clinical use of drugs* (8th ed.). Philadelphia: Lippincott Williams & Wilkins.

Mills, J.L., et al. (2004). Long-term mortality in the United States cohort of pituitary-derived growth hormone recipients. *J Pediatrics, 144,* 430-436.

Mosby's drug consult (15th ed.). (2005). St. Louis: Mosby.

Parker, K.L., & Schimmer, B.P. (2001). Pituitary Hormones and Their Hypothalamic Releasing Factors. In: Hardman, J.G., & Limbird, L.E. (Eds.), *Goodman & Gilman's The pharmacological basis of therapeutics* (10th ed.). New York: McGraw-Hill.

Rennie, M.J. (2003). Claims for the anabolic effects of growth hormone: a case of the emperor's new clothes? *British Journal of Sports Medicine, 37,* 100-105.

USP DI: Drug information for the health care professional (25th ed.). (2005). Greenwood Village, CO: MICROMEDEX Thomson Healthcare.

Wenzel, V., Krismer, A.C., Arntz, H.R., Sitter, H., Stadlbauer, K.H., Lindner, K.H., and the European Resuscitation Council Vasopressor during Cardiopulmonary Resuscitation Study Group. (2004). A comparison of vasopressin and epinephrine for out-of-hospital cardiopulmonary resuscitation. *New England Journal of Medicine, 350,* 105-113.

e-LEARNING SUPPLEMENTS

Student CD-ROM
- Final Exam questions
- NCLEX® Examination review questions
- Pharmacology animations
- Printable chapter summary

Evolve Website (http://evolve.elsevier.com/mckenry)
- Case study on drugs affecting the pituitary

- Content updates, including information on new drugs
- WebLinks corresponding to this chapter
- Answers to the critical thinking questions in this chapter
- *Elsevier ePharmacology Update* newsletter
- Mosby's Drug Consult Internet Edition
- Supplemental and reference information

47

DRUGS AFFECTING THE PARATHYROID AND THYROID GLANDS

CHAPTER FOCUS

Disorders of the parathyroid and thyroid have far-reaching effects because as part of the endocrine system they influence growth and development, metabolic rate, energy level, and reproductive systems. The nurse needs to be knowledgeable about the various drugs that affect the parathyroid and thyroid system to provide direct care to clients, and educate clients regarding safe and effective self-management of the therapeutic regimen.

LEARNING OBJECTIVES

- Describe the clinical complications associated with hypothyroidism, hyperthyroidism, hypoparathyroidism, and hyperparathyroidism.
- Describe the dose and action of calcium and vitamin D products in the treatment of hypoparathyroidism.
- Implement the nursing management for clients receiving agents for the prophylaxis or treatment of osteoporosis.
- Describe the primary therapy for and the agents available to treat hypothyroidism.
- Describe the actions of iodine (iodide ion), radioactive iodine, and thioamide drugs in treating hyperthyroidism.
- Implement the nursing management for clients receiving drugs affecting the parathyroid or thyroid gland.

▲ KEY TERMS
iodine, p. 844
myxedema, p. 839
primary hyperparathyroidism, p. 833

▪⌐▪ KEY DRUGS
etidronate, p. 835
levothyroxine, p. 840
propylthiouracil, p. 846

This chapter will review the wide variety of medications available to treat the various conditions of the parathyroid and thyroid glands.

✳ What are the clinical features and treatments of hypoparathyroidism?

In idiopathic hypoparathyroidism, serum calcium levels are decreased and serum phosphate levels are increased. Vitamin D levels are usually low. The administration of calcium and vitamin D supplements usually restores levels of calcium and phosphorus to normal (Table 47-1). Calcitriol (Rocaltrol) is an active metabolite form of vitamin D that is also used to elevate serum calcium levels, and commonly utilized in clients with renal failure who cannot convert other forms of vitamin D to their active forms. Gallstones and kidney stones, more common in women and obesity (Taylor, Stampfer, & Curhan, 2005), are contraindications to calcium and vitamin D; hypercalcemia is also a contraindication. Table 47-2 lists the drugs used to treat hypocalcemia. Chapter 35 discusses calcium and phosphate management in renal failure, which utilizes many of the same modalities (calcium and vitamin D supplementation).

❋ What are the important aspects to consider with the treatment of hyperparathyroidism?

Primary hyperparathyroidism is a hyperactivity of the parathyroid glands typically resulting in significant hypercalcemia. The excessive secretion of parathyroid hormone results in increased resorption of calcium from the skeletal system and increased absorption of calcium by the kidneys and gastrointestinal (GI) system. Serious dehydration may result from hypercalcemic-induced renal impairment of urine concentrating capacity. The urine phosphate is high (the serum level is low to normal), which can lead to renal stones, bone pain with skeletal lesions, and possibly pathologic fractures. Because adenomas or tumors may cause this syndrome; surgery is usually the primary treatment.

Another important etiology of hypercalcemia is noted in clients with neoplasms with or without bone metastasis. Although not directly related to hyperparathyroidism, hypercalcemia is often treated in a similar manner. In clients with mild hypercalcemia or mild hyperparathyroidism, a thorough examination by a physician determines whether or not surgery is indicated. High serum levels of calcium may require immediate treatment with drugs and fluids (see the following section).

❋ **L.B. is a 42-year-old woman with an elevated serum calcium level of 11.2 mg/dL (normal range 8.6-10.3 mg/dL) and normal albumin level at 4.1 g/dL (normal range 3.5-5 g/dL). The endocrinologist diagnoses hyperparathyroidism, which will be managed with surgery scheduled the next week. In the interim, she is to receive 1 liter of normal saline at 200 mL/hour and one dose of furosemide (Lasix) 40 mg intravenously (IV) at clinic today. She will also receive calcitonin (Miacalcin) 240 units (4 units/kg) every 12 hours subcutaneously for four doses with follow-up calcium levels daily at clinic.**

❋ What drugs are used to reduce serum calcium levels?

Drugs to treat hypercalcemia include modalities to increase calcium excretion (e.g., hydration, diuretics) and drugs to alter calcium resorption from bone (e.g., calcitonin, bisphosphonates

---

TABLE 47-1 CALCIUM SUPPLEMENTS

The activity of calcium depends on calcium ion (elemental) content. The following calcium salts are listed by milligrams per gram, milliequivalents per gram, and percent of calcium in the preparations.

Preparation	Calcium (mg/g)*	Calcium (mEq/g)†	Percentage of Preparation as Elemental Calcium
calcium glubionate	65	3.3	6.5
calcium gluconate	90	4.5	9
calcium lactate	130	6.5	13
calcium citrate	211	10.5	21.1
tricalcium phosphate	390	19.3	39
calcium carbonate	400	20.0	40

Modified from *Drug facts and comparisons* (58th ed.). (2005). St. Louis: Facts and Comparisons.
*mg elemental calcium per gram of calcium salt.
†mEq elemental calcium per gram of calcium salt.

TABLE 47-2 DRUGS USED IN THE MANAGEMENT OF HYPOCALCEMIA

Drug	Usual Adult Dosage
calcium gluconate	IV: 970 mg given slowly at a rate not exceeding 1.5 mL per minute
Vitamin D analogs	
• calcifediol (Calderol)	Oral: 300-350 mcg per week administered daily or alternate days; adjust dose monthly if necessary
• calcitriol (Rocaltrol)	Oral: 0.25 mcg daily, increased every 2 to 4 weeks if necessary IV: 0.5 mcg three times a week, increased every 2 to 4 weeks if necessary
• dihydrotachysterol (Hytakerol)	Oral: 0.1-2.5 mg daily
• ergocalciferol (Calciferol)	Oral: individualized dosing; prophylaxis dose is 5-15 mcg daily in the United States or 2.5-5 mcg in Canada, depending on age
• paricalcitol (Zemplar)	Usual adult dose: 0.04-0.1 mcg/kg IV three times weekly

such as pamidronate [Aredia]). Diuretics result in renal elimination of excessive calcium and aggressive hydration is necessary to help prevent calcium salt deposits in tissues and the kidney. The use of diuretics is discussed in Chapter 33. Calcitonin and bisphosphonates alter the balance of osteoblastic/osteoclastic activity resulting in increased serum calcium being laid down in bone. Calcitonin and representative bisphosphonates are presented in the following monographs and are discussed further in the management of osteoporosis. Plicamycin (Mithramycin) is a cytotoxic agent used for testicular cancer that is also used for nonresponsive cases of hypercalcemia associated with malignancies, as is gallium nitrate (Ganite). Cinacalcet (Sensipar) affects the sensitivity of chief cells of the parathyroid gland to extracellular calcium and thereby reduces parathyroid hormone secretion (Block et al., 2004). Table 47-3 describes typical recommendations for the treatment of hypercalcemia.

calcitonin [kal sih **toe** nin]
(Miacalcin, Caltine✹)
Indications
Calcitonin is administered subcutaneously or intramuscularly (IM) to treat hypercalcemia, osteoporosis, and Paget's disease. An intranasal formulation is also available for osteoporosis.

Pharmacokinetics/Dosing
The half-life of calcitonin is 60 to 90 minutes. The usual adult dosage of salmon calcitonin for Paget's disease is 100 International Units (IM or subcutaneous) daily, decreasing to 50 International Units daily, every other day, and then three times weekly. For postmenopausal osteoporosis, the parenteral dosage is 100 International Units (IM or subcutaneous) daily; the nasal dosage is 200 International Units intranasally daily, alternating nostrils each day.

Adverse Effects
The adverse effects of calcitonin as a nasal spray include rhinitis, nasal irritation and redness, muscle and back pain, epistaxis, and headache. The parenteral dosage form of the drug may cause flushing or a tingling sensation of the face, ears, hands, and feet; gastric distress, anorexia, nausea, and vomiting; and pain or swelling at the injection site. To reduce the nausea or flushing adverse effects, bedtime administration is suggested, or a reduction in dosage may be required.

✱ **L.B. asks for information about her prescribed calcitonin.**

Assessment Because L.B. has no history of allergies, skin testing is recommended before initiating L.B.'s calcitonin therapy to determine her sensitivity to calcitonin or foreign proteins. During her diagnostic workup, serum calcium and

TABLE 47-3 TREATMENTS FOR HYPERCALCEMIA

Drug	Class/Rationale	Typical Adult Dose	Comment
normal saline (NS; 0.9% sodium chloride)	Rehydration and prevention of calcium deposits; increase calcium excretion	100-200 mL/hr continuous IV	Monitor for fluid overload
furosemide (Lasix)	Diuretic to increase calcium excretion	20-40 mg IV two to four times daily	Monitor hydration status, typically used with hydration
calcitonin (Miacalcin)	Calcitonin to inhibit bone resorption	4-8 International units/kg IM or subcutaneous q12h	Concurrent corticosteroids may be used to prevent tolerance if used beyond 48-72 hr
etidronate (Didronel)*	Bisphosphonates to inhibit bone resorption	7.5 mg/kg in 250 mL normal chloride over 2 hours IV daily × 3 days	Oral formulation available for Paget's disease of bone or chronic hypercalcemic conditions
pamidronate (Aredia)		30-90 mg IV in 1 L normal saline infused over 24 hr	Effective as a single 24-hr infusion
zoledronic acid (Zometa)		4 mg IV over at least 15 min	Higher doses or rapid administration associated with renal toxicity
plicamycin (Mithramycin)*	Cytotoxic antibiotic to inhibit bone resorption in malignancy associated hypercalcemia	25 mcg/kg in 500 mL of dextrose 5% or normal saline IV over 4-60 hr	More toxic than other interventions
cinacalcet (Sensipar)	Increases sensitivity of parathyroid to extracellular calcium thereby decreasing parathyroid hormone secretion	Secondary hyperparathyroidism: 30 mg PO daily up to 180 mg PO daily Hypercalcemia secondary to parathyroid cancer: 30-90 mg PO twice daily	Administer with food Metabolized by P450 3A4, strong inhibitor of P450 2D6. Multiple drug interactions possible

*Brand name product no longer marketed in the United States.

serum alkaline phosphatase concentrations were determined that can be used for baseline criteria. Urinary hydroxyproline (24-hour) levels may be determined but, as with all 24-hour urine samples, levels may be difficult to obtain with accuracy. Additionally, a baseline assessment of L.B.'s underlying condition is noted, such as bone pain, previous fractures, and bone loss as measured by bone density studies.

Nursing Diagnosis While L.B. is receiving calcitonin, she is at risk for the following nursing diagnosis/collaborative problem: impaired comfort (anorexia, nausea and vomiting; abdominal cramping; flushing or redness of the face, ears, hands, or feet; redness or swelling at the injection site; increased urinary frequency) and the potential complication of hypersensitivity (skin rash, urticaria).

Planning While receiving calcitonin, L.B. will:
- Demonstrate lower serum calcium concentrations without experiencing adverse drug effects
- Effectively manage the therapeutic regimen, including administering her injections, medication compliance, and reporting adverse drug effects appropriately.
- Collaborate with health care providers for monitoring and follow-up care.

Implementation

Monitoring Monitor results of periodically drawn serum calcium levels until her surgery. Monitor L.B. for the nursing diagnosis and potential complication mentioned previously, and for an improvement in baseline indicators.

Intervention L.B.'s dosage is twice daily; for others, administration at bedtime helps to reduce the nausea and facial flushing sometimes experienced with this drug.

Education Instruct L.B. on the correct method of administering her calcitonin, subcutaneous or IM, whichever is easier for her. Keep the solution refrigerated.

Evaluation The expected outcome is that L.B.'s serum calcium concentrations will be lowered until surgery. She will be compliant with her drug therapy, correctly administer her medication, report adverse effects (e.g., nausea, vomiting, abdominal cramping, increased urinary frequency) to her prescriber, and maintain appointments for serum calcium levels and other follow-up care until her surgery.

Parenteral Bisphosphonates

The bisphosphonates are incorporated into bone to inhibit normal and abnormal resorption of bone primarily by decreasing activity of osteoclasts. Among the bisphosphonates, etidronate is unique in also reducing osteoblastic activity as well. Multiple mechanisms may be involved. Their action is postulated to result from binding to hydroxyapatite in bone, decreasing the dissolution of mineral bone content, or their effect on bone resorbing cells. The use of bisphosphonates for clients with metastatic bone disease secondary to cancer is associated with reduced fracture risk and reduced rates of

hypercalcemia (Ross et al., 2003). Pamidronate is similar to etidronate with the exception that it has greater selectivity to inhibit osteoclasts without much effect on the bone-building osteoclasts. Zoledronic acid is a third bisphosphonate used for management of hypercalcemia. Osteonecrosis of the jaw has been noted with IV bisphosphonate therapy (Novartis, May 2005). Renal dysfunction has also been noted with zoledronic acid (Novartis, December 2004). Oral bisphosphonates, including alendronate (Fosamax), ibandronate (Boniva), risedronate (Actonel), and tiludronate (Skelid), are primarily used to manage osteoporosis.

✱⊓ etidronate [eh **tye** droe nate]
(Didronel)

Indications
Intravenous etidronate is indicated for the treatment of hypercalcemia associated with malignancy, but is used for other types of hypercalcemic states. The oral formulation is indicated for Paget's disease of bone, and heterotrophic ossification.

Dosing
For hypercalcemia, it is dosed 7.5 mg/kg by IV infusion daily for 3 consecutive days. Orally for other indications, the dose is 5 to 20 mg/kg PO daily (2 hours before or after food) for 1 to 6 months depending on indication.

Adverse Effects
Bone pain (and perhaps bone fractures, osteomalacia), nausea, diarrhea, metallic taste and, rarely, hypersensitivity occur with etidronate.

pamidronate [pam ih **droe** nate]
(Aredia)

Indications
Pamidronate is indicated for hypercalcemia associated with malignancy, osteolytic bone lesions secondary to multiple myeloma or metastatic breast cancer, and moderate to severe Paget's disease of bone.

Pharmacokinetics/Dosing
The onset of action of pamidronate is 24 to 48 hours with peak effect observed about a week after infusion. The adult dosage of pamidronate for hypercalcemia is 60 to 90 mg diluted in saline or dextrose to be infused over 2 to 24 hours. At least 7 days should elapse before repeating doses. Many clients respond well to repeat doses every 2 to 3 weeks up to every 2 to 3 months.

Adverse Effects
The adverse effects of pamidronate include fever, nausea, vomiting, anorexia, leukopenia, hypocalcemia (more common with doses of 90 mg), and muscle stiffness. Osteonecrosis of the jaw has also been reported in clients with cancer, and the risk may be highest with concurrent invasive dental procedures (Novartis, May 2005).

zoledronic acid [zole **droe** nik **as** id]
(Zometa)

Indications
Zoledronic acid in indicated for the treatment of hypercalcemia and bone metastasis of solid tumors.

Dosing
The dosage of zoledronic acid doses is at 4 mg IV infused over at least 15 minutes. Dosage reductions are recommended for clients with creatinine clearance (CrCl) values below 60 mL/min, and use is not recommended for clients with a CrCl of less than 30 mL/min.

Adverse Effects
The most serious adverse effect is renal dysfunction. This risk is minimized by not exceeding the 4-mg dose, assuring adequate hydration with use, and administering over 15 minutes or longer. Other adverse effects include leg edema, fatigue, fever, agitation, hy-

pophosphatemia, nausea, vomiting, diarrhea, constipation, muscle and joint pain, dyspnea, and coughing. Hypotension and rigors have also been reported. The risk for osteonecrosis of the jaw is also possible, and the precautions cited for pamidronate also pertain here.

Calcimimetic Agents: Parathyroid Gland Sensitivity Modulators

Cinacalcet (Sensipar) is the first in a class of calcimimetic agents, which affects the sensitivity of the parathyroid gland to extracellular calcium. This modulation results in reduced secretion of parathyroid hormone secretion and may be useful for both secondary hyperparathyroid states (e.g., renal failure) and parathyroid cancer.

cinacalcet [sin a **kal** cet]
(Sensipar)
Indications
Cinacalcet is used in the treatment of secondary hyperparathyroidism for clients on dialysis and for treating hypercalcemia secondary to parathyroid cancer.

Pharmacokinetics/Dosing
Cinacalcet is fairly well absorbed orally with high fat intake improving the extent of absorption. Peak effects are noted between 2 and 6 hours after administration. Cinacalcet is extensively metabolized by P450 3A4, 1A2, and 2D6 to inactive metabolites. The elimination half-life is 30 to 40 hours and is not affected by renal function. Table 47-3 presents dosing.

Adverse Effects
Nausea and vomiting are the most frequently reported adverse effects. Risk for seizures may be greater with cinacalcet therapy. Hypocalcemia is an expected effect of cinacalcet therapy; if present, discontinuation or dosage reduction is indicated.

Drug Interactions
Cinacalcet is metabolized by a number of the P450 enzymes, including 3 A4. Use of other drugs that inhibit 3 A4 (e.g., azole antifungals) may result in elevated levels of cinacalcet and cause reductions in parathyroid hormone and calcium levels. Concurrent use of drugs metabolized by P450 2D6 may result in elevated levels of those drugs (e.g., antidepressants, antipsychotics, β-adrenergic blockers, stimulants, procainamide, protease inhibitors, calcium channel blockers). Particular caution is recommended for use of agents in which prolonged QT interval is possible and metabolism may be affected (e.g., thioridazine, haloperidol, procainamide). A number of other interactions are possible (*Mosby's Drug Consult*, 2005).

✱ **S.L. is a 61-year-old postmenopausal woman with newly diagnosed osteoporosis. Despite intake of three servings of dairy products daily, a recent bone density assessment confirms moderately severe osteoporosis. Her history is negative for other medical conditions other than osteoarthritis for which she takes glucosamine sulfate 500 mg PO three times daily. She is evaluated by her nurse practitioner and is started on alendronate (Fosamax) 70 mg PO once weekly on Sunday mornings.**

✱ **What therapies increase calcium levels in bone?**
Calcitonin (most often intranasally) and some of the bisphosphonates are also used to manage osteoporosis and Paget's disease. Additionally, estrogen agonists (e.g., estrogens) and estrogen receptor modulators (e.g., Chapter 51 discusses raloxifene [Evista]) used for osteoporosis in women). The recombi-

nant parathyroid hormone derivative (teriparatide [Forteo]) is also used to treat osteoporosis, although it is not considered a first-line therapy due in part to its expense. Calcium supplements and vitamin D are also routine treatments for osteoporosis to help preserve bone density (Trivedi, Doll, & Khaw, 2003), but adherence may be problematic and benefit may be limited (Grant et al., 2005; Bischoff-Ferrari et al., 2005; Porthouse et al., 2005), and they are obviously contraindicated in the management of hypercalcemia. Table 47-4 outlines treatments for osteoporosis. These bone-strengthening interventions are sometimes used to help reverse osteopenias secondary to other drug therapy, including the osteopenia associated with chronic use of corticosteroids and/or heparin.

Oral Bisphosphonates

The oral bisphosphonates, like the parenteral agents described previously, inhibit osteoclasts in bone and thereby serve to decrease bone resorption. These agents are poorly absorbed orally, yet enough drug reaches bone tissue to be effective by this route of administration. Benefit is observed for clients with existing fractures, but the role of bisphosphonates in prevention has been questioned (Quandt et al., 2005; Schousboe, Nyman, Kane, & Ensrud, 2005). Orally administered bisphosphonates are associated with a relatively high risk of esophageal irritation or ulcers, and must be administered in the fasting state with clients remaining upright for a period of time after administration. With the exception of risk for esophageal irritation, these agents appear safe and effective with long-term use (Bone et al., 2004), but some researchers recommend limiting their use to 5 years' duration (Odvina et al., 2005; Ott, 2005). The oral bisphosphonates used clinically are alendronate, ibandronate, risedronate, and tiludronate.

alendronate [ah **len** drew nate]
(Fosamax)
Indications
Alendronate is used to treat osteoporosis in men and women, and to prevent osteoporosis in women. It is also indicated for clients with symptomatic Paget's disease of bone.

Pharmacokinetics/Dosing
Only 0.7% of the dose of orally administered alendronate is systemically absorbed. What is absorbed, however, has a high affinity for bone tissue. Alendronate is dosed at 10 mg PO daily or 70 mg PO once weekly for the treatment of osteoporosis. The dose for prophylactic management of osteoporosis is 5 mg PO daily or 35 mg PO once weekly. Doses for Paget's disease of bone are 40 mg PO daily × 6 months. Alendronate must be administered with water only in the fasting state on arising, and no other food or drink should be administered for at least 30 minutes. Clients must remain in the upright position for at least 30 minutes after dosing to minimize the risk for esophageal ulcers.

Adverse Effects
The adverse effects of alendronate include gas production, acid regurgitation, esophageal ulcer, gastritis, dysphagia, muscle pain, headaches, constipation, or diarrhea.

ibandronate [eye **ban** droe nate]
(Boniva)
Indications
Ibandronate is indicated for the prevention and treatment of postmenopausal osteoporosis. It is avoided for clients with significant renal impairment (CrCl <30 mL/min).

TABLE 47-4 TREATMENTS FOR OSTEOPOROSIS AND/OR OTHER BONE DISEASE

Drug	Class	Typical Adult Dose for Osteoporosis Treatment	Comment
calcitonin*† (Miacalcin)	Calcitonin	100 International units subcutaneous/IM daily 200 International units (one spray) via nasal inhalation daily (alternate nostrils each day)	For osteoporosis, requires supplemental calcium to prevent hypocalcemia
alendronate *† (Fosamax)	Bisphosphonate	10 mg PO daily OR 70 mg PO weekly (Prophylaxis: 50% of above dose)	Requires client to take with only water on arising in the morning, maintaining upright in the fasting state for 30-60 min (120 min for tiludronate) Contraindicated if significant GI disease
ibandronate (Boniva)		150 mg PO once monthly	
risedronate *† (Actonel)		5 mg PO daily OR 35 mg PO weekly	
tiludronate† (Skelid)		400 mg PO daily × 3 months	
conjugated estrogen‡ (Premarin)	Estrogen	Dose varies	See Chapter 51 for contraindications and role of estrogens
raloxifene‡ (Evista)	Estrogen Receptor Modulator	60 mg PO daily	See Chapter 51
teriparatide* (Forteo)	Recombinant PTH	20 mcg subcutaneous daily for up to 2 years	Available as injector pen for autoinjection
calcium salts*	Mineral	Supplement + diet = 1000-1500 mg elemental calcium daily	See Table 47-1 and Chapter 67
vitamin D* supplement	Fat-soluble vitamin	Recommended dose: 400-800 units daily	See Table 47-2 and Chapter 67

*Indicated for osteoporosis.
†Indicated for Paget's disease of the bone.
‡Indicated for osteoporosis in women.

Pharmacokinetics/Dosing

The pharmacokinetics for ibandronate are similar to other bisphosphonates. It is dosed at 150 mg orally once a month. It must be taken with water upon waking in the morning. The client must avoid taking any other food, drink, or medication for 60 minutes and must not lie down for 60 minutes.

Adverse Effects

Similar to alendronate.

risedronate [rih **she** droe nate]
(Actonel)
Indications

Risedronate is indicated for the treatment of Paget's disease of bone, treatment and prevention of corticosteroid-induced osteoporosis, and treatment and prevention of osteoporosis in postmenopausal women.

Pharmacokinetics/Dosing

Oral bioavailability of risedronate is approximately 0.5% to 0.7%, but, like other orally administered bisphosphonates, has a high affinity for bone. Dosing for Paget's disease is 30 mg PO daily for 2 months. Doses for osteoporosis prevention and treatment are 5 mg PO daily or 35 mg PO once weekly. A dose of 5 mg PO daily is recommended for the prevention of glucocorticoid-induced osteoporosis. It must be administered with water 30 to 60 minutes before intake of any food or drink, and the client must remain upright.

Adverse Effects

Similar to alendronate.

tiludronate [tye **loo** droe nate]
(Skelid)
Indications

Tiludronate is indicated for clients with Paget's disease of bone.

Pharmacokinetics/Dosing

Similar to alendronate and risedronate. For Paget's disease, the adult dosage of tiludronate is 400 mg PO at least 2 hours before or after food, beverages, or other medications.

Adverse Effects

Tiludronate may cause an upper respiratory or flu-like syndrome (e.g., fever, nasal congestion, sore throat), back or body pain, abdominal distress, nausea, headache, diarrhea, arthralgia, conjunctivitis, pharyngitis, rash, nausea, vomiting, cataract, glaucoma, and chest pain.

Recombinant Parathyroid Hormone

Via genetic technology, a recombinant formulation of parathyroid hormone is available.

teriparatide [ter ih **par** ah tide]
(Forteo)
Like the physiologic parathyroid hormone, teriparatide stimulates osteoblasts and increases gastric absorption and renal tubular reabsorption of calcium. Increased bone density has been associated with teriparatide use.

Indications
Teriparatide is indicated for the treatment of osteoporosis.

Pharmacokinetics/Dosing
Administered subcutaneously, teriparatide has an elimination half-life of about 1 hour. It is dosed at 20 mcg daily for up to 2 years. A pen-like device delivering 20 mcg/dose is available for client self-administration.

Adverse Effects
The most common adverse effects are transient hypercalcemia, joint pain, rhinitis, weakness and dizziness.

✱ What are the nursing management issues with bisphosphonate therapy for S.L.?

Assessment Alendronate is contraindicated when the creatinine clearance is less than 35 mL/min. It should be used cautiously in any client with some degree of renal impairment. (Etidronate and pamidronate therapy is contraindicated in clients with renal insufficiency when serum creatinine is greater than 5 mg/dL; tiludronate, ibandronate, and risedronate are contraindicated when creatinine clearance is less than 30 mL/min.) If S.L. has a preexisting hypocalcemia or vitamin D deficiency, it is corrected before beginning bisphosphonate therapy, because this therapy may worsen these conditions. The use of alendronate (and tiludronate) would be contraindicated if S.L. has a GI disease such as esophagitis, esophageal ulcers, or gastric ulcers because they could be made worse. Assess for sensitivity to any of the bisphosphonates. Take a history of dietary calcium and vitamin D and any supplements that are taken.

Review S.L.'s current drug regimen for potential drug interactions, such as would occur with calcium, iron, or other mineral supplements and antacids; if taken at the same time, these substances decrease bisphosphonate absorption. Avoid concurrent use of salicylates and alendronate because of the increased risk of upper GI irritation. Bisphosphonates and estrogen may be prescribed concurrently to significantly increase bone mass in postmenopausal osteoporosis (Parent-Stevens & Sagraves, 2005).

A baseline assessment of the client with osteoporosis includes serum calcium levels and bone density studies to determine bone mass. A history of fractures, particularly vertebral fractures, is documented. Clients with Paget's disease require documentation of their symptoms (bone pain, headache, skull size) and serum alkaline phosphatase before beginning therapy; assess for pain, weakness, and loss of function.

Nursing Diagnosis While receiving bisphosphonate therapy, S.L. may experience the following nursing diagnoses/collaborative problems: risk for injury related to the preexisting condition and the ineffectiveness of therapy; impaired comfort (headache, abdominal discomfort, bloating, nausea, heartburn, musculoskeletal pain, metallic taste); diarrhea or constipation; impaired skin integrity (rash, erythema); and the potential complications of allergic reaction, hypercalcemia (nausea, vomiting, anorexia, weakness, constipation, thirst, cardiac dysrhythmias), hypocalcemia (paresthesia, muscle twitching, colic, cardiac dysrhythmias), and gastritis or esophageal ulceration.

Planning During alendronate therapy, S.L. will:
- Demonstrate increases in bone density without adverse effects of alendronate.
- Remain compliant with medication regimen and supportive measures.
- Collaborate with health care providers, reporting adverse symptoms appropriately and maintaining scheduled appointments for monitoring and treatment.

Implementation
Monitoring Monitor results of bone scans for bone density, serum creatinine and serum calcium determinations, which are performed periodically for clients being treated for osteoporosis. Additionally, clients with Paget's disease require periodic alkaline phosphatase determinations.

Intervention Administer alendronate first thing in the morning with 8 ounces of water 30 minutes (60 minutes with ibandronate) before meals or other medications. Have S.L. sit or stand upright for 30 minutes (60 minutes with ibandronate) after ingesting the drug to minimize esophageal irritation. The other oral bisphosphonates are administered on an empty stomach at least 2 hours before or after food, milk or milk products, antacids, other medications high in iron, or other mineral supplements.

Education Instruct S.L. to take the drug as previously discussed. This drug is NOT to be taken at bedtime or before arising for the day as this may result in severe esophageal irritation, pain or ulceration. Beverages other than water will decrease absorption of the drug. Encourage S.L. to engage in supportive lifestyle changes, such as smoking cessation, reduction of alcohol intake, and participation in regular exercise with weight-bearing on the long bones (e.g., walking). Instruct her about dietary sources of calcium and vitamin D. Consult with the prescriber about calcium and vitamin D supplementation, but S.L. needs to have an adequate intake of calcium (1 to 1.5 g of elemental calcium a day) and vitamin D (400 to 800 units a day).

Evaluation The expected outcome of bisphosphonate therapy is that S.L. will experience decreased progression of osteoporosis and reduced risk for vertebral and nonvertebral fractures. Serum calcium, serum creatinine, and bone density studies will be within the normal limits for age. She will remain compliant with her medication, state the importance of taking it as prescribed, state adverse effects reportable to the prescriber, practice nonpharmacologic supportive measures (e.g., walking), and maintain scheduled appointments for monitoring and treatment.

Drugs Affecting the Thyroid Gland

✱ How are hypothyroidism and hyperthyroidism differentiated?

Chapter 45 discusses regulation of the thyroid gland by the interplay of hypothalamic, pituitary, and thyroid gland activity and Box 47-1 depicts this interplay graphically. The thyroid produces two iodine-containing active hormones, thyroxine (T_4) and triiodothyronine (T_3), that are essential for human growth and development and the maintenance of metabolic homeostasis. These hormones are released from the thyroid based on a feedback loop with thyroid-releasing hormone from the hypothalamus and thyroid-stimulating hormone from the pituitary. Hypothyroidism classically presents with dry skin, cold intolerance, lethargy, depression, and weight gain, and is related to reduced levels of T_4 and T_3. Hyperthyroidism has a number of potential etiologies, and presents with exophthalmos (protruding eyes), thin hair, intolerance to heat, nervousness and tachycardia or tachydysrhythmias. Table 47-5 presents the differentiation of hyperthyroidism and hypothyroidism.

✱ B.T. is a 61-year-old school teacher who presents to her physician with fatigue, depression, and cold/dry skin, and complains of never being warm enough despite wearing layered clothing. Her endocrine labs demonstrate an elevated TSH (8.1 mU/L [normal range: 0.4-5.5 mU/L]) and low T4 (2.8 mcg/L [normal range: 4.5-12.5 mcg/L]). She is diagnosed with primary hypothyroidism.

✱ What agents are available to treat hypothyroidism?

Individuals with hypothyroidism require thyroid replacement therapy. Natural or desiccated thyroid was used for replacement therapy for many years, but the synthetic thyroid preparations available today are more standardized and stable and therefore are usually prescribed. Thyroid (United States Pharmacopeia [USP]) is derived mainly from hog thyroid glands, but cattle and sheep thyroid glands have also historically been used. The available synthesized hormones in current use are liothyronine (for T_3), levothyroxine (for T_4), and liotrix (both T_3 and T_4). Table 47-6 summarizes the equivalent and usual adult dosages of the thyroid products.

The goal of treatment of clients with hypothyroidism or **myxedema** (adult hypothyroidism) is to eliminate symptoms and restore a normal emotional and physical state. For women who are pregnant, correcting thyroid status helps reduce risk for low birth weight, abnormal development of the fetus, placental abruption, and preterm delivery (Blazer, Moreh-Waterman, Miller-Lotan, Tamir, & Hochberg, 2003; Casey et al., 2005). The clinical response is more important than the blood hormone level; nevertheless, laboratory assessments of T_3, T_4, serum cholesterol, and thyroid-stimulating hormone (TSH) are used as criteria for adequacy of therapy. Thyroid supplements are indicated for the treatment of hypothyroidism, the treatment and prevention of goiter and thyroid carcinoma, and thyroid function diagnostic tests. Pregnancy safety for all thyroid products has been established at U.S. Food and Drug Administration (FDA) Category A.

Levothyroxine (T_4) is the most commonly used treatment in North America for hypothyroidism. Liothyronine (T_3) and mixtures of levothyroxine and liothyronine are also used, although they offer no advantage over levothyroxine in the treatment of primary hypothyroidism (Clyde, Harari, Getka, & Shakir, 2003). Thyroid and levothyroxine are incompletely absorbed from the GI tract (50% to 75%) and may vary by brand, whereas liothyronine is nearly completely absorbed (95%). Thyroid preparations are highly protein bound, with a peak effect in 3 to 4 weeks and a duration of action of 1 to 3 weeks for thyroid, thyroglobulin, and levothyroxine after withdrawing chronic therapy. Lio-

---

BOX 47-1 THYROID FEEDBACK MECHANISM

The relationship of the hypothalamus, pituitary, and thyroid gland under normal conditions is depicted in the following figure.

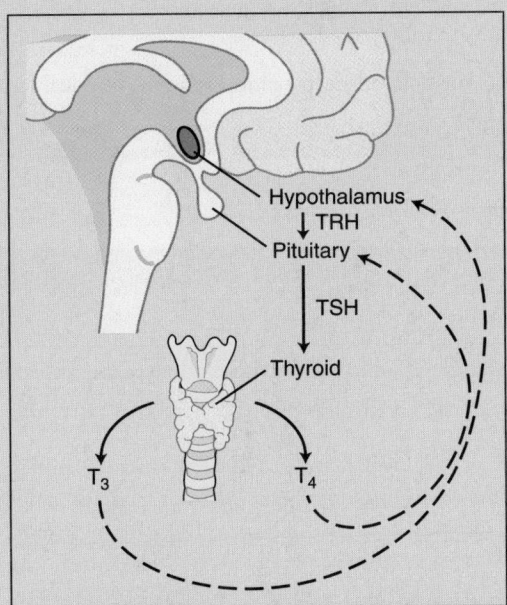

When serum levels of T_3 and T_4 are increased, the release of thyrotropin-releasing hormone (TRH) from the hypothalamus and TSH from the anterior pituitary gland is reduced, thus inhibiting their effects on the thyroid gland.

When serum levels of T_3 and T_4 are decreased, TRH release triggers the release of TSH from the pituitary. TSH affects the thyroid by increasing the size and number of its follicular cells in the thyroid. The cells are then able to absorb more iodide and increase thyroglobulin breakdown, which releases T_3 and T_4 hormones from the thyroid gland into the bloodstream. This process increases the blood levels of the thyroid hormones.

thyronine peaks in 2 to 3 days and has a duration of action of up to 3 days after withdrawal. These agents are metabolized the same as endogenous thyroid hormone—some in peripheral tissues, smaller amounts in the liver—and are then excreted in bile.

The adverse effects of thyroid hormone therapy are dose related and may occur more rapidly with liothyronine than with the other products, mainly because it has a faster onset of action. The general signs of an underdose or hypothyroidism are dysmenorrhea, ataxia, coldness, dry skin, constipation, lethargy, headaches, drowsiness, tiredness, weight gain, and muscle aching. Hair loss may occur in children during the early period of treatment, but normal hair growth resumes with chronic therapy.

A rare adverse reaction is an allergic skin rash. An overdose of thyroid products results in hyperthyroidism—alterations in appetite and menstrual periods, elevated temperature, diarrhea, hand tremors, increased irritability, leg cramps, increased nervousness, tachycardia, irregular heart rate, increased sensitivity to heat, chest pain, respiratory difficulties, increased sweating, vomiting, weight loss, and insomnia.

✱▐▔ **levothyroxine** [lee voe thye **rox** een]
(Levothroid, Synthroid, Eltroxin✦, Novothyrox✦)
Indications
Levothyroxine is indicated as replacement therapy in hypothyroidism.
Pharmacokinetics/Dosing
The bioavailability of levothyroxine is erratic with differences noted between different formulations and among different clients. Once a

---

TABLE 47-5 CLINICAL FEATURES OF HYPERTHYROIDISM AND HYPOTHYROIDISM

	Hyperthyroidism	Hypothyroidism
Eyes	Prominent (exophthalmus)	Eyelids edematous, ptosis
Hair	Thin, fine texture	Dry, brittle, thin
Temperature	Intolerance to heat	Intolerance to cold
Weight	Appetite increases, weight loss	Appetite decreases, weight gain
Emotional	Increased nervousness, irritability, insomnia	Lethargic, depressed, increase in sleeping needs
Gastrointestinal	Diarrhea	Constipation
Neuromuscular	Fast deep-tendon reflexes, tremor	Slow or delayed deep-tendon reflexes, physical lethargy
Extremities	Hot, moist skin	Cold, dry skin

TABLE 47-6 THYROID SUPPLEMENTS

Drug	Equivalent Dose	Usual Adult Dosage
levothyroxine (Synthroid)	100 mcg (0.1 mg)	Orally: 12.5-50 mcg daily (older adults or those with cardiovascular disease, dose range is 12.5-25 mcg daily), adjusting dose every 2-3 weeks as necessary up to a maximum of 300 mcg daily. Injection: 50-100 mcg IM or IV daily. The dose is 200-500 mcg IV initially for myxedema, stupor, or coma, even in older clients. If improvement is not noted by the second day, an additional 100-200 mcg (0.1-0.2 mg) may be given. Switch to oral dose form as soon as possible.
liothyronine (Cytomel)	25 mcg (0.025 mg)	Orally: 25-50 mcg daily, adjusting dose every 1-2 weeks as needed up to 100 mcg daily. For myxedema and simple, nontoxic goiter, dose is 2.5-5 mcg daily (increasing at 5- to 10-mcg increments every 7-14 days) as necessary. Maintenance myxedema dose is 25-50 mcg daily; for simple goiter, it is 50-100 mcg daily.
liotrix (Thyrolar)	50-60 mcg of levothyroxine and 12.5-15 mcg liothyronine	Orally: myxedema, 50-60 mcg of levothyroxine and 12.5-15 mcg of liothyronine daily; increase monthly if necessary. Dose for older adults is 25%-50% of the usual adult dose, adjusted as necessary at 6- to 8-week intervals.
Thyroid	60 mg	Orally: 60-120 mg daily. For myxedema or hypothyroidism with cardiovascular disease, initial dose is 15 mg daily, increased as necessary every 2 weeks. Older adults: 7.5-15 mg daily, doubled every 6-8 weeks if necessary.

client is stabilized on a particular brand of levothyroxine, any changes in formulation should be conducted only under close medical supervision. The dosage ranges for hypothyroidism vary based on client need and response to therapy. Response to therapy is evaluated by monitoring T4 levels every 1 to 3 months with dosage adjustments as needed until stable. Levels of TSH, although useful for screening for thyroid function, may be a less reliable indicator for severity of hypothyroidism and response to levothyroxine (Meier, Trittibach, Guglielmetti, Staub, & Muller, 2003). The typical adult dose ranges from 25 mcg (0.025 mg) to 200 mcg (0.2 mg) daily, although higher doses are occasionally required. Increased requirement for levothyroxine of approximately 50% is noted during pregnancy for many women, with dose adjustments based on thyroid function (Alexander et al., 2004).

Adverse Effects

The most common adverse effects of levothyroxine mimic the symptoms of hyperthyroidism, including tachycardia, dysrhythmias (including atrial fibrillation), angina, anxiety, nervousness, diaphoresis, heat intolerance, flushing, alopecia, menstrual irregularities, and GI upset. Overaggressive thyroid supplementation can also predispose to osteoporosis. Choking and gagging on tablet formulations have been reported when levothyroxine (Levoxyl) was taken without adequate water (Pamplin, 2004).

Drug Interactions

When thyroid supplementation is administered to a client on warfarin therapy, excessive anticoagulation may be observed. Additive stimulation, tachycardia and/or hypertension can occur when dosed with tricyclic antidepressants or ketamine. Absorption of levothyroxine may be reduced by bile acid sequestrants (e.g., cholestyramine), iron, antacids, and sucralfate. Enzyme-inducing drugs, (including rifampin, phenytoin, phenobarbital, and carbamazepine) may result in increased metabolism and decreased levels of levothyroxine. A number of other drugs may affect thyroid function and/or conversion of T_4 to T_3, including lithium, amiodarone, iodine-based contrast dyes, β-adrenergic blockers, thiazide diuretics, and glucocorticoids.

✴ **B.T. is started on levothyroxine 0.05 mg (50 mcg) orally daily for her hypothyroidism and is scheduled for follow-up thyroid function tests in 6 weeks.**

✴ **What are the nursing management issues involved in the use of thyroid supplements for B.T.?**

Assessment Because B.T. is 61 years of age, levothyroxine is used with care, because older adults are more sensitive to the effects of thyroid hormones. A 25% reduction in the dosage of the thyroid hormone replacement may be required

for clients older than 60 years of age (see the Special Considerations for Older Adults box below). The use of thyroid hormonal therapy is carefully considered if B.T. were to have preexisting adrenocortical or pituitary insufficiency (thyroid hormonal replacement increases the physiologic need for adrenocortical hormone), cardiovascular disease (too-rapid thyroid hormonal replacement increases metabolic demand), a history of hyperthyroidism, or thyrotoxicosis. An increased sensitivity may exist in cases of chronic hypothyroidism or myxedema. Pregnancy in women with previously diagnosed hypothyroidism may require an increased dosage of replacement therapy (Dong, 2005).

Review B.T.'s current medication regimen for the risk of significant drug interactions, such as those that may occur when thyroid preparations are given concurrently with oral anticoagulants. The thyroid preparation may alter the therapeutic effects of the oral anticoagulant; an increase in thyroid hormone may require a decrease in the oral dosage of anticoagulant. Monitor coagulation time closely using the prothrombin time (PT) or International Normalization Ratio (INR). Cholestyramine (Questran) or colestipol (Colestid) may bind thyroid hormones, delaying or decreasing their absorption from the GI tract. A 4- to 5-hour interval is recommended between the administration of these drugs. With sympathomimetics, the effects of one or both medications may be increased. This may result in an increased risk of coronary insufficiency if B.T. has coronary artery disease (see the levothyroxine monograph for other drug interactions).

A baseline assessment of B.T. will include her general status (weakness, fatigue, cold intolerance, weight change, dry skin), mental status, bowel status, menorrhagia, hoarseness; bradycardia; deep tendon reflexes, complete blood count (CBC) for anemia, electrolytes for hyponatremia, T_4, and TSH.

Nursing Diagnosis While receiving thyroid hormones, B.T. is at risk for the following complications related to an underdose (hypothyroidism) or overdose (hyperthyroidism). Selected nursing diagnoses/collaborative problems associated with hypothyroidism are excess fluid volume, edema related to retention of fluids secondary to slowed metabolism; activity intolerance related to weakness

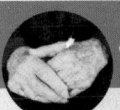

Special Considerations for Older Adults | THYROID HORMONES

- Because older adults are usually more sensitive to thyroid hormones and experience more adverse effects to them than other age groups, it is recommended that thyroid replacement dosages be individualized. In some clients, the dosage should be 25% lower than the usual adult dosage.
- Hypothyroidism, the second most common endocrine disease in older adults, is often misdiagnosed. Only one third of older adults exhibit the typical signs and symptoms of cold intolerance and weight gain. Most often

the symptoms are nonspecific and include failure to thrive, stumbling and falling episodes, and incontinence; if neurologic involvement has occurred, the client may also be misdiagnosed with dementia, depression, or a psychotic episode (*USP DI*, 2005).
- Laboratory tests for serum T_4 and TSH are used to confirm hypothyroidism.
- Levothyroxine (Synthroid, others) is usually the drug of choice for thyroid replacement.

and fatigue secondary to a decreased metabolic rate; imbalanced nutrition: more than body requirements related to decreased need; constipation related to decreased peristalsis; risk for ineffective breathing pattern, hypoventilation related to decreased respiratory drive; and the potential complication of myxedema coma. Selected nursing diagnoses/collaborative problems related to hyperthyroidism are imbalanced nutrition: less than body requirements related to hypermetabolism; disturbed sleep pattern; anxiety related to sympathetic nervous system stimulation; and the potential complication of thyrotoxic crisis. There is the potential complication of allergic reaction. (See the Nursing Care Plan below.)

Planning During thyroid hormone therapy, B.T. will:
- Demonstrate a euthyroid status.
- Remain compliant with medication regimen and supportive measures.

NURSING CARE PLAN SELECTED NURSING DIAGNOSES RELATED TO THYROID THERAPY

Nursing Diagnosis	Outcome Criteria	Nursing Interventions
Deficient knowledge related to thyroid dysfunction	Client will: • Express understanding of normal thyroid function and the effects of altered thyroid function	• Assess client's level of understanding. • Determine educational needs of client and family. • Instruct client in function of the thyroid gland and thyroid hormones. • Instruct client in specific effects of the client's alteration in thyroid function. • Provide opportunity for client to ask questions and verbalize concerns.

Deficient knowledge related to drug regimen (thyroid drug)	Client will:
	• Relate the purpose of drug therapy and identify adverse effects of the medication
	• Take thyroid drugs as prescribed
		• Teach the client:
		  • Purpose and action of the drug
		  • Proper administration
		  • The need for continued therapy throughout lifetime, even after euthyroid state is obtained
		  • Signs and symptoms of hypothyroidism and hyperthyroidism
		  • Adverse effects and which are reportable
		• Provide the client with a list of drugs or conditions that interact with or alter the drug requirements.
		• Explain the benefit of wearing or carrying a medical identification tag, bracelet, or card.

Disturbed body image related to thyroid dysfunction	Client and family will: • Express concerns regarding body image changes • State the basis for body changes related to thyroid function and identify the benefit of drug therapy	• Assess the client and family for perceptions and concerns related to body image. • Encourage open communication and talking about perceived body image. • Encourage adequate rest periods. • Encourage good grooming and attractive dress to promote self-confidence and positive self-image.
Imbalanced nutrition related to altered metabolic needs	Client will: • Move toward and maintain an ideal body weight • Show evidence of maintaining a well-balanced diet	• Assess normal dietary patterns. • Instruct client to monitor his or her weight weekly. • Instruct client to adjust diet to match caloric needs. • Encourage a high-bulk diet, fluids, and exercise to prevent or limit constipation. • Assist client in planning meals and dietary modifications.
Risk for impaired skin integrity related to altered thyroid function	Client will: • Maintain intact skin • Demonstrate proper skin care	• Assess skin for dryness, itching, or altered integrity. • Monitor client for development of skin disruption. • Keep skin clean and well lubricated. • Apply moisturizer as needed. • Use skin massage and position changes. • Instruct client in proper skin care.

• Collaborate with health care providers, reporting adverse symptoms appropriately and maintaining scheduled appointments for monitoring and treatment.

Implementation

Monitoring Assess B.T. for decreased symptoms of hypothyroidism; she should show weight loss, relief from constipation, and an increased activity level, appetite, sense of well-being, deep tendon reflexes, and pulse rate.

Monitor thyroid function studies throughout therapy. Such studies may include serum free T_4 index determinations (total T_3 or T_4 resin uptake determinations), and TSH determinations. Monitor apical pulse and blood pressure before and periodically during therapy.

B.T. is at risk for altered cardiac output related to the thyroid's cardiovascular effects. If the resting pulse is greater than 100 beats/min mm Hg, withhold the dose and notify the prescriber. For clients with preexisting cardiovascular disease, observe closely for cardiac ischemia (chest pain) and tachydysrhythmias. If B.T. were a child, she would be assessed periodically for growth, bone age, and psychomotor development.

Intervention Because clients with hypothyroidism respond rapidly to replacement doses, B.T. is started on the lowest possible dosage, with increases titrated over several weeks in accordance with her clinical response and laboratory data until the optimal clinical response is obtained. Once the maintenance dosage has been established, it is administered daily, preferably before breakfast.

However, in neonates with congenital hypothyroidism, the full dosage of hormone replacement therapy is started as soon as possible after birth. Replacement therapy started after 3 months of life may reverse many of the physical symptoms of hypothyroidism but not all of the mental effects.

Levothyroxine is preferred for thyroid replacement therapy. It is recommended that levothyroxine be taken on an empty stomach. In its parenteral form, levothyroxine sodium is reconstituted with sodium chloride injection (without preservative) to a solution of 100 mcg (0.1 mg)/mL. It should be reconstituted immediately before use.

Education Lifelong therapy is a possibility with thyroid hormonal replacement. Counsel B.T. accordingly. This means regular consultations with the prescriber to monitor the effectiveness of the therapy and compliance with the prescribed regimen. To simulate the natural process of the body, B.T. should take the medication at the same time every day. Morning administration will help to prevent insomnia.

Inform B.T. that a missed dose should be taken as soon as possible. Caution her not to take the missed dose if it is close to the next dose, because this will have the effect of doubling doses. Contact the prescriber if two or more consecutive doses are missed.

Instruct B.T. to alert other health care providers about her thyroid hormonal replacement, particularly if any type of surgery is required (including dental surgery). She should wear a medical identification tag or bracelet. Advise her to

consult with the prescriber before taking other medications concurrently with thyroid replacement.

Advise B.T. to inform the prescriber if the pulse rate increases or if palpitations or chest pain occur. Irritability, nervousness, heat intolerance, and excessive sweating may indicate the need for a dosage reduction; insomnia is usually the earliest sign. If such symptoms occur, drug withdrawal may be indicated for a few days before resuming it at a lower dosage.

Advise B.T. not to change brands of thyroid replacement therapy, because different brands of the same drug are not bioequivalent.

Alert the parents of a child taking thyroid hormones that a partial but temporary hair loss sometimes occurs during the first few months of therapy with children; the hair will usually return, even if hormonal replacement is continued.

Evaluation The expected outcome of thyroid hormone replacement therapy is that B.T. is independent in activities of daily living without becoming overtired. She maintains a euthyroid state as evidenced by thyroid function studies within the normal limits. B.T. effectively maintains her therapeutic regimen that includes remaining compliant with her medication, stating the importance of taking it as prescribed, stating adverse effects reportable to the prescriber and maintaining scheduled visits to her health care provider for monitoring and treatment.

✱ **T.L. is a 59-year-old truck driver with tachycardia, who presents to his physician with restlessness and insomnia. His physician observes exophthalmos, elevated heart rate, hyperactive deep tendon reflexes, and moist, warm skin. Endocrine lab results demonstrate a suppressed TSH at 0.2 mU/L and elevated T4 at 12.8 mcg/L. T.L. is diagnosed with Graves' disease. The tachycardia is managed with a β-adrenergic blocker, atenolol (Tenormin) 25 mg PO daily. He is referred to the endocrinologist who will evaluate the role of drugs and surgery.**

✱ **What pharmacologic agents are available for treating hyperthyroidism?**

The goal in treating hyperthyroidism is to both manage the systemic complications of hyperactive thyroid function and to manage the disease at its source. The primary options for treatment of hyperthyroidism are antithyroid drugs (thioamides), radioiodine, and surgery. In addition to antithyroid drugs, β-adrenergic blockers (e.g., propranolol [Inderal]) are often used concurrently with other interventions because the complications of hyperthyroid states often involve tachydysrhythmias. Antithyroid drugs are chemical agents that lower the basal metabolic rate by interfering with the formation, release, or action of thyroid hormones. Agents that interfere with the synthesis of the thyroid hormones are known as goitrogens. A variety of compounds are included in this category of antithyroid drugs; iodine (iodide ion), radioactive iodine, and thioamide derivatives are discussed in the following sections.

Iodine, Iodides

Iodine, an essential micronutrient, is the oldest of the antithyroid drugs. Almost 80% of the iodine in the body is found in the thyroid gland. Although a small amount of iodine is necessary for normal thyroid function and for the synthesis of thyroid hormones, the response of the client with thyrotoxicosis to iodine administration is inhibition of thyroid hormone synthesis and thyroid release from the hyperfunctioning thyroid gland.

Iodide from dietary sources is rapidly absorbed into the bloodstream. Approximately one third of it is removed from the blood by the iodide pump in the thyroid. The initial iodide removed from the blood is usually sodium or potassium iodide. The enzyme peroxidase converts the iodides to iodine; iodine is then used to form monoiodotyrosine (MIT) and diiodotyrosine (DIT), which are the components of T_3 and T_4. The synthesized hormones (T_3, T_4) are stored within thyroglobulin until they are released into the circulation. These activities involve a complex negative feedback mechanism between the thyroid gland and the hypothalamus-pituitary gland. Low levels of circulating thyroid hormone increase the release of TSH from the pituitary and appear to influence the secretion of thyrotropin-releasing factor (TRF) from the hypothalamus. Increased levels of TSH increase iodide trapping by the gland that results in an increase in synthesis and circulating thyroid hormones. As thyroid hormone levels increase, the hypothalamic and pituitary centers stop the release of TRF and TSH. This process is repeated if thyroid hormone levels decrease again in response to the declining levels of circulating thyroid hormones (see Box 47-1).

The inhibition of thyroid hormone release for several weeks leads to an increase in TSH secretion that can overcome this blockade. Thus large dosages of iodides are generally used for 7 to 14 days before thyroid surgery to decrease the size and vascularity of the thyroid, resulting in diminished blood loss and a less complicated surgical procedure.

Radioactive iodine (RAI) is preferred for clients with diffuse toxic goiter (Graves' disease) or toxic nodular goiter who are poor surgical risks (e.g., debilitated clients, clients with advanced cardiac disease, and older adults). It is the treatment of choice for clients with multinodular toxic goiter (Dong, 2005). It is also used for clients who have not responded adequately to drug therapy or who have had recurrent hyperthyroidism after surgery. In addition to the risk involved with surgery and postsurgical complications, the primary disadvantage of surgery or RAI therapy is the induction of hypothyroidism. Radioactive iodine is absolutely contraindicated in pregnant clients. Radioactive iodine is a substance of potential use as a weapon of terrorism (see the Pharmacologic Issues in an Age of Terrorism box on p. 845).

Iodine Products

potassium iodide [poe **tass** ee um **eye** oh dide]
(Thyro-Block)
Indications
Iodine is indicated to protect the thyroid gland from radiation before and after the administration of radioactive isotopes of iodine or in radiation emergencies; it may also be used with an antithyroid drug in clients with hyperthyroidism in preparation for thyroidectomy.

Pharmacokinetics/Dosing
Therapeutic effects may be noted within 24 hours, with the maximum effects achieved within 10 to 14 days of continuous therapy. Potassium iodide liquid or tablets are also commonly known as KI or SSKI. The adult oral dosage is 60 to 250 mg 24 hours before radiation, then daily for 3 to 10 days afterward. For children 3 to 12 years of age, the postexposure oral dose is 65 mg daily; for children 1 month to 3 years of age, the oral dose is 32 mg daily. Doses may continue for up to 10 days after exposure to radioactive iodine.

Adverse Effects
The adverse effects of iodine therapy include diarrhea, nausea, vomiting, stomach pain, rash, and swelling of the salivary gland. With prolonged usage there may be severe headaches, sore gums or teeth, increased salivation, a burning sensation in the mouth or throat, or a metallic taste in the mouth. Potassium iodide is Pregnancy Category D when used long term or close to term; it does cross the placenta and may produce abnormal thyroid function in infants. Short-term use (e.g., 10 days) does not carry this risk.

strong iodine solution
(Lugol iodine solution)
Indications
As with potassium iodide.

Pharmacokinetics/Dosing
Strong iodine solution is a combination of 5% iodine and 10% potassium iodide. The iodine is converted to iodide in the GI tract before systemic absorption. The adult oral dosage is 2 to 6 drops three times daily.

Adverse Effects
Similar to potassium iodide.

Nursing Management
These substances are not commonly used in the treatment of hyperthyroidism, but the nurse should be familiar with their use in response to a radiation emergency. Ensure client is not allergic to seafood or other iodine-containing agents. However, the administration of the drug is quite different the other medications. To improve taste, dilute Lugol's iodine solution and saturated solutions of sodium or potassium in 240 mL of fruit juice, carbonated beverage, broth, or other substance. Because the medication evaporates rapidly, do not leave it open to air for long periods before administration. Do not use if the solution has turned brownish yellow. If crystals form in the solution, warm the closed container and shake it gently until dissolved. Administer iodine products through a straw to prevent tooth discoloration. Administer after meals to minimize gastric irritation.

sodium iodide
(^{131} I, Iodotope)
Sodium iodide, a radioactive isotope of iodine, accumulates in the thyroid tissue and selectively damages or destroys it.
Indications
Sodium iodide is indicated for the treatment of hyperthyroidism and thyroid carcinoma.

Pharmacokinetics/Dosing
Administered orally, this drug has an onset of effect within 2 to 4 weeks and a peak therapeutic effect between 2 and 4 months. It is mainly excreted by the kidneys. Up to 20% of the dose may appear in breast milk within 24 hours. Sodium iodide has a radionuclide half-life of approximately 8 days; the principal types of radiation are beta and gamma rays.

Adverse Effects
The adverse effects of sodium iodide therapy may include a sore throat, a temporary loss of taste, nausea, vomiting, and painful and swollen salivary glands. Signs of hypothyroidism may follow treatment. Pregnancy safety is classified as Category X by the Food and Drug Administration (FDA).

Drug Interactions
Although no significant drug interactions are noted with this product, many drugs are capable of interfering with test results. Refer to

Pharmacologic Issues in an Age of Terrorism

Radiation Exposure and the Thyroid

Small exposures to radiation in the environment occur daily from environmental sources (e.g., sun, soil elements), electronics (e.g., televisions, microwave ovens), and health care facilities (x-rays, diagnostics and treatments). Additional small doses may be secondary to nuclear weapons testing or, in rare cases, nuclear generating power plants. The risks associated with these low, long-term exposures may include a slightly higher risk for cancers and other ailments in future years, although genetics probably also plays a part.

High amounts to radiation pose significant risks, depending on dose and duration of exposure. Moderate doses of radiation are directly linked to future cancer development or other adverse effects, whereas high doses can be lethal in days to weeks.

Sources of radiation from a terrorist attack could include contamination of water or food supply, use of a "dirty bomb" (conventional explosives used to scatter radioactive material), bombing a nuclear facility, or detonating a nuclear device. Each potential scenario could result in different risks with different doses of radiation. Dirty bombs, for example, would not likely cause serious acute radiation sickness, but could increase cancer risk in some individuals and result in a large geographic area with low to moderate radiation contamination. Bombing a nuclear facility or detonating a nuclear device could result in both acute and long-term radiation sickness.

The types of radioactive isotopes may also differ. Nuclear devices and explosion of a nuclear plant typically will generate radioactive iodine, whereas other types of exposures (e.g., dirty bombs) may involve different radioisotopes.

High doses of radioactive iodine pose a significant risk for future thyroid cancer because they will accumulate in high doses in the thyroid. In the event of a significant nuclear exposure to radioactive iodine (e.g., nuclear device, nuclear plant bomb), individuals with a high exposure risk may benefit from the administration of potassium iodide. Potassium iodide serves to saturate the thyroid with iodine and thereby reduces the degree to which radioactive iodine is incorporated into thyroid tissue. Unfortunately, potassium iodide does not offer protection to other tissue, and is only effective for radioactive iodine. Potassium iodide is less likely to be of benefit for a dirty bomb because the radioactive isotope is unlikely to be iodine.

Potassium iodide therapy in response to a nuclear incident should only be instituted under the direction of local emergency management officials. This assures an assessment of risk, the nature of the radioactive isotope, dose, and prevailing wind patterns. Once the risk is quantified and believed responsive to potassium iodide, emergency management officials will alert health care providers and the public regarding the use of potassium iodide. Many communities within a 10-mile radius of nuclear power plants have developed programs to provide potassium iodide to the community in advance of a nuclear threat. In such circumstances, many clients at high risk may already have potassium iodide at home.

Potassium iodide should be taken immediately after a radiation release occurs if possible, although protective benefits are still realized if KI is taken up to 3 to 4 hours postexposure. Typically a single dose is all that is required, as radioactive iodide decays quickly. It is important to remember that potassium iodide will not reduce risk for forms of radiation other than radioactive iodine, and that potassium iodide itself may pose some risks.

Children and adolescents have the highest risk of developing cancer secondary to high doses of radioactive iodine. As such, they are routinely given potassium iodine in an emergency that warrants its use. Young adults also have a significant risk, and are often treated in low to moderate exposure risk circumstances. Women who are pregnant or breastfeeding are also typically administered potassium iodide. Adults older than 40 years of age have a lower risk for developing thyroid cancer and the use of potassium iodide is reserved for large doses of radioactive iodine. Those with a history of allergy to shellfish or iodine should avoid taking potassium iodide. Similarly, those with hyperthyroidism, thyroid nodules, and those with significant dermal conditions should use caution with potassium iodide, and consultation with their health care provider is recommended if feasible.

The dose of potassium iodide for adults is a 130-mg tablet. Children between 3 and 18 years of age should take 65 mg (one half tablet), although if the child is of adult size, the adult dose is recommended. Children aged 1 month to 3 years should take 32 mg (one fourth tablet). A liquid formulation compounded from KI crystals may be given in drop form to infants and children. This formulation affords a more accurate dose than attempting to break the KI tablet into multiple pieces. Higher doses do not offer additional protection and increase the risk for hypersensitivity reactions. A second dose is recommended if the exposure is significant for a period greater than 24 hours, and dosed every 24 hours while the exposure risk is high. Most forms of potassium iodide are stable for at least 5 years. Health care practitioners should be aware of local emergency response programs in advance of an emergency to help expedite the effective dissemination of potassium iodide in an emergency.

Data from Emergency Preparedness and Response: Center for Disease Control. (2005). Retrieved February 22, 2005, from http://www.bt.cdc.gov; Potassium Iodide: Emergency Preparedness and Response: Center for Disease Control. (2005). Retrieved February 22, 2005, from http://www.bt.cdc.gov/radiation/ki.asp; Frequently Asked Questions on Potassium Iodide. (2005). Retrieved February 22, 2005, from http://www.fda.gov/cder/drugprepare/KI_Q&A.htm.

a current reference for possible drug interferences and current dosage recommendations.

Nursing Management

Sodium iodide ^{131}I therapy was a consideration for treatment of T.L., however, his age probably made the difference in the treatment. ^{131}I therapy is usually used in older clients for whom surgery would be a risk. Although ^{131}I therapy is administered by nuclear medicine departments, nursing is responsible for care of the client (Box 47-2).

Thioamide Derivatives

Thioamide derivatives, or antithyroid agents, inhibit thyroid hormone synthesis by inhibiting the incorporation of iodide into tyrosine and inhibiting the coupling of iodotyrosines. They do not affect exogenous thyroid hormones. Propylthiouracil (but not methimazole) also inhibits the conversion of thyroxine (T_4) to triiodothyronine (T_3),

which may make it more effective for the treatment of thyroid crisis or thyroid storm. Thioamides cross the placenta and can cause fetal hypothyroidism and goiter; pregnancy safety has been established as FDA Category D.

✱☜ propylthiouracil [proe pill thye oh **yoor** ah sill] (Propyl-Thyracil✤)

Indications

Propylthiouracil is indicated for the treatment of hyperthyroidism, before surgery or radiotherapy, or as adjunct therapy for the treatment of thyrotoxicosis or thyroid storm.

Pharmacokinetics/Dosing

The half-life of propylthiouracil is 1 to 2 hours, and peak effect is observed at 17 weeks. Propylthiouracil is metabolized hepatically and renally eliminated. The adult dosage of propylthiouracil is 300 to 900 mg PO daily in divided doses. Children between 6 and 10 years of age receive 50 to 150 mg PO daily, whereas children over 10 years of age receive 50 to 300 mg PO daily. For neonatal thyrotoxicosis, the dosage is 10 mg/kg PO daily in divided doses.

BOX 47-2 CARE OF CLIENT RECEIVING ^{131}I THERAPY

NURSING MANAGEMENT

Assessment

Thyroid function studies should be performed before and after therapy. Do not give radioactive iodine to pregnant women or nursing mothers. In women with childbearing potential, therapy begins the first few days after the onset of menses.

Nursing Diagnosis

Most clients experience deficient knowledge and anxiety related to the administration of radioactive materials. The client may also experience temporary impaired comfort following a course of ^{131}I therapy as evidenced by a loss of taste, nausea and vomiting, and tenderness of the salivary glands. Additionally, there is the potential complication of hypothyroidism with therapeutic dosages. Other potential complications may include leukopenia as evidenced by fever, chills, and sore throat, and thrombocytopenia with symptoms of unusual bleeding or bruising.

Planning

During ^{131}I therapy, the client will:
- Demonstrate decreased symptoms of hyperthyroidism without experiencing adverse effects of the agent.
- Relate the purpose of the therapy and identify adverse effects and which are reportable.
- Implement safety measures associated with ^{131}I use.

Implementation

Monitoring After therapy, assess thyroid function with serum thyroxine examinations.

Intervention The client should take nothing by mouth after midnight before a morning dose, because food slows the absorption of the drug. Increase the fluid intake of the client to 2500 mL daily to enhance excretion of the isotope.

If the dose is administered for hyperthyroidism, institute

full radiation precautions for 24 hours. If the dose is for thyroid cancer, isolate the client for 3 days. Check the institution's protocol for radiation precautions. Pregnant women (personnel or visitors) should not have contact with the client. Use disposable utensils with the client. Consult with nuclear medicine personnel about limitations for individual staff contact with the client. To avoid exposure to the radioactive products of the iodine, wear rubber gloves when giving ^{131}I to clients and when disposing of their excreta. Limit the exposure of individuals by limiting the time of contact with the client and increasing the distance from the source of radiation.

Education To prevent radiation contamination of others and the environment, instruct the client in the appropriate methods for disposing of urine and feces (e.g., double-flushing the toilet, washing hands after using the toilet) until radiation precautions are no longer needed. If the client is discharged but radiation precautions are still necessary, ensure that personnel from the nuclear medicine department provide the client with specific instructions for visitor contact and the disposal of utensils and excreta.

If the client received a dose of ^{131}I for the treatment of hyperthyroidism or thyroid carcinoma, 48- to 72-hour precautions may include the following: avoiding close contact with others, especially children; not kissing anyone or sharing other persons' eating or drinking utensils; not engaging in sexual activities; sleeping alone; washing the sink and tub after use; and using separate clothes, towels, and linens and washing them separately.

Evaluation

The expected outcome of sodium iodide ^{131}I therapy is that the client will experience a euthyroid state as evidenced by thyroid function study values that are within the normal range. The client will relate the purpose of the therapy and report adverse effects appropriately. Safety precautions such as limited visitor contact and disposal of utensils and excreta will be taken.

Adverse Effects

The adverse effects of the thioamide derivatives include a loss of taste, nausea, vomiting, dizziness, skin rash, fever, and other signs of infection secondary to leukopenia or agranulocytosis.

methimazole [meth **im** a zole]

(Tapazole)

Indications

Methimazole is used to treat hyperthyroidism before surgery or radiation.

Pharmacokinetics/Dosing

The half-life of methimazole is 5 to 6 hours. The peak effect is 7 weeks with methimazole. Methimazole is metabolized in the liver and excreted by the kidneys. The adult dosage of methimazole is 15 to 60 mg PO daily for hyperthyroidism; the maintenance dosage is 5 to 30 mg PO daily in 1 or 2 divided doses. To treat thyrotoxic crisis, the dosage is 15 to 20 mg PO every 4 hours for 24 hours as an adjunct to other therapies. The pediatric dosage for hyperthyroidism is 0.4 mg/kg PO daily; the maintenance dosage is 0.2 mg/kg PO daily. The dosage in children should not exceed 30 mg daily.

Adverse Effects

See propylthiouracil.

✳ **T.L. is scheduled for surgery, and is also started on thioamides as adjunctive short-term therapy to produce euthyroidism before surgery or radioactive iodine.**

✳ **What are the nursing management issues with T.L.'s thioamide therapy?**

Assessment Determine if T.L. has a history of allergic reaction to these preparations, propylthiouracil or methimazole. Review T.L.'s health status to ascertain that he does not have a condition for which the administration of these drugs would entail a greater risk (e.g., hepatic function impairment). Propylthiouracil is the drug of choice for pregnant women who require antithyroid therapy.

Review T.L.'s current drug regimen for the risk of significant drug interactions, such as those that may occur when methimazole or propylthiouracil is given concurrently with amiodarone, iodinated glycerol, iodine, or potassium iodide. Amiodarone contains 37% iodine by weight. Increased or excess amounts of amiodarone, iodide, or iodine may result in a decreased response to the antithyroid drugs. However, iodine deficiency may result in an increased response to the antithyroid medications. Monitor the client closely. If antithyroid agents are administered with oral anticoagulants, the response to anticoagulants may decrease as thyroid status approaches normal. If the thioamide produces a drug-induced hypoprothrombinemia, the anticoagulant response may increase. Monitor closely, because dosages of anticoagulants are adjusted according to PT or INR results. If T.L. takes digoxin, serum levels of digoxin may increase as thyroid status approaches normal. Monitor closely, because dosage adjustments may be necessary. The thyroid uptake of ^{131}I may be decreased by the antithyroid agents. Monitor. T.L.'s BP and pulse rate closely, because his dose of propranolol may need to be decreased as he becomes euthyroid.

A baseline assessment of T.L. will include his general status (weakness, fatigue, heat intolerance, increased sweating. weight change [usually loss]), mental status (restlessness,

nervousness), frequent bowel movements, palpitations or angina pectoris, hyperreflexia, ophthalmopathy, CBC, T_4, and TSH.

Nursing Diagnosis While T.L. is receiving thioamide derivative therapy, he is at risk for the following nursing diagnoses/ collaborative problems: impaired comfort (nausea, loss of taste, itching, stomach cramping, dizziness); ineffective protection related to the bone marrow depressant effects of the drug (delayed healing, gingival bleeding, leukopenia); and the potential complications of agranulocytosis (fever, chills, throat infection, chills, mouth sores or hoarseness), arthralgias, systemic lupus erythematous–like syndrome, and peripheral neuropathy, and hyperthyroidism as a result of ineffectiveness of the therapeutic regimen or hypothyroidism because of overdose.

Planning During thioamide derivative therapy, T.L. will:
- Demonstrate decreased symptoms of hyperthyroidism toward an euthyroid status without adverse effects of the drug.
- Remain compliant with medication regimen.
- Collaborate with health care providers, reporting adverse symptoms appropriately and maintaining scheduled appointments for monitoring and treatment.

Implementation

Monitoring For these antithyroid products, observe the CBC results periodically during therapy to detect blood dyscrasias such as agranulocytosis, leukopenia, or thrombocytopenia. Propylthiouracil may reduce thrombin and result in bleeding; monitor PT/INR (prothrombin time/ International Normalized Ratio) during therapy.

Assess T.L. for effectiveness of the therapeutic regimen. Signs of thyrotoxicosis (e.g., fever, tachycardia, irritability, weakness, diarrhea, and vomiting) indicate inadequate therapy. Signs of hypothyroidism (e.g., intolerance to cold, constipation, lethargy, weight gain) indicate overdose. TSH and T_4 assays are important in monitoring T.L.'s status.

Intervention Administer thioamide derivatives with meals to minimize gastric irritation. Use the smallest effective dose for pregnant clients. Propylthiouracil crosses the placental barrier; therefore large doses can cause goiter in the newborn or hypothyroidism in the fetus.

Although T.L.'s therapy will only be continued until his surgery, for some other clients compliance may become an issue because therapy to obtain a prolonged remission may take 6 months to several years. For the greatest effectiveness, the doses should be divided into evenly spaced intervals throughout the day. To improve compliance and decrease the incidence of adverse effects, a once- or twice-daily dosage schedule may be used; however, this schedule is less effective. Antithyroid medications need to be taken at the same time every day in relation to meals, because food may alter the response to the drug by affecting its absorption.

Because of the risk of thyroid storm, T.L. should consult with the prescriber if his health status changes because of infection, injury, or other illness, or if surgery, dental surgery, or emergency treatment is required.

Education Instruct T.L. to report a sore throat, head cold, skin eruptions, or malaise immediately to his prescriber, because these symptoms signal the onset of agranulocytosis. This condition may occur too quickly to be determined by periodic blood testing. Instruct T.L. to consult with the prescriber about the restriction of iodized salt and seafood. Caution T.L. against taking over-the-counter (OTC) medications, because many contain iodine preparations or sympathomimetics, which could aggravate hyperthyroidism. Alert breastfeeding mothers to take these drugs with caution and ensure thyroid function monitoring for their infants, because these drugs are excreted in the milk.

Evaluation The expected outcome of thioamide derivative therapy is that T.L. will experience a decrease in his symptoms of hyperthyroidism in preparation for surgery or for other clients, a euthyroid state with thyroid function study values that are within the normal range. He effectively manages his therapeutic regimen including remaining compliant with his medication, stating the importance of taking it as prescribed, stating adverse effects reportable to the prescriber and maintaining scheduled visits to his health care provider for monitoring and treatment.

Summary

As with other endocrine glands, parathyroid and thyroid functioning may increase or decrease resulting in pathologic conditions for the client. With hypoparathyroidism, the administration of vitamin D and calcium supplements will usually restore the calcium and phosphorus levels to normal. Surgery is usually the primary treatment for hyperparathyroidism but may require management of hypercalcemia with calcitonin or bisphosphonates. Calcitonin and bisphosphonates are also used in the management of osteoporosis.

With hypothyroidism, the clinical goal is to eliminate the client's symptoms by thyroid replacement therapy, for which a number of preparations are available. Hyperthyroidism is managed by large doses of iodides, which inhibit the release of thyroid hormones and decrease the size of the thyroid; thioamide derivatives, which inhibit the synthesis of thyroid hormone; radioactive iodine; or surgery.

During all the therapies associated with hormonal replacement or inhibition, the client requires support and explanation to understand the many body and mood changes that may occur with these therapies. Because the clinical manifestations of the therapies are as important as laboratory studies in determining the efficacy of treatment, ongoing skilled assessment of the client's health status is essential.

✳ Critical Thinking Questions

• Grace Smith examines the label on the OTC calcium supplement she takes each day. It indicates that two tablets taken daily provide 3000 mg of calcium carbonate. How much elemental calcium is Grace taking?

• Why is clinical response more important than blood hormone level in thyroid preparation therapy? What signs and symptoms should the nurse monitor to determine the effectiveness of the therapy?

Bibliography

Alexander, E.K., Marqusee, E., Lawrence, J., Jarolim, P., Fischer, G.A., & Larsen, P.R. (2004). Timing and magnitude of increases in levothyroxine requirements during pregnancy in women with hypothyroidism. *New England Journal of Medicine, 351*, 241-249.

Anderson, D.M., Keith, J., & Novak, P.D. (Eds.) (2002). *Mosby's medical, nursing, and allied health dictionary* (6th ed.). St. Louis: Mosby.

Bischoff-Ferrari, H.A., Willett, W.C., Wong, J.B., Giovannucci, E., Dietrich, T., & Dawson-Hughes, B. (2005). Fracture prevention with vitamin D supplementation: A meta-analysis of randomized controlled trials. *Journal of the American Medical Association, 293*, 2257-2264.

Blazer, S., Moreh-Waterman, Y., Miller-Lotan, R., Tamir, A., & Hochberg, Z. (2003). Maternal hypothyroidism may affect fetal growth and neonatal thyroid function. *Obstetrics and Gynecology, 102*, 232-241.

Block, G.A., Martin, K.J., de Francisco, A.L., Turner, S.A., Avram, M.M., & Suranyi, M.G., et al. (2004). Cinacalcet for secondary hyperparathyroidism in patients receiving hemodialysis. *New England Journal of Medicine, 350*, 1516-1525.

Bone, H.G., Hosking, D., Devogelaer, J.P., Tucci, J.R., Emkey, R.D., & Tonino, R.P., et al., and the Alendronate Phase III Osteoporosis Treatment Study Group. (2004). Ten years' experience with alendronate for osteoporosis in postmenopausal women. *New England Journal of Medicine, 350*, 1189-1199.

Bosker, G. (Ed.). (2004). *Primary and acute care medicine: Practice, protocols, pathways,* (2nd ed.). Atlanta: Thomson American Health Consultants.

e-LEARNING SUPPLEMENTS

Student CD-ROM
• Final Exam questions
• NCLEX® Examination review questions
• Pharmacology animations
• Printable chapter summary

Evolve Website (http://evolve.elsevier.com/mckenry)
• Case study on drugs affecting the parathyroid and thyroid glands

• Content updates, including information on new drugs
• WebLinks corresponding to this chapter
• Answers to the critical thinking questions in this chapter
• *Elsevier ePharmacology Update* newsletter
• Mosby's Drug Consult Internet Edition
• Supplemental and reference information

Casey, B.M., Dashe, J.S., Wells, C.E., McIntire, D.D., Byrd, W., Leveno, K.J., et al. (2005). Subclinical hypothyroidism and pregnancy outcomes. *Obstetrics and Gynecology, 105,* 239-245.

Clyde, P.W., Harari, A.E., Getka, E.J., & Shakir, K.M. (2003). Combined levothyroxine plus liothyronine compared with levothyroxine alone in primary hypothyroidism: A randomized controlled trial. *Journal of the American Medical Association, 290,* 2952-2958.

Dong, B.J. (2005). Thyroid disorders. In M.A. Koda-Kimble, L.Y. Young, W.A. Kradian, B.J. Guglielmo, B.K. Alldredge, & R.L. Corelli (Eds.), *Applied therapeutics: The clinical use of drugs* (8th ed.). Philadelphia: Lippincott Williams & Wilkins.

Drug facts and comparisons (58th ed.). (2005). St. Louis: Facts and Comparisons.

Farwell, A.P., & Braverman, L.E. (2001). Thyroid and Antithyroid Drugs. In: J.G. Hardman & L.E. Limbird (Eds.), *Goodman & Gilman's The pharmacological basis of therapeutics* (10th ed.). New York: McGraw-Hill.

Fitzgerald, P.A. (2003). Endocrinology. In L.M. Tierney, Jr., S.J. McPhee & Papadakis, M.A. (Eds.), *Current Medical Diagnosis & Treatment.* New York: Lange Medical Books/McGraw-Hill.

Grant, A.M., Avenell, A., Campbell, M.K., McDonald, A.M., MacLennan, G.S., McPherson, G.C., et al; RECORD Trial Group. (2005). The RECORD Trial Group: Oral vitamin D3 and calcium for secondary prevention of low-trauma fractures in elderly people (Randomised Evaluation of Calcium or Vitamin D, RECORD): A randomised placebo-controlled trial. *Lancet, 365,* 1621-1628.

Lacy, C.F., Armstrong, L.L., Goldman, M.P., & Lance, L.L. (2004). *Lexi-Comp's Drug Information Handbook* (12th ed.). Hudson, Ohio: Lexi-Comp.

Lau, A.H. (2005). Fluid and electrolyte disorders. In M.A. Koda-Kimble, L.Y. Young, W.A. Kradian , B.J. Guglielmo, B.K. Alldredge, & R.L. Corelli (Eds.), *Applied therapeutics: The clinical use of drugs* (8th ed.). Philadelphia: Lippincott Williams & Wilkins.

Meier, C., Trittibach, P., Guglielmetti, M., Staub, J.J., & Muller, B.(2003). Serum thyroid stimulating hormone in assessment of severity of tissue hypothyroidism in patients with overt primary thyroid failure: Cross sectional survey. *British Medical Journal, 326,* 311-312.

Mosby's drug consult (15th ed.). (2005). St. Louis: Mosby.

Novartis. (December 2004) Dear Doctor Letter: Zometa. Retrieved July 17, 2005, from http:www.fda.gov/medwatch/safety/2005.

Novartis. (May 2005) Dear Doctor Letter: Bisphosphonates and osteonecrosis of the jaw. Retrieved July 17, 2005, from http:www.fda.gov/medwatch/safety/2005.

Odvina, C.V., Zerwekh, J.E., Rao, D.S., Maalouf, N., Gottschalk, F.A., & Pak, C.Y. (2005). Severely suppressed bone turnover: A potential complication of alendronate therapy. *Journal of Clinical Endocrinology and Metabolism, 90,* 1294-1301.

Ott, S.M. (2005). Editorial: Long-term safety of bisphosphonates. *Journal of Clinical Endocrinology and Metabolism, 90,* 1897-1899.

Pamplin C. (2004). Dear Health Care Professional Letter. Retrieved January 7, 2005, from http://www.fda.gov/medwatch/SAFETY/2004/Levoxyl_HCPletter.pdf.

Parent-Stevens, L., & Sagraves, R. (2005). Gynecologic and other disorders of women. In M.A. Koda-Kimble, L.Y. Young, W.A. Kradian, B.J. Guglielmo, B.K. Alldredge, & R.L. Corelli (Eds.), *Applied therapeutics: The clinical use of drugs* (8th ed.). Philadelphia: Lippincott Williams & Wilkins.

Peacock, M. (2005). Cinacalcet hydrochloride maintains long-term normocalcemia in patients with primary hyperthyroidism. *Journal of Clinical Endocrinology and Metabolism, 90*(1), 135-141.

Porthouse, J., Cockayne, S., King, C., Saxon, L., Steele, E., Aspray, T., et al. (2005). Randomised controlled trial of calcium and supplementation with cholecalciferol (vitamin D3) for prevention of fractures in primary care. *British Medical Journal, 330,* 1003-1005.

Quandt, S.A., Thompson, D.E., Schneider, D.L., Nevitt, M.C., Black, D.M.; Fracture Intervention Trial Research Group. (2005). Effect of alendronate on vertebral fracture risk in women with bone mineral density T scores of -1.6 to -2.5 at the femoral neck: The Fracture Intervention Trial. *Mayo Clinic Proceedings, 80,* 343-349.

Reasner, C.A. III, & Talbert, R.L. (2002). In J.T. DiPiro, R.L. Talbert, G.C. Yee, G.R. Matzke, B.G. Wells & L.M. Posey (Eds.), *Pharmacotherapy: A Pathophysiological Approach* (5th ed.). New York: McGraw-Hill.

Ross, J.R., Saunders, Y., Edmonds, P.M., Patel, S., Broadley, K.E., & Johnston, S.R. (2003). Systematic review of role of bisphosphonates on skeletal morbidity in metastatic cancer. *British Medical Journal, 327,* 469-472.

Schousboe, J.T., Nyman, J.A., Kane, R.L., & Ensrud, K.E. (2005). Cost-effectiveness of alendronate therapy for osteopenic postmenopausal women. *Annals of Internal Medicine, 142,* 734-741.

Taylor, E.N., Stampfer, M.J., & Curhan, G.C. (2005). Obesity, weight gain, and the risk of kidney stones. *Journal of the American Medical Association, 293,* 455-462.

Trivedi, D.P., Doll, R., & Khaw, K.T. (2003). Effect of four monthly oral vitamin D$_3$ (cholecalciferol) supplementation on fractures and mortality in men and women living in the community: Randomised double blind controlled trial. *British Medical Journal, 326,* 469-472.

USP DI: Drug information for the health care professional (25th ed.). (2005). Greenwood Village, CO: MICROMEDEX Thomson Healthcare.

48

DRUGS AFFECTING THE ADRENAL CORTEX

CHAPTER FOCUS

A number of pathologic conditions associated with hyposecretion or hypersecretion of the adrenal cortex are pharmacologically managed. The glucocorticoids are widely used in pharmacologic doses for their antiinflammatory and immunomodulating effects. However, clients receiving systemic corticosteroid preparations for nonendocrine disorders are at risk for adverse effects. Nurses need to be skillful at assessing not only the steroid-responsive disorder but also the client's individual responses to corticosteroid therapy.

LEARNING OBJECTIVES

- Compare and contrast glucocorticoids and mineralocorticoids.
- Describe the major pharmacologic effects of the corticosteroids.
- Identify five significant drug interactions of the glucocorticoids.
- Describe the advantages for an alternate-day dosing schedule.
- Explain a recommended method for corticosteroid drug withdrawal.
- Identify four major adverse effects associated with the use of adrenocorticoids.
- Implement the nursing management of drug therapy for clients receiving agents affecting the adrenal cortex.

 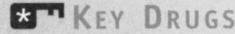

✳ What hormones are secreted by the adrenal cortex?
The adrenal cortex secretes two classes of steroids: the **corticosteroids** (glucocorticoids and mineralocorticoids) and the androgens; Chapter 53 discusses androgens. In humans, hydrocortisone, or cortisol, is the primary (prototype) **glucocorticoid,** and aldosterone is the main **mineralocorticoid.**

The glucocorticoid cortisol has multiple functions in the body, including regulating carbohydrate metabolism. Cortisol is secreted in times of physiologic stress. The mineralocorticoid aldosterone regulates sodium and other electrolytes and fluid in the body. Therapeutically, drugs with cortisol-like glucocorticoid effects and/or aldosterone-like mineralocorticoid are administered to augment natural physiologic actions.

The glucocorticoids are often administered for their antiinflammatory activity (e.g., control of asthma, inflammatory swelling, and edema). Dexamethasone (Decadron) represents an agent with almost pure glucocorticoid activity and is used to treat a number of inflammatory states. The mineralocorticoids are less frequently used clinically, although fludrocortisone (Florinef), an almost pure mineralocorticoid, is sometimes used to augment mineralocorticoid activity in adrenal insufficiency or to increase fluid retention and blood pressure in clients with symptomatic orthostatic hypotension. Most corticosteroids used in clinical practice (e.g., prednisone, prednisolone, hydrocortisone) possess both glucocorticoid and mineralocorticoid effects, and result in a wide array of short- and long-term adverse effects.

Corticosteroids are synthesized from cholesterol and stored in the adrenal cortex. Corticosteroid synthesis depends on pituitary adrenocorticotropic hormone (ACTH), which is governed by the corticotropin-releasing hormone (CRH) from the hypothalamus. Increased levels of corticosteroids can inhibit the adrenal glucocorticoid system by inhibiting the release of CRH from the hypothalamus and by inhibiting the release of ACTH from the pituitary. When exogenous corticosteroids are administered for sustained periods of time (e.g., beyond 10-14 days), it leads to the suppression of CRH and ACTH resulting in minimal or no synthesis and release of endogenous corticosteroids. Such inhibition with chronic corticosteroids is referred to as suppression of the hypothalamic-pituitary axis (HPA) and can result in addisonian crisis if chronic exogenous corticosteroid administration is halted abruptly.

✳ **P.G. is a 13-year-old boy with severe persistent asthma. His condition has worsened, and he is started on prednisone 50 mg (1 mg/kg) today that will be tapered by 10 mg daily until discontinued.**

✳ **What are the actions of glucocorticoids?**
Cortisone and prednisone are inactive substances until they are metabolized in the body to hydrocortisone and prednisolone, respectively. Hydrocortisone and prednisolone possess both glucocorticoid and mineralocorticoid activity, but clinically the glucocorticoid activity produces the predominant desired effect of reducing inflammatory states.

Glucocorticoids are used in replacement therapy for adrenocortical insufficiency. They are also used to treat severe allergic reactions, anaphylactic reactions not responsive to other therapies, collagen disorders such as systemic lupus erythematosus (SLE), dermatologic conditions, hematologic disorders, neoplastic disease (adjunct treatment), ophthalmic disorders, respiratory disorders, rheumatic disorders, and septic shock (Box 48-1). Glucocorticosteroid use to reduce inflammation following head trauma has been questioned and may be associated with negative outcomes (Roberts et al., 2004).

Glucocorticoids have the following pharmacologic actions:

Antiinflammatory Action Glucocorticoids, especially cortisol in larger than normal dosages, can stabilize lysosomal membranes and prevent the release of proteolytic en-

---

BOX 48-1 SEPTIC SHOCK

Septic shock usually results from a gram-negative bacteremia that leads to circulatory insufficiency. The inadequate tissue perfusion generally results in hypotension, oliguria, tachycardia, elevated temperature, and tachypnea.

MECHANISM

Septic shock may be caused by bacterial substances that interact with body cell membranes and systems, especially coagulation and the complement system, resulting in injury to cells and alterations in blood flow in the body.

TREATMENT

Treatment may consist of volume replacement, antibiotics, surgery (if the client has an abscessed or necrotic bowel or organs/tissues), vasoconstricting agents (dopamine, norepinephrine, or levarterenol), diuretics, and glucocorticoids (steroids). Use of steroids is somewhat controversial, but low dose corticosteroids may offer benefit with their use if used early in the treatment of shock (Annane et al., 2004). Drotrecogin alfa (Xigris), a human recombinant form of activated protein C, may also be used but is not helpful in children and may be associated with increased risk for intracranial hemorrhage (U.S. Food and Drug Administration, 2005).

STEROID BENEFICIAL EFFECTS

Beneficial effects of steroids in septic shock may be secondary to adrenal insufficiency induced by stress, or the actions of corticosteroids, or both. Actions of cortisol and the corticosteroids include protecting cellular membranes from injury, decreasing platelet aggregation, reducing extracellular release of leukocyte enzymes, and preventing the formation of vasoactive substances in the body.

---

zymes during inflammation. They can also potentiate vasoconstrictor effects.

Maintenance of Normal Blood Pressure Glucocorticoids potentiate the vasoconstrictor action of norepinephrine. When glucocorticoids are absent, the vasoconstricting action of the catecholamines is diminished, and blood pressure falls.

Carbohydrate and Protein Metabolism Glucocorticoids help to maintain the blood glucose level and the glycogen content of liver and muscle. They facilitate protein breakdown in muscle and extrahepatic tissues that leads to increased plasma levels of amino acids. Glucocorticoids increase the trapping of amino acids by the liver and stimulate amino acid deamination. They also increase the activity of enzymes important to gluconeogenesis and inhibit glycolytic enzymes; this can produce hyperglycemia and glycosuria. They are diabetogenic; their effects can aggravate diabetes, bring on latent diabetes, and cause insulin resistance. The inhibition of protein synthesis can delay wound healing and cause muscle wasting and osteoporosis. These effects may inhibit growth in young persons.

Fat Metabolism Glucocorticoids promote mobilization of fatty acids from adipose tissue, increasing their concentration in the plasma and their use for energy. Despite this effect, clients taking glucocorticoids may accumulate fat stores (rounded face, buffalo hump). The effect of glucocorticoids on fat metabolism is complex and poorly understood.

Thymolytic, Lympholytic, and Eosinopenic Actions Glucocorticoids can cause atrophy of the thymus and decrease the number of lymphocytes, plasma cells, and eosinophils in the blood. By blocking the production and release of cytokines, corticosteroids interfere with the integrated role of T and B lymphocytes, macrophages, and monocytes in the immune response and thus ultimately interfere with immune and allergic responses. This response, along with their antiinflammatory action, makes them useful immunosuppressants for delaying rejection in clients with organ or tissue transplants, and useful antiallergenics for treating acute allergic reactions such as urticaria, bronchial asthma, and anaphylactic shock. For infections in which inflammation and/or inflammatory mediators are a major source of pathology (e.g., septic shock, some cases of meningitis, some types of interstitial pneumonia), the antiinflammatory effects of glucocorticoids can be helpful (see Box 48-1). However, steroids can also be a source of danger in many other types of infections by limiting useful protective inflammation. This is particularly true for tuberculosis (TB), in which corticosteroid therapy can result in reactivation of otherwise stable TB. These hormones also inhibit the activity of the lymphatic system, causing lymphocytopenia and reducing the size of enlarged lymph nodes.

Stress Effects During stressful situations (e.g., injury, major surgery), corticosteroids are suddenly released or are necessary to help maintain homeostasis (Figure 48-1). This sudden release is believed to be a protective mechanism. Hypotension and shock may occur without steroid administration. During stress, epinephrine and norepinephrine are released from the adrenal medulla, and these catecholamines have a synergistic action with the corticosteroids.

Central Nervous System Corticosteroids affect mood and behavior and possibly cause neuronal or brain excitability. Some persons report euphoria, insomnia, anxiety, depression, or increased motor activity, or they may become psychotic.

★ ◼◻ prednisone [**pred** ni sone]

(Deltasone, Prednisone Intensol, Apo-Prednisone✦, Winpred✦)
Prednisone is considered the prototype corticosteroid with primarily glucocorticoid effect, but also possessing some mineralocorticoid activity.

Indications
Prednisone is indicated for a number of conditions, including adrenocortical insufficiency states, inflammatory disorders, and organ transplant. Prednisone is used to treat a great number of respiratory, gastrointestinal (GI), rheumatologic, dermatologic, ocular, and neoplastic conditions in which moderate to severe inflammation is a component.

Pharmacokinetics/Dosing
Prednisone, like many other glucocorticoids, is well absorbed orally. Rectally, approximately 20% of the drug is absorbed normally; if the

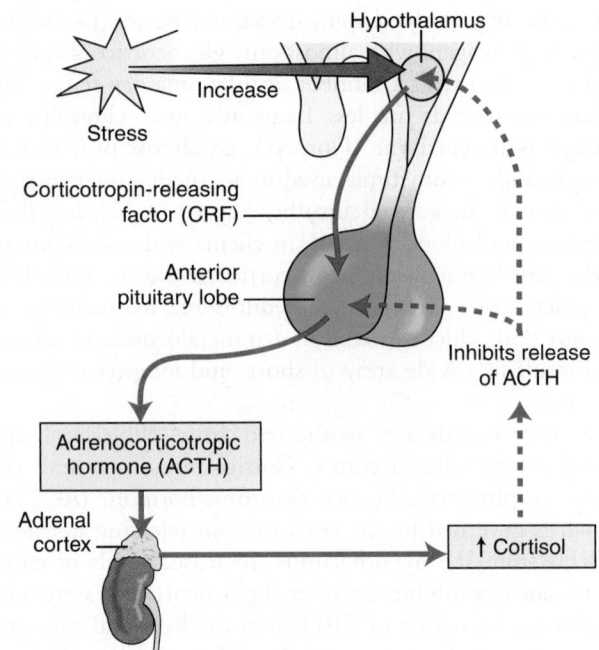

Figure 48-1 Glucocorticoid secretion.

rectum is inflamed, absorption may increase up to 50%. Prednisone is metabolized in the liver to the active prednisolone and excreted by the kidneys. See Table 48-1 for the onset of action, peak effect, and duration of action for the prednisone and other glucocorticoids. See Table 48-2 for the relative potency of prednisone and the major short-acting, intermediate-acting, and long-acting adrenocorticoids. Abrupt withdrawal with chronic dosing must be avoided because of hypothalamic-pituitary axis (HPA) suppression of endogenous cortisol release.

Adverse Effects
The corticosteroids share a number of significant adverse effects, including insomnia, nervousness, increased appetite, and GI upset. These drugs can cause dizziness, glucose intolerance, joint discomfort, seizures, mood changes, hallucinations, edema, hypertension, nose bleed, and the potential to aggravate cataracts and glaucoma. Osteoporosis is a common finding with chronic corticosteroid use. Other adverse effects (more commonly associated with chronic use) include fat redistribution, pancreatitis, pituitary axis suppression, hepatitis, growth suppression and muscle wasting. Long-term use of higher dose corticosteroids (most often used in treatment of cancers and organ transplant) is noted in some clients with genetic markers (see the Special Considerations for Pharmacogenetics box on p. 854).

Drug Interactions
Prednisone metabolism can be accelerated with concurrent barbiturate, phenytoin, or rifampin therapy. The addition of such drugs to clients stabilized on chronic prednisone therapy could induce addisonian crisis.

✷ **P.G. is instructed to take his prednisone in the morning.**

✷ **What is the natural pattern of secretion of glucocorticoids?**
Two rhythms appear to influence glucocorticoid function: circadian (daily) rhythm and ultradian rhythm.

TABLE 48-1 PHARMACOKINETICS OF CORTICOSTEROIDS

Drug (route)	Onset of Action	Peak Effect	Duration of Action
betamethasone			
• PO	—	1-2 hr	3.25 days
• IM, IV	Rapid	—	—
acetate/sodium phosphate			
• IM	1-3 hr	—	7 days
corticotropin repository			
• IM	—	—	12-24 hr
cortisone acetate (PO)			
• PO	Rapid	2 hr	30-36 hr
• IM	Slower	20-48 hr	—
dexamethasone			
• PO	—	1-2 hr	66 hr
• IM	—	8 hr	6 days
• IV	Rapid	—	—
hydrocortisone			
• PO	—	1 hr	30-36 hr
• IM	—	4-8 hr	—
• Rectal enema (retention)	3-5 days	—	—
• Rectal foam	5-7 days	—	—
cypionate			
• PO	Slow	1-2 hr	—
• IM	Rapid	1 hr	Varies
methylprednisolone			
• PO	—	1-2 hr	30-36 hr
• IM	6-48 hr	4-8 days	1-4 wk
• Intraarticular, intralesion, soft tissue	Very slow	7 days	1-5 wk
sodium succinate			
• IV, IM	Rapid	—	—
prednisolone			
• PO	—	1-2 hr	30-36 hr
acetate/sodium phosphate			
• IM	—	—	Up to 4 wk
• Intrabuccal, intrasynovial, intraarticular, soft tissue	—	—	3-28 days
sodium phosphate			
• IV, IM	Rapid	1 hr	—
prednisone			
• PO	—	1-2 hr	30-36 hr
triamcinolone			
• PO	—	1-2 hr	52 hr
• IM	1-2 days	—	1-6 wk

Data from *USP DI: Drug information for the health care professional* (25th ed.). (2005). Greenwood Valley, CO: MICROMEDEX Thomson Healthcare.

Drug names in **bold** indicate active drugs.

—, Not available; *PO*, orally; *IA*, intraarticularly; *IB*, intrabursal; *IL*, intralesion; *IM*, intramuscularly; *IS*, intrasynovial; *ST*, in soft tissue.

TABLE 48-2 RELATIVE POTENCY AND HALF-LIFE OF CORTICOSTEROIDS

Adrenocorticoids	Equivalent Glucocorticoid Dose (mg)*	Relative Glucocorticoid Potency†	Relative Mineralocorticoid Potency‡	Half-life (hr) Serum	Half-life (hr) Tissue
SHORT-ACTING					
cortisone	25	0.8	2	0.5	8-12
hydrocortisone	20	1	2	1.5-2	8-12
INTERMEDIATE-ACTING					
methylprednisolone	4	5	0§	>3.5	18-36
prednisolone	5	4	1	2.1-3.5	18-36
prednisone	5	4	1	3.4-3.8	18-36
triamcinolone	4	5	0§	2 to >5	18-36
LONG-ACTING					
betamethasone	0.6	20-30	0§	3-5	36-54
dexamethasone	0.5-0.75	20-30	0§	3-4.5	36-54

*Approximate dosages, applies to oral and IV only.
†Refers to antiinflammatory, immunosuppressant, and metabolic-type effects.
‡Potassium excretion, sodium and water retention.
§Some hypokalemia and/or sodium and water retention may occur, depending on dose and individual response.

Special Considerations for Pharmacogenetics | CORTICOSTEROIDS

PHARMACODYNAMICS

Gene expression in inflammatory states is affected by glucocorticoid administration and may explain variation in client responses to corticosteroids (Benson, 2005). Approximately 30% of clients with inflammatory bowel disease respond to corticosteroids (Ho, Lees, & Satsangi, 2004). The ability of prednisone and other corticosteroids to penetrate cell membranes and therefore be active in Crohn's disease is related to genetic markers for the drug membrane pump p-glycoprotein (Dilger, Schwab, & Fromm, 2004).

PHARMACOKINETICS

The potential for enzyme-inducing agents such as phenytoin, phenobarbital or carbamazepine to increase metabolism of corticosteroids and reduce corticosteroid levels has been well established. The genetic variation in these enzyme systems, however, likely contributes significantly to the variation in the clinical importance of this interaction in different individuals (Anderson, 2004).

ADVERSE EFFECTS

A genetic link between corticosteroid use and glaucoma risk has been identified (Challa, 2004), although it is not clear whether this would be useful clinically in identifying individuals at higher risk for glaucoma with glucocorticoid use. The risk for osteonecrosis, a rare bone complication related to prolonged use of high dose corticosteroids (Koo et al, 2002), may be predictable based on genetics (Relling et al, 2004; Asano et al, 2003).

Circadian rhythm is a pattern based on a 24-hour cycle with the repetition of certain physiologic phenomena; it is controlled by the dark/light and sleep/wakefulness cycles. Sleeping in the dark at night normally increases plasma cortisol levels in the early morning hours. These levels reach a peak after awakening and then slowly fall to very low levels in the evening and during the early phase of sleep. Corticosteroid therapy may have more pronounced effects when given at midnight than when given at noon, but in general corticosteroid therapy is administered in the morning to mimic natural circadian rhythm of cortisol.

Ultradian rhythms are periodic or intermittent functions more frequently than once every 24 hours. In human beings, four to eight adrenal glucocorticoid bursts occur every 24 hours, which may follow bursts in the release of CRH and ACTH. These bursts are clustered close together and are very pronounced during the circadian rise in plasma glucocorticoid levels in the early morning hours. At other times these bursts are so widely spaced that adrenal secretion is zero. Consequently, the adrenal cortex secretes glucocorticoids only approximately 25% of the time in unstressed individuals.

✱ **P.G. notes an improved sense of well-being and states he feels hungry more often while on prednisone.**

✱ **What adverse effects are common among these agents?**

The adverse effects of the glucocorticoids include euphoria, increased appetite, insomnia, restlessness, anxiety, gas, hyperpigmentation, hypertension, headache, hirsutism, lowered resistance to infections, visual disturbances (cataracts), increased urination or thirst, and decreased growth in children. Anorexia may occur with triamcinolone. Redness, swelling, rash, pain, tingling, or numbness may occur at the injection site. Chronic use may result in abdominal pain, acne, GI bleeding, and peptic ulcers, round face (Cushing's syndrome), hypertension, edema, weight gain, muscle cramps, weakness, irregular heart rate, nausea, vomiting, bone pain, increased bruising, and wounds that are difficult to heal.

✱ **How are corticosteroids dosed?**

Most corticosteroids have a relatively long duration of action and can be dosed once daily (usually in the morning). When a shorter acting agent (e.g., cortisone or hydrocortisone) is used as replacement therapy, the drug should be scheduled according to the normal endogenous secretion of corticosteroid in the body; give two thirds of the dose in the morning and one third in the evening.

An alternate-day schedule may be used with chronic corticosteroid therapy to reduce the potential of suppressing the hypothalamic-pituitary-adrenal (HPA) axis and producing adverse effects. A short- or intermediate-acting corticosteroid is used to stabilize the client's condition. The dosage on one day is tapered and the dosage on the alternate day is increased; this continues until the client is taking approximately two to three times the daily dose every other day. A gradual dosage reduction is recommended when discontinuing these drugs. Table 48-3 provides additional information on corticosteroid drug dosing.

✱ **What are the nursing implications in using glucocorticoids for P.G.?**

Assessment Before P.G. begins systemic corticosteroid therapy with prednisone, assess him for preexisting conditions that would contraindicate the drug or would warrant caution in its use. Glucocorticoids are contraindicated for clients with the following conditions (or the risk-benefit ratio is carefully considered): systemic infections (acquired immunodeficiency syndrome [AIDS], human immunodeficiency virus [HIV], chickenpox, measles, fungal infection, *Strongyloides*, tuberculosis) or ocular herpes, because these infections may be exacerbated. Clients with diabetes mellitus may experience an exacerbation of their condition. Symptoms of the progression or reactivation of active or latent esophagitis, gastritis, or peptic ulcer may be masked, and clients may bleed or perforate without warning. Monitor carefully those clients for whom edema may be hazardous (e.g., those with cardiac disease, heart failure, hyper-

TABLE 48-3 CORTICOSTEROID PREPARATIONS AND DOSING*

| Drug | Usual Dosage | |
	Adult	Child
dexamethasone (Decadron and others)	PO: 0.5-10 mg daily	Adrenocortical insufficiency: 0.03-0.3 mg/kg/day in 3 divided doses
hydrocortisone (Cortef and others) enema (Cortenema)	PO/IM: 15-20 mg, up to 240 mg daily Rectal: 100 mg retention enema nightly for 3 weeks	Oral: 0.56 mg/kg/day IM: 0.56-4 mg/kg/day Not established
methylprednisolone (Medrol)	PO: 4-48 mg daily	Adrenocortical insufficiency: 0.5-1.7 mg/kg/day in 3 divided doses
prednisolone (Delta-Cortef and others)	PO: 5-60 mg daily (maximum 250 mg daily)	Adrenocortical insufficiency: 0.14-2 mg/kg/day in 3 divided doses
prednisone (Deltasone and others)	PO: 5-60 mg daily	Dosage varies; refer to current drug references
triamcinolone (Aristocort, Kenacort, Kenalog)	PO: 4-40 mg daily	Adrenocortical insufficiency: 1.17 mg/kg/day

From *USP DI: Drug information for the health care professional* (25th ed.). (2005). Greenwood Valley, CO: MICROMEDEX Thomson Healthcare.
*Dexamethasone, methylprednisolone, prednisolone, and triamcinolone are also available in short-acting and long-acting preparations; refer to a current drug reference for dosing information.

tension, or renal function impairment). Note that a myasthenic crisis may be induced if these drugs are administered to clients with myasthenia gravis. Clients with acute psychosis may have the condition aggravated.

Use glucocorticoids with caution in pregnant women, because adrenal insufficiency in both mother and child is possible at delivery. Fetal abnormalities can also occur. If the drug is administered maternally to help prevent neonatal respiratory distress syndrome, there is an increased risk of maternal infection (tuberculosis, herpes type II), uterine bleeding, placental insufficiency, and premature membrane rupture. Older adults are more likely to develop hypertension during glucocorticoid therapy, and postmenopausal women are more likely to develop osteoporosis.

If P.G. were receiving the corticosteroid as an intraarticular injection, the joint should not be infected, bleeding, fractured, or have had recent surgery, because the condition will be aggravated and/or healing will be inhibited. Juxtaarticular nonarthritic osteoporosis may be worsened.

Rectal administration of the drug is avoided in instances of bowel obstruction, recent GI surgery, or infection, because healing will be delayed.

Review P.G.'s current medication regimen for significant drug interactions, such as those that may occur when corticosteroids are given concurrently with the following:

- Aminoglutethimide (Cytadren) suppresses adrenal function; therefore do not administer corticotropin concurrently. Although glucocorticoid supplements are often prescribed when aminoglutethimide is given, be aware that aminoglutethimide can increase the metabolism of dexamethasone and reduce its half-life significantly. Hydrocortisone is recommended, because its metabolism does not appear to be affected by aminoglutethimide.
- Amphotericin B parenteral (Fungizone) may result in severe hypokalemia. If given concurrently, monitor serum potassium levels closely. It may also decrease the adrenal gland response to corticotropin.
- Antacids may decrease absorption of prednisone or dexamethasone and a decrease in steroid absorption may result. Monitor closely, because steroid dosage adjustments may be necessary.
- Antidiabetic drugs (oral) or insulin may require a dosage adjustment of one or both drugs. Glucocorticoids may elevate serum glucose levels (both during therapy and after, if the glucocorticoid is stopped).
- Cyclosporine administered concurrently with high doses of methylprednisolone has resulted in seizures.
- Digoxin administration may result in an increased potential for toxicity (dysrhythmias) associated with hypokalemia.
- Diuretics may have their effectiveness reduced because of the sodium and fluid-retaining effects of the adrenocorticoids. Monitor closely for edema and fluid retention. Potassium-depleting diuretics given with adrenocorticoids may result in severe hypokalemia. Monitor potassium serum levels.

- Hepatic enzyme-inducing agents, such as barbiturates, carbamazepine, phenytoin, and others, may decrease the adrenocorticoid effect because of increased metabolism. Dosage adjustments may be necessary. Monitor serum cortisol levels closely.
- Mitotane (Lysodren) will decrease the response of the adrenal gland to corticotropin. Adrenocorticoids are usually necessary during mitotane administration and higher than normal dosages of glucocorticoids are usually needed.
- Potassium supplements reduce the effect of the supplements and/or the corticosteroids on serum potassium levels. Monitor serum levels if given concurrently.
- Ritodrine (Yutopar) is given to inhibit premature labor in the pregnant woman and the long-acting glucocorticoids are given to enhance fetal lung maturity, the result may be pulmonary edema in the mother. Monitor pregnant women closely for the first signs of pulmonary edema (shallow, rapid, difficult breathing; anxiety; restlessness; increased heart rate and blood pressure; enlarged peripheral and neck veins; edema of the extremities; lung rales; and diaphoresis); early detection and treatment are necessary to prevent a potentially serious adverse effect or fatality.
- Sodium-containing foods or medications may result in edema and hypertension. Monitor weight, intake and output, and blood pressure closely.
- Somatrem or somatropin effect on growth rate may be inhibited with concurrent chronic therapy with corticotropin or with daily doses of glucocorticoids above certain levels, such as daily doses of prednisone or prednisolone above 2.5 to 3.75 mg/m^2 of body surface. Refer to Chapter 46 for the dosages of other glucocorticoids.
- Vaccines, live virus, and other immunizations are not recommended for clients who are receiving pharmacologic or immunosuppressant doses of glucocorticosteroids. Because corticosteroids inhibit the antibody response, the immunization effect will be reduced or ineffective and the client may develop neurologic complications. Avoid concurrent use or a potentially serious drug interaction may occur. If live virus vaccines are given to individuals receiving immunosuppressant glucocorticoid therapy, the client may develop the viral disease or at least have a reduced response to the vaccine. Avoid concurrent use or a potentially serious drug interaction may occur.

Because a variety of adverse effects can occur with corticosteroid administration, a comprehensive baseline assessment is essential. Because there is a risk for fluid volume excess related to sodium and fluid retention, obtain P.G.'s weight before initiating therapy. Obtain baseline data for hematologic values, serum electrolytes, and blood glucose. Check the stool for occult blood. If therapy is anticipated to last more than 6 weeks, P.G. should obtain a baseline ophthalmologic examination for the presence of cataracts, glaucoma, and ocular infections. These determinations are monitored during therapy. Obtain a baseline assessment of P.G.'s asthma, for which the glucocorticoid is being prescribed. See respiratory assessment in Chapter 37. Because P.G. is 13 and still growing, assess height before and periodically during therapy, because there is a risk for altered growth and development with glucocorticoid therapy.

Nursing Diagnosis While P.G. is undergoing what is hoped to be short-term therapy with glucocorticoids, long-term therapy (which is a common occurrence with adolescents with asthma) will put him at risk for the following nursing diagnoses/collaborative problems: disturbed sleep pattern because of drug-induced insomnia; disturbed body image related to physical changes with long-term therapy (moon face, central obesity, striae, acne, hirsutism); activity intolerance related to muscle wasting; sexual dysfunction related to physiologic limitations secondary to abnormal hormone levels; risk for infection related to immunosuppression; risk for trauma related to osteoporosis; disturbed thought processes related to the central nervous system (CNS) effects (euphoria, psychotic behavior, restlessness); imbalanced nutrition: more than body requirements related to increased appetite; excess fluid volume related to sodium and water retention; and the potential complications of cataracts, mental depression, anaphylaxis, heart failure and hypertension related to cardiovascular effects, peptic ulcer related to GI effects, and hypokalemia, hyperglycemia, and hyperlipidemia related to metabolic effects.

Planning While P.G. is on corticosteroid therapy, he will:
- Experience a remission of his asthmatic symptoms with minimal complications of his drug therapy.
- Remain free of infection, body image disturbances, fluid retention, and changes in sensorium.
- Effectively manage his therapeutic regimen by maintaining compliance with his medications, employing supportive measures to minimize adverse effects, and reporting adverse symptoms appropriately to his prescriber.
- Collaborate with his health care providers by maintaining scheduled appointments for monitoring and treatment.

Implementation

Monitoring Instruct P.G. to weigh himself daily and report to the prescriber any sudden weight increase that may indicate fluid retention. Monitor intake and output ratios daily. Correlate these findings with physical findings of edema. Assess for the following when long-term or excessive doses are given: CNS symptoms (anxiety, depression/stimulation), elevated blood pressure, hematologic values, serum electrolytes, changes in growth pattern and Cushing's syndrome (Box 48-2). If therapy is more than 6 weeks, P.G. should obtain an ophthalmologic examination at periodic intervals. Check the stool for occult blood.

Closely monitor P.G.'s blood glucose level, because these drugs can cause hyperglycemia. Clients with diabetes may need changes in diet or insulin dosage to maintain blood glucose control.

Remember that not only the total daily dose but also frequent individual doses during the day must be adjusted to

---

BOX 48-2 BODY IMAGE ALTERATIONS WITH GLUCOCORTICOID THERAPY

Alterations in body image may be a major concern in clients receiving glucocorticoid therapy. Among the body changes that may occur are the following:

- Abdominal distention
- Acneiform eruptions
- Fat deposits on upper back ("buffalo hump")
- Fluid retention
- Hirsutism
- Hyperpigmentation
- Loss of muscle mass
- Lupus erythematosus–like lesions
- Petechiae and ecchymosis
- Purpura
- Round face ("moon face")
- Striae
- Thin fragile skin
- Thinning of extremities, thickening of torso
- Weight gain

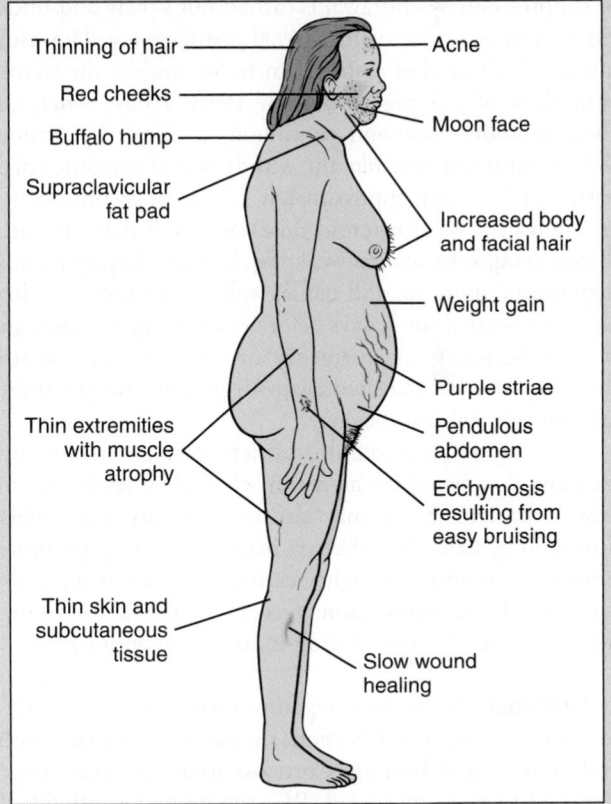

From Lewis, S.L., Heitkemper, M.M., & Dirksen, S.R. (2004). *Medical-surgical nursing: Assessment and management of clinical problems* (6th ed.). St. Louis: Mosby.

---

meet the client's needs. Notify the prescriber of P.G.'s varying responses to the drugs.

Intervention Give glucocorticoids as a single daily dose in the morning (before 9 AM if possible) and with food or milk. Glucocorticoids suppress adrenal activity the least when it is at its peak, which is early morning. Note that an alternate-day dosing regimen may be valuable when considering the long-term use of glucocorticoids in less severe disease processes, especially when an intermediate range–acting agent (methylprednisolone, prednisolone, prednisone) is used, because it diminishes suppression of the HPA axis. The alternate-day dose given every other morning before 9 AM is at least twice the daily dose equivalent. This therapy requires that a client's pituitary axis be responsive and stabilized initially on the alternate-day schedule.

Administer IM injections of suspensions deep in the gluteal muscle to avert local tissue atrophy at the injection sites. Note that injections into the deltoid muscle can cause atrophy.

Clients taking cortisone who require surgery should receive a preoperative dose of a rapid-acting corticosteroid. The drug is continued postoperatively in decreasing doses for several days. Clients with atrophy of the adrenal gland may be unable to cope with the stress of surgery if cortisone treatment is interrupted.

Be prepared to perform an HPA axis suppression test after high dosages or long-term therapy to determine the level of suppression. Withdrawal is carried out slowly and under close supervision to avoid adrenal insufficiency. The usual rate of withdrawal of systemic corticosteroids is the steroid equivalent of 2.5 mg prednisone every 4 days when the client is under close and continuous medical supervision. When this is not possible, the withdrawal of systemic corticosteroids is slower, approximately 2.5 mg of prednisone (or an equivalent corticosteroid dose) every 10 days. If withdrawal symptoms such as weakness, lethargy, hypoglycemia, depression, anorexia, and nausea appear, the previous dose may be resumed for 7 days before continuing the decrease. If a medical-surgical emergency or stressful event occurs, the drug may be increased again to prevent the possibility of acute adrenal insufficiency.

P.G. may require sodium restriction or potassium supplementation based on his serum electrolyte levels. An increased protein intake may also be necessary, particularly during long-term drug therapy because the drug promotes protein catabolism. Weight-bearing exercises (e.g., walking), and the administration of calcium and vitamin D may help to reduce the risk of drug-induced osteoporosis.

Education With systemic administration, instruct P.G. to report any signs of infection, such as a sore throat, fever, and poor wound healing. Corticosteroids can mask infection and increase its spread. P.G. should avoid individuals with known contagious illnesses. Also advise him and his parents that glucocorticoids impair the antibody response and that the response to immunizations may be reduced.

Instruct P.G. to report any visual disturbances. Long-term glucocorticoid therapy can cause cataracts, glaucoma, or optic nerve damage.

Because these drugs can cause gastric distress, instruct P.G. to report any persistent GI symptoms. Instruct him to take the drug with meals or milk in the morning.

Warn P.G. and his family self-concept disturbances may occur as the result of changes in appearance (see Box 48-2). Assist him in dealing with the changes that occur, and reassure them that these changes will disappear when the drug is stopped.

Most clients receiving glucocorticoids, including P.G. should follow a high-potassium, low-sodium diet to counter the potassium-depleting and sodium-retaining effects of the drug. To minimize peptic ulceration, he is to limit his intake of alcohol, caffeine, aspirin, and other gastric irritants. Caution him to report any symptoms of abdominal pain, infection, bone pain, tiredness, bruising, or tarry stools. Because altered thought processes may occur, have P.G. report changes in mental status (euphoria, mood swings, depression) or insomnia to the prescriber.

Inform female clients that they may experience menstrual irregularities while taking glucocorticoids. Additionally, inform them that cortisone, dexamethasone, hydrocortisone, methylprednisolone, and prednisolone are unsafe to take during pregnancy because of their effects on the fetus. (See the Pregnancy Safety box below.)

Have P.G. carry a card describing his medical condition and drug therapy. Remember that any client who has received a significant amount of cortisone or related glucocorticoid is likely to experience some atrophy of the adrenal cortex. It is not known how much hormone produces atrophy and how long the atrophy persists, but acute adrenal insufficiency may result from too-rapid withdrawal of therapy. Instruct P.G. to report withdrawal symptoms, including weakness, lethargy, malaise, restlessness, hypoglycemia, psychologic despondency, anorexia, and nausea.

Instruct the client not to overuse the injected joint after intraarticular injection. Weight-bearing joints should be rested 24 to 48 hours after injection.

Evaluation The expected outcome of corticosteroid therapy is that P.G. will experience an improvement in the signs and symptoms of the asthma for which the glucocorticoid was administered without experiencing any adverse effects of the drug. He eats adequate foods and maintain his

PREGNANCY SAFETY — DRUGS AFFECTING THE ADRENAL CORTEX	
Category	**Drug**
C	betamethasone, corticotropin, dexamethasone, fludrocortisone, hydrocortisone, methylprednisolone, prednisolone, prednisone, triamcinolone
D	aminoglutethimide, cortisone

Data from *Mosby's drug consult* (15th ed.). (2005). St. Louis, Mosby.

weight, does not experience a weight gain of greater than 2 pounds/week or experience edema. He remains free of infection, body image disturbances, and changes in sensorium. P.G., and his parents report weight gain greater than 2 pounds week, shortness of breath, edema, signs and symptoms of infection, or lightheadedness to the prescriber. He experiences minimal problems as he weans off corticosteroid drugs. P.G.'s parents maintain scheduled appointments for the monitoring and treatment of his asthma.

What are the important actions of mineralocorticoids?

Mineralocorticoids such as aldosterone are secreted by the adrenal cortex to increase the rate of sodium reabsorption by the kidneys, thereby increasing blood levels of sodium. This results in increased water reabsorption by the kidneys and increased blood volume. Mineralocorticoids also increase the excretion of potassium and hydrogen ions into the urine, thereby decreasing blood levels of potassium and hydrogen ions. In adrenal cortex insufficiency, it is necessary to replace a glucocorticoid and, in some individuals, a mineralocorticoid such as fludrocortisone.

fludrocortisone [floo droe **kor** tih sone]
(Florinef)
Fludrocortisone has potent mineralocorticoid activity with minimal glucocorticoid effects. It acts primarily on the renal distal tubule to reabsorb sodium and enhance the excretion of potassium and hydrogen.

Indications
Fludrocortisone is used to treat Addison disease (chronic primary adrenocortical insufficiency) and congenital adrenogenital syndrome. It has also been used to treat symptomatic orthostatic hypotension.

Pharmacokinetics/Dosing
Fludrocortisone has good oral absorption, a half-life of approximately 3.5 hours in the plasma, and a biologic half-life of activity in the body of 18 to 36 hours. The duration of action is 24 to 48 hours. It is metabolized in the liver and kidneys and excreted by the kidneys. The oral dosage for adults and adolescents is 0.1 mg daily. The usual dosage for children is 50 to 100 mcg daily.

Adverse Effects
The adverse effects of fludrocortisone include severe or persistent headaches; hypertension; dizziness; edema of the lower extremities; joint pain; hypokalemia; increased weakness; tingling or numbness in legs that may progress to the arms, trunk, and face; heart failure; and anaphylaxis. Such adverse effects should be reported immediately to the prescriber.

Drug Interactions
Concurrent use of P450 enzyme inducers (rifampin, phenobarbital, phenytoin, and carbamazepine) may result in increased metabolism and reduced efficacy of fludrocortisone.

Nursing Management
Assessment
Determine that the client does not have hypertension, heart failure, cardiac disease, or renal function impairment (except when the drug is used to treat type IV renal tubular acidosis). Mineralocorticoid therapy is administered with caution in the presence of these conditions.

Review the client's current medication regimen for the risk of significant drug interactions, such as those that may occur when fludrocortisone is given concurrently with digoxin because hypokalemic effect of fludrocortisone may potentiate the risk for cardiac dysrhythmias or digoxin toxicity. Monitor closely with electrocardiogram (ECG) and pulse readings. With concurrent use of hepatic enzyme inducers,

the effectiveness of fludrocortisone may be decreased and a dosage requirement may be required. The concurrent use of potassium-depleting diuretics or hypokalemic-inducing medications may produce severe hypokalemia. Monitor serum potassium levels and cardiac function closely. Potassium supplementation may be necessary. In type IV renal tubular acidosis, the concurrent use of sodium-containing foods or medications with fludrocortisone may result in hypertension, hypernatremia, and edema. To avoid hypernatremia, monitor sodium intake closely and advise clients on the safe consumption of foods and medications. Instruct clients to read the labels on foods and medications regarding sodium content.

Because clients receiving mineralocorticoid therapy are at risk for fluid volume excess related to sodium and fluid retention, establish the client's baseline serum electrolytes, weight, and blood pressure.

In addition obtain baseline information of symptoms of Addison's disease for which mineralocorticoid therapy is administered: weakness; fatigue; anorexia; weight loss; nausea and vomiting; diarrhea; abdominal, joint and abdominal pain; and, plasma cortisol and plasma ACTH levels.

Nursing Diagnosis
Clients receiving fludrocortisone are at risk for the following nursing diagnoses/collaborative problems: impaired comfort (headache, dizziness); excess fluid volume (peripheral edema); and the potential complications of anaphylaxis, altered cardiac output related to heart failure, and hypokalemic syndrome (weakness, anorexia, nausea, dysrhythmia, muscle cramps).

Planning
The client on mineralocorticoid therapy will:
- Experience a remission of his addisonian symptoms with minimal complications of drug therapy.
- Effectively manage the therapeutic regimen by maintaining compliance with his medications, employing supportive measures to minimize adverse effects, and reporting adverse symptoms appropriately to his prescriber.
- Collaborate with his health care providers by maintaining scheduled appointments for monitoring and treatment.

Implementation
Monitoring
Weigh daily, and report weight increases of 1 kg in 24 hours to the prescriber. Monitor intake and output ratios. Periodically assess the client's blood pressure, and check for evidence of edema. If hypertension develops, adjust the salt intake and consult with the prescriber to modify the dosage of the steroid.

Periodic serum electrolyte determinations are recommended. Because there is a potential for hypokalemia, be aware that the excessive loss of potassium can cause dysrhythmias and sudden weakness, palpitations, paresthesia, or nausea.
Intervention
Provide the client with a diet that is low in sodium and high in potassium and protein. The use of a potassium supplement may be necessary.
Education
Advise the client to maintain scheduled visits with the prescriber to check serum electrolyte levels at periodic intervals, especially during prolonged therapy, and to implement dietary salt restrictions. Alert the client to report symptoms of Addison's disease or hypokalemia. Instruct the client to weigh daily and to report a sudden weight gain to the prescriber. Consult with the prescriber for specific weight gain limitations for each client. Advise the client to carry medical identification and to notify health care providers of the medication regimen.

Evaluation
The expected outcome of fludrocortisone therapy is that the client does not show any signs of Addison's disease, fluid volume deficit, other signs and symptoms of mineralocorticoid insufficiency, or any adverse effects of fludrocortisone therapy. The

client remains compliant with the medication regimen, institutes a low-sodium, high-potassium diet and states reportable adverse symptoms prescriber.

Scheduled appointments will be maintained for monitoring and treatment.

✳ What agents inhibit adrenal function?

As discussed above, chronic administration of corticosteroids suppresses the HPA axis and endogenous release of cortisol. Acute withdrawal of chronically administered corticosteroids can lead to acute addisonian crisis (see above and Chapter 45).

Clients with certain adrenal cancers that secrete excessive amounts of cortisol may respond to an agent that inhibits adrenal cortex function like aminoglutethimide (Cytadren).

aminoglutethimide [ah mee noe glue **teh** tha mide] (Cytadren)

Aminoglutethimide is an antiadrenal or adrenal steroid inhibitor that inhibits or suppresses adrenal cortex function. It inhibits the enzyme conversion of cholesterol or pregnenolone (hormone precursor), thereby blocking the synthesis of adrenal steroids. It also may have other suppression effects in the synthesis and metabolism of the steroids. It also inhibits estrogen production from androgens by blocking an enzyme in the peripheral tissues and may also enhance the metabolism of estrone; thus it is investigationally used to treat breast cancer.

Indications

Aminoglutethimide is indicated for the treatment of Cushing's syndrome associated with adrenal carcinoma, ectopic adrenocorticotropic hormone tumors, or adrenal gland hyperplasia.

Pharmacokinetics/Dosing

Aminoglutethimide is absorbed orally and has a half-life of 13 hours, which is reduced to 7 hours after chronic therapy. The time to peak concentration is 1.5 hours, with adrenal function suppression occurring within 3 to 5 days of therapy. Aminoglutethimide is metabolized in the liver and excreted by the kidneys. The adult oral dosage of aminoglutethimide is 250 mg two or three times daily for approximately 14 days; the maintenance dosage is 250 mg every 6 hours (four times daily). A pediatric dosage has not been established.

Adverse Effects

The adverse effects of aminoglutethimide therapy include the CNS effects of ataxia, dizziness, sedation, loss of energy, uncontrolled eye movements, anorexia, nausea, vomiting, a maculopapular rash on the face and/or the palms of the hands and, rarely, fever, chills, sore throat caused by leukopenia or agranulocytosis, jaundice of the eyes and skin, increased bleeding episodes, or unusual bruising (thrombocytopenia). The CNS effects are usually dose related and may decline in with 2 to 6 weeks of continuous therapy; however, the drug may need to be discontinued if these effects are severe.

Drug Interactions

Aminoglutethimide may interfere with the effect of warfarin.

Nursing Management

Assessment

Use antiadrenals cautiously in clients undergoing stresses such as surgery, infection, trauma, and acute illness. Aminoglutethimide is not to be administered to clients with chickenpox and herpes zoster or other infections (or who have had a recent exposure to these conditions), because the disease may become more generalized.

Do not give aminoglutethimide to pregnant women, because it causes increased fetal deaths and teratogenic effects; see the Pregnancy Safety box on p. 858. Older adults may be more sensitive

to the CNS effects of the drug and become lethargic. Ensure that the client is not also taking dexamethasone. Aminoglutethimide increases the metabolism of dexamethasone, thus reducing its effectiveness. If a glucocorticoid is necessary for a client receiving aminoglutethimide, hydrocortisone is usually the drug of choice.

Obtain baseline lying and standing blood pressures, serum electrolyte levels, thyroid function studies, stool determinations for occult blood, and AST concentrations. Document client's symptoms of Cushing's syndrome as baseline for assessing the therapeutic effects of the drug.

Nursing Diagnosis

The client receiving aminoglutethimide is at risk for the following nursing diagnoses/collaborative problems: risk for injury related to the CNS effects of hypotension, drowsiness, dizziness, and clumsiness; imbalanced nutrition related to GI effects as evidenced by anorexia and nausea; disturbed body image related to masculinization and hirsutism in females; impaired comfort (measles-like rash, headache, and muscle pain); and the potential complications of allergic response, hypoglycemia, mental depression, hypothyroidism and goiter, thrombocytopenia, leukopenia, and agranulocytosis.

Planning

The client on aminoglutethimide therapy will:
- Experience a remission of Cushing's syndrome with minimal complications of drug therapy.
- Effectively manage the therapeutic regimen by maintaining compliance with medications, employing supportive measures to minimize adverse effects, and reporting adverse symptoms appropriately to his prescriber.
- Collaborate with health care providers by maintaining scheduled appointments for monitoring and treatment.

Implementation

Monitoring

Monitor thyroid function studies periodically during therapy. Because this drug can cause blood dyscrasias and liver and electrolyte abnormalities, routinely monitor serum electrolytes and hematologic and liver function studies. Monitor blood pressure (BP), because hypotension (weakness, dizziness) is caused by aldosterone suppression. If amino-glutethimide is administered for adrenal disorders, plasma cortisol or 24-hour urinary 17-hydroxycorticosteroid concentrations are monitored to determine if steroid supplementation is required. In prostatic carcinoma, serum acid phosphatase concentrations indicate the client's response to therapy; concentrations should decrease.

Intervention

Clients receiving aminoglutethimide should be under the care of an oncologist or endocrinologist. Consult with the prescriber about lowering the dosage of aminoglu-tethimide if CNS adverse effects occur.

Education

Because the client may experience orthostatic hypotension, advise him or her to change position or to stand slowly to minimize this effect. Advise the client to avoid activities that require alertness until a response to the drug has been determined. Instruct the client to carry a medical identification card and to alert other health care providers that the drug is being taken. The prescriber should be notified if injury, infection, or illness occurs, because a steroid supplement may be needed.

Evaluation

The expected outcome of aminoglutethimide therapy is that the client will experience an improvement in the signs and symptoms of Cushing's syndrome without any adverse effects of the drug. Complete blood count (CBC), electrolytes, and hepatic function studies will be within the normal limits. The client will remain compliant with the medication regimen, change position slowly, and describe adverse symptoms that are reportable to the prescriber. Scheduled appointments will be maintained for monitoring and treatment.

Summary

Corticosteroids affect the adrenal cortex and are divided into the two following groups: glucocorticoids and mineralocorticoids. Glucocorticoids have many pharmacologic actions: antiinflammatory effects; fat, carbohydrate, and protein metabolism; thymolytic, lympholytic, and eosinopenic actions; and stress effects. Mineralocorticoids act on the renal distal tubules to reabsorb sodium and enhance the excretion of potassium and hydrogen.

Because the actions of both of these groups affect all aspects of the body's physiology, it is particularly important to evaluate the client for the therapeutic effects and adverse effects of their administration. Aminoglutethimide, an antiadrenal or adrenal steroid inhibitor, is used for the treatment of Cushing's syndrome and in some instances for the treatment of breast and prostate cancer; however, it is has not been approved by the FDA for oncology therapy.

✳ Critical Thinking Questions

- A 28-year-old man is brought to the emergency department 2 hours after a motorcycle accident. He is conscious on admission, with stable vital signs and with minimal abrasions to the left side of his body. A neurologic examination reveals an absence of light touch and pinprick sensation in both lower extremities, lower-extremity paralysis, and no reflexes below the groin. High-dose IV methylprednisolone is initiated. Why is a corticosteroid used? What is the current evidence regarding efficacy? What observations and interventions by the nurse will be necessary?

- Misunderstandings about steroid use, which have been generated by recent publicity about steroid abuse by athletes, have contributed to a widespread "steroid phobia." Why would that be so? How would you counter this impression in a newly diagnosed client with asthma who has been prescribed corticosteroid inhalers?

Bibliography

Anderson, D.M., Keith, J., & Novak, P.D. (Eds.) (2002). *Mosby's medical, nursing, and allied health dictionary* (6th ed.). St. Louis: Mosby.

Anderson, G. (2004). Pharmacogenetics and enzyme induction/inhibition properties of antiepileptic drugs. *Neurology, 63*(10) Supplement 4, S3-S8.

Annane, D., Bellissant, E., Bollaert, P.E., Briegel, J., Keh, D., & Kupfer, Y. (2004). Corticosteroids for severe sepsis and septic shock: A systematic review and meta-analysis. *British Medical Journal, 329*, 480-484.

Asano, T., Takahashi, K.A., Fujioka, M., Inoue, S., Okamoto, M., & Sugioka, N., et al. (2003). ABCB1 C3435 T and G2677 T/A polymorphism decreased the risk for steroid-induced osteonecrosis of the femoral head after kidney transplantation. *Pharmacogenetics, 13*(11), 675-682.

Benson, M. (2005). Pathophysiological effects of glucocorticoids on nasal polyps: an update. *Current Opinion in Allergy & Clinical Immunology, 5*(1), 31-35.

Bosker, G. (Ed.). (2004). *Primary and acute care medicine: Practice, protocols, pathways,* (2nd ed.). Atlanta: Thomson American Health Consultants.

Challa, P. (2004). Glaucoma Genetics: Advancing New Understandings of Glaucoma Pathogenesis. *International Ophthalmology Clinics, 44*(2), 167-185.

Dilger, K., Schwab, M., & Fromm, M.F. (2004). Identification of Budesonide and Prednisone as Substrates of the Intestinal Drug Efflux Pump P-glycoprotein. *Inflammatory Bowel Diseases, 10*(5), 578-583.

Drug facts and comparisons (58th ed.). (2005). St. Louis: Facts and Comparisons.

Fitzgerald, P.A. (2003). Endocrinology. In L.M. Tierney, Jr., S.J. McPhee & Papadakis, M.A. (Eds.), *Current Medical Diagnosis & Treatment.* New York: Lange Medical Books/McGraw-Hill.

Gong, W.C. (2005). Connective tissue disorders: The clinical use of corticosteroids. In M.A. Koda-Kimble, L.Y. Young, W.A. Kradian, B.J. Guglielmo, B.K. Alldredge, & R.L. Corelli (Eds.), *Applied therapeutics: The clinical use of drugs* (8th ed.). Philadelphia: Lippincott Williams & Wilkins.

Gums, J.G., & Terpening, C.M. (2002). Adrenal gland disorders. In J.T. DiPiro, R.L. Talbert, G.C. Yee, G.R. Matzke, B.G. Wells, & L.M. Posey (Eds.), *Pharmacotherapy: A Pathophysiological Approach* (5th ed.). New York: McGraw-Hill.

e-LEARNING SUPPLEMENTS

Student CD-ROM
- Final Exam questions
- NCLEX® Examination review questions
- Pharmacology animations
- Printable chapter summary

Evolve Website (http://evolve.elsevier.com/mckenry)
- Case study on drugs affecting the adrenal cortex
- Content updates, including information on new drugs
- WebLinks corresponding to this chapter
- Answers to the critical thinking questions in this chapter
- *Elsevier ePharmacology Update* newsletter
- Mosby's Drug Consult Internet Edition
- Supplemental and reference information

Ho, G.T., Lees, C., & Satsangi, J. (2004). Pharmacogenetics and Inflammatory Bowel Disease: Progress and Prospects. *Inflammatory Bowel Diseases, 10*(2),148-158.

Koo, K.H., Kim, R., Kim, Y.S., Ahn, I.O., Cho, S.H., & Song, H.R., et al. (2002). Risk period for developing osteonecrosis of the femoral head in patients on steroid treatment. *Clinical Rheumatology, 21*(4), 299-303.

Lacy, C.F., Armstrong, L.L., Goldman, M.P., & Lance, L.L. (2004). *Lexi-Comp's Drug Information Handbook* (12th ed.). Hudson, Ohio: Lexi-Comp.

Mosby's drug consult (15th ed.).(2005). St. Louis: Mosby.

Relling, M.V., Yang, W., Das, S., Cook, E.H., Rosner, G.L., & Neel, M., et al. (2004). Pharmacogenetic Risk Factors for Osteonecrosis of the Hip Among Children With Leukemia. *Journal of Clinical Oncology, 22*(19), 3930-3936.

Roberts, I., Yates, D., Sandercock, P., Farrell, B., Wasserberg, J., & Lomas, G., et al., and the CRASH trial collaborators. (2004). Effect of intravenous corticosteroids on death within 14 days in 10,008 adults with clinically significant head injury (MRC CRASH trial): Randomised placebo-controlled trial. *Lancet, 364*, 1321-1328.

Schimmer, B.P., & Parker, K.L. (2001). Adrenocorticotropic Hormone: Adrenocortical Steroids and Their Synthetic Analogs; Inhibitors of the Synthesis and Actions of Adrenocortical Hormones. In J.G. Hardman & L.E. (Eds.), *Goodman & Gilman's The pharmacological basis of therapeutics* (10th ed.). New York: McGraw-Hill.

U.S. Food and Drug Administration. (2005). 2005 Safety Alert: Xigris (drotrecogin alfa [activated]). Retrieved July 17, 2005, http://www.fda.gov/medwatch/SAFETY/2005/xigris_dearHCP_4-21-05.htm.

USP DI: Drug information for the health care professional (25th ed.). (2005). Greenwood Village, CO: MICROMEDEX Thomson Healthcare.

49

DRUGS AFFECTING CONDITIONS OF THE PANCREAS

CHAPTER FOCUS

Diabetes mellitus is the most important disease involving the pancreas. It affects over 6% of the U.S. population, half of whom are undiagnosed. The incidence is equal in males and females and increases with age. Clients with diabetes must manage their lives effectively to maintain a balance between lifestyle and treatment. To assist them in this process, nurses need to be knowledgeable about diabetes mellitus and the drugs affecting the disease process.

LEARNING OBJECTIVES

- Describe type 1 and type 2 diabetes mellitus.
- Compare and contrast the different insulin preparations.
- Discuss oral antidiabetic agents and related nursing management of the client's therapeutic regimen.
- List hyperglycemic agents and their mechanisms of action.
- Implement the nursing management for clients receiving agents affecting the pancreas.

▲ KEY TERMS

diabetes mellitus (DM), p. 863
endogenous insulin, p. 864
euglycemia, p. 865
exogenous insulin, p. 864
glucagon, p. 863
gluconeogenesis, p. 884
glycogenesis, p. 863
glycogenolysis, p. 863
insulin, p. 863
type 1 diabetes, p. 864
type 2 diabetes, p. 864

KEY DRUGS

acarbose, p. 880
glucagon, p. 884
glyburide, p. 877
insulin, p. 866
metformin, p. 879
repaglinide, p. 880
rosiglitazone, p. 881

✳ What hormones are secreted by the pancreas?

Insulin and glucagon are the primary hormones released by the pancreas. When serum blood glucose declines, **glucagon,** which is synthesized in the alpha cells of the pancreatic islets, facilitates the catabolism of stored glycogen in the liver. The result is **glycogenolysis,** the conversion of glycogen to glucose; this leads to an increase in blood glucose (Figure 49-1). The release of glucagon stimulates the secretion of insulin, which then inhibits the release of glucagon. This feedback mechanism serves to keep glucose within a desired serum level. Alternately, the conversion of excess glucose to glycogen for storage in skeletal muscle and the liver (**glycogenesis**) occurs when blood glucose increases.

✳ What are the key features of DM?

Diabetes mellitus (DM) is the most important endocrine disease involving the pancreas. It is a disorder of carbohydrate metabolism that involves an insulin deficiency (most

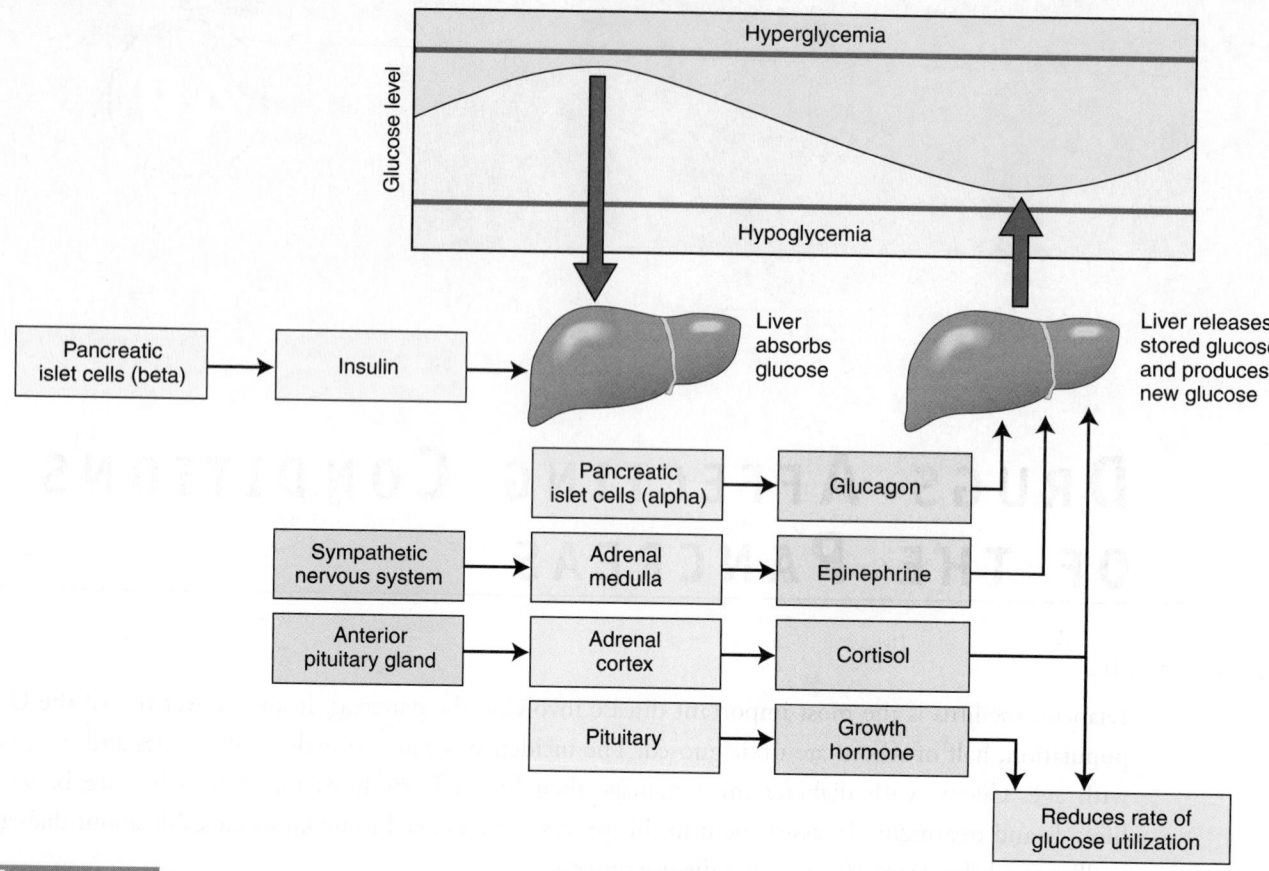

FIGURE 49-1 Physiologic response to changes in blood glucose levels.

typical of type 1), insulin resistance (most typical of type 2), or both. It is briefly reviewed in Chapter 45.

There are 18.2 million people in the United States, or 6.3% of the population, who have diabetes. Although an estimated 13 million have been diagnosed, unfortunately, 5.2 million people (or nearly one third) are unaware that they have the disease (American Diabetes Association, 2004). According to the Centers for Disease Control and Prevention (CDC), the incidence of diabetes has jumped nearly 50% in the past 10 years. In Canada there are an estimated 60,000 new cases of diabetes every year (National Statistics and Opportunities for Improved Surveillance, Prevention, and Control, 1999). Uncontrolled diabetes is a devastating disease that is the leading cause of new cases of blindness, end-stage renal disease, and lower limb amputations. It was also the sixth leading cause of death in the United States in 2002 (National Center for Health Statistics, 2004). Aggressive interventions to treat related risks with DM, including blood pressure (BP) control, lipid management, diet and exercise, can contribute significantly to reduced morbidity and mortality (Gaede et al., 2003). DM affects males and females equally, and the incidence increases with age.

✸ How are type 1 and type 2 DM differentiated?
The two general classifications for DM are type 1 and type 2. Clients with **type 1 diabetes** have very little or usually no **endogenous insulin** capacity, that is their bodies do not pro-

duce insulin. The pathogenesis of type 1 DM is related to an autoimmune attack on pancreatic beta cells and may be responsive to gene therapy in the future (Nakayama et al., 2005; Kent et al., 2005). This type of diabetes usually occurs before age 30 and was previously called insulin-dependent diabetes mellitus (IDDM) or juvenile-onset diabetes. Clients with type 1 diabetes are prone to ketosis and require **exogenous insulin** therapy for survival, insulin from an external source.

Type 2 diabetes was previously known as non–insulin dependent diabetes mellitus (NIDDM) or maturity-onset diabetes because the age of onset is usually after 40 years of age. Approximately 90% of the diabetes cases are type 2 (Carlisle, Kroon & Koda-Kimble, 2005). In general, clients with type 2 diabetes have some insulin function and thus are not fully dependent on insulin for survival. The vast majority of individuals with type 2 diabetes are obese, and ketosis is rare. Clients who frequent fast-food establishments appear to be at increased risk for developing insulin resistance and type 2 diabetes (Pereira et al., 2005). Weight reduction through dietary adjustments often helps to reduce hyperglycemia in clients with type 2 diabetes. Controlling other factors, such as obstructive sleep apnea, may also improve blood sugar levels (Babu, Herdegen, Fogelfield, Shott, & Mazzone, 2005).

Although insulin resistance may occasionally occur with type 1 diabetes, it is believed to be more common in type 2 diabetes because of insulin receptor and postreceptor defects.

Table 49-1 compares the primary features of both types of diabetes. The treatment of DM usually includes diet, exercise and, if necessary, oral antidiabetic agent(s) or insulin to help control blood glucose levels, or reach **euglycemia** (blood glucose levels within the normal limits). Control of blood sugar in combination with smoking cessation and management of blood pressure and dyslipidemias is important in reducing long-term renal and cardiovascular complications for clients with DM (Tesfave et al., 2005).

✷ **M.M. is a 6-year-old girl with no prior medical history admitted to the emergency department (ED) with altered mental status, vomiting, abdominal pain and dehydration. On examination, she has fruity smelling breath, dry mucous membranes, and tachycardia. Her blood glucose level is 940 g/dL (normal range: less than 200 g/dL nonfasting), her serum potassium is 5.4 mEq/L (normal range: 3.5-5.1 mEq/L) and her urine is positive for ketone bodies. Arterial blood gases reveal a pH of 7.15 and are consistent with metabolic acidosis. She is diagnosed with diabetic ketoacidosis.**

✷ **What are the symptoms and pathophysiology of ketoacidosis?**
Diabetic ketoacidosis is a result of altered energy metabolism in the cell because of a lack of insulin.

In the absence of insulin, glucose cannot enter the cell to be used for energy. As such, free fatty acids are used in metabolism resulting in acidosis and ketosis. Significant acido-sis can result in an extracellular shift of potassium. Potassium ions move out of cells as hydrogen ions move in. Intracellular potassium levels decline, often with elevated serum potassium levels initially. Elevated blood glucose levels are secondary to the absence of insulin and glucose is eliminated in the urine. The high urine glucose serves as an osmotic diuretic leading to dehydration and electrolyte disturbances. Ketone bodies in the serum also contribute to nausea and vomiting, which exacerbate the dehydration.

Clients with diabetic ketoacidosis typically present with polyuria, gastrointestinal (GI) upset and abdominal pain. Dehydration and orthostatic hypotension are common. In response to metabolic acidosis, the client may exhibit slow, deep respirations (Kussmaul breathing) in an attempt to "blow off" carbon dioxide. Acetone, a ketone, is often noted on the breath, lending to a "fruity" odor. Uncorrected, diabetic ketoacidosis can lead to shock, coma, and increase the risk for death (Figure 49-2).

✷ **M.M. is treated with normal saline and regular insulin 0.1 unit/kg × 1 IV, then 0.1 unit/kg/hr by continuous infusion. Her electrolytes are monitored hourly.**

✷ **How is diabetic ketoacidosis treated?**
Routinely, clients with diabetic ketoacidosis are treated with aggressive rehydration. Initially, this rehydration is with normal saline, at least until blood glucose levels return to 250 or 300 mg/dL, at which point, a dextrose/saline combination is often used. Insulin is administered intravenously (IV) with a

	Type 1	**Type 2**
Older terms	Insulin-dependent diabetes mellitus (IDDM), juvenile onset	Non–insulin-dependent diabetes mellitus (NIDDM), adult onset
Age of onset	Usually <30 years	Usually >35 years
Onset of symptoms	Sudden (symptomatic)	Gradual (usually asymptomatic)
Body weight	Usually not obese	Obese (80%)
Family history	Often negative	Often positive
Incidence	5%-10%	90%-95%
Insulin levels	Low, then absent	May be low, normal, or high (insulin resistance)
Insulin dependent	Yes	May be required if not responsive to oral agents
Insulin resistance	No	Yes
Receptors	Normal	Usually decreased or defective
Plasma insulin	Decreased	Decreased, normal, or increased
Complications	Common	Common
Ketoacidosis	Prone to this condition	Usually resistant to this condition
Dietary modifications	Mandatory	Mandatory

TABLE 49-1 FEATURES OF TYPE 1 AND TYPE 2 DIABETES MELLITUS

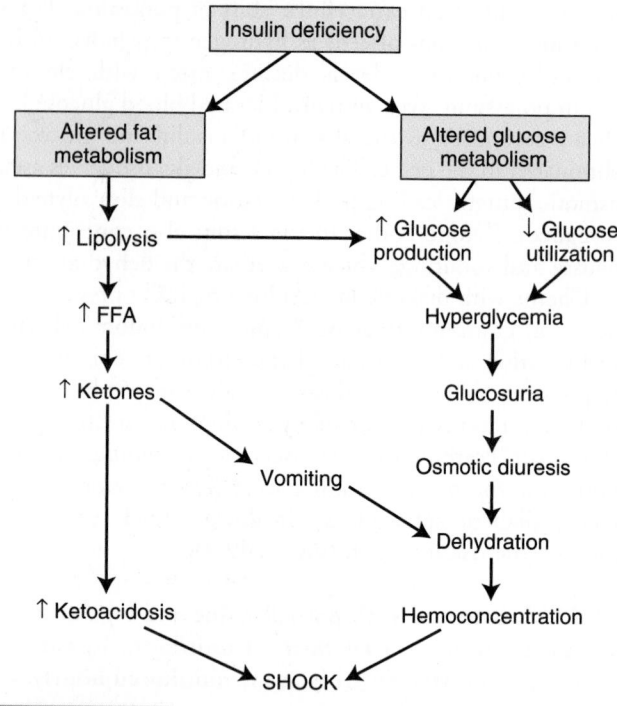

Figure 49-2 Factors leading to shock in diabetic ketoacidosis.

goal of slow and steady decreases in serum glucose levels (e.g., not more than 100 mg/dL decline per hour). Rapid declines in blood glucose should be avoided, because large shifts in glucose levels can result in osmotic shifts of fluid in tissues. This may be particularly concerning with rapid fluid shifts in the central nervous system (CNS) and may result in altered level of consciousness or respiratory arrest.

Electrolyte monitoring is also required. Initially in the acidotic state, serum potassium levels may be high. As insulin is administered, however, and the acidosis is corrected, potassium ions shift intracellularly. The osmotic diuresis leading up to ketoacidosis typically results in excessive depletion of body stores of potassium, which must be corrected. As such, frequent evaluation of electrolytes is necessary, and routinely dilute solutions of potassium chloride are administered to replenish losses once serum potassium is below 5 mEq/L. Potassium MUST be diluted and administered slowly via an infusion pump to prevent cardiac arrest. Most institutions have a standard protocol regarding maximum potassium concentrations and rates of administration (often not more than 80 mEq/L and no faster than 10 mEq/hr unless monitored in a critical care setting).

What is insulin?

Insulin is composed of two amino acid chains, A (acidic) and B (basic), which are joined together by disulfide linkages. It is synthesized in the beta cells of the pancreas, which are located in the islets of Langerhans; these cells secrete insulin when blood glucose levels are elevated.

Insulin controls the storage and metabolism of carbohydrate, protein, and fat that binds to receptor sites on cellular plasma membranes, especially in the liver, muscle, and adipose tissues. Although the exact molecular mechanism of action for insulin is still being investigated, it is known that it influences cell membrane transport, cell growth, enzyme activation and inhibition, and the metabolism of protein and fats.

Insulin is used to treat type 1 DM. It is also used in type 2 DM during emergencies or in specific situations, such as supplementation in the client with low physiologic endogenous insulin during high fevers, severe infection, ketoacidosis, or severe burns or after major surgery and severe trauma.

Insulin is also the drug of choice to control diabetes during pregnancy. Insulin requirements may drop for 24 to 72 hours after delivery and slowly return to prepregnancy levels in approximately 6 weeks.

How are insulin preparations differentiated?
Insulins can be classified by source and by onset and duration of action. Each is briefly discussed below.

Sources of Insulin

Historically, insulin preparations were derived from animals, being extracted from beef or pork pancreas. Beef insulin differs from human insulin by three amino acids, whereas pork insulin differs from human insulin by only one amino acid. These animal source insulins had a higher degree of immunogenicity, and resulted in a greater potential for insulin resistance, insulin allergies or lipoatrophy (a breakdown of subcutaneous fat occurring after repeated injections at the same insulin injection sites).

Today, insulin is synthesized in the laboratory via recombinant deoxyribonucleic acid (DNA) technology that uses strains of *Escherichia coli* to form biosynthetic human insulin. Human (or recombinant) insulin is identical to the insulin produced by the pancreas. It is much less antigenic than the animal-based insulin. Subcutaneous human insulin may also be absorbed faster and has a shorter duration of action than the animal insulins. It is standard practice now to prescribe human insulin whenever possible.

Newer insulin analogues are also available. These agents are nearly identical to human insulin, but have minor alterations in amino acid sequencing that affects onset and duration of action. Such agents are the fast-acting insulin analogs insulin aspart (NovoLog), insulin glulisine (Apidra), and insulin lispro (Humalog); and the long-acting insulins glargine (Lantus) and insulin detemir (Levemir). The fast-acting analogs have the advantage of a more rapid onset of action and can be administered immediately before (or in some cases, during or immediately after) a meal. The long-acting glargine and detemir formulations are considered "peak-less" insulins.

Onset and Duration of Action of Insulins

Insulin preparations are usually chosen by their pharmacokinetic profile. Available for use are products with rapid action, intermediate action, and prolonged action. Combinations of insulins with differing pharmacokinetics are also used.

Within each profile, individual agents are further differentiated regarding sources, onsets, and durations of action. The wide variety of available insulins (including combination mixtures) allow for sufficient blood glucose control to meet the need and lifestyle of a client with diabetes. Maintaining glucose levels as close as possible to normal will help to improve the client's quality of life and will also reduce the progression of complications associated with diabetes. Table 49-2 compares the pharmacokinetics of different insulins.

✳ **M.M. is managed in the ED and in the hospital with fluids, potassium, and insulin. On day two, she is euglycemic and is diagnosed with type 1 DM by the endocrinology team. She is started on an insulin sliding scale with insulin lispro (Humalog) and frequent blood glucose monitoring.**

✳ **How are blood glucose levels monitored?**
To maintain euglycemia, blood glucose levels are determined at frequent intervals by blood glucose monitoring. This process has been simplified by the availability of both visual test strips and strips used in blood glucose meters or instruments. Such devices allow clients to monitor their diabetes and make the necessary adjustments with medication, diet, and exercise as instructed by their health care provider. The visual glucose testing strips are less expensive than the testing instruments, but strips have been largely replaced by glucose meters. The meter readings of the testing instruments are much more precise (assuming they are properly calibrated) and are easier to use for clients with visual problems. The appropriate dosage of insulin for the client is indicated by the maintenance of normal fasting serum glucose levels within 70 to 105 mg/dL for adults less than 60 years of age and 80 to 115 mg/dL for adults 60 years of age and over.

Urine glucose testing is primarily of historic interest only because it is an indirect measurement of the client's glycemic status. The spillage of glucose into the urine usually occurs at blood levels of 160 to 180 mg/100 mL, but may be higher in older adults or lower in children and pregnant women. Therefore it may not correlate well with

TABLE 49-2 INSULIN PHARMACOKINETICS AFTER SUBCUTANEOUS INJECTION

Insulins	Onset (hr)	Peak Effect (hr)	Duration of Action (hr)
RAPID-ACTING			
insulin injection (regular insulin, Humulin R)*	0.5-1	2-4	5-7
insulin aspart (NovoLog)	0.5	1-3	3-5
insulin lispro (Humalog)	0.25	1	4
insulin glulisine (Apidra)	0.25	1	2-3
INTERMEDIATE-ACTING			
isophane insulin suspension (NPH insulin, Humulin N)	3-4	6-12	18-28
insulin zinc suspension (Lente Insulin)	1-3	8-12	18-28
LONG-ACTING			
extended insulin zinc suspension (Ultralente)	4-6	18-24	36
insulin glargine (Lantus)	1-5	Plateau	24
insulin detemir (Levemir)	3-4	"Peakless"	24
COMBINATIONS			
isophane human insulin (50%) & regular human insulin (50%) (Humulin 50/50)	0.5	3	22-24
isophane human insulin (70%) & regular human insulin (30%) (Humulin 70/30, Novolin 70/30)	0.5	4-8	24
insulin lispro protamine/insulin lispro (Humalog Mix 75/25)	0.25	0.5-6	24
insulin aspart protamine/insulin aspart (NovoLog Mix 70/30)	0.25	1-4	24

*Regular insulin may be administered IV. Intravenously, the onset of action is within 10 minutes to 30 minutes, the peak effect is within 20 minutes to 30 minutes, and the duration of action is within 30 minutes to 60 minutes.

serum glucose levels. In contrast, type 1 diabetic clients are taught to test the urine for ketones as needed for early detection of ketoacidosis, which can occur during times of stress, illness, or other situations in which blood glucose levels are not controlled.

Another evaluation test involves determining the client's glycosylated hemoglobin (hemoglobin A1C). The level of A1C increases when individuals have prolonged hyperglycemic serum levels. Red blood cells have a life span of 4 months; therefore a measurement of A1C will give the prescriber an evaluation of the client's long-term diabetic control. An elevated A1C indicates inadequate diabetic control for the previous 2 to 3 months (Carlisle, Kroon & Koda-Kimble, 2005). For clients with diabetes, the usual target goal for A1C is 7% or less.

✴ How is insulin dosed?

There is no average dosage of insulin; each client's needs must be determined individually to attain euglycemia and avoid hypoglycemia and hyperglycemia. Cumulative daily doses in the range of 0.5 to 1.5 units/kg/day are used as guideposts, but significant variation in insulin requirement is noted based on age, growth pattern, diet, exercise, concurrent illness or infection, or other conditions. Clients who are newly diagnosed often experience a "honeymoon" period early in treatment in which only very low doses of insulin are required (e.g., in the range of 0.2-0.5 units/kg/day).

Insulin dosages are expressed in units standardized by the United States Pharmacopeia (USP) rather than in milliliters. Most formulations of insulin are standardized so that each milliliter contains 100 USP units, although there is a formulation of 500 units/mL for regular insulin. Insulin is classified according to its duration of action (short- or rapid-acting, intermediate-acting, and long-acting) (Figure 49-3). In general, meals should occur at the same time that administered insulin reaches its peak effect. Insulin requirements can vary widely among clients, so dosages must be adjusted to individual need.

Clients with diabetes who become hyperglycemic, perhaps because of hospitalization or an infection, may need insulin coverage in addition to their regular insulin. The amount of insulin given will vary with the blood glucose values; this titration is known as the "sliding-scale" administration of insulin. Today urine testing is rarely used to monitor blood glucose

and should not be used to determine insulin doses. However, if this method is used, different brands of urine glucose testing products should not be used interchangeably and product directions should be followed carefully.

The client's dietary intake, physical activity, ability to manage the therapeutic regimen, and glucose tolerance are taken into consideration when establishing insulin dosages. Insulin dosages are not considered to be a fixed regimen; dosages may need to be adjusted as a result of physical growth (child growing into adulthood), illness, stress, the development of antiinsulin antibodies, concomitant administration of certain medications, or changes in exercise and diet. Specific instructions should be obtained regarding insulin administration for the preoperative client because of the alteration in the client's dietary patterns and metabolic requirements as the result of the surgical procedure. Treatment programs need to be reviewed and adjusted as necessary, with the prescriber, nurse, and client working closely to manage hypoglycemia and hyperglycemia and, if possible, avoid their complications. Research is supporting closer management for euglycemia. The concept is to mimic normal insulin secretion as closely as possible. This can be accomplished by either insulin pump therapy or multiple daily doses of insulin.

Portable insulin pumps have improved the metabolic state of some clients with type 1 diabetes who do not have adequate diabetic control with intensive dietary restrictions and multiple daily insulin injections. The insulin pump is battery-operated and connected to a small computer that is programmed to release small amounts of insulin per hour (see Figure 5-8). It does not analyze the blood glucose level, but it is programmed according to the client's daily insulin needs, diet, and physical exercise. The client can also push a button that releases a bolus dose to cover each meal consumed.

Although insulin pumps are effective and useful for clients who are properly trained, health care professionals need to be aware of several problems associated with them. Malfunction of the insulin infusion may occur because of battery failure, and defects in the tubing may cause leakage of insulin solution or blockage of the infusion tubing. Therefore it is vitally important to teach the client to change the infusion set and battery. Clients must be highly motivated and educated in the handling of insulin pumps. Clients should be capable of keeping records and following specific procedures and should be willing to perform blood tests daily or more often.

Insulin is given subcutaneously (or intravenously [IV] for regular insulin only). It cannot be given by mouth because digestive enzymes destroy it. Regular insulin is usually given approximately 15 to 30 minutes before meals whereas insulin aspart is usually given 5 to 10 minutes before meals. Insulin injectors such as NovoPen PenMate and NovoPen Junior hide the needle before injection, and a single button press triggers the PenMate to insert the needle automatically. Needleless injectors, such as the Vitajet, Medi-Jector, and others are also available. These devices are expensive and appear to have limited usefulness in practice. Many devices are also available for the visually impaired client with diabetes. Information on injection aids for the blind may be obtained from state and national associations, such as the

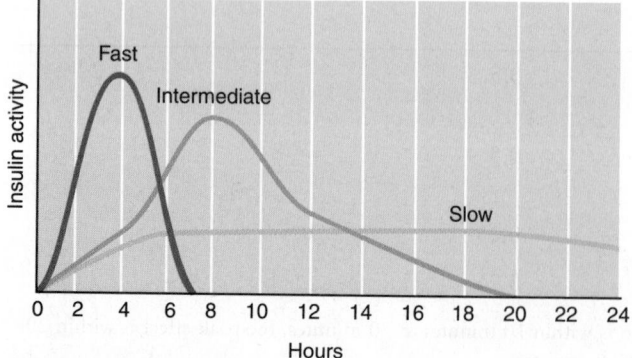

FIGURE 49-3 Insulin pharmacokinetics.

American Foundation for the Blind and the American Diabetes Association (ADA).

✱ **The nurses' role in managing M.M.'s insulin therapy and assisting her and her parents to effectively manage a life-long drug regimen is essential.**
Teaching M.M. and her family about diabetes, diet, insulin and its administration, and other related care is a long process and cannot be accomplished during this hospitalization. The client educator should meet with M.M. and her family to determine knowledge needs, schedules, settings, and resources and plan accordingly. Over the course of that program, a comprehensive view of diabetes and the relevant care will be discussed. Here the focus will be on insulin.

Assessment A comprehensive nursing history is necessary in helping M.M. and her parents to manage her diabetes. This assessment is as essential for clients newly diagnosed with diabetes and for clients seeking reassurance they are managing their diabetes appropriately or who have readjusted insulin dosage because of stress, illness, change of lifestyle, or ineffective management of the therapeutic regimen.

Assess M.M.'s blood glucose level before beginning or adjusting insulin therapy; also include a baseline assessment of her skin (lesions and color), orientation, peripheral sensation, reflexes, blood pressure, pulse, respirations, lung sounds, urinalysis, blood glucose levels, and A1C.

Determine her ideal body weight, present weight, daily exercise, dietary management and preferences, and the family's understanding of diabetes and its control. Also note any physical impairments (e.g., developmental delays, decreased manual dexterity, or limitations of vision) that would impede the self-administration of insulin. Because the cost of insulin, injection equipment, and blood testing equipment can be considerable, assess M.M.'s parents' financial status and health insurance coverage, and locate alternative resources if necessary. After hospitalization, ophthalmologic testing should be obtained for baseline. Ascertain M.M.'s religion; although the use of pork insulin is no longer common, clients with certain religious affiliations (e.g., Jewish or Islamic clients) prefer not to use it because their dietary codes involve the avoidance of pork.

Although M.M. is only 6 years old, interview her and her parents to identify any medications that might place her at increased risk of significant drug interactions; also see Box 49-1. For older clients, there would be a need to discuss the effects of commonly abused drugs on diabetic management; see Box 49-2. Corticosteroids may increase blood glucose levels; a dosage adjustment of insulin may be necessary. Many over-the-counter (OTC) cough and cold remedies contain alcohol that may increase the hypoglycemic effect of insulin. If possible, avoid the concurrent use of alcohol. Although more relevant for older diabetic clients, it is important for all clients with diabetes to know that β-adrenergic blocking agents (including eye preparations) may mask symptoms of hypoglycemia, such as increased pulse rate and decreased blood pressure. They may also prolong hypoglycemia by blocking gluconeogenesis. Dosage adjustments

---

BOX 49-1 DRUGS REPORTED TO CAUSE HYPERGLYCEMIA OR HYPOGLYCEMIA

HYPERGLYCEMIA	HYPOGLYCEMIA
atypical antipsychotics (e.g., olanzepine, risperidol)	ACE inhibitors
β blockers	anabolic steroids
calcium channel blocking agents	alcohol
clonidine	β-adrenergic blocking agents
corticosteroids	β blockers
danazol	bromocriptine
diuretics	clofibrate
epinephrine	ketoconazole
estrogen	lithium
estrogen-progestin–containing hormonal contraceptives	mebendazole
glucagon	NSAIDs
growth hormone	octreotide
heparin	pyridoxine
H_2 receptor blockers	sulfonamides
morphine	theophylline
phenytoin	
sulfinpyrazone	
thyroid hormones	

Data from *USP DI: Drug information for the health care professional* (25th ed.). (2005). Greenwood Village, CO: MICROMEDEX Thomson Healthcare.

---

of insulin may be necessary. Selective β blockers in low dosages, such as metoprolol and atenolol, cause fewer problems than the other β-adrenergic blocking agents. Propranolol may cause hyperglycemia or hypoglycemia when given concurrently with insulin. Periodic blood glucose tests are recommended to monitor the combined effects and allow for a dosage adjustment for insulin if necessary.

Nursing Diagnosis See the Nursing Care Plan on p. 870 for nursing diagnoses that commonly apply to the client receiving insulin.

Planning See Box 49-3. Relate these goals to M.M. and her family realizing that as M.M. grows older, her need for information and support will change.

Implementation
Monitoring Monitor the effectiveness of insulin therapy by obtaining blood glucose levels at frequent intervals—more often if the client is under stress, is pregnant, or has been recently diagnosed. The appropriate dosage of insulin

Nursing Diagnosis	Outcome Criteria	Nursing Interventions
Deficient knowledge related to newly diagnosed diabetes	Client and family will: • Demonstrate an understanding of diabetes, its therapy and complications, and measures to minimize or prevent complications	• Assess the understanding/learning ability of the client/family. • Determine educational needs and desires. • Provide information regarding the pathophysiology of diabetes and the function of insulin. • Explain goals and methods of diet and drug therapy. • Explain the function and purpose of tests. • Answer questions and clarify misconceptions. • Provide resources for further learning and support (American Diabetes Association [ADA], Juvenile Diabetes Foundation [JDF], and others).

Deficient knowledge related to newly prescribed diabetic medication (insulin)	Client and family will:
	• Demonstrate correctly the appropriate storage, handling, and administration of insulin
	• Be familiar with the signs and symptoms of insulin/hypoglycemic reaction and the appropriate response
	• State the different insulin preparations and appropriate adjustment of drug therapy
	• Be aware of possible adverse effects of insulin
		• Teach the client and family:
		  • The function and importance of therapy and the name and dosage of insulin
		  • The technique of blood (or urine) glucose monitoring and adjusting insulin appropriately
		  • The proper technique of administration
		  • The need for life-long dietary and drug management
		  • The differences among the various forms of insulin
		  • How to calculate dosages correctly
		  • The proper storage and handling of insulin
		  • The importance of rotating sites to minimize adverse local reactions
		  • The signs and symptoms of insulin/hypoglycemic reaction and appropriate management
		• Help the client establish and maintain a monitoring record of blood (or urine) glucose and insulin administration.
		• Advise the client to wear or carry a medical identification tag, bracelet, or card.
		• Provide the client with a list of drugs and conditions that may alter insulin requirements.

Risk for injury related to hyperglycemia or hypoglycemia related to insulin administration	Client will:
	• Achieve control of blood glucose and maintain desired nutritional intake
	Client and family will:
	• Demonstrate knowledge of appropriate diabetic diet and modifications of dietary practices
		• Administer insulin as prescribed.
		• Teach client and family:
		  • The correct method of blood glucose monitoring
		  • The signs, symptoms, and treatment for hyperglycemia and hypoglycemia
		  • The importance of a balanced diabetic diet to control diabetes
		• Provide dietary instruction and counseling regarding the appropriate diet; refer the client to a dietitian.
		• Assist client and family in planning a sample diet.

Disturbed body image related to insulin dependence	Client and family will: • Verbalize feelings and concerns • Understand disease and measure of control Client will: • Maintain, as much as possible, prediagnosis activities	• Encourage the client and family to express feelings and concerns. • Determine assets and strengths. With the client and family, determine strategies for managing areas of difficulty or concern. • Provide resources for further learning and support (ADA, JDF, others). • Be alert for signs of nonacceptance or difficulties such as denial or ineffective management of therapeutic regimen.
Powerlessness related to perceived lack of personal control	Client and family will: • Identify those areas of diabetes that are possible to control, and participate in decision making related to diabetic management	• Assess the client's and family's coping patterns and support mechanisms. • Assess the client's and family's perceptions related to diagnosis. • Allow and encourage the expression of concerns and fears. • Encourage client and family participation in therapy planning and implementation.

Many drugs can increase or decrease blood glucose levels, but rarely are the commonly abused drugs reviewed in relation to diabetes. Because substance abuse by the client with diabetes can be very problematic, the most commonly abused drugs are reviewed here.

ALCOHOL

Alcohol promotes hypoglycemia and blocks the formation, storage, and release of glycogen. It may also interact with many other drugs, including oral hypoglycemic agents such as chlorpropamide. In individuals with alcoholism who have decreased their food intake, alcohol can cause a serious drop in blood glucose levels, which leads to a need for acute intervention.

CNS STIMULANTS

Amphetamines, sympathomimetics, anorexics, cocaine, psychedelic drugs, and others may result in hyperglycemia and an increase in the breakdown of liver glycogen. Large amounts of caffeine in products such as coffee, tea, and cola drinks can also increase blood glucose levels.

MARIJUANA

Marijuana may increase appetite and food consumption. Heavy use may produce a glucose intolerance, which leads to hyperglycemia.

CIGARETTES

The nicotine in cigarettes is a potent vasoconstrictor. It can decrease the absorption of subcutaneous insulin or increase an individual's insulin requirements by 15% to 20%. Cigarette smoking can cause a drop of 1 to 2 degrees in skin temperature. It also is a risk factor for the development of diabetic nephropathy.

ABUSE OF CNS-ACTING DRUGS

CNS-acting drugs (e.g., stimulants, depressants, sedative-hypnotics, opioids, marijuana, alcohol) can impair judgment and alter perceptions (time, place) and thus interfere with the individual's control of the diabetic state.

BOX 49-3 GOALS FOR ANTIDIABETIC DRUG THERAPY

During antidiabetic drug therapy, the client will:

- Remain free from adverse effects of the drug therapy and the complications of diabetes.
- Describe the effects and complications of diabetes and reportable symptoms for the health care provider (hypoglycemia, hyperglycemia, ketoacidosis).
- State the action and adverse effects of the antidiabetic agent.
- Effectively manage the therapeutic regimen including compliance with medication, dietary program, exercise, self-monitored blood glucose testing and interpretation, sick day management, cardiovascular risk factors, and other monitoring.

See the Nursing Care Plan on p. 870 for additional outcome criteria.

tion sites for impaired tissue integrity, such as lipoatrophy or lipohypertrophy (a buildup of subcutaneous fat tissue) after she begins to have subcutaneous injections.

M.M. and other clients with diabetes are evaluated periodically in the primary care setting for complications of DM related to the ineffectiveness of insulin therapy, including visual impairment (ophthalmic examination), nephropathy (complete urinalysis [including protein], blood urea nitrogen, serum creatinine), neuropathy (neurologic examination), increased atherosclerotic disease (serum cholesterol, high-density lipoprotein cholesterol, serum triglycerides, electrocardiogram, peripheral pulses, bruits), and foot and skin examinations for problem areas (American Diabetes Association, 2004).

Intervention Note that all insulin preparations are stable as long as the vials are protected from heat or excessive cold; store them in a cool place, but do not freeze them. Two strengths of insulin are available, 100 units/mL and 500 units/mL. Regular (concentrated) Iletin II is available as U-500 for clients who have developed insulin resistance and require large dosages. See the Medication Safety Alert box on p. 872 for safety issues in insulin ordering and administration.

Vials of insoluble preparations (all except regular insulin) should be rotated between the hands and inverted end-to-end several times before withdrawing a dose. The vial should not be shaken vigorously or the suspension will foam. Do not interchange human, beef-pork combination, or pork insulins, because species differences may require a dosage change. Do not use insulin that has become clumped or granular in appearance.

Use a properly calibrated syringe for insulin. For doses of less than 50 units of U-100, use a low-dose syringe (50 units of U-100/0.5 mL). The decreased diameter of the barrel of the syringe results in the calibrations being further apart, which enhances accuracy of the measurement. Avoid bubbles in the solution; the displacement of a few units of insulin, particularly with U-500 insulin, can alter the actual dose received by the client.

for M.M. is indicated by the maintenance of normal fasting serum glucose levels within 60 to 100 mg/dL (75-110 mg/dL for adults; 80 to 115 mg/dL for adults 60 years of age; 75-120 mg/dL for adults older than 90 years of age) (Schnell, Van Leeuwen, & Kranpitz, 2003). For frail older adults or those living alone where monitoring for hypoglycemic events is problematic, maintaining fasting glucose levels above this range may be appropriate. Hemoglobin A_{1c} determinations are performed to evaluate the adequacy of diabetic control more comprehensively because the result is not age-dependent and is not effected by exercise, diabetic medications, or nonfasting state before specimen collection.

Monitor M.M. for signs and symptoms of hyperglycemia, hypoglycemia, and ketoacidosis. Observe injec-

Medication Safety Alert

Insulin and Medication Errors

Insulin has been identified as one of several medications that deserve particular concern in quality assessment programs. It has been reported that glucose control is inadequate in in-patient settings (Metchick, Petit, Jr., & Inzucchi, 2002). Additionally, clients taking unintentional overdoses of insulin were more likely to be hospitalized than those with other adverse drug effects. Warfarin and insulins were associated with 16% of adverse drug events overall (Budnick, 2005). Hypoglycemia may result from drug-dispensing errors, including administration errors of hypoglycemic agents to nondiabetic clients. For diabetic clients, prescribing errors, the use of trailing zeros after decimal points, or misinterpreted abbreviations for insulin contribute to client risk (Bates, 2002; Ragone & Lando, 2002). Because the capital "U" can be mistaken for a numeral when handwritten, the word "units" should be spelled out in physician orders (Clement et al, 2004). The erroneous administration of a large dose of rapid-acting insulin in place of insulin glargine can easily occur, because insulin glargine and rapid-acting insulins look clear in the vial; bar-coding of drugs could help reduce this type of error.

Take care not to store U-500 insulin in the same area as other insulin preparations because of the possibility of a massive overdose if it is accidentally administered to a client.

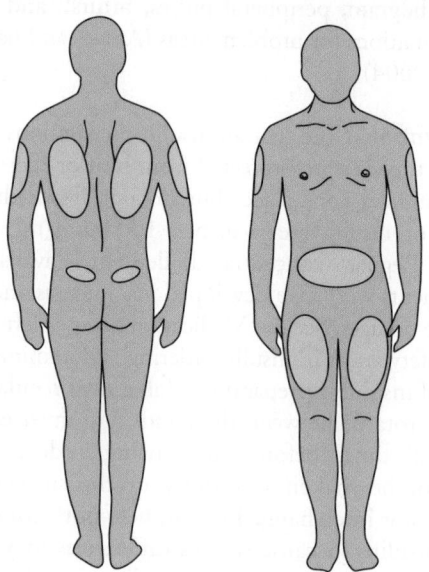

FIGURE 49-4 Common sites for subcutaneous injections.

From Perry, A.G., & Potter, P.A. (2006). *Clinical nursing skills & techniques* (6th ed.) St. Louis: Mosby.

Administer insulin subcutaneously using a 25- or 26-gauge needle; the length of the needle is determined by the client's size. A $^3/_8$ to $^5/_8$-inch needle is usually used, with the injection administered at a 90-degree angle in a large fold of skin that has been gently pinched up. The injection may also

BOX 49-4 INTRASITE ROTATION OF INSULIN INJECTION SITES

A good approach to administering insulin is to instruct the client to mark the first injection site with a spot bandage and give future injections around the bandage. The client should imagine each circle as a clock, administering injections at the 12 o'clock, 3 o'clock, 6 o'clock, and 9 o'clock points before starting a new circle more than an inch away from the previous sites (see below).

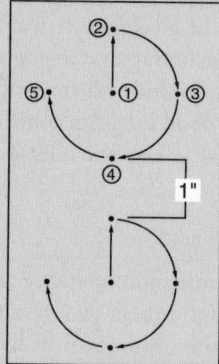

Following this plan, the client can administer five injections per circle. The spot bandage also works as a convenient memory jogger. After going through two or three showers, the bandage is usually ready to be removed and a new one applied; this occurs at the approximate time the circle is complete.

Figure modified with permission from Drass, J. (1992). What you need to know about insulin injections. *Nursing 22*(11), 40-43.

be inserted at a 30- to 45-degree angle at the base of the fold of skin. Apply pressure after the injection; do not rub the site, because doing so alters the absorption rate. Rotate injection sites; see Figure 49-4. Because of the differences in absorption from different anatomic sites, rotate injections with a pattern (e.g., morning injections rotated within the abdominal region, evening injections rotated in the thighs). Rotate injection sites within an anatomical area also, see Box 49-4.

Understand that only the regular form of insulin may be administered by the IV route. Regular insulin is compatible with dextrose injection, 0.9% sodium chloride injection and combinations of these. Insulin adsorption occurs onto the surfaces of vinyl and plastic IV infusion containers and tubing (Dunn, 2002). Such adsorption is unpredictable. Depending on availability of infusion pumps that accurately deliver very low hourly volumes, IV insulin therapy is conducted with regular crystalline insulin in a solution of 1 unit per 1 mL normal saline. The concentrated infusion is piggy-backed into a dedicated running IV line. Highly concentrated solutions may be reserved for clients requiring volume restriction; otherwise, solutions as dilute as 1 unit insulin per 10 mL normal saline may be used. When the more dilute solutions are used, at least 50 mL of the insulin-containing solution should be allowed to run through the tubing and stored for 30 minutes before use, then flushed again before use to stabilize the amount of insulin adsorbed and ensure optimal results (Clement et al., 2004). Afterwards adjust the dosage per protocol to meet M.M.'s targeted blood glucose concentration. Saturation of the adsorption sites on the tubing requires special care when changing the tubing, because exposure of the new tubing to insulin may result in decreased insulin dosing and the need for more frequent monitoring of client needs. Adsorption can be minimized by injecting directly into the vein, by using an intermittent infusion device, or by using a port close to the IV access site. Use an IV pump for accuracy when administering insulin as an infusion.

Education Instruct M.M. and her parents with age-appropriate levels of explanation on the relationship of diabetes to the administration of insulin, blood glucose monitoring, and the necessity to maintain euglycemia. Teach M.M. and her parents about blood glucose monitoring so they can adjust her insulin dosages when her blood levels are above normal limits. Results of blood tests are described as "high," "low," or "normal"; never "good" or "bad." There are various models of glucometers. At M.M.'s age, it would be better to help her parents select one that was simple to operate and only required a small drop of blood. At M.M.'s age, offer her the choice of picking which finger to use for testing or site for insulin injection. In teaching M.M. to help prevent soreness associated with finger sticks, she may rotate them by using the left thumb, then the left index finger, and so on; when the left hand is finished she should use the same sequencing on the right. This more evenly distributes the finger sticks. Some new glucometers may also use other areas of the body, such as the forearm that may be less sensitive.

Instruct M.M. and her parents in the administration of insulin, including the type of insulin, the injection technique, onset and peak action times of insulin, proper storage of insulin, the disposal of syringes, and the rotation of injection sites. Have M.M. agitate the vial (unless using regular insulin) and properly cleanse the top with 70% isopropyl alcohol. To draw insulin out of a vial, inject the vial with an amount of air equal to the insulin dose. This prevents a negative pressure from occurring in the vial, which would make the withdrawal of the insulin difficult. Teach M.M. and her parents to eliminate air bubbles from the syringe because they decrease the dose.

Although there are premixed combinations of insulins, there are occasions when clients or nurses must mix insulins. When mixing insulins, first inject air (equal to the volume of the dose to be withdrawn) into the vial of NPH insulin. Then inject air into the vial of the regular insulin. Keep the needle in the vial, and draw the regular insulin into the syringe first; this prevents contamination of the regular insulin vial with the other insulin admixture. Then return to the NPH vial and withdraw the dose of NPH insulin. The onset of action of regular insulin is delayed when mixed with other insulins. The interaction of regular and NPH insulin occurs within 15 minutes of mixing and remains at this stability for 30 days at room temperature and 90 days if refrigerated. The interaction of regular and Lente

Community and Home Health Considerations

Prefilling of Insulin Syringes by Home Health Nurses

The timing of the chemical interaction following the combination of different types of insulins modifies the clinical effectiveness of the insulins by delaying the onset of action of regular insulin. Home health nurses who prefill insulin syringes with different insulins in the same syringe for future use by their clients should ensure that clients are not using insulin mixed the same day. The insulin should be administered so that there is a consistency of dosage in the insulin therapy. Administering a "fresh" syringe (one mixed within the previous 15 minutes) will produce the same reaction as if administering the insulins separately, and this may significantly alter the client's blood glucose levels and glycemic response. Due to the potential for variable response, insulin glargine (Lantus) syringes should not be prefilled.

mixtures requires up to 24 hours before reaching a stable level of consistent response; if premixed in the same syringe, the onset of the regular insulin is delayed. This activity is stable for 30 days at room temperature and 90 days under refrigeration. Clients stabilized on this premixed insulin may have a different response (e.g., the onset of insulin effect will be shortened) if they inject the insulin separately from each component (see the Community and Home Health Considerations box above).

The use of the longer-acting insulins may increase the risk for hypoglycemia, particularly with longer-acting insulins that peak late in the day. Hypoglycemia, particularly at night, is a major concern for families with children with diabetes. An insulin regimen of either multiple daily injections, using "peak-less" insulin glargine (Lantus) as a basal and either insulin aspart (NovoLog or insulin lispro [Humalog] to cover food, or insulin pump therapy, results in good glycemic control with a reduced risk of nocturnal hypoglycemia compared to NPH/regular insulin (Murphy et al., 2002; Ratner et al., 2000).

Different brands of syringes have sufficient differences in "dead space" (the unmeasured volume between the needle point and the bottom calibration) to cause improper dosages. Dosage errors are avoided by not changing the injection order of mixing insulins and by not changing the model of needles, brands of syringes, or sources of insulins.

Instruct M.M. and her parents in how to plan the rotation of injection sites and to observe for lipodystrophies, the occurrence of which may be minimized by rotation. Note that insulin is most rapidly absorbed from the abdomen, followed by the upper arm and then the thigh. Physical activity in the client accelerates absorption, especially in the injected limb; alert joggers and walkers.

Teach M.M. and her parents that alternating the insulin injection sites from the leg to the abdomen or arm has the effect of accelerating the absorption of insulin and diminishing the postprandial rise in plasma glucose. Varying injection sites within the same anatomic region rather than between different regions may diminish daily fluctuations or variations in insulin absorption and in metabolic control in clients who are insulin dependent. For example, if the abdomen is used for a morning injection, subsequent morning injections should also be given in the abdomen. Injections at another time of day should always be given in the same part of the body, for example, use thigh sites for before-dinner injections. Each injection should be administered an inch away from any previously used site, and a site should not be used more often than once a month (see Box 49-4).

Be sure M.M. and her parents understand that frequent serum glucose monitoring is necessary to achieve insulin control. Reinforce compliance with the understanding that insulin helps to control hyperglycemia but is not a cure for diabetes.

Instruct them about the signs and symptoms of hypoglycemia that can occur secondary to the dosage of insulin (Box 49-5). A dosage adjustment downward may be necessary to prevent repeated episodes of hypoglycemia. If M.M. develops hypoglycemia, she should promptly ingest a carbohydrate with high sugar content, and the prescriber should be notified. Orange juice, candy, a lump of sugar, or a complex carbohydrate such as milk or cheese and crackers can be given if the individual is conscious (Box 49-6). Early symptoms of hypoglycemia are fatigue, headache, drowsiness, lassitude, tremulousness, or nausea. Late symptoms are weakness, sweating, tremors, or nervousness. Have M.M.'s parents observe her at night for excessive restlessness and profuse sweating or obtain an insulin pump system with an alarm for abnormal blood glucose levels.

Advise M.M.'s parents to always read bottle labels or check with their pharmacies before purchasing OTC medications. Manufacturers often change the sugar content of OTC medications. The best advice is to check the list of ingredients every time a medication is purchased. Ask the pediatrician for a list of sugar-free antipyretics and cough and cold preparations for children.

Teach M.M. and her parents to assess for signs of hyperglycemia: thirst, polyuria, flushed skin, fruity odor to the breath, and drowsiness that progresses to unconsciousness. Instruct the family to have regular insulin available for administration and to observe M.M. closely after insulin has been given.

Diabetic ketoacidosis is acidosis accompanied by an accumulation of ketones in the body, which results from faulty carbohydrate metabolism. It is evidenced by the symptoms of hyperglycemia (see Box 49-5) and, if left untreated, may result in coma. Discuss the following with M.M. and her family to prevent recurrences of ketoacidosis:

- Use a regimented pattern of diabetic control.
- Never omit antidiabetic drugs, particularly when a secondary illness is manifested (e.g., infection).
- Consume clear liquids and eat smaller meals when illness occurs.

BOX 49-5 SYMPTOMS OF HYPOGLYCEMIA AND HYPERGLYCEMIA

Persons administering insulin should be aware of the symptoms of hypoglycemia and hyperglycemia and know what actions to take if they occur.

Hypoglycemia: Increased anxiety,* blurred vision, chilly sensation, cold sweating,* pallor, confusion, difficulty concentrating, drowsiness, headache, nausea, increased pulse rate,* shakiness,* increased weakness, increased appetite.

PLASMA GLUCOSE LEVEL	RESPONSE/SYMPTOM†
>70 mg/dL	None
70 mg/dL	Counterregulation (decreased insulin secretion, increased glucagon secretion, initial epinephrine release)
60 mg/dL	Autonomic response (sweating, increased heart rate secondary to epinephrine release)
50 mg/dL	Neuroglycopenic (lightheadedness)
40 mg/dL	Lethargy
30 mg/dL	Coma
20 mg/dL	Seizures
10 mg/dL	Permanent brain damage/death
0 mg/dL	Death

Hyperglycemia: Drowsiness, red/dry skin, fruity breath odor, anorexia, abdominal pain, nausea, vomiting, dry mouth, increased urination, rapid/deep breathing, unusual thirst, rapid weight loss

*Symptoms masked by β-adrenergic blockers.
†Variation among individuals is expected with hypoglycemia.

BOX 49-6 QUICK FIXES FOR CLIENTS WITH MILD HYPOGLYCEMIA

Clients who have the potential to develop hypoglycemia should have ready access to a source of rapid-acting carbohydrate. The following substances contain 10 to 15 g of such a carbohydrate, which will stabilize a client who is having a mild hypoglycemic reaction—usually within 15 minutes. Monitor the blood glucose, if it remains low, take another snack from the foods below. As the blood glucose begins to return to normal, then eat a snack containing carbohydrate and protein such as crackers and cheese or peanut butter. Some forms of carbohydrate are easier to carry on a daily basis, such as the glucose tablets or a tube of cake frosting:

3 glucose tablets
4 ounces orange juice
6 ounces regular soda
6-8 ounces 2% fat or skim milk
6-8 Lifesavers
3 graham cracker squares
6 jelly beans
2 tablespoons of raisins
1 small (2-ounce) tube of cake frosting

Modified from American Diabetes Association (2004), Alexandria, VA.

- When ill, test blood glucose levels at frequent intervals because stress increase blood glucose.
- Notify the prescriber of secondary illness, nausea and vomiting, fever, an inability to eat, or an inability to control blood glucose levels.

Inform M.M. and the family that the following factors may lead to diabetic ketoacidosis: type 1 DM, omission of insulin, infections, cerebrovascular accidents (stroke), myocardial infarction, pregnancy, trauma, surgery, and stress (especially emotional).

Inform M.M. and her family that diet therapy is an important part of glucose control. The dietitian and the meal preparer must be included in the total care of clients with diabetes. Before M.M. is discharged, the family must be able to verbalize a basic understanding of her diet therapy and be willing to participate in meal planning.

Caution clients against the ingestion of alcohol, because hypoglycemia can result. Alcohol may be found in many liquid cough and cold preparations. If alcohol is consumed, the dosage of insulin may need to be reduced, because alcohol potentiates the hypoglycemic effect of insulin.

M.M. should carry medical identification at all times to identify herself as a person with diabetes and to describe the therapeutic regimen. The family will need to work with M.M.'s school to ensure her safety related to her diabetic condition.

Refer to a general nursing text for other aspects of diabetes education not directly related to insulin therapy, such as skin care, foot care, stress reduction, and dietary regimen. (See also the Special Considerations for Children box below). Teach the parents about current electronic sources of information on DM, such as outlined in the Technology Link box below.

Evaluation The expected outcome of insulin therapy is that M.M.'s blood glucose level will remain within normal limits and that she and her family will manage the therapeutic insulin regimen effectively; see the Nursing Care Plan on p. 870 for additional outcome criteria to be evaluated.

✪ **On day three, M.M. is noted to be shaking, weak, irritable, diaphoretic, tachycardic and is very hungry. Her blood glucose is checked with bedside monitoring and reveals a level of 52 g/dL.**

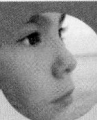 ## Special Considerations for Children | DIABETES

- Children with type 1 diabetes produce little or no insulin; therefore they generally require a daily combination of a short-acting and long-acting insulin.
- Carefully planned and scheduled meals, exercise, and insulin dosages are necessary to control the child's blood glucose level.
- Inform the child's teachers (including the gym teacher), teacher's aides, bus drivers, and anyone in regular contact with the child about diabetes and the signs, symptoms,

and treatment of hypoglycemia. These people should also be aware that late or skipped meals or snacks or unplanned exercise can be potentially dangerous for the child.
- Because many medications interact with insulin, alert the family to check with the prescriber before administering any new prescription or nonprescription medications.
- The child should carry or wear a MedicAlert identification tag at all times.

 ## Technology Link

Diabetes

American Diabetes Association (www.diabetes.org/home.jsp)

This site is dedicated to the prevention and cure of diabetes. It provides information for clients with diabetes and their families. It provides information on children's camps to recipes for the consumer and research opportunities and information for health care professionals.

CDC's Diabetes and Public Health Resource (www.cdc.gov/diabetes/index.htm)

This site presents research findings, statistics, special projects, publications, and other information on diabetes.

Diabetes Exercise & Sports Association (www.diabetes-exercise.org/)

Although this site charges a fee to join, it provides healthy and safe strategies for the treatment of type 1 and type 2 diabetes and the prevention of type 2 diabetes, included is an online support component. Without a fee. The site allows viewing of inspirational stories of the athletic accomplishments of people with diabetes.

Diabetes Mall (www.diabetesnet.com)

This site provides information on diabetes, including tools and technologies to make management of diabetes more effective, such as cookbooks, sleep sentries, glucometers, identification jewelry, and more. It also has a Diabetes Forum component for group discussion.

✳ **What are the symptoms of hypoglycemia?**

Hypoglycemia is a common complication of insulin therapy and is often manifested by anxiety, blurred vision, sweating, tachycardia and hunger pains. Box 49-5 lists the symptoms of hypoglycemia and hyperglycemia. Of note, clients of β-adrenergic blocking agents (e.g., propranolol) may not present with classic symptoms of hypoglycemia, because the tachycardia, tremors and diaphoresis are adrenergic responses and are inhibited by β blockers.

✳ **M.M. is treated with 3 ounces of orange juice and her follow up blood glucose level in 30 minutes is 116 g/dL.**

✳ **How is mild hypoglycemia managed?**

The management of hypoglycemia depends in part on the blood glucose concentration, what symptoms the client has including mental status, and the causes of the hypoglycemia. In mild cases in which consciousness in maintained, oral administration of a rapidly acting carbohydrate or glucose tablets (described in the following section) is indicated (see Box 49-6). In severe cases, or in which consciousness is impaired, parenteral dextrose and/or glucagon are used. These agents are discussed later in this chapter.

glucose [**gloo** koes]

(Glutose, Insta-Glucose)

Glucose is a monosaccharide that is absorbed from the intestine and then either used or stored by the body. It is indicated to treat or manage hypoglycemia. As a nutrient, glucose provides 4 calories/g.

Indications

Oral glucose is used to reverse mild hypoglycemic events secondary to insulin or oral hypoglycemics in conscious clients.

Pharmacokinetics/Dosing

In adults approximately 10 to 20 g PO are administered and repeated in 15 minutes if necessary.

Adverse Effects

The only adverse effects are some reports of nausea. No significant drug interactions have been reported.

✳ **M.M.'s pattern of insulin use and blood glucose readings are evaluated for the first three days and her treatment team is considering beginning a regimen of regularly administered insulin with a cumulative daily dose of 0.5 units/kg/day. On day four, M.M. is started on lispro (Humalog) and NPH insulin as follows: 2 units insulin lispro/1 unit NPH before breakfast, 1.5 units lispro before lunch, and 2 units insulin lispro/1 unit NPH before dinner with a total insulin dose each day of about 0.5 units/kg/day with supplemental sliding scale insulin for blood glucose levels in excess of 200 g/dL.**

•   •   •

✳ **T.L. is a 58-year-old woman who is 5' 7", weighs 95 kg, and reports to her nurse practitioner complain-**

ing of fatigue, polydipsia, and polyuria. Her fasting blood glucose is 155 g/dL and her hemoglobin A_{1c} is at 9.5%. She is diagnosed with type 2 DM. She is hesitant to start insulin because of her fear of injections.

✳ **What oral agents are available for the treatment of type 2 DM?**

Clients with type 2 DM are usually treated initially with diet and exercise. A number of oral agents are available and include the sulfonylureas, the biguanides, the thiazolidinedione derivatives (or "glitazones"), the α-glucosidase inhibitors, and the meglitinides. The older term "Oral Hypoglycemics" for oral agents is misleading, because many of these agents work to control type 2 disease and blood glucose levels by mechanisms other than directly inducing hypoglycemia. The oral agents do not replace insulin for clients with type 1 DM and therefore have no role in type 1 disease. Instead these agents work by different mechanisms to increase insulin secretion from the pancreas, improve insulin sensitivity at the cellular level, decrease hepatic glucose production, and/or decrease absorption of glucose in the GI tract. Adverse effects widely vary as well and include hypoglycemia, hepatic injury, lactic acidosis, and GI complaints. Variation in response and in metabolism to many of these agents may in part be explained by genetics (see Special Considerations for Pharmacogenetics box on p. 877).

Choice of oral agent or combination of agents is based on matching client needs with demonstrated efficacy of each class and adverse effect profile. For example, the sulfonylureas like glyburide (DiaBeta, Micronase) are often used as first line agents because they improve secretion of insulin from the pancreas. However, the risk for hypoglycemia may not render these a good choice for clients with irregular eating patterns that would predispose them to low blood glucose levels. The meglitinides (repaglinide [Prandin] and nateglinide [Starlix]) are short acting agents much like the sulfonylureas that may be appropriate for clients who eat irregularly, but require dosing before each meal. For clients with significant obesity, the biguanide metformin (Glucophage) may be preferred because of its demonstrated efficacy in this population and low potential for hypoglycemia. Metformin is contraindicated, however, in clients at risk for renal insufficiency as it may increase the risk for lactic acidosis. The thiazolidinedione derivatives ("glitazones") like pioglitazone (Actos) or rosiglitazone (Avandia) are effective in controlling diabetes in many clients, but they cause fluid retention and would be inappropriate choices for clients with uncontrolled heart failure (HF). In addition the glitazones may have a higher risk for hepatic injury. The α-glucosidase inhibitors (acarbose [Precose], miglitol [Glyset]) interfere with GI absorption of carbohydrates and offer some improved control as "add on" therapy, but are associated with significant diarrhea, flatulence and abdominal discomfort. Balancing the beneficial effects with their adverse effect profiles is an important aspect of implementing oral drug management of type 2 DM.

Two noninsulin polypeptide analogues, pramlintide (Symlin) and exenatide (Byetta), were approved by the U.S.

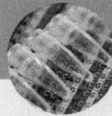 Special Considerations for Pharmacogenetics | **TREATMENTS FOR DIABETES MELLITUS**

PHARMACODYNAMICS

Both type 1 and type 2 DM have a strong genetic component in the pathophysiology of each disease (Altshuler et al., 2000). Variation in the *GNB3* gene, which codes for insulin receptor sensitivity and action, is noted across populations (Fernandez-Real et al., 2003; Rosskopf, Manthey, & Siffert, 2002) and may predict responders to insulin and therapies that target insulin receptors. The risk for cardiovascular events associated with type 2 diabetes is also correlated with genetic markers (Doney, Fischer, Leese, Morris, & Palmer, 2004). Genetics has a strong influence in the development of diabetes, the link of obesity with diabetes, and activity at the receptors where pioglitazone and rosiglitazone act (Meirhaeghe et al., 2000).

PHARMACOKINETICS

Significant variation in genes coding for drug metabolism via the P450 enzyme systems is noted. Glipizide, glimepiride,

nateglinide, pioglitazone, and rosiglitazone are each highly metabolized by P450 2 C8/9 (Lacy, Armstrong, Goldman, & Lance, 2004). About one third of Caucasian North Americans display variation in the gene which codes for this enzyme, whereas variation in this gene in African-Americans, Chinese, Japanese, and Koreans is less than 5% of the population (Lee, Goldstein, & Pieper, 2002). This may account for variable drug dose and response, particularly in Caucasians, with many oral agents to treat type 2 DM.

ADVERSE EFFECTS

Troglitazone, a thiazolidinedione similar to pioglitazone and rosiglitazone, was removed from the market in 2000 after over 90 reports of serious hepatotoxicity of which 68 were fatal (Lee, 2003). It is unclear if genetic variation in metabolism of these agents, all extensively metabolized by P450 enzyme systems, can predict likelihood of hepatotoxicity.

Food and Drug Administration (FDA) in 2005. Their use is limited to clients with poorly controlled DM despite other therapy, and they require subcutaneous injection.

✳ How are the oral agents differentiated?

As suggested above, each of these agents differ by mechanism and by adverse effect profiles. Each class is discussed individually with a representative agent or agents from each class presented in monograph format. Table 49-3 differentiates each agent and class.

Sulfonylureas

Although the sulfonylureas are sometimes called "oral insulins," this description is incorrect because chemically they are completely different from insulin. They also differ from insulin in their mode of action. The sulfonylureas enhance the release of insulin from the beta cells in the pancreas, decrease liver glycogenolysis (the breakdown of glycogen stored in the liver to glucose) and gluconeogenesis (the formation of glycogen from fatty acids and proteins rather than from carbohydrates), and increase cellular sensitivity to insulin in body tissues. Therefore they reduce the concentration of blood glucose in people with a functioning pancreas (Figure 49-5). Additionally, chlorpropamide has an antidiuretic effect; it increases the effect of low levels of antidiuretic hormone present in persons with central diabetes insipidus.

The first-generation sulfonylureas include acetohexamide (Dymelor), chlorpropamide (Diabinese), tolazamide (Tolinase), and tolbutamide (Orinase); they are considered to be equally effective but differ in pharmacokinetics and some adverse effects. The second-generation sulfonylureas include glimepiride (Amaryl), glipizide (Glucotrol), and glyburide (DiaBeta, Micronase), which are much more potent than the previous generation but probably have similar

efficacy. The advantages in using the second-generation sulfonylureas are that they have a long duration of action and fewer adverse effects.

The most common adverse effect of the sulfonylureas is hypoglycemia. Others are diarrhea or constipation, dizziness, gas, anorexia, headache, nausea, vomiting, or abdominal distress. Less common adverse effects are photosensitivity or rash. Rare adverse effects include respiratory difficulties, especially in persons with cardiac problems and HF; sedation; muscle cramping; seizures; edema of the face, hands, or ankles; comatose state, increased weakness (antidiuretic effect); pruritus, jaundice, light-colored stools, dark urine (impairment of liver function); or increased fatigue, sore throat, increased temperature, increased bleeding or bruising (blood dyscrasias).

The most frequently used sulfonylureas are glyburide and glipizide.

✳🔲 glyburide [**glye** byoo ride]
(DiaβBeta, Glynase, Micronase, Daonil✤, Euglucon✤)
Indications
Glyburide is indicated alone or in combination with other agents in the management of type 2 DM.
Pharmacokinetics/Dosing
Increased insulin levels are noted 15 to 60 minutes after oral administration with reductions in blood glucose observed within 2 hours. For clients with normal renal function, the duration of action is less than 24 hours. It is metabolized to an active metabolite, which accumulates in renal insufficiency and may lead to nocturnal hypoglycemic episodes in such clients. The usual initial adult dose is 2.5 to 5 mg daily administered with the first meal of the day. Doses up to 20 mg daily have been used.

The initial adult oral dose for micronized glyburide (Glynase) is 0.75 to 3 mg daily. The typical dosage is 0.75 to 12 mg daily divided in one or two doses.
Adverse Effects
Hypoglycemia is the most frequently observed adverse effect of glyburide. Hypoglycemia is most likely to be observed 3 to 4 hours af-

TABLE 49-3 ORAL AGENTS FOR TYPE 2 DIABETES MELLITUS

Agent	Peak (hr)*	Duration (hr)	Usual Oral Adult Dose	Comment
FIRST-GENERATION SULFONYLUREA				
acetohexamide (Dymelor)	1.5-6*	8-24	250 mg daily to 750 mg twice daily	Avoid with older clients or with renal insufficiency
chlorpropamide (Diabinese)	2-4*	24-72	100-500 mg daily	Long duration of action with potential for hypoglycemia; avoid in older clients
tolazamide (Tolinase)	3-4*	10-20	100-500 mg daily	Active metabolites may accumulate in renal failure
tolbutamide (Orinase)	3-4*	6-12	250 mg daily to 1000 mg twice daily	Short duration of action
SECOND-GENERATION SULFONYLUREA				
glimepiride (Amaryl)	2-3*	24	1-2 mg daily	Dose with first main meal of day
glipizide (Glucotrol, Glucotrol XL)	1-3* (XL 6-12*)	12-24	2.5-20 mg twice daily XL: 5-20 mg daily	Administer 30 minutes before meals
glyburide (DiaBeta, Micronase)	3-4*	24	1.25-20 mg daily	Active metabolite that may accumulate in renal failure
BIGUINIDE				
metformin (Glucophage)	2-3†	12-24†	500-1000 mg daily or twice daily (Maximum daily dose: 2550 mg)	Avoid in renal failure because of risk of lactic acidosis
α-GLUCOSIDASE INHIBITOR				
acarbose (Precose)	Not absorbed	8-12	50-100 mg three times daily	Initiate dose slowly to reduce gastrointestinal adverse effects
miglitol (Glyset)		8	25-100 mg three times daily	
MEGLITINIDE				
nateglinide (Starlix)	1*	<4	60-120 mg three times daily before meals	Administer 15 minutes before meals, weight gain, HF
repaglinide (Prandin)	1*	4	0.5-4 mg three times daily before meals	
THIAZOLIDINEDIONE				
pioglitazone (Actos)	2†	16-24†	15-45 mg daily	Monitor liver function, monitor for edema, weight gain, HF
rosiglitazone (Avandia)	1†	12-24†	2-4 mg twice daily (alt: 4-8 mg daily)	

*Also most likely period to experience hypoglycemia after dose, although may be prolonged in renal failure.
†Full therapeutic effect not noted for up to 3 months.

ter dosing, but may be delayed for clients in renal failure. Other adverse effects of the class are listed above.

Drug Interactions
Glyburide and glipizide are metabolized by cytochrome P450 2 C8/9 and may be affected by concurrently administered azole antifungals (itraconazole, fluconazole) or other drugs. Clinicians should check with appropriate references for interacting agents.

glipizide [glip ih zide]
(Glucotrol, Glucotrol XL)
Indications
Indications for glipizide are identical to glyburide.
Pharmacokinetics/Dosing
Insulin release and reductions in serum glucose are noted between 90 and 120 minutes after oral administration of immediate-release

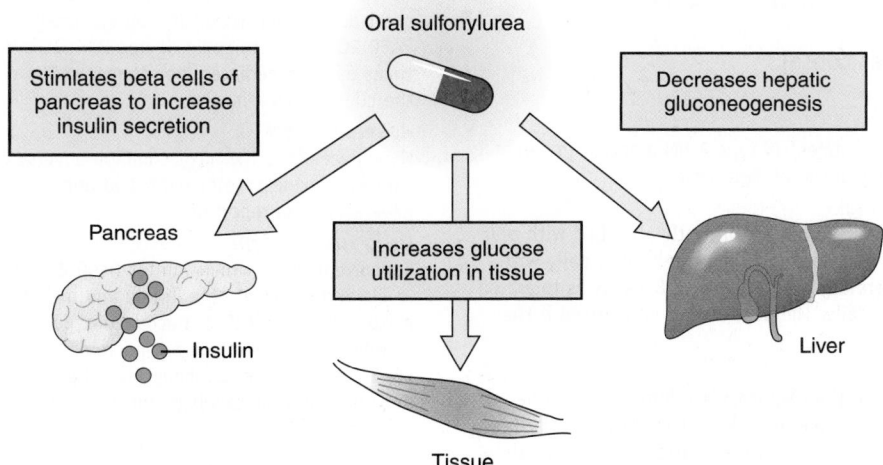

FIGURE 49-5 Mechanism of action of sulfonylureas.

FIGURE 49-5 Mechanism of action of sulfonylureas.

glyburide. Its duration of action is 18 to 24 hours and it is metabolized to inactive metabolites. Unlike with glyburide, glipizide is less likely to produce nocturnal hypoglycemia in clients with renal insufficiency.

Adverse Effects
As with glyburide, hypoglycemia is the most common adverse effect.

Drug Interactions
See glyburide.

Biguanides

The biguanides work to decrease hepatic glucose production. They also serve to improve the action of insulin at the cellular level and reduce GI carbohydrate absorption. Clients with obesity often respond well to biguanides. The first drug released in this chemical category was phenformin, but it was withdrawn from the market because of its association with lactic acidosis. Metformin (Glucophage) is the only biguanide currently available; it has been associated only rarely with lactic acidosis, which may be more likely in clients with renal insufficiency. Metformin, when used alone, rarely causes hypoglycemia. However, combination with other agents (e.g., sulfonylureas) can result in low blood glucose levels.

⭐ metformin [met **for** min]
(Glucophage, Glycon✤, Novo-Metformin✤)
Indications
Metformin is indicated as monotherapy or combined therapy with insulin or sulfonylureas for clients with type 2 DM. It is contraindicated for clients with renal insufficiency and is avoided in clients with uncontrolled HF. Metformin is also available combined with glyburide (Glucovance) and with glipizide (Metaglip).

Pharmacokinetics/Dosing
Metformin has a slow onset of action with response not noted for up to 14 days after initiation of therapy. Initial dosing is typically 500 mg once or twice daily with increases every 2 weeks until adequate response or maximum dose is reached (850 mg three times daily for immediate release or 1000 mg twice daily for sustained release).

Adverse Effects
The most serious (but rare) adverse effect of metformin is lactic acidosis. The risk is highest for clients with some degree of renal impairment. Symptoms of lactic acidosis include severe nausea, vomiting, abdominal pain, malaise, loss of appetite, and difficulty breathing. Such a constellation of symptoms should be reported to the prescriber at once. Other adverse effects include diarrhea, nausea/vomiting, and muscle weakness. Vitamin B_{12} deficiency has been occasionally reported with chronic therapy.

Drug Interactions
Use of contrast dyes in diagnostic imaging may increase the potential for lactic acidosis. Holding metformin doses prior to use of contrast dyes through 48 hours after completion of procedure is recommended. A number of other drugs have the potential to increase metformin levels, including furosemide, cimetidine, digoxin, morphine, procainamide, ranitidine, and vancomycin, but the clinical importance of these interactions is not clear. Drugs known to induce hyperglycemia such as corticosteroids, diuretics, and sympathomimetics may contribute to loss of glucose control with metformin therapy.

α-Glucosidase Inhibitors

Acarbose and miglitol are oral α-glucosidase inhibitors that delay the digestion and absorption of carbohydrates in the small intestine, thereby causing a smaller rise in blood glucose levels after food is ingested. These drugs do not increase insulin secretion or cause hypoglycemia, lactic acidosis, or weight gain. They may be given alone or in combination with a sulfonylurea to lower blood glucose.

The major drawback of these agents is GI effects including flatulence, abdominal cramping, and diarrhea, which are troublesome early in therapy for the majority of clients. Acarbose and miglitol are better tolerated if dosed at the beginning of meals and if therapy is started at low doses with dosage increases every 4 to 8 weeks as tolerated. Of note: the use of oral carbohydrates to treat hypoglycemia related to other drug therapy is often ineffective because these drugs inhibit intestinal absorption of carbohydrates. For clients on these agents, treatment of mild hypoglycemia may require higher doses of oral carbohydrates, or may require subcutaneous glucagon or IV dextrose.

✴🔳 acarbose [ah **kar** bohse]
(Precose, Prandase✤)

Indications
Acarbose is indicated for treatment of type 2 DM alone or in combination with insulin, sulfonylureas, or metformin.

Pharmacokinetics/Dosing
The α-glucosidase inhibitors are not significantly absorbed with oral administration. Typical initial dose is 25 mg three times daily with first bite of meal. Doses are adjusted every 4 to 8 weeks as tolerated up to 100 mg three times daily. The dose should be omitted if the client skips a meal.

Adverse Effects
The major adverse effects of the α-glucosidase inhibitors may be seen in the majority of clients and include abdominal pain, diarrhea and flatulence. These often improve over the first few weeks of therapy. Elevated liver enzymes have been rarely reported.

Drug Interactions
Acarbose may result in decreased absorption of digoxin. When used alone, hypoglycemia is rare. However, clients receiving agents which can produce hypoglycemia (e.g., insulin, sulfonylureas), hypoglycemia may be more likely and refractory to oral glucose replacement.

miglitol [**mig** lih toll]
(Glyset)

Indications
Miglitol is indicated as treatment for type 2 DM. It can be used alone or in combination with a sulfonylurea.

Pharmacokinetics/Dosing
Miglitol acts locally in the GI tract. It is dosed at 25 mg three times daily with the first bite of each meal, and doses are increased up to 100 mg three times daily as tolerated over 2 to 4 months. As with acarbose, omit dose if client misses a meal.

Adverse Effects
Adverse effects are similar to acarbose.

Drug Interactions
Interactions are similar to those with acarbose. Decreased absorption of digoxin, ranitidine, and propranolol is possible with the use of miglitol. Pancreatic enzymes reduce the efficacy of miglitol.

Meglitinides

Nateglinide and repaglinide are nonsulfonylurea hypoglycemic agents that stimulate pancreatic beta cells to produce insulin. They also improve insulin secretion in response to increased glucose levels by regulating the ATP-sensitive potassium channels on pancreatic beta cells. The drugs are shorter acting and are excreted faster than the oral sulfonylurea drugs; they produce a glucose control similar to therapy with glyburide. The rapid onset and short duration of action make them ideal for clients with irregular eating patterns, as the drug can be dosed immediately before meals. Adverse effects are similar to oral sulfonylureas with the exception of potential cardiovascular effects (e.g., hypertension, dysrhythmias) with repaglinide.

nateglinide [nah **teg** glih nide]
(Starlix)

Indications
Nateglinide is indicated for the management of type 2 DM as monotherapy or in combination with metformin or a glitazone.

Pharmacokinetics/Dosing
Nateglinide has a rapid onset of action (within 20 minutes) and a short duration of action (4 hours). Nateglinide is metabolized by P450 2C8/9 and to some degree 3A4. It is dosed at 60-120 mg three times daily immediately before meals. The dose should be omitted if the client skips a meal.

Adverse Effects
Hypoglycemia is the most common adverse effect of the meglitinides. Dizziness, joint pain, and upper respiratory tract infections have also been reported.

Drug Interactions
Concurrent drugs which inhibit P450 2 C8/9 may result in increased levels and effect of nateglinide and include nonsteroidal antiinflammatory drugs (NSAIDs), fluconazole, gemfibrozil, nicardipine, pioglitazone, and sulfonamide antimicrobials. Drugs that induce P450 2 C8/9 (carbamazepine, phenytoin, phenobarbital, rifampin) can produce increased metabolism and reduced levels and effect of nateglinide.

✴🔳 repaglinide [reh **pah** glih nide]
(Prandin)

Indications
Repaglinide indications are similar to nateglinide.

Pharmacokinetics/Dosing
Repaglinide produces increased insulin levels within the first hour after administration, and has a duration of action of about 4 hours. It is highly bound to plasma proteins. Repaglinide is primarily metabolized by P450 3A4 with some metabolism by 2 C8/9. Adult dosing is 0.5 to 4 mg three times daily immediately before each meal. Like with nateglinide, the dose is skipped for missed meals.

Adverse Effects
Like with nateglinide, hypoglycemia is possible. Other adverse effects include headache, respiratory tract infections, and altered liver function tests. Cardiac effects, including hypotension, chest pain, and cardiac dysrhythmias, have also been reported.

Drug Interactions
Drugs that inhibit P450 3A4 (fluconazole, erythromycin, clarithromycin) can result in increased levels and increase risk for hypoglycemia. Increased effect may also be noted when other highly plasma protein bound drugs (phenytoin, NSAIDS, warfarin) displace bound repaglinide. Increased effect of repaglinide is also noted with concurrent gemfibrozil. Cytochrome P450 3A4 enzyme inducers (carbamazepine, phenytoin, phenobarbital, rifampin) can result in reduced levels and effect of repaglinide.

Thiazolidinediones (Glitazones)

Troglitazone (Rezulin) was the first agent in a new classification of drugs that lowers insulin resistance in poorly controlled, type 2 DM. It was removed from the market because severe liver toxicity and fatalities were associated with its use. The other two drugs in this category, pioglitazone and rosiglitazone, appear to have the same benefits as troglitazone but produce less risk for severe liver toxicity. They are also equal in efficacy to metformin but are associated with edema and weight gain (Schernthaner, Matthews, Charbonnel, Hanefeld, Brunetti, 2005).

The mechanism of action of thiazolidinediones is totally different from all the other hypoglycemic agents. Pioglitazone and rosiglitazone appear to resensitize the body to its own insulin; they decrease insulin resistance in the periphery and liver, which results in an increase in glucose processing in the body. Be aware, however, that these agents are only indicated for clients with type 2 diabetes who can produce insulin.

Pioglitazone and rosiglitazone are potent agonists for peroxisome proliferator-activated receptors that are found in adipose tissue, skeletal muscle, and the liver. Activation of these receptors ultimately results in control of glucose production, transport and use in the body, and lipid metabolism. These actions are also likely contributory to its adverse effect profile.

Among the adverse effects of these agents are fluid retention, weight gain, and altered lipid levels. Fluid retention can precipitate or worsen HF and requires careful monitoring in clients who are predisposed to HF (Nesto et al., 2003). Headache, muscle discomfort, and hypoglycemia have also been reported. Although rare, the risk for serious hepatotoxicity is a concern for use. Blood testing for liver function should be performed before the start of therapy, every 2 months during the first year, and periodically thereafter (*Mosby's Drug Consult*, 2005).

✳⬛ rosiglitazone [rose ih **glit** ah zone]
(Avandia)
Indications
Rosiglitazone is indicated for monotherapy of type 2 DM. It is also used in combination with sulfonylureas, metformin, and/or insulin.
Pharmacokinetics/Dosing
Rosiglitazone is well absorbed orally and reaches peak serum levels in approximately 1 hour. It has a half-life between 3 and 4 hours and is excreted primarily by the kidneys. The usual adult monotherapy dosage for rosiglitazone is 4 mg daily or 2 mg twice daily. Full therapeutic effect of these agents may not be realized for up to 3 months. When rosiglitazone is combined with metformin, the initial dosage is 4 mg daily (or 2 mg twice daily), which may be increased if necessary after 3 months of therapy.
Adverse Effects
The most serious adverse effect of this class of drugs is hepatotoxicity which can potentially be life threatening. Although rare, hepatotoxicity may occur. Liver function should be monitored for clients receiving drugs in this class. Fluid retention is a troublesome adverse effect of rosiglitazone and may contribute to HF in some clients. Headache, muscle and back pain, upper respiratory tract infection, and anemia are also possible.
Drug Interactions
Rosiglitazone is metabolized by cytochrome P450 2 C8/9. Interactions with delavirdine, fluconazole, gemfibrozil, sulfonamides, antiepileptic drugs, and other drugs may be noted. Consult appropriate references.

pioglitazone [pie oh **glit** ah zone]
(Actos)
Indications
Pioglitazone shares the same indications as rosiglitazone.
Pharmacokinetics/Dosing
Pioglitazone is rapidly absorbed orally in the fasting state and reaches peak serum levels in 2 hours. It is highly protein bound to serum albumin. It is metabolized in the liver via P450 enzyme systems to active metabolites. Although a small amount of the drug is excreted by the kidneys unchanged, the primary source of excretion of the drug and metabolites is in bile and, ultimately, the feces. The usual adult dosage of pioglitazone is 15 to 45 mg once daily.
Adverse Effects
The adverse effects of pioglitazone are similar to rosiglitazone, and include the risk for hepatotoxicity. Other potential adverse effects include edema and HF, headache, myalgia, sinusitis, and upper respiratory infections.
Drug Interactions
Pioglitazone is metabolized by cytochrome P450 2C8/9, 3A4, inhibits the metabolism of other drugs metabolized by 2 C8/9 and

may induce the metabolism of drugs metabolized by 3A4. As such, a number of potential interactions exist. Increased levels and effect of pioglitazone may be noted when administered with fluconazole, itraconazole, gemfibrozil, nicardipine, NSAIDs, and sulfonamide antimicrobials. Reduced pioglitazone levels may be expected with concurrent enzyme inducers such as carbamazepine, phenytoin, phenobarbital, and rifampin Consult appropriate references for specific interactions.

Noninsulin Polypeptide Analogues

Two injectable polypeptide analogues were approved by the FDA in 2005 for additional glycemic control in clients with poorly controlled DM.

Pramlintide acetate (Symlin) is a synthetic analogue of amylin, a neuroendocrine hormone synthesized by pancreatic beta cells and released shortly after eating. Amylin slows gastric emptying time, suppresses the release of glucagon, and appears to suppress appetite. As a polypeptide, it is not stable in gastric acid and requires subcutaneous injection. Serious hypoglycemic events in combination with insulin have been reported in clients with type 1 DM. Overall changes in A1C levels in both type 1 and type 2 DM are modest (typically in the range of a decline of 0.3% to 0.6% at 6 months) (Ratner et al., 2005). Given its risks for acute hypoglycemic reactions, modest overall benefit with ongoing use, and three-times-daily subcutaneous injection, its role in treatment appears limited to clients who do not obtain glycemic control with conventional therapy.

Exenatide (Byetta) is a glucagon-like peptide-1 (GLP-1) receptor agonist. Incretin, including GLP-1, assists in the control of blood glucose via augmentation of gastric emptying time, hepatic gluconeogenesis, appetite, and secretion of both insulin and glucagon. Exenatide was originally identified from venom found in the saliva of the Gila monster lizard, which eats only four times per year and secretes exenatide to stimulate pancreatic action. As with pramlintide, its benefit is modest (typical decline of 0.4% to 0.9% in A1C, and dosing is subcutaneous (DeFronzo et al., 2005; Kendall et al., 2005; Buse et al., 2004). It is indicated only for clients with type 2 DM not controlled with conventional oral therapy.

pramlintide acetate [**pram** lin tide]
Symlin
Indications
Pramlintide is indicated as adjunct treatment in type 1 DM for clients who have not obtained adequate glycemic control with insulin therapy and for clients with type 2 DM who have not obtained adequate glycemic control with insulin with or without oral therapy. Because of its ability to slow gastric emptying time, it is contraindicated for clients with diabetic gastroparesis. It is also avoided in clients who have exhibited significant hypoglycemic reactions or who are not able to recognize and manage hypoglycemic reactions.
Pharmacokinetics/Dosing
After subcutaneous injection to the abdomen or thigh, about 30% to 40% of the administered dose is absorbed systemically with a maximum effect observed in 20 minutes. Pramlintide is metabolized in the kidney with an elimination half-life of about 50 minutes. For clients with type 1 DM, pramlintide is initiated at a dose of 15 mcg subcutaneously immediately before major meals, and concurrent short-acting insulin doses are reduced by 50%. Further doses of in-

sulin are pramlintide are titrated, with doses of pramlintide increased to 30 mcg, 45 mcg, or 60 mcg as tolerated. For clients with type 2 DM, initial doses of 60 mcg subcutaneously immediately before major meals are used. As with type 1 clients, concurrent short-acting insulin doses are reduced by 50%, and doses of insulin and pramlintide are titrated to effect. Doses as high as 120 mcg subcutaneously before meals have been used with type 2 DM. Pramlintide must be administered separately from insulin. It is not compatible when mixed with insulins. Its use in children has not been established.

Adverse Effects
The most serious adverse effect of pramlintide is hypoglycemia and limits its use. Other adverse effects include nausea, vomiting, headache, joint pain, and hypersensitivity reactions.

Drug Interactions
Increased risk for hypoglycemia is noted when pramlintide is administered with insulin. Hypoglycemia may be more pronounced when used with other hypoglycemic agents such as oral sulfonylureas. The use of other drugs that slow gastric emptying time should be used cautiously for clients receiving pramlintide. Such agents include metoclopramide and drugs with anticholinergic (antimuscarinic) activity. Delayed absorption of other orally administered drugs is possible.

exenatide [ex **en** ah tide]
(Byetta)
Indications
Exenatide is indicated for clients with type 2 DM who are not adequately controlled with oral therapy. It is not indicated for clients with type 1 DM.

Pharmacokinetics/Dosing
Peak plasma levels are achieved 2 hours after subcutaneous injection of exenatide. It is eliminated primarily via glomerular filtration with an elimination half-life of 2.4 hours.

The initial adult dose is 5 mcg administered subcutaneously twice daily within 60 minutes before breakfast and again before the evening meal. Doses of concurrently administered sulfonylureas should be reduced with initial dosing to prevent hypoglycemia, with subsequent doses of sulfonylureas titrated to response. Based on response, the dose can be increased up to 10 mcg twice daily after 1 month. It is available as a 5 mcg/1.2 mL and a 10 mcg/2.4 mL prefilled injection pen. Data are not available for compatibility when mixed with insulins. As such, exenatide should be administered separately from insulin.

Adverse Effects
As with pramlintide, hypoglycemia is the most common adverse effect. Other adverse outcomes with therapy include nausea, vomiting, hypersensitivity reactions, and headache.

Drug Interactions
Concurrent insulin or sulfonylurea therapy may lead to increased risk for hypoglycemic reactions. As with pramlintide, gastric emptying time may be reduced. Precautions should be observed for clients receiving metoclopramide or anticholinergic therapy or drugs for which delay in oral absorption may be important.

✱ **T.L. is started on metformin (Glucophage) 500 mg daily with increases to 1000 mg twice daily over the following 8 weeks. Hemoglobin A1C levels decline from 9.5% to 7.9% by 3 months time. After an additional month of monitoring, glyburide (Micronase) 5 mg daily is added.**

Assessment Determine T.L.'s level of knowledge for health maintenance related to DM and the prescribed oral antidiabetic. Provide or reinforce information related to compliance with the appropriate ADA diet for ideal weight attainment, weight monitoring, activity program, stress management, cardiovascular risk factors, and adverse signs and symptoms

to report to the health care provider.

The oral hypoglycemic agents are contraindicated for clients who have rapidly changing insulin needs or conditions that cause severe blood glucose fluctuations such as those undergoing major surgery or those with diabetic coma, ketoacidosis, significant ketosis or acidosis, severe burns, infection, or trauma. The sulfonylureas are used with caution in clients with conditions causing delayed food absorption (severe diarrhea, gastroparesis, intestinal obstruction, prolonged vomiting), hyperglycemia-causing conditions (hyperadrenalism, fever, infection), hypoglycemia-causing conditions (adrenal or pituitary insufficiency, malnutrition), or impairment of thyroid, renal, or hepatic function. Because of the antidiuretic effects of chlorpropamide and tolbutamide, the use of other oral hypoglycemic agents should be considered in clients with cardiac impairment or fluid retention. Metformin is not used if T.L. has any condition that may contribute to lactic acidosis, such as hepatic disease, uncontrolled HF, or decreased renal function.

For younger female clients, pregnancy or potential for pregnancy is an important consideration in both the etiology of DM and its management. See the Pregnancy Safety box below.

T.L.'s sensitivity to sulfonylurea agents, sulfonamides, or thiazide-type diuretics needs to be determined because of their cross-sensitivity with the sulfonylureas or to metformin.

Review T.L.'s current medication regimen for the risk of significant drug interactions, such as those that may occur when the oral hypoglycemic agents are given with alcohol; it may result in increased risk of hypoglycemia and the combination of alcohol and metformin may predispose her to increased blood lactate levels. Oral anticoagulants may prolong the half-life of sulfonylureas causing hypoglycemia, but less of this effect is seen with glyburide. Monitor closely, because one or both drugs may require a dosage adjustment. β-adrenergic blocking agents (including ophthalmics) may inhibit insulin-secretion. This may increase the risk of hyperglycemia or blunt the symptoms of hypoglycemia with the sulfonylureas. Antifungals, chloramphenicol (Chloromycetin), guanethidine (Ismelin), insulin, monoamine oxidase (MAO) inhibitors, cimetidine or ranitidine, fluoroquinolones, sulfonamides and large doses of salicylates or sulfonamides may result in an increase in the hypoglycemic effect of the sulfonylureas; monitor closely, because dosage adjustments may be necessary. As-

PREGNANCY SAFETY DRUGS AFFECTING THE PANCREAS	
Category	**Drug**
B	acarbose, glucagon, insulin, miglitol
C	acetohexamide, chlorpropamide, diazoxide, exenatide, glimepiride, glipizide, glyburide, metformin, nateglinide, pioglitazone, pramlintide, repaglinide, rosiglitazone, tolazamide, tolbutamide

Data from *Mosby's drug consult* (15th ed.). (2005). St. Louis, Mosby.

paraginase, corticosteroids, thiazide diuretics, and lithium have hyperglycemic activity and may require higher dosages of sulfonylurea antidiabetic agents. A baseline assessment of the client is the same as for insulin administration.

Nursing Diagnosis While T.L. is receiving sulfonylurea oral hypoglycemic agents, she may experience the following nursing diagnoses/collaborative problems: diarrhea or constipation; impaired comfort such as headache, heartburn, nausea, vomiting, abdominal discomfort, rash, and photosensitivity; and the potential complications of hypoglycemia, agranulocytosis, aplastic or hemolytic anemia, eosinophilia, thrombocytopenia, and hepatic function impairment. With metformin, impaired comfort (heartburn, flatulence, headache, metallic taste, anorexia) and the potential complications of anemia and lactic acidosis (diarrhea, shortness of breath, muscle pain, fatigue) may occur.

Planning See Box 49-3.

Implementation

Monitoring Remember that T.L. requires close supervision, especially when an oral hypoglycemic agent is tried for the first time. When converting from insulin to an oral hypoglycemic agent for the control of diabetic status, monitor T.L.'s blood glucose levels at least three times daily before meals. A1C is recommended every 3 months.

No transition period is usually required when changing from one sulfonylurea agent to metformin or another sulfonylurea agent (except with chlorpropamide). With chlorpropamide, caution should be exercised during the first 2 weeks because of its prolonged half-life of 25 to 60 hours. Older adults tend to be more sensitive to the effects of the sulfonylureas as oral hypoglycemic agents. Because hypoglycemia may be more difficult to recognize in these clients, they require lower dosages and closer monitoring.

Observe for hypoglycemia in T.L. who is taking sulfonylureas and if she has irregular meal patterns, exercises more than usual, or ingests significant amounts of alcohol; hypoglycemia is more likely. A moderate lifestyle is essential to diabetes management. Periods of physiologic or psychologic stress may necessitate a temporary use of insulin. See the section for client monitoring of insulin therapy on pp. 869-871.

Intervention See Table 49-3 for the pharmacokinetics, typical doses and peak effects of the oral agents. Metformin may be added to maximum-dose sulfonylurea therapy and vice versa, with the dosage of the new drug gradually titrated upward. If high-dose combination therapy is not effective in controlling T.L.'s blood glucose in 3 months, the prescriber and T.L. may consider other oral agents, but the addition of insulin to oral therapy may be needed to improve glycemic control (Janka, 2005; Raskin, 2005).

Education Recognize that the need for instruction that stresses dietary restriction is important for all clients with DM. Diets low in refined carbohydrates may help control blood glucose, but clients should be cautioned against diets high in saturated fats, which could contribute to increased cardiovascular risk. Clients who are more than 20% over their ideal weight may not respond to oral hypoglycemic agents. T.L. should keep a weight record and weigh in once a week at the same time using the same scale. Teach T.L. about blood glucose testing, proper skin care, and the signs and symptoms of hypoglycemia and hyperglycemia.

Caution T.L. about excessive alcohol intake (and medications containing alcohol) when sulfonylurea therapy is begun. Alcohol can increase the rate of metabolism of these drugs when there is long-term consumption of excessive quantities of these drugs. Additionally, a disulfiram-like reaction with nausea and flushing on ingestion of alcohol may occur with the sulfonylureas. Also alert T.L. that some complementary and alternative therapies may interact with her medication regimen and so affect her blood glucose values. See the Complementary and Alternative Considerations box below.

Blood glucose testing should be performed at frequent intervals as recommended by the prescriber. during the transition period when clients are switched from insulin to oral hypoglycemic agents. Teach T.L. to carry or have access to some form of glucose at all times.

Have T.L. take her glyburide in the morning to minimize the risk of nocturnal hypoglycemia; it may be given with food to decrease any gastric upset.

Evaluation The expected outcome of T.L.'s oral antidiabetic agent therapy is that her blood glucose level will remain within normal limits, and she will manage the therapeutic oral hypoglycemic regimen effectively. See the Nursing Care Plan on p. 870 for additional outcome criteria.

✳ **K.S. is a 34-year-old male with a 28-year history of type 1 DM. He is admitted to the ED in a nonresponsive state accompanied by his wife. His wife states he gave himself an injection of insulin about 1 hour ago, and missed his breakfast. He has no history of ethanol abuse. His blood glucose level is 24 g/L. The ED physician orders dextrose 25 grams IV as a 50% solution and glucagon 1 mg IV × 1.**

✲ Complementary and Alternative Considerations

Herbal Interactions with Hypoglycemics

Insulin, acetohexamide, chlorpropamide, glipizide, metformin, tolazamide, tolbutamide, pioglitazone, and rosiglitazone may interact with the following to enhance hypoglycemic effects. Monitor closely:

bilberry	garlic
bitter melon	*Panax ginseng*
Coccinia indica	

Data from Memorial Sloan-Kettering Cancer Center. (2005). About herbs. Retrieved July 25, 2005, from http://www.mskcc.org.

✷ What agents are available to treat severe hypoglycemia?

Box 49-5 presented symptoms of hypoglycemia. As noted above, treatment of mild hypoglycemia can be achieved by the administration of rapidly absorbed carbohydrates (see Box 49-6), although this intervention is not appropriate if the client has altered mental status, and may be less successful if the client is receiving an α-glucosidase inhibitor like acarbose or miglitol.

For significant hypoglycemic reactions, glucagon or IV dextrose is indicated. In Canada, oral diazoxide is also available.

✷💊 glucagon [**gloo** ka gon]

Glucagon (for injection) is a natural polypeptide hormone secreted by pancreatic alpha cells in response to hypoglycemia. It is released to maintain plasma levels of glucose by stimulating hepatic glycogenolysis and **gluconeogenesis** (the conversion of glycerol and amino acids to glucose) and by the inhibition of glycogen synthesis. The effect of glucagon is accelerated by stimulating the synthesis of cyclic adenosine monophosphate (cAMP). Hepatic and adipose tissue lipolysis is enhanced by activating adenyl cyclase, which produces free fatty acids and glycerol and stimulates ketogenesis and gluconeogenesis.

Indications

Glucagon is indicated for the treatment of severe hypoglycemia in clients with diabetes and as an adjunct for GI radiography. It is useful in hypoglycemia only if liver glycogen is available; thus it is ineffective in chronic hypoglycemia, starvation, and adrenal insufficiency. Glucagon is also used as an adjunct to barium in GI radiography. It decreases peristalsis and produces relaxation of the esophagus, stomach, duodenum, small bowel, and colon (hypotonicity), thus improving outcome of the examination. It is also used as a cardiac stimulant for overdose of β-adrenergic blockers.

Pharmacokinetics/Dosing

Parenterally administered (intramuscular [IM], IV, or subcutaneous), glucagon has a half-life of 10 minutes. The onset of action (hyperglycemic) depends on the route of administration: IV, 5 to 20 minutes; IM, 15 minutes; subcutaneous, 30 to 45 minutes. The duration of action is 1.5 hours. It is metabolized in the liver and excreted by the kidneys. The adolescent and adult dosage of glucagon for hypoglycemia is 0.5 to 1 mg IM, IV, or subcutaneous, repeated in 20 minutes when necessary. The pediatric dosage is 0.5 to 1 mg (IM, IV, or subcutaneous).

Adverse Effects

The adverse effects of glucagon are not usually severe and may include nausea or vomiting and an allergic reaction. No significant drug interactions have been reported.

dextrose 50% (25 grams/50 mL)

Indications

Intravenous dextrose 50% is indicated for management of hypoglycemia in clients with altered mental status.

Pharmacokinetics/Dosing

Dextrose 50% is a hypertonic solution that reverses hypoglycemia almost immediately. The adult dose is 12.5 to 25 grams IV at 10 mL/min with repeat doses as indicated. It can be irritating to the vein, and is administered by slow IV in the largest vein possible. Aspiration of blood during set up for the administration of dextrose 50% is recommended to assure vein patency.

Adverse Effects

Extravasation to surrounding tissue may lead to tissue necrosis. In clients who are thiamine deficient (e.g., history of ethanol abuse), it may precipitate Wernicke encephalopathy. For such clients, concurrent administration of thiamine 100 mg IV is indicated.

diazoxide [dye ah **zocks** eyd]
(Proglycem✤)

Oral diazoxide produces a prompt, dose-related increase in blood glucose levels by inhibiting the release of pancreatic insulin. It may also have an extrapancreatic effect.

Indications

Oral diazoxide is indicated for the treatment of hypoglycemia caused by hyperinsulinism, secondary to an inoperable islet cell adenoma or carcinoma, an extrapancreatic malignancy, or an islet cell hyperplasia. It is not indicated for treatment in functional hypoglycemia. It is also available in Canada as a parenteral dosage form to treat hypertensive emergencies.

Pharmacokinetics/Dosing

Under normal conditions, diazoxide is rapidly absorbed orally, has an onset of action within 1 hour, a duration of effect less than 8 hours, and a half-life between 20 and 36 hours. It is highly protein bound, metabolized in the liver, and excreted by the kidneys. The adult dosage of diazoxide is 1 mg/kg PO every 8 hours, with dosage adjustments as necessary. The maintenance dosage is 3 to 8 mg/kg PO daily, which is divided into 2 or 3 equal doses and administered every 8 or 12 hours. The maximum dosage is usually 15 mg/kg/day.

Adverse Effects

The adverse effects of diazoxide include taste alterations, constipation, anorexia, nausea, vomiting, and abdominal pain. With chronic use it may cause increased hair growth on the arms, legs, back, and forehead (hypertrichosis). The most commonly reported adverse effects include a decrease in urine output that results in edema of the hands, feet, or lower extremities; weight gain; and possibly HF in susceptible individuals. Hyperglycemia or ketoacidosis are typical symptoms of a diazoxide overdose.

✷ The nurse for K.S. prepares and administers dextrose 25 grams IV as a 50% solution and glucagon 1 mg IV × 1.

✷ What are the nursing management issues with the use of these agents to reverse hypoglycemia?

Assessment It is important to recognize the symptoms of hypoglycemia: anxiousness, irritability, altered mood, nervousness, weakness, shakiness, inability to concentrate, perspiration, cool/pale skin, hunger, nausea, headache before the client loses consciousness. A rapid blood glucose level may be obtained to confirm the hypoglycemia. In K.S.'s case, his hypoglycemia progressed rapidly to unconsciousness.

Nursing Diagnosis The client may develop impaired comfort (nausea and vomiting) as a result of the underlying hypoglycemia or glucagon overdose, and there is also the potential complication of allergic reaction or severe hypoglycemia because of ineffectiveness of the drug.

Planning While having glucagon therapy, K.S. will:
- Remain free of symptoms of hypoglycemia.
- Describe the effects and complications of diabetes and reportable symptoms for the health care provider (hypoglycemia, hyperglycemia, ketoacidosis).
- State the management of glucagon for hypoglycemia.
- Effectively manage the therapeutic regimen including self-monitored blood glucose testing and interpretation, and other monitoring.

Implementation

Monitoring Check K.S.'s blood glucose level throughout the hypoglycemic episode, after administration, and for 3 to 4 hours after he regains consciousness. Note his clinical response; monitor his vital signs and level of consciousness.

Intervention Glucagon is administered for hypoglycemia in the unconscious client as directed by the prescriber. After administering, turn the individual on one side to prevent choking and/or aspiration. If hypoglycemia occurs out of the hospital setting, emergency medical assistance should be obtained as quickly as possible. If the client does not regain consciousness in 5 to 20 minutes, administer a second dose and transport the client to the hospital. IV glucose needs to be started if the individual does not respond to the second dose of glucagon. Glucagon and glucose may be given at the same time.

When K.S. regains consciousness and can swallow, offer some oral form of sugar followed by a more complex carbohydrate, such as crackers and cheese or a glass of milk. This helps to prevent a recurrence of hypoglycemia before the next meal. If K.S. is experiencing nausea and vomiting that prevents food intake for more than an hour after the administration of glucagon, notify the physician.

Medical follow-up is necessary for all clients who experience a hypoglycemic episode as a result of oral antidiabetic agents.

Education Before the need arises to use glucagon, teach the family and the client how to mix the drug and how to inject it properly. A standard insulin syringe may be used for injection unless the dose is greater than the capacity of the syringe. The injection should be made at a 90-degree angle instead of the usual subcutaneous approach. Advise the client and family to keep supplies on hand and check the expiration dates frequently. If used, replace the client's supply of glucagon as soon as possible.

Instruct the client and family about the symptoms of hypoglycemia and the importance of ingesting some form of sugar when symptoms first occur, such as orange juice, honey, syrup, hard candy, sugar cubes, or milk.

Evaluation The expected outcome of glucagon therapy is that K.S.'s blood glucose level will be within normal limits. The client and family will state an understanding of the effective management of glucagon therapy and will successfully demonstrate administration techniques. See the Nursing Care Plan for additional outcome criteria on p. 870.

Summary

The two primary hormones released by the pancreas are insulin and glucagon. When blood glucose falls, glucagon is released; this facilitates the catabolism of glycogen stored in the liver, which increases blood glucose. The release of glucagon stimulates the secretion of insulin, which inhibits the release of glucagon and maintains the homeostasis of carbohydrate metabolism.

DM is a disorder of carbohydrate metabolism that results from an insulin deficiency, a resistance, or both. DM is classified as type 1 (formerly insulin-dependent) DM, and type 2 (formerly non–insulin-dependent) DM. Although type 2 may require insulin at some time, it is usually managed by dietary treatment, weight reduction, client education and, if necessary, oral hypoglycemic agents.

Insulin may be rapid-, intermediate-, or long-acting. Therapeutic dosages are not fixed but are set in response to blood glucose levels, considering the client's dietary intake and physical activity. Client education is essential so the client can participate in ascertaining the necessary insulin dosage through blood testing and can self-administer insulin safety and accurately.

Oral antidiabetic agents have a variety of mechanisms of action. They can encourage the release of insulin from the pancreas, decrease glycogenolysis and gluconeogenesis, increase the sensitivity of body tissues to insulin, and decrease the absorption of carbohydrates from the gastrointestinal tract, but all are used for type 2 DM. Choice of agent is based on likely client response and tolerability of therapy.

Hyperglycemic agents are used in the treatment of hypoglycemia in which the client is unable to ingest sufficient amounts of glucose to meet body requirements.

✴ Critical Thinking Questions

- Sally Milton, 59 years old, was diagnosed with type 2 DM 6 years ago. In the past, her blood glucose control has been managed by weight loss and diet. She has just started treatment with glipizide (Glucotrol XL), 5 mg PO daily. She confides in you, "I'm pleased to be starting on the pills. I was tired of watching my diet." How should you respond?

- Loretta Baxter, 45 years old with type 1 DM, is admitted to the hospital. She is placed on a 1500-calorie ADA diet and prescribed 30 units of NPH insulin to be taken at 7 AM each morning. At 4 PM, she becomes diaphoretic, weak, and pale. What action should you take? What explanation will you provide Ms. Baxter about what has occurred?

Bibliography

Altshuler, D., Hirschhorn, J.N., Klannemark, M., Lindgren, C.M., Vohl, M.C., & Nemesh, J., et al. (2000). The common PPARgamma Pro12 Ala polymorphism is associated with decreased risk of type 2 diabetes. *Nature Genetics, 26,* 76–80.

American Diabetes Association. (2004). *Diabetes Statistics.* Retrieved July 25, 2005, from www.diabetes.org/diabetes-statistics.jsp.

Anderson, D.M., Keith, J., & Novak, P.D. (Eds.) (2002). *Mosby's medical, nursing, and allied health dictionary* (6th ed.). St. Louis: Mosby.

Babu, A.R., Herdegen, J., Fogelfeld, L., Shott, S., & Mazzone, T. (2005). Type 2 diabetes, glycemic control, and continuous positive airway pressure in obstructive sleep apnea. *Archives of Internal Medicine, 165,* 447-452.

Bates, D.W. (2002). Unexpected hypoglycemia in a critically ill patient. *Annals of Internal Medicine, 137,* 110-116.

Bosker, G. (Ed.). (2004). *Primary and acute care medicine: Practice, protocols, pathways,* (2nd ed.). Atlanta: Thomson American Health Consultants.

Budnick, D.S., Pollack, D.A., Memdelsohn, A.B., Weidenbach, K.N., McDonald, A.K., & Aunest, J.L. (2005). Emergency department visits for outpatient adverse drug events: Demonstration for a national surveillance system. *Annals of Emergency Medicine, 45*(2), 197-206.

Buse, J.B., Henry, R.R., Han, J., Kim, D.D., Fineman, M.S., Baron, A.D., et al.; Exanatide-113 Clinical Study Group. (2004). Effects of exenatide (exendin-4) on glycemic control over 30 weeks in sulfonylurea-treated patients with type 2 diabetes. *Diabetes Care, 27,* 2628-2635.

Carlisle, B.A., Kroon, L.A., & Koda-Kimble, M.A. (2005). Diabetes mellitus. In M.A. Koda-Kimble, L.Y. Young, W.A. Kradian & B.J. Guglielmo (Eds.), *Applied therapeutics: The clinical use of drugs* (8th ed.). Vancouver, WA: Applied Therapeutics.

Clement, S., Braithwaite, S.S., Magee, M.F., Ahmann, A., Smith, E.P., & Schafer, R.G., et al. (2004). Management of diabetes and hyperglycemia in hospitals, *Diabetes Care, 27,* 553-591.

Davis, S.N., & Granner, D.K. (2001). Insulin, Oral Hypoglycemic Agents, and the Pharmacology of the Endocrine Pancreas. In: J.G. Hardman & L.E. Limbird (Eds.), *Goodman & Gilman's The pharmacological basis of therapeutics* (10th ed.). New York: McGraw-Hill.

DeFronzo, R.A., Ratner, R.E., Han, J., Kim, D.D., Fineman, M.S., & Baron, A.D., (2005). Effects of exenatide (exendin-4) on glycemic control over 30 weeks in metformin-treated patients with type 2 diabetes. *Diabetes Care, 28,* 1092-1100.

Doney, A., Fischer, B., Leese, G., Morris, A.D., & Palmer, C. (2004). Cardiovascular Risk in Type 2 Diabetes Is Associated With Variation at the PPARG Locus: A Go-DARTS Study. *Arteriosclerosis, Thrombosis & Vascular Biology, 24*(12), 2403-2407.

Drug facts and comparisons (58th ed.). (2005). St. Louis: Facts and Comparisons.

Dunn, C.M. (2002). Assessing and Preventing Medication Interactions. *Home Healthcare Nurse, 20*(2), 104-112.

Fernandez-Real, J.M., Penarroja, G., Richart, C., Castro, A., Vendrell, J., & Broch, M., et al. (2003). G Protein β3 Gene Variant, Vascular Function, and Insulin Sensitivity in Type 2 Diabetes. *Hypertension, 41*(1), 124-129.

Fitzgerald, P.A. (2003). Endocrinology. In L.M. Tierney, Jr., S.J. McPhee & M.A. Papadakis (Ed.), *Current Medical Diagnosis & Treatment.* New York: Lange Medical Books/McGraw-Hill.

Gaede, P., Vedel, P., Larsen, N., Jensen, G.V., Parving, H.H., & Pedersen, O. (2003). Multifactorial intervention and cardiovascular disease in patients with type 2 diabetes. *New England Journal of Medicine, 348,* 383-393.

Janka, H.U., Plewe, G., Riddle, M.C., Kliebe-Frisch, C., Schweitzer, M.A., Yki-Jarvinen, H. (2005). Comparison of basal insulin added to oral agents versus twice-daily premixed insulin as initial insulin therapy for type 2 diabetes. *Diabetes Care, 28,* 254-259.

Kendall, D.M., Riddle, M.C., Rosenstock, J., Zhuang, D., Kim, D.D., Fineman, M.S., et al. (2005). Effects of exenatide (exendin-4) on glycemic control over 30 weeks in patients with type 2 diabetes treated with metformin and a sulfonylurea. *Diabetes Care, 28,* 1083-1091.

Kent, S.C., Chen, Y., Bregoli, L., Clemmings, S.M., Kenyon, N.S., Ricordi, C., et al. (2005). Expanded T cells from pancreatic lymph nodes of type 1 diabetic subjects recognize an insulin epitope. *Nature, 435,* 224-228.

Lacy, C.F., Armstrong, L.L., Goldman, M.P., & Lance, L.L. (2004). *Lexi-Comp's Drug Information Handbook* (12th ed.). Hudson, Ohio: Lexi-Comp.

Lee, C.R., Goldstein, J.A., & Pieper, J.A. (2002). Cytochrome P450 2 C9 polymorphisms: a comprehensive review of the in-vitro and human data. *Pharmacogenetics, 12*(3), 251-263.

Lee, W.M. (2003). Medical Progress: Drug-Induced Hepatotoxicity. *New England Journal of Medicine, 349*(5), 474-485.

Meirhaeghe, A., Fajas, L., Helbecque, N., Cottel, D., Auwerx, J., & Deeb, S.S., et al. (2000). Impact of the Peroxisome Proliferator Activated Receptor gamma2 Pro12 Ala polymorphism on adiposity, lipids and non-insulin-dependent diabetes mellitus. *International Journal of Obesity and Related Metabolic Disorders, 24,* 195–199.

Metchick, L.N., Petit, Jr., W.A., & Inzucchi, S.E. (2002). Inpatient management of diabetes mellitus. *American Journal of Medicine, 113*(4), 317-323.

Mosby's drug consult (15th ed.). (2005). St. Louis: Mosby.

Murphy, N.P., Keane, S.M., Ong, K.K., Ford-Adams, M., Edge, J.A. & Acerini, C.L., et al. (2003). Randomized cross-over trial of insulin glargine plus lispro or NPH insulin plus regular human insulin in adolescents with type 1 diabetes on intensive insulin regimens. *Diabetes Care, 26,* 799-804.

Nakayama, M., Abiru, N., Moriyama, H., Babaya, N., Liu, E., Miao, D., et al. (2005). Prime role for an insulin epitope in the development of type 1 diabetes in NOD mice. *Nature, 435,* 220-223.

National Center for Health Statistics. (2004). Access July 25, 2005, at http://www.cdc.gov/nchs/fastats/deaths.htm.

National Statistics and Opportunities for Improved Surveillance, Prevention, and Control. (1999). Diabetes in Canada. Retrieved July 25, 2005, from http://www.phac-aspc.gc.ca/publicat/dic-dac99/d16_e.html.

Nesto, R.W., Bell, D., Bonow, R.O., Fonseca, V., Grundy, S.M., & Horton, E.S., et al., and the American Heart Association; American Diabetes Association. (2003). Thiazolidinedione use, fluid retention, and congestive heart failure: A consensus statement from the American Heart Association and American Diabetes Association. *Circulation, 108,* 2941-2948.

e-LEARNING SUPPLEMENTS

Student CD-ROM
- Final Exam questions
- NCLEX® Examination review questions
- Pharmacology animations
- Printable chapter summary

Evolve Website (http://evolve.elsevier.com/mckenry)
- Case study on drugs affecting the pancreas
- Interactive concept map on type 2 diabetes

- Content updates, including information on new drugs
- WebLinks corresponding to this chapter
- Answers to the critical thinking questions in this chapter
- *Elsevier ePharmacology Update* newsletter
- Mosby's Drug Consult Internet Edition
- Supplemental and reference information

Oki, J.C., & Isley, W.L. (2002). Diabetes mellitus. In J.T. DiPiro, R.L. Talbert, G.C. Yee, G.R. Matzke, B.G. Wells, & L.M. Posey (Eds.), *Pharmacotherapy: A Pathophysiological Approach* (5th ed.). New York: McGraw-Hill.

Pereira, M.A., Kartashov, A.I., Ebbeling, C.B., Van Horn, L., Slattery, M.L., Jacobs, D.R., et al. (2005). Fast-food habits, weight gain, and insulin resistance (the CARDIA study): 15-year prospective analysis. *Lancet, 365,* 36-42.

Ragone, M., & Lando, H. (2002). Errors of insulin commission? *Clinical Diabetes, 20,* 221-222.

Raskin, P., Allen, E., Hollander, P., Lewin, A., Gabbay, R.A., Hu, P., et al; INITIATE Study Group. (2005). Initiating insulin therapy in type 2 diabetes: A comparison of biphasic and basal insulin analogs. *Diabetes Care, 28,* 260-265.

Ratner, R.E., Hirsch, I.B., Neifing, J.L., Garg, S.K., Mecca, T.E., & Wilson, C.A. (2000). Less hypoglycemia with insulin glargine in intensive insulin therapy for type 1 diabetes. U.S. Study Group of Insulin Glargine in Type 1 Diabetes. *Diabetic Care, 23,* 639-643.

Ratner, R., Whitehouse, F., Fineman, M.S., Strobel, S., Shen, L., Maggs, D.G., et al. (2005). Adjunctive therapy with pramlintide lower HbA$_{1c}$ without concomitant weight gain and increased risk of severe hypoglycemia in patients with type 1 diabetes approaching glycemic targets. *Experimental and Clinical Endocrinology and Diabetes, 113*(4), 119-204.

Rosskopf, D., Manthey, I., & Siffert, W. (2002). Identification and ethnic distribution of major haplotypes in the gene GNB3 encoding the G-protein β3 subunit. *Pharmacogenetics, 12*(3), 209-220.

Schernthaner, G., Matthews, D.R., Charbonnel, B., Hanefeld, M., Brunetti, P.; Quartet Study Group. (2004). Efficacy and safety of pioglitazone versus metformin in patients with type 2 diabetes mellitus: A double-blind, randomized trial. *Journal of Clinical Endocrinology and Metabolism, 89,* 6068-6076.

Schnell, Z.B., Van Leeuwen, A.M., & Kranpitz. (2003). *Davis' Comprehensive handbook of laboratory and diagnostic tests with nursing implications.* Philadelphia: F.A. Davis Company.

Tesfave, S., Chaturvedi, N., Eaton, S.E., Ward, J.D., Manes, C., Ionescu-Tirgoviste, C., et al.; EURODIAB Prospective Complications Study Group. (2005). Vascular risk factors and diabetic neuropathy. *New England Journal of Medicine, 352,* 341-350.

USP DI: Drug information for the health care professional (25th ed.). (2005). Greenwood Village, CO: MICROMEDEX Thomson Healthcare.

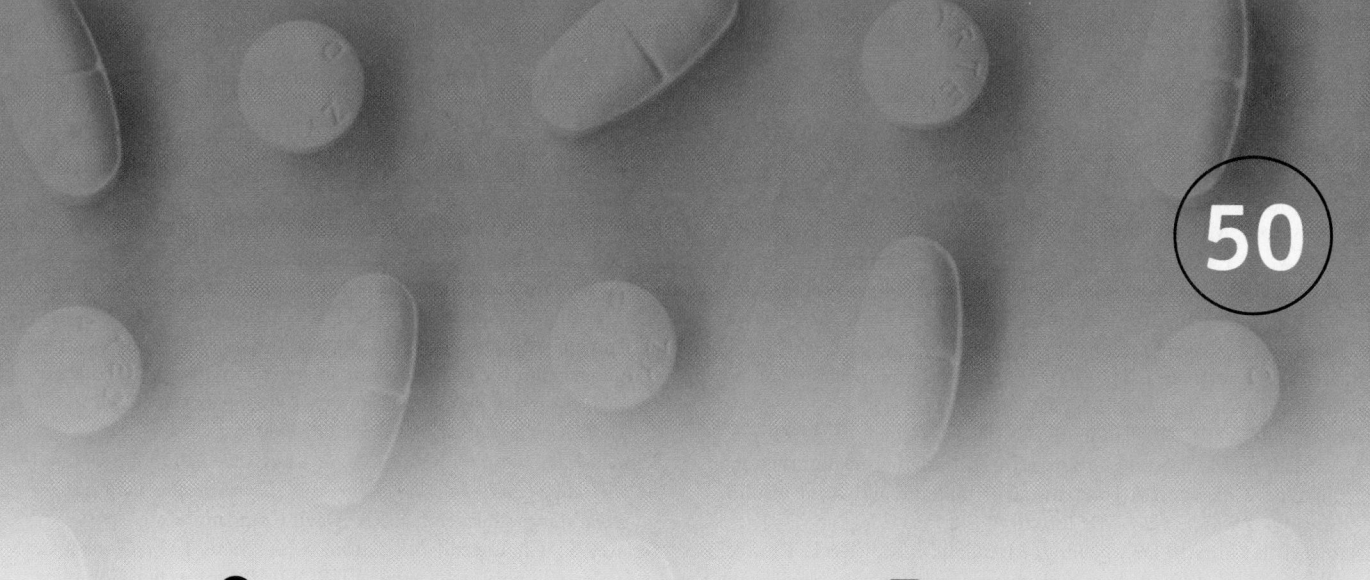

50

OVERVIEW OF THE FEMALE AND MALE REPRODUCTIVE SYSTEMS

CHAPTER FOCUS

Because secrecy and cultural sensitivity often influence perceptions of reproductive disorders, caring for clients with dysfunctions of the reproductive system is particularly challenging for the nurse. The client may experience a disturbance of self-esteem, altered sexual patterns, or sexual dysfunction; this requires the nurse to apply knowledge of reproductive anatomy and physiology and associated drugs for sensitive and appropriate teaching and counseling. This chapter reviews the anatomy and physiology of the female and male reproductive systems as background for the next four chapters, which discuss the drugs affecting the reproductive system.

LEARNING OBJECTIVES

- Identify the anterior pituitary gland hormones that influence the female and male reproductive systems.
- Describe hormonal influences on uterine function during the menstrual cycle.
- Identify the primary male and female hormones.
- Describe the effects of estrogen and progesterone during the proliferative stage.
- Trace the transport of sperm in the male body from production to ejaculation.

▲ KEY TERMS

androgens, p. 888
estrogens, p. 888
follicle-stimulating hormone (FSH), p. 888
luteinizing hormone (LH), p. 888

ovulation, p. 890
progestogens, p. 888
testosterone, p. 892

✷ What are the key features of the male and female reproductive systems?

Reproduction is the sum of genetic and hormonal influences that originate from members of a species to perpetuate the species. In human beings, the reproductive process in both genders is highly complex. It involves the following: (1) **follicle-stimulating hormone (FSH),** which stimulates the growth and maturation of graafian follicles in the ovary and spermatogenesis in the testes; and (2) **luteinizing hormone (LH),** which stimulates the secretion of sex hormones by the

ovary and the testes and is involved in the maturation of the spermatozoa and ova. Both follicle-stimulating hormone and luteinizing hormone are secreted from the anterior pituitary gland. The hormones from the reproductive systems of the male (**androgens**) and the female (**estrogens** and **progestogens**) are also involved in the reproductive process.

The reproductive system of the human female consists of the ovaries, fallopian tubes, uterus, and vagina. The male reproductive system consists of the testes, seminal vesicles, prostate gland, bulbourethral glands, and penis. The reproductive organs of both the male and female are mainly under the control of the endocrine glands. The ovaries and testes, known as gonads, not only produce ova and sperm cells but also form endocrine secretions that initiate and maintain the secondary sexual characteristics of men and women. Chapter 46 reviews the structure and physiologic functions of the pituitary gland; the discussion of the pituitary gland in this chapter is limited to its effect on the female and male reproductive systems.

✳ What are the pituitary gonadotropic hormones?

The following gonadotropins or pituitary hormones are responsible for the development and maintenance of sexual gland functions:

- Follicle-stimulating hormone (FSH) stimulates the development of the ovarian (graafian) follicles up to the point of ovulation in the female. In the male, FSH stimulates the development of the seminiferous tubules and promotes spermatogenesis.

- Luteinizing hormone (LH), or interstitial cell–stimulating hormone (ICSH), acts in the female to promote the growth of the interstitial cells in the follicle and the formation of the corpus luteum. In the male, LH stimulates the growth of interstitial cells in the testes and promotes the formation of the hormone androgen (testosterone).

In the female, FSH initiates the cycle of events in the ovary. Under the influence of both FSH and LH, the graafian follicle grows, matures, secretes estrogen, ovulates, and forms the corpus luteum. LH promotes the secretory activity of the corpus luteum and the formation of progesterone. In the absence of LH the corpus luteum undergoes regressive changes and fails to make progesterone.

✳ What are the important anatomic and physiologic components of the female reproductive system?

The female reproductive system is illustrated in Figure 50-1. Figure 50-2 illustrates the effects of the pituitary hormones,

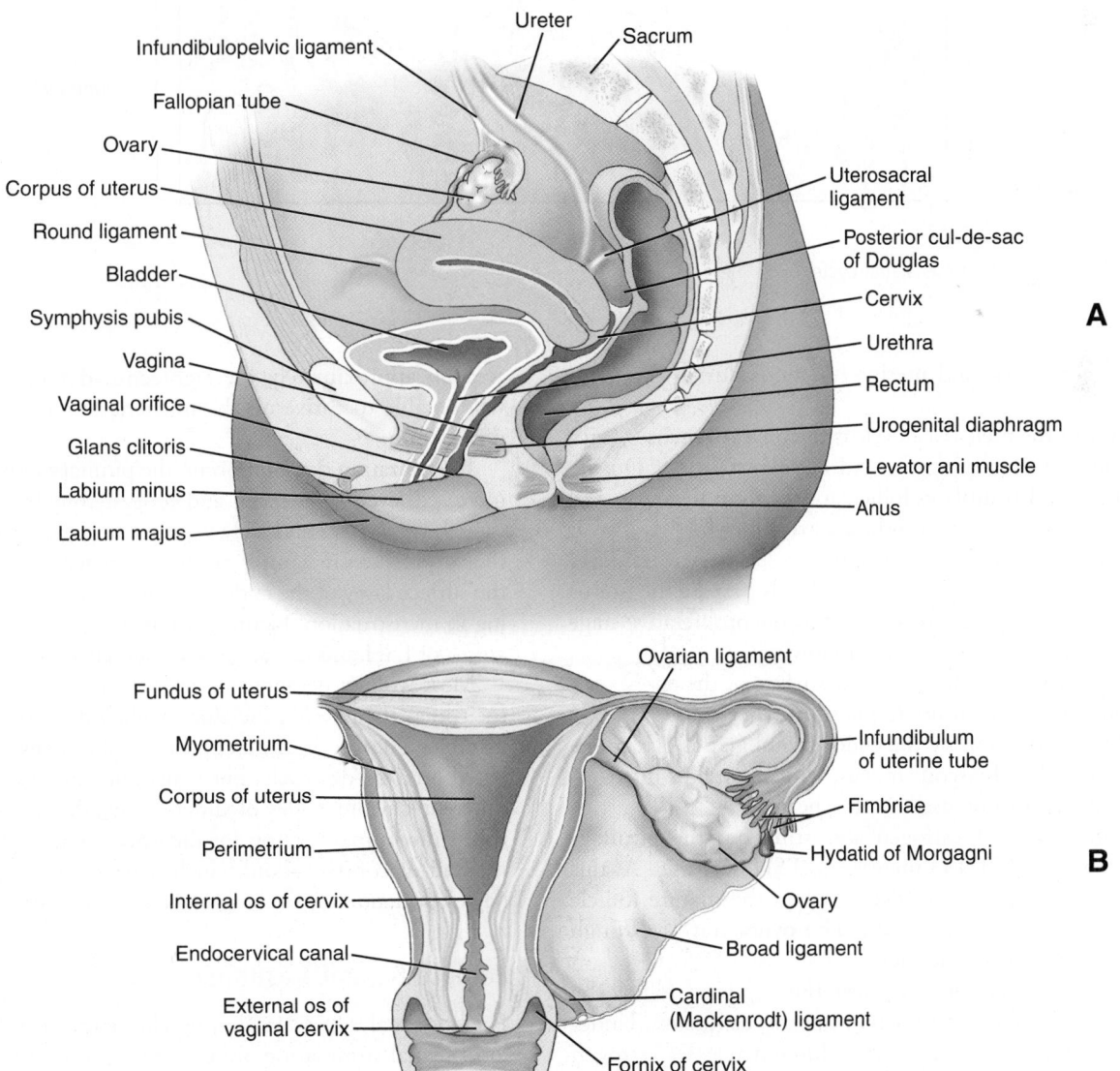

FIGURE 50-1 **A,** Female reproductive system. **B,** Cross section of the uterus, adnexa, and upper vagina.

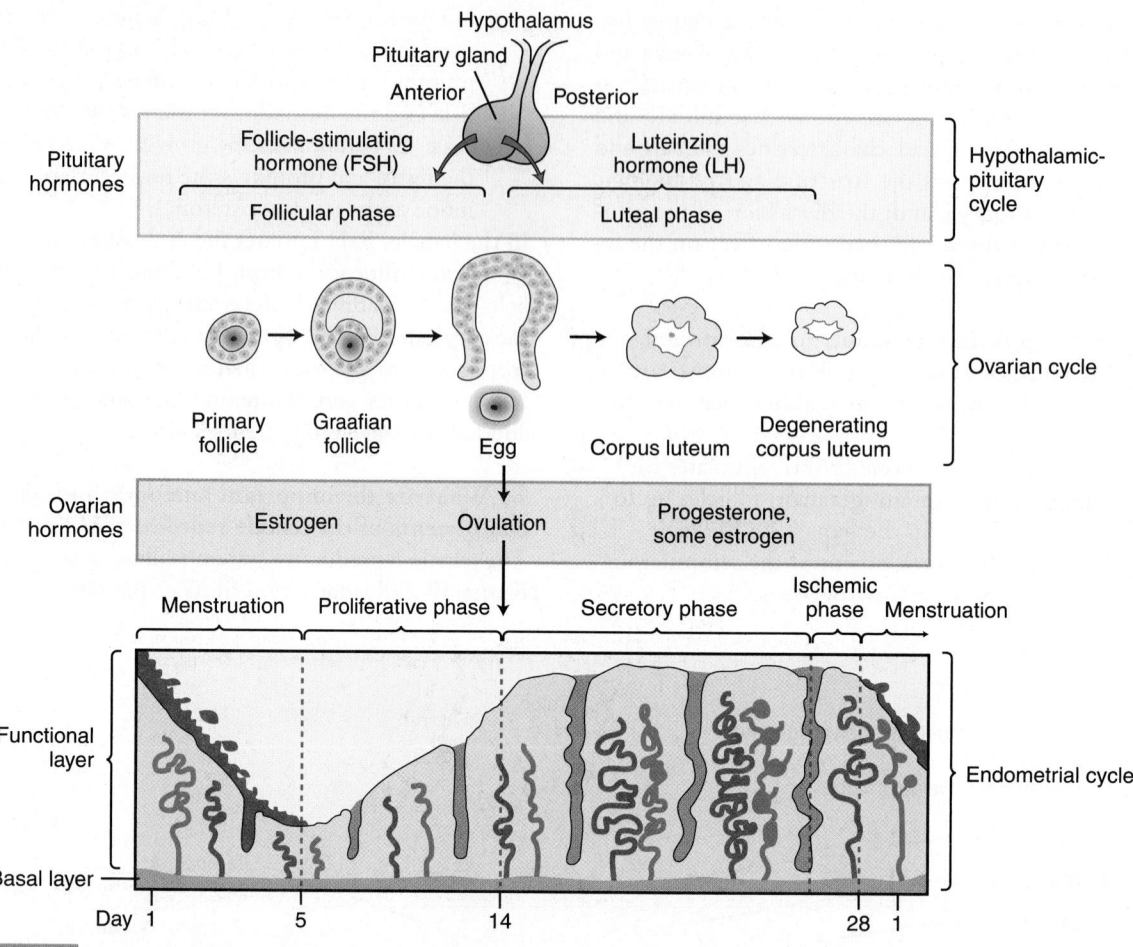

FIGURE 50-2 The menstrual cycle.

ovarian hormones, and uterine functions during the menstrual cycle.

Day 1 of the menstrual cycle is the onset of menses, with day 5 usually signifying the end of menstruation. During this time, FSH stimulates follicular growth in the ovary and stimulates the ovary to produce estrogen, which is low at the beginning of the cycle. As estrogen levels increase, FSH levels decrease. The rising estrogen levels prepare the uterus for a fertilized ovum; this is known as the proliferative stage of the uterus and results in the following:

- The growth of the glandular surface of the endometrium, or inner lining of the uterus
- The production by the endocervical glands of a more plentiful and viscous mucus, which contains nutrients that can be used by the sperm

Increasing levels of estrogen also stimulate the pituitary gland to release LH. LH increases as FSH decreases. At this time (day 14), **ovulation** occurs when the mature follicle ruptures and releases its ovum. The ovum travels through the fallopian tube to the uterus.

Increasing levels of LH affect the ruptured follicle by changing the follicle capsule into the corpus luteum. Under the influence of LH, the corpus luteum releases estrogen and progesterone. In the second phase, or secretory phase, both uterine hormones increase the secretion of the endometrial glands. If the ovum is fertilized and reaches this

area on approximately the eighteenth day of the cycle, it will be able to thrive on the nutrient secretions of the endometrium.

If fertilization does not occur, the pituitary responds to the increased levels of estrogen and progesterone by shutting off the release of FSH and LH. Without the central stimulation, the corpus luteum cannot produce estrogen or progesterone; the surface layer of the endometrium then sloughs off, resulting in menstruation. Figure 50-3 depicts the feedback mechanism of FSH and LH and their main effects on the ovaries.

Most women demonstrate month-to-month variations in their menstrual cycles; therefore ovulation is not always predictable. The previous description of the menstrual cycle is based on a 28-day cycle, but ovulation varies and occurs on different days in cycles of different lengths. Physiologically, this is the primary reason for the unreliability of the rhythm method of contraception, which depends on predicting the day of ovulation on the basis of previous menstrual cycles.

Female Sexual Response

For both males and females, psychological stimulation and local sexual stimulation are necessary for a satisfactory sexual experience. Psychological stimulation may be aided by an individual's erotic thoughts, but sexual desire is also affected by increasing levels of estrogen secretion, especially

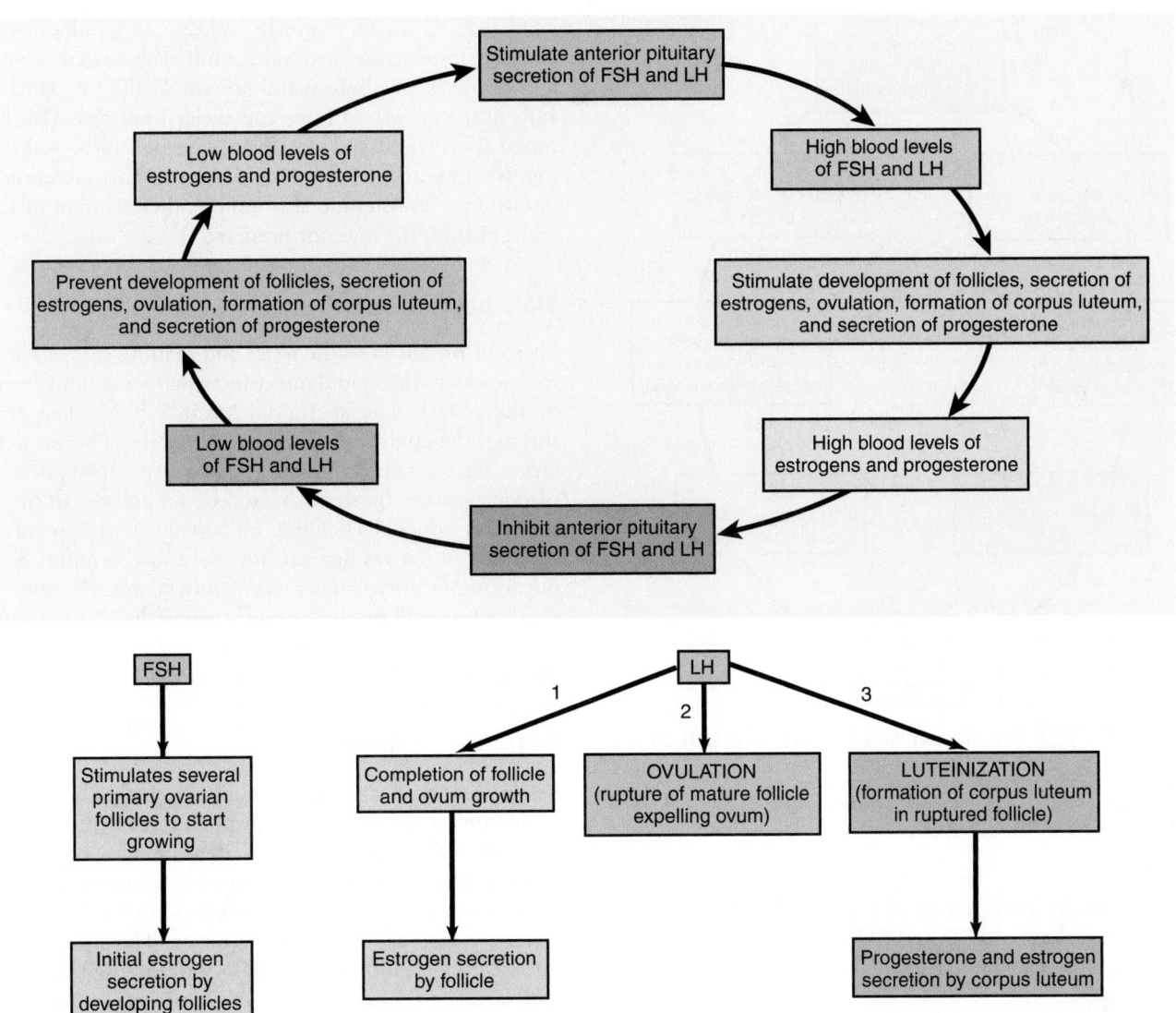

FIGURE 50-3 Feedback mechanisms of follicle-stimulating hormone (FSH) and luteinizing hormone (LH) and their main effects on the ovaries.

Modified from Thibodeau, G.A., & Patton, K.T. (2003). *Anatomy and physiology* (5th ed.). St. Louis: Mosby.

during the preovulatory period. Androgens (e.g., testosterone) also plays a role in libido for women, particularly after menopause (Bachmann & Leiblum, 2004).

Local sexual stimulation causes similar responses in both genders; massage, increasing stimulation, or irritation of the perineal region or sexual organs can result in an enhancement of sexual sensations. In the female, the clitoris is very sensitive, and its stimulation can initiate a sexual sensation. Erectile tissue is located in the introitus (vaginal opening) and clitoris. This tissue is under parasympathetic nerve control; in early stimulation, the parasympathetic nerves dilate the arteries in the erectile tissues. Blood collects in the erectile tissue so that the introitus tightens around the penis; this aids in male satisfaction of sexual stimulation, thus leading to ejaculation.

The parasympathetic nerves also signal the Bartholin glands situated near the labia minora, which results in increased mucus secretion inside the introitus. This secretion, in addition to mucus from the vaginal epithelium, serves as a lubricant during sexual intercourse.

The female climax, or orgasm, is reached when the local sexual stimulation reaches the maximum sensation or intensity. It is considered similar to emission and ejaculation in the male and may also help to promote fertilization of the ovum. It has been theorized that orgasm produces a rhythm in the female tract from spinal cord reflexes; this rhythm increases both uterine and fallopian tube motility and may result in cervical canal dilation for up to 30 minutes. This allows for easy sperm transport in the female.

The intense sexual sensations that develop during orgasm also result in an increase in muscle tension throughout the body. After the sexual act, this tension subsides into relaxation or feelings of satisfaction, sometimes referred to as resolution.

✷ What are the key anatomic and physiologic functions of the male reproductive system?

The effects of FSH and LH in the male were described on p. 889. FSH from the anterior pituitary gland stimulates the seminiferous tubules to increase the production of spermatozoa, and LH stimulates the interstitial cells to increase

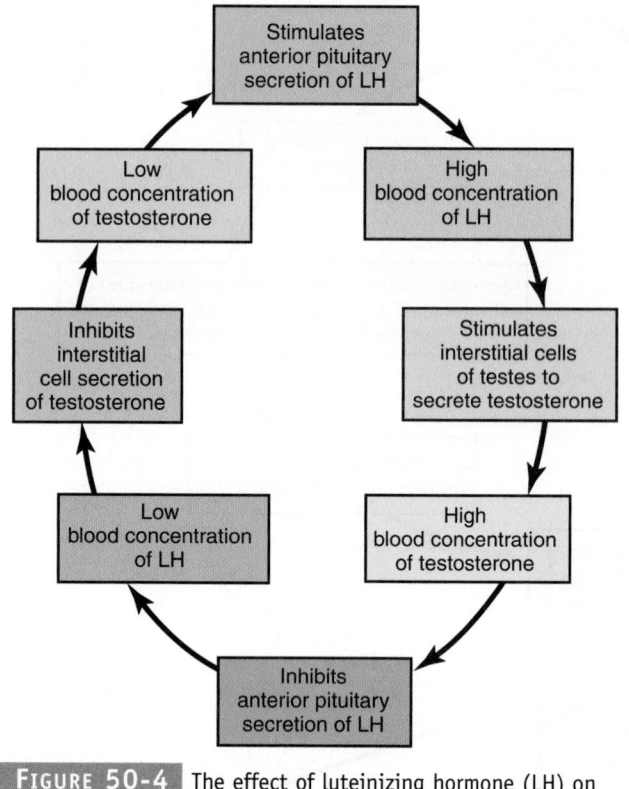

FIGURE 50-4 The effect of luteinizing hormone (LH) on testosterone.

Modified from Anthony, C., & Thibodeau, G. (1987). *Textbook of anatomy and physiology* (12th ed.). St. Louis: Mosby.

the secretion of testosterone. A high level of testosterone inhibits the release of FSH and LH from the pituitary. Figure 50-4 illustrates the effects of LH on the secretion of testosterone.

Testosterone, an androgen, performs numerous functions in the male. It aids in developing and maintaining the male secondary sex characteristics and male accessory or-

gans (e.g., prostate, seminal vesicles, and bulbourethral glands). Testosterone promotes adult male sexual behavior and regulates metabolism and protein anabolism, which results in the growth of bone and skeletal muscles. This hormone affects fluid and electrolyte metabolism by reabsorbing sodium and water and increasing the excretion of potassium. Testosterone also inhibits the secretion of FSH and LH from the anterior pituitary.

Transport of Sperm in the Male

Sperm is produced in the testes and matures by spending 1 to 3 weeks in the epididymis (ducts that lie around the top of the testes). The sperm, in seminal fluid, then travel through the epididymis to the vas deferens. The vas deferens, a duct extension of the epididymis, extends over the bladder surface (posteriorly) to the ampulla to form the ejaculatory duct. Depending on sexual activity, sperm can be stored in the vas deferens for more than 1 month without losing fertility. Thus a vasectomy, or a severing of the vas deferens, will produce sterility primarily by interrupting the journey of sperm to the ejaculatory duct and urethra. The male reproductive system is illustrated in Figure 50-5.

Male Sexual Response

Penile erection is a parasympathetic response that consists of dilation of the arteries and arterioles in the penis, which compresses the veins in this area. Because more blood is entering than leaving the penis, the penis becomes larger and erection occurs. Emission and ejaculation of the sperm and secretions (semen) is a reflex response. The stimulus that initiated the erection also helps to move the sperm and secretions from the genital ducts to the prostatic urethra. Orgasm, the climax of the sexual act, moves the semen through the ejaculatory ducts. Sperm can be transferred from the male to the female during coitus.

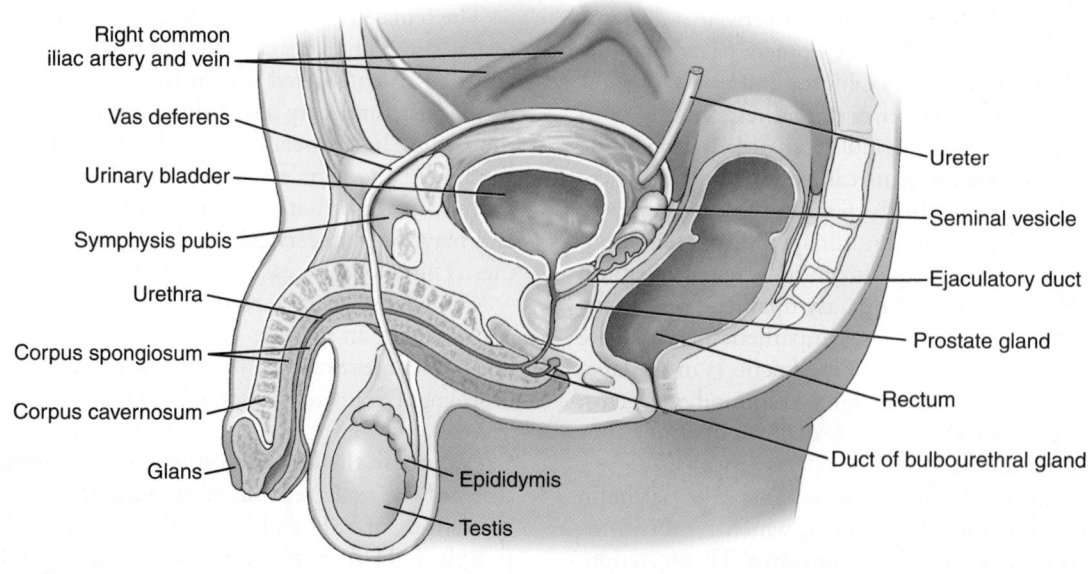

FIGURE 50-5 Male reproductive system.

Gonadal function ceases later in life. Women undergo menopause (the cessation of menses), and men experience a decrease in the production of sex hormones (sometimes called the male climacteric).

Summary

Disorders of the reproductive system of men and women result in acute and chronic physical and emotional stress. The nurse needs to have a sound knowledge of the anatomy and physiology of the reproductive system to assess clients for health adaptations and alterations and to assist them with complex health issues in this area.

✳ Critical Thinking Questions

- If you wanted to develop a birth control pill for men, how would you want that pill to influence the male hormonal system?

- Because of the positive-feedback mechanism of hormonal influences in the menstrual cycle, what hormonal changes take place if fertilization does not occur?

Bibliography

Anderson, D.M., Keith, J., & Novak, P.D. (Eds.) (2002). *Mosby's medical, nursing, and allied health dictionary* (6th ed.). St. Louis: Mosby.

Bachmann, G.A., & Leiblum, S.R. (2004). The impact of hormones on menopausal sexuality: a literature review. *Menopause, 11*(1), 120-130.

Guyton, A.C., & Hall, J.E. (2000). *Textbook of medical physiology* (10th ed.). Philadelphia: W.B. Saunders.

Herlihy, B., & Maebius, N.K. (2003). *The human body in health and illness* (2nd ed.). Philadelphia: W.B. Saunders.

Loose-Mitchell, D.S., & Stancel, G.M. (2001). In J.G. Hardman & L.E. Limbird (Eds.), *Goodman and Gilman's The pharmacological basis of therapeutics* (10th ed.). New York: McGraw-Hill.

McCance, K.L., & Huether, S.E. (2002). *Pathophysiology: The biological basis for disease in adults and children.* (4th ed.). St. Louis: Mosby.

Snyder, P.J. (2001). Androgens In J.G. Hardman & L.E. Limbird (Eds.), *Goodman and Gilman's The pharmacological basis of therapeutics* (10th ed.). New York: McGraw-Hill.

Thibodeau, G.A., & Patton, K.T. (2003). *Anatomy and physiology* (5th ed.). St. Louis: Mosby.

e-LEARNING SUPPLEMENTS

Student CD-ROM
- Final Exam questions
- NCLEX® Examination review questions
- Pharmacology animations
- Printable chapter summary

Evolve Website (http://evolve.elsevier.com/mckenry)
- Content updates, including information on new drugs
- WebLinks corresponding to this chapter
- Answers to the critical thinking questions in this chapter
- *Elsevier ePharmacology Update* newsletter
- Mosby's Drug Consult Internet Edition
- Supplemental and reference information

DRUGS AFFECTING WOMEN'S HEALTH AND THE FEMALE REPRODUCTIVE SYSTEM

CHAPTER FOCUS

Drugs that affect the female reproductive system therapeutically are synthetic or natural analogues of homogenous hormones. They are administered to mimic the biologic effects of endogenous hormones, to supplement inadequate production (e.g., menopause), to correct hormonal balance (e.g., dysfunctional bleeding), to reverse an abnormal process (e.g., hirsutism), and for contraception. Some of these same agents also may be used to treat conditions in males (e.g., diagnosis of hypogonadism, central precocious puberty, male infertility, and advanced prostate cancer). Whatever the indication, the nurse needs to be knowledgeable about these drugs to support the client's need for intervention and instruction.

LEARNING OBJECTIVES

- Describe the source and action of chorionic gonadotropin.
- Explain the function of the primary female sex hormones.
- List drugs affecting the female reproductive system.
- Identify the adverse effects of estrogens and progestins.
- Compare and contrast monophasic, biphasic, and triphasic hormonal contraceptives.
- Implement the nursing management of clients receiving drug therapy affecting the female reproductive system.

▲ **KEY TERMS**

anovulation, p. 915
biphasic, p. 909
estrogens, p. 899
hormonal contraception, p. 907
monophasic, p. 909
progestogens, p. 899
triphasic, p. 909

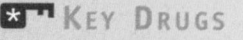 **KEY DRUGS**

estrogen, p. 900
medroxyprogesterone, p. 905

Synthetic and natural substances that affect the female reproductive system include gonadotropin-releasing hormones, nonpituitary chorionic gonadotropin, menotropins, female sex hormones, hormonal contraceptives, ovulatory stimulants, and drugs used for infertility.

✴ **What drugs affect gonadotropin-releasing hormone?**
Gonadotropin releasing hormone (GnRH) stimulates the synthesis and release of luteinizing hormone (LH) and follicle-stimulating hormone (FSH) from the anterior pituitary (Figure 51-1). Synthetic GnRH is available as gonadorelin

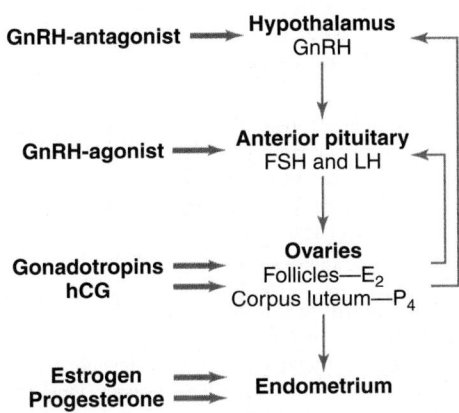

FIGURE 51-1 Hormonal relationships and sites of action of medications. *GnRH*, Gonadotropin-releasing hormone; *FSH*, follicle-stimulating hormone; *LH*, luteinizing hormone; *hCG*, human chorionic gonadotropin hormone.

From DiPiro, J.T., et al. (Eds.). (2002). *Pharmacotherapy: A pathophysiological approach* [5th ed.]. New York: McGraw-Hill. Reproduced with permission of The McGraw-Hill Companies.

(Factrel) and is used for diagnosing hypogonadism. Nafarelin is an agonist of GnRH and is used in the treatment of endometriosis and precocious puberty. Histrelin (Supprelin) is also a GnRH agonist used to treat precocious puberty in young girls and boys. Ganirelix (Antagon) is a GnRH antagonist used as part of an infertility treatment protocol to prevent ovulation until follicles reach maturity.

Leuprolide (Lupron) and goserelin (Zoladex) are GnRH analogs that inhibit gonadotropin release and thereby suppress ovarian and testicular hormone release. They are both used in the treatment of prostate cancer; goserelin is also used in the treatment of endometriosis. They are reviewed in Chapter 56.

Synthetic GnRH

gonadorelin [goe nad oh **rell** in]
(Factrel)
Gonadorelin is chemically identical to natural GnRH and stimulates the synthesis and release of luteinizing hormone (LH) and, to a lesser extent, follicle-stimulating hormone (FSH) from the anterior pituitary.

Indications
Gonadorelin is a synthetic GnRH used as an adjunct to other tests to diagnose hypogonadism in males and females. When diagnosing hypogonadism, multiple dosing may be more valuable than a single-dose test in differentiating between hypothalamic function impairment and pituitary function impairment. It has also been used in the treatment of primary hypothalamic amenorrhea in adult women.

Pharmacokinetics/Dosing
Intravenously, gonadorelin has an initial half-life of 2 to 10 minutes, followed by a terminal half-life of 10 to 40 minutes. It is metabolized rapidly in the body and excreted by the kidneys. For adults and children 12 years of age and older, the dose for diagnosing hypogonadism is 100 mcg subcutaneous or intravenous (IV). In females, the drug should be administered in the early follicular phase of the menstrual cycle, preferably within the first week. For the treatment of primary hypothalamic amenorrhea, the adult dose of gonadorelin acetate (Lutrepulse) is 5 mcg every 90 minutes for a 21-day cycle

using a specified pump for delivery (Lutrepulse pump). See specific referencing for dosing of gonadorelin in primary hypothalamic amenorrhea.

Adverse Effects
Adverse effects include anaphylaxis, pain, or inflammation at the injection site, and multiple pregnancies.

Drug Interactions
Variable response to androgen, estrogen, progestin, glucocorticoid, and hormonal contraceptive agents may be observed with the use of gonadorelin. Increased levels or effect of spironolactone and levodopa are occasionally observed. Reduced digoxin levels and levels of phenothiazines have also been reported with its use.

Nursing Management
Assessment
A thorough health history and physical examination, including a gynecologic examination, is done before initiating gonadorelin testing to determine that the client is in good general health and is not allergic to gonadorelin or any components of the product. The client should not have a preexisting GnRH adenoma or any other condition that might be worsened by reproductive hormones.

To determine a baseline serum concentration of LH, a sample or two of venous blood is drawn 15 to 20 minutes before administering gonadorelin, and if two samples were drawn the results are averaged. After administering the drug, other blood samples are drawn at regular intervals for diagnostic purposes. An ultrasound of the ovaries is accomplished before drug administration.

Nursing Diagnosis
Once gonadorelin has been administered, assess the client for the following nursing diagnoses/collaborative problems: impaired comfort (abdominal discomfort, transient flushing, headaches, light-headedness, nausea); impaired skin integrity related to a generalized skin rash or itching and swelling at the injection site; and the potential complication of sensitization following multiple doses (anaphylaxis).

Planning
While receiving gonadorelin, the client will:
- Be diagnosed regarding hypothalamic-pituitary-gonadal axis function, if the drug is used as an adjunctive diagnostic agent.
- Have normal LH levels and menses, if the drug is administered for primary amenorrhea.
- Conceive, if the drug is used as an infertility agent.
- Effectively manage the therapeutic regimen, including supportive, nonpharmacologic measures.
- Collaborate with health care providers for monitoring and treatment.

Implementation
Monitoring
If the client is self-administering gonadorelin, monitor injection technique. Monitor client's temperature for infection. The client should receive an ovarian ultrasound on the seventh and fourteenth day of treatment.
Intervention
Discard any unused reconstituted solution being used for diagnosis after 24 hours.
Education
If the gonadorelin is administered as a diagnostic agent, explain the test procedure to the client. Alert the client to the symptoms of hypersensitivity reaction (e.g., hives, wheezing, and dyspnea), and indicate that these are to be reported immediately.

Stress the need for regular visits to the prescriber for the necessary monitoring.

Evaluation
The expected outcome of gonadorelin therapy is that the normal baseline serum LH concentration will be 0.0 to 1.6 mIU/mL for prepubertal children, 1 to 10.2 mIU/mL for men, and 0.9 to 14 mIU/mL for women, depending on the laboratory. The test will determine the client's functional capacity and response to gonadotropic hormones without the client experiencing any untoward effects of the procedure. If used for infertility, the client will conceive.

Gonadotropin-Releasing Hormone Agonists

nafarelin [naf ah **rell** in]
(Synarel)

Nafarelin is a potent agonist of GnRH that initially stimulates the release of LH and FSH but results in a decreased secretion of the gonadotropins with continued dosing. The continuous stimulation of the GnRH receptors results in desensitization and ultimately decreased production of LH and FSH.

Indications

Nafarelin is indicated for the treatment or management of endometriosis and central precocious puberty (CPP).

Pharmacokinetics/Dosing

Nafarelin is administered nasally, with maximum serum levels reported in 10 to 40 minutes. It has a half-life of 3 hours and a maximum effect within 1 month. The dosage for endometriosis is one nasal spray of 200 mcg in one nostril in the morning and one spray in the other nostril at night. It is usually administered for a period of 6 months. For clients with CPP, the 1600-mcg dose is administered by two sprays into each nostril two times daily for a total of 8 sprays daily; this dosage may be increased to 1800 mcg by a daily dose of 9 sprays (three sprays into alternating nostrils three times daily). In CPP, treatment is continued until puberty is desired.

Adverse Effects

Adverse effects of nafarelin include hot flashes, increased or decreased libido, vaginal dryness, headaches, insomnia, oily skin, acne, edema, hirsutism, hypersensitivity, and paresthesia, and emotional lability.

Nursing Management
Assessment

Assist in determining before therapy that the client is not pregnant, breastfeeding, or experiencing any undiagnosed abnormal vaginal bleeding. Some bone density loss has been demonstrated with the use of this drug. Use caution if more than one 6-month course is considered for women who are at high risk for osteoporosis (a strong family history of osteoporosis, chronic alcohol or tobacco use, or chronic use of drugs that can reduce bone mass [antiepileptic drugs or corticosteroids]). Obtain a baseline assessment of the client's endometriosis before therapy.

CPP should be confirmed in children who develop secondary sex characteristics at an earlier stage than their cohorts and have significant advanced bone age. This diagnosis is confirmed by measuring serum sex steroids and basal levels of gonadotropins, testing the response to GnRH, assessing diagnostic imaging of the brain (including the pituitary and hypothalamus), and a pelvic ultrasound (in girls). Before initiating a course of therapy for clients with CPP, determine the parents' willingness to comply with dosing and the frequent monitoring by the prescriber, which is necessary for the first 6 to 8 weeks of therapy. Determine the client's sensitivity to nafarelin or any other gonadotropin-releasing agonists or hormones.

Nursing Diagnosis

Assess the client with endometriosis for development of the following nursing diagnoses/collaborative problems related to adverse effects of nafarelin: impaired comfort (hot flashes, headaches, eye pain, and galactorrhea); ineffective sexuality patterns related to a libido increase or decrease and vaginal dryness; disturbed sleep pattern (insomnia); fatigue; ineffective coping related to emotional lability or depression; disturbed body image related to acne, weight gain/weight loss, and hirsutism; and the potential complications of osteoporosis, arthralgia, ovarian enlargement or overstimulation, and breakthrough bleeding, menorrhagia, or amenorrhea.

The child being treated for CPP may experience several nursing diagnoses/collaborative problems. Girls may experience a situational low self-esteem related to changes in menstrual patterns, acne, hirsutism, or body odor; and ineffective coping related to emotional lability. Boys may experience a disturbed self-esteem related to the growth of pubic hair, body odor, acne, and dandruff.

All clients receiving nafarelin may experience impaired comfort (nasal irritation from the dosage form) and are at risk for the potential complication of allergic reaction.

Planning

If administered for endometriosis, the client will experience:
- A decrease in pelvic pain and a reduction in the size and number of endometriotic implants on ultrasound.

If administered for CPP, the client will experience:
- Regression of secondary sexual development.
- A return of LH levels to prepubertal levels within 1 month of therapy.
- Slowing of linear growth to 5 to 6 cm/year or less.

In both instances, the client (and family) will:
- Effectively manage the therapeutic regimen, including medication compliance, stating reportable symptoms to prescriber, undertaking supportive interventions to the drug.
- Collaborate with health care providers for monitoring and treatment.

Implementation
Monitoring

Assess the client with endometriosis at regular intervals for improvement of the condition. Pregnancy tests are required if therapy does not begin during menstruation or if the client has an irregular menses cycle. A bone density determination is recommended if a second course of therapy is considered.

For clients with CPP, bone linear growth and bone age velocity determinations, imaging studies of the left (or nondominant) hand and wrist, magnetic imaging of the brain, and pelvic sonography (for females) should be performed 3 to 6 months after initiating therapy. Blood studies for various hormones are also performed. Document the evaluation of the secondary sex characteristics.

Assess all clients receiving nafarelin for discomfort of the nasal passages, dryness, and irritation related to administration of the drug.

Intervention

Administer one spray (200 mcg) of nafarelin into one nostril in the morning and one spray into the other nostril in the evening for endometriosis. Treatment is initiated between days 2 and 4 of the menstrual cycle for females with endometriosis. For CPP the dose is more variable, two to nine sprays daily. After administration of the nasal dose, instruct the client to tilt the head backward for 30 seconds to allow the medication to reach the back of the nose. The client should try to avoid sneezing during or immediately after administration, because drug absorption may be decreased.

The prescriber may also recommend a nasal decongestant if the client develops rhinitis during therapy. Instruct the client to use the decongestant at least 30 minutes after the nafarelin spray to minimize the possibility of decreasing drug absorption.

Dietary calcium and calcium supplements have not been shown to help prevent bone calcium loss associated with the administration of GnRH.

Education

Alert the client that menstruation will cease with effective nafarelin therapy; the prescriber needs to be notified if regular menstruation continues. Although nafarelin will usually inhibit ovulation and menstruation, advise the client that it is not a reliable contraceptive and that a nonhormonal or barrier form of contraception should be used. The client should discontinue the drug and notify her prescriber immediately if she suspects she is pregnant.

Instruct the child with CPP and his or her parents to notify the prescriber if prepubertal symptoms are not suppressed within 6 to 8 weeks.

Evaluation

The expected outcome of nafarelin therapy is that the client with endometriosis will experience pain relief and a reduction in endometrial lesions. If administered for CPP, secondary sexual development of breasts in girls and genital enlargement in boys will diminish; additionally, linear bone growth will slow to 5 to 6 cm per year or less, thereby improving the possibility of attaining the predicted adult height. The client will maintain medication compliance, demonstrate the appropriate method of administering nafarelin, report adverse symptoms to the prescriber appropriately, and maintain scheduled visits to the prescriber for monitoring and treatment.

histrelin [his **trel** in]
(Supprelin in United States, not available in Canada)
Histrelin is a synthetic GnRH agonist that is more potent than the natural hormone. It controls the secretion of pituitary gonadotropin, which results in a decrease in sex steroid levels and a regression of secondary sexual characteristics in children with CPP.

Indications
Histrelin is used for clients with CPP—before 8 years of age in girls and age 9.5 years of age in boys. It decreases estradiol levels in females and inhibits testosterone in males. Decreases in LH, FSH, and sex steroid serum levels are noted within 3 months of therapy. It is also used in the palliative treatment of advanced carcinoma of the prostate, for the treatment of intermittent porphyria, and in the management of endometriosis, leiomyomata uteri (uterine fibroids), and severe premenstrual syndrome.

Pharmacokinetics/Dosing
The usual dosage for CPP is 10 mcg/kg subcutaneous daily. A 50 mg insert is planted subcutaneously for a 12-month period in the palliative treatment of prostate cancer.

Adverse Effects
The adverse effects of histrelin include vasodilation, vaginal dryness, breast edema and pain, gastric distress, headaches, fever, arthralgia, anxiety, and reactions at the site of injection. Transient vaginal bleeding usually occurs within the first 3 weeks of initial therapy.

Nursing Management
Histrelin therapy is similar to the use of nafarelin, but it is used only for CPP. However, instead of being administered by nasal spray, clients must be able to maintain compliance with a daily regimen of subcutaneous injections. In addition to the nursing diagnoses with nafarelin, the client may experience impaired tissue integrity at the injection site (redness, swelling, and itching). To minimize these reactions, the daily injections are rotated through different body sites. Instruct the child and family in the proper administration of injections and the proper disposal of needles, syringes, and vials. The pubertal process may be reactivated if injections are not given daily. Stress the importance of administering the daily injection at the same time each day and in complying with daily administration. Allow the solution to come to body temperature before injecting. Discard any unused portion in the vial as it contains no preservative. Report to the prescriber if the skin reactions are severe or if the client demonstrates any signs of allergy (skin rash, urticaria, or difficulty in breathing).

Gonadotropin-Releasing Hormone Antagonists

ganirelix [gah **nih** reh licks]
(Antagon)
Ganirelix (Antagon) is a GnRH antagonist that competitively blocks GnRH receptors in the pituitary. Its administration suppresses LH and gonadotropic secretion and prevents premature ovulation.

Indications
Ganirelix is used to inhibit premature LH increase in women receiving controlled ovarian hyperstimulation.

Pharmacokinetics/Dosing
It is administered subcutaneously and has an elimination half-life of about 16 hours. It is dosed at 250 mcg daily by subcutaneous injection as part of an infertility treatment protocol with FSH. See package insert for additional dosing information.

Adverse Effects
Adverse effects include abdominal pain, headache, vaginal bleeding, and nausea. It is a Pregnancy Category X drug that may cause fetal death and therefore should not be used during pregnancy.

Nursing Management
Assessment
Determine that the client is not sensitive to ganirelix, gonadotropin-releasing hormone, or any other GnRH analog. Given ganirelix is FDA Pregnancy Category X, ensure that the client is not pregnant before use and that the duration of use is carefully evaluated to prevent fetal harm. There are no listed drug interactions for this drug, but if the client wishes to conceive, see Box 51-1 for drugs for the client to avoid taking. The packaging contains natural rubber latex; determine if client has latex sensitivity.

Nursing Diagnosis
While taking ganirelix, the client is at risk for the following nursing diagnoses: altered comfort (headache, nausea, abdominal or gastrointestinal [GI] pain) and impaired tissue integrity (injection site reaction); and the potential complications of ovarian hyperstimulation syndrome (OHS) (severe abdominal pain, rapid weight gain, nausea and vomiting) and fetal death.

BOX 51-1 MEASURES TO INCREASE FERTILITY

- Men and women should avoid certain medications, products or activities:

Alcohol	Organic solvents
Chlorinated hydrocarbons	Perchloroethylene
Cigarette smoking	Pesticides
Ethylene oxide (gas in sterilization of instruments, etc.)	Radiant heat "Recreational" drugs (e.g., marijuana, cocaine)
Heavy metals	Solvent mixtures
Nitrous oxide	Toluene

- Women with body mass index (BMI) greater than 30 should be advised to lose weight.
- Women should avoid excessive dieting or exercising.
- Women should avoid all teratogenic drugs, NSAIDs, and aspirin before or around the time of ovulation.
- Before attempting contraception, all medications, including OTC and complementary/alternative medications, should be evaluated by the prescriber for fetal risk.
- Medications that cause hyperprolactinemia or impair spermatogenesis should be avoided:

chlorpromazine	methyldopa
cimetidine	metoclopramide
estrogen	phenothiazine derivatives
fluphenazine	pimozide
haloperidol	reserpine
medroxyprogesterone acetate	tricyclic antidepressants verapamil

- Women should be advised to eat a balanced diet and take folic acid and multivitamin supplementation.
- Males with subfertility may benefit from antioxidant therapy (e.g., vitamins C and E, selenium).

Planning

While undergoing ganirelix therapy, the client will:

- Conceive without experiencing adverse effects of the drug.
- Effectively manage the therapeutic regimen, including administering subcutaneous injections appropriately, medication compliance, stating reportable symptoms to prescriber, undertaking supportive interventions to the drug.
- Collaborate with health care providers for monitoring and treatment.

Implementation

Monitoring

Clients receiving ganirelix should be under the direct supervision of a physician experienced in the treatment of infertility. Discontinue ganirelix and notify physician if severe abdominal pain occurs.

Intervention

Administer 250 mcg once daily during the early to mid follicular phase following FSH therapy on day 2 or 3 of the client's cycle.

Education

Instruct client on correct subcutaneous injection techniques, proper dosing, storage of medication, and proper disposal of used syringes. Have client give a return demonstration of injection technique. Stress the importance of following the physician's instructions for recording basal body temperature, if requested, and the timing of intercourse. Maintain regular visits to prescriber to check progress.

Evaluation

The client will conceive without experiencing adverse effects of the drug. The client will effectively manage the therapeutic regimen, including administering subcutaneous injections appropriately and on the prescribed days, reporting severe abdominal pain to the prescriber if it occurs, and undertaking supportive interventions to the drug (see Box 51-1). The client will maintain scheduled visits to the prescriber for monitoring and treatment.

❋ **What are the gonadotropins and how are they used?**

The two types of gonadotropins are those secreted by the placenta during pregnancy (nonpituitary chorionic gonadotropin) and those secreted by the pituitary (purified FSH and LH; sometimes referred to as the human menopausal gonadotropins or menotropins).

Nonpituitary Chorionic Gonadotropin

chorionic gonadotropin [kor **ee** on ick goe nad oh **troe** pin]
(APL, Pregnyl)

The chorionic gonadotropins formed by the placenta during pregnancy are extracted from the urine of pregnant women. The action of human chorionic gonadotropin (hCG) is nearly equivalent to that of LH in the pituitary, with little or no follicle-stimulating effects.

Indications

Chorionic gonadotropin is administered to make up for a deficiency in LH. They are used for prepubertal cryptorchidism and hypogonadotropic hypogonadism to stimulate androgen production in the testes. This may enhance the descent of testes and increase the development of the secondary male sex characteristics. They are also used to treat male and female infertility alone, or in combination with the menotropins or other drugs. It is also used as part of combination therapy to stimulate multiple oocytes in ovulatory women.

Pharmacokinetics/Dosing

Administered intramuscularly (IM), this drug has a half-life between 11 and 23 hours, and ovulation usually occurs within 32 to 36 hours of administration. It is excreted by the kidneys within 24 hours. The adult dosage for male hypogonadotropic hypogonadism is 1000 to 4000 units IM two to three times weekly for several weeks or months (in some cases, indefinitely). For the induction of ovulation, 5000 to 10,000 units IM is administered after the last dose of menotropins or from 5 to 9 days after the last dose of clomiphene. For children with prepubertal cryptorchidism, the dosage is 1000 to 5000 units IM two or three times weekly for a maximum of 10 doses; the therapy is discontinued when the desired response is achieved.

Adverse Effects

The adverse effects of chorionic gonadotropin include headaches, anxiety, depression, breast enlargement, weakness, abdominal bloating/pain, increased incidence of multiple births, and possible arterial thromboembolism. Ovarian cysts, nausea, vomiting, and pain at injection site are also noted.

Pituitary Gonadotropin

menotropins [**men** oh troe pins]
(Pergonal, Repronex)

Menotropins is a preparation of human pituitary gonadotropin; it is a purified preparation of FSH and LH obtained from the urine of postmenopausal women. It is sometimes called human menopausal gonadotropins (HMG). The mechanism of action of menotropins is equivalent to the effects produced by FSH and LH; menotropins stimulates the development of the ovarian follicle, causes ovulation, and may stimulate the development of the corpus luteum. It stimulates sperm production in males.

Indications

In combination with chorionic gonadotropin, menotropins are indicated for female infertility caused by ovulatory dysfunction. It is considered the treatment of choice for clients with hypothalamic hypogonadism or for those who did not respond to clomiphene. It is also used in combination with chorionic gonadotropin for male infertility to stimulate spermatogenesis in primary or secondary hypogonadotropic hypogonadism (male infertility) and to stimulate multiple oocyte development in ovulatory clients who are using other technologies to conceive (e.g., gamete intrafallopian transfer [GIF] or in vitro fertilization [IVF]).

Pharmacokinetics/Dosing

Menotropins preparation is administered IM, and it is excreted by the kidneys. The adult dosage of menotropins for the induction of ovulation is 1 ampule (75 units of FSH and LH activity) IM daily for one week or more; this is followed by 5000 to 10,000 units of chorionic gonadotropin 1 day after the last dose of menotropins. If necessary, the ampule dose may be increased every 4 to 5 days, up to a maximum of 6 ampules. For the treatment of male infertility, 1 ampule is administered IM three times weekly (in addition to chorionic gonadotropin twice weekly) for a minimum of 4 months after pretreatment with chorionic gonadotropin for 4 to 6 months.

Adverse Effects

The adverse effects of menotropins include gastric distress, severe pelvic pain, weight gain, edema, shortness of breath, decreased urine output, abdominal bloating or pain (usually in females), and breast enlargement and erythrocytosis in males.

❋ **What are the nursing implications for the use of gonadotropins?**

Assessment It should be determined whether the client has a preexisting pituitary hypertrophy or tumor, because the medication will stimulate growth of the tumor. Gonadotropin should not be used for clients with prostatic cancer, undiagnosed abnormal vaginal bleeding, uterine fibroids, ovarian cysts, active thrombophlebitis, or cryptorchidism related to precocious puberty. In female clients an ultrasound examination is recommended before therapy to determine a baseline assessment of the ovaries. Baseline serum testosterone levels and sperm counts are determined for male clients.

Nursing Diagnosis The following nursing diagnoses may be appropriate in clients receiving gonadotropins: impaired comfort (headache, irritability, pain at injection site, tiredness, enlargement of breasts); excess fluid volume (rapid weight gain, pedal edema) and disturbed body image related to physical changes in the secondary sexual characteristics of young male clients, such as precocious puberty (rapid height increase, acne, growth of pubic hair, enlargement of penis or testes. The potential complications of mental depression, ovarian cysts, or ovarian hyperstimulation syndrome (severe pelvic pain, moderate to severe bloating, rapid weight gain, decreased amount of urine, pedal edema) may also occur.

Planning If the gonadotropins are administered for:
- Cryptorchidism without anatomical obstruction, the client will experience the descent of both testicles negating the need for surgery.
- Male infertility, the client will experience increased testosterone levels and an adequate sperm count of with normal motility.
- Female infertility, the client will experience serum estradiol within normal limits without ovarian overstimulation.

All clients will effectively manage their therapeutic regimen.

Implementation

Monitoring Assess the client's progress periodically. Because the regimen is lengthy and time-consuming, continue to support and encourage the client to cooperate over the course of therapy.

Estradiol serum determinations are performed to monitor the female client receiving chorionic gonadotropin for induction of ovulation. Hyperstimulation of the ovaries may be indicated by abdominal or pelvic pain and should be reported to the prescriber immediately. A pelvic examination and/or ultrasound examination may be performed to evaluate ovarian size and minimize the risk of ovarian hyperstimulation syndrome.

To monitor the male client receiving gonadotropin therapy for hypogonadism, inspect the genitalia for signs of puberty. Serum testosterone may be measured periodically to assess progress. If the drug is administered for male infertility, testosterone levels, sperm counts, and determinations of sperm mobility are also performed.

Intervention Reconstitute gonadotropins with the diluent provided by the manufacturer. After reconstitution the solution is stable for 60 to 90 minutes in the refrigerator.

Education When used to treat infertility, provide support for the client and partner throughout their attempt to achieve fertility. Societal and familial pressures create stress for them both as a couple and individually. They should be

advised that gonadotropin-induced ovulation is expensive and may result in multiple births. Because success is difficult to achieve, the couple should be counseled on alternatives such as adoption.

If the prescriber has requested a daily record of the woman's temperature, inform the client about the relationship of temperature to ovulation and its importance for the appropriate timing of intercourse to enhance the chance of pregnancy. Daily or every-other-day intercourse or insemination should be attempted beginning the day after chorionic gonadotropin is given until ovulation is thought to have occurred. Therapy should be reconsidered after three cycles of nonovulatory menses.

In treating prepubertal cryptorchidism, prepubertal males receiving chorionic gonadotropin should be prepared for acceleration of their sexual development and supported through self-image changes.

Evaluation The expected outcome of gonadotropin therapy for prepubertal cryptorchidism and hypogonadotropic hypogonadism is that the male experiences a descent of the testes into the scrotum and the normal development of secondary male sex characteristics. If administered for infertility, conception occurs without ovarian hyperstimulation. The client will maintain medication compliance, demonstrate the appropriate method of administering the drug, report adverse symptoms to the prescriber appropriately, and maintain scheduled visits to the prescriber for monitoring and treatment.

✪ How are the ovarian hormones (estrogens and progestins) differentiated?

In addition to providing ova, the ovaries manufacture and secrete female hormones that control secondary sex characteristics, the reproductive cycle, and the growth and development of the accessory reproductive organs in the female. Two main types of hormones are secreted by the ovary: (1) the follicular or estrogenic hormones (estrogens) produced by the cells of the developing graafian follicle, and (2) the luteal or progestational hormones (progestogens) derived from the corpus luteum that is formed in the ovary from the ruptured follicle. The periodic cycling of the female sex hormones depends on an interaction between FSH and LH and the ovarian hormones, estrogen and progesterone. This results in a menstrual cycle that normally continues throughout life until meno-pause (except during pregnancy). Estrogens are primarily secreted by the ovarian follicles, but some may also be secreted by the adrenals, corpus luteum, placenta, and testes.

✪ M.B. is a 49-year-old perimenopausal woman who is experiencing vasomotor menopausal symptoms of hot flashes, insomnia and changes in mood. She had a partial hysterectomy (removal of her uterus with both ovaries remaining intact) at age 42. She receives a prescription from her health care provider for the estrogen patch (estradiol transdermal 0.025 mg daily) to be worn continuously and changed twice weekly.

✳ What are the key features of estrogens?

Estrogens are available from natural sources in conjugated dosage forms and from synthetic formulations. One of the most common sources of estrogens historically has been pregnant mare urine, which may explain the derivation of one brand name for conjugated estrogens—Premarin (**PRE**gnant **MAR**e ur**IN**e). Examples of natural steroidal estrogens include estradiol, estrone, and esterified estrogens; nonsteroidal estrogens include diethylstilbestrol (DES), dienestrol, and chlorotrianisene. Estrogen increases the synthesis of deoxyribonucleic acid (DNA), ribonucleic acid (RNA), and protein in estrogen-responsive tissues. Elevated estrogen serum levels inhibit the secretion of FSH and LH from the pituitary, which results in the inhibition of lactation and ovulation, and the development of a proliferative endometrium. Estrogen supplementation in women produces a number of physiologic responses, including both beneficial effects and the risk of serious complications.

The beneficial effects of supplemental estrogen include improving vasomotor symptoms of menopause. Although estrogens are effective in improving "hot flashes," over 80% of women with menopausal symptoms do not experience frequent flashes (Barnabei et al., 2002) and would not likely achieve significant benefit from estrogen therapy. Additionally, estrogen therapy does not contribute to significant improvement in quality of life for most menopausal women (Hays et al., 2003). Alternatives to estrogens for treating hot flashes include phytoestrogens, for which there is conflicting data regarding efficacy and safety. Similar concerns have been raised with black cohosh (North American Menopause Society, 2004), but recent data suggest benefit (Osmers et al., 2005). See the Evidence-Based Practice box on p. 901. Selective serotonin reuptake inhibitor (SSRI) antidepressants, also studied for the management of postmenopausal symptoms, yield conflicting but generally disappointing results (Suvanto-Luukkonen et al., 2005). Estrogens also slow the decline in bone mineral density, but safer alternatives are available (see Chapter 47). In lower or similar doses, they are also used in combination with progestins in birth control (hormonal contraception). The role of estrogen in preventing Alzheimer's dementia has been long debated and largely refuted (Shumaker et al., 2004), as has its purported benefit for urinary incontinence (Hendrix et al., 2005). DES is a synthetic nonsteroidal estrogen primarily used as an antineoplastic agent.

Unfortunately, supplemental estrogen has significant risk, including increased thromboembolic events, and increased risk for certain cancers including breast cancer and if used alone (without progestins) endometrial cancer. Estrogens and raloxifene should be avoided in clients with a history of thromboembolism or coronary artery disease (CAD), and in smokers, all of whom may experience a higher risk for a new thromboembolic event (Grady et al., 2004; Manson et al., 2003). Estrogen use increases the risk for breast cancer (Beral, Million Women Study Collaborators, 2003; Chlebowski et al., 2003) and is also contraindicated in women with a history of estrogen-dependent neoplasms (particularly breast cancer) (Holmberg & Anderson,

and the HABITS steering and data monitoring committees, 2004). Supplemental estrogen use is also associated with increased risk for migraine headache and increased triglyceride levels. The risk for gallbladder disease is significantly elevated with estrogen use (Cirillo et al., 2005). Nausea, vomiting, breast tenderness, mental depression, changes in weight, and changes in menstrual flow are also effects of supplemental estrogen use. Estrogen use is correlated with increased risk for symptomatic gastroesophageal reflux, particularly in obese women (Nilsson, Johnsen, Ye, Hveem, Lagergren, 2003). Present or past estrogen use also increases the potential for false positive mammogram results (Banks et al., 2004). A brief discussion of the role of genetics in estrogen risks is presented in the Special Considerations for Pharmacogenetics box on p. 902.

These risks have been debated and evaluated for many years, but most clinicians now favor limiting supplemental estrogen and prescribe it only for women who have had a hysterectomy and require supplemental estrogen therapy or for short term use (e.g., under 2-5 years) in women who have significant intolerable vasomotor symptoms of menopause. These recommendations are supported by the U.S. Preventive Services Task Force (USPSTF, 2005). The use of lower dose estrogen in combination with progestins for hormonal contraception also has some risks, and its use will be discussed later in the chapter. Significant education of the client and client participation in the decision to use estrogen or estrogen/progestin combinations are key in the safe and effective use of these agents. A number of estrogen formulations and brands are available and include the following:

- estrogen, conjugated/equine (Premarin, others alone or in combination with progestins)
- estrogen, conjugated/synthetic (Cenestin, C.E.S.✽, Congest✽)
- estrogens, esterified (Menest, Estratab✽)
- estradiol (Alora, Climara, many other alone and in combination with progestins)
- ethinyl estradiol (Estinyl, many others in combination with progestins)
- estropipate (Ogen, Ortho-Est)

✳◨ estrogen [**ess** troe jin]
(various manufacturers)

Indications

Indications for estrogens include treatment of estrogen deficiency, atrophic vaginitis, female hypogonadism, insufficient primary ovarian function, severe vasomotor symptoms in menopause. Estrogens are typically used in combination with a progestin for women with an intact uterus to lower the risk for endometrial cancer. Estrogens have been used in the treatment of abnormal uterine bleeding, but only when the cause of bleeding has been identified and cancer has been ruled out. Historically, estrogens have been used with progestins in the treatment of postmenopausal osteoporosis, but this is no longer considered a treatment of choice (see Chapter 47 for a discussion of treatments for osteoporosis). Rarely, estrogens are used in the treatment of selected metastatic breast carcinomas in postmenopausal women with tumor estrogen-negative receptors, and for selected cases of breast carcinomas or advanced prostate cancer in men. Estrogens in combination with progestins are also used for

Evidence-Based Practice

When clients inquire about the use of complementary/alternative medications, they should be provided with the most current data, just as with any other drug.

According to an analysis conducted in the United States (Bair et al., 2005), three out of four women in midlife report regular use of complementary/alternative therapies. It is expected that concerns regarding estrogens and their risks will prompt perimenopausal women to see alternatives, including phytoestrogens and black cohosh.

Phytoestrogens/Isoflavones for Menopausal Symptoms

The safety concerns of estrogens have prompted many women to seek alternatives for the treatment of menopausal symptoms. Interest in plant-derived estrogen-like substances, including soy and clover products, phytoestrogens and isoflavones, have been promoted as effective treatments for controlling these symptoms. Unfortunately, conflicting data leave clinicians and clients confused regarding their benefits.

A year-long trial of one phytoestrogens, genistein, was compared with estrogen and placebo in 90 postmenopausal women. After a year, daily flushes were reduced 24% with genistein compared with placebo, although benefits were not as significant as with estrogen (Crisafulli et al., 2004). A review of available trials of soy-based isoflavones for vasomotor symptoms by the North American Menopause Society suggests only modest positive findings with statistically significant benefit noted in only 4 of the 16 studies evaluated. Similar findings were identified for clover-based phytoestrogens (North American Menopause Society, 2004).

An 8-month trial of isoflavonoids in 56 postmenopausal breast cancer survivors revealed no difference between drug and placebo for improving menopausal symptoms, anxiety, or depression (Nikander et al., 2003). A 12-week randomized double blind evaluation of isoflavone supplements in 246 menopausal women yielded no difference between two different doses and placebo in relief of hot flashes (Tice et al., 2003). Isoflavone enriched soy protein therapy for one year failed to yield meaningful differences in cognition, bone mineral den-

sity, or cholesterol levels in a trial with 175 older postmenopausal women (Kreijkamp-Kaspers et al., 2004). A similar lack of response was noted when soy milk with phytoestrogens was used in 202 postmenopausal women (Kok, Kreijkamp-Kaspers, Grobbee, Lampe, & van der Schouw, 2005).

The safety of phytoestrogens/isoflavones has not been well studied. One case report of male breast cancer has been attributed to phytoestrogen therapy (Dimitrakakis, Gosselink, Gaki, Bredakis, Keramopoulos, 2004), although it appears premature to generalize this observation to the population at large.

Black Cohosh for Menopausal Symptoms

Extracts derived from the plant root of black cohosh have long been advocated for the treatment of vasomotor symptoms of menopause. A number of poorly designed studies have suggested promising results, but researchers have questioned their methodology (North American Menopause Society, 2004). A more rigorous randomized double-blind trial of 304 postmenopausal women in Germany revealed that 2.5 mg of isopropanolic extract—equivalent to 20 mg of root stock—taken twice daily over 12 weeks resulted in the improvement of hot flashes, vaginal dryness, mood, and memory compared with placebo (Osmers et al., 2005). Women who were in their early menopause years appear to respond better to cohosh according to this evaluation. Although short-term use did not result in altered liver enzyme levels, it is not clear if black cohosh possesses activity at estrogen receptors. As such, the long-term safety of black cohosh remains in question.

Critical Thinking Questions

- What recommendations should the nurse make to a postmenopausal woman who inquires about the benefits of phytoestrogens or black cohosh?
- How should the nurse respond to questions regarding the safety of these agents?

---

hormonal contraception (see the discussion on pp. 912 to 915). Estrogens are contraindicated in women who are pregnant (because of risk of fetal malformation), have a history of CAD, thromboembolic events or have a history of estrogen dependent neoplasms. Estrogens should be avoided unless the benefit outweighs risk for clients who smoke, have a family history of breast cancer, history of gallstones, hypertension, heart failure, hypercalcemia or hypertriglyceridemia, or who are breastfeeding.

Pharmacokinetics/Dosing

Estrogen is protein bound, metabolized in the liver, and excreted by the kidneys.

The lowest effective dosage of estrogens is administered for the shortest time period to reduce the possibility of serious adverse effects. When continuous therapy is required, the prescriber should reevaluate the client at least annually.

Estradiol and estrone are naturally occurring steroidal estrogens that are principal endogenous estrogens. Estradiol is available alone

or synthetically as estradiol cypionate, estradiol valerate, ethinyl estradiol, and polyestradiol phosphate. The primary pharmacologic effects of all estrogens are similar. Conjugated estrogens (Premarin), a mixture of estrogenic substances (especially estrone and equilin), are available in oral, parenteral, and vaginal cream dosage forms. The dosage must be individualized according to diagnosis and therapeutic response (e.g., vasomotor symptoms associated with menopause). The usual oral adult dosage for esterified estrogens is 0.3 to 1.25 mg daily, either cyclically or continuously. Some women may require higher dosages.

A cyclic dosing schedule of 3 weeks of estrogen administration and 1 week off or the addition of a progestin for the last 10 to 13 days of the cycle most closely approximates the natural hormonal cycle and prevents overstimulation of estrogen-sensitive tissues. This is not the schedule for clients who have had an oophorectomy or for clients who have cancer and are receiving hormonal therapy. Prempro, a combination of conjugated estrogen and medroxyproges-

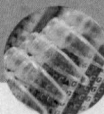

Special Considerations for Pharmacogenetics | ESTROGENS AND PROGESTINS

PHARMACODYNAMICS

The estrogen receptors are regulated by genetically determined factors and account for a variety of effects in different individuals (Draper & Chin, 2003). This variation may result in different responses and risks associated with estrogen use and drugs that act at estrogen receptors (Herrington, 2003).

Synthesis of progestins and androgens in both men and women may be affected by genetic variation in glutathione transferase. Some African populations may be display more variation in the gene which codes for this enzyme (Tetlow, Coggan, Casarotto, & Board, 2004). The clinical significance of this finding is unclear, but may be linked increased risk for endometrial cancer (Modugno, 2004).

PHARMACOKINETICS

A number of genetically determined enzymes are involved in estrogen metabolism, including P450 1 A2 and 3 A4 and subtypes of uridine diphospho-gluronosyltransferases (UGT) (Lepine et al., 2004) and may explain varying responses to estrogen doses across populations.

Disparity in both endogenous estrogen levels and administered estrogens is observed in clients for enzyme inducing agents such as the antiepileptic drugs carbamazepine, phenobarbital, and phenytoin. Variation in enzyme function, being genetically determined, is likely to explain why some women taking antiepileptic drugs experience reduced fertility and hyposexuality compared to the general population (Anderson, 2004).

ADVERSE EFFECTS

The ability of estradiol (the endogenous estrogen) to induce platelet aggregation is genetically determined (Tanus-Santos et al., 2002) and may explain variable risk for deep vein thrombosis and other clotting disorders with estrogen use. Additionally, thromboembolic events may be up to eleven times higher for women who have inherited thrombophilia as manifest by the deficiencies in the endogenous anticoagulants protein C and protein S (Martinelli, Battaglioli, & Mannucci, 2003). Cancer risks associated with estrogen use may be higher in some women with genetic predisposition for altered metabolism of estrogens or altered estrogen receptors. Markers identifying a genetic risk for endometrial cancer with estrogen use remain elusive (Paynter, Hankinson, Colditz, Hunter, De Vivo, 2004). Cholestasis of pregnancy is related to genetic markers (Pauli-Magnus et al., 2004). It is unclear if these markers could also predict for the risk of cholestasis associated with estrogen use.

Identification of high risk clients utilizing pharmacogenomics may allow for safer use of estrogen therapy in the future (Krauss, 2002).

---

terone, is indicated for the treatment of menopausal symptoms and vulvae/vaginal atrophy.

Transdermal estradiol (Estraderm) is as effective for women with estrogen deficiency as oral hormone replacement therapy. Applied topically to intact skin, the reservoir-type patch is available in 25 (Canada only), 50 (United States and Canada), and 100 mcg (United States and Canada) and is replaced twice weekly. The matrix-type estradiol (Fem Patch, Climara) is available in 25, 50, or 100 mcg for once-weekly dosing; the twice-weekly transdermal system (Vivelle, Alora) is available in 25, 50, 75, or 100 mcg. The strengths listed are released daily from the transdermal patch. The patch should be replaced according to schedule. Usually no patch is worn on the fourth week, although continuous application may be appropriate for some clients.

Adverse Effects

The most serious adverse effects include thromboembolic events, and increased risk for breast or endometrial cancers. Thromboembolic events are more likely in clients who are smokers, and/or who have a history of thromboembolic disease (e.g., deep vein thrombosis, pulmonary embolism [PE], thromboembolic cerebrovascular accident), or who have CAD. The risk for breast cancer is highest for clients with a history or strong family history of breast cancer. The risk for endometrial cancer may be lower when progestin is used in combination with estrogen, but this combination may increase the risk for breast cancer. Modest elevations in blood pressure may also be noted with estrogen use. Other adverse effects of estrogen include gallstones, stomach cramps or gas, anorexia, chloasma (facial hyperpigmentation), headaches, nausea, vomiting, change in female libido, decrease in male sex drive, edema of the lower extremities, breast pain and enlargement, and changes in menstrual bleeding. Nausea and stomach discomfort are often minimized by dosing at bedtime.

Drug Interactions

Estrogens are metabolized by cytochrome P450 1 A2 and 3 A4 and interact with a number of different medications affecting these enzyme systems. Drugs that may increase estrogen metabolism (and result in decreased estrogen levels) include many of the antiepileptic drugs (e.g., phenobarbital, carbamazepine, phenytoin) and antiinfectives (e.g., rifampin, rifabutin), azole antifungals like fluconazole, macrolides (e.g., erythromycin), and human immunodeficiency virus (HIV) therapies (e.g., efavirenz). Consult with appropriate references for more interacting drugs. See the assessment of concurrent drug therapy in the following nursing assessment.

⚬ **M.B. is concerned about the use of an estrogen-containing product and asks the clinic office nurse what she should do.**

⚬ **What nursing management is appropriate in the use of supplemental estrogens?**

Assessment Estrogen therapy is contraindicated for M.B. if breast cancer is known or suspected, because there is the possible promotion of tumor growth. It is also contraindicated for her, if she has abnormal or undiagnosed vaginal bleeding; such bleeding may indicate endometrial hyperplasia or carcinoma, which would be promoted by estrogen use. Active thromboembolic disorders are also a contraindication for estrogen therapy.

Estrogens are to be used with caution in M.B. if she has hypercalcemia associated with metastatic breast disease or a history of gallstones, hypertension, heart failure, hypertriglyceridemia, endometriosis, uterine fibroids, or thrombophlebitis secondary to estrogen use; these conditions may be aggravated by estrogen use. In males for whom estrogens may be administered for the treatment of prostatic or breast cancer, there is an increased risk for myocardial infarction (MI), PE, and thrombophlebitis; therefore care should be exercised in clients with a past or active history of these conditions.

Review M.B.'s current medication regimen for the risk of significant drug interactions, such as those that may occur when estrogens are given concurrently with the following drugs: bromocriptine (Parlodel) as concurrent use may result in amenorrhea and may also interfere with the therapeutic effect of bromocriptine. Monitor closely, because a dosage adjustment may be required. Calcium supplementation used concurrently with estrogens may increase calcium absorption and increase the risk for nephrolithiasis, but it may also be used to therapeutic advantage by increasing bone mass. Use of estrogens with corticosteroids may decrease the clearance of corticosteroids, increasing the therapeutic and toxic effects of corticosteroids; dosage adjustments of corticosteroids may be necessary. Concurrent use of cyclosporine (Sandimmune) may inhibit its metabolism resulting in increased cyclosporine plasma levels and an increased risk of hepatotoxicity and nephrotoxicity. Use estrogen only with very close monitoring of cyclosporine serum levels and liver and kidney function. Estrogens increase the risk of inducing hepatotoxicity with hepatotoxic drugs, with women older than 35 years of age at increased risk. Avoid concurrent use of hepatotoxic drugs to avoid potentially serious drug interactions. Protease inhibitors, such as ritonavir (Norvir) decrease plasma levels of estrogens; dosage adjustments may be necessary. Tobacco smoking increases the risk of serious cardiac adverse effects such as cerebrovascular accident (CVA), transient ischemic attacks (TIAs), thrombophlebitis, and PE. The risk is higher in women over 35 years of age who smoke; avoid concurrent use. Concurrent use with tamoxifen (Nolvadex) may interfere with the therapeutic effect of tamoxifen.

Depending on M.B.'s health status, some of the following assessments are performed as a baseline before therapy: a physical examination that includes blood pressure, a serum lipid profile, and hepatic function determinations. Additionally, a Papanicolaou (Pap) smear, breast examination, and mammogram are required for female clients; if appropriate, an endometrial biopsy is performed to rule out malignancy.

Nursing Diagnosis While M.B. is receiving estrogen therapy, she may experience the following nursing diagnoses/collaborative problems: impaired comfort related to anorexia, nausea, vomiting, abdominal cramping, breast tenderness, headaches, mild dizziness or skin irritation (transdermal patches); impaired skin integrity related to the development of acne; disturbed sensory perception (vision) related to a steepening of the corneal curvature and contributing to an intolerance of contact lenses; excess fluid volume (peripheral edema, sudden weight gain); disturbed body image related to chloasma (brown, blotchy skin changes), gynecomastia (men), increased libido (women), or decreased libido (men); and the potential complications of gallbladder obstruction, hepatitis, pancreatitis, breast tumors, and thrombophlebitis and thromboembolism.

Planning While taking estrogen therapy, the client will, if being treated for:

- Breast carcinoma (selected men and postmenopausal or oophorectomized women), experience palliation such as a decrease in the size of the tumor or less rapid growth and improved quality of life during the remission.
- Prostatic carcinoma, experience palliation such as a decrease in size of tumor and spread of metastases without gynecomastia, hot flushes, thromboembolic disease, or erectile dysfunction.
- Estrogen deficiency, experience a decrease in vasomotor symptoms of menopause, atrophic vaginitis, vulvar atrophy, and reduced rate of bone loss.

All clients will:

- Effectively manage the therapeutic regimen, including medication compliance, stating reportable symptoms to prescriber, undertaking supportive interventions to the drug.
- Collaborate with health care providers for monitoring and treatment.

Implementation

Monitoring Assess M.B.'s blood pressure periodically. Hepatic function studies are performed every 6 to 12 months for clients with hepatic dysfunction. Males treated with estrogens are checked regularly for the development of breast carcinomas. At least annually, M.B. will undergo a physical examination that includes a Pap smear, mammogram, and serum lipid profile. Breast self-examinations are done monthly. Hand and wrist radiographs for bone age determinations are recommended every 6 months for children and adolescents.

Intervention Estrogens are administered at the lowest effective dosage and M.B. is evaluated annually to determine continuance of therapy. To reduce the risk of endometrial hyperplasia or cancer, the concurrent use of a progestin for 10 to 14 days of the cycle is recommended for women with an intact uterus. Estrogens may be administered on a cycle of 3 weeks on and 1 week off or continuously, except in males, who take them continuously. Some prescribers recommend the continuous use of estrogen and progestin in a combination tablet for women who do not want to resume menses.

Clients who have been taking oral estrogens should wait a week after the last oral dose to start transdermal dosage forms. For women with a uterus, the transdermal dosage system is used 3 weeks on and 1 week off; again progestin is recommended for 10 to 14 days of the cycle. For women without a uterus, the patch may be used in a continuous fashion.

Other forms of administration: Administer the IM forms slowly to minimize client discomfort. Use large muscles, such as the gluteus maximus, for injection to maximize absorption. For oil-based preparations, use at least a 21-gauge needle and a dry syringe.

Administer IV estrogens slowly; vaginal burning occurs if they are administered too rapidly.

Administer vaginal forms at bedtime to enhance absorption. Sanitary napkins or panty shields may be used to protect clothing from stains.

Education Assist M.B. in exploring concerns about the risks of taking estrogens. Provide her with information regarding the occurrence of cardiovascular disease and cancer in relationship to age, smoking habits, and other health characteristics. Encourage her to carefully read the package insert that is required to be given to every client and then discuss any concerns. Advise M.B. to have regular physical examinations every 6 to 12 months during treatment that would include a pelvic and breast examination, mammogram, and a Pap smear. Provide instructions for monthly self-examination of the breasts; any lumps found should be reported to the prescriber. M.B. has no uterus, but other clients are to be advised to stop the medication immediately and contact their prescriber if they suspect they are pregnant.

Caution M.B. that smoking increases the incidence of serious adverse cardiovascular effects, particularly in women older than 35 years of age. Instruct her to notify the health provider in the instance of severe headache, blurred or lost vision (which may signal possible stroke), or symptoms of chest pain, shortness of breath, or leg pain (which may indicate thromboembolism elsewhere in the body). She should also inform the prescriber of a severe abdominal pain or mass, jaundice, severe mental depression, or unusual bleeding.

If M.B. is considering the use of phytoestrogens/isoflavones or black cohosh in addition to or in place of estrogen replacement, she should be provided with current information in the same manner as the nurse would provide information about any drug. Refer again to Evidence-Based Practice box.

Nausea often occurs at the beginning of therapy and usually ceases after 1 or 2 weeks. It is seldom severe and can be controlled by taking the medication once a day with food or at bedtime.

Advise M.B. to weigh one or two times weekly and to report a sharp increase in weight or other signs of fluid retention, such as swollen ankles, puffy eyelids, and "tight" rings. A low-sodium diet and diuretic may be prescribed to control these symptoms.

Encourage M.B. to maintain a program of good oral hygiene, including teeth cleaning by a professional and thorough brushing and plaque control by her to minimize any gingival hyperplasia that may occur during estrogen therapy. Warn her that exposure to the sun or tanning devices

may result in a brown, blotchy discoloration of the skin. For other clients with an intact uterus, bleeding after estrogen withdrawal is expected. Explain to postmenopausal women that such bleeding does not indicate that a state of fertility has returned.

Instruct M.B. that while taking estrogen for osteoporosis prophylaxis (no longer considered a primary indication for use), she should increase her intake of calcium and vitamin D and to engage in regular weight-bearing exercise such as walking.

When applying the transdermal form of the drug, teach M.B. to wash her hands before and after applying the patch. Apply the system immediately after removing it from the pouch and its protective liner. Apply it to the trunk below the waist on clean, dry, intact skin without hair. Rotate the sites to prevent application to any site more frequently than every 7 days. Do not apply the patch to the breasts or to the waistline, where clothing might cause the patch to become loose. Press the patch into place for 10 seconds and then examine it to ensure that all the edges are tight. If the patch loosens or falls off, it may be reapplied or a new one applied as long as the original schedule is maintained, either a patch every 7 days or two times a week as prescribed.

Instruct clients with diabetes to report elevated blood glucose tests so the dosage of their antidiabetic medications can be adjusted.

Forewarn male clients of estrogen-induced feminization and impotence, which will disappear when therapy terminates. Advise male clients of the increased risk of MI, PE, and thrombophlebitis while undergoing estrogen therapy.

Instruct clients using the estradiol vaginal insert in the proper technique for insertion and removal.

Evaluation The expected outcome of estrogen therapy is that M.B. will demonstrate an improvement in the underlying condition for which the drug was prescribed without experiencing any adverse effects related to drug therapy; see planning. She will maintain medication compliance, demonstrate the appropriate method of administering the drug, report adverse symptoms to the prescriber appropriately, institute supportive measures, and maintain scheduled visits to the prescriber for monitoring and treatment.

✱ **S.J. is a 27-year-old woman with a history of significant vaginal bleeding in irregular cycles. S.J. has become anemic and requires iron supplementation. She is evaluated carefully by her gynecologist who evaluates the bleeding and rules out cancer. She is diagnosed with dysfunctional uterine bleeding and is started on the progestin medroxyprogesterone (Provera) 5 mg daily for 10 days beginning on day 16 of her cycle. She will continue therapy for 3 months at which time she will return to the gynecologist for a follow-up evaluation.**

✱ **What are the primary actions and uses of progesterone and progestins?**
Progesterone produced by the ovaries is a naturally occurring progestin. Anterior pituitary LH stimulates the synthe-

sis and secretion of progesterone from the corpus luteum, mainly during the latter half of the menstrual cycle. Progesterone may also be formed from steroid precursors available in the ovaries, testes, adrenal cortex, and placenta.

Progesterone and progestins vary in potency. Chemically, progesterone and the progestins are similar in structure to estrogens and androgens, and possess varying estrogen-like and androgen-like properties. Unlike estrogens, however, progestins do not appear to increase the risk for breast cancer (Strom et al., 2004). Progesterone and progestins produce biochemical changes in the endometrium to prepare for the implantation and nourishment of the embryo. They also perform the following functions: (1) supplement the action of estrogen in its effects on the uterus and mammary glands, (2) suppress ovulation during pregnancy, (3) cause relaxation of the uterine smooth muscles, (4) increase the synthesis of DNA and RNA, and (5) inhibit, in large doses, the secretion of LH from the anterior pituitary.

Progesterone and synthetic progestins have similar pharmacologic effects in the body. A micronized formulation of progesterone (Prometrium) is available for oral use. Progestins are synthetic progesterone derivatives with greater potency, longer durations of action and some improvement in bioavailability.

Available progestin-only products include levonorgestrel (Minera, Norplant Implant, Plan B), medroxyprogesterone (Depo-Provera, Provera), norethindrone acetate (Aygestin). Progestins that are available in combination with estrogens for hormonal contraception include desogestrel, ethynodiol diacetate, etonogestrel, levonorgestrel, norethindrone, norgestrel, norgestromin, and norgestimate. Megestrol acetate (Megace) is pharmacologically classified as a progestin, but its use is limited to treatment of breast and endometrial cancers, and to treat anorexia and cachexia of acquired immune deficiency syndrome (AIDS). Medroxyprogesterone is considered the typical progestin and is discussed in the following section.

✱⚕ medroxyprogesterone
[meh drocks ee pro **jess** ter one]
(Depo-Provera, Provera, Novo-Medrone✤)
Indications
Medroxyprogesterone and other progestins are indicated for the treatment of female hormonal imbalance of amenorrhea, dysmenorrhea, and endometriosis. They are also used for hyperventilation disorders and specific carcinomas. Other progestins are combined with estrogen to lower the risk of breast and endometrial cancer with hormone replacement therapy. Progestins are also used to diagnose endogenous estrogen deficiency and to prevent pregnancy. _Precautions_: When used to treat dysfunctional uterine bleeding, other causes of bleeding (e.g., cancer) must first be ruled out, as progestins will arrest the bleeding, but not treat the underlying condition. Progesterone-only products, including medroxyprogesterone, are used for hormonal contraception and are also discussed later. Caution is recommended when used for clients with depression, migraines, cardiac dysfunction, history of thromboembolic events, or hyperlipidemias. Progestins should be avoided in pregnancy.
Pharmacokinetics/Dosing
Oral absorption of medroxyprogesterone is fairly rapid with an extensive metabolism by the liver immediately after absorption (high first-pass effect). The IM formulation is slowly absorbed and released from IM sites. Medroxyprogesterone is metabolized by P450 3 A4.

Medroxyprogesterone (Provera) is dosed at 2.5 to 10 mg PO daily for 5-10 days (day 16 and after for 10 days or day 21 and after for 5 days) each cycle for amenorrhea or abnormal uterine bleeding. For hormonal therapy with estrogens, medroxyprogesterone is dosed 2.5 to 10 mg PO daily for 12 to 14 days starting on day 16 or 21 of menstrual cycle. In some regimens medroxyprogesterone is dosed concurrently with estrogens throughout the month; in others it is used for 14 days once every 3 months. Medroxyprogesterone acetate as an injectable suspension (Depo-Provera) is typically dosed at 150 mg IM every 3 months. Its use is discussed later in the chapter.
Adverse Effects
Adverse effects of medroxyprogesterone include weight gain, stomach pain/cramps, swelling of the face and lower extremities, headache, mood alterations, anxiety, increased weakness, amenorrhea, breakthrough bleeding, hyperglycemia, menorrhagia, galactorrhea, rash, acne, insomnia, and breast pain. Like with estrogens, dosing at bedtime can reduce gastrointestinal complaints. Significant loss in bone density, possibly irreversible, has been reported with the use of Depo-Provera. The risk is highest for women who receive prolonged therapy. Prompted by the FDA, the manufacturer (Pfizer) has revised labeling to limit long-term therapy (e.g., 2 years or longer) to women for whom alternate forms of contraception are inadequate (FDA Talk Paper T04-50, November 17, 2004).
Drug Interactions
Enzyme inducing drugs (e.g., carbamazepine, phenobarbital, phenytoin, rifampin, and rifabutin) may result in increased metabolism (and reduced effect) of progestins.

✱ **S.J. asks the nurse about how to use the medroxyprogesterone (Provera).**

✱ **What are the nursing management issues in the use of progestins?**

Assessment Determine before progestin therapy begins that S.J. does not have preexisting cancer of the breast or reproductive tract, suspected pregnancy, incomplete abortion, abnormal and undiagnosed vaginal or urinary tract bleeding, a history of or active thrombophlebitis or thromboembolic disorder, hepatic dysfunction, or sensitivity to progestins, or peanuts (oral or parenteral progesterone), which are conditions for which progestins are contraindicated. If used for controlling excessive menstrual bleeding, a hematologic assessment for anemia or for platelet for coagulation abnormalities may also be indicated (Philipp et al., 2005). Progestins should be used cautiously in clients with asthma, migraine headaches, epilepsy, cardiac insufficiency, or renal dysfunction because of their tendency to cause fluid retention. Progestins may aggravate existing hepatic disease. Metabolism of progestins may also be impaired in clients with hepatic insufficiency. Clients with a history of diabetes should also be monitored carefully for a mild decrease in glucose tolerance. Mental depression may be worsened. Because some progestins elevate levels of low-density lipoproteins (LDLs) and lower high-density lipoproteins (HDLs), hyperlipidemia may be aggravated.

Congenital anomalies have been reported with the use of progestins during the first 4 months of pregnancy. They should not be used as diagnostic tests for pregnancy (see the Pregnancy Safety box on p. 906). Progestins are also excreted in breast milk and therefore are not recommended for use by nursing women.

When progestins are given concurrently with aminoglutethimide (Cytadren), the absorption of oral medroxyprogesterone may be decreased, and serum concentrations are significantly lowered. Hepatic enzyme-inducing drugs, such as carbamazepine (Tegretol), phenobarbital (Barbita), phenytoin (Dilantin), rifabutin (Mycobutin), or rifampin (Rifadin) may cause decreased serum concentrations of progestins; dosage adjustments may be necessary.

Nursing Diagnosis Clients undergoing progesterone/progestin therapy are at risk for the following nursing diagnoses/collaborative problems: impaired comfort (headache, nausea, breast tenderness, cramping, hot flashes, or irritation at the injection site); excess fluid volume (peripheral edema, weight gain); disturbed sleep pattern (insomnia); fatigue; disturbed body image related to increased facial and body hair, loss of scalp hair, weight gain, or melasma; impaired skin integrity (acne); disturbed sensory perception related to neuroocular lesions (double vision or loss of vision); and the potential complications of changed vaginal bleeding pattern, mental depression, hyperglycemia, adrenal suppression, hepatitis, ovarian enlargement, or ovarian cyst formation and, in high-dose therapy for noncontraceptive uses, thrombophlebitis, retinal thrombosis, or thromboembolism.

Planning While taking progestin therapy, the client will, if being treated for:

- Secondary amenorrhea or induction of menses, experience endometrial shedding 3 to 7 days after discontinuance of progestin.
- Advanced hormonally dependent breast carcinoma (postmenopausal or oophorectomized women), experience a decrease in the size of the tumor or less rapid growth, and improved quality of life during the remission.
- Endometrial or renal cancer, experience decrease in tumor size and spread of metastases, and improved quality of life.

- Prostatic carcinoma, experience palliation such as a decrease in size of tumor and spread of metastases without gynecomastia, hot flushes, thromboembolic disease, or erectile dysfunction.
- Prevention of pregnancy, not conceive.

All clients will:

- Effectively manage the therapeutic regimen, including medication compliance, stating reportable symptoms to prescriber, undertaking supportive interventions to the drug.
- Collaborate with health care providers for monitoring and treatment.

Implementation

Monitoring Undesirable effects are usually mild or absent during short-term use. However, the number and severity of adverse effects increase as the duration of progestin therapy increases. Assess for these effects as long as therapy continues. A physical examination at least every 6 to 12 months should include a breast and pelvic examination, Pap smear, lipid profile, and hepatic function studies. S.J. needs to perform a breast self-exam monthly.

Intervention Give oil preparations by deep IM injection. A low-sodium diet and diuretic may be prescribed to control symptoms of fluid retention, such as swollen ankles and puffy eyelids.

Education Regulations require that a package insert be given to every client who is dispensed a progestin unless the drug is being used as an antineoplastic adjunct. Encourage S.J. to read the package insert carefully and then discuss with the health care provider any concerns. Advise her to have regular physical examinations as described previously.

Instruct S.J. to notify the prescriber in the instance of severe headache, blurred or lost vision (which may possibly signal stroke), and symptoms of chest pain, shortness of breath, or leg pain (which may indicate thromboembolism elsewhere in the body). She should also inform the prescriber of severe abdominal pain or mass, jaundice, severe mental depression, or unusual bleeding. Changes in vaginal bleeding may include irregular cycle time, spotting, breakthrough bleeding, or a complete lack of bleeding. Provide instruction for monthly self-examination of the breasts; and report any changes.

Advise S.J. to discontinue the medication immediately and notify the prescriber if she suspects she is pregnant. Pregnancy should be avoided during the first month of progestin administration and for at least 3 months after they are discontinued. Barrier contraceptives should be used during this time.

Because progestins may cause glucose intolerance, instruct users with diabetes to report elevated glucose tests so that an adjustment in their insulin or oral hypoglycemic dosage may be prescribed.

If progestins are used for contraceptive purposes, instruct the client to take the drug at the same time of day, every day of the year. The tablets need to be kept in their original containers. It is best to keep an extra month's supply, replacing it with the new container of tablets purchased each month. This will always ensure a fresh supply.

Evaluation The expected outcome is that the client will demonstrate an improvement in the underlying condition for which the drug was prescribed without experiencing untoward effects; see planning. S.J. will maintain medication compliance, demonstrate the appropriate method of administering the drug, report adverse symptoms to the prescriber appropriately, institute supportive measures, and maintain scheduled visits to the prescriber for monitoring and treatment.

⚙ **P.L. is an 18-year-old college freshman who reports to the university health service for contraception. She is thinking of hormonal contraception and asks the nurse which choices are safe and effective.**

⚙ **What are the important issues involved in choosing hormonal contraceptives?**

Many forms of contraception are available to clients and most are effective (Table 51-1). **Hormonal contraception** delivery systems are among the most effective forms of birth control available. The experience of millions of women who have used oral and transdermal hormonal contraceptives has yielded an enormous amount of information about the safety and effectiveness of estrogen-progestin combinations and progestin-only agents. In the late 1950s and early 1960s, early forms of hormonal contraception (oral contraceptives, or "the pill") used fairly high doses of estrogen to prevent pregnancy in sexually active women. The newer, low-dose estrogen-progestin combinations and the progestin-only agents are highly effective with fewer adverse effects than early formulations of oral contraceptives. Although highly effective for most clients, failure of these lower dose hormonal contraceptives appears 60% to 70% higher for obese women compared to controls (Holt,

TABLE 51-1 COMPARATIVE EFFICACY OF CONTRACEPTIVE METHODS

Method	Unintended Pregnancies Within First Year of Use (%)		Frequency of Use
	Typical Use*	Ideal Use†	
None	85	85	
Spermicide	29	15	Each time
Withdrawal	27	4	Each time
Periodic abstinence: Calendar method	25	9	Each time
Periodic abstinence: Ovulation method	25	3	Each time
Cervical cap with spermicide: parous women	32	26	Each time
Cervical cap with spermicide: nulliparous women	16	9	Each time
Diaphragm with spermicide	16	6	Each time
Female condom	21	5	Each time
Male condom	15	2	Each time
Oral contraceptive pill	8	0.3	Taken daily
Contraceptive patch	Unknown	0.3	Applied weekly
Vaginal ring	Unknown	0.3	Inserted every 4 weeks
Medroxyprogesterone depot IM	3	0.3	Given every 12 weeks
Copper-containing intrauterine device	0.8	0.6	Inserted every 10 years
Levonorgestrel intrauterine system	0.1	0.1	Inserted every 5 years
Female sterilization	0.5	0.5	Done once
Male sterilization	0.15	0.10	Done once

Modified from Herndon, E.J., & Zieman, M. (2004). New Contraceptive Options. *American Family Physician* 69:853-60. Retrieved August 1, 2004, from http://www.aafp.org/afp/20040215/853.html (this has been adapted from Hatcher, R.A. (2000). *A pocket guide to managing contraception.* 5th ed. Tiger, Ga.: Bridging the Gap Foundation, 44-141, (www.managingcontraception.com).

*Percentage of typical couples who experience an accidental pregnancy during the first year of use if they continue intervention for one full year.

†Percentage of couples who experience an accidental pregnancy during the first year of ideal, as intended use of intervention if they continue intervention for one full year.

Scholes, Wicklund, Cushing-Haugen, & Daling, 2005). This may be related to altered metabolism of estrogen in obese women or an increased dose requirement for tissue distribution, but may be more common with use of newer low-dose agents.

Trials of testosterone and combinations of testosterone/progestins in suppressing male LH and spermatogenesis have

not been successful, which suggests that a hormonally based contraceptive for men is not likely to be effective (Grimes, Gallo, Grigorieva, Nanda, & Schulz, 2005).

A great number of estrogen/progestin and progestin only agents and formulations are currently available for use to prevent pregnancy (Table 51-2). The hormonal contraceptives require sustained levels of estrogen and/or progestin to sup-

TABLE 51-2 SELECTED HORMONAL CONTRACEPTIVES*

Brand Name Drug	Route	Typical Adult Dose	Estrogen Content	Progestin Content
Brevicon	Monophasic oral	One tablet active drug PO daily on days 1-21 of cycle; some systems include placebo or low dose iron tablets for days 22-28	ethinyl estradiol 35 mcg	norethindrone 500 mcg
Demulen 1/35			ethinyl estradiol 35 mcg	ethynodiol 1 mg
Lo/Ovral			ethinyl estradiol 30 mcg	norgestrel 300 mcg
Ovral			ethinyl estradiol 50 mcg	norgestrel 500 mcg
Ortho-Novum 10/11	Biphasic oral		ethinyl estradiol 35 mcg	norethindrone: 0.5 mg days 1-10 1 mg days 11-21
Ortho Tri-Cyclen	Triphasic oral		ethinyl estradiol: 35 mcg days 1-21 placebo days 22-28	norgestimate: 180 mcg days 1-7 215 mcg days 8-14 250 mcg days 15-21 placebo days 22-28
Estrostep Fe			ethinyl estradiol: 20 mcg days 1-5 30 mcg days 6-12 35 mcg days 13-21	norethindrone acetate: 1 mg days 1-21 [ferrous fumarate 75 mg days 22-28]
Ovrette	Progestin only oral			norgestrel 75 mcg
NuvaRing	Vaginal ring	Insert vaginally on day 5, remove after 3 weeks; insert new 1 week later	ethinyl estradiol: 15 mcg daily delivered	etonogestrel: 120 mcg daily delivered
Ortho Evra	Transdermal	Transdermal 1 patch/ week × 3 weeks; 1 week off	ethinyl estradiol 20 mcg daily	norelgestromin 150 mcg daily
Depo-Provera	Depot IM	150 mg IM q3 months		medroxyprogesterone 150 mg
Plan B	Postcoital oral	One tablet PO q12h × 2 up to 72 hr postcoitus		levonorgestrel 750 mcg
Preven		Two tablets PO q12h × 2 up to 72 hr postcoitus	ethinyl estradiol: 50 mcg/tab	levonorgestrel: 250 mcg/tab
RU486/Mifeprex	Early oral pregnancy termination (Limited access)	600 mg PO × 1 with misoprostol (Cytotec) up to 49 days from last menstrual period		Progesterone antagonist mifepristone 600 mg

*This table represents selected agents only. There are at least 50 different monophasic estrogen/progestin formulations, 11 triphasic estrogen/progestin formulations and 6 oral progestin-only formulations marketed in North America.

press LH and FSH, and thereby prevent ovulation. Additionally, changes in the endometrium impair ova implantation, and an increase in cervical mucus impedes the passage of sperm. The oral tablets are usually packaged in a 21- or 28-day packaging system to improve adherence. Many offer variations in estrogen/progestin concentrations throughout the cycle for 21 days of active drug (and 7 days of placebo or low dose iron supplementation for the last 7 days). The formulations with identical concentrations of estrogen/progestin for 21 days are often referred to as "monophasic." Those which offer two or three different concentrations of progestin (and sometime estrogen) through the cycle to more closely mimic endogenous changes are referred to as "biphasic" or "triphasic" formulations respectively.

Oral tablet formulations must be administered daily, and nonadherence for even 2 or 3 consecutive days poses a risk for pregnancy. Transdermal formulations (e.g., ethinyl estradiol/norelgestromin transdermal [Ortho-Evra]), vaginal ring formulations (e.g., ethinyl estradiol/etonogestrel vaginal [NuvaRing], and progesterone depot injections (medroxyprogesterone acetate [Depo-Provera]) and intradermal implants (levonorgestrel implants [Norplant]) offer alternatives to daily oral therapy and may improve adherence.

The estrogen/progestin and progestin-only contraceptives carry the same risks as that observed with the use of these agents for other indications and are discussed previously. The estrogen containing products in particular carry risks for thromboembolic events, which are highest in smokers and women older than 35 years of age. They are also contraindicated in pregnancy, in clients with a history of breast cancer or other estrogen-dependent tumors, and clients with a history of cardiovascular or thromboembolic disorders. Women with a history of gallstones, liver disorders, or migraine headaches should also avoid hormonal contraception, particularly agents containing estrogen. Also, the estrogens (and to some degree the progestins) interact with a number of drugs metabolized by cytochrome P450 systems. Many of these interacting drugs may result in subtherapeutic estrogen and/or progestin levels and increase pregnancy risk (see drug interactions under individual agents).

The progestin-only formulations (often referred to as the "mini-pill") do not contain estrogen. They are generally prescribed for 28 days of the menstrual cycle and are usually slightly less effective than the combination products. They also involve a higher incidence of spotting and breakthrough bleeding. One advantage, however, is that they are less likely to cause the more serious adverse effects associated with estrogen therapy.

Clients must understand that, unlike male condoms, hormonal contraceptives offer no protection against sexually transmitted infections (including HIV and herpes). Performing a thorough history and physical examination, selecting an appropriate contraceptive method with the individual/couple, and instituting a client teaching and monitoring program are basic for the development of a good family planning program. Table 51-3 presents recommendations for particular circumstances.

Hormonal Contraceptives

estrogen and progestin contraceptives (various manufacturers [see Table 51-2])

Indications
Estrogens and progestins are indicated for the prevention of pregnancy and for the treatment of hypermenorrhea. Some agents are also indicated for dysmenorrhea, endometriosis, polycystic ovary syndrome, and the agents with less androgenic progestin activity (e.g., ethinyl estradiol/norgestimate [Ortho Tri-Cyclen, TriNessa]) can improve acne. These agents share the same contraindications and precautions as outlined with estrogens, pp. 900 and 901.

Pharmacokinetics/Dosing
The hormonal contraceptives are protein bound, metabolized mainly in the liver, and excreted primarily by the kidneys. Dosing for each agent varies, but they are typically dosed once daily. Although it is often recommended to begin a new package on the first Sunday after onset of menses, they can probably be initiated at any time (Westhoff, Morroni, Kerns, & Murphy, 2003). Therapy is continued for 21 or 28 days, with a new package begun every 28 days. Some monthly packages have tablets that have the same medication dosages in every active drug tablet (**monophasic**). Some vary the dosages in the active tablets twice in the month (**biphasic**), and others have three different dosages during the month (**triphasic**) to more closely mimic the natural cycle of hormones (see Table 51-2 for examples).

Levonorgestrel and ethinyl estradiol (Levlen, Levora 0.15/30, Nordette, Preven) or norgestrel and ethinyl estradiol (Lo/Ovral, Ovral), are used as systemic postcoital contraceptives. Depending on formulation, two to four tablets are taken as soon as possible after unprotected coitus, preferably within 12 hours but no more than 72 hours later. Two to four more tablets are taken 12 hours after the first dose. Although it is debatable whether the availability of postcoital emergency contraception reduces pregnancy rates, such use does not appear to result in altered use of regular contraception or increased risky sexual behavior (Raine et al., 2005; Litt, 2005). Consult with package insert for more specific dosing information related to emergency contraceptive use.

Transdermal ethinyl estradiol/norelgestromin (OrthoEvra) is available as a transdermal patch administered as one patch weekly for three weeks, then a 1-week drug free interval (Figure 51-2, A). Vaginal administration of ethinyl estradiol/etonogestrel via a vaginal ring (NuvaRing) is also available for contraceptive use (Figure 51-2, B). The 2-inch diameter ring is an ethylene vinyl acetate complex impregnated with ethinyl estradiol and etonogestrel. The continuous slow absorption of the estrogen/progestin allow for lower estrogen dosing than with oral formulations. The ring is placed deep into the vagina once every 3 weeks and is removed on day 21. After a 7-day drug free interval, a new ring is inserted for an additional 21 days. Like the oral formulations, vaginal and transdermal formulations require an additional form of contraception for the first 7 days of therapy. Transdermal and vaginal ring estrogen/progestin administration shares the same risks, adverse effects, contraindications, precautions, and drug interactions as the oral formulations.

Adverse Effects
Hormone-related adverse effects are caused by an excess or a deficiency in estrogen or progestin or by an excess of androgen. Androgen effects are more common with norgestrel and levonorgestrel than with the other progestins. Reporting adverse effects to the prescriber is useful because it allows for the choice of a more appropriate hormonal contraceptive for the individual.

Excesses and deficiencies of estrogen and progestins produce a variety of symptoms. The adverse effects of estrogen excess include nausea, dizziness, abdominal bloating, leg pain, chloasma, hypertension, cyclic weight gain, hypertension, breast tenderness, and an increase in breast size. A deficiency in estrogen may produce an increase in anxiety, hot flashes, mid-cycle spotting, a decrease in menstrual flow, and a possible decrease in libido. An excess in prog-

TABLE 51-3 RECOMMENDATIONS FOR HORMONAL CONTRACEPTION IN SPECIFIED CONDITIONS

Conditions	Recommendations
AGE	
Sexually active teenagers to 35 years of age	Low estrogen (30-35 mcg)/low progestin Discourage smoking
Heavy smokers* and nonsmokers older than 35 years of age and nonsmokers older than 40 years of age	Increased risk of serious cardiovascular adverse effects; advise alternate methods of contraception
CONCURRENT DISEASE STATES	
Cancer (breast, uterus, cervix, liver)	Hormonal contraceptives contraindicated
Cerebrovascular disease, coronary artery disease, and thromboembolic disorders	Hormonal contraceptives contraindicated
Liver impairment; smokers older than 35 years of age; history of cardiovascular accident (CVA), uncontrolled hypertension, and migraine	Progestin only mini-pill is recommended
ADVERSE EFFECTS	**MANAGEMENT OF ADVERSE EFFECTS**
Acne, oily skin, hirsutism, sebaceous cysts, weight gain	Trial with hormonal contraceptives with lower progestin dose
Breakthrough bleeding	Early to mid-cycle bleeding or bleeding that never completely stops after menses is usually due to estrogen deficiency, whereas late breakthrough bleeding is due to progestin deficiency Prescribers often continue with the same hormonal contraceptive for 3 to 4 months because intermenstrual bleeding usually decreases with continued use; if bleeding continues, estrogen and/or progestin dosage may be adjusted to minimize effects
Withdrawal bleeding absent	First rule out pregnancy; if not pregnant, then a hormonal contraceptive with a lower progestin dose may be prescribed; some prescribers use ethinyl estradiol 20 mcg for 3 months in addition to the hormonal contraceptive (Hardman, 2005)
Missed dosing or adherence issues	Weekly transdermal estrogen/progestin Monthly vaginal ring estrogen/progestin Quarterly intramuscular medroxyprogesterone Yearly intrauterine progesterone system

Data from *Drug facts and comparisons* (58th ed.). (2005). St. Louis: Facts and Comparisons; Hardman, J.L. (2005). Contraception. In M.A. Koda-Kimble, L.Y. Young, W.A. Kradian, B.J. Guglielmo, B.K. Alldredge, & R.L. Corelli (Eds.), *Applied therapeutics: The clinical use of drugs* (8th ed.). Philadelphia: Lippincott Williams & Wilkins; and *USP DI: Drug information for the health care professional* (25th ed.). (2005). Greenwood Village, CO: MICROMEDEX Thomson Healthcare.
*More than 15 cigarettes/day.

estins may result in alopecia, oily skin (acne) and scalp, increased fatigue, increased appetite, and weight gain that is noncyclic, decrease in length of menstrual flow, breast tenderness, and increased breast size. A progestin deficiency may manifest itself as dysmenorrhea, heavy menstrual flow, weight loss, and/or a delayed onset of menses. An excess of androgen may result in hirsutism, oily skin or skin rash, acne, pruritus, increased appetite and weight gain (noncyclic), and cholestatic jaundice.

Drug Interactions
Refer to drug interactions for estrogens and medroxyprogesterone above.

progestin contraceptives (Various manufacturers [see Table 51-2])

Indications
The progestin-only preparations are indicated for contraception. They are also used for dysmenorrhea, endometriosis, polycystic ovarian syndrome, and dysfunctional uterine bleeding when the cause of bleeding is identified. Contraindications and precautions are listed under medroxyprogesterone, p. 905.

Pharmacokinetics/Dosing
Although systemic absorption of orally administered progesterone may be variable, the progestins (levonorgestrel [Plan B], norethin-

A

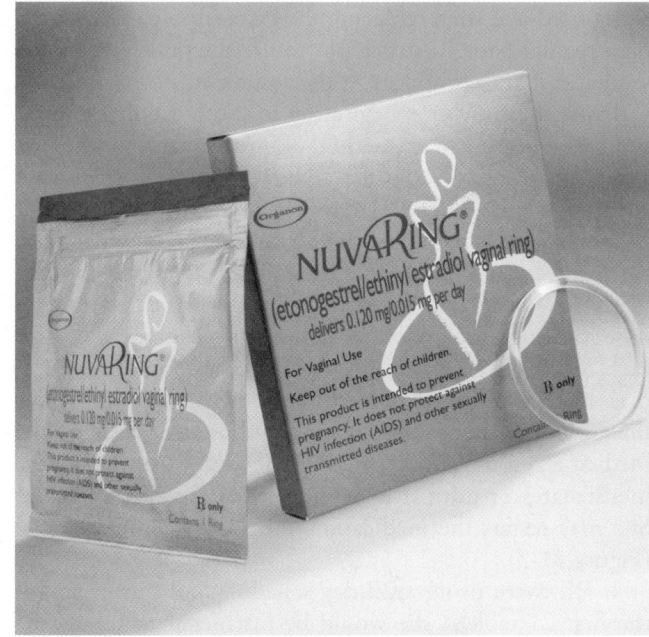

B

drone [Camila, Errin, Jolivette, Nor-QD, Ortho-Micronor], norgestrel
[Ovrette]) are well absorbed orally. With the exception of levonorgestrel, they are dosed once daily for 21 days with a drug free
or placebo interval for 7 days. Levonorgestrel (Plan B) is used for
emergency contraception administered as one 750 mcg tablet within
72 hours of unprotected intercourse, and a second dose taken 12
hours later.

Long-acting progestin-only contraceptives include intrauterine
progesterone (Progestasert) and medroxyprogesterone injection
(Depo-Provera). The intrauterine progesterone system is a unit that
contains 38 mg of progesterone and is inserted in the uterine cavity.
It is indicated for women in a stable, monogamous relationship who
have had at least one child and do not have any history of pelvic
inflammatory disease (PID). This system releases an average of 65
mcg daily of progesterone for 1 year. Medroxyprogesterone IM is ad-

BOX 51-2 DRUGS USED IN ABORTION PROCEDURES

Carboprost tromethamine (Hemabate) and dinoprostone
or prostaglandin E₂ (Prepidil, Cervidil, Prostin E₂) are abortifacient prostaglandins used to induce abortion. They have
other indications, including postpartum bleeding.

When used for pregnancy termination, carboprost is
used between 13 and 20 weeks of gestation, which is calculated from the first day of the last normal menstruation. It
is an injectable for IM use only. The initial dose is 250 mcg,
followed by the same dose every 1.5 to 3.5 hours depending on the client's response. Carboprost is also used to manage postpartum bleeding and is dosed at 250 mcg IM, with
doses repeated every 15 to 90 minutes up to a cumulative
dose of 2 mg.

Dinoprostone is primarily used near-term for cervical
ripening and is presented in Chapter 52. When used for
pregnancy termination, it is used between 12 and 20 weeks
of gestation, which again is calculated from the first day of
the last normal menstruation. It is available as a suppository
(Prostin E₂), a gel (Prepidil), and a vaginal insert (Cervidil).
These agents are inserted in the vagina following the specific instructions available in the package insert or *Drug
Facts and Comparisons* (2005).

The adverse effects of these agents include leg cramps,
fever, eye pain, rash, blurred vision, cardiac dysrhythmias,
flushing nausea, vomiting, diarrhea and, possibly, uterine
rupture.

ministered to women every 3 months to inhibit gonadotropin secretion, thereby resulting in contraception.

Adverse Effects
Adverse effects include vaginal bleeding, muscle pain, stomach distress, vaginitis, chloasma, breast discharge, and weight gain. Rarely
reported is thrombus formation or thromboembolism, but the risk
with progestin-only products is believed to be much lower than with
estrogen-containing formulations. Refer to progestins above for a
further discussion.

Drug Interactions
See medroxyprogesterone, p. 905.

Progesterone Antagonist

mifepristone [mih feh **pris** tone]
(Mifeprex, also known as RU-486)
The availability of the progesterone antagonist mifepristone (RU-
486) has been considered controversial since its availability in 1988
in France. It was adopted in the United Kingdom in 1991 and Swe-
den in 1992. It became available for limited access use in the
United States in the year 2000.

Mifepristone is a progesterone antagonist used as an abortifacient
under very strict guidelines. As an antagonist to progesterone, it induces contractions in the myometrium. Access is limited to prescribers
enrolled with the manufacturer (Danco Laboratories 1-877-432-7596)
and is not to be used for women who report their last menstrual period
greater than 49 days (7 weeks) ago. Protocol requires close medical supervision and ongoing evaluation. Misoprostol (Cytotec) is used concurrently with mifepristone to stimulate uterine contractions. Other
drugs used for abortion are outlined in Box 51-2.

Indications
Mifepristone is indicated for medical termination of pregnancy
through day 49 of pregnancy. Concurrent misoprostol (Cytotec) is

recommended, and possible surgery may be required to complete therapy.

Pharmacokinetics/Dosing

Mifepristone is moderately well absorbed orally and is metabolized by cytochrome P450 3 A4 to three active metabolites. It reaches a peak effect 90 minutes after dosing, and is eliminated predominately within 72 hours after dosing. It is dosed orally at 600 mg (three 200-mg tablets). On day 3, clients must return to the health care provider for evaluation and ultrasound with possible use of misoprostol (Cytotec) 400 mcg (2 doses of 200 mcg) if termination of pregnancy cannot be confirmed. Clients are required to return to clinic on day 14 for follow-up evaluation and ultrasound.

Adverse Effects

Vaginal bleeding and cramping are expected with this therapy. If severe, it may require medical intervention. Other adverse effects commonly observed are nausea, vomiting, headache, diarrhea, dizziness, fatigue, and back pain. Refer to package insert for more complete information.

Drug Interactions

Although not well studied, concurrent agents which inhibit P450 3A4 might result in increased levels and response to mifepristone. These include grapefruit juice, erythromycin, clarithromycin, fluconazole, itraconazole, diltiazem, fluoxetine, and a number of the drugs used to treat HIV. Enzyme inducers (e.g., carbamazepine, phenobarbital, phenytoin, rifampin) may result in reduced mifepristone levels and response. Refer to package labeling for additional information.

✳ **P.L. tests negative for pregnancy, has no history of thromboembolic events, cancer history, or gallbladder/liver problems. She smokes an occasional cigarette at a party and reports occasional alcohol and marijuana use. She receives a prescription for Ortho-Novum 10/11.**

✳ **What are the nursing management issues involved in the use of hormonal contraception?**

Assessment See the assessment for estrogens and progestins. Other drug interactions that need to be considered are corticosteroids (concurrent administration may decrease the clearance and increase the effects of corticosteroids and necessitate lower dosages) and theophylline (concurrent use increases serum concentrations of both drugs, but only the theophylline effect is clinically significant; lower dosages of theophylline may be required).

Nursing Diagnosis In addition to the nursing diagnoses and collaborative problems previously cited in the material for estrogens and progestins, see the Nursing Care Plan on p. 913.

Planning While taking hormonal contraceptive therapy, the client will:
- Not conceive or experience any adverse effects of drug therapy.
- Effectively manage the therapeutic regimen, including medication compliance, stating reportable symptoms to prescriber, undertaking supportive interventions to the drug.
- Collaborate with health care providers for monitoring and treatment.

Implementation

Monitoring Assess P.L. for the development of adverse effects. Among the more common reactions are fluid retention, breakthrough bleeding, thromboembolic disorders, hypertension, and nausea. If significant adverse effects occur, a different birth control pill formula or alternate birth control method should be used. For other monitoring considerations, see the nursing management of progesterone/progestin therapy on p. 905.

Education Instruct P.L. to take the medications as prescribed. The tablets are taken at the same time each day, preferably in association with another daily routine (e.g., brushing of teeth, cleansing of face in the morning or at night). Nausea occurs in some clients during the first cycle but tends to subside after the third or fourth month. Nighttime administration or dosing with a meal may be preferable to decrease nausea.

Caution P.L. never to let her tablet supply run out and always to keep an extra month's supply on hand. Rotate the packages by using the extra package after the pills currently being used and then replacing the extra supply each month on a regular basis. Instruct P.L. to use the pills in the same sequence that they appear in the container.

Instruct J.L. who is beginning to use hormonal contraceptives to use a barrier method of birth control for the first cycle until the body adjusts to the medication. If she misses a dose for 1 day of the 21-day schedule, she should take it as soon as she remembers. If she does not remember until the next day, tell her to take the missed tablet and the regularly scheduled one together. If she does not remember a dose for 2 days in a row, she should take 2 tablets a day for each of the next 2 days. Additionally, she should use a second method of birth control for full protection. If she misses 3 or more doses in a row, she should stop taking the medicine and use another method of birth control until she menstruates or until it is determined she is not pregnant. She may restart the medication with the appropriate cycle (Figure 51-3).

If P.L. were using a 28-day schedule and misses any of the first 21 tablets, she would be instructed to follow the preceding instructions. If she misses any of the last 7 tablets of the 28-dose cycle, which are inactive, there is no hazard of pregnancy; however, the first tablet of the next month's series must be taken on the regularly scheduled day. Be sure to review the literature provided with the medication with P.L. to ensure understanding.

Assist P.L. in exploring her concerns about the risks of taking oral contraceptives. Provide her with information regarding the occurrence of cardiovascular disease and cancer in relationship to her age, smoking habits, and other health characteristics. Encourage the client to read the package insert carefully and then to discuss with her health care provider any concerns she might have.

Advise P.L. to have physical examinations, which should include a pelvic and breast examination and a Pap smear, every 6 to 12 months during treatment. Instruct her to notify her prescriber immediately in the instance of severe

NURSING CARE PLAN SELECTED NURSING DIAGNOSES RELATED TO HORMONAL THERAPY AND CONTRACEPTIVE USE

Nursing Diagnosis	Outcome Criteria	Nursing Interventions
Deficient knowledge related to female hormone therapy	Client will: • Verbalize action, use, dose, and adverse effects of hormonal therapy. • Demonstrate a reduction in symptoms without adverse effects.	• Instruct client to take medication as prescribed. • Advise client using in vaginal cream form to administer at bedtime to increase absorption. Use a sanitary napkin, not tampons, to protect clothing. • Advise client that the medication may be taken with food to minimize or prevent nausea. • Alert client to stop taking her medication and consult with the prescriber if she suspects she is pregnant. • Advise client to report to the prescriber any symptoms of thromboembolism (sudden, severe headache, sudden change in vision, sudden pain, weakness, or numbness); liver impairment (yellow eyes or skin, dark urine, pale stools); or mental depression. • Alert client that cigarette smoking while on this medication increases the risk of thromboembolism (deep-vein thrombosis, pulmonary embolism [PE], heart attack, stroke), particularly after age 35. • Stress the importance of regular visits to the prescriber for follow-up care every 6-12 months.
Deficient knowledge related to hormonal contraceptive regimen	Client will: • Demonstrate compliance with medication regimen (hormonal contraception) without adverse effects.	• Instruct client to take medication as prescribed. • Advise client to use an additional method of birth control during the 3 weeks of the initial cycle. • Encourage client to take the medication at the same time each day, not more than 24 hours apart. • Alert client that although nausea may occur in the first few weeks of therapy, it is usually temporary and may be minimized by taking the dose with food or dosing at bedtime. • Advise client to always keep a month's supply on hand. Replace the extra supply each month. • Provide specific information regarding appropriate action to be taken by the client when "missed" doses occur. • Stress the importance of regular visits to the prescriber for follow-up care every 6 to 12 months. • Advise client to alert other health care providers that she is taking hormonal contraceptives, because they may cause serious symptoms and interact with other drugs to less contraceptive effectiveness. • Alert client to stop taking her medication and consult with the prescriber if she suspects she is pregnant. • Advise client to report to the prescriber any symptoms of thromboembolism (sudden severe headache, sudden change in vision, sudden pain, weakness, or numbness); liver impairment (yellow eyes or skin, dark urine, pale stools); or mental depression. • Alert client that cigarette smoking while on this medication increases the risk of thromboembolism (deep-vein thrombosis, PE, heart attack, stroke), particularly after 35 years of age.

headache, blurred or lost vision (which may signal possible stroke), and symptoms of chest pain, shortness of breath, or leg pain (which may indicate thromboembolism elsewhere in the body). See Table 51-4 for symptoms of hormonal contraceptive complications, using the *ACHES* mnemonic.

She should also inform the health care provider of severe abdominal pain or mass, jaundice, severe mental depression, or unusual bleeding. Instructions should be provided for monthly self-examination of the breasts, and any lumps should be reported to the prescriber.

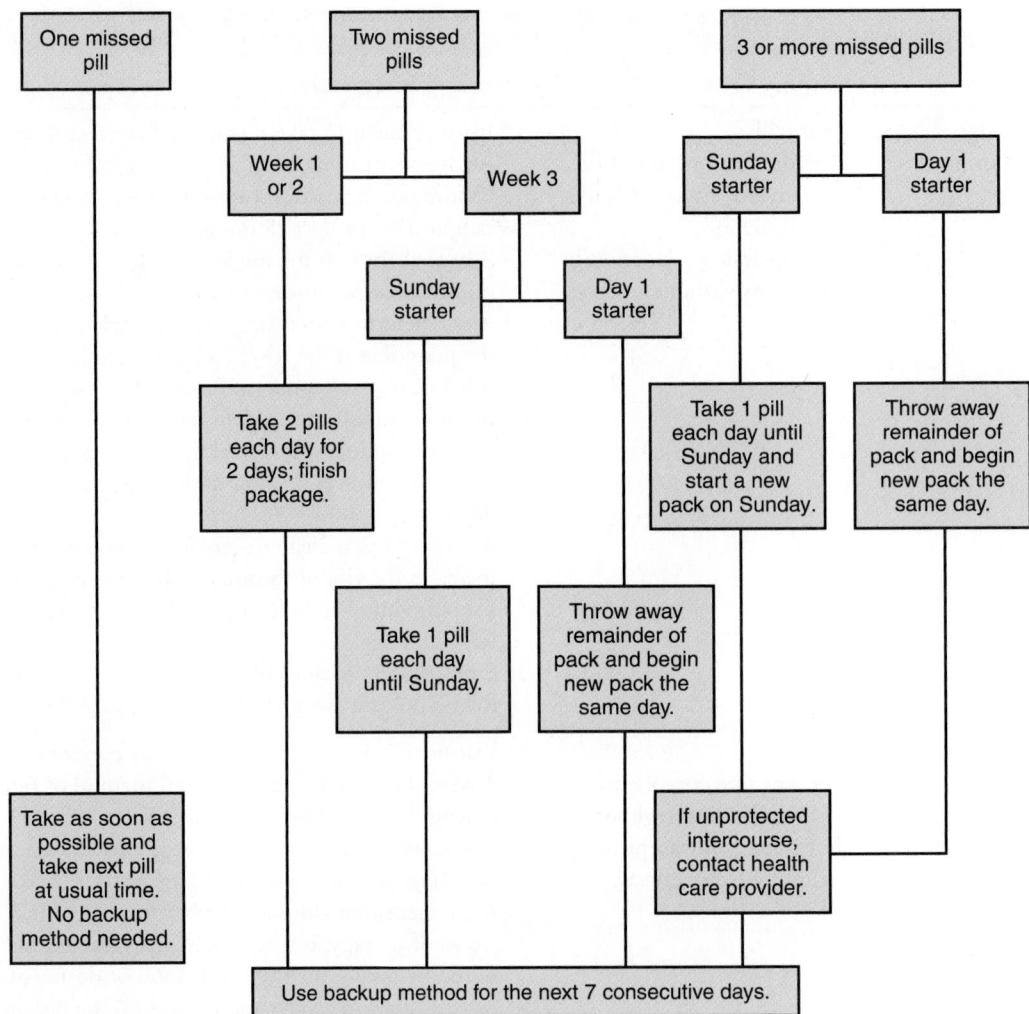

FIGURE 51-3 An example of a flow chart for missed oral contraceptive pills.

TABLE 51-4 ACHES: SIGNS OF HORMONAL CONTRACEPTIVE COMPLICATIONS

Symptom	Possible Problem
Abdominal pain (sharp or severe)	Thrombus in mesenteric vein, gallbladder disease, pancreatitis, hepatic tumor
Chest pain (severe), shortness of breath, or coughing of blood	Blood clot in lungs or myocardial infarction (MI)
Headaches (severe)	Stroke, hypertension, or migraine
Eye problems: flashing lights, blurred vision, or blindness	Stroke, hypertension, or blood clot
Severe leg pain (calf or thigh)	Deep vein thrombosis in legs

Modified from Venous thromboembolism and combination OCPs containing desogestrel orgestodenene. Where are we now? (1999). *Contraception Report 10*(1), 4.

Medical intervention is necessary for various changes in menstrual bleeding pattern, increased and painful urination, jaundice, abdominal cramping, ocular changes (double vision, partial or complete loss of vision, bulging eyes), increased blood pressure, breast alterations (lumps, secretions), depression, or pain or numbness in the fingers or toes.

Compliance with therapy is especially important if hormonal contraceptives are to be effective. Periodically review with the client the appropriate use and importance of taking the drug daily. Ensure that the client knows the proper procedure to follow should one or more doses be missed. Advise P.L. about smoking cessation programs in her area and reinforce with her that hormonal contraception will prevent pregnancy, but offers no protection against sexually transmitted diseases.

Evaluation The expected outcome of hormonal contraceptive therapy is that P.L. will not become pregnant and will not show evidence any untoward effects of the drug. P.L. will maintain medication compliance, report adverse symptoms to the prescriber appropriately, institute supportive measures, and maintain scheduled visits to the prescriber for monitoring and treatment.

✱ What drugs are used for infertility?

Anovulation, the absence of ovulation, is physiologic in women who are pregnant, breastfeeding, or postmenopausal. It becomes a suspected pathologic condition in women with abnormal bleeding or infertility. The incidence of anovulation is unknown and cannot be ascertained, but diagnostic tests may determine its presence. Clomiphene and urofollitropin are ovulation stimulants used to treat infertility in the female.

clomiphene citrate [**kloe** mih feen]
(Clomid, Serophene)

Clomiphene has both antiestrogenic effects and estrogen effects. Although its exact mechanism of action is unknown, it has been postulated that its competition with estrogen for receptor sites in the hypothalamus causes an increased secretion of FSH and LH. The result is ovarian stimulation, maturation of the ovarian follicle, and development of the corpus luteum.

Indications

Clomiphene is indicated to treat female infertility.

Pharmacokinetics/Dosing

Clomiphene is well absorbed orally and recirculated in the enterohepatic system, which may account for its prolonged duration of action in the body. It has a plasma half-life of 5 to 7 days, with ovulation usually occurring between 4 to 10 days after the first day of treatment. It is metabolized in the liver and excreted in the feces and bile. The adult dosage for female infertility is 50 mg PO daily for 5 days, starting on the fifth day of the menstrual period if bleeding occurs or at any time in women who have no recent uterine bleeding. This cycle is repeated until conception occurs, up to three or four cycles. If ovulation does not occur, the dosage is increased to 75 to 100 mg daily for 5 days, which may be repeated if necessary.

Adverse Effects

Adverse effects include hot flashes, abdominal pain or gas, visual disturbances, headache, nausea, vomiting, depression, anxiety, and weakness.

Nursing Management

Assessment

Determine whether the client has preexisting conditions for which clomiphene would be contraindicated before the initiation of therapy, such as mental depression, active hepatic dysfunction, or thrombophlebitis. If the client has ovarian cysts, clomiphene may cause them to enlarge. Clients with polycystic ovary syndrome may experience an exaggerated response to the drug. The presence of an ovarian cyst or ovarian enlargement not associated with polycystic ovarian disease is a contraindication for the use of this drug because of the risk of further enlargement. Risk benefit is considered if the client has abnormal and undiagnosed vaginal bleeding, endometriosis, fibroid tumors, a history of hepatic function impairment, or a sensitivity to clomiphene.

Nursing Diagnosis

Clients receiving clomiphene therapy are at risk for the following nursing diagnoses/collaborative problems: impaired comfort related to premenstrual syndrome, hot flashes, headache, breast tenderness,

nervousness, nausea and vomiting; disturbed sleep pattern (insomnia); disturbed sensory perception—visual (blurred vision, afterimages, diplopia, floaters, phosphenes, scotoma, or photophobia); and the potential complications of development or enlargement of ovarian cysts, enlargement of uterine fibroids, menorrhagia, mental depression, hepatotoxicity, or thromboembolism.

Planning

As a result of clomiphene therapy, the client will:
- Conceive if infertility is the result of anovulation or oligo-ovulation without experiencing any adverse effects of the drug.
- Effectively manage the therapeutic regimen, including medication compliance, stating reportable symptoms to prescriber, and undertaking supportive interventions to clomiphene therapy.
- Collaborate with health care providers for monitoring and treatment.

Implementation

Monitoring

A pelvic examination to assess ovarian size is completed before each course of the drug. Immunologic assay for human chorionic gonadotropin (hCG) is recommended for the detection of pregnancy if menses does not occur before the next course of clomiphene is to begin. Urinary LH surge testing may be used to predict ovulation. An ophthalmologic examination is recommended if treatment with clomiphene is continued for more than 1 year or if visual disturbances occur.

Intervention

Women who have been hypoestrogenic for a long time may require pretreatment with estrogen therapy to ensure a better environment for ovum implantation. To increase the efficacy of clomiphene, a single injection of 5000 to 10,000 USP units of hCG may be given 5 to 9 days after the last dose of clomiphene to simulate the mid-cycle LH surge that results in ovulation. If three or four cycles of clomiphene therapy do not result in pregnancy, or if pregnancy does not occur after a treatment interval of 3 to 6 months with documented ovulation, review the course of therapy with the client and her partner to ensure understanding. If the regimen is being managed effectively by the client, the client's diagnosis should be reconsidered.

Education

Couples are advised to have frequent intercourse at or around the time that ovulation is anticipated, usually approximately 7 days (range 5 to 10 days) after the last dose of clomiphene to enhance fertilization.

If the medication is to start on day 5, count the first day of the menstrual period as day 1. Advise the client that taking the medication at the same time every day maintains drug levels and helps in remembering the daily dose. Advise the client to take a missed dose as soon as possible. If the dose is not remembered until it is time for the next dose, both should be taken together. If more than one dose is missed, consult the prescriber.

Inform the client and her partner about the possibility of multiple births with this drug. Advise her that abdominal pain is an indication for immediate medical attention, because such pain may be symptomatic of the formation or enlargement of an ovarian cyst. Counsel the client to report visual disturbances to the prescriber at once. Alert her to be cautious with tasks that require alertness, because clomiphene may cause visual disturbances, vertigo, and lightheadedness.

Evaluation

The expected outcome of clomiphene therapy is that the client will become pregnant without experiencing any adverse effects of the drug (e.g., hot flashes, abdominal pain or gas, visual disturbances, headache, nausea, vomiting, depression). The client will maintain medication compliance, report adverse symptoms to the prescriber appropriately, institute supportive measures, and maintain scheduled visits to the prescriber for monitoring and treatment.

urofollitropin [yoor oh **foe** lih troe pin]
(Bravelle, Fertinex, Metrodin)
follitropin alfa [foe lih **troe** pin **al** fa]
(Gonal-F)

follitropin beta [foe lih **troe** pin **bee** tah]
(Follistim)

Indications

The follitropins, including urofollitropin, follitropin alpha and follitropin beta, are used to treat female infertility. Follitropin alpha and beta are also used to induce spermatogenesis in men. Urofollitropin is obtained from the urine of postmenopausal women and contains FSH whereas follitropin alpha and beta are derived from recombinant DNA technology. Human chorionic gonadotropin (hCG) is administered after follitropin therapy to simulate natural ovulation in women. Human chorionic gonadotropin is used as pretreatment in men to normalize testosterone levels before initiating follitropin.

Pharmacokinetics/Dosing

These agents are slowly absorbed by IM or subcutaneous injection depending on formulation and indication. Each possesses an elimination half-life between 15 and 36 hours. The usual adult dosages for urofollitropin and follitropin alpha vary based on indication but range from 75 to 300 units daily by subcutaneous injection with a duration of 10 to 12 days.

Adverse Effects

The most commonly reported adverse effects of follitropins in women are ovarian cysts or ovarian enlargement, and severe pelvic pain as a result of severe ovarian hyperstimulation syndrome. Pain and redness at the injection site can be noted with all formulations in both men and women. Other effects include severe stomach pain, bloating, decreased urination, severe nausea, vomiting or diarrhea, weight gain, swelling of the lower extremities, breathing difficulties, skin rash, elevated temperature, and chills.

Nursing Management

Assessment

Assess that the client does not have a medical condition for which follitropins would be contraindicated, such as undiagnosed vaginal bleeding, ovarian cyst or enlargement not associated with polycystic ovary syndrome, or sensitivity to follitropins or other gonadotropins. No significant drug interactions have been reported with its use. A baseline ultrasound examination is recommended to determine the number and size of mature follicles.

Nursing Diagnosis

The client receiving follitropin therapy is at risk for the following nursing diagnoses/collaborative problems: impaired comfort (breast tenderness, nausea, vomiting, chills, rash, mild diarrhea); imbalanced body temperature (fever); impaired tissue integrity (pain, swelling, and tenderness at the injection site); and for women the potential complications of ovarian enlargement or ovarian cysts and severe ovarian hyperstimulation syndrome exist.

Planning

As for clomiphene.

Implementation

Monitoring

Serum estradiol concentrations are monitored to determine the best dosing levels and to decrease the risk of ovarian hyperstimulation syndrome. A periodic ultrasound examination to follow follicular development is recommended. Daily basal body temperatures may be taken to determine if ovulation has occurred.

Intervention

The dosage of urofollitropin varies considerably and is based on the client's clinical response. The series may be once a day, usually for 7 or more days or once a day beginning in the early follicular phase (cycle day 2 or 3) until sufficient follicular development occurs. In either case the series is followed by 5000-10,000 units of hCG 1 day after the last dose of follitropins.

Education

Intercourse or insemination is performed daily beginning the day after the hCG is administered until ovulation is thought to have occurred. After three to six cycles of nonovulatory menses, the appropriateness of continuing the use of follitropins is to be considered.

Instruct the client to take her basal body temperature daily and record it on a flow chart. This determines when ovulation occurs and assists in properly timing coitus to enhance fertilization. Easy-to-read oral thermometers are available that register 96° F to 100° F; some prescribers prefer rectal temperatures for accuracy. The temperature is taken from day 1 of the menstrual period and every morning on awakening—before the client engages in any activity such as drinking coffee, brushing her teeth, smoking, or intercourse. Oral body temperature is low (approximately 97.5° F) and stable for 2 weeks after menstruation. There is a slight decrease at ovulation followed the next day by an increase (approximately 98.5° F), which continues if progesterone levels are normal. The temperature decreases again just before menstruation. If this decrease does not occur, the client may be pregnant.

Evaluation

The expected outcome of follitropin therapy is that the client will become pregnant without experiencing any ill effects of the drug (e.g., abdominal pain, visual disturbances, nausea and vomiting, headache, depression). The client will maintain medication compliance, report adverse symptoms to the prescriber appropriately, institute supportive measures, and maintain scheduled visits to the prescriber for monitoring and treatment.

Summary

Drugs used for diagnostic purposes, to treat disorders, or to alter the normal functioning of the female reproductive system include many substances, such as GnRH, nonpituitary chorionic gonadotropin, menotropins, female sex hormones, hormonal contraceptives, ovulatory stimulants, and drugs used for infertility. GnRH, or gonadorelin, is used for the diagnosis of hypogonadism in both males and females and, investigationally, for the treatment of primary hypothalamic amenorrhea. Nafarelin, a GnRH agonist, is used in the management of endometriosis and CPP. A deficiency in LH is the indication for chorionic gonadotropin. Menotropins are used in the treatment of both male and female infertility.

Estrogens, progesterone, and progestins are the more commonly used drugs that affect the female reproductive system. Although historically used for a number of indications, estrogen use is primarily limited to treating significant vasomotor symptoms of menopause and for hormonal contraception. Progesterone/progestins are indicated for hormonal replacement, the treatment of endometriosis and specific carcinomas, and the prevention of pregnancy.

Hormonal contraception with progestins or combinations of estrogens and progestins are among the most effective forms of birth control currently available. Because these drugs are primarily for self-administration, the emphasis for the nurse is on client education for safe and accurate administration and for early recognition of adverse effects. Clomiphene and urofollitropin are indicated for the treatment of infertility.

Because all of these drugs affect sexual identity, the nurse must be sensitive to the client's needs as a sexual being and must be alert to cues that reflect problems such as a disturbance of self-concept.

- Lillian Taylor, a college freshman, was seen in the University Health Center in September by the nurse practitioner, who prescribed Ortho-Novum birth control pills for her. In February, Ms. Taylor calls the Center and states that she thinks she is pregnant even though she has consistently taken her birth control pills. What instructions should the nurse give her?

- Mary Ann Gilbert, 51 years old, has been experiencing distressing menopausal symptoms for which her health care provider has prescribed estrogen replacement. As she is leaving the office, she seems concerned about filling her prescription because her neighbor has said that "those pills cause cancer." What action should the nurse take?

Bibliography

Anderson, G. (2004). Pharmacogenetics and enzyme induction/inhibition properties of antiepileptic drugs. *Neurology, 63*(10) Supplement 4, S3-S8.

Anderson, D.M., Keith, J., & Novak, P.D. (Eds.) (2002). *Mosby's medical, nursing, and allied health dictionary* (6th ed.). St. Louis: Mosby.

Bair, Y.A., Gold, E.B., Azari, R.A., Greendale, G., Sternfeld, B., Harkey, M.R., et al. (2005). Use of conventional and complementary health care during the transition to menopause: Longitudinal results from the Study of Women's Health Across the Nation (SWAN). *Menopause, 12,* 31-39.

Banks, E., Reeves, G., Beral, V., Bull, D., Crossley, B., & Simmonds, M., et al. (2004). Impact of use of hormone replacement therapy on false positive recall in the NHS breast screening programme: Results from the Million Women Study. *British Medical Journal, 328,* 1291-1292.

Barnabei, V.M., Grady, D., Stovall, D.W., Cauley, J.A., Lin, F., & Stuenkel, C.A., et al.(2002). Menopausal symptoms in older women and the effects of treatment with hormone therapy. *Obstetrics and Gynecology, 100,* 1209-18.

Beral, V., and the Million Women Study Collaborators. (2003). Breast cancer and hormone-replacement therapy in the Million Women Study. *Lancet, 362,* 419-427.

Bosker, G. (Ed.). (2004). *Primary and acute care medicine: Practice, protocols, pathways,* (2nd ed.). Atlanta: Thomson American Health Consultants.

Chlebowski, R.T., Hendrix, S.L., Langer, R.D., Stefanick, M.L., Gass, M., & Lane, D., et al., and the WHI Investigators. (2003). Influence of estrogen plus progestin on breast cancer and mammography in healthy postmenopausal women: The Women's Health Initiative randomized trial. *Journal of the American Medical Association, 289,* 3243-3253.

Cirillo, D.J., Wallace, R.B., Rodabough, R.J., Greenland, P., LaCroix, A.Z., Limacher, M.C., et al. (2005). Effect of estrogen therapy on gallbladder disease. *Journal of the American Medical Association, 293,* 330-339.

Crisafulli, A., Marini, H., Bitto, A., Altavilla, D., Squadrito, G., & Romeo, A., et al. (2004) Effects of genistein on hot flushes in early postmenopausal women: a randomized, double-blind EPT- and placebo-controlled study. *Menopause, 11*(4), 400-404.

Dickerson, L.M., & Bucci, K.K. (2002). Contraception. In J.T. DiPiro, R.L. Talbert, G.C. Yee, G.R. Matzke, B.G. Wells & L.M. Posey (Eds.), *Pharmacotherapy: A Pathophysiological Approach* (5th ed.). New York: McGraw-Hill.

Dimitrakakis, C., Gosselink, L., Gaki, V., Bredakis, N., & Keramopoulos, A. (2004). Phytoestrogen supplementation: a case report of male breast cancer. *European Journal of Cancer Prevention, 13*(6), 481-484.

Draper, M.W., & Chin, W.W. (2003). Molecular and Clinical Evidence for the Unique Nature of Individual Selective Estrogen Receptor Modulators. *Clinical Obstetrics and Gynecology, 46*(2), 265-297.

Drug facts and comparisons (58th ed.). (2005). St. Louis: Facts and Comparisons.

FDA Talk Paper T04-50 (November 17, 2004). Black Box Warning Added Concerning Long-Term Use of Depo-Provera Contraceptive Injection. Washington DC: Food and Drug Administration. Retrieved January 12, 2005, from http://www.fda.gov/bbs/topics/ANSWERS/2004/ANS01325.html.

Grady, D., Ettinger, B., Moscarelli, E., Plouffe, L. Jr, Sarkar, S., & Ciaccia, A., et al. and the Multiple Outcomes of Raloxifene Evaluation Investigators. (2004). Safety and adverse effects associated with raloxifene: Multiple Outcomes of Raloxifene Evaluation. *Obstetrics and Gynecology, 104,* 837-844.

Grimes, D.A., Gallo, M.F., Grigorieva, V., Nanda, K., Schulz, K.F. (2005). Steroid hormones for contraception in men: Systematic review of randomized controlled trials. *Contraception, 71,* 89-94.

Hardman, J.L. (2005). Contraception. In M.A. Koda-Kimble, L.Y. Young, W.A. Kradian, B.J. Guglielmo, B.K. Alldredge, & R.L. Corelli (Eds.), *Applied therapeutics: The clinical use of drugs* (8th ed.). Philadelphia: Lippincott Williams & Wilkins.

Hays, J., Ockene, J.K., Brunner, R.L., Kotchen, J.M., Manson, J.E., & Patterson, R.E., et al., and the Women's Health Initiative Investigators. (2003). Effects of estrogen plus progestin on health-related quality of life. *New England Journal of Medicine, 348,* 1839-1854.

Hendrix, S.L., Cochrane, B.B., Nygarrd, I.E., Handa, V.L., Barnabei, V.M., Iglesia, C., et al. (2005). Effects of estrogen with and without progestin on urinary incontinence. *Journal of the American Medical Association, 293,* 935-948.

e-LEARNING SUPPLEMENTS

Student CD-ROM
- Final Exam questions
- NCLEX® Examination review questions
- Pharmacology animations
- Printable chapter summary

Evolve Website (http://evolve.elsevier.com/mckenry)
- Case study on drugs affecting women's health and the female reproductive system

- Content updates, including information on new drugs
- WebLinks corresponding to this chapter
- Answers to the critical thinking questions in this chapter
- *Elsevier ePharmacology Update* newsletter
- Mosby's Drug Consult Internet Edition
- Supplemental and reference information

Herndon, E.J., & Zieman, M. (2004). New contraceptive options, *American Family Physician 69*:853-60. Retrieved August 1, 2004, from http://www.aafp.org/afp/20040215/853.html.

Herrington, D.M. (2003). Role of estrogen receptor-α in pharmacogenetics of estrogen action. *Current Opinion in Lipidology, 14*(2), 145-150.

Holmberg, L., & Anderson, H., and the HABITS steering and data monitoring committees. (2004). HABITS (Hormonal replacement therapy after breast cancer – Is it safe?), a randomised comparison: Trial stopped. *Lancet, 363*, 453-455.

Holt, V.L., Scholes, D., Wicklund, K.G., Cushing-Haugen, K.L., & Daling, J.R. (2005). Body mass index, weight, and oral contraceptive failure risk. *Obstetrics and Gynecology, 105*(1), 46-52.

Kok, L., Kreijkamp-Kaspers, S., Grobbee, D.E., Lampe, J.W., & van der Schouw, Y.T. (2005). A randomized, placebo-controlled trial on the effects of soy protein containing isoflavones on quality of life in postmenopausal women. *Menopause, 12*, 56-62.

Krauss, R.M. (2002). Individualized Hormone-Replacement Therapy? *New England Journal of Medicine, 346*(13), 1017-1018.

Kreijkamp-Kaspers, S., Kok, L., Grobbee, D.E., de Haan, E.H., Aleman, A., & Lampe, J.W., et al. (2004). Effect of soy protein containing isoflavones on cognitive function, bone mineral density, and plasma lipids in postmenopausal women: A randomized controlled trial. *Journal of the American Medical Association, 292*, 65-74.

Lacy, C.F., Armstrong, L.L., Goldman, M.P., & Lance, L.L. (2004). *Lexi-Comp's Drug Information Handbook* (12th ed.). Hudson, Ohio: Lexi-Comp.

Lepine, J., Bernard, O., Plante, M., Tetu, B., Pelletier, G., & Labrie, F., et al. (2004). Specificity and Regioselectivity of the Conjugation of Estradiol, Estrone, and Their Catecholestrogen and Methoxyestrogen Metabolites by Human Uridine Diphosphoglucuronosyltransferases Expressed in Endometrium. *Journal of Clinical Endocrinology and Metabolism, 89*(10), 5222-5232.

Lieu, C.L., & Yoshida, T. (2002). Infertility. In J.T. DiPiro, R.L. Talbert, G.C. Yee, G.R. Matzke, B.G. Wells & L.M. Posey (Eds.), *Pharmacotherapy: A Pathophysiological Approach* (5th ed.). New York: McGraw-Hill.

Litt, I.F. (2005). Placing emergency contraception in the hands of women. *Journal of the American Medical Association, 293*, 98-99.

Loose-Mitchell, D.S., & Stancel, G.M. (2001). Estrogens and Progestins. In: J.G. Hardman & L.E. Limbird (Eds.), *Goodman & Gilman's The pharmacological basis of therapeutics* (10th ed.). New York: McGraw-Hill.

MacKay, H.T. (2003). Gynecology. In L.M. Tierney, Jr., S.J. McPhee & M.A. Papadakis, (Eds.), *Current Medical Diagnosis & Treatment.* New York: Lange Medical Books/McGraw-Hill.

Manson, J.E., Hsia, J., Johnson, K.C., Rossouw, J.E., Assaf, A.R., & Lasser, N.L., et al., and the Women's Health Initiative Investigators. (2003). Estrogen plus progestin and the risk of coronary heart disease. *New England Journal of Medicine, 349*, 523-534.

Martinelli, I., Battaglioli, T., & Mannucci, P.M. (2003). Pharmacogenetic aspects of the use of oral contraceptives and the risk of thrombosis. *Pharmacogenetics, 13*(10), 589-594.

Million Women Study Collaborators.(2003). *Breast cancer and hormone-replacement therapy in the Million Women Study. Lancet, 362*, 419-427.

Modugno, F. (2004). Ovarian cancer and polymorphisms in the androgen and progesterone receptor genes: a HuGE review. *American Journal of Epidemiology, 159*, 319–335.

Mosby's drug consult (15th ed.). (2005). St. Louis: Mosby.

Nikander, E., Kilkkinen, A., Metsa-Heikkila, M., Adlercreutz, H., Pietinen, P., & Tiitinen, A., et al. (2003). A randomized placebo-controlled crossover trial with phytoestrogens in treatment of menopause in breast cancer patients. *Obstetrics and Gynecology, 101*, 1213-1220.

Nilsson, M., Johnsen, R., Ye, W., Hveem, K., & Lagergren, J. (2003). Obesity and estrogen as risk factors for gastroesophageal reflux symptoms. *Journal of the American Medical Association, 290*, 66-72.

North American Menopause Society. (2004). Treatment of menopause-associated vasomotor symptoms: position statement of The North American Menopause Society. *Menopause, 11*(1), 11-33.

Osmers, R., Friede, M., Liske, E., Schnitker, J., Freudenstein, J., Henneicke-von Zepelin, H.H. (2005). Efficacy and safety of isopropanolic black cohosh extract for climacteric symptoms. *Obstetrics and Gynecology, 105*, 1074-1083.

Parent-Stevens, L., & Sagraves, R. (2005). Gynecologic and other disorders of women. In M.A. Koda-Kimble, L.Y. Young, W.A. Kradian, B.J. Guglielmo, B.K. Alldredge, & R.L. Corelli (Eds.), *Applied therapeutics: The clinical use of drugs* (8th ed.). Philadelphia: Lippincott Williams & Wilkins.

Pauli-Magnus, C., Lang, T., Meier, Y., Zodan-Marin, T., Jung, D., & Breymann, C., et al. (2004). Sequence analysis of bile salt export pump (ABCB11) and multidrug resistance p-glycoprotein 3 (ABCB4, MDR3) in patients with intrahepatic cholestasis of pregnancy. *Pharmacogenetics, 14*(2), 91-102.

Paynter, R.A., Hankinson, S.E., Colditz, G.A., Hunter, D.J., & De Vivo, I. (2004). No evidence of a role for PPAR[gamma] Pro12 Ala polymorphism in endometrial cancer susceptibility. *Pharmacogenetics, 14*(12), 851-856.

Philipp, C.S., Faiz, A., Dowling, N., Dilley, A., Michaels, L.A., Ayers, C., et al. (2005). Age and the prevalence of bleeding disorders in women with menorrhagia. *Obstetrics and Gynecology, 105*, 61-66.

Raine, T.R., Harper, C.C., Rocca, C.H., Fischer, R., Padian, N., Klausner, J.D., et al. (2005). Direct access to emergency contraception through pharmacies and effect on unintended pregnancy and STIs: A randomized controlled trial. *Journal of the American Medical Association, 293*, 54-62.

Schildkraut, J.M., Calingaert, B., Marchbanks, P.A., Moorman, P.G., & Rodriguez, G.C. (2002). Impact of progestin and estrogen potency in oral contraceptives on ovarian cancer risk. *Journal of National Cancer Institute, 94*(1), 32-38.

Schnell, Z.B., Van Leeuwen, A.M., & Kranpitz, T.R. (2003). *Davis' Comprehensive handbook of laboratory and diagnostic tests with nursing implications.* Philadelphia: F.A. Davis Company.

Shumaker, S.A., Legault, C., Kuller, L., Rapp, S.R., Thal, L., & Lane, D.S., et al., and the Women's Health Initiative Memory Study. (2004). Conjugated equine estrogens and incidence of probable dementia and mild cognitive impairment in postmenopausal women: Women's Health Initiative Memory Study. *Journal of the American Medical Association, 291*, 2947-2958.

Strom, B.L., Berlin, J.A., Weber, A.L., Norman, S.A., Bernstein, L., & Burkman, R.T., et al. (2004). Absence of an effect of injectable and implantable progestin-only contraceptives on subsequent risk of breast cancer. *Contraception, 69*, 353-360.

Suvanto-Luukkonen, E., Koivunen, R., Sundstrom, H., Bloigu, R., Karjalainen, E., Haiva-Mallinen, L., et al. (2005). Citalopram and fluoxetine in the treatment of postmenopausal symptoms: A prospective, randomized, 9-month, placebo-controlled, double-blind study. *Menopause, 12*, 18-26.

Tanus-Santos, J.E., Desai, M., Deak, L.R., Pezzullo, J.C., Abernethy, D.R., & Flockhart, D.A., et al. (2002). Effects of endothelial nitric oxide synthase gene polymorphisms on platelet function, nitric oxide release, and interactions with estradiol. *Pharmacogenetics, 12*(5), 407-413.

Tetlow, N., Coggan, M., Casarotto, M.G., & Board, P.G. (2004). Functional polymorphism of human glutathione transferase A3:

effects on xenobiotic metabolism and steroid biosynthesis. *Pharmacogenetics, 14*(10), 657-663.

Tice, J.A., Ettinger, B., Ensrud, K., Wallace, R., Blackwell, T., & Cummings, S.R.(2003). Phytoestrogen supplements for the treatment of hot flashes. The Isoflavone Clover Extract (ICE) Study: A randomized controlled trial. *Journal of the American Medical Association, 290,* 207-214.

USP DI: Drug information for the health care professional (25th ed.). (2005). Greenwood Village, CO: MICROMEDEX Thomson Healthcare.

U.S. Preventive Services Task Force. (2005). Hormone therapy for the prevention of chronic conditions in postmenopausal women: Recommendations from the U.S. Preventive Services Task Force. *Annals of Internal Medicine, 142,* 855-860.

Westhoff, C., Morroni, C., Kerns, J., & Murphy, P.A. (2003). Bleeding patterns after immediate vs. conventional oral contraceptive initiation: A randomized, controlled trial. *Fertility and Sterility, 79,* 322-329.

52

DRUGS FOR LABOR AND DELIVERY

CHAPTER FOCUS

Labor and delivery are the culmination of the childbearing cycle and constitute an intense experience for all involved. To implement nursing care, the nurse must understand the essential processes of labor, maternal and fetal adaptations, and the effects of the drugs used for labor and delivery.

LEARNING OBJECTIVES

- Describe the altered pharmacokinetic pattern of drugs during labor and delivery.
- Explain the pharmacologic action of oxytocics on the uterus.
- Identify the three primary indications for the use of oxytocin.
- Explain the two primary actions of ergonovine.
- Describe the mechanism of action and use of ritodrine.
- Explain the action of lactation inhibitors.
- Implement nursing management of drug therapy for a client experiencing labor and delivery.

▲ KEY TERMS

oxytocics, p. 920
tocolytics, p. 920

❂ KEY DRUGS

dinoprostone, p. 921
oxytocin, p. 922
ritodrine, p. 925

Because many drugs are available for use during labor and delivery, it is important to consider the benefit versus the risk to the fetus. The pharmacokinetics of drugs may be altered during labor and delivery. For example, gastric emptying is delayed during labor, and vomiting may result; this alters drug absorption. Vomiting may also be exacerbated by the use of opioid analgesics. Because oral drug absorption is unpredictable at this time, parenteral routes are used. Drug metabolism and excretion may be altered and prolonged during labor; and although clinical data are currently sparse, the potential for inducing adverse or undesirable effects is always a concern. If a drug such as an opioid analgesic or sedative may be potentially harmful to the fetus and if alternate methods are not available, then the smallest possible dose is used.

Chronic health problems or complications of pregnancy may also dictate the use of additional medications, such as those to treat diabetes, hypertension, preeclampsia, eclampsia, and systemic infections. These medications and their proper use are discussed in the appropriate pharmacologic sections of this text. For example, the use of magnesium sulfate specifically for toxemia of pregnancy is reviewed in Chapter 17. Discussion in this chapter is limited to the drugs used to induce labor (oxytocics), inhibit premature labor (tocolytics), and suppress lactation.

❂ What drugs affect the uterus?

The uterus is a highly muscular organ that exhibits a number of characteristic properties and activities. The smooth muscle fibers of the uterus extend longitudinally, circularly, and obliquely. The uterus has a rich blood supply; blood flow is diminished when the uterine muscle contracts. Profound changes occur in the uterus during pregnancy: It increases in weight from approximately 50 g to approximately 1000 g, its capacity increases tenfold in length, and new muscle fibers may be formed. These changes are accompanied by changes in the response to drugs. Drugs that act on the uterus include oxytocics and tocolytics.

✴ **K.E. is a 21-year-old in labor with her first pregnancy and has made little progress. Her cervix is only slightly dilated at 2 cm. She is becoming exhausted and her uterine contractions have decreased in strength.**

✴ **What drugs affect the cervix and stimulate uterine contractions?**

Oxytocics are agents that stimulate contraction of the smooth muscle of the uterus, resulting in contractions and spontaneous labor. Oxytocin, the most commonly used agent in the group, also induces cervical ripening (dilation of the cervix) in low doses. Other oxytocics are alkaloids of synthetic oxytocin and ergot, although many other drugs may have some effect on uterine contractility. Prostaglandin analogs like PGE$_2$ dinoprostone (Cervidil, Prepidil) are administered vaginally or endocervically for cervical ripening, usually before full doses of oxytocic agents. A similar prostaglandin analog misoprostol (PGE$_1$ Cytotec) is primarily indicated for prevention of nonsteroidal antiinflammatory drugs (NSAID)-induced peptic ulcers (see Chapter 40), but is also used for cervical ripening, and part of a protocol with mifepristone for medical termination of early pregnancy (see Chapter 51 and Box 51-2).

✴▪▪ dinoprostone [dye noe **pros** tone] (also known as PGE2 or prostaglandin E2)
(Cervidil, Prepidil, Prostin E$_2$)
Indications
Dinoprostone is indicated to promote cervical ripening prior to labor induction. A suppository formulation has been used as part of protocols to terminate pregnancy. Also see Box 51-2.
Pharmacokinetics/Dosing
Dinoprostone cervical gel (Prepidil) contains 0.5 mg PGE$_2$ per 2.5 mL prefilled syringe and is administered at 0.25 to 1 mg intracervically. Prostin E$_2$ is available as a vaginal gel in Canada and as a vaginal suppository in the United States. Higher doses are required if dinoprostone is used intravaginally than intracervically. Dinoprostone vaginal system (a suppository within a retrieval device) (Cervidil) contains 10 mg of PGE$_2$ per insert and is delivered slowly at a release rate of about 300 mcg/hr and remains in place until onset of labor or 12 hours have passed. Typically a response is observed initially within one hour and peak effect within 4 hours with gel use.
Adverse Effects
The most common adverse effects with dinoprostone are headache, nausea, vomiting, and diarrhea. Bradycardia, fever, and back pain have also been reported. Rarely bronchospasm, cardiac dysrhythmia, and hypotension have been reported.

✴ **K.E. receives a dose of dinoprostone by placement of a 10-mg sustained-release vaginal system to augment her labor.**

✴ **What nursing management accompanies the administration of dinoprostone to K.E.?**

Assessment It is determined that K.E. is not allergic to dinoprostone or other prostaglandin E2 analogs such as misoprostol. Conditions that would contraindicate a vaginal delivery for K.E., such as a hypertonic uterus, significant cephalopelvic disproportion, fetal distress without imminent delivery, fetal malpresentation, history of multiparity greater than six, acute pelvic inflammatory disease, or unexplained uterine or vaginal bleeding would contraindicate the use of dinoprostone for her. Preexisting cardiovascular disease would also put K.E. at risk because, in doses that stimulate the uterus, dinoprostone decreases blood pressure (BP) and may also cause bradycardia. The major drug interaction is with oxytocin and other oxytocics; dinoprostone is not to be administered if K.E. were already receiving oxytocin. It is recommended that a delay occur between the use of dinoprostone and the administration of oxytocin (30 minutes after the removal of the vaginal system, 6-12 hours after the insertion of the cervical gel or vaginal suppository, and 12-24 hours after the insertion of the vaginal gel). However, studies have found that concurrent use of the two drugs have significantly shortened induction-to-delivery times with a higher proportion of vaginal deliveries with no apparent adverse effects (Christensen, Tehranifar, Gonzalez, Qualls, Rappaport, & Rayburn, 2002; Kill, 2002). K.E.'s baseline assessment includes BP, pulse and temperature; fetal heart rate; vaginal examination for cervical dilation and effacement; and the frequency, duration, and force of her contractions.

Nursing Diagnosis While K.E. is receiving dinoprostone, she is at risk for the following nursing diagnoses: altered comfort (flushing, headache, nausea and vomiting, increased abdominal cramping); diarrhea; hyperthermia; and the potential complications of anaphylaxis, bradycardia, bronchoconstriction, tachycardia, and uterine hypertonus. Clients in whom this drug is used to facilitate abortion may experience acute pain related to uterine contractions, deficient knowledge regarding drug therapy and ineffective coping related to abortion or fetal death and the potential complications of endometritis or increased uterine bleeding.

Planning During dinoprostone therapy, K.E. will:
- Experience a shortened time from induction to delivery without adverse effects of dinoprostone.
- State the rationale for the use of the drug, reportable adverse effects, and a realistic expectation for the drug's action.

Implementation
Monitoring Monitor maternal vital signs and report significant differences in BP and pulse. As in 50% of clients, K.E.'s temperature may increase greater than 2° F (1.1° C) 15 to 45 minutes after the placement of the vaginal system; it will normalize 2 to 6 hours after therapy is discontinued. If it does not, consider endometritis as the etiology. Con-

tinue to monitor K.E.'s contractions, cervical dilation and effacement, and the fetal heart tone. Contractions usually begin within 1 hour and peak within 4 hours.

Intervention Use a minimal amount of water-soluble lubricant to assist in the insertion of the dinoprostone vaginal system, as excessive amounts may cause premature release of the drug. Warming of the system is not necessary. Instruct K.E. to remain in a supine position for 2 hours after insertion of the vaginal system (10-30 minutes after the cervical gel, 30 minutes after the vaginal gel). Avoid skin contact with dinoprostone; wash hands immediately with soap and water after administration of the drug. Prevent contamination of the drug and work area while administering the drug. Carefully dispose of the system and other contaminated equipment after use.

Education Prepare K.E. for the insertion of the vaginal system and indicate it is to augment her labor and that her contractions will become more intense, but her labor will be shorter. Inform her that the dinoprostone vaginal system will be removed when she begins active labor.

Evaluation After receiving dinoprostone, K.E. will advance her labor without uterine hyperstimulation. She will continue to collaborate in the labor experience.

✹ **One hour after the placement of the dinoprostone system, K.E.'s labor becomes more active. Thirty minutes after the dinoprostone system is removed, a low-dose oxytocin IV infusion (2 milliunits/min with 2 milliunits/min with increases every 20 minutes) is started to augment her labor.**

Oxytocin is one of two hormones secreted by the posterior pituitary gland, the other hormone being vasopressin, or antidiuretic hormone (ADH). Oxytocin means "rapid birth," a term derived from its ability to contract the pregnant uterus. It also facilitates milk ejection during lactation.

The nonpregnant uterus is relatively insensitive to oxytocin; uterine sensitivity to oxytocin gradually increases during pregnancy, with the uterus being most sensitive at term. The secretion of oxytocin may precede and possibly trigger delivery of the fetus. Large amounts of oxytocin have been detected in the blood during the expulsive phase of delivery. A positive feedback mechanism may be operating; more forceful contractions of uterine muscle and greater stretching of the cervix and vagina result in the release of more oxytocin. Oxytocin acts directly on the myometrium and has a stronger effect on the fundus than on the cervix. This activity is the rationale for its use for the induction of labor. Oxytocin has been associated with a significant shortening of labor without any demonstrable adverse fetal or neonatal effects or a significant difference in cesarean birth rates.

Oxytocin also transiently impedes uterine blood flow and stimulates the mammary gland to increase the excretion of milk from the breast; it does not increase the production of milk.

✹▅ **oxytocin** [ox i **toe** sin]
(Pitocin, Syntocinon)
Indications
Oxytocin is used to induce labor for women who are at term. It is also used to control postpartum and postabortion hemorrhage and to stimulate lactation.
Pharmacokinetics/Dosing
Oxytocin is available parenterally and in a rapidly absorbed nasal dosage form (Syntocinon). Because the intranasal product may be erratic, it is primarily used before nursing or pumping of the breasts rather than during delivery. Oxytocin has a half-life of 1 to 6 minutes. The onset of action is as follows: nasal, within a couple of minutes; intramuscularly (IM), within 3 to 5 minutes; intravenously (IV), immediate, with uterine contractions increasing gradually over 15 to 60 minutes before stabilizing. The duration of action is as follows: nasal, 20 minutes; IM, 30 to 60 minutes; IV, within an hour after stopping the infusion. Oxytocin is metabolized and excreted by the kidneys. The dosage to induce labor is 0.5 to 2 milliunits/min by IV infusion, increased every 15 to 60 minutes by 1 to 2 milliunits/min until a contraction pattern that simulates normal labor is established (up to a maximum of 20 milliunits/min). For the control of postpartum uterine bleeding, the dosage is 10 units at a rate of 20 to 40 milliunits infused intravenously after birth of the infant. The dosage for the nasal solution is 1 spray in one or both nostrils 2 or 3 minutes before nursing or pumping the breasts.
Adverse Effects
The adverse effects of parenteral oxytocin include nausea, vomiting, tachycardia, and an irregular heart rate. It may occasionally cause fetal bradycardia, dysrhythmias, neonatal jaundice, postpartum excessive bleeding and, rarely, hematoma in the pelvic area. Prolonged therapy may result in water intoxication and possible maternal death because of its slight antidiuretic effects.

✹ **What is the nursing management of oxytocin for K.E.?**

Assessment Before administering oxytocin, ascertain that K.E. is not experiencing any contraindications to a vaginal delivery, such as cord presentation or prolapse, placenta previa or vasa previa, or fetal distress, as was done with the dinoprostone. Oxytocin would also be contraindicated if K.E. had a history of allergy to the drug or if she had hypertonic uterine patterns. Prolonged use of oxytocin is not recommended with uterine inertia; a course of oxytocin therapy is usually limited to 6 to 8 hours.

Oxytocin is used cautiously if K.E. were to exhibit grand multiparity (several prior births), overdistention of the uterus, or a past history of trauma or major surgery on the cervix or uterus (such clients are predisposed to uterine rupture); invasive cervical carcinoma (vaginal delivery is contraindicated); partial placenta previa; prematurity of the fetus; or an unfavorable fetal position. Caution is also recommended for women over 35 years of age or for those having an abortion using hypertonic saline because of the higher risk for water intoxication. When oxytocin is used as an adjunct to drugs that cause abortion (e.g., intraamniotic sodium chloride or urea or other oxytocics), it is not administered until the oxytocic effect of the abortifacient has diminished to decrease the risk of uterine hyperactivity and cervical laceration. (See the Pregnancy Safety box on p. 923.)

Before administering oxytocin to induce labor, it is determined that K.E. has pelvic adequacy for vaginal delivery and that there is fetal maturity. Record K.E.'s baseline data including BP and other vital signs; the characteristics, frequency, and duration of her contractions; and fetal heart rate.

Nursing Diagnosis While K.E. is receiving oxytocin, she is at risk for the following nursing diagnoses/collaborative problems: excess fluid volume related to the antidiuretic effect of the drug (hypertension, water intoxication); impaired comfort with nasal use related to nasal irritation and tearing of the eyes; and the collaborative problems of anaphylaxis and other allergic reactions, cardiac dysrhythmias, hypotension, hypertension, or postpartum hemorrhage. The fetus may also be at risk because of the potential for injury related to fetal trauma (cardiac dysrhythmias, intracranial hemorrhage, asphyxia), fetal bradycardia, and neonatal jaundice.

Planning While receiving oxytocin therapy, K.E. will:
• Experience a labor that will progress satisfactorily without adverse effects.
• Collaborate with health care providers in the birthing process and use nonpharmacologic strategies to ease delivery (e.g., controlled breathing, water tubs).

Implementation
Monitoring Check K.E.'s blood pressure and pulse at least every 15 minutes, during the infusion; also assess the frequency, duration, and force of uterine contractions. Assess the myometrium for tonus during and between contractions, and report hypertonic uterine contractions or a period of uterine relaxation. Continuous fetal monitoring is performed while the client is receiving oxytocin, and the infusion should be discontinued at any sign of uterine hyperactivity or fetal distress. The dosage is titrated for each client depending on maternal and fetal response.

Determine fluid intake and output ratio and assess lung sounds because oxytocin has a slight antidiuretic effect that could result in severe water intoxication with prolonged IV infusion. Hypochloremia and hyponatremia may occur because of water intoxication.

Intervention Parenteral administration should occur only in a hospital setting and under medical supervision. IV infusion is preferred for the induction or stimulation of labor be-

cause absorption from IM administration is difficult to regulate and could result in uterine hyperactivity and fetal distress. Accurate administration by infusion pump is mandatory, as is using a Y connection so the oxytocin solution may be discontinued while access to the vein is maintained. Administer oxytocin for no longer than 6 to 8 hours in instances of uterine inertia. At the first sign of uterine hypertonicity or fetal distress, decrease the rate of oxytocin infusion, or discontinue it.

Education Because K.E. contractions will become stronger, nonpharmacologic interventions are instituted to reduce her discomfort. Controlled breathing, relaxation through biofeedback methods, massage and the use of different body positions may reduce the sensation of pain. Techniques, such as hypnosis and acupuncture have been used with variable success, but require skilled personnel. Some birthing centers may use cutaneous electric nerve stimulation (TENS) or hydrotherapy (laboring in a bath of warm water).

Evaluation While receiving oxytocin to induce or stimulate labor, K.E.'s labor will progress normally without indications of fluid volume excess, uterine hypertonicity, or fetal distress. When oxytocin is administered after expulsion of the placenta, postpartum bleeding will be reduced. K.E. will collaborate with health care providers and actively participate in the birthing process.

Oxytocin for Breastfeeding If the nasal spray is indicated for pain related to postpartum breast engorgement, obtain a baseline assessment of the client's breastfeeding status before initiating therapy. After the client uses the spray, monitor milk ejection and the client's comfort level. Before the client takes the nasal spray, instruct her to clear her nasal passages. Then, with the client's head in a vertical position and the bottle upright, spray the solution into the nostril. Use the spray before breastfeeding or pumping the breasts. Do not administer oxytocin by more than one route simultaneously. If oxytocin is being administered as a lactation stimulant, teach the client the proper technique for self-administration. She should also be aware of the possibility that oxytocin may not be effective. When oxytocin is administered for postpartum breast engorgement, the expected outcome is that the client will experience pain relief and diminished swelling.

•　　　•　　　•

Clients who experience postpartum bleeding or those at high risk for postpartum bleeding are candidates for ongoing oxytocin or may receive ergot alkaloids (ergonovine, methylergonovine) or carboprost (Hemabate).

ergonovine [er goe **noe** veen]
(Ergotrate)
Ergonovine increases the force and frequency of uterine contractions by direct stimulation of the smooth muscle of the uterine wall.
Indications
Ergonovine is indicated to prevent and treat postpartum hemorrhage.
Pharmacokinetics/Dosing
Ergonovine is administered either orally or parenterally. The onset of action is as follows: orally, within 6 to 15 minutes; IM, within 2 to 3

minutes; and IV, within 1 minute. The duration of uterine contraction is as follows: orally and IM, approximately 3 hours; and IV, approximately 45 minutes (rhythmic contractions can persist for up to 3 hours). This drug is metabolized in the liver and excreted by the kidneys. The oral dosage for ergonovine maleate tablets is 0.2 to 0.4 mg two to four times daily (on a schedule of every 6 to 12 hours). The usual treatment course is 48 hours. Parenterally, 0.2 mg is administered intramuscularly or intravenously and repeated in 2 to 4 hours if necessary for up to five doses. The IV route is usually recommended only in emergencies or in cases of excessive uterine bleeding.

Adverse Effects

The adverse effects include nausea, vomiting, diarrhea, dizziness, tinnitus, increased sweating, confusion, hypertension, chest pain and, rarely, respiratory difficulties, pruritus, cold hands or feet, leg weakness, and pain in the arms, legs, or lower back.

methylergonovine [meth ill er goe **noe** veen]
(Methergine)

Indications

Methylergonovine direct stimulates of the smooth muscle of the uterine wall, which results in hemostasis. It is indicated to prevent and treat postpartum hemorrhage.

Pharmacokinetics/Dosing

Methylergonovine may be administered orally or parenterally; the onset of a postpartum uterine contraction effect is as follows: orally, within 5 to 10 minutes; IM, 2 to 5 minutes; IV, immediately. The duration of action is approximately 3 hours for oral or IM dosage forms; and approximately 45 minutes for the IV dosage form. This drug is metabolized in the liver and excreted by the kidneys. The oral dosage of methylergonovine is 200 to 400 mcg two to four times daily (spaced every 6 to 12 hours) until uterine bleeding and atony are under control. Oral dosing usually follows the administration of an initial parenteral dose.

Adverse Effects

The adverse effects of methylergonovine are similar to ergonovine.

✳ **Three hours later, K.E. delivers a healthy 8-pound, 5-ounce girl. After delivery of the placenta, she is given ergonovine 200 mcg PO q12hours for 4 doses.**

✳ **What are the nursing implications of the ergot alkaloids for K.E.?**

Assessment If K.E. cannot tolerate other ergot derivatives, she may not tolerate ergonovine. Assess K.E. for preexisting conditions that may contraindicate the use of ergonovine, such as unstable angina or recent myocardial infarction (MI), because ergonovine-induced vasospasm may precipitate another attack. Because ergonovine causes coronary vasospasm, it should be used cautiously in clients who have coronary artery disease, cardiovascular disease, mitral valve stenosis, or venoatrial shunts; ergonovine increases susceptibility to angina and MI. Clients with occlusive peripheral vascular disease or Raynaud's phenomenon may experience an exacerbation of their ischemia. Ergonovine may also increase blood pressure; its use should be limited in clients with hypertension, preeclampsia, eclampsia, and a history of transient ischemic attacks and cerebrovascular accidents. As with most drugs, administer ergonovine with care to clients with hepatic or renal function impairment. Clients who are septic may have an increased sensitivity to the drug.

The administration of ergonovine is contraindicated before delivery of the placenta, because it may result in entrapment of the placenta. It is not to be used to induce labor or in cases of threatened spontaneous abortion.

Determine a baseline assessment for the pulse, blood pressure, and uterine response. If indicated for the diagnosis of variant angina pectoris, obtain a baseline BP and electrocardiogram (ECG).

Nursing Diagnosis While she is receiving ergonovine, K.E. is at risk for the following nursing diagnoses/collaborative problems: impaired comfort (severe uterine cramping, dizziness, sweating, nausea and vomiting); diarrhea; disturbed sensory perception (ringing in the ears); and the potential complications of severe hypertension, coronary vasospasm (chest pain), bradycardia, MI, peripheral vasospasm, allergic reaction, and overdose (ergotism), with such symptoms as severe headache, diarrhea, nausea and vomiting, peripheral vasospasm, respiratory depression, and seizures.

Planning As the result of taking ergonovine therapy, K.E. will:

- Not experience postpartum bleeding because of uterine atony and not experience any adverse effects of the drug.
- Collaborate with health care providers by implementing nonpharmacologic measures to ease delivery and reporting adverse effects if they occur.

Implementation

Monitoring Monitor K.E.'s BP and pulse, fundal tone and placement; and character and amount of vaginal bleeding. If K.E. has chest pain, notify the physician or nurse-midwife immediately and an ECG should be obtained. ECG monitoring is also essential if the drug is used to diagnose variant angina pectoris.

If K.E. does not respond to ergonovine, serum calcium levels should be determined. The correction of hypocalcemia with IV calcium salts will restore the oxytocic action of the drug. Observe K.E. for signs of ergotism, such as headache, nausea and vomiting, peripheral ischemia, and paresthesia.

Intervention When given IV, administer ergonovine slowly over a minimum of 1 minute. Because the risk of severe adverse effects is increased, IV administration is reserved for emergencies, such as excessive uterine bleeding.

Education Alert K.E. that discomfort may result from ergonovine-related uterine contractions and instruct her about appropriate analgesics and nonpharmacologic methods to alleviate the discomfort as in the oxytocin discussion above. Instruct her also to avoid smoking, because nicotine enhances the effects of ergonovine.

Evaluation The expected outcome of ergonovine therapy is that K.E. will experience a reduction in or an absence of uterine bleeding and will have stable vital signs. She will report adverse effects if they occur (e.g., dizziness, nausea and vomiting, chest pain, pain in legs and lower back).

Nursing management [for methylergonovine] is the same as for ergonovine therapy.

⊛ **P.F. is a 27-year-old lawyer in her first pregnancy at 32 weeks gestation. She is admitted to the hospital for observation with backache and uterine contractions that vary in intensity and are approximately 8 to 10 minutes apart. Her cervix is dilated less than 2 cm and less than 80% effaced without signs of premature rupture of membranes. She is hydrated with 1000 mL Ringer's lactate solution over 30 to 60 minutes and then maintained with dextrose 5% in 0.45% NaCl at 100 mL/hr. She is placed on bed rest on her left side.**

⊛ **What drugs are used to inhibit premature labor?**
Preterm labor, or labor that occurs before the thirty-seventh week of pregnancy, is a major problem in obstetrics; it is responsible for 85% of neonatal illnesses and death (Crombleholme, 2003). It is defined as regular uterine contractions, every 5 to 10 minutes or 6 to 10 in one hour, occurring before the 37 weeks' gestation associated with progressive cervical effacement or dilatation, greater than 2 cm dilation or greater than 80% effacement. Preterm labor occurs in approximately 10% to 15% of all pregnancies. Premature birth increases the possibility of neonatal morbidity and mortality.

Drugs that inhibit premature labor are often referred to as tocolytics. The goal of tocolysis is to stop contractions and prolong delivery for at least 48 to 72 hours in most women. This prolongation of labor allows time for the administration of glucocorticoids to women who are between 24 and 34 weeks' gestation to improve fetal pulmonary status, allow time for antibiotic treatment of infections, and/or allow time for transport of the mother to a tertiary facility prepared to care for a preterm infant (Hatzopoulos, 2005). Tocolysis is less likely to be effective in women with cervical dilation of greater than 3 cm and is usually unsuccessful if cervical dilation is greater than 5 cm. There is presently no evidence that tocolytic therapy alone improves neonatal morbidity or mortality rates. The β-adrenergic agonist ritodrine has been the prototype for premature labor inhibitors. Terbutaline (Brethine, Bricanyl), also a β-adrenergic agonist (see Chapters 22 and 37), is also used to inhibit premature labor, but its use is considered investigational by the FDA and its delivery by pump maintenance therapy has not been shown to decrease the risk of preterm birth by prolonging pregnancy (Nanad, Cook, Gallo, & Grimes, 2004). Other classifications of drugs are being used with more frequency. The calcium channel blocker, nifedipine, exhibits modest tocolytic properties (see Chapter 27) and can be considered safer and more effective than β adrenergic agonists (King, Fienady, Papatsonis, Dekker, & Carbonne, 2003). Magnesium sulfate is given in doses of 2 to 4 grams intravenously over 12 to 24 hours in the management of premature labor, see also Chapters 17 and 27. However, a Cochrane Review concluded that it is ineffective at delaying

birth or preventing preterm birth, and its use is associated with an increased mortality for the infant (Crowther, Hiller & Hoyle, 2004). Clinical trials have shown that only one agent, indomethacin, an NSAID, significantly prolongs gestation for more than 7 days. However, because indomethacin may decrease urine output and amniotic fluid volume and there are concerns about premature closure of the ductus arteriosus, its use should be restricted to 48-hour courses.

⊛⫿ ritodrine [**rih** toe dreen]
(Yutopar)
Ritodrine is a β₂-adrenergic stimulant that relaxes uterine muscle by inhibiting uterine contractions.
Indications
Ritodrine is indicated to prevent and treat uncomplicated premature labor in pregnancies of 20 or more weeks' gestation.
Pharmacokinetics/Dosing
Ritodrine is available orally and parenterally. With oral administration, the drug has an onset of action within 30 minutes to 60 minutes; the onset of action of the IV form is within 5 minutes. The time to peak serum concentration by both routes is within 1 hour. The half-life of the oral form is biphasic: 1.3 and 12 hours (in male testing); the IV half-life has three phases: 6 to 9 minutes, 1.7 to 2.6 hours, and 15 to 17 hours in nonpregnant females. This drug is metabolized in the liver and excreted by the kidneys. The IV dosage of ritodrine is 50 to 100 mcg/min, which is increased in 50 mcg increments every 10 minutes (as necessary) to an effective dosage. The maintenance dosage is 150 to 350 mcg/min IV, which is continued for 12 to 24 hours after labor contractions have stopped. Oral ritodrine therapy is then instituted. The initial oral dosage is 10 mg 30 minutes before the ritodrine infusion is stopped, then 10 mg every 2 hours for 24 hours. The maintenance dosage is 10 to 20 mg PO every 4 to 6 hours until birth or as directed by the prescriber. The maximum recommended daily dose is 120 mg. Although the use of oral ritodrine for the treatment of preterm labor is approved in Canada, the United States Pharmacopeia Obstetrics and Gynecology Advisory Panel does not recommend its use because its efficacy has not been established. Bed rest at home and early admission are considered better alternatives than oral ritodrine.
Adverse Effects
The adverse effects of IV ritodrine include increased maternal heart rate and increased systolic and decreased diastolic maternal blood pressure. The oral dosage forms may cause small increases in maternal heart rate but do not affect maternal blood pressure or fetal heart rate. Both dosage forms may cause trembling or tremors, anxiety, or restlessness. Nausea, vomiting, headaches, tachycardia, irregular heart rate and, rarely, chest pain and respiratory difficulties are reported with IV administration.
Drug Interactions
Ritodrine is contraindicated with monoamine oxidase (MAO) inhibitors. Its use is generally avoided with other drugs that could result in vasoconstriction, including ergot alkaloids, other sympathomimetics including amphetamines, stimulants, and decongestants. As with other sympathomimetics, ritodrine may reduce the efficacy of insulin and oral hypoglycemic agents. Refer to package labeling for more complete information.

⊛ **Two hours later, P.F.'s cervical examination reveals 3 cm dilation and tocolysis is initiated. Despite recent emerging evidence, the provider determines that current therapy should prevail and P.F. is given a loading dose of magnesium sulfate 6 g of a 10% solution IV over 30 minutes, followed by a maintenance dose of**

2 g/hr continuous infusion through a controlled infusion pump. Additionally, P.F. is given betamethasone 12 mg IM with a second dose in 24 hours to facilitate fetal lung maturation.

⚙ **What are the nursing management issues in the use of tocolytics for P.F.?**

Assessment Pretreatment considerations for tocolysis include maternal-fetus status, gestational age, and the clinical resources. With maternal-fetus status, the concern is for infection, intrauterine growth retardation, preeclampsia, or other conditions in which tocolysis would be ill-advised. The use of tocolytics in clients with ruptured membranes may lead to intrauterine infection. Preterm labor should not have progressed more than 4 cm of cervical dilation or 80% effacement, or the drugs may be ineffective. Tocolytic therapy is considered for P.F. because her length of gestation is 32 weeks. Such therapy is not recommended for use before the twenty-fourth week of pregnancy. Necessary clinical resources include the equipment, professional expertise and personnel to monitor the fetus during labor and provide neonatal care if tocolysis is not successful.

Preexisting health conditions that would contraindicate the various tocolytics are: impaired renal function, recent myocardial infarct, or myasthenia gravis for magnesium sulfate; renal or hepatic disease, active peptic ulcer, NSAID-associated asthmatic episodes, coagulation disorders or poorly controlled hypertension for indomethacin; heart failure, or aortic stenosis with nifedipine; and cardiovascular disorders, eclampsia, pulmonary hypertension, or hyperthyroidism for ritodrine. Immediate delivery is required if P.F. should develop intrauterine infection, nonreassuring fetal status, or intrauterine fetal death. Caution is indicated if P.F. has abruptio placentae, maternal hemorrhage, placenta previa, diabetes, or mild to moderate preeclampsia.

Review P.F.'s current medication regimen for the risk of significant drug interactions. Nifedipine given concurrently with antihypertensive agents may cause excessive hypotension or if given with negative inotropic agents may lead to prolongation of the QT interval because nifedipine also has negative inotropic properties. Indomethacin is contraindicated if P.F. were also taking a medication to prolong coagulation time or cause hypoprothrombinemia; it will also make antihypertensive medications less effective because of its ability for sodium retention. Ritodrine given concurrently with the following drugs may cause serious drug interactions: ß-adrenergic agonists (may cause an increased sympathomimetic response, such as hypertension or cardiac problems); ß-adrenergic blocking agents (labetalol, nadolol, propranolol, and others are not recommended because the two drugs are antagonistic toward each other) and long-acting corticosteroids (betamethasone and dexamethasone), which have resulted in pulmonary edema and death in pregnant women. Avoid concurrent use, or if concurrent drug administration is absolutely necessary, monitor closely and discontinue both drugs at the first sign of pulmonary edema.

Obtain a baseline assessment of P.F.'s labor patterns before initiating ritodrine therapy. Determine P.F.'s beliefs, attitudes, and values regarding the possible premature birth to enhance the educational and emotional support provided by the nurse.

Nursing Diagnosis While P.F. is receiving magnesium sulfate, she is at risk for the potential complication of hypermagnesemia. If she received other tocolytics and was administered the following drugs, P.F. would be at risk for:

- indomethacin: excess fluid volume (increased BP, pedal edema, rapid weight gain), altered comfort (indigestion, nausea, headache, dizziness) and the potential complication of premature closure of the ductus arteriosus.
- nifedipine: excess fluid volume (pedal edema), altered comfort (flushing, headache, nausea) and disturbed sleep pattern (drowsiness).
- ritodrine: altered comfort (headache, nausea, trembling, palpitations) and the potential complications of pulmonary edema, hypotension, cardiac dysrhythmias, agranulocytosis, and hepatic function impairment.

Planning While receiving tocolytic therapy, P.F. will:

- Experience diminished contractions and cessation of premature labor.
- Postpone delivery long enough to reduce the incidence of problems associated with prematurity of the infant.
- Collaborate with health care providers in implementing supportive measures and reporting adverse symptoms appropriately.

Implementation

Monitoring Check P.F.'s BP, heart rate, ECG, breath sounds, uterine activity, and fetal heart rate and rhythm periodically; every 15 minutes during loading doses, with dosage increases, or with unstable vital signs and every hour during maintenance. Minimize digital examinations. Urinary output should be at least 100 mL for 4 hours. Monitor her for early signs and symptoms of hypermagnesemia: bradycardia, diplopia, flushing, headache, hypotension, nausea, vomiting, shortness of breath, slurred speech, and weakness. Assess deep tendon reflexes and level of consciousness every hour. The effects of the drug relate to serum magnesium concentrations (mEq/L) (Box 52-1).

For clients taking indomethacin, monitor BP, pulse, lung sounds, and weight for signs of fluid retention. For those taking nifedipine, measurements of BP, ECG, and heart rates are needed; monitor for fluid retention.

Increases in maternal fluid retention, heart rate, and systolic blood pressure are common with IV ritodrine. Oral doses do not affect maternal blood pressure. If the maternal heart rate is greater than 120 beats/min mm Hg or the fetal heart rate is greater than 170 or 180 beats/min mm Hg, the IV rate may be slowed or the dosage decreased without reducing the effectiveness of ritodrine. It is recommended

BOX 52-1 EFFECTS OF HYPERMAGNESEMIA IN RELATION
TO SERUM MAGNESIUM CONCENTRATIONS

EFFECT	SERUM MAGNESIUM CONCENTRATION (mEQ/L)
Deep tendon reflexes present, but possibly hypoactive	4 to 7
Prolonged PQ interval; widened QRS interval on ECG	5 to 10
Loss of deep tendon reflexes	8 to 10
Respiratory paralysis	10 to 13
Altered cardiac conduction	15
Cardiac arrest	25

Data from *USP DI: Drug information for the health care professional* (25th ed.). (2005). Greenwood Village, CO: MICROMEDEX Thomson Healthcare.

that ritodrine therapy be discontinued if labor persists after administration of the maximum dosage.

Intervention When administering tocolytics IV, a controlled infusion device is used to better enable dosage titration. Avoid the use of sodium chloride for infusion because of the risk of pulmonary edema. Place P.F. on bed rest in lateral recumbent position to increase uterine blood flow. IV administration is usually continued for 12 to 24 hours after contractions stop. With magnesium sulfate, ensure that the antidote calcium gluconate is available at P.F.'s bedside. If indicated, antenatal corticosteroids are given to enhance fetal pulmonary function. If labor is irreversible, the drug is discontinued before delivery. IV antibiotics should be given for group B *Streptococcus* prophylaxis.

Education Caution P.F. to watch for and report: increased abdominal tightening, increased backache, pelvic pressure, vaginal spotting or bleeding or if her water breaks. If P.F.'s contractions do not recur, she may gradually resume ambulation and other activities of daily living after 36 to 48 hours.

Evaluation The expected outcome of tocolytic therapy is that P.F. will experience diminished contractions and an absence of premature labor. If P.F. continues to labor, the delivery will be delayed sufficiently to reduce the incidence of problems associated with prematurity of the infant. P.F. will actively participate in therapy by restricting her activities of daily living as advised by the prescriber and by promptly reporting increased contractions, vaginal spotting or bleeding, or rupture of her membranes.

What drugs are used to inhibit lactation?
Androgens have been used to treat postpartum breast engorgement (methyltestosterone, fluoxymesterone, and testosterone propionate) and to inhibit lactation (bromocriptine [Parlodel]). The use of estrogens for breast engorgement has declined over the years, mainly because the incidence of painful engorgement is considered low, and studies have indicated that analgesics or other supportive therapies are quite effective.

Bromocriptine directly inhibits the release of prolactin from the anterior pituitary gland, resulting in the suppression of lactation. For further information on bromocriptine, refer to the drug monograph for dopamine agonists in Chapter 23.

Summary

Although many drugs are available for use during the process of labor and delivery, it is essential to consider the possible alteration of drug pharmacokinetics during labor and to weigh the risks and benefits to the fetus. The drugs discussed in this chapter focus on uterine contractility, which controls the labor process. Drugs that increase or decrease the contractility of the uterus also enhance or inhibit labor.

Oxytocics are drugs that increase uterine motility to induce labor, augment labor, control postpartum hemorrhage, and facilitate milk ejection during lactation. The most commonly used oxytocics are oxytocin, ergonovine, and methylergonovine. When oxytocics are used to induce or augment labor, the nurse should perform a baseline assessment of fetal heart tones, uterine status, and maternal vital signs. These indicators should be monitored every 15 to 30 minutes during the administration of these drugs. Low doses of oxytocin and prostaglandin analogs are used to enhance cervical ripening for women at full term prior to inducing labor with higher doses of oxytocics.

Premature labor (labor that occurs before the thirty-seventh week of pregnancy) increases the possibility of neonatal morbidity and mortality. Ritodrine may be prescribed once a determination is made that it is in the best interest of the mother and the fetus to halt the labor process. Ritodrine, a β_2-adrenergic stimulant that relaxes uterine muscle and inhibits uterine contractions, is used to prevent and treat premature labor in pregnancies of at least 20 weeks gestation.

The role of the nurse in the administration of these drugs is to facilitate a healthy outcome for both the fetus and the mother.

Critical Thinking Questions

- Shirley Demas is admitted to labor and delivery in possible preterm labor at 30 weeks' gestation. She is to be treated with ritodrine. What observations will be most relevant to determine the maternal adverse effects of this drug? Mrs. Demas' contractions do not abate, and betamethasone is ordered. The client asks you why she is receiving this drug. What is your response?

- Lillian Chandler is admitted to the hospital for the birth of her first child. The nurse-midwife assesses that Mrs. Chandler is experiencing irregular contractions and decides to stimulate her labor by administering oxytocin. What assessments are required before such therapy can begin?

Bibliography

Anderson, D.M., Keith, J., & Novak, P.D. (Eds.) (2002). *Mosby's medical, nursing, and allied health dictionary* (6th ed.). St. Louis: Mosby.

Christensen, F.C., Tehranifar, M., Gonzalez, J.L., Qualls, C.R., Rappaport, V.J., & Rayburn, W.F. (2002). Randomized trial of concurrent oxytocin with sustained-release dinoprostone vaginal insert for labor induction at term, *American Journal of Obstetrics & Gynecology, 186*(1), 61-65.

Corrine, L., Bailey, V., Valentin, M., Morantus, E., & Shirley, L. (1992). The unheard voices of women: Spiritual interventions in maternal-child health. *Maternal Child Nursing, 17*(3), 141-145.

Crombleholme, W.R. (2003). Obstetrics. In L.M. Tierney, Jr., S.J. McPhee & M.A. Papadakis(Ed.), *Current Medical Diagnosis & Treatment.* New York: Lange Medical Books/McGraw-Hill.

Crowther, C.A., Hiller, J.E., & Hoyle, L.W. (2004). Magnesium sulphate for preventing preterm birth in threatened preterm labor (Cochrane Review). Retrieved September 11, 2004, from http: www.cochrane.org/cochrane/revabstr/ab001060.htm.

Drug facts and comparisons (58th ed.). (2005). St. Louis: Facts and Comparisons.

Hatzopoulos, F.K. (2005). Obstetric drug therapy. In M.A. Koda-Kimble, L.Y. Young, W.A., Kradian, B.J. Guglielmo, B.K. Alldredge, & R.L. Corelli (Eds.), *Applied therapeutics: The clinical use of drugs* (8th ed.). Philadelphia: Lippincott Williams & Wilkins.

Kelly, A.J., Kavanagh, J., & Thomas, J. (2004). Vaginal prostaglandin (PGE2 and PGF2) for induction of labor at term (Cochrane Review). Retrieved September 11, 2004, from http:www.cochrane.org/cochrane/revabstr/ab003101.htm.

Kill, J. (2002). Does use of oxytocin and dinoprostone inserts shorten labor more than use of oxytocin after removal of dinoprostone? Patient-oriented evidence that matters. *Journal of Family Practice.*

Retrieved September 11, 2004, from http:www.findarticles.com/p/articles/mi_m0689/is_5 _5/ai_86127301.

King, J.F., Fienady, V., Papatsonis, D., Dekker, G., & Carbonne, B. (2003). Calcium channel blockers for inhibiting preterm labour; a systematic review of the evidence and a protocol for administration of nifedipine. *Australian and New Zealand Journal of Obstetrics and Gynaecology, 43*(3), 192-198.

Lacy, C.F., Armstrong, L.L., Goldman, M.P., & Lance, L.L. (2004). *Lexi-Comp's Drug Information Handbook* (12th ed.). Hudson, Ohio: Lexi-Comp.

Mosby's drug consult (15th ed.). (2005). St. Louis: Mosby.

Nanad, K., Cook, L.A., Gallo, M.F., & Grimes, D.A. (2004). Terbutaline pump maintenance therapy after threatened preterm labor for preventing preterm birth (Cochrane Review). Retrieved September 11, 2004, from http:www.cochrane.org/cochrane/revabstr/ab003933.htm.

Parker, K.L., & Schimmer, B.P. (2001). Pituitary Hormones and Their Hypothalamic Releasing Factors. In: J.G. Hardman & L.E. Limbird (Eds.), *Goodman & Gilman's The pharmacological basis of therapeutics* (10th ed.). New York: McGraw-Hill.

Parsons, M.T., & Spellacy, W.N. (2003). Preterm labor. In J.R. Scott, R.S. Gibbs, A.F. Haney & B.Y. Karlan. (Eds.), *Danforth's Obstetrics and Gynecology.* Philadelphia: Lippincott, Williams & Wilkins.

Pigarelli, D.L.W., & Kraus, C.K. (2002). Pregnancy and lactation: Therapeutic considerations. In J.T. DiPiro, R.L. Talbert, G.C. Yee, G.R. Matzke, B.G. Wells, & L.M. Posey (Eds.), *Pharmacotherapy: A Pathophysiological Approach* (5th ed.). New York: McGraw-Hill.

Schwab, R. (2004). Preeclampsia/Eclampsia. In I.G. Bosker. (Ed.), *Primary and acute care medicine: Practice, protocols, pathways,* (2nd ed.). Atlanta: Thomson American Health Consultants.

USP DI: Drug information for the health care professional (25th ed.). (2005). Greenwood Village, CO: MICROMEDEX Thomson Healthcare.

e-LEARNING SUPPLEMENTS

Student CD-ROM
- Final Exam questions
- NCLEX® Examination review questions
- Pharmacology animations
- Printable chapter summary

Evolve Website (http://evolve.elsevier.com/mckenry)
- Case study on drugs for labor and delivery
- Content updates, including information on new drugs
- WebLinks corresponding to this chapter
- Answers to the critical thinking questions in this chapter
- *Elsevier ePharmacology Update* newsletter
- Mosby's Drug Consult Internet Edition
- Supplemental and reference information

DRUGS AFFECTING THE MALE REPRODUCTIVE SYSTEM

CHAPTER FOCUS

Androgens are usually prescribed for androgen deficiency. When they are prescribed for other conditions, their most common undesirable effect is virilism—the development of masculine characteristics. Body image disturbance may be of concern for clients who have an androgen deficiency or are receiving androgen therapy. The nurse must be prepared to encourage the client to express perceptions of self and provide reliable information about health concerns.

<table>
<tr><td>LEARNING
OBJECTIVES</td><td>
• Compare the pharmacokinetics of three preparations of testosterone.
• Identify the approved indications for androgen (testosterone) therapy.
• List the adverse effects of androgen therapy.
• Implement the nursing management of clients undergoing androgen therapy.
• Describe the use of finasteride for benign prostatic hyperplasia.
• Implement nursing management of clients receiving finasteride therapy and other drugs affecting the male reproductive system.
</td></tr>
</table>

▲ **KEY TERMS**
androgens, p. 929
hypogonadism, p. 929
testosterone, p. 929

✴⬚ **KEY DRUGS**
testosterone, p. 930

Androgens, primarily testosterone, are male sex hormones necessary for the normal development and maintenance of male sex characteristics. Testosterone and its derivatives and synthetic agents are commonly used as replacement therapy for males who lack the hormone. In individuals with hypogonadism or eunuchoidism (a deficiency of male hormone), the androgens produce marked changes in the growth of the male sex organs, body contour, voice, and other secondary sex characteristics. Chapter 54 reviews drugs that affect sexual behavior and impotence, such as sildenafil (Viagra). Chapter 56 describes testosterone antagonists that are used primarily as antineoplastic agents.

Hypertrophy of glandular and connective tissue in the portions of the prostate that surround the urethra, or benign prostatic hyperplasia (BPH), is considered a normal age-related change in men. Finasteride (Proscar) is a welcome addition to the treatment of BPH, which until recently had been almost exclusively surgical.

✴ **R.S. is a 48-year-old man who has been attending the human immunodeficiency virus (HIV) clinic for 10 years. He has been treated with antiretroviral therapy for the past 5 years. He is also treated with intermittent fluconazole for chronic oral *Candida albicans* in-**

fection. His last CD4 count was 102 (normal, approximately 1000). R.S. is on a monthly visit schedule to the clinic. Over the last 2 months his weight has dropped from 150 to 125 pounds. He reports intermittent fevers and diarrhea, and anorexia and activity intolerance for the past 6 weeks. The physician decides to treat R.S.'s HIV wasting with testosterone because it has been shown to increase muscle mass and strength in clients with this syndrome. Oxandrolone (Oxandrin) 10 mg PO twice daily is selected from the available androgens because most weight gain is lean body mass with a lower risk for hepatotoxicity and it is available in oral dosing for increased compliance.

✷ What are the actions and uses of testosterone and testosterone derivatives?

Testosterone, a naturally occurring androgenic hormone produced primarily by the testes, regulates male development. As a natural hormone in normal males, androgens are responsible for the stimulation of spermatogenesis, the development of secondary male sex characteristics and, at puberty, sexual maturity. Testosterone also stimulates the synthesis and activity of ribonucleic acid (RNA), which results in increased production of protein. Androgens are also potent anabolic agents; they stimulate the formation and maintenance of muscular and skeletal protein. They bring about the retention of nitrogen (essential to the formation of protein in the body) and enhance the storage of inorganic phosphorus, sulfate, sodium, and potassium.

Athletes have used androgens to increase weight, musculature, and muscle strength. Weight gain may be caused by fluid retention, an adverse effect of androgen therapy. The potential risk of developing major serious adverse effects from androgens far outweighs the advantages to be gained in athletic events. Many major sporting events disqualify athletes who have documented use of such products. Most androgens are classified as Schedule III drugs (less abuse potential than schedule II drugs and moderate dependence liability) in the United States. Chapter 9 presents additional information on the abuse of androgens.

Testosterone is available in combination with esters to prolong its duration of action. For example, testosterone propionate is formulated in an oily solution that produces hormonal effects for 2 or 3 days. Testosterone cypionate and testosterone enanthate in oil have a much longer duration of action and are usually administered once every 2 to 4 weeks. Testosterone pellets are available for subcutaneous implantation. This form also provides an extended duration of action; depending on the number of pellets used, replacement pellets may not be necessary for 2 to 6 months.

Testosterone may also be administered transdermally. One transdermal testosterone system (Testoderm) is applied to scrotal skin, where testosterone is highly absorbed at a rate at least five times greater than other skin sites. Another transdermal testosterone system (Androderm) is applied to nonscrotal skin. This system requires the application of two patches nightly, every 24 hours. Oral testosterone is absorbed but is highly metabolized by the liver before it reaches

the systemic circulation. Administering methyltestosterone (Android, Oreton Methyl, Testred, Virilon) by the buccal route of administration increases its serum level and effectiveness. Fluoxymesterone (Halotestin) and oxandrolone (Oxandrin) are synthetic androgens that are effective orally in tablet form. Fluoxymesterone is also infrequently used for postpartum breast engorgement.

Androgens

✦⌐ testosterone [tess **toss** ter one]

(Androderm, AndroGel, Delatestryl✤, Depo-Testosterone, Striant, Testim, Testoderm, Testopel, Depotest 100✤, Virilon IM✤)

Indications

The androgens are indicated for androgen deficiency in men (e.g., testicular failure caused by cryptorchidism [failure of one or both testes to descend into the scrotum], orchitis [inflammation of the testes], orchidectomy [surgical removal of one or both testes], or pituitary-hypothalamic insufficiency.) They are also used to treat breast carcinoma; palliative or secondary treatment for inoperable metastatic breast cancer in postmenopausal women who have demonstrated a previous response to hormone therapy. Historically, androgens were used in the treatment of anemias, but their use has largely been replaced by erythropoietin. While not Food and Drug Administration (FDA) approved, testosterone in combination with estrogen appears to improve libido and sexual satisfaction for postmenopausal women (Alexander et al., 2004; Buster et al., 2005).

Pharmacokinetics/Dosing

The half-life of intramuscular (IM) testosterone in plasma is 10 to 20 minutes. The duration of action depends on the dose and the ester formulation administered. The longest duration of action is for testosterone enanthate preparations, followed by cypionate and then propionate; the base form has the shortest duration of action. Testosterone is metabolized in the liver and excreted by the kidneys.

The choice of dosage, route of administration, drug delivery system and length of therapy depend on the diagnosis, the client's age and gender, and the intensity of adverse effects. For delayed puberty and males with hypogonadism (a decrease in androgen secretion from the gonads), dosage regimens are started in the lower ranges and gradually increased according to the client's needs and response. With delayed puberty, androgens are discontinued for 1 to 3 months after 4 to 6 months of therapy, and radiograph examinations are evaluated to determine the drug's effect on bone growth. Males with hypogonadism will receive androgens throughout puberty, with dosage adjustments as required. Lower maintenance dosages are usually used after puberty. Androgen antineoplastic therapy usually requires a 3-month period to evaluate effectiveness. Women with metastatic breast cancer should receive a shorter-acting androgen, especially during the initial therapies. It has been reported that androgens occasionally increase the progression of breast cancer. Consult with standard compendium for specific dosing regimens for each product and indication.

Adverse Effects

Serious complications of testosterone therapy include accelerated bone maturation, altered glucose regulation, fluid retention, aggressive behavior, anxiety, elevated low-density lipoprotein (LDL) and reduced high-density lipoprotein (HDL) cholesterol, and liver injury. Many of these effects are often dose related and may be observed more frequently with higher doses or in individuals who are abusing these agents (see Chapter 9). Adverse effects of testosterone in females are an increase in oily skin or acne, a deepening of the voice, increased body hair growth (hirsutism) or alopecia (baldness), an enlarged clitoris, and irregular menses. The deep voice or hoarseness may be irreversible, even when the medication is stopped. Adverse effects reported in males include urinary urgency, breast swelling or tenderness (gynecomastia), and frequent or continuous erections. Less common adverse effects of testosterone that occur in both genders include abdominal pain, insomnia, diarrhea or constipation, dizziness, increased weakness, red skin or changes in skin color, redness at the site of injection, mouth soreness, frequent headaches, confusion, respiratory difficulties, depression, nausea, vomiting, pruritus, jaundice, an increase in bleeding episodes, and an unusual increase or decrease in libido. Priapism (persistent, abnormal penile or clitoral erection) is an indication of excessive dosing of the androgen and temporary withdrawal of the drug is indicated. Testosterone and other androgens are Pregnancy Category X drugs and should not be used in women who are pregnant or who could become pregnant.

Testosterone plays a role in the development of prostate cancer, but it is unclear to what extent supplemental testosterone therapy increases cancer risk (Parnes, Thompson, & Ford, 2005). The risks for prostate cancer with testosterone and the pharmacogenetic implications for androgens is presented in the Special Considerations for Pharmacogenetics box below.

Drug Interactions
Androgens may enhance the anticoagulant effects of warfarin and hypoglycemic effects of insulin and oral hypoglycemics. Fluid retention or peripheral edema may be more pronounced with concurrent corticosteroids, calcium channel blockers, or nondiuretic vasodilators.

oxandrolone [ox **an** droe lone]
(Oxandrin)
Indications
Oxandrolone shares many of the indications with testosterone. It is also indicated for weight gain in severe conditions with involuntary weight loss (HIV, burns, postsurgery, catabolic states) and for bone pain associated with osteoporosis.
Pharmacokinetics/Dosing
Oxandrolone is well absorbed and hepatically metabolized. Full effects may not be observed for up to 1 month of therapy. Doses in adults vary from 2.5 mg once or twice daily up to 5 mg four times daily.
Adverse Effects
Adverse effects are identical to those noted above for testosterone. Oxandrolone is a controlled substance Schedule III.
Drug Interactions
See testosterone. Oxandrolone may result in significant increases in anticoagulant effects for clients on warfarin, and usually requires

dramatic reductions in warfarin dose (as much as 80% to 85%) in addition to careful monitoring (Ottery, 2004).

What nursing management occurs with androgen therapy for R.S.?

Assessment Ascertain that R.S. has no preexisting conditions for which oxandrolone may be contraindicated or require increased surveillance during its administration. Assess whether R.S. has breast cancer or known or suspected prostatic cancer, because androgens will stimulate tumor growth and are thus contraindicated. Androgens are used with caution in clients with cardiac impairment, severe cardiorenal disease, or nephrosis because they may cause fluid retention. Clients with prostatic hyperplasia may experience further enlargement. Impaired hepatic dysfunction may result in an increased half-life and so increase the incidence of gynecomastia. Because of the hypercholesterolemic effects of androgens, clients with a history of myocardial infarction or coronary artery disease may experience a worsening of their condition. If R.S. had diabetes mellitus, his medications for diabetes management might need to be adjusted as androgens may decrease blood glucose concentrations.

Review R.S.'s current medications to determine if there could be significant drug interactions. Drug interactions have been reported with the concurrent use of testosterone and oral anticoagulants (increased anticoagulant activity), nonsteroidal antiinflammatory drugs (NSAIDs) (increased risk for bleeding) and hepatotoxic medications (increased risk of hepatotoxicity).

For R.S., a baseline assessment includes height and weight, and a description of his underlying symptoms of diarrhea, anorexia, and activity intolerance associated with his

Special Considerations for Pharmacogenetics | ANDROGENS AND DRUGS AFFECTING MALE REPRODUCTION

PHARMACODYNAMICS

A wide variation in the androgen synthesis or androgen receptors is believed to be correlated with differences in genetic makeup. Genetically determined glutathione transferase activity required for androgen synthesis is noted to be more diverse in some African populations (Tetlow, Coggan, Casarotto, & Board, 2004). Genetic variation in markers for androgen receptors is correlated with height, testicular size, presence and degree of gynecomastia (Zitzmann, Depenbusch, Gromoll, & Nieschlag, 2004). This may in part explain the wide variation in dosing of testosterone required to achieve therapeutic goals.

PHARMACOKINETICS

Testosterone metabolism is genetically determined (Chang & Altman, 2004) and has implications for both desired drug response and adverse effects. A potential for drugs like es-

omeprazole (Nexium) to increase testosterone metabolism may be genetically linked (Rosenshein, Flockhart, & Ho, 2004).

ADVERSE EFFECTS

Testosterone metabolism and its link to prostate cancer appear to be influenced by genetics (Makridakis & Reichardt, 2004). Glucuronidation of testosterone (a phase-II metabolic process in the metabolism of testosterone) is governed by UDP-glucuronosyltransferases (UGTs) that are genetically determined and correlated with prostate cancer risk (Desai, Innocenti, & Ratain, 2003). Other genetic markers for testosterone metabolism via 5-α-reductase appear predictive of age of onset of prostate cancer (Soderstrom et al., 2002). Higher rates of prostate cancer are observed in black men compared with white and Asian men. This finding correlates with altered genetically mediated testosterone metabolism (Parnes, Thompson, & Ford, 2005).

viral infection. A hemoglobin level, hematocrit and lipid profile would serve as baseline to assess development of polycythemia, and increased LDLs (that would increase his risk for atherosclerosis). If androgens were being used as a treatment adjunct for growth failure for children, a baseline assessment includes height, weight, radiographs to determine bone age, and a description of their sexual development.

Nursing Diagnosis While R.S. is receiving androgen therapy, he is at risk for the following nursing diagnoses/collaborative problems: disturbed body image related to gynecomastia and priapism (virilism in female clients and prepubertal males), or increased or decreased libido; excess fluid volume (rapid weight gain, edema of the feet and lower legs, shortness of breath); impaired comfort (gastric irritation); disturbed sleep pattern (insomnia); impaired skin integrity (acne); diarrhea; and the potential complications of benign prostatic hyperplasia, hepatic impairment, hypercalcemia, erythrocytosis, and polycythemia. For clients receiving androgen injections or transdermal systems, there is the risk of impaired tissue integrity (pain, redness, and swelling at the injection site; irritation at patch site).

Planning While taking androgen therapy, R.S. will:
- Experience an increase in lean body mass, increased activity tolerance and improved mood.
- Effectively manage his therapeutic regimen, including medication compliance and appropriately reporting adverse effects to the prescriber.
- Collaborate with health care providers including scheduled visits for treatment and monitoring.

Implementation

Monitoring Monitor R.S.'s weight, bowel status, and activity tolerance at each clinical visit. Check results of serum cholesterol levels to ascertain his risk of cardiovascular disease as the result of androgen administration. Hepatic function is also monitored for hepatotoxicity; hemoglobin and hematocrit are evaluated for polycythemia. Observe R.S. for increasing difficulty or frequency of urination, which may indicate enlargement of the prostate secondary to the drug. Total serum testosterone levels help to determine appropriate dosages. If R.S. had been prescribed a transdermal system, wait until the patch has been worn for 3 to 4 weeks. Draw the blood specimen 2 to 4 hours after patch application.

For other uses of androgen, such as for growth failure, bone age determinations are performed every 6 months to assess the rate of bone maturation in children and adolescents. If androgens are administered for gender change androgen therapy, it is suggested that luteinizing hormone serum levels be determined every 6 months to monitor the success of therapy. For clients being treated for breast cancer, monitor the client's serum calcium carefully. Promptly report indications of hypercalcemia: such as nausea and vomiting, lethargy, loss of muscle tone, polyuria, and increased urine and serum calcium levels. Hypercalcemia in clients with metastatic breast cancer usually indicates bone metastasis. Tumor growth should be monitored by radiography.

Intervention Administer the oral preparations with food to minimize gastric distress. For other forms of dosage, administer IM testosterone deep within the gluteal muscle. Be aware that testosterone cypionate and testosterone enanthate are not interchangeable with testosterone propionate and suspension forms of the drug because of the difference in duration and action. With testosterone cypionate, the preparation may be warmed and shaken to dissolve the crystals. It may turn cloudy if a wet needle or syringe is used, but this does not affect its potency.

Note, too, that there is also a difference between the transdermal systems. The matrix type of patch is adhered to the scrotum and may be removed for swimming, bathing, or sexual activity. In contrast, the reservoir type of patch is placed on the abdomen, back, thighs, or upper arms and is not removed for those activities.

An implant form of testosterone can be inserted subcutaneously using local anesthesia. This implant is a crystalized form of testosterone that dissolves over 3 to 6 months.

Be sensitive to the emotional responses of clients taking androgens. Female clients may have changes in secondary sex characteristics, such as unnatural hair growth or heightened libido; these subside with cessation of the drug. Other changes that may occur, such as enlarged clitoris or hoarseness or deepening of the voice, may not be reversible. Adolescent male clients may need support to deal with deepening of the voice and rapid changes in height, size of sex organs, and hair growth patterns; these changes may occur more rapidly with testosterone than with normal growth and development. Frequent or continuing erection may be a concern.

Education Work with R.S. and/or appropriate family member to develop a diet that is high in protein, calories, vitamins, and minerals and is individualized to his food preferences. Instruct him to weigh daily to monitor for fluid retention. Sodium restriction and/or diuretics may be required if edema occurs. Advise R.S. to maintain regular visits to the prescriber for monitoring progress.

Encourage R.S. to drink at least 3 to 4 L of fluids to ensure adequate urinary output to prevent urinary calculi. Encourage him, because he is active, to perform weight-bearing exercise, such as walking daily. Clients confined to bed should perform range-of-motion exercises at least daily. This exercise inhibits the mobilization of calcium from bone. Monitor the client with diabetes closely. Antidiabetic agents may require a dosage adjustment with concurrent administration of androgens.

Instruct the male client using the matrix type of transdermal patch to apply the patch to a clean, dry, and dry-shaved skin area of the scrotum. Caution the client not to use chemical depilatories. Additionally, advise him that there is the potential to transfer testosterone to his female sexual partner, which might result in mild virilization. The reservoir-type patch site should be rotated between the abdomen, back, thighs, or upper arms and not applied to the scrotum, bony prominences, or any body area that would be subject to pressure when sitting or sleeping. If a patch from either system falls off and cannot be reapplied, do not use a new patch at that time, but return to the usual dosing schedule.

Evaluation The expected outcome of R.S.'s androgen therapy is that he increase his lean body mass, have less activity intolerance, and report a better sense of well-being without adverse effects of the drug. If the androgen was prescribed as a growth failure adjunct, the child will demonstrate an improved growth rate without ill effects of the drug. Those with breast carcinoma will demonstrate slowed tumor growth and bone metastases. For hypogonadal men, the mean number of sexual events (sexual intercourse, orgasm, erections) increased per week compared to baseline.

✱ **P.T. is a 72-year-old male living at home with his wife. His medications include lisinopril (Prinivil), an angiotensin-converting enzyme (ACE) inhibitor, 10 mg daily in the AM and hydrochlorothiazide, a thiazide diuretic, 25 mg daily in the AM for hypertension. He also takes an over-the-counter (OTC) Sominex, diphenhydramine 50 mg, at bedtime to help him sleep. He is scheduled for a home visit by the visiting nurse after a recent fall. P.T. reports he fell while trying to get to the bathroom during the night. He reports frequent awakenings at night to urinate. On arriving at the bathroom, he reports difficulty in initiating a urine stream, that it is slower than it used to be, and some postvoiding dribbling.**

✱ **What are the key pathologic features in benign prostatic hyperplasia?**
Benign prostatic hyperplasia (BPH) with enlargement of the glandular and connective tissue in the portions of the prostate that surround the urethra, is considered a normal age-related change that begins in men around 40 years of age. By 70 years of age, approximately 75% of males will develop BPH symptoms severe enough to require professional intervention.

BPH obstructs the bladder neck and compresses the urethra, which results in urinary retention and increases the risk of bacteriuria. If left untreated, it may affect the ureters and kidneys and result in hydroureter, hydronephrosis, and renal impairment. The pathophysiology of BPH may also include impaired detrusor contractility, sensory abnormalities of the bladder wall, and contractility of the smooth muscle of the prostatic urethra innervated by α_1-adrenergic receptors.

Symptoms of BPH include hesitancy (difficulty starting the urinary stream), a decrease in the diameter and force of the stream, an inability to terminate urination abruptly that results in post void dribbling, and a sensation of incomplete bladder emptying that results in frequency and nocturia. Nocturia usually prompts frequent trips to the bathroom for men with BPH and increases risk for falls.

✱ **What drugs worsen symptoms of BPH?**
Drugs with antimuscarinic properties increase the risk for urinary retention and reduce urine stream flow for men with BPH. Obviously, the antimuscarinics like atropine, scopol-

amine, benztropine (Cogentin) and trihexyphenidyl (Artane), and some of the agents used to treat bladder spasms like oxybutynin (Ditropan), hyoscyamine (Levbid), and tolterodine (Detrol) can all make symptoms of BPH worse (see Chapter 21). Similarly, drugs with significant antimuscarinic effects like the H_1 receptor antagonists (e.g., diphenhydramine [Benadryl, Sominex, Extra Strength Tylenol PM]) and tricyclic antidepressants (e.g., imipramine [Tofranil]) should also be avoided. Diuretics dosed late in the day can contribute to nocturnal urinary frequency, but in and of itself, they do not affect the initiation or rate of urine flow.

✱ **P.T. sees his health care provider, who requests that he discontinue the diphenhydramine (Sominex). He is to report back to clinic in 1 week to see if symptoms improve.**

✱ **What drugs are used in the management of BPH?**
Given the involvement of α_1-adrenergic receptors in the pathology of BPH, it is not surprising that nonselective adrenergic blockers have been tried. Tamsulosin (Flomax) and alfuzosin (Uroxatral) are the classic peripheral acting α_{1A} blocker used to manage BPH because of selectivity for α_1 receptors in the genitourinary tract, reducing smooth muscle tone of the prostatic urethra, thereby reducing the functional component of urethral constriction and obstruction with less effect on blood pressure. Other α_1 blockers used include prazosin (Minipress), doxazosin (Cardura) and terazosin (Hytrin) which also are more pronounced in lowering blood pressure and typically result in a hypotensive state on initial dosing. See Chapters 22 and 27 for a discussion of these agents. Finasteride (Proscar) and dutasteride (Avodart) are 5-α reductase inhibitors available for the treatment of BPH. (See the Complementary and Alternative Considerations box on p. 934 and Chapter 12 for a discussion of saw palmetto in the management of BPH.)

5-α Reductase Inhibitors

Finasteride and dutasteride inhibit 5-α reductase, the enzyme that converts testosterone into the potent androgen 5-α dihydrotestosterone (DHT), a substance responsible for prostate gland growth. Finasteride decreases serum DHT by nearly 70%, which causes shrinkage of the enlarged prostate gland. Clinical improvement in urine flow rates have been reported in clients with BPH treated with finasteride and benefits persist for at least 6 years (Roehrborn et al., 2004). At lower doses, the inhibition of serum DHT production results in an improvement in male pattern hair loss. Finasteride has been used in the treatment and has also been studied in the prevention of prostate cancer (Thompson et al., 2003).

finasteride [fih **nas** teer ide]
(Proscar, Propecia)
Indications
Finasteride is used to manage symptoms of BPH in symptomatic men. In lower doses, it is used to treat male pattern hair loss in men age 18 to 41 years. It has been used investigationally in the treatment of prostate cancer, and for treatment of female hirsutism.

Complementary and Alternative Considerations

Saw Palmetto

Saw palmetto has been used traditionally to treat genitourinary problems such as chronic or subacute cystitis, decreased sperm production, and testicular atrophy. In recent years, saw palmetto has been investigated primarily for its therapeutic use in BPH. Increased DHT synthesis in the prostate and a shift in the androgen and estrogen ratio contribute to BPH. It is thought that the beneficial effect of saw palmetto—alleviating the symptoms of BPH—results from two actions: inhibition of the enzyme 5-α-reductase (inhibition prevents testosterone from converting to DHT) and the blocking of DHT binding at the androgen receptors. Use of the saw palmetto berry in clients with BPH has demonstrated improvements in urinary flow rates and ultrasound-determined residual urine volumes. Its use has also been demonstrated to decrease the frequency of nocturia. *Clinical Evidence* classifies it as beneficial for the treatment of benign prostatic hyperplasia.

Saw palmetto is considered safe when used in recommended dosages on a short-term basis. Adverse effects seem to be limited to headache and mild gastrointestinal (GI) upset. Because of its antiandrogenic and estrogenic properties, its use should be avoided in pregnancy and lactation and in clients taking oral contraceptives and hormone therapy. In client education, stress that urinary or prostate problems are not to be self-treated and that the diagnosis and management of therapy by a health care provider is essential.

Standardized extracts are available, which contain 80% to 95% fatty acids; the common dosage is 160 mg twice daily. Allow 8 weeks before seeing therapeutic benefit.

Data from Gerber, G.S., Kuznetsov, D., Johnson, B.C., & Burstein, J.D. (2001). Randomized, double-blind, placebo-controlled trial of saw palmetto in men with lower urinary tract symptoms. *Urology* 58, 960-964; and Webber, R. (2004). Benign prostatic hyperplasia. In F. Godlee (Ed.), *Clinical evidence concise*. London: British Medical Journal.

Pharmacokinetics/Dosing
Finasteride is 90% protein bound to plasma proteins, with maximum plasma concentrations reached 1 to 2 hours after oral administration. Three to 6 months of ongoing therapy is required to observe clinical results. The dosage for BPH is 5 mg (Proscar) PO once daily. For male pattern baldness, 1 mg PO daily (Propecia) is recommended.

Adverse Effects
The adverse effects of finasteride include decreased libido, impotency, and decreased amount of ejaculate. Finasteride is a Pregnancy Category X drug for which use in pregnant women must be avoided.

Drug Interactions
Concurrent use of St. John's wort may result in decreased finasteride levels.

dutasteride [doo **tas** teer ide]
(Avodart)

Indications
Dutasteride is indicated for the treatment of symptomatic BPH.

Dosing
The typical adult dose for BPH is 0.5 mg once daily. Like with finasteride, meaningful clinical response is not observed for 3 to 6 months.

Adverse Effects
See finasteride.

✱ **P.T. returns to clinic with ongoing symptoms of nocturia. He is started on finasteride (Proscar) 5 mg PO daily.**

✱ **What are the nursing management issues for finasteride therapy for P.T.?**

Assessment Assess P.T. for preexisting conditions that might contraindicate the use of finasteride therapy or require more careful surveillance. Finasteride is contraindicated in individuals with a hypersensitivity to any component of the drug. There is no indication for use in women and children. It is used with caution in clients with liver function impairment. Determine whether P.T. has been evaluated for prostate cancer, because finasteride may interfere with the serum prostate-specific antigen (PSA) test, a test used to screen for prostatic cancer. Drugs with antimuscarinic activity may precipitate or worsen urinary retention and so reduce the effectiveness of finasteride, but no significant drug interactions have been determined for finasteride. Saw palmetto may augment its effectiveness.

A baseline assessment of P.T. includes liver function studies, prostatic status, and an evaluation of his urinary elimination pattern.

Nursing Diagnosis While receiving finasteride therapy, P.T. is at risk for sexual dysfunction related to impotence and decreased libido; impaired comfort (headache, abdominal or back pain, dizziness, gynecomastia); diarrhea; and the potential complication of a hypersensitivity reaction.

Planning While on finasteride therapy, P.T. will:
* Experience an improvement in his symptoms of BPH, including decreased nocturia, stronger urinary stream that starts without hesitation and an absence of urinary dribbling.
* Effectively manage his therapeutic regimen including medication compliance, implementing supportive measures, and appropriately reporting adverse effects to the prescriber.
* Collaborate with health care providers for monitoring and treatment.

Implementation
Monitoring Continue to monitor P.T.'s urinary hesitancy, force of urinary stream, postvoid dribbling, nocturia, and frequency, urgency, and burning with urination. Review results of periodic liver function tests. A periodic digital rectal examination will assist in detecting possible prostate cancer.

Intervention Finasteride may be given with or without meals, because bioavailability is not affected by food. Women who are or may become pregnant should avoid handling the crushed tablets to avoid the possibility of transdermal absorption.

Education Inform P.T. that finasteride does not cure, but helps to control BPH and that it takes at least 6 months for its full effect to occur in relieving symptoms. There may be the possibility of life long therapy. P.T. should limit his fluid intake, especially coffee and alcohol, in the evening to reduce nocturia. Alert any client taking finasteride that if his sexual partner is pregnant or to become pregnant, he should avoid exposing her to his semen because a small amount of the drug is present in semen (see the Pregnancy Safety box above).

If finasteride is prescribed for male-pattern baldness, alert the client that it will take at least 3 months to see an effect and that any improvement will only last as long as the medication is taken.

Evaluation The expected outcome of finasteride therapy. For P.T. is that his prostate will decrease in size, and he will not experience urinary hesitancy, urinary dribbling, nocturia, or frequency and urgency of urination. He will effectively manage his finasteride regimen including medication compliance, evening restriction of fluids, and reporting to his prescriber appropriately for monitoring and treatment. If finasteride is taken for male-pattern baldness, the client will experience hair growth.

Summary

Androgens, the male sex hormones, are responsible for the normal development and maintenance of male sex charac-teristics. Testosterone is most commonly used for hormonal replacement therapy in males and is also indicated for the treatment of breast carcinoma and anemia. Clients receiving androgen therapy require additional support because of their risk for self-concept disturbance as a result of the drug's effects on secondary sex characteristics. Although testosterone may be essential for an improvement in health status, the development of virilism in female clients, gynecomastia and priapism in male clients, and a change in libido may be distressing for clients of both genders. The androgens are schedule III substances and have the potential for abuse.

Management of BPH includes avoiding muscarinic antagonists (e.g., atropine-like drugs) and considering treatments to improve symptoms of urine flow and frequency/urgency. The α_{1A}-adrenergic antagonists (alfuzosin, tamsulosin), the 5-α-reductase inhibitors (finasteride, dutasteride) and the complementary agent saw palmetto have all demonstrated improved symptom control for men with BPH. Finasteride has also been used to treat male pattern baldness in lower doses.

⊛ Critical Thinking Questions

- Althea Johnson, who is 54 years old and 3 years post-menopause, has an estrogen-dependent tumor. The physician has prescribed testosterone for her condition. What do you need to teach Ms. Johnson about the effects of testosterone in women?

- Ed Taylor, who is 56 years old and a widower of 2 years, has just been placed on finasteride. What assessments of his sexuality and sexual functioning pattern will be necessary?

Bibliography

Alexander, J.L., Kotz, K., Dennerstein, L., Kutner, S.J., Wallen, K., & Notelovitz, M. (2004). The effects of postmenopausal hormone therapies on female sexual functioning: a review of double-blind, randomized controlled trials. *Menopause, 11*(6) Supplement, 749-765.

Anderson, D.M., Keith, J., & Novak, P.D. (Eds.) (2002). *Mosby's medical, nursing, and allied health dictionary* (6th ed.). St. Louis: Mosby.

Bosker, G. (Ed.). (2004). *Primary and acute care medicine: Practice, protocols, pathways,* (2nd ed.). Atlanta: Thomson American Health Consultants.

Buster, J.E., Kingsberg, S.A., Aguirre, O., Brown, C., Breaux, J.G., Buch, A., et al. (2005). Testosterone patch for low sexual desire in surgically menopausal women: A randomized trial. *Obstetrics and Gynecology, 105,* 944-952.

e-LEARNING SUPPLEMENTS

Student CD-ROM
- Final Exam questions
- NCLEX® Examination review questions
- Pharmacology animations
- Printable chapter summary

Evolve Website (http://evolve.elsevier.com/mckenry)
- Content updates, including information on new drugs
- WebLinks corresponding to this chapter
- Answers to the critical thinking questions in this chapter
- *Elsevier ePharmacology Update* newsletter
- Mosby's Drug Consult Internet Edition
- Supplemental and reference information

Chang, J.T., & Altman, R.B. (2004). Extracting and characterizing gene-drug relationships from the literature. Pharmacogenetics. 14(9):577-586. Retrieved December 2, 2004, from http://bionlp.stanford.edu/genedrug/gene_drug_predictions.html.

Desai, A., Innocenti, F., & Ratain, M. (2003). UGT pharmacogenomics: implications for cancer risk and cancer therapeutics. *Pharmacogenetics, 13*(8), 517-523.

Drug facts and comparisons (58th ed.). (2005). St. Louis: Facts and Comparisons.

Fitzgerald, P.A. (2003). Endocrinology. In L.M. Tierney, Jr., S.J. McPhee & M.A. Papadakis (Eds.), *Current Medical Diagnosis & Treatment*. New York: Lange Medical Books/McGraw-Hill.

Kalantaridou, S.N., Davis, S.R., & Calis, K.A. (2002). Hormone replacement therapy. In J.T. DiPiro, R.L. Talbert, G.C. Yee, G.R. Matzke, B.G. Wells & L.M. Posey (Eds.), *Pharmacotherapy: A pathophysiological approach* (5th ed.). Norwalk, CT: Appleton & Lange.

Lacy, C.F., Armstrong, L.L., Goldman, M.P., & Lance, L.L. (2004). *Lexi-Comp's Drug Information Handbook* (12th ed.). Hudson, Ohio: Lexi-Comp.

Makridakis, N., & Reichardt, J.K. (2004). Molecular Epidemiology of Androgen-Metabolic Loci in Prostate Cancer: Predisposition and Progression. *Journal of Urology, 171*(2, Part 2 of 2), S25-S29.

Mosby's drug consult (15th ed.). (2005). St. Louis: Mosby.

Ottery, F. (April 20, 2004). Dear Health Care Professional Letter. East Brunswick, NJ: Savient Pharmaceuticals, Inc. Retrieved January 12, 2005, from http://www.fda.gov/medwatch/SAFETY/2004/oxandrin.htm.

Parnes, H.L., Thompson, I.M., & Ford, L.G. (2005). Prevention of Hormone-Related Cancers: Prostate Cancer. *Journal of Clinical Oncology, 23*(2), 368-377.

Roehrborn, C.G., Bruskewitz, R., Nickel, J.C., McConnell, J.D., Saltzman, B., & Gittelman, M.C., et al., and the Proscar Long-Term Efficacy and Safety Study Group. (2004). Sustained decrease in incidence of acute urinary retention and surgery with finasteride for 6 years in men with benign prostatic hyperplasia. *Journal of Urology, 171*, 1194-1198.

Rosenshein, B.B., Flockhart, D.A., & Ho, H. (2004). Induction of Testosterone Metabolism by Esomeprazole in a CYP2 C19*2 Heterozygote. *American Journal of the Medical Sciences, 327*(5), 289-293.

Soderstrom, T., Wadelius, M., Andersson, S.O., Johansson, J.E., Johansson, S., & Granath, F., et al. (2002). 5 α-Reductase 2 polymorphisms as risk factors in prostate cancer. *Pharmacogenetics, 12*(4), 307-312.

Snyder, P.J. (2001) Androgens. In J.G. Hardman & L.E. Limbird (Eds.), *Goodman & Gilman's The pharmacological basis of therapeutics* (10th ed.). New York: McGraw-Hill.

Tetlow, N., Coggan, M., Casarotto, M.G., & Board, P.G. (2004). Functional polymorphism of human glutathione transferase A3: effects on xenobiotic metabolism and steroid biosynthesis. *Pharmacogenetics, 14*(10),657-663.

Thompson, I.M., Goodman, P.J., Tangen, C.M., Lucia, M.S., Miller, G.J., & Ford, L.G., et al. (2003). The influence of finasteride on the development of prostate cancer. *New England Journal of Medicine, 349*, 215-224.

Thompson, J.F. (2005). Geriatric urologic disorders. In M.A. Koda-Kimble, L.Y. Young, W.A. Kradjan, B.J. Guglielmo, B.K. Alldredge, & R.L. Corelli (Eds.), *Applied therapeutics: The clinical use of drugs* (8th ed.). Philadelphia: Lippincott Williams & Wilkins.

USP DI: Drug information for the health care professional (25th ed.). (2005). Greenwood Village, CO: MICROMEDEX Thomson Healthcare.

Zitzmann, M., Depenbusch, M., Gromoll, J., & Nieschlag, E. (2004). X-Chromosome Inactivation Patterns and Androgen Receptor Functionality Influence Phenotype and Social Characteristics as Well as Pharmacogenetics of Testosterone Therapy in Klinefelter Patients. *Journal of Clinical Endocrinology & Metabolism, 89*(12), 6208-6217.

DRUGS AFFECTING SEXUAL BEHAVIOR

CHAPTER FOCUS

Sexuality is an integral part of one's identity; it is a reflection of how one feels about oneself and how one interacts with others. Sexual function refers to the psychologic and physiologic ability to perform in a sexually satisfying manner, with or without a partner (Carpenito-Moyet, 2004). Drugs can influence both sexuality and sexual function. The nurse should be able to discuss sexual health with clients and provide information about medications and their effects on sexual behavior.

LEARNING OBJECTIVES

- Describe the effect of drugs on sexual behavior.
- Identify the effect of commonly prescribed drugs, such as antihypertensives, antihistamines, antispasmodics, sedatives and tranquilizers, antidepressants, ethyl alcohol, barbiturates, steroid hormones, and methadone, on the libido.
- List drugs that may affect sexual behavior to enhance libido or sexual gratification.
- Identify client cues about problems related to drug use and sexuality.
- Provide appropriate client education about drugs that have the potential to cause sexual dysfunction.

▲ **KEY TERMS**
impotence, p. 938
libido, p. 938
premenstrual dysphoric disorder (PMDD), p. 940

✶ **KEY DRUGS**
sildenafil, p. 943

Sexuality and sexual behavior have psychological, social, and physiologic dimensions that reflect a complexity beyond drug-related effects. Contributing factors include self-esteem, general health, availability of a partner, appropriate environment, and perhaps age. Because drugs can affect sexual activities or sexual identity, nurses must be sensitive to their clients' needs as sexual beings and alert to cues that reflect problems. Clients may present these cues if given the chance, such as confusion or embarrassment about a lack of interest in sexual activities, about a lack of arousal despite desire, or about other phenomena they consider unusual. Nurses need to be aware

of the potential sexual adverse effects of common drugs; with this knowledge, they can ask clients about sexual function as part of a routine drug history to determine issues that might influence the client's adherence to therapy.

✳ What are the types of sexual dysfunction?

Sexual dysfunction is common among adults and is classified based on symptoms and etiology. Both men and women can experience decreased libido, difficulty in sexual arousal, or inability to have an orgasm. Both men and women may also experience pain with sexual stimulation.

Decreased libido or reduced sex drive is common in both genders and may be secondary to depression, drug therapy or other factors. Difficulty in arousal may manifest in men as erectile dysfunction. It may also present as premature or delayed ejaculation. For women, arousal difficulties may result in reduced vaginal lubrication. Both men and women may have difficulty in obtaining an orgasm. Pain associated with sexual stimulation may be related to a physical cause. Priapism for men and clitoral priapism or spasms of the vagina for women may also cause significant discomfort.

The causes of sexual dysfunction may be physical, hormonal, or psychosocial. Among the physical factors affecting sexual dysfunction are clinical depression, chronic disease, and medication. Many clients with depression report a diminished interest in sexual relations, and the drugs used in treating depression are among the most frequently observed medications contributing to sexual dysfunction. Men with vascular complications of chronic diseases (particularly those with diabetes) report a higher incidence of erectile dysfunction. Recent surgery or pain syndromes also contribute to changes in sexual health.

Hormonal changes may affect libido or may contribute to pain. This is particularly true for women who are undergoing menopause. The changes in estrogen contribute to altered vaginal structure and reduced vaginal elasticity and lubrication making vaginal intercourse more painful (dyspareunia). Reduced testosterone levels (for both men and women) are also associated with reduced libido.

Sexual dysfunction is quite common, affecting 22% of men and 40% of women in one cross-sectional analysis of primary care clients in London (Nazareth, Boynton, & King, 2003). Loss of libido was noted frequently in both men and women. Men also experienced erectile dysfunction frequently and women noted failure of orgasmic response. Psychosocial issues are large contributors to sexual dysfunction. The stress of work, home, relationships or other factors are common factors in many clients with sexual dysfunction. Trauma or history of sexual abuse can have lasting effects on sexual function. Cultural and religious beliefs also impact on sexual health.

✹ What is the role of the autonomic nervous system in sexual response?

Many physiologic functions significant to sexual pleasure are controlled by the psyche and the autonomic nervous system or ANS (see also Chapter 20). The ANS comprises two parts—the sympathetic (adrenergic) and parasympathetic (cholinergic) systems—and its functional units are nerves, nerve plexuses, and ganglia. Although viewed as physiologic antagonists, the two systems often have synergistic effects on sexual functioning.

The male and female sexual organs are composed of homologous tissues; although the shapes of the organs differ, they correspond part for part in structure, position, and embryologic origin. The genital protuberance of the embryo appears identical in both genders. The embryo is characteristically female initially and does not differentiate until fetal androgens begin to masculinize tissues (seventh to twelfth weeks of pregnancy). Thus it is not surprising that the mature analogous organs function similarly.

In the male, sympathetic (adrenergic) impulses produce ejaculation by causing contraction of the prostate and seminal vesicles along with effects on the bulbocavernous and ischiocavernous muscles. Impotence, or impotency, is the inability of the adult male to achieve or maintain a penile erection, along with decreased sexual function. Drugs that block adrenergic impulses may affect ejaculatory function through sympathetic blockade.

Parasympathetic (cholinergic) stimulation controls penile erection. This response results from congestion of the vascular sinuses in the penile corpora caused by parasympathetic nerve action in the venous channels. Drugs that interfere with parasympathetic nerve transmitters (cholinergic nerves) can cause defects in erection. Ganglionic blocking agents, which may block both sympathetic and parasympathetic nerve transmission, can cause complete impotence and impaired sexual functioning.

In the female, parasympathetic (cholinergic) impulses cause arterial dilation and venoconstriction, which produce clitoral erection and vasocongestion of the vulva, transudation (oozing of a fluid through pores) of lubricating secretions from the vaginal walls, and swelling of the introitus (vaginal opening). Continued stimulation of the clitoris, and/or the Graefenberg spot that is located on the anterior wall of the vagina, may produce orgasm and, for some, a miniature facsimile of ejaculation from glands that surround the female urethra.

✹ **L.P. is a 46-year-old woman who serves as the office manager at her local church. She is married with two teenage children, and reports to the nurse that she has diminished interest in sexual relations with her husband. She indicates that she started fluoxetine (Prozac) 18 months ago for clinical depression.**

✹ What drugs adversely affect sexual functioning?

A number of drugs can cause sexual dysfunction. Chief among these are drugs that impact the ANS, those that affect androgen production, and those that produce more global central nervous system (CNS) depressant effects. Such drugs include the antihypertensives, diuretics, histamine 1 and 2 blockers, anxiolytics, phenothiazines, antidepressants, ethanol, barbiturates, and hormones.

Antihypertensives

Propranolol (Inderal) and other β-adrenergic blockers have been associated with decreased libido and erectile dysfunction. The calcium channel blockers, including nifedipine (Adalat, Procardia), diltiazem (Cardizem), and verapamil (Calan, Isoptin) may cause erectile dysfunction.

Central-acting α_2 agonists such as methyldopa (Aldomet), clonidine (Catapres), guanabenz (Wytensin), and guanfacine (Tenex) have been associated with more frequent reports of impotence and sexual dysfunction. Difficulty in ejaculation has been reported with the infrequently used guanethidine (Ismelin), and reserpine (Serpasil) may induce impotence or a decreased interest in sex. Failure to ejaculate without a concomitant alteration of erection or orgasm has been reported in individuals treated with phenoxybenzamine (Dibenzyline), an α-adrenergic blocking agent once used to supplement psychiatric therapy. This drug has sometimes been referred to, mistakenly, as the male contraceptive, and was historically used to treat premature ejaculation (Montague et al., 2004). Ganglionic blockers, although rarely used, may also produce impotence and other untoward effects on sexual function. Guanethidine falls into this category. Other agents include mecamylamine (Inversine) and trimethaphan (Arfonad), which are rarely used as antihypertensive agents. Because these drugs may block both sympathetic and parasympathetic innervation of the sex organs, both erectile capability and ejaculatory function may be affected during their use.

Diuretics

The thiazide diuretics may induce sexual dysfunction, and spironolactone (Aldactone) has been associated with a decrease in libido, impotence, and gynecomastia. Spironolactone is associated with considerably more reports of sexual dysfunction than the thiazides; this effect appears to be dose related.

Histamine 1 and 2 Blockers

Antihistaminic drugs act as competitive inhibitors of histamine at physiologic receptor sites to prevent histaminic effects. Well-known examples of such drugs include diphenhydramine (Benadryl), promethazine (Phenergan), and chlorpheniramine (Chlor-Trimeton). These drugs are consumed by millions as antiemetics, as mild sedatives, and for the control of allergy symptoms. Most antihistamines display anticholinergic effects such as dry mouth, urinary retention, and constipation. Continuous use of these drugs may interfere with sexual activity. This effect is presumably mediated by the blockade of parasympathetic nerve impulses to the sex glands and organs.

H_2 receptor antagonists such as cimetidine (Tagamet) and ranitidine (Zantac) have been reported to cause antiandrogenic effects (impotence, gynecomastia) when administered in high doses for a prolonged period.

Phenothiazines/Antipsychotics

Phenothiazines such as chlorpromazine (Thorazine), prochlorperazine (Compazine), thioridazine (Mellaril), and mesoridazine (Serentil) induce a sedative effect that may partly account for the decreased sexual interest of persons undergoing phenothiazine therapy. In addition to their CNS effects, the peripheral effects of phenothiazines may contribute to the inhibition of sexual function. These drugs decrease skeletal muscle tone and block cholinergic synapses at both muscarinic and nicotinic receptors. Various adrenergic impulses may also be inhibited. Impotence, decreased libido, ejacula-

tion disorders, and prolonged amenorrhea have been reported in individuals taking phenothiazines. Failure to ejaculate has been reported in men treated with thioridazine, but erection and orgasm do not appear to be affected. Thioridazine has a significantly greater peripheral α-adrenergic blocking effect than the other phenothiazines and results in a higher incidence of ejaculation failure. Ejaculation problems have also been reported with the use of chlorprothixene (Taractan) and mesoridazine (Serentil). Haloperidol (Haldol), an antipsychotic, can adversely affect libido in men.

Anxiolytics

Benzodiazepine compounds are commonly prescribed antianxiety medications. Diazepam (Valium) is used for treating anxiety, seizure activity and as a skeletal muscle relaxant. The sedative and relaxing effects of this drug may account for the decreased interest in sexual activity. There have been several reports of anorgasmia in males and females, and ejaculation failure. Alternatively, the judicious use of these tranquilizers has been considered to be of value in the treatment of sexual impotence and other problems involving sexual performance when excessive anxiety is a factor.

Antidepressants

Depression is often associated with diminished sexual interest, drive, and activity (see Chapter 19), and the drugs used to treat depression often compound the negative effects on sexual function. Although antidepressants generally elevate mood and thus increase sexuality, they can cause impotence and have an adverse effect on sexual behavior. The effect of tricyclic antidepressants on sexuality may be related to peripheral anticholinergic effects, such as those produced by some antihypertensives. Examples of these drugs include imipramine (Tofranil) and amitriptyline (Elavil). Although monoamine oxidase (MAO) inhibitors may be used as antihypertensives and antidepressants, the impotence that can result may be caused by their tendency to block peripheral ganglionic nerve transmission. The selective serotonin reuptake inhibitors are also known to decrease libido and sexual function. Only bupropion (Wellbutrin) appears to be devoid of inducing sexual dysfunction in men and women.

Many antidepressants are associated with delayed ejaculation. Four antidepressants are actually recommended by the American Urological Association for the treatment of men with problematic premature ejaculation: clomipramine, fluoxetine, paroxetine and sertraline (Montague et al., 2004) (Table 54-1).

Ethanol

As a drug of individual and unique notoriety, ethyl alcohol is considered for its effects on human sexual function and behavior. Revered for centuries as a sexual stimulant and a cure for all illnesses, alcohol is in fact a depressant and is recognized today to have far greater social than therapeutic value. Although a sedative, alcohol in moderate amounts

TABLE 54-1 AMERICAN UROLOGICAL ASSOCIATION RECOMMENDATIONS FOR PHARMACOLOGIC MANAGEMENT OF MALE PREMATURE EJACULATION

Agent	Typical Dose for Intermittent Management of Premature Ejaculation	Typical Daily Dose for Management of Premature Ejaculation
clomipramine (Anafranil)	25 mg PO 4-24 hr before intercourse	25-50 mg PO daily
fluoxetine (Prozac)	NA	5-20 mg PO daily
paroxetine (Paxil)	20 mg PO 3-4 hr before intercourse	10-40 mg PO daily
sertraline (Zoloft)	50 mg PO 4-8 hr before intercourse	25-200 mg PO daily
lidocaine 2.5%/prilocaine 2.5% cream (EMLA)	Applied locally 20-30 min before intercourse	NA

Modified from Montague, D.K., Jarow, J., Broderick, G.A., Dmochowski, R.R., Heaton, J.P., & Lue, T.F., et al., for the American Urological Association Erectile Dysfunction Guideline Update Panel (2004). AUA Guideline on the pharmacologic management of premature ejaculation. *Journal of Urology,* 172(1), 290-294.
NA, Not applicable.

may enhance sexual activity by relieving anxieties and loosening the inhibitions that often shroud sexual behavior.

Beyond a certain limit, however, neither desire nor potency overcome the depressed physical capability that occurs under its influence. Studies on the pharmacologic action of alcohol show that the CNS is more affected by alcohol than is any other system of the body. Electrophysiologic studies suggest that alcohol initially depresses the part of the brain responsible for integrating the various activities of the nervous system. The result is that various processes related to thought and motor activities become disrupted. The first mental processes affected are related to sobriety and self-restraint, which produces a less inhibited and less restrained approach to sexual behavior and other activities normally inhibited by previous training or experience. With continued alcohol consumption, the brain becomes narcotized, reflexes become slowed, blood vessels are dilated, and the capacity for sexual function is diminished. Additionally, alcohol produces a severe diuretic effect, which may also interfere with sexual function. Alcohol intoxication may also contribute to increased participation in risky sexual behavior, thus increasing the potential for pregnancy and sexually transmitted infections.

Typically, the male client with alcoholism experiences delayed ejaculation during intoxication; impotence can occur after years of chronic alcoholism. Vascular changes, peripheral neuropathy, and lower testosterone levels because of liver damage are thought to cause the impotence. The problem is compounded by body image changes such as testicular atrophy and gynecomastia.

Barbiturates

Barbiturates, such as amobarbital (Amytal), pentobarbital (Nembutal), secobarbital (Seconal), and thiopental (Pentothal), are sedative-hypnotic drugs that have general depressant effects on all nervous tissues. As with alcohol, these drugs in their prescribed dosage produce relaxation, hypnosis, and sleep with depression of various body functions, in-

cluding sexual performance and ability. Barbiturates can cause respiratory failure and death with prolonged use or overdose. Withdrawal after long-term, heavy consumption of barbiturates may result in seizures. There is no rationale for their use in altering sexual behavior in human beings.

Androgens/Estrogens/Progestins

Sex hormones act on the CNS and other body organs to influence sexual and aggressive behavior, and mood and emotional outlook. Variations in female hormones may play a role in **premenstrual dysphoric disorder (PMDD),** a mental health condition that begins 1 or 2 weeks before menstrual flow and characterized by anxiety, irritability, and depression, whereas male hormones are associated with aggression and increased sexual interest. Evidence indicates that sexual drive may be influenced by treatment with sex hormones.

The anabolic steroids are derived from or are related to the male sex hormone testosterone. They have been misused by athletes and other postpubertal persons to promote muscle growth and endurance. These androgens can cause (1) virilization, hirsutism, libido changes, and clitoral enlargement in females, and (2) testicular atrophy, impotence, chronic priapism, and oligospermia in males (see Chapters 9 and 53). Androgens, including testosterone, are sometimes used with postmenopausal women in combination with estrogens for the treatment of reduced libido and sexual dysfunction (Alexander et al., 2004; Buster et al., 2005).

Other Medications

A number of other medications have been reported to cause sexual dysfunction. Ketoconazole (Nizoral), an antifungal agent, may cause oligospermia and decreased libido in males. Opioids have also been associated with sexual dysfunction (Thompson, 2005).

✱ **L.P. asks the nurse if her loss of libido is related to antidepressant use. The nurse confirms that this is** likely, and explores with her the significance of sexual dysfunction on her life. Although the Prozac that L.P. is taking has been effective, it would seem that this adverse effect may cause L.P. to become noncompliant. Together they explore with the prescriber the possibility to changing her drug to bupropion (Wellbutrin) that does not have sexual dysfunction as an adverse effect.

❄ **What is the role of the nurse in assessing drug induced sexual dysfunction?**

An appreciation of the serious effects of sexual dysfunction on client's lives can produce a special sensitivity to their concerns. Clients often find it easier to confide in and discuss such important personal information with a nurse (male or female), than with anyone else. Therefore high-quality professional nursing should be directed toward achieving the following goals:

- Gaining an understanding of and accepting feelings about one's own sexuality. It takes time and effort to be comfortable enough to be therapeutic with others who are having sexual problems.
- Being open to clients' discussions about sexual concerns.
- Allowing clients to hold any belief or sexual practice they choose that is not overtly harmful.
- Recognizing that it is probably impossible to be truly comfortable with all clients or all related topics. It may be necessary to refer some clients to more adequately prepared personnel. This might be a clinical nurse specialist or a social worker with expertise in dealing with sexual issues.
- Keeping current with the constantly changing data about drugs with the potential for causing sexual dysfunction. This becomes more complex with the discovery that certain combinations of drugs elicit unusual sexual responses. Drugs that are currently suspect include antihypertensives, antidepressants, antihistamines, sedatives and tranquilizers, ethyl alcohol, barbiturates, steroid hormones and derivatives, opioids and psychoactive drugs, and certain natural substances.
- Being able to identify and interpret client cues about problems dealing with sexuality, such as unexplained noncompliance with medication instructions, certain subjective data from the nursing history, avoidance of the topic, or other subtle cues.
- Discussing clients' medication with them (casual use of drugs and over-the-counter [OTC] and prescribed drugs), including information about potential adverse effects.
- Consulting with the prescriber when adverse effects do appear and suggesting alternate forms or dosages of drug therapy, if feasible. Such changes may be the route to enhanced compliance.
- Listening with sensitivity to expressed feelings of frustration, anger, anxiety, or fear that may accompany body image changes or perceptions of aging and waning sexual ability and/or attractiveness; some of these feelings may result from the effects of prescribed drugs.

❄ T.J. is a 17-year-old high school junior who mentions to a fellow classmate how "sexually free" she felt on ecstasy (MDMA) at a party the prior evening. The school nurse overhears the conversation and gently questions T.J. about her experience. The nurse offers guidance to the two students regarding the effects of MDMA on sexual decision making.

❄ **What drugs are reported to enhance libido or sexual gratification?**

Substances to increase sexual potency or drive have been sought throughout history. Inscriptions in the ruins of ancient cultures have described the preparation of "erotic potions," and an endless number of "aphrodisiacs" have been described since then. In contemporary society many drugs and chemicals that modify mood and behavior are claimed to have aphrodisiac properties, including drugs of abuse, and both prescription and OTC products. In reality, no known drugs specifically increase libido or sexual performance; chemicals taken for this purpose without medical advice (especially in combination with other drugs) pose the danger of adverse effects, drug interactions, or overdose. However, many pharmacologically active agents do temporarily modify both physiologic responsiveness and subjective perception to enhance the enjoyment, if not the fulfillment, of the sex act. Chapter 53 presents testosterone and androgens. Other agents are briefly discussed here.

Ecstasy/MDMA and Other Amphetamines

Ecstasy (MDMA or methylene-dioxymethamphetamine) is widely used and has often been nicknamed the "love drug." Among other effects, MDMA induces feelings of closeness with others, and reduces feelings of defensiveness. Individuals who have taken MDMA often display limited judgment under its influence and may be much more likely to engage in unsafe or risky sexual activity (Taylor et al., 2004). Chapter 9 discusses additional risks for MDMA, including the risk for life-threatening rhabdomyolysis.

Other amphetamines such as dextroamphetamine (Dexedrine) and crystal methamphetamine ("crystal meth") have also been used to stimulate sexual function. These drugs have a powerful central stimulant action in addition to peripheral α and β sympathomimetic effects. Their main effects are wakefulness and alertness, mood elevation, increased motor and speech activity, and often elation and euphoria. Physical performance is usually improved, and fatigue can be prevented or reversed. The effects of amphetamines on sexual performance, however, are inconsistent.

Other Drugs of Abuse

Other drugs such as morphine, heroin, cocaine, marijuana, lysergic acid diethylamide (LSD) are also used by some as aphrodisiacs. For some individuals, these agents can enhance the enjoyment of the sexual experience under certain circumstances, but individual response is often not predictable. Responsiveness varies because these agents have no particular properties that specifically increase sexual potency; instead they tend to affect the user according to expectations. Thus the user's state of mind and the amount consumed contribute considerably to the effect achieved. Like alcohol, these drugs act on the CNS to weaken inhibitions, which are often the cause of problems involving sexual behavior. If taken in excess or too often, these drugs have the opposite effect and inhibit sexual drive and function. Because of these variations, researchers are skeptical of their value.

Marijuana (cannabis), an extract of the *Cannabis sativa* plant, is considered by many to be a sexual stimulant. However, like alcohol, its effect results indirectly from relaxation and the release of inhibitions surrounding sexual activity. The active ingredient in marijuana is tetrahydrocannabinol (THC). The pharmacologic effects resulting from smoking marijuana depend on the expectations and personality of the user, the dose, and the prevailing circumstances. The usual effects of marijuana are time distortion and enhanced suggestibility, which produces the illusion that sexual climax is somewhat prolonged. The expectation that marijuana is an aphrodisiac may enhance enjoyment of the sex act. However, studies on the properties of marijuana for a specific effect on sexual behavior have revealed no such properties. On the contrary, there is evidence that marijuana smokers have a higher incidence of decreased libido and impaired potency than nonusers. Additionally, chronic intensive use of marijuana depresses plasma testosterone levels in healthy males and produces gynecomastia in some users. Chromosomal breaks have also occurred.

LSD is another drug that, although considered an aphrodisiac by some, has potentially untoward effects on sexual function and behavior. As with marijuana, any alteration of sexual performance produced by LSD is principally subjective. This drug acts almost entirely on the CNS. Little response, if any, has been noted in other organ systems that can be attributed to the direct effect of LSD, and no biochemical or pharmacologic evidence supports the contention that LSD or similar drugs contain any sex-stimulating properties. In fact, the repeated use of LSD may produce serious psychologic problems, which overall could have an adverse affect on sexual interest or activity. Women who use LSD during pregnancy may have a higher rate of malformed babies or stillbirths than women who do not use LSD.

Most of these agents do little to promote the enjoyment of sexual activity and over time may produce adverse psychologic and physical effects that reduce sexual interest and capability.

cantharis [**kan** thar is]

Cantharis (cantharidin, Spanish fly), a legendary sexual stimulant, is a powerful irritant and potent systemic poison. This substance is a powder made from dried beetles *(Cantharis vesicatoria)* found in southern Europe, and it can produce severe illness characterized by vomiting, diarrhea, abdominal pain, and shock. When taken internally, it causes irritation and inflammation of the genitourinary tract and dilation of the blood vessels of the penis and clitoris, sometimes producing prolonged erections (priapism) or engorgement, usually without increased sexual desire. Deaths have been reported from the promiscuous use of cantharis as an aphrodisiac. It is currently recognized that cantharis is not an effective sexual stimulant.

yohimbe [yo **him** bee]

Another natural substance with purported aphrodisiac properties is yohimbe, an alkaloid derived from the West African tree *Corynanthe yohimbe*. Yohimbe produces a competitive α-adrenergic block of limited duration and antidiuresis, probably from the release of antidiuretic hormone. It can cause respiratory depression, urinary retention, hyperglycemia, tachycardia, tremors and irritability. Although yohimbe stimulates the lower spinal nerve centers controlling erection, there is no convincing evidence that it is effective as a sexual stimulant. When used for impotence, it is dosed at $1/_2$ to 1 tablet (each tablet is 5.4 mg) up to three times daily for up to 10 weeks.

levodopa [lee voe **doe** pa]
(L-dopa)

Levodopa (L-dopa) is a natural intermediate in the biosynthesis of catecholamines in the brain and peripheral adrenergic nerve terminals. In the biologic sequence of events it is converted to dopamine, which in turn serves as a substrate of the neurotransmitter norepinephrine. Levodopa is used successfully in treating parkinsonism, a disease characterized by dopamine deficiency. When levodopa is administered to an individual with this syndrome, the symptoms of Parkinson's disease are ameliorated, presumably because the drug is converted to dopamine and thereby counteracts the deficiency.

Individuals treated with levodopa, especially older men, have been observed to experience a sexual rejuvenation. This effect has led to the belief that levodopa stimulates sexual prowess. Consequently, studies with younger men complaining of decreased erectile ability have shown that levodopa increases libido and the incidence of penile erections. Overall, however, these effects are short-lived and do not reflect continued satisfactory sexual function and potency. Thus levodopa is not a true aphrodisiac. The increased sexual activity experienced by parkinsonian clients treated with levodopa may reflect improved well-being and partial recovery of normal sexual functions that were impaired by Parkinson's disease. (See Chapter 23 for a further discussion.)

amyl nitrite [**am** il]

Amyl nitrite, a drug used in the past to treat angina pectoris, is alleged to enhance sexual activity in humans. As a vasodilator and smooth muscle stimulant, amyl nitrite has been reported to intensify the orgasmic experience for men if inhaled at the moment of orgasm. This effect is probably the result of relaxation of smooth muscles and consequent vasodilation of the genitourinary tract. No effects of amyl nitrite on libido have been reported, but a loss of erection or delayed ejaculation may result. Women generally experience negative effects on orgasm when taking this drug. Concurrent use of amyl nitrite with phosphodiesterase type 5 inhibitors (e.g., sildenafil [Viagra]) may result in significant hypotension and is absolutely contraindicated.

vitamin E

Much has been said about the positive effects of vitamin E (alpha tocopherol) on sexual performance and ability in human beings. Unfortunately, there is little scientific rationale to substantiate such claims. The primary reasons for attributing a positive role in sexual performance to vitamin E come from experiments on vitamin E deficiency in laboratory animals. In such experiments the principal manifestation of this deficiency is infertility, although the reasons for this condition differ in males and females. In female rats there is no loss in ability to produce apparently healthy ova, nor is there any defect in the placenta or uterus. However, fetal death occurs shortly after the first week of embryonic life, and fetuses are reabsorbed. This situation can be prevented if vitamin E is administered any time up to the fifth or sixth day of embryonic life. In the male rat the earliest observable effect of vitamin E deficiency is immobility of spermatozoa, with subsequent degeneration of the germinal epithelium. Secondary sex organs are not altered and sexual vigor is not diminished, but vigor may decrease if the deficiency continues. Because of experimental results such as these, vitamin E has been conjectured to restore potency or to preserve fertility, sexual interest, and endurance in humans. No evidence supports these contentions, but because sexual performance is often influenced by mental attitude, a person who believes vitamin E may improve sexual prowess may actually find improvement. The only established therapeutic use for vitamin E is for the prevention or treatment of vitamin E deficiency, a condition that is rare in humans. A meta-analysis of 19 clinical trials involving approximately 135,000 participants determined that taking high doses (400 international units or more) of vitamin E may actually increase overall mortality and should be avoided (Miller III et al., 2004).

⚙ **B.Y. is a 56-year-old truck driver with type 2 diabetes mellitus in fair control. He reports to his health care provider that he has difficulty in getting an erection and asks for sildenafil (Viagra), which the physician prescribes.**

⚙ **What drugs are used to treat erectile dysfunction in men?**

A number of agents are used to treat erectile dysfunction in men. The most frequently used agents are the inhibitors of phosphodiesterase 5: sildenafil (Viagra), tadalafil (Cialis) and vardenafil (Levitra). Other agents occasionally used to treat erectile dysfunction are the prostaglandin E1 analogs (alprostadil [Caverject, Edex, Muse]), and yohimbe (briefly discussed above).

Many other drug and herbal products are marketed to men with a number of claims, including improved libido, increased penile size, and improved sexual endurance or performance. The safety and efficacy of such treatments remain unsubstantiated.

Phosphodiesterase Inhibitors

The phosphodiesterase inhibitors have revolutionized the treatment of erectile dysfunction. Although their legitimate use requires a prescription, they are heavily marketed directly to consumers and can be easily obtained by many on the Internet. Sildenafil (Viagra) was originally studied for its antihypertensive effects but its efficacy for that purpose was not pursued. The mechanism of action in treating erectile dysfunction is secondary to sexual stimulation, which increases the release of nitric oxide and increases the levels of cyclic guanosine monophosphate (cGMP), a smooth muscle relaxant. Sildenafil enhances the effects of nitric oxide by inhibiting phosphodiesterase 5, a substance that degrades cGMP and is found primarily in the penis. As a result, increased levels of cGMP in the corpus cavernosum enhance smooth muscle relaxation, the inflow of blood, and erection. Sildenafil has no effect in the absence of sexual stimulation. Tadalafil (Cialis) and vardenafil (Levitra) have similar pharmacology.

The phosphodiesterase inhibitors are effective in the treatment of sexual dysfunction secondary to a number of causes, including antidepressants (Nurnberg et al., 2003).

Phosphodiesterase inhibitors are contraindicated with the use of nitrates. The combination causes severe hypoten-sion and possibly a decrease in coronary perfusion, which may result in myocardial ischemia and infarction. Health care providers should be aware that a man without a history of angina who takes one of these agents for sexual impotence and develops his first angina attack should not receive any nitrate products in the emergency department. This includes nitroglycerin and nitroprusside. Concerns for ophthalmic toxicity prompted a U.S. Food and Drug Administration (FDA) warning for users of these agents in 2005.

Use of the phosphodiesterase type 5 inhibitors in women is under study, particularly for their role in improving libido with antidepressant use. However, their use in women is not currently recommended.

⚙🔲 sildenafil [sill **den** ah fill]
(Viagra)
Indications
Sildenafil is indicated for the treatment of erectile dysfunction in men.

Pharmacokinetics/Dosing
The onset of action of sildenafil is approximately 60 minutes with a duration of 2 to 4 hours. It is hepatically metabolized by cytochrome P450 3 A4, which may account for a number of potential drug interactions (see below). The typical initial dose is 50 mg PO approximately one hour before sexual activity (range 4 hours to 30 minutes before). For older clients (older than 65 years of age), clients with hepatic or renal impairment, or those receiving drugs that inhibit 3 A4 activity, an initial dose of 25 mg orally is recommended. Future doses are adjusted based on response and tolerance with a dosage range of 25 to 100 mg per dose.

Adverse Effects
The adverse effects of sildenafil include headache, nausea, facial flushing, nasal congestion, gastric distress, back pain, flu syndrome, arthralgia, allergic reaction, and cardiovascular events (e.g., angina pectoris, tachycardia, hypotension). At higher doses, this drug may cause some visual changes, including a bluish tinge in the field of vision for some men. Of most concern is the risk for nonarteritic anterior ischemic optic neuropathy (NAION) due to ischemia to the optic nerve (FDA, July 2005). Risk is highest in clients who smoke, are over 50 years of age, or have existing cardiovascular disease, diabetes mellitus, hypertension, elevated cholesterol, or existing eye complications. This concern also exists for tadalafil (Cialis) and vardenafil (Levitra). Although sildenafil is not FDA approved for administration in women, it is categorized as Pregnancy Category B.

Drug Interactions
The major contraindication to the use of sildenafil is concurrent nitrate therapy (including the use of amyl nitrate, sublingual or topical nitroglycerin, and oral nitrate derivatives like isosorbide mononitrates and dinitrates) and can result in severe hypotension. Concurrent use with other drugs that lower blood pressure (e.g., antihypertensives) may also result in additive hypotension. Drugs and foods that inhibit cytochrome P450 3 A4 activity (e.g., grapefruit juice, azole antifungals, macrolide antimicrobials, and many other drugs) may result in excessive effects and should be avoided. Clinicians should refer to current drug compendia for interactions and their management.

tadalafil [tha **da** la fil]
(Cialis)
Indications
See sildenafil.

Pharmacokinetics/Dosing
Tadalafil has an onset of action within 1 hour, but the duration of action persists up to 36 hours. Like sildenafil, it is metabolized by cytochrome P450 3 A4 and shares the same drug interaction risks.

Typical initial dosing is 10 mg orally prior to anticipated sexual activity and is not to be dosed more frequently than once daily. For older clients, those with renal or hepatic impairment, or with concurrent drugs that affect 3 A4 metabolism, initial doses of 5 mg are often recommended. Future doses are based on response and tolerance and range from 5 mg to 20 mg as needed, not to exceed one dose per day.

Adverse Effects
See sildenafil.

Drug Interactions
See sildenafil.

vardenafil [var **deh** na fil]
(Levitra)
Indications
See sildenafil.

Pharmacokinetics/Dosing
Pharmacokinetics and dosing of vardenafil are similar to tadalafil. It has a rapid onset of action but a more rapid elimination half-life of about 4 to 5 hours. It is also metabolized by 3 A4 and shares the same interaction risks as the other two agents in the class. Initial doses are 10 mg PO as needed not to exceed one dose daily, with 2.5 to 5 mg doses used for those with interacting drugs, those with hepatic impairment, or those older than 65 years of age. Future doses are titrated to a range of 2.5 to 20 mg.

Adverse Effects
Similar to sildenafil.

Drug Interactions
Similar to sildenafil. Concurrent higher doses of indinavir, itraconazole, ketoconazole or ritonavir may result in elevated vardenafil levels and the maximum dose of vardenafil recommended with these drugs is 2.5 mg.

Prostaglandin E1 Analog

alprostadil [al **pros** ta dill]
(Caverject, Edex, Muse, Prostin VR Pediatric)
The prostaglandin E1 agent alprostadil is sometimes used for clients who cannot tolerate the phosphodiesterase type 5 inhibitors (e.g., those on nitrates or other interacting drugs). Alprostadil is not considered first-line therapy for erectile dysfunction, however, because it requires intracavernous injection or urethral pellet insertion. Alprostadil is also used in neonates with certain congenital cardiac states to maintain patency of the ductus arteriosus.

Indications
Alprostadil is used in the treatment of erectile dysfunction in men. The intracavernous injection is also used as a single injection in the diagnosis of erectile dysfunction. The pediatric formulation is indicated for temporary control of patent ductus arteriosus in neonates.

Pharmacokinetics/Dosing
The onset of action of alprostadil for erectile dysfunction rapid and the duration of effect is under one hour. For erectile dysfunction, the dose is individualized and range from 1.25 to 10 mcg per dose by intracavernous injection or 125 to 250 mcg inserted as a pellet intraurethrally per dose.

Adverse Effects
Penile pain is the most common complaint with the injection and urethral pellets. Urethral burning is also noted with pellet use. Other effects include hypertension, headache, prolonged erection and penile edema.

Drug Interactions
Rarely, concurrent antihypertensives may result in additive hypotension.

✳ **What are B.Y.'s nursing management issues related to phosphodiesterase inhibitors?**

Assessment Assess B.Y. for preexisting health conditions that may preclude the use of sildenafil or make it necessary for closer monitoring of his drug regimen. Clients with cirrhosis or severe hepatic or renal function impairment receive lower initial doses of sildenafil. A history of B.Y.'s cardiovascular status is important because clients with hypertension, hypotension, cardiac dysrhythmia, angina, cardiac failure, history of stroke and myocardial infarct may be affected by the vasodilatory effects of sildenafil. Check B.Y.'s medication regimen for drugs that may cause serious drug interactions when administered concurrently, such as nitrates (for reasons previously cited) and hepatic enzyme inhibitors for cytochrome P450, such as cimetidine (Tagamet), erythromycin (E-Mycin), itraconazole (Sporanox), ketoconazole (Nizoral), mibefradil (Posicor), ritonavir (Norvir), and saquinavir (Fortovase). Both nitrates and hepatic enzyme inhibitors increase serum levels of sildenafil and necessitate lower doses of the drug. A thorough assessment of B.Y.'s cardiac status, including electrocardiogram (ECG), blood pressure, and cardiovascular risk factors and vision status is essential before the initiation of therapy. A baseline assessment of B.Y.'s underlying condition includes the frequency, firmness, and maintenance of erections; frequency of orgasm; frequency, satisfaction, and enjoyment of sexual activities; and satisfaction with the sexual relationship.

Nursing Diagnosis While B.Y. is taking sildenafil, he is at risk for the following nursing diagnoses/collaborative problems: sexual dysfunction related to ineffectiveness of drug; impaired comfort (heartburn, headache, flushing, nasal congestion); disturbed sensory perception (mild and transient blurred vision, sensitivity to light, color tinge to vision); diarrhea; risk for infection (urinary); risk for injury related to dizziness; and the potential complications of risk for myocardial infarction, dysrhythmia, sudden cardiac death, and cerebrovascular hemorrhage and other cardiovascular conditions associated with sexual activity.

Planning While B.Y. is taking sildenafil therapy, he will:
- Report satisfactory sexual performance without adverse effects of the drug.
- Effectively manage his therapeutic regimen including medication compliance and stating reportable adverse effects.
- Collaborate with health care providers for monitoring and treatment.

Implementation
Monitoring Have B.Y. maintain a diary related to the use of sildenafil and his sexual response to the drug, and any cardiovascular symptoms that may occur (transient chest pain, palpitations, throbbing headache). Monitor blood pressure and other cardiovascular risk factors during visits to the office.

Education Advise B.Y. that a delay in the response to the medication may occur when sildenafil is taken with a high-fat meal. Avoid grapefruit, grapefruit juice, and alcohol (e.g., beer, wine, liquor). Alert him to seek emergency treatment for chest pain, severe palpitations, and a sudden, sharp headache and to report vision disturbances to the prescriber. Alert him to avoid activities that require alertness until the sensory-perceptual responses to the drug are known. Increasing fluid intake to 2000 mL daily may help prevent the adverse effect of urinary tract infection.

Evaluation The expected outcome of sildenafil therapy is that B.Y. will report satisfaction with the firmness and maintenance of erections, frequency of orgasm, and enjoyment of sexual activities without experiencing vision and adverse cardiac effects of the drug. He will effectively manage his therapeutic regimen by medication compliance, maintenance of diary, stating reportable symptoms and their management, and maintaining scheduled visits to the prescriber for monitoring and treatment.

✱ How is female sexual dysfunction treated?

As with men, avoidance of drugs that contribute to dysfunction and psychosocial support are first steps in treatment. However, effective pharmacologic treatment options for sexual dysfunction for women are lacking (Modelska & Cummings, 2003). Declines in libido in both men and women are occasionally treated with low dose androgen therapy (e.g., testosterone) (see Chapter 53). Transdermal testosterone delivery systems for the treatment of female sexual dysfunction are under development and are most often considered for postmenopausal women (Alexander et al., 2004; Buster et al., 2005). The role of the phosphodiesterase type 5 inhibitors in women is not yet clear, but may offer limited benefit for select postmenopausal women (Berman, Toler, Gill, Haughie, and the Sildenafil Study Group, 2003). Many other products are directly marketed to consumers for treating sexual dysfunction, but do not have demonstrated safety and efficacy.

Summary

Drugs that affect the ANS or alter levels of consciousness often have a negative impact on sexual response. A number of legal and illegal substances are purported to enhance sexual response but have varying effects in different individuals.

Treatment of sexual dysfunction in both men and women includes ruling out drugs that impair libido or response, and providing psychosocial support. Drug therapy for men is primarily limited to the phosphodiesterase type 5 inhibitors (e.g., sildenafil [Viagra]), although prostaglandin E1 (alprostadil [Caverject, Muse]) has been used. Pharmacologic therapy for women is primarily limited to low dose testosterone.

Because drug therapy has many dimensions that affect sexuality and sexual behavior, nurses must be sensitive in their assessment of clients' needs as sexual beings and able to intervene to promote health in this area.

✱ Critical Thinking Questions

- What are some appropriate assessment questions that will elicit client responses related to diminished libido secondary to a medication?
- What would be your response if a nonnursing student at your school asked about the sexual effects of "crystal meth," cannabis, or alcohol?

Bibliography

Alexander, J.L., Kotz, K., Dennerstein, L., Kutner, S.J., Wallen, K., & Notelovitz, M. (2004). The effects of postmenopausal hormone therapies on female sexual functioning: a review of double-blind, randomized controlled trials. *Menopause, 11*(6) Supplement, 749-765.

Anderson, D.M., Keith, J., & Novak, P.D. (Eds.) (2002). *Mosby's medical, nursing, and allied health dictionary* (6th ed.). St. Louis: Mosby.

Berman, J.R., Berman, L.A., Toler, S.M., Gill, J., & Haughie, S. and the Sildenafil Study Group. (2003). Safety and efficacy of sildenafil citrate for the treatment of female sexual arousal disorder: A double-blind, placebo controlled study. *Journal of Urology, 170,* 2333-2338.

Bosker, G. (Ed.). (2004). *Primary and acute care medicine: Practice, protocols, pathways,* (2nd ed.). Atlanta: Thomson American Health Consultants.

Buster, J.E., Kingsberg, S.A., Aguirre, O., Brown, C., Breaux, J.G., Buch, A., et al. (2005). Testosterone patch for low sexual desire in surgically menopausal women: A randomized trial. *Obstetrics and Gynecology, 105,* 944-952.

Carpenito-Moyet, L.J. (2004). *Nursing diagnosis: Application to clinical practice* (10th ed.). Philadelphia: Lippincott, Williams & Wilkins.

e-LEARNING SUPPLEMENTS

Student CD-ROM
- Final Exam questions
- NCLEX® Examination review questions
- Pharmacology animations
- Printable chapter summary

Evolve Website (http://evolve.elsevier.com/mckenry)
- Content updates, including information on new drugs
- WebLinks corresponding to this chapter
- Answers to the critical thinking questions in this chapter
- *Elsevier ePharmacology Update* newsletter
- Mosby's Drug Consult Internet Edition
- Supplemental and reference information

Cleary, J.D., Chapman, S.W., & Pearson, M. (2005). Fungal infections. In M.A. Koda-Kimble, L.Y. Young, W.A. Kradian, B.J. Guglielmo, B.K. Alldredge, & R.L. Corelli (Eds.), *Applied therapeutics: The clinical use of drugs* (8th ed.). Philadelphia: Lippincott Williams & Wilkins.

Drug facts and comparisons (58th ed.). (2005). St. Louis: Facts and Comparisons.

Hardman, J.G., & Limbird, L.E. (Eds.). (2001). *Goodman & Gilman's The pharmacological basis of therapeutics* (10th ed.). New York: McGraw-Hill.

Hardman, J.L. (2005). Contraception. In M.A. Koda-Kimble, L.Y. Young, W.A. Kradian, B.J. Guglielmo, B.K. Alldredge, & R.L. Corelli (Eds.), *Applied therapeutics: The clinical use of drugs* (8th ed.). Philadelphia: Lippincott Williams & Wilkins.

Lacy, C.F., Armstrong, L.L., Goldman, M.P., & Lance, L.L. (2004). *Lexi-Comp's Drug Information Handbook* (12th ed.). Hudson, Ohio: Lexi-Comp.

Lee, M. (2002). Erectile dysfunction. In J.T. DiPiro, R.L. Talbert, G.C. Yee, G.R. Matzke, B.G. Wells & L.M. Posey (Eds.), *Pharmacotherapy: A pathophysiological approach* (5th ed.). Norwalk, CT: Appleton & Lange.

Miller, III, E.R., Pastor-Barriuso, R., Dalal, D., Riemersma, R.A., Appel, L.J., & Guallar, M.D. (2004). Meta-analysis: High-Dosage Vitamin E Supplementation May Increase All-Cause Mortality. *Annals of Internal Medicine, 142*(1), 37-46.

Modelska, K., & Cummings, S. (2003). Female sexual dysfunction in postmenopausal women: Systematic review of placebo-controlled trials. *American Journal of Obstetrics and Gynecology, 188*, 286-293.

Montague, D.K., Jarow, J., Broderick, G.A., Dmochowski, R.R., Heaton, J.P., & Lue, T.F., et al., for the American Urological Association Erectile Dysfunction Guideline Update Panel. (2004). AUA Guideline on the Pharmacologic Management of Premature Ejaculation. *Journal of Urology, 172*(1), 290-294

Mosby's drug consult (15th ed.). (2005). St. Louis: Mosby.

Nazareth, I., Boynton, P., & King, M. (2003). Problems with sexual function in people attending London general practitioners: Cross sectional study. *British Medical Journal, 327*, 423-426.

Nurnberg, H.G., Hensley, P.L., Gelenberg, A.J., Fava, M., Lauriello, J., & Paine, S. (2003). Treatment of antidepressant-associated sexual dysfunction with sildenafil: A randomized controlled trial. *Journal of the American Medical Association, 289*, 56-64.

Stoller, M.L., & Carroll, P.R. (2003). Urology. In L.M. Tierney, Jr., S.J. McPhee & M.A. Papadakis (Ed.), *Current Medical Diagnosis & Treatment*. New York: Lange Medical Books/McGraw-Hill.

Taylor, J., et al. (2004). MDMA Frequently Asked Questions. *The Vaults of Erowid*. Retrieved August 4, 2004, from http://www.erowid.org/chemicals/mdma/mdma_faq.shtml#safety2.

Thompson, J.F. (2005). Geriatric urologic disorders. In M.A. Koda-Kimble, L.Y. Young, W.A. Kradian, B.J. Guglielmo, B.K. Alldredge, & R.L. Corelli (Eds.), *Applied therapeutics: The clinical use of drugs* (8th ed.). Philadelphia: Lippincott Williams & Wilkins.

U.S. Food and Drug Administration. (July 2005). FDA Alert: Viagra (sildenafil citrate) information. Retrieved July 17, 2005, from http://www.fda.gov/cder/consumerinfo/viagra/vIAGRA.htm.

USP DI: Drug information for the health care professional (25th ed.). (2005). Greenwood Village, CO: MICROMEDEX Thomson Healthcare.

PRINCIPLES OF ANTINEOPLASTIC CHEMOTHERAPY

CHAPTER FOCUS

Progress in antineoplastic chemotherapy has helped in providing palliation and a longer life expectancy for many persons with a diagnosis of cancer. Unfortunately, however, the cure for most cancers is unknown. Many of the commonly used antineoplastic agents also have undesirable adverse effects such as fatigue, nausea, vomiting, stomatitis, and bone marrow depression. Nurses not only administer antineoplastic agents as part of their role in many health care agencies but also are primarily responsible for providing care for clients receiving these agents, for promoting comfort, and for minimizing the risk for injury associated with these agents.

LEARNING OBJECTIVES
- Identify four major developmental stages of normal and malignant cells.
- List common antineoplastic drugs and their effects on the cell cycle.
- Explain the major principles of chemotherapy.
- Describe the common toxicities of antineoplastic chemotherapy.
- Describe age-related considerations for cancer in older adults and children.
- Implement a plan of care using nursing management common to all antineoplastic drug therapy.

▲ **KEY TERMS**
cancer, p. 947
combination chemotherapy, p. 952
dose-limiting effects, p. 953
Gompertzian growth, p. 950

metastasis, p. 950
micrometastases, p. 950
myelosuppression, p. 958

Cancer refers to a group of more than 300 diseases characterized by the uncontrolled growth and spread of abnormal cells. Many people fear cancer, and it is difficult to accept that a small lump or mole that has the potential for rapid growth may lead to serious illness or death. Therefore education and early treatment are imperative to manage the care of cancer, which is second only to cardiovascular disease as a cause of death.

In the *Annual Report to the Nation on the Status of Cancer, 1975-2001* (ARNSC), a collaboration among the American Cancer Society (ACS), the Centers for Disease Control and Prevention (CDC), the National Cancer Institute (NCI), and the North American Association of Central Cancer Registries (NAACCR), it is reported that Americans' risk of getting and dying from cancer continues to decline and survival rates for many cancers continue to improve. The percentage of individuals who have survived more than 5 years after being diagnosed with cancer has increased over the past two decades.

The U.S. data find overall observed cancer incidence rates dropped 0.5% per year from 1991 to 2001, whereas death rates from all cancers combined dropped 1.1% per year from 1993 to 2001. According to the ARNSC report's authors, the new data reflect progress in prevention, early detection, and treatment; however, not all segments of the U.S. population have benefited equally from the advances (see the Cultural Considerations box below).

Cultural Considerations

Racial Differences in Cancer Statistics

The *Annual Report to the Nation on the Status of Cancer, 1975-2001* identifies wide variations in survival associated with race and ethnicity. In every racial and ethnic population, with the exception of Asian/Pacific Islander (API) women, the risk of cancer death from all cancer sites combined was higher than the risk of death for non-Hispanic white clients. Black men were at higher risk of dying of 12 cancers compared to white men, with the increased risk ranging from 9% (lung cancer) to a high of 67% (oral cavity). Black women experienced higher risks of death from 12 cancers, with the increase ranging from 7% (lung cancer) to 82% (corpus uterus and melanoma). Additionally, non-Hispanic white and API clients tended to have higher survival rates than other racial and ethnic groups except for clients with brain cancer and leukemia (American Cancer Society et al., 2004). The extent which genetics, lifestyle, or early access to care account for these discrepancies is unclear.

Death rates in the United States from all cancers combined have been decreasing since the early 1990s. Death rates decreased for 11 of the top 15 cancers in men, and 8 of the top 15 cancers in women. Lung cancer deaths rates among women leveled off for the first time between 1995 and 2001, after continuously increasing for many decades (American Cancer Society et al., 2004).

Among men, cancer incidence rates have recently declined for 7 of the top 15 cancer sites: lung, colon, oral cavity, leukemia, stomach, pancreas, and larynx. Incidence rates increased only for melanoma and cancers of the prostate, kidney, and esophagus. For men, large gains in cancer survival rates (more than 10%) were seen in cancers of the prostate, colon and kidney, and non-Hodgkin lymphoma, melanoma, and leukemia. Modest gains (5% to 10%) were found for cancers of the bladder, stomach, liver, brain, and esophagus; see Figure 55-1 (American Cancer Society et al., 2004).

For the first time, lung cancer incidence rates among women are on the decline. Incidence rates decreased for 5 additional cancers out of the top 15 in women (colon, cervix, pancreas, ovary, and oral cavity). Only breast, thyroid, bladder, and kidney cancer and melanoma rates are rising among women. For women, large gains in cancer survival rates were seen for colon, kidney, and breast cancers and non-Hodgkin lymphoma. Modest gains were found for bladder, oral cavity, stomach, brain, esophageal, and ovarian cancers and melanoma and leukemia; see Figure 55-1 (American Cancer Society et al., 2004).

Limited survival improvement was noted for the most fatal forms of cancer in adults including cancers of the lung, pancreas, and liver, which are characterized by late stage at diagnosis and relatively poor survival rates even when these cancers are diagnosed at a localized stage. There was also lit-

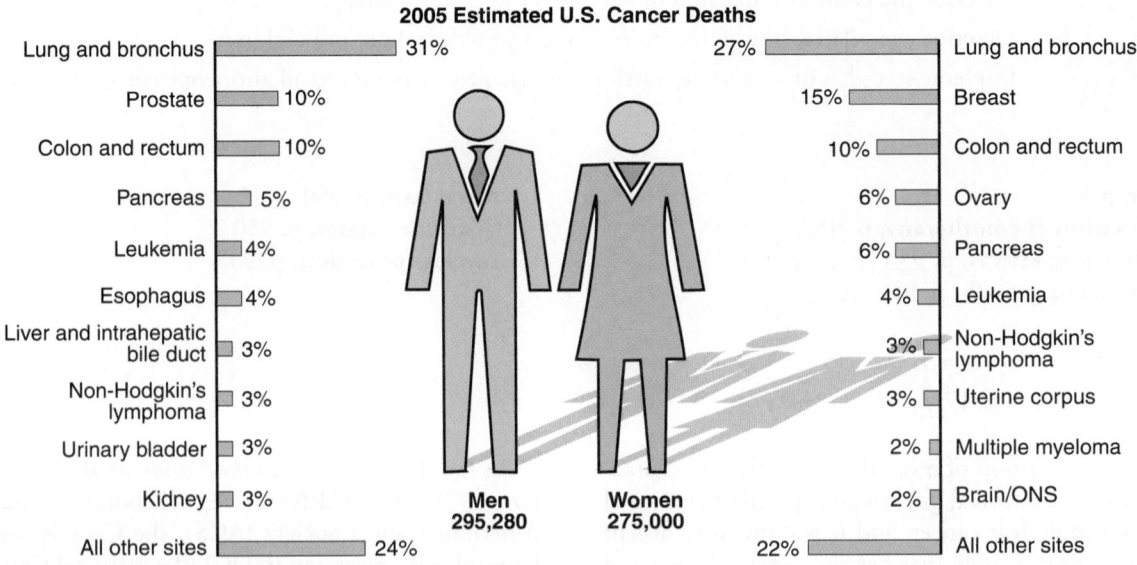

FIGURE 55-1 2005 estimated cancer deaths.

Data from American Cancer Society. (2005). Cancer Statistics 2005: A Presentation from the American Cancer Society. Retrieved September 13, 2004, from http://www.cancer.org.

Technology Link

Cancer Statistics

American Cancer Society
(http://www.cancer.org)

This site provides statistics by year, type of cancer, and other variables. It also provides the most requested graphs and figures to be used in presentations, including a power point presentation of cancer statistics for 2005.

National Center for Chronic Disease Prevention and Health Promotion, Cancer Prevention and Control (http://www.cdc.gov/cancer)

This is an online source for statistical information related to cancer. It provides an interactive version of the United States Cancer Statistics 2001 Incidence and Mortality Data and 2004/2005 Cancer Fact Sheets on various types of cancer.

National Center for Health Statistics
(http://www.cdc.gov/nchs/about/major/dvs/mortdata.htm)

This website provides a source of information about the nation's health to guide actions and policies to improve the health of individuals in the United States.

tle or no gain in several cancers that already have high survival rates, including larynx, thyroid, and uterine cancers (American Cancer Society et al., 2004). For additional information on the statistics related to various cancers, see the Technology Link box above.

Childhood cancers showed some of the largest improvements in cancer survival during the past 20 years, with an absolute survival rate increase of 20% in boys and 13% in girls. The current 5-year survival rate of over 75% confirms substantial progress made since the early 1960s, when childhood cancers were nearly always fatal (American Cancer Society et al., 2004).

In Canada, the *Canadian Cancer Statistics 2002* by the National Cancer Institute of Canada reports that incidence and mortality rates for the majority of cancer sites have stabilized or declined over the past decade. Among men, the cancer mortality rate, after reaching a peak in 1988 is declining slowly because of decreases in mortality rates for lung, colorectal, and other cancers. In contrast, the cancer incidence rate rose slightly in the early 1990s because of the sharp increase in incidence of prostate cancer, and more recently has begun to level off or decline sharply. Among women, since 1989, cancer incidence has risen slightly whereas mortality rates have declined slightly. Among women, lung cancer incidence and mortality rates continue their increase and are now almost four times as high as the rates in 1973; however, in 2002 they were still much lower than that of men. Among men, lung cancer rates leveled off in the mid-1980s and have consis-

tently declined, reflecting a drop in tobacco consumption beginning in the mid-1960s. After years of steady increases, incidence rates of prostate cancer rose, particularly from 1989 to 1993. This probably is the result of increased early detection with the Prostate Specific Antigen (PSA) test, but mortality rates have declined from the mid 1990s. Since 1993 incidence rates for breast cancer among women have stabilized, and mortality rates have declined steadily since 1990. The incidence of just two cancers among men and one among women has increased at an average rate greater than 2% annually. These were cancers of the thyroid (+2.8%) and melanoma (+2.8%) in men, and thyroid cancer (+3.9%) in women (National Cancer Institute of Canada, 2002).

Although these data indicate some progress in the early detection and treatment of cancer, note that the actual number of cases and deaths will increase because of population growth and the aging of the population in North America.

This chapter discusses the principles of antineoplastic chemotherapy and the use of chemotherapeutic drugs in the treatment of cancer.

What interventions are used to treat cancers?

A number of modalities are used in the treatment of cancer. Choices include pharmacologic interventions, radiation, and surgery. Choice of treatment depends on cancer type, stage of disease, client age, and other client factors. Surgery and radiation are often used for solid cancers or localized tumors responsive to these interventions. Drug therapy may be utilized for a number of types of disease, and are often used in combination with surgery and radiation.

Pharmacologic interventions include cytotoxic chemotherapy, hormonal interventions, targeted therapies that block specific enzyme or receptor function, antiangiogenesis agents, and the biologic response modifiers. Cytotoxic chemotherapy targets rapidly dividing cancer cells and may or may not be specific for a particular point in the dividing cell cycle. The chemotherapeutic agents are often classified according to mechanism of action (e.g., alkylating agents, antibiotics, antimetabolites, or inhibitors of mitosis). Hormonal agents are used in a number of cancers, but are most often used in cancers with receptors for estrogens or androgens. Agents that block specific receptors or enzymes, including inhibition of tyrosine kinase (imatinib [Gleevec], gefitinib [Iressa], erlotinib [Tarceva], or 26 S proteasome bortezomib [Velcade]), result in cell death. Some agents, including gefitinib, also inhibit angiogenesis (new blood vessel formation) and serve to "starve" tumor cells. Drugs with specific antibody affinity for tumor cells (e.g., rituximab [Rituxan], trastuzumab [Herceptin]) are used in certain lymphomas or breast cancers respectively. Biologic response modifiers including the interferons, are used for many cancer types, including Kaposi's sarcoma and bladder cancer. Research using RNA targeting of genes also looks promising for effective treatment in the future. RNA interference (RNAi) at specific cell sites may activate tumor suppressor genes or suppress genes known to be correlated with undesirable cell growth (oncogenes) (He et al., 2005; O'Donnell, Wentzel, Zeller, Dang, & Mendell, 2005; Song et al., 2005). Other similar targeted properties have suppressed tumors in mice (Oltersdorf et al., 2005).

A number of agents may be classified under one or more categories. For example, the aromatase inhibitors, which might be considered targeted therapy by blocking the enzyme that produces estrogen, is most often considered a hormonal agent. Many of the monoclonal antibodies have various effects including angiogenesis inhibition (bevacizumab [Avastin]), binding to CD20 or CD52 surface antigen on lymphocytes (ibritumomab tiuxetan [Zevalin], alemtuzumab [Campath]), or inhibiting cell growth via binding to epidermal growth factor (cetuximab [Erbitux]). They therefore may also rightly be considered angiogenesis inhibitors or targeted therapies depending on their actions.

To better understand the mechanisms and sites of action of the cancer chemotherapeutic agents, it is important to understand the kinetics of both normal cells and cancer cells.

✴ What are the characteristics of growth and division in cancer cells?

The interplay of genetics and environment typically predisposes to cancer. Cancer cells often display altered deoxyribonucleic acid (DNA) as a result of genetic mutation, exposure to chemical carcinogens, irradiation, viruses, or other insults. This altered DNA results in changes in growth and division patterns for cancer cells. The important distinguishing characteristics of cancer cell growth include persistent proliferation, immortality, invasive growth, and formation of metastasis.

Persistent proliferation, or unrestrained growth and division, is probably the most distinguishing characteristic of cancer cells. Normal cells contain feedback mechanisms that recognize environmental cues for adequate resources of space and nutrients. Such feedback mechanisms regulate cellular proliferation. Malignant cancer cells are typically unresponsive to these feedback mechanisms, leaving cell division and growth to continue unchecked. Cancer cells also seem to be *immortal*. Such cells do not demonstrate a typical cell life cycle, but instead undergo perpetual cell division. Alterations in telomerase (an enzyme that permits infinite cell doublings), or other factors have been suggested as explanations for this observation.

Invasive growth is also a hallmark of cancer cells. Normal cells grow and divide in an orderly fashion. Normal cells also typically remain identical in morphology, and segregated in localized tissue. In general, neoplastic cells lack the cellular differentiation of the tissues in which they originate and are unable to function like the normal cells around them. Malignant cells are disorganized, have variations in cell morphology, and often penetrate into adjacent tissue.

Cancer growth is enhanced by an increased rate of cell proliferation that lacks the normal body control system on cellular growth patterns. The growth of a cancer is usually rapid in the early stages. However, as the tumor enlarges, it nearly outgrows its blood and nutrient supply, and the growth rate pattern decreases or reaches the plateau phase

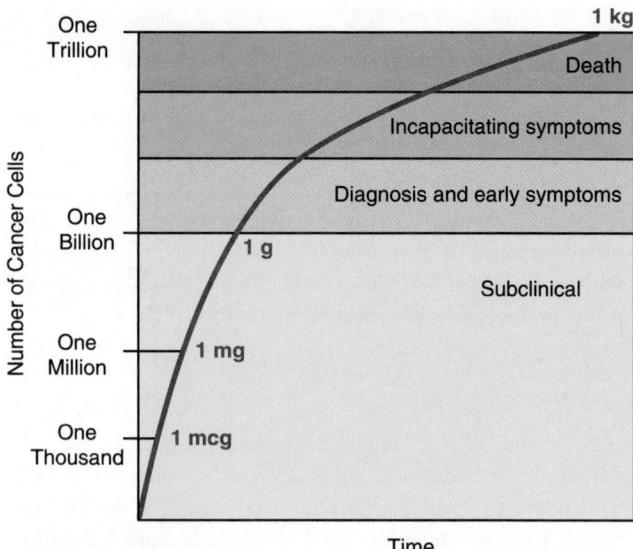

FIGURE 55-2 Cancer cell growth (Gompertzian). The size and weight of a typical tumor is in red.

for the tumor. This is referred to as **Gompertzian growth** kinetics (Figure 55-2). A cell burden of 10^9 is usually the smallest tumor burden (quantitative size) that is physically detectable (palpated). At this point the client has approximately 1 billion cancer cells, which is equal to a tumor that is approximately the size of a small grape and weighs 1 g. This is the point at which clinical symptoms usually first appear. The Papanicolaou (Pap) smear is a cytologic test capable of detecting carcinoma of the cervix and endometrium in an earlier subclinical stage. The early detection and treatment of small cancer lesions that are not detectable by visual examination has dramatically reduced mortality from cervical cancer in the United States and Canada.

Some cancer cells will *metastasize*. In normal cells, the body process of cell adhesion inhibits the movement of newly formed cells. Because of the genetic differences, cancer cells lack the cell adhesive property of normal cells, which may lead to **metastasis,** or spreading of the cancer. A cancer cell or a number of cancer cells can become dislodged from the original site. If the cells migrate via the lymphatic or vascular system, a new metastasis or cancer can form at a distant site (**micrometastases**). The potential for metastasis varies by both type of cancer and staging of cancer. Advanced cancers are more commonly associated with metastasis and make treatment much more problematic. Common sites for such metastasis include the liver, brain, and bone.

✴ How do drugs interfere with cancer cell growth?

The reproductive cycles of normal and cancer cells are essentially the same (Figure 55-3). Ribonucleic acid (RNA) and protein synthesis may occur during the presynthesis phase (G_1). The decision for cell replication or cell differentiation is also determined during this phase. The cell progresses to the synthesis phase (S), which is the replication phase; DNA doubles in preparation for cell division. DNA

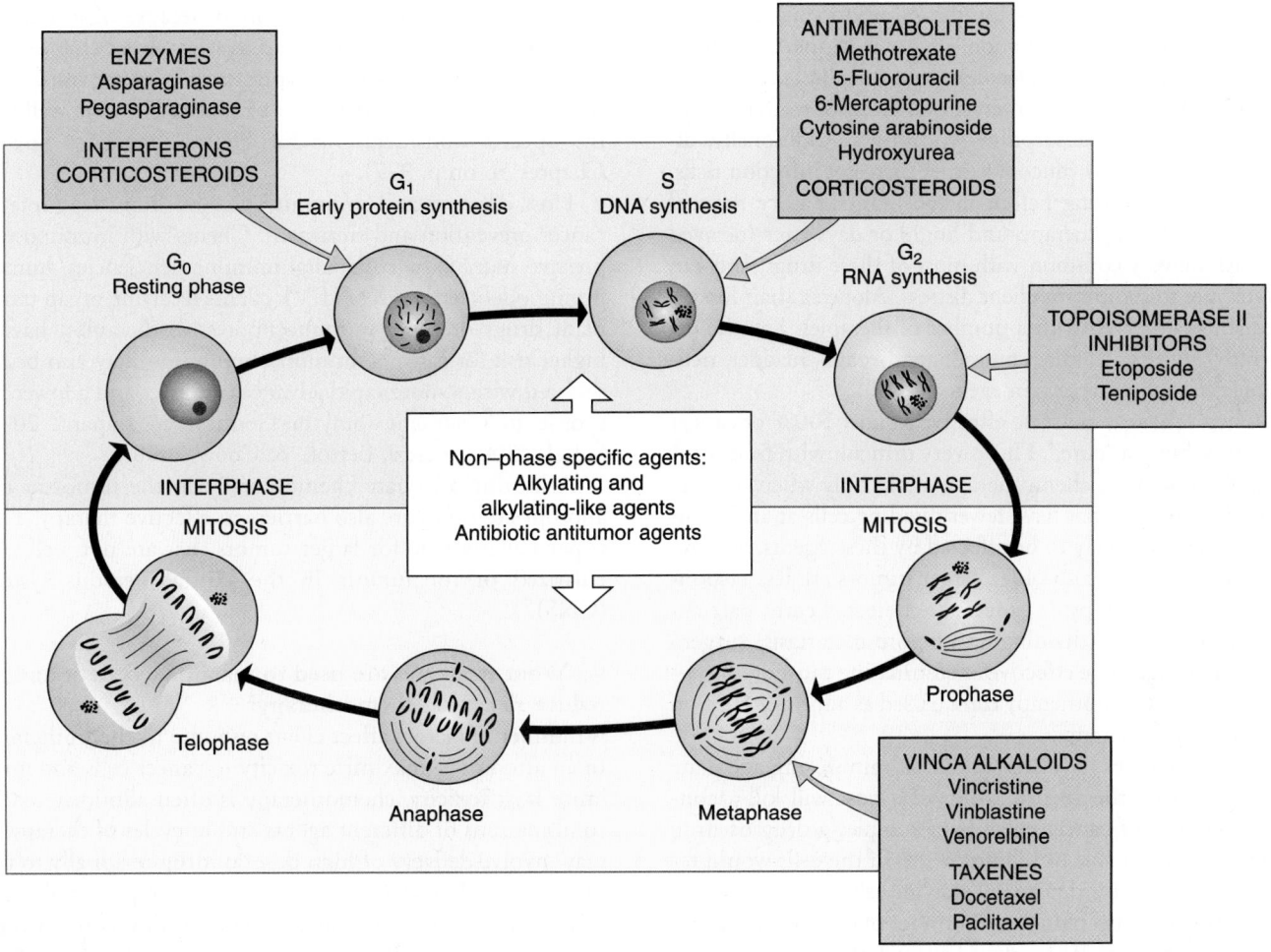

FIGURE 55-3 Phases of the cell cycle.

synthesis ceases during the postsynthesis or premitotic phase (G_2), but RNA and protein synthesis continues to prepare the cell for mitosis (M), or spindle formation. During the M phase, cells divide into two completely new cells. These two new cells may leave the cell cycle to do the following: (1) develop into differentiated cells that perform a specialized function (e.g., neuron, epithelium) and can no longer undergo cell division; or (2) become either temporarily or permanently nonproliferative (G_0 phase). Cells in the G_0 (or resting) phase may remain in this phase, reenter the cell cycle in time, or mature and die.

Cytotoxic chemotherapeutic agents have different sites of action on the dividing cell cycle. Agents that are most effective in one specific phase are referred to as cell-cycle–specific agents. Asparaginase, pegasparaginase, and interferons are specific for the G_1 phase of the cell cycle. The antimetabolites methotrexate, 5-fluorouracil, 6-mercaptopurine, cytosine arabinoside, and hydroxyurea work primarily by interfering with S-phase activity. Corticosteroids exert their action at both G_1 and S phases. The topoisomerase II inhibitors etoposide and teniposide are specific for the G_2 phase, whereas the vinca alkaloids and taxanes affect the metaphase.

Antineoplastic agents that are active against both proliferating and resting cells are called cell cycle–nonspecific agents.

Many commonly used agents are phase nonspecific in action, including the nitrogen mustards (cyclophosphamide, chlorambucil, ifosfamide), platinum agents (carboplatin, cisplatin), and most of the antitumor antibiotics (dactinomycin, daunorubicin, doxorubicin, plicamycin, valrubicin).

Hormonal and targeted therapies bind to specific receptors, affect specific enzyme function or inhibit angiogenesis. The timing of administration of most of these agents in relation to cell division is not as critical as with the cell cycle–specific cytotoxic chemotherapeutic agents.

✴ What are obstacles to successful treatment with chemotherapy?

A number of issues become problematic in the use of chemotherapy for treating cancer. Among them are drug toxicity, the need to kill 100% of cancer cells, growth fraction of tumor, absence of early detection, drug resistance and heterogeneity of tumors, host defenses, and pharmacokinetics of delivery of drug to tumor sites.

Among these hurdles, toxicity to chemotherapy is considered by many to be the most troublesome. By impacting on rapidly dividing cells, cancer chemotherapy is usually toxic to bone marrow and epithelial cells in the gastrointestinal (GI) tract. Most of these agents result in neutropenia after therapy, and many also pose risks for thrombocytopenia and suppressed erythrocyte production. As a result, there is significant risk for infection, bleeding, and anemias respectively. The GI toxicities may manifest at oral ulcers or stomatitis, diarrhea, and/or malabsorption syndromes. Additionally, altered integrity of GI mucosa further increases infection risks. Nausea and vomiting before therapy (anticipatory nausea/vomiting), during therapy, and hours or days later (delayed emesis) are very common with most of these drugs, and can contribute to significant client distress. Alopecia (hair loss) is frequently observed with a number of therapies. Specific organ toxicity (e.g., cardiac, pulmonary, hepatic, bladder, neurologic) is seen with certain agents as well.

Chemotherapy must be effective against 100% of cancer cells to achieve a "cure." This is very difficult with most cancers. Because most chemotherapy works only when cells are dividing, tumors that have fewer dividing cells at any point in time are less likely to be affected by these agents. As a result, solid tumors, and older, larger tumors are less responsive to chemotherapy. If cancers are detected early, particularly when rapidly dividing and before metastasis, surgery and radiation can be effective at eliminating most or all cancer cells, and chemotherapy can be used as adjuvant (add on or "mop up") therapy.

Animal studies have shown that administering adequate doses of chemotherapeutic drugs to a host will kill a constant fraction of cancer cells. For example, a drug or drug combination capable of killing 99.9% of the cells would reduce a 10^{10} cell burden to 10^7 cancer cells. Each course of chemotherapy may reduce the number of cancer cells; eventually, cell levels may be reduced enough that the remaining cancer cells can be controlled by the client's immune system (Figure 55-4). This reduction may produce a remission. However, if further therapies are not instituted or the immune system is inadequate, the remaining cells may grow into another detectable tumor.

Resistance to chemotherapy is common with repeated

cycles of drug therapy. This is often because of mutations that occur in the tumor, and lead to selection of chemotherapy resistant cells. Genetics appears to play an important role in the successful treatment of some cancers as well (see the Special Considerations for Pharmacogenetics box in Chapter 56 on p. 977).

Host defenses and immunity play an important role in cancer prevention and treatment. Clients with immunosuppressive states (e.g., congenital immune deficiencies, human immunodeficiency virus [HIV], clients receiving organ transplant drugs or other immunosuppressive therapies) have a higher risk for cancers. Immunosuppression may also be associated with a more rapid advance of cancer and a lower response to treatment (Smyth, Godfrey, & Trapani, 2001; Soloski, 2001; Berczi, Bertok, & Chow, 2000).

Achieving adequate chemotherapy to the tumor at the appropriate times are also barriers to effective therapy. This is particularly true for larger tumors that are not well vascularized or for tumors in the central nervous system (CNS).

✴ What strategies are used to maximize benefit and reduce risk with chemotherapy?

A number of factors affect client response to chemotherapy. In an attempt to maximize toxicity to cancer cells and minimize host toxicity, chemotherapy is often administered in combinations of different agents and in cycles of therapy. It may involve delivery of high doses of drug regionally to the tumor site. High-dose systemic chemotherapy is also used when risk can be controlled. Specific additions to therapy are used to counteract organ specific toxicity.

In the late 1960s, **combination chemotherapy** (the use of two or more anticancer drugs at the same time) was initiated to treat acute lymphoblastic leukemia and Hodgkin disease. When the complete response rates for single agents were compared with the response rates for combination drugs, the results were enlightening. The response rates for the "MOPP" treatment of advanced Hodgkin disease are a classic illustration as presented in the following table:

DRUG	COMPLETE RESPONSE RATES
M—mechlorethamine (Mustargen)	20%
O—vincristine (Oncovin)	<10%
P—procarbazine (Matulane)	<10%
P—prednisone	<5%
MOPP combination	80%

Mechlorethamine (Mustargen) is an alkylating agent that can interfere with the replication, transcription, and translation of DNA. Vincristine (Oncovin) inhibits mitosis by interfering with the mitotic spindle. Procarbazine (Matulane) is a weak monoamine oxidase (MAO) inhibitor, and its antineoplastic action is believed to occur during the S phase. It inhibits the synthesis of DNA, RNA, and protein. Prednisone has lympholytic properties and may produce an antifibrotic effect that would be useful in treating cancer

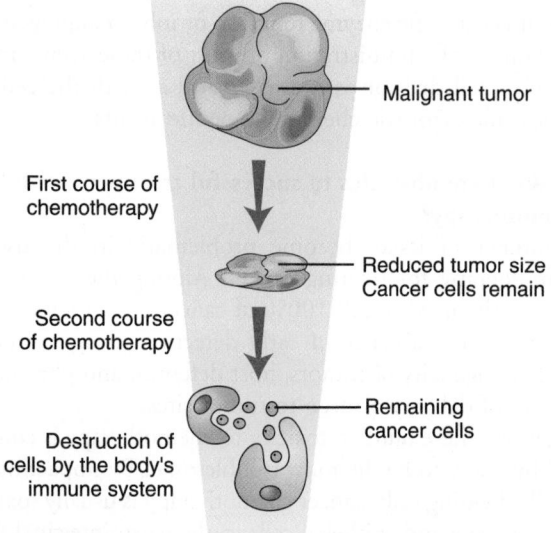

First course of chemotherapy

Second course of chemotherapy

Destruction of cells by the body's immune system

Malignant tumor

Reduced tumor size Cancer cells remain

Remaining cancer cells

FIGURE 55-4 Cancer cell response to chemotherapy.

metastases surrounded by fibrous materials. It also improves appetite and general feelings of well-being. By using drugs with different activities and toxicities, therapeutic response is improved and toxicity is balanced.

Combination therapy with multiple agents is most often used according to carefully developed protocols. These combinations offer different modes of action for superior tumor cell kill and reduced drug resistance. They may also be sequenced with agents that enhance tumor cell differentiation that are administered prior to cell cycle–specific agents. Additionally, combinations are often chosen to offset toxicity of a single agent. The toxicities may either be different, or may occur at different times during use. In the case of MOPP therapy, the dose-limiting toxicity of bone marrow suppression is a property of both mechlorethamine and procarbazine. However, the nadir (the lowest depression point for this effect) occurs approximately 10 days after the administration for mechlorethamine and 21 days after the administration of procarbazine. Thus additive myelosuppressive effects from this combination are essentially avoided. Vincristine does not have bone marrow suppression effects but does exhibit a dose-limiting neurotoxicity. **Dose-limiting effects** are adverse effects that prevent a drug from being administered in higher doses or that indicate caution in continuing to administer the drug at the current dosage. Prednisone does not demonstrate bone marrow suppression or neurotoxicity.

Protocols for combined chemotherapy are also usually administered in a specified sequence, for an established duration and dosage (many of the drugs may be administered daily for 2 to 5 days), and in cycles that may repeat every 3 to 6 weeks. Such sequencing is important to assure that drug is delivered at cell cycle–specific times, and to control for immediate and delayed toxicities. The nature of protocols, however, may be confusing and lead to a risk for medical errors. Important communication and understanding is imperative in ordering, preparing, administering, monitoring, and documenting chemotherapy use. In addition to the risks for the client receiving chemotherapy, there are potential exposure risks for personnel who work with these agents. See the Medication Safety Alert box above for occupational safety concerns with these agents.

Strategies to control or minimize client toxicity may include use of drug formulations with less toxic effect. Such an example is the administration of liposomal doxorubicin (Doxil) (e.g., liposomal preparations), in which the active drug doxorubicin is encapsulated in a phospholipid bilayer sphere and administered intravenously.

Another strategy is the addition of fluids or drugs that may preserve or affect organs that are targeted for toxicity. The kidney, bladder, heart, and bone marrow are particular targets for which strategies to reduce risk are available.

Renal Toxicity Aggressive prehydration with 1 to 2 liters of intravenous (IV) fluid is standard therapy before administration of cisplatin to prevent renal toxicity. Amifostine (Ethyol) administration can help preserve renal tissue and reduce cisplatin-induced renal toxicity as well.

Medication Safety Alert

Occupational Safety Concerns with Chemotherapy

Personnel policies regarding working with chemotherapy during pregnancy are quite varied, despite OSHA's suggestion that appropriate protective practices should reduce any potential reproductive hazards. Although OSHA recommends that employees be informed of potential risks and, if necessary, reassigned to other duties, it is not uncommon to find institutional policies that prohibit pregnant or lactating women from working with cytotoxic drugs, particularly in drug preparation. These precautionary measures are undertaken to protect the mother and developing fetus from the potential effects of drug exposure and the institution from potential liability. Another personnel issue is medical surveillance, which usually includes a preemployment health assessment, a baseline CBC, and thorough documentation of any risk factors in the health history. More extensive testing is becoming less common, for there are no data to support a cause-and-effect relationship between precautionary cytotoxic drug handling and abnormal physical or laboratory findings.

Bladder Toxicity Mesna (Mesnex) is routinely administered with ifosfamide to reduce the risk of hemorrhagic cystitis.

Cardiac Toxicity Cardiac toxicity is reported with both doxorubicin (Adriamycin) and daunorubicin (Cerubidine). Cardiotoxicity increases in clients who receive more than 550 mg/m^2 of body surface (total accumulated dose given throughout therapy). Toxicity is also greater in older adults and in children younger than 2 years of age. Because this effect is cumulative if either drug is given, the amount of one drug already received by the client must be considered when planning therapy with the other drug. Dexrazoxane (Zinecard) administered concurrently with doxorubicin can help prevent doxorubicin-induced cardiomyopathy.

Bone Marrow Toxicity Filgrastim (G-CSF, Neupogen), pegfilgrastim (Neulasta), and sargramostim (GM-CSF, Leukine) are administered to stimulate granulocytes after chemotherapy in nonmyelogenous cancers. Similarly, epoetin alfa (Epogen, Procrit) and darbepoetin alfa (Aranesp) stimulate erythrocyte production and oprelvekin (Neumega) stimulates platelet production in clients with anemia and thrombocytopenia toxicities associated with chemotherapy.

What considerations should be made when using chemotherapy in the young and old?

Older Clients Cancer increases sharply with age. Over 50% of all cases of cancer in the United States occur in persons older than 65 years of age. When compared with younger cancer victims, older adults have more concurrent illnesses, which may decrease their ability to withstand the effects of cancer or the antineoplastic therapies. Additionally, decreased pulmonary and renal function and decreased bone marrow cellularity may interfere with treatment. The possibility of reduced income and the loss of loved ones and family support need to be considered when managing regimens for older adults.

Compromises in treatment are often made because of a client's advanced age; however, data suggest that a dosage reduction of chemotherapy based on age alone is not always appropriate. A treatment approach should be based on the individual cancer and the biologic and physiologic differences noted in the older adult. More clinical trials are needed to further examine the relationship between responsiveness to cancer chemotherapy and the person's age.

Younger Clients Although cancer in children is relatively uncommon for North American children (between the ages of 1 and 14 years), it is the most common cause of death from disease. However, cancer-related mortality has been decreasing in children ages 0 to 14 steadily for more than two decades, although the rate of decrease appears to have slowed since the mid 1990s. Incidence rates have stabilized since the 1980s (National Cancer Institute, 2002). Acute leukemias are the most common cancers in children. Carcinomas, which are common in adults, are rare in children; sarcomas are much more common in children.

Because tumors grow rapidly in children, childhood cancer is generally more responsive than adult cancer to chemotherapy. Children also tend to tolerate the acute toxicity of chemotherapy better than adults. Fifty percent of children with cancer are long-term survivors or are actually cured (see the Special Considerations for Children box below).

Among the 12 major types of childhood cancers, leukemias (blood cell cancers) and brain and other CNS tumors account for over one half of the new cases. About one third of childhood cancers are leukemias; approximately 2700 children (younger than 15 years) were diagnosed with leukemia in 2001. The most common type of leukemia in children is acute lymphocytic leukemia. The most common solid tumors are brain tumors (e.g., gliomas and medulloblastomas), with other solid tumors (e.g., neuroblastomas, Wilms tumors, and rhabdomyosarcomas) being less common (National Cancer Institute, 2002).

Over the past 20 years, there has been some increase in the incidence of children diagnosed with all forms of invasive cancer; from 11.4 cases per 100,000 children in 1975 to 15.2 per 100,000 children in 1998. During this same time, however, death rates declined dramatically and sur-

vival increased for most childhood cancers. For example, the 5-year survival rates for all childhood cancers combined increased from 55.7% in 1974 to 1976 to 77.1% in 1992 to 1997. This improvement in survival rates is a result of significant advances in treatment, resulting in cure or long-term remission for a substantial proportion of children with cancer (National Cancer Institute, 2002).

✳ What are the key nursing management issues with the use of antineoplastic chemotherapy?

The role of the nurse is to ensure safe and effective administration of antineoplastic agents. This responsibility becomes more complex as a greater proportion of these therapies is administered during shorter hospital stays and within the client's home setting. Because there is such a need to identify the knowledge and skills required of the nurse when administering and monitoring antineoplastic agents, nursing organizations such as the Oncology Nursing Society and the Intravenous Nurses Society have established recommendations and guidelines for practice (Box 55-1).

Assessment Nursing care for clients receiving drug therapy with antineoplastic agents is complex and is inseparable from nursing care of the family. The client may be in any state of the disease process and may be facing impending death. In assessing the client and family, give special considerations to their coping abilities. Use an approach that is sensitive and appropriate to the individual needs of the client and family. Assess the client's degree of acceptance of chemotherapy, and be prepared to help the client deal with mixed emotions about chemotherapy. Assess also the client's and family's knowledge of the chemotherapy and their expectations for treatment.

A baseline assessment includes a complete history and physical examination, including weight, complete blood count (CBC), vital signs, blood chemistry, and renal and hepatic function studies. Evaluate the client for preexisting health conditions that may contraindicate the use of antineoplastic therapy, such as hypersensitivity to the drug, radiation therapy within the previous 4 weeks, severe bone marrow depression, breastfeeding, and pregnancy. Diagnostic procedures that are specific to the type of neoplasm and its location are performed.

Nursing Diagnosis See the Nursing Care Plan on pp. 956 and 957 for selected nursing diagnoses related to the use of antineoplastic agents. Other nursing diagnoses related to

---

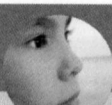 Special Considerations for Children | INCIDENCE OF CANCER IN CHILDREN

- About 130 out of 1 million children are found to have cancer each year; childhood cancer is the leading cause of death from diseases for children ages 1 to 19 years (U.S. Environmental Protection Agency [EPA], 2003). However, mostly because of improvements in treatment, childhood mortality due to cancer has decreased in recent years (EPA, 2003).

- Despite a dramatic decline in the childhood cancer mortality rate since 1971, cancer still represents the second leading cause of death among Canadian children aged 1 to 14 years (Public Health Agency of Canada, 2005).

BOX 55-1 THE NURSE'S ROLE IN ADMINISTRATION OF ANTINEOPLASTIC AGENTS

The role of the nurse is dynamic, increasing in its competencies to meet the needs of the increasing technology and the health care of society. Certainly this evolution of role is being demonstrated in the administration of antineoplastic agents and the monitoring of clients receiving them. Because these types of changes in the responsibilities of the nurse frequently come about by custom and practice rather than law, nurses must ensure that their health care agencies have in place policies and procedures to protect them and their clients. Nursing organizations often provide guidance for health care agencies by indicating their position in relation to the new responsibilities that nurses are to assume.

The Intravenous Nurses Society maintains the standard that the administration of antineoplastic agents requires a physician's order. Knowledge and technical expertise of both administration and specific interventions are required to administer these agents.

To maintain this standard the administration of antineoplastic agents should be established in organizational policy and procedure. Written consent by the client or legally authorized representative should be obtained prior to the administration of these agents. This therapy requires client education. The client must be informed of all aspects of this therapy, including physical and psychological effects, adverse effects, risks and benefits. The administration of these agents requires knowledge and understanding of the cell cycle and malignant cell growth. Prior to administration, laboratory data should be reviewed and assessed for appropriateness of prescribed therapy. The nurse's responsibilities for administering these agents include knowledge of the disease process, drug classifications, pharmacological indications, actions, side effects, adverse reactions, method of administration (e.g., intravenous push, continuous), rate of delivery, treatment goal (e.g., palliative or curative), and drug properties (e.g., vesicant, nonvesicant, and irritant).

The nurse must understand the vascular system. Preservation of venous access is crucial. To avoid serious complications of this therapy, technical expertise of cannula placement is mandatory. Selection of appropriate equipment will enhance therapy and help prevent potential complications. Cannula types should be selected based on the overall aspects of prescribed therapy and client condition. Electronic infusion devices are a consideration in specific types of antineoplastic administration. When an electronic infusion device is indicated to administer a vesicant medication, a nonpressure device is the instrument of choice. A new access site is initiated immediately prior to any peripheral vesicant administration. Access device patency is verified prior to the administration of each antineoplastic agent. Knowledge of drug calculation regarding dose and volume relative to age, height and weight or body surface area is required.

Nurses must anticipate potential complications of administering this therapy and be skilled at performing immediate interventions. As with any IV drug administration, the possibility of extravasation should be anticipated, but not expected, and its occurrence requires immediate recognition with intervention and investigation. Technical expertise in cannula placement is required.

Vesicant extravasation can lead to short-term complications, such as blistering, ulceration, infection, impaired venous access, delay in receiving prescribed infusion therapy, tissue necrosis, and eschar formation. As a result of tissue damage, the client may need surgical interventions, such as debridement, excision, amputation, and skin grafting. Additionally, long-term sequelae, including joint stiffness, neuropathy, and deformity may occur.

The nurse may note extravasation immediately following vesicant infusion with both peripheral and central vascular access devices or may not discover the problem right away. Nurses administering such solutions and medications need to understand vesicant administration and be able to recognize and manage associated complications. Box 56-5 for the actions to be taken with specific vesicants and irritants.

Knowing how best to manage this serious complication and swiftly intervening can significantly lessen the progression of tissue damage.

- Stop the infusion immediately.
- Assess the affected area for swelling, erythema, warmth, taut skin, or altered sensation like pain, numbness, or tingling. Swelling may not be an accurate assessment tool once extravasation has taken place. The absence of pain or discomfort does not rule out extravasation.
- Do not rely on the presence or absence of a blood return as a determining factor for extravasation because of possible migration of the catheter tip.
- Always rate extravasation as Grade 4, which is the highest score, on the Infusion Nursing Standards of Practice Infiltration Scale.
- Notify a physician, and obtain any specific treatment orders.
- Treat the injury according to physician's orders and manufacturer's recommendations.
- Apply moist compresses. Use cold, moist compresses for extravasation from all medications or solutions except vinca alkaloids (vincristine sulfate, vinblastine sulfate, and vinorelbine tartrate). Apply warm, moist compresses for extravasation from vinca alkaloids. Compliance with the manufacturer's recommendations regarding the use of compresses for extravasated medications is the best policy.
- Evaluate the venous access device (VAD) for possible removal.
- Evaluate the client for new VAD placement, according to the physician's orders.

The risk of extravasation increases with vein wall injury, such as through unskilled or multiple venipuncture attempts, accidental VAD dislodgment, inadequate device securement,

Continued

and excessive catheter manipulation. The following steps can help minimize its occurrence:

- Use the smallest gauge and shortest length catheter in the largest appropriate vein.
- Use long-term central VADs when possible, especially if the client will receive irritant or vesicant therapies for several weeks to months.
- Select the site carefully, and use a meticulous, skilled device insertion technique. Avoid areas of flexion found in the antecubital fossa and wrist, the dorsal veins of the hand, or the lower extremities.
- Locate each venipuncture location proximal to previous sites.
- Request that after two unsuccessful venipuncture attempts, a more experienced clinician assess the client for adequate peripheral vascular access sites and perform the venipuncture.
- Stabilize and secure catheter, allowing for frequent site inspection.
- Establish and confirm catheter patency; check for positive blood return before, during, and after medication or solution administration.
- Check dressing integrity for compromise, such as evidence of moisture or nonadherence.
- Consider the client's physical condition and mental alertness. Clients who have extremities with poor circulation, such as those with lymphedema, postsurgical treatments like mastectomy, or peripheral vascular disease or neuropathy are at greater risk for extravasation. Clients who are unable to indicate early warning signs are also at greater risk of significant injury from extravasation. This includes very young children and clients who are comatose, intubated, undergoing cardiac resuscitation, experiencing violent vomiting or coughing, and those suffering from paralysis, stroke, confusion, or impaired communication ability as a result of sedation from anesthesia or other medications.

When extravasation does occur, it's imperative to thoroughly document in the client's medical record. Documentation should include the following:

- Date and time of discovery
- Time of medication or solution administration and estimated time elapsed since onset of extravasation
- Particulars of the administration: vein location; type, gauge, and size of catheter; medication or solution type and name; sequence and dose, amount infused; route and mode of delivery (e.g., IV push, pump); client complaints of pain, stinging, or burning with administration
- Recording of all venipunctures and attempts, as vesicants may seep into the tissue surrounding previous insertion sites, enlarging the area of damage
- Clinical signs of extravasation: estimated size and extent of extravasation. Photograph the injury for the medical record
- Primary physician notified, with date, time, and orders received
- Interventions taken once discovery occurred
- Follow-up care
- Client education

The greater the nurse's knowledge of extravasation, the sooner this complication can be discovered and remedial interventions initiated. The extent of the damage may in turn be minimized, and permanent disability for the client averted.

CRITICAL THINKING QUESTIONS

- How could a nursing standard statement serve to protect the public? How would it serve to protect nurses?
- If you were the nurse manager on an oncology unit, how could you use this standard?

NURSING CARE PLAN SELECTED NURSING DIAGNOSES RELATED TO ANTINEOPLASTIC AGENTS

Nursing Diagnosis	Outcome Criteria	Nursing Interventions
Impaired oral mucous membrane related to drug-induced stomatitis, mouth ulcers, or poor oral hygiene	Client will: • Demonstrate knowledge of oral hygiene • Maintain adequate nutrition and hydration • Maintain normal oral mucosa or have decreasing inflammation and/or ulceration	• Instruct client to complete all dental work before beginning chemotherapy. • Teach optimal oral hygiene to prevent stomatitis. • Inspect oral cavity with a tongue blade and light daily and before each administration of the antineoplastic drug • Implement appropriate mouth care if inflammation is present. • Encourage soothing foods: bland foods, cool liquids, cool foods (popsicles). • Instruct client to avoid alcohol and tobacco, spicy or acidic foods, very hot or very cold foods, and abrasive foods or those difficult to chew. • Consult with prescriber if oral pain relief solution is needed. • Instruct client to report any ulcers in or around the mouth.

Nursing Diagnosis	Outcome Criteria	Nursing Interventions
Risk for infection related to bone marrow depression,	Client will: • Remain free of infection	• Instruct client in reading a thermometer. Teach client to take temperature daily in leukopenia the afternoon and report any elevation over 101° F. • Teach client to avoid being immunized with live virus vaccines, having contact with people with infections, and contact with pet excreta, including cat boxes and fish tanks. • Instruct the client to avoid antipyretics (aspirin, nonsteroidal antiinflammatory drugs [NSAIDs], acetaminophen), which may mask fever, unless specifically instructed to use such agents by the prescriber. • Instruct client to report any signs of infection, such as cough, sore throat, and burning on urination.
Risk for injury related to bone marrow depression, thrombocytopenia	Client will: • Exhibit no signs of bleeding or excessive bruising	• Avoid performing invasive procedures such as IM injections and rectal temperatures. • Inspect IV sites, skin, and mucous membranes for signs of bleeding and bruising. • Instruct client to report easy bruising, bloody urine, and bleeding from nose or gums. • Test urine, emesis, and stool for occult blood. • Instruct client to exercise care in oral hygiene and in using safety razors and nail clippers. • Teach client measures to help avoid constipation. • Encourage the use of caution to prevent falls.
Risk for diarrhea or constipation	Client will: • Maintain a normal bowel pattern • Have less constipation or diarrhea	• Assess client's normal bowel pattern as baseline. If client is constipated, increase fluid intake and fiber in diet. If client has diarrhea, decrease fiber, increase fluids, and give small feedings. • Consult with a prescriber if stool softener, laxative, or antidiarrheal is needed. • Assess client for fluid and electrolyte status. • Monitor bowel movements; record diarrhea as output. • Clean and dry the perianal area after each bowel movement. • Test stools for occult blood.
Disturbed body image related to alopecia	Client will: • Demonstrate progress toward coping with altered body image	• Allow client to express apprehensions related to alopecia. • Encourage client to obtain cap or hairpiece before treatment begins. • Reassure client that hair growth should begin 8 weeks after therapy, but the new growth may be of a different color and texture.
Deficient fluid volume related to nausea and vomiting	Client will: • Experience decreased incidence of nausea and vomiting • Regain normal fluid balance	• Administer antiemetic drugs 1-3 hr before the administration of the antineoplastic drugs; or administer antineoplastic therapy before bedtime with an antiemetic and a sedative. • Provide the client with frequent, small amounts of liquids of the client's preference (at least 3 L daily).

chemotherapy might be imbalanced nutrition: less than body requirements related to anorexia and GI distress; impaired gas exchange related to anemia or pulmonary fibrosis; disturbed sensory perception (tactile, auditory) related to neurotoxicity; impaired skin integrity related to extravasation or drug-induced skin pathology; ineffective tissue perfusion (cardiopulmonary) related to drug-induced cardiotoxicity; and ineffective coping related to the stress of antineoplastic chemotherapy.

Planning While receiving antineoplastic therapy, the client will:

- Experience the greatest malignant cell death with the least adverse effects of the drugs.
- Effectively manage the therapeutic regimen including interventions to minimize adverse effects.
- Collaborate with health care providers by reporting early symptoms of toxicities and maintaining scheduled visits for monitoring and treatment.

Implementation

Monitoring and Intervention The nurse has many responsibilities in dealing with the inevitable toxic effects of antineoplastic drugs. Many protocols for chemotherapy include criteria for holding or reducing future doses based on the degree of toxicity. One of the most common means to quantify the degree of toxicity is to use a grading scale as is established by the Cancer Therapy Evaluation Program of the National Cancer Institute (http://ctep.cancer.gov/reporting/ctc.html). This authoritative set of guidelines establishes definitions of a great number of toxicities on a grading scale from 1 (low grade toxicity) to 5 (death). Table 55-1 presents a brief example of some of the grade definitions for the more common toxicities.

Myelosuppression is an expected and significant adverse effect of most antineoplastic therapy. The extent of the hematopoietic depression depends on the nadir of the cell line and the survival of the cells. Because red blood cells (RBCs) survive approximately 120 days in the peripheral blood, clinically significant anemia is not likely to occur if the course of antineoplastic therapy is of short duration; however, it will develop slowly after several courses of therapy. On the other hand, granulocytes survive approximately 6 to 8 hours and platelets, 10 days. For this reason, granulocytopenia generally occurs before thrombocytopenia. Both of these conditions may be life-threatening, so some action must be taken to minimize the risk of adverse effects with additional chemotherapy. In the past, the dose of the causative antineoplastic agent was usually reduced. Now with the availability of colony-stimulating factors (CSFs) and interleukin-11, there are alternatives to minimizing myelosuppressive effects of antineoplastic agents (Lindley, 2005).

The risk for infection is increased because of bone marrow depression. Use strict aseptic technique during contact with the hospitalized client, who should also be protected from persons harboring harmful microorganisms. Monitor the client's temperature, and observe for signs of infection.

Antipyretics (e.g., aspirin, nonsteroidal antiinflammatory drugs [NSAIDs], and acetaminophen) are typically avoided so as not to mask fever, which may be the only indication of infection. Frequent blood counts are necessary; ensure that these lab tests are drawn and monitor results for early signs of bone marrow depression. A client with an absolute neutrophil count below 500 cells/mm³ is at high risk for infection. Clients with granulocytopenia should maintain scrupulous oral hygiene and receive topical antibiotics for abrasions and scratches. Encourage fluids and avoid indwelling catheters and other invasive procedures. Caution the client to avoid crowds and individuals with infectious diseases (e.g., colds, influenza, chickenpox, measles) and pet excreta including fish tanks. Avoid exposure to fresh fruit, vegetables, flowers, and live plants. No one in the client's household should be vaccinated with a live attenuated virus, such as oral polio or live nasal influenza vaccine. Instruct those who come into contact with the client to wash their hands before touching the client. Instruct clients to report to the health care provider any signs of infection, such as fever (greater than 100° F), chills, sweating, sore throat, cough, dyspnea, mouth ulcerations, diarrhea, flu-like symptoms, or burning on urination.

Ineffective protection occurs for clients with thrombocytopenia when platelet levels are less than 150,000 cells/mm³, with highest risk less than 50,000 cells/mm³. Avoid taking rectal temperatures and administering vaginal douches, rectal suppositories or enemas to such clients. Protective care for these clients might include the administration of stool softeners and the use of soft-bristled toothbrushes, electric razors, and the use of nail file rather than nail clippers. Avoid flossing. Avoid soft tissue injury; decrease activity to prevent falls and maintain a safe environment. Instruct menstruating clients to avoid tampon use and monitor pad count and saturation. Use oral preparations of analgesics and other medications to avoid the tissue damage resulting from IM injections; however, avoid aspirin and NSAID use because of the risk for prolonged bleeding. As noted above, also avoid acetaminophen for clients with neutropenia because it may suppress fever, which may be the only indication of infection. Venipunctures should be performed carefully by experienced personnel using strict sterile technique and pressure applied to site for 5 to 10 minutes afterward. Monitor for hypotension and tachycardia. Neurological changes may indicate intracranial bleeding. Test urine and stool for occult blood. Instruct the client to report signs that indicate decreased platelets, such as petechiae, easy bruising, hemorrhage, bleeding from the gums, epistaxis, menstrual irregularities, and blood in the stool and urine.

Anemia, a late occurring adverse effect after many courses of antineoplastic therapy, distresses clients because of weakness and fatigue, the overwhelming sustained sense of exhaustion and decreased capacity for physical and mental work that is not relieved by rest. The client demonstrates an inability to maintain usual routines and usually verbalizes an unremitting and overwhelming lack of energy and distress related to fatigue. The goal of care is that the client

TABLE 55-1 EXAMPLES OF NATIONAL CANCER INSTITUTE CRITERIA FOR ADVERSE EVENTS

	Grade 1	Grade 2	Grade 3	Grade 4	Grade 5
Hemoglobin	LLN to 10 g/dL	8-9.99 g/dL	6.5-7.99 g/dL	<6.5 g/dL	Death
Leukocytes (total WBC)	LLN to 3000 cells/mm³	2000-2999 cells/mm³	1000-1999 cells/mm³	<1000 cells/mm³	Death
Absolute neutrophil count (ANC)*	LLN to 1500 cells/mm³	1000-1499 cells/mm³	500-999 cells/mm³	<500 cells/mm³	Death
Platelets	LLN to 75,000 cells/mm³	50,000-74,999 cells/mm³	25,000-49,999 cells/mm³	<25,000 cells/mm³	Death
Fever	38°-39° C	39.1°-40° C	>40° C for 24 hr or less	>40° C for more than 24 hr	Death
Nausea	Loss of appetite, no change in eating habits	Oral intake decreased without significant weight loss, dehydration or malnutrition and/or IV fluids indicated for less than 24 hr	Inadequate oral caloric or fluid intake and/or IV fluids, enteral or parenteral nutrition indicated for 24 hr or more	Life-threatening consequences	Death
Vomiting	1 episode in 24 hr	2-5 episodes in 24 hr and/or IV fluid indicated for <24 hr	6 or more episodes in 24 hr and/or IV fluids or parenteral nutrition indicated for 24 hr or more	Life-threatening consequences	Death
Mucositis or stomatitis	Erythema of mucosa	Patchy ulceration or pseudomembranes	Confluent ulceration or pseudomembranes and/or bleeding with minor trauma	Tissue necrosis and/or significant spontaneous bleeding and/or life-threatening consequences	Death

Modified from Common Terminology for Adverse Events V3.00 (CTCAE) as published by the National Cancer Institute. Retrieved January 28, 2005, from http://ctep.cancer.gov/forms/CTCAEv3.pdf.
LLN, Lower limit of normal.
*See Box 29-2 for an example of how to calculate ANC.

participates in activities of importance to the client. Discuss the causes of fatigue and allow the client to express the effects of fatigue on his or her life and analyze the pattern of the client's fatigue. Assist the client to determine priorities and activities that may be delegated or eliminated. Plan priority tasks when the client's energy is high and teach ways to conserve energy, such as resting before energy-consuming tasks and stopping before fatigue occurs; distribute these tasks throughout the week. If further support is required, refer to community services for home maintenance and Meals on Wheels.

Nausea and vomiting that accompany the use of antineoplastic drugs can be relieved by the following: (1) administering an antiemetic drug 1 to 3 hours before administration of the antineoplastic drugs, or (2) administering the antineoplastic drug at night with an antiemetic and a hypnotic, so that the client sleeps all night and experiences less nausea. Delayed nausea and vomiting may occur 1 to 4 days after antineoplastic chemotherapy and requires antiemetics scheduled for that period. Additional antiemetics may be prescribed for breakthrough nausea. Refer to Chapter 40 for a discussion of various antiemetic agents and their role in preventing and treating chemotherapy induced nausea and vomiting. Chapter 56 describes the emetic potential of various chemotherapeutic agents.

Speeding the passage of food through the stomach sometimes solves the problem of nausea, vomiting, and feelings of fullness. Small quantities of carbohydrates eaten at frequent intervals help to achieve this effect. Clients should not drink liquids at mealtime but instead should take them at frequent intervals throughout the day and up to 30 to 60 minutes before eating. Because hot foods have been reported to contribute to nausea, foods should be served at room temperature or cooler. Resting for 1 to 2 hours after eating is advised, because activity can slow the digestive process. Some clients lose their appetite or complain of a bitter or metallic taste in the mouth. Their desire for red meat or other protein foods may be reduced, because these foods are most commonly perceived as bitter tasting. Because protein is essential for good nutrition (greater than 1 g/kg of body weight), alternative sources for red meat should be pursued. Cold cooked turkey, fish, eggs, and dairy products may be suitable substitutes. The biggest meal of the day should be planned for the time the client is usually hungriest, even if that time is early morning or midnight. The client is instructed to report anorexia, taste changes, and weight loss. Weigh the client to monitor nutritional status.

Impaired oral mucous membranes following antineoplastic therapy may be xerostomia (dryness of the mouth), stomatitis (an inflammatory condition of the mouth), or mouth ulcers. In the last two instances, the client reports a burning sensation before tissue changes, and a sensitivity to heat, cold and salty and spicy foods. The goal is to provide nutritional intake with minimum discomfort. Small, frequent servings of foods that are cold or at room temperature, bland, and nonirritating are best tolerated by the client. See dietary advice above. Remove dentures to prevent further irritation. Good oral hygiene is important to maintain proper nutritional intake and decrease the possibility that oral infections will become systemic. Avoid the use of commercial mouthwash products containing alcohol, lemon/glycerin swabs, or hydrogen peroxide combinations to minimize irritation. Use sugar-free gum or sugar-free candies to stimulate salivation. Monitor the client's oral cavity at least every 24 hours, gently using a tongue blade and flashlight. Some antineoplastic agents are titrated on the severity of mouth ulceration. An antifungal or antiviral medication may be prescribed to minimize further tissue injury.

The client's body image may be disturbed as a result of *alopecia*. This adverse effect is extremely distressing to women, even when they have been prepared for it, have cosmetic aids available, and are aware that it is reversible. Clients, even those who experience only thinning of the hair, need assurance that the hair will begin to grow back in approximately 3 to 5 months after the last antineoplastic treatment, although it may have a different texture or color. Because the hair may be more fragile, the client should avoid permanents, hair coloring, curling irons, or electric rollers until the regrowth is long enough to have had two haircuts. Clients who are purchasing a wig are advised to do so before therapy begins when their energy levels are still high. Treatment with hormones may necessitate support for the client in the event of effects such as masculinization in a female client, feminization in a male client or cushingoid symptoms. These clients need assistance in coping with body image problems.

As an adverse effect of antineoplastic drugs, *diarrhea* results from the death of rapidly dividing cells of the bowel mucosa. Assess the client's bowel status (number of stools, amount, and consistency), hydration, and electrolyte levels, and record diarrhea as output. Encourage the intake of clear fluids between meals and if the diarrhea is severe, a liquid diet may be necessary; IV therapy may be needed to replace lost fluids if diarrhea is severe enough. Because of the client's frequent defecation, give special attention to skin care in the perianal area; warm sitz baths promote comfort. Modification of the diet will prevent or decrease diarrhea. Instruct the client to avoid foods that may cause gas and cramping, such as cabbage, beans, and highly spiced foods or irritating foods, such as alcohol. Foods that decrease tone of the lower esophageal sphincter, including coffee, wine, and chocolate, may also contribute to nausea or gastric distress. Hot, spicy foods should be avoided because they increase peristalsis, which reduces nutrient absorption and may cause diarrhea. Reducing high-fiber foods in the diet (e.g., raw fruits and vegetables, popcorn, bran, and whole grain cereals and bread) may help to control diarrhea. A low-residue, high-protein, high-calorie diet is recommended. Foods that are high in potassium (to replace the potassium lost through diarrhea) and that usually do not worsen diarrhea include bananas, apricot or pear nectar, red meat, saltwater fish, boiled or mashed potatoes, and orange juice. An antidiarrheal medication may be prescribed to reduce the frequency and volume of stools.

Constipation may also be a problem with some clients. This may be an early symptom of CNS toxicity or impaired intestinal motility from drug therapy (e.g., opioid analgesics), or it may result from eating mostly soft and liquid foods. High-fiber foods and prune juice have a laxative effect; 1 or 2 tablespoons of bran may be added to cooked cereals, casseroles, and homemade baked goods. Encourage the client to drink plenty of fluids, preferably 8 to 10 glasses daily. A cup of hot water in the morning usually stimulates bowel activity. The prescriber may order a laxative or stool softener as needed. Avoid enemas, because they may injure intestinal mucosa and increase the risk for bleeding in clients with thrombocytopenia.

Pain commonly occurs in clients receiving antineoplastic drugs. The treatment of pain associated with cancer, especially chronic pain, requires careful assessment of the client, consideration of appropriate nursing interventions, and skillful application of pharmacologic agents. Nonpharmacologic techniques for pain relief (e.g., relaxation therapy, guided imagery, aromatherapy, and diversional activities) may assist the client. Chronic pain may progress in a cycle to anxiety or depression, insomnia, fatigue, and increased pain. Figure 14-1 lists the factors that modify pain threshold. See Chapter 14 for the treatment of chronic pain.

The kidneys are at risk for injury because of the *nephrotoxicity* of some antineoplastic drugs. There may be direct damage to the glomerulus and nephron and/or precipitation of metabolites. Purines are released through cell destruction, including cancer cells, and converted to uric acid. The possibility of renal failure may result from the precipitation of uric acid crystals in the kidneys. Monitor the client's intake and output, serum uric acid, blood urea nitrogen (BUN), serum creatinine, creatinine clearance, and serum electrolytes. Alert the oncologist if the BUN is greater than 22 mg/dL and/or the serum creatinine is greater than 2 mg/dL. Allopurinol may be prescribed to prevent the accumulation of uric acid in the kidneys from high cell kill. (Note that allopurinol itself is renally eliminated and may require a dosage adjustment. Refer to Chapter 34 for further discussion of allopurinol.) Fluid intake should be 3 L daily to minimize renal damage. Cold, clear liquids, such as tea, unsweetened apple juice or other juices, and soft drinks or carbonated beverages such as ginger ale may be well tolerated. Freezing a favorite beverage into ice cubes or popsicles is also recommended. Instruct the client to report anorexia, fatigue, reddish or dark urine or lumbar discomfort. Acute tubular necrosis is also possible with some agents (e.g., cisplatin), and the risk is reduced with aggressive hydration before and during chemotherapy infusion.

When chemotherapy agents undergo metabolism, they may damage the metabolic processes in the liver resulting in *hepatotoxicity*. Clients with a history of previous liver disease are at higher risk for its occurrence. Monitor the client for impaired liver function studies (serum transaminases, alkaline phosphatase, and bilirubin levels), and anorexia, nausea, vomiting, fatigue, jaundice, ascites and upper right quadrant abdominal pain. The oncologist will determine whether the abnormal liver function studies are because of tumor involvement of the liver or drug toxicity. If the hepatic dysfunction is because of chemotherapy, it may be withheld until the liver function studies are normal or an alternative (nonhepatotoxic) chemotherapy may be considered. Inform the client about signs and symptoms of liver failure and advise the client to avoid alcohol-containing beverages.

Cardiotoxicity is an expected toxic effect of daunorubicin, doxorubicin, and related anthracycline cytotoxic agents, usually occurring 24 hours to 4 to 5 weeks after drug administration. Prevention of cardiomyopathy is achieved primarily by limiting the total cumulative dose; however, this dose may vary by individual or clinically. It may be necessary to exceed the dose limit to achieve a positive therapeutic outcome. Maintain documentation of the client's cumulative dose. A chemoprotectant drug, dexrazoxane, may be administered to reduce the incidence and severity of cardiomyopathy. Many cardiac monitoring methods are too nonspecific or measure changes that come late in the clinical course. Current state-of-the-art monitoring is done using radionuclide ventriculography (RNV) and endomyocardial biopsy (Lindley, 2005). However, be alert for signs and symptoms of heart failure (HF), such as dyspnea, crackles at the lung bases, wheezing and rhonchi, ascites, bilateral pitting edema of the lower extremities, chest pain, and electrocardiogram (ECG) changes.

Pulmonary toxicity may occur with a number of antineoplastic agents. The most frequent pathology is interstitial pneumonitis followed by pulmonary fibrosis. Monitor the client for dyspnea, nonproductive cough, and fine bibasilar crackles progressing to coarse crackles. Arterial blood gases generally indicate hypoxia, with worsening results of pulmonary function studies. If pulmonary toxicity occurs, responsible agents are discontinued and symptomatic support, such as oxygen, is provided. In many cases, the pulmonary toxicity is irreversible and progressive. Have the client report dyspnea and chest pain immediately. Assist the client to decrease symptoms of dyspnea through positioning, pursed-lipped breathing, and the appropriate use of oxygen. Opioid analgesics may be used to decrease the fear of air hunger.

Hemorrhagic cystitis is an adverse effect of ifosfamide and cyclophosphamide; it is characterized by tissue edema and ulceration of the bladder wall followed by sloughing of mucosal epithelial cells, necrosis of smooth muscle fibers and arteries, and culminating in focal hemorrhage (Lindley, 2005). Monitor the client for episodes of painful urination, frequency, and hematuria. With cyclophosphamide, forced hydration prevents hemorrhagic cystitis by flushing the toxic metabolites out of the bladder so that they have minimal contact with the bladder wall. Advise the client to drink 6 to 8 glasses of fluid daily and to empty bladder every 4 to 6 hours. With ifosfamide, which is more urotoxic, the uroprotective agent mesna (Mesnex) is administered to prevent bladder toxicity. Forced hydration is contraindicated with administration of mesna because it will increase the elimination of mesna from the bladder and decrease its protective properties. Once hemorrhagic cystitis occurs, the responsible agent is discontinued. Alert the client to report urinary frequency and burning, and blood in the urine to the oncologist.

Neurotoxicities are dose and schedule related; their prevalence is higher in subsequent doses rather than initial courses of therapy. Older clients are more susceptible than younger ones. These toxicities may be caused by the direct action of the drug on nervous tissue, metabolic encephalopathy, or intracranial bleeding related to decreased capacity for clotting. The toxicity may evidence as encephalopathy (headache, lethargy, confusion, disorientation, drowsiness, stupor, coma, hallucination, severe depression), cerebellar neuropathy (ataxia, limb incoordination, dysarthria, nystagmus), peripheral neuropathy (paresthesias, depressed deep tendon reflexes, motor weakness, foot drop), cranial neuropathy (ptosis, ophthalmoplegia, trigeminal neuralgia, facial palsy, depressed corneal reflexes, vocal cord paralysis, hearing loss), or autonomic neuropathy (constipation, urinary retention, impotence, orthostatic hypotension). Instruct the client about reportable symptoms for the particular antineoplastic agent. Clients with suspected neurotoxicity should be examined by a neurologist and, if warranted, their antineoplastic therapy should be discontinued.

Antineoplastic therapy has an effect on oogenesis and spermatogenesis (*gonadotoxicity*) and so affects fertility. In women, drug-induced injury to ova and follicular elements reduces hormone secretion and may also cause ovarian fibrosis and follicular destruction. If the toxicity is severe and/or prolonged, permanent ovarian failure may occur secondary to depletion of ova and follicles. Clients may experience signs and symptoms of menopause. However, the risk of pregnancy still exists early in therapy, and the client should be encouraged to use contraception because these agents are teratogenic. Loss of reproductive capacity is a major toxicity of chemotherapy for men. However, in contrast to women who are born with their full complement of ova, spermatogenesis is a continuous cycle of regeneration, so many men experience a return to pretreatment sexual function and spermatogenesis is nearly always regained (Lindley, 2005). Men may also bank sperm before therapy is initiated; women may also bank oocytes or embryos, but the technology is expensive and not always successful.

Universal nursing interventions may include physical activity to help prevent further deterioration resulting from inactivity. Deep breathing, turning the client, and skin care are some of the actions that reduce complications. In addition to physical and pharmacologic interventions, the client may need psychosocial, intellectual, and spiritual support. The holistic approach of carefully assessing the client's current needs and anticipating and planning for continued care is important in the care of many illnesses but is crucial for a client with a neoplasm. A variety of home-care programs are available. Additionally, hospice programs have been developed throughout the United States and Canada to help provide the supportive and palliative services necessary for clients with life-threatening illness and their families. The American Cancer Society and the Canadian Cancer Society offer a variety of resources for the client with cancer and his or her family.

Systemic antineoplastic agents are most commonly administered by the IV route, either as a bolus (less than 15 minutes), a short infusion (greater than 15 minutes to several hours) or a continuous infusion (lasting 24 hours to several weeks) (Davis & Lindley, 2005). Many of the antineoplastic agents are vesicants (drugs that cause severe necrosis if they leak from the blood vessels into the tissues). Extreme care is taken to prevent extravasation. Avoid placing a peripheral IV site over joints, bony prominences, tendons, neurovascular bundles or the antecubital fossa. Assess the patency of the IV line and observe the IV site every 30 minutes for swelling, leakage, inflammation, burning, or pain. If extravasation occurs, follow the institutional policy for antidote and local care to the site. This usually involves stopping the administration of the drug, leaving the needle in place, gently aspirating residual drug or blood in the tubing, giving the antidote per protocol, applying heat or cold depending on the agent, and elevating the limb for 24 hours. Currently, most clients receive chemotherapy through a central venous catheter to reduce the risk associated with recurrent administration of these agents. Monitor the central line every hour; assess for swelling, leakage, inflammation, and pain.

Remember that anticancer drugs are potent drugs that are mutagenic and carcinogenic in animals and may be carcinogenic in humans. Nurses and pharmacists who prepare antineoplastic drugs should institute safety measures such as using proper technique; wearing gloves, mask, and protective clothing; and preparing the solutions in a vertical laminar flow, biologically safe hood whenever possible. All unused solutions and associated vials, needles, syringes, tubing, gloves, and other equipment and materials used to clean up spills should be processed as hazardous materials; the waste should be properly incinerated. Wear gloves when in contact with all body substances; dispose of them according to institutional policies. For further detail, check the policies related to hazardous waste for the health agency. See Home Spill Kit procedure within the Community and Home Health Considerations box on p. 963 for a sample procedure.

Education In addition to the client teaching discussed previously in relation to specific interventions, discuss with the client all aspects of drug administration before initiating chemotherapy, including any adverse symptoms that could occur during or after the injection and throughout therapy. Printed materials should be used to reinforce the verbal instructions. An assessment should reveal the expectations of the client and the family; they may need assistance in accepting a realistic view of the results of chemotherapy. Expectations of total cure may be unrealistic and should not be reinforced, whereas expectations of remission are often appropriate. One of the most important nursing interventions is providing emotional support to a client who is receiving physically and psychologically distressing therapy. The long periods of therapy, with frequent interruptions and sporadic progress, may compound the client's anxieties.

Caution any client receiving cancer chemotherapy not to take any over-the-counter (OTC) medication before checking with the oncologist. Many OTC preparations contain aspirin, alcohol, or other substances that could interfere with the antineoplastic agents, increase the risk for toxicity, or mask symptoms of infection such as fever. See the Nursing Care Plan on p. 957 for specific areas of client instruction related to selected nursing diagnoses.

Clients commonly return home after a few hours of receiving chemotherapy, or they receive chemotherapeutic agents at home administered by home health nurses. Home chemotherapy allows clients to be active participants in administering their own therapy, and it provides them the opportunity to regain the sense of control they may believe they lost to their cancer. In addition to learning the technical skills to maintain these therapies at home, clients and their families need to practice the safe handling of cytotoxic drugs and body waste. The client and family need to know that these chemotherapeutic agents are eliminated from the body through vomitus, urine, and feces. Direct contact with these waste products can expose a person to the drug during chemotherapy and for up to 48 hours after the drug has been discontinued. If precautions are not taken, the effects of these drugs may accumulate in the body of the caregiver who is routinely exposed over a period of time. For example, this may occur if the caregiver regularly changes and washes the bed linens of a client who is receiving these agents and is wetting the bed. Soiled bedpans and containers contaminated with vomitus need to be handled with gloves, emptied directly into the toilet, and washed with de-

---

Community and Home Health Considerations

Handling Chemotherapy Drugs Safely at Home

Handling Chemotherapy Drugs

- Wash your hands before and after handling chemotherapy drugs.
- Wear disposable latex gloves when handling any type of IV or IM drug. If the chemotherapy drugs are taken by mouth, be careful not to touch the drugs with your hands. Some oral medications may require that gloves are worn while administering.
- After each use, discard gloves in specially marked chemotherapy waste bags.
- Place a plastic-backed, absorbent pad under the work area when changing pump cassettes, tubing, or when handling chemotherapy medications.
- Check IV connections regularly to ensure that they are secure.
- Place all supplies for giving or preparing chemotherapy drugs in specially marked chemotherapy waste bags.
- Seal the waste bags securely using rubber bands or zip-lock tops. Return these bags to the hospital for proper disposal.

Storing Chemotherapy Drugs

- Keep chemotherapy drugs out of the reach of children and pets.
- If the drugs need refrigeration, separate them from other food by placing them in a container, or using a clean crisper bin for only these medications. Do not freeze chemotherapeutic drugs.

Disposal of Body Waste While Taking Hazardous Drugs

- You may use the toilet as usual. Wash your hands with soap and water after using the toilet.

- All caregivers must wear gloves when handling your blood, urine, stool, or emesis while you receive chemotherapy medications. After using any devises for bodily waste, thoroughly wash your hands and the devises with soap and water.
- Your caregivers at home will wear gloves while caring for you for 2 days after you receive chemotherapy.

Chemotherapy Drug Spills

- Clean small drug spills (less than a teaspoon) immediately. Wear two pairs of latex gloves, and wipe up the spill with a gauze pad. Wash the area three times with soap and water.
- For larger spills, follow the instructions on the spill kit. Clean the spill area three times, and dispose of the gauze pads in specially marked chemotherapy waste bags. Immediately remove any clothing soiled with the chemotherapy medications.
- Do not touch the soiled areas of bed linens or clothing with your bare hands. Wear latex gloves and immediately place the soiled articles in the washing machine. Wash these items separately from other laundry in hot water. If you are unable to wash them immediately, place them in a sealed bag until they can be washed. Throw this bag away in the specially marked chemotherapy waste bag with the gloves.

Skin Care for Accidental Splashes

- Chemotherapy drugs spilled on your skin will may cause irritation. Wash the area thoroughly with soap and water; then dry the area. Watch the area for the next 7 days, if redness or skin irritation occurs, contact your physician.
- If the chemotherapy drugs get into your eyes, flush them with tap water for at least 5 minutes and then contact your physician immediately.

---

tergent and water without splashing (with the rinse water discarded directly into the toilet); the toilet is then flushed three times. Hands are always washed after removing the gloves. Skin surfaces contaminated by body wastes or antineoplastic drugs should be washed with detergent and water for 5 minutes. If an eye is involved, it is washed with water for 5 minutes, and the oncologist is notified.

A spill of antineoplastic agents may occur in the home if IV fluid bags are defective or if IV lines leak or get disconnected accidentally. Although the client is usually provided a commercially available spill kit that fulfills the requirement of the Occupational Safety and Health Administration (OSHA), reinforce instruction on the spill kit procedure to prevent undue exposure of the client and caregivers (see the Community and Home Health Considerations box above).

Evaluation Evaluation of drug effects is an integral nursing function in antineoplastic chemotherapy. Often no dosage schedule for antineoplastic agents is universally ther-

apeutic, and the dosage is changed according to the client's response and the toxic effects of the drug. Thus it is essential that the nurse evaluates progress toward therapy goals and communicates both drug toxicity and client response. In evaluating toxic effects, the nurse should be vigilant for early signs, because the progression of toxic effects may have severe and irreversible consequences.

Summary

Cancer is a major health issue today. Although many people fear cancer, more people are cured of cancer than ever before. Education for cancer prevention, early detection, and early treatment are essential to combating this disease. It is essential that nurses have knowledge of cell kinetics so they can understand the mechanisms and sites of action of the cancer chemotherapeutic agents and appropriately manage the nursing care of clients receiving such agents.

✳ Critical Thinking Questions

• Mr. Matsui, a 56-year-old client with Hodgkin's disease, is questioning his therapy with four different drugs. He is concerned about the cost of his health care and wants to know why so many drugs are needed to treat him. What will be your response to Mr. Matsui?

• Mrs. Hayes has been receiving a course of antineoplastic therapy. Her laboratory results show a platelet count of 46,000 cells/mm³ and an absolute granulocyte count of 86 cells/mm³. What assessments should be obtained? How should she be monitored on a daily basis? What safety precautions will you take with her care?

Bibliography

American Cancer Society (ACS), Centers for Disease Control and Prevention (CDC), the National Cancer Institute (NCI), & North American Association of Central Cancer Registries (NAACCR). (2004). *Annual report to the nation on the status of cancer, 1975-2001.* Retrieved September 13, 2004, from http://www.cancer.gov/statistics.

Anderson, D.M., Keith, J., & Novak, P.D. (Eds.) (2002). *Mosby's medical, nursing, and allied health dictionary* (6th ed.). St. Louis: Mosby.

Balmer, C.M., & Valley, A.W. (2002). Cancer treatment and chemotherapy. In J.T. DiPiro, R.L. Talbert, G.C. Yee, G.R. Matzke, B.G. Wells & L.M. Posey (Eds.), *Pharmacotherapy: A pathophysiological approach* (5th ed.). Norwalk, CT: Appleton & Lange.

Berczi, I., Bertok, L., & Chow, D.A. (2000). Natural immunity and neuroimmune host defense. *Annals of the New York Academy of Science, 917,* 248.

Bosker, G. (Ed.). (2004). *Primary and acute care medicine: Practice, protocols, pathways,* (2nd ed.). Atlanta: Thomson American Health Consultants.

Common Terminology for Adverse Events V3.00 (CTCAE) as published by the National Cancer Institute. Retrieved January 28, 2005, from http://ctep.cancer.gov/forms/CTCAEv3.pdf.

Davis, L., & Lindley, C. (2005). Neoplastic disorders and their treatment: General principles. In M.A. Koda-Kimble, L.Y. Young, W.A. Kradjan, B.J. Guglielmo, B.K. Alldredge, & R.L. Corelli (Eds.), *Applied therapeutics: The clinical use of drugs* (8th ed.). Philadelphia: Lippincott Williams & Wilkins.

Drug facts and comparisons (58th ed.). (2005). St. Louis: Facts and Comparisons.

Hardman, J.G., & Limbird, L.E. (Eds.). (2001). *Goodman & Gilman's The pharmacological basis of therapeutics* (10th ed.). New York: McGraw-Hill.

He, L., Thomson, J.M., Hemann, M.T., Hernando-Mongue, E., Mu, D., Goodson, S., et al. (2005). A microRNA polycistron as a potential human oncogene. *Nature, 435,* 828-833.

Lacy, C.F., Armstrong, L.L., Goldman, M.P., & Lance, L.L. (2004). *Lexi-Comp's Drug Information Handbook* (12th ed.). Hudson, Ohio: Lexi-Comp.

Lindley, C. (2005). Adverse effects of chemotherapy. In M.A. Koda-Kimble, L.Y. Young, W.A. Kradjan, B.J. Guglielmo, B.K. Alldredge, & R.L. Corelli (Eds.), *Applied therapeutics: The clinical use of drugs* (8th ed.). Philadelphia: Lippincott Williams & Wilkins.

Mosby's Drug Consult (15th ed.). (2005). St. Louis: Mosby.

National Cancer Institute. (2002). Surveillance, Epidemiology, and End Results Program, 1975-2001, Bethesda, Maryland: Division of Cancer Control and Population Sciences, National Cancer Institute.

National Cancer Institute of Canada. (2004). *Canadian cancer statistics 2002.* Retrieved September 13, 2004, from http://www.hc-sc.gc.ca/pphb-dgspsp/publicat/ccs-scc02/pdf/stats2002 _e.pdf.

O'Donnell, K.A., Wentzel, E.A., Zeller, K.I., Dang, C.V., Mendell, J.T. (2005). c-Myc-regulated microRNAs modulate E2F1 expression. *Nature, 435,* 839-843.

Oltersdorf, T., Elmore, S.W., Shoemaker, A.R., Armstrong, R.C., Augeri, D.J., Belli, B.A., et al. (2005). An inhibitor of Bcl-2 family proteins induces regression of solid tumors. *Nature, 435,* 677-681.

Public Health Agency of Canada. (2005). Measuring up: A health surveillance update on Canadian children and youth. Retrieved July 29, 2005, from http://www.phac-aspc.gc.ca/publicat/meas-haut/mu_h_e.html.

Rugo, H.S. (2003). Cancer. In L.M. Tierney, Jr., S.J. McPhee & Papadakis, M.A. (Eds.), *Current Medical Diagnosis & Treatment.* New York: Lange Medical Books/McGraw-Hill.

Smyth, M.J., Godfrey, D.I., & Trapani, J.A. (2001). A fresh look at tumor immunosurveillance and immunotherapy. *Natural Immunology, 2,* 293.

Soloski, M.J. (2001). Recognition of tumor cells by the innate immune system. *Current Opinion in Immunology, 13,* 154.

Song, E., Zhu, P., Lee, S.K., Chowdhury, D., Kussman, S., Dykxhoorn, D.M., et al. (2005). Antibody-mediated in vivo delivery of small interfering RNAs via cell-surface receptors, *Nature Biotechnology, 23,* 709-717.

U.S. Environmental Protection Agency. (2003). Childhood cancer. Retrieved July 29, 2005, from http://yosemite.epa.gov/ochp/ochpweb.nsf/content/childhood_cancer.htm.

USP DI: *Drug information for the health care professional* (25th ed.). (2005). Greenwood Village, CO: MICROMEDEX Thomson Healthcare.

 *e-*LEARNING SUPPLEMENTS

Student CD-ROM
• Final Exam questions
• NCLEX® Examination review questions
• Pharmacology animations
• Printable chapter summary

Evolve Website (http://evolve.elsevier.com/mckenry)
• Case study on principles of antineoplastic chemotherapy
• Interactive concept map on cancer

• Content updates, including information on new drugs
• WebLinks corresponding to this chapter
• Answers to the critical thinking questions in this chapter
• *Elsevier ePharmacology Update* newsletter
• Mosby's Drug Consult Internet Edition
• Supplemental and reference information

ANTINEOPLASTIC CHEMOTHERAPY AGENTS

CHAPTER FOCUS

The efficacy of antineoplastic agents as both primary and adjunctive treatment for cancer has greatly increased the use of this therapy. The high level of toxicity associated with many of these agents requires that the nurse possess specialized knowledge and skills when administering them and monitoring the client who is receiving them.

<table>
<tr><td>

LEARNING OBJECTIVES

</td><td>

- Classify antineoplastic agents based on their major mechanism of action.
- List the common adverse effects of antineoplastic drugs.
- Describe the use of "leucovorin rescue" with methotrexate treatments.
- Explain precautions in the preparation and administration of antineoplastic drugs.
- Implement nursing management of clients receiving therapy with various antineoplastic agents.

</td></tr>
</table>

▲ KEY TERMS

alkylating agents, p. 966
**antibiotic antitumor
  agents,** p. 966
antimetabolites, p. 966
immunomodulators,
  p. 988
leucovorin rescue, p. 973

mitotic inhibitors,
  p. 966
nadir, p. 971
topoisomerase
  inhibitors, p. 966

ꙮ KEY DRUGS

anastrozole, p. 987
cyclophosphamide, p. 968
doxorubicin, p. 973
interferon alfa-2a, p. 988
leucovorin, p. 973

methotrexate, p. 973
paclitaxel, p. 975
tamoxifen, p. 986
topotecan, p. 977
vincristine, p. 975

Antineoplastic agents do not directly kill tumor cells; they act by interfering with cell reproduction or replication at some point in the cell cycle. (See Chapter 55 for a discussion on cell cycle.) For cells to proliferate, deoxyribonucleic acid (DNA) must be replicated once every cell cycle. DNA is the genetic substance in body cells that transfers information to produce ribonucleic acid (RNA), which is needed to produce enzymes and synthesize protein (Figure 56-1). Enzymes determine the structure, biochemical activity, growth rate, and functions of the cell.

ꙮ How are the antineoplastic agents classified?

The antineoplastic agents used to treat cancer include cytotoxic chemotherapy, hormonal interventions, targeted therapies that block specific enzyme or receptor function, antiangiogenesis agents, and the biologic response modifiers. The cytotoxic drugs are directly toxic to cells and include the alkylating and alkylating-like agents, antimetabolites, antibiotic antitumor agents, mitotic inhibitors, and topoisomerase inhibitors. Many of these groupings for cytotoxic agents are further subdivided by action or chemical structure, or may

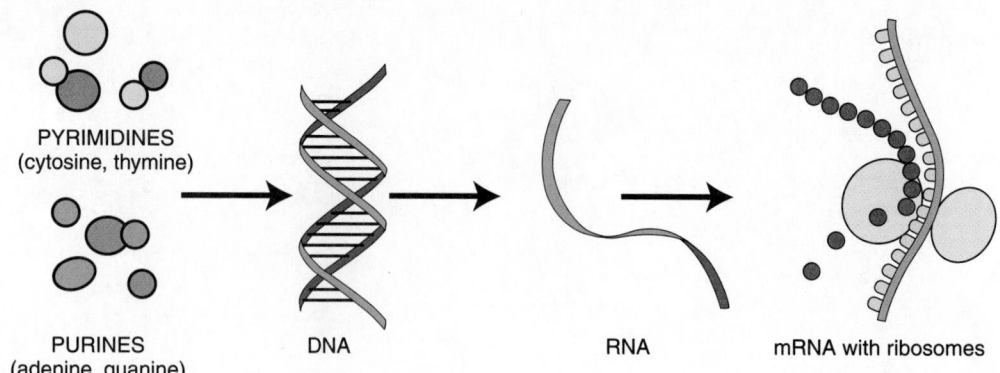

PYRIMIDINES (cytosine, thymine)

PURINES (adenine, guanine)

DNA

RNA

mRNA with ribosomes

FIGURE 56-1 Protein synthesis.

have overlapping classifications. Agents that modify normal biologic responses (often immune based), and those with hormonal action are also used to treat cancer and are discussed later in the chapter. Drugs that inhibit development of blood vessels (angiogenesis inhibitors) are currently being evaluated in the treatment of some types of cancer as well.

✳ What are the major actions of the cytotoxic drugs?

Alkylating agents are drugs that substitute an alkyl chemical structure for a hydrogen atom in DNA. This results in a cross-linking of each strand of DNA, thus preventing cell division. Alkylator-like drugs are chemically different agents that are believed to have an action similar to the alkylating agents.

The formation of the nucleic acids, DNA and ultimately RNA, requires pyrimidines and purines (nitrogen compounds) as the basic building block materials. **Antimetabolites** have a structure similar to a necessary building block for the formation of DNA. Antimetabolites are accepted by the cell as the necessary ingredient for cell growth but, because they are impostors, they interfere with the normal production of DNA.

Antibiotic antitumor agents interfere with DNA functioning by blocking the transcription of new DNA or RNA. They also delay or inhibit mitosis. The term *antibiotic,* used in this sense as an antineoplastic, is not to be confused with its more widespread use in describing antibacterial drugs.

The **mitotic inhibitors,** vinblastine, and vincristine, are plant alkaloids that block cell division in metaphase. Vinorelbine (Navelbine) is a semisynthetic vinca alkaloid that also has antitumor activity in metaphase. The mitotic inhibitors probably have other major sites of action, because these agents differ from each other pharmacologically and in therapeutic application. Vinblastine has been used in the treatment of various lymphomas and in carcinoma of the breast and testes, and vincristine is often used to treat acute leukemias and Hodgkin's disease. Vinorelbine is indicated for nonsmall-cell lung cancer.

The **topoisomerase inhibitors** (topotecan, irinotecan, etoposide, teniposide) interfere with the enzyme involved in repairing breaks in DNA and ultimately maintaining DNA helix flexibility. They are used for various cancer types depending on the particular agent.

❊ Evidence-Based Practice

Cancer Chemotherapy Research

Cancer chemotherapy research is a priority area of study in the United States and Canada. Many new drugs are being studied with the hope of overcoming resistance and improving the treatment and survival of clients with cancer (Shah et al, 2004). The use of targeted drug therapy, angiogenesis inhibitors, and biologic response modifiers has evolved over the past decade. The role of genetics, and the use of agents that are customized to the genetic profile of the client and/or the tumor may hold the greatest hope in advances in therapy over the next decade. (See Special Considerations for Pharmacogenetics box on p. 977.) The reader is encouraged to monitor professional literature for information on the release of new drugs for the treatment of cancer and for other related research. Box 56-1 lists the classifications for investigational drugs.

✳ How are the combination and dosage of drugs and sequencing of use determined?

As reviewed in Chapter 55, careful combinations and sequencing of chemotherapy can improve client response and offset toxicity. The health care professional should be aware that clinical trials are constantly being conducted to optimize drug combinations and treatment regimens for cancer. Current indications may not always be listed in the package insert of the drug or in the *Physician's Desk Reference,* but the *USP DI: Drug Information for the Health Professional* often lists unapproved indications (see the Evidence-Based Practice box above). Investigational agents not yet approved for use by the U.S. Food and Drug Administration (FDA) must be administered under strict investigational protocols (Box 56-1).

A number of collaboratives exist to identify optimal clinical trials and combination therapy. One such group is the Eastern Cooperative Oncology Group (ECOG), which was established in 1955 as a network of physicians, health care professionals, and researchers to evaluate and document the safety and efficacy of cancer chemotherapeutic and radiation protocols (http://ecog.dfci.harvard.edu/). ECOG serves as a clear-

BOX 56-1 INVESTIGATIONAL DRUG CLASSIFICATIONS

Investigational drugs are agents that have not been released for marketing by the FDA. Although responsibility for regulating drugs rests with the FDA, the National Cancer Institute (NCI) is the largest developer of antineoplastic agents in the United States. The NCI has established stringent regulations to monitor the receipt, use, and disposal of investigational drugs. It also requires that investigators report adverse effects on an established time schedule. For example, anaphylactic reactions to an investigational drug must be reported by phoning a specific branch office that is available on a 24-hour basis. This call must be followed up with a written report within 10 working days.

Investigational drugs are studied in three phases as outlined below:

	DRUG GROUP	PURPOSE
Phase I	A	To determine maximum tolerated dosage
		To detect toxicities associated with various dosage schedules
		To determine pharmacokinetics and optimum dosing schedule
Phase II	B	To identify antineoplastic activity in specific cancers affecting humans
		To determine client's response to various drug dosages and schedules
Phase III	C	New agent now compared with previously marketed drugs to ascertain effectiveness, effect on quality of life, mortality, and morbidity

Some clients elect to participate in clinical trials involving investigational drugs when available standard therapies fail or are inappropriate. The nurse should be familiar with such agents, their likely effects, and protocols for their use when caring for clients taking investigational agents.

TABLE 56-1 EASTERN COOPERATIVE ONCOLOGY GROUP (ECOG) PERFORMANCE STATUS

These scales and criteria are used by physicians and researchers to assess disease progression and its effect on the daily living activities of the client and to determine appropriate treatment and prognosis.

Grade	ECOG Performance Status
0	Fully active, able to carry on all predisease performance without restriction
1	Restricted in physically strenuous activity but ambulatory and able to carry out work of a light or sedentary nature, e.g., light house work, office work
2	Ambulatory and capable of all self-care but unable to carry out any work activities. Up and about more than 50% of waking hours
3	Capable of only limited self-care, confined to bed or chair more than 50% of waking hours
4	Completely disabled. Cannot carry on any self-care. Totally confined to bed or chair

From Oken, M.M., Creech, R.H., Tormey, D.C., Horton, J., Davis, T.E., & McFadden, E.T., et al. (1982). Toxicity and response criteria of the Eastern Cooperative Oncology Group. *American Journal of Clinical Oncology, 5,* 649-655.

inghouse for protocol development, registration, and evaluation. ECOG has also established standardized ratings for client performance status, which assist clinicians in determining the likely tolerability of chemotherapy regimens (Table 56-1). Another excellent site to review current protocols and combinations is via the National Cancer Institute (http://www.cancer.gov/clinicaltrials). Because dosage of each drug varies widely based on indication, concurrent drugs, protocol, sequence, and other factors, the clinician is referred to protocols or other drug information sources for dosing information. Box 56-2 presents an example of a chemotherapy protocol.

Each of the classifications of cytotoxic drugs, the alkylating agents, antimetabolites, antibiotic antitumor agents, mitotic inhibitors, and topoisomerase inhibitors, vary regarding mechanism of action and cell cycle–specificity.

⚙ How do the alkylating agents work?

Alkylating drugs are often used as anticancer agents and are believed to be the first class of medications applied clinically in the modern era of antineoplastic drug therapy. Various groups of alkylating agents are available, including the nitrogen mustards and nitrosoureas. Drugs that work similar to alkylating agents include the platinum drugs. These drugs work to form a strong covalent bond with DNA or RNA. A number of these agents form a cross-link with a bond at two locations. By binding to DNA or RNA, miscoding of information and/or DNA replication is inhibited. This binding results in cell death.

The binding of alkylating agents occurs throughout the cell cycle rendering these agents cell cycle phase nonspecific, although cells undergoing division may be more prone to damage. Compared to cell cycle–specific agents that require prolonged levels to achieve damage (e.g., only damage cells in the specific cycle when administered), these non-cell cycle–specific agents are effective as a single one-time dose. Mutations are able to survive in the presence of alkylating agents, as with other chemotherapeutic agents; this activity is fairly common so these agents are rarely used alone.

Alkylating agents are toxic to rapidly dividing cells and almost all the agents are associated with significant neu-

BOX 56-2 EXAMPLE OF CHEMOTHERAPY PROTOCOL

BRITISH COLUMBIA CANCER AGENCY (BCCA) PROTOCOL SUMMARY FOR ADJUVANT THERAPY FOR BREAST CANCER USING DOXORUBICIN AND CYCLOPHOSPHAMIDE FOLLOWED BY PACLITAXEL (TAXOL)

- Protocol Code: BRAJACT
- Tumor Group: Breast

ELIGIBILITY

- Women with one or more axillary lymph node metastasis(es), or node negative but with high risk of recurrence (see Cancer Management Guidelines for categories of risk [http://www.bccancer.bc.ca/HPI/CancerManagementGuidelines/Breast/Management/AdjuvantSystemicTherapy.htm])
- A "Class II Drug Registration Form" must be submitted at the time of initiation of treatment. For other indications, an "Individual use of Benefit Drug List Medication for an Undesignated Indication" form must be approved.

EXCLUSIONS

- Pregnancy
- Severe cardiovascular disease with left ventricle ejection fraction (LVEF) less than 55%

TESTS

- Baseline: CBC and differential, platelets, bilirubin, AST (AST and bilirubin should be measured prior to first cycle of AC [anthracycline] and first cycle of paclitaxel)
- Before each treatment: CBC and differential, platelets
- If clinically indicated: creatinine; multiple gated acquisition (MUGA) scan or echocardiogram, bilirubin, AST

PREMEDICATIONS

- For the four cycles of doxorubicin and cyclophosphamide: Antiemetic protocol for High/Moderate emetogenic chemotherapy (see protocol SCNAUSEA)
- For the four cycles of paclitaxel: **Paclitaxel must not be started unless the following drugs have been given:**
  - 45 minutes prior to paclitaxel give dexamethasone 20 mg IV in 50 mL NS over 15 minutes
  - 30 minutes prior to paclitaxel give diphenhydramine 50 mg IV and ranitidine 50 mg IV in 50 mL over 20 minutes (compatible up to 3 hours when mixed in bag)
- Additional antiemetics are not usually required

TREATMENT

- 4 consecutive cycles of doxorubicin and cyclophosphamide

DRUG	DOSE	BCCA ADMINISTRATION GUIDELINE
doxorubicin	60 mg/m²	IV push
cyclophosphamide	600 mg/m²	IV in 100-250* mL NS over 20-60 min

Repeat every 21 days × 4 cycles.

*Use 250 mL for dose ≥1000 mg

From Chia, S. (2005). BCCA protocol summary for adjuvant therapy for breast cancer using doxorubicin and cyclophosphamide followed by paclitaxel (Taxol). Retrieved September 23, 2005, from http://www.bccancer.bc.ca/HPI/ChemotherapyProtocols/Breast/BRAJACT.htm.
ANC, Absolute neutrophil count (see Box 29-2).

tropenia, thrombocytopenia, and anemias. The alkylating agents vary widely in their ability to induce nausea and vomiting, with higher doses of most drugs resulting in significant nausea and vomiting. Table 56-2 compares the alkylating and related drugs and their major toxicities. An example from each class is presented below:

Nitrogen Mustard

A number of nitrogen mustard products are available and include cyclophosphamide, chlorambucil, ifosfamide, melphalan, and methchloramine. Cyclophosphamide, considered the prototype nitrogen mustard, is presented here. Table 56-2 presents each of these drugs briefly.

cyclophosphamide [sye kloe **foss** fa mide] **(Cytoxan, Procytox✦)**
Cyclophosphamide is a cell cycle–nonspecific agent that cross-links DNA and RNA strands and also inhibits protein synthesis.

Indications
Cyclophosphamide is indicated for acute and chronic leukemias, carcinomas of the ovary and breast, neuroblastomas, retinoblastomas, Hodgkin's and non-Hodgkin's lymphomas, multiple myeloma, and mycosis fungoides. It is also used as an immunosuppressant for a number of conditions, including prevention of organ transplant rejection, severe autoimmune states (e.g., rheumatoid arthritis, lupus) nephritic syndrome, and idiopathic thrombocytic purpura (ITP).

Pharmacokinetics
Cyclophosphamide is well absorbed orally and has limited crossing of the blood-brain barrier. It undergoes hepatic metabolism to active and inactive metabolites, has a half-life between 3 and 12 hours, and is excreted primarily by the kidneys. Dosage varies based on indication, concurrent therapy, and protocol.

Adverse Effects
Bone marrow suppression is noted with all alkylating agents. Other adverse effects of cyclophosphamide include anorexia, nausea, vomiting, diarrhea, abdominal pain, flushing of the face, headache, increased sweating, swollen lips, rash, alopecia, darkening of the skin and nails, gonadal suppression, missed menstrual periods, leukopenia, anemia, and thrombocytopenia. With high-dose therapies or long-term treatment, there may be car-

BOX 56-2 EXAMPLE OF CHEMOTHERAPY PROTOCOL—*cont'd*

- 4 consecutive cycles of paclitaxel to start **21 days after** final cycle of doxorubicin and cyclophosphamide

DRUG	DOSE	BCCA ADMINISTRATION GUIDELINE
paclitaxel	175 mg/m²	IV in 500 mL NS over 3 hr (use non-PVC, in line filter)

Repeat cycle every 21 days × 4 cycles.

DOSE MODIFICATIONS

1. **Hematologic (for Day 1 counts)**

For cycles of doxorubicin and cyclophosphamide only:

ANC (× 10⁹/L)		PLATELETS (× 10⁹/L)	DOSE (BOTH DRUGS)
≥1.5	and	>90	100%
1.0-1.49	or	70-90	75%
<1.0	or	<70	Delay

For cycles of paclitaxel only:

ANC (× 10⁹/L)		PLATELETS (× 10⁹/L)	DOSE (PACLITAXEL)
≥1.5	and	>90	175 mg/m²
1.0-1.49	or	70-90	150 mg/m²
<1.0	or	<70	Delay

2. **Renal dysfunction:** Dose modification may be required for cyclophosphamide. Refer to BCCA Cancer Drug Manual.

3. **Hepatic dysfunction:** Dose modification required for doxorubicin and for paclitaxel. Refer to BCCA Cancer Drug Manual.

4. **Arthralgia and/or myalgia:** If arthralgia and/or myalgia from paclitaxel of grade 2 (moderate) or higher is not relieved by adequate doses of nonsteroidal antiinflammatory drugs (NSAIDS) or acetaminophen with codeine (Tylenol #3) a limited number of studies report a possible therapeutic benefit from the following:
   - Prednisone 10 mg PO twice daily × 5 days starting 24 hours post paclitaxel
   - Gabapentin 300 mg PO on day prior to paclitaxel, 300 mg PO twice daily on treatment day and then 300 mg PO three times daily × 7 to 10 days

5. **Neuropathy:** Dose modification or discontinuation for paclitaxel may be required. Refer to BCCA Cancer Drug Manual.

PRECAUTIONS

1. **Neutropenia:** Fever or other evidence of infection must be assessed promptly and treated aggressively.

2. **Extravasation:** Doxorubicin and paclitaxel causes pain and tissue necrosis if extravasated. Refer to BCCA Extravasation Guidelines.

3. **Cardiac Toxicity:** Doxorubicin is cardiotoxic and must be used with caution, if at all, in clients with severe hypertension or cardiac dysfunction. Cardiac assessment recommended if lifelong dose of 450 mg/m² to be exceeded. Refer to BCCA Cancer Drug Manual.

4. **Hypersensitivity:** Reactions are common with Paclitaxel. Refer to BCCA Hypersensitivity Guidelines.

---

diotoxicity, hemorrhagic cystitis, hyperuricemia, nephrotoxicity, pneumonitis, or interstitial pulmonary fibrosis, and a condition that resembles the syndrome of inappropriate antidiuretic hormone (SIADH), with symptoms of confusion, agitation, increased weakness, and dizziness.

Platinum Agent

Although the exact mechanism of action of cisplatin, carboplatin, and oxaliplatin is unknown, they are believed to be cell cycle–nonspecific agents with an action similar to the alkylating agents. They each cross-link DNA, thus interfering with its function. Cisplatin is presented here in greater depth. Table 56-2 briefly outlines each agent.

cisplatin [**sis** pla tin]
(Platinol)

Indications

Cisplatin is used to treat a number of cancers including bladder, ovarian, head and neck, breast, lung, gastric, cervical, testicular, esophageal, and small-cell lung cancer. It is also used in the treatment of Hodgkin's and non-Hodgkin's lymphomas, neuroblastoma, sarcomas, myelomas, mesothelioma, melanoma, and osteosarcoma.

Pharmacokinetics

The IV form of cisplatin does not significantly cross the blood-brain barrier; its half-life is biphasic. It is metabolized to inactive metabolites that are renally excreted after 5 days, although platinum has been detected in body tissues for 4 months or longer.

Adverse Effects

The adverse effects of cisplatin include anorexia, severe nausea and vomiting, bone marrow suppression, nephrotoxicity, neurotoxicity (peripheral neuropathies), ototoxicity, anaphylaxis, and extravasation. Rare adverse effects include optic neuritis (blurred vision) and SIADH secretion.

Nursing Management

The nursing management for cisplatin is as for other antineoplastic agents, is generally described in Chapter 55, with the following additions. Because ototoxicity may occur with cisplatin, test hearing status before the initial dose and each subsequent dose. Ringing in the ears and difficulty in hearing high frequencies may indicate ototoxicity. Hearing loss is cumulative and may be unilateral. Discontinue the administration of cisplatin at the first indication of pe-

TABLE 56-2 CYTOTOXIC ANTINEOPLASTIC MEDICATIONS: ALKYLATING AND ALKYLATING TYPE AGENTS

Drug	Route	Major Toxicity		
		Bone Marrow Suppression	**Emetogenic Potential***	**Other Toxicities**
ALKYLATING AGENT				
Nitrogen Mustard				
chlorambucil (Leukeran)	PO	X	NE	
cyclophosphamide (Cytoxan)	PO, IV	X	M-H-VH	hemorrhagic cystitis
ifosfamide/mesna (Ifex/Mesnex)	IV	X	M	psychiatric/cognitive dysfunction hemorrhagic cystitis (mesna reduces risk)
melphalan (Alkeran)	PO, IV	X	L-VH	
methchlorethamine (Mustargen)	IV, topical	X	VH	
Other				
busulfan (Myleran)	PO	X	NE	pulmonary toxicity
dacarbazine (DTIC-Dome)	IV	X	VH	
procarbazine (Matulane)	PO	X	H	
temozolomide (Temodar)	PO	X	M	
thiotepa (TESPA, Thioplex)	IV, IT, Local	X	L	
ALKYLATING-LIKE AGENT				
Nitrosurea				
carmustine (BiCNU, Gliadel)	IV, surgical implant	X	H-VH	
lomustine (CeeNU)	PO	X	VH	
streptozocin (Zanosar)	IV		VH	renal toxicity
Platinum				
carboplatin (Paraplatin)	IV	X	H	CNS, peripheral neuropathy, ototoxicity
cisplatin (Platinol-AQ)	IV	X	H-VH	renal toxicity
oxaliplatin (Eloxatin)	IV	X	M-H	neuropathy
Other				
altretamine (Hexalen)	PO	X	M	

VH, Very high (frequency greater than 90%); *H*, high (frequency 60% to 90%); *M*, moderate (frequency 30% to 60%); *L*, low (frequency 10% to 30%); *NE*, not emetogenic (frequency less than 10%); *IT*, intrathecal.
*Emetogenic potential varies with dose and concurrent drug therapy.

ripheral neuropathy, because it may be irreversible. Symptoms to watch for are a loss of taste and numbness or tingling in the fingers, toes, or face. Perform regular neurologic examinations.

Do not use aluminum needles or other equipment containing aluminum. Cisplatin is incompatible with aluminum; the interaction causes a black precipitate and a loss of potency.

Nitrosourea

Nitrosoureas are highly lipophilic agents that easily cross the blood-brain barrier. They differ from other alkylating agents, but are often considered to act in a similar manner. In general, these agents are very useful for the treatment of primary brain tumors.

lomustine [loe **mus** teen]
(CeeNU)
Indications
Lomustine is used to treat primary brain tumors and Hodgkin's lymphomas. It is also indicated for non-Hodgkin's lymphoma, melanoma, lung cancer, renal carcinoma, and colon cancer.
Pharmacokinetics
It is well absorbed orally, has a half-life of approximately 90 minutes (the half-life of active metabolites is 16 to 48 hours), and is metabolized in the liver and excreted primarily by the kidneys.
Adverse Effects
The adverse effects of lomustine include anorexia, nausea, vomiting, bone marrow suppression (leukopenia, thrombocytopenia, anemia), neurotoxicity, nephrotoxicity and, rarely, hepatotoxicity, pulmonary infiltrates, and/or fibrosis. Drug toxicity is cumulative; thus

drug dosage is adjusted regularly on the basis of the **nadir** (the lowest point) blood count from the previous dose administered. Because of the seriousness of this effect, blood counts are closely monitored.

Other Alkylating or Alkylating-Like Agents

Additional alkylating agents include busulfan, dacarbazine, procarbazine temozolomide, and thiotepa. Alkylating-like agents include carmustine, streptozocin, and altretamine. Dacarbazine, procarbazine, and altretamine are presented here. Table 56-2 briefly outlines each agent.

dacarbazine [da **kar** ba zeen]
(DTIC-Dome, DTIC✦)
Dacarbazine is a cell cycle–nonspecific agent that inhibits DNA and RNA synthesis and appears to be more active in the late G_2 phase of the cell cycle.

Indications
Dacarbazine is indicated for the treatment of malignant melanoma and Hodgkin's disease. It is also used in the treatment of soft tissue sarcomas, islet cell carcinoma, neuroblastoma, thyroid cancer.

Pharmacokinetics
The onset of action after intravenous (IV) dosing is 18 to 24 hours. It is extensively metabolized with active metabolites.

Adverse Effects
The adverse effects of dacarbazine include flu-like syndrome, anorexia, nausea, vomiting, and diarrhea.

procarbazine [proe **kar** ba zeen]
(Matulane, Natulan✦)
Procarbazine is an alkylating agent and a weak MAO inhibitor that appears to have its greatest impact on the S phase of cell division and is believed to inhibit DNA, RNA, and protein synthesis.

Indications
Procarbazine is prescribed for the treatment of Hodgkin's disease.

Pharmacokinetics
Procarbazine is well absorbed after oral administration and easily crosses the blood-brain barrier. It is highly metabolized and primarily eliminated in the urine.

Adverse Effects
Adverse effects include bone marrow suppression, pneumonitis, nausea, vomiting, weakness, drowsiness, myalgia, muscle twitching, insomnia, nightmares, and nervousness.

altretamine [al **tre** ta meen]
(Hexalen)
Altretamine has an unknown mechanism of action, but chemically it resembles the alkylating agents

Indications
Altretamine is a cytotoxic agent for the palliative treatment of persistent or recurrent ovarian cancer. Clinically, it is effective for ovarian tumors that are resistant to the previously marketed alkylating agents.

Pharmacokinetics
Altretamine is well absorbed orally with high concentrations delivered to the liver and kidney. It is excreted in the urine as active metabolites.

Adverse Effects
The adverse effects of altretamine include nausea and vomiting, neurotoxicity, myelosuppression, and central nervous system (CNS) changes (ataxia, dizziness, mood alterations). Avoid the most significant drug interactions, which include cimetidine (increases the half-life of altretamine) and monoamine oxidase (MAO) inhibitors (results in severe hypotension).

❇ How are antimetabolites effective in treating cancer?
The antimetabolites mimic naturally occurring substances in cells and thereby interfere with enzyme function or DNA synthesis. Antimetabolites are classified as purine analogs, pyrimidine analogs or antagonists of folic acid. Purine and pyrimidine are naturally occurring building blocks of nucleic acids. The purine and pyrimidine analogs are similar enough to disrupt DNA or RNA synthesis. The most commonly used folic acid antagonist is methotrexate, which interferes with the enzyme that converts folic acid to its active form. When high-dose methotrexate is used, a form of folic acid not impacted by methotrexate, leucovorin, is administered as a "rescue" to noncancer cells.

Hydroxyurea is an antimetabolite that interferes with DNA synthesis during the S phase of cell division. In lower doses, it is sometimes used for sickle cell anemia, and in higher doses, in the treatment of a number of cancers, including chronic myelocytic leukemia.

The antimetabolites (particularly methotrexate) are sometimes used for other indications in lower doses, including autoimmune states like rheumatoid arthritis. Other antimetabolites (e.g., trimethoprim, sulfamethoxazole) interfere with bacterial use of folic acid and are used in the treatment of infectious diseases (see Chapter 58).

Examples from each group will be discussed briefly. Table 56-3 compares these agents.

Purine Analog

Analogs of purine used in the treatment of cancers include cladribine, fludarabine, mercaptopurine, pentostatin, and thioguanine. Cladribine and fludarabine are presented here in greater detail. Table 56-3 presents the remaining agents.

cladribine [**kla** dri been]
(Leustatin)
Cladribine enters the cell and is phosphorylated to a deoxyadenosine concentration that accumulates in these cells, interfering with DNA repair and eventually causing cell death.

Indications
Cladribine is used to treat hairy cell leukemia, chronic lymphocytic leukemia, and chronic myelogenous leukemia.

Pharmacokinetics
Administered intravenously, cladribine is metabolized to an active metabolite.

Adverse Effects
The adverse effects of cladribine include headache, anorexia, nausea, vomiting, severe anemia, infection, skin rash, bleeding or bruising, and fatigue.

fludarabine [floo **dah** rah a been]
(Fludara)
Fludarabine inhibits two enzymes (DNA polymerase and RNA reductase) and thereby inhibits DNA synthesis. It has specific activity during the S phase of cell division.

Indications
Fludarabine is indicated for the adult treatment of chronic lymphocytic leukemia and non-Hodgkin's lymphoma. It is also used in treating non-Hodgkin's lymphoma and acute leukemias in children.

Pharmacokinetics
Fludarabine is widely distributed to tissue with IV dosing, and is metabolized to an active metabolite that enters tumor cells.

TABLE 56-3 CYTOTOXIC ANTINEOPLASTIC MEDICATIONS: ANTIMETABOLITES

Drug	Route	Major Toxicity Bone Marrow Suppression	Emetogenic Potential*	Other Toxicities
PURINE ANALOG				
cladribine (Leustatin)	IV	X	NE	
fludarabine (Fludara)	IV	X	NE	
mercaptopurine (Purinethol)	PO	X	NE	
pentostatin (Nipent)	IV	X	H-VH	CNS
thioguanine	PO, IV	X	NE	
PYRIMIDINE ANALOG				
capecitabine (Xeloda)	PO	X	M	GI, diarrhea
cytarabine (Cytosar-U)	IV, subcutaneous, IT	X	H	
floxuridine (FUDR)	Intraarterial	X	NQ	GI
fluorouracil (Adrucil)	IV	X	L-M	
gemcitabine (Gemzar)	IV	X	L	
FOLATE ANTAGONIST				
methotrexate (Rheumatrex, Trexall)	IV, IM, PO, IT	X	M-H (Low dose: NE)	GI
pemetrexed (Alimta)	IV	X	NQ	
OTHER				
hydroxyurea (Droxia, Hydrea)	PO	X	L	

VH, Very high (frequency greater than 90%); *H*, high (frequency 60% to 90%); *M*, moderate (frequency 30% to 60%); *L*, low (frequency 10% to 30%); *NE*, not emetogenic (frequency less than 10%); *CNS*, central nervous system; *GI*, gastrointestinal; *IT*, intrathecal; *NQ*, not quantified.
*Emetogenic potential varies with dose and concurrent drug therapy.

Adverse Effects

Fludarabine produces significant bone marrow suppression with neutropenia, thrombocytopenia and anemias commonly observed. The full impact of bone marrow suppression, or nadir, is typically observed 10 to 14 days after treatment, and recovery is noted over 5 to 7 weeks. Unlike other chemotherapy, fludarabine causes little or no nausea or vomiting.

Pyrimidine Analog

Pyrimidine analogs used in the cancer treatment include capecitabine, cytarabine, floxuridine, fluorouracil, and gemcitabine. Fluorouracil and gemcitabine are presented in greater depth here. Table 56-3 briefly presents each analog.

fluorouracil [flure oh **yoor** a sill]

(Adrucil, 5-FU; Topical: Efudex, Fluoroplex)
Fluorouracil is a pyrimidine antagonist that interferes with the synthesis of DNA and RNA. It is a cell cycle–specific agent that produces its effect in the S phase of cell division.

Indications

Fluorouracil is indicated for treatment of carcinomas of the colon, rectum, breast, head, neck, stomach, and pancreas. Topically, it is used in the treatment of keratoses and superficial basal cell carcinomas.

Pharmacokinetics

With IV administration, fluorouracil is metabolized rapidly (within 1 hour) in the tissues to the active metabolite floxuridine. Final metabolic degradation occurs in the liver. This drug is distributed throughout the body and also crosses the blood-brain barrier. The half-life for the alpha phase is 10 to 20 minutes; the beta phase is prolonged up to 20 hours because of tissue storage of metabolites. The route of excretion is primarily respiratory as carbon dioxide (60% to 80%).

Adverse Effects

The adverse effects of fluorouracil include anorexia, esophagopharyngitis, diarrhea, ulceration of the gastrointestinal (GI) tract (severe nausea and vomiting, black stools, abdominal cramps), dermatitis on the extremities (less often on the trunk), leukopenia, thrombocytopenia, weakness, loss of hair, and dry skin. A wide variety of doses and schedules of this agent is used, which often influences the extent and type of adverse effect.

gemcitabine [jem **sigh** tah been]
(Gemzar)
Gemcitabine interferes with cell synthesis (S phase) and also blocks cell progression through the G_1/S part of the cycle.

Indications
Gemcitabine is indicated for treatment of non–small-cell lung cancer and for adenocarcinoma of the pancreas in clients with nonresectable or metastatic pancreatic cancer who have been previously treated with 5-FU.

Pharmacokinetics
Gemcitabine is metabolized to active and inactive metabolites after IV administration.

Adverse Effects
The adverse effects of gemcitabine include nausea, vomiting, diarrhea, dyspnea, peripheral edema, flu-like syndrome, rash, paresthesia, and stomatitis.

Folate Antagonist

Methotrexate is an antimetabolite that is cell cycle–specific for the S phase. To synthesize DNA, folic acid must be reduced to tetrahydrofolate by the enzyme dihydrofolate reductase. Methotrexate binds with dihydrofolate reductase, thereby inhibiting the synthesis of DNA and RNA. Because the growth of malignant cells is usually greater than the cell growth of normal tissues, cancer growth may be impaired by methotrexate.

Methotrexate and pemetrexed are both antagonists of folic acid. Methotrexate, also used for the treatment of advanced rheumatoid arthritis and psoriasis, is presented in greater depth here. Table 56-3 briefly presents both.

★▢▥ methotrexate [meth oh **trex** ate]
(MTX, Folex PFS)

Indications
Methotrexate is indicated for a number of conditions, including breast, head, neck, and lung cancers; trophoblastic tumors; renal, ovarian, bladder, and testicular carcinomas; acute lymphocytic leukemia and non-Hodgkin's lymphomas; and the prevention and treatment of meningeal leukemia. It is also used for advanced cases of mycosis fungoides, osteosarcoma, and for the noncancerous, selected cases of severe psoriasis and rheumatoid arthritis that are unresponsive to standard therapies

Pharmacokinetics
Methotrexate is administered orally or parenterally (intramuscular [IM], IV, and intrathecal). The oral preparation reaches peak serum levels within 1 to 2 hours. Limited amounts of methotrexate can cross the blood-brain barrier, but significant quantities pass into the systemic circulation after intrathecal drug administration. It is metabolized intracellularly and in the liver, with the unchanged drug excreted by the kidneys.

Adverse Effects
The adverse effects of methotrexate include dose-related anorexia, nausea, and vomiting. Other effects include acne, boils, skin rash or itching, loss of hair, GI ulcers and bleeding, leukopenia, infections, thrombocytopenia, stomatitis, pharyngitis and, with prolonged daily therapy, liver toxicity, pneumonitis, or pulmonary fibrosis. Renal failure, hyperuricemia, and cutaneous vasculitis may occur with high-dose therapy.

Folate Replacement with Folate Antagonist

★▢▥ leucovorin [loo koe **vor** in]
(folinic acid, Wellcovorin)
Leucovorin, or folinic acid, is a form of folic acid that does not require dihydrofolate reductase to produce folic acid. Therefore it is used to prevent or treat toxicity induced by folic acid antagonists.

Indications
Leucovorin is indicated as an antidote (prophylaxis and treatment) for folic acid antagonists (e.g., methotrexate, pyrimethamine, and trimethoprim) and as a treatment for megaloblastic anemia caused by nutritional deficiencies, sprue, or pregnancy and whenever oral folic acid therapy is not appropriate. **Leucovorin rescue** is a term used to describe the use of leucovorin to reduce the time that sensitive (normal) cells are exposed to the toxic effects of high-dose methotrexate treatments.

Pharmacokinetics
Leucovorin is rapidly absorbed orally and converted by the intestinal mucous membrane and liver to 5-methyltetrahydrofolate, an active metabolite. The onset of action is as follows: oral, between 20 and 30 minutes; IM, 10 to 20 minutes; IV, less than 5 minutes. The duration of action by all routes is between 3 and 6 hours. It is primarily excreted by the kidneys.

Adverse Effects
Serious adverse effects to leucovorin are rare, but include allergic reactions (rash, hives, itching, wheezing) and seizures. No significant drug interactions are reported with leucovorin.

Other Antimetabolite

hydroxyurea [hye **drox** ee yoo ree ah]
(Hydrea)
Hydroxyurea inhibits DNA synthesis without affecting the synthesis of RNA or protein.

Indications
Hydroxyurea is indicated for the treatment of head, neck, and ovarian carcinoma; chronic myelocytic leukemia; and malignant melanoma. It is also used in lower doses for the treatment of sickle cell anemia.

Pharmacokinetics
Hydroxyurea is well absorbed orally. It undergoes enterohepatic cycling and is metabolized by intestinal bacteria.

Adverse Effects
The adverse effects of hydroxyurea include anorexia, nausea, vomiting, diarrhea, drowsiness, and bone marrow suppression.

✸ What issues surround the use of the antitumor antibiotics?
The antitumor antibiotics are cytotoxic agents that directly bind DNA, thus inhibiting the synthesis of DNA and RNA. The early agents in this class (the anthracyclines) cause the clinically limiting adverse effect of irreversible cardiomyopathy with cumulative dosing. Newer agents that lack this cardiac toxicity are being sought. See Table 56-4 for drugs in this classification and their toxicities.

★▢▥ doxorubicin [dox oh **roo** bi sin]
(Adriamycin)
doxorubicin liposome [dox oh **roo** bi sin lip oh **sohm**]
(Doxil, Caelyx✤)
Doxorubicin binds to DNA base pairs and obstructs DNA and RNA synthesis. It may have greater activity during the S phase of cell division. Liposomal versions of doxorubicin are available and may increase penetration of the drug at the tumor site. Liposomal preparations contain the active drug in a phospholipid bilayer envelope, which prolongs action and may affect the ability of active drug to cross membranes.

Indications
Doxorubicin is used to treat acute leukemia, Wilms' tumor, soft tissue and bone sarcomas, Hodgkin's disease, lymphomas, and breast and various other carcinomas. The liposomal formulations have a more limited FDA-approved indication listing including treatment of

TABLE 56-4 CYTOTOXIC ANTINEOPLASTIC MEDICATIONS: ANTIBIOTIC ANTITUMOR AGENTS

| Drug | Route | Major Toxicity | | |
		Bone Marrow Suppression	Emetogenic Potential*	Other Toxicities
ANTHRACYCLINE				
daunorubicin (Cerubidine, DaunoXome)	IV	X	M	Cardiac, GI
doxorubicin (Adriamycin, Rubex), doxorubicin liposomal (Doxil)	IV	X	M-H	Cardiac, GI
epirubicin (Ellence)	IV	X	M	Cardiac
idarubicin (Idamycin)	IV	X	M	Cardiac (↓ risk compared to other anthracyclines), but monitoring is necessary (Serono, 2005)
mitoxantrone (Novantrone)	IV	X	M-H	
valrubicin (Valstar)†	Intravesicular		NE	Local bladder irritation
OTHER				
bleomycin (Blenoxane)	IV, IM, subcutaneous, intrapleural		NE	Pulmonary
dactinomycin (Cosmegen)	IV	X	H	GI
mitomycin (Mutamycin)	IV	X	L	
plicamycin (Mithracin)	IV	X	NQ	Hemorrhage

VH, Very high (frequency greater than 90%); *H*, high (frequency 60% to 90%); *M*, moderate (frequency 30% to 60%); *L*, low (frequency 10% to 30%); *NE*, not emetogenic (frequency less than 10%); *GI*, gastrointestinal; *NQ*, not quantified.
*Emetogenic potential varies with dose and concurrent drug therapy.
†Discontinued in the United States.

acquired immunodeficiency syndrome (AIDS)-related Kaposi's sarcoma, breast and ovarian cancer, and certain solid tumors.

Pharmacokinetics
Doxorubicin does not cross the blood-brain barrier and is highly tissue bound. It is metabolized in the liver to produce adriamycinol, an active metabolite. The half-life of doxorubicin is biphasic: 0.6 hours and 16.7 hours. The active metabolite has a half-life of 3.3 hours and 31.7 hours. It is metabolized in the liver and excreted primarily in the bile. The liposomal formulation is distributed to vascularized tissue and has a more prolonged elimination pattern. Doxorubicin and doxorubicin liposomal are not interchangeable and do not have the same dosing schedules.

Adverse Effects
The adverse effects of doxorubicin include severe nausea and vomiting; esophagitis; diarrhea; darkening of the soles, palms, or nails (especially in children and blacks); alopecia; red urine; leukopenia; thrombocytopenia; stomatitis; cardiotoxicity (usually heart failure); extravasation leading to cellulitis or tissue necrosis; hyperuricemia; nephropathy; and dark or red skin.

✸ How are the mitotic inhibitors different from other agents?

The primary mitotic inhibitors, vinblastine and vincristine (vinca alkaloids derived from a periwinkle plant), are cell cycle–specific agents that inhibit mitosis during the M phase. Vinorelbine is a semisynthetic vinca alkaloid. The vinca alkaloids are similar chemically but have different therapeutic indications and different adverse effects. Other agents that inhibit mitotic function include the taxanes, including paclitaxel (Taxol) and docetaxel (Taxotere). The taxanes are commonly used in breast and other forms of cancer by interfering with mitosis and cell division. Table 56-5 briefly compares examples from each group.

Vinca Alkaloid

vinblastine [vin **blast** een]
(Velban)
Indications
Vinblastine is used to treat breast and testicular carcinoma, Hodgkin's and non-Hodgkin's lymphomas, Kaposi's sarcoma, and mycosis fungoides.
Pharmacokinetics
Administered intravenously, vinblastine binds to peripheral tissue but does not distribute to the CNS. The triphasic half-life reflecting distribution, then elimination is 3.7 minutes, 1.6 hours, and 25 hours. It is metabolized by the liver and excreted in bile.

TABLE 56-5 CYTOTOXIC ANTINEOPLASTIC MEDICATIONS: MITOTIC INHIBITORS

| Drug | Route | Major Toxicity | | Other Toxicities |
		Bone Marrow Suppression	Emetogenic Potential*	
VINCA ALKALOIDS				
vinblastine (Velban)	IV	X	NE	
vincristine (Oncovin) vincristine liposomal (Marqibo)	IV		NE	Peripheral neuropathy
vinorelbine (Navelbine)	IV	X	NE	
TAXANES				
docetaxel (Taxotere)	IV	X	M-H	GI
paclitaxel (Onxol, Taxol)	IV	X	L	GI

VH, Very high (frequency greater than 90%); *H*, high (frequency 60% to 90%); *M*, moderate (frequency 30-60%); *L*, low (frequency 10% to 30%); *NE*, not emetogenic (frequency less than 10%); *GI*, gastrointestinal; *NQ*, not quantified.
*Emetogenic potential varies with dose and concurrent drug therapy.

Adverse Effects

Bone marrow suppression is the major adverse effect of vinblastine and often limits dosing. Nausea, vomiting, stomatitis, alopecia, extravasation at the injection site, cellulitis, muscle pain hyperuricemia, rectal bleeding, and hemorrhagic colitis have also been reported with vinblastine.

★⊓ vincristine [vin **kris** teen]

(Oncovin)
vincristine liposomal
(Marqibo)
Indications

Vincristine is used to treat acute lymphoblastic leukemia, Hodgkin's and non-Hodgkin's lymphomas, rhabdomyosarcoma, neuroblastoma, Wilms' tumor, and various other carcinomas.
Pharmacokinetics

Vincristine is administered intravenously and does not cross the blood-brain barrier. It is highly tissue bound and has a triphasic half-life of 0.07 hour, 2.27 hours, and 85 hours. Metabolites of vincristine are eliminated in the bile. Vincristine and vincristine liposomal formulations are not interchangable.
Adverse Effects

Peripheral neuropathy is the major adverse effect of vincristine. It is most common in clients over 40 years of age and may limit use. Vincristine may also induce anorexia, nausea and vomiting, rash, autonomic toxicity (abdominal cramping, constipation, bed-wetting, orthostatic hypotension, lack of sweating, and increased, decreased or painful urination), hyperuricemia, a progressive neurotoxicity (blurred or double vision, difficulty in walking, drooping eyelids, headache, jaw pain, numbness and pain in the fingers and toes, weakness), and SIADH secretion.
Nursing Management

Although the nursing management of the antineoplastic chemotherapy agents is discussed in detail in Chapter 55, the neurotoxicity of vincristine deserves special mention. The use of vincristine in clients with neuromuscular disease should be carefully considered. The client's baseline assessment includes the status of the underlying condition, bowel and bladder function, muscle tone and reflexes, serum uric acid concentrations, hematocrit, hemoglobin, platelet count, total and differential white blood cell (WBC) count, and liver function studies. With vincristine, impaired urinary elimination related to autonomic toxicity is also a possibility and is evidenced by bed-wetting, increased or decreased urination, and painful or difficult urination; impaired comfort (headache, rash, bloating) is also possible. Monitor the client's neuromuscular status. Watch for ataxia, numbness, tingling, or pain in the fingers or toes, headache, double vision, depression of deep tendon reflexes, and other early signs of neurotoxicity. Monitor the client's bowel status for early signs of autonomic toxicity, such as constipation.

Taxanes

The taxanes are antimicrotubule agents that stabilize microtubule bundles, thereby interfering with the late G_2 mitotic and metaphase cell cycle and resulting in the inhibition of cell replication.

★⊓ paclitaxel [pac li **tax** el]

(Taxol)
Paclitaxel is a natural substance extracted from the yew tree and marketed for the treatment of metastatic ovarian cancer that is refractory to other drug treatments.
Indications

Paclitaxel is used for the treatment of breast, lung, and ovarian cancers.
Pharmacokinetics

Paclitaxel is widely distributed to tissues following IV infusion. It is metabolized by cytochrome P450 2C8/9 and 3A4, which may account for its increased toxicity when dosed with other drugs, including cisplatin, and azole antifungals; and its reduced efficacy when dosed with phenobarbital, carbamazepine, rifampin, and phenytoin.
Adverse Effects

The adverse effects of paclitaxel include severe allergic reactions that may be prevented by pretreatment with a steroid and an H_1 and H_2 antagonist. Other toxicities include bone marrow suppression, peripheral neuropathy, muscle pain, alopecia, and gastric distress.

docetaxel [dok i **tax** el]

(Taxotere)
Docetaxel is also a taxane, a semisynthetic product originating from the yew plant. It may produce its effect by binding and stabilizing microtubule bundles, thus inhibiting cell mitosis.

It is indicated for the treatment of advanced breast cancer and advanced non–small-cell lung cancer.

Pharmacokinetics
The pharmacokinetics of intravenously administered docetaxel are similar to paclitaxel. It is metabolized by cytochrome P450 3A4 and may interact with drugs metabolized by this system.

Adverse Effects
The adverse effects of docetaxel include nausea, diarrhea, stomatitis, fever, skin reactions, myalgia, and bone marrow suppression.

✱ What other drugs are used as cytotoxic agents in the treatment of cancer?

Rounding out drugs that are toxic to cancer cells are the topoisomerase inhibitors, enzymes, an adrenal gland suppressant, and arsenic trioxide; these are presented in Table 56-6. A number of other agents that modify biologic responses, affect hormonal action, or impact blood flow to tumors may also have effects that benefit cancer treatment and will be discussed later.

Topoisomerase Inhibitors

Topoisomerases are enzymes that are involved in making reversible breaks in DNA strands and later repairing them to allow for flexibility in DNA during replication. Topoisomerase 1 and 2 are each involved in repairing these reversible breaks in DNA. Irinotecan and topotecan are topoisomerase 1 inhibitors whereas etoposide and teniposide are topoisomerase 2 inhibitors.

Etoposide is a type 2 topoisomerase inhibitor affecting S phase and early G_2 phase activity by causing DNA strand breaks. Irinotecan is a type 1 topoisomerase inhibitor that binds to the type 1 topoisomerase DNA complex, resulting in double-stranded DNA breaks that cause tumor cell death. Topotecan is also a topoisomerase type 1 inhibitor.

etoposide [e toe **poe** side]
(Toposar, VePesid)
etoposide phosphate [e toe **poe** side **fos** fate]
(Etopophos)
Indications
Etoposide is indicated for a wide number of cancer types including lymphomas, acute nonlymphocytic leukemia, and prostate, lung, testicular, bladder, uterine, and other cancers. Etoposide phosphate is indicated for refractory small cell lung and testicular cancers.

Pharmacokinetics
Etoposide is available as an oral formulation, and has variable absorption on oral administration. Both etoposide and etoposide phosphate are available as IV preparations, distribute poorly to the CSF, and are metabolized by cytochrome P450 3A4.

Adverse Effects
Hematologic adverse effects can be significant with the nadir for granulocytes observed 1 to 2 weeks after dosing. Alopecia, and dose-related nausea, vomiting, and stomatitis are common.

irinotecan [eye ri **noe** te can]
(Camptosar)
Indications
Irinotecan is indicated for the treatment of metastatic colorectal cancer or rectal cancer that has occurred or progressed after 5-FU, another chemotherapeutic agent.

TABLE 56-6 MISCELLANEOUS CYTOTOXIC ANTINEOPLASTIC MEDICATIONS

Drug	Route	Major Toxicity		
		Bone Marrow Suppression	Emetogenic Potential*	Other Toxicities
TOPOISOMERASE INHIBITOR				
Topoisomerase I inhibitor				
irinotecan (Camptosar)	IV	X	H-VH	GI, diarrhea
topotecan (Hycamtin)	IV	X	L	
Topoisomerase II inhibitor				
etoposide (VePesid)	IV, PO	X	L	
teniposide (Vumon)	IV	X	L-M	
MISCELLANEOUS				
Enzymes				
asparaginase (Elspar)	IV, IM		L	
pegaspargase (Oncospar)	IM, IV		M	
Antiadrenal				
mitotane (Lysodren)	PO		M	CNS
Heavy Metal				
arsenic trioxide (Trisenox)	IV	X†	H	Cardiac, renal, GI, CNS, hepatic

VH, Very high (frequency greater than 90%); *H,* high (frequency 60% to 90%); *M,* moderate (frequency 30% to 60%); *L,* low (frequency 10% to 30%); *NE,* not emetogenic (frequency less than 10%); *CNS,* central nervous system; *GI,* gastrointestinal; *NQ,* not quantified.
*Emetogenic potential varies with dose and concurrent drug therapy.
†Leukocytosis may also be seen.

Pharmacokinetics
Irinotecan is administered intravenously and is metabolized by cytochrome P450 2B6 and 3A4.

Adverse Effects
Irinotecan may cause severe diarrhea, which requires immediate treatment with loperamide (Imodium). Severe myelosuppression, nausea, and vomiting may also occur. Genetic variation among individuals is correlated with the potential for adverse effects with irinotecan (see the Special Considerations for Pharmacogenetics box below).

★⊓ topotecan [toe poe **tee** kan]
(Hycamtin)
Indications
Topotecan is indicated for the treatment of ovarian and small lung cell cancers. It is also used for the treatment on non–small-cell lung cancer and pediatric sarcomas.

Pharmacokinetics
Intravenously administered topotecan is metabolized in the plasma to an inactive metabolite.

Adverse Effects
The adverse effects of topotecan include headache, nausea, vomiting, neutropenia (a dose-limiting toxicity), leukopenia, thrombocytopenia, anemia, diarrhea, stomach pain, alopecia, fatigue, dyspnea, and neuromuscular pain.

Enzymes

Two drugs that affect asparagines levels are used in treating leukemias. Asparagine is necessary for cell survival, but because normal body cells are capable of synthesizing appropriate supplies of asparaginase, they are not affected by an asparagine deficiency. Certain cancer cells, however, depend on a circulating supply of asparagine within the blood; when this supply is decreased, the cancer cells will die. Asparaginase and pegaspargase (modified asparaginase) reduce asparagine to aspartic acid and serve to deprive cells of asparagine. They are considered cell-cycle specific at the G_1 phase.

asparaginase [a **spar** a gi nase]
(Elspar, Kidrolase✦)
Indications
Asparaginase is used to treat acute lymphocytic leukemia (ALL) and lymphoma.

Pharmacokinetics
Asparaginase is administered intravenously or intramuscularly. It is extensively metabolized with an elimination half-life of 8 to 30 hours.

Adverse Effects
The adverse effects of asparaginase are hyperammonemia (headache, anorexia, nausea, vomiting, abdominal cramps), a decrease in the

---

Special Considerations for Pharmacogenetics | TREATMENTS FOR CANCER

PHARMACODYNAMICS

Many cancers have a strong genetic basis, including breast, prostate, and oral cancers. Profiling of tumor genes may have enormous potential to successfully identify prevention and treatment strategies (Mocellin et al., 2005). Genetic determinants for testosterone or estrogen metabolism may assist in identification of those at high risk for prostate or breast cancer respectively and who will likely benefit from hormonal targeted therapies (Parnes, Thompson, & Ford, 2005). Genetic markers for oral cancers have been identified and may play a role in identifying high risk individuals and targeted treatments (Lippman, Sudbo, & Hong, 2005). The potential for metastasis is correlated with the amount of extracellular matrix degrading metalloproteinase (MMP) levels, which are coded by a number of genes and may display considerable variation across populations (Spitz, Wu, & Mills, 2005).

Many targeted therapies and monoclonal antibody treatments are primarily effective only for those individuals with significant genetic-based receptor presence. This is demonstrated by the response of trastuzumab for clients with the presence of the HER-2 receptor in metastatic breast cancer (Elkin et al., 2004).

PHARMACOKINETICS

Genetically determined enzyme systems are responsible for metabolism of substances to carcinogens. Cytochrome P450 2D6 and 3A4 is involved in metabolic conversion of substances like nicotine to carcinogens (Dally et al., 2003). Individuals with high degree of 2D6 activity may be at a higher risk for cancer related to tobacco habituation compared to those with lower 2D6 activity (Spitz et al., 2005).

Metabolism of chemotherapy is also largely influenced by the presence of genetically determined enzyme function. Many

tumors themselves are capable of drug metabolism and may display variation from the host in genetics that code for enzyme function. Cytotoxic drug resistance can be partially explained by genetic mutations in tumors that affect drug metabolism or drug transfer across tumor membranes. Significant variation is noted both across populations, and with different tumor types. Most frequently studied are breast, gastrointestinal, lung, and hematologic cancers with drug metabolism often significantly different within tumors (Michael & Doherty, 2005).

Genetic differences are noted in the metabolism of fluorouracil (via P450 2 A6), cyclophosphamide (via P450 2 B6), paclitaxel (via P450 2 C8), methotrexate (via DHFR), busulfan (via GSTA1), carmustine (via MGMT), mitomycin c (via NQO1), 6-mercaptopurine/thioguanine (via TPMT), and irinotecan (via UGT1 A1) (Chang & Altman, 2004). Glutathione is involved in cisplatin metabolism and its activity is correlated with successful outcomes (Spitz et al., 2005). Similar correlations between specific enzyme function and drug response has been also observed with fluorouracil, docetaxel, irinotecan, and cyclophosphamide (Michael & Doherty, 2005).

ADVERSE EFFECTS

Given the strong influence of genetics in metabolism of many cytotoxic agents, it should not be surprising that genetics influences the likelihood of adverse effects and therapeutic response (Donnelly, 2004). Significant bone marrow suppression and diarrhea are correlated with genetic markers for irinotecan toxicity (Kitagawa et al., 2005; Innocenti et al., 2004). Strong correlations between CYP 2 B6 and cyclophosphamide toxicity, and CYP 2 C8 and paclitaxel toxicity have also been reported (van Schaik, 2004).

blood-clotting factors, allergic reactions, liver toxicity, pancreatitis, and anaphylaxis.

pegaspargase [peg ah **spar** gaze]
(Oncaspar)
Indications
Pegaspargase is used in combination chemotherapies for acute lymphoblastic leukemia in clients unable to take L-asparaginase and for the treatment of crisis of chronic lymphocytic leukemia. It is also occasionally used in non-Hodgkin's lymphoma.
Pharmacokinetics
Pegaspargase displays prolonged activity (e.g., beyond 2 weeks) after IM injection. Intravenous administration may also be used, but is not routinely recommended.
Adverse Effects
The adverse effects of pegaspargase include hypersensitivity reactions, hepatotoxicity, and coagulopathies.

Antiadrenal Agents

mitotane [**mye** toe tane]
(Lysodren)
Mitotane is an adrenal gland suppressing agent producing adrenal cortex atrophy. With ongoing use, it suppresses cortisol production and alters peripheral steroid metabolism.
Indications
Mitotane is indicated for the treatment of inoperable carcinoma of the adrenal cortex.
Pharmacokinetics
Administered orally, it is distributed throughout the body but is mainly stored in fat. The onset of effect is reported within 48 to 72 hours of starting therapy; the tumor response is usually within 6 weeks.
Adverse Effects
Significant adverse effects of mitotane include adrenal gland insufficiency: dark skin, diarrhea, anorexia, depression, nausea, vomiting, weakness, drowsiness, and light-headedness.

Other Cytotoxic Agents

arsenic trioxide [**ar** se nik tri **oks** ide]
(Trisenox)
Arsenic trioxide causes changes to DNA in human leukemic cells and degrades the fusion protein PML-RAR-alpha. Its toxicity renders this drug limited for clinical use in cases in which other therapies have not been effective.
Indications
Arsenic trioxide is used to in the treatment of acute promyelocytic leukemia. Its use is primarily limited to those with PML/RAR-alpha gene or a t(15;17) translocation and who have not responded to retinoid and anthracycline therapy.
Pharmacokinetics
Arsenic trioxide is hepatically metabolized and excreted in urine.
Adverse Effects
Among the most serious and common adverse effects of arsenic trioxide are cardiac dysrhythmias, prolongation of QT intervals, edema, chest pain, and hypotension. Nausea, vomiting, abdominal pain, fever, fatigue, headache, dermatitis, rigors, joint pain, cough, dyspnea, leukocytosis, thrombocytopenia, and elevated liver function tests are also common. Multiple other toxicities, including renal failure and encephalopathy, are also observed with arsenic therapy.

⊛ **M.S., a 65-year-old woman with recently diagnosed breast cancer, had a lumpectomy. The surgery is to be** followed by radiation therapy and chemotherapy to minimize the risk of recurrence. She is in the oncology treatment center today to receive the first of four cycles of doxorubicin (Adriamycin) and cyclophosphamide (Cytoxan) over the next 12 weeks to be followed by four cycles of paclitaxel (Taxol) (see Box 56-2). M.S. expresses fear of "receiving so many drugs" and "what will happen to me?"

⊛ **What are the nursing management issues for M.S. with the use of a combination antineoplastic chemotherapy regimen including these agents?**
The cytotoxic combination of agents included in M.S.'s therapeutic regimen is cyclophosphamide, an alkylating agent; doxorubicin, an antibiotic antitumor agent; and paclitaxel, a mitosis inhibitor. Combination therapy is characterized by each drug being effective against this particular cancer, having a different site of action, acting at a different point of the cell cycle, and having different organ toxicities (or if they are the same toxic effect, at least it occurs at different times for each drug).

- Cyclophosphamide, a cell cycle—nonspecific agent that cross-links DNA and RNA strands and inhibits protein synthesis, is effective against carcinomas of the breast. Although thrombocytopenia is rare, bone marrow suppression is evidenced by a marked leukopenia with the nadir in 2 to 8 days after first dose, but may be as late as 1 month after a series of daily doses. Other adverse effects are interstitial pulmonary fibrosis, hemorrhagic cystitis, and Stevens-Johnson syndrome.
- Doxorubicin, a cytotoxic antibiotic, blocks effective DNA and RNA transcription, is also effective against carcinoma of the breast. It also causes bone marrow suppression with the nadir of leukopenia occurring 10 to 14 days after a single dose. Cardiotoxicity is also a concern.
- Paclitaxel, a taxane, inhibits mitosis and is effective for ovarian, breast, and lung cancers and a treatment for Kaposi's sarcoma associated with advanced HIV disease. Bone marrow suppression is associated with paclitaxel therapy. Allergic reactions related to histamine release occur frequently during the first hour of infusion. Neuropathies and myopathies are common with higher doses.

M.S. will need to be prepared for these specific toxicities and the ones that are common to all antineoplastic agents, such as anorexia, nausea, vomiting, diarrhea, and alopecia.

Assessment Determine sensitivity to any agent of the combination. The use of cyclophosphamide and paclitaxel is carefully considered if M.S. has renal or hepatic function impairment (may require dosage reduction); existing or recent infection, chickenpox, or herpes zoster (risk of severe generalized disease); and bone marrow depression, tumor cell infiltration of the bone marrow, or previous cytotoxic drug or radiation therapy (dosage reduction by one half or one third is recommended) as the bone marrow is already compromised. These precautions are true of doxorubicin also but with added concern if M.S. had a history of cardiac disease because of its cardiotoxicity. If M.S. were of childbearing age, her pregnancy status would be determined. See the Pregnancy Safety box below.

Review M.S.'s current medication regimen for the risk of significant drug interactions, such as those that may occur when this combination of drugs is given with radiation therapy and other bone marrow depressants (additive bone marrow suppression may occur), other immunosuppressants (increased risk of infection), and antigout agents (cell death from the combination of drugs may increase blood uric acid, dosages of these medications may need adjustment). Because of immunosuppression, M.S. will need to avoid viral vaccines, live or killed, until she has the ability to respond to the vaccine, 3 months to 1 year after her last chemotherapy. If M.S. had received a course of daunorubicin, there would be increased risk of cardiotoxicity. The inhibition of cholinesterase activity by cyclophosphamide reduces cocaine metabolism and excretion and may lead to cocaine toxicity, and the use of cytarabine (Cytosar-U) in preparation for bone marrow transplant may result in increased cardiomyopathy with subsequent death.

Obtain a baseline assessment of M.S.'s general health status (particularly her mouth for ulceration), hematocrit or hemoglobin, platelet count, total and differential WBC count, serum uric acid and creatinine levels, blood urea nitrogen (BUN), urinalysis for hematuria (cyclophosphamide, hemorrhagic cystitis) and specific gravity (cyclophosphamide, SIADH), and liver function studies. Radionuclide angiography determination of ejection fraction and echocardiography are recommended before doxorubicin therapy.

Nursing Diagnosis While receiving this combination therapy, M.S. is at risk for the following nursing diagnoses: risk for infection related to compromised immune system evidenced by leukopenia; altered protection related to an increased tendency for bleeding secondary to thrombocytopenia; impaired tissue integrity related to extravasation; disturbed body image related to gonadal suppression, darkening of the skin and nails, or alopecia; fatigue; impaired comfort (headache, rash); deficient fluid volume and imbalanced nutrition: less than body requirements related to anorexia, nausea, and vomiting; diarrhea; impaired oral mucous membrane related to stomatitis and ulceration; and the potential complications of allergic reaction, altered cardiac output (cardiotoxicity), hepatitis, SIADH-like symptoms (dizziness, confusion, edema, decreased urinary output), hemorrhagic cystitis, nephropathy (a result of hyperuricemia from rapid cell breakdown), pneumonitis, and interstitial pulmonary fibrosis. (unusual bleeding or bruising, petechiae, blood in urine or stool); or disturbed body image related to alopecia and palmar-plantar erythrodysesthesia syndrome or hand-foot syndrome (tingling, swelling, and reddening of the nail beds and the skin of the soles of the feet and the palms of the hands). The client is also at risk for the complication of GI ulceration and complications related to the prolonged use of an arterial catheter to administer the drug, such as thrombosis, embolism, thrombophlebitis, abscesses, and bleeding, leakage, or infection at the catheter site.

Planning During this combination antineoplastic therapy, M.S. will:
- Maintain comfort levels that are acceptable to her.
- Regain normal or prechemotherapy level of intact oral mucosa.

PREGNANCY SAFETY
ANTINEOPLASTIC CHEMOTHERAPY AGENTS

Category	Drug
B	mesna, prednisone, trastuzumab
C	aldesleukin, alemtuzumab, amifostine, asparaginase, bevacizumab, cetuximab, dacarbazine, dactinomycin, denileukin diftitox, dexamethasone, dexrazoxane, interferon alfa-2 a, interferon alfa-2 b, filgrastim, leucovorin, levamisole, mitomycin, mitotane, nilutamide, pegaspargase, pegfilgrastim, rasburicase, rituximab, sargramostim, testolactone, tretinoin, valrubicin
D	altretamine, anastrozole, arsenic trioxide, bleomycin, bortezomib, busulfan, capecitabine, carboplatin, carmustine, chlorambucil, cisplatin, cladribine, cyclophosphamide, cytarabine, daunorubicin, docetaxel, doxorubicin, epirubicin, estramustine, etoposide, exemestane, floxuridine, fludarabine, fluorouracil, flutamide, fulvestrant, gefitinib, gemcitabine, gemtuzumab ozogamicin, hydroxyurea, ibritumomab tiuxetan, idarubicin, ifosfamide, imatinib, irinotecan, letrozole, lomustine, megestrol acetate, melphalan, mercaptopurine, methchlorethamine, methotrexate, mitoxantrone, oxaliplatin, paclitaxel, pemetrexed, pentostatin, pipobroman, procarbazine, streptozocin, tamoxifen, temozolomide, teniposide, thioguanine, thiotepa, topotecan, toremifene, vinblastine, vincristine, vinorelbine
X	bexarotene, bicalutamide, diethylstilbestrol, ethinyl estradiol, fluoxymesterone, goserelin, leuprolide, medroxyprogesterone, methotrexate, plicamycin, polyestradiol, raloxifene, testosterone, triptorelin

Data from *Mosby's drug consult* (15th ed.). (2005). St. Louis: Mosby.

- Maintain normal or prechemotherapy body weight with minimal GI adverse effects.
- Remain free of infection.
- Regain normal or prechemotherapy bowel pattern.
- Maintain healthy body image while experiencing alopecia.
- Remain free from injury related to IV administration of antineoplastic therapy and its organ specific adverse effects (bone marrow suppression [anemia, neutropenia, thrombocytopenia], cardiotoxicity, hemorrhagic cystitis, interstitial pulmonary fibrosis, SIADH syndrome).

Implementation

Monitoring Monitor for myelosuppression as evidenced by leucopenia, thrombocytopenia, and anemia evidenced by decreased hematocrit, platelet count, and total and differential WBC count. Lowest levels of leukopenia with cyclophosphamide generally occur 7 to 12 days after the first dose and the WBC count recovers 17 to 21 days after the last dose. With doxorubicin, the lowest WBC count usually occurs 10 to 14 days after dosage and recovers within 21 days. In general, the lowest levels of WBC counts occur day 11 with recovery day 15 to 20 and the lowest platelet counts occur 8 to 9 days after the first day of paclitaxel therapy. Monitor WBC and platelet counts, and watch the client for signs of bruising and bleeding, particularly GI bleeding. Test stools for occult blood. Monitor M.S.'s temperature and observe for signs of infection, such as fever, chills, sore throat, low back pain, or painful urination.

Monitor BUN and creatinine determinations; a decrease in creatinine clearance and an increase in the other test values may indicate nephrotoxicity. Perform a urinalysis for microscopic hematuria to determine hemorrhagic cystitis (cyclophosphamide). Monitor serum uric acid levels and intake and output ratios to ensure that M.S. is adequately hydrated to prevent hyperuricemia.

Observe M.S. for symptoms of SIADH-like syndrome: reduced urinary output, increased urine specific gravity, weight gain over several days, and edema of the feet and lower legs, flank pain, pruritus, urine odor on the breath, anorexia, nausea, and vomiting (cyclophosphamide).

Monitor vital signs. For doxorubicin, monitor echocardiography, electrocardiography (ECG), and radionuclide angiography reports for evidence of cardiopathy; observe for swelling of the feet and lower legs and shortness of breath. Cardiotoxicity usually occurs within 1 to 6 months after initiating therapy and is more common in adults older than 70 years of age and in children younger than 2 years of age. The risk of cardiotoxicity is also dose related and is estimated to be 1% to 2% at a total cumulative dose of 300 mg/m² of body surface area, 3% to 5% at 400 mg/m², 5% to 8% at 450 mg/m², and 6% to 20% at 500 mg/m². Cardiotoxicity may develop suddenly and may be irreversible; it is critical that it be detected early, when it usually responds to therapy. With cyclophosphamide, observe for cardiotoxicity such as myopericarditis as evidenced by tachycardia, fever, chills, and shortness of breath. Pneu-

monitis or other respiratory complications may result in a cough and shortness of breath (cyclophosphamide).

Examine M.S.'s mouth for ulceration with a tongue blade and flashlight before therapy is initiated and before each dose (cyclophosphamide, doxorubicin). Stomatitis is a sign of toxicity; it usually occurs 5 to 10 days after administration and may be severe enough to place M.S. at risk for infection. Check also for oral candidiasis and herpes.

Watch for signs of toxicity and indications for discontinuing the drug, including intractable vomiting, diarrhea, severe stomatitis, WBC count below 3500/mm³, thrombocytopenia (below 10,000/mm³), and gastrointestinal (GI) bleeding. The leukopenia and thrombocytopenia associated with the pharmacologic action of these drugs are used as measures for the titration of M.S.'s dosage.

Intervention Antiemetics are administered concurrently to reduce nausea and vomiting. Maintain M.S.'s fluid intake at 3000 mL daily before treatment and for 72 hours following cyclophosphamide treatment to ensure frequent voiding, including at least once during the night; this minimizes the risk of hemorrhagic cystitis and promotes the excretion of uric acid. Adequate hydration minimizes uric acid nephropathy. Alkalinization of urine or allopurinol administration may also be used to prevent uric acid nephropathy.

It is best to administer cyclophosphamide early in the day so that most of the drug's metabolites have been excreted before bedtime; this prevents continued contact of the metabolites with the bladder mucosa. The drug should be discontinued at the first sign of hemorrhagic cystitis; symptomatic treatment may be instituted through routes such as blood replacement, cryosurgery, or formaldehyde bladder instillation. Continuation of cyclophosphamide therapy is done cautiously because recurrence is common.

Doxorubicin may be administered over 1 to 2 minutes or IV piggyback (IVPB). Continuous infusions may be administered via a central line. Flush with 5 to 10 mL of IV solution before and after drug administration. However, M.S.'s dose of doxorubicin will be IV push according to the protocol (see Box 56-2). In that case, the double syringe method may be used to decrease pain at the injection site (Box 56-3).

Take precautions against IV extravasation. If extravasation occurs, the IV line should be moved to another site for completion of the dose. Ice packs should be applied, and the extremity should be elevated to minimize injury. Surgical excision of the area may be required if inflammation is extensive. Do not administer doxorubicin intramuscularly or subcutaneously, because it will cause tissue necrosis (*USP DI*, 2005).

To prevent severe hypersensitivity reactions to paclitaxel, M.S. should be premedicated with dexamethasone, diphenhydramine and ranitidine (see protocol in Box 56-2).

Because of the hazards in preparing the doses, consult the institution guidelines for the handling of antineoplastic agents (Box 56-4).

Take precautions against IV infiltration. Administration should be stopped immediately if extravasation occurs, with the remaining dose injected into another vein. See Box 56-5 for treatment of extravasation of antineoplastic agents.

BOX 56-3 DOUBLE SYRINGE METHOD

Some antineoplastic agents have vesicant properties (causing blisters) and require careful handling. The following are common vesicant agents:

dactinomycin

carmustine (BiCNU)

daunorubicin

doxorubicin

mechlorethamine

mithramycin

mitomycin C

vinblastine

vincristine

If these agents are administered by bolus dose a double-syringe technique is used as follows:

1. Select site for administration according to following order of preference: forearm, dorsum of hand, wrist, or antecubital fossa.
2. Use 20- or 21-gauge "butterfly" needle for drug administration. Use one syringe to administer 5-mL normal saline solution and withdraw small amount of blood into tubing to test vein patency. If blood return is poor, select site other than distal location.
3. Use another syringe to administer vesicant agent for a least 3 minutes, drawing blood back into tubing after every 2- to 3-mL solution.
4. Flush with 3- to 5-mL saline solution after administration.
5. If client has pain at site of injection or an unusual sensation during drug administration, extravasation may have occurred, and a new site for drug injection should be selected. The health agency's procedure/protocol for extravasation should be followed.

Take safety precautions if the platelet count is low. Precautions include avoiding invasive procedures or using extreme care in such procedures; regularly examining the skin, mucous membranes, and injection sites for bruising or bleeding; testing emesis, urine, and stool for signs of occult bleeding; exercising care in the use of grooming implements, toothbrushes, toothpicks, razors, and nail clippers; preventing constipation; and preventing physical injury. Platelet transfusions may be required. Protective isolation may be instituted if the WBC count falls below $3500/mm^3$. Broad-spectrum antimicrobials may be administered pending appropriate culture results.

Education Instruct M.S. to avoid intake of excessive amounts of alcohol or any aspirin because of the risk of GI bleeding. Caution her against being immunized with live viral vaccines during therapy, because it may cause rather than prevent the disease. Persons in close contact with the client should not receive immunization with the nasal influenza vaccine, because the live virus is excreted by the vaccine recipient and can be transmitted to the immunocompromised client. The client should avoid being exposed to infections. Other immunizations should ideally be completed before initiating chemotherapy because the immunosuppression caused by chemotherapy lasts for 3 months to 1 year and may limit the vaccination's benefit. Inform M.S. that alopecia may occur but is reversible; hair regrowth may be different in texture or color. Instruct the client on the previously mentioned safety precautions. See the Community and Home Health Considerations box on p. 983 for information about working with clients who are receiving antineoplastic agents at home.

Advise M.S., if she is taking the oral form of cyclophosphamide therapy, that nausea and vomiting often occurs, but stress that the medication needs to be taken despite these symptoms. M.S.'s urine may become reddish for 1 or 2 days after the administration of doxorubicin, but it generally clears in 48 hours. Alert her that a discoloration of the skin and nails may also occur.

As with the nursing management of antineoplastic agents discussed in Chapter 55, observe safety precautions for invasive procedures.

Evaluation The expected outcome of doxorubicin therapy is that the client will demonstrate signs of clinical improvement, with decreased tumor size and metastases and a normal complete blood count (CBC), and no bleeding, infection, stomatitis, mouth ulcers, local tissue damage at the infusion site, adverse GI effects, or signs and symptoms of cardiotoxicity, interstitial pulmonary fibrosis, SIADH syndrome, or hemorrhagic cystitis. The client and family will demonstrate the effective management of the antineoplastic regimen including: pharmacologic and nonpharmacologic measures to control pain, and measures to enhance skin integrity, minimize alterations of the oral mucous membranes, risk for infection, self-concept disturbances, and self-injury.

✳ **What hormonal agents are used in the treatment of cancers?**

Hormonal agents are used in the treatment of neoplasms that are sensitive to hormonal growth controls in the body. The exact mechanism of action of hormonal agents against neoplasms is unknown, but apparently they interfere with growth-stimulating receptors on target tissues. Such agents are more selective and less toxic than other antineoplastics and include corticosteroids, androgens, androgen antagonists, gonadotropic releasing hormone agonists, estrogens, antiestrogens, progestins, and aromatase inhibitors. Table 56-7 reviews these agents.

Corticosteroids

Because corticosteroids slow lymphocytic proliferations, their greatest value lies in the treatment of lymphocytic leukemias and lymphomas. They are also used in conjunction with radiation therapy to decrease the occur-

BOX 56-4 PRECAUTIONS FOR HANDLING ANTINEOPLASTIC AGENTS

All persons handling cytotoxic (hazardous) drugs, such as antineoplastic agents, should be properly trained in safety procedures and have access to policies and procedures that follow current government and professional practice standards.

DRUG PREPARATION AND ADMINISTRATION

- Wash hands thoroughly and wear a disposable gown, surgical latex gloves, and eye protection when preparing or administering cytotoxic drugs.
- Whenever possible, it is highly recommended that preparation of injectable antineoplastic agents be performed in the clean-air work station or biohazard cabinet in the pharmacy.
- Use areas for the preparation of drugs only for that purpose. Limit access to that area.
- Remove only the required amount of the drug into the syringe. If more is withdrawn accidentally, inject the excess back into the vial and dispose of it properly.
- Vent vials with a 20-gauge needle to avoid the creation of aerosol particles.
- Nurses should not prepare or administer IV chemotherapy if they are pregnant because of suspected risk to the fetus from these agents.

DISPOSAL OF ANTINEOPLASTIC DRUGS AND EQUIPMENT

- All antineoplastic drugs and all vials, needles, syringes, tubing, and equipment used in their administration need to be discarded with caution. Special leak-proof, puncture-proof, double-bagged containers should be used and labeled "biohazard" for disposal by incineration.

- Needles and syringes should not be broken and/or separated before disposal because leakage of the medication may occur.

SPILLAGE OR ANTINEOPLASTIC DRUG CONTACT WITH NURSE OR CLIENT

Spillage

- Wear two pairs of gloves when cleaning up an antineoplastic drug spill. Wash hands before and after.
- Wear a mask and eye protection if the medication is powdered.
- Place the spilled substance in a plastic bag. Wipe up the remainder with a damp cloth and also place in the plastic bag.
- Seal the bag and place it inside of a second bag, and seal the second bag. Label it BIOHAZARD and send it for disposal by incineration.

Drug Contact with Nurse or Client

- Thoroughly wash the affected area with soap and water. If clothing was contaminated, remove clothing immediately.
- If eye contact was made, flush the eyes with copious amounts of water, holding the eyelids open during flushing.

DISPOSAL OF CLIENT EXCRETA

- Urine, vomitus, and other body fluids from clients receiving antineoplastic drugs should be handled with caution. Flush excreta down the toilet; wear gloves to avoid contact. Wash containers thoroughly.

Try to prevent extravasation if at all possible. The vein selected for the chemotherapy infusion should be large, intact, and have a good flow. The best administration site is in the forearm veins (basilic, cephalic, and median antebrachial). Avoid sites in the hand, wrist, etc., because extravasation at these sites could permanently damage nerves, tendons, and muscles. Veins in the vicinity of joints (e.g., the antecubital space) should be avoided to minimize the potential for inadvertent dislodging of the catheter. Dilate veins by wrapping the extremity in warm towels or soaking in warm water rather than using a tourniquet, particularly in older adults or frail clients, because the pressure it creates may rupture the vein wall when you release the tourniquet. Avoid puncturing the same vein more than once; multiple venipunctures promote extravasation if the vein used to administer the drug is distal to the previous site. If unsuccessful in your attempt at venipuncture, select a different vein, preferably in the other arm. If no other vein is available, use an insertion site in the same vein that is proximal to the previous one to prevent extravasation occurring at the so-called upstream venipuncture. The patency of the IV line should be verified before drug administration by flushing with 5 to 10 mL of an isotonic saline or 5% dextrose.

The use of a central venous catheter for infusion of vesicant drugs provides reliable venous access, high flow rates, and rapid drug infusion. However, these vascular access devices are subject to a number of complications, including drug extravasation. The catheter tip may not be properly positioned in the superior vena cava or right atrium, it may migrate out of position, the needle may be improperly inserted into the injection port, or it may rupture.

If extravasation is suspected, stop administration of the chemotherapeutic agent immediately. Leave the IV in place and begin your agency's extravasation procedure. Attempt to aspirate any residual vesicant agent and blood from the IV. Prepare and instill the antidote. Remove the needle. If you are unable to aspirate residual agent from the IV tubing, do not instill the antidote through the existing IV. The amount of antidote used will depend on the size of the extravasation and the amount of the drug believed to be extravasated. Avoid applying direct pressure to the site. Cover lightly with a sterile occlusive dressing. Apply heat or cold as determined by the protocol for the agent that has extravasated. Take measurements of the affected area to use as a point of reference during the healing process. Elevate and rest the area. Notify the physician of the extravasation and the actions taken. The dose should be completed in another vein.

Data from *USP DI: Drug information for the health care professional* (25th ed.). (2005). Greenwood Village, CO: MICROMEDEX Thomson Healthcare.; and Selkin, B.A., & Savarese, D.M.F. (2005). Cutaneous complications of chemotherapy. I. Wellesley, MA: UptoDate.

Data from Catania, P.N. (1999). When patients ask: Home chemotherapy: Basic concepts. *Home Care Provider, 4*(20), 60-61.

Community and Home Health Considerations

Home Administration of Antineoplastic Therapy

Home health care nurses are finding that antineoplastic chemotherapy administration has increased as oncologists have discovered it as a cost-effective means of providing cancer care. However, not all chemotherapeutic agents are appropriate for home administration. Some agents such as cisplatin require rigorous hydration, which might not be feasible at home. Some chemotherapeutic agents commonly administered at home include bleomycin, doxorubicin, etoposide, fluorouracil, methotrexate, plicamycin, and vincristine.

The nurse should be qualified to administer chemotherapy (see guidelines in Chapter 55) and follow the specific policies established by the home health care agency. The client to receive home chemotherapy should also be carefully selected. A client receiving an antineoplastic agent for the first time, one who is historically noncompliant, and the client who has multiple, chronic, unstable health problems are not good candidates for home chemotherapy. The client's support system and physical environment need to be adequate: a qualified care giver is present should the client experience debilitating adverse effects and plumbing and telephone services are available. All chemotherapeutic agents should be prepared by a pharmacist using established guidelines and packaged in a leak-proof container for transport by the nurse. Supplies need to be available in the home to manage extravasation, anaphylaxis, or a chemical spill. For chemical spill instructions, see Chapter 55.

The nurse should review with the client and family the antineoplastic agent to be administered and the planned treatment schedule, and signs and symptoms to report and how to care for the client if they occur. Instruction should be provided about any posttreatment care, such as hydration or medication administration. A 24-hour resource should be available in case the client requires assistance. All of this can be provided in written form to serve as a reference in the home.

The nurse should establish an environment conducive to safe administration, without distractions. The client may be comfortably situated in bed or a reclining chair. It is recommended that the nurse obtain written orders for the treatment of extravasation at the time the chemotherapy orders are received so that the antidote can be administered without delay.

Nurses should reduce their exposure to these agents as much as possible. Latex gloves are preferred to polyvinyl chloride gloves because they are more resistant to needle punctures. Masks and gowns are not required for administration, but a plastic-backed barrier should cover the work surface. All supplies used should be bagged and labeled as toxic waste and returned to the agency or equipment supplier.

Documentation should be done in accordance with agency policy. It is particularly important for the site of the chemotherapy injection and its condition be recorded because the effects of infiltration may not be evident until hours later. If extravasation occurs, record any actions taken to treat the infiltration and the client's response. Record any instructions provided to the client and family to care for the area. If possible, a photograph of the affected area should be obtained to document the degree of tissue damage and provide a guideline for monitoring the site. Recording the client and family response to the therapies will assist in the decision making regarding whether therapy should be continued in the home or moved to another setting.

Antineoplastic chemotherapy can be provided safely in the home through preparation and knowledge of administration and symptom management for the benefit of clients and their families.

---

rence of radiation edema in critical areas such as the superior mediastinum, brain, and spinal cord. Dexamethasone in low doses is also used as part of many antiemetic regimens.

Prednisone has a demonstrated lympholytic and antiinflammatory effect that is useful in the treatment of leukemias, lymphomas, and breast carcinomas. Steroids, especially dexamethasone, are useful in reducing cerebral edema induced by the increasing growth of a brain tumor or from radiation therapy. Chapter 48 discusses individual drugs belonging to this category.

Androgens

Androgens such as testosterone and fluoxymesterone (Halotestin) are used to treat advanced breast carcinoma if surgery, radiation, and other therapies are inappropriate or ineffective. Chapter 53 discusses androgens more fully.

Androgen Antagonists

Androgen antagonists specifically block androgenic activity and are primarily used to treat prostate cancer.

Flutamide is an oral antiandrogenic product that inhibits the uptake and/or the binding of androgens at the target site. The result is suppression of ovarian and testicular steroidogenesis, which induces a medical castration. Bicalutamide competitively inhibits androgens from binding to receptors in target tissues. Nilutamide is an antiandrogen that blocks testosterone effects at the androgen receptor in vitro, and it interacts with the androgen receptor in vivo to prevent normal androgen responses.

flutamide [floo ta myde]
(Eulexin, Euflex✤, Novo-Flutamide✤)
Indications
Flutamide is used in combination with leuprolide (Lupron), a luteinizing hormone–releasing hormone agonist, to treat metastatic

TABLE 56-7 HORMONAL AGENTS USED IN TREATING CANCER

Drug	Route	Indication Breast Cancer	Prostate Cancer	Other Cancer Related Indications
CORTICOSTEROIDS				
prednisone (Deltasone)	PO			Lymphomas, leukemias
dexamethasone (Decadron)	PO, IV			Antiemetic, cerebral edema
ANDROGENS				
fluoxymesterone (Halotestin)	PO	X		
testosterone	PO	X		
testolactone (Teslac)	PO	X		
ANDROGEN ANTAGONISTS				
bicalutamide (Casodex)	PO		X	
flutamide (Eulexin)	PO		X	
nilutamide (Nilandron)	PO		X	
GONADOTROPIC RELEASING HORMONE AGONISTS				
leuprolide (Lupron, others)	Implanted sub-cutaneous, IM		X	
goserelin (Zoladex)	Subcutaneous	X	X	
triptorelin (Trelstar)	IM		X	*Ovarian cancer
ESTROGENS				
diethylstilbestrol (DES, Stilphostrol)	PO, IV		X	
polyestradiol (Estradurin),	PO		X	
ethinyl estradiol (Estinyl)	PO		X	
ESTROGEN-NITROGEN MUSTARD				
estramustine (Emcyt)	PO		X	
SELECTIVE ESTROGEN RECEPTOR MODULATORS (SERMs)				
raloxifene (Evista)	PO	X*		
tamoxifen (Nolvadex)	PO	X		
toremifene (Fareston)	PO	X		
ESTROGEN ANTAGONISTS				
fulvestrant (Faslodex)	IM	X		
AROMATASE INHIBITORS				
anastrozole (Arimidex)	PO	X		
exemestane (Aromasin)	PO	X		
letrozole (Femara)	PO	X		
PROGESTINS				
medroxyprogesterone (Depo-Provera)	PO, IM			Endometrial, renal cancer
megestrol acetate (Megace)	PO	X		Endometrial cancer

*Not an FDA-approved indication.

prostate carcinomas. This combination has been reported to prolong survival by at least 25% as compared with leuprolide therapy alone.

Pharmacokinetics
Flutamide is well absorbed orally, highly protein bound, and eliminated in the urine primarily as metabolites.

Adverse Effects
Adverse effects include diarrhea, impotence, and hepatotoxicity.

bicalutamide [bi kah **loo** tah mide]
(Casodex)
Indications
Bicalutamide is indicated in combination with a luteinizing hormone–releasing hormone for the treatment of advanced prostate cancer.

Pharmacokinetics
Bicalutamide is well absorbed following oral administration and is highly plasma protein bound. It is slowly eliminated via hepatic metabolism.

Adverse Effects
The most common adverse effects observed with bicalutamide are hot flashes, gynecomastia, and breast tenderness.

nilutamide [nye **loo** ta mide]
(Nilandron, Anandron✦)
Indications
Nilutamide is used in conjunction with surgery or chemical castration for the treatment of metastatic prostate cancer. For maximum effect it must be started on the same day as surgical castration.

Pharmacokinetics
Nilutamide is well absorbed orally with active metabolites excreted in the urine and feces.

Adverse Effects
Adverse effects are similar to flutamide and bicalutamide.

Gonadotropic-Releasing Hormone Agonists

The gonadotropin-releasing hormone agonists indirectly serve as antiandrogens by suppressing testicular production of androgens. These drugs are most often used in the treatment of advanced prostate cancer, although occasionally have other indications.

Leuprolide is a synthesized form of luteinizing hormone-releasing hormone or gonadotropic releasing hormone. It suppresses further gonadotropic secretion and serves to suppress luteinizing hormone (LH), follicle stimulating hormone (FSH) levels and subsequently decreases testosterone and estrogen levels. Goserelin is a potent inhibitor of pituitary gonadotropins; the serum levels of testosterone usually drop to the range seen in surgically castrated men within 2 to 4 weeks of initiating drug therapy. Triptorelin, like leuprolide and goserelin, is an analog of gonadotropin releasing hormone and suppresses LH and FSH with a resulting suppression of estrogen and androgen levels.

leuprolide [loo **proe** lide]
(Lupron, Lupron Depot, Viadur, Eligard)
Indications
Leuprolide is indicated for the palliative treatment of advanced prostate cancer and management of endometriosis. It is also used in the treatment of uterine leiomyomata (fibroids) and in the treatment of precocious puberty.

Pharmacokinetics
Leuprolide is administered as a subcutaneous or IM injection depending on formulation. The active drug is metabolized to inactive

metabolites. Formulations are available for monthly, every 3-month, or every 12-month administration.

Adverse Effects
Adverse effects vary depending on gender and age of client and formulation used. Hot flashes, changes in libido, or sexual function, and bone pain are commonly observed effects.

goserelin [gos **er** e lin]
(Zoladex, Zoladex LA✦)
Indications
Goserelin is used for a number of indications, including palliative treatment of advanced breast and prostate cancer, treatment of endometriosis, and dysfunctional uterine bleeding.

Pharmacokinetics
Subcutaneous implant formulations are available for every 1- or 3-month administration. The drug is well absorbed from these implants and peak effects are observed at 1 to 3 weeks after dosing.

Adverse Effects
Adverse effects of goserelin are related to lowered testosterone levels and may include hot flashes, sexual dysfunction, and decreased erections.

triptorelin [trip **tor** e lyn]
(Trelstar)
Indications
Triptorelin is indicated for palliative treatment of advance prostate cancer. It has also been used in the treatment of endometriosis, growth hormone deficiency, hyperandrogenism, ovarian and pancreatic cancer, precocious puberty, treatment of fibroids, and as part of an in vitro fertilization protocol.

Pharmacokinetics
Depot IM injections are available for every 28-day or every 84-day administration.

Adverse Effects
Adverse effects for triptorelin are similar to leuprolide and goserelin.

Estrogens

Estrogens may be used to treat androgen-sensitive prostatic carcinomas in men or advanced breast carcinoma in postmenopausal women. Estrogens such as diethylstilbestrol (DES, Stilphostrol), polyestradiol (Estradurin), and ethinyl estradiol (Estinyl) are used to treat advanced prostate cancer; Chapter 51 discusses estrogens. Estramustine (Emcyt) is a combination of estradiol and nitrogen mustard that provides both a weak hormone effect and an alkylating action. It is used to treat advanced prostatic carcinoma. In this combination, estrogen helps to carry the drug into estrogen receptor cells, thus enhancing the nitrogen mustard cytotoxic effects in these cells.

estramustine [ess tra **muss** teen]
(Emcyt)
Indications
Estramustine is indicated for the palliative treatment of advanced prostate cancer.

Pharmacokinetics
Estramustine is reasonably well absorbed orally and metabolized extensively. Estramustine is taken orally with water preferably an hour before meals. Avoid concurrent consumption of milk, dairy products, or any calcium-containing products.

Adverse Effects
The main precaution in monitoring estramustine is an increased risk of inducing thrombosis, especially in clients with a history of throm-

bophlebitis or thromboembolic disease. Avoid immunizations unless specifically ordered by the prescriber. The client and others in the household should avoid immunization with a live vaccine, such as nasal influenza vaccine.

Antiestrogens

Most breast cancer growth is stimulated by high levels of estrogen; such breast cancers are referred to as estrogen receptor positive or hormone receptor positive. Blocking the effects of estrogens or decreasing estrogen production is a goal of much of the hormonal treatment of breast cancer.

The estrogen antagonists bind to estrogen receptors and display multiple effects. The four antiestrogen agents available are tamoxifen, toremifene, raloxifene, and fulvestrant. Each agent has varying affinity for different estrogen receptors and possesses variable agonist and antagonist activity. As such, these agents are often referred to as selective estrogen receptor modulators (SERMs) and their indications are based on pharmacologic activity.

Tamoxifen (Nolvadex) represents the classic SERM. It is believed to bind to estrogen receptors in breast cancer cells and act as a competitive inhibitor of estrogen. It is effective for tumors that contain high concentrations of estrogen receptors. It is an estrogen agonist in the liver, which has desirable effects on serum lipids in postmenopausal women; it also helps to preserve bone mineral density, which may decrease the risk for osteoporosis in these women. Tamoxifen use is associated with an increased risk for endometrial adenocarcinoma and endometriosis (Chalas et al., 2005). Raloxifene (Evista) is a SERM with lower risk for endometrial cancer than tamoxifen and is indicated for osteoporosis in postmenopausal women. Long-term studies evaluating the effect of raloxifene in breast cancer are underway.

Toremifene (Fareston) is a SERM indicated for metastatic breast cancer. Toremifene is similar to tamoxifen chemically and has a similar pharmacologic effect. The major difference between the agents is that the chronic use of large doses of tamoxifen is hepatotoxic in rats, whereas toremifene does not appear to produce this effect. Both products have a hypocholesterolemic effect after chronic administration. The effect of toremifene on bone mineral density, thromboembolic events, and the risk for endometrial cancer is unknown because of the lack of long-term clinical studies.

Fulvestrant (Faslodex) is a pure antiestrogen compound indicated for hormone receptor positive metastatic breast cancer in postmenopausal women. Fulvestrant is an estrogen antagonist at multiple estrogen receptors. Unlike the SERMs, fulvestrant does not possess any estrogen agonist activity.

✱🎞 tamoxifen [ta **mox** i fen]
(Nolvadex, Apo-Tamox✽, Nolvadex-D✽, Novo-Tamoxifen✽, Tamofen✽, Tamone✽)
Indications
Tamoxifen is indicated as a treatment for breast cancer. It has also been approved to prevent breast cancer in women who are at high risk. *High risk* is defined as women at least 35 years of age with a 5-year predicted risk of breast cancer of at least 1.67% as calculated by the Gail Model Risk Assessment Tool *(Drug Facts and Comparisons,* 2005). The Gail model, first developed and used in 1989, is probably

the most widely employed and quoted risk assessment instrument. In the Gail model, factors affecting breast cancer risk are used to calculate a woman's 5-year and lifetime risk for breast cancer. These factors include age, race, number of first-degree relatives with a history of breast cancer, age at first live birth or nulliparity, age at menarche, number of breast biopsies, and a history of atypical hyperplasia. The relative risk for each of these factors is multiplied to produce a composite risk, i.e., the Gail index.
Pharmacokinetics
Tamoxifen is well absorbed following oral administration and is metabolized by cytochrome P450 3A4.
Adverse Effects
The adverse effects of tamoxifen include hot flashes, weight gain, and endometriosis in women; impotence in men, and nausea, vomiting, and headache in both men and women. Other rare adverse effects include an increased risk for endometrial carcinoma, thromboembolism, and ocular toxicity.

raloxifene [ra **lox** ih feen]
(Evista)
Indications
Raloxifene is currently used to prevent postmenopausal osteoporosis but is also being studied for the treatment of breast cancer (Martino et al., 2004)
Pharmacokinetics
Raloxifene is reasonably well absorbed after oral administration and is extensively metabolized with a high first-pass effect.
Adverse Effects
Adverse effects of raloxifene are similar to tamoxifen and include the risk for thromboembolic events.

toremifene [tor **em** ih feen]
(Fareston)
Indications
Toremifene is an antiestrogen product released in 1998 for the treatment of metastatic breast cancer in postmenopausal women. Toremifene is used to treat estrogen-receptor (ER) positive or ER unknown-type tumors.
Pharmacokinetics
Toremifene is well absorbed orally and metabolized by cytochrome P450 3A4.
Adverse Effects
The adverse effect profile for toremifene is similar to tamoxifen and raloxifene, including hot flashes and the risk for thromboembolic events.

fulvestrant [ful **ves** trant]
(Faslodex)
Indications
Fulvestrant is used for hormone receptor-positive metastatic breast cancer in postmenopausal women.
Pharmacokinetics
Fulvestrant is administered intramuscularly at 1-month intervals. Following IM administration, plasma levels of the drug are sustained for at least 30 days. Like the other agents in this class, it is metabolized by cytochrome P450 3A4.
Adverse Effects
Adverse effects are similar to the SERMs, although the risk for thromboembolic events may be lower.

Aromatase Inhibitors

Aromatase is an enzyme that converts adrenal androgens to estrogen. Although estrogen is produced primarily in the ovary in premenopausal women, estrogen is primarily synthesized in postmenopausal women via aromatase. As such, inhibitors of aromatase are used to reduce estrogen production in post-menopausal women with breast cancer. Numerous studies are indicating these agents may be used as first-line therapy, with results equaling or surpassing the efficacy of the estrogen antagonists or SERMs (Coombes et al, 2004; Piccart-Gebhart, 2004). However, aromatase inhibitors are not indicated for premenopausal women who produce ovarian estrogen. Compared with the selective estrogen receptor modulators (e.g., tamoxifen, raloxifene), the use of aromatase inhibitors is associated with an increased risk for osteoporosis.

✱▥ anastrozole [ah **nas** troe zole]
(Arimidex)
Indications
Anastrozole is indicated for the treatment of advanced and metastatic breast cancer in postmenopausal women.
Pharmacokinetics
Anastrozole is well absorbed orally and metabolized to primarily inactive metabolites. Estradiol reductions are observed during the first week of therapy.
Adverse Effects
Flushing, headache, nausea, muscle weakness, and joint pain are the most commonly observed adverse effects of anastrozole.

exemestane [ex eh **mes** tane]
(Aromasin)
Indications
As with anastrozole.
Pharmacokinetics
Oral absorption of exemestane is variable and improves when taken with a high-fat meal. It is metabolized by cytochrome P450 3A4 but does not appear to interact with other drugs metabolized by this system.
Adverse Effects
As with anastrozole.

letrozole [**le** troe zole]
(Femara)
Indications
As with anastrozole.
Pharmacokinetics
Letrozole is well absorbed and not affected by food. It is metabolized by cytochrome P450 2 A6 and 3A4, but interactions have not been well studied.
Adverse Effects
Adverse effects for letrozole are similar to anastrozole, although coronary and thromboembolic events have been rarely reported.

Progestins

Progestins such as medroxyprogesterone (Depo-Provera) and megestrol (Megace) are used to treat advanced endometrial cancer. It is primarily a palliative approach that seeks tumor regression and an increase in the client's survival time. Megestrol is also indicated for advanced carcinoma of the breast and for the treatment of cachexia in advanced AIDS. Medroxyprogesterone is also used in clients with advanced renal carcinoma. These agents are discussed in Chapter 51.

✱ **R.T., a 72-year-old man, is diagnosed with prostate cancer. Although he is asymptomatic, a magnetic resonance imaging (MRI) of the pelvis reveals prostatic le-sions with several enlarged lymph nodes consistent with metastatic prostate cancer. A bone scan reveals lesions in the lumbar region of the spine. His prostate-specific antigen (PSA) level is 100 mg/mL. R.T. refuses a bilateral orchidectomy that would permanently remove the source of testosterone production. Given the status of R.T.'s cancer, a combined androgen blockage approach is prescribed with leuprolide 22.5 mg IM every 3 months and flutamide 250 mg three times daily.**

Assessment Assess R.T. for preexisting health conditions that would require special monitoring while he was on leuprolide and flutamide. Although his age should be a consideration, neither medication has evidence that its use would be limited in the older adults. Hypersensitivity to either agent must be determined. If R.T. had hepatic function impairment, the use of flutamide is not recommended as he would be at increased risk for hepatotoxicity. Because one of the metabolites of flutamide is a methylaniline derivative, conditions predisposing to aniline toxicity should be identified such as G6PD deficiency, hemoglobin M disease, and smoking, which provide increased risk of aniline exposure. If R.T. has urinary tract obstruction or vertebral metastases, these may worsen in the first few weeks of therapy. R.T. will receive daily injections of leuprolide, rather than the depot injection for the first 2 weeks to gauge his response because this worsening of symptoms sometimes requires discontinuation of therapy; in which case another therapy would be chosen. R.T.'s medication regimen is reviewed for significant interactions. Careful monitoring of R.T. for bleeding, including prothrombin time (PT) or International Normalized Ratio (INR), would be required if he were taking oral anticoagulants; dosages may have to be adjusted. A baseline assessment includes the bone scan and imaging studies that established his diagnosis, hepatic function impairment studies (ALT, AST), serum prostate-specific antigen (PSA) concentrations, and serum testosterone concentrations.

Nursing Diagnosis While R.T. is receiving his current therapy, he is at risk for the following nursing diagnoses: altered comfort (hot flashes, nausea or vomiting, gynecomastia [leuprolide and flutamide]); disturbed sleep pattern (insomnia [leuprolide]); disturbed body image (weight gain, decreased size of testicles [leuprolide]); constipation [leuprolide]; diarrhea [flutamide]; fatigue (anemia related to flutamide); sexual dysfunction (impotence) [both drugs]; and potential complications of leuprolide (anaphylaxis, dysrhythmias, thrombophlebitis, angina or myocardial infarction, pulmonary embolism, and a transient flare up of his prostatic carcinoma) and flutamide (neuropathy, leucopenia, and skin rash).

Planning
During his therapy with leuprolide and flutamide, R.T. will:
- Maintain comfort levels that are acceptable to him.
- Maintain normal body weight with minimal GI adverse effects.
- Remain free of infection.
- Maintain normal bowel pattern.

- Maintain healthy body image while experiencing hot flashes, gynecomastia, testicular changes, and sexual dysfunction.
- Collaborate with health care providers by maintaining scheduled visits for monitoring and treatment and appropriately reporting adverse drug effects.

Implementation

Monitoring Monitor hepatic function tests monthly for the first 4 months of flutamide therapy and every 3 months afterwards. Observe for jaundice, pruritus, persistent anorexia, fatigue, upper right quadrant abdominal tenderness, dark urine, nausea, vomiting, and "flu-like" symptoms as indicators of hepatotoxicity. The PSA is helpful in monitoring response to therapy; if it continues to rise, R.T. should be re-evaluated for disease progression. Periodic bone scans and imaging studies also monitor progress of the disease.

Intervention In the beginning of leuprolide therapy, if R.T. experiences bone pain, treat with analgesics appropriate to his pain level and, if he experiences urinary obstruction, catheterization should be available. These symptoms should subside after the first 2 weeks. His depot injections are given every 3 to 4 months. These formulations are not equivalent to the daily or monthly injections; be cautious in the preparation of this drug for administration. Flutamide should begin simultaneously with, or 24 hours prior to leuprolide therapy.

Education Alert R.T. to report any persistent anorexia, shortness of breath, fever, chills, nausea, vomiting, edema, or jaundice to the prescriber. Stress the importance of complying with the daily schedule for flutamide and the every-3-month schedule for leuprolide depot injections. Caution R.T. that photosensitivity of skin is a possibility with flutamide and to take precautions: avoid sunlight 10 AM to 3 PM, wear sunscreen, long sleeve shirts, and a hat when in the sun. Alert R.T. to changes in body image (gynecomastia, changes in testicular size) and sexual function (decreased libido, impotence) and ensure he receives appropriate counseling.

Evaluation The expected outcome of leuprolide and flutamide therapy is that R.T. will demonstrate signs of clinical improvement, with decreased tumor size and metastases and a normal CBC, and no signs and symptoms of hepatotoxicity. He will remain free of infection, maintain a normal bowel pattern, maintain normal body weight, and experience minimal hot flashes, gynecomastia or sexual dysfunction. R.T. and his family will demonstrate the effective management of the antineoplastic regimen including: pharmacologic and nonpharmacologic measures to control pain, and measures to minimize risk for infection, self-concept disturbances, and sexual dysfunction. R.T. and his family will maintain scheduled visits with the prescriber for monitoring and further treatment.

✲ What are the biologic response modifiers and their role in cancer treatment?

The newest strategies in the treatment of cancers involve the use of agents that modify existing immune or other cellular functions and serve to augment treatment of cancers. These agents vary widely in pharmacologic action, indication, and role in treatment. Selected agents will be briefly discussed. Table 56-8 compares a number of these agents, their class, and major adverse effect profiles.

Immunomodulators

It is well established that the immune system plays an important role in the prevention and development of cancer (Soloski, 2001). **Immunomodulators,** a subtype of biologic response modifiers, typically increase a specified action in the immune system. Agents that stimulate the immune system, including interferon and interleukin-2, are used for a number of cancers, including Kaposi's sarcoma, which is noted in some clients with advanced human immunodeficiency virus (HIV) disease. Levamisole (Ergamisol) is also used to stimulate immune function. These agents are also discussed in Chapter 63.

aldesleukin [al dess **lew** kin]
(interleukin 2, IL-2, T-cell growth factor, Proleukin)
Aldesleukin activates the development and action of T and B cells and natural killer cells. These responses may contribute to the body's response to cancer. Aldesleukin is usually reserved, however, for clients with significant disease not responsive to other interventions and is prescribed with close supervision because of significant complications associated with its use.

Indications
Aldesleukin is indicated for the treatment of metastatic renal cell cancer and melanoma. It is also used investigationally in a number of other conditions, including multiple myeloma, HIV, colorectal cancer, and non-Hodgkin's lymphoma.

Pharmacokinetics
Administered intravenously or by subcutaneous injection, aldesleukin displays an elimination half-life of about 100 minutes.

Adverse Effects
The adverse effect profile of aldesleukin is significant and death has been noted with use. One of the most serious consequences of treatment with aldesleukin is capillary leak syndrome (CLS) with hypotension and diminished organ perfusion. Clients who have reduced cardiac, renal or pulmonary function may be at higher risk for this complication. CLS may present with life-threatening cardiovascular complications (e.g., dysrhythmias, pulmonary congestion, angina), respiratory failure, or renal dysfunction. Numerous other adverse effects are noted with aldesleukin and clinicians should consult appropriate references before use.

✲ interferon alfa-2a [in ter **feer** on **al** fa too aye]
(Roferon-A)
interferon alfa-2b [in ter **feer** on **al** fa too bee]
(Intron-A)
Interferons have a number of actions in the body, including inhibiting cell growth, affecting cell differentiation, and blocking the expression of oncogenes. They also stimulate macrophage and lymphocyte action. In addition to their use in oncology, they are used in the treatment of hepatitis B and C.

Indications
Interferon alfa-2a is indicated for hairy cell leukemia, Kaposi's sarcoma, and hepatitis C in adults and chronic myelogenous leukemia (CML) in children. Interferon alfa 2-b is used in the treatment of hairy cell leukemia, hepatitis C, and Kaposi's sarcoma in adults and in the treatment of hepatitis B in children and adults. Peginterferon alfa-2a is a longer acting injectable form only indicated for hepatitis C in clients with existing hepatic disease.

TABLE 56-8 BIOLOGIC RESPONSE MODIFIERS USED IN TREATING CANCER

Drug	Route	Major Toxicity		Other Toxicities
		Bone Marrow Suppression	**Emetogenic Potential***	
IMMUNOMODULATOR				
Interleukin				
aldesleukin (Proleukin)	IV, subcutaneous	X	M	Cardiotoxicity, capillary leak syndrome
Interferon				
interferon alfa-2a (Roferon-A)	IM	X	NE-L	Clinical depression
interferon alfa-2b (Intron-A)	Subcutaneous, IM, local	X	NE-L	Clinical depression
Immunostimulant				
levamisole (Ergamisol)	PO		L	
MONOCLONAL ANTIBODY				
Binds to CD52 on lymphocytes, monocytes, macrophages, granulocytes				
alemtuzumab (Campath)	IV	X	H	Hypertension, fever
Angiogenesis Inhibitor				
bevacizumab (Avastin)	IV	X	NE	GI, thromboembolic events (Barron, 2004), CVA, hypertension, nephrotoxicity, cardiotoxicity
Epidermal Growth Factor Inhibitor				
cetuximab (Erbitux)	IV		L	Rash
trastuzumab (Herceptin)	IV		L-M	Cardiotoxicity
Binds to CD33 on leukemic blasts				
gemtuzumab ozogamicin (Mylotarg)	IV	X	M-H	GI
Binds to CD20 on B lymphocytes				
ibritumomab tiuxetan (Zevalin)	IV	X	L-M	
rituximab (Rituxan)	IV	X	L	Angioedema
MISCELLANEOUS				
Proteasome Inhibitor				
bortezomib (Velcade)	IV	X	M-H	Edema, fever
Diphtheria Toxin-Interleukin 2				
denileukin diftitox (Ontak)	IV	X	H	Capillary leak syndrome
Tyrosine Kinase Inhibitor				
gefitinib (Iressa)†	PO		L	Rash
imatinib (Gleevec)	PO	X	M-H	Hemorrhage
Retinoid				
bexarotene (Targretin)	PO, topical	X	NE	Fever, weight gain, GI bleeding, teratogenic
tretinoin (Vesanoid)	PO		NE	

CVA, Cardiovascular accident; *GI,* gastrointestinal; *H,* high (frequency 60% to 90%); *L,* low (frequency 10% to 30%); *M,* moderate (frequency 30% to 60%); *NE,* not emetogenic (frequency less than 10%); *VH,* very high (frequency greater than 90%).
*Emetogenic potential varies with dose and concurrent drug therapy.
†Distribution is limited based on conflicting data regarding efficacy (U.S. Food and Drug Administration, 2005).

Pharmacokinetics

Interferon alfa-2a and alfa-2b are each administered by subcutaneous or intramuscular injection and demonstrate elimination half-lives of between 2 and 5 hours.

Adverse Effects

The interferons are commonly associated with psychiatric disturbances (particularly clinical depression and suicidal ideation), fatigue, headache, and dizziness. Hypertension, edema, and chest pain have also been reported. Neutropenia and thrombocytopenia are common, but may be related to concurrent disease in the population receiving the drug. Multiple adverse effects have been attributed to interferon, and clinicians should consult the package insert for a more complete listing of effects.

levamisole [leave **ah** mih sole]
(Ergamisol)
Indications

Levamisole is biologic response modifier (immunostimulant) and is used in combination with fluorouracil (5-FU) to treat colorectal carcinoma (Dukes stage C adenocarcinoma). This combination has resulted in an increased survival time (decreased mortality) and a decreased risk of cancer recurrence.

Pharmacokinetics

Levamisole is well absorbed orally and is metabolized by the liver.

Adverse Effects

Significant adverse effects of levamisole include bone marrow suppression, nausea, diarrhea, metallic taste, arthralgia, and flu-like syndrome.

Monoclonal Antibodies

The use of monoclonal antibodies in a number of medical fields has grown dramatically over the past decade. This technology has allowed specific agents with targeted affinity for a unique receptor type to modulate a limited physiologic response. Monoclonal antibody therapy is used in cardiovascular medicine (abciximab [ReoPro]), GI medicine and rheumatology (infliximab [Remicade]), transplant medicine (OKT3 and daclizumab [Zenapax]), and pulmonary medicine (omalizumab [Xolair]). Their use in oncology is more frequent than other fields, and the target receptors vary with each agent. Multiple monoclonal antibodies are marketed and more or expected over the next decade. Table 56-8 highlights a number of these drugs. Two more commonly used agents will be presented here.

rituximab [rit **ux** ih mab]
(Rituxan)

Rituximab is a genetically made monoclonal antibody that is directed against an antigen (CD20) located on the surface of both normal and malignant B lymphocytes. The CD20 antigen governs the early steps in cell-cycle initiation and differentiation and is found on more than 90% of B-cell non-Hodgkin's lymphomas.

Indications

Rituximab is indicated for the treatment of clients who have relapsed or have a refractory low-grade or follicular, CD20-positive, B-cell, non-Hodgkin's lymphoma.

Pharmacokinetics

Rituximab is administered intravenously. Prolonged action is observed for 3 to 6 months after in IV dose.

Adverse Effects

Adverse effects include fever, chills, weakness, headache, angioedema, hypotension, myalgia, nausea, vomiting, leukopenia, pruritus, and rash.

trastuzumab [tra **stew** zoo mab]
(Herceptin)

Trastuzumab is a monoclonal antibody that binds HER-2, a growth factor identified in approximately 25% to 30% of women with breast cancer. The HER-2 growth factor receptor was identified in certain types of breast cancer and may also be present in other cancers. The use of trastuzumab combined with chemotherapy for the treatment of breast cancer has resulted in an increase in clinical response rate and survival.

Indications

Trastuzumab is indicated for the treatment of metastatic breast cancer in which there is overexpression of the HER-2 protein.

Pharmacokinetics

Trastuzumab is administered via IV infusion and displays a wide variation in elimination half-lives (range, 1 to 32 days)

Adverse Effects

The adverse effects of trastuzumab include chills, fever (usually with the first infusion dose), diarrhea, leukopenia, and infections. One adverse reaction is an increased risk of cardiac dysfunction (heart failure, tachycardia) in approximately 25% of women receiving the combination of trastuzumab and an anthracycline (e.g., doxorubicin [Adriamycin]) and in approximately 7% of women receiving only trastuzumab. Monitor closely for signs and symptoms of cardiovascular dysfunction.

Miscellaneous Biologic Response Modifiers

A number of other agents that modify cell response in cancer are available. Table 56-8 presents many of these, but two are briefly discussed here.

Denileukin diftitox is a recombinant DNA-derived drug that is composed of diphtheria toxin fragments A & B amino acid sequences plus the sequence of interleukin-2. This combination results in higher concentrations of the diphtheria toxin reaching affected malignant T cells in T-cell lymphoma.

Tretinoin is a retinoid that appears to enhance the maturation of primitive promyelocytes from the leukemic clone; this is followed by reseeding the bone marrow and blood with normal blood cells.

denileukin diftitox [den ih **loo** kin **dif** tee tox]
(Ontak)
Indications

It is indicated for the treatment of persistent or recurrent cutaneous T-cell lymphoma.

Pharmacokinetics

Administered intravenously, it is rapidly distributed and eliminated.

Adverse Effects

Denileukin diftitox shares the adverse effect profile and risk for capillary leak syndrome noted above with interleukin-2.

tretinoin [**tret** i noyn]
(Vesanoid, Stieva-A✤, Vitamin A Acid✤)
Indications

Tretinoin is used to treat acute promyelocytic leukemia. Its topical use is described in Chapter 65.

Pharmacokinetics

Orally administered tretinoin is metabolized via the cytochrome P450 system.

Adverse Effects

Adverse effects include headaches, fever, increased weakness, malaise, shivering, infections, hemorrhage, and peripheral edema. Retinoids are contraindicated in pregnancy and women of childbearing age.

What agents are used to reduce toxicity of antineoplastic therapy?

Treatment with antineoplastic agents usually results in significant toxicities including bone marrow suppression with the resultant neutropenia, thrombocytopenia and anemia. It is common to use colony stimulating factors G-CSF, GM-CSF, oprelvekin, and erythropoietin to stimulate neutrophils, macrophages, platelets, and erythrocytes respectively. For drugs with specific toxicities to the bladder, kidney, or heart, specified agents are sometimes used to reduce target organ damage secondary to drug therapy. Such agents include ifosfamide (Ifex) with mesna (Mesnex) to reduce hemorrhagic cystitis. Amifostine (Ethyol) is sometimes used with hydration to reduce cisplatin induced renal damage. Dexrazoxane (Zinecard) may be used with anthracycline therapy to lower the risk of cardiomyopathy. Rasburicase (Elitek) or allopurinol (Zyloprim) is sometimes used to prevent hyperuricemia associated with tumor lysis in some treatments. Chapter 35 discusses erythropoietin (epoetin alfa, recombinant [Epogen]), which is used to treat anemia associated with cancer and Chapter 36 presents allopurinol. The remaining agents are briefly presented here.

Colony Stimulating Factors

filgrastim [fil **gras** tim]
(granulocyte colony-stimulating factor [G-CSF] Neupogen)
pegfilgrastim [peg fil **gras** tim]
(Neulasta)
Filgrastim and pegfilgrastim accelerate neutrophil production, maturation, and activation.

Indications
Both drugs are used to decrease the risk for infection in clients with chemotherapy-induced neutropenia. They are contraindicated in clients who have myeloid cancers because these agents may activate the disease.

Pharmacokinetics
These agents are administered subcutaneously. The elimination half-life of filgrastim is approximately 2 to 4 hours whereas pegfilgrastim has an elimination half-life of 15-80 hours. Increases in neutrophils are expected within 24 to 72 hours of filgrastim therapy, and within the first week of pegfilgrastim.

Adverse Effects
The major adverse effects of G-CSF include nausea, vomiting, alopecia, diarrhea, fevers, mucositis, anorexia, and fatigue. Bone pain is reported approximately 2 to 3 days before the increase in neutrophil count and is usually controlled with nonopioid-type analgesics. Neutrophil counts are closely monitored; the drug should be discontinued when the absolute neutrophil count is 1000/mm³ or more for 3 or more days after the nadir induced by the chemotherapy.

sargramostim [sar **grah** mos tim]
(granulocyte-macrophage colony stimulating factor [GM-CSF], Leukine)
Sargramostim stimulates both granulocytes and macrophage production and maturation. Unlike filgrastim, sargramostim inhibits neutrophil migration.

Indications
Sargramostim is used to accelerate myeloid recovery in persons with acute lymphoblastic leukemia (ALL), Hodgkin's disease, and non-Hodgkin's lymphoma who are undergoing bone marrow transplantation. CBCs are performed to monitor the hematologic response to this drug.

Investigationally this drug has been used to increase the WBC count in clients with AIDS who are receiving zidovudine (AZT) and to correct neutropenia in aplastic anemia. Closely monitor clients who are receiving lithium or corticosteroids concurrently, because the myeloproliferative action of this drug may be increased.

Pharmacokinetics
Increases in WBC are noted in the first 1 to 2 weeks of therapy after IV or subcutaneous injection.

Adverse Effects
Adverse effects of sargramostim are similar to filgrastim, but hypotension, flushing and syncope are often observed on initial dosing. Bone pain may also be more pronounced with sargramostim.

oprelvekin [oh **prel** ve kin]
(Neumega)
Oprelvekin stimulates megakaryocyte production and promotes their proliferation and maturation. This results in increases in platelet levels. Unfortunately, oprelvekin is associated with significant plasma volume expansion and often precipitates edema and the risk for HF. Such concerns limit the use of this agent.

Indications
Oprelvekin is used to prevent severe thrombocytopenia secondary to chemotherapy.

Pharmacokinetics
It is administered subcutaneously and has an elimination half-life of about 6 hours.

Adverse Effects
Cardiovascular effects are the most common and serious with this agent and include peripheral edema, cardiac dysrhythmias, tachycardia, dyspnea, and syncope. Fluid overload is common and may precipitate HF. A decline in erythrocytes is almost universally observed in all clients and may be secondary to altered fluid balance. Other effects include a high rate of nausea and vomiting, rash, dizziness, fever, headache, and insomnia.

Cytoprotective Agents

amifostine [am i **foss** teen]
(Ethyol)
Amifostine is a cytoprotective agent administered before cisplatin to reduce the potential for renal toxicity. It is converted in tissue to an active free thiol metabolite that binds to reactive metabolites of cisplatin.

Indications
Amifostine is used to reduce renal toxicity with concurrent cisplatin therapy. It is also used to reduce xerostomia in clients receiving head and neck radiation therapy.

Pharmacokinetics
Amifostine is administered intravenously and is eliminated quickly with an elimination half-life of 9 minutes.

Adverse Effects
The most common adverse effect is hypotension, noted in approximately two out of three clients receiving therapy. Hypotension is noted early in the course of therapy (usually within 10 to 15 minutes of onset of administration). Other adverse effects include flushing, chills, dizziness, nausea and vomiting, and hiccups.

dexrazoxane [dex ra **zox** ane]
(Zinecard)
Dexrazoxane is an intracellular chelating agent, but its mechanism of action is not clearly defined. There are some reports that the concurrent use of this product with the FAC (5-FU, doxorubicin [Adriamycin], and cyclophosphamide) regimen for breast cancer results in a lower response rate to therapy.

Indications
Dexrazoxane is a cardioprotective substance used with doxorubicin to reduce drug-induced cardiomyopathy. It is only recommended for

clients who have received the cumulative 300 mg/m² dose of dox-orubicin and are continuing to receive anthracycline therapy

Pharmacokinetics
Dexrazoxane is administered intravenously and has an elimination half-life of approximately 2 hours.

Adverse Effects
The adverse effects of dexrazoxane include myelosuppression effects, alopecia, nausea, vomiting, tiredness, anorexia, stomatitis, fever, diarrhea, neurotoxicity, phlebitis, and dysphagia. Refer to a current package insert for more information.

mesna [**mess** na]
(Mesnex, Uromitexan✤)
Mesna is typically used in combination with the alkylating agent ifosfamide to prevent hemorrhagic cystitis associated with ifosfamide therapy.

Indications
Mesna is used to prevent hemorrhagic cystitis caused by ifosfamide therapy.

Pharmacokinetics
Administered orally or intravenously, it has a relatively short elimination half-life of about 30 to 75 minutes.

Adverse Effects
Mesna is well tolerated, although nearly all clients complain of a bad taste in the mouth after dosing.

rasburicase [ras **byoor** ih kayse]
(Elitek)
Rasburicase is a recumbent enzyme that facilitates the conversion of uric acid to an inactive and soluble metabolite. It is used to manage elevated uric acid levels in clients with hyperuricemia secondary to chemotherapy tumor lysis.

Indications
Rasburicase is indicated for the management of uric acid levels in pediatric clients undergoing chemotherapy for leukemia, lymphoma, and solid tumor malignancies.

Pharmacokinetics
Administered intravenously, it displays an elimination half-life of 18 hours.

Adverse Effects
Fever and headache, nausea and vomiting are the most commonly reported adverse effects. Mucositis, abdominal pain, rash, and constipation have also been reported.

✪ **T.C., a 7-year-old boy, is receiving an antineoplastic combination of vincristine, dactinomycin, and cyclophosphamide. Because of the high risk for infection related to neutropenia, each course of the chemotherapy is to be followed by filgrastim (Neupogen) 5 mcg/kg/day subcutaneously for 14 days or until the absolute neutrophil count (ANC) is greater than 1000.**
Filgrastim is used to minimize neutropenia so that the chemotherapy dose intensity can be maintained (Goodin & Henry, 2005). The nursing management of T.C.'s drug regimen will include all of the previous nursing care discussed for the immunocompromised client, in addition to the following.

Assessment A contraindication to filgrastim therapy would be hypersensitivity to the agent, hypersensitivity to *E. coli* proteins, or the presence of excessive leukemic myeloid blasts in the bone marrow or peripheral blood (10% or more). Filgrastim therapy is used in clients with serious underlying disease. A causal relationship between the drug and the adverse effects is not clear, because many adverse effects have been reported in both clients receiving this drug and in clients not receiving the drug. Perform a complete baseline assessment with T.C. to facilitate detecting any change in signs and symptoms that may occur. Hepatic and renal function studies are performed to ensure that there are no underlying impairments. A CBC with differential and platelet counts are done.

Nursing Diagnosis In addition to the nursing diagnoses secondary to T.C.'s antineoplastic therapy, T.C. is at risk for the following nursing diagnoses while receiving filgrastim: impaired comfort (pain at injection site, headache, arthralgias, myalgias,); impaired tissue integrity (thrombophlebitis at the infusion site); impaired skin integrity (vasculitis); and the potential complications of allergic reaction, splenomegaly, dysrhythmias, and pericarditis (dose-limiting).

Planning During his therapy with filgrastim, T.C. and his family will:

- Maintain comfort levels that are acceptable to him.
- Remain free of infection.
- Collaborate with health care providers by maintaining scheduled visits for monitoring and treatment and appropriately reporting adverse drug effects.

Implementation
Monitoring CBCs and platelet counts should be performed twice weekly. Filgrastim therapy is usually discontinued if the absolute neutrophil count (ANC) exceeds 1000/mm³ for 3 or more days. (See Box 29-2 for determination of ANC.) Check T.C.'s blood pressure, because a transient hypotension may occur. Monitor T.C.'s general health status to provide for supportive care.

Intervention If administered to a client receiving chemotherapy, immunomodulator therapy is usually begun at least 24 hours after the last dose of chemotherapy and is discontinued at least 24 hours before the next dose of chemotherapy. With radiotherapy, the timing is 12 hours before and after therapy.

Examine the vial to ensure that the solution is clear and does not contain particulate matter. Do not shake the vial. Keep the medication refrigerated, although it is stable for 6 hours at room temperature. Filgrastim injection is incompatible with sodium chloride-containing solution and may precipitate.

Education If it is determined that T.C. and/or his caregiver can administer the drug in the home safely and effectively, give them the client information supplied by the manufacturer. Give them also instructions on the proper dosage and administration of the drug, including aseptic technique. Provide instruction on the proper safe disposal of needles, syringes, and any unused drug. Reportable symptoms to the prescriber are redness or pain at the injection site, wheezing, fever, sores on the skin, chest pain, irregular or rapid heart rate, and bone pain.

Evaluation The expected outcome of filgrastim therapy for T.C. is that his ANC will exceed 1,000/mm³. T.C. and his family will manage the therapeutic regimen effectively. They will demonstrate measures to minimize risk for infection and other care specific to his other medications.

Summary

The antineoplastic agents act by various mechanisms. Most agents interfere with cell reproduction or replication at some point in the cell cycle. They are classified into various groups based on their probable mechanisms of action: antimetabolites, alkylating agents, mitotic inhibitors, antibiotic antitumor agents, hormones, cytoprotective and immunomodulator agents, and miscellaneous agents. Because the drugs are nonselective and affect all cells in the body as they replicate, there is always some degree of injury to normal cells. Cells with a high rate of growth (e.g., bone marrow, GI epithelium, and hair follicles) are particularly susceptible. Bone marrow depression with the resultant anemia, leukocytopenia, and thrombocytopenia is unavoidable, and therefore laboratory values for blood counts are used to titrate the individual client's dosage and to determine when the client is most susceptible to infection and hemorrhage.

Much of the nursing management of antineoplastic therapy is to prevent injury and infection; promote comfort; provide care for the GI effects of stomatitis, nausea, and vomiting and changes in bowel elimination; and assess for the development of bone marrow suppression, nephrotoxicity, neurotoxicity, cardiotoxicity, pulmonary toxicity, and dermatologic effects. Although short-term and long-term toxicities occur, the potential for cure or a reduction of symptoms is a benefit that most often outweighs the risk and discomfort of the administration.

Bibliography

American Cancer Society (ACS), Centers for Disease Control and Prevention (CDC), the National Cancer Institute (NCI), & North American Association of Central Cancer Registries (NAACCR). (2004). *Annual report to the nation on the status of cancer, 1975-2001.* Retrieved March 1, 2005, from http://www.cancer.gov/statistics.

⊛ **Critical Thinking Questions**

- Mr. Alan Hale, 48 years old, suddenly develops a high fever and petechiae on his chest and arms. After bone marrow aspiration, he is diagnosed with acute lymphocytic leukemia. The oncologist puts Mr. Hale on a regimen that contains vincristine (Oncovin). For what nursing diagnoses is Mr. Hale at risk? What laboratory values should the nurse monitor? If Mr. Hale develops a tingling in his fingers and toes, what might be occurring?

- Mrs. Hextall is returning home after a series of antineoplastic chemotherapies. In discussing her home arrangements for care, she indicates that there should be no problem. Her daughter, who has moved back in with her along with her 3-month-old granddaughter, will care for her. Given Mrs. Hextall's altered protection status, what concerns might the nurse have about this arrangement?

- Given that the antineoplastic agents have a number of potential complications, how would the nurse monitor the client receiving a relevant antineoplastic agent for cardiotoxicity? For neurotoxicity? For nephrotoxicity?

Anderson, D.M., Keith, J., & Novak, P.D. (Eds.) (2002). *Mosby's medical, nursing, and allied health dictionary* (6th ed.). St. Louis: Mosby.

Balmer, C.M., & Valley, A.W. (2002). Cancer treatment and chemotherapy. In J.T. DiPiro, R.L. Talbert, G.C. Yee, G.R. Matzke, B.G. Wells & L.M. Posey (Eds.), *Pharmacotherapy: A pathophysiological approach* (5th ed.). Norwalk, CT: Appleton & Lange.

Barron, H. (January 5, 2004). Important Drug Warning - Dear Health Provider Letter. South San Francisco: Genentech, Inc. Retrieved January 22, 2005, from http://www.fda.gov/medwatch/SAFETY/2005/Avastin_dearhcp.pdf.

Berczi, I., Bertok, L., & Chow, D. A. (2000). Natural immunity and neuroimmune host defense. *Annals of the New York Academy of Science, 917,* 248.

Bosker, G. (Ed.). (2004). *Primary and acute care medicine: Practice, protocols, pathways,* (2nd ed.). Atlanta: Thomson American Health Consultants.

Catania, P.N. (1999). When patients ask: Home chemotherapy: Basic concepts. *Home Care Provider, 4*(2), 60-61.

Chalas, E., Costantino, J.P., Wickerham, D.L., Wolmark, N., Lewis, G.C., Bergman, C., et al. (2005). Benign gynecologic conditions

---

 e-**LEARNING SUPPLEMENTS**

Student CD-ROM
- Final Exam questions
- NCLEX® Examination review questions
- Pharmacology animations
- Printable chapter summary

Evolve Website (http://evolve.elsevier.com/mckenry)
- Case study on antineoplastic chemotherapy agents
- Content updates, including information on new drugs

- WebLinks corresponding to this chapter
- Answers to the critical thinking questions in this chapter
- *Elsevier ePharmacology Update* newsletter
- Mosby's Drug Consult Internet Edition
- Supplemental and reference information

among participants in the Breast Cancer Prevention Trial. *American Journal of Obstetrics and Gynecology, 192,* 1230-1237.

Chang, J.T., & Altman, R.B. (2004). Extracting and characterizing gene-drug relationships from the literature. *Pharmacogenetics, 14*(9):577-586, retrieved December 2, 2004, from http://bionlp.stanford.edu/genedrug/gene_drug_predictions.html.

Coombes, R.C., Hall, E., Gibson, L.J., Paridaens, R., Jassem, J., & Delozier, T., et al., and the Intergroup Exemestane Study. (2004). A randomized trial of exemestane after two to three years of tamoxifen therapy in postmenopausal women with primary breast cancer. *New England Journal of Medicine, 350,* 1081-1092.

Dally, H., Edler, L., Jager, B., Schmezer, P., Spiegelhalder, B., & Dienemann, H., et al. (2003). The CYP3 A4*1 B allele increases risk for small cell lung cancer: effect of gender and smoking dose. *Pharmacogenetics, 13*(10), 607-618.

Davis, L., & Lindley, C. (2005). Neoplastic disorders and their treatment: General principles. In M.A. Koda-Kimble, L.Y. Young, W.A. Kradjan, B.J. Guglielmo, B.K. Alldredge, & R.L. Corelli (Eds.), *Applied therapeutics: The clinical use of drugs* (8th ed.). Philadelphia: Lippincott Williams & Wilkins.

Donnelly, J.G. (2004). Pharmacogenetics in cancer chemotherapy: Balancing toxicity and response. *Therapeutic Drug Monitoring, 26*(2), 231-235.

Drug facts and comparisons (58th ed.). (2005). St. Louis: Facts and Comparisons.

Elkin, E.B., Weinstein, M.C., Winer, E.P., Kuntz, K.M., Schnitt, S.J., & Weeks, J.C. (2004). HER-2 testing and trastuzumab therapy for metastatic breast cancer: A cost-effectiveness analysis. *Journal of Clinical Oncology, 22*(5), 854-863.

Goodin, S., & Henry, D.W. (2005). Solid tumors. In M.A. Koda-Kimble, L.Y. Young, W.A. Kradjan, B.J. Guglielmo, B.K. Alldredge, & R.L. Corelli (Eds.), *Applied therapeutics: The clinical use of drugs* (8th ed.). Philadelphia: Lippincott Williams & Wilkins.

Hardman, J.G., & Limbird, L.E. (Eds.). (2001). *Goodman & Gilman's The pharmacological basis of therapeutics* (10th ed.). New York: McGraw-Hill.

Innocenti, F., Undevia, S.D., Iyer, L., Chen, P.X., Das, S., & Kocherginsky, M., et al. (2004). Genetic variants in the UDP-glucuronosyltransferase 1 A1 gene predict the risk of severe neutropenia of irinotecan. *Journal of Clinical Oncology, 22*(8), 1382-1388.

Kitagawa, C., Ando, M., Ando, Y., Sekido, Y., Wakai, K., & Imaizumi, K., et al. (2005). Genetic polymorphism in the phenobarbital-responsive enhancer module of the UDP-glucuronosyltransferase 1 A1 gene and irinotecan toxicity. *Pharmacogentics & Genomics, 15*(1), 35-41.

Lacy, C.F., Armstrong, L.L., Goldman, M.P., & Lance, L.L. (2004). *Lexi-Comp's Drug Information Handbook* (12th ed.). Hudson, Ohio: Lexi-Comp.

Lammers, L. (April 2005). Dear Healthcare Professional letter: Novantrone. Rockland, MA: Serono.

Lindley, C. (2005). Adverse effects of chemotherapy. In M.A. Koda-Kimble, L.Y. Young, W.A. Kradjan, B.J. Guglielmo, B.K. Alldredge, & R.L. Corelli (Eds.), *Applied therapeutics: The clinical use of drugs* (8th ed.). Philadelphia: Lippincott Williams & Wilkins.

Lippman, S.M., Sudbo, J., & Hong, W.K. (2005). Oral cancer prevention and the evolution of molecular-targeted drug development. *Journal of Clinical Oncology, 23*(2), 346-356.

Martino, S., Cauley, J.A., Barrett-Connor, E., Powles, T.J., Mershon, J., & Disch, D., et al., and the CORE Investigators. (2004). Continuing outcomes relevant to Evista: Breast cancer incidence in postmenopausal osteoporotic women in a randomized trial of raloxifene. *Journal of the National Cancer Institute, 96,* 1751-1761.

Michael, M., & Doherty, M.M. (2005). Tumoral drug metabolism: Overview and its implications for cancer therapy. *Journal of Clinical Oncology, 23*(1), 205-229.

Mocellin, S., Provenzano, M., Rossi, C.R., Pilati, P., Nitti, D., & Lise, M. (2005). DNA array-based gene profiling: From surgical specimen to the molecular portrait of cancer. *Annals of Surgery, 241*(1), 16-26.

Mosby's drug consult (15th ed.). (2005). St. Louis: Mosby.

National Cancer Institute of Canada. (2004). *Canadian cancer statistics 2002.* Retrieved September 13, 2004, from http://www.hc-sc.gc.ca/pphb-dgspsp/publicat/ccs-scc02/pdf/stats2002 _e.pdf.

Parnes, H.L., Thompson, I.M., & Ford, L.G. (2005). Prevention of hormone-related cancers: Prostate cancer. *Journal of Clinical Oncology, 23*(2), 368-377.

Piccart-Gebhart, M.J. (2004). New stars in the sky of treatment for early breast cancer. *New England Journal of Medicine, 350,* 1140-1142.

Rugo, H.S. (2003). Cancer. In L.M. Tierney, Jr., S.J. McPhee & Papadakis, M.A. (Eds.), *Current Medical Diagnosis & Treatment.* New York: Lange Medical Books/McGraw-Hill.

Shah, N.P., Tran, C., Lee, F.Y., Chen, P., Norris, D., & Sawyers, C.L. (2004). Overriding imatinib resistance with a novel ABL kinase inhibitor. *Science, 305,* 399-401.

Smyth, M.J., Godfrey, D.I., & Trapani, J.A. (2001). A fresh look at tumor immunosurveillance and immunotherapy. *Natural Immunology, 2,* 293.

Soloski, M.J. (2001). Recognition of tumor cells by the innate immune system. *Current Opinion in Immunology, 13,* 154.

Spitz, M.R., Wu, X., & Mills, G. (2005). Integrative epidemiology: From risk assessment to outcome prediction. *Journal of Clinical Oncology, 23*(2), 267-275.

U.S. Food and Drug Administration. (2005). FDA Public Health Advisory: New labeling and distribution program for gefitinib (Iressa). Retrieved July 17, 2005, from http://www.fda.gov/cder/drug/advisory/iressa.htm.

USP DI: *Drug information for the health care professional* (25th ed.). (2005). Greenwood Village, CO: MICROMEDEX Thomson Healthcare.

van Schaik, R.H. (2004). Implications of cytochrome P450 genetic polymorphisms on the toxicity of antitumor agents. *Therapeutic Drug Monitoring, 26*(2), 236-240.

57

OVERVIEW OF INFECTIONS, INFLAMMATION, AND FEVER

CHAPTER FOCUS

Fever, inflammation, and infection have been a concern to those caring for the ill and injured since ancient times. The majority of clients are at risk for infection, not only as a direct result of injury or illness, but also as an indirect consequence of multiple invasive devices, surgical procedures, and immunosuppression. Nurses have the responsibility of assessing these clients, decreasing their risk for infection, palliating symptoms of infection through drug therapy and nonpharmacologic interventions, and the evaluating the effectiveness of these therapies.

LEARNING OBJECTIVES

- Describe the mediators of the inflammatory system.
- Identify different types of fever.
- Explain the body's set point temperature mechanism.
- Describe the goal and mechanisms of action of antimicrobial therapy.
- Identify the general adverse effects of antimicrobial drugs.
- Describe general guidelines for the optimal use of antimicrobial agents.
- Implement the nursing management for a client receiving antimicrobial therapy.

▲ KEY TERMS

bacteremia, p. 997
bactericidal agents, p. 1001
bacteriostatic agents, p. 1001
colonization, p. 997
empiric therapy, p. 1004
infection, p. 995
inflammation, p. 997

microorganisms, p. 997
phagocytosis, p. 998
resistance, p. 1004
sepsis, p. 997
septicemia, p. 997
superinfection, p. 997

✳ What constitutes an infection?

Infectious diseases comprise a wide spectrum of illnesses caused by pathogenic microorganisms. Table 57-1 lists some common pathogens and their most likely sites of infection in the body. These pathogens are responsible for a number of conditions, including pneumonia, urinary tract infections (UTI), upper respiratory tract infections (UTIs), gastroenteritis, venereal disease, vaginitis, tuberculosis (TB), and candidiasis.

Infection is the invasion and multiplication of pathogenic microorganisms in body tissues; these microorganisms cause disease by local cellular injury, secretion of a toxin, or an

TABLE 57-1 COMMON PATHOGENS AND MOST LIKELY SITES OF INFECTION

Organism	Likely Infection Site
GRAM-POSITIVE COCCI	

Staphylococcus aureus
   Nonpenicillinase producing
   Penicillinase producing
   Methicillin resistant
 Staphylococcus epidermidis
   Nonpenicillinase producing
   Penicillinase producing
	Burns, skin, decubital and surgical wounds, paranasal and middle ear (chronic sinusitis and otitis), lungs, lung abscess, pleura, endocardium, bone (osteomyelitis), and joints

Streptococcus pneumoniae	Paranasal area and middle ear, lungs, pleura
Streptococcus pyogenes (group A β-hemolytic)	Burns, skin infections, pressure ulcers and surgical wounds, paranasal and middle ear, throat, bone (osteomyelitis), and joints
Streptococcus viridans group	Endocardium
GRAM-POSITIVE BACILLI	
Clostridium tetani (anaerobe)	Puncture wounds, lacerations, and crush injuries; toxins affecting nervous system
Corynebacterium diphtheriae	Throat, upper part of respiratory tract
GRAM-NEGATIVE COCCI	
Neisseria gonorrhoeae	Urethra, prostate, epididymis and testes, joints
Neisseria meningitides	Meninges
ENTERIC GRAM-NEGATIVE BACILLI	
As a group (*Bacteroides, Enterobacter, Escherichia coli, Klebsiella pneumoniae, Proteus mirabilis, other Proteus, Salmonella, Serratia, Shigella*)	Peritoneum, biliary tract, kidney and bladder, prostate, decubital and surgical wounds, bone
Bacteroides	Brain abscess, lung abscess, throat, peritoneum
Enterobacter	Peritoneum, biliary tract, kidney and bladder, endocardium
Escherichia coli	Peritoneum, biliary tract, kidney and bladder
Klebsiella pneumoniae	Lungs, lung abscess
OTHER GRAM-NEGATIVE BACILLI	
Haemophilus influenzae	Meninges, paranasal and middle ear, lungs, pleura
Pseudomonas aeruginosa	Burns, paranasal area and middle ear, (chronic otitis media), decubital and surgical wounds, lungs, joints, kidney, bladder
ACID-FAST BACILLI	
Mycobacterium avium *Mycobacterium tuberculosis*	Lungs, pleura, peritoneum, meninges, kidney and bladder, testes, bone, joints
MYCOPLASMAS	
Mycoplasma pneumoniae	Lungs

TABLE 57-1 COMMON PATHOGENS AND MOST LIKELY SITES OF INFECTION—*cont'd*	
Organism	**Likely Infection Site**
SPIROCHETES	
Treponema pallidum (syphilis)	Any tissue or vascular organ of the body
FUNGI	
Aspergillus	Paranasal area and middle ear, lungs
Candida species *Cryptococcus*	Skin infections, throat, lungs, endocardium, kidney and bladder, vagina
VIRUSES	
Human immunodeficiency virus (HIV)	T cells and macrophages (see Chapter 59)
Herpes virus or varicella-zoster virus	Skin infections (herpes simplex or zoster)
Enterovirus, mumps virus, and others	Meninges, epididymis, and testes
Respiratory viruses (including Epstein-Barr virus)	Throat, lungs
ANAEROBES	

Gram-positive
  Clostridium difficile*
  Clostridium perfringens
  Clostridium tetani**
  Peptococcus species
  Peptostreptococcus species***
Gram-negative
  Bacteroides fragilis
  Fusobacterium species***
	Deep wounds, gut, crush injuries.
	*Antibacterial-associated colitis
	**Toxins affect nervous system
	***More common as oral/dental pathogens and in aspiration pneumonia

antigen-antibody reaction in the host. An infection can be classified primarily as either local or systemic. A localized infection may involve the skin or internal organs and may progress to a systemic infection. A systemic infection involves the entire body rather than a localized area of the body. Several terms describe the degree of local or systemic infection.

Colonization is the localized presence of microorganisms in body tissues or organs, which can be pathogenic or part of the normal flora. Colonization alone is not necessarily an infection but rather signifies the potential for infection depending on multiplication of the microorganisms or reduction in the defense mechanisms of the host. When flora at their normal colonization site are altered (e.g., by administration of an antimicrobial that affects pathogens and some but not all normal microorganisms), unaffected microorganisms within that environment may grow uninhibited and cause a secondary infection. This secondary infection is sometimes referred to as a **superinfection.**

Inflammation is a protective mechanism of body tissues in response to invasion or toxins produced by colonizing microorganisms. This reaction consists of cytologic and histologic tissue responses for the localization of phagocytic activity and the destruction or removal of injurious material, leading to repair and healing.

Bacteremia is the presence of viable bacteria in the circulatory system. **Septicemia** refers to a systemic infection caused by the multiplication of microorganisms in the circulation. Although bacteremia may lead to septicemia in the immunocompromised host, it is usually a short-lived, self-limited process (depending on the pathogen). In an immunocompromised host, bacteremia may rapidly produce an overwhelming systemic disease. **Sepsis** is a syndrome in which multiple organ systems are involved as a result of the circulation of microorganisms or their toxins in the blood.

In immunocompetent hosts, antimicrobial therapy is seldom required to treat the colonization of nonpathogenic organisms or transient bacteremia without tissue invasion; however, prophylactic antimicrobial therapy may be required in immunocompromised hosts. In most cases of localized inflammation (e.g., wound infections, pneumonia, or UTI), antimicrobials reduce the number of viable pathogens. This permits the immune system to eliminate the microorganisms. Antimicrobials are also an essential part of the treatment of septicemia and sepsis.

Microorganisms are divided into several groups: bacteria, mycoplasmas, spirochetes, fungi, and viruses. Bacteria are classified according to their shape (e.g., bacilli, spirilla, and cocci) and their capacity to be stained. The specific identification of bacteria requires a Gram stain and culture with chemical testing. A Gram stain is a sequential procedure that involves crystal violet and iodine solutions followed by alcohol. It allows the rapid identification of organisms into groups, such as gram-positive or gram-negative rods or cocci. Culture procedures require at least 24 to 48 hours for completion to identify specific organisms. For a few slow-growing pathogens, like tuberculosis, gram stain is particularly important in initial identification, because 6 to 12 weeks may be required for identification using culture techniques.

Often the initial or empiric antibacterial selection is based on the prescriber's clinical impression plus the Gram stain procedure; if necessary, the antibacterial may be changed once culture and sensitivity results are available. The purpose of culture and sensitivity testing is to ensure correct identification of the microorganism and its sensitivity or resistance to various antiinfectives.

✳ What is the role of inflammation in infections?

Inflammation is the reaction of body tissues to injury, such as physical trauma, foreign bodies, chemical substances, surgery, radiation, and electricity. The affected area undergoes a series of changes as bodily processes attempt to wall off, heal, and/or replace the injured tissue. For example, after an injury the body releases chemical substances into the tissue to form a wall called a chemotactic gradient. Fluids and cells begin to move toward this area.

Blood vessels dilate within 30 minutes of the insult, which provides for increased blood flow and exudation of fluid from blood vessels into the injured tissues. The exudate includes protein-rich fluids that are high in fibrinogen and attract other substances to the area, such as complement, antibodies, and leukocytes. The collection of fluids in this area results in edema or swelling. In general, this occurs within 4 hours of the injury. The degree and site of this response can lead to further pathology. Inflammation in lung infection, for example, leads to the classic fluid accumulation of pneumonia and contributes to worsening gas exchange.

✳ What are the cellular mediators of infection?

Neutrophils, monocytes (macrophages), and lymphocytes (which arrive later) are the cells that affect the injured area. During the cellular phase, granulocytes migrate from the dilated blood vessels toward the chemotactic site and accumulate in the area of injury. If the injury is a foreign substance or bacteria, they will engulf and destroy the foreign material (**phagocytosis**). The phagocytosis process tends to localize or wall off the foreign material to prevent its spread through the tissues. Large numbers of phagocytes lead to the accumulation of pus and the eventual destruction and removal of the foreign material.

Some pathogens are resistant to destruction and are only walled off; an example is the tuberculosis bacillus, which can live for many years within confined areas in the body. Other pathogens may transform from a local infection into a systemic infection and require antimicrobial treatment.

✳ What are the chemical mediators of infection?

The complement system is composed of complement components (18 distinct proteins and their cleavage products) that are present in the blood in the form of inactive proteins called zymogens. Complement is essential in reacting to an acute inflammatory state caused by bacteria, certain viruses, and immune complex diseases. Complement enhances chemotaxis, increases blood vessel permeability, and eventually causes cell lysis.

Histamine, prostaglandins, arachidonic acid, and leukotrienes are other mediators capable of producing local reactions, smooth muscle contraction, increased chemotaxis, blood vessel vasodilation, and other inflammatory effects. When the foreign agent is destroyed, the resulting debris is removed by the macrophages and neutrophils, and the inflammatory reaction is resolved.

In severe infection, as is sometimes seen in overwhelming sepsis, the combination of triggered complement bacterial endotoxins and/or other mediators can lead to septic shock and may progress to disseminated intravascular coagulation (DIC). These conditions require management in a critical care setting and carry a high risk for multiorgan failure and death.

✳ What is the role of fever?

The hypothalamic thermoregulatory center is responsible for setting body core temperature. It is influenced by action at α-adrenergic, dopaminergic, and serotonergic receptors. The hypothalamus sets the point at which body temperature is maintained, but body temperature regulation depends on a balance between heat production and heat loss. Fever may result from an infection or an inflammatory process or it may be caused by release of endogenous pyrogens from microorganisms or macrophages. These pyrogens, or fever-producing substances, interfere with the temperature-regulating centers located in the hypothalamus, which raises the thermostat set point. The body may respond to pyrogens by increasing the formation of cytokines. A number of cytokines, including tumor necrosis factor, interferon, interleukin 1 (α and β), and interleukin 6 may be involved (Table 57-2). The interplay of cytokines and epithelial cells lead to increased synthesis of prostaglandin (PGE_2), which then increases the hypothalamic set point (Cuddy, 2004). The body reacts by conserving heat through vasoconstriction, piloerection (goose flesh), and shivering—all of which increase the body temperature.

Normal body temperature is 98.6°F (37°C); the normal range is 97°F to approximately 99°F when measured orally; it is 1°F higher when measured rectally. Hyperthermia occurs when the temperature of the body rises above normal. Seizures often result when body temperature reaches 106°F, and any elevated temperature can increase seizure risk in predisposed individuals with a history of seizure activity. If the body's thermoregulatory mechanisms have trouble returning the body temperature to normal, body metabolism may increase so rapidly that the body cannot regulate its own heat production. At 108°F, tissue damage occurs and cells begin to die; this results in irreversible brain damage.

TABLE 57-2 EXAMPLES OF CYTOKINES INVOLVED IN INFLAMMATION AND FEVER		
Cytokine	**Source**	**Function**
Interferon Gamma (INF-γ)	Natural killer cells T-helper cells	Activates macrophages Promotes T-cell differentiation
Interleukin-1 (IL-1)	Macrophages	Prostaglandin synthesis T-cell production Enhances production of other cytokines
Interleukin-6 (IL-6)	Macrophages Monocytes	Protein synthesis B cell differentiation T-cell production
Tumor Necrosis Factor (TNF)	Macrophages Monocytes	Increases endothelial permeability Enhances neutrophil release from bone marrow toxic to cells

Modified from Gosain, A., Gamelli, R. (2005). A primer in cytokines. *Journal of Burn Care & Rehabilitation,* 26(1), 7-12.

Several types of fever are known. For example, a *constant* fever that rises or falls only a few degrees above or below a specified point is seen with typhoid fever. An *intermittent* fever may return to normal once or several times in 24 hours. This type of fever is associated with pyogenic infections, abscesses, lymphomas, tuberculosis, and drug reactions. A *remittent* fever fluctuates but does not usually return to normal; this occurs in many viral and bacterial infections. A *relapsing* fever consists of afebrile episodes of one or more days between fevers, such as in malaria and Hodgkin's disease.

Fever of unknown origin (FUO) is described as a temperature greater than 103°F that is recorded daily for more than 2 weeks in a client with an uncertain diagnosis after a week's evaluation in a hospital setting. Most clients with FUO are later found to have an infection, neoplasm, or connective tissue disease.

Body temperature is regulated by feedback mechanisms of the nervous system through a temperature-regulating center in the hypothalamus. When the hypothalamus is no longer in contact with the pyrogens, it resets the temperature to the normal set point. Prostaglandins of the E series produced in response to endogenous pyrogens act on the anterior hypothalamus to increase the set point, resulting in fever. Drugs that inhibit the synthesis of E prostaglandins have antipyretic activity (e.g., acetaminophen, salicylates). Salicylates reduce fever by causing the hypothalamic center to reestablish a normal set point. Heat production will not be inhibited, but heat loss will be increased by an increase in cutaneous blood flow and sweating caused by the lowered thermostat (Figure 57-1). Antibacterials indirectly reduce temperature by destroying the bacteria that are causing the fever. As such, fever is a common monitoring parameter in judging the success of antimicrobial therapy (Cuddy, 2004).

⚙ **What agents are available to treat infectious diseases?**
Treatment of an infectious disease depends on the microorganism; different groups of antimicrobial agents are used to

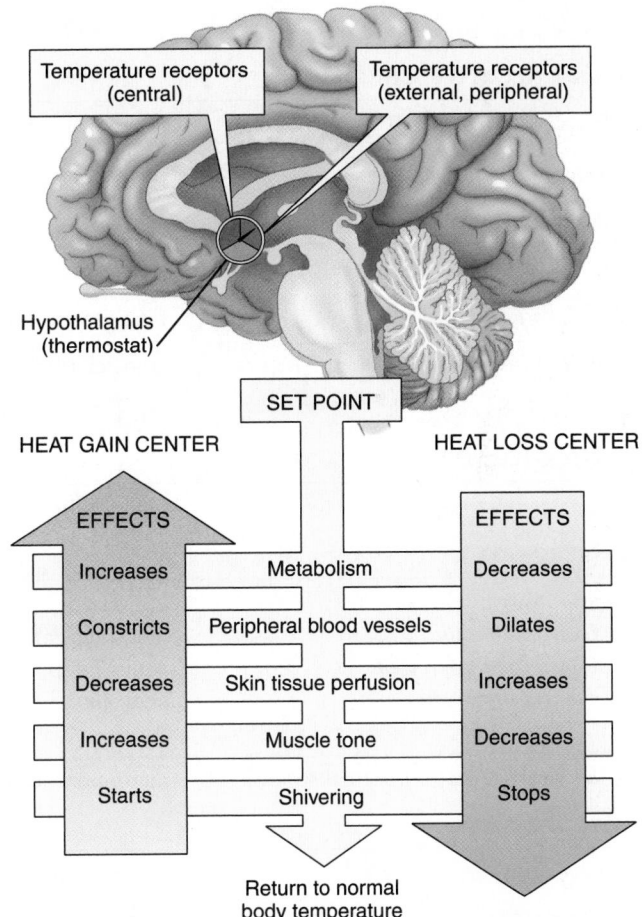

FIGURE 57-1 Set-point temperature mechanism.

treat different groups of microorganisms. Table 57-3 lists some antimicrobial agents used in the treatment of infectious diseases. Antimicrobial drugs can help cure or control most infections caused by microorganisms, but they alone do not necessarily produce the cure. They are adjuncts to methods such as surgical incision and drainage or wound debridement, which remove nonviable, infected tissue.

TABLE 57-3 ANTIMICROBIAL AGENTS TO TREAT VARIOUS GROUPS OF MICROORGANISMS

Organism	Antimicrobial Agent
GRAM-POSITIVE COCCI	
Staphylococcus aureus	
Nonpenicillinase producing	penicillin G or V
Penicillinase producing	First-generation cephalosporins, cloxacillin, dicloxacillin, methicillin,
Methicillin resistant	vancomycin
Streptococcus pneumoniae	penicillin G or V, ampicillin, first-generation cephalosporins
Streptococcus pyogenes (group A)	penicillin G or V
Streptococcus (group B)	penicillin G, ampicillin
Streptococcus viridans	penicillin G ± gentamicin
GRAM-POSITIVE BACILLI	
Bacillus anthracis	penicillin G, erythromycin
Corynebacterium diphtheriae	erythromycin
Corynebacterium, JK strain	vancomycin, erythromycin
Listeria monocytogenes	ampicillin
GRAM-NEGATIVE COCCI	
Neisseria gonorrhoeae	ceftriaxone, cefixime
Neisseria meningitides	penicillin G, cefotaxime
GRAM-NEGATIVE ENTERIC BACILLI	
Escherichia coli	First-generation cephalosporins, fluoroquinolones, sulfamethoxazole/trimethoprim
Klebsiella pneumoniae	First-generation cephalosporins, fluoroquinolones, sulfamethoxazole/trimethoprim
Proteus mirabilis	amoxicillin/clavulanate, second and third generation cephalosporin
Salmonella species	ceftriaxone, fluoroquinolone
OTHER BACILLI	
Pseudomonas aeruginosa	piperacillin, ticarcillin, tobramycin, + fluoroquinolone
ANAEROBES	
Gram-positive	
Clostridium difficile	metronidazole, vancomycin
Clostridium perfringens	penicillin G, metronidazole
Clostridium tetani	penicillin G, tetracycline
Gram-negative	
Bacteroides (gastrointestinal strains)	metronidazole, clindamycin, piperacillin, ticarcillin
MYCOPLASMAS	
Mycoplasma pneumoniae	azithromycin, erythromycin, tetracycline, clarithromycin, fluoroquinolone
SPIROCHETES	
Treponema pallidum (syphilis)	penicillin G
FUNGI	
Aspergillus, Candida species	amphotericin B, fluconazole, itraconazole
VIRUSES	
Herpes simplex	acyclovir

Modified from Gilbert, D.N., Moellering, R.C., Eliopoulos, G.M., & Sande, M.A. (2004). *The Sanford Guide to Antimicrobial Therapy* 2004 (34th ed.). Hyde Park, VT: Antimicrobial Therapy, Inc.

The first major antimicrobial agents were the sulfonamides, whereas the second group consisted of true antibiotics such as penicillin. Antibiotics are natural substances derived from certain organisms (e.g., bacteria, fungus) that are used against infections caused by other organisms. The term antibiotic (literally "against life") is also used for other agents that are used to cause cell lysis (e.g., in the treatment of cancers). As such, the term "antibiotic" can sometimes be confusing. For the remainder of this unit, terms more reflective of the action of these agents will be used. These terms include antimicrobial (drugs deterring growth or causing lysis of microorganisms), antibacterial (drugs with activity against bacteria), antiprotozoan, antiviral, and antifungal. Agents that alter the ability of organisms to grow in a specific localized area are often termed antiseptics (e.g., topical antiseptics, urinary tract antiseptics). As a result of research, there are now many synthetic and semisynthetic antimicrobial agents.

✱ **What are the mechanisms of action of antimicrobials?**
The goal of antimicrobial therapy is to destroy or suppress the growth of infecting microorganisms so that normal host defenses and other supporting mechanisms can control the infection, resulting in its cure. To exert their effects, antimicrobial agents must first gain access to target sites. Usually this is accomplished by absorption of the drug into the body and its distribution via the circulatory system. More specific antimicrobial agents are capable of penetrating to the site and having an affinity for target proteins on the pathogen. Local application to the infected area is sometimes necessary, such as with infections of the eyes. Once the drug has reached its site of action, it can cause death to the organism (-cidal) or prevent the pathogen from growing and dividing (-static). The specific mechanisms that are -cidal or -static activities vary with different agents. Because bacteria, viruses, fungi and other pathogens differ in structure and physiology, the mechanisms of action of antimicrobials differ significantly. A drug that is effective against bacteria is not effective against viral or fungal pathogens. Antivirals most often work to reduce viral replication, but usually do not produce absolute eradication of all viral particles, and are not effective against bacteria or fungi. Similarly, antifungal agents are useless against bacteria or viral pathogens. Table 57-4 presents examples of antimicrobials classified by mechanism of action.

Antibacterial Agents

Bacteriostatic agents inhibit bacterial growth, which allows the host's defense mechanisms additional time to remove the invading microorganisms. In contrast, **bactericidal agents** cause bacterial cell death and lysis. Antibacterial agents may be divided into bacteriostatic (e.g., sulfonamides) and bactericidal (e.g., penicillins) categories. However, such categorization is not always valid or reliable, because the same antimicrobial agent may have either effect depending on the dose administered, the concentration achieved at its site of action, and the particular species of bacteria. For example, tetracycline is generally bacteriostatic but may be bactericidal in high concentrations. Chloramphenicol, which is often listed as a bacteriostatic drug, has bactericidal effects against *Streptococcus pneumoniae* and *Haemophilus influenzae* in the cerebrospinal fluid (CSF).

Antibacterial agents may exert their bacteriostatic or bactericidal effects in one of four major ways:
1. Inhibit bacteria cell wall synthesis. Unlike host cells, bacteria are not isotonic with body fluids; therefore their contents are under high osmotic pressure and their viability depends on the integrity of the cell walls. Any compound that inhibits any step in the synthesis of this cell wall weakens it and causes the cell to lyse. Antimicrobial agents having this mechanism of action are bactericidal.
2. Disrupt or alter membrane permeability, resulting in the leakage of essential bacterial metabolic substrates. Agents causing these effects can be either bacteriostatic or bactericidal.
3. Inhibit protein synthesis. Antimicrobial agents may induce the formation of defective protein molecules; such agents are bactericidal in their action. Antimicrobial agents that inhibit specific steps in protein synthesis are bacteriostatic.
4. Inhibit the synthesis of essential metabolites. Antimicrobial agents that work in this manner structurally resemble physiologic compounds and act as competitive inhibitors in a metabolic pathway. In general, they are bacteriostatic agents.

Antiviral Agents

Agents with activity against viruses are typically subdivided into those agents that target retroviruses (e.g., human immunodeficiency virus [HIV]) and those that do not. The nonretroviral agents target deoxyribonucleic acid (DNA) and ribonucleic acid (RNA) viruses and typically interfere with one of the steps involved in viral entry into host cells or a step that leads to viral replication within the host cell. The retroviral agents used in treating HIV work by similar mechanisms, but are primarily effective for retroviral infections only. Targets of action of nonretroviral antiviral therapy include affecting entry into the cell, mistranscription of viral genome or mistranslation of viral proteins, assembly of components of the virus, or release of newly formed virus particles from the host cell. The antiviral agents typically are not "curative," but instead slow viral action or reproduction, and rely heavily on host defense mechanisms to respond. A number of naturally occurring cytokines (e.g., interferons) assist in the host response to viral infections and are administered as treatment for some viral infections (e.g., hepatitis C).

The treatment of HIV involves the use of combinations of drugs that inhibit various enzyme functions in the HIV replication processes. Agents currently used include nucleoside reverse transcriptase inhibitors, nonnucleoside reverse transcriptase inhibitors, and protease inhibitors. A newer

| Table 57-4 Antimicrobial Classification by Mechanism of Action and Overall Spectrum |

Mechanism	Spectrum of Activity			
	Antibacterial	**Antiviral**	**Antifungal**	**Other**
Inhibit cell wall synthesis	bacitracin carbapenems cephalosporins cycloserine penicillins teicoplanin vancomycin			
Alter membrane permeability	colistin polymyxin		amphotericin B azoles nystatin	
Inhibit protein synthesis via impeding replication genetic information	metronidazole nalidixic acid rifampin	acyclovir foscarnet ganciclovir interferons vidarabine	flucytosine griseofulvin	metronidazole pyrazinamide rifabutin rifampin

Inhibit protein synthesis via impairing translation genetic information	aminoglycosides
	chloramphenicol
	clindamycin
	fluoroquinolones
	lincomycin
	linezolid
	macrolides
	quinupristin/dalfopristin
	tetracyclines
		interferons
		nucleoside/nonnucleoside
		  reverse transcriptase
		  inhibitors
		protease inhibitors
		ribavirin
				aminoglycosides
				fluoroquinolones

Antimetabolites	sulfonamides trimethoprim			ethambutol isoniazid (INH) paraaminosalicylic acid (PAS)
Altered fusion of virus to cell		enfuvirtide (T-20)		
Alter uncoating of virus		amantadine interferons rimantadine		
Impair budding and release of virus		interferons oseltamivir zanamivir		

agent targeted at decreasing fusion of HIV with host cells is also available.

Antifungal Agents

Agents with activity against fungi work by different mechanisms to affect fungi or yeast functioning. Most act by interfering with membrane function in some way. Other mechanisms noted with specific agents include affecting DNA or RNA synthesis and inhibiting mitosis. The anti-

fungals are often categorized as those used topically for superficial fungal infections and those used systemically for deep-seated fungal infection. A few agents are used for both topical and systemic fungal infection.

Other Agents

Drugs used for protozoan, parasitic, mycobacterial (e.g., tuberculosis) or other infections vary regarding mechanism of action and include inhibition of cell wall structures, inhibi-

TABLE 57-5 SELECTED ADVERSE EFFECTS TO ANTIMICROBIALS

Effect	Drug
Anaphylaxis	penicillin
Hematologic effects	chloramphenicol (low incidence but high mortality)
Nephrotoxicity	polymyxins
	aminoglycosides
	sulfonamides (low incidence with newer preparations)
	amphotericin
	vancomycin (low incidence with newer preparations)
Potential for neuro-muscular blockade	polymyxins
	aminoglycosides
Injury to eighth cranial nerve	aminoglycosides
Photosensitivity	selected fluoroquinolones
	tetracyclines
Seizures	carbapenems
Cardiac dysrhythmias	erythromycin

tion of enzymes, and interference with DNA or RNA synthesis. The treatment of various protozoan, mycobacterial and parasitic infections varies, and may often include use of drugs with antibacterial activity. Chapter 60 discusses these agents more fully.

✳ What adverse effects are attributed to antibacterial drugs?

Although the development of antimicrobial agents represents one of the most important advances in drug therapy, these drugs can have adverse and toxic effects. The list of adverse effects and toxic effects of each specific drug group is long and varied. Table 57-5 identifies some of the major adverse effects of a few antimicrobial agents. In addition to other adverse effects, all antimicrobial agents are capable of producing the following two general types of adverse reactions of which the nurse must be aware: (1) allergic or hypersensitivity reactions, or (2) superinfection.

Allergic or Hypersensitivity Reactions

Allergic or hypersensitivity reactions may occur with all available antimicrobial agents. Hypersensitivity is a state of altered reactivity in which the body reacts with an exaggerated immune response. Such responses may include rash, fever, urticaria with pruritus, chills, generalized erythema, anaphylaxis, and Stevens-Johnson syndrome. Stevens-Johnson syndrome is a form of toxic epidermal necrolysis in which the epidermis separates from the dermis, leaving the client with a skin loss similar to a second-degree burn. Stevens-Johnson syndrome has a high risk for mortality.

A minor rash may be easily tolerated, but a generalized rash or erythema accompanied by chills and fever needs

medical intervention. Rapid administration of IV vancomycin, for example, may result in localized histamine release, causing temporary discomfort for the client. This "pseudo" allergic reaction is often called "red man" or "red neck" syndrome due to facial or neck flushing. The use of histamine-1 antagonists may help, but administering vancomycin at a slower infusion rate typically prevents the problem.

Type IV hypersensitivity reactions aer commonly noted with ampicillin and produce a body rash 2 to 5 days into therapy. The mechanism of this type of reaction involves sensitized lymphocyte migration to dermal tissue where ampicillin is present. While uncomfortable, this reaction is not considered life threatening and may fade with continued treatment.

Type I hypersensitivity reactions involving IgE are the most serious and are most common with penicillins. These range from hives/urticaria seen within minutes of administration to full-blown anaphylaxis. With IgE reactions, the offending drug is discontinued and is avoided in the future. Any respiratory distress, drop in blood pressure, or anaphylaxis requires immediate medical attention.

Sensitization can occur through indirect exposure to a drug, such as drinking milk from cows treated with antimicrobials or eating poultry or beef from livestock treated with antimicrobials. Previous topical application of antimicrobials may also cause sensitization.

The treatment of allergic reactions includes the use of antihistamines and epinephrine, which block or counteract the effects of the vasoactive mediators of allergy, and the use of corticosteroids, which may reduce tissue injury and edema in the inflammatory response. The use of corticosteroids is controversial in the face of systemic infection because of their prolonged inhibition of normal host defense responses, but corticosteroids are used when inflammation is significant.

Superinfection

Superinfection is an infection that occurs during the course of therapeutic or prophylactic antimicrobial therapy. Most antimicrobials reduce or eradicate the normal microbial flora of the body, which is then replaced by resistant exogenous or opportunistic endogenous bacteria. If the number of these replacement organisms is large and the host conditions are favorable, clinical superinfection can occur.

The risk of superinfection is greater when large doses of antimicrobials are used, when more than one antimicrobial is administered concurrently, and when broad-spectrum drugs are used. Superinfections are more commonly associated with certain antimicrobials than with others. For example, *Pseudomonas* organisms often colonize in and infect clients who are taking cephalosporins. In a similar manner, clients taking tetracyclines may become infected with *Candida albicans.*

In general, superinfections are caused by microorganisms that are resistant to the drug the client is receiving. In the past, penicillinase-producing staphylococci were the most common cause of superinfection. *Staphylococcus aureus* and *S. epidermidis* superinfections, especially with methicillin-resistant strains, are again on the rise. Gram-negative enteric bacilli and fungi are also common offenders. *Clostridium difficile* infection of the colon has become quite problematic in many institutional settings, and can be potentially life-threatening.

The proper management of superinfections includes the following: (1) discontinue the drug being given or replace it with another drug to which the organism is sensitive, (2) culture the suspected infected area, and (3) possibly, administer an antimicrobial agent effective against the new offending organism. Use of "pro-biotics" or administration of active microorganisms to replenish normal flora in the affected area is also an effective strategy for prevention of some types of superinfections, but does not appear effective for preventing vulvovaginal candidiasis (Pirotta et al., 2004). For infants, probiotics—even in the absence of antimicrobial therapy—are associated with reduced frequency of diarrhea and fever (Weizman, Asli, & Alsheikh, 2005; Lin et al., 2005).

✳ What general guidelines for use of antimicrobials should be considered?

Several important principles guide the judicious and optimal use of antimicrobial agents. Adverse effects and therapeutic failures are often related to a lack of adherence to the following principles of antimicrobial therapy. The principles include identifying the infecting pathogen, preventing resistance by limiting antimicrobial use, utilizing culture and sensitivity data to guide therapy, considering the client's existing defense mechanisms, and choosing optimal dose, duration and route of administration. Chapter 58 through 60 discuss specific conditions or drugs that require special consideration.

Identification of the Infecting Pathogen

Because most antimicrobial agents have a specific effect on a limited range of microorganisms, the prescriber must formulate a specific diagnosis about the potential pathogens or organisms most likely causing the infection. The drug most likely to be specifically effective against the suspected microorganism can then be selected.

This objective is most reliably accomplished by obtaining specimens from the infected area if possible (e.g., urine, sputum, wound drainage) or by obtaining venous blood specimens and sending them to the laboratory for culture and identification of the causative organism. The recovery of a specific microorganism from appropriate specimens is a significant factor in determining antimicrobial therapy. When a significant microorganism has been isolated, laboratory tests for antimicrobial susceptibility to various antimicrobial agents are performed. Urine specimens are routinely obtained for potential UTIs; sputum cultures can be used in guiding drug selection for community-acquired pneumonia but appear most useful in nosocomial pneumonia (Garcia-Vazquez et al., 2004).

It is desirable to receive culture and sensitivity reports before initiating antimicrobial therapy. In most situations, however, it is not practical to wait for these laboratory results. Antimicrobial therapy must be initiated without delay in acute, life-threatening situations such as peritonitis, septicemia, or pneumonia. In such circumstances the choice of the initial antimicrobial agent used must be based on likely pathogens observed in similar clients for similar infections and/or on tentative identification of the pathogen and a Gram stain. This is often referred to as empiric therapy, since the choice of agent is based on a likely but not isolated pathogen or pathogens. It is known, for example, that microorganisms commonly isolated in acute adult infections of the lung include pneumococci, *Haemophilus* strain streptococci, and staphylococci. Antimicrobial agents specifically toxic to those organisms may be administered temporarily. The drugs can be changed, if necessary, when laboratory reports are received.

When even tentative identification is difficult, broad-spectrum antimicrobials (which are effective against a wide range of microorganisms) can be prescribed, or several antimicrobial agents may be prescribed for simultaneous administration.

Most infections are treated most effectively with the use of only one antimicrobial. Combined antimicrobial drug therapy may be indicated for other situations. Indications for the simultaneous use of two or more antimicrobial agents include the following: (1) the treatment of mixed infections, in which each drug may act on different pathogens; (2) the need to delay rapid emergence of bacteria that are resistant to one drug (as is seen with HIV, tuberculosis, and *H. pylori* infections); and (3) the need to reduce the incidence or intensity of adverse effects by decreasing the dosage of a potentially toxic drug. Indiscriminate use of combined antimicrobial drug therapy, however, should be avoided because of expense, toxicity, and a higher incidence of superinfections and resistance.

Sensitivity and Resistance

A discrepancy often exists between in vitro testing and the activity of the drug within the body. The activity of a drug in the body depends on a number of variables, such as affinity for antimicrobial active sites and penetration into the bacteria, pH, temperature, and the ability of a drug to reach the site of an infection. For example, with meningitis it would be inappropriate to use a drug that does not cross the blood-brain barrier, even though the organism tested may be sensitive to the drug.

Resistance refers to the ability of a particular microorganism to resist the effects of a specific antimicrobial. Resistance occurs in one of the three following ways:

1. The antimicrobial is unable to reach the potential target site of its action. Some organisms, such as *Pseudomonas,* form a protective membrane (a glycocalyx or slime) that prevents the antimicrobial from reaching the cell wall.

2. The microorganism may produce an enzyme that reduces or eliminates the toxic effect of the antimicrobial on the cell wall. Examples of these enzymes are the β lactamases that cleave the β-lactam ring on penicillins and cephalosporins, forming inactive compounds; acylases that acetylate chloramphenicol to yield inactive derivatives; and enzymes that inactivate aminoglycosides by phosphorylation, adenylation, and acetylation.

The microorganism may also be altered in the individual through several biochemical changes so that the drug no longer is effective. In this case a specific organism is said to have "become resistant" to an antimicrobial to which it was previously susceptible. As a rule, microorganisms that are resistant to a certain drug will tend to be resistant to other chemically related antimicrobial agents; this phenomenon is known as *cross-resistance*. For example, bacteria that are unresponsive to tetracycline will also be resistant to doxycycline and minocycline. Of major concern is the rapid, worldwide increase in multiple drug-resistant organisms in response to current antimicrobial therapies (Purssell, 2005).

3. Host Defense Mechanisms. No antimicrobial agent will cure an infection if the host's defense mechanisms are inadequate. Such drugs act only on the causative organisms of infectious disease and have no effect on the defense mechanisms of the body, which need to be assessed and supported. Many infections do not require drug therapy and are adequately combated by individual defense mechanisms, including antibody production, phagocytosis, interferon production, or gastrointestinal (GI) rejection (vomiting, diarrhea). However, the host's defense mechanisms may be diminished, such as with diabetes mellitus, neoplastic disease, and immunologic suppression. A client who is very ill may require supportive care to ensure adequate oxygenation, fluid and electrolyte balance, and optimal nutrition so that antimicrobial therapy can be effective. Surgical intervention is also necessary in some situations. In general, in the presence of a substantial amount of pus, necrotic tissue, or foreign bodies, the most effective treatment is a combination of an antimicrobial agent and an appropriate surgical procedure.

Antimicrobial-resistant pathogens, including methicillin-resistant *Staphylococcus aureus* (MRSA) and vancomycin-resistant enterococcus (VRE), are now widespread in acute, long-term, and community-care settings (Francis et al., 2005; Begier et al., 2004; Frazee et al., 2005). Even drugs used to treat superinfections have lost effectiveness in some areas (Musher et al., 2005; Pepin et al., 2005). The development of resistant strains is correlated with widespread use of antimicrobials (Goossens, Ferech, Vander Stichele, Elseviers, ESAC Project Group, 2005) and may also be a function of antimicrobial additives in cattle, pig, and poultry feed (Ramchandani, 2005; Johnson, Kuskowski, Smith, O'Bryan, Tatini, 2005).

The status of the host's defense mechanisms also influences the choice of therapy, route of administration, and dosage. For example, if an infection is fulminating, parenteral (preferably IV) administration of a bactericidal drug will be selected rather than the oral administration of a bacteriostatic drug. To achieve maximum blood concentrations rapidly, large "loading" doses of antimicrobial agents are often administered at the beginning of treatment for severe infections.

Factors influencing drug dosage are also related to the status of a client's renal function. Because many antimicrobial agents are excreted by the kidneys, a major management problem exists with individuals who have compromised renal function. Drug dosages are then generally reduced in parallel with the client's creatinine clearance levels. Hemodialysis may further alter the therapeutic regimen. In some disease states (such as burns and cystic fibrosis) the dosage of the antimicrobial may need to be increased to achieve therapeutic levels.

In short, administration of an antimicrobial agent based on culture and sensitivity results is not the only important measure in antimicrobial therapy. An equally important determinant of antimicrobial effectiveness is the functional state of the host's defense mechanisms.

Dosage, Duration, and Route of Administration

To achieve therapeutic goals, antimicrobial drugs must be administered in adequate dosages and for long enough periods of time. Fortunately, serum levels of some of the antimicrobials with a narrow therapeutic index (e.g., aminoglycosides) can be monitored to prevent or minimize the risk of toxicity. Be sure to assess for alterations in renal and hepatic functions, because both can affect drug dosage, the dosing interval, and/or drug toxicity.

Failures in antimicrobial therapy are often the result of drug dosages that are too small or are given for too short of a time. For some infections, orally administered agents do not achieve adequate tissue levels and therefore require IV administration. Topically applied antimicrobials rarely are effective for deep-seated tissue infections. In general, antimicrobial therapy should not be discontinued until the client has been afebrile and clinically well for 48 to 72 hours. Follow-up cultures may be necessary to assess the effectiveness of therapy.

Inadequate drug therapy may lead to remissions and exacerbations of the infection and contribute to the development of resistance. When antimicrobials are used prophylactically, they are usually given for short periods of time to enhance the host's defense mechanisms. With perioperative antibacterials, for example, a loading dose is given immediately before surgery and adequate blood levels maintained through the surgical procedure. In some cases, therapy may continue for up to 48 hours after surgery.

Antimicrobial agents in current use are discussed as chemically related groups of drugs in the following chapters. Become familiar with the general characteristics of each drug group or category and with one or two prototype drugs in each group. Because the dosage for any given antimicrobial varies with the type of infection, the site of infection, and the age of the client, only general dosages or dosage ranges are given in this text. Consult the manufacturer's package insert or a formulary for specific dosages.

✳ What are the nursing implications in the use of antimicrobials?

The antimicrobial agents available today destroy or inhibit the growth of most bacteria, many fungi, and some viruses. Some antimicrobial agents are derived from living organisms, whereas others are synthetic and semisynthetic chemical compounds. Nurses need to have knowledge of both host defenses and antimicrobial drugs to safely and effectively care for clients who are taking antimicrobials.

The primary defense mechanisms against infection are intact skin and mucous membranes, the chemical composition and pH of specific body secretions, phagocytic cells, mechanical movements of certain cells or tissues (e.g., cilia action, coughing, peristalsis), and the inflammatory process. Many factors can impair host defenses and thereby increase the risk for the development of infection by virulent organisms.

Any disruption in the integrity of skin or mucous membranes becomes a portal of entry for disease-producing organisms. Relatively minor breaks in the skin or mucosa can lead to fatal infections in very ill, hospitalized clients or in those who are immunocompromised (e.g., individuals who have acquired immunodeficiency syndrome [AIDS] or are receiving immunosuppressive therapies). Provision of good dental care has been projected to reduce the risk of nursing home pneumonia by as much as 40% (Quagliarello et al., 2005). Avoid vigorous teeth cleaning, tube insertions, and injections, if possible. Supporting appropriate lifestyle and nutrition decisions by the client may also improve immune function. For example, vitamin and mineral supplementation is associated with reduced infection risk in older adults (El-Kadiki & Sutton, 2005). Also correct environmental hazards such as furniture obstructions, wet flooring, or the presence of irritating agents to prevent injury.

Impaired blood supply to body tissues will also reduce host defenses by reducing the overall resistance of tissues to injury, by preventing migration of inflammatory cells to the area of injury, and by limiting the distribution of antimicrobial therapy to infected tissue. Other factors that impair the body's defenses against infection include neutropenia, anemia, protein malnutrition, and autoimmune and antiinflammatory agents such as antineoplastic agents and corticosteroids. Persons with chronic preexisting cardiopulmonary, renal, or metabolic disease and those at the extremes of age are susceptible to the development of infection because of altered organ function. Poor personal hygiene and the suppression of normal bacterial flora by antimicrobials create conditions in which normal defenses

are overwhelmed; this results in pathogen overgrowth (superinfection).

Hundreds of antimicrobial agents are marketed currently, and it is impossible to have infinite knowledge about each drug. However, despite the numerous and varied drugs available, there are significantly fewer drug categories to remember. Knowledge of the general characteristics of each drug category and of the general principles of antimicrobial drug therapy enable the nurse to function effectively. In addition to the antibacterials, which include penicillins, cephalosporins, macrolides, lincomycins, vancomycin, aminoglycosides, tetracyclines, chloramphenicol, fluoroquinolones, sulfonamides, and polymyxins, major groups of antiinfective drugs include urinary tract antiseptics, and antimycobacterial, antifungal, and antiviral agents. Refer to Table 57-5 for a brief summary of the major allergic and toxic effects of certain antimicrobial agents.

Nursing interventions in antimicrobial drug therapy generally relate to (1) assessing the client, (2) assisting in the identification of the infecting organism, (3) administering the drug, (4) monitoring the client's response to the drug, (5) educating the client, (6) providing comfort, and (7) preventing and treating adverse effects, including pharmacologic and chemical drug interactions.

Assessment In the initial assessment of the client, document the client's temperature, pulse, respiratory status, and blood pressure to detect fever and systemic responses to fever. Diaphoresis and flushing may also occur. Make note of the client's general behavior; a slumped posture, slow and unsteady posture, and careless grooming may indicate fatigue and malaise. Listen to the client's nonspecific symptoms, such as "aching all over," loss of appetite, headache, change of mental status, generalized discomfort, and "not feeling one's self" or "up-to-snuff." Ask the client about specific indicators, such as night sweats, pain, dyspnea, or arthralgia. Inspect the client's skin for heat, erythema, lesions, moisture, and swelling. Inspect and palpate the lymph nodes in the area of a suspected localized infection. Examine all the lymph nodes for a generalized infection. Additionally, perform a history and physical examination, including a review of all systems.

Cultures are ordered if an area of suspected infection is found. Obtaining the cultures to determine the source and type of infection is often the nurse's responsibility. If there is an order to give an antimicrobial agent before an infective source is determined, obtain cultures before administering the first dose of the drug ordered.

Send specimens obtained for culture directly to the laboratory and do not allow them to stand. Delay may cause the death of fastidious organisms and allow contaminating organisms to overgrow the pathogen. If subsequent culture specimens are obtained while the client is receiving antimicrobials, send to the laboratory information regarding the drug(s) being administered. The appropriate selection of laboratory tests for the identification of offending organisms often depends on this knowledge.

Be sure to assess a client's previous reactions to drugs and to antimicrobial agents, which is especially important in avoiding allergic reactions to drugs. Carefully question the individual regarding drugs previously taken and the client's exact clinical responses to them; this is an important part of the client's history. Some clients equate common adverse effects such as nausea and diarrhea with a drug allergy. Although these drug responses are important, their appearance may not be as sufficient a reason to withhold a specific antimicrobial as would a true allergy. Once drug allergies are known, warnings are prominently displayed on the client's record or hospital chart. The following actions are additional precautions: (1) ask the client if he or she has drug allergies before administering any medications; (2) tell the client what drug he or she is receiving; (3) observe the client for at least half an hour after drug administration (penicillin in particular), especially if the drug is administered parenterally and the client has never taken the drug previously; and (4) know what drugs are used to treat allergic responses and where they are kept.

Because most hospitalized clients receive more than one medication, review the client's current medication regimen for significant drug interactions; this is necessary if antimicrobial therapy is to be optimally effective. Be alert to drugs that interact biologically with antimicrobial agents, and chemical incompatibilities between antimicrobial drugs and other agents when they are mixed for IV administration. Resources (written or computerized) on each unit provide accurate and current information about these interactions.

In addition to a careful history of allergies and other adverse effects to drugs and a review of the current medication regimen for potential significant drug interactions, include in the pretherapy assessment the baseline signs and symptoms of the client's infection, and the white blood cell (WBC) count, serum electrolytes, and relevant culture and sensitivity.

Nursing Diagnosis Clients receiving antimicrobial therapy are at risk for the following nursing diagnoses/collaborative problems: risk for infection and hyperthermia related to the ineffectiveness of antimicrobial therapy and/or the development of superinfection with another organism; risk for deficient fluid volume related to antimicrobial-induced adverse GI reactions or anorexia, nausea, and vomiting related to gastric irritation by the drug; and the potential complications of allergic reaction, sepsis, ototoxicity, blood dyscrasias, and nephrotoxicity caused by specific antimicrobial agents.

Planning The planning process includes setting goals for the client both during and after antimicrobial therapy. Following antimicrobial therapy, the client will be free of the signs and symptoms of infection. During the antimicrobial therapy, the client will:

- Experience a decrease in signs and symptoms of the infection.
- Experience minimal adverse effects of drug therapy.
- Effectively manage the therapeutic regimen, including being compliant with medications, and implementing nonpharmacologic supportive measures.

- Collaborate with health care providers by appropriately reporting untoward symptoms and maintaining scheduled visits for monitoring and treatment.

Implementation

Monitoring Assess for the effectiveness of drug therapy by monitoring signs and symptoms of the client's infection, including WBC count and culture results. In most instances, the client's condition should improve within 48 hours after drug administration. Be alert for early signs of allergic or other adverse responses to therapy, and signs of superinfection, such as diarrhea and white patches in the oral cavity and vaginal area (see the following discussion of the management of adverse responses). Serum antimicrobial concentrations can be monitored throughout therapy to assess for therapeutic and toxic levels of some individual antimicrobials.

In addition to monitoring the therapeutic effects of antimicrobials, monitor the client for the development of common adverse effects of individual drugs. Fluid and electrolyte imbalances can occur during the course of administering many antimicrobials, either from the drug itself, the mode of administration, or adverse effects such as diarrhea. For example, extracellular volume excess may result from administering multiple IV drugs, each of which is diluted in 100 mL of saline. Edema, pulmonary congestion with subsequent shortness of breath, and an increase in body weight indicate the presence of extracellular volume excess.

Hypokalemia resulting from severe diarrhea or the IV administration of an antimicrobial containing large quantities of sodium produces no obvious clinical signs or symptoms until the potassium deficit is significant. At this point, widespread muscular weakness and cardiac conduction abnormalities appear. In the client whose cardiac function is being monitored, the appearance of U waves may be an earlier indication of low serum potassium (McCance & Huether, 2002). Laboratory demonstration of hypokalemia is often the only way to detect this disorder.

Hypernatremia, another electrolyte imbalance commonly seen with use of antimicrobials that have a sodium base, is also associated with few early clinical signs or symptoms, with the exception of a high serum sodium value. In general, periodic serum electrolyte studies may be ordered for clients who must take prolonged courses of IV antimicrobials that can cause fluid and electrolyte imbalances.

Intervention Because the constant and consistent administration of an antimicrobial drug at prescribed dosage intervals is necessary to maintain therapeutic blood levels, administer such a drug according to the prescribed times as accurately as possible. This may mean awakening sleeping clients and ensuring that tests or therapies do not interrupt this schedule.

When IV antimicrobial agents are administered, observe the following additional precautions: (1) dilute the drugs as recommended in package literature (usually in neutral solutions [pH 7 to 7.2] of isotonic sodium chloride [0.9%] or 5% dextrose in water), (2) administer the drugs without the admixture of any other drug to avoid chemical or physical incompatibilities, (3) administer the drugs by intermittent IV infusions to avoid inactivation (e.g., by temperature) and prolonged vein irritation from high drug concentration, (4) change the infusion site every 48 hours to reduce the risk of chemical phlebitis, and (5) inject intramuscular (IM) antimicrobials deeply into large muscle masses (e.g., gluteal muscles), and rotate injection sites to prevent tissue irritation.

The establishment of automatic stop and renewal orders in many hospitals is another precaution against adverse effects and also ensures that a particular drug's effectiveness is evaluated. Such orders restrict the administration of a prescribed antimicrobial agent to a definite time period (e.g., 7 days); its continued use past that time requires a new prescription.

Education Teach clients principles of antimicrobial therapy, including that these drugs should never be taken without medical supervision and should be taken in strict accordance with their prescriptions. This is especially important because many individuals receiving antimicrobial drugs are not hospitalized and are responsible for self-medication. Specifically, teach clients:

- Not to stop taking these drugs as soon as symptoms abate, because an ineffective course of antimicrobial therapy will provide an opportunity for microbes to mutate and develop resistance to the drug.
- Not to share these drugs with family and friends, because they may have allergies and the drug may not be appropriate for their illness.
- Not to take "leftover" antimicrobial drugs for new illnesses, even if the symptoms appear similar. Many infections may have the same symptoms but are caused by different organisms or by organisms that have developed a resistance to the drug. Additionally, some drugs become toxic as they degenerate past their expiration date.

Teach clients who are allergic to an antimicrobial agent how to protect themselves from future treatment with the drug in question, such as by using Medic Alert wallet cards or tags.

Give "drug information sheets" containing special administration considerations, expected effects, and adverse effects of individual antimicrobials to clients so they may refer to them at home while taking antimicrobial therapy. Also include a telephone number to call when questions arise, which conveys the message that it is expected and desirable for clients to discuss their medication concerns with health care workers.

Evaluation The expected outcome of antimicrobial therapy is a decrease in the severity or a disappearance of the clinical and laboratory manifestations of infection. Redness, heat, edema, and pain should decrease with local infections. In the case of a systemic infection, temperature, heart rate, respiratory rate, and WBC count should return to normal, and appetite and a sense of well-being should improve. Purulent drainage, if present, should decrease in amount and change to a more normal appearance and consistency. In

clients who are seriously ill, an improvement in organ function should accompany other signs of infection resolution. While self-administering antimicrobial therapy, the client will be compliant with medications, completing the prescription unless directed otherwise by the prescriber, and will use nonpharmacologic measures to minimize adverse drug effects and maximize good health. The client will appropriately report adverse effects to the prescriber and will maintain scheduled visits for monitoring and treatment.

✸ How are adverse effects of antimicrobials prevented and managed?

Anaphylaxis

The most serious allergic reaction to antimicrobials is anaphylaxis. This IgE-mediated reaction can occur anywhere from a few seconds to 30 minutes after an antimicrobial injection. This reaction usually begins with diffuse flushing, itching, and a feeling of warmth. Hives may appear on the client's face, neck, and chest. Generalized body edema develops as the syndrome progresses. Massive facial edema signals the possibility of upper airway edema, with impending obstruction and respiratory difficulty from pulmonary involvement. These problems are manifested as a choking sensation, stridor, chest tightness and pain, wheezing, shortness of breath, and restlessness.

The initial step in the emergent management of anaphylaxis is to stop the antimicrobial immediately if it is still being infused. If the individual is not in a medical facility, immediate transport to one should be arranged, preferably by a vehicle staffed with paramedics, who can establish an artificial airway if the client's airway becomes totally obstructed.

Drug therapy is used to reverse anaphylaxis. Epinephrine 1:1000 is injected subcutaneously and will reverse the vascular effects of anaphylaxis. If the individual is in anaphylactic shock, the administration of IV epinephrine and IV fluids is necessary. The antihistamine diphenhydramine (Benadryl) is administered parenterally or orally. Corticosteroids (methylprednisolone) may be administered to prevent protracted symptoms in severe reactions.

Superinfection

The emergence of superinfection may be suspected in the presence of diarrhea or recurrent fever in clients taking antimicrobial drugs. Stomatitis is indicated by the presence of a sore mouth or white patches on the oral mucosa. Monilial vaginitis may produce a vaginal discharge or perineal rash. Increasing redness, heat, edema, pain, and possibly drainage may herald localized superinfections. *Clostridium difficile* as a nosocomial infection may manifest as a pseudomembranous colitis. Children, older adults, and others whose normal host defense mechanisms may be weakened should be especially observed for signs of superinfection. In the course of prolonged antimicrobial drug therapy, periodic cultures of the upper respiratory tract and of the feces may be indicated to determine changes in bacterial flora that may be subsequently responsible for secondary infection. Be careful not to introduce new microorganisms and emphasize aseptic technique in those who are in contact with clients receiving antimicrobial therapy.

Summary

Infectious disease has been a major health concern for humans even before recorded history. It comprises a variety of illnesses caused by pathogenic microorganisms, bacteria, fungi, and viruses. Inflammation is a reaction of the body tissues, not only to infection but also to physical, chemical, and thermal injuries. Fever is a sign of inflammation. All reactions present challenges for nursing care and antimicrobial therapy.

Depending on the concentration at the site of action, antimicrobial agents may be -static (inhibiting growth), -cidal (causing pathogen death and lysis), or both. These agents are effective by a number of potential mechanisms and include inhibiting synthesis of the bacterial cell wall, altering membrane permeability, inhibiting protein synthesis, or inhibiting the synthesis of essential metabolites. Antimicrobials are generally well tolerated by humans. However, with all antimicrobials there is the possibility of an allergic or hypersensitive response or a superinfection (an infection that occurs during the course of antimicrobial therapy because of a reduction in the normal microbial flora of the body).

The following are guidelines for the use of antimicrobials: identification of the infecting organism, which allows for the selection of the most effective antimicrobial for the specific infecting organism; determination of the ability of a specific antimicrobial to limit the growth of or kill microorganisms in vitro; supportive therapy for the host's defense mechanisms; and administration of the agent in an adequate dosage and for long enough periods to be effective. Judicious use of antimicrobials may help curtail drug resistance.

Nursing management of antimicrobial therapy includes assessing the client's ability to deal with the stressor of infection, administering antimicrobial drugs safely and accurately, educating the client to do the same regarding self-administration of the drug, preventing and managing adverse effects, and evaluating the client's response to the drug and progress toward the goal of resolution of the infection.

✴ Critical Thinking Questions

- Susan Brooks is a 71-year-old resident in a skilled nursing facility who choked one morning while drinking her coffee but seemed to recover fully. Some days later, however, you notice that Ms. Brooks has become more restless and agitated than usual and cannot sleep. She has no cough or sputum production, but her temperature is over 102°F. A chest radiograph examination shows right lower lobe infiltrate, a common finding in aspiration pneumonia. What nursing actions should occur before initiating antimicrobial therapy? After 3 days of antibacterial therapy, Ms. Brooks develops diarrhea. What do you suspect has occurred? How will you validate your suspicions? How will this change your plan of care for Ms. Brooks? What outcome criteria would be appropriate for her plan of care?

- Nick Nicholson, a 78-year-old man with Alzheimer's disease, is also a resident of the skilled nursing facility. He has frequent urinary incontinence and wears an external catheter at night. One evening Mr. Nicholson vomits but otherwise does not seem unwell. The next day he has a fever of 101°F. He has no cough or sputum production, and his chest radiograph is negative. However, a urine culture shows greater than 100,000 colonies of *Escherichia coli* per milliliter with WBCs present, which indicates a UTI. What aspects of Ms. Brooks and Mr. Nicholson's plans of care will be the same, and how will they differ? How will you evaluate the effectiveness of your plan of care for Mr. Nicholson?

Bibliography

Abate, B.J., & Barriere, S.L. (2002). Antimicrobial regimen selection. In J.T. DiPiro, R.L. Talbert, G.C. Yee, G.R. Matzke, B.G. Wells & L.M. Posey (Eds.), *Pharmacotherapy: A pathophysiological approach* (5th ed.). Norwalk, CT: Appleton & Lange.

Anderson, D.M., Keith, J., & Novak, P.D. (Eds.) (2002). *Mosby's medical, nursing, and allied health dictionary* (6th ed.). St. Louis: Mosby.

Begier, E.M., Frenette, K., Barrett, N.L., Mshar, P., Petit, S., Boxrud, D.J., et al. (2004). A high-morbidity outbreak of methicillin-resistant *Staphylococcus aureus* among players on a college football team, facilitated by body shaving and turf burns. *Clinical Infectious Disease, 39,* 1446-1453.

Bosker, G. (Ed.). (2004). *Primary and acute care medicine: Practice, protocols, pathways,* (2nd ed.). Atlanta: Thomson American Health Consultants.

e-LEARNING SUPPLEMENTS

Student CD-ROM
- Final Exam questions
- NCLEX® Examination review questions
- Pharmacology animations
- Printable chapter summary

Evolve Website (http://evolve.elsevier.com/mckenry)
- Content updates, including information on new drugs
- WebLinks corresponding to this chapter
- Answers to the critical thinking questions in this chapter
- *Elsevier ePharmacology Update* newsletter
- Mosby's Drug Consult Internet Edition
- Supplemental and reference information

Cuddy, M.L. (2004). The effects of drugs on thermoregulation. *AACN Clinical Issues, 15*(2), 238-253.

Drug facts and comparisons (58th ed.). (2005). St. Louis: Facts and Comparisons.

El-Kadiki, A., & Sutton, A.J. (2005). Role of multivitamins and mineral supplements in preventing infections in elderly people: Systematic review and meta-analysis of randomised controlled trials. *British Medical Journal, 330*, 871-874.

Francis, J.S., Doherty, M.C., Lopatin, U., Johnston, C.P., Sinha, G., Ross, T. et al. (2005). Severe community-onset pneumonia in healthy adults caused by methicillin-resistant *Staphylococcus aureus* carrying the Panton-Valentine leukocidin genes. *Clinical Infectious Disease, 40*, 100-107.

Frazee, B.W., Lynn, J., Charlebois, E.D., Lambert, L., Lowery, D., Perdreau-Remington, F. (2005). High prevalence of methicillin-resistant *Staphylococcus aureus* in emergency department skin and soft tissue infections. *Annals of Emergency Medicine, 45*, 311-320.

Garcia-Vazquez, E., Marcos, M.A., Mensa, J., de Roux, A., Puig, J., & Font, C., et al. (2004). Assessment of the usefulness of sputum culture for diagnosis of community-acquired pneumonia using the PORT predictive scoring system. *Archives of Internal Medicine, 164*, 1807-1811.

Gilbert, D.N., Moellering, R.C., Eliopoulos, G.M., & Sande, M.A. (2004). The Sanford Guide to Antimicrobial Therapy 2004 (34th ed). Hyde Park, VT: Antimicrobial Therapy.

Goossens, H., Ferech, M., Vander Stichele, R., Elseviers, M.; ESAC Project Group. (2005). Outpatient antibiotic use in Europe and associate with resistance: A cross-national database study. *Lancet, 365*, 579-587.

Gosain, A., & Gamelli, R. (2005) A primer in cytokines. *Journal of Burn Care & Rehabilitation, 26*(1), 7-12.

Guglielmo, B.J. (2005). Principles of infectious diseases. In M.A. Koda-Kimble, L.Y. Young, W.A. Kradjan, B.J. Guglielmo, B.K. Alldredge, & R.L. Corelli (Eds.), *Applied therapeutics: The clinical use of drugs* (8th ed.). Philadelphia: Lippincott Williams & Wilkins.

Hardman, J.G., & Limbird, L.E. (Eds.). (2001). *Goodman & Gilman's The pharmacological basis of therapeutics* (10th ed.). New York: McGraw-Hill.

Jacobs, R.A. (2003). General problems in infectious disease. In L.M. Tierney, Jr., S.J. McPhee & Papadakis, M.A. (Eds.), *Current Medical Diagnosis & Treatment*. New York: Lange Medical Books/McGraw-Hill.

Johnson, J.R., Kuskowski, M.A., Smith, K., O'Bryan, & Tatini, S. (2005). Antimicrobial-resistant and extraintestinal pathogenic *Escherichia coli* in retail foods. *Journal of Infectious Disease, 191*, 1040-1049.

Lacy, C.F., Armstrong, L.L., Goldman, M.P., & Lance, L.L. (2004). *Lexi-Comp's Drug Information Handbook* (12th ed.). Hudson, Ohio: Lexi-Comp.

Lin, H.C., Su, B.H., Chen, A.C., Lin, T.W., Tsai, C.H., Yeh, T.F. (2005). Oral probiotics reduce the incidence and severity of necrotizing enterocolitis in very low birth weight infants. *Pediatrics, 115*, 1-4.

McCance, K.L., & Huether, S.E. (2002). *Pathophysiology: the biologic basis for disease in adults and children* (4th ed). St. Louis: Mosby.

Mosby's drug consult (15th ed.). (2005). St. Louis: Mosby.

Musher, D.M., Aslam, S., Logan, N., Nallacheru, S., Bhaila, I., Borchert, F., et al. (2005). Relatively poor outcome after treatment of *Clostridium difficile* colitis with metronidazole. *Clinical Infectious Disease, 40*, 1586-1590.

Pepin, J., Alary, M.E., Valiqueete, L., Raiche, E., Ruel, J., Fulop, K., et al. (2005). Increasing risk of relapse after treatment of *Clostridium difficile* colitis in Quebec, Canada. *Clinical Infectious Disease, 40*, 1591-1597.

Pirotta, M., Gunn, J., Chondros, P., Grover, S., O'Malley, P., & Hurley, S., et al. (2004). Effect of lactobacillus in preventing post-antibiotic vulvovaginal candidiasis: A randomised controlled trial. *British Medical Journal, 329*, 548-551.

Purssell, E. (2005). Evolutionary nursing: the case of infectious diseases. *Journal of Advanced Nursing, 49*(2):164-172.

Quagliarello, V., Ginter, S., Han, L., Van Ness, P., Allore, H., Tinetti, M. (2005). Modifiable risk factors for nursing home–acquired pneumonia. *Clinical Infectious Disease, 40*, 1-6.

Ramchandani, M., Manges, A.R., DebRoy, C., Smith, S.P., Johnson, J.R., & Riley, L.W. (2005). Possible animal origin of human-associated, multidrug-resistant, uropathogenic *Eshcherichia coli*. *Clinical Infectious Disease, 40*, 251-257.

Rybak, M.J., & Aeschlimann, J.R. (2002). Laboratory tests to direct antimicrobial pharmacotherapy. In J.T. DiPiro, R.L. Talbert, G.C. Yee, G.R. Matzke, B.G. Wells & L.M. Posey (Eds.), *Pharmacotherapy: A pathophysiological approach* (5th ed.). Norwalk, CT: Appleton & Lange.

USP DI: Drug information for the health care professional (25th ed.). (2005). Greenwood Village, CO: MICROMEDEX Thomason Healthcare.

Weizman, Z., Asli, G., Alsheikh, A. (2005). Effect of a probiotic infant formula on infections in child care centers: Comparison of two probiotic agents. *Pediatrics, 115*, 5-9.

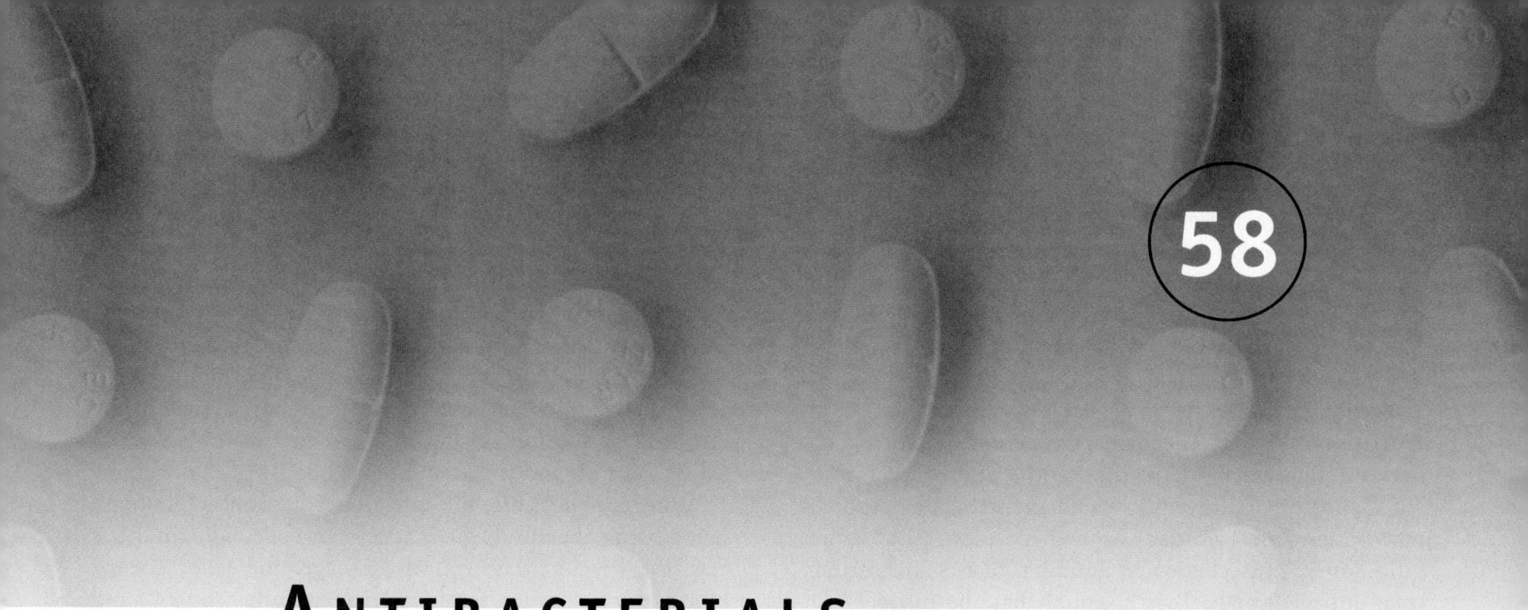

58

ANTIBACTERIALS

CHAPTER FOCUS

Infectious disease has always held a special threat for humans. There have been eras in which uncontrolled plague and pestilence have shaped the course of humankind. However, not until the advent of the sulfonamides, penicillin, and other antibacterials in the twentieth century was there an effective treatment for those with infectious diseases. Nurses have a major role in minimizing the risk for infection of individual clients and populations. When a client develops an infection, the nurse ensures that pharmacologic and nonpharmacologic therapies are implemented, client education is provided, and evaluation of the therapy occurs. Today, with the occurrence of drug-resistant strains of microorganisms and opportunistic bacterial infections, the importance of disease prevention and the use of antibacterial agents cannot be overlooked.

LEARNING OBJECTIVES

- Explain the nursing management of antibacterial therapy.
- Differentiate among peak, trough, and mean serum levels.
- List four major classifications of antibacterials.
- Compare different antibacterials within the same general classification.
- Explain the role of antibacterials, sulfonamides, urinary antiseptics, and urinary tract analgesics in the treatment of urinary tract infections (UTI).
- Implement the nursing management of clients receiving antibacterial therapy.

▲ KEY TERMS

antibiotics, p. 1012
antimicrobial, p. 1012
β-lactams, p. 1015
cephalosporins, p. 1022
fluoroquinolones, p. 1039
macrolides, p. 1028
penicillins, p. 1015
tetracyclines, p. 1034

KEY DRUGS

cefazolin, p. 1022
ciprofloxacin, p. 1039
clindamycin, p. 1032
erythromycin, p. 1030
metronidazole, p. 1033
penicillin V potassium, p. 1015
sulfamethoxazole-trimethoprim, p. 1047
tetracycline, p. 1037
tobramycin, p. 1042
vancomycin, p. 1027

Antibiotics are chemical substances produced from various microorganisms (bacteria, fungus) that kill or suppress the growth of other microorganisms. This term is also used for a number of natural and synthetic antimicrobial agents, such as sulfonamides and quinolones. As discussed in Chapter 57, the more precise term antimicrobial and more specific term antibacterial will be used for the remainder of this chapter.

Although hundreds of available antibacterials vary in spectrum of activity, mechanism of action, potency, toxicity, and pharmacokinetic properties, this chapter is divided into penicillins and related agents, cephalosporins, macrolides, lincosamides, aminoglycosides, tetracyclines, quinolones, miscellaneous antimicrobials, and urinary tract antimicrobials. It is essential that the nurse understand the general principles of antimicrobial therapy as discussed in Chapter 57. Additionally, before administering an antimicrobial, the nurse must be familiar with the specific drug and its actions and effects for the individual client. There are, however, some principles for antibacterial therapy that apply to all clients (Box 58-1).

✱ **T.L. is a 34-year-old kitchen worker who cut his hand with a sharp knife 4 days ago. He presents to the clinic with a history of worsening pain, redness, and swelling of his hand and lower arm. Purulent fluid can be expressed from the wound. The area around the wound is warm to the touch. Mild lymphadenopathy is present and T.L. has a temperature of 101° F (38.2° C).**

✱ **What are the nursing management issues to consider in treating infections with antibacterials?**

Assessment The nursing assessment is particularly important when an infection is suspected. Obtain detailed information regarding T.L.'s general health, and the symptoms indicating an infection, such as elevated temperature, chills, sweats, redness, pain, or swelling in a previously unaffected area, fatigue, anorexia, weight loss, cough, a change in the character or amount of sputum, increased white blood cell (WBC) count, and the amount and quality of drainage.

Whenever possible, the infecting organism is identified before drug therapy begins. Specimen collection (in T.L.'s case the specimen is wound drainage, for other clients, blood, urine, sputum, fecal material, and other sources) and cultures should be completed before initiating antibiotic therapy. Obtain specimens carefully adhering to agency guidelines to ensure test accuracy and to protect personnel from exposure to infectious organisms. Prompt treatment is imperative in serious infections; in such cases antimicrobial drugs are not withheld pending laboratory study and culture results.

Antibacterials, particularly penicillins, have been associated with serious hypersensitivity and allergic reactions. A complete drug history of T.L. and his family helps to identify possible hypersensitivity or cross-sensitivity to the drugs. Cross-sensitivity often exists between drugs of the same class (e.g., penicillins) or related classes (e.g., penicillins and cephalosporins). Clients who are intolerant of

---

BOX 58-1 PRINCIPLES OF ANTIBACTERIAL USE

To assess the appropriateness of antibacterial therapy in all clients, the following criteria are generally accepted:

1. In choosing empiric therapy, the selected antimicrobial should have documentation of both adequate penetration at the site and proven effectiveness against the common organisms usually isolated from that specific site.
2. Multiple drug therapy may be indicated if a broad range of possible microorganisms is suspected or if multiple organisms have been isolated from an infection site. In most cases, the minimum number of drugs necessary to treat the infection should be used whenever possible. Exceptions include infections where monotherapy may lead to treatment failure (e.g., treatment of *Pseudomonas* infections, tuberculosis [see Chapter 60] and *H. pylori* in peptic ulcer disease [see Chapter 40]). Combination therapy is also used in the treatment of HIV infection (see Chapter 59).
3. If no contraindication is present, the drug of first choice should be selected. The drug dosage regimen should be within the accepted range of current usage for the individual client, taking into account body surface area (height, weight), organ function, and concurrent disease processes.
4. Unless the benefit far outweighs the risk, no antibiotic should be used in clients who have prior documentation of an allergic or adverse reaction to the specific medication.
5. Drug plasma levels are warranted for ongoing therapy with aminoglycosides and intravenous vancomycin to both establish efficacy and reduce toxicity.
6. Whenever possible, cultures should be drawn before the initiation of antibiotic therapy. The usual sites cultured include sputum, urine, blood, wound, or nonhealing topical sites.
7. Antimicrobial therapy should be continued until the infection is no longer present. However, time periods should not exceed the usual treatment time established for suspected infection.
8. Prophylactic antimicrobial therapy given immediately before and during uncomplicated surgery to achieve high tissue levels of drug during the high risk surgical period. Repeated intraoperative doses are sometimes used for prolonged procedures if the levels from the original dose are reduced. Prophylactic antibacterial therapy is rarely continued postoperatively in otherwise uncomplicated surgical cases unless indwelling catheters or other devices pose an ongoing risk for infection.
9. Consider using an antibacterial with a "B" pregnancy category rating for all women of childbearing years.

one antimicrobial may be intolerant of similar antibiotics. Information regarding possible contraindications, cautions, potential drug interactions, and drug-taking patterns is also obtained.

Nursing Diagnosis Many antibacterials are administered prophylactically. In such cases, the nursing diagnosis of risk for infection would pertain. But once the client has an infection, such as with T.L., the risk for infection transmission is an appropriate diagnosis along with other nursing diagnoses specific to the client. See Chapter 57 and the Nursing Care Plan below for other selected nursing diagnoses.

✳ **A specimen of wound drainage is sent to the lab for culture and sensitivity (C&S). T.L.'s wound is cleansed and a dressing applied. The physician initiates antibacterial therapy with dicloxacillin 250 mg PO every 6 hours without waiting for the culture and sensitivity results. The prescriber has determined that penicillinase-resistant penicillin is likely to be effective in most cases of soft tissue infection. If the results of the C&S demonstrate otherwise, T.L.'s prescription will be changed.**

Planning Following the antibacterial therapy, T.L. will be free of the signs and symptoms of wound infection. During the antibacterial therapy, T.L. will:

- Experience a decrease in the signs and symptoms of his wound infection.
- Experience minimal adverse effects of the drug therapy.
- Effectively manage the therapeutic regimen, including compliance with the antibacterial, and implementation of nonpharmacologic supportive measures (e.g., wound care).
- Collaborate with health care providers by appropriately reporting untoward symptoms and maintaining scheduled visits for monitoring and treatment.

Implementation

Monitoring When an antibacterial is administered for prophylaxis, monitor the client for signs indicating the absence or development of infection. When a specific infection is treated, as with T.L., therapeutic response will be indicated by a decrease in the specific signs of infection identified in the baseline assessment (fever, malaise, elevated WBC count, redness, inflammation, drainage, pain, positive cultures). Evaluation of the therapeutic response is im-

NURSING CARE PLAN SELECTED NURSING DIAGNOSES RELATED TO ANTIMICROBIAL THERAPY

Nursing Diagnosis	Outcome Criteria	Nursing Interventions

Deficient knowledge related to antimicrobial drug therapy	Client will:
	• Express an understanding of the purpose, function, and adverse effects of drug therapy
	• Demonstrate an understanding of proper drug handling and administration
		• Assess the client's level of knowledge and understanding.
		• Determine the education needs of the client.
		• Provide information related to the following:
		  The specific problem being treated with the antimicrobial agent
		  The purpose and function of drug therapy
		  The adverse effects of the drug
		  The methods of reducing adverse effects
		• Answer questions and clarify misconceptions.
		• If the drug is to be self-administered, instruct the client in the following:
		  The proper route and method of administration
		  Proper storage and handling
		  The importance of taking all of the prescribed drug
		  Alert the client to possible drug interactions
		  Instruct the client not to take additional medications without first checking with the prescriber

Imbalanced nutrition: less than body requirements related to gastrointestinal effects of antimicrobial drugs	Client will: • Maintain desired nutritional status	• Assess the client's normal dietary patterns and intake. • Assess the normal pattern of bowel function. • Emphasize the importance of adequate nutrition. • Instruct the client to report any gastrointestinal changes (nausea, vomiting, cramping, gas, diarrhea, constipation). • Administer the drug in relation to meals and food to minimize adverse effects (with meals, before or after, depending on the specific drug) yet maintain effectiveness of therapy. • Encourage the intake of active culture yogurt or buttermilk to maintain or restore intestinal flora. • Report adverse effects to the prescriber.

portant, because T.L.'s antibacterial therapy may be ineffective for several reasons, including incorrect route of administration, inappropriate wound care, and poor antibacterial penetration of infected tissues, subtherapeutic serum levels, or bacterial resistance to the antibacterial agent.

As discussed in Chapter 57, reducing or eliminating normal flora by antibacterial therapy provides an environment conducive to the growth of undesirable bacteria, fungi, or yeasts in a condition known as superinfection. Examples commonly seen include diarrhea from altered intestinal flora or, in female clients, vaginal yeast infections resulting from a reduction in normal vaginal flora, which suppress yeast growth.

Adverse effects vary widely and depend on the drug, dose, route of administration, and client-related factors. Refer to the nursing management sections of specific antimicrobials for the adverse effects and the nursing evaluation related to those drugs.

Allergic reactions are always possible following the first or successive doses. In general, it is important to monitor for allergic reactions such as anaphylaxis, skin rashes, urticaria, and bronchospasm. Stop administration immediately at the first sign of an allergic reaction, and notify the prescriber (see Chapter 57 for more information).

Intervention Dosages and routes of administration of antibacterials are highly individualized and are based on the organism or infection being treated and on a variety of T.L.'s individual client factors such as age, weight, general health, and preexisting diseases or organ or system dysfunction. Antibacterials are available in various dosage forms for topical, oral, or parenteral use. Dosage adjustments between different forms or routes of administration are necessary because of differences in absorption, distribution, metabolism, or excretion. For example, if T.L. were to be prescribed penicillin G, the oral dose of penicillin G would need to be five times the amount of the parenteral dose to achieve the same serum levels.

Special attention must be given to the interactions of oral antibacterials with food or other drugs. Some agents should not be administered with food. Dicloxacillin is to be taken on an empty stomach (at least 1 hour before or 2 hours after meals). Food interferes with the rate and extent of drug absorption. Other antimicrobials are administered with food to minimize gastric irritation.

The times of antibacterial drug administration should be spaced as evenly as possible over a 24-hour period to ensure stable and consistent serum levels. Antibacterials that are to be given four times daily should be administered every 6 hours; those administered three times daily are given every 8 hours. T.L. determines that it will be best for him to take his dicloxacillin on a 6 AM, 12 PM, 6 PM, and 12 AM schedule because he is an early riser. However, ensuring that his medication will be taken on an empty stomach is a bit more challenging. He decides that if he has breakfast at 7 AM, and has a coffee break snack at 10 AM, he will be able to lunch at 1 PM with dinner at 7 PM. It is important to administer antibacterials at the scheduled time with an equal time between dosing to maintain a consistent blood level. Allowable variation differs with specific drugs and institutional

policy. As a general rule, antibacterials should be administered within 15 minutes of the scheduled time.

The serum levels of some antibacterials are monitored to determine if the concentration is at the correct (therapeutic) level, a high (toxic) level, or a low (subtherapeutic) level. The timing of serum determinations is also important. To determine the lowest serum level, or trough concentration, the blood is drawn immediately before administering a dose. Mean serum levels are determined at some point between doses, and the highest serum level, or peak level, is determined shortly after dose administration. The desired serum concentration may vary with different drugs and the infecting organism. The exact timing of peak, mean, or trough serum concentrations is determined by each particular drug and route of administration. Consult with the pharmacist or laboratory for specific recommendations.

Education Inform T.L. about the nature of his wound and his treatment plan. He should understand the medication regimen, including the name of the medication (generic and trade names) and its general action, purpose, proper handling, dosage, and correct administration. Provide T.L. with a list of adverse effects, drug-drug interactions, and food-drug interactions; advise him of the proper response to take if these interactions occur. Difficulty breathing or wheezing are adverse effects requiring immediate contact with a health care provider. Nausea, diarrhea, rash, itching, hives, fever, chills, joint pain or swelling are also signs of an adverse effect. The drug should be stopped and the prescriber contacted immediately.

Discuss with T.L. how to integrate his therapeutic regimen into his lifestyle, e.g., to take the medication exactly as prescribed, at evenly spaced intervals, and for the full length of time prescribed or until all the drug is gone. Even if his wound begins to heal, the infection may return if the full course of therapy is not completed. Any leftover medication should be appropriately discarded.

Evaluation If T.L.'s antibacterial therapy is administered therapeutically, he will maintain or achieve an infection-free state as evidenced by an absence of wound drainage, negative cultures, a body temperature within normal limits, a WBC count within the normal limits for age, a well-healed wound, and the resolution of the lymphadenopathy or any other infection-related symptoms that he might be experiencing. T.L. will also manage the therapeutic regimen effectively and demonstrate practices to prevent the spread of infection. If the antibacterial were to be administered prophylactically, the expected outcome is that the client will remain free of infectious processes and will demonstrate appropriate practices to prevent infection.

✱ **J.K., a 13-year-old male weighing 50 kg, presents to the pediatrician with pharyngeal pain, low grade fever, and erythema noted on the back of his throat. A throat culture is obtained and sent to the lab. An office-based test for hemolytic streptococci is positive, and penicillin V potassium 250 mg PO every 8 hours for 10 days is prescribed.**

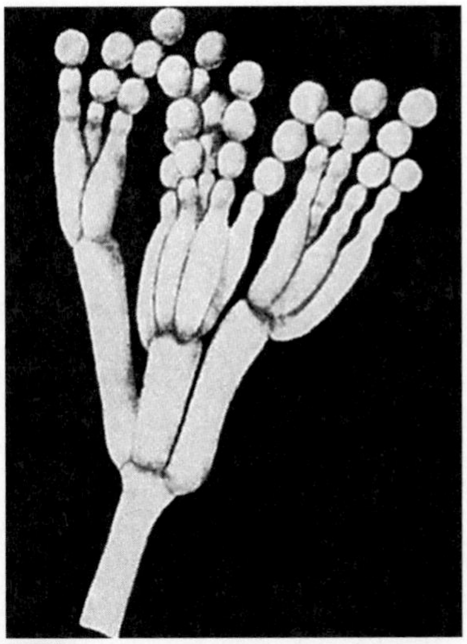

FIGURE 58-1 Typical penicillus of *Penicillus notatum*, Flemming triple stain.

From Raper, K.B., & Alexander, D.F. (1945). *J Elisha Mitchell Sc Soc, 61,* 74.

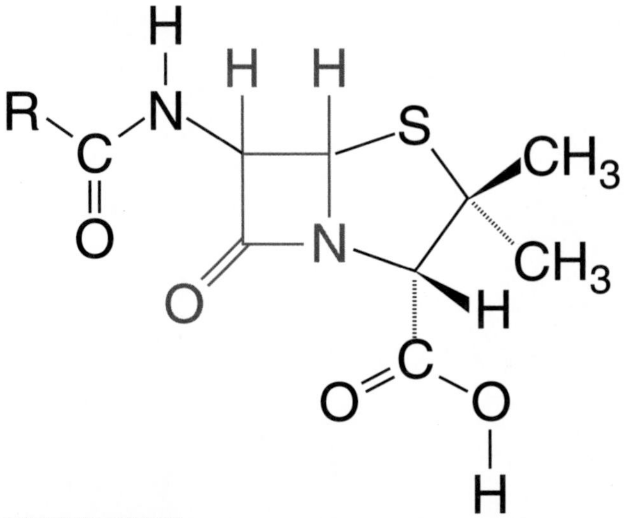

FIGURE 58-2 Chemical structure of penicillins with β-lactam ring highlighted. Variations in chemical structures of different penicillins occur at "R" in the chemical structure.

Courtesy of the Chemical Heritage Foundation, Philadelphia, PA.

What is penicillin?

Penicillins are antimicrobials derived from a number of strains of common molds often seen on bread or fruit (Figure 58-1). Introduced into clinical practice in the 1940s, penicillin and related agents constitute a large group of antimicrobial agents that remain the most effective and least toxic of all available antimicrobial drugs.

Penicillins are among a broad group of agents that share a β-lactam ring in their chemical structure (Figure 58-2). There are now four different classifications of antibacterials that contain the β-lactam ring: penicillins, cephalosporins, monobactams, and carbapenems. These agents are sometimes classified together as **β-lactams** because of their similar chemical structures. A great number of β-lactam antimicrobials are available for use. Each of these classes share similar mechanisms of action and share the potential for adverse effects and allergic reactions. Table 58-1 presents an overview of the β-lactams.

What is the mechanism of action of penicillins?

The cell walls of bacteria are permeable and rigid to protect cellular cytoplasm. Penicillins weaken the cell wall by inhibiting the transpeptidase enzymes responsible for cross-linking the cell wall strands, which results in cell lysis and death. Penicillins are therefore bactericidal because they inhibit the synthesis of the bacterial cell wall.

Many β-lactams are not useful in the presence of bacterial enzymes that are capable of destroying penicillins, such as penicillinase strains of the β-lactamase enzymes. Alteration of the β-lactam rings has resulted in the formulation of drugs that are more active against gram-negative cell wall organisms and are less susceptible to β-lactamases that inactivate the drug. The β-lactam-altered penicillins nafcillin, oxacillin, and dicloxacillin are stable in the presence of β-lactamases, whereas ampicillin and/or amoxicillin must be combined with β-lactamase inhibitors such as clavulanate, sulbactam, or tazobactam to improve their effectiveness.

Most penicillins are much more active against gram-positive than gram-negative bacteria. However, the extended spectrum penicillins (e.g., ticarcillin), monobactams (e.g., aztreonam) and carbapenems (e.g., imipenem), and the combination of penicillins with β-lactamase inhibitors are more effective against gram-negative bacteria *(Escherichia coli, Klebsiella pneumoniae,* and others*)*. Prophylactically, penicillin is indicated for the prevention of diphtheria, bacterial endocarditis, and rheumatic fever.

What penicillins are available and how are they differentiated?

Penicillins are divided into the following categories. Each category is presented below and includes a brief monograph on a selected agent in the group:

1. **Natural penicillins.** This category includes penicillin G and penicillin V. Penicillin G and penicillin V are comparable therapeutically, but oral penicillin V is more stable in stomach acid and therefore reaches higher serum levels than oral penicillin G. Penicillin G is available in intramuscular (IM), and intravenous (IV) dosage forms in various salt formulations: sodium penicillin G, potassium penicillin G, procaine penicillin G, benzathine penicillin G, and a parenteral combination of the latter two formulations.

penicillin V potassium [pen i **sill** in vee poe **tass** ee um]
(Veetids, Apo-Pen-VK✱, Novo-Pen-VK✱)

Indications

Penicillin V potassium is used treat infections caused by susceptible organisms in the respiratory tract and other areas, and for the prophylaxis of rheumatic fever.

TABLE 58-1 β-LACTAMS

Class	Subclass	Agents
Penicillin	Natural penicillins	penicillin G penicillin V
	Penicillinase-resistant penicillins	cloxacillin dicloxacillin methicillin nafcillin oxacillin
	Aminopenicillins	amoxicillin amoxicillin-clavulanate ampicillin ampicillin-sulbactam bacampicillin
	Extended spectrum penicillins	carbenicillin mezlocillin* piperacillin piperacillin-tazobactam ticarcillin ticarcillin-clavulanate
Cephalosporin	First generation	cefadroxil cefazolin cephalexin cephalothin cephradine
	Second generation	cefaclor cefmetazole cefotetan cefoxitin cefprozil cefuroxime loracarbef
	Third generation	cefdinir cefditoren cefixime cefoperazone cefotaxime cefpodoxime ceftazidime ceftibuten ceftizoxime ceftriaxone
	Fourth generation	cefepime
Monobactam		aztreonam
Carbapenem		ertapenem imipenem-cilastatin meropenem

*No longer marketed; generic name product may be available in the United States; not commercially available in Canada.

Pharmacokinetics/Dosing

Orally administered penicillin V potassium is stable in gastric acid and approximately 65% of the drug is absorbed into systemic circulation. It has a short elimination half-life of approximately 30 minutes. The adult dose is usually 125 to 500 mg orally every 6 to 8 hours, with twice daily dosing sometimes used for prophylaxis.

Adverse Effects

The most serious adverse effect of penicillins is hypersensitivity reactions, including anaphylaxis. Acute interstitial nephritis, hemolytic anemia, and seizures are rare but serious events as well. More commonly, penicillin produces nausea, vomiting, mild diarrhea, and may result in oral candidiasis.

2. **Penicillinase-resistant penicillins.** This category includes the parenterally administered nafcillin and oxacillin, and the orally administered cloxacillin, dicloxacillin. Methicillin, also a member of this group, is no longer marketed for clinical use, but is used by laboratories to identify resistant strains of staphylococcus aureus (e.g., methicillin-resistant *Staphylococcus aureus* or MRSA).

A chemical alteration of the penicillin structure results in penicillins resistant to β-lactamase inactivation; these penicillins are used to treat penicillinase-producing staphylococci. These antimicrobials are not effective against methicillin-resistant bacteria.

nafcillin [naf **sil** in]
(Unipen)
Indications

Nafcillin is used IV to treat osteomyelitis, septicemia, endocarditis, cellulitis, and central nervous system (CNS) infections caused by susceptible strains of staphylococci. It is not effective against MRSA.

Pharmacokinetics/Dosing

On IV administration, it is distributed well to body tissues. Penetration to the cerebrospinal fluid (CSF) is limited, but may be adequate when the meninges are inflamed. It is eliminated in the feces and urine. Dosing varies based on indication. The typical adult dose is 500 mg to 2000 mg IV every 4 to 6 hours. It can also be administered IM, but frequency of dosing makes IM administration undesirable.

Adverse Effects

Nafcillin shares the same risks for hypersensitivity, seizures, and gastrointestinal (GI) upset with other penicillins. Phlebitis is common at the IV site and can be reduced with dilution and slower administration rates.

3. **Aminopenicillins or broader-spectrum penicillins.** This category includes amoxicillin, amoxicillin and potassium clavulanate, ampicillin, ampicillin and sulbactam, and bacampicillin. Although these agents have the spectrum of activity of penicillin in addition to efficacy against selected gram-negative bacteria, the single agents are usually not very effective against *S. aureus* (β-lactamase-producing) bacteria. The penicillin is protected from inactivation by β-lactamase enzymes when combined with β-lactamase inhibitors such as potassium clavulanate and sulbactam.

amoxicillin/potassium clavulanate
[a moks i **sil** in/poe **tass** ee um klav yoo **lan** ate]
(Augmentin)
Indications

Amoxicillin/clavulanate is used to treat otitis media, sinusitis, and infections involving susceptible pathogens. The addition of the β-lactamase inhibitor, clavulanate, improves activity against strains of *H. influenzae, B. catarrhalis, N. gonorrhoeae,* and *S. aureus* (although not MRSA). The use of amoxicillin/clavulanate or other antibacterials in the treatment of otitis media is typically limited to children under 2 years of age or with severe infection accompanied by fever (McCormick et al., 2005).

Pharmacokinetics/Dosing

Amoxicillin and clavulanate are both well absorbed orally and eliminated renally. A number of dosing combinations are available, and dose and schedule varies widely based on indication and dosage form. A typical adult dose is 250 to 500 mg amoxicillin/125 mg clavulanate every 8 hours or 500 to 875 mg amoxicillin/125 mg clavulanate every 12 hours.

Adverse Effects

Amoxicillin/clavulanate shares the risk for hypersensitivity reactions with penicillins. Diarrhea is a frequent complication to amoxicillin/clavulanate and may be more common with higher doses of clavulanate. A rash is also observed frequently 2 to 5 days into therapy. It is important to differentiate this delayed rash (type IV hypersensitivity reaction) from immediate onset urticaria or hives which are type I, IgE-based reactions. Type IV reactions are uncomfortable, but not life threatening; and future β-lactam therapy could be considered if absolutely necessary. Type I reactions pose a risk for anaphylaxis and all β-lactams should be avoided if these reactions are noted.

4. **Extended-spectrum penicillins.** This category includes parenterally administered mezlocillin, piperacillin, piperacillin/tazobactam, ticarcillin, and ticarcillin/clavulanate potassium. Carbenicillin is an orally administered agent in the class that is occasionally used for bladder and prostate infections, but inadequate tissue levels are achieved for more serious infections. These drugs have a broader spectrum of antimicrobial activity that includes *Pseudomonas aeruginosa, Enterobacter, Proteus,* and others. Because *P. aeruginosa* is such an important hospital acquired pathogen, these agents are often referred to as the anti-*pseudomonal* penicillins. In this category, only the combination agents are effective against *S. aureus* (β-lactamase-producing) bacteria.

piperacillin/tazobactam [pi **per** a sil in/ta zoe **bak** tam]
(Zosyn, Tacozin✚)
Indications

Piperacillin/tazobactam is indicated for serious infections due to susceptible pathogens, including pneumonias, urinary tract, gynecologic, bone, intraabdominal, and blood-borne infections. The addition of the β-lactamase inhibitor, tazobactam, extends coverage for strains of *H. influenzae, S. aureus,* and *Bacteroides.*

Pharmacokinetics/Dosing

Piperacillin/tazobactam is administered IV and is eliminated renally. Dosing varies based on indication. The typical adult dose is piperacillin 2 to 4 g/tazobactam 250 to 500 mg IV every 6 to 8 hours. Dosage adjustment is recommended for renal impairment.

Adverse Effects

Adverse effects are similar to other penicillins. GI upset and diarrhea are relatively common adverse effects.

TABLE 58-2 PENICILLINS: PHARMACOKINETICS AND USUAL ADULT DOSAGE

Drug	Oral Absorption	Renal Excretion*	Usual Adult Dose*
NATURAL PENICILLINS			
penicillin G			
IV	NA	60%-90%	1-5 million units IV q4-6h
IM benzathine	NA	60%-90%	1.2-2.4 million units IM single dose
IM procaine	NA	60%-90%	600,000 units-1.2 million units IM daily
penicillin V (Veetids)			
Oral	60%-73%	20%-40%	125-500 mg PO q6-8h
PENICILLINASE-RESISTANT PENICILLINS			
cloxacillin (Tegopen)			
Oral	50%	30%-60%	250-500 mg PO q6h
dicloxacillin (Dynapen)			
Oral	37%-50%	50%-70%	125-500 mg PO q6h
nafcillin (Unipen)			
IV	NA	10%-30%	0.5-1.5 g IV q4h
IM	NA	10%-30%	500 mg IM q4-6h
oxacillin (Prostaphlin)			
IV	NA	55%-60%	250 mg-1 g IV q4-6h
IM	NA	55%-60%	250 mg-1 g IM q4-6h
AMINO-PENICILLINS (BROADER-SPECTRUM)			
amoxicillin (Amoxil)			
Oral	75%-90%	60%-75%	250-500 mg PO q8h or 500-875 mg PO q12h
amoxicillin/clavulanate (Augmentin, Clavulin✤)			
Oral	90%	50%-78%	250-500 mg amoxicillin/125 mg clavulanate PO q8h OR 500-875 mg amoxicillin/125 mg clavulanate q12h
ampicillin (Polycillin)			
IV	NA	75%-90%	250-500 mg IV q6h
IM	NA	75%-90%	250-500 mg IM q6h
Oral	35%-50%	75%-90%	250-500 mg PO q6h
ampicillin/sulbactam (Unasyn)			
IV	NA	75%-85%	1.5-3 g IV q6h
IM	NA	75%-85%	1.5-3 g IM q6h
bacampicillin (Penglobe✤)			
Oral	35%-50% (as ampicillin)	70%-75% (as ampicillin)	400-800 mg PO q12h

Modified from Lacy, C.F., Armstrong, L.L., Goldman, M.P., & Lance, L.L. (2004). *Lexi-Comp's Drug Information Handbook* (12th ed.). Hudson, Ohio: Lexi-Comp, and *USP DI: Drug Information for the Health Care Professional* (24th ed.). (2004). Greenwood Village, CO: MICROMEDEX Thomson Healthcare.
*Dosage reduction is required for clients with renal dysfunction for most agents—refer to package labeling for more details.

TABLE 58-2 PENICILLINS: PHARMACOKINETICS AND USUAL ADULT DOSAGE—CONT'D

Drug	Oral Absorption	Renal Excretion*	Usual Adult Dose*
EXTENDED-SPECTRUM PENICILLINS (ALSO REFERRED TO AS ANTI-*PSEUDOMONAL* PENICILLINS)			
carbenicillin (Geocillin)			
Oral	30%	36%	0.5-1 g PO q6h
piperacillin (Pipracil)			
IV	NA	60%-80%	3-4 g IV q4-6h
IM	NA	60%-80%	3-4 g IM q4-6h
piperacillin/tazobactam (Zosyn)			
IV	NA	60%-80%	3.375-4.5 g IV q4-6h
ticarcillin (Ticar)			
IV	NA	60%-80%	3-4 g IV q4-6h
IM	NA	60%-80%	3-4 g IM q4-6h
ticarcillin/clavulanate (Timentin)			
IV	NA	60%-70%	3.1 g IV q4-6h

Table 58-2 summarizes pharmacokinetics and the usual adult dosages of the penicillins.

✻ What are the adverse effects of penicillins?

The adverse effects of penicillins include diarrhea, nausea, vomiting, headache, sore mouth or tongue, and oral and vaginal candidiasis, some of which may be related to superinfection. Less commonly reported, but potentially serious, are allergic reactions, anaphylaxis, serum sickness–type reaction (rash, joint pain, fever), hives, and pruritus.

✻ J.K. receives a prescription for penicillin V potassium. He and his mother talk with the office nurse about the use of penicillin.

✻ What are the important nursing implications in the use of penicillins for T.L.?

Although general nursing management of antibacterials was discussed in the previous case of T.L. and as general principles related to antimicrobials in Chapter 57, the penicillins present some unique nursing management issues.

Assessment Ascertain J.K.'s history of sensitivity to penicillins. Because allergic reactions are a significant problem in the use of penicillins, meticulously assess his previous drug experiences, giving special attention to the development of prior drug-related rashes. For infants less than 3 months of age, assess for a history of penicillin allergy in the mother. If at all possible, no penicillin preparation of any type should be prescribed for or administered to a client with a history of allergic reaction to the drug. Because of possible cross-sensitization, it is also wise to avoid the use of cephalosporins in clients with severe or immediate allergic reactions to penicillins. (See the Special Considerations for

Children box on p. 1020 regarding how to assess the appropriate antimicrobial therapy in children.)

Assess J.K.'s health status for conditions in which the administration of penicillin might be contraindicated or need cautious use. Clients with a history of bleeding disorders require monitoring for bleeding tendencies with the administration of carbenicillin, piperacillin, and ticarcillin because they may cause platelet dysfunction. Clients with a history of GI disease, particularly ulcerative colitis, and regional enteritis, are more at risk for pseudomembranous colitis as an adverse effect. Although J.K. will not be administered parenteral forms of penicillin, the sodium content of high doses of parenteral carbenicillin and ticarcillin should be considered with clients who may have sodium restrictions, such as those with heart failure and hypertension. Skin rash may occur in 43% to 100% of clients who have infectious mononucleosis and are receiving ampicillin or bacampicillin. Clients with cystic fibrosis who are administered piperacillin are at greater risk for fever and skin rash. Clients with renal function impairment may require lower dosages. See the Pregnancy Safety box on p. 1020 for the Food and Drug Administration (FDA) pregnancy categories for the penicillins.

Review J.K.'s medications for the risk of significant drug interactions. For orally administered penicillins, such as with J.K., a number of interactions are possible. Cholestyramine (Questran) or colestipol (Colestid) may decrease the absorption of oral penicillins. Concurrent use of estrogen-containing contraceptives with ampicillin, amoxicillin, or penicillin V may reduce the effectiveness of the hormonal contraceptive.

For either orally or parenterally administered penicillins, methotrexate (Folex) toxicity may be noted because penicillins decrease methotrexate clearance. Probenecid (Benemid) decreases renal tubular secretion of penicillins, result-

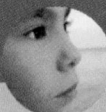

Special Considerations for Children | ANTIMICROBIALS

To assess the appropriateness of antimicrobial therapy in children, the following criteria are generally accepted:

1. In choosing empiric therapy, the selected antimicrobial should have documentation of both adequate penetration at the site and proven effectiveness against the common organisms usually isolated from that specific site.
2. Multiple drug therapy may be indicated if a broad range of possible microorganisms is suspected or if multiple organisms have been isolated from an infection site. However, the minimum number of drugs necessary to treat the infection should be used whenever possible.
3. If no contraindication is present, the drug of first choice should be selected. The drug dosage regimen should be within the accepted range of current usage for the individual client, taking into account the child's body surface area (height, weight), organ function, and concurrent disease processes.
4. Unless the benefit far outweighs the risk, no antimicrobial should be used in clients who have prior documen-

tation of an allergic or adverse reaction to the specific medication.
5. Children receiving potentially dangerous drugs (e.g., gentamicin, amikacin, tobramycin, or vancomycin) for more than 2 days should have steady state drug serum concentrations drawn at the appropriate times for evaluation.
6. Whenever possible, cultures should be drawn before the initiation of antimicrobial therapy. The usual sites cultured include sputum, urine, blood, wound, or nonhealing topical sites.
7. Antimicrobial therapy should be continued until the infection is no longer present. However, time periods should not exceed the usual treatment time established for suspected infection. Prophylactic antimicrobial therapy given after uncomplicated surgery is usually discontinued within 48 hours with few exceptions, such as cardiac surgery.

PREGNANCY SAFETY
ANTIBACTERIALS

Category	Drug
B	azithromycin, cephalosporins, clindamycin, ertapenem, erythromycin, meropenem, penicillins, penicillins + β-lactamase inhibitors, metronidazole, nitrofurantoin
C	chloramphenicol, clarithromycin, colistin, fluoroquinolones (ciprofloxacin, ofloxacin, levofloxacin, gatifloxacin, moxifloxacin), imipenem/cilastatin, linezolid, sulfamethoxazole-trimethoprim, vancomycin
D	aminoglycosides (e.g., gentamicin, tobramycin), tetracyclines

Data from *Mosby's drug consult* (15th ed.) (2005). St. Louis: Mosby.

ing in elevated serum levels and an increased half-life. Several combinations of penicillin and probenecid are marketed to take advantage of this effect. Concurrent use of antibacterial agents that are bacteriostatic (e.g., tetracyclines, macrolides) slow bacterial multiplication and may inhibit the penicillins that act against rapidly multiplying bacteria. Such combinations, although not absolutely contraindicated, are generally avoided if possible.

For penicillins administered IV, a number of potentially significant interactions are also possible. Aminoglycosides (e.g., gentamicin, tobramycin) are often used with the penicillinase resistant agents (e.g., nafcillin) against enterococci and *S. aureus* or the extended spectrum agents (e.g., piperacillin) against *P. aeruginosa*. In such cases, the penicillin must not be mixed in the same syringe or IV infusion as the aminoglycoside, because inactivation of both drugs is possible. Instead, their administration should be separated by up to 1 hour, and IV lines flushed between the administration of each. High doses of IV potassium salts of penicillin (e.g., penicillin G potassium) can lead to potential hyperkalemia if given to clients with renal failure, or who are receiving angiotensin-converting enzyme (ACE) inhibitors, potassium-sparing diuretics, potassium-containing drugs, or potassium supplements. Sodium salts of high dose parenteral penicillins (e.g., penicillin G sodium, piperacillin, piperacillin/tazobactam, ticarcillin, ticarcillin/clavulanate) present a significant sodium load and may contribute to heart failure in clients with underlying cardiovascular or renal disease. Use of oral anticoagulants, heparin or thrombolytic agents can lead to increased risk of bleeding when given with high doses of parenteral piperacillin, or ticarcillin, because these drugs inhibit platelet aggregation. Similarly, nonsteroidal antiinflammatory drugs (NSAIDs), platelet aggregation inhibitors (e.g., salicylates, dextran, dipyridamole [Persantine], valproic acid [Depakote], and sulfinpyrazone [Anturane]) increase the risk for bleeding or hemorrhage with high doses of parenteral piperacillin, or ticarcillin.

A baseline assessment as described in Chapter 57 is necessary for J.K. who will be receiving penicillin therapy.

Nursing Diagnosis While receiving penicillin therapy, J.K. is at risk for the following nursing diagnoses/collaborative problems: ineffective protection related to a reduction in normal flora (superinfection) as evidenced by a darkened tongue (fungal superinfection) and white oral plaques and creamy vaginal discharge (*Candida* superinfection); diarrhea (watery and severe) related to the development of antibiotic-associated pseudomembranous colitis (AAPMC); deficient fluid volume related to nausea, vomiting, and/or diarrhea; impaired skin integrity (exfoliative dermatitis, urticaria, rash); and the potential complications of allergic response, interstitial nephritis, hepatotoxicity, leukopenia or neutropenia, thrombocytopenia, mental disturbances, seizures, or a cross-sensitivity to cephalosporins, cephamycins, griseofulvin, or penicillamine.

Planning Following penicillin therapy, J.K. will be free of the signs and symptoms of his pharyngeal infection. During the penicillin therapy, J.K. will:

- Experience diminished signs and symptoms of infection with minimal or no adverse effects of drug therapy.
- Effectively manage the therapeutic regimen with his family, including being compliant with the penicillin, and implementing nonpharmacologic supportive measures (e.g., hydration, rest, good nutrition, proper hygiene with soiled handkerchiefs, hand washing).

- Collaborate with health care providers with his family by appropriately reporting untoward symptoms and maintaining scheduled visits for monitoring and treatment.

Implementation

Monitoring Assess J.K.'s temperature along with his clinical symptoms of pharyngeal discomfort and redness. His C&S should confirm the office Quik-Strep test. If it does not, his medication regimen will be altered to cover the responsible pathogen. Because of the possibility of bacterial and fungal superinfection, observe J.K. carefully for unusual weight loss (AAPMC), abdominal cramps and diarrhea, a darkened or discolored tongue, and sore mouth; although older adults and debilitated clients are at higher risk. See Box 58-2 for a discussion of AAPMC.

In addition for other penicillins, serum electrolytes should be monitored for hyperkalemia and/or hypernatremia when the client is receiving mezlocillin, parenteral penicillin G, piperacillin, and ticarcillin. Monitor also a client's vital signs, total and differential WBC count, culture results and bowel function. If significant diarrhea is noted and/or *Clostridium difficile* colitis is suspected, stool cytotoxic assays may be warranted. Bleeding times (partial thromboplastin time [PTT] and prothrombin time [PT]) should be monitored with the administration of piperacillin or ticarcillin for high-risk clients (e.g., those with a history of bleeding and those with concurrent antiplatelet, anticoagulant, or fibrinolytic therapy).

Box 58-2 ANTIBACTERIAL ASSOCIATED PSEUDOMEMBRANOUS COLITIS (AAPMC)

During or after treatment with a number of antibacterial agents, some clients may develop antibacterial associated pseudomembranous colitis (AAPMC), caused by the *C. difficile* toxin. Although any antibacterial can lead to AAPMC, β-lactams, some fluoroquinolones, and clindamycin that disrupt gut anaerobes may pose the highest risk (Gaynes et al., 2004). Concurrent use of proton pump inhibitors (e.g., omeprazole) may also increase risk (Dial, Alrasadi, Manoukian, Huang, & Menzies, 2004). AAPMC is characterized by inflammation and necrosis of the mucosal and submucosal layers of the bowel wall as evidenced by two to five semisolid or liquid stools per day in mild cases and 30 or more watery stools per day in severe disease. Fluid and electrolyte loss, abdominal tenderness, cramping, and fever also occur. AAPMC is fatal in up to 14% of cases (Pepin et al., 2004) and the risk for fatalities is up to ten times more likely in older adults compared to younger clients (Eggertson, 2004). It is called pseudomembranous because the inflammation causes the formation of exudative plaques or "pseudomembranes" on the mucosal wall.

Two types of clients develop AAPMC: those who are carriers of *C. difficile* and are given antibacterial agents and noncarriers who are given antibacterials and then are exposed to the organism through environmental conditions. Spores of the organism have been known to persist for long periods of time

and are not killed by alcohol hand gels (Loo et al., 2004). The Centers for Disease Control and Prevention (CDC) recommends judicious use of antimicrobials, institution of contact precautions for clients with known or suspected *C. difficile*–associated disease, and environmental cleaning with a hypochlorite-based (e.g., household bleach) disinfectant. In 23% of cases, symptoms resolve in 2 to 3 days after discontinuation of the offending antibacterial (CDC Fact Sheet, September 2004).

Moderate to severe cases may require the replacement of fluid and electrolytes. In clients nonresponsive to discontinuing the caustic antibacterial, and in more severe cases, oral metronidazole or vancomycin is used. Unfortunately, metronidazole-resistant strains have been noted (Musher et al., 2005; Pepin et al., 2005). Cholestyramine may occasionally be used to bind the toxin (Poutanen & Simor, 2004), but must be dosed hours apart from metronidazole or vancomycin so regarding reduce binding of those drugs to cholestyramine.

Recurrences are not common and can be treated with a second round of drugs. Watery diarrhea in AAPMC may occur for up to several weeks after completion of metronidazole or vancomycin therapy. Antidiarrheals are not recommended because they can retain the toxin within the bowel and prolong or worsen damage to the colon (Wolfson & Kahana, 2004).

Intervention In addition to performing nursing measures common to all types of antibacterial drug therapy (as discussed previously in this chapter and Chapter 57), be especially cognizant of the following factors when penicillins are prescribed.

Although penicillin V potassium for J.K. is to be taken after a meal rather than on an empty stomach for better absorption, most oral penicillins are bound to food and are poorly absorbed in acid media. Therefore their administration should not be preceded or followed by food for at least 1 hour to minimize binding. Table 58-3 lists the effect of food on oral penicillin absorption. Ampicillin, bacampicillin oral suspension, carbenicillin, cloxacillin, and dicloxacillin, should be taken when the stomach is empty. Amoxicillin, bacampicillin, and penicillin V may be taken either on an empty stomach or with food to decrease GI distress.

Although J.K. is taking oral penicillin, the nurse should note that when administering penicillins IV, most penicillins in clinical use are sodium or potassium salts. Significant amounts of cations can be administered when these drugs are given IV in a massive dose. For example, 20 million units of potassium penicillin G contain 34 mEq of potassium ion. Fatalities have occurred because of the toxic effect of potassium on the heart following the administration of such large doses in the presence of renal insufficiency. High-dose parenteral ticarcillin can provide 2 to 3 grams of sodium per day—a potential concern for clients with sodium restrictions because of heart failure or renal disease (Gilbert, Moellering, Eliopoulos, & Sande, 2004). Monitor serum electrolytes and cardiac status closely when the client is receiving IV penicillins. Signs and symptoms of hyperkalemia (e.g., cardiac dysrhythmias) and hypernatremia (e.g., edema) should be duly noted and reported. To prevent blood vessel irritation and phlebitis when administering penicillins IV, do so intermittently. The IV site should be changed at least every 48 hours.

Education Instruct J.K. to take the full course of medication, even if he is feeling better and is symptom free. Emphasize the importance of taking evenly spaced doses to maintain therapeutic blood levels. Prescriptions for penicillins or other antimicrobials should never be shared with others or saved and taken for a different episode of illness. Instruct J.K. and his mother to report to his prescriber if his condition fails to improve in a few days or if he develops severe diarrhea, sore mouth, rash, fever, or chills, which may indicate a delayed sensitivity reaction or superinfection.

Caution women taking penicillins, especially ampicillin, amoxicillin, and penicillin V, to use an alternate form of contraception if they are using estrogen-containing contraceptives. The loss of effectiveness of the contraceptive is thought to be because of a reduction in enterohepatic circulation of estrogens resulting in lower serum levels.

Evaluation The expected outcome of J.K.'s penicillin therapy is that J.K. will achieve an infection-free state as evidenced by negative throat cultures and an absence of his symptoms, sore and reddened pharyngeal tissue, without any adverse effects of the penicillin. He will have a body temperature within normal limits and a WBC count within the normal limits. J.K. will be compliant with his penicillin therapy. With the assistance of his family, he will maintain scheduled visits with his health care provider and implement nonpharmacologic supportive measures (e.g., 1500-mL fluid intake, adequate diet).

✳ **M.T. is a 19-year-old construction worker who reports to the clinic with cellulitis of the left hand and upper arm. He receives one dose of ceftriaxone 2 grams IM now, and is discharged to home with a prescription of cephalexin (Keflex) 500 mg PO q6h × 10 days.**

✳ **What are the cephalosporins?**
Cephalosporins and related products are chemical modifications of the penicillin structure. These modifications create compounds with different microbiologic and pharmacologic activities. To classify the differences in antimicrobial activity, cephalosporins are divided into four generations. Also included in this section is loracarbef (Lorabid), a β-lactam antibacterial (carbacephem); it is chemically similar to second-generation cephalosporins.

Cephalosporins inhibit cell wall synthesis in a manner similar to penicillin; they are also bactericidal. They are effective in numerous situations, with first-generation agents being used for skin/soft tissue infections and third- and fourth-generation agents used for broader indications.

First-generation cephalosporins are primarily active against gram-positive bacteria. The initial prototype drug for this category was cephalothin (Keflin), but cefazolin (Ancef, Kefzol) is now referred to as the key or prototype drug because of its more widespread use.

■✳▔ **cefazolin** [sef **a** zoe lin]
(Ancef, Kefzol)
Indications
Cefazolin is indicated for the treatment of infections caused by gram-positive and some gram-negative pathogens. It is most commonly used for surgical prophylaxis during clean surgical procedures.

TABLE 58-3 EFFECT OF FOOD ON ORAL PENICILLIN ABSORPTION

Drug	Food Effect
amoxicillin	No effect
amoxicillin/clavulanate	No effect
ampicillin	Decreased absorption
bacampicillin	No effect
carbenicillin indanyl sodium	Increased absorption
cloxacillin	Decreased absorption
dicloxacillin	Decreased absorption
penicillin V potassium	Slightly decreased absorption

Data from *Mosby's drug consult* (15th ed.). (2005). St. Louis: Mosby.

Pharmacokinetics/Dosing

Cefazolin is most often administered IV, although IM administration is also used. It is widely distributed to most body tissue but does not cross well into the CSF. It is hepatically metabolized and has an elimination half-life of approximately 2 hours. It is usually dosed at 1 to 2 grams IV every 8 hours. Surgical prophylaxis doses are usually 1 to 2 grams IV immediately before surgery, with repeat doses after 4 to 6 hours for prolonged procedures.

Adverse Effects

Cefazolin is usually well tolerated. Pain at the injection site and diarrhea are occasionally reported. There is a low, but real chance for significant hypersensitivity reactions for clients with allergies to other β-lactams, including the penicillins. The cross-reactivity between penicillins and cephalosporins is estimated between 2% and 10%. Kelkar and Li (2001) concluded that the risk of an allergic reaction to a cephalosporin was up to eight times higher in clients with a history of penicillin allergy versus nonallergic clients.

The second-generation cephalosporins (cefamandole, cefotetan, and others) have increased activity against gram-negative microorganisms, and a few in this group cover some anaerobes.

cefotetan [**sef** oh tee tan]
(Cefotan)
Indications

Cefotetan is less active against staphylococci and streptococci than the first-generation agents, but has activity against *Bacteroides fragilis*, *E. coli*, *Proteus*, and *Klebsiella*. It is used for gynecologic infections, and some infections of the respiratory tract, urinary tract, bone, joint and skin, and soft tissue.

Pharmacokinetics/Dosing

Cefotetan is administered IV and IM. It possesses a relatively long elimination half-life of 3-5 hours and is usually dosed at 1 to 2 grams every 12 hours in adults.

Adverse Effects

In addition to the risk for hypersensitivity reactions, cefotetan and other second-generation agents contain a methylthiotetrazole (MMT) side chain on the chemical structure. Cephalosporins with this MMT side chain pose a risk for hypoprothrombinemia and bleeding.

The third-generation agents are more active against gram-negative bacteria; ceftazidime (and to some extent, cefoperazone) are also effective against *P. aeruginosa* and β-lactamase-producing microbial strains. However, the third generation is less effective against gram-positive cocci.

ceftriaxone [sef trye **aks** one]
(Rocephin)
Indications

Ceftriaxone is indicated for a number of infections, including pneumonia, UTIs, and infections of the skin, bone, and soft tissue. Because ceftriaxone penetrates well into the CSF, it is also commonly used to treat bacterial meningitis caused by sensitive bacteria.

Pharmacokinetics/Dosing

Ceftriaxone is usually administered IV. IM administration is also used, but is quite painful. Discomfort may be minimized by preparing ceftriaxone with a 1:1 mixture of sterile water for injection and 1% lidocaine prior to IM administration as long as the client has no hypersensitivity to lidocaine. Ceftriaxone is widely distributed to tissue including the CSF. It is highly plasma protein bound (up to 95%) and is often avoided in neonates because it may displace bilirubin from albumin binding sites and lead to icterus. Ceftriaxone is also associated with high levels in bile and may contribute to the risk of cholestasis. Ceftriaxone has a long elimination half-life of 5

to 9 hours and is often dosed once daily. Typical adult dosing is 1 to 2 grams every 24 hours, although doses as high as 2 grams every 12 hours are used in the treatment of meningitis.

Adverse Effects

Pain on injection is the most commonly observed adverse effect. Other adverse effects are similar to those of other cephalosporins. As noted above, icterus in neonates and cholestasis in all clients is possible.

ceftazidime [**sef** tay zi deem]
(Fortaz, Tazidime)
Indications

Ceftazidime is indicated for the treatment of aerobic gram-negative infections and infections with sensitive strains of *P. aeruginosa*. It is also used for the treatment of febrile neutropenia in granulocytopenic clients (e.g., postcancer chemotherapy).

Pharmacokinetics/Dosing

Ceftazidime is administered IV and IM and is distributed widely. Penetration to the CSF is not as high as with ceftriaxone, but it can penetrate CSF with inflamed meninges. The elimination half-life is 1 to 2 hours and is prolonged in renal failure. It is typically dosed at 1 to 2 grams every 8 to 12 hours intravenously in adults.

Adverse Effects

Ceftazidime is well tolerated, and shares the risks for hypersensitivity and superinfection with other cephalosporins.

A fourth-generation cephalosporin that has antimicrobial effects comparable to the third generation and is also more resistant to some β-lactamases is cefepime (Maxipime). It has the advantage of coverage against many *Pseudomonas* species and activity against gram-positive pathogens.

cefepime [**sef** e pim]
(Maxipime)
Indications

Cefepime is indicated for serious infections caused by streptococcus species as well as *P. aeruginosa* and other gram-negative pathogens. Types of infections treated with cefepime include complicated UTIs, pneumonias, and skin and soft tissue infections.

Pharmacokinetics/Dosing

Cefepime is usually administered IV, but IM administration is also possible. It is well distributed to tissue and achieves reasonably high levels in the CSF. It has an elimination half-life of approximately 2 hours and is eliminated via the kidney. The usual adult dose for clients with normal renal function is 500 mg to 2 grams every 8 to 12 hours, with lower doses or longer intervals used in renal insufficiency.

Adverse Effects

Adverse effects of cefepime are similar to ceftazidime, although a high rate of Coombs positive testing without hemolysis is noted.

The initial advantage of cephalosporins over penicillins was their resistance to enzymatic degradation by penicillinase (β-lactamase). However, resistance has now been reported with drugs from all generations, possibly through four mechanisms: (1) the microorganisms lack an outer cell membrane permeability, which causes poor drug penetration in the bacteria; (2) the bacteria lack a receptor for the specific drug; (3) the bacteria produce a β-lactamase enzyme that can split the β-lactam ring in the cephalosporin (many such enzymes have been isolated); or (4) the bacteria develop a type of tolerance in which bacterial strains are inhibited but not killed by the cephalosporins. The reason for this effect is the lack of, or deficiency in, autolytic enzymes in the bacterial cell wall. This class of drugs has historically been overused. As a result, reports of bacterial resistance have increased.

Because cephalosporins inhibit cell wall synthesis, cell division and growth, rapidly dividing bacteria are most affected by them. These agents are indicated for the treatment of a variety of infections and as prophylactic agents before surgery. Combinations of ceftazidime or cefepime and aminoglycosides are used synergistically to treat *P. aeruginosa, Serratia marcescens,* and other susceptible organisms.

✳ What are the adverse effects of cephalosporins?
The adverse effects of cephalosporins include diarrhea, abdominal cramps or distress, oral and/or vaginal candidiasis, rash, pruritus, redness, or edema. An increase in bleeding episodes and bruising because of hypoprothrombinemia is reported with cefamandole, cefmetazole, cefoperazone, and cefotetan.

Cephalosporins are often prescribed for clients who are allergic to penicillins. They should be used with caution, because the possibility of a cross reaction is 2% to 10%. The cephalosporins should not be used if the client reports a serious reaction or anaphylaxis to penicillin.

Table 58-4 summarizes the pharmacokinetics and usual adult dosages for the cephalosporins.

✳ M.T. is counseled by the nurse on the management of his cephalosporin therapy.

✳ What are the nursing management issues with the use of cephalosporins for M.T.?
In addition to the measures taken in the discussion of the nursing management of antibacterials on pp. 1012-1014, the following is of importance with the nursing management of cephalosporins.

Assessment Assess M.T. for preexisting health conditions that may cause cephalosporin therapy to be contraindicated or managed with caution. The use of cephalosporins is contraindicated if M.T. had a history of sensitivity to cephalosporins, penicillin, penicillin derivatives, or penicillamine. Cephalosporins should be used with caution if M.T. had a history of bleeding disorders, because all may cause hypoprothrombinemia and, potentially, bleeding. As with penicillins, clients with a history of GI disease, particularly ulcerative colitis and regional enteritis, are at higher risk for pseudomembranous colitis. It is recommended that clients with renal and hepatic function impairment receive lower dosages.

Review M.T.'s current medication regimen for the risk of significant drug interactions, such as anticoagulants and thrombolytics (increased risk of bleeding and hemorrhage when given concurrently with cefamandole, cefoperazone, or cefotetan as these cephalosporins interfere with vitamin K metabolism in the liver resulting in hypoprothrombinemia); NSAIDs, especially aspirin, sulfinpyrazone (Anturane) and other platelet aggregation inhibitors (an increased risk of hemorrhage exists when given with cefamandole, cefoperazone, or cefotetan, because of the additive effect on platelet inhibition); probenecid (Benemid) (decreases renal tubular secretion of the cephalosporins that are excreted by this mechanism, which can result in increased serum levels, an extended half-life, and an increased potential for toxicity); iron (interferes with the absorption of cefdinir); and other nephrotoxic drugs (increases the risk for nephrotoxicity).

Although not a concern with the cephalexin M.T. has been prescribed, a social history for alcohol consumption is important with cephalosporins. Alcohol is not recommended with cefamandole, cefoperazone, or cefotetan. An increase in acetaldehyde in the blood may result, producing a disulfiram (Antabuse)–type reaction (e.g., stomach pain, nausea, vomiting, headaches, low blood pressure, tachycardia, respiratory difficulties, increased sweating, or flushing of the face). Clients should avoid the use of alcoholic beverages, medications containing alcohol, or IV alcohol solutions during the administration of these drugs and for 3 days afterward.

A baseline assessment as described in Chapter 57 should be obtained before initiating cephalosporin therapy.

Nursing Diagnosis While M.T. is taking cephalosporin therapy, he is at risk for any of the following nursing diagnoses/collaborative problems: impaired comfort (headache, abdominal cramping, mild diarrhea, nausea, and vomiting); diarrhea related to AAPMC; risk for infection (oral candidiasis); ineffective protection related to hypoprothrombinemia; and the potential complications of hypersensitivity (fever, rash), allergic reactions (anaphylaxis, Stevens-Johnson syndrome, drug-induced immune hemolytic anemia, renal dysfunction, serum sickness–like reaction), and seizures (with high doses or renal impairment).

Planning Following cephalosporin therapy, M.T. will be free of the signs and symptoms of his cellulitis. During the cephalosporin therapy, M.T. will:
- Experience minimal adverse effects of the drug therapy.
- Effectively manage the therapeutic regimen, including being compliant with the cephalexin, and implementing nonpharmacologic supportive measures (e.g., hydration, rest, good nutrition, handwashing).
- Collaborate with health care providers by appropriately reporting adverse drug effects and maintaining scheduled visits for monitoring and treatment.

Implementation
Monitoring Because of the possibility of superinfection, observe M.T. for symptoms of bacterial and fungal overgrowth. Monitor WBC counts and culture results. Cytotoxic assays of stool samples to document the presence of *C. difficile* are needed if M.T. develops significant diarrhea. If he were going to be on the drug long term or if M.T. develops abnormal bruising, bleeding gums, or other signs of abnormal bleeding, then bleeding time and PT/INR should be monitored, because hypoprothrombinemia may occur with cephalosporins, especially cefamandole, cefoperazone, or cefotetan. In clients with renal impairment, most cephalosporins require dosage adjustment (especially if primarily excreted renally (see Table 58-4).

TABLE 58-4 CEPHALOSPORINS: PHARMACOKINETICS AND USUAL ADULT DOSAGE

Drug	IV	IM	PO	Renal Excretion*	Usual Adult Dose*
FIRST GENERATION					
cefadroxil (Duricef)			X	93%	500 mg PO q12h
cefazolin (Ancef)	X	X		80%-100%	250 mg-2 g IM/IV q6-12h
cephalexin (Keflex, Ancef)			X	80%-90%	250-500 mg PO q6-12h
cephradine (Velosef, Anspor)			X	~ 80%	250-500 mg PO q6h
SECOND GENERATION					
cefaclor (Ceclor)			X	60%-85%	250-500 mg PO q8h
cefamandole (Mandol)	X	X		65%-85%	500 mg IM/IV q6h
cefotetan (Cefotan)	X	X		50%-80%	500 mg-3 g IM/IV q12h
cefoxitin (Mefoxin)	X	X*		~ 85%	1-2 g IM/IV q6-8h (IM is painful)
cefprozil (Cefzil)			X	>60%	250-500 mg PO q12h
cefuroxime (Zinacef, Ceftin)	X	X		32%-48%	0.75-1.5 g IM/IV q8h
loracarbef (Lorabid)			X	87%-97%	200-400 mg PO q12h
THIRD GENERATION					
cefdinir (Omnicef)			X	12%-18%	300 mg PO q12h
cefditoren (Spectracef)			X	>80%	200-400 mg PO q12h
cefixime (Suprax)			X	50%	400 mg PO q24h
cefoperazone (Cefobid)	X	X		20%-30%	1-2 g IM/IV q12h
cefotaxime (Claforan)	X	X		60%	1-2 g IM/IV q6-8h
cefpodoxime (Vantin)			X	29%-33%	100-400 mg PO q12h
ceftazidime (Fortaz)	X	X		80%-90%	1-2 g IM/IV q8-12h
ceftibuten (Cedax)			X	56%	400 mg PO q24h
ceftizoxime (Cefizox)	X	X		85%-95%	1-2 g IM/IV q8-12h
ceftriaxone (Rocephin)	X	X*		33%-67%	1-2 g IM/IV q24h (IM is painful)
FOURTH GENERATION					
cefepime (Maxipime)	X	X		85%	0.5-2 g IM/IV q8-12h

Modified from Lacy, C.F., Armstrong, L.L., Goldman, M.P., & Lance, L.L. (2004). *Lexi-Comp's Drug Information Handbook* (12th ed.). Hudson, Ohio: Lexi-Comp, and *USP DI: Drug Information for the Health Professional* (25th ed.). (2005). Greenwood, Village CO: MICROMEDEX Thomson Healthcare.

*Dose adjustment is necessary for renal impairment with most agents. Exceptions include those with renal excretion less than 50%. Refer to package labeling for more complete information.

Intervention In addition to performing nursing measures common to all types of antimicrobial drug therapy (as discussed in Chapter 57), be aware of the following factors when cephalosporins are prescribed.

Most cephalosporins may be taken on a full or empty stomach. Taking them with food may help to prevent any GI irritation. However, cefaclor extended-release tablets, cefpodoxime proxetil, and cefuroxime axetil oral suspension should be taken with food. Ceftibuten oral suspension is the only cephalosporin that needs to be taken on an empty stomach, either 1 hour before or 2 hours after taking food.

Shake oral suspensions well before pouring. Administer IM cephalosporins deep into a large muscle mass, because they are irritating to tissues and can cause pain, induration, and sterile abscesses following injection. IM ceftriaxone is sometimes prepared with a dilute solution of lidocaine to reduce pain, but the addition of lidocaine must be reviewed by the prescriber (see monograph for ceftriaxone).

The perioperative parenteral administration of cephalosporins for prophylaxis is usually discontinued 24 hours after surgery.

Education Instruct M.T. to take the full course of medication, even though he may feel better and be symptom free. Stress the importance of taking evenly spaced doses to maintain therapeutic blood levels.

If M.T. were taking cefamandole, cefoperazone, or cefotetan, caution him not to drink alcoholic beverages or take alcohol-containing medications, because abdominal cramps, nausea, vomiting, hypotension, tachycardia, shortness of breath, sweating, and facial flushing may occur. Instruct him to read over-the-counter (OTC) labels, because many cough and cold remedies contain alcohol.

Evaluation The expected outcome of cephalosporin therapy is that M.T. will achieve an infection-free state as evidenced by resolution of his symptoms of cellulitis (e.g., absence of swelling, redness, and tenderness of left arm and hand) without adverse effects of the drug (e.g., absence of nausea, vomiting, abdominal cramping, diarrhea, oral candidiasis, excessive bruising, bleeding). He will also have a temperature within normal limits and a WBC count within the normal limits for age. He will use his entire prescription and evidence adequate hydration, rest, and nutrition. M.T. will wash his hands frequently to prevent the risk of transmission of his infection. He will state three reportable adverse drug effects and how to contact his prescriber. He will also maintain scheduled prescriber visits during the course of his illness.

⚙ **What other β-lactams are available for use?**
The monobactam, aztreonam (Azactam), and the carbapenems, ertapenem (Invanz), imipenem/cilastatin (Primaxin), and meropenem (Merrem), are used to treat serious infections. Although these agents have broad coverage, including activity against *P. aeruginosa*, widespread use increases the potential for microorganisms to develop resistance.

Monobactam

aztreonam [az **tree** oh nam]
(Azactam)
Aztreonam, the first drug in a monobactam class, is a synthetic bactericidal agent with an activity similar to penicillin. It binds to the penicillin-binding protein, resulting in inhibition of bacterial cell wall synthesis, cell lysis, and death. It is active against many gram-negative microorganisms and is used in the treatment of bronchitis and urinary tract, intraabdominal, gynecologic, and skin infections. Coverage against *P. aeruginosa* may be unreliable in many geographic regions.
Indications
Aztreonam is used for treating serious urinary tract, lower respiratory, and skin infections due to sensitive pathogens.

Pharmacokinetics/Dosing
Aztreonam is well distributed after parenteral administration. It is eliminated via hepatic metabolism and excreted primarily as unchanged drug in the urine. The adult dosage is 0.5 to 2 g IV or IM every 8 to 12 hours.
Adverse Effects
The adverse effects of aztreonam include gastric distress, diarrhea, nausea, vomiting, hypersensitivity, and thrombophlebitis at the site of injection.

Carbapenem

Imipenem/cilastatin, is a member of the carbapenem class and is structurally related to the β-lactams. The carbapenems have a wide spectrum of activity against gram-positive and gram-negative aerobic and anaerobic organisms. Imipenem binds to penicillin-binding proteins, thus inhibiting bacterial cell wall synthesis. It is very resistant to degradation by β-lactamases. Cilastatin inhibits renal dehydropeptidase and blocks the tubular secretion of imipenem, thus preventing renal metabolism of this drug. Therefore cilastatin is combined with imipenem to prevent its inactivation by renal dehydropeptidase. Meropenem and ertapenum are bactericidal, broad-spectrum carbapenems similar to imipenem that inhibit cell wall synthesis.

imipenem/cilastatin [i mi **pen** em/sye la **stat** in]
(Primaxin IM, Primaxin IV)
Indications
Imipenem/cilastatin is indicated for treatment of bone, joint, skin, and soft tissue infections, bacterial endocarditis, intraabdominal bacteria infections, pneumonia, urinary tract and pelvic infections, and bacterial septicemia when caused by susceptible bacterial organisms.
Pharmacokinetics/Dosing
When imipenem/cilastatin is administered IM, the time to peak serum level is within 2 hours, with a half-life of 2 to 3 hours. When administered IV, the half-life is approximately 60 minutes. Forms of IM and IV preparations differ and are not interchangeable. Excretion is primarily by the kidneys. No significant drug interactions have been reported to date with this product. The usual adult dosage for IV infusion is 250 to 500 mg every 6 hours for mild infections and 500 mg every 6 to 8 hours for moderate to severe infections. The maximum dosage is 50 mg/kg daily. The IM adult dosage is 500 to 750 mg every 12 hours, up to a maximum of 1500 mg daily. The dosage for children up to age 12 has not been determined; older children may receive the adult dosage.
Adverse Effects
The adverse effects of imipenem/cilastatin include gastric distress, nausea, vomiting, diarrhea, allergic-type reactions, confusion, lightheadedness, seizures, and tremors. Pseudomembranous colitis has also been reported with this product. The risk for seizures is highest when dose is not adjusted for renal dysfunction.

meropenem [mer oh **pen** em]
(Merrem IV)
Indications
Meropenem is used to treat susceptible intraabdominal infections (complicated appendicitis and peritonitis) and bacterial meningitis.
Pharmacokinetics/Dosing
After IV dosing, meropenem distributes well to tissue including the CSF. It has an elimination half-life of approximately 60 to 90 minutes and is eliminated renally after some hepatic metabolism. The typical adult dose is 1 gram IV every 8 hours. Reconstituted doses are only stable at room temperature for 1 to 2 hours after reconstitution so fresh doses must be prepared immediately before administration.

Adverse Effects

Pseudomembranous colitis, hypersensitivity, and the adverse effects of diarrhea, nausea, vomiting, headache, and rash have been reported with its use.

✳ What are the nursing management issues for these β-lactams?

The nursing management of aztreonam, imipenem-cilastatin, and meropenem is the same as for the penicillins, except that there are no cautions for significant drug interactions.

✳ F.G. is a 78-year-old resident of a nursing home who is admitted to the hospital with confusion and low-grade fever. The emergency room staff members assess F.G., obtain blood, urine and sputum cultures, and identify MRSA in the urine. F.G. has moderately impaired renal function with an estimated creatinine clearance of 25 mL/min. She weighs 55 kg and is started on vancomycin 750 mg IV every 24 hours.

✳ In addition to the β-lactams, what other drugs interfere with bacterial cell wall structure?

The most commonly used non-β-lactam in use that interferes with bacterial cell wall structure is vancomycin. It is most often used to treat MRSA, but is also used orally to treat *C. difficile* infection. Widespread use of vancomycin has led to resistant strains of enterococcus (vancomycin resistant enterococcus [VRE]), which has become problematic in North America over the past decade. Other agents with similar activity to vancomycin include bacitracin, cycloserine, and teicoplanin, but these agents are rarely used systemically.

✳🔲 vancomycin [van koe **mye** sin]
(Vancocin)

Vancomycin inhibits bacterial cell walls by binding to a cell wall precursor, a mechanism that differs from penicillin or cephalosporins. This action leads to cell lysis, so it is bactericidal for many organisms. Vancomycin may also inhibit RNA synthesis.

Indications

Parenteral vancomycin is indicated for treatment of bone and joint infections, bacterial septicemia caused by *Staphylococcus* species, and for the prevention and treatment of bacterial endocarditis caused by staphylococcus, including methicillin-resistant strains. Vancomycin is ineffective for treatment of gram-negative or anaerobic infections. Because oral vancomycin is not systemically absorbed, it is only indicated for treatment of AAPMC produced by *C. difficile* and for the treatment of staphylococcal enterocolitis.

Pharmacokinetics/Dosing

The absorption of vancomycin from the intestinal tract is poor. It is excreted mainly in the feces. Parenteral vancomycin has a half-life of 6 hours in adults and approximately 2 to 3 hours in children. It is primarily excreted by the kidneys and requires dosage adjustment with renal dysfunction. The oral adult dosage of vancomycin for the treatment of *C. difficile* colitis or diarrhea is 125 to 500 mg every 6 hours for 7 to 10 days, repeated if necessary. In children, the dosage is 10 mg/kg (up to 125 mg) every 6 hours for 7 to 10 days, repeated if necessary. With IV infusion, the adult dosage is 15 mg/kg every 12 hours, although doses may vary significantly based on condition treated, renal function and serum levels. For IV dosing in children, refer to the package insert or a current reference.

Adverse Effects

The significant adverse effects for oral doses include nausea, vomiting, and taste alterations. Less often or rarely, adverse effects with parenteral administration include ototoxicity and nephrotoxicity. Reported after bolus or too-rapid drug injection is "red-neck syndrome" or "red man syndrome," a response that results in histamine release and chills, fever, tachycardia, pruritus, rash, or a red face, neck, upper body, back, and arms. It can be minimized by the slow infusion of vancomycin over 60 to 120 minutes.

✳ A student nurse is preparing the first dose of vancomycin for F.G. and asks the charge nurse how to safely administer the drug.

✳ What are the nursing issues involved in vancomycin therapy for F.G.?

In addition to the previous discussions about the nursing management of antibacterials in general, vancomycin involves the following care:

Assessment Because F.G. is 78 years old, she is more likely to have an age-related decrease in renal function as demonstrated by her creatinine clearance estimate. To avoid excessive vancomycin serum concentrations, she may require an increase in dosing interval. Renal function impairment is noted at baseline before the initiation of IV vancomycin therapy. Because of decreased renal function as demonstrated by the creatinine clearance, she is at greater risk for vancomycin-related ototoxicity. Assess her for hearing loss as a baseline assessment. Ascertain if F.G. has a sensitivity to vancomycin.

Review F.G.'s current medication regimen for the risk of significant interactions, such as those that may occur when vancomycin is given concurrently with aminoglycosides, amphotericin B parenteral (Fungizone), aspirin, bacitracin, parenteral bumetanide (Bumex), capreomycin (Capastat), cisplatin (Platinol), cyclosporine (Sandimmune), ethacrynate sodium parenteral (Edecrin), furosemide parenteral (Lasix), paromomycin (Humatin), polymyxins, or streptozocin (Zanosar), because the risk for ototoxicity and/or nephrotoxicity. If vancomycin is given with anesthetics, the client may experience vancomycin-related hypotension or with vecuronium, enhancement of neuromuscular depression. Although concurrent dexamethasone may result in less penetration of vancomycin into CSF for clients with bacterial meningitis, adequate levels of vancomycin can be achieved (Feigin, Watson, & Gerber, 2004), and the administration of dexamethasone in bacterial meningitis significantly reduces mortality (van de Beek et al., 2004).

In addition to the baseline assessment described in Chapter 57 for nursing management of antibacterials, some issues are unique to UTIs. Part of that assessment was the C&S that determined the causative organism, MRSA. In addition are the intake and output ratio, F.G.'s temperature, WBC, and her subjective report of frequency, urgency, dysuria, and suprapubic pain associated with the condition. The urinalysis will determine WBCs, RBCs, and the presence of protein in the urine.

Nursing Diagnosis While F.G. is receiving vancomycin therapy, she is at risk for the following nursing diagnoses/collaborative problems: risk for injury related to "red neck syndrome" or "red man syndrome"—histamine release common with bolus or rapid injection (chills, fever, tachycardia, flushing of the face and/or upper body, syncope, tingling, unpleasant taste); deficient fluid volume related to nausea and vomiting; ineffective protection related to neutropenia or thrombocytopenia; impaired tissue integrity related to extravasation; disturbed sensory perception related to ototoxicity (loss of hearing and tinnitus); and the potential complications of pseudomembranous colitis and nephrotoxicity (blood in urine, greatly increased or decreased frequency of urination, and amount of urine).

Planning Following vancomycin therapy, F.G. will be free of the signs and symptoms of her UTI. During the vancomycin therapy, F.G. will:

- Experience minimal adverse effects of the drug therapy.
- Cooperate with nursing personnel to effectively manage her therapeutic regimen, including participating in nonpharmacologic supportive measures (e.g., hydration, rest, good nutrition, proper hygiene).
- Collaborate with health care providers by appropriately reporting adverse drug effects and understanding her role in the prevention of future infections.

Implementation

Monitoring Renal function studies may be needed periodically if F.G. has high-dose or prolonged therapy. Urinalyses should be monitored for the presence of albumin, casts, and cells in the urine, and for decreased specific gravity. Serum concentrations of vancomycin may need to be determined for F.G., as a client with renal impairment and a client over 60 years of age; peak concentrations should not exceed 40 mcg/mL. Trough levels are typically maintained between 5 and 15 mcg/mL depending on the indication for vancomycin. Older adults excrete vancomycin more slowly and therefore should be assessed for hearing loss over the course of therapy. The IV site should be monitored for extravasation. Oral vancomycin, poorly absorbed systemically, is limited to the treatment AAPMC produced by *C. difficile*, and is virtually free of systemic toxicity.

Intervention The IV dosage as calculated for F.G. is based on her creatinine clearance (CrCl), 750 mg/24 hr is a reasonable dosage for a CrCl of 25 mL/min, but further dose adjustments may be required based on vancomycin serum levels. Parenteral vancomycin is primarily administered IV because it is so irritating to the tissues. Take care to avoid extravasation. To avoid adverse effects such as hypotension, thrombophlebitis, and "red-neck syndrome," do not administer this drug as a bolus injection. Vancomycin may be administered intermittently in at least 100 mL of 0.9% sodium chloride injection or 5% dextrose injection over at least 60 minutes. If intermittent IV administration is not feasible, vancomycin may be given by continuous IV infusion, using sufficient 5% dextrose injection, 0.9% sodium chloride, or other injection solutions to run over 24 hours. Rotation of the IV sites will help to prevent local irritation. Vancomycin is also incompatible with alkaline solutions, heavy metals, and a wide variety of substances.

Consult the package insert before combining with other drugs, or administer it alone.

For other clients taking oral vancomycin for *C. difficile*-related AAPMC, ensure the suspension is well mixed before pouring. Alert the client that the suspension may have an unpleasant taste. It may be administered undiluted or through a nasogastric tube to minimize the unpleasant taste.

Education Alert F.G. to possible adverse effects, and instruct her to alert the nursing staff should they occur.

Evaluation The expected outcome of vancomycin therapy is that F.G. will achieve an infection-free state as evidenced by negative urine culture results and an absence of the frequency, urgency, and burning, and without adverse effects of the drug (e.g., absence of "red man syndrome," nausea, vomiting, ototoxicity, further renal damage). Her temperature and WBC will be within normal limits. She will return to her preinfection mental status and will alert caregivers to any nausea and/or hearing loss during the course of her vancomycin therapy.

✱ **A.J. is a 48-year-old smoker who presents to his health care provider with 4 weeks of purulent sputum production, coughing, and wheezing. A 2-week trial of inhaled albuterol, ipratropium, and fluticasone offered some benefit, but symptoms persist. He also presents with a mild confusion and a low-grade fever. Pulse oximetry is at 93%. He is diagnosed with acute exacerbation of chronic bronchitis and is being considered for oral macrolide therapy.**

✱ **What are the macrolide and related antibacterial agents and their use?**

The **macrolides** are bacteriostatic because they inhibit RNA-dependent protein synthesis; they may be bactericidal in high concentrations with selected organisms. The macrolides include azithromycin (Zithromax, Zithromax Z-Pak), clarithromycin (Biaxin), erythromycin, dirithromycin (Dynabac), and troleandomycin (Tao). Dirithromycin is a prodrug that is activated during intestinal absorption to erythromycylamine, an active metabolite. Telithromycin (Ketek) is officially a ketolide, but is structurally related to macrolides. It has a similar mechanism of action, and shares many of the risks associated with macrolide therapy.

Erythromycin is the first macrolide and key drug for this classification. Table 58-5 compares macrolides.

With the exception of troleandomycin, these agents have similar antimicrobial action (against gram-positive and selected gram-negative microorganisms) and are used for respiratory, GI tract, skin, and soft tissue infections when β-lactams are contraindicated (*Drug Facts and Comparisons*, 2005). Azithromycin and clarithromycin offer improved coverage of *H. influenzae* and *M. catarrhalis* compared to erythromycin and are therefore more commonly used for upper respiratory tract infections. Despite its lack of consistent efficacy against *P. aeruginosa* (Gilbert et al., 2004), azithromycin may also be helpful for some clients with cystic fibrosis (Saiman, 2004).

TABLE 58-5 MACROLIDES/KETOLIDES: PHARMACOKINETICS AND USUAL ADULT DOSAGE

Drug	Oral Absorption	Renal Excretion	Usual Adult Dose
azithromycin (Zithromax)			
IV	NA	5%-12%	500 mg IV q24h × 2 days, then 500 mg PO q24h
PO	37%	5%-12%	Varies/500 mg PO day 1, then 250 mg PO q24h
clarithromycin (Biaxin)			
PO	50%	20%-40%	Varies/250-500 mg PO q12h
dirithromycin (Dynabac)			
PO	10%	2%	500 mg PO q24h
erythromycin			
IV	NA	2%-5%	250 mg to 1 g IV q6h
PO	30-65	2%-5%	Varies/250-500 mg PO q6h
troleandomycin (Tao)			
PO	Unknown	10%-25%	250-500 mg PO q6h
telithromycin (Ketek)			
PO	57%	13%	800 mg PO q24h

Modified from Lacy, C.F., Armstrong, L.L., Goldman, M.P., & Lance, L.L. (2004). *Lexi-Comp's Drug Information Handbook* (12th ed.). Hudson, Ohio: Lexi-Comp, and *USP DI: Drug Information for the Health Professional* (25th ed.). (2005). Greenwood Village, CO: MICROMEDEX Thomson Healthcare.

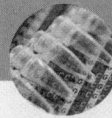

Special Considerations for Pharmacogenetics | ANTIBACTERIALS

PHARMACODYNAMICS

The potential for antibacterial drug resistance is directly related to the genetic variation exhibited by the pathogen, but little data are available to suggest genetic variation in the host is correlated with pharmacodynamic response to antibacterials.

PHARMACOKINETIC

Clients with cystic fibrosis (an inherited condition) display considerable variation in pharmacokinetics for β-lactams and aminoglycosides, and typically require dramatically larger doses than those without cystic fibrosis to attain similar tissue drug levels (Beringer, 1999).

ADVERSE EFFECTS

The potential for macrolides and ketolides (specifically erythromycin) induced ECG changes cardiac dysrhythmias and sudden death risk is correlated with P450 3A4 activity and interactions (Ray et al., 2004). Considerable variation in P450 3A4 activity is correlated with genetic markers and varies considerably across populations (Lamba et al., 2002; Ozedemir et al., 2000). Some clients may also be more genetically predisposed to ECG changes before administration of macrolides (Yang et al, 2002) and addition of these drugs likely further increases risk. Some antimicrobials (specifically rifampin, penicillins, and tetracyclines) result in considerable but variable changes in estradiol levels with hormonal contraceptives (Dickinson, Altman, Nielsen, & Sterling, 2001). Risk for antimicrobial-induced contraceptive failure may be genetically determined. (Altman, Nielsen, Sterling, & Dickinson, 2002).

Troleandomycin is the only macrolide drug indicated for the treatment of *Streptococcus pneumoniae* and *Streptococcus pyogenes*.

The most serious of adverse effect of erythromycin is prolonged QT interval on electrocardiogram with a risk for life-threatening ventricular dysrhythmias and sudden cardiac death (Ray et al., 2004). This risk appears highest among clients taking other drugs that inhibit cytochrome P450 3A4 (e.g., azole antifungals, diltiazem, verapamil, nefazodone, protease inhibitors, and cimetidine). Whether this risk extends to other macrolides and ketolides (particularly clarithromycin and telithromycin that are also metabolized by P450 3A4) is not clear, but genetics probably also plays a role (see the Special Considerations for Pharmacogenetics box above). Telithromycin is also associated with QT interval prolongation, and interacts with a wide variety of drugs including those metabolized by P450 3A4. Other adverse effects of macrolides include nausea, vomiting, and increased GI peristalsis. Erythromycin, a prokinetic agent, is used to improve gastric peristalsis in clients with diabetic gastroparesis because of this effect. Other adverse effects vary by agent, but can include hepatic injury, allergic reactions, and *C. difficile* colitis (see Box 58-2).

Macrolides

✱▪▪ erythromycin [er ith roe **mye** sin]
(EES, E-Mycin, Ery-Tab, Erybid✤, Erythromid✤)
Indications
Erythromycin and its salts are indicated for the treatment of systemic infections involving susceptible strains of *S. pyogenes, S. pneumoniae, S. aureus, M pneumonia, Legionella pneumophila, H. pertussis,* and other pathogens. Used topically, erythromycin is used in the treatment of superficial conjunctivitis, neonatal ophthalmia, and acne vulgaris. An unlabeled use is in the treatment of gastroparesis.

Pharmacokinetics/Dosing
Erythromycin is not particularly stable in acid medium. It is variably absorbed with oral administration and the rate and extent of absorption differs regarding dosage form, salt formulation, and concurrent gastric contents. It is widely distributed to tissue and has an elimination half-life of about 2 hours. It is primarily excreted in the feces after biliary excretion.

A typical adult dose is 250 to 500 mg of erythromycin base orally every 6 to 12 hours, but doses vary based on indication and dosage form. IV dosing for *Legionella pneumophila* infection can be as high as 1 gram every 6 hours; such high dosing of IV erythromycin may result in phlebitis and requires significant dilution and fluid administration. Clients on high-dose erythromycin should be monitored for fluid and cardiac status.

Adverse Effects
GI symptoms are the most commonly reported adverse effect with erythromycin and its salts. Oral and/or vaginal candidiasis and, less commonly, hypersensitivity and hepatotoxicity have also been reported. Erythromycin in high doses has been associated with prolonged QT interval on electrocardiogram (ECG).

Drug Interactions
Erythromycin interacts with a number of agents because of inhibition of cytochrome P450 1A2 and 3A4. Additive QT interval prolongation is also possible when administered with other drugs that affect cardiac conduction (refer to discussion above). A great number of drugs are implicated, and references should be consulted to identify risk.

azithromycin [az ith roe **mye** sin]
(Zithromax, Z-PAK)
Indications
Azithromycin is indicated for treatment of infections involving *H. influenzae, M. catarrhalis, Mycoplasma pneumonia,* and *S. pneumonia,* including otitis media, upper and lower respiratory tract infections, community acquired pneumonia, and acute exacerbation of chronic obstructive pulmonary disease (COPD). It is also used in the treatment of chlamydial urethritis. Because of low plasma levels of azithromycin, it is not recommended for use in septicemias or bloodborne infections.

Pharmacokinetics/Dosing
Azithromycin is rapidly absorbed on oral administration and widely distributed to tissues. Because of extensive tissue binding, azithromycin has an extensive elimination half-life of about 3 days. This offers an advantage in dosing and improving adherence to therapy, but may provide prolonged low levels of drug, which may contribute to drug resistance. Dose and duration of therapy vary based on indication. A typical adult oral dose for the treatment of mild to moderate respiratory infection is 500 mg on day 1, followed by 250 mg PO every 24 hours for 4 days.

Adverse Effects
Nausea, vomiting, and diarrhea are the most common adverse effects reported, but are significantly less frequently observed compared to erythromycin. Allergic reactions and acute interstitial nephritis are rare adverse effects.

Drug Interactions
Interactions with azithromycin are possible when administered concurrently with other drugs metabolized by cytochrome P450 systems, but they are much less likely compared to erythromycin.

clarithromycin [kla **rith** roe mye sin]
(Biaxin, Biaxin XL)
Indications
Clarithromycin is indicated for a number of respiratory and skin infections due to sensitive strains of *H. influenzae, Mycoplasma pneumonia, S. pneumonia,* and *Chlamydia pneumoniae*. It is indicated in combination with amoxicillin and/or other antimicrobials along with acid suppression in the treatment of *H. pylori* peptic ulcer disease. It is also used in the prevention and treatment of *M. avium complex* infections seen in advanced HIV disease.

Pharmacokinetics/Dosing
Clarithromycin is reasonably well absorbed orally and widely distributed to tissues outside of the CNS. It is metabolized to an active metabolite and has a 6-hour elimination half-life. The adult dosage varies significantly based on indication, but a typical dose for most indications is 250-500 mg PO every 12 hours.

Adverse Effects
Clarithromycin is generally better tolerated compared with erythromycin. Adverse effects include anorexia, nausea, vomiting, headache, lethargy, severe anemia, fever, infection, rash, abnormal taste sensations and, rarely, *C. difficile* colitis, hepatotoxicity, hypersensitivity, and thrombocytopenia.

Drug Interactions
Clarithromycin inhibits cytochrome P450 3A4 and to some extent 1 A2 and has the potential to interact with a number of drugs. It may also prolong QT intervals and should be used cautiously with other drugs having this effect.

Ketolides

telithromycin [tel ith roe **mye** sin]
(Ketek)
Telithromycin is the first marketed ketolide. It is structurally similar to macrolides, and also inhibits protein synthesis. The spectrum of activity is similar to azithromycin.

Indications
Telithromycin is used to treat community acquired pneumonia, and acute bacterial bronchitis and sinusitis. Because of the potential for significant interactions and the potential for prolongation of QT interval, it is typically reserved for clients not responsive to other therapies.

Pharmacokinetics/Dosing
Telithromycin is moderately well absorbed orally. It may be administered without regard to meals. It is extensively metabolized by P450 3A4 and other pathways. The typical adult dose is 800 mg orally once daily for 5 to 10 days depending on indication.

Adverse Effects
Among the most serious adverse effects is the potential for prolongation of QT interval and risk for sudden cardiac death. This risk may be higher for individuals with concurrent drugs metabolized by P450 3A4. In addition to the risk for cardiac dysrhythmias, telithromycin may be associated with hypersensitivity reactions or hepatic dysfunction. Other adverse events appear similar to macrolides, including GI upset.

Drug Interactions
Telithromycin interacts with a number of other drugs metabolized by the cytochrome P450 enzyme systems including azole antifungals, simvastatin, midazolam, cisapride, carbamazepine, and a great number of other drugs. Significant interaction may pose increased risk for rhabdomyolysis, prolonged QT interval and risk for potentially

life-threatening cardiac dysrhythmias. Consult appropriate references to review the complete list of interacting drugs.

⊛ **A.J. is started on azithromycin 500 mg PO daily for 3 days.**

⊛ **What are the nursing implications in the use of macrolides for A.J.?**

In addition to the general nursing management of antimicrobials as discussed in Chapter 57, nursing management of macrolide therapy includes the following:

Assessment Ascertain if A.J. has preexisting health conditions that may preclude the use of a macrolide antibacterial or indicate caution in his care. Determine if A.J. has a hypersensitivity to azithromycin, erythromycin, or other macrolides. Because the macrolides have biliary excretion as a major route of elimination, determine if A.J. has hepatic impairment, in which case the drug will be used with caution. Although less of a concern with azithromycin, the prototype drug erythromycin may place clients with a history of cardiac dysrhythmias at risk for a recurrence with high doses because erythromycin, and possibly clarithromycin, prolong QT interval and may lead to sudden cardiac death.

Review A.J.'s current medication regimen for the risk of significant drug interactions, such as those that may occur when macrolides are given concurrently with the following drugs: aluminum and magnesium-containing antacids (decreases azithromycin's peak serum concentration; administer azithromycin at least 1 hour before or 2 hours after antacids); carbamazepine (Tegretol), cyclosporine (Sandimmune), digoxin (Lanoxin), phenytoin (Dilantin) (may result in drug toxicity of these agents), hepatotoxic medications (increased risk for liver toxicity); warfarin (Coumadin) (may result in decreased warfarin metabolism and excretion, leading to an increased risk of bleeding or hemorrhage); and theophylline (may increase theophylline levels).

A baseline assessment as described in Chapter 57 should be obtained before initiating macrolide antibiotic therapy.

Nursing Diagnosis The client receiving erythromycin, azithromycin, or clarithromycin may experience the following nursing diagnoses/collaborative problems: diarrhea; impaired tissue integrity related to inflammation or phlebitis at the injection site; deficient fluid volume related to nausea and vomiting; impaired comfort (abdominal cramping); disturbed sensory perception related to hearing loss (erythromycin only); ineffective protection related to the loss of normal flora and the development of *Candida albicans* (sore mouth or tongue, vaginal itching and discharge); and the potential complications of hypersensitivity, hepatotoxicity (dark urine, pale stools, tiredness, and yellowing of the sclera and skin), acute interstitial nephritis (azithromycin only), thrombocytopenia (clarithromycin only), pancreatitis (erythromycin only), and cardiotoxicity (dysrhythmia, bradycardia, fainting, sudden death).

Planning As for vancomycin.

Implementation

Monitoring Complete temperature measurement, WBC counts, cultures, and a focal examination of the infection. If A.J. was on high-dose or prolonged erythromycin therapy, then periodic hepatic function studies and an ECG may be required.

Intervention Azithromycin capsules and the pediatric suspension, as with most macrolide antibiotics, should be administered with a full glass of water on an empty stomach (1 hour before or 2 hours after meals) to obtain the maximum effect. Azithromycin tablets and clarithromycin may be taken with or without food. When administering oral suspensions, ensure that they have been refrigerated and shaken well and that the calibrated liquid-measuring device is used for accurate dosing.

Continuous infusion is preferable to intermittent infusion for the macrolide antibiotics; they are not to be administered by bolus or IM. If intermittent infusion is considered, azithromycin should be administered over 1 to 3 hours and erythromycin over 20 to 60 minutes depending on the strength. Intravenously administered erythromycin is very irritating to the vein and requires dilution. Extensive dilution of erythromycin may result in excessive IV fluid intake that may not be tolerated by clients with renal insufficiency or heart failure.

Education With erythromycin, clarithromycin, and other antibiotics, stress the importance of complying with a full course of therapy, sometimes 7 to 14 days, even though the client feels better or is symptom free. However, the dosing of azithromycin may be quite short, a single dose in the case of gonococcal urethritis, or 3 to 5 days for other infections. A.J. may still have symptoms at the end of his drug therapy regimen (3 days). Inform him that his symptoms will continue to resolve after his medication is regimen is completed, but he should report ongoing or worsening symptoms after 5 days. Review proper inhaler use. Provide A.J. with smoking cessation information, and discuss local services for support.

The decreased frequency of dosing and fewer adverse GI effects experienced with the newer, longer-acting macrolide antibiotics (e.g., azithromycin, clarithromycin, and dirithromycin) may offset their higher prices and increase client adherence.

Evaluation The expected outcome of macrolide antibiotic therapy is that A.J. will achieve an infection-free state as demonstrated by an absence of sputum or negative sputum cultures. He will also demonstrate a body temperature within normal limits, a WBC count within the normal limits for age, and the resolution of his respiratory symptoms (e.g., absence of coughing and wheezing, pulse oximetry 98% to 100%) without experiencing adverse effects of the drug (e.g., nausea, vomiting, diarrhea). A.J. will return to his preinfection mental status, demonstrate proper inhaler use, and express an interest in smoking cessation.

⊛ **K.P. is a 41-year-old administrative assistant who seeks care with her dentist for severe toothache. She is** diagnosed with a dental abscess and undergoes incision and drainage (I&D) of the abscess via a root canal. The dentist is about to order an antibacterial with coverage for oral anaerobes and strep species and is thinking of using penicillin V potassium. KP reports a history of hives with penicillin.

✴ What agents are available for treating anaerobic infections?

Pathogenic anaerobes are believed to be responsible for a number of infectious states. Anaerobes that are found in the mouth and are responsible for many dental abscesses and aspiration pneumonias include *Peptostreptococcus* and other species. Intraabdominal infections are often complicated by *Bacteroides* species, particularly *B. fragilis*.

Many of the penicillins (e.g., penicillin G, penicillin VK, and amoxicillin) are effective for oral anaerobes and are often a first choice in dental or oral infections, or when oral flora (including the aerobe *Streptococcus*) poses a risk for systemic infection. Amoxicillin, in particular, is used in treating dental abscesses. It is also used as a standard treatment as a single 2-gram oral dose 1 hour before dental and surgical procedures for preventing subbacterial endocarditis (SBE prophylaxis) in clients with a history of heart valve problems. The extended penicillins (e.g., piperacillin, ticarcillin) are effective for both the oral anaerobes and for treating intraabdominal infections where *Bacteroides* species are problematic. A few of the second generation cephalosporins (e.g., cefotetan, cefoxitin) also cover *Bacteroides* species and are used for intraabdominal infections.

When penicillin is contraindicated (e.g., for clients with a history of type I hypersensitivity reactions to β-lactams as is seen with K.P.), alternatives are considered. The most common alternative for treating oral anaerobes in such clients is clindamycin (Cleocin), which covers oral anaerobes, bacteroides, and many gram-positive cocci (including staph and strep species). Clindamycin is an alternative for SBE prophylaxis in clients with penicillin allergy. It is also used in combination with other antimicrobials for treating anaerobic infections elsewhere (e.g., intraabdominal infection, diabetic foot ulcers). Clindamycin is a semisynthetic derivative of lincomycin and inhibits protein synthesis by binding to bacterial ribosomes and prevents peptide bond formation. Unfortunately, clindamycin use may pose a higher risk for AAPMC with *C. difficile*, because it disrupts gut anaerobe flora.

Metronidazole (Flagyl) is also frequently used to cover bacteroides and is used as part of a regimen for treating intraabdominal infections. Metronidazole is reduced intracellularly to a short-acting, cytotoxic agent that interacts with DNA, thus inhibiting bacteria synthesis and resulting in cell death (microbicidal). Unlike clindamycin, metronidazole is effective against *C. difficile* and is used as a first-line treatment for AAPMC. Metronidazole is also used in the treatment of protozoan infections, but it is not reliable as treatment for oral infections or aspiration pneumonia because it lacks coverage for many common oral aerobic and anaerobic pathogens.

✴▥ clindamycin [klin da **mye** sin]
(Cleocin, Dalacin✤)
Indications
Clindamycin is indicated for the treatment of bone and joint infections, pelvic (female) and intraabdominal infections, bacterial septicemia, pneumonia, and skin and soft tissue infections caused by susceptible bacteria. It is also used widely for the treatment of oral or dental infections where β-lactams are contraindicated.
Pharmacokinetics/Dosing
Oral clindamycin is well absorbed and is administered with food or with a full glass (8 ounces) of water. It is rapidly distributed to most body fluids and tissues, with the exception of CSF; the highest concentrations are noted in bone, bile, and urine. The half-life of clindamycin in adults is 2 to 3 hours. It reaches peak blood levels within 45 minutes to 1 hour after oral administration, 1 hour in children (IM), 3 hours in adults (IM), and by the end of the infusion with IV injection. It is metabolized in the liver and excreted primarily by the kidneys. The usual adult dosage of clindamycin is 150 to 450 mg PO, IM, or IV every 6 hours. For infants aged 1 month and older, the oral dosage is 2 to 5 mg/kg body weight every 6 hours.
Adverse Effects
The most significant adverse and limiting effect for clindamycin is AAPMC secondary to *C. difficile* (see Box 58-2). With oral administration, clindamycin is also associated with dose related GI upset, phlebitis on IV injection, and a risk for sterile abscess formation with IM administration.

✴ Because of the risks associated with K.P.'s drug sensitivities with β-lactams, she is started on clindamycin (Cleocin) 300 mg orally every 6 hours.

✴ What are the important nursing implications with the use of clindamycin for K.P.?

Assessment Determine if K.P. has a history of GI disease, particularly ulcerative colitis or regional enteritis, because pseudomembranous colitis may occur with therapy. Severe hepatic or renal function impairment will require a dosage reduction. Ascertain K.P.'s sensitivity to lincomycins because of cross-sensitivity between clindamycin and lincomycins.

Review K.P.'s current medication regimen for the risk of significant drug interactions, such as those that may occur when clindamycin is administered with the following drugs: anesthetics (hydrocarbon inhalation) or neuromuscular blocking agents (may result in enhanced neuromuscular blockade, skeletal muscle weakness, respiratory depression, or paralysis if this combination is used during or immediately after surgery); adsorbent type antidiarrheals (kaolins, attapulgite) (decreases the absorption of oral clindamycin; take the antidiarrheal 2 hours before or 3 to 4 hours after the oral clindamycin); and chloramphenicol (Chloromycetin) or erythromycins (may antagonize the therapeutic effect of clindamycin).

Perform a baseline assessment as described in Chapter 57 before initiating clindamycin prophylaxis.

Nursing Diagnosis While K.P. is on clindamycin prophylaxis, assess her for the following nursing diagnoses/collaborative problems: diarrhea related to the development of AAPMC; deficient fluid volume related to nausea, vomiting, and diarrhea; ineffective protection related to neutropenia (infection), thrombocytopenia (bleeding), and loss of normal flora (superinfection); and the potential complication of hypersensitivity.

Planning During clindamycin prophylaxis, K.P. will:
- Be compliant with her medication regimen.
- Experience an absence of symptoms of infection and, minimal adverse effects of the drug therapy.
- Collaborate with health care providers by appropriately reporting untoward symptoms.

Implementation

Monitoring During therapy, have K.P. report abdominal cramps, diarrhea, weight loss, or weakness, which might be indications of pseudomembranous colitis, to her prescriber. If the clindamycin were prescribed for antiinfective therapy, rather than prophylaxis, her temperature, WBC counts, cultures, and cytotoxin assays of stool samples would be monitored. Perform a focal assessment related to her risk for infection.

Intervention Administer clindamycin capsules with a full glass of water or with meals to prevent esophageal ulceration.

Education Stress the importance of complying with a full course of the medication, even though K.P. feels well and is symptom-free. Instruct her to take the medication at evenly spaced times to ensure that serum levels are maintained. Alert K.P. to adverse effects and to report them to the prescriber.

Evaluation The expected outcome of clindamycin prophylaxis is that K.P. will remain infection-free after the incision and drainage of her dental abscess. She will be compliant with her medications, taking the drug every 6 hours with a full glass of water until her prescription is complete. She states she will report to the dentist if she experiences abdominal cramping, diarrhea, or an increase in swelling and tenderness over the surgical site. If clindamycin is administered therapeutically, the client will also demonstrate a body temperature within normal limits, a WBC count within the normal limits for age, and the resolution of any other infection-related symptoms without experiencing adverse effects of the drug.

⚙ **S.J. is a 19-year-old, sexually actively woman with a 2-week history of a moderate vaginal discharge that is malodorous. She has no complaints of vaginal itching or burning. On examination by her nurse practitioner, the discharge is grayish and frothy, with a pH of 5.3. A "fishy" odor is present when a drop of the discharge is alkalinized with 10% potassium hydroxide. A wet mount of the vaginal secretion contained few leucocytes and numerous epithelial cells are covered with bacteria to such an extent that cell borders are obscured (clue cells). S.J. is diagnosed with bacterial vaginosis and she is prescribed metronidazole 500 mg PO twice daily for 7 days.**

⚙🗎 **metronidazole** [me troe **ni** da zole]
(Flagyl, Flagyl IV, Apo-Metronidazole✦, Nida-Gel✦, Novonidazol✦)

Indications
Metronidazole is indicated for the treatment of amebiasis (intestinal and extraintestinal), AAPMC, bone infections, brain abscesses, CNS infections, bacterial endocarditis, genitourinary tract infections, septicemia, trichomoniasis, and other infections caused by organisms susceptible to the action of metronidazole.

Pharmacokinetics/Dosing
Oral metronidazole is well absorbed and distributed throughout the body. It reaches peak serum levels within 1 to 2 hours and has a half-life of 8 hours. It is metabolized in the liver and primarily excreted in the kidneys. The usual oral adult dosage is 7.5 mg/kg, up to maximum of 1 g, every 6 hours for a week or longer. The adult dosage for IV infusion is 15 mg/kg initially, then 7.5 mg/kg up to a maximum of 1 g every 6 hours for a week or longer. The maximum daily dose is 4 g.

Adverse Effects
The adverse effects of metronidazole include dizziness, headache, gastric distress, anorexia, nausea, vomiting, diarrhea, peripheral neuropathy, CNS toxicity, leukopenia, thrombophlebitis, and vaginal candidiasis.

Drug Interactions
Metronidazole inhibits cytochrome P450 3A4 (and to some extent 2 C8/9) activity. Other drugs metabolized by these systems, notably warfarin, may be affected. The combination of metronidazole and ethanol leads to a disulfiram-like reaction including flushing, nausea, and vomiting. Clients should avoid alcoholic beverages, and alcohol-containing products (e.g., mouth rinses) while on metronidazole therapy.

⚙ **What are the nursing issues for S.J.'s metronidazole therapy?**

Assessment Assess S.J. for preexisting health conditions that may contraindicate metronidazole therapy or be cause for caution during its administration. Because metronidazole may cause CNS toxicity, any individual with active organic CNS disease, such as epilepsy, should be carefully evaluated before treatment. Determine whether S.J. has a history of blood dyscrasias as she would require careful monitoring, because metronidazole may cause leukopenia. Reduced dosages may be required if S.J. has hepatic dysfunction. Metronidazole is contraindicated if S.J. is hypersensitive to it.

Review S.J.'s current medication regimen for the risk of significant drug interactions, such as those that may occur when metronidazole is given concurrently with the following drugs: alcohol may result in disulfiram (Antabuse)-type effects: flushing, headaches, nausea, vomiting, and abdominal distress); warfarin (Coumadin) (may enhance anticoagulant effects by inhibiting warfarin metabolism); disulfiram (Antabuse) (avoid concurrent use, or use within 14 days of disulfiram administration; confusion and psychosis have been reported); and lithium (may increase serum lithium concentrations).

Perform a baseline assessment as described in Chapter 57 before initiating metronidazole therapy.

Nursing Diagnosis While S.J. is receiving metronidazole therapy, assess her for the following nursing diagnoses/ collaborative problems: impaired comfort (headache and unpleasant metallic taste); deficient fluid volume related to anorexia, nausea, vomiting, and diarrhea; ineffective protection related to leukopenia and the loss of normal flora (fungal overgrowth); disturbed sensory perception related to peripheral neuropathy (numbness, tingling, and pain in the hands and feet); disturbed thought processes related to CNS toxicity (confusion, mood changes); and the potential complications of hypersensitivity (rash, itching), seizures related to high doses, and pancreatitis (severe abdominal pain, nausea, and vomiting).

Planning Following metronidazole therapy, S.J. will be free of the signs and symptoms of her vaginal infection. During her therapy, S.J. will:

- Experience minimal adverse effects of the drug therapy.
- Effectively manage the therapeutic regimen, including being compliant with the metronidazole, and implementing nonpharmacologic supportive measures (e.g., hydration, rest, good nutrition, proper perineal hygiene, handwashing).
- Collaborate with health care providers by appropriately reporting untoward symptoms and maintaining scheduled visits for monitoring and treatment.

Implementation

Monitoring If S.J. were to be on metronidazole for a longer time, CBCs would be monitored at frequent intervals for blood dyscrasias. As it is, instruct M.T. to report immediately to the prescriber any symptoms of sore throat, unusual tiredness or weakness, or unusual bleeding or bruising.

With prolonged use, assess clients periodically for symptoms of peripheral neuropathy such as numbness and tingling of the hands or feet. Mood changes and irritability also indicate CNS toxicity.

If metronidazole is administered for giardiasis, three stool examinations (taken several days apart) should be performed to determine the success of therapy; these should begin 3 to 4 weeks after treatment. Additional specimens may be required if GI symptoms persist.

Intervention The oral form of metronidazole is taken with meals to minimize GI irritation. If S.J. were on the extended-release form of the drug, it would be just the opposite; it is taken at least 1 hour before meals or 2 hours afterward. Parenteral metronidazole is administered by slow IV infusion. It may be administered continuously or intermittently over a 1-hour period. If administered concurrently with a primary IV, the primary IV should be discontinued while the metronidazole is infused. The sodium content of the parenteral forms of the drug should be considered as part of sodium intake in clients for whom sodium intake is restricted.

Education Advise S.J. that this drug may cause an unpleasant taste in the mouth, diminished taste sensation, and a dry mouth. The use of sugar-free candies, ice cubes, and frequent mouth rinses may bring some relief. If therapy is long-term, dry mouth may contribute to dental caries and gum disease, and the client should receive regular dental checkups.

Stress the importance of completing a full course of therapy, even though S.J. may be feeling well and be symptom-free. The doses should be evenly spaced to ensure that therapeutic serum levels are maintained.

Advise S.J. not to ingest alcoholic beverages while taking metronidazole, because a disulfiram-like effect may result (flushing, nausea, and vomiting, and abdominal cramping). Advise her that her urine may turn a darker color but that this change is not clinically significant.

If metronidazole were being prescribed for trichomoniasis, the client will need to prevent reinfection from her male partner. The partner will need to undergo concurrent drug therapy and use a condom until the infection is resolved in both partners.

Evaluation The expected outcome of metronidazole therapy is that S.J. will maintain or achieve an infection-free state as evidenced by a negative wet mount for clue cells and an absence of grayish, frothy vaginal discharge and vaginal bleeding. She will not experience any adverse drug effects (e.g., headache, nausea, vomiting, diarrhea, CNS toxicity, peripheral neuropathy). S.J. will effectively manage her therapeutic regimen by taking her complete prescription in a timely fashion and using proper perineal hygiene, hand washing, and avoiding alcoholic beverages. She will report adverse effects of metronidazole to her prescriber appropriately and maintain scheduled visits for follow up. If the metronidazole is administered for other types of infections, the client will also demonstrate a body temperature within normal limits, a WBC count within the normal limits for age, and the resolution of any other infection-related symptoms without experiencing adverse effects of the drug.

✴ **T.L. is a 15-year-old male with significant cystic acne not responsive to topical treatments. His dermatologist is considering the addition of a tetracycline.**

✴ **What tetracyclines are available and what is their role?**

Tetracyclines include a large group of drugs that have a common basic structure and similar chemical activity. Among the tetracyclines available for use are demeclocycline (Declomycin), doxycycline (Vibramycin), minocycline (Minocin), oxytetracycline (Terramycin), and tetracycline (Achromycin V). Tetracyclines are bacteriostatic for many gram-negative and gram-positive organisms; they exhibit cross-sensitivity and cross-resistance. Tetracyclines inhibit protein synthesis by blocking the binding of transfer RNA to the messenger RNA ribosome. Demeclocycline is also used to treat the syndrome of inappropriate diuretic hormone (SIADH); it inhibits antidiuretic hormone (ADH)–induced water reabsorption in the kidneys, resulting in diuresis.

The tetracyclines are commonly used to treat many infections such as acne vulgaris, actinomycosis, bacterial UTIs, bronchitis, rickettsial infection (Rocky Mountain spotted fever, typhus, Q fever), Lyme disease, and numerous systemic bacterial infections sensitive to the tetracyclines. They are also alternatives to fluoroquinolones (discussed later in this chapter) for the management of anthrax exposure (see the Pharmacologic Issues in an Age of Terrorism box below). Tetracycline does not appear to offer benefits over topical treatments for mild to moderate acne

(Ozolins et al., 2005); therefore oral tetracycline is often reserved for more serious acne. The effects of tetracyclines on the treatment of acne may relate to mechanisms other than antimicrobial because low doses appear to be effective (Skidmore et al., 2003).

 Pharmacologic Issues in an Age of Terrorism

Bacterial Agents and Related Toxins

A number of bacterial agents and their toxins could pose a potential grave risk to the public if widely disseminated in air, water or food by terrorists. Unlike chemical or radiation exposures, a delay between exposure and symptoms may be noted with agents used for bioterrorism. Vigilance by health care personnel is critical in the timely identification and management of a bioterrorist threat.

The CDC has stratified agents used for bioterrorism according to risk as Category A, B, or C agents. Category A agents are the most dangerous and have the following characteristics:

- Pose the greatest risk for public health
- May spread across a large area or need public awareness
- Need a great deal of planning to protect the public's health

Category A bacterial agents include anthrax (*Bacillus anthracis*), plague (*Yersinia pestis*), tularemia (*Francisella tularensis*), and botulism (*Clostridium botulinum* toxin). Chapter 59 discusses Category A viral agents, including smallpox and viral hemorrhagic fever. Information on other potential bioterrorist threats, including brucellosis, and Q fever can be found at the CDC website for bioterrorism (http://www.bt.cdc.gov/agent/agentlist.asp).

Anthrax (Bacillus anthracis)

Bacillus anthracis is a spore forming gram-positive bacillus, which itself is dangerous, and produces toxins that produce edema and other effects. Anthrax can be highly lethal and its spores can be aerosolized. Anthrax can present as a cutaneous, GI, or pulmonary disease. Anthrax is found in infected livestock and can be transmitted by consumption of contaminated meat or contact with animal hides, bone, or hair/wool that are infected. Between 20,000 and 100,000 cases are observed worldwide, but it is rare in North America. Most of these cases are the less severe cutaneous form, with a more severe GI condition accounting for most of the remaining cases. The pulmonary form of the disease is the most dangerous of all forms, and left untreated, has a mortality rate approaching 100%.

Presentation

Bacillus anthracis has a usual incubation period of 1 to 6 days, but spores have been noted to survive for over a month in the lung before symptoms appear. Anthrax can cause dermal, oropharyngeal, or GI lesions depending on the route of exposure. Several deaths have occurred as a result of exposure to anthrax mailed in envelopes. The cost to decontaminate a facility contaminated by anthrax spores can run into the tens of millions of dollars.

Cutaneous

Initially a small sore develops into a blister than an ulcer with a black center. All lesions are generally painless.

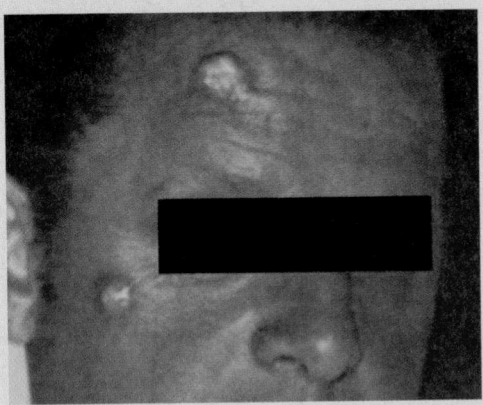

Typical Anthrax cutaneous lesions.

Courtesy Centers for Disease Control and Prevention. Retrieved August 17, 2005, from http://phil.cdc.gov/Phil/home.asp.

Gastrointestinal

Nausea, anorexia, bloody diarrhea, fever, and stomach pain are typically noted.

Inhalation

Initial symptoms are cold or flu-like symptoms with a sore throat, mild fever, and muscle aches. Cough, dyspnea, and fatigue are also common. Full symptoms may be noted within days or may not be noted for up to 6 weeks after exposure.

Management

Postexposure prophylaxis with ciprofloxacin 500 mg orally twice daily × 60 days or 10 to 15 mg/kg orally twice daily for children is recommended. Other fluoroquinolones or doxycycline may also be considered if ciprofloxacin is not available. Some strains may be responsive to penicillins or amoxicillin. Treatment of active disease is similar to postexposure prophylaxis, but may require higher doses with IV therapy and the addition of clindamycin or rifampin. Prophylaxis or treatment should be initiated as soon as possible. A vaccine is available for military use, but is not available for use in the general public; it is discussed in Chapter 62.

Plague (Yersinia pestis)

Y. pestis or plague is a gram-negative bacillus harbored by rodents and transmitted to humans by fleas. The history of plague dates to biblical times, and accounted for millions of deaths due to "black death" in fourteenth-century Europe.

Modified from Emergency Preparedness and Response: Centers for Disease Control and Prevention. Retrieved March 6, 2005, from http://www.bt.cdc.gov.

Continued

Bacterial Agents and Related Toxins—cont'd

Two forms of plague can be observed; the bubonic plague transmitted only by the bite of an infected flea, and the pneumonic plague that can be transmitted from person to person. The pneumonic form can also be transmitted by inhaling respiratory droplets from an infected person and thus poses the more likely risk in a terrorist attack.

Presentation

The incubation period for pneumonic plaque is 1 to 6 days and for bubonic plague, 2 to 10 days. The pneumonic form is much more likely to be observed in a terrorist event, because its transmission is more efficient from aerosol forms and from person to person. The delay between exposure and symptoms may contribute to more widespread infection as those exposed may travel during the incubation period.

Bubonic

Swollen, tender lymph nodes (known as buboes) present within 24 hours. Fever and malaise are also typical. Septicemia is also common and can involve necrosis to fingers and toes.

Pneumonic

Fever, weakness, and rapidly developing pneumonia are common with this disease. Pneumonia often presents with dyspnea, cough, chest pain, and may include bloody sputum. Nausea, vomiting, and abdominal pain are also common. Respiratory symptoms quickly lead to respiratory failure, shock, and death.

Management

Left untreated, plague is fatal. Prophylaxis with ciprofloxacin 500 mg PO twice daily or doxycycline 200 mg PO twice daily for 7 days is recommended. Treatment of active disease may include aminoglycosides (streptomycin, gentamicin, tobramycin), fluoroquinolones (ciprofloxacin), and/or doxycycline. Rapid initiation of treatment is associated with improved outcomes. The CDC recommends the use of tight fitting disposable surgical masks by those in direct or close contact to infected individuals to help prevent further transmission. Currently, no vaccine for the pneumonic form of plague is available.

Tularemia (F. tularensis)

Tularemia, also known as rabbit fever, is caused by the gram-negative coccobacillus *F. tularensis*. It is typically isolated in animals with rodents and rabbits being the most frequent reservoir. Tularemia presents both an airborne threat and a potential contaminant in food and water. Human infection can occur via a bite by a vector (e.g. flea, tick), direct contact with infected animals, ingestion of contaminated food or water, or inhaling airborne bacteria. Tularemia is highly infectious with only a small number of airborne organisms required for infection, but transmission from person to person is not likely.

Presentation

Presenting signs and symptoms vary based on the nature of exposure. The incubation period can vary from 1 to 14 days, but is most often 3 to 5 days. Dermal and perioral ulcers, swollen and painful lymph nodes, sore throat, and diarrhea can be noted. With inhaled exposures, pneumonia, fever, chills, headache, muscle and joint pain, weakness, and dry cough are more common. Pneumonia typically involves dyspnea, may include bloody sputum, and can progress to respiratory failure. Between 30% and 60% of cases result in death if not treated.

Management

Postexposure prophylaxis includes the use of doxycycline 100 mg PO twice daily or ciprofloxacin 500 mg PO twice daily for 14 days. Treatment of active disease includes IV aminoglycosides (streptomycin, gentamicin) and may involve IV doxycycline and/or ciprofloxacin. Early treatment is associated with improved outcomes. A live, attenuated vaccine is being investigated, but it is not readily available for use.

Botulism (Clostridium botulinum toxin)

C. botulinum is a spore-forming anaerobic bacteria which produces botulinum toxin. This toxin is responsible for neurotoxicity and risk for death. Three manifestations of botulism are possible. Food-borne botulism is caused by ingestion of botulism toxin contained in food. Wound botulism results from wounds infected with *C. botulinum,* which produces the toxin. Finally, infants who consume spores of *C. botulinum* (e.g., in honey) can manifest intestinal disease, which can become systemic. Food-borne disease is the major risk for a bioterrorist attack of botulism.

Presentation

Botulism classically presents 3 to 4 days (range, 6 hours to 10 days) after exposure with difficulty in swallowing, cold-like symptoms, and blurry vision. This rapidly progresses to mental numbness, reduced eye movement, dilated pupils, slurred speech, unsteady gait, and muscle weakness. A descending flaccid paralysis soon follows with respiratory arrest. Its presentation may appear similar to that observed with nerve agents or atropine overdose (see the Pharmacologic Issues in an Age of Terrorism: Chemical Warfare box in Chapter 21 on pp. 432 and 433), but is slower in onset. It may also be confused with the Guillain-Barre syndrome, myasthenia gravis, or stroke.

Management

Administration of botulinum antitoxin is helpful if treatment is initiated before the onset of symptoms. A vaccine is also under development (see the Pharmacologic Issues in an Age of Terrorism: Role of Vaccines and Antitoxins in Response to a Bioterrorism Threat box in Chapter 62 on pp. 1146 and 1147). Respiratory support is required in advanced cases of botulism. Ultimate recovery may be slow. A major concern in a mass exposure is a lack of a sufficient number of ventilators to provide needed respiratory support.

Modified from Emergency Preparedness and Response: Centers for Disease Control and Prevention. Retrieved March 6, 2005, from http://www.bt.cdc.gov.

Oral tetracyclines are fairly well absorbed and distributed to most body fluids. CSF levels vary and can range from 10% to 25% of the plasma drug concentration following parenteral administration. Tetracyclines localize in the teeth, liver, spleen, tumors, and bone. As such, tetracyclines are avoided in pregnancy or in women who are likely to become pregnant (Category D). They are also avoided in children younger than 8 years of age unless absolutely necessary (e.g., anthrax exposure) because they can deposit in and discolor teeth. Doxycycline can reach clinical concentrations in the eye and prostate, and minocycline results in high levels in saliva, sputum, and tears. Doxycycline and minocycline are inactivated in the liver, but most tetracyclines are excreted by the kidneys. Table 58-6 lists the half-life and usual adult dosages for the tetracyclines.

✱▀▔ tetracycline [tet ra **sye** kleen]
(Achromycin V, Novotetra✦)
Indications
Tetracycline is indicated for the treatment of a number of gram-positive and gram-negative infections, for the treatment of acne, for infections with *Chlamydia*, *Mycoplasma*, and *Rickettsia*. It is also used to treat exacerbations of chronic bronchitis, gonorrhea, and syphilis in penicillin allergic clients, and as part of regimens for peptic ulcer disease with *H. pylori*.
Pharmacokinetics/Dosing
Tetracycline is fairly well absorbed orally as long as it is administered on an empty stomach. Divalent and trivalent cations (e.g., magnesium salts, calcium salts, aluminum salts, iron) dosed within 2 to 4 hours will chelate with tetracycline and prevent absorption. Likewise, dairy products administered with tetracycline will reduce absorption. Tetracycline is dosed in adults at 250 to 500 mg orally every 6 hours.
Adverse Effects
Tetracyclines cause frequent GI upset. All tetracyclines are contraindicated in children younger than the age of 8 years because the drug deposits in bone and teeth enamel and can result in permanent discoloration of developing teeth. Tetracycline is avoided in pregnant women (category D) because of its effects on fetal development. Hepatotoxicity as the result of tetracycline is rare, but a metabolite of tetracycline produced in an expired or poorly stored product (e.g., in a humid environment such as a medicine cabinet in a bathroom) can increase the risk of hepatotoxicity. Phototoxicity is also a potential adverse effect of tetracyclines.
Drug Interactions
As noted above, tetracycline should not be dosed within 2 to 4 hours of antacids, dairy products, calcium supplements, iron therapy, or any divalent or trivalent cation.

doxycycline [dox i **sye** kleen]
(Doxychel, Vibramycin, Apo-Doxy✦, Doxycin✦)
Indications
Indications for doxycycline are similar to tetracycline. It is also indicted as a treatment for anthrax exposure.
Pharmacokinetics/Dosing
Doxycycline is well absorbed orally; dosing with food or milk reduces absorption by about 20%. Chelation with divalent and trivalent cations is also observed with doxycycline. The elimination half-life of doxycycline is 12 to 15 hours, which allows for less frequent dosing and improved adherence to therapy. Doses vary based on indication, but are typically in the range of 50-200 mg PO once or twice daily.
Adverse Effects
Adverse effects and risks for doxycycline are similar to tetracycline.
Drug Interactions
Doxycycline shares the same drug interactions with tetracycline.

✱ **T.L. is started on a regimen of 50 mg of doxycycline (Vibramycin) twice daily.**

✱ **What are the nursing implications regarding the use of tetracyclines for T.L.?**
Implement the following measures with clients who are receiving drugs of the tetracycline family.

TABLE 58-6 TETRACYCLINES: PHARMACOKINETICS AND USUAL ADULT DOSAGE

Drug	IV	IM	PO	Normal Half-Life	Half-Life in Renal Failure	Usual Adult Dose
demeclocycline (Declomycin)			X	10-17 hr	40-60 hr	300 mg PO q12h*
doxycycline (Vibramycin)	X		X	12-22 hr	12-22 hr	100 mg IV/PO q12h × 1 day, then 100 mg q24h†
minocycline (Minocin)	X		X	11-23 hr	11-23 hr	200 mg IV/PO × 1 dose, then 100 mg q12h
oxytetracycline (Terramycin IM)		X		6-10 hr	47-66 hr	250 mg IM q24h or 100 mg IM q8h*
tetracycline (Sumycin)			X	6-11 hr	57-108 hr	125-500 mg PO q6h*

Modified from Lacy, C.F., Armstrong, L.L., Goldman, M.P., & Lance, L.L. (2004). *Lexi-Comp's Drug Information Handbook* (12th ed.). Hudson, Ohio: Lexi-Comp, and *USP DI: Drug Information for the Health Care Professional (25th ed.).* (2005). Greenwood Village, CO: MICROMEDEX Thomson Healthcare.
*Adjust dose or avoid in renal impairment.
†See the Pharmacologic Issues in an Age of Terrorism box on p. 1035 for alternate dosing related to anthrax exposure.

Assessment Doxycycline is appropriate drug therapy for acne for T.L. given his age and gender and the fact that topical medications have not been efficacious. Tetracyclines are contraindicated in women of childbearing age, who are sexually active and not using consistent contraception, pregnant women, breastfeeding women, and children younger than the age of 8 years of age because they cause permanent mottling and discoloration of the teeth and decrease the linear skeletal growth rate in fetuses or children. Acne is not an infectious disease, but the antimicrobial will decrease *P. acnes* colonization and so prevents future lesions by decreasing sebaceous fatty acid metabolic byproducts that stimulate inflammation (Seaton, 2005).

Determine T.L.'s allergy history. If he is hypersensitive to one tetracycline, he may also be hypersensitive to others. Additionally, clients with hypersensitivities to "caine-type" drugs, such as lidocaine or procaine, may be intolerant of the lidocaine in an oxytetracycline injection or to the procaine in a tetracycline IM injection.

With the exception of doxycycline and minocycline, the use of tetracyclines in clients with renal impairment is not recommended

Review T.L.'s current medication regimen for the risk of significant drug interactions, such as those that may occur when tetracyclines are given concurrently with antacids, calcium supplements, choline and magnesium salicylates, iron supplements, magnesium salicylate or magnesium laxatives, foods containing milk, and milk products. These combinations may result in a nonabsorbable complex, thus reducing the absorption and serum levels of the antibiotic. Antacids may also increase gastric pH, which further decreases the absorption of tetracyclines. If given concurrently, advise clients to separate medications by 1 to 3 hours from the oral tetracyclines. If colestipol (Colestid) or cholestyramine (Questran) is given concurrently, it may bind oral tetracyclines, thus decreasing its absorption. Separate drugs by at least 2 hours. If tetracyclines are given with estrogen-containing contraceptives, concurrent long-term therapy may reduce the effectiveness of contraceptives and may also result in breakthrough bleeding.

Perform a baseline assessment as described in Chapter 57 before initiating tetracycline therapy.

Nursing Diagnosis While T.L. is receiving doxycycline therapy, he is at risk for the following nursing diagnoses/collaborative problems: impaired comfort (heartburn, abdominal cramping, anorexia, nausea, vomiting); diarrhea; ineffective protection related to the loss of normal flora (fungal overgrowth); and the potential complications of hypersensitivity, increased sensitivity of the skin to sunlight, CNS toxicity (dizziness, syncope), nephrogenic diabetes insipidus, hepatotoxicity, and pancreatitis.

Planning While on doxycycline therapy, T.L. will experience:
- Relief from the discomfort of acne.
- Compliance with doxycycline regimen.

- Effective management of the therapeutic regimen, including appropriate skin cleansing and care, reporting of adverse drug effects to physician appropriately.

Implementation

Monitoring Monitor the condition of T.L.'s acne lesions. Cultures, temperature, WBC count, and other symptoms of the infection would be monitored if T.L. were receiving tetracycline therapy for a different type of infection. Because the risk for superinfection is greater with tetracycline therapy than with other antimicrobial agents, observe clients carefully for signs and symptoms of secondary infections, especially *Candida* infections. Meticulous oral and perineal hygiene is helpful in preventing a *Candida* superinfection.

Intervention Tetracyclines should be taken with a full glass of water to prevent esophageal erosion and GI irritation. With the exception of doxycycline and minocycline, the tetracyclines should be taken on an empty stomach (1 hour before or 2 hours after meals) for maximum effectiveness. Consult with the prescriber about ordering an oral suspension if a client would have difficulty swallowing and administer the oral suspension using the calibrated liquid-measuring device provided by the manufacturer.

Parenteral administration of tetracyclines is varied. Doxycycline may be administered IV (not IM or subcutaneous) in concentrations not less than 100 mcg/mL or greater than 1 mg/mL over a period of 1 to 4 hours. With IV oxytetracycline, dilute in at least 100 mL of the appropriate IV solution and avoid rapid administration; do not give the IV preparation IM or subcutaneous. Avoid the rapid administration of IV minocycline. Tetracycline may be administered IM but not IV or subcutaneous; the amount should not exceed 2 mL in each site. With IM preparations of oxytetracycline and tetracycline, serum levels are lower than with oral administration; the client should be switched to oral forms of the drugs as soon as possible.

Education Stress the importance of taking the full course of the medication in evenly spaced doses to maintain serum levels. Photosensitivity may occur and persist for some time after discontinuing the drug. Instruct T.L. to avoid direct sunlight and ultraviolet light. If exposure is unavoidable, a sunscreen may help to prevent a reaction. Although T.L. does not need to avoid eating in association with his doxycycline (or minocycline), alert other clients, taking other tetracyclines, to the appropriate dosing schedule in relation to food and to drug-drug and drug-food interactions. Instruct T.L. to discard outdated tetracyclines (show him where the expiration date is found), because they become toxic as they decompose.

For nonpharmacologic interventions, instruct T.L. to wash the affected twice daily with warm water and mild, nonmoisturizing soap to remove excess sebum. Aggressive skin washing with antibacterial or abrasive cleansers is not recommended. Discourage T.L. from manipulating (e.g., picking, squeezing) his acne lesions. Discourage clients from using cosmetics or other preparations that would irritate the skin (Seaton, 2005).

Evaluation The expected outcome of T.L.'s doxycycline therapy is that T.L.'s acne will show improved skin appearance with minimal pitting or scarring and without adverse drug effects (e.g., hypersensitivity, CNS toxicity, hepatotoxicity). He will remain compliant with his therapy, taking the drug with a full glass of water on an empty stomach and completing his full prescription. He will use nonpharmacologic measures to support his medication therapy (e.g., appropriate cleansing techniques, not picking at or squeezing lesions, taking sunlight precautions with skin). For other clients taking tetracyclines, the client will maintain or achieve an infection-free state as evidenced by negative culture results and/or lack of symptoms related to infection without adverse drug effects. If administered therapeutically, the client will also demonstrate a body temperature within normal limits, a WBC count within the normal limits for age, and the resolution of any other infection-related symptoms without experiencing adverse effects from the drug.

⚹ **J.B. is a nonsmoking 63-year-old male, who lives at home with his wife, and visits his health care provider with dyspnea, fever, chills, and malaise. On physical examination, J.B. presents with a respiratory rate of 28 breaths/min, crackles at both lung bases, and a pulse oximetry of 92%. Chest radiograph findings are consistent with community-acquired pneumonia and a sputum culture is obtained. His prescriber is considering initiating J.B. on fluoroquinolone therapy.**

⚹ **What are the fluoroquinolones and their role in therapy?**

Fluoroquinolones are synthetic, broad-spectrum agents with bactericidal activity. They alter DNA by interfering with the DNA gyrase, an enzyme necessary for duplication, transcription and repair of bacterial DNA. A number of fluoroquinolones are available for use, including ciprofloxacin (Cipro), enoxacin (Penetrex), gatifloxacin (Tequin), gemifloxacin (Factive), levofloxacin (Levaquin), lomefloxacin (Maxaquin), moxifloxacin (Avelox), ofloxacin (Floxin), and sparfloxacin (Zagam). Cinoxacin (Cinobac), nalidix acid (NegGram), and norfloxacin (Noroxin) have limited roles in the treatment of UTIs. Two other agents, trovafloxacin (Trovan) and alatrofloxacin (Trovan IV) are available for limited use, but pose a serious risk for hepatic injury and are limited to the treatment of serious infections.

Except as noted above, the fluoroquinolones are indicated for the treatment of bone and joint infections, bronchitis, gastroenteritis, gonorrhea, pneumonia, UTIs, and many other infections caused by susceptible microorganisms. Fluoroquinolones, specifically levofloxacin, are also effective for the treatment of Legionnaires' disease (Blazquez Garrido et al., 2005). Individual fluoroquinolones may vary in their spectrum of activity and penetration to tissue sites.

For example, whereas most of the fluoroquinolones are indicated for the treatment of UTIs, but only ciprofloxacin is approved to treat bone and joint infections. The antimicrobial spectrum for fluoroquinolones includes gram-positive and gram-negative aerobes. Most quinolones have some activity against *P. aeruginosa* and other gram-negative pathogens, but significant resistance has developed over the past decade (Neuhauser et al., 2003). Fluoroquinolones, particularly ciprofloxacin, are considered the drugs of choice for the treatment of anthrax or anthrax exposure (see the Pharmacologic Issues in an Age of Terrorism box on p. 1035). Refer to current references for approved individual drug indications.

The oral bioavailability of fluoroquinolones is good, although reduced when administered with divalent or trivalent cations (as is seen with the tetracyclines). These agents are metabolized in the liver (minimally for ofloxacin and lomefloxacin) and excreted primarily by the kidneys.

The significant adverse effects of fluoroquinolones include dizziness, drowsiness, restlessness, stomach distress, nausea, vomiting diarrhea, and vaginitis (trovafloxacin). Rare adverse effects include psychosis, confusion, hallucinations, tremors, hypersensitivity, and interstitial nephritis. Tendon rupture has also been associated with fluoroquinolone therapy, and this risk may be highest for older adults receiving ofloxacin or levofloxacin (van der Linden et al., 2003). A number of the fluoroquinolones have produced prolonged QT intervals on ECG and predispose to serious cardiac dysrhythmias, including the life-threatening *torsades de pointes*. Trovafloxacin and alatrofloxacin are associated with rare but life-threatening hepatic failure and so their use is limited to the treatment of life-threatening infections where other therapy is not indicated. Use of fluoroquinolones in children is generally not recommended because of a potential risk for cartilage damage, but they are occasionally used in children and adolescents when the benefit outweighs the risk.

Most of the fluoroquinolones interact with divalent or trivalent cations (as noted above) and concurrent antacids, calcium salts, iron preparations and mineral therapy will decrease oral bioavailability. Many of the fluoroquinolones impact on cytochrome P450 enzyme function and may result in decreased metabolism and increased levels of a number of substances, including warfarin, theophylline and caffeine. Clinicians should consult current package insert or other references for a complete list of interacting drugs and foods.

Table 58-7 presents comparative pharmacokinetics and dosing of available agents. The prototype fluoroquinolone is ciprofloxacin.

⚹▭ **ciprofloxacin** [sip ro **flocks** a sin]
(Cipro)
Indications
Ciprofloxacin is indicated for a number of infectious states, including infections of the lower respiratory tract, sinuses, bone and joints, prostate, and other areas where susceptible pathogens are present. Ciprofloxacin is also the drug of choice for the treatment of anthrax and anthrax exposure.

TABLE 58-7 FLUOROQUINOLONES: PHARMACOKINETICS AND USUAL ADULT DOSING

Agent	Half-Life (hours)	Routes of Administration	Typical Adult Dose	Comment
cinoxacin (Cinobac)	1-2	PO	250 mg PO q6h or 500 mg PO q12h*	Use limited to uncomplicated urinary tract infection. Avoid caffeine and divalent/trivalent cations.
ciprofloxacin (Cipro)	3-5	PO, IV (also ophthalmic)	250-750 mg PO q12h* 200-400 mg IV q8-12h*	Avoid caffeine and divalent/trivalent cations.
enoxacin (Penetrex)	3-6	PO	200-400 mg PO twice daily*	Avoid caffeine and divalent/trivalent cations.
gatifloxacin (Tequin)	7-14	PO, IV	400 mg PO/IV q24h*	May prolong QT interval. Avoid divalent/trivalent cations.
gemifloxacin (Factive)	4-12	PO	320 mg PO q24h*	May prolong QT interval. Avoid divalent/trivalent cations.
levofloxacin (Levaquin)	6-8	PO, IV (also ophthalmic)	250-750 mg PO/IV q24h*	May prolong QT interval. Avoid divalent/trivalent cations and caffeine.
lomefloxacin (Maxaquin)	5-8	PO	400 mg PO q24h*	Avoid divalent/trivalent cations and caffeine.
moxifloxacin (Avelox)	12-15	PO, IV	400 mg PO/IV q24h	May prolong QT interval. Avoid divalent/trivalent cations and caffeine.
nalidixic acid (NegGram)	6-7	PO	500-1000 mg PO q6h*	Use limited to uncomplicated urinary tract infection where pathogen is known to be sensitive. Avoid divalent/trivalent cations and caffeine.
norfloxacin (Noroxin)	3-4	PO	400 mg PO q12h*	Use limited to uncomplicated urinary tract infection, gonorrhea, and prostatitis. Avoid divalent/trivalent cations and caffeine.
ofloxacin (Floxin)	4-7	PO, IV	200-400 mg PO/IV q12h*	Avoid divalent/trivalent cations and caffeine.
sparfloxacin (Zagam)	20	PO	400 mg PO × 1, then 200 mg q24h*	Higher risk to prolong QT interval. Avoid divalent/trivalent cations and caffeine.
trovafloxacin (Trovan)	9-12	PO	200 mg PO q24h	Rare but serious risk for hepatotoxicity; limit use to serious or life-threatening infections.
alatrofloxacin (Trovan IV)	9-12	IV	300 mg IV, usually as a single dose before starting oral therapy	

* Adjust dose for renal impairment.

Pharmacokinetics/Dosing
Ciprofloxacin is reasonably well absorbed orally if not administered with calcium, dairy products, antacids, or iron. It is partially metabolized to mildly active metabolites and eliminated in the urine and feces. Table 58-7 presents doses.

Adverse Effects
Ciprofloxacin is fairly well tolerated. The most common adverse effects are nausea, diarrhea, and elevated results in liver function tests. The prolongation of QT intervals that is noted with other fluoroquinolones is not a frequent complication of ciprofloxacin.

Drug Interactions
In addition to reduced oral absorption when dosed with divalent or trivalent cations, ciprofloxacin also affects cytochrome P450 enzyme systems, include 3A4 and 1A2. Ciprofloxacin can affect the clearance of a number of drugs, including caffeine, theophylline, and warfarin. Consult the package insert or other references for a full listing of interacting drugs and their management.

✷ J.B. is started on levofloxacin (Levaquin) 500 mg orally once daily for 2 weeks and will receive daily telephone contact with the office to review his status and progress.

✷ What are the nursing management issues involved in the use of fluoroquinolones for J.B.?

Assessment Determine J.B.'s allergy history. If he has had an allergic reaction to any of the fluoroquinolones, all of them are contraindicated because of cross-sensitivity. Clients with hepatic or renal impairment may require reduced dosages. With CNS disorders such as cerebral arteriosclerosis or epilepsy, use the fluoroquinolones with caution because of the risk of CNS toxicity.

Review J.B.'s current medication regimen for the risk of significant drug interactions, such as those that may occur when fluoroquinolones are given concurrently with antacids, ferrous sulfate or sucralfate because they may decrease the absorption of ciprofloxacin, enoxacin, levofloxacin, lomefloxacin, norfloxacin, and trovafloxacin/alatrofloxacin, reducing drug effectiveness; administer fluoroquinolones at least 2 hours before these medications. With concurrent caffeine ingestion, ciprofloxacin, enoxacin, and norfloxacin significantly decrease the hepatic metabolism of caffeine, which increases its half-life and the risk for caffeine-related CNS stimulation. Avoid sources of caffeine while taking these drugs. When ciprofloxacin is administered with phenytoin, it reduces phenytoin serum levels by 34% to 80%. Administering quinolones to clients who are stabilized on phenytoin may lower serum levels and result in seizures; monitor phenytoin levels when discontinuing fluoroquinolones. Fluoroquinolones (with the possible exception of lomefloxacin and ofloxacin) may result in increased theophylline plasma levels and toxicity when administered with theophylline and other xanthines. Monitor theophylline plasma levels closely, because dosage adjustments may be necessary. Concurrent administration of quinolones with warfarin (Coumadin) may result in an increase in anticoagulant effect and the potential for bleeding. Although not currently reported with all quinolones, it is recommended that PT/INR be monitored closely whenever these drugs are administered concurrently.

Perform a baseline assessment as described in Chapter 57 before initiating fluoroquinolone therapy.

Nursing Diagnosis While J.B. is receiving fluoroquinolone therapy, assess him for the following nursing diagnoses/collaborative problems: altered comfort related to anorexia, nausea, and vomiting, cramps; impaired tissue integrity related to phlebitis (IV ciprofloxacin and ofloxacin only); diarrhea; altered sensory perception (visual) related to ocular effects of fluoroquinolones; disturbed thought processes related to CNS stimulation (confusion, acute psychosis, hallucinations); and the potential complications of hypersensitivity (rash, itching, swelling of face), interstitial nephritis (blood in the urine, lower back pain, rash, edema), photosensitivity (increased sensitivity of skin to sunlight), hepatotoxicity (dark urine, pale stools, anorexia, weakness), pseudomembranous colitis (severe watery stools, fever, abdominal pain), tendonitis or tendon rupture (pain and swelling in calves), and CNS toxicity (dizziness, headache, insomnia).

Planning During his levofloxacin therapy, J.B. will:
- Experience decreased symptoms of pneumonia.
- Experience minimal adverse effects of the drug therapy.

- Effectively manage the therapeutic regimen, including being compliant with the levofloxacin, and implementing nonpharmacologic supportive measures (e.g., hydration, rest, good nutrition, handwashing).
- Collaborate with health care providers by appropriately reporting untoward symptoms and maintaining scheduled visits for monitoring and treatment.

Implementation

Monitoring Monitor J.B.'s temperature, WBC counts, cultures, and the symptoms of infection, such as breath sounds, pulse oximetry, and chest radiographs. Monitor him for signs and symptoms of adverse effects. Monitor urinary pH because ciprofloxacin becomes more insoluble in an alkaline medium (greater than 6.8), resulting in crystalluria. Assess for signs and symptoms of superinfection.

Intervention Clients with community-acquired pneumonia, such as J.B., who are able to eat and are ambulatory can often be treated with oral antimicrobials at home (Carratala et al., 2005). Administer fluoroquinolones with a full glass of water. Ensure that J.B. maintains a urinary output of at least 1200 to 1500 mL daily (for adults) to minimize the occurrence of crystalluria. Enoxacin or norfloxacin are to be taken on an empty stomach; ciprofloxacin, lomefloxacin, ofloxacin, and sparfloxacin may be taken either with or without food.

IV ciprofloxacin and ofloxacin should be infused slowly into a large vein over 60 minutes to minimize discomfort and venous irritation.

Education Stress the importance of taking a full course of therapy, taking all doses at evenly spaced intervals as prescribed to maintain therapeutic serum levels. Restrict caffeine because of effects such as anxiety, nervousness, tachycardia, or insomnia.

Advise J.B. to report dizziness, light-headedness, or depression; these signs indicate CNS toxicity. Visual disturbances such as blurred or double vision and increased light sensitivity should be reported for the same reason. Because visual disturbances, dizziness, light-headedness, or drowsiness may occur, advise J.B. to limit activities that require alertness and dexterity until his response to the drug has been determined. Alert J.B. to report GI symptoms, e.g., nausea, vomiting, diarrhea, and abdominal cramping. Caution J.B. that photosensitivity is a possible effect of these drugs; avoid exposure to sun and sunlamps.

Take fluoroquinolones 2 hours before antacids. Photophobia is a concern with norfloxacin; advise J.B. to wear sunglasses and avoid exposure to bright light.

Evaluation The expected outcome of J.B.'s fluoroquinolone therapy is that he will achieve an infection-free state as evidenced by an absence of symptoms (e.g., dyspnea, fever, chills, malaise, crackles at both lung bases, sputum) related to his pneumonia. He will demonstrate a body temperature within normal limits, a WBC count within the normal limits for age, pulse oximetry 98% to 100%, and

1042 CHAPTER 58 Antibacterials

negative chest radiograph without experiencing adverse effects from the drug (e.g., GI distress, dizziness, headache, insomnia, pain or swelling in calves, bloody urine). He will remain compliant with his drug therapy and effectively manage his therapeutic regimen.

✳ **A.L. is a 38-year-old female who has recently undergone chemotherapy and comes to the emergency department with fever and an absolute neutrophil count of 300 cells/mm³. After providing blood, urine, and sputum samples for culture, she is started on ceftazidime 2 grams every 8 hours IV. After the first day of therapy, the initial lab reports suggest *P. aeruginosa* in the urine. The addition of aminoglycoside therapy is recommended by the Infectious Disease Service of the hospital.**

✳ **What are the aminoglycosides and their role?**

Aminoglycosides are potent bactericidal agents that are usually reserved for serious or life-threatening infections. They are very effective against many bacteria but are generally reserved for gram-negative infections where *P. aeruginosa* is a likely pathogen (e.g., institutionally acquired infections, clients with cystic fibrosis). Safer and less toxic agents are available to treat the majority of less serious infections. Currently available aminoglycosides include amikacin (Amikin), gentamicin (Garamycin), kanamycin (Kantrex), netilmicin (Netromycin), spectinomycin (Tobicin), streptomycin, and tobramycin (Nebcin). Paromomycin (Humatin), an orally available aminoglycoside, is occasionally used to treat intestinal amebiasis and hepatic coma.

The mechanism of action for aminoglycosides is to irreversibly bind ribosomes of the susceptible bacteria, thus inhibiting protein synthesis (interferes with the complex between messenger RNA and the bacteria ribosomes) and leading to eventual cell death (bactericidal). The aminoglycosides are indicated for the treatment of serious or life-threatening infections when other agents are ineffective or contraindicated. They are used with extended spectrum penicillins and antipseudomonal cephalosporins, for their synergistic effects in the treatment of gram-negative infections such as those caused by *Pseudomonas* species, *E. coli*, *Proteus* species, *Klebsiella* species, *Serratia* species, and others. Concurrent use with other penicillins or vancomycin is sometimes used to improve bactericidal activity against gram-positive pathogens (e.g., staph and strep species) in serious infections like endocarditis.

Aminoglycosides are very water soluble compounds and are poorly absorbed from an intact intestinal tract. They are reasonably absorbed IM, but most commonly administered IV. Local or topical application or irrigation may lead to absorption from most areas of the body, with the exception of the bladder. Aminoglycosides are eliminated almost completely in the urine and clearance is dependent on renal function. Interestingly, clients with cystic fibrosis often require higher doses of β-lactams and aminoglycosides to achieve therapeutic serum and tissue levels. This may be because of altered metabolism, distribution and/or renal elimination in such clients (Beringer, 1999).

Significant adverse effects of the aminoglycosides include nephrotoxicity, neurotoxicity, ototoxicity (auditory and vestibular), and hypersensitivity. The risk for ototoxicity and nephrotoxicity are directly related to sustained elevations in tissue concentration. The risk for such toxicity can be reduced when the drug levels are allowed to decline to very low levels. Unlike other antimicrobials that require sustained elevations in levels for therapeutic response, the aminoglycosides can penetrate into tissue (and bacteria) and continue to be toxic to bacteria when blood and tissue levels have declined. As such, dosing of aminoglycosides is different from other therapies and is aimed at achieving a relatively high peak serum level and to allow trough levels to become quite low. This is often achieved by dosing aminoglycosides only once every 24 hours and has become a more routine manner of dosing these agents. The therapeutic levels of aminoglycosides reported by standard laboratories are listed below but they are not particularly indicative of efficacy or toxicity when using once daily aminoglycoside dosing.

Therapeutic aminoglycoside serum levels as reported by many laboratories:
- amikacin: 15-25 mcg/mL
- gentamicin: 4-10 mcg/mL

The post-infusion peak level is sometimes used to establish efficacy and is drawn 30 minutes after the completion of the infusion. With once-daily dosing of aminoglycosides, postdistribution peak levels are often expected to be well above the "therapeutic range" reported by the laboratory and therefore are infrequently obtained with this regimen. The trough, or lowest level of the day, drawn right before the next dose, should ideally be less than 1 mcg/mL for tobramycin or gentamycin to reduce the risk for nephrotoxicity and ototoxicity. These elevated peak levels and low trough levels are often a source of confusion for many clinicians, but should be interpreted in relation to the dosing regimen used, times of infusion, and client response. Many hospital settings offer a clinical pharmacokinetic service to assist clinicians with aminoglycoside dosing and monitoring. Tobramycin is the most commonly used aminoglycoside and is presented in the following monograph.

✳▀ **tobramycin** [toe bra **mye** sin]
(Nebcin)

Indications

Tobramycin is indicated for the treatment of gram-negative infections caused by *P. aeruginosa*, or other gram-negative pathogens. An inhaled formulation is available for adjunct management of clients with cystic fibrosis and *P. aeruginosa* colonization or infection. The inhaled route of tobramycin alone is not adequate for the treatment of pneumonia. An ophthalmic formulation is also available for topical use in the eye. It has also been used in low doses for synergy with β-lactam therapy in the treatment of gram-positive endocarditis.

Pharmacokinetics/Dosing

Tobramycin, like the other aminoglycosides, is poorly absorbed orally and must be administered parenterally for the treatment of systemic infections. Dosing varies based on indications. Weight-based dosing is typically based on a calculated body weight based on lean body weight. For morbidly obese clients, the weight used for dosing is typically the ideal body weight plus 40% of the difference between actual and ideal body weight. Historically, dosing of 1.5 to 2.5 mg/kg per dose at every 8 to 12 hour intervals has been used. More commonly, once daily dosing of 2.5 to 7 mg every 24 hours has been utilized for many clients with normal renal function. Such dosing may be associated with good therapeutic response and lower toxicity. For such dosing, the goal postdistribution peak levels are usually significantly above 8 to 10 mcg/mL (although not routinely monitored), and trough levels should be ideally less than 1 mcg/mL (range less than 0.5 to 2 mcg/mL) to achieve therapeutic response with reduced toxicity (Olsen, 2004). Once daily dosing has not been studied extensively for clients with cystic fibrosis (Smyth et al., 2001).

Adverse Effects
The major adverse effects of aminoglycosides, including tobramycin, are nephrotoxicity and ototoxicity. Other adverse effects include pain on injection, nausea, and confusion. Impaired neuromuscular function has been reported and may be more likely with concurrent use of neuromuscular blocking agents.

Drug Interactions
Concern for cumulative or additive toxicity with concurrent neuromuscular blockers, or other nephrotoxic or ototoxic drugs is an ongoing concern when using aminoglycosides. Concurrent amphotericin B, or loop diuretics may increase the risk for nephrotoxicity.

✴ **A.L. is started on tobramycin 300 mg IV every 24 hours (5 mg/kg/day) with a follow-up trough tobramycin level, serum creatinine, and BUN levels over the next 2 days.**

✴ **What are the nursing management issues involved in the use of aminoglycosides for A.L.?**

Assessment Obtain weight and height of A.L. before treatment for the calculation of the dose. Determine A.L.'s allergy history; a previous history of an allergic response to one aminoglycoside would contraindicate the use of another because of cross-sensitivity. Renal function impairment increases the risk of toxicity. Assess for impairment of the eighth cranial nerve as auditory and vestibular toxicity might occur with aminoglycosides. Infants with botulism and clients with myasthenia gravis and parkinsonism may experience greater muscle weakness because of neuromuscular blockade with the aminoglycosides.

Review A.L.'s current medication regimen for the risk of significant drug interactions, such as those that may occur when aminoglycosides are given concurrently with other aminoglycosides (two or more concurrently) or the antitubercular capreomycin (Capastat), which increases the potential for ototoxicity, nephrotoxicity, and neuromuscular blockade. Hearing loss may progress to deafness even after the drug is stopped. In some cases, hearing loss may be irreversible. Giving aminoglycosides with anesthetics (halogenated hydrocarbon), citrate-anticoagulated blood by massive transfusions, or neuromuscular blocking agents may increase neuromuscular blockade; avoid concurrent use or a potentially serious drug interaction may occur. With methoxyflurane (Penthrane) or parenteral polymyxins there may be an increased possibility for nephrotoxicity and/or neuromuscular blockade. Nephrotoxic drugs and other oto-

toxic drugs, such as amphotericin B parenteral (Fungizone), aspirin, bumetanide, parenteral (Bumex), cisplatin (Platinol), cyclosporine (Sandimmune), ethacrynate sodium parenteral (Edecrin), furosemide parenteral (Lasix), or vancomycin (Vancocin) increase the risk for ototoxicity and/or nephrotoxicity. Hearing loss may be permanent. If drugs are given concurrently, serial audiometric hearing determinations are suggested. Maintaining trough tobramycin or gentamicin levels below 1 mg/L reduces the risk for ototoxicity and nephrotoxicity by allowing the drug to be cleared from otic and renal tissues.

Perform a baseline assessment as described earlier in this chapter before initiating aminoglycoside therapy. Additionally, a urinalysis, audiogram, and renal and vestibular function determination should occur before the start of therapy.

Nursing Diagnosis While A.L. is receiving aminoglycoside therapy, assess her for the following nursing diagnoses/collaborative problems: disturbed sensory perception related to auditory ototoxicity (loss of hearing and tinnitus), vestibular ototoxicity (dizziness and loss of balance) and, for streptomycin only, peripheral neuritis (tingling of the fingers and toes, facial burning); and the potential complications of hypersensitivity, nephrotoxicity (blood in urine, greatly increased or decreased frequency of urination and amount of urine), neurotoxicity (muscle twitching, numbness, or seizures), or neuromuscular blockade (weakness, difficulty breathing).

Planning During her aminoglycoside therapy, A.L. will:
- Experience decreased symptoms of urinary infections.
- Not experience adverse effects of aminoglycoside therapy.
- Collaborate with health care providers by appropriately reporting untoward adverse effects.

Implementation
Monitoring Older adults are at greater risk of nephrotoxicity and ototoxicity because of reduced renal function, and they generally require smaller daily doses. However, a loss of hearing may occur in clients with normal renal function. Audiograms, renal function studies, and vestibular function studies should be performed periodically during high-dose therapy or therapy that lasts more than 10 days. Urinalyses should be monitored for the presence of albumin, casts, and cells, and for decreased specific gravity.

Monitor trough drug levels routinely, because evidence suggests that the incidence of ototoxicity and nephrotoxicity with aminoglycosides correlates with even slight elevations in trough levels. The trough concentration is believed to be a more sensitive indicator of renal function than serum creatinine levels. Peak levels, when used, are drawn 30 minutes after a 30-minute infusion, and trough levels are drawn immediately before the next dose.

With streptomycin only, caloric stimulation tests may be required during and after prolonged therapy to detect vestibular toxicity.

Vancomycin and aminoglycosides may be ordered to prevent bacterial endocarditis or to treat specific infections (e.g., carditis caused by organisms such as streptococci and corynebacteria). Frequent determinations of drug serum levels and renal function are recommended in such instances, because dosage adjustments or other interventions may be necessary.

Intervention For IV administration, dilute appropriately and administer slowly over a 20- to 60-minute period to prevent neuromuscular blockade as the result of toxic serum levels. Clients should be well hydrated while taking these medications to minimize chemical irritation of the urinary tubules. Monitor intake and output ratios. A daily urinalysis may be required during therapy for signs of renal irritation.

Inject the IM dosage forms of these drugs deeply into large muscle. Rotate sites.

Education Instruct A.L. to report any loss of hearing or any ringing or buzzing in the ears, which indicates ototoxicity; any change in urinary pattern or blood in the urine, which indicates nephrotoxicity; dizziness, which indicates vestibular toxicity; or numbness, tingling, or twitching, which indicates neurotoxicity. Stress the importance of taking the full course of medication as prescribed.

Evaluation The expected outcome of aminoglycoside therapy is that A.L. will maintain or achieve an infection-free state as evidenced by negative cultures and an absence of fever and of frequency, urgency, and burning associated with urination. She will not experience any adverse effects of aminoglycoside therapy (e.g., nephrotoxicity, neurotoxicity, ototoxicity) and will report adverse effects appropriately (e.g., tinnitus, vertigo, oliguria).

✴ **E.S. is an 18-year-old female college student who presents to the college health service with urinary frequency and burning. E.S. denies fever, cramps, or back tenderness. A urine sample is collected, and is tested with a dip stick which is positive for leukocytes and nitrites. The sample is forwarded to the laboratory for culture and sensitivity.**

✴ **What are the important considerations in evaluating a client for a UTI?**
UTIs occur much more frequently in females. The incidence of UTI greatly increases in late adolescence and during the third and fourth decades of life. Approximately one third of women 20 to 40 years of age develop signs and symptoms suggestive of UTI. During the reproductive years, women are 20 to 50 times more likely to acquire UTI than men. It is more common in sexually active women, and its incidence increases with age. The difference in the incidence of UTI between men and women diminishes in later life. In the older age group, hospitalization for other illnesses is frequently associated with urinary catheterization

and increases the risk of nosocomial UTI (Noble et al., 2001).

Differentiating between an upper UTI (pyelonephritis) and lower UTI (cystitis) is usually based on the presenting signs and symptoms. An upper UTI usually causes pain in the lower back, flank, or stomach, and fever, sweating, nausea, vomiting, weakness, and headache. A lower UTI leads to frequent but small amounts on urination, urgency, dysuria and, perhaps, incontinence. However, the infection may be present both in the upper and lower urinary tract in approximately one third of UTIs.

UTIs are primarily caused by bacteria. *E. coli* is by far the most common cause of UTI, accounting for 85% of community-acquired and 50% of hospital-acquired infections. Other gram-negative Enterobacteriaceae including *Proteus* and *Klebsiella,* and gram-positive *E. faecalis* and *Staphylococcus saprophyticus* are responsible for the remainder of most community-acquired infections. Complicated or nosocomial infections are frequently caused by *E. coli* and *E. faecalis* and by *Klebsiella, Enterobacter, Citrobacter, Serratia, P. aeruginosa, Providencia,* and *S. epidermidis* (Walsh, 2002).

Drug therapies for lower UTIs are often started before culture and sensitivity reports are known. The most probable infecting organism and the antibiotic sensitivity can be predicted from the information discussed in the previous paragraph.

✴ **What are the nursing management issues with E.S. for antimicrobial therapy for UTIs?**

Assessment The initial assessment of E.S. provides baseline information and includes her history of UTIs and the signs and symptoms of the current UTI. Drug allergies, concurrent drug therapy, or the altered function of any body system may affect the drug therapy.

Obtaining urine specimens to determine the causative organism for a UTI is often the nurse's responsibility. Through client education, most clients can obtain a clean-catch urine sample of the appropriate quantity and quality for laboratory testing. The health care provider will specify whether a midstream clean-catch or catheterized specimen is required. Specimens for culture should be taken directly to the laboratory to prevent the death of the suspect organisms and to prevent the growth of contaminating ones. However, there is economic value in empiric treatment without urine cultures in young women with dysuria and frequency.

Nursing Diagnosis While E.S. is receiving urinary antimicrobial therapy, she is at risk for the following nursing diagnoses: risk for injury related to a preexisting health condition, drug interaction, or adverse effect of the drug; deficient knowledge related to the antimicrobial therapy; and ineffective therapeutic regimen management. (See the Nursing Care Plan on p. 1045 for other selected nursing diagnoses.)

NURSING CARE PLAN SELECTED NURSING DIAGNOSES RELATED TO THE ADMINISTRATION
OF URINARY TRACT ANTIMICROBIALS

Nursing Diagnosis	Outcome Criteria	Nursing Interventions
Risk for infection	Client will: • Have infection prevented or symptoms of infection resolved • Maintain temperature within the normal range. • Maintain white blood cell count within normal range. • Be free of pathogens in urine cultures. • Have clear and odorless urine. • Increase fluid intake to 3000 mL/24 hr.	• Monitor and record temperature at least every 4 hours. Report elevations. • Monitor white blood cell count. Report significant changes. • Culture urine as ordered, and monitor results. • Use strict aseptic technique when inserting urinary catheters. • Encourage a fluid intake of at least 3000 mL daily.
Deficient knowledge related to medication regimen	• Client will describe underlying conditions and how the drug relates to the condition, how and when to take the medication, common drug interactions, safety precautions, common adverse effects, and which of these warrant reporting. • Client will self-administer medication safely and accurately.	• Assess learning needs and learning readiness. • Plan with the client for the achievement of realistic goals. • Provide information to meet outcome criteria. • Administer medication with food or milk to decrease gastrointestinal distress. • Alert the client that medication may cause a discoloration of the urine. • Instruct the client to take the medication as ordered and to consult with the prescriber if no improvement is seen within a few days.

Planning As the result of urinary antimicrobial therapy, E.S. will:
- Experience an absence of signs and symptoms of UTI.
- Have a negative urine culture.
- Have effectively managed her therapeutic regimen.

Implementation

Monitoring Periodically assess E.S.'s health status regarding fever, chills, flank pain, nausea and vomiting, frequency and urgency of urination, dysuria, costovertebral tenderness, gross hematuria and pyuria, and general well-being. Monitor urinalyses for WBCs, red blood cells (RBCs), casts, protein, crystals, and bacteria. Urine culture and sensitivity examinations indicate the efficacy of the drug. Also monitor CBC. If needed, serum antibiotic concentrations of selected drugs can be monitored during the course of therapy to assess for therapeutic and toxic levels of specific antimicrobials. In addition to monitoring the therapeutic effects of these antimicrobials, assess E.S. for the development of common adverse effects of individual drugs (see the discussions of specific drugs for these effects).

Intervention Chapter 57 discussed nursing interventions relative to antimicrobial drug therapy in greater detail. In general, these interventions relate to the following: (1) assistance in the identifying the infecting organism, (2) actual administration of the drug, (3) assessment of the client's response to the drug, (4) client education, and (5) prevention and treatment of adverse effects, including pharmacologic and chemical drug-drug interactions. If an antimicrobial agent is ordered before the infecting organism has been identified, it is important that the urine sample for initial culture be obtained before the first dose of the drug is administered. With subsequent specimens for culture, it is important to describe the client's antimicrobial regimen for the laboratory, because the selection and interpretation of laboratory tests often depend on this information.

Around-the-clock administration of antimicrobial drugs at prescribed intervals is required for maintaining therapeutic blood and urine levels of these drugs, and it is the nurse's responsibility to see that this occurs. This is accomplished by providing the necessary client education, which may entail waking sleeping clients and ensuring that tests or therapies do not interrupt the dosing schedule.

Education Instruct E.S. relative to the principles of antimicrobial therapy so that these drugs can be self-administered safely. The necessity of adhering to an inconvenient around-the-clock schedule may require special reinforcement. Compliance for the full course of therapy is essential to prevent the possible development of resistant strains of microorganisms even if marked improvement occurs within a few days. "Leftover" antimicrobial medications should not be used for new bouts of UTI but disposed of properly. The prescriber should be consulted for any new bouts of infection. Refer to the text for specific instructions for each drug. Instruct E.S. to notify the prescriber if her symptoms do not significantly improve in the first 3 days of therapy.

Advise E.S. to avoid coffee, tea, juices with a high citric acid content, cola, alcohol, chocolate, and spices, which often irritate a sensitive bladder. The daily fluid intake for a client with a UTI should be at least 3000 mL (unless contraindicated) to help flush organisms from the urinary tract. Acidification of the urine inhibits the growth of many urinary tract microorganisms. Thus when clients with UTIs are encouraged to consume large volumes of fluids, they should select fluids that increase urine acidity, such as cranberry juice or prune juice. Vitamin C will also acidify the urine and can enhance antiinfective therapy. Cranberry juice contains a compound that prevents bacteria from anchoring themselves in the bladder. Suggest cranberry sauce if E.S. considers cranberry juice unpalatable to increase compliance. Eating more protein, plums, or prunes will also help to make the urine more acidic. Most fruits, particularly citrus fruits and juices, milk and other dairy products, and other alkalinizing foods should be avoided. Alka-Seltzer and sodium bicarbonate, which alkalinize the urine, should be avoided.

Instruct E.S. about health practices that may reduce the chance of developing another UTI (Box 58-3).

Evaluation An expected outcome of urinary tract antimicrobial therapy is that E.S. will experience a decreased severity or a disappearance of the clinical and laboratory manifestations of the UTI (e.g., absence of pathogen on cultures, normothermia, WBC count within the normal range, and an absence of urgency, frequency, and burning of urination) without adverse effects of drug. She will effectively manage her therapeutic regimen by completing her full prescription,

---

BOX 58-3 CLIENT EDUCATION TO REDUCE OCCURRENCE OF UTIs

UTIs often occur as a result of contamination of the lower urinary tract with perineal bacteria. Preventive measures attempt to do the following: reduce perineal bacteria and prevent bacteria from entering the lower urinary tract. Client education should focus on these two measures and include the following instructions:

1. Good perineal hygiene helps to reduce bacterial growth.
2. Female clients should always wipe from the front to the back to prevent contamination of the urinary tract with fecal bacteria.
3. Emptying the bladder soon after intercourse helps to flush out bacteria that may have entered the urethra.
4. Cotton undergarments (or synthetics with a cotton crotch) that "breathe" are preferred to synthetics that foster bacterial growth.
5. Drinking six to eight glasses of fluids per day and urinating often help to cleanse the urinary tract of bacteria.

---

increasing her fluid intake to 2000 mL daily, practicing perineal hygiene, and appropriately reporting adverse effects.

✱ **E. S. is diagnosed with simple cystitis and is started on a 3-day course of trimethoprim-sulfamethoxazole double strength (trimethoprim 160 mg/sulfamethoxazole 800 mg) [Bactrim DS, Septra DS] twice daily.**

✱ **What agents are used to treat UTIs?**
A number of drugs are used to treat UTIs, including the aminopenicillins (e.g., amoxicillin, ampicillin), cephalosporins, and fluoroquinolones. The choice of empiric therapy before culture results are available is based on community-resistance patterns (Hooton et al., 2005). For serious infections, IV extended penicillins, aminoglycosides, or vancomycin are used depending on the pathogen. Phenazopyridine (Pyridium) is used primarily as a urinary tract analgesic.

A very widely used class of agents to treat UTIs is the sulfonamide group. The most frequently used sulfonamide, sulfamethoxazole, is routinely combined with trimethoprim for synergistic activity against gram-negative and limited gram-positive pathogens. Rather than being bactericidal, these agents are primarily bacteriostatic in concentrations that are normally useful in controlling infections. All of the sulfonamides used therapeutically are synthetically produced.

Because the sulfonamides are structurally similar to paraaminobenzoic acid (PABA), they inhibit a bacterial enzyme (dihydropteroate synthetase) necessary to incorporate PABA into dihydrofolic acid. Blocking dihydrofolic acid synthesis results in a decrease in tetrahydrofolic acid, which interferes with the synthesis of purines, thymidine, and DNA in the microorganism. Therefore the bacteria most sensitive to sulfonamides are those that synthesize their own folic acid. The presence of purulence, necrotic tissue, and serum interferes with the activities of the sulfonamides because PABA is present in such materials. Among the microorganisms highly susceptible to the sulfonamides are group A (-hemolytic streptococci, pneumococci, *N. meningitides*, *N. gonorrhoeae*, *E. coli*, *Pasteurella pestis*, *Bacillus anthracis*, *Shigella species*, *H. influenzae*, and *Pneumocystis carinii*.

The absorption of sulfonamides is good. For most sulfonamides, peak serum levels are reached between 2 and 6 hours; for sulfamethoxazole, the intermediate-acting sulfonamide, peak levels are reached in 6 to 12 hours. These agents are acetylated in the liver and excreted primarily by the kidneys.

Although the newer sulfonamides, such as sulfisoxazole and sulfacetamide, are quite soluble, even in acid urine, and so have a decreased risk of crystalluria; it is still recommended that clients increase their fluid intake to maintain a urine output of at least 1200 mL daily *(USP DI, 2005)*.

✱⌐ **sulfamethoxazole-trimethoprim** [sul fa meth **oks** a zole/trye **meth** oh prim]
(SMZ-TMP, TMP-SMZ, co-trimoxazole, Bactrim, Bactrim DS, Septra, Septra DS)
Sulfamethoxazole is commonly combined with the trimethoprim to target two different steps in folate metabolism of the bacterial cell. The efficacy of this combination over the use of single agents has

rendered this combination far and away the most frequently used of the sulfonamides agents. This combination in fixed dosage is often referred by other names such as co-trimoxazole, SMZ-TMP, TMP-SMZ, Trim-Sulf, Sulf-Trim, and others.

Indications

SMZ-TMP is used to treat UTIs due to susceptible pathogens including *E. coli, Enterobacter, Proteus, Providentia, Klebsiella, Morganella,* and other gram-negative pathogens. It is also used for the treatment of chronic bronchitis and otitis media, although its reliability against *H. influenzae* is variable. SMZ-TMP has activity against *Pneumocystis carinii* pneumonitis (PCP) (as seen in advanced HIV disease), strains of *E. coli* and *Cyclospora* (e.g., traveler's diarrhea), and is used for treating typhoid, shigellosis, and *Nocardial asteroides* infections.

Pharmacokinetics/Dosing

SMZ-TMP is usually administered orally, but an IV formulation is available for use. It is fairly well absorbed orally and each agent has a half-life of approximately 10 to 11 hours. The drugs are primarily cleared renally. The adult dose and duration vary based on indication. A typical dose for treating UTIs in adults is one double-strength tablet (sulfamethoxazole 800 mg/trimethoprim 160 mg) twice daily for 10 to 14 days. Single-dose, three-, and seven-day regimens are also used for uncomplicated cystitis.

Adverse Effects

SMZ-TMP most frequently causes anorexia, nausea, vomiting, and rash or urticaria. Occasional rare reactions include hepatotoxicity, confusion and seizures. Stevens-Johnson syndrome, toxic epidermal necrolysis, and exfoliative dermatitis are all possible with SMZ-TMP and have been observed most frequently in clients with advanced HIV or other immunocompromised states. SMZ-TMP may also predispose to hemolytic anemia in clients with glucose-6-phosphate dehydrogenase (G6PD) deficiency.

Drug Interactions

SMZ-TMP is metabolized by and inhibits cytochrome P450 2 C8/9 and may result in interactions with a number of agents, including warfarin, carbamazepine, phenobarbital, phenytoin, and rifampin. Hyperkalemia may be more likely with concurrent potassium-sparing diuretics or use of ACE inhibitors or angiotensin receptor blockers.

✳ What are the nursing implications in the use of sulfonamides?

Assessment Although cross-sensitization reactions with sulfonamides is not as severe as with penicillins, it is safer to avoid all sulfonamides in clients who develop a hypersensitivity to any one agent. Cross-sensitivity also exists with some diuretics (e.g., furosemide, acetazolamide, and the thiazides) and with sulfonylurea antidiabetic agents; therefore, as always, obtain an accurate history of E.S.'s sensitivities. Avoid the use of sulfonamides in clients with hepatic and renal dysfunction, blood dyscrasias, glucose-6-phosphate dehydrogenase (G6PD) deficiency, and porphyria. The risk-benefit ratio should be considered for clients with blood dyscrasias and anemia because of folate deficiency, because these drugs may cause blood dyscrasias. The administration of sulfonamides is contraindicated in neonates. (See the Pregnancy Safety box on p. 1020.)

Review E.S.'s current medication regimen for the risk of significant drug interactions. SMZ-TMP frequently prolongs the prothrombin time in clients who are receiving the anticoagulant warfarin. Keep this interaction in mind when SMZ-TMP is given to clients already on anticoagulant

therapy, and the PT/INR should be reassessed. SMZ-TMP may inhibit the hepatic metabolism of phenytoin (Dilantin). SMZ-TMP, given at a common clinical dosage, increased the phenytoin half-life by 39% and decreased the phenytoin metabolic clearance rate by 27%. When administering these drugs concurrently, be alert for possible excessive phenytoin effect. Sulfonamides can also displace methotrexate from plasma protein binding sites, thus increasing free methotrexate concentrations. In older adult clients concurrently receiving certain diuretics, primarily thiazides, an increased incidence of thrombocytopenia with purpura has been reported. There have been reports of marked but reversible nephrotoxicity with coadministration of SMZ-TMP and cyclosporine in renal transplant recipients. Increased digoxin blood levels can occur with concomitant SMZ-TMP therapy, especially in older adults. Monitor serum digoxin levels. Increased sulfamethoxazole blood levels may occur in clients who are also receiving indomethacin. The efficacy of tricyclic antidepressants can decrease when coadministered with SMZ-TMP. Like other sulfonamide-containing drugs, SMZ-TMP potentiates the effect of oral hypoglycemics (*Mosby's Drug Consult,* 2005).

Obtain a baseline assessment of E.S.'s symptoms related to the UTI, and a CBC and urinalysis, before initiating sulfonamide therapy.

Nursing Diagnosis While receiving sulfonamide therapy, assess E.S. for the development of the following nursing diagnoses/collaborative problems: impaired comfort related to CNS effects (dizziness, headache); altered comfort related to anorexia, nausea, and vomiting; diarrhea; and the potential complications of hypersensitivity (rash, fever), photosensitivity (increased sensitivity of skin to sunlight), blood dyscrasias (unusual bruising or bleeding, sore throat, fever, unusual fatigue), hepatitis (yellow eyes or skin), toxic epidermal necrolysis, interstitial nephritis, hematuria, or crystalluria.

Planning Planning is as previously discussed for E.S. within the general discussion of urinary antimicrobial therapy.

Implementation

Monitoring Because E.S. is on short-term sulfonamide therapy, the risk for adverse effects is low. However, renal toxicity is a potentially serious problem with long-term sulfonamides, so monitor the hospitalized client's urinary output and ensure that it totals at least 1200 mL in 24 hours. The maintenance of urinary output at this level decreases the tendency for crystals to form. The urine should be examined visually for the presence of crystals; periodic urinalyses should be performed with long-term sulfonamide therapy to determine if crystals are present. Monitor the urinalysis to determine the status of the UTI and for early detection of crystalluria. Carefully observe the client for toxic effects, such as a rash, sore throat, or purpura. Monitor immunosuppressed clients, especially for Stevens-Johnson syndrome.

With prolonged sulfonamide therapy, the client requires periodic blood counts to assess for the occurrence of hematologic adverse effects (anemia, granulocytopenia, and thrombocytopenia).

Intervention Administer sulfonamides on an empty stomach with a full glass of water to enhance absorption. If the common adverse effect of nausea and vomiting occurs, administer the drug with food to decrease GI distress.

Education Advise E.S. to drink at least 3 L of fluids per day unless contraindicated for renal or cardiac conditions. Liquids and vitamins that produce acid urine (e.g., ascorbic acid) should be avoided. Inform E.S. of the importance of completing a full course of drug therapy, even though she may feel better after several days of therapy. Instruct her to observe for and report any dermatologic reactions after initiating the sulfonamide. Fever may occur after 7 to 10 days of therapy, indicating a serum sickness–like reaction. Fever may be accompanied by joint pain, urticaria, and leukopenia. All of these responses are indications for discontinuation of the drug and a follow-up referral to the prescriber. Advise E.S. to avoid direct skin exposure to the sun and sunlamps, because skin photosensitivity may be present.

Evaluation The expected outcome of sulfonamide therapy is that E.S. will experience a decrease in the severity or a disappearance of the clinical and laboratory manifestations of the UTI (e.g., absence of pathogen on cultures, normothermia, WBC count within the normal range, and an absence of urgency, frequency, and burning of urination) without adverse drug effects of sulfonamides (e.g., nausea, vomiting, diarrhea, photosensitivity, rash, blood dyscrasias).

✸ What is the role of urinary tract antiseptics and analgesics?

Cinoxacin and nalidixic acid are fluoroquinolones, which are sometimes used to treat UTIs (see Table 58-7). Methenamine mandelate and nitrofurantoin are also used as urinary tract antiseptics. The role of cranberries and cranberry juice is also noted to reduce UTI risk. Urinary tract antiseptics are drugs that exert antibacterial activity in the urine but have little or no systemic antibacterial effects. Their usefulness is limited to the treatment of UTI.

Urinary Tract Antiseptics

methenamine mandelate [meth **en** a meen]
(Mandelamine)
methenamine hippurate
(Hiprex, Urex, Hip-Rex)
Methenamine, which is used to treat UTI, combines the action of methenamine and mandelic acid or hippurate acid salts. Its effectiveness depends on the release of formaldehyde, which requires an acid medium. The acids released from the mandelate or hippurate salts contribute to this acidity. Formaldehyde may be bactericidal or

bacteriostatic, and its effects are believed to be the result of denaturation of bacteria protein. It is ineffective in alkaline urine.

Indications
Because of its fairly wide bacterial spectrum, low toxicity, and low incidence of resistance, methenamine is often used for long-term suppression of infections.

Pharmacokinetics/Dosing
Methenamine is absorbed orally and takes 30 minutes to 2 hours to reach peak urinary formaldehyde levels at a urinary pH of 5.6; the enteric-coated methenamine mandelate reaches its urinary peak in 3 to 8 hours. Excretion is via the kidneys. The typical oral adult dose is 1 gram two to four times daily.

Adverse Effects
Methenamine is well tolerated, but bladder irritation, GI upset, and rash have been reported.

Drug Interactions
Drugs that may result in alkalinization of the urine render methenamine ineffective. Such agents include antacids, calcium and magnesium salts, carbonic anhydrase inhibitors, sodium bicarbonate, citrates, and thiazide diuretics. Concurrent use of sulfonamides may increase the risk for urine crystal formation.

Nursing Management
Give after meals and at bedtime to minimize gastric distress. Methenamine is most effective when the urine pH is 5.5 or less. Urine pH is easily monitored at the bedside and at home with commercially available test strips.

nitrofurantoin [nye troe **fyoor** an toyn]
(Furadantin, Macrodantin, Macrobid, Apo-Nitrofurantoin✢, Novo-Furan✢)
Nitrofurantoin is a broad-spectrum bactericidal agent at therapeutic serum levels. It is reduced by bacteria to reactive substances that inactivate or alter bacterial ribosomal proteins.

Indications
It is indicated for the treatment of UTIs caused by organisms such as *E. coli* and *S. aureus* or the *Klebsiella, Enterobacter,* and *Proteus* species.

Pharmacokinetics/Dosing
After oral administration, nitrofurantoin is absorbed and has a half-life of 20 to 60 minutes. Approximately 65% of the drug is rapidly metabolized and inactivated in the liver and body tissues and excreted by the kidneys. The usual adult dose is 50 to 100 mg twice daily or four times daily depending on dosage used. A low dose of 50 mg once daily has been used for chronic UTI suppression but monitoring for pulmonary toxicity is indicated with long-term use. Inadequate urine levels are noted for clients with renal dysfunction; as such, it is not effective for clients with a creatinine clearance below 30 mL/min.

Adverse Effects
The most serious adverse effects of nitrofurantoin include pulmonary toxicity (most often seen with chronic use) and hemolytic anemia (usually limited to clients with G6PD deficiency). Other adverse effects include GI upset, confusion, dizziness, and *C. difficile* colitis. Rarely, hepatic or other hematologic problems have been reported.

Nursing Management
Use nitrofurantoin cautiously in clients with peripheral neuropathy (because it may be worsened) and also in clients with pulmonary disease (because the drug may cause a pulmonary reaction, including interstitial pneumonitis). Pulmonary studies may be indicated to monitor for adverse drug effects. Give with food to minimize gastric distress. Avoid crushing the tablets because of the risk of staining teeth; use dilute oral suspension, and rinse mouth thoroughly after taking preparation. The client taking nitrofurantoin should be advised that urine may be brown in color. Nitrofurantoin is discolored by alkalis and strong light. The client should not use metal pillboxes unless they are stainless steel or aluminum, because this drug decomposes on contact with other metals.

Urinary Tract Analgesics

phenazopyridine [fen az oh **peer** i deen]
(Pyridium, Phenazo✤, Pyronium✤)

Phenazopyridine is an azo dye most commonly used as a urinary tract analgesic. Its exact mechanism of action is unknown, but it appears to have a topical analgesic or local anesthetic effect on the mucosa of the urinary tract.

Indications

Phenazopyridine is used for urinary tract irritation, such as urinary frequency and pain and burning on urination. It is indicated only for short-term use; the underlying reason for the irritation should be determined and treated appropriately.

Pharmacokinetics/Dosing

Phenazopyridine is metabolized by the liver and other body tissues and is excreted by the kidneys. It is typically dosed at 100 to 200 mg three times daily after meals for the first 2 days of the UTI. It should be avoided for clients with significant renal impairment.

Adverse Effects

The most pronounced effect of phenazopyridine is that it produces an orange to red urine that may stain clothing. Clients will often be alarmed about this effect unless educated that this is a normal reaction because phenazopyridine is an azo dye. Other infrequent reactions include stomach cramps and headache. Rarely, hepatic or renal damage have been reported with its use.

Nursing Management

Phenazopyridine is contraindicated in clients with G6PD deficiency, impaired renal or hepatic function, or a history of sensitivity to the drug. The client receiving phenazopyridine therapy is at risk for the nursing diagnosis of impaired comfort (headache, heartburn, abdominal cramps) and the potential complications of hemolytic anemia (fatigue), renal function impairment, methemoglobinemia, allergic dermatitis, and hepatotoxicity (yellow eyes or skin). Monitor the client's progress after 24 hours for decreased symptoms of urgency and burning on urination. Phenazopyridine is usually prescribed in conjunction with an antimicrobial or urinary antiseptic. Administer with food to decrease GI distress. Phenazopyridine may be discontinued after 2 days if the client's discomfort has resolved. Instruct the client to observe for yellowness of the skin and sclera, which may indicate an accumulation of the drug as a result of renal impairment. If this occurs, the drug is discontinued and the prescriber is notified. Alert the client not to wear soft contact lenses during therapy or they may be permanently stained. The expected outcome of phenazopyridine therapy is that the client will experience an absence of urgency, frequency, and burning on urination within 2 days, although the drug may be administered for as long as 15 days.

✳ **What other systemically administered drugs are available to treat bacterial infections?**

A number of miscellaneous agents round out the antibacterial agents used to treat bacterial infections. These include chloramphenicol, spectinomycin, linezolid, and quinupristine/dalfopristine, and have focused roles in therapy. Occasionally used to treat skin infections, daptomycin (Cubicin) interferes with intracellular protein synthesis.

chloramphenicol [klor am **fen** i kole]
(Chloromycetin)

Chloramphenicol (Chloromycetin), a broad-spectrum antibacterial, is a potent inhibitor of protein synthesis. It is a bacteriostatic agent for a wide variety of gram-negative and gram-positive organisms. However, its approved indications are limited because it is potentially seriously toxic to bone marrow (aplasia leading to aplastic anemia and possibly death).

Although chloramphenicol is usually bacteriostatic, it may be bactericidal in high doses with highly susceptible organisms. It penetrates bacteria cell membranes and reversibly prevents peptide bond formation, thus inhibiting protein synthesis.

Indications

Chloramphenicol is indicated for the treatment of meningitis (*Haemophilus influenzae, S. pneumoniae,* and *Neisseria meningitidis*), paratyphoid fever, Q fever, Rocky Mountain spotted fever, typhoid fever *(Salmonella typhi),* typhus infections, brain abscesses, and bacterial septicemia when other agents are not indicated or effective.

Pharmacokinetics/Dosing

Chloramphenicol has good oral and parenteral bioavailability, with highest concentrations reported in the liver and kidneys. Concentrations of up to 50% of serum levels have been noted in cerebrospinal fluid. Chloramphenicol is metabolized in the liver to glucuronide (an inactive metabolite). The immature liver of fetuses and neonates cannot conjugate chloramphenicol, which may result in toxic levels or an accumulation of the active drug resulting in "gray syndrome" (blue-gray skin, hypothermia, irregular breathing, coma, cardiovascular collapse).

The half-life of chloramphenicol in an adult is 1.5 to 3.5 hours. Peak serum levels are reached in 1 to 1.5 hours via the IV route or in 1 to 3 hours after an oral dose. Chloramphenicol is excreted mainly by the kidneys. The oral dosage forms of chloramphenicol were withdrawn from the U.S. market in 1998. The IV adult dosage is 12.5 mg/kg every 6 hours. The dosage for infants 2 weeks old and older is 12.5 mg/kg every 6 hours. Chloramphenicol is not recommended for use during pregnancy or breastfeeding.

Adverse Effects

The common adverse effects of chloramphenicol include nausea, vomiting, or diarrhea. More serious adverse effects include blood dyscrasias, optic neuritis and, possibly, irreversible bone marrow depression that may result in aplastic anemia.

Nursing Management

Assessment

Bone marrow depression or a history of previous cytotoxic drug or radiation therapy increases the client's risk for adverse effects because chloramphenicol may cause a dose-related bone marrow depression, aplastic anemia, and other blood dyscrasias. CBCs are necessary for a baseline assessment before therapy. Clients with hepatic and renal function impairment require a dosage reduction. Chloramphenicol is a contraindicated if the client has had a previous allergic or toxic response to the drug. Use caution if the client has a G6PD deficiency.

Review the client's current medication regimen for the risk of significant drug interactions, such as those that may occur when chloramphenicol is given concurrently with other blood dyscrasia-causing drugs, bone marrow depressants, or radiation therapy as it may result in enhanced bone marrow depressant effects. A dosage reduction may be necessary. Monitor CBCs closely for leukopenia. Chloramphenicol may inhibit the metabolism of antidiabetic drugs, resulting in increased serum levels and hypoglycemic effects of tolbutamide and chlorpropamide. Monitor blood glucose levels closely, because a dosage adjustment may be necessary. Concurrent drug administration with phenobarbital (Luminal), phenytoin (Dilantin), or warfarin (Coumadin) may result in elevated drug serum levels and toxicity of these agents. Monitor all drugs metabolized by the liver enzyme system (chloramphenicol inhibits the cytochrome P450 system), because toxicity may result.

A baseline assessment as described in Chapter 57 should be performed before initiating chloramphenicol therapy.

Nursing Diagnosis

Assess clients receiving chloramphenicol therapy for the following nursing diagnoses: altered comfort related to anorexia, nausea, and vomiting; ineffective protection related to dose-related bone marrow depression (leukopenia, thrombocytopenia, anemia); diarrhea; disturbed thought processes (confusion, delirium) related to neurotoxic reactions; disturbed sensory perception related to optic neuritis (blurred vision, loss of vision, eye pain) and peripheral neuritis (tingling, numbness, and burning pain of the hands and feet); and the potential complications of hypersensitivity (rash, fever, dyspnea) and "gray syndrome" if used in neonates.

Planning
Are as for other antimicrobial therapy.

Implementation
Monitoring
Monitor periodic CBCs for dose-related, reversible bone marrow depression, reticulocytopenia, leukopenia, thrombocytopenia, and decreased RBCs. Observe the client for pale skin, sore throat and fever, unusual bruising or bleeding, or unusual fatigue. CBCs are not helpful in predicting drug-related aplastic anemia, which usually occurs after the completion of treatment.

Monitor serum chloramphenicol levels weekly or more frequently with hepatic impairment and in clients receiving therapy for longer than 2 weeks; it should be in the range of 10 to 20 mg/mL (the most effective concentration). Concentrations higher than 30 mg/mL increase the risk for bone marrow depression and gray syndrome.

Check the client's temperature every 4 hours; the drug is usually discontinued if the temperature remains normal for 48 hours. If the client is on oral antidiabetic agents, monitor the serum glucose more frequently. Monitor for signs and symptoms of Gray syndrome, usually occurring 2 to 9 days after high doses of the drug in premature infants, neonates, and children younger than 2 months. Report early symptoms (e.g., failure to feed, pallor, changes in vital signs). Early diagnosis and discontinuation of the drug may prevent a potentially fatal adverse effect.

Intervention
Chloramphenicol that is administered IV should be infused over at least a 1-minute period. Check the IV site daily for local irritation. If chloramphenicol is administered IM, inject it deeply.

Education
Because the bone marrow depressant effects of chloramphenicol may increase gingival bleeding and delay healing, instruct the client to delay dental work until blood counts return to normal. Instruct all clients in proper oral hygiene and the cautious use of toothbrushes, dental floss, and toothpicks.

Advise the client to report to the prescriber immediately any symptoms of blood dyscrasia, such as sore throat, fever, extreme fatigue, or unusual bleeding or bruising. Alert clients to report activity intolerance and other signs of anemia that may occur weeks or months after therapy, because these symptoms are indicative of drug-related aplastic anemia.

Evaluation
The expected outcome of chloramphenicol therapy is that the client will maintain or achieve an infection-free state as evidenced by negative cultures. If administered therapeutically, the client will also demonstrate a body temperature within normal limits, a WBC count within the normal limits for age, and the resolution of any other infection-related symptoms without experiencing adverse effects of the drug without the development of adverse drug effects.

linezolid [lin **neh** zoe lid]
(Zyvox)
Linezolid (Zyvox) belongs to a class of agents chemically known as oxazolidinones. Its spectrum of activity is limited to gram-positive infections and its use is primarily limited to the treatment of VRE and MRSA infections. It binds to bacterial 23 S ribosomal RNA and inhibits bacterial protein synthesis and is considered bacteriostatic for VRE and MRSA.

Indications
Linezolid is used to treat VRE, MRSA, and other serious gram-positive infections including diabetic foot infections, community acquired pneumonia and skin and skin structure infections.

Pharmacokinetics/Dosing
Linezolid is rapidly and completely absorbed with oral administration. It is metabolized to inactive metabolites and eliminated in the urine as active and inactive drug. The elimination half-life is approximately 4 hours in adults. The dosage for adults is typically 400 to 600 mg PO or IV every 12 hours.

Adverse Effects
The most common adverse effects include GI upset, diarrhea, and pseudomembranous colitis. Most concerning is the risk for thrombocytopenia and other bone marrow suppression that is more likely for clients who remain in linezolid for more than 2 weeks. Hypertension is also possible.

Nursing Management
Because of the pressor effects of linezolid, assess the client for hypertension and the concurrent administration of adrenergic drugs, particularly those taken for coughs and cold. Linezolid also interacts with serotonergic drugs, such as, serotonin reuptake inhibitors or monoamine oxidase (MAO) inhibitors. Assess for previous thrombocytopenia as it places the client at higher risk for that adverse drug effect. Monitor for hypertension, bleeding, diarrhea (pseudomembranous colitis) or any symptoms of lactic acidosis (nausea and vomiting, unexplained acidosis). Advise a low tyramine diet; avoidance of foods that are aged, pickled, fermented, or smoked in preparation. The drug may be taken without regard to food.

quinupristin/dalfopristin [kwi **nyoo** pris tin/dal **foe** pris tin]
(Synercid)
The combination of quinupristin/dalfopristin is used primarily in the treatment of serious gram-positive infections and its use is usually limited to life-threatening *Enterococcus faecium* and staphylococcal infections, including VRE and MRSA. Each individual agent is a streptogramin in a fixed ratio. These agents inhibit protein synthesis in a manner similar to the macrolide antimicrobials.

Indications
Quinupristin/dalfopristin is used to treat serious or life-threatening gram-positive infections, including VRE and MRSA.

Pharmacokinetics/Dosing
The quinupristin/dalfopristin combination is administered IV and has short elimination half-lives of under 1 hour for each drug. Both drugs are metabolized to active metabolites and are primarily excreted in the feces and urine. The usual dose for adults is 7.5 mg/kg (combined product) every 8 to 12 hours. The drug is available in 500 mg vials (quinupristin 150 mg/dalfopristin 350 mg).

Adverse Effects
Quinupristin/dalfopristin poses a risk for hepatic or renal injury and very commonly produces pain, inflammation and edema at the infusion site. Allergic reactions, bone marrow suppression, and cardiac dysrhythmias have also been attributed to these drugs.

Drug Interactions
Quinupristin/dalfopristin are weak inhibitors of cytochrome P450 3A4 and may prolong the action of a number of other agents. Quinupristin/dalfopristin inhibits the metabolism of cyclosporine, midazolam, and nifedipine. It has the potential to increase the levels of protease inhibitors, vincristine, vinblastine, docetaxel, paclitaxel, diazepam, cisapride, tacrolimus, carbamazepine, quinidine, lidocaine, and disopyramide as the result of inhibition of CYP3A4 metabolism. Consult the package insert for more complete information.

Nursing Management
Assess concurrent medication regimen. Monitor IV site for extravasation and thrombophlebitis. Alert the client to report any discomfort at IV infusion site, or any rash, pruritus, or redness of upper body.

spectinomycin [spek ti noe **mye** sin]
(Trobicin)
Spectinomycin is a bacteriostatic agent that inhibits protein synthesis in the bacteria cell and has activity against *N. gonorrhea*.

Indications
The therapeutic indication for spectinomycin is the treatment of infections caused by *N. gonorrhoeae*. It is for IM use only and gener-

ally is recommended as an alternate regimen for clients with gonorrhea who have antibiotic resistance or cannot take ceftriaxone. Spectinomycin is not effective for treating syphilis and should not be used for mixed infections (gonorrhea and syphilis), because it can mask the symptoms of syphilis.

Pharmacokinetics/Dosing

Spectinomycin is administered by deep IM injection and has a duration of action of 6 to 8 hours. It is dosed at 2 to 4 grams as a single dose. Doses greater than 2 grams should be administered at separate injection sites. It is usually dosed concurrently with doxycycline 100 mg PO twice daily for 7 days as coverage for chlamydial infection.

Adverse Effects

The adverse effects of spectinomycin include nausea, chills, fever, dizziness, and urticaria.

Nursing Management

Spectinomycin was formerly used for the treatment of gonococcal infections in children; however, the diluent to reconstitute spectinomycin contains 0.945% benzyl alcohol, which has been associated with fatal gasping syndrome in infants. Observe the client for 45 to 60 minutes after injection, because anaphylaxis has been reported. At the beginning of therapy and after 3 months, perform a serologic examination to monitor the client with a gonococcal infection for concurrent syphilis. Obtain cultures of gonococcal infection sites to monitor for effectiveness of therapy. Spectinomycin is for IM use only. Agitate the vial thoroughly to ensure even suspension of the drug. Administer the IM injection deep into the ventrogluteal site or vastus lateralis site. Inject the suspension using a 20-gauge needle, and inject only 5 mL in each site. Caution the client that dizziness may occur and to avoid operating hazardous equipment until the vertigo effects of the drug are known. The client should be instructed to use a condom to prevent infection, and it may be necessary to treat the partner concurrently to prevent reinfection. The expected outcome of spectinomycin therapy is that the client's gonococcal infection sites will show negative culture results after 3 to 7 days.

with DNA, is effective against anaerobic bacteria and protozoa. Tetracyclines block the binding of transfer RNA complex to the ribosome and are therefore bacteriostatic for a wide range of gram-positive and gram-negative organisms. Fluoroquinolones inhibit bacterial RNA synthesis and are bactericidal. Aminoglycosides are bactericidal agents that are usually held in reserve for serious or life-threatening infections. Chloramphenicol inhibits protein synthesis and is bacteriostatic for a wide range of organisms; however, its use is limited because of its toxicity to bone marrow.

UTIs are a common reason for seeking medical care in the community and a major result of nosocomial infection transmission in institutions; their incidence increases with age. Antimicrobial therapy for UTIs includes aminopenicillins, sulfonamides, urinary tract antiseptics, and fluoroquinolones. Urinary tract analgesics may also be used.

Although a repertoire of antimicrobials can be used in the treatment of infections, health care professionals cannot become complacent in their use. The risk of infection in certain populations has increased with the emergence of newly recognized pathogens, drug resistance in known strains of organisms, the use of immunosuppressive agents, and the increase in invasive procedures for diagnosis and treatment.

Summary

Antibacterials (also known as antimicrobials or antibiotics) are chemical substances that kill or suppress the growth of microorganisms. Once the nurse has acquired an understanding of the principles of antimicrobial therapy, the particular drugs may be classified by groups, actions, and effects for familiarization. Penicillins are derived from molds and inhibit the synthesis of bacterial cell walls; they are bactericidal for a wide range of gram-positive and some gram-negative organisms. Cephalosporins, now in their fourth generation, are chemical modifications of the penicillin structure and are bactericidal by inhibiting cell wall synthesis. Vancomycin is bactericidal for most gram-positive organisms and bacteriostatic for enterococci by inhibiting RNA synthesis and bacterial cell wall synthesis, causing lysis. Macrolides, including erythromycin, are bacteriostatic by inhibiting protein synthesis; they are bactericidal in higher concentrations with selected organisms. Clindamycin inhibits protein synthesis in bacteria by binding the ribosomes of susceptible organisms, are primarily bacteriostatic (except in higher concentrations with selected organisms, in which case they are bactericidal). Metronidazole, a short-acting cytotoxic agent that interacts

Critical Thinking Questions

- Why is the assessment phase so important in the nursing process for antimicrobial therapy?
- Kevin Reardon, 27 years old, has been prescribed oral Augmentin for sinusitis. On the third day of Augmentin therapy, Mr. Reardon telephones the clinic to indicate he has developed diarrhea. What might be occurring with Mr. Reardon's therapy? What action should the nurse take?
- In many countries where prescription regulations are not as restrictive as in the United States and Canada, many antibiotics are OTC drugs, including chloramphenicol. What might be the consequences of this lack of regulation?
- Why is it important to monitor urinary output with the administration of the various antimicrobials?
- Molly Ellis, 22 years old, has an acute lower UTI. Her health care provider prescribes the sulfonamide sulfisoxazole for 10 days. What instruction may be required to enable Ms. Ellis to manage her drug therapy effectively? What instruction should be reviewed with the client to assist her in preventing recurrences of the UTI?

Bibliography

Abate, B.J., & Barriere, S.L. (2002). Antimicrobial regimen selection. In J.T. DiPiro, R.L. Talbert, G.C. Yee, G.R. Matzke, B.G. Wells & L.M. Posey (Eds.), *Pharmacotherapy: A pathophysiological approach* (5th ed.). Norwalk, CT: Appleton & Lange.

Altman, R., Nielsen, N., Sterling, M.L., & Dickinson, B.D. (2002). The Council on Scientific Affairs Drug Interactions Between Oral Contraceptives and Antibiotics. *Obstetrics and Gynecology, 99*(5, Part 1), 842.

Anderson, D.M., Keith, J., & Novak, P.D. (Eds.) (2002). *Mosby's medical, nursing, and allied health dictionary* (6th ed.). St. Louis: Mosby.

Aspen, O.Q., & Stern, R.S. (2004). Acne vulgaris and rosacea. In R.E. Rakel & E.T. Bope (Eds.), *Conn's Current Therapy 2004: Latest Approved Method of Treatment* (56th ed). Philadelphia: Elsevier.

Beringer, P. (1999). New approaches to optimizing antimicrobial therapy in patients with cystic fibrosis. *Current Opinion in Pulmonary Medicine, 5*(6), 371.

Blazquez Garrido, R.M., Espinosa Parra, F.J., Alemany Frances, L., Ramos Guevara, R.M., Sanchez-Nieto, J.M., Segovia Hernandez, M., et al. (2005). Antimicrobial therapy for Legionnaires disease: Levofloxacin versus macrolides. *Clinical Infectious Disease, 40,* 800-806.

Bosker, G. (Ed.). (2004). *Primary and acute care medicine: Practice, protocols, pathways,* (2nd ed.). Atlanta: Thomson American Health Consultants.

Carratala, J., Fernandez-Sabe, N., Ortega, L., Castellsague, X., Roson, B., Dorca, J., et al. (2005). Outpatient care compared with hospitalization for community-acquired pneumonia: A randomized trial in low-risk patients. *Annals of Internal Medicine, 142,* 165-172.

CDC Fact Sheet (September 23, 2004). *Clostridium difficile* information for healthcare providers. Centers for Disease Control and Prevention. Retrieved January 24, 2005, from http://www.cdc.gov/ncidod/hip/gastro/ClostridiumDifficileHCP_print.htm.

Dial, S., Alrasadi, K., Manoukian, C., Huang, A., & Menzies, D. (2004). Risk of *Clostridium difficile* diarrhea among hospital inpatients prescribed proton pump inhibitors: cohort and case-control studies. *CMAJ Canadian Medical Association Journal, 171*(1),33-38.

Dickinson, B., Altman, R.D., Nielsen, N.H., & Sterling, M.L. (2001). Drug interactions between oral contraceptives and antibiotics. *Obstetrics and Gynecology, 98,* 853-860.

Drug facts and comparisons (58th ed.). (2005). St. Louis: Facts and Comparisons.

Eggertson, L. (2004). *C. difficile* hits Sherbrooke, Que., hospital: 100 deaths. *CMAJ Canadian Medical Association Journal, 171*(5), 436.

Feigin, R., Watson, J.T., & Gerber, S.I. (2004). Use of corticosteroids in bacterial meningitis. *Pediatric Infectious Disease Journal, 23*(4), 355-357.

Gaynes, R., Rimland, D., Killum, E., Lowery, H.K., Johnson, II T.M., & Killgore, G., et al. (2004). Outbreak of *Clostridium difficile* infection in a long-term care facility: association with gatifloxacin use. *Clinical Infectious Diseases, 38,* 640-645.

Gilbert, D.N., Moellering, R.C., Eliopoulos, G.M., & Sande, M.A. (2004). The Sanford guide to antimicrobial therapy (34th ed). Hyde Park, VT: Antimicrobial Therapy, Inc.

Guglielmo, B.J. (2005). Principles of infectious diseases. In M.A. Koda-Kimble, L.Y. Young, W.A. Kradjan, B.J. Guglielmo, B.K. Alldredge, & R.L. Corelli (Eds.), *Applied therapeutics: The clinical use of drugs* (8th ed.). Philadelphia: Lippincott Williams & Wilkins.

Hardman, J.G., & Limbird, L.E. (Eds.). (2001). *Goodman & Gilman's The pharmacological basis of therapeutics* (10th ed.). New York: McGraw-Hill.

Hooton, T.M., Scholes, D., Gupta, K., Stapleton, A.E., Roberts, P.L., & Stamm, W.E. (2005). Amoxicillin-clavulanate vs. ciprofloxacin for the treatment of uncomplicated cystitis in women: A randomized trial. *Journal of the American Medical Association, 293,* 949-955.

Jacobs, R.A. (2003). General problems in infectious disease. In L.M. Tierney, Jr., S.J. McPhee & Papadakis, M.A. (Eds.), *Current Medical Diagnosis & Treatment.* New York: Lange Medical Books/McGraw-Hill.

Kelkar, P.S., & Li, J.T. (2001). Cephalosporin allergy. *New England Journal of Medicine, 345*(11), 804-809.

Lacy, C.F., Armstrong, L.L., Goldman, M.P., & Lance, L.L. (2004). *Lexi-Comp's Drug Information Handbook* (12th ed.). Hudson, Ohio: Lexi-Comp.

Lamba, J.K., Lin, Y.S., Thummel, K., Daly, A., Watkins, P.B., & Strom, S., et al. (2002). Common allelic variants of cytochrome P4503 A4 and their prevalence in different populations. *Pharmacogenetics, 12*(2):121-132.

Loo, V.G., Libman, M.D., Miller, M.A., Bourgault, A.M., Frenette, C.H., & Kelly, M., et al. (2004). Clostridium difficile: a formidable foe. *CMAJ Canadian Medical Association Journal, 171*(1), 47-48.

McCormick, D.P., Chonmaitree, T., Pittman, C., Saeed, K., Friedman, N.R., Uchida, T., et al. (2005). Nonsevere acute otitis media: A clinical trial comparing outcomes of watchful waiting versus immediate antibiotic treatment. *Pediatrics, 115,* 1455-1465.

Mosby's drug consult (15th ed.) (2005). St. Louis: Mosby.

Musher, D.M., Aslam, S., Logan, N., Nallacheru, S., Bhaila, I., Borchert, F., et al. (2005). Relatively poor outcome after treatment of *Clostridium difficile* colitis with metronidazole. *Clinical Infectious Disease, 40,* 1586-1590.

e-LEARNING SUPPLEMENTS

Student CD-ROM
- Final Exam questions
- NCLEX® Examination review questions
- Pharmacology animations
- Printable chapter summary

Evolve Website (http://evolve.elsevier.com/mckenry)
- Case study on antibacterials
- Interactive concept map on lower UTI

- Content updates, including information on new drugs
- WebLinks corresponding to this chapter
- Answers to the critical thinking questions in this chapter
- *Elsevier ePharmacology Update* newsletter
- Mosby's Drug Consult Internet Edition
- Supplemental and reference information

Neuhauser, M.M., Weinstein, R.A., Rydman, R., Danziger, L.H., Karam, G., & Quinn, J.P. (2003). Antibiotic resistance among gram-negative bacilli in U.S. intensive care units: Implications for fluoroquinolone use. *Journal of the American Medical Association, 19*;289:885-888.

Noble, J., Greene, H.L., Levinson, W., Modest, G.A., Mulrow, C.D., & Scherger, J. et al. (2001). *Textbook of Primary Medicine.* (3rd ed.). St. Louis: Mosby.

Olsen, K.M., Rudis, M.I., Rebuck, J.A., Hara, J., Gelmont, D., & Mehdian, R., et al. (2004). Effect of once-daily dosing vs. multiple daily dosing of tobramycin on enzyme markers of nephrotoxicity. *Critical Care Medicine, 32*(8), 1678-1682.

Ozolins, M., Eady, E.A., Avery, A.J., Cunliffe, W.J., Po, A.L., O'Neill, C., et al. (2004). Comparison of five antimicrobial regimens for treatment of mild to moderate inflammatory facial acne vulgaris in the community: Randomised controlled trial. *Lancet, 364,* 2188-2195.

Özdemir, V., Kalow, W., Tang, B.K., Paterson, A.D., Walker, S.E., & Endrenyi, L., et al. (2000). Evaluation of the genetic component of variability in CYP3 A4 activity: a repeated drug administration method. *Pharmacogenetics, 10,* 373–388.

Pepin, J., Alary, M.E., Valiquette, L., Raiche, E., Ruel, J., Fulop, K., et al. (2005). Increasing risk of relapse after treatment of *Clostridium difficile* colitis in Quebec, Canada. *Clinical Infectious Disease, 40,* 1591-1597.

Pepin, J., Valiquette, L., Alary, M.E., Villemure, P., Pelletier, A., & Forget, K., et al. (2004). Clostridium difficile-associated diarrhea in a region of Quebec from 1991 to 2003: a changing pattern of disease severity. *CMAJ Canadian Medical Association Journal, 171*(5), 466-472.

Poutanen, S.M., & Simor, A.E. (2004). Clostridium difficile-associated diarrhea in adults. *CMAJ Canadian Medical Association Journal, 171*(1), 51-58.

Ray, W., Murray, K.T., Meredith, S., Narasimhulu, S.S., Hall, K., & Stein, C.M. (2004). Oral erythromycin and the risk of sudden death from cardiac causes. *New England Journal of Medicine, 351*(11), 1089-1096.

Rybak, M.J., & Aeschlimann, J.R. (2002). Laboratory tests to direct antimicrobial pharmacotherapy. In J.T. DiPiro, R.L. Talbert, G.C. Yee, G.R. Matzke, B.G. Wells & L.M. Posey (Eds.), *Pharmacotherapy: A pathophysiological approach* (5th ed.). Norwalk, CT: Appleton & Lange.

Saiman, L. (2004). The use of macrolide antibiotics in patients with cystic fibrosis. *Current Opinion in Pulmonary Medicine, 10*(6), 515-523.

Seaton, T.L. (2005). Acne. In M.A. Koda-Kimble, L.Y. Young, W.A. Kradjan, B.J. Guglielmo, B.K. Alldredge, & R.L. Corelli (Eds.), *Applied therapeutics: The clinical use of drugs* (8th ed.). Philadelphia: Lippincott Williams & Wilkins.

Skidmore, R., Kovach, R., Walker, C., Thomas, J., Bradshaw, M., & Leyden, J., et al. (2003). Effects of subantimicrobial-dose doxycycline in the treatment of moderate acne. *Archives of Dermatology, 139,* 459-464.

Smyth, A., Doherty, C., Govan, J., Tan, K., Hyman-Taylor, P., & Stableforth, D., et al. (2001). Once daily tobramycin achieves cidal levels against pseudomonas aeruginosa in patients with cystic fibrosis. *Thorax, 56*(Supplement iii), 84-87.

Spencer, R.C. (1998). The role of antimicrobial agents in the aetiology of *Clostridium difficile*-associated disease. *The Journal of Antimicrobial Chemotherapy, 41*(Suppl C), 21-27.

USP DI: Drug information for the health care professional (25th ed.). (2005). Greenwood Village, CO: MICROMEDEX Thomson Healthcare.

van de Beek, D., de Gans, J., Spanjaard, L., Weisfelt, M., Reitsma, J., & Vermeulen, M. (2004). Clinical features and prognostic factors in adults with bacterial meningitis. *New England Journal of Medicine, 351*(18), 1849-1859.

van der Linden, P.D., Sturkenboom, M.C., Herings, R.M., Leufkens, H.M., Rowlands, S., & Stricker, B.H. (2003). Increased risk of Achilles tendon rupture with quinolone antibacterial use, especially in elderly patients taking oral corticosteroids. *Arch Intern Med, 163,* 1801-1807.

Walsh, P.C. (Ed.). (2002). *Campbell's Urology.* Philadelphia: W.B. Saunders.

Wolfson, R.K., & Kahana, M.D. (2004). Double jeopardy- clindamycin and loperamide in an adolescent with clostridium difficile colitis: 633. *Critical Care Medicine, 32*(12) Supplement, A178.

Yang, P., Kanki, H., Drolet, B., Yang, T., Wei, J., & Viswanathan, P.C., et al. (2002). Allelic variants in long-QT disease genes in patients with drug-associated torsades de pointes. *Circulation, 105*(16), 1943-1948.

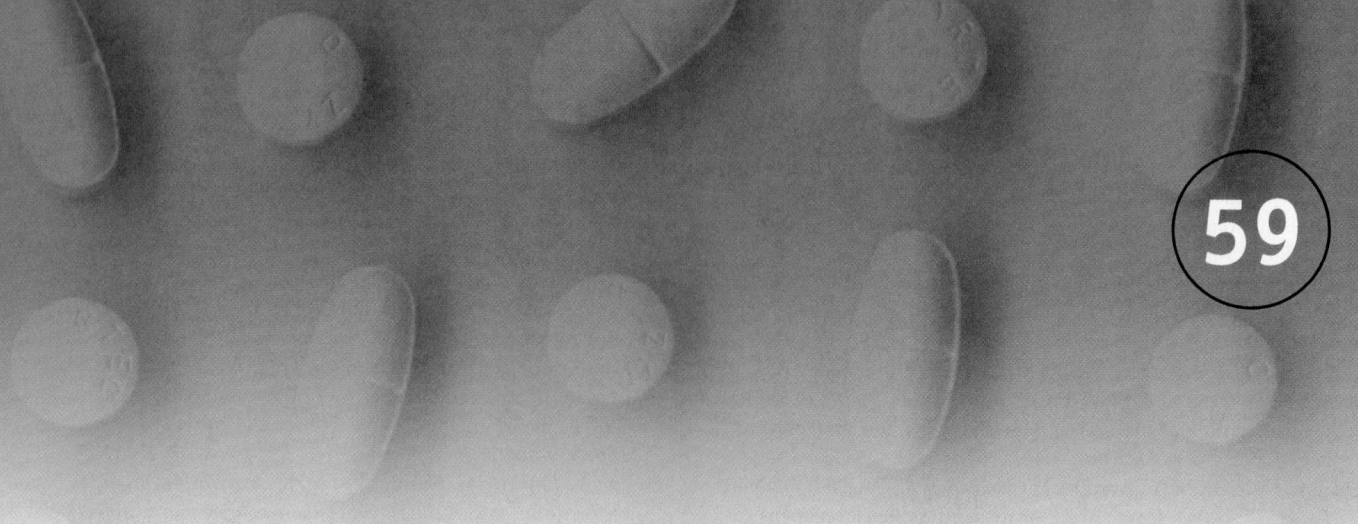

59

ANTIFUNGAL AND ANTIVIRAL DRUGS

CHAPTER FOCUS

All clients who are receiving broad-spectrum antibacterials for an infection, immunosuppressed as the result of a transplant or antineoplastic therapy, or with acquired immunodeficiency syndrome (AIDS) are at risk for the developing superinfection with fungal or viral organisms. The growth of the worldwide AIDS epidemic has fostered pharmaceutical research for agents to combat the diseases caused by these organisms. The nurse needs to remain current in the knowledge of antifungal and antiviral drugs.

LEARNING OBJECTIVES

- List four commonly used antifungal agents.
- Describe five adverse effects of antifungal agents.
- Implement the nursing management of clients receiving antifungal agents.
- Identify two reasons why effective antiviral drug therapy is more limited than antibacterial and antifungal therapy.
- List four commonly used systemic antiviral agents.
- Implement the nursing management of clients receiving antiviral therapy.

▲ KEY TERMS

candidiasis, p. 1055
chemoprophylactic, p. 1064
fungi, p. 1054
mycoses, p. 1054

✱▰ KEY DRUGS

acyclovir, p. 1067
amantadine, p. 1074
amphotericin B, p. 1055
delavirdine, p. 1086
enfuvirtide, p. 1089

fluconazole, p. 1058
saquinavir, p. 1088
zidovudine, p. 1081

Antifungal Therapy

✱ **What fungal pathogens are observed in human disease?**

Human infections with fungi can be caused by any of approximately 50 species of plantlike, parasitic microorganisms. These simple, parasitic plants lack chlorophyll; as a result, they are unable to make their own food and are dependent on other life forms. Infections with fungi, or mycoses, can range from mild and superficial to severe and life-threatening. Infecting organisms can be ingested orally, implanted under the skin after injury, or inhaled if the fungal spores are airborne. One species of fungi, *Candida albicans*, is usually part of the normal flora of the skin, mouth, intestines, and vagina; overgrowth and systemic infection may result from antibacterial, antineoplastic, and corticosteroid drug therapy. This is referred to as an opportunistic infection. Oral candidiasis (thrush) is common in newborn infants and immunocompromised clients. Its management with topical therapies was reviewed in Chapter 40. Vaginal candidiasis is common in women who are pregnant, have diabetes mellitus, or take hormonal contraceptives. Immunodeficiency greatly increases the likelihood of serious opportunistic mycoses. Nonopportunistic fungal infections such as blastomycosis, histoplasmosis, and others are usually rare.

✱ **T.K. is a 34-year-old female who recently underwent chemotherapy for breast cancer. She is neutropenic (absolute neutrophil count of 200), is febrile, and has not responded to a 2-day course of intravenous (IV) ceftazidime and vancomycin. The infectious disease service is contacted and is concerned that T.K. may have a systemic fungal infection.**

✱ **What are the risk factors for developing a systemic fungal infection?**
Among the most common risk factors for systemic fungal infection is an immunocompromised state. This can occur in clients who are neutropenic for various reasons, including receipt of bone marrow suppressing agents like cancer chemotherapy. Also at risk are clients receiving immunosuppressive agents to manage organ transplant or autoimmune disease; such drugs include methotrexate, cyclosporine, mycophenolate, etanercept, adalimumab, infliximab, and others. Clients with advanced human immunodeficiency virus (HIV) disease are also at a high risk for developing systemic fungal infections.

For clients with normal immune states, serious systemic fungal infections are uncommon. For such individuals, use of antibacterial agents may alter oral/pharyngeal or vaginal flora and predispose to localized yeast infections that are rarely life-threatening.

✱ **What agents are available to treat systemic fungal infections?**
The list of agents available to treat systemic fungal infections is relatively short. Many of the agents that have been studied for their antifungal properties are toxic to human cells. The two most frequently used categories of systemically administered antifungals are amphotericin B and the azole antifungals. Other agents with systemic activity include caspofungin and flucytosine. Griseofulvin, nystatin, and terbinafine are also used for specific fungal indications and are presented here as well. Table 59-1 compares systemically administered antifungals. Chapters 40 and 65 discuss topical antifungals that are used for superficial or localized fungal infections.

Amphotericin and Related Formulations

✱▣ **amphotericin B** [am foe **ter** i sin]
(Fungizone IV)
Amphotericin B has broad antifungal activity against many fungal pathogens, including *Aspergillus, Blastomyces dermatidis, Candida* species, *Cryptococcus* species, *Histoplasma capsulatum,* and *Zygomycetes*. It can be fungistatic or fungicidal depending on the concentrations achieved clinically. This drug does not have a therapeu-

tic effect on bacteria or viruses. Amphotericin B binds to sterols in the fungus cell membrane, which increases cell permeability and results in a loss of potassium and other elements from the cell. It is associated with significant toxicity and is therefore reserved for serious or life-threatening fungal infections.

Indications
Amphotericin B is effective for treating aspergillosis, blastomycosis, candidiasis (moniliasis), coccidioidomycosis, cryptococcosis, fungal endocarditis, histoplasmosis, cryptococcal meningitis, fungal septicemia, and many other systemic fungal infections.

Pharmacokinetics/Dosing
Administered parenterally, amphotericin B is widely distributed in the body. The initial half-life in adults is 24 hours, and the elimination half-life is approximately 15 days. The site of metabolism is unknown, but it is excreted by the kidneys. Approximately 40% of the drug is excreted over 7 days, but it can be detected in the urine for at least 7 weeks after it is discontinued. The adult dosage for a systemic fungus infection is usually a 1-mg test dose in 5% dextrose solution administered over 10 to 30 minutes. If tolerated, this is followed by a 0.25 to 1 mg/kg/day infusion (maximum per day of 1.5 mg/kg/day) given slowly over 2 to 6 hours depending on the infection and the client's tolerance of the medication. Often the daily dose is started at 0.25 mg/kg/day and increased to the full daily dose over a few days as tolerated (MICROMEDEX Healthcare Series, 2005). The initial pediatric dosage is 0.25 mg/kg/day in 5% dextrose administered over 6 hours. The dosage may be increased gradually (up to 1 mg/kg/day), depending on the infection and the child's tolerance of the medication.

Adverse Effects
Amphotericin B is associated with both infusion related reactions, and significant risk for renal injury. The common infusion related reactions include fever, hypotension, chills, and rigors. Concurrent use of ibuprofen or acetaminophen, diphenhydramine, meperidine, and/or hydrocortisone has been administered to reduce infusion-related reactions with various results.

Common and serious reactions with continued use include renal impairment, hypokalemia, and hypomagnesemia. Regular monitoring of renal function (creatinine and blood urea nitrogen [BUN]) and electrolytes is required with amphotericin B therapy. These risks are reduced when adequate hydration is maintained (often 1 L of normal saline is infused in advance of amphotericin B to reduce renal toxicity). Concurrent use of mannitol has not demonstrated benefit in reducing risk for nephrotoxicity of amphotericin therapy (Goldman & Koren, 2004). Use of alternate amphotericin formulations may reduce these renal toxicity risks (see the following section). Aggressive potassium and magnesium replacement is also required for a number of clients who receive ongoing amphotericin B therapy. Other adverse effects include headache, nausea, vomiting, phlebitis with IV infusion, hypo or hypertension, flushing, tachypnea, and hypersensitivity reactions.

amphotericin B cholesteryl sulfate complex [am foe **ter** i sin bee kole **les** te ril **sul** fate **kom** plecks]
(Amphotec)
amphotericin B deoxycholate [am foe **ter** i sin bee dee oxi **kole** ate]
(Amphocin)
amphotericin B lipid complex [am foe **ter** i sin bee **lip** id **kom** plecks]
(Abelcet)
amphotericin B liposomal [am foe **ter** i sin bee lye po **soe** mal]
(AmBisome)
Alternative formulations of amphotericin B are available that reduce the risk for nephrotoxicity. Amphotericin B cholesteryl sulfate complex (Amphotec) is a mixture of amphotericin and a cholesteryl sulfate. Amphotericin B deoxycholate (Amphocin) uses a different lipid-like complex (deoxycholate) to carry the active drug. Amphotericin B lipid complex injection (Abelcet) is a liposomal encapsula-

TABLE 59-1 COMPARISON OF SYSTEMIC ANTIFUNGALS

Agent	Typical Adult Dose	Comments
CONVENTIONAL AMPHOTERICIN B		
amphotericin B (Fungizone)	0.3-1 mg/kg IV daily	Significant risk for nephrotoxicity, potassium and magnesium wasting. Infusion reactions common
LIPOSOMAL AND RELATED FORMULATIONS OF AMPHOTERICIN B		
amphotericin B cholesteryl sulfate complex (Amphotec)	3-4 mg/kg IV daily	Dose and infusion rates differ from conventional amphotericin B
amphotericin B lipid complex (Abelcet)	5 mg/kg IV daily	Reduced risk for nephrotoxicity
amphotericin B liposomal (AmBisome)	3-5 mg/kg IV daily	Infusion and hypersensitivity reactions also possible
AZOLE ANTIFUNGALS		
fluconazole (Diflucan)	200 mg IV/PO × 1, then 100 mg IV daily	Generally better tolerated than amphotericin
itraconazole (Sporanox)	200 mg IV twice daily or 200 mg PO three times daily	Significant drug interaction potential
ketoconazole (Nizoral)	200-400 mg PO daily	Typically require dose adjustment for renal dysfunction
miconazole (Monistat IV)	400-1200 mg IV q8h	
voriconazole (Vfend)	6 mg/kg IV q12h × 2, then 4 mg/kg IV q12h	
MISCELLANEOUS SYSTEMIC ANTIFUNGALS		
caspofungin (Cancidas)	70 mg IV daily × 1, then 50 mg IV daily	Nephrotoxicity and hypokalemia, but less frequent than with amphotericin
flucytosine (Ancobon)	12.5-37.5 mg/kg PO q6h	Typically used in combination with other agents
ANTIFUNGALS WITH LIMITED INDICATIONS		
griseofulvin microsize (Grifulvin V)	500 mg PO daily	Use limited to dermal tineal infection and/or onychomycosis
griseofulvin ultramicrosize (Gris-PEG)	375 mg PO daily	Griseofulvin often better absorbed if dosed with fatty meal
terbinafine (Lamisil)	250 mg PO daily	
clotrimazole (Mycelex troche)	10 mg slowly dissolved in mouth five times daily	For oral candidiasis. Presented in Chapter 40
nystatin (Mycostatin, Nystatin)	400,000-600,000 units (4-6 mL suspension) swish and swallow four times daily	

tion of amphotericin. Amphotericin B liposomal (AmBisome) is a slightly different formulation with lipid/amphotericin layers. Each of these formulations is a considerably more expensive agent than conventional amphotericin B.

Indications

Each of these formulations is used to treat aspergillosis or other life-threatening fungal infections in clients who are refractory to or unable to tolerate standard amphotericin B therapy.

Pharmacokinetics/Dosing

The specific pharmacokinetic parameters of these agents vary, and they are not interchangeable. The dosage is different from conventional amphotericin B, and confusion about formulations could result in a potential medication error. The dose of Amphotec ranges from 3 to 4 mg/kg/day (up to 7 mg/kg/day) at a rate of 1 mg/kg/hour. Abelcet is usually dosed at 2.5 to 5 mg/kg/day while AmBisome is administered in doses ranging from 3 to 6 mg/kg/day.

Adverse Effects
These formulations provide a therapeutic effect with significantly less nephrotoxicity than amphotericin B. They do share infusion related adverse effects including fever, chills, nausea, hypotension, vomiting, dyspnea, and also may produce hypersensitivity reactions. As with conventional amphotericin, significant hypokalemia and hypomagnesemia are also frequently observed with these products. Concurrent use of ibuprofen, acetaminophen, diphenhydramine, meperidine, and/or hydrocortisone is also used with these formulations with variable results. Nephrotoxicity is also possible with these agents, but appears to be lower than with conventional amphotericin B.

✷ **After 48 hours, T.K.'s fever persists and the infectious disease team starts her on IV amphotericin B 0.25 mg/kg/day after a test dose of the drug caused no significant adverse effect.**

Assessment Amphotericin B is used with caution if renal function is impaired. Although it is not renally excreted, amphotericin B is nephrotoxic and can worsen any preexisting renal pathologic condition. It is also administered with caution if there is intolerance to the drug or if T.K. were receiving other nephrotoxic agents. If renal function is significantly impaired, use of one of the liposomal products might be considered. Care must always be taken to assure the correct dose of amphotericin or one of the liposomal-type amphotericin B agents. Dosages vary significantly with each product, and confusion about dosing may lead to a serious underdosage and lack of response or overdosage and renal injury.

Leukocyte transfusions should not be administered concurrently with amphotericin B lipid complex (Abelcet); acute pulmonary toxicity has been reported. Review T.K.'s current medication regimen for the risk of significant drug interactions, such as the following:

- Adrenocorticoids, glucocorticoids, mineralocorticoids (ACTH), and potassium-depleting diuretics may further worsen hypokalemia associated with amphotericin. If such agents are given concurrently, even more attention to frequent serum potassium determinations is warranted.
- Bone marrow depressants and radiation therapy may produce increased bone marrow depressant effects; monitor blood cell counts closely because dosage adjustments may be necessary if anemia, leukopenia, or thrombocytopenia become extreme.
- Amphotericin B–induced hypokalemia may increase the potential for digoxin toxicity; monitor closely for dysrhythmias, anorexia, nausea, vomiting, or other indications of possible toxicity.
- Nephrotoxic medications increase the risk of nephrotoxicity; monitor closely for edema and oliguria, because dosage adjustments may be necessary.

For a baseline, assess T.K.'s general health status including the status of her underlying infection, weight, blood urea nitrogen (BUN), serum creatinine concentrations, electrolyte levels (particularly potassium), and complete blood and platelet counts.

Nursing Diagnosis While T.K. is receiving amphotericin B, she is at risk for the following nursing diagnoses/collaborative problems: deficient fluid volume related to anorexia, nausea, and vomiting; activity intolerance related to anemia or hypokalemia; hyperthermia; ineffective protection related to leukopenia and thrombocytopenia; impaired tissue integrity related to extravasation or thrombophlebitis at the infusion site; disturbed sensory perception related to polyneuropathy (numbness, tingling, or burning in the hands and feet), hearing loss, or a change in vision; and the potential complications of infusion-related reaction (fever, chills, nausea, vomiting, headache, hypotension), seizures, electrolyte imbalances (hypokalemia, hypomagnesemia), hypersensitivity, cardiac dysrhythmias, and nephrotoxicity (increased or decreased urinary output).

Planning Following antifungal therapy, T.K. will be free of the signs and symptoms of infection. During antifungal therapy, she will:

- Experience minimal adverse effects of the drug therapy.
- Effectively manage the therapeutic regimen, including being compliant with medications, and implementing nonpharmacologic supportive measures.
- Collaborate with health care providers by appropriately reporting untoward symptoms and maintaining scheduled visits for monitoring and treatment.

Implementation
Monitoring If a test dose (1 mg over 20 to 30 minutes) is given, monitor vital signs every 30 minutes for at least 4 hours. Febrile reactions (fever, chills, headache, nausea, and vomiting) occur in the majority of clients, usually 1 to 2 hours after initiating the infusion and subside within 4 hours after the drug is discontinued.

BUN and serum creatinine values should be determined every other day as the dosage is increased to its optimal level and then weekly once the maintenance dosage is achieved and until the drug is discontinued. If BUN levels exceed 40 mg/dL or serum creatinine increases to 3 mg/dL, the dosage should be decreased or discontinued until renal function improves. Under such circumstances, one of the alternative liposomal-like products is often considered in place of conventional amphotericin, particularly if the infection is life-threatening and therapy must continue. With both conventional and liposomal-type amphotericin, serum potassium and magnesium levels should be monitored at least twice a week. Monitor blood counts at least weekly in anticipation of bone marrow suppression, which could be critical given T.K.'s preexisting neutropenia.

Pain at the site of infusion may indicate extravasation. Be cautious, because the drug causes local tissue irritation and thrombophlebitis. Assess T.K. for gastrointestinal (GI) disturbances such as anorexia, indigestion, nausea and vomiting, and diarrhea. Daily weight monitoring will determine if these symptoms are associated with weight loss. Monitor fluid intake and output ratios to determine fluid loss and renal status. Report oliguria, any unusual weight gain, or change in input and output (I&O) ratios or appearance of the urine (sediment, pink) to the physician; nephrotoxicity is usually reversible if identified early. Observe for signs of hypokalemia and hypomagnesemia (e.g., muscle cramps, irregular pulse, and weakness or lethargy). Monitor for symptoms of bone marrow suppression (fever, sore throat, and unusual bleeding or bruising), and report them to the prescriber.

Intervention Do not use amphotericin B if there is any evidence of precipitate or foreign matter in the vial. Before administering, read the package insert for the major points of safe delivery. Because of a variation in formulations, some will use in-line filters of different sizes, and others will not. Because amphotericin B is incompatible with a wide range of drugs, confirm its compatibility with other drugs before preparing the infusion. Wear gloves while preparing the drug. Because the reconstituted preparation of the lipid complex is a colloidal suspension, gently shake the hanging solution every half hour during administration to keep it in suspension.

Administering amphotericin B on alternate days and over a 6-hour period may reduce the incidence of adverse effects. If therapy is interrupted for more than 7 days, the dosage should be restarted at the lowest level and increased to the appropriate therapeutic level. The duration of the course of amphotericin B should be sufficient to prevent a relapse.

Febrile reactions during administration may be minimized by administering a small dose of IV corticosteroid just before the infusion of amphotericin B. Antipyretics and antihistamines are also used. Nephrotoxicity may be minimized by saline infusion just before the administration of amphotericin B. Heparin may be added to the IV infusion of amphotericin B to help prevent thrombophlebitis at the IV site. The infusion site should be changed with each dose to minimize the development of thrombophlebitis.

If T.K. has GI symptoms during the administration of amphotericin B, provide a pleasant and relaxed atmosphere for mealtimes; encourage small, frequent feedings of high-protein, high-calorie foods of her choice; and assist her to maintain good oral hygiene. Palliative medication may be necessary if T.K. experiences indigestion, vomiting, or diarrhea.

Education Instruct T.K. on appropriate oral hygiene, including the gentle use of soft toothbrushes and the avoidance of toothpicks. Advise her to alert the nursing staff at the first indication of pain at the IV site. Alert T.K. to the adverse effects of the drug and the need to report these promptly.

Evaluation The expected outcome of amphotericin B therapy is that T.K. will experience symptomatic improvement (e.g., decreased fever), with clinical and laboratory evidence of decreased fungal infection, and will experience no adverse effects of amphotericin B (e.g., fever, chills, vomiting, hypokalemia, hypomagnesemia). She will maintain her schedule for infusions for treatment, laboratory tests for monitoring, and will report adverse effects appropriately.

Azole Antifungals

The azole antifungals are better tolerated than amphotericin, but are less broad is spectrum than amphotericin B. They also possess significant interactions with other agents. Although they possess activity against *Histoplasma capsulatum, Cryptococcus species,* and many *Candida* species, they vary in active against *Aspergillus*, and are not active against *Zygomycetes* (mucor), and some *Candida* species. They may be fungistatic or fungicidal agents depending on the dosage and systemic levels achieved. Ergosterol is the primary sterol in fungus cell membranes. Azole antifungals affect the biosynthesis of the fungal sterols by interfering with the cytochrome P450 enzyme system. The result is impaired or depleted ergosterol biosynthesis that inhibits fungus growth.

Fluconazole and itraconazole have a greater affinity for fungal cytochrome P450 activity than for the human liver cytochrome P450 system. Fluconazole has good penetration in cerebrospinal fluid (CSF) and therefore is used for the treatment of cryptococcal meningitis; itraconazole has poor CSF penetration but is widely distributed in the body and is indicated for the treatment of aspergillosis, blastomycosis, and histoplasmosis.

Resistance to the azole antifungals has been noted, but therapeutic failures related to poor adherence, incorrect dosing, or other factors have also been reported (Stevens, 2004).

■ fluconazole [floo **con** a zole]
(Diflucan, Apo-Fluconazole✦)
Indications
Fluconazole is the most widely used of the azole antifungals. It is used to treat oral and vaginal candidiasis not responsive to topical nystatin or clotrimazole, for non–life-threatening *Candida* infections, treatment and prophylaxis of cryptococcal infections, and antifungal prophylaxis in bone marrow transplant recipients. They are also useful in the treatment of *H. capsulatum* and *Coccidioides immitis* infection.

Pharmacokinetics/Dosing
Fluconazole is well absorbed orally, distributes throughout the body including into the CSF and is primarily eliminated in the urine unchanged. The half-life of fluconazole is 24 to 30 hours for clients with normal renal function and can be dosed once daily. Fluconazole has been used in neonates, infants, children and adults. The usual adult dose depends on indication, but is in the range of 50 to 400 mg IV or orally once daily. Often a higher dose is administered on the first day of therapy and lower doses are administered for clients with renal insufficiency.

Adverse Effects
Fluconazole is well tolerated. Adverse effects include headache, GI upset, and diarrhea. Hepatotoxicity, including elevated liver function tests (ALT/AST) and more rarely hepatitis, cholestasis, jaundice and even hepatic failure have been reported. Hypersensitivity reactions and Stevens-Johnson syndrome are possible, and appear to be more frequently observed in clients with advanced HIV disease.

Drug Interactions

Fluconazole and the other azole antifungals are strong inhibitors of the cytochrome P450 enzyme systems, including 2 C19, 2 C8/9, and 3 A4. As such, toxicity may occur with a great number of drugs metabolized by these systems. Box 59-1 presents a partial listing of drugs that interact with the azole antifungals.

itraconazole [eye trah **con** a zole]

(Sporanox)

Indications

Oral itraconazole is used to treat superficial mycoses (including vaginal candidiasis), and systemic candidiasis, non–central nervous system (CNS) cryptococcal infections, and other fungal infections. IV itraconazole is used to treat blastomycosis, histoplasmosis, aspergillosis, and empiric treatment of febrile neutropenic fever.

Pharmacokinetics/Dosing

Oral absorption is dependent on the presence of gastric acid, although an oral solution currently available is reasonably well absorbed with reduced gastric acidity. Because of these differences in bioavailability, the oral capsule should be taken after meals whereas the oral solution is best taken on an empty stomach. It is widely distributed to many tissues, but penetration to the CSF is low. It is hepatically metabolized by cytochrome P450 3 A4 and eliminated primarily as metabolites. The typical adult dose depends on indication, and ranges from 100 mg once daily to 200 mg three times daily.

Adverse Effects

Adverse effects are similar to fluconazole. Heart failure has also been reported. Rash is more commonly reported with itraconazole.

Drug Interactions

See fluconazole and Box 59-1. Additionally, drugs that increase gastric pH (antacids, histamine-2 antagonists, proton pump inhibitors) can reduce systemic absorption of orally administered capsule form of itraconazole.

ketoconazole [kee toe **con** a zole]

(Nizoral, Apo-Ketoconazole✚)

Indications

Ketoconazole is also used to treat candidiasis, coccidiomycosis, and histoplasmosis.

Pharmacokinetics/Dosing

Ketoconazole is fairly well absorbed orally, but bioavailability is reduced with elevated gastric pH. (See Drug Interactions.) The oral adult dose is 200 to 400 mg daily. It is also available as a topical cream and shampoo.

Adverse Effects

Similar to fluconazole. Ketoconazole can cause gynecomastia and impotency because of the inhibition of adrenal steroid and testosterone synthesis, but these reactions are rare. Menstrual irregularities have also been reported.

Drug Interactions

See fluconazole and Box 59-1. Additionally, concurrent use of antacids, histamine 2 blockers (e.g., cimetidine, ranitidine, famotidine), or proton pump inhibitors (e.g., omeprazole) result in significantly reduced absorption of ketoconazole and potential therapeutic failures.

BOX 59-1 DRUG INTERACTIONS WITH AZOLE ANTIFUNGALS

Azole antifungals inhibit the cytochrome P450 enzyme systems and result in reduced metabolism of a number of other drugs metabolized by these enzymes. Drugs most affected are agents metabolized by cytochrome P450 2 C8/9, 2 C19, 3 A4 and 1 A2. The following list of drugs represents some (although not all) drugs that may have impaired metabolism (and therefore potential risk of toxicity) when administered with the azole antifungals:

alfentanil	cisapride	glyburide	omeprazole	simvastatin
almotriptan	cyclosporine	griseofulvin	oxcarbazepine	sirolimus
alprazolam	digoxin	imatinib	paclitaxel	sufentanil
amiodarone	diltiazem	indinavir	phenobarbital	tacrolimus
amlodipine	disopyramide	lansoprazole	phenytoin	tadalafil
amprenavir	docetaxel	lopinavir	pimozide	theophylline
aripiprazole	dofetilide	lovastatin	pioglitazone	tinidazole
atorvastatin	eletriptan	metformin	prednisone	tolterodine
bepridil	eplerenone	methadone	propafenone	trazodone
bortezomib	ergotamine	methylprednisolone	quetiapine	triazolam
bosentan	estrogen	midazolam	quinidine	vardenafil
bromocriptine	ethosuximide	mifepristone	ranitidine	verapamil
budesonide	fentanyl	modafinil	repaglinide	vinblastine
buprenorphine	fluticasone	nateglinide	rifabutin	vincristine
buspirone	fluvastatin	nefazodone	rifampin	warfarin
carbamazepine	fosamprenavir	nelfinavir	ritonavir	ziprasidone
celecoxib	gefitinib	nevirapine	saquinavir	zonisamide
cimetidine	glipizide	nifedipine	sildenafil	

Management of interactions with azoles includes avoiding concurrent use, or dosage adjustment of the affected drug. Consult package inserts for detailed management strategies.

miconazole [my **con** a zole] injection
(Monistat IV, Micozole✿, Monistat✿)

Indications
IV miconazole is primarily indicated for the treatment of disseminated and chronic mucocutaneous candidiasis.

Pharmacokinetics/Dosing
Adult dosing is 400 to 1200 mg IV every 8 hours.

Adverse Effects
See fluconazole. Miconazole may cause phlebitis at the injection site; nausea, vomiting, and cardiorespiratory arrest have been reported with an injection that is too rapid.

Drug Interactions
See fluconazole and Box 59-1.

voriconazole [vor i **con** a zole]
(Vfend)

Indications
Voriconazole is indicated for invasive aspergillosis, and other serious fungal infections for clients intolerant to other therapy.

Pharmacokinetics/Dosing
Voriconazole is well absorbed orally and is metabolized by the cytochrome P450 enzymes 2 C19 and others. It has a variable elimination half-life. In adults, it is dosed at 3 to 6 mg/kg IV (200 to 400 mg PO) every 12 hours with specific dosing based on indication, tolerability, and drug interactions. Refer to package insert for more data.

Adverse Effects
Adverse effects are similar to other azole antifungals. Additionally, voriconazole has been associated with prolongation of QT intervals on ECG and may increase the risk for cardiac dysrhythmias. This risk may be greater when administered with other drugs that affect the metabolism of voriconazole.

Drug Interactions
See fluconazole and Box 59-1.

✪ **After receiving amphotericin for 2 weeks, clinical improvement of T.K.'s condition is subjectively and objectively documented. To facilitate returning to her home, the physician changes her antifungal regimen to itraconazole 200 mg orally three times daily for 3 days and then 200 mg twice daily for at least 3 months.**

✪ **What are the nursing management issues with the use of systemic azole antifungals for T.K.?**
Because fungi are plant-like parasitic organisms, high chemical concentrations of antifungal drugs are required. Therefore there are limited systemic forms available and their administration requires careful monitoring.

Assessment T.K. will be receiving an azole antifungal, itraconazole. It was probably selected for T.K. because, unlike fluconazole and other azole antifungals, it has a broader spectrum of activity for non-CNS fungal infections, including coverage for *Aspergillus*. It also is less toxic than amphotericin B. Hypersensitivity to itraconazole or other azole antifungal agents would be a contraindication for use of the drug. Assess T.K. for heart failure (HF) or ventricular dysfunction because itraconazole has negative inotropic effects and poses a risk for edema and worsening HF. Clients with achlorhydria or hypochlorhydria, which is common with AIDS, may experience a reduced absorption of these drugs.

Use azole antifungals (especially ketoconazole) cautiously if T.K. has hepatic function impairment (including late stage ethanol abuse), because there may be a higher risk for drug-induced hepatotoxicity. Although there are no renal impairment precautions with itraconazole, there is with fluconazole and its doses may need to be decreased or the dosage interval increased.

Review T.K.'s current medication regimen for the risk of significant drug interactions. Refer back to Box 59-1 for a listing of drugs that interact with the azole antifungals.

For baseline, assess T.K.'s general health status including symptoms of the underlying infection, weight, and liver function tests. Ensure that serum potassium levels are within normal limits as hypokalemia in clients taking itraconazole has resulted in ventricular fibrillation. Appropriate specimens should be taken to identify the causative fungi before initiating therapy. BUN and serum creatinine values are important for clients taking fluconazole, another azole antifungal. Obtain appropriate specimens before initiating therapy to identify the causative fungi when indicated.

Nursing Diagnosis While receiving an azole antifungal agent, T.K. is at risk for the following nursing diagnoses/collaborative problems: impaired tissue integrity because of IV administration (phlebitis); impaired comfort related to the central nervous system (CNS) effects of the drug (headache, dizziness, photophobia); deficient fluid volume related to anorexia, nausea, or vomiting; sexual dysfunction (menstrual irregularities [for male clients, gynecomastia, or impotence]) related to the inhibition of testosterone and adrenal steroid synthesis and the potential complications of photosensitivity, anemia, agranulocytosis, thrombocytopenia, hypersensitivity (fever, chills, skin rash, and itching), Stevens-Johnson syndrome (blistering or peeling of skin), and hepatotoxicity.

Planning Goals for T.K.'s azole antifungal therapy are the same as they were for her amphotericin B antifungal therapy.

Implementation

Monitoring Monitor the infection for improvement, because the dosage and length of treatment are determined by this and by T.K.'s general response to therapy. Her treatment may continue for weeks or months until she has clinically improved and her laboratory tests indicate that active fungal infection has subsided. Assess T.K. for GI disturbances such as anorexia, indigestion, nausea and vomiting, and diarrhea. Daily weights will determine if these symptoms are associated with weight loss. Monitor fluid intake and output ratios to determine fluid loss and renal status. T.K. requires periodic serum potassium determinations because hypokalemia may result in ventricular fibrillation. Liver function studies need to be monitored; although a mild, transient increase in transaminases may occur with therapy, it may, on rare occasion, progress to hepatotoxicity. Observe T.K. for anorexia, dark urine, jaundice, and right upper quadrant abdominal pain.

Intervention T.K.'s dosage form is capsular; however, the oral capsules and oral solution cannot be used interchangeably because of differences in bioavailability. Administer itraconazole capsules with food to increase absorption; itraconazole solution is to be taken on an empty stomach for the same reason. If T.K. were receiving IV itraconazole, it would be prepared by adding the dose to the 50 mL bag of normal saline (NS) provided, infusing over an hour using a flow control device and the infusion set provided. When the infusion is complete, flush the set with 15 to 20 mL of NS over 5 to 15 minutes, and then discard the entire infusion set. If T.K. were receiving itraconazole for oropharyngeal or esophageal candidiasis, the solution is to be swished vigorously in the mouth, and then swallowed.

Education Instruct T.K. to take itraconazole capsules with meals or food to minimize nausea and enhance absorption. Avoid the concurrent use of alcohol as it may result in hepatotoxicity. Advise T.K. to avoid exposure to bright light and to wear sunglasses because of the photophobic effects of the drug. Because itraconazole causes drowsiness, caution her to avoid activities that require mental alertness until her response has been determined. Instruct T.K. to report any symptoms of anorexia, nausea, vomiting, dark urine, abdominal tenderness, yellow skin or eyes, and any blistering or peeling of skin. Advise T.K. to complete the full course of medication even if she is feeling better, to maintain regular visits with the prescriber for monitoring, and to be alert for significant adverse effects to report to the provider. Taking the drug at the same time every day increases compliance.

Evaluation The expected outcome of azole antifungal therapy is that T.K. will experience symptomatic improvement (e.g., normal body temperature), with clinical and laboratory evidence of decreased fungal infection and without experiencing any adverse effects of itraconazole (e.g., headache, GI upset, diarrhea, hepatotoxicity).

Other Systemic Antifungals

Caspofungin and flucytosine are occasionally used to treat certain systemic fungal infections in addition to or in place of azole antifungal or amphotericin. Caspofungin inhibits synthesis of an essential component of the growing cell wall of fungi and is generally well-tolerated. Flucytosine enters fungus cells, in which it is converted to the antimetabolite fluorouracil. Flucytosine interferes with the metabolism of pyrimidine, thus preventing the synthesis of nucleic acids and protein. Because flucytosine is not converted to fluorouracil in humans, it possesses selective toxicity against susceptible strains of fungi and is not particularly toxic to the host.

caspofungin [kas poe **fung** in]
(Cancidas)
Indications
Caspofungin is used to treat invasive *Aspergillus* infection and *Candida* infections.

Pharmacokinetics/Dosing
Caspofungin is administered IV and is slowly metabolized. Its elimination half-life is 40 to 50 hours. It is typically dosed in adults at 50 to 70 mg daily. Dosage in hepatic dysfunction is often reduced.
Adverse Effects
Among the most serious adverse effects of caspofungin are nephrotoxicity and hypokalemia. Other adverse effects include headache, flushing, facial edema, fever, chills, reduced hemoglobin, hypertension, and elevated liver enzymes.
Drug Interactions
Levels of caspofungin may be increased by concurrent cyclosporine use, and decreased with use of enzyme-inducing agents (e.g., rifampin, carbamazepine, efavirenz, nevirapine, and phenytoin).

flucytosine [floo **sye** toe seen]
(Ancobon)
Indications
Flucytosine is indicated for the treatment of fungal endocarditis caused by *Candida* species, fungal meningitis caused by *Cryptococcus* species, and fungal pneumonia, septicemia, or urinary infections caused by *Candida* or *Cryptococcus* species. It is most often used in combination with other antifungal agents.
Pharmacokinetics/Dosing
Flucytosine is well absorbed orally and widely distributed in the body, including the CSF, with CSF levels reaching 60% to 90% of serum concentrations. Flucytosine has a half-life of 2.5 to 6 hours, is not significantly metabolized, and is excreted by the kidneys, mostly as unchanged drug. The adult and pediatric oral dosage is 12.5 to 37.5 mg/kg every 6 hours.
Adverse Effects
The common adverse effects of flucytosine include gastric distress, anemia, hepatitis, hypersensitivity, and bone marrow suppression.
Nursing Management
The nursing considerations are similar to those for the azole antifungals. However, the serum level of flucytosine may be measured to ascertain whether it is being maintained in the therapeutic range (25 to 120 mg/mL). Serum concentrations are also used to assess renal excretion and prevent drug accumulation in clients with renal function impairment.

Antifungals with Limited Indications

A few systemically or regionally administered antifungal agents are available for limited use in the treatment of nailbed or localized fungal infections. Griseofulvin is an oral fungistatic agent that inhibits fungus cell mitosis during metaphase. It is also deposited in the keratin precursor cells in the skin, hair, and nails, thus inhibiting fungal invasion of the keratin. When infested keratin is shed, healthy keratin replaces it. Orally administered terbinafine interferes with the biosynthesis of fungal ergosterol, which interferes with cell wall synthesis and results the death of fungal cells, and is also used for nailbed infections. Applied locally to cutaneous or mucocutaneous tissue, nystatin and clotrimazole adhere to sterols in the fungal cell membrane, altering cell membrane permeability and resulting in the loss of essential intercellular contents. Chapter 40 presents these agents in the context of treating oral candidiasis.

griseofulvin microsize [gri see oh **ful** vin]
(Grisactin, Grifulvin V, Fulvicin-U/F, Grisovin-FP)
griseofulvin tablets, ultramicrosize
(Fulvicin P/G)

Indications

Griseofulvin is indicated for the treatment of susceptible organisms for onychomycosis (nail fungal infection). It is also used for tinea capitis (ringworm of the scalp), tinea corporis (body ringworm), tinea cruris (groin ringworm or "jock itch"), and tinea pedis (ringworm of the feet, "athlete's foot") not responsive to topical therapy. Griseofulvin is not indicated for severe or life-threatening fungal infections.

Pharmacokinetics/Dosing

The oral absorption of microsize griseofulvin varies from 25% to 70% of the oral dose, whereas the ultramicrosize form is nearly completely absorbed. Absorption is significantly enhanced if griseofulvin is administered with or after a fatty meal. Griseofulvin is distributed in keratin layers in the skin, hair, and nails; very little is distributed in body tissues and fluids. It has a half-life of 24 hours and reaches peak serum levels in approximately 4 hours. This drug is metabolized in the liver and excreted primarily unchanged in the feces. The oral adult dosage of microsize griseofulvin is 500 mg daily; the dose may be divided in 2 doses. To treat tinea pedis or onychomycosis, the dosage is 500 mg twice daily. The pediatric dosage is 5 mg/kg every 12 hours (*USP DI*, 2005). The adult dosage for ultramicrosize is 250 to 375 mg daily.

Adverse Effects

The most commonly reported adverse effect of griseofulvin is headache; less commonly noted is hypersensitivity, confusion, gastric distress, oral thrush, weakness, and photosensitivity.

Nursing Management

Assessment

Administer griseofulvin with caution if a client has preexisting porphyria, lupus erythematosus, hepatic function impairment, or sensitivity to griseofulvin. Review the client's current medication regimen for the risk of significant drug interactions, especially when griseofulvin is given concurrently with the following drugs: anticoagulants (decreased anticoagulant effect may be noted; monitor prothrombin [PT])/international normalized ratio [INR] closely) and oral estrogen-containing contraceptives (decreased effectiveness of contraceptive; use alternative method of contraception when taking griseofulvin).

To establish a baseline, assess the client's underlying condition for which the griseofulvin is prescribed, a mental status examination, a complete blood count (CBC), serum creatinine concentration, urinalysis, and hepatic function studies.

Nursing Diagnosis

While the client is receiving griseofulvin, assess for the following nursing diagnoses/collaborative problems: impaired comfort (headache, nausea, abdominal cramping); fatigue; risk for injury related to dizziness; impaired oral mucous membrane related to oral thrush; disturbed sleep pattern (insomnia) related to CNS effects; disturbed sensory perception related to peripheral neuritis (numbness and tingling of the hands and feet); disturbed thought processes (confusion) related to CNS effects; and the potential complications of hypersensitivity, photosensitivity, leukopenia, agranulocytopenia, or the development of hepatitis (jaundiced skin and sclera).

Planning

As for antifungals discussed above.

Implementation

Monitoring

Monitor blood counts and hepatic and renal function studies periodically during therapy. Therapy is continued until clinical signs or laboratory confirmation indicates that the causative organism has been eradicated.

Intervention

Administer griseofulvin with meals to help prevent GI distress and to enhance absorption. Therapy is even more effective if the meal is fatty. Consult the prescriber if the client is on a low-fat diet. The concurrent use of an appropriate topical agent maximizes the therapeutic effect of griseofulvin and reduces the possibility of relapse tinea pedis.

Education

Encourage the client to comply with the full course of therapy, even if feeling better. Regular visits to the prescriber are necessary to check progress. Advise the client that the treatment period is lengthy: 8 to 10 weeks for tinea capitis, 2 to 4 weeks for tinea corporis, and 4 to 8 weeks for tinea pedis. For onychomycosis, the treatment is at least 4 months for fingernails and at least 6 months for toenails. Even with treatment, the recurrence rate is very high for onychomycosis of the toenails.

Frequent shampoos and clipping of the hair and nails, and keeping affected skin areas clean and dry, will support the therapeutic effect of griseofulvin. Advise the client that skin may be more sensitive to sunlight; recommend that the client use sunscreen and avoid direct sunlight.

Advise the client to report any symptoms of fever and sore throat to the prescriber; such symptoms may indicate blood dyscrasias. Because the drug may cause dizziness, the client should avoid tasks that require mental alertness until the response to the drug can be ascertained. Instruct the client about good oral hygiene and to report any soreness or irritation of the mouth, which might indicate a fungal overgrowth (oral thrush). Advise the client not to ingest alcoholic beverages while taking griseofulvin, because it may potentiate the effects of alcohol, causing tachycardia and flushing.

Evaluation

The expected outcome of griseofulvin therapy is that the client will experience symptomatic improvement without evidence of any adverse effects of the drug.

terbinafine [ter **bin** a feen]
(Lamisil)

Indications

Oral terbinafine is an antifungal agent indicated for the treatment of onychomycosis. Topical and oral terbinafine are used to treat tinea capitis, tinea corporis, tinea cruris, and tinea pedis.

Pharmacokinetics/Dosing

Orally administered terbinafine is well absorbed in the GI tract and has an elimination half-life (plasma) of 11 to 17 hours. In sebum and stratum corneum, the elimination half-life is 3 to 5 days. It reaches a peak serum level in 2 hours and a steady state in 10 days to 2 weeks. It is metabolized in the liver and excreted primarily by the kidneys. The usual dosage for adolescents and adults is 125 mg PO twice daily (or 250 mg daily). The course of therapy is 6 weeks to 3 months for onychomycosis, 4 to 6 weeks for tinea capitis, 2 to 4 weeks for tinea corporis and tinea cruris, and 2 to 6 weeks for tinea pedis. Chapter 65 discusses topical terbinafine.

Adverse Effects

Elevated liver function tests and lymphocytopenia are not uncommon with systemic terbinafine therapy, but fortunately, serious hepatic injury (including hepatic failure) and bone marrow suppression are rare. Stevens-Johnson syndrome and toxic epidermal necrolysis are rare, but very serious complications of terbinafine therapy. Other adverse effects of terbinafine include anorexia, skin rash, gastric distress (nausea, vomiting, pain, diarrhea) and taste alterations.

Nursing Management

The nursing considerations are similar to griseofulvin.

Antiviral Therapy

⊛ **What viral diseases are considered treatable with drugs?**

A number of conditions are related to viral infection. Viruses play a clear role in a number of inflammatory states, including hepatitis, encephalitis and meningitis. Viral agents, including smallpox and viral hemorrhagic fever, may also be involved in a terrorist attack (see the Pharmacologic Issues in an Age of Terrorism box on pp. 1063 and 1064). Many

Pharmacologic Issues in an Age of Terrorism

Viral Agents

According to the Centers for Disease Control and Prevention (CDC), among the highest risk viral agents for bioterrorism are smallpox and viral hemorrhagic fever (VHF). They are classified as Category A agents by the CDC. A description of the CDC risk categories for bioterrorism agents is discussed in the Pharmacologic Issues in an Age of Terrorism: Bacterial Agents and Related Toxins box in Chapter 58.

Smallpox (variola major smallpox virus)

Smallpox is highly contagious and is caused by the poxvirus, variola major or variola minor. Its use in bioterrorism dates back to the French and Indian War in the eighteenth century when Sir Jeffrey Amherst knowingly gave smallpox-infected blankets to Native Americans. It has also been studied or used as a potential weapon since that time.

Vaccine development against smallpox was begun by Edward Jenner in the late eighteenth century. A worldwide vaccination program was implemented by the World Health Organization (WHO) in 1966. By 1980, WHO declared smallpox eradication efforts completed. Unfortunately, smallpox has been produced in very large quantities by some countries to be used as a potential weapon of mass destruction.

Smallpox is primarily transmitted by direct contact with infected bodily fluids or infected bedding or clothing. Transmission by prolonged close contact or airborne routes is less likely, but may occur in enclosed settings. Infected individuals are most contagious when the rash is present and remains contagious until all scabs have been shed. Humans are the only natural hosts, and it is not transmitted by animals or insects.

Presentation

Smallpox infection classically presents with an asymptomatic incubation period, a prodromal phase, an early rash, a pustular rash period, pustular scab period, and finally a resolving scab phase. It is sometimes mistaken for varicella (chickenpox).

Incubation

The incubation period for smallpox is between 7 and 17 days. Smallpox is not contagious during this incubation period.

Prodromal Phase

The prodromal phase is then observed for 2 to 4 days in which fever, malaise, headache, body ache, and high fever are noted.

Early Rash

Small red spots containing the virus on the tongue and mouth soon break open and pose the greatest risk for transmission to others. Distribution of rash for smallpox differs from varicella (chickenpox). Smallpox lesions typically start on the face and spread primarily to limbs over 24 hours. Unlike varicella, fewer lesions are noted on the trunk (see figure). Fever begins to decline at this time and individuals begin to feel more comfort-

able. By day 3 or 4 of this phase, the rash is raised and filled with a thick, opaque fluid with a central depression resembling a bellybutton. Fever may rise again until scabs form.

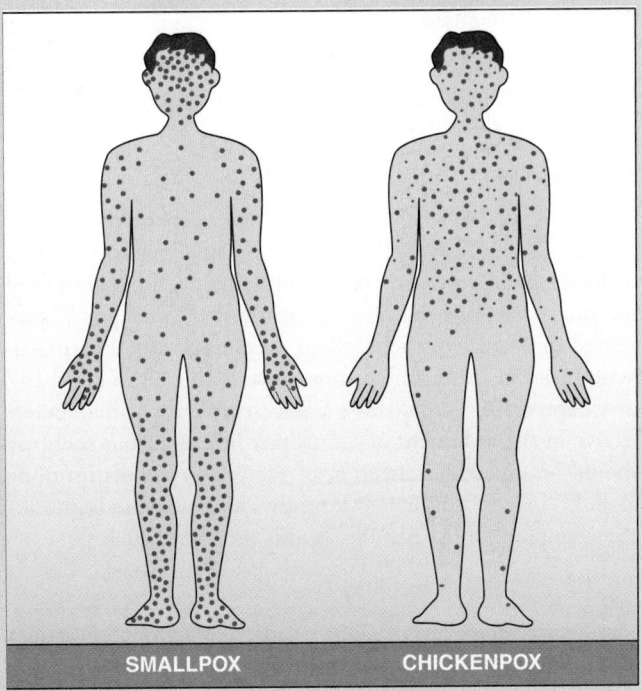

SMALLPOX   CHICKENPOX

Pustular Rash

The rash becomes pustular (see figure). Each pustule becomes hard and is often described as a BB pellet. This phase may persist for up to 5 days. Although not as contagious as in the early rash state, smallpox is still contagious at this state.

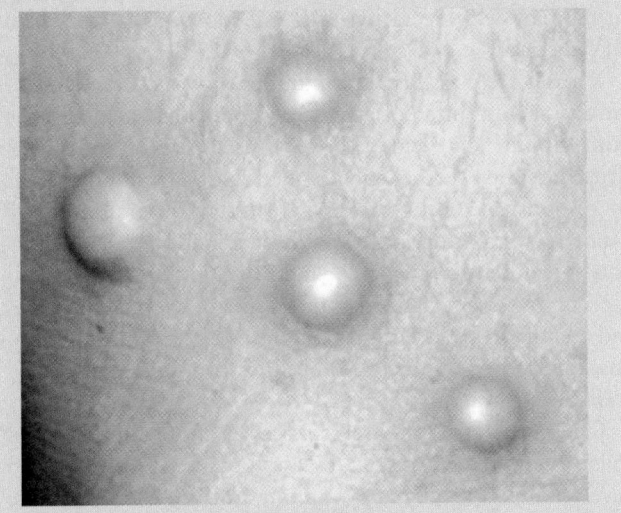

Data from Emergency Preparedness and Response: Center for Disease Control. Retrieved March 6, 2005, from http://www.bt.cdc.gov.

Continued

Pharmacologic Issues in an Age of Terrorism—cont'd

Viral Agents—cont'd

Pustular/Scab Phase

Scabs begin to form over pustules. This phase may persist for 5 to 7 days. The client remains contagious.

Resolving Scab Phase

Scabs eventually fall off within 3 weeks of developing the rash. Pitted scars remain after scabs fall off. The client remains contagious until all scabs have fallen off.

Management

Mortality rates vary from 30% to 100% depending on viral subtype. No definitive treatment is available. Supportive care, including fluid, fever, and pain management, and treatment of secondary bacterial infection are warranted. Smallpox is prevented by the use of the smallpox vaccine (see the Pharmacologic Issues in an Age of Terrorism box on pp. 1146 and 1147 in Chapter 62). Some data suggest that cidofovir may be effective in the treatment of a smallpox infection, but such use should be under the direction of the CDC. Variola immune globulin may be considered for individuals who are immunocompromised, but availability of this product is limited.

Viral Hemorrhagic Fever

Viral hemorrhagic fever (VHF) is caused by a group of distinct RNA viruses, which produce life-threatening multisystem disease. In most cases, these agents produce vascular injury and often are accompanied by hemorrhage. A number of viral pathogens cause VHF, including Ebola, Marburg, Junin, Lassa, Hanta, yellow fever, and Argentine hemorrhagic fever. Natural reservoirs for most of these pathogens are rodents, and arthropods serve as vectors. Transmission to humans is initially by contact with the infected animal or the result of an insect bite. In some cases, direct person to person transmission occurs, and in such cases, very strict public health measures must be enforced to contain the threat.

Presentation

The incubation period for most VHF pathogens is between 3 and 16 days. Signs and symptoms of VHF vary with different pathogens, but most often include fever, dizziness, fatigue, muscle ache, and loss of strength. In severe cases, internal hemorrhage, massive cutaneous ecchymosis, or spontaneous bleeding from the mouth, eyes, or ears may be noted. These bleeding episodes are quite frightening but are often not fatal. Mortality rates vary with agent, and are most commonly due to shock, neurotoxicity, or organ failure. Altered mental status, including delirium, seizures, and coma are also noted.

Management

Management of VHF primarily involves supportive care for those infected, and institution of public health measures to contain the disease. Ribavirin has some efficacy in treating Lassa infection, but cannot routinely be recommended for treating other forms of VHF. Vaccines have been developed for yellow fever and Argentine hemorrhagic fever (see the Pharmacologic Issues in an Age of Terrorism box on pp. 1146 and 1147 in Chapter 62).

---

viruses have also been linked with cancers (e.g., human papillomavirus and cervical cancer). Host defense mechanisms may be affected by virus infections, as is seen with HIV disease.

Viruses are classified in a number of ways. One classification scheme differentiates deoxyribonucleic acid (DNA) from ribonucleic acid (RNA) viruses. DNA and RNA viruses are then further subclassified. Not all viral infections are responsive to drug therapy. Treatment of viral infection is not as straightforward as with bacterial or fungal infection. Treatment strategies include prevention (e.g., avoidance of risk, vaccination), prevention of viral replication, and treatment to assist host response (e.g., immunoglobulins, interferons). Table 59-2 outlines common viruses and available treatment strategies.

Chemotherapy for viral diseases is more limited than chemotherapy for bacterial diseases because it is difficult to develop and clinically apply antiviral drugs. Most antiviral agents work by inhibiting viral replication. In many viral infections, virus replication in the body reaches its peak before any clinical symptoms appear. The multiplication of the virus is ending by the time signs and symptoms of illness appear, and the subsequent course of the illness has been determined. Thus, to be clinically effective in many viral conditions, antiviral drugs must be administered in a chemoprophylactic manner as preventive agents before disease appears or early in the disease process.

A second factor limiting the development of antiviral drugs is that viruses are true parasites; they replicate within the mammalian cell and use the enzyme systems of the host cells. Drugs that would inhibit virus replication would also disturb the host cells and may therefore be toxic.

⬡ **P.K. is an 18-year-old high school senior who reports to his health care provider with upper respiratory congestion, runny nose, and moderately sore throat. He is requesting an "antibiotic" to treat his symptoms. His nurse practitioner assesses his condition, which is consistent with a viral upper respiratory infection (a common cold).**

Many clients seek medical attention and drug therapy for viral conditions. Pharmacotherapy, when indicated, is based on the specific viral pathogen. The herpes-related viruses are treated with a number of agents, including acyclovir (Zovirax), famciclovir (Famvir), valacyclovir (Valtrex), penciclovir (Denavir), foscarnet (Foscavir), cidofovir (Vistide), ganciclovir (Cytovene), and valganciclovir (Valcyte). Agents with activity against the hepatitis B or C include adefovir (Hep-

TABLE 59-2 CLASSIFICATIONS OF COMMON VIRUSES AND TREATMENT STRATEGIES

Virus Class	Examples	Prophylaxis	Treatment
adenoviruses	Common cold	zinc, *Echinacea**	zinc
hepadnaviruses— hepatitis B	Acute and chronic hepatitis B	hepatitis B immune globulin, hepatitis B vaccine	interferons, lamivudine, adefovir
herpes viruses	Herpes simplex (HSV type 1 & 2) Herpes zoster (type 3)		ganciclovir, cidofovir, foscarnet, valganciclovir
	Epstein-Barr (type 4)		
	Cytomegalovirus (CMV) (type 5)		acyclovir, famciclovir, valacyclovir, foscarnet
coronaviruses	Upper respiratory tract infections, common cold	zinc, *Echinacea**	zinc
flaviviruses	Acute and chronic hepatitis C		ribavirin, interferons
myxoviruses	Influenza A	influenza vaccine, amantadine, rimantadine, oseltamivir, zanamivir	oseltamivir, zanamivir
	Influenza B	influenza vaccine, oseltamivir, zanamivir	amantadine, oseltamivir, rimantadine, zanamivir
paramyxoviruses	Measles, mumps	MMR vaccine	
	Respiratory syncytial virus	palivizumab	ribavirin
picornaviruses	Acute hepatitis A	immunoglobulin, hepatitis A vaccine	
	Polio	polio vaccine	
	Rhinoviruses Common cold	zinc, *Echinacea**	zinc
retroviruses	HIV	*Postexposure*: nucleosides, non-nucleosides, protease inhibitors	nucleosides, nonnucleosides, protease inhibitors, fusion inhibitors

Modified from Holt, C.D. (2005). Viral hepatitis. In M.A. Koda-Kimble, L.Y. Young, W.A. Kradjan, B.J. Guglielmo, B.K. Alldredge, & R.L. Corelli (Eds.), *Applied therapeutics: The clinical use of drugs* (8th ed.). Philadelphia: Lippincott Williams & Wilkins; and Nahata, M.C., O'Mara, N.B., & Benavides, S. (2005). Viral infections. In M.A. Koda-Kimble, L.Y. Young, W.A. Kradjan, B.J. Guglielmo, B.K. Alldredge, & R.L. Corelli (Eds.), *Applied therapeutics: The clinical use of drugs* (8th ed.). Philadelphia: Lippincott Williams & Wilkins.
*The role of *Echinacea* for prophylaxis is controversial (Caruso & Gwaltney, 2005).

sera), ribavirin (Copegus, Virazole), and the interferons (see Chapter 63). Drugs used to prevent or treat influenzae infections include amantadine (Symmetrel), rimantadine (Flumadine), oseltamivir (Tamiflu), and zanamivir (Relenza). Zinc supplements are also frequently used to treat the common cold with varying effects. These drugs have specific roles in treating particular viral infections, although occasionally agents effective against one virus group are helpful in treating a different pathogen. Table 59-3 compares these drugs. Other strategies to prevent or manage viral disease in individuals and populations include vaccines, immunomodulators and immunoglobulin therapy; Chapters 62 and 63 discuss these agents in greater detail.

For the sake of clarity, we will consider the antiretroviral agents for HIV disease separately. The agents effective for HIV are rarely indicated for other viral infections, although there are exceptions (e.g., lamivudine for hepatitis B infection). Four antiretroviral classes are available for managing HIV infection and include the nucleoside reverse transcriptase inhibitors, the nonnucleoside reverse transcriptase inhibitors, the protease inhibitors and fusion inhibitors. Since the advent of highly active antiretroviral therapy (HAART) in the mid-1990s, mortality rates related to HIV declined by 42% between 1996 and 1997, and 15% further between 1998 and 2000 (Centers for Disease Control & Prevention [CDC], 2004). Although treatment is more successful in recent years, ongoing research on alternative modalities, including vaccines to prevent or treat HIV disease have been disappointing.

TABLE 59-3 COMPARISON OF ANTIVIRALS (NON-HIV)

Agent	Typical Systemic Adult Dose	Comments
ANTI-HERPES AGENTS		
acyclovir (Zovirax)	400 mg PO three times daily* 5-10 mg/kg IV q8h*	Indicated for herpes infections Risk for renal toxicity with high dose reduced with adequate hydration.
famciclovir (Famvir)	125-500 mg PO q12h*	
valacyclovir (Valtrex)	500-1000 mg PO q8-12h*	
ANTI-CMV AGENTS		
cidofovir (Vistide)	5 mg/kg IV once weekly × 2 weeks, then 5 mg/kg IV every 2 weeks	Significant toxicity, including renal, CNS, bone marrow, hepatic. Oral probenecid is frequently administered concurrently. Contraindicated in renal dysfunction.
foscarnet (Foscavir)	90-120 mg/kg IV daily	May also be used for acyclovir resistant herpes infection. Significant toxicity includes renal, CNS, and bone marrow. Dose reduction required for renal dysfunction.
ganciclovir (Cytovene)	5 mg/kg IV q12h × 7-14 days, then 5 mg/kg q24h Prophylaxis: 1000 mg PO three times daily	Significant toxicity includes CNS effects and bone marrow suppression. Implant form available for CMV retinitis. Dose reduction required for renal dysfunction.
valganciclovir (Valcyte)	900 mg PO twice daily × 21 days, then 900 mg PO daily	Absorption best if taken with food. Same toxicity risks as ganciclovir. Dose reduction required for renal dysfunction.
ANTI-HEPATITIS AGENTS		
adefovir (Hepsera)	10 mg PO daily	Treatment for chronic hepatitis B. Adverse effects include renal and GI toxicity. Dose reduction required for renal dysfunction.
ribavirin (Rebetol, Virazole, others)	400 mg PO in AM, 600 mg PO in PM* (600 mg PO twice daily if greater than 75 kg) Inhaled form available for RSV	For treatment of chronic Hepatitis C and RSV. Toxicities include teratogenicity (category X), bone marrow suppression, GI, CNS.
interferons (Intron A, Wellferon, others)	Vary based on formulation	For treatment of hepatitis C, some specific cancers. Clinical depression is major concern. Other toxicities, roles discussed in Chapter 63.
lamivudine (Epivir HBV)	100 mg PO daily	Used for chronic hepatitis B. Higher doses used for HIV. Dose reduction required for renal dysfunction.
TRICYCLIC AMINES FOR INFLUENZA A		
amantadine (Symmetrel)	100 mg PO twice daily	Used for Influenzae A prophylaxis and treatment, (amantadine also for Parkinson's disease). Toxicities include CNS, GI.
rimantadine (Flumadine)	100 mg PO twice daily	Dose reduction required for renal dysfunction.

CNS, Central nervous system; GI, gastrointestinal; HIV, human immunodeficiency virus.
*Dose varies based on indication.

TABLE 59-3 COMPARISON OF ANTIVIRALS (NON-HIV)—cont'd

Agent	Typical Systemic Adult Dose	Comments
NEURAMINIDASE INHIBITORS FOR INFLUENZA TYPE A OR B		
oseltamivir (Tamiflu)	Treatment: 75 mg PO twice daily × 5 days Prophylaxis: 75 mg PO daily	GI is most common adverse effect. Dose reduction required for renal dysfunction.
zanamivir (Relenza)	Treatment: 10 mg (2 puffs, each providing 5 mg) by inhalation q12h × 5 days	May exacerbate chronic obstructive pulmonary disease (COPD), asthma. GI upset also noted.
ZINC FOR COMMON COLD		
zinc supplements (Zicam, others)	Based on formulation	Reports of efficacy vary

✳ **P.K. is treated symptomatically with fluids, rest, anesthetic throat drops, and the decongestant pseudoephedrine (Sudafed) 60 mg orally every 4 to 6 hours. He is to avoid others and use frequent handwashing to reduce the transmission of his cold to others during that time. Because his symptoms began within the past 24 hours, he will also start zinc nasal swabs (zincum gluconicum [Zicam]) every 4 hours for until 48 hours after symptoms resolve.**

✳ **What is the role of zinc in the treatment of the common cold?**

Formulations of zinc administered as lozenges or nasal swabs have become popular over the past decade as a treatment for the common cold. Reports of efficacy of zinc preparations vary. When administered early (within 24 to 48 hours of first symptoms), severity and duration of cold symptoms appear to be diminished in some studies. One trial of zincum gluconicum nasal swabs administered four times daily was associated with reduced nasal drainage, congestion and sore throat, and shortened average duration of cold from an average of 6 days with placebo to 4.3 days with zinc therapy (Mossad, 2003). Similar findings were observed with zinc acetate lozenges administered every two to three hours in one study (Prasad, Fitzgerald, Bao, Beck, & Chandrasekar, 2000), but a systematic review of a number of zinc trials failed to note benefit from zinc lozenges (Jackson, Lesho, & Peterson, 2000). Zinc lozenges and nasal swabs are not associated with serious adverse effects, although altered taste and localized irritation may occur.

✳ **J.S. is a 31-year-old female with a recent outbreak of genital herpes infection as manifested by multiple, painful, small, grouped, vesicular lesions on her labia. She consults her health care provider seeking intervention.**

✳ **What drugs are available to treat genital herpes, herpes simplex, and herpes zoster infections?**

Agents primarily effective against the herpes simplex, genital herpes and herpes zoster infections include acyclovir (Zovirax), famciclovir (Famvir), valacyclovir (Valtrex). Chapter 65 discusses penciclovir (Denavir), a related antiviral used topically to treat herpes simplex infections.

Acyclovir is selectively taken up by herpes simplex virus (HSV)-infected cells and is eventually converted via a number of cellular enzymes to an active triphosphate form that is incorporated into growing DNA chains produced by the virus; this results in the inhibition of viral DNA replication. Famciclovir, a pro-drug of penciclovir, the active antiviral substance, has inhibitory action against herpes simplex viruses (types 1 and 2) and varicella zoster virus. Valacyclovir is a pro-drug that is converted to acyclovir by first-pass intestinal and liver metabolism.

⬛ acyclovir [ay **sye** kloe veer]
(Zovirax, Avirax✚)

Indications
Oral acyclovir is used in the prophylaxis and treatment of genital herpes infections in both immunocompromised and immunocompetent clients. It is also used to treat varicella (chickenpox) infections in immunocompetent children if used within 24 hours of the appearance of the rash. Injectable acyclovir is used to treat initial severe herpes genitalis in immunocompromised and immunocompetent clients who are unable to take or absorb the oral dosage form. The parenteral dosage form is also used to treat herpes simplex encephalitis and herpes zoster infections, the latter being caused by the varicella-zoster virus (VZV).

Pharmacokinetics/Dosing
The oral dosage form of acyclovir is poorly absorbed (20%), but therapeutic serum levels are achieved. It is widely disseminated to various body fluids and tissues, including CSF and herpetic vesicular fluid. CSF levels are approximately 50% of the serum drug concentration. The half-life is approximately 2.5 hours; the drug is metabolized in the liver and excreted primarily in the urine. The usual initial oral adult dosage for a herpes genital infection is 400 mg three times daily for up to 10 days. For use as a chronic suppressant in a client with recurrent infection, the typical dosage is 400 mg three times daily for 5 days. Other dosing regimens are also used. For children 2 to 12 years of age who weigh up to 40 kg, the dosage to treat varicella is 20 mg/kg (up to 800 mg/dose) four times daily for 5 days.

The parenteral adult dosage for severe genital herpes is 5 mg/kg IV every 8 hours for 5 days. Refer to the current package insert for other dosage recommendations. Topical acyclovir is commonly used to treat herpes simplex infections, but the systemic dosage form is much more effective in immunocompromised persons.

Adverse Effects

The adverse effects of the oral dosage form of acyclovir include nausea, headache, diarrhea, vomiting, and dizziness. When administered parenterally, phlebitis at the injection site or acute renal failure with rapid injection may occur. High-dose acyclovir may also result in crystallization of the drug in the urine, particularly in clients who are dehydrated. Burning and irritation are associated with the topical use of acyclovir. Rarely, acyclovir is associated with potentially life-threatening reactions including Stevens-Johnson syndrome, thrombocytopenia, and thrombocytopenic purpura/hemolytic uremic syndrome. Use of high doses of acyclovir in clients who are immunocompromised may increase risk for these serious reactions.

famciclovir [fam **sye** kloe veer]
(Famvir)

Indications

Famciclovir is indicated for the treatment of genital herpes and acute herpes zoster.

Pharmacokinetics/Dosing

Administered orally, famciclovir is well absorbed and converted in the intestinal wall to the active penciclovir. It reaches peak serum levels in approximately 1 hour and has a half-life of 2 to 3 hours. It is excreted primarily unchanged in the urine and feces. The usual adult dosage for herpes zoster is 500 mg PO every 8 hours for 1 week.

Adverse Effects

The adverse effects of famciclovir include headaches, weakness, nausea, vomiting, diarrhea, abdominal pain, and fatigue.

valacyclovir [val a **sye** kloe veer]
(Valtrex)

Indications

Valacyclovir is indicated for the treatment of herpes zoster (shingles) caused by VZV and herpes genitalis in immunocompetent persons. When compared to acyclovir, valacyclovir is reported to be more significant in reducing the pain and postherpetic neuralgia associated with herpes zoster in persons older than 50 years of age. Valacyclovir has not been studied in children, immunocompromised individuals, or persons with disseminated zoster (*USP DI*, 2005).

Pharmacokinetics/Dosing

Administered orally, valacyclovir is well absorbed and is converted to acyclovir, the active substance. It reaches peak serum levels in 1.6 to 2 hours and has a half-life of 2.5 to 3.3 hours. Valacyclovir is converted to inactive metabolites by alcohol and aldehyde dehydrogenase and is excreted primarily in the urine. The usual adult dosage for herpes zoster is 1 g three times daily for 1 week.

Adverse Effects

Adverse effects of valacyclovir are similar to acyclovir and famciclovir, and include nausea, headache, weakness, gastric distress, and dizziness.

✱ **J.S. receives a prescription for valacyclovir (Valtrex) 1000 mg PO twice daily × 10 days.**

✱ **What are the nursing management issues involved in using these antiviral agents with J.S.?**

Assessment Assess J.S. for hypersensitivity to antiviral agents. Use these agents with caution in clients with renal function impairment; they are at greater risk for nephrotoxicity. A history of neurologic abnormalities or a previous neurologic reaction to cytotoxic agents may indicate a tendency for such responses. Assess J.S.'s immune status; immunosuppressed clients (those with bone marrow or renal transplantation or advanced HIV) have developed thrombotic, thrombocytopenia purpura/hemolytic uremic syndrome (TTP/HUS) with prolonged high-dose therapy, however, TTP/HUS has not been seen in immunocompetent clients. With obese clients, antiviral dosage is calculated on ideal body weight rather than actual weight.

Review J.S.'s current medication regimen. Renal clearance of valacyclovir is reduced by cimetidine and probenecid. The potential for nephrotoxicity is increased when parenteral acyclovir, another antiviral in this class, is given concurrently with other nephrotoxic drugs. Maintaining adequate hydration may decrease this risk. Monitor renal function closely.

Assess lesions before administering the drug and daily throughout therapy. Determine a baseline BUN and serum creatinine concentration to effectively monitor for the risk of developing renal impairment.

Nursing Diagnosis While J.S. is receiving antiviral therapy, assess for the following nursing diagnoses/collaborative problems: impaired comfort (headache, abdominal pain, arthralgia, nausea); risk for injury related to dizziness; diarrhea; risk for transmission of infection; and the potential complications of hypersensitivity, depression, nephrotoxicity (oliguria, thirst, anorexia, nausea, vomiting, fatigue) and encephalopathic effects (confusion, tremors, seizures).

Planning During the antiviral therapy, J.S. will:
- Experience decreased symptoms of herpes genitalis, particularly pain, with minimal adverse effects of the drug therapy.
- Effectively manage the therapeutic regimen, including being compliant with medications, and implementing nonpharmacologic supportive measures.
- Collaborate with health care providers by appropriately reporting untoward symptoms and maintaining scheduled visits for monitoring and treatment.

Implementation

Monitoring Monitor J.S. for the development of the nursing diagnoses/potential complications discussed above. Monitor the client's lesions for resolution. Valacyclovir and famciclovir have greater oral availability than acyclovir allowing for more infrequent dosing, however, if a client requires a parenteral antiviral, acyclovir is given. With acyclovir, monitor the client closely for nephrotoxicity; rapid bolus administration has been linked to precipitation of the drug in the renal tubules, resulting in acute renal insufficiency.

Intervention Oral forms of antivirals may be administered with meals to minimize GI distress. When dispensing acyclovir oral suspension, shake it well and use the calibrated measuring device supplied by the manufacturer.

IV acyclovir should be administered via an infusion pump at a constant rate for at least 1 hour; this prevents the precipitation of drug crystals in the renal tubules. The client should also receive hydration during the infusion and for 2 hours afterward to prevent this effect. Avoid rapid or bolus injection of the drug. Rotate infusion sites to prevent phlebitis. The IV solution is not to be used topically or orally or administered intramuscularly or subcutaneously.

Education J.S. needs accurate information about herpes, its symptoms and transmission, and the course of the illness and treatment. Because herpes genitalis is sexually transmitted, misinformation about it is prevalent. J.S. should avoid sexual activity if either participant has symptoms of herpes. Condom use may help to prevent the spread of the infection, but spermicidal jellies or diaphragms probably will not. Antivirals will neither prevent the transmission of the disease nor cure it.

Caution J.S. that valacyclovir may shorten the outbreak duration, but that it does not affect the frequency of subsequent recurrences, which tend to be substantially less severe. However, if she has a recurrence of the infection, she may want to discuss being placed on suppressive antiviral therapy.

The medication should be initiated as soon as possible after symptoms appear. To minimize the episode of herpes, instruct J.S. to begin taking the medication as soon as itching, tingling, or pain develops at the site. Instruct her regarding comfort measures, such as wearing loose-fitting clothing to minimize irritation of the lesions. The infected areas should be kept clean and dry.

Caution J.S. to obtain a Papanicolaou (Pap) smear at least annually, because women with genital herpes are at higher risk for cervical cancer than women without genital herpes.

Evaluation The expected outcome of acyclovir therapy is that J.S.'s infection will go into remission with a decrease in pain and in time to full crusting and a decrease in vesicles, ulcers, and crusts, and she will not experience any adverse effects of the drug (e.g., nausea, vomiting, headache, diarrhea, dizziness, nephrotoxicity). She will wear loose-fitting clothing, keep the infected area clean and dry, use condoms, and avoid sexual activity if either partner has symptoms of herpes. J.S. will collaborate with her health care provider by keeping her scheduled appointments, taking the antiviral at the first symptom of recurrence, and appropriately reporting adverse symptoms.

✴ **L.S. is a 29-year-old male with advanced HIV and cytomegalovirus (CMV) retinitis. His therapies are being managed by the infectious disease service and an ophthalmologist.**

✴ **What agents are effective against CMV infection?**
CMV is common, but only produces disease in clients who are immunocompromised (including clients who have un-

dergone organ transplant and are receiving chronic immunosuppressive therapy). Available treatments for advanced CMV infection include foscarnet (Foscavir), cidofovir (Vistide), ganciclovir (Cytovene), and valganciclovir (Valcyte). Because the advent of HAART with these agents in the mid-1990s, the incidence of HIV complications has decreased by 50% (CDC, 2004).

Cidofovir inhibits DNA synthesis and thereby reduces CMV replication. Foscarnet is a virustatic agent acting to inhibit viral replication of all known herpes viruses in vitro, including CMV, herpes simplex virus types 1 and 2, Epstein-Barr virus, and VZV. Foscarnet acts by selective inhibition at the pyrophosphate-binding site of viral DNA polymerase. Ganciclovir is a pro-drug; it is converted intracellularly to the active, antiviral triphosphate form. In the presence of the CMV, ganciclovir is rapidly phosphorylated to ganciclovir-triphosphate, which then inhibits viral DNA polymerase and suppresses viral DNA synthesis. Valganciclovir is a pro-drug that is rapidly converted to ganciclovir and offers improved bioavailability on oral administration.

These agents also may have some activity against other viral infections, but indications are primarily limited to CMV. When these drugs are discontinued, viral replication resumes. As such, uninterrupted therapy to maintain consistent tissue levels is required for optimal treatment.

cidofovir [sye **dof** oe veer]
(Vistide)
Indications
Cidofovir is indicated for the treatment of CMV retinitis in clients with advanced HIV. It is dosed concurrently with probenecid to reduce renal toxicity.
Pharmacokinetics/Dosing
Cidofovir is administered IV and does not distribute to the CSF. It is eliminated renally. Adult dose is typically 5 mg/kg IV over 1 hour once weekly for 2 weeks, then once every other week. Two grams of oral probenecid are administered 3 hours before infusion, and an addition one gram of oral probenecid is administered 2 and 8 hours after completion of the infusion. Doses are reduced in renal impairment
Adverse Effects
Nephrotoxicity, the major adverse effect of cidofovir, is reduced with concurrent probenecid therapy. Other effects include mental confusion, fever, chills, insomnia, alopecia, rash, GI upset, muscle weakness, respiratory distress, hepatic dysfunction, pancreatitis, and bone marrow suppression.

foscarnet [fos **kar** net]
(Foscavir)
Indications
Foscarnet is currently used to treat CMV retinitis in clients with AIDS.
Pharmacokinetics/Dosing
This drug is administered by IV infusion, has an elimination half-life of 3.3 to 6.8 hours, reaches peak serum levels at the end of the infusion, is not metabolized, and is excreted primarily unchanged in the urine. For induction, the usual adult dosage by IV infusion is 60 mg/kg every 8 hours for 2 to 3 weeks. The maintenance dosage is 90 to 120 mg/kg daily.
Adverse Effects
Common adverse effects of foscarnet include nephrotoxicity, gastric distress, and neurotoxicity. It may also cause anemia and leukopenia.

ganciclovir [gan **sye** kloe vir]
(Cytovene, Cytovene-IV)

Indications

Parenteral ganciclovir is indicated for the prophylaxis and treatment of CMV retinitis in immunocompromised clients. The oral form is used to manage CMV retinitis in clients whose condition has stabilized after parenteral therapy.

Pharmacokinetics/Dosing

Ganciclovir is administered by IV infusion or intravitreal injection. The serum half-life is 2.5 to 3.6 hours; the half-life in vitreous fluid is approximately 13 hours. This drug is primarily excreted unchanged by the kidneys.

The oral dosage form has a half-life of 3 to 5.5 hours and reaches peak serum concentrations in 3 hours if administered with food. An intravitreal ganciclovir implant (Vitrasert Implant) has been found to be more effective in delaying the progression of retinitis than IV ganciclovir. The implant releases ganciclovir for a period of 5 to 8 months.

The usual adult dosage of ganciclovir by IV infusion for induction is 5 mg/kg every 12 hours for 2 to 3 weeks. The maintenance dosage is 5 mg/kg daily. With oral ganciclovir, the maintenance dosage is 1000 mg three times daily with food.

Adverse Effects

The common adverse effects of ganciclovir include granulocytopenia, thrombocytopenia and, possibly, gastric distress. Rash, fever, headache, confusion, insomnia, and gastric upset are also fairly frequently observed adverse effects. GI bleeding, seizures, Stevens-Johnson syndrome, ventricular dysrhythmias, psychosis, and renal failure are also possible. Ganciclovir may be mutagenic to both sperm and ova. Both men and women should be informed about using contraception for at least 3 months after completion of therapy.

valganciclovir [val gan **sye** kloh veer]
(Valcyte)

Indications

Valganciclovir is used to prevent and treat CMV retinitis in high-risk clients including those with kidney, heart, and kidney-pancreas transplants. It is not indicated for clients who have a history of liver transplant, and safety for other solid organ transplantation has not been established (Lange, 2003).

Pharmacokinetics/Dosing

Valganciclovir absorption is improved when taken with a fatty meal. It is converted to ganciclovir and dosed at 900 mg twice daily × 21 days, then 900 mg daily.

Adverse Effects

See ganciclovir.

✳ **L.S. receives ganciclovir by slow IV infusion, 5 mg/kg/dose every 12 hours for 3 weeks, followed by valganciclovir 900 mg orally daily.**

✳ **What are the nursing implications for using these anti-CMV therapies with L.S.?**

Assessment Determine if L.S. has a hypersensitivity to antiviral agents. If L.S. has impaired renal function, the dosage must be modified on the basis of his creatinine clearance. The risk-benefit ratio must be determined for L.S. if he has an absolute neutrophil count less than 500 cells/mm³ or a platelet count less than 25,000/mm³ given that granulocytopenia and thrombocytopenia may be caused by ganciclovir. Review L.S.'s current medication regimen for the risk of significant drug interactions, such as those that may

occur when antiretrovirals are given with other nephrotoxic drugs, blood dyscrasia-causing drugs or bone marrow depressants. For baseline, assess L.S.'s CD4⁺ cell count and other symptoms of his underlying HIV infection. Ascertain renal function using creatinine clearance determinations. Evaluate L.S.'s fluid status because he should be well hydrated before initiating therapy to help prevent renal toxicity. A baseline ophthalmologic examination is required because L.S. is being treated for CMV retinitis.

Nursing Diagnosis While L.S. is receiving anti-CMV therapy, assess him for the following nursing diagnoses/collaborative problems: impaired comfort related to phlebitis (pain at the site of infusion); deficient fluid volume related to anorexia, nausea, or vomiting; disturbed sensory perception related to CMV retinitis secondary to the ineffectiveness of the drug; and the potential complications of neurotoxicity (anxiety, confusion, dizziness, headache, tremor, seizures, pain, or numbness in the hands and feet), hepatotoxicity, anemia, granulocytopenia, thrombocytopenia, and nephrotoxicity.

Planning The goals of L.S.'s anti-CMV therapy are that he will:

- Experience no further loss of vision without adverse drug effects.
- Effectively participate in the therapeutic regimen by appropriately reporting untoward symptoms and implementing nonpharmacologic supportive measures.

Implementation

Monitoring Monitor L.S.'s vision status, CBCs, platelet counts, BUN, serum creatinine concentration, liver function studies, signs and symptoms of his HIV infection, and ophthalmologic examinations.

Intervention IV infusions of ganciclovir should be administered using a controlled infusion device over at least a 1 hour time period. It may be administered via a central or peripheral vein. Rapid or direct IV injection may cause potentially toxic serum concentrations. L.S. should be adequately hydrated to prevent renal toxicity. Use the same precautions as when handling cytotoxic solutions; consult the procedure manual of the institution. All safety precautions should be taken with the client during periods of low blood counts. Intravitreal injection may be used if L.S. is unresponsive to IV therapy or has severe myelosuppression because of ganciclovir therapy.

Education Alert L.S. to report any change in urinary elimination pattern or a worsening vision in the involved eye(s). Maintain an adequate fluids intake. Valganciclovir should be taken with food for maximum absorption. Do not break or crush valganciclovir tablets. If contact does occur, wash the area thoroughly with soap and water; rinse the eyes copiously with plain water. Alert L.S. to reportable drug-induced signs and symptoms, and signs of infection (fever or chills). Encourage him to remain compliant with his medication regimen to help prevent a worsening of his vision and maintain his appointment schedule with his provider for frequent hematologic monitoring. L.S. should use barrier contraception during treatment and for at least 90 days after therapy. Instruct females of reproductive age who are taking ganciclovir to use effective contraception, because this drug has mutagenic and teratogenic potential (see the Pregnancy Safety box below).

Evaluation The expected outcome of L.S.'s anti-CMV therapy is that he will not have further vision loss and that his CMV retinitis will be alleviated without his experiencing any untoward effects of the drugs (e.g., fever, chills). He will report these symptoms, take his medications with meals, use barrier contraceptive measures for 90 days after therapy, and maintain his scheduled appointments for monitoring and therapy. If these anti-CMV drugs had been prescribed for clients at risk for CMV, the disease would be prevented.

✴ **J.A. is a 42-year-old developmentally disabled client who resides in a group home and is being followed by his health care providers for chronic hepatitis B infection.**

✴ **What treatments are available to treat hepatitis?** Each type of hepatitis is prevented and managed with different modalities. Hepatitis A is prevented by using good hygiene and considering the use of hepatitis A vaccine. Hepatitis A is a usually a self-limiting disease and treatment of acute hepatitis A is supportive.

Hepatitis B is best prevented with the use of hepatitis B vaccine and hepatitis B immune globulin (see Chapters 62

and 63), and treatment options are somewhat helpful but the risk/benefit of these treatments are still undergoing evaluation. Treatment options for the management of chronic hepatitis B include the use of interferons (see Chapters 56 and 63) and two nucleoside reverse transcriptase inhibitors: adefovir (Hepsera), discussed below, and lamivudine (Epivir, Epivir-HBV), discussed later in this chapter with treatments for HIV.

Currently, there is not a vaccine to prevent hepatitis C, and its treatment, like hepatitis B, is being refined. Treatment of hepatitis C involves the use of interferons (particularly the pegylated versions which provide a more even pharmacokinetic profile) and to some degree, ribavirin (Copegus, Virazole), which has some efficacy for other viral conditions as well.

adefovir [a **def** oe veer]
(Hepsera)
Adefovir is a nucleoside reverse transcriptase inhibitor similar in activity to a number of the drugs used to treat HIV disease. It inhibits DNA polymerase, thereby inhibiting replication of hepatitis B virus.

Indications
Adefovir is used to treat chronic hepatitis B in clients with existing hepatic injury secondary to infection.

Pharmacokinetics/Dosing
Adefovir is converted to an active metabolite in the intestines and is fairly well absorbed after oral administration. It is eliminated in the urine and has an elimination half-life of approximately 8 hours. The typical adult dose is 10 mg once daily. Dosage is adjusted for clients with renal dysfunction.

Adverse Effects
Adefovir is associated with hematuria, fever, headache, and GI upset. Nephrotoxicity has been reported as well and should be used cautiously if at all for clients with renal impairment. Exacerbations of hepatitis have been reported on discontinuation of the drug.

Drug Interactions
Concurrent use of ibuprofen (and possibly other nonsteroidal antiinflammatory agents [NSAIDs]) results in increased absorption of adefovir. Use of drugs which are potentially nephrotoxic (e.g., NSAIDs, aminoglycosides, amphotericin B) may increase the potential for nephrotoxicity with adefovir.

✴ **J.A. is treated with adefovir 10 mg PO daily to eradicate the viral carriage. The goal of this therapy is to resolve ongoing hepatocellular damage and help prevent the development of cirrhosis and hepatocellular carcinoma.**

✴ **What are the nursing management issues for the treatment of J.A.'s chronic hepatitis B with adefovir?**

Assessment Use adefovir with caution in clients with nephrotoxicity; dosage adjustment is required for renal dysfunction. Assess J.A.'s serum creatinine and BUN for a baseline to monitor for adefovir's nephrotoxicity. Review J.A.'s concurrent medication regimen because aminoglycosides, immunosuppressants (cyclosporine, tacrolimus), NSAIDS, vancomycin, and other nephrotoxic drugs increase his risk for nephrotoxicity with adefovir. Establish a baseline for J.A.'s hepatitis with a review of ALT, AST, alka-

Category	Drug
PREGNANCY SAFETY **ANTIFUNGAL AND ANTIVIRAL DRUGS**	
B	amphotericin B, didanosine, emtricitabine, enfuvirtide, famciclovir, nelfinavir, penciclovir, ritonavir, saquinavir, tenofovir, valacyclovir
C	abacavir, acyclovir, adefovir, amantadine, amprenavir, caspofungin, cidofovir, delavirdine, fluconazole, flucytosine, foscarnet, ganciclovir, griseofulvin, indinavir, itraconazole, ketoconazole, lamivudine, lopinavir, miconazole, nevirapine, nystatin, oseltamivir, rimantadine, taurine, valganciclovir, zalcitabine, zanamivir, zidovudine
D	efavirenz, voriconazole
X	ribavirin

Data from *Mosby's drug consult* (15th ed.). (2005). St. Louis: Mosby.

line phosphatase, prothrombin time/International Normalized Ratio (PT/INR), serum albumin, and total protein determinations. Document any clinical symptoms that he may have such as anorexia, malaise, abdominal discomfort, and jaundice.

Nursing Diagnosis While J.A. is receiving adefovir therapy, he is at risk for the following nursing diagnoses: altered nutrition: less than required related to anorexia; fatigue; impaired comfort (dyspepsia, abdominal pain, headache); risk for transmission of disease; and the potential complications of nephropathy, lactic acidosis, coagulopathy, cirrhosis, and hepatocellular carcinoma.

Planning The goals of J.A.'s adefovir therapy are that he will:

- Experience no further progression of liver impairment.
- Effectively manage the therapeutic regimen with the assistance of his caregiver, including being compliant with medications, and implementing nonpharmacologic supportive measures.
- Collaborate with health care providers with the assistance of his caregivers, by appropriately reporting untoward symptoms and maintaining scheduled visits for monitoring and treatment.

Implementation

Monitoring Monitor J.A. for the nursing diagnoses and potential complications above. Monitor ALT/AST for disease progression, serum creatinine determinations for nephrotoxicity, creatinine kinase, and serum amylase for lactic acidosis.

Intervention Adefovir may be given without regard to food.

Education Instruct J.A. and his caregiver to report blood in his urine, increased and unexplained weakness, or a return of his symptom of hepatitis. Stress the importance of compliance with the medication regimen to obtain the optimal clinical result. Avoid strenuous physical exercise and avoid alcohol use. Caution against herbal preparations as some have been found to contain hepatotoxic substances. Small frequent meals may assist to avoid nausea and prevent altered nutrition: less than body requirements.

Evaluation The expected outcome of J.A.'s adefovir therapy is that he will not experience progression of hepatitis B to cirrhosis or hepatocellular carcinoma. With his caregiver's assistance, he will be able to effectively maintain his therapeutic regimen completing his full prescription every 30 days, eating small frequent meals to prevent nausea, avoiding the use of alcoholic beverages, and reporting symptoms of hematuria, fever, headache, and GI distress. J.A., with the assistance of his caregiver, will maintain scheduled visits for monitoring disease progression.

✱ **H.S., an 8-month-old infant with a history of immunosuppression, is brought into the emergency department (ED) by his mother. He is lethargic, cyanotic, febrile, and tachypneic. Respiratory syncytial virus (RSV) is present in his respiratory secretions. He is placed on oxygen and ribavirin aerosol 2 g over 2 hours three times daily for 3 to 7 days.**

✱ **What is the role of ribavirin in the treatment of RSV?**

Respiratory syncytial virus (RSV) is a common viral pathogen responsible for bronchiolitis in infants and toddlers during the late fall, winter, and early spring in North America. RSV is also common in older adults (Falsey, Hennessey, Formica, Cox, & Walsh, 2005). It is particularly problematic for those younger than 2 years of age who are immunocompromised, were born prematurely (below 28 to 32 weeks gestational age) and/or have a history of chronic lung disease or congenital heart disease. In these high-risk individuals, the use of palivizumab (Synagis), a monoclonal antibody directed against RSV, is commonly used during the winter months (see Chapter 62). Occasionally, ribavirin is used in the treatment of RSV as well.

Ribavirin is a purine nucleoside analog with virustatic activity. Its mechanism of action is diverse and not completely understood. It rapidly penetrates viral infected cells and is believed to reduce the storage of intracellular guanosine triphosphate (GTP). It inhibits viral RNA and protein synthesis, thus inhibiting viral duplication, viral spread to other cells, or both. The use of ribavirin in children is controversial. At one time, it was thought to decrease fever and increase oxygen saturation in nonimmunocompromised children. However, a systematic evaluation of published studies failed to find consistent benefit of its routine use in RSV (King et al., 2004), although it is of some benefit for critically ill infants (Davison, Ventre, Luchetti, & Randolph, 2004). The American Academy of Pediatrics recommends that the decision of its use be made on the basis of particular circumstances, such as underlying congenital heart disease, lung disease, or immunosuppression, or on physician experience (American Academy of Pediatrics Committee on Infectious Disease, 1999).

ribavirin [rye ba **vye** rin]
(Virazole)
Indications
Oral ribavirin is used in combination with interferon or peginterferon in the treatment of hepatitis C. Inhaled ribavirin is indicated for serious viral pneumonia caused by RSV.

Pharmacokinetics/Dosing
The oral formulation of ribavirin is moderately well absorbed and has an elimination half-life of 24 to 48 hours. It is dosed orally based on client weight (typically 400 mg in the AM, and 600 mg in the PM, if less than 75 kg; 600 mg twice daily, if greater than 75 kg).

Following oral inhalation, ribavirin is well absorbed and rapidly distributed to plasma, respiratory tract secretions, and erythrocytes. The half-life is 9.5 hours after oral inhalation and approximately 40 days in erythrocytes. Ribavirin is metabolized in the liver and excreted primarily by the kidneys. The adult dosage of ribavirin for inhalation aerosol has not been established. For RSV infection in children, this drug is administered by oral inhalation via a Viratek small-particle aerosol generator, with a ribavirin concentration of 20 mg/mL in the reservoir. Administer over 12 to 18 hours per day for 3 to 7 days.

Adverse Effects
Ribavirin is teratogenic (Category X) and should be avoided in women who are pregnant or may become pregnant. Other serious adverse effects include bone marrow suppression, anemia, and psychiatric disturbances (particularly irritability, emotional lability, confusion and inability to concentrate). Headache, depression, dizziness, fever and fatigue hair loss, nausea, vomiting, muscle and joint pain, and dyspnea are also commonly reported for clients on combined ribavirin and interferon therapy (of which interferon is likely the greater contributor). Bolus IV administration can result in rigors similar to that seen with amphotericin B. The adverse effects of inhaled ribavirin are less frequent but may include skin rash or lung/eye irritation with chronic administration. Health care workers exposed to aerosolized ribavirin may experience headache, conjunctivitis, and tearing. Aerosolized ribavirin may also pose a teratogen risk for pregnant health care providers.

✳ What are the nursing implications of ribavirin for H.S.?

Assessment Assess H.S. for hypersensitivity to ribavirin. Determine if H.S. has severe anemia because ribavirin may cause anemia, however, it is reversible when the drug is discontinued. For a baseline, document H.S.'s vital signs, lung sounds, and oxygen saturation. Zidovudine and ribavirin are antagonistic and should not be used together.

Nursing Diagnosis While H.S. is receiving ribavirin therapy, he is at risk for impaired comfort related to direct contact chemical irritation as evidenced by conjunctivitis and/or rash and anorexia, nausea and headache; and fatigue and the potential complication of fatigue.

Planning The goal of H.S.'s ribavirin therapy is that he will:
* Experience resolution of his respiratory infection without adverse effects of the drug.

Implementation
Monitoring Monitor H.S.'s respiratory status before and after the administration of ribavirin. If administered to clients receiving ventilation assistance, observe for increased positive-end expiratory pressure (PEEP) and increased positive inspiratory pressure, which occur if ribavirin precipitates within the ventilator apparatus. Check the equipment at least every half hour to prevent fluid accumulation in the tubing. Therapy is generally effective if begun within the first 3 days of RSV infection. If H.S. were receiving IV or oral ribavirin, his hematocrit would be monitored for the development of anemia.

Intervention Therapy with ribavirin may begin before the diagnosis is confirmed by diagnostic tests; however, treatment should not continue if the presence of RSV is not confirmed.

Administer ribavirin aerosol only with the Viratek SPAG Model (SPAG-2); refer to the SPAG-2 manual for exceptions. After preparation of ribavirin solution according to

package directions, ensure that the final solution is free of particulate matter. Always discard the remaining solution when its level gets low and add freshly reconstituted solution to the reservoir. The solution retains its potency at room temperature for 24 hours. Do not administer ribavirin concurrently with any other medication by aerosolization.

Monitor for hypotension (faintness, light-headedness, unusual fatigue); transient increases in AST, ALT, and bilirubin; abdominal cramps; and jaundice.

Health care workers in the client's environment may experience headache and conjunctivitis. Health care providers who are pregnant should avoid exposure to inhaled ribavirin.

Education Instruct H.S.'s parents about ribavirin therapy and its action, route of administration, equipment involved, frequency of treatments, and adverse effects. Although not indicated for use in adults, health care workers and visitors who spend time at the bedside may become environmentally exposed. There is a risk of teratogenic and/or embryocidal effects in women who are pregnant. Female health care workers and visitors that are pregnant or may become pregnant should be advised of the potential risk of exposure.

Evaluation The expected outcome of ribavirin therapy is that H.S. will experience improved airway clearance as evidenced by a normal respiratory rate, pink color, an absence of adventitious lung sounds, and a pulse oximetry of 98% to 100%; and that the RSV pneumonia will resolve without adverse drug effects (e.g., bone marrow suppression, headache, fatigue, psychiatric disturbances).

✳ K.F. is a nurse manager for a long-term care facility who is concerned about an outbreak of influenza in his facility. During October, most clients received influenza vaccination. During the first week of December, two cases of influenza were noted in two health care workers at the facility. K.F. questions the medical director about additional modalities to prevent or treat influenza.

✳ What agents are available to prevent or treat influenza A and B infection?
Individuals at risk for complications associated with influenza (e.g., children 6 to 24 months, those older than 65 years of age and those with chronic medical conditions) are candidates for annual influenzae vaccination. The CDC (www.cdc.gov) provides annual updates in predicting strains of influenza during the influenza season, availability of vaccine and recommendations regarding which individuals should receive vaccination. Refer to Chapter 62 for a discussion of the vaccines available for use.

Drug therapy to prevent influenza infections has a more limited role compared to vaccination. The tricyclic amines, amantadine (Symmetrel) and rimantadine (Flumadine) are both effective in preventing the most commonly observed strains of influenza, influenza A types. Unfortunately, they offer limited benefit if infection is underway.

Two other agents, oseltamivir (Tamiflu) and zanamivir (Relenza) inhibit the enzyme neuraminidase in influenza type A and B strains and are effective for both prophylaxis and early treatment. Cost may prohibit their widespread use for prophylaxis, and treatment must be initiated within 24 to 48 hours of symptoms to achieve an adequate client response.

Tricyclic Amines for Influenza A Prophylaxis

Amantadine appears to block the uncoating of the influenza A virus and the release of viral nucleic acid into the respiratory epithelial cells of the host. It also increases the release of dopamine and inhibits the reuptake of dopamine and norepinephrine centrally. Rimantadine, an analogue of amantadine, inhibits viral replication by blocking or reducing the uncoating of viral RNA in host cells.

✦⌐ amantadine [a **man** ta deen]
(Symmetrel, Symadine, Endantadine❀, PMS-Amantadine❀)

Indications
Amantadine is indicated for the prevention and early treatment of influenza A and for treatment of Parkinson's disease and drug-induced, extrapyramidal reactions.

Pharmacokinetics/Dosing
Amantadine is rapidly absorbed orally, distributed to saliva and nasal secretions, and crosses the blood-brain barrier. It has a half-life of 11 to 15 hours and reaches a peak serum level within 2 to 4 hours. Its onset of action as an antidyskinetic is usually within 2 days. It is excreted mostly unchanged by the kidneys. The adult dosage of the oral antiviral is 200 mg daily or 100 mg every 12 hours. The usual antidyskinetic dosage is 100 mg PO once or twice daily (up to 400 mg daily). Dosage must be reduced in clients with renal insufficiency to reduce the risk of CNS toxicity.

Adverse Effects
The adverse effects of amantadine include CNS toxicity (anxiety, insomnia, hallucinations), gastric distress and, with chronic therapy, livedo reticularis (a vasospastic disorder worsened by exposure to cold and evidenced by a reddish blue mottling of the legs and, sometimes, the arms). It also may cause anticholinergic adverse effects and orthostatic hypotension.

Drug Interactions
Drugs with antimuscarinic (anticholinergic) activity may increase the likelihood of CNS toxicity. Such agents include atropine, benztropine, trihexyphenidyl, antihistamines, tricyclic antidepressants, cimetidine, and ranitidine. Quinidine, triamterene, thiazide diuretics, and trimethoprim/sulfamethoxazole may also be associated with increased levels and toxicity of amantadine.

rimantadine [ri **man** ti deen]
(Flumadine)

Indications
Rimantadine is indicated for the prevention and early treatment of influenza type A respiratory tract infections.

Pharmacokinetics/Dosing
Rimantadine is well absorbed orally and reaches a peak concentration in 1 to 4 hours. The half-life is 13 to 38 hours in children (4 to 8 years of age), 25 to 30 hours in younger adults (22 to 44 years of age), and 32 hours in older adults (71 to 79 years of age). It is metabolized in the liver and primarily excreted by the kidneys. For adults and children over 10 years of age, the dosage of rimantadine for prophylaxis and treatment is 100 mg PO twice daily. The recommended dosage is 100 mg PO daily for older adults in nursing homes or in persons with severe liver or renal impairment.

Adverse Effects
The adverse effects of rimantadine are uncommon, with older adults having a higher incidence of these effects than younger adults. Adverse effects include CNS toxicity (as with amantadine) and gastric distress.

Drug Interactions
As with amantadine. Additionally, cimetidine use may result in increased levels and potential for toxicity of rimantadine whereas aspirin and acetaminophen may result in reduced rimantadine levels.

Neuraminidase Inhibitors to Prevent or Treat Influenza Types A and B

Oseltamivir and zanamivir are two neuraminidase inhibitors released for use in North America in 1999. Oseltamivir is metabolized to oseltamivir carboxylate and inhibits the influenza enzyme neuraminidase. Such inhibition results in reduced release of the virus from infected cells. Zanamivir also inhibits influenza neuraminidase and works in a manner similar to oseltamivir. It is administered by inhalation.

oseltamivir [oh sel **tam** i veer]
(Tamiflu)

Indications
Oseltamivir is used to treat influenza infection types A and B for children older than 1 year of age. It is also used as prophylaxis for influenza in at-risk adults and adolescents older than 13 years of age.

Pharmacokinetics/Dosing
Oseltamivir is well absorbed orally and metabolized to the active metabolite oseltamivir carboxylate. The parent compound and its active metabolite are eliminated in the urine. Treatment must be initiated within 2 days of the onset of symptoms and is dosed at 75 mg orally twice daily for adults. Prophylaxis dosing for adults is 75 mg once daily. Dosage reduction is recommended for clients with renal dysfunction.

Adverse Effects
Oseltamivir is fairly well tolerated with GI complaints (particularly nausea and vomiting) being the most frequently observed adverse effects. Oseltamivir is not indicated for children under the age of 1 year because of potential for toxicity in this population (Iacuzio, 2003).

Drug Interactions
Concurrent use of probenecid may result in increased levels of oseltamivir, but no adjustment of dose is recommended.

zanamivir [za **na** mi veer]
(Relenza)

Indications
Zanamivir is indicated for treatment of influenza in adults and children older than 7 years of age provided that therapy is initiated within 2 days of onset of symptoms. Its role in preventing influenza infection is considered investigational.

Pharmacokinetics/Dosing
The dry power for inhalation is available as a blister pack in a Rotadisk delivery system. Systemic absorption is low with inhaled administration. The adult dose for treatment is two inhalations twice daily for 5 days.

Adverse Effects
The most frequently observed adverse effects of zanamivir are GI upset and respiratory irritation. Use of inhaled zanamivir is not recommended for clients with asthma, chronic obstructive pulmonary dis-

ease, or other chronic lung disease because of increased potential for bronchospasm.

⚙ **Because of the severity of the flu symptoms in the affected personnel, the Medical Director of the long-term care facility decides to provide amantadine prophylaxis for the residents and staff of the institution.**

⚙ **What are the nursing implications of the use of amantadine and the other antivirals indicated for influenza?**

Assessment The following health problems necessitate the cautious use of amantadine: heart failure and/or peripheral edema (the drug may worsen the condition), epilepsy (the drug may increase seizure activity), untreated angle closure glaucoma (the drug has anticholinergic effects), suicide attempts (drug increases the risk of suicide ideation), hepatic impairment, and renal impairment (accumulation of the drug increases the risk of adverse CNS effects). Adults older than 65 years of age are more prone to confusion and difficulty in urination as common effects of amantadine because of its antimuscarinic activity and may require lower dosages. In particular, lower doses are required for all clients with any degree of renal dysfunction because of accumulation of the drug and higher potential for CNS toxicity. Assess for hypersensitivity to the specific antiviral agent as well.

Review the client's current drug regimen for the risk of significant drug interactions, such as those that may occur when amantadine is coadministered with anticholinergics (may result in an increase in anticholinergic adverse effects, such as hallucinations, dry mouth, blurred vision, confusion, and nightmares) and CNS-stimulating agents (may cause increased CNS stimulation, resulting in insomnia, increased irritability, nervousness, cardiac dysrhythmias and seizures). Quinidine, triamterene, thiazide diuretics, and trimethoprim/sulfamethoxazole coadministered with amantadine may result in higher plasma amantadine concentrations.

If amantadine is used for the treatment of active influenza infection, document a baseline assessment of the client's infection and neurologic status before initiating amantadine therapy.

Although the other drugs used for influenza do not have the contraindications that amantadine does, except for careful dosing in adults older than 65 years of age, rimantadine does have the same cautions for epilepsy, renal, and hepatic impairment. When rimantadine is coadministered with aspirin and acetaminophen, its plasma concentrations are reduced, and cimetidine increases its plasma concentrations. No clinically important drug interactions are reported for oseltamivir and zanamivir.

Nursing Diagnosis Assess the client receiving amantadine for the possibility of the following nursing diagnoses/collaborative problems: impaired comfort (rash, headache,

dry mouth, anorexia, and nausea); disturbed sleep pattern (insomnia); risk for injury related to lightheadedness secondary to orthostatic hypotension; fatigue; disturbed thought processes (confusion, hallucinations, severe mental or mood changes) related to the anticholinergic effects; impaired verbal communication related to the CNS effects (slurred speech); risk for self-harm; impaired urinary elimination (retention); constipation; and the potential complications of CNS toxicity (seizures), corneal opacity, heart failure, and livedo reticularis (purplish spots on the skin; occurs with chronic therapy only). The administration of rimantadine requires assessment for impaired comfort (dyspepsia, nausea, dry mouth, abdominal pain); disturbed sleep pattern (insomnia); diarrhea; and the potential complications of CNS toxicity (seizure) and the development of rimantadine-resistant virus. The administration of zanamivir may result in ineffective airway clearance (cough, asthma); diarrhea and impaired comfort (headache, nausea). Oseltamivir is similar to zanamivir with the addition of the nursing diagnosis of risk for injury related to vertigo.

Planning The goals for the use of these drugs are to:
- If given prophylactically, prevent or abort an occurrence of influenza without drug adverse effects.
- If given therapeutically, mitigate the client's symptoms of influenza (fever, chills, malaise, muscular aching, headache, nasal stuffiness, nausea) without adverse effects of the drug.

Implementation
Monitoring Closely monitor clients for the nursing diagnoses and potential complications listed above. Monitor blood pressure, temperature, pulse, and respirations to record the progress of the illness and the effectiveness of therapy.

Monitor the client throughout the course of therapy if taking amantadine for parkinsonism or for dyskinetic symptoms such as tremors, rigidity, and gait disturbances. Clients with Parkinson's disease should not discontinue drug therapy abruptly; to do so may result in a parkinsonian crisis, rigidity, tremor, and psychic disturbances.

Intervention If these antiviral agents are administered as chemoprophylactic agents, they should be started in anticipation of contact with, or as soon after exposure to, individuals with influenza infections and continued for at least 10 days after exposure. Continue therapy for 2 to 3 weeks if given concurrently with the influenza vaccine; this allows immunity from the influenza vaccine to develop.

Changing from a once-daily dosage to a twice-daily schedule of amantadine may minimize syncope, insomnia, and nausea. Administering the last daily dose several hours before bedtime helps to minimize insomnia.

Education Caution the client to avoid alcoholic beverages while taking these antivirals, because alcohol increases the risk of CNS effects such as dizziness, syncope, and confusion. Mental confusion, hallucinations, and difficulty sleeping are indications of CNS toxicity; report them to the prescriber promptly. Because amantadine may cause dizziness, alert the client to avoid tasks such as driving until the response to the drug has been determined. Because of the orthostatic effects, advise the client to use caution when changing positions from lying to sitting or standing and from sitting to standing. To decrease the discomfort of mouth dryness, clients may use ice, sugarless gum, or candy. The client should complete the full course of therapy and should notify the prescriber if viral infection symptoms do not decrease within a few days.

Clients taking amantadine as an antidyskinetic medication should complete the course of therapy as prescribed and not take more than the prescribed dosage. Advise the client that it may require 2 or more weeks to obtain the full benefit of the drug. Counsel the client to resume physical activities gradually. The drug should be discontinued gradually. Alert the client to the possible occurrence of a purplish red rash, which disappears 2 to 12 weeks after the drug is discontinued.

Evaluation If administered for its antiviral effect, the expected outcome will be decreased risk for infection of the susceptible client. If given therapeutically, the client will experience fewer symptoms of influenza for less time without adverse effects of the drug (e.g., headache, nausea, insomnia, confusion, fatigue). If amantadine therapy is administered for extrapyramidal symptoms, the expected outcome is that the client will experience improved motor control with decreased tremor.

Acquired Immunodeficiency Syndrome

HIV is the etiologic agent in AIDS (Box 64-1). As of the end of 2003, an estimated 37.8 million people worldwide, 35.7 million adults and 2.1 million children younger than 15 years of age, were living with HIV/AIDS. Approximately two thirds of these people (25 million) live in Sub-Saharan Africa; another 20% (7.4 million) live in Asia and the Pacific. Worldwide, approximately 11 of every 1000 adults aged 15 to 49 are HIV-infected. In Sub-Saharan Africa, about 7.5% of all adults in this age group are HIV-infected. Women account for nearly half of all people worldwide living with HIV/AIDS (UNAIDS, 2004).

⚹ **T.P. is a 32-year-old female with a 4-year history of HIV infection. She has regular visits with her health care provider and visits the lab for a viral load and CD4⁺ count every 3 months. Her latest HIV-1 RNA count is about 5000 copies/mL and her CD4⁺ count is 625 cells/mm³. T.P. and her health care provider have elected to hold off on using antiretroviral drug therapy until her viral load is above 20,000 plasma HIV-1 RNA copies/mL or her CD4⁺ count is below 350 cells/mm³.**

⚹ **What is the burden of HIV/AIDS in the United States?**
The CDC in the United States estimate that 850,000 to 950,000 U.S. residents are living with HIV infection, one-quarter of who are unaware of their infection. Approximately 40,000 new HIV infections occur each year in the United States, about 70% among men and 30% among women. Of these newly infected people, half are younger than 25 years of age. Of new infections among men in the United States, CDC estimates that approximately 60% of men were infected through homosexual sex, 25% through injection drug use, and 15% through heterosexual sex. Of newly infected men, approximately 50% are black, 30% are white, 20% are Hispanic, and a small percentage is members of other racial/ethnic groups (CDC, 2001). The estimated annual number of AIDS-related deaths in the United States fell approximately 14% from 1998 to 2002, from 19,005 deaths in 1998 to 16,371 deaths in 2002 (CDC, 2002). However, HIV infection is the fifth leading cause of death for people who are 25 to 44 years old in the United States, and is the leading cause of death for African American men ages 35 to 44 (National Center for Health Statistics [NCHS], 2004).

⚹ **What is the burden of HIV/AIDS in Canada?**
The U.S. pattern also holds for Canada in which the number of deaths among reported AIDS cases peaked in 1995 at 1500 per year and has been declining annually until it was 93 per year in 2003 (Centre for Infections Disease Prevention and Control [CIDPC], 2004). This change in AIDS-related deaths is largely a result of new drugs (especially the protease inhibitors) and, perhaps, more effective prevention programs. In Canada, an estimated 49,800 people were living with HIV or AIDS at the end of 1999. Although many infected individuals are living longer, healthier lives, and the rate of deaths from AIDS and AIDS-related illnesses has declined, Canada's HIV/AIDS epidemic has evolved in unforeseen and alarming ways. Most disturbing is the fact that the virus continues to spread. The annual number of positive HIV tests declined from 2996 in 1995 to 2187 in 2001 and has since increased to 2504 in 2002 and 2482 in 2003 (CIDPC, 2004). Despite evidence that Canadians generally have a good understanding of modes of HIV transmission, risk factors, and prevention options, about 4200 new infections occur in Canada each year. Although men who have sex with men and injection drug users continue to be hit hardest by the epidemic, HIV/AIDS is increasingly spreading through heterosexual transmission (Public Health Agency of Canada, 2002).

⚹ **What are the concerns about the transmission of HIV?**
The early worldwide spread of HIV disease was primarily among homosexual men, IV substance abusers, and persons receiving contaminated blood products. Over the past decade, an increased incidence has been reported in heterosexuals, especially females and infants. Most AIDS cases in children are a result of perinatal transmission. Although

AIDS can affect all populations, current statistics indicate that the incidence of cases in children is much more common in black and Hispanic children than in Caucasian children.

HIV is transmitted sexually, via blood and blood products, or from a mother with AIDS to her child during birth. Transmission through commercial blood transfusion is considered rare today, but transmission via IV substance abuse is still very common. HIV is transmitted by intimate contact with the body fluids of an infected person, which can occur through sex, sharing of contaminated needles and syringes, blood or blood products, and from mother to child, before, during, or shortly after birth. Health care providers are at increased risk because of their exposure to human blood and body secretions. Following universal precautions with all clients greatly reduces health care worker risk.

The CDC has issued guidelines for health care workers to follow to minimize the possibility of virus exposure and transfer. Postexposure prophylaxis (PEP) is recommended when health care personnel are exposed to HIV in the workplace and it is a high-risk exposure (punctured skin). Similar recommendations are endorsed to prevent sexually transmitted HIV (Smith et al., 2005). Recommendations for HIV PEP include a basic 4-week regimen of two drugs (zidovudine and lamivudine; lamivudine and stavudine; or didanosine and stavudine) for most HIV exposures and an expanded regimen that includes the addition of a third drug for HIV exposures that pose an increased risk for transmission. When the source person's virus is known or suspected to be resistant to one or more of the drugs considered for the PEP regimen, the selection of drugs to which the source person's virus is unlikely to be resistant is recommended. Additionally, some special circumstances, such as delayed exposure report, unknown source person, pregnancy in the exposed person, resistance of the source virus to antiretroviral agents, or toxicity of the PEP regimen, then consultation with local experts and/or the National Clinicians' Post-Exposure Prophylaxis Hotline (PEPline) at 1-888-448-4911 is advised. Occupational exposures should be considered urgent medical concerns to ensure timely postexposure management (United States Public Health Service, 2001).

AIDS is a deadly disease and there is no known cure for it at this time; therefore client teaching should focus on disease prevention.

HIV Life Cycle

Although the pathogenesis of AIDS is not fully understood, HIV is an intracellular infection that primarily infests CD4+ T lymphocytes (Figure 59-1). The virus is a retrovirus that has RNA in its core; after it binds to CD4+ T lymphocyte receptor cells in the body, it releases its RNA into the cytoplasm. It also has the potential of infecting monocytes and macrophages. Reverse transcriptase, an enzyme carried by HIV, assists in transcribing the HIV RNA into viral DNA strands in the host body. Thereafter, activation of this DNA will result in the production of viral substances that infect other CD4+ T lymphocyte cells; this leads to the eventual loss of functioning CD4+ lymphocytes.

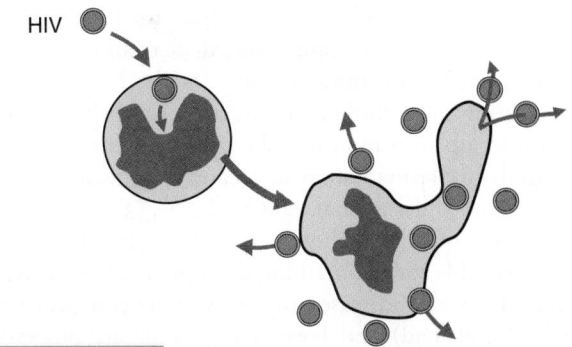

FIGURE 59-1 Infection of CD4+ T lymphocytes by HIV is followed by viral replication and spread to other cells.

The CD4+ helper cells are destroyed by the virus, which eventually leads to the immunodeficiency disease known as AIDS. The CD4+ cells are needed directly and indirectly for proper functioning of the human immune system. Both the humoral immune response, which involves antibodies produced by B lymphocytes, and the cellular immune response involving stimulation of the cytotoxic T cells are mediated by the helper-inducer T cells. Therefore a severe decline or destruction of CD4+ T cells by HIV is responsible for the multiple symptoms of AIDS—severe suppression of the immune system leading to opportunistic infections and cancers.

The revised CDC classification for HIV infection emphasizes the importance of the CD4+ T lymphocyte count. This system includes all symptomatic and asymptomatic persons:

- Category 1: CD4+ T cell count greater than 500 cells/mm³ (or CD4+% greater than 28%)
- Category 2: CD4+ T cell count 200 to 499 cells/mm³ (or CD4+% 14% to 28%)
- Category 3: CD4+ T cell count less than 200 cells/mm³ (or CD4+% less than 14%)

The presence of particular symptoms further differentiates these categories into more refined clinical categories A, B, or C. This expanded definition has been estimated to result in an increased number of AIDS cases reported initially, thus allowing for better surveillance and earlier interventions for this devastating disease state.

As CD4+ T cells decline, the risk and severity of opportunistic infections increases; therefore the use of this system helps to identify persons in need of close medical attention. Instituting antiviral therapy and antimicrobial prophylaxis in correlation with HIV immunosuppression levels as measured by CD4+ T lymphocytes has slowed the rate of progression from HIV status to AIDS-defined clinical conditions.

✴ How are viral loads and CD4+ counts used to evaluate antiviral therapy and the progression of HIV disease?

The viral load, or number of copies of HIV-1 RNA in the plasma, is indicative of the degree of viral replication in the client. During initial infection (immediately after exposure), the viral load is high and may remain elevated for weeks or months. Viral load then declines for 12 months or years until later stage disease is noted. Screening for HIV antibodies has been routine for two decades but may miss early infection since antibody production lags behind initial infection by up to 6 months. The measurement of HIV-1 RNA levels in plasma is now advocated to screen for early HIV infection (Pilcher et al., 2005).

The target of HIV is the CD4+ cell (a type of lymphocyte) responsible for maintaining defenses against infection and cancer. As HIV disease progresses, more copies of viral particles (viral load) and fewer CD4+ cells are observed. These levels are now routinely used both to assess client disease status and to evaluate response to any given drug therapy. The decision regarding when to begin antiretroviral therapy is complex, and relates to the client's status, the likelihood that the client will strictly adhere to therapy, and whether the HIV-1 strain is sensitive or resistant to existing therapy. Resistance has become more commonplace because short interruptions in therapy (e.g., greater than 24 hours) allows for an interruption in viral suppression and the potential for the development of mutant strains to flourish without competition. Up-to-date information about treatment decisions, monitoring parameters, and when to start and stop therapy are published at www.aidsinfo/nih/gov.

✹ What drugs are available for treating HIV disease?

Drugs used in the treatment of HIV disease include those that target the HIV virus itself (antiretrovirals), and those used to prevent or treat opportunistic infections associated with advanced AIDS. The antiretrovirals are divided into four categories: (1) nucleoside reverse transcriptase inhibitors, (2) nonnucleoside reverse transcriptase inhibitors, (3) protease inhibitors, and (4) fusion inhibitors. These agents, when used alone, quickly become ineffective due to HIV resistance. As such, they are always used in combination of at least two, and more often three or four, agents and are often referred to by clients as "drug cocktails." In addition to combining agents with different actions or resistance patterns, it is critical that therapy remain uninterrupted to prevent HIV resistance from developing.

Resistance to HIV therapies has become more common, and newly infected clients may acquire an HIV-resistant strain (Markowitz et al., 2005). Frequently, infectious disease specialists test the HIV strain to establish resistance before using an initial regimen with a client. Once a client is maintained on a drug regimen, regular monitoring of CD4+ and viral load counts help clinicians to establish efficacy or resistance to therapy. Factors including tolerability, ease of dosing, adherence, and cost are also considerations in choice of combination therapies. Aggressive education and support is required for clients to adhere to these regimens, and the nurse is essential to helping the client understand the disease, the therapy, and how the disease and drug therapy interface with the client's psychosocial well-being.

Chapter 58 and this chapter discuss the drugs used to treat opportunistic infections. Table 59-4 lists common opportunistic infections associated with advanced HIV and the drugs used to treat them.

✹ **T.P. is 6 years into her HIV infection and reviews her viral load (22,000 HIV-1 RNA copies/mL) and CD4+ count (390 cells/mm³) with her health care providers. After discussion of regimen choices, their adverse effects, and dosing regimens, T.P. and her provider start highly active antiretroviral therapy (HAART) with lopinavir/ritonavir 400 mg/100 mg twice daily, lamivudine 150 mg twice daily, and zidovudine 300 mg twice daily. Her health care providers counsel her about the use of these drugs.**

✹ What are the principles of use for antiretroviral therapy in the management of HIV in adults?

Guidelines for the management of HIV with antiretroviral therapy are continuously evolving. The Panel on Clinical Practices for Treatment of HIV Infection, under the support of the U.S. Department of Health and Human Services, published updated guidelines in October 2004 to assist clinicians and clients in the effective and evidence based use of drug therapy in HIV management (Bartlet & Lane, 2004). Goals of therapy are to suppress viremia to below the level of detection of viral particles in blood, prevent further deterioration of the immune system, and avoid HIV-related morbidity and mortality.

To achieve these goals, the Panel recommends that use of combinations of HAART be initiated before CD4+ counts fall below 200 cell/mm³, and that some clients benefit from initiation of therapy when HIV-RNA loads are greater than 100,000 copies/mL even if CD4+ counts are above 350 cells/mm³. Combination of two nucleotide reverse transcriptase inhibitors (NRTIs) and either a nonnucleoside reverse transcriptase inhibitor (NNRTI) or protease inhibitor (PI) is preferred for initial therapy. Drug combinations involving similar mechanisms of action, additive toxicities, or antagonistic actions are generally avoided. Limitations to the use of HAART include difficulty in drug adherence for some clients, short- and long-term toxicities, and significant drug interactions. Women who are pregnant or of childbearing potential, clients with concurrent opportunistic or other infections (e.g., hepatitis B, hepatitis C, tuberculosis), and children or adolescents often require special consideration. For any client who experiences treatment failure, resistance testing is often utilized. Current guidelines, including specific recommendations for combination therapies are available at http://www.aidsinfo.nih.gov.

✹ What are the key nursing issues involved in the use of HIV drug treatments for T.P.?

Assessment Assess T.P. and document her physical and psychologic status. For some viral illnesses, such as herpes zoster or viral pneumonia, the disease episode is acute and self-limiting, but many more emotional and social issues complicate a diagnosis of HIV. The baseline assessment includes nutritional, respiratory, neurologic, and fluid and electrolyte status; a description of the skin and mucous membranes; and the client's level of knowledge and emotional response to the diagnosis (Box 59-2). Potential risk

Table 59-4 Examples of Potential Opportunistic Infections Observed with Advanced HIV Disease and Possible Therapeutic Agents

Opportunistic Infection	Agents Used for Possible Prophylaxis and/or Treatment*
Cryptococcus neoformans	amphotericin B fluconazole flucytosine itraconazole
Cytomegalovirus (CMV)	cidofovir foscarnet ganciclovir valganciclovir
Hepatitis A virus	hepatitis A vaccine
Hepatitis B virus	hepatitis B vaccine
Hepatitis C virus	hepatitis A vaccine (to prevent co-infection) peginterferon ribavirin
Histoplasma capsulatum	amphotericin B fluconazole itraconazole
Mycobacterium avium complex	azithromycin clarithromycin ethambutol rifabutin
Mycobacterium tuberculosis	ethambutol isoniazid/pyridoxine pyrazinamide rifabutin rifampin
Pneumocystis jiroveci pneumonia (PCP)	atovaquone clindamycin corticosteroids often added for severe disease dapsone pentamidine primaquine sulfamethoxazole/trimethoprim trimethoprim trimetrexate/leucovorin
Toxoplasma gondii	atovaquone azithromycin clindamycin dapsone pyrimethamine/leucovorin sulfadiazine sulfamethoxazole/trimethoprim
Varicella zoster virus	acyclovir famciclovir foscarnet valacyclovir varicella zoster immune globulin

Modified from Benson, C.A., Kaplan, J.E., Masur, H., Pau, A., Holmes, K.K. (December 17, 2004). Treating Opportunistic Infections Among HIV-Infected Adults and Adolescents – Recommendations from CDC, the National Institutes of Health, and the HIV Medicine Association/Infectious Diseases Society of America. *Morbidity and Mortality Weekly Report, 53*, (RR15), 1-112. Retrieved February 4, 2005, from http://www.cdc.gov/mmwr/preview/mmwrhtml/rr5315 a1.htm.

*Combinations of agents sometimes used in treatment and occasionally in prophylaxis. Refer to http://www.cdc.gov/mmwr/preview/mmwrhtml/rr5315 a1.htm for additional opportunistic infections and more details on treatments.

BOX 59-2 ASSESSMENT OF THE CLIENT WITH AIDS

STATUS OF ILLNESS

- CD4$^+$ lymphocyte count
- HIV viral load
- Testing of drug sensitivity of HIV strain

NUTRITIONAL STATUS

- Height and weight
- Oral intake
- Weight loss
- Factors that could interfere with oral intake (anorexia, nausea, vomiting, mouth ulcers, gingival disease, difficulty swallowing)
- Serum protein, BUN, albumin, transferrin levels

RESPIRATORY STATUS

- Presence and quality of breath sounds
- Cough, sputum production, shortness of breath, tachypnea, chest pain
- Chest radiograph examination findings, arterial blood gases, pulmonary function test results

NEUROLOGIC STATUS

- Level of consciousness, orientation, memory lapses, mental status
- Sensory deficits (visual disturbances, numbness and tingling in the extremities)

- Motor involvement (weakness, altered gait, paralysis)
- Seizure activity

SKIN AND MUCOUS MEMBRANES

- Evidence of breakdown, ulceration, infection
- Mouth ulcerations, stomatitis, thrush
- Perianal excoriation, infection
- Wound cultures

FLUID AND ELECTROLYTE STATUS

- Fever, night sweats
- Turgor and dryness of skin and mucous membranes
- Thirst; urinary output; hypotension; irregular, weak, and rapid pulse
- Nausea, vomiting, diarrhea
- Decreased mental status, muscle twitching or cramps
- Serum electrolytes: sodium, potassium, calcium, magnesium, chloride

RESPONSE TO DIAGNOSIS

- Level of knowledge: disease and methods of transmission
- Reaction to illness: denial, anger, fear, shame, depression
- Identifiable sources of social support

Modified from Smeltzer, S.C., & Bare, B.G. (2003). *Brunner and Suddarth's textbook of medical-surgical nursing* (10th ed.). Philadelphia: J.B. Lippincott.

---

factors are identified with T.P. (e.g., sexual practices and IV drug use). A physiologic baseline includes a CBC with WBC differential and platelets, CD4$^+$ counts, measures of viral load, serum electrolytes and lipids, and renal and hepatic function studies. As with any medication, impaired renal and hepatic function places her at higher risk for drug toxicities; this is especially true with the antivirals. T.P.'s hypersensitivity to the drugs should be determined and documented.

Nursing Diagnosis Although many nursing diagnoses/collaborative problems are related to the viral diseases themselves, some are directly related to the antiviral medications: activity intolerance related to weakness and fatigue; ineffective protection related to blood dyscrasias (anemia, leukopenia, thrombocytopenia); and the potential complication of CNS toxicity (confusion, dizziness). The protease inhibits also have the potential complications of hyperglycemia and peripheral neuropathy.

Planning The goals of T.P.'s antiviral therapy are that she will:

- Experience no further progression of HIV disease with minimal adverse drug effects.
- Effectively manage the therapeutic regimen, including being compliant with medications, and implementing nonpharmacologic supportive measures.

- Collaborate with health care providers by appropriately reporting untoward symptoms and maintaining scheduled visits for monitoring and treatment.

Implementation

Monitoring Document an ongoing assessment of T.P.'s clinical status, including the signs and symptoms of HIV infection, CD4$^+$ count, viral load, and the presence of opportunistic infection. Also monitor the results of CBCs, serum electrolytes, lipids, and glucose and renal and hepatic function tests.

Intervention Timeliness is important in administering antiviral medications. If these antiviral drugs were to be given prophylactically, it is important to initiate the medications as soon as possible. Because of the adverse effect profiles of the antivirals, T.P. and her provider have decided to initiate HAART therapy later in the course of her illness. Once the drug therapy is begun, it is essential that they be administered on time and around-the-clock to maintain therapeutic serum levels, to reduce viral load, and to prevent viral resistance to the drug.

Education Instruct T.P. to self-manage a complex medication regimen, including the use of a written drug regimen for the 24 hours and an alarm clock to assist in maintaining compliance. Stress the importance of not taking more medication than prescribed. Many clients may increase their dosage with the erroneous belief that doing so will provide a "cure"; instead they experience greater drug toxicities. It is also important that T.P. not discontinue the antiviral medication without consulting with the prescriber. Many drugs have discomforting adverse effects but may be managed with changes of dosages, schedules, antiemetics, or other palliative measures. Stress to T.P. the importance of complying with the medication regimen, taking the drugs at evenly spaced times and not missing doses. Because many of the antivirals have serious drug interactions with a number of drugs, caution her not to take other medications, even over-the-counter (OTC) medications, without checking with the prescriber. See individual drug monographs for specific administration measures.

Stress the importance of regular visits to the prescriber for blood tests to monitor the progress of therapy and to detect any adverse effects from drug therapy as early as possible. Encourage T.P. to report any adverse effects to the prescriber as soon as possible.

Caution T.P. that antiviral therapy does not cure HIV or prevent its spread to others. Instruct in the avoidance of sexual contact, the use of condoms, the avoidance of sharing needles or giving blood to prevent the spread of the infection to others, and breastfeeding. See the Pregnancy Safety box on p. 1071 for individual drugs.

Advise T.P. to alert her dentist so that dental work may be planned around the bone marrow depressant effects of the drugs that may result in gingival bleeding and delayed healing. Teach appropriate oral hygiene, including the gentle use of toothbrushes and floss and the avoidance of toothpicks.

Evaluation The expected outcome of antiviral therapy is that T.P. will experience a decrease in symptoms related to the underlying viral infection. She should experience a slowed progression of the HIV infection, increased CD4$^+$ counts, decreased viral loads, and an absence of opportunistic infections and other adverse drug effects (e.g., confusion, blood dyscrasias, peripheral neuropathy). She will effectively manage her complex medication regimen and collaborate with health providers for life-long monitoring and treatment.

Nucleoside Reverse Transcriptase Inhibitors

The NRTIs were among the first agents used to treat HIV infection. These drugs inhibit the activity of reverse transcriptase, an early step in HIV infection in CD4$^+$ cells. They act by mimicking naturally occurring nucleosides and become incorporated in the conversion of viral RNA to DNA. Table 59-5 compares agents in this class, including abacavir, didanosine, emtricitabine, lamivudine, stavudine, tenofovir, zalcitabine, and zidovudine. Many of these products may be found in combination formulations to enhance client adherence (e.g., Combivir is a combined formulation

of lamivudine and zidovudine; Epzicom combines abacavir and lamivudine in the same tablet; Trizivir is a formulation of abacavir, lamivudine and zidovudine; Trivia is a combination of emtricitabine and tenofovir).

Zidovudine was the first available agent in the treatment of HIV and is considered the prototype agent. It is converted in the CD4$^+$ cell to monophosphate, diphosphate, and then zidovudine triphosphate by cellular enzymes. The triphosphate form competes with natural thymidine triphosphate for incorporation into growing chains of viral RNA-dependent DNA polymerase (reverse transcriptase), thus inhibiting viral DNA replication. It has a greater affinity for retroviral reverse transcriptase than for the human α-DNA polymerase; thus it selectively inhibits viral replication.

Abacavir is a synthetic nucleoside with inhibitory effects against HIV. Abacavir inhibits reverse transcriptase by two mechanisms: (1) competing with the natural substrate dGTP, and (2) being incorporated into the viral DNA. The result is the termination of viral DNA growth. Didanosine is converted intracellularly to its active form, ddA-TP; this in turn inhibits HIV DNA reverse transcriptase and results in the suppression of HIV replication. Emtricitabine is an analog of cytosine that undergoes alteration in the cell to inhibit viral RNA dependent DNA polymerase. Lamivudine is converted in the body to an active metabolite (L-TP), which then inhibits HIV reverse transcription by terminating the viral DNA chain. Lamivudine also inhibits RNA and DNA-dependent DNA polymerase functions of reverse transcriptase. Stavudine is converted to stavudine triphosphate, which then competes with deoxythymidine triphosphate and results in the inhibition of HIV replication and DNA synthesis. Tenofovir is an adenosine mono-phosphate analog that acts as a reverse transcriptase inhibitor. Zalcitabine, an antiviral agent, is converted by cellular enzymes to its active form (ddC-TP), which inhibits viral reverse transcriptase, thereby inhibiting viral replication.

Each of these agents differ in adverse effect profiles, although they all share the risk of lactic acidosis and hepatomegaly with steatosis that may be more pronounced with chronic use or in clients who are obese.

★⬛⬛ zidovudine [zye **doe** vue deen]

(AZT, Retrovir, Apo-Zidovudine✦)

Indications

Zidovudine is indicated for the treatment of HIV infection and AIDS in combination with at least two other agents. It is available in combination with other agents, including lamivudine/zidovudine (Combivir) and abacavir/lamivudine/zidovudine (Trizivir).

It is also indicated for monotherapy in the prevention of HIV transmission to the fetus in mothers who are HIV-positive. It is used in combination with other antiretrovirals to prevent HIV immediately after exposure (e.g., needle sticks), although this is not an officially FDA-approved indication.

Pharmacokinetics/Dosing

Administered orally, zidovudine is rapidly absorbed and distributed in the plasma and CSF. It reaches a peak serum level in 0.5 to 1.5 hours and has a half-life of approximately 1 hour (in serum, 3.3 hours intracellularly). It is metabolized in the liver and excreted by

TABLE 59-5 COMPARATIVE AGENTS FOR HIV

Agent	Typical Adult Dose*	Major Adverse Effects	Comments
NUCLEOSIDE REVERSE TRANSCRIPTASE INHIBITORS (NRTIs)			
abacavir (Ziagen)	300 mg PO twice daily OR 600 mg PO once daily	Hypersensitivity reactions, nausea, vomiting, diarrhea	Hypersensitivity reaction may be fatal.
didanosine (ddI, Videx)	167-250 mg PO q12h OR 400 mg PO once daily	Peripheral neuropathies, CNS toxicity	Degraded by gastric acid.
emtricitabine (Emtriva)	200 mg PO daily	Lactic acidosis, headache, cough, GI upset	
lamivudine (3TC, Epivir, Epivir-HBV)	150 mg PO twice daily OR 300 mg PO once daily	Headache, GI upset, anorexia, peripheral neuropathies, depression, muscle pain, insomnia	Also used for hepatitis B infection.
stavudine (d4 T, Zerit)	30-40 mg PO q12h OR 75-100 mg extended release PO once daily	Peripheral neuropathies, anemia	Hold dose if peripheral neuropathy noted. Contraindicated with zidovudine.
tenofovir (Viread)	300 mg PO daily	Nausea, GI upset	Dosing with high fat meal increases bioavailability.
zalcitabine (ddC, HIVID)	0.75 mg PO q8h	Peripheral neuropathy, GI upset, headache	
zidovudine (AZT, Retrovir)	300 mg PO twice daily OR 200 mg PO three times daily	Nausea, GI upset, anemia, bone marrow suppression, headache, insomnia, myalgia	IV formulation available. Contraindicated with stavudine.
NONNUCLEOSIDE REVERSE TRANSCRIPTASE INHIBITORS (NNRTIs)			
delavirdine (Rescriptor)	400 mg PO three times daily	Nausea, GI upset, fatigue, rash, joint/muscle pain	
efavirenz (Sustiva)	600 mg PO daily at bedtime	Rash, nausea, GI upset, insomnia, fatigue, confusion	Avoid with fatty meal. Numerous drug interactions.
nevirapine (Viramune)	200 mg PO daily × 2 weeks, then 200 mg PO twice daily	Nausea, headache, Stevens-Johnson syndrome	Severe rash could indicate Stevens-Johnson syndrome.
PROTEASE INHIBITORS (PIs)			
amprenavir (Agenerase)	Capsule: 1200 mg PO twice daily Liquid: 1400 mg PO three times daily	Hyperglycemia, hyperlipidemia, altered body fat, hepatic injury, rash, GI upset, depression, Stevens-Johnson syndrome	Numerous significant drug interactions possible, and dosage adjustment may be necessary. See package labeling for complete information.
atazanavir (Reyataz)	400 mg PO daily		
fosamprenavir (Lexiva)	700-1400 mg PO twice daily		
indinavir (Crixivan)	800 mg PO q8h		
lopinavir/ ritonavir (Kaletra)	400 mg/100 mg PO twice daily		

CNS, Central nervous system; *GI*, gastrointestinal; *HIV*, human immunodeficiency virus.

*Dosing represents typical adult dose with normal renal and hepatic function. Dose recommendation may be based on concurrent drug therapy. Always check updated reference for more complete information.

†Lower doses are sometimes used to enhance levels of other protease inhibitors.

TABLE 59-5 COMPARATIVE AGENTS FOR HIV—cont'd

Agent	Typical Adult Dose*	Major Adverse Effects	Comments
PROTEASE INHIBITORS (PIs)—cont'd			
nelfinavir (Viracept)	1250 mg PO twice daily OR 750 mg PO three times daily	Hyperglycemia, hyperlipidemia, altered body fat, hepatic injury, rash, GI upset, depression, Stevens-Johnson syndrome	Numerous significant drug interactions possible, and dosage adjustment may be necessary. See package labeling for complete information.
ritonavir (Norvir)	Titrate up to 600 mg PO twice daily over 5 days†		
saquinavir (Fortovase, Invirase)	Dependent on formulation Invirase: 600 mg PO three times daily		
FUSION INHIBITOR			
enfuvirtide (Fuzeon)	90 mg subcutaneously twice daily	Injection site reactions, hypersensitivity, pneumonia, peripheral neuropathy, anorexia, hyperlipidemias	Restricted access in United States. 1-866-694-6670 for information.

the kidneys. Dosage varies based on client age/weight and indication. The typical adult dose for treatment of HIV or prevention of fetal transmission in a pregnant woman is 300 mg PO twice daily or 200 mg PO three times daily. For prevention of HIV after needle sticks, it is often dosed with lamivudine (e.g., zidovudine 300 mg twice daily plus lamivudine 130 mg twice daily), adding a protease inhibitor for high-risk exposures.

An IV formulation is also available for use during labor and delivery or when oral access is not available. The parenteral adult dosage for symptomatic HIV infection is 1 to 2 mg/kg by IV infusion, administered over 60 minutes every 4 hours around-the-clock until oral therapy can be used. The pediatric dosage is 120 mg/m² every 6 hours.

Adverse Effects
The most serious adverse effects of zidovudine include bone marrow suppression, hepatotoxicity, lactic acidosis and hypersensitivity reactions, including Stevens-Johnson syndrome and toxic epidermal necrolysis. Nausea and severe headaches are quite common with zidovudine. Other adverse effects include myalgia, insomnia, cardiotoxicity (rare), gynecomastia, and muscle/joint pain and weakness.

Drug Interactions
Stavudine and zidovudine should not be used together because efficacy of both agents is reduced in combination. Increased risk for bone marrow suppression is possible with concurrent interferon, acyclovir, ganciclovir, and dapsone, or immunosuppressant agents. Elevated zidovudine levels and/or risk for toxicity are associated with a number of drugs, including those that are nephrotoxic (e.g., aminoglycosides, amphotericin B), or interfere with elimination (acetaminophen, cimetidine, indomethacin). Valproic acid may result in elevated zidovudine levels, as may lamivudine. Risk for lactic acidosis in increased with concurrent ribavirin therapy and other NRTIs.

Nursing Management
See the case of T.P. beginning on p. 1076 for general nursing management related to antiviral therapy with HIV. In addition to general nursing management with antivirals, IV zidovudine is given at a constant rate over 1 hour. Zidovudine should not be admixed with biological or colloidal solutions (e.g., blood or protein-containing solutions).

abacavir [ah **ba** ka veer]
(Ziagen)
Indications
Abacavir is used in the treatment of HIV infection in combination with other agents active against HIV, such as the combination of abacavir/lamivudine/zidovudine, Trizivir.

Pharmacokinetics/Dosing
Abacavir is a pro-drug that is converted in the cell to carbovir triphosphate, an active metabolite. Administered orally, abacavir is rapidly absorbed and is distributed in the blood and erythrocytes. It has an elimination half-life of 1 to 2 hours. It is metabolized by alcohol dehydrogenase and excreted primarily in urine. See Table 59-5 for adult dosing. Children 3 months to 16 years of age receive 8 mg/kg PO twice daily (up to a maximum of 300 mg twice daily) in combination with other antiretroviral agents.

Adverse Effects
The most severe adverse effects of abacavir are hypersensitivity reactions, which can be life threatening and are manifested by fever, skin rash, respiratory, or abdominal distress. Under such circumstances, abacavir must be discontinued immediately and not reinstituted. The likelihood of this reaction appears to be genetically influenced (see the Special Considerations for Pharmacogenetics box on p. 1084). Other adverse effects of abacavir in adults include hepatotoxicity, nausea/vomiting (if severe, consider hypersensitivity), diarrhea, anorexia, and insomnia.

Drug Interactions
Toxicity is more likely with ingestion of ethanol. Abacavir may result in increased levels of methadone or the protease inhibitor amprenavir.

Nursing Management
See the case of T.P. beginning on p. 1076. But additionally, abacavir may be taken with or without food. Because of the life-threatening adverse effects to abacavir, ensure that the client understands the guide that comes with each prescription and that the client carries the warning card from the package summarizing the symptoms of hypersensitivity. Advise client that the long-term effects of abacavir are not yet known.

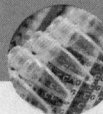

Special Considerations for Pharmacogenetics | ANTIRETROVIRALS AND HIV

PHARMACODYNAMICS

The host's response to HIV is largely influenced by genetics. Transmission, disease progression, and drug response have all been correlated with various genetic markers, including those that code for receptors on CD4+ cells, production of various cytokines, and receptors to which cytokines act (Tang & Kaslow, 2003). Genetics is also used in establishing drug resistance in the use of genotypic and phenotypic assays (Bartlet & Lane, 2004).

PHARMACOKINETICS

A number of antivirals, specifically the NNRTIs and the protease inhibitors, are metabolized by the P450 enzyme systems. Genetic markers for the metabolism of nelfinavir and ritonavir, including the significant variation in expression of the cytochrome P450 enzymes based on genetics, are well-established (Wojnowski, 2004) and likely explain much of the variation in metabolism, response, and toxicity with these agents across populations.

ADVERSE EFFECTS

Much of the toxicity of many of the antiretroviral therapies is dose related, including the potential for peripheral neuropathy, CNS toxicity, and pancreatitis. The likelihood of efavirenz and nevirapine to produce changes in mood, sleep, and fatigue were directly correlated with genetic markers for cytochrome P450 2 B6 (*CYP2 B6* 516 TT) affecting their metabolism (Rotger et al., 2005). Similar findings are presented by different researchers and help explain variation in drug response and toxicity of efavirenz in African Americans compared to European Americans (Haas et al., 2004).

Abacavir hypersensitivity is potentially life-threatening, and if predictable by genetics, could result in improved safety with this agent. Potential for hypersensitivity with abacavir is predicted by presence of a genetic marker (HLA-B*5701) (Hughes et al., 2004), but the cost-effectiveness of routine screening for this marker has been questioned (Watson, Pimenta, Spreen, & Hernandez, 2004).

Correlation of other serious toxicities with genetics for clients with advanced HIV has been less fruitful to date. A genetic marker that is predictive of which individuals will likely demonstrate significant adverse metabolic effects with protease inhibitors has remained elusive (Yang et al., 2003). Although there appears to be a genetic basis for the degree of drug transport in the liver (Pauli-Magnus & Meier, 2003), no genetic markers have yet been identified which predict hepatotoxicity for antiretroviral drugs. Use of sulfonamides (e.g., sulfamethoxazole-trimethoprim) in clients with advanced HIV disease is associated with an increased risk for Stevens-Johnson syndrome, but searching for genetic predictors has not been successful (Pirmohamed et al., 2000).

Given that much of the antiretroviral drug metabolism is genetically determined, it is likely that genetics will play a larger role in predicting and preventing some adverse effects associated with antiretroviral drug therapy in the future.

---

didanosine [dye **dah** noe seen]
(ddI, Videx)

Indications
Didanosine is indicated for the treatment of AIDS and advanced HIV in clients who are unable to take zidovudine or who exhibit a decreased response to it.

Pharmacokinetics/Dosing
This product, which is available in oral dosage forms, is considered to be acid labile (broken down by gastric acid). Therefore oral formulations are buffered to increase gastric pH and thus protect this drug from gastric acid destruction. Didanosine crosses the blood-brain barrier, has a half-life of 1.5 hours in adults, and reaches peak serum concentrations in 30 to 60 minutes. It is excreted primarily by the kidneys. The usual adult dosage for clients weighing less than 60 kg is 167 mg PO every 12 hours; for clients weighing more than 60 kg, the dosage is 250 mg PO every 12 hours. For the pediatric dosing schedule, check the current package insert or drug reference for didanosine (buffered oral suspension).

Adverse Effects
Among the more serious adverse effects of didanosine are pancreatitis, peripheral neuropathies, hepatotoxicity (including liver failure), rhabdomyolysis, bone marrow suppression, and seizures. Other adverse effects include anorexia, nausea, vomiting, diarrhea, elevated uric acid and the potential for gout, and muscle pain.

Drug Interactions
Use of other drugs which have the potential to cause pancreatitis (e.g., valproic acid, hydroxyurea, other antiretrovirals) or peripheral neuropathies (e.g., isoniazid, other antiretrovirals) may increase potential for toxicity. Increased toxicity of didanosine has also been noted with concurrent ganciclovir, ribavirin, and tenofovir. The buffers used in didanosine formulations may impair absorption of quinolone antimicrobials, tetracyclines, azole antifungals, and dapsone. Methadone use may be associated with reduced levels of didanosine.

Nursing Management
See the case of T.P. beginning on p. 1076 for general nursing management related to antiviral therapy with HIV. In addition to general nursing management with antivirals, determine that the client does not currently have a history of pancreatitis, active alcoholism, or hypertriglyceridemia. Didanosine has caused pancreatitis, which on rare occasion has been fatal. These conditions place the client at higher risk for pancreatitis. Many drugs if coadministered with didanosine will increase this risk; check the most current package insert. Have the client report abdominal pain. Obtain a baseline assessment of the client's infection and serum amylase, lipase, and triglycerides.

Cautious use is also required for clients on sodium restrictions, because each dose of 2 chewable/dispersible tablets contains 529 mg of sodium; each single-dose packet for powder for oral solution contains 1380 mg of sodium. Have clients report sudden weight gain, pedal edema, or increasing shortness of breath.

Because of the high risk of peripheral neuropathy with didanosine, document any preexisting neuropathy and monitor carefully for the worsening of, or the development of, peripheral neuropathy. Again, many drugs that have been shown to cause peripheral neuropathy, if coadministered with didanosine will increase the risk of its occurrence; check current package insert for list of drugs. Monitor for vision changes; ophthalmic examinations should be performed in children every 3 to 6 months. Have clients report vision disturbances and tingling of the fingers and toes.

Didanosine should be administered on an empty stomach at least 1 hour before or 2 hours after a meal. The tablets should not be swallowed whole but thoroughly chewed, crushed, or dissolved in water before administration. The tablets are hard and may need to be crushed by hand. Dissolve the tablets in at least 30 mL of water, stir, and have the client swallow the solution immediately. To produce adequate buffering and prevent gastric acid degradation, clients older than 1 year of age must take two tablets at each dose. Pediatric dosages are calculated according to body surface area, and adult dosages are calculated based on weight.

emtricitabine [em trye **sye** ta been]
(Emtriva)
Indications
Emtricitabine is used to treat HIV in combination with at least two other antiretroviral agents.
Pharmacokinetics/Dosing
Emtricitabine is well absorbed orally and primarily excreted in the urine as unchanged drug. The adult dose is 200 mg orally once daily.
Adverse Effects
The most serious (but rare) adverse events reported with emtricitabine are lactic acidosis and liver injury, as may be seen with other agents of this class. Other adverse effects include headache, dizziness, insomnia, rash, nausea, gastric discomfort, diarrhea, cough, muscle weakness, and elevated CPK levels.
Drug Interactions
The use of ribavirin with emtricitabine and other NRTIs may increase risk for lactic acidosis.
Nursing Management
See the case of T.P. beginning on p. 1076 for general nursing management related to antiviral therapy with HIV. Additionally, monitor the client for the adverse effect of lactic acidosis (rapid onset over a few hours) with hyperventilation, low plasma bicarbonate and blood pH, hyperphosphatemia, and elevated plasma levels of lactic acid.

lamivudine [lam i **vue** deen]
(3TC, Epivir, Epivir-HBV, Heptovir✤)
Indications
Lamivudine is used in combination with zidovudine (Combivir), or in combination with abacavir and zidovudine (Trizivir), for the treatment of HIV infection based on evidence of disease progression. It is also used in combination with pegylated interferon to treat chronic hepatitis B infection in which liver inflammation is present, but the sustained benefit of lamivudine has been questioned (Janssen et al., 2005).
Pharmacokinetics/Dosing
Lamivudine is rapidly absorbed after oral administration. It has an intracellular half-life of 10 to 15 hours and is excreted primarily unchanged by the kidneys. The usual dosage of lamivudine for HIV in adolescents (12 to 16 years of age) and adults is 150 mg PO twice daily or, in combination form, 150 mg of lamivudine and 300 mg of zidovudine twice daily. The dose for treating chronic hepatitis B is 100 mg once daily. Dosage reduction is recommended with renal impairment.
Adverse Effects
The most serious adverse effects of lamivudine include pancreatitis, peripheral neuropathies, and hepatotoxicity. Lactic acidosis, rhabdomyolysis, hepatomegaly, splenomegaly, steatosis, bone marrow suppression and hypersensitivity reactions are additional serious reactions associated with lamivudine therapy. Additional adverse effects include headache, cough, fatigue, fever, anorexia, nausea,

vomiting, gastric pain or distress, diarrhea, insomnia, depression, and skeletal muscle pain.
Drug Interactions
Lamivudine is associated with elevated zidovudine levels, although these two agents are frequently dosed together (e.g., Combivir). Lamivudine levels are increased with trimethoprim/sulfamethoxazole therapy. Lactic acidosis risk may be increased with concurrent ribavirin therapy or use of other NRTIs.
Nursing Management
See the case of T.P. beginning on p. 1076 for general nursing management related to antiviral therapy with HIV. In addition to general nursing management with antivirals, avoid the use of lamivudine with children with a history of pancreatitis; use lamivudine only if there is no alternative and only with extreme caution. Monitor clients, particularly children, for symptoms of pancreatitis (e.g., nausea, vomiting, and abdominal pain); discontinue the drug and contact the prescriber immediately.

Review the client's current drug regimen for potential drug interactions, such as with trimethoprim/sulfamethoxazole (Bactrim, TMP/SMX), which increases the blood levels of lamivudine; and zidovudine (AZT), which has its blood levels increased by lamivudine. Administer lamivudine without regard to food.

stavudine [**sta** vue deen]
(d4 T, Zerit)
Indications
Stavudine is an antiviral agent indicated for the treatment of advanced HIV infection or AIDS in clients who have not responded to or are unable to take zidovudine and proven therapeutic agents.
Pharmacokinetics/Dosing
Oral stavudine is rapidly absorbed and reaches peak serum levels in 0.5 to 1.5 hours. It has a half-life of 1 to 1.6 hours and is excreted primarily unchanged by the kidneys. The usual adult oral dosage of stavudine is 30 mg every 12 hours for persons weighing less than 60 kg; for persons weighing more than 60 kg, the dosage is 40 mg every 12 hours.
Adverse Effects
Toxicity associated with stavudine may be more frequent than with other NRTIs and has resulted in this agent as not recommended as first line therapy (Bartlet & Lane, 2004). Serious adverse effects of stavudine include peripheral neuropathies (often dose-related), hepatotoxicity (including hepatomegaly and liver failure), lactic acidosis, pancreatitis and bone marrow suppression. Other adverse effects include headache, insomnia, anxiety, depression, nausea, vomiting, diarrhea, abdominal pain, muscle, and joint pain.
Drug Interactions
Use of other agents associated with peripheral neuropathy (especially concurrent didanosine) may increase the potential for neuropathies with stavudine. Concurrent ribavirin may increase risk for lactic acidosis.
Nursing Management
See the case of T.P. beginning on p. 1076 for general nursing management related to antiviral therapy with HIV. In addition to general nursing management with antivirals, stavudine is similar to didanosine with special nursing management related to the development of pancreatitis, hepatotoxicity, and peripheral neuropathy.

tenofovir [te **noe** fo veer]
(Viread)
Indications
Tenofovir is used to manage HIV infection in combination with other antiretroviral agents.
Pharmacokinetics/Dosing
Tenofovir exhibits fair bioavailability that increases with a fatty meal. It is eliminated in the urine primarily as active drug. It is dosed in adults at 300 mg orally once daily.

Adverse Effects

Tenofovir has the potential to produce the same serious reactions as other agents in the class, including lactic acidosis, hepatotoxicity (including hepatomegaly and liver failure), and pancreatitis. Peripheral neuropathies are less commonly observed than with other agents in the class. Other common adverse effects include nausea, vomiting, diarrhea, flatulence, and weakness. Bone marrow suppression has been reported rarely.

Drug Interactions

Increased didanosine levels and toxicity (lactic acidosis, peripheral neuropathies, pancreatitis) is associated when tenofovir is used with didanosine. A number of non-HIV antiviral agents (acyclovir, ganciclovir, cidofovir, and others) may result in increased levels of tenofovir. Concurrent use of tenofovir with the protease inhibitors atazanavir, lopinavir, and ritonavir may result in reduced protease inhibitor levels and therapeutic failure.

Nursing Management

See the case of T.P. beginning on p. 1076 for general nursing management related to antiviral therapy with HIV. In addition to general nursing management with antivirals, monitor the client for the adverse effect of lactic acidosis (rapid onset [over a few hours]) hyperventilation, low plasma bicarbonate and blood pH, hyperphosphatemia, and elevated plasma levels of lactic acid.

zalcitabine [zal **sit** a been]
(ddC, HIVID)
Indications

Zalcitabine is indicated for the treatment of advanced HIV infection and AIDS in clients who either cannot take zidovudine or who experience a disease progression while taking zidovudine.

Pharmacokinetics/Dosing

Administered orally, zalcitabine is metabolized intracellularly to ddC-TP; it reaches peak serum levels in 1 to 2 hours and has a half-life of 1 to 3 hours. It is excreted primarily by the kidneys. The usual adult oral dosage of zalcitabine is 0.75 mg, alone or in combination with 200 mg of zidovudine every 8 hours.

Adverse Effects

The most frequent serious effect associated with zalcitabine is peripheral neuropathy. As with other agents in the class, serious adverse effects of zalcitabine also include hepatotoxicity, hypersensitivity reactions, lactic acidosis and pancreatitis. Other adverse effects include gastric distress, and headache.

Drug Interactions

Zalcitabine toxicity and dose related peripheral neuropathies are more likely with concurrent amphotericin B, foscarnet, or aminoglycoside therapy. Other agents that increase the potential for peripheral neuropathy include isoniazid, ethionamide, metronidazole, and ribavirin. Concurrent use of didanosine should be avoided because this combination is very frequently associated with peripheral neuropathy. Concurrent use of stavudine and lamivudine should likewise be avoided. Absorption of zalcitabine is reduced by concurrent antacid therapy.

Nursing Management

The nursing management of the client receiving zalcitabine is the same as didanosine except that zalcitabine should be administered 1 hour before or 2 hours after meals to enhance absorption. Zalcitabine is often administered in conjunction with zidovudine.

Nonnucleoside, Reverse Transcriptase Inhibitors

The nonnucleoside reverse transcriptase inhibitors (NNRTIs) are diverse chemicals that inhibit reverse transcriptase similar to the nucleoside agents. Unlike the nucleoside agents, however, they act by binding directly to, or very near, the active site of the enzyme and render it inactive. These agents only display activity against HIV-1 replication, and do not appear to be effective for HIV-2 infection. Included among the NNRTIs are delavirdine, efavirenz, and nevirapine.

★🔲 delavirdine [del ah **vir** deen]
(Rescriptor)

Delavirdine binds noncompetitively to HIV-1 reverse transcriptase to block RNA-dependent and DNA-dependent polymerase activities. It does not affect human DNA polymerase activities. Despite different chemical structures, efavirenz and nevirapine work by similar mechanisms of action.

Indications

Delavirdine is used in combination with other antiretroviral agents to treat HIV.

Pharmacokinetics/Dosing

Administered orally, delavirdine is rapidly absorbed and is highly protein bound (98%). It reaches peak serum levels in 1 hour and has a half-life of approximately 6 hours (range, 2 to 11 hours). It is metabolized in the liver by the cytochrome P450 3 A (CYP3 A) system and can reduce the action of CYP3 A—an action that may be reversed in 7 days after discontinuing the drug. It is excreted both in the feces (44%) and by the kidneys (51%). The usual adult dosage is 400 mg PO three times daily.

Adverse Effects

The most frequently observed adverse effect of delavirdine is rash that is often serious enough to require discontinuation of delavirdine therapy. Serious, but infrequent, adverse effects include renal failure, hypersensitivity reactions (angioedema, Stevens-Johnson syndrome), hepatotoxicity or hepatic failure, hallucinations, bone marrow suppression, pancreatitis, and hallucinations. Other adverse effects include nausea, vomiting, diarrhea, fatigue, and, uncommonly or rarely, conjunctivitis, blisters, fever, joint and muscle pain, oral lesions, and dyspnea.

Drug Interactions

Drugs that affect the action of P450 3 A4 may affect delavirdine levels. Concurrent clarithromycin, azole antifungals, and fluoxetine are among the drugs associated with elevated delavirdine levels and potential toxicity. Delavirdine inhibits a number of the P450 isoenzymes, including benzodiazepines, amiodarone, flecainide, HMG-CoA reductase inhibitors (e.g., "statins"), amphetamines, amprenavir, calcium channel blockers, cisapride, clarithromycin, methadone, indinavir, saquinavir, sildenafil, and warfarin. Reduced delavirdine levels (and the potential for therapeutic failure) are possible with a number of enzyme inducers including carbamazepine, phenytoin, phenobarbital, rifampin, rifabutin, didanosine, and saquinavir. Agents that alter gastric pH (e.g., antacids, histamine 2 receptor blockers, and proton pump inhibitors) may reduce bioavailability of delavirdine.

Nursing Management

See the case of T.P. beginning on p. 1076 for general nursing management related to antiviral therapy with HIV. In addition to general nursing management with antivirals, review the client's current medication regimen for the risk of significant drug interactions: antacids and H₂ receptor blockers reduce absorption; delavirdine needs to be taken 1 hour apart so as not to decrease delavirdine levels; clarithromycin, fluoxetine, and ketoconazole may increase delavirdine levels; carbamazepine, phenobarbital, phenytoin, rifabutin, and rifampin may decrease delavirdine levels. In turn, delavirdine may increase serum levels of clarithromycin, astemizole, indinavir, saquinavir, dapsone, rifabutin, alprazolam, midazolam, triazolam, dihydropyridine, calcium channel blockers, cisapride, quinidine, and warfarin.

Although impaired skin integrity is a common nursing diagnosis, a diffuse, maculopapular, erythematous and pruritic rash usually occurring in the first to third weeks of therapy, delavirdine should be discontinued and the prescriber notified if it is accompanied by fever, blistering, muscle, or joint pain.

efavirenz [eh **fah** vye renz]
(Sustiva)
Indications
Efavirenz is used in combination with other agents to treat HIV-1 infection.

Pharmacokinetics/Dosing
Administered orally, efavirenz reaches peak plasma levels in 3 to 5 hours and steady-state plasma levels in 6 to 10 days. It is highly protein bound (99.5%) and is metabolized by the cytochrome P450 system to inactive metabolites. Efavirenz can also increase P450 enzyme activity, which results in an increase in its own metabolism (autoinduction). It has a half-life of 52 to 76 hours and is excreted in the urine and feces. The usual adult dosage is 600 mg daily (at bedtime) in combination with other antiviral agents.

Adverse Effects
Serious adverse effects of efavirenz include depression, insomnia, vivid dreams, anxiety, and hallucinations, aggression, mania, paranoid agitation, and suicidal ideation. Its use is generally avoided for clients with a history of mental illness or those with a history of use of illicit psychostimulants. Serious but rare nonpsychiatric adverse effects include hepatotoxicity, seizures, fat redistribution, seizures, Stevens-Johnson syndrome, and visual changes. CNS toxicity appears to be influenced by genetics (see the Special Considerations for Pharmacogenetics box on p. 1084). Other adverse effects of efavirenz include skin rashes (usually within the first 2 weeks of therapy), fatigue, headache, nausea, vomiting, diarrhea, and elevated cholesterol levels (with favorable increases in high-density lipoprotein [HDL] cholesterol).

Drug Interactions
Many of the interactions between efavirenz and other drugs relate to P450 isoenzyme activity. Efavirenz is metabolized by P450 2 B6 and 3 A4 and its metabolism is affected by other drugs that are inducers or inhibitors of these systems. It may inhibit or induce other drugs metabolized by 3 A4 and other isoenzymes. Potentially life-threatening adverse effects can be noted if combined with cisapride, midazolam, or ergotamine. Levels of some of the protease inhibitors (particularly nelfinavir and ritonavir) are elevated with efavirenz use, whereas with others, levels may be reduced (saquinavir, amprenavir). Enzyme inducers including carbamazepine, phenobarbital, phenytoin, rifampin, rifabutin, and St. John's Wort can result in decreased efavirenz levels and potential therapeutic failure. Warfarin effects may be increased or decreased with efavirenz therapy. Efavirenz may produce decreased levels of methadone (and induce withdrawal), and lower levels of some selective serotonin reuptake inhibitor (SSRI) antidepressants (particularly sertraline).

Nursing Management
See the case of T.P. beginning on p. 1076 for general nursing management related to antiviral therapy with HIV. In addition to general nursing management with antivirals, review the client's current medication regimen for the risk of significant drug interactions: efavirenz levels are decreased by saquinavir and rifampin, and increased by ritonavir and fluconazole. Efavirenz decreases serum levels of clarithromycin, indinavir, nelfinavir and saquinavir and increases serum levels of ritonavir, azithromycin and ethinyl estradiol.

Monitor more for CNS adverse effects; these may decreased by using a bedtime dosing of efavirenz.

nevirapine [neh **vir** ah peen]
(Viramune)
Indications
Nevirapine is used to treat HIV-1 infection when combined with other antiretroviral agents. Its use is not recommended for women with CD4$^+$ counts above 250 because of the risk for serious hepato-

toxicity and the availability of safer agents (FDA Advisory, January 2005).

Pharmacokinetics/Dosing
Administered orally, nevirapine is well absorbed, reaches peak serum levels in 4 hours, and is distributed in CSF (45% of serum concentration). Nevirapine is metabolized in the liver and is also an inducer of hepatic cytochrome P450 metabolic enzymes; therefore autoinduction or an increased clearance and a decreased half-life occurs within 2 to 4 weeks of therapy. The initial therapy is 200 mg PO daily for 2 weeks; the maintenance dosage is 200 mg twice daily in combination with another antiretroviral agent. The use of initially lower doses reduces the potential for hypersensitivity reactions.

Adverse Effects
The most serious adverse effect of nevirapine is the potential for life-threatening skin reactions, such as Stevens-Johnson syndrome. The other serious adverse effect of nevirapine is hepatotoxicity, which may progress to hepatic necrosis or hepatic failure. These risks appear highest in women. Discontinue nevirapine in clients who develop a severe rash, rash accompanied by other symptoms such as fever, myalgia, fatigue, oral lesions, and conjunctivitis, rash with elevated liver function tests (ALT, AST), symptoms of hepatitis (e.g., jaundice, flank pain), or persistently or severely elevated liver function tests (Boehringer Ingelheim, January 2004). Additional adverse effects include headache, bone marrow suppression, ulcerative stomatitis, and peripheral neuropathies. A revised label for the client is provided by the manufacturer to explain risks associated with nevirapine.

Drug Interactions
Like the other NNRTIs, nevirapine is metabolized by and affects the P450 enzyme systems. It is primarily metabolized by P450 3 A4 and may induce the metabolism of other drugs metabolized by 3 B6 and 3 A4. Other pharmacokinetic interactions are also possible. Elevated nevirapine levels may be noted with a number of P450 3 A4 inhibitors, including cimetidine, azole antifungals, clarithromycin, and erythromycin. Nevirapine levels are reduced by rifampin, rifabutin, and other enzyme inducers (e.g., carbamazepine, phenytoin, phenobarbital). Nevirapine may result in reduced levels of a number of protease inhibitors, including indinavir, lopinavir, nelfinavir, and saquinavir and contribute to therapeutic failure. Hormonal contraceptives may be less effective with concurrent nelfinavir therapy.

Nursing Management
See the case of T.P. beginning on p. 1076 for general nursing management related to antiviral therapy with HIV. In addition to general nursing management with antivirals, review the client's current medication regimen for the risk of significant drug interactions. Nevirapine decreases serum concentrations of protease inhibitors, hormonal contraceptives and methadone (resulting in opioid withdrawal). Monitor for skin and CNS adverse effects as with delavirdine and efavirenz. Instruct the client to use or add a barrier contraceptive.

Protease Inhibitors

Although its complete mechanism of action is unknown, the protease inhibitors appear to inhibit the replication of retroviruses (HIV types 1 and 2) by interfering with HIV protease. They affect the replication cycle of HIV and are active in both acute and chronically infected cells, which in general are not affected by dideoxynucleoside reverse transcriptase inhibitors (e.g., didanosine, lamivudine, stavudine, zalcitabine, and zidovudine). This inhibition results in the formation of immature, noninfectious viral particles. Unfortunately, their use as monotherapy quickly results in resistant strains of HIV.

Protease inhibitors are associated with altered body fat distribution, hyperglycemia, and other metabolic effects, which may predispose to the development of type 2 diabetes mellitus. Hepatotoxicity and hypersensitivity reactions (including the risk for Stevens-Johnson syndrome) are possible as well. They are also highly metabolized by the cytochrome p450 enzyme systems and are associated with many significant interactions with other drugs.

Available protease inhibitors include amprenavir, atazanavir, fosamprenavir, indinavir, lopinavir/ritonavir, nelfinavir, ritonavir, and saquinavir. The combination of lopinavir and ritonavir combines two HIV-1 protease inhibitors to provide potentially improved benefit to clients. The primary role of ritonavir in this combined formulation is to reduce metabolism of lopinavir and allow for more sustained levels of the drug, thereby allowing for more even viral suppression.

✱▚ saquinavir [sa **kwin** a veer]
(Fortovase, Invirase)

Indications
Saquinavir is used in combination with the nucleoside analogues to treat advanced HIV infection in selected individuals.

Pharmacokinetics/Dosing
Oral absorption of the Invirase formulation of saquinavir is improved when administered with a high fat meal. Absorption of the Fortovase formulation is improved over the Invirase formulation. Administered orally, saquinavir has extensive first-pass metabolism, is highly protein bound, is metabolized in the liver, and is excreted primarily in the feces. Dosage varies based on formulation and interacting drugs. Clinicians should consult the package insert.

Adverse Effects
Similar to the other protease inhibitors, hepatic injury and metabolic changes with ongoing use are possible. Other serious adverse effects include confusion, hypersensitivity reactions (e.g., Stevens-Johnson syndrome), seizures, bone marrow suppression, and hepatotoxicity. Diarrhea, abdominal distress, headache, and weakness have also been noted.

Drug Interactions
Saquinavir, like the other protease inhibitors, is metabolized by 3 A4 and other isoenzymes of the P450 system. Levels of saquinavir may be affected by other drugs that impact on 3 A4 activity. Likewise, saquinavir may alter the metabolism of other drugs metabolized by 3 A4. Although usually less dramatic than ritonavir, significant interactions are possible. Consult package insert for drug interactions and dosing recommendations.

Nursing Management
See the case of T.P. beginning on p. 1076 for general nursing management related to antiviral therapy with HIV. In addition to general nursing management with antivirals, instruct the client to take saquinavir with a meal or within 2 hours after a meal.

amprenavir [am **pren** a veer]
(Agenerase)

Indications
Amprenavir is indicated in combination with other antiretroviral therapy for the treatment of HIV.

Pharmacokinetics/Dosing
Amprenavir is moderately well absorbed administered orally. Administration with a high fat meal dramatically increases absorption. It is available as a capsule and oral solution, each having different bioavailability and dosing. Amprenavir, like other protease inhibitors, is extensively metabolized by the cytochrome P450 enzyme systems (particularly 3 A4) and is eliminated in the feces and urine. The dosage of amprenavir varies widely based on age, formulation, concurrent drugs, and hepatic function.

Adverse Effects
All of the protease inhibitors have the potential to produce metabolic changes, including hyperlipidemias, altered body fat metabolism, hepatic injury, hyperglycemia, and risk for development of type 2 diabetes mellitus. Amprenavir shares these risks. It is also associated with rash, nausea, vomiting, diarrhea, and depression.

Drug Interactions
Each of the protease inhibitors, including amprenavir, is metabolized by cytochrome P450 and also inhibits the action of P450 enzymes. Amprenavir interacts with a great number of drugs which are metabolized or interact with these systems, including cisapride, pimozide, quinidine, benzodiazepines, ergot alkaloids, estrogens, and hormonal contraceptives. Other drugs that interact include the HMG-CoA reductase inhibitors ("statins"), azole antifungals, antidysrhythmics, calcium channel blockers, antidepressants, warfarin, rifampin, rifabutin, estrogen-containing products (including hormonal contraceptives, and a number of other antiretroviral agents). The oral solution is only used when absolutely necessary, and may produce toxic reactions when used with disulfiram or metronidazole. Practitioners should consult the package insert for a complete listing of interacting drugs.

Nursing Management
See the case of T.P. beginning on p. 1076 for general nursing management related to antiviral therapy with HIV. In addition to general nursing management with antivirals, assess clients for diabetes mellitus as amprenavir causes increases in glucose blood levels; monitor with blood glucose determinations and HbA_{1c}. Amprenavir capsules and oral solution are not interchangeable. Instruct the client that amprenavir may be taken without regard to food, but not to take it with a high fat meal as absorption will be reduced. Take 1 hour before or after an antacid.

indinavir [in **din** a veer]
(Crixivan)

Indications
Indinavir is used to treat HIV in combination with at least two other antiretroviral agents.

Pharmacokinetics/Dosing
Administered orally, indinavir reaches a peak serum level in approximately 1 hour; it is metabolized in the liver and excreted primarily by the kidneys. The usual adult dosage of indinavir is 800 mg PO every 8 hours, but dosage adjustment is required when dosing concurrently with other interacting drugs (see Drug Interactions).

Adverse Effects
The most serious acute onset adverse effect observed with indinavir is nephrolithiasis, and has been noted in up to 29% of pediatric and 12% of adult clients (Lacy, Armstrong, Goldman, & Lance, 2004). Other adverse effects of indinavir include nausea, vomiting, gastric distress, diarrhea, headache, dizziness, fatigue, fever, flu-like syndrome, and chest pain. As with other protease inhibitors, indinavir is associated with metabolic changes, including fat redistribution, elevated cholesterol and triglyceride levels, and increased risk for type 2 diabetes mellitus.

Drug Interactions
Indinavir is metabolized by cytochrome P450 3 A4 and to a lesser extent 2D6. It also inhibits 3 A4 and other isoenzymes. As such, a significant number of interactions are possible. Refer to package insert or current data if dosing with other agents, particularly with delavirdine, efavirenz, indinavir, itraconazole, ketoconazole, lopinavir, nevirapine, rifabutin, rifampin, or ritonavir.

Nursing Management
See the case of T.P. beginning on p. 1076 for general nursing management related to antiviral therapy with HIV. In addition to general nursing management with antivirals, monitor the client for the onset of kidney stones (flank pain, hematuria). Advise the client to increase fluid intake to at least 2 L to minimize the risk of stones. Inform the client that indinavir is best taken on an empty stomach (1 hour before or 2 hours after a meal) with a full glass of water. If the

client is taking indinavir and didanosine concurrently, separate the doses by 1 hour and take each on an empty stomach.

lopinavir/ritonavir [lop i **na** veer/rit oe **na** veer]
(Kaletra)
Indications
Lopinavir/ritonavir is used in combination with other antiretroviral agents in the treatment of HIV infection.
Pharmacokinetics/Dosing
Administered as an oral capsule or solution, lopinavir/ritonavir is metabolized extensively and eliminated primarily in the feces as metabolized drug. The elimination half-life of lopinavir in combination with ritonavir is about 5 hours. The adult dose is typically lopinavir 400 mg/ritonavir 100 mg by mouth twice daily.
Adverse Effects
The metabolic complications of hyperglycemia, hyperlipidemia, and hepatotoxicity are also observed with this combination. Other adverse effects include diarrhea, nausea, neutropenia, and headache.
Drug Interactions
See ritonavir.
Nursing Management
See the case of T.P. beginning on p. 1076 for general nursing management related to antiviral therapy with HIV. In addition to general nursing management with antivirals, see ritonavir.

nelfinavir [nel **fin** ah veer]
(Viracept)
Indications
Nelfinavir is used to treat HIV infection in combination with other antiretroviral agents.
Pharmacokinetics/Dosing
Nelfinavir is available as an oral powder and tablet. It has a half-life in plasma of 3.5 to 5 hours and reaches peak plasma levels in 2 to 4 hours. Nelfinavir is metabolized to active and inactive metabolites in the liver (cytochrome P450) and is excreted primarily in the feces. The oral powder is for use in children only; children 2 to 13 years of age receive 20 to 30 mg/kg PO three times daily with food. The tablet dosage form is used for adolescents and adults; the dosage is usually 750 mg three times daily or 1250 mg twice daily with food and in combination with other nucleoside agents.
Adverse Effects
Metabolic effects, including the development of diabetes mellitus, have been reported protease inhibitors, including nelfinavir. Other adverse effects of nelfinavir include diarrhea, bloating, nausea, skin rash, hyperglycemia and, possibly, ketoacidosis.
Drug Interactions
Nelfinavir is metabolized by 3 A4 and other isoenzymes of cytochrome P450, and, like indinavir, inhibits the metabolism of drugs metabolized by 3 A4 and others. Consult the package insert or other references for a full listing of affected drugs and management.
Nursing Management
See the case of T.P. beginning on p. 1076 for general nursing management related to antiviral therapy with HIV. In addition to general nursing management with antivirals, monitor the client for diarrhea that is common with this drug. It may be managed with OTCs that slow GI motility such as loperamide. Nelfinavir comes both as a powder and tablets. Both forms of the drug must be taken with food. The oral powder may be mixed with a small amount of water, milk, formula, soy formula, soy milk, or dietary supplements. It should not be mixed with acidic food or juices because the result will have a bitter taste. Once the powder is reconstituted, it should be taken within 6 hours.

ritonavir [ri **ton** ah veer]
(Norvir)
Indications
Ritonavir is indicated for the management of HIV infection in combination with other agents. It is often used in combination with lopinavir (Kaletra); see the monograph earlier.

Pharmacokinetics/Dosing
Administered orally, ritonavir reaches peak serum levels within 2 to 4 hours (fasting or nonfasting); five metabolites have been identified with ritonavir, but only the M-2 metabolite has antiviral activity. Most of this drug is excreted in the feces. The usual dosage is 600 mg twice daily with meals. Doses of 100 to 200 mg PO once or twice daily are sometimes used to increase levels of other protease inhibitors (often referred to as pharmacokinetic "boosting").
Adverse Effects
Ritonavir shares the risk for metabolic effects and hepatic injury with the other protease inhibitors. Additional adverse effects of ritonavir include weakness, nausea, vomiting, GI distress, diarrhea, taste alterations, peripheral paresthesias, allergic reactions, back or chest pain, chills, facial edema, flu-like symptoms, and many other potential adverse effects. Refer to current references for a complete list of adverse effects.
Drug Interactions
Ritonavir is metabolized by the cytochrome P450 enzymes, particularly 2D6 and 3A4. It also inhibits the metabolism of other drugs metabolized by these systems. As with the other protease inhibitors, numerous drug interactions are possible, even probable, with ritonavir. The long list of interacting drugs includes benzodiazepines, the ergot alkaloids, HMG-CoA reductase inhibitors ("statins"), meperidine, rifampin, rifabutin, drugs used to treat sexual dysfunction like sildenafil (Viagra), saquinavir, ß-adrenergic blockers, calcium channel blockers, anticonvulsants, antidepressants, antidysrhythmics, corticosteroids, and immunosuppressants. Clinicians should consult the package insert or other references to evaluate risk and management.
Nursing Management
See the case of T.P. beginning on p. 1076 for general nursing management related to antiviral therapy with HIV. In addition to general nursing management with antivirals, monitor the client for both central and peripheral neurologic symptoms. Instruct the client to take ritonavir with food; the oral solution may be mixed with chocolate milk or liquid food supplements to improve its palatability. Use within an hour of mixing.

Fusion Inhibitors

To date, fusion inhibitors have a limited role in the management of HIV disease. The first available agent with this mechanism is enfuvirtide (Fuzeon).

★⌐▀⌐ enfuvirtide [en fu **veer** tide]
(Fuzeon)
Enfuvirtide binds to a subunit (gp41) of the HIV viral envelope and reduces the ability of HIV to fuse with CD4$^+$ cells. By inhibiting entry of HIV to the CD4$^+$ cells, HIV replication is reduced.
Indications
Use of enfuvirtide is limited to clients with HIV who have not achieved adequate control of their disease despite alternate therapy. It is used in combination with other antiretroviral agents.
Pharmacokinetics/Dosing
Enfuvirtide is administered by subcutaneous injection and has an elimination half-life of about 4 hours. Typical adult dose is 90 mg subcutaneously twice daily.
Adverse Effects
In addition to the common injection site reactions of pain, erythema, induration, and ecchymosis, there is a potentially increased risk for pneumonias and hypersensitivity reactions with this drug. Other adverse effects include insomnia, depression, anxiety, neuropathy, anorexia, and elevated triglyceride levels.
Nursing Management
See the case of T.P. beginning on p. 1076 for general nursing management related to antiviral therapy with HIV. In addition to general nursing management with antivirals, administer the subcutaneous

form of enfuvirtide, carefully rotating injection sites. The drug is slow to dissolve in the vial; rotate vial to mix and let stand for up to 45 minutes for it to dissolve. Ensure that the preparation is fully dissolved, colorless and without bubbles or particular matter before withdrawing it from the vial. Instruct the client to report promptly any signs of infection at injection sites, paresthesia, or skin rash.

Summary

Mycoses, infections of humans by fungi, range from very mild to life-threatening conditions. Some occur as the result of overgrowth during treatment with antibacterials whereas others present as opportunistic infections secondary to immunocompromised states (e.g., postantineoplastic therapy, advanced HIV disease, immunosuppressive or corticosteroid therapy). Systemic antifungal therapy is required for life-threatening fungal infections. Amphotericin B is the most effective systemic agent available for use, with a broad antifungal spectrum of activity. Unfortunately, amphotericin B is associated with significant toxicity. Less toxic systemic antifungals include the azole antifungals fluconazole, itraconazole, and ketoconazole, which are often to avoid the toxicity of amphotericin if the pathogen is susceptible. Additional systemic antifungal agents used for specific indications include flucytosine, griseofulvin, nystatin, and terbinafine.

Antiviral chemotherapy has limited benefit because these drugs act primarily to prevent viral replication. Unfortunately, by the time symptoms of the illness appear, extensive viral replication has usually occurred, and the antiviral may have lesser impact on the course of the disease. Antiviral agents used to treat nonretroviral infections are best administered prophylactically or early in the course of disease to be most effective. The nonretroviral antiviral agents include are acyclovir, amantadine, famciclovir, foscarnet, ganciclovir, oseltamivir, ribavirin, rimantadine, and valacyclovir. The antiretrovirals for the treatment of HIV infection are grouped in four categories: nucleoside reverse transcriptase inhibitors (including zidovudine), nonnucleoside reverse transcriptase inhibitors (e.g., nevirapine), protease inhibitors (e.g., saquinavir) and fusion inhibitors (enfuvirtide); numerous agents are available in the first three of these categories. Adherence to therapy and the prevention and management of adverse effects are major nursing responsibilities for both antiviral and antifungal agents.

Critical Thinking Questions

- Why is antiviral therapy more limited than antibacterial or antifungal therapy?
- Alice Mild, a 20-year-old college student, has been admitted to the hospital with histoplasmosis. The physician has prescribed amphotericin B to be administered 0.25 mg/kg IV. If Alice weighs 154 pounds, how many milligrams will her dose be? What precautions will the prescriber take before beginning the infusion to minimize the adverse effects of the drug? How will the nurse monitor Alice's health status during the infusion?

Bibliography

American Academy of Pediatrics Committee on Infectious Disease. (1999). Reassessment of the indications for ribavirin therapy in respiratory syncytial virus infections, *Pediatrics, 97*(1), 137-40.

Anderson, D.M., Keith, J., & Novak, P.D. (Eds.) (2002). *Mosby's medical, nursing, and allied health dictionary* (6th ed.). St. Louis: Mosby.

Balmer, C.M., & Valley, A.W. (2002). Cancer treatment and chemotherapy. In J.T. DiPiro, R.L. Talbert, G.C. Yee, G.R. Matzke, B.G. Wells & L.M. Posey (Eds.), *Pharmacotherapy: A pathophysiological approach* (5th ed.). Norwalk, CT: Appleton & Lange.

Bartlet, J.G., & Lane, H.C. and the Panel on Clinical Practices for Treatment of HIV Infection. (October 29, 2004). Guidelines for the Use of Antiretroviral Agents in HIV-1-Infected Adults and Adolescents. Retrieved February 4, 2005, from http://aidsinfo.nih.gov/guidelines/adult/AA_102904.html.

Bennett, J.E. (2001). Antimicrobial agents (continued): Antifungal agents. In Hardman, J.G. & Limbird, L.E. (Eds.), *Goodman & Gilman's The pharmacological basis of therapeutics* (10th ed.). New York: McGraw-Hill.

Benson, C.A., Kaplan, J.E., Masur, H., Pau, A., & Holmes, K.K. (December 17, 2004). Treating opportunistic infections among HIV-infected adults and adolescents – Recommendations from CDC, the National Institutes of Health, and the HIV Medicine Association/Infectious Diseases Society of America. *Morbidity and Mortality Weekly Report, 53*(RR15), 1-112. Retrieved February 4, 2005, from http://www.cdc.gov/mmwr/preview/mmwrhtml/rr5315 a1.htm.

Berczi, I., Bertok, L., & Chow, D. A. (2000). Natural immunity and neuroimmune host defense. *Annals of the New York Academy of Science, 917*, 248.

Boehringer, I. (January 2004). Guidelines: Management of rash/hepatic events with viramune. Retrieved February 5, 2005, from

e-LEARNING SUPPLEMENTS

Student CD-ROM
- Final Exam questions
- NCLEX® Examination review questions
- Pharmacology animations
- Printable chapter summary

Evolve Website (http://evolve.elsevier.com/mckenry)
- Case study on antifungal and antiviral drugs
- Interactive concept map on the client with HIV/AIDS

- Content updates, including information on new drugs
- WebLinks corresponding to this chapter
- Answers to the critical thinking questions in this chapter
- *Elsevier ePharmacology Update* newsletter
- Mosby's Drug Consult Internet Edition
- Supplemental and reference information

http://www.fda.gov/medwatch/SAFETY/2004/viramune_guidelines.pdf.

Bosker, G. (Ed.). (2004). *Primary and acute care medicine: Practice, protocols, pathways,* (2nd ed.). Atlanta: Thomson American Health Consultants.

Caruso, T.J., & Gwaltney, J.M., Jr. (2005). Treatment of the common cold with echinacea: A structured review. *Clinical Infectious Disease, 40*(6), 807-810.

Centers for Disease Control and Prevention (CDC). (2001). HIV and AIDS - United States, 1981-2001, *Morbidity and Mortality Weekly Report, 50,* 430-434.

Centers for Disease Control and Prevention (CDC). (2002). *HIV/AIDS Surveillance Report 2002* 14:1-40. Retrieved February 4, 2005, from http://www.cdc.gov/hiv.

Centers for Disease Control and Prevention (CDC). (2004). *HIV/AIDS Surveillance Report 1985-2003*. Retrieved February 4, 2005, from http://www.cdc.gov/hiv.

Centre for Infectious Disease Prevention and Control (CIDPC) Canada. (2004). HIV and AIDS in Canada. Surveillance Report. Ottawa: CIDPC.

Cleary, J.D., Chapman, S.W., & Pearson, M. (2005). Fungal infections. In M.A. Koda-Kimble, L.Y. Young, W.A. Kradjan, B.J. Guglielmo, B.K. Alldredge, & R.L. Corelli (Eds.), *Applied therapeutics: The clinical use of drugs* (8th ed.). Philadelphia: Lippincott Williams & Wilkins.

Davison, C., Ventre, K.M., Luchetti, M., & Randolph, A.G. (2004). Efficacy of interventions for bronchiolitis in critically ill infants: A systematic review and meta-analysis. *Pediatric Critical Care Medicine, 5*(5), 482-489.

Drug facts and comparisons (58th ed.) (2005). St. Louis: Facts and Comparisons.

Falsey, A.R., Hennessey, P.A., Formica, M.A., Cox, C., & Walsh, E.E. (2005). Respiratory syncytial virus infection in elderly and high-risk adults. *New England Journal of Medicine, 352,* 1749-1759.

FDA Advisory (January, 2005). FDA Public Health Advisory for Nevirapine (Viramune) Washington DC: U.S. Food and Drug Administration. Retrieved February 5, 2005, from http://www.fda.gov/cder/drug/advisory/Nevirapine.htm.

Goldman, R.D., & Koren, G. (2004). Amphotericin B Nephrotoxicity in Children. *Journal of Pediatric Hematology/Oncology, 26*(7), 421-426.

Haas, D.W., Ribaudo, H., Kim, R.B., Tierney, C., Wilkinson, G.R., & Gulick, R.M., et al. (2004). Pharmacogenetics of efavirenz and central nervous system side effects: an Adult AIDS Clinical Trials Group study. *AIDS, 18*(18), 2391-2400.

Hayden, F.G. (2001). Antimicrobial Agents (Continued) – Antiviral Agents (Nonretroviral) In Hardman, J.G. & Limbird, L.E. (Eds.), *Goodman & Gilman's The pharmacological basis of therapeutics* (10th ed.). New York: McGraw-Hill.

Hughes, D.A., Vilar, F.J., Ward, C.C., Alfirevic, A., Park, B.K., & Pirmohamed, M. (2004). Cost effectiveness analysis of HLA B*5701 genotyping in preventing ABC hypersensitivity. *Pharmacogenetics, 14,* 335-342.

Iacuzio, D. (December 2003) Dear Health Care Professional Letter. Nutley, NJ: Hoffmann-La Roche Inc. Retrieved February 5, 2005, from http://www.fda.gov/medwatch/SAFETY/2003/tamiflu_deardoc.pdf.

Jackson, J.L., Lesho, E., & Peterson, C. (2000). Zinc and the common cold: a meta-analysis revisited. *Journal of Nutrition, 130*(Suppl 5), 1512-1515.

Janssen, H.L., van Zonneveld, M., Senturk, H., Zeuzem, S., Akarca, U.S., Cakaloglu, Y., et al. (2005). Pegylated interferon alfa-2b alone or in combination with lamivudine for HbeAg-positive chronic hepatitis B: A randomised trial. *Lancet, 365,* 123-129.

Kashuba, A.D.M., & Robinson, M.D. (2005). Opportunistic infections in HIV-infected patients. In M.A. Koda-Kimble, L.Y. Young, W.A. Kradjan, B.J. Guglielmo, B.K. Alldredge, & R.L. Corelli (Eds.), *Applied therapeutics: The clinical use of drugs* (8th ed.). Philadelphia: Lippincott Williams & Wilkins.

King, V.J., Viswanathan, M., Bordley, W.C., Jackman, A.M., Sutton, S.F., & Lohr, K.N., et al. (2004). Pharmacologic treatment of bronchiolitis in infants and children: a systematic review. *Archives of Pediatric and Adolescent Medicine, 158,* 127-137.

Lacy, C.F., Armstrong, L.L., Goldman, M.P., & Lance, L.L. (2004). *Lexi-Comp's Drug Information Handbook* (12th ed.). Hudson, Ohio: Lexi-Comp.

Luber, A.D. (2005). Pharmacotherapy of human immunodeficiency virus infection. In M.A. Koda-Kimble, L.Y. Young, W.A. Kradjan, B.J. Guglielmo, B.K. Alldredge, & R.L. Corelli (Eds.), *Applied therapeutics: The clinical use of drugs* (8th ed.). Philadelphia: Lippincott Williams & Wilkins.

Lange, W.R. (September 2003). Dear Healthcare Professional Letter. Nutley, NJ: Roche Laboratories, Inc. Retrieved February 5, 2005, from http://www.fda.gov/medwatch/SAFETY/2003/valcyte.htm.

Markowitz, M., Mohri, H., Mehandru, S., Shet, A., Berry, L., Kalyanaraman, R., et al. (2005). Infection with multidrug resistant, dual-tropic HIV-1 and rapid progression to AIDS: A case report. *Lancet, 365,* 1031-1038.

MICROMEDEX Healthcare Series. (2005). Amphotericin B. Retrieved July 25, 2005, from http://www.thomsonhc.com/hcs/librarian/PFPUI/my4m3nMRUExHB/ND_PG/PRIH.

Mosby's drug consult (15th ed.). (2005). St. Louis: Mosby.

Mossad, S.B. (2003). Effect of zincum gluconicum nasal gel on the duration and symptom severity of the common cold in otherwise healthy adults. The Quarterly Journal of Medicine, 96(1), 35-43.

Nahata, M.C., O'Mara N.B., & Benavides, S.(2005). Viral infections. In M.A. Koda-Kimble, L.Y. Young, W.A. Kradjan, B.J. Guglielmo, B.K. Alldredge, & R.L. Corelli (Eds.), *Applied therapeutics: The clinical use of drugs* (8th ed.). Philadelphia: Lippincott Williams & Wilkins.

National Center for Health Statistics (NCHS), Health, United States, 2004, Table 33. Age-adjusted death rates according to race, sex, region, and urbanization level. United States, average annual 1994-1996, 1997-1999, and 2000-2002. Retrieved August 5, 2005, from http://www.cdc.gov/nchs/data/hus/hus0.4pdf.

Osmond, D.H. (1998). *Classification and Stages of HIV Infection.* Retrieved November 10, 2004, from http://hivsite.ucsf.edu/InSite?page=kb-01-01#52 x.

Panel on Clinical Practices for Treatment of HIV Infection, Department of Health and Human Services (DHHS). (2004). *Guidelines for the use of antiretroviral agents in HIV-1-infected adults and adolescents.* Retrieved August 29, 2004, from http://aidsinfo.nih.gov.

Patel, R. (1998). Antifungal agents. Part I. Amphotericin B preparations and flucytosine, *Mayo Clinic Proceedings, 73*(12), 1205-1225.

Pauli-Magnus, C., Meier, P.J. (2003). Pharmacogenetics of hepatocellular transporters. *Pharmacogenetics, 13*(4), 189-198.

Pilcher, C.D., Fiscus, S.A., Nguyen, T.Q., Foust, E., Wolf, L., Williams, D., et al. (2005). Detection of acute infections during HIV testing in North Carolina. *New England Journal of Medicine, 352,* 1873-1883.

Pirmohamed, M., Alfirevic, A., Vilar, J., Stalford, A., Wilkins, E.G., & Sim, E., et al. (2000). Association analysis of drug metabolizing enzyme gene polymorphisms in HIV-positive patients with co-trimoxazole hypersensitivity. *Pharmacogenetics, 10*(8), 705-713.

Prasad, A.S., Fitzgerald, J.T., Bao, B., Beck, F.W., & Chandrasekar, P.H. (2000). Duration of symptoms and plasma cytokine levels in patients with the common cold treated with zinc acetate. A randomized, double-blind, placebo-controlled trial. *Ann Intern Med, 133,* 245–252.

Public Health Agency of Canada. (2002). *HIV/AIDS: Canada's Report on HIV/AIDS.* Ottawa: Public Health Agency of Canada.

Raffanti, S., & Haas, D.W. (2001). Antimicrobial agents (continued): Antiretroviral agents. In Hardman, J.G. & Limbird, L.E. (Eds.), *Goodman & Gilman's The pharmacological basis of therapeutics* (10th ed.). New York: McGraw-Hill.

Rotger, M., Colombo, S., Furrer, H., Bleiber, G., Buclin, T., & Lee, B.L., et al. (2005). The Swiss HIV Cohort Study Influence of CYP2 B6 polymorphism on plasma and intracellular concentrations and toxicity of efavirenz and nevirapine in HIV-infected patients. *Pharmacogenetics & Genomics, 15*(1), 1-5.

Smith, D.K., Grohskopf, L.A., Black, R.J., Auerbach, J.D., Veronese, F., Struble, K.A., et al. (2005). Antiretroviral postexposure prophylaxis after sexula, injection-drug use, or other nonoccupational exposure to HIV in the United States: Recommendations from the U.S. Department of Health and Human Services. *Morbidity and Mortality Weekly Report, 54,* 1-20.

Smyth, M. J., Godfrey, D. I., & Trapani, J. A. (2001). A fresh look at tumor immunosurveillance and immunotherapy, *Natural Immunology, 2,* 293.

Stevens, D.A. (2004). Azoles in the management of systemic fungal infections. *Infectious Diseases in Clinical Practice, 12*(2), 81-92.

Tang, J., & Kaslow, R.A. (2003). The impact of host genetics on HIV infection and disease progression in the era of highly active antiretroviral therapy. AIDS, 17 Supplement 4, S51-S60.

UNAIDS. (July 2004). 2004 Report on the Global AIDS Epidemic. Retrieved August 5, 2005, from http://www.unaids.org/bangkok2004/report.html.

United States Public Health Service. (2001). USPHS guidelines for management of occupational exposures to HBV, HCV, and HIV for postexposure prophylaxis. *Morbidity and Mortality Weekly Report, 50*(RR-11), 1-42.

U.S. Food and Drug Administration. (2005). FDA Public Health Advisory for nevirapine (Viramune). Retrieved July 17, 2005, from http://www.fda.gov/cder/drug/advisory/Nevirapine.htm.

USP DI: Drug information for the health care professional (25th ed.). (2005). Greenwood Village, CO: MICROMEDEX Thomson Healthcare.

Watson, M.E., Pimenta, J.M., Spreen, W.R., & Hernandez, J.E. (2004). HLA-B*5701 and abacavir hypersensitivity. *Pharmacogenetics, 14*(11), 783.

Wojnowski, L. (2004). Genetics of the variable expression of CYP3 A in humans. *Therapeutic Drug Monitoring, 26*(2), 192-199.

Yang, A., King, M., Han, L., Isaacson, J.D., Mueller, T., & Grimm, D.R., et al. (2003). Lack of correlation between SREBF1 genotype and hyperlipidemia in individuals treated with highly active antiretroviral therapy. *AIDS, 17*(14), 2142-2143.

OTHER ANTIMICROBIAL DRUGS AND ANTIPARASITIC DRUGS

CHAPTER FOCUS

Many of the diseases discussed in this chapter were thought to be eradicable within the past century. The teaching of good health practices and the use of effective drugs held promise to end malaria and tuberculosis (TB), which are endemic in many parts of the world. The World Health Organization (WHO) believed that malaria might be eradicated by 1964 with the combined use of DDT and antimalarial drugs; however, DDT was found to be harmful, and the *Anopheles* mosquito that carries the organism became resistant to the insecticide. Additionally, the ability of pathogens to become drug resistant to the treatments for both TB and malaria has made health officials less optimistic. TB has returned in the United States, with the resurgence of the disease peaking in 1992. Although rates remain high in the United States, there has been a decrease in the number of reported cases of TB, down 44.2% from 1992 (Centers for Disease Control and Prevention, 2004). In Canada, 1694 cases (5.5 per 100,000) of new active and relapsed TB were reported in 2000, with incidence highest among the foreign-born population (Centre for Infectious Disease Prevention and Control, 2003). There has been a growth of ideal environments for the resurgence of TB in the United States and Canada—the homeless, the impoverished, the immunosuppressed, and recent immigrants from countries in which the disease is still endemic. These diseases will continue to challenge health care providers for some time.

LEARNING OBJECTIVES

- Describe the life cycle of the malarial parasite in the human body.
- Implement the nursing management of clients receiving antimalarial drug therapy.
- Implement the nursing management of clients receiving antituberculous drug therapy.
- Describe the life cycle of the ameba, and intestinal and extraintestinal amebiasis in humans.
- Explain antiamebiasis agents and their nursing management.
- Identify other protozoan diseases and the drugs used in their treatment.

▲ KEY TERMS

amebiasis, p. 1112
Hansen's disease, p. 1120
helminths, p. 1115
malaria, p. 1094
tuberculosis (TB), p. 1100

☼ KEY DRUGS

chloroquine, p. 1097
dapsone, p. 1121
isoniazid, p. 1102
mebendazole, p. 1116
paromomycin, p. 1113
pyrazinamide, p. 1103

Antimicrobial and antiparasitic agents discussed in this chapter include antimalarial, antituberculous, amebicidal, anthelmintic, and leprostatic medications. Chapter 58 reviews sulfonamides.

Antimalarials

✳ **J.L. is a 27-year-old engineer traveling to Ghana, West Africa to consult on a 3-week project. She approaches the travel clinic seeking advice on malaria prevention.**

✳ **What are the key pathologic and epidemiologic issues with malaria?**

Malaria is the most important of the parasitic diseases in humans. Some 2.24 billion people, more than 41% of the world's population, are at risk of acquiring malaria. Each year 300 to 500 million people develop malaria and 1.5 to 3 million—mostly children—die, according to WHO (Vincent, 2000). Approximately 30,000 travelers from industrialized countries contract malaria each year. The risk for acquiring malaria for the traveler not taking chemoprophylaxis and residing in an endemic malarial area for 1 month varies by region. Oceania and sub-Saharan Africa have the highest risk (1:30 and 1:500, respectively), followed by the Indian Subcontinent (1:250), Southeast Asia (1:1000), South America (1:2500), and Central America (1:10,000) (Leder & Weller, 2004). In the United States, about 1200 malaria cases are reported annually, which are mostly attributed to imported malaria; in Canada, the per capita rate is about 10 times that reported in the United States (Kain et al., 2001). Most cases involved persons who acquired this infection abroad because they either were not taking antimalarial chemoprophylaxis or were taking an inappropriate drug regimen. Four species of the genus *Plasmodium* are responsible for human malaria: *P. vivax*, *P. malariae*, *P. ovale*, and *P. falciparum*. In the U.S. cases, *P. vivax* is the most commonly reported. *P. falciparum* malaria is the most lethal form of malaria and is usually resistant to chloroquine.

Malaria may be transmitted to humans by the bite of an infected female *Anopheles* mosquito, by blood transfusion (usually *P. malariae*), congenitally, or by contaminated needles used by those who abuse IV drugs.

To understand the chemotherapy of malaria, it is essential to review the life cycle of the malarial parasite, the plasmodium (Figure 60-1).

P. vivax is the most common form of malaria; this infestation is usually mild. Drug resistance is uncommon, and this form is suppressed easily with antimalarial medications. The *P. falciparum* strain of malaria is less common but is much more severe than *P. vivax*. Drug-resistant strains of *P. falciparum* are reported; symptoms of this infestation occur at irregular intervals and can cause very serious complications. If left untreated or if treatment is delayed, the disease may progress to irreversible cardiovascular shock and death. Relapses are reported with *P. vivax*, but no dormant forms

remain in the liver once *P. falciparum* is eliminated; therefore no relapses are reported with *P. falciparum*.

Persons who harbor the sexual forms of plasmodia are called carriers; it is from carriers that mosquitoes receive the parasite forms that perpetuate the disease. The asexual forms cause the clinical symptoms of malaria. Carriers should avoid giving blood, because it is possible that the recipient of this blood will contract malaria or become a carrier. An increasing number of malaria cases (some fatal) have occurred from transfusions of infected blood (Blood Centers of the Pacific, 2002). Some infected individuals who donated blood may have once lived in an area with malaria. Therefore any traveler who is a resident of a nonmalarious area may be accepted as a donor one year after return to the nonmalarious area (irrespective of the use of chemoprophylaxis) if free of malaria symptoms. Immigrants or visitors from malarious areas may be accepted for donors three years after departure from the area if they have been asymptomatic. A person who has had malaria is deferred from giving blood for 3 years after full recovery (American Associations of Blood Banks, 2002).

✳ **What drugs are available for preventing or treating malaria?**

There are a few different types of agents used to either prevent or treat malaria. Unfortunately, resistance to agents is problematic. Agents that are used to prevent or treat malaria include the cinchona alkaloids (e.g., quinine), aminoquinolines and related drugs, and the diaminopyrimidines. Other drugs used include doxycycline (see Chapter 58) and the artemisinin derivatives, which are not used in North America.

Cinchona Alkaloids

quinine [kwye nine]

Quinine was the first drug used to treat malaria. It is derived from natural sources of the South American cinchona tree. Quinidine, used more commonly in cardiovascular medicine, is derived from the same source and also possesses antimalarial properties. As a schizonticidal agent quinine concentrates in parasitized erythrocytes, which may be why it has selective toxicity during the erythrocytic stages of plasmodial infections. It can also bind to deoxyribonucleic acid (DNA), thus inhibiting ribonucleic acid (RNA) synthesis and DNA replication.

Indications

Quinine sulfate was indicated for use in combination with other drugs for the treatment of chloroquine-resistant malaria caused by chloroquine-resistant *P. falciparum*, but today it is rarely used for malaria because more effective and less toxic drugs are available. It has also been used historically for treating nocturnal leg cramps, but this use is typically discouraged.

Pharmacokinetics/Dosing

Quinine is well absorbed orally and undergoes hepatic metabolism. Adult doses to treat chloroquine-resistant malaria are 650 mg every 8 hours dosed with an additional agent (tetracycline, sulfadoxine/pyrimethamine, clindamycin, or doxycycline). Suppressive doses are 325 mg once daily with therapy continuing for 6 weeks after exposure.

Adverse Effects

Classic adverse effects of quinidine (often referred to as cinchonism) include nausea, vomiting, diarrhea, dizziness, tinnitus, and headache. It also predisposes to hemolytic anemia for clients with glucose-6-phosphate dehydrogenase (G6PD) deficiency. Quinine has

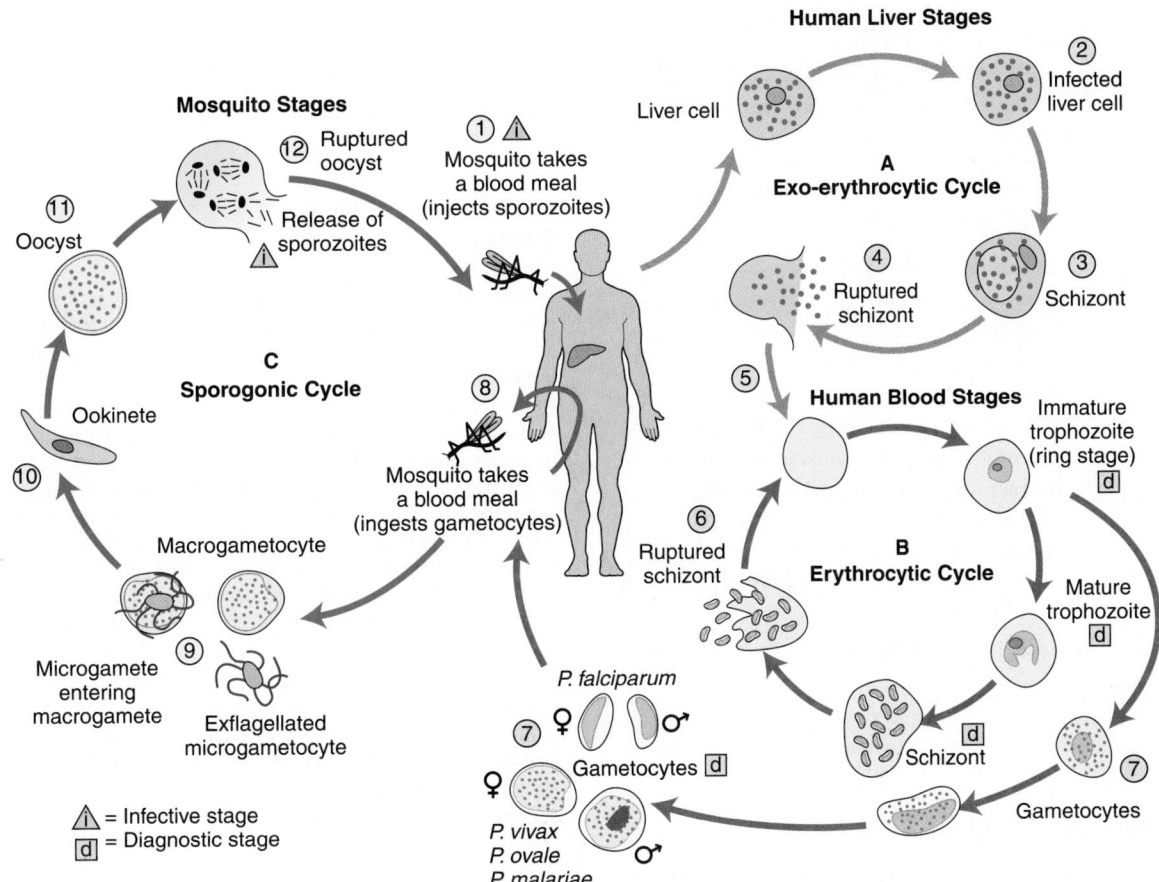

FIGURE 60-1 The life cycle of malaria. The malaria parasite life cycle involves two hosts. During a blood meal, a malaria-infected female *Anopheles* mosquito inoculates sporozoites into the human host (1). Sporozoites infect liver cells (2) and mature into schizonts (3), which rupture and release merozoites (4). (Of note, in *P. vivax* and *P. ovale* a dormant stage [hypnozoites] can persist in the liver and cause relapses by invading the bloodstream weeks or even years later.) After this initial replication in the liver (exo-erythrocytic schizogony [A]), the parasites undergo asexual multiplication in the erythrocytes (erythrocytic schizogony [B]). Merozoites infect red blood cells (5). The ring stage trophozoites mature into schizonts, which rupture releasing merozoites (6). Some parasites differentiate into sexual erythrocytic stages (gametocytes) (7). Blood stage parasites are responsible for the clinical manifestations of the disease.

The gametocytes, male (microgametocytes) and female (macrogametocytes), are ingested by an *Anopheles* mosquito during a blood meal (8). The parasites' multiplication in the mosquito is known as the sporogenic cycle (C). While in the mosquito's stomach, the microgametes penetrate the macrogametes, generating zygotes (9). The zygotes in turn become motile and elongated (ookinetes) (10), which invade the midgut wall of the mosquito where they develop into oocysts (11). The oocysts grow, rupture, and release sporozoites (12), which make their way to the mosquito's salivary glands. Inoculation of the sporozoites (1) into a new human host perpetuates the malaria life cycle.

Modified from Centers for Disease Control and Prevention. (2004). Schema of the life cycle of malaria. Retrieved April 5, 2005, from http://www.cdc.gov/malaria/biology/life_cycle.htm.

been reported to cause congenital malformations and stillbirths and therefore should not be taken by pregnant women (see the Pregnancy Safety box on p. 1096).

Nursing Management

Assess the client for hypersensitivity to quinine or quinidine; G6PD deficiency (may result in hemolytic anemia); hypoglycemia (may worsen), myasthenia gravis (may increase muscle weakness); purpura thrombocytopenia (may exacerbate); or blackwater fever (may increase complications). Assess concurrent medications; use with mefloquine may result in an increased incidence of seizures and electrocardiogram (ECG) abnormalities. A baseline assessment of

complete blood count (CBC) and blood glucose is determined. For long-term therapy, vision and hearing tests are recommended. In addition to the nursing diagnoses noted for mefloquine in J.L.'s antimalarial case below, the client is at risk for disturbed sensory perception, visual and auditory. Planning and client education is as for J.L.'s case below. Monitor the client's CBC for agranulocytosis, leukopenia, and/or thrombocytopenia, and the client's vision and hearing status. Administer with meals to minimize GI distress. The outcome of the client's quinine therapy is negative blood smears without adverse effects of the drug (e.g., cinchonism, hemolytic anemia).

Aminoquinolines and Related Agents

Among the aminoquinolines and related agents are chloroquine, hydroxychloroquine, mefloquine, primaquine, and atovaquone.

The mechanisms of action of chloroquine as an antiprotozoal to treat malaria are unknown but may be a result of its ability to bind or alter DNA properties. It increases the pH of acid vesicles, thereby interfering with the functions of DNA. During suppressive therapy, chloroquine inhibits the erythrocytic stage of development of plasmodia; during acute malarial attacks, it interferes with the erythrocytic schizogony of parasites. As chloroquine selectively accumulates in parasitized erythrocytes, it has a selective toxicity in the erythrocytic stages of plasmodial infestation. Hydroxychloroquine is chemically very similar to chloroquine, and possesses the same pharmacologic properties.

Mefloquine is a blood schizonticide; it prevents the replication of asexual erythrocytic parasites but has no effect on the gametocytes of *P. falciparum*. Its exact mechanism of action is unknown, but it is believed to inhibit protein synthesis (bind DNA), increase the intravascular pH of acid vesicles in the parasite, and have a variety of other actions. It is not effective in eliminating the exoerythrocytic or intrahepatic stages of *P. vivax* or *P. ovale* infections.

The mechanism of action of primaquine is unknown, but it can bind and alter DNA. It is very effective in the exoerythrocytic stages of *P. vivax* and *P. ovale* malaria and against the primary phase (exoerythrocytic stage) of *P. falciparum* malaria. It is also effective against the sexual forms (gametocytes) of plasmodia (especially *P. falciparum*).

Atovaquone is chemically similar to aminoquinolines and is closely related to ubiquinone (Co-enzyme Q-10 [see

Chapter 12]). It inhibits electron transport in mitochondria in malarial parasites. It also displays activity against *Pneumocystis carinii* and *Toxoplasma gondii*, and is used to treat these infections in immunocompromised clients (e.g., those with advanced HIV disease).

mefloquine [**me** floe kwin]
(Lariam)
Indications
Mefloquine is indicated for the prevention and treatment of chloroquine-resistant malaria and multiple drug-resistant strains of *P. falciparum*. It is also used to prevent malaria caused by *P. vivax*, *P. ovale*, and *P. malariae*.
Pharmacokinetics/Dosing
Mefloquine is well absorbed orally. It is widely distributed in the body and reaches peak serum levels in 7 to 24 hours. It has an elimination half-life of 13 to 33 days, is partially metabolized in the liver, and is excreted primarily in the bile and feces. The usual adult dosage for prophylaxis is 250 mg PO once weekly, beginning 1 week before travel, then weekly during traveling, and for 1 month after leaving the endemic areas. The therapeutic dosage for chloroquine-resistant *P. falciparum* malaria is 1250 mg PO as a single dose.
Adverse Effects
The adverse effects of mefloquine are uncommon and dose-related. They occur more commonly in therapeutic than in prophylaxis drug regimens and include vomiting, headache, dizziness, insomnia, gastric distress, visual disturbances, anxiety, depression, and psychosis.
Nursing Management
See the continuation of J.L.'s case below.

❋ In addition to the various immunizations that J.L. needs before she can travel to Ghana, her physician prescribes mefloquine (Lariam) 250 mg once a week, starting a week before she leaves for Ghana and continuing for 4 weeks after she returns.

❋ What are the nursing management issues in the use of antimalarials for J.L.?

Assessment Assess J.L. for allergies; mefloquine is used with caution in the presence of hypersensitivity to mefloquine, quinidine, quinine, or related medications. Mefloquine is well tolerated and rarely has been associated with serious adverse effects when used for prophylaxis. However, assess J.L. for epilepsy or a history of seizures as mefloquine may rarely cause seizures. Because an adverse effect of mefloquine is dysrhythmia, assess her cardiovascular status for first- or second-degree heart block. A mental health history is taken because the drug may cause anxiety, depression and psychosis. Determine J.L.'s pregnancy status. Malaria in pregnant women results in a higher mortality rate and greater morbidity than in other adults. Although mefloquine is Food and Drug Administration (FDA) Pregnancy Category C, the risks of malaria far outweigh any harmful effects of chemoprophylaxis.

Review J.L.'s medication regimen for the risk of significant drug interactions, such as those that may occur when mefloquine is given with quinidine or quinine. Concurrent use may result in an increased risk of sinus bradycardia, prolonged Q-T intervals, or cardiac arrest. The risk of seizures is also increased with quinine and chloroquine. Avoid concurrent use or a potentially serious drug interaction may occur. If concurrent use cannot be avoided, monitor closely and also advise J.L. to take mefloquine at least 12 hours after the last dose of quinidine or quinine. Divalproex (Depakote) or valproic acid (Depakene) taken concurrently may result in decreased serum levels of valproic acid with a loss of seizure control.

A baseline assessment should include a description of J.L.'s health status, CBC, alanine aminotransferase (ALT), and aspartate aminotransferase (AST) (may be transiently increased while J.L. is taking mefloquine) and, if J.L. has an existing cardiovascular problem, an ECG.

Nursing Diagnosis

While J.L. is taking mefloquine, she is at risk for the following nursing diagnoses/collaborative problems: impaired comfort (anorexia, nausea, vomiting, headache, arthralgia and/or myalgia); diarrhea; ineffective protection related to blood dyscrasias (leukopenia, thrombocytopenia); disturbed body image related to alopecia; anxiety; disturbed thought processes related to the development of psychosis or depression; and the potential complications of cardiovascular toxicity (dysrhythmia, QT prolongation) or seizures.

Planning

The goals for J.L.'s mefloquine therapy are that she will:

- Not contract malaria or experience adverse effects of the drug.
- Effectively manage her therapeutic regimen, including reporting adverse effects, medication compliance, and practicing measures to prevent exposure to malaria.
- Contact a physician immediately if fever of "flu-like" symptoms develop while traveling in, or within several months after departure from Ghana.

Implementation

Monitoring Observe J.L. for drug resistant strain of the parasite; failure to prevent or cure clinical malaria may require treatment with other drugs.

Intervention Administer with food and a full glass of water. Starting the drug in advance of travel also allows J.L. to determine her tolerance to the medication. Drug substitutions can be made before exposure if she is intolerant.

Education Oral preparations are taken once a week. Suppressive therapy is initiated 1 week before exposure, and the medication is continued while J.L. is staying in the malarious area and for 4 weeks after leaving the region. Alert J.L. to notify a physician if fever develops while traveling or within 2 months after leaving the endemic area. In addition to taking this medication to avoid contracting malaria, advise J.L. to stay indoors in well-screened areas between dusk and dawn; sleep under mosquito netting impregnated with the insecticide permethrin or deltamethrin at night, unless staying in an air-conditioned or well-

screened housing; wear trousers, long-sleeved shirts and a hat; use insect repellents that contain DEET (diethylmethyltoluamide) on exposed skin surfaces being careful to read and follow the directions and precautions on the product label (CDC, 2005). For additional information about staying healthy while abroad, advise her to consult the Centers for Disease Control and Prevention (CDC)'s Travelers' Health site (www.cdc.gov/travel/). Because J.L. is of childbearing age, she is advised to take reliable contraceptive precautions while taking mefloquine and for 2 months after the last dose.

Evaluation

The expected outcome of J.L.'s mefloquine prophylaxis is that she will not contract malaria or experience adverse effects of the drug. If she were being treated for malaria with mefloquine, the expected outcome would be that she would be free of malarial infection (negative blood smears) without experiencing adverse effects of the drug (e.g., GI disturbance, mental changes, blood dyscrasias). J.L. will practice lifestyle measures to avoid getting malaria effects (e.g., medication compliance, use of well-screened areas between dusk and dawn, use of insect repellant and appropriate clothing). She will report any "flu-like" symptoms occurring within 4 months of her return from travel to Ghana.

★🔲 chloroquine [**klor** oh kwin]
(Aralen)

Indications
Chloroquine is indicated for the prevention and treatment of malaria for the four strains of plasmodium. Curing *P. vivax* and *P. ovale* malaria also requires the administration of primaquine. Its use in treating malaria is typically limited to uncomplicated cases or clients with mild to moderate disease. It is sometimes used in the treatment of rheumatoid arthritis.

Pharmacokinetics/Dosing
Chloroquine is fairly well absorbed orally and widely distributed. Peak levels are achieved in about 3 hours. The terminal half-life of chloroquine is 1 to 2 months. It is partially metabolized in the liver and excreted by the kidneys. The usual oral adult dosage of chloroquine for malaria prophylaxis in chloroquine-sensitive areas is 500 mg once every 7 days begun 2 weeks before entering area and continuing for 8 weeks after leaving area. The pediatric dosage is 8.3 mg/kg PO daily (not to exceed the adult dosage) every 7 days. The parenteral adult dosage is 200 to 250 mg intramuscularly (IM) repeated in 6 hours if needed. Do not exceed 1000 mg in the first day.

Adverse Effects
The adverse effects of chloroquine are usually dose related and reversible. Gastric distress; headaches; pruritus; blurred vision; difficulty reading; headache and itching (reported mostly in black clients); hair loss or hair bleaching; blue-black discoloration of the skin, nails, or inside mouth; corneal opacities; and retinopathy have been reported. Blood disorders, cardiac dysrhythmia, mood alterations, ototoxicity, muscle weakness, and seizures are rare.

Nursing Management
Assessment
Assess the client for hypersensitivity to chloroquine and hydroxychloroquine. Use with caution in clients with liver disease (who may require reduced dosages) and in clients with G6PD deficiency and hematologic disorders (they may cause blood dyscrasias). Avoid use in clients with psoriasis or porphyria, because these conditions may become exacerbated. Polyneuritis, ototoxicity, seizures, or neuromyopathy may further compromise clients with severe neurologic disor-

ders with the use of chloroquine. Clients with retinal or visual field changes are at greater risk for corneal opacities, keratopathy, or retinopathy. Long-term therapy in children is also contraindicated. The concurrent use of mefloquine may cause seizures.

A baseline assessment of the client taking chloroquine therapeutically should include a history of foreign travel and exposure, the cyclic symptoms of fever and chills and other symptoms, and the findings of a CBC, ophthalmologic examination, and neuromuscular examination, including deep tendon reflexes of the knee and ankle reflexes.

Nursing Diagnosis
The client receiving chloroquine therapy is at risk for the following nursing diagnoses/collaborative problems: impaired comfort (anorexia, nausea, vomiting, headache and itching, particularly in black clients); diarrhea; ineffective protection related to blood dyscrasias (agranulocytosis, aplastic anemia, neutropenia, thrombocytopenia); disturbed body image related to blue-black discoloration of the skin and fingernails or alopecia; disturbed sensory perception related to ototoxicity (tinnitus and hearing loss) or ocular toxicity (retinopathy, keratopathy, or cataracts evidenced by blurred vision); disturbed thought processes related to the development of psychosis (mood and mental changes); and the potential complications of cardiovascular toxicity (hypotension, QRS prolongation), neuromyopathy, or seizures.

Planning
The goals for chloroquine therapy are that the client will:

- Have negative blood smears and not experience adverse effects of the drug.
- Effectively manage the therapeutic regimen, including reporting adverse effects, medication compliance, and practicing measures to prevent exposure to malaria.
- Collaborate with members of the health team by maintaining appointments for monitoring and ongoing treatment.

Implementation
Monitoring
Review periodic CBC results for abnormalities. Clinical symptoms of blood dyscrasia are fever, sore throat, fatigue, and easy bruising. Perform periodic tests of muscle strength and reflexes, particularly in clients who are undergoing long-term therapy. Consult with the prescriber to discontinue therapy if positive signs occur. Discontinue drugs at the first sign of retinal changes and/or visual disturbances, and continue to observe the client for possible progression even after therapy has been discontinued. Observe the client for drug resistance of the parasite. Failure to prevent or cure clinical malaria may require treatment with other drugs.

Intervention
Administer oral drug with milk or meals to minimize gastric irritation. Parenteral therapy may be IM or intravenous (IV), switch to an oral dosage as soon as possible. For IV use, the drug should be diluted and administered very slowly, over at least 4 hours.

Education
Chloroquine malarial prophylaxis is taken once a week, starting 2 weeks before exposure, and is continued while the client is staying in the malarious area. The client maintains the drug regimen for 4 weeks after leaving the region. For other lifestyle measures to prevent malaria, see J.L.'s case on p. 1097.

Instruct the client to take the drug for the full course of treatment, even if he or she is feeling better. This will ensure that the infection is completely eradicated and that symptoms will not return. To obtain the full effect of the drug, inform the client to follow a regular schedule by taking it the same day each week. Keep this drug out of reach of children. Fatalities in children have occurred after the ingestion of one 300-mg tablet.

Instruct the client to keep regularly scheduled visits for ophthalmoscopic and audiometric examinations and to report to the prescriber any signs of visual and auditory disturbances. This is to prevent irreversible retinopathy, which may occur even after therapy is discontinued.

When chloroquine is administered for rheumatoid arthritis (RA), inform the client that therapeutic benefits usually do not occur until 6 to 12 months after initiating therapy.

Caution the client to avoid alcoholic beverages while taking this drug. Because the medication may cause dizziness, advise the client to avoid tasks that require mental alertness until the response to the medication has been determined.

Evaluation
The expected outcome of chloroquine therapy is that the client will be free of malarial infection (negative blood smears) without experiencing adverse effects of the drug (e.g., headache, GI disturbances, itching, ototoxicity, ocular toxicity, mental changes). The client will be compliant with the medication regimen and will practice measures to avoid exposure to malaria. The client will appropriately report adverse drug effects to the health care provider.

hydroxychloroquine [hye drox ee **klor** oh kwin]
(Plaquenil)
Indications
Hydroxychloroquine shares the same indications as with chloroquine. It is also approved for the treatment of RA and for discoid and systemic lupus erythematosus (SLE).

Pharmacokinetics/Dosing
Hydroxychloroquine has similar pharmacokinetics as observed with chloroquine. The adult oral dosage of hydroxychloroquine for malaria prophylaxis is 400 mg once every 7 days begun 2 weeks before entering area and continuing for 4 weeks after leaving area. The pediatric dosage is 6.4 mg/kg/day PO repeated weekly. For treating SLE it is dosed at 400 mg once or twice daily. When used to treat RA, an initial oral adult dose of 400 to 600 mg daily is often used, then decreased to 200 to 400 mg PO dailiy.

Adverse Effects
As with chloroquine.

Nursing Management
Hydroxychloroquine therapy management is the same as for chloroquine, except that hydroxychloroquine tablets may be crushed and placed in gelatin capsules or mixed with jam or gelatin to make them easier to swallow.

primaquine [**prim** a kween]
Indications
Primaquine is indicated to prevent malaria relapses (radical cure) caused by *P. vivax* and *P. ovale* and is also effective against gametocytes of *P. falciparum*.

Pharmacokinetics/Dosing
Primaquine is absorbed orally and reaches a peak level within 2 to 3 hours. It has a half-life of approximately 6 hours and is rapidly metabolized in an unspecified site. A small amount is excreted by the kidneys. The adult oral dosage of primaquine is 26.3 mg daily for 2 weeks. The pediatric dosage is 680 mcg/kg daily for 2 weeks. Primaquine is not recommended for use during pregnancy.

Adverse Effects
The adverse effects of primaquine include gastric distress, hemolytic anemia and, rarely, leukopenia.

Nursing Management
Assessment
The more serious adverse effects of primaquine involve clients with a genetically determined G6PD deficiency, which can cause a lethal hemolysis of red blood cells. Review the client's current medication regimen for the risk of significant drug interactions, such as when primaquine is given concurrently with other hemolytic agents or bone marrow depressants that increase the risk of toxic drug effects. Quinacrine taken concurrently increases the toxicities of antimalarial agents. A baseline assessment includes the client's history of exposure, underlying condition, CBC, hemoglobin, and G6PD determinations.

Nursing Diagnosis
The client receiving primaquine is at risk for the following nursing diagnoses/collaborative problems: deficient fluid volume related to anorexia, nausea, and vomiting; ineffective protection related to leukopenia; and the potential complications of hemolytic anemia and methemoglobinemia.

Planning

See chloroquine therapy above.

Implementation

Monitoring

Review CBC and hemoglobin determinations weekly for a sudden decrease in hemoglobin concentration, erythrocyte count, or leukocyte count; discontinue medication if this occurs. Monitor for the signs of hemolytic anemia: fatigue; fever; pallor; anorexia; darkened urine; and back, leg, or abdominal pain. Additionally, monitor for the less commonly occurring methemoglobinemia, with cyanosis, dizziness, dyspnea, and fatigue.

Intervention

Primaquine can be administered with meals or antacids to minimize gastric irritation.

Education

Encourage the client to comply with the full course of medication and to report promptly any symptoms of adverse effects.

Evaluation

The expected outcome of primaquine therapy is that client will be free of malaria infection (negative blood smears) without any experiencing adverse effects of the drug.

atovaquone [a **toe** va kwone]
(Mepron)
atovaquone/proguanil [a **toe** va kwone/pro **gwa** nil]
(Malarone)

Indications

Atovaquone alone is indicated for the treatment of *Pneumocystis carinii* pneumonia (PCP) and *Toxoplasma gondii* infections in advanced HIV disease. In combination with proguanil (an inhibitor of folic acid), it is used for chemoprophylaxis and to treat acute uncomplicated malaria.

Pharmacokinetics/Dosing

Oral absorption of atovaquone is improved with a high-fat meal. It enterohepatic circulation and is primarily excreted in the feces as unchanged drug. The adult dose of atovaquone for prevention of PCP in HIV is 1500 mg orally once daily with food; it is dosed at 750 mg twice daily for active treatment of mild to moderate PCP in adults. Combined with proguanil it is dosed at atovaquone/proguanil 250 mg/100 mg once daily for 1 to 2 days prior to entering a malarial area through 7 days after returning in adults. Adult treatment of mild to moderate malaria is atovaquone 1000 mg/400 mg once daily for 3 days.

Adverse Effects

GI complaints (nausea, vomiting, abdominal pain) are the most common adverse effects reported with atovaquone or atovaquone/proguanil. Other effects include headache, insomnia, diarrhea, and muscle pain.

Nursing Management

In general, the nursing management for atovaquone/proguanil is as for J.L.'s case on pp. 1096 and 1097, except that it is recommended *not* to give atovaquone/proguanil concurrently with rifampin, metoclopramide, and tetracycline (decreases atovaquone serum levels). It is taken daily (starting 2 days before travel through 7 days after leaving malarial area) and with food to enhance absorption and prevent GI distress. The oral suspension and tablets are not bioequivalent and are not to be substituted for each other.

Diaminopyrimidines

Among the diaminopyrimadines are pyrimethamine (discussed here) and trimethoprim (reviewed in combination with sulfamethoxazole in Chapter 58). Pyrimethamine binds to and inhibits the protozoal enzyme dihydrofolate reductase, thus inhibiting the conversion of dihydrofolic acid to tetrahydrofolic acid. This results in a depletion of folate, which is essential for nucleic acid synthesis and protein production. When used, diaminopyrimidines are often combined with a sulfonamide or sulfone to provide improved antifolate activity.

pyrimethamine tablets [peer i **meth** a meen]
(Daraprim)
pyrimethamine with sulfadoxine
(Fansidar)

Indications

Pyrimethamine is used to treat malaria and toxoplasmosis. Pyrimethamine in combination with mefloquine and sulfadoxine (Fansidar) is indicated for the treatment of chloroquine-resistant *P. falciparum* malaria. This drug is also combined with a sulfonamide to treat toxoplasmosis caused by *Toxoplasma gondii*.

Pharmacokinetics/Dosing

Pyrimethamine is absorbed orally and is widely distributed in the body; it concentrates mainly in the blood cells, kidneys, liver, and spleen. It reaches peak plasma levels in 3 hours and has a half-life of 80 to 123 hours. It is metabolized in the liver and excreted by the kidneys. The adult oral dosage in specific world areas (e.g., Southeast Asia, East Africa, or the Amazon) is 75 mg of pyrimethamine in combination with 750 mg mefloquine and 1.5 g of sulfadoxine as a single dose. For additional dosing recommendations, refer to a current package insert.

Adverse Effects

The adverse effects of pyrimethamine are usually rare, but gastric distress, atrophic glossitis, and blood dyscrasias are reported with high dosages.

Nursing Management

Assessment

Determine the G6PD deficiency status of the client as pyrimethamine may precipitate a hemolytic anemia in such clients. Use pyrimethamine with caution in clients with anemia or bone marrow depression, because its use may cause folic acid deficiency and result in megaloblastic anemia and blood dyscrasias. Do not use this drug for the treatment of resistant forms of the parasite.

Review the client's concurrent drug regimen. An increase in leukopenia and/or thrombocytopenia may occur when pyrimethamine is administered concurrently with other bone marrow depressants. A baseline assessment should include a CBC and platelet count, and a history of exposure to malaria and a description of the client's malarial symptoms.

Nursing Diagnosis

The client receiving pyrimethamine should be assessed for the following nursing diagnoses/collaborative problems: deficient fluid volume related to anorexia, nausea, vomiting, and diarrhea; ineffective protection related to blood dyscrasias (agranulocytosis, megaloblastic anemia, thrombocytopenia); impaired oral mucous membrane related to folic acid deficiency (pain and inflammation of the tongue [atrophic glossitis]); and the potential complications of hypersensitivity (rash) and neurotoxicity (excitability, seizures).

Planning

As for chloroquine.

Implementation

Monitoring

The high dosage required for treating toxoplasmosis could approach the toxic level. Monitor CBCs and platelet counts. The dosage may be reduced if folic acid deficiency develops. The clinical symptoms of folic acid deficiency are soreness, redness, or burning of the tongue; pharyngitis; mouth ulcers; or diarrhea. Therapy should be discontinued if these symptoms occur; folic acid deficiency may be prevented by the administration of leucovorin. The administration of folinic acid (leucovorin) restores the depressed platelet or white blood counts to normal levels.

Intervention

Administer pyrimethamine with milk or food to minimize gastric irritation. To prevent possible central nervous system (CNS) toxicity in clients with seizure disorders, use a small initial dose for the treatment of toxoplasmosis.

If used to prevent malaria, pyrimethamine should be taken 2 weeks before entering a malarious area and continued for 6 weeks after leaving it. Besides building tissue stores of the drug, early administration allows assessment of the client's tolerance of the drug before travel.

Education
Advise the client to have weekly blood counts and platelet counts if undergoing high-dose therapy. If taken as a malaria suppressant, instruct the client to follow the dosage schedule as prescribed by taking the drug on the same day each week. For lifestyle measures to help prevent malaria, see J.L.'s case.

Instruct the client to report to the prescriber any signs of possible blood dyscrasia (fever, sore throat, unusual bleeding or bruising, extreme weakness, and fatigue). Alert the client to use caution when performing dental hygiene, such as using soft toothbrushes, no dental floss, and no toothpicks. Dental work is postponed until blood counts are within normal limits.

Because of the risk of severe skin reactions, Fansidar (pyrimethamine with sulfadoxine) should be used only when the client is planning to stay longer than 3 weeks in an area in which chloroquine-resistant malaria is prevalent. The drug should be discontinued and a health care provider notified at the first sign of a rash.

Evaluation
The expected outcome of pyrimethamine therapy is that the client is free of infection, with negative blood smears without adverse effects of the drug (e.g., GI disturbances, blood dyscrasias). The client will practice lifestyle measures to avoid getting malaria.

✳ How are the antimalarial agents chosen?
The choice of drug for treating malaria is based on the particular malarial strain involved and the stage of the *Plasmodium* life cycle. It is the plasmodia that cause malaria that develop resistance to antimalarial drugs not the mosquitoes that transmit the disease.

Resistance to antimalarial drugs is proving to be a challenging problem in malaria control in most parts of the world. Since the early 1960s the sensitivity of the parasites to chloroquine (Aralen), the best and most widely used drug for treating malaria, has been on the decline. Drug resistance is the ability of a parasite species to survive and multiply despite the administration of a drug in doses equal to or higher than those usually recommended but within the limit of tolerance. Drug resistance is most commonly seen in *P. falciparum*. Only sporadic cases of resistance have been reported in *P. vivax* malaria. Resistance to chloroquine is most prevalent, but resistance to most other antimalarials has also been reported. In areas containing chloroquine-resistant *P. falciparum*, mefloquine (Lariam) is used for prophylaxis; doxycycline is recommended if the client cannot take mefloquine.

Newer antimalarials have been developed in an effort to tackle this problem, but all these drugs are either expensive or have undesirable drug effects. Moreover after a variable length of time, the parasites, especially the falciparum species, have started showing resistance to these new drugs.

Travelers to endemic areas should receive malaria chemoprophylaxis. Details on prevalence of both malaria and chloroquine-resistant *P. falciparum* malaria are reported by country by the CDC in both an annual publication, *Health Information for International Travel*, and at http://

www.cdc.gov. Within "Travelers Health," this CDC site includes an online version of *Health Information for International Travel* and updates on travel-related infections, including the regional prevalence of malaria and chloroquine-resistant *P. falciparum*. Likewise, recommendations for malaria prophylaxis provided by U.K. malariologists are available at http://www.hpa.org.uk/infections/topics_az/malaria/menu.htm.

The emergence of drug-resistant strains of malaria, particularly that caused by *P. falciparum*, poses a major public health problem throughout the world. Despite the combined efforts of many countries to eradicate malaria, it remains the most devastating infectious disease in the world because of the many lives lost and the economic burdens it imposes. Fortunately, endemic malaria has been completely eradicated in the United States and Canada.

Malaria exists in Africa, Central and South America, the Middle East, Haiti, Mexico, the Far East, and many other countries. It is essential that travelers contemplating a trip to malarious areas of the world be aware of the need to obtain information from their health care provider about measures for reducing exposure to the disease.

Antituberculosis Drugs

✳ J.L. returned from Ghana without contracting malaria. However, 6 months after her return, she visits her primary care physician for a routine physical examination. She asks him if there is any testing for tuberculosis (TB) because two of the engineers that she worked with in Ghana have been diagnosed with TB. She is asymptomatic but receives a Mantoux purified protein derivative (PPD) skin test of 5 tuberculin units (TU).

✳ What are the key pathologic and epidemiologic issues to consider with TB infection?
Tuberculosis (TB) is a chronic granulomatous infection caused by the acid-fast bacillus *Mycobacterium tuberculosis*. The incidence of TB of the lungs in the United States and Canada declined from the 1950s until 1984; sanatoriums were closed and routine screening was abandoned. Then, between 1984 and 1992, the incidence increased by 20%, chiefly because of immigration from countries in which it is common and because of acquired immunodeficiency syndrome (AIDS), which leaves people particularly vulnerable to the disease. Renewed efforts at control and advances in treatment have been rewarded with incidence declines each year.

Worldwide the outlook has been far less encouraging. The largest number of cases occurs in the South-East Asia region, which accounts for 33% of incident cases globally. However, the estimated prevalence per capita in sub-Saharan Africa is nearly twice that of the South-East Asia, at 350 cases per 100,000 population.

It is estimated that 2 million deaths resulted from TB in 2002. As with cases of disease, the highest total number of estimated deaths is in the South-East Asia region, but the highest mortality per capita is in the Africa region, in which HIV has led to rapid increases in the incidence of TB and increased the likelihood of dying from TB.

In 1993, the WHO declared TB a global health emergency; approximately one third of the world's population is infected, and an estimated 3 million die each year (World Health Organization [WHO], 2004). Spread of TB is especially rapid in areas with poor public health services and crowded living conditions. In homeless shelters and prisons, crowded conditions and inadequate treatment often go together. Areas in which living conditions are disrupted by wars, famine, and natural disasters also are heavily affected. In Canada and the United States, TB is largely attributed to high-risk individuals, such as those with AIDS, those living on the street, homeless persons, undernourished or malnourished persons, or those taking immunosuppressant drugs or suffering from cancer.

Especially alarming has been the spread of drug-resistant strains of TB. By the late 1990s scientific experts and international health officials warned that drug-resistant strains were spreading faster than had been anticipated. Bacteria can survive and become drug resistant in individuals whose treatment is not properly monitored and seen to completion. Some believe that unless major new treatment strategies are initiated in source countries, drug-resistant TB will eventually become epidemic even in areas with good control programs, such as Europe and America (WHO, 2004). Resistance to two or more drugs is referred to as multidrug-resistant TB (MDR TB), and outbreaks have been noted in institutional facilities. Fortunately, MDR-TB declined from 2.5% of total TB cases in 1993 to 1.0% in 2001 in the United States (CDC, 2003a). In Canada, 1.2% of cases of TB were MDR (Health Canada, 2000). This may indicate progress in early detection and the use of appropriate therapies as factors that contributed to this decline.

M. tuberculosis, the bacteria that causes TB, most commonly affects the lungs, but other body areas can also be infected, such as the bones, joints, skin, meninges, or genitourinary tract. This bacterium is an aerobic bacillus that needs a highly oxygenated organ site for growth; thus the lungs, the growing ends of the bones, and the cerebral cortex are ideal sites. Tubercle bacilli may be transmitted by airborne droplets but cannot be transmitted on objects such as dishes, clothing, or sheets and bedding (Figure 60-2). Sharing an enclosed environment with an infected person is associated with a high risk of developing this infection, especially in facilities that provide less than optimum health care.

The development of drug-resistant TB continues to be a major concern. Tubercle bacilli droplets are transmitted when an infected person coughs or sneezes. In general, persons who produce sputum have many bacilli and are more infectious than infected persons who do not cough. The three primary types of tubercle bacilli that are pathogenic to humans are human to human, bovine to human, and avian to human. Avian TB is rare in the United States and Canada; bovine TB is much less prevalent with the pasteur-

ization of milk and testing of cows. Thus the primary source of transmission is human to human.

When tubercle bacilli enter the lungs, infection can spread to other body organs through the blood and lymph system. Usually, however, the infection becomes dormant and is walled off by calcified and fibrous tissues. The bacilli become inactive, perhaps for the lifetime of the host. However, the bacilli may be reactivated if host defenses break down or if the host receives an immunosuppressive drug.

⊛ What drugs are used to prevent and treat TB?

Effective drug regimens are available to prevent and treat TB. Choice of agents is based on efficacy and toxicity. Those agents that are most effective and least toxic are considered first line agents by the CDC (CDC, 2003b). The two most frequently used first-line agents to prevent or treat TB in North America are isoniazid (INH) and rifampin. Other first-line agents to treat active TB include ethambutol, pyrazinamide, rifabutin, and rifapentine. In cases in which resistant strains of TB are likely or have been isolated, combinations of alternative agents (sometimes referred to as second line agents), including aminosalicylic acid (PAS), capreomycin, cycloserine, ethionamide, and streptomycin, are used. Ciprofloxacin or ofloxacin is sometimes also added to other agents in the treatment of drug resistant TB (see Chapter 58 for a discussion of these agents). In other countries, Bacillus of Calmette and Guérin (BCG) vaccine may be used as a prevention strategy, but its use in North America is limited (http://www.cdc.gov/nchstp/tb/pubs/ corecurr/Chapter9/Chapter_9_Recommendations.htm).

The treatment of active TB requires consistently administered combinations of antitubercular agents to prevent drug resistance and treatment failures. Methods to achieve these ends include implementing strict public health strategies in identification and case management of active cases of TB, and implementing direct observation of therapy (DOT) systems. Additional public health strategies are outlined by the WHO (http://www.who.int/tb/dots/en/). Specific protocols and dosing regimens fluctuate based on resistance patterns and are beyond the scope of this text. Clinicians are referred to the CDC (http://www.cdc.gov) and the WHO (http://www.who.org) for updated treatment recommendations.

Primary First-Line Agents for Prevention and Treatment of TB

Isoniazid and rifampin are the mainstay agents used in the prevention and treatment of TB. Isoniazid is an antimycobacterial (bactericidal) agent that affects mycobacteria in the division phase. The exact mechanism of action is unknown, but it is believed to inhibit mycolic acid synthesis and cause cell wall disruption in susceptible organisms. Its metabolism via acetylation is highly influenced by genetics (see the Cultural Considerations box on p. 1103). Rifampin is a broad-spectrum bactericidal antibiotic (antimycobacterial) that blocks RNA transcription.

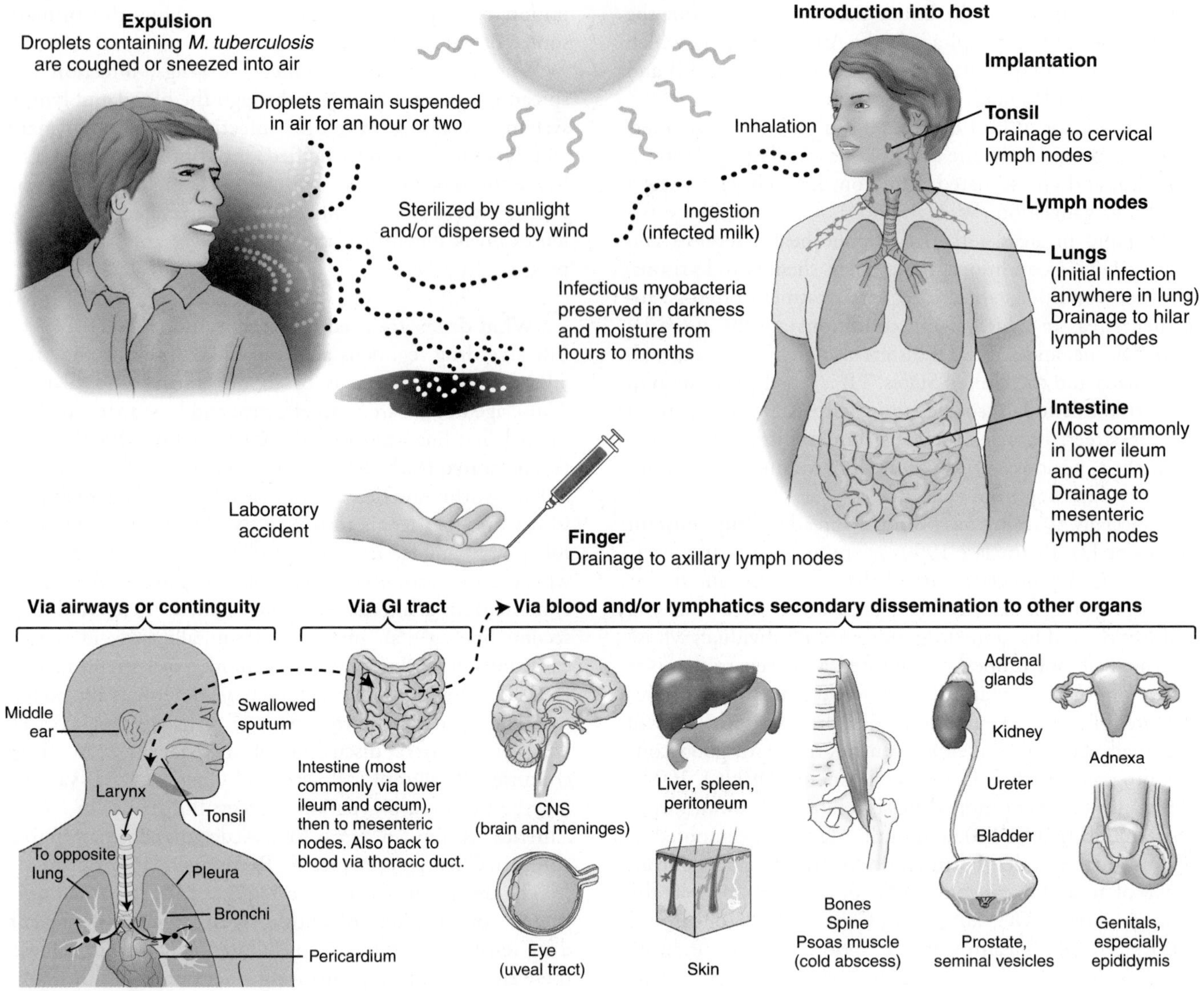

Expulsion
Droplets containing *M. tuberculosis*
are coughed or sneezed into air

Droplets remain suspended
in air for an hour or two

Inhalation

Introduction into host

Implantation

Tonsil
Drainage to cervical
lymph nodes

Lymph nodes

Sterilized by sunlight
and/or dispersed by wind

Ingestion
(infected milk)

Lungs
(Initial infection
anywhere in lung)
Drainage to hilar
lymph nodes

Infectious myobacteria
preserved in darkness
and moisture from
hours to months

Intestine
(Most commonly
in lower ileum
and cecum)
Drainage to
mesenteric
lymph nodes

Laboratory
accident

Finger
Drainage to axillary lymph nodes

Via airways or continuity | **Via GI tract** | **Via blood and/or lymphatics secondary dissemination to other organs**

Middle
ear

Swallowed
sputum

Larynx

Tonsil

To opposite
lung

Pleura

Bronchi

Pericardium

Intestine (most
commonly via lower
ileum and cecum),
then to mesenteric
nodes. Also back to
blood via thoracic duct.

CNS
(brain and meninges)

Eye
(uveal tract)

Liver, spleen,
peritoneum

Skin

Adrenal
glands

Kidney

Ureter

Bladder

Bones
Spine
Psoas muscle
(cold abscess)

Prostate,
seminal vesicles

Adnexa

Genitals,
especially
epididymis

FIGURE 60-2 Dissemination of TB.

★▪▪ isoniazid [eye soe **nye** a zid]
(Nydrazid, INH, Iodamine✦, PMS Isoniazid✦)

Indications
Isoniazid is indicated for the treatment and prevention of TB.

Pharmacokinetics/Dosing
Isoniazid is well absorbed orally and is widely distributed throughout the body. The time to peak serum levels is 1 to 2 hours for fast drug acetylators (metabolism) or 4 to 6 hours for slow drug acetylators. The half-life in fast acetylators is 0.5 to 1.6 hours; the half-life in slow acetylators is 2 to 5 hours. Isoniazid is metabolized in the liver, primarily by acetylation to inactive metabolites, some of which may be hepatotoxic. The rate of acetylation by the liver is genetically determined; slow acetylators have a decrease in hepatic *N*-acetyltransferase. Excretion is primarily by the kidneys. The adult oral and parenteral (IM) prophylactic dosage of isoniazid is 300 mg daily. When administered in combination with other agents, the parenteral (IM) treatment dosage is 5 mg/kg, up to 300 mg once daily. When given in combination with other agents to treat TB, the oral dosage is 300 mg daily. The pediatric dosage for prophylaxis orally and parenterally (IM) is 10 mg/kg, up to 300 mg daily.

Adverse Effects
The most serious adverse effect associated with isoniazid is hepatic injury and on rare occasions, has been fatal. Other adverse effects of isoniazid include gastric distress, anorexia, nausea, vomiting, weakness, and peripheral neuritis. Neuritis risk may be reduced with concurrent use of pyridoxine 50 mg PO daily.

Drug Interactions
Isoniazid interacts with a number of other hepatically metabolized drugs including warfarin, antiepileptic drugs, cycloserine, and benzodiazepines and may lead to elevated or toxic levels of these drugs.

rifampin [**rif** am pin]
(Rifadin, Rofact✦)

Indications
Rifampin is indicated for the treatment of TB and for asymptomatic meningococcal carriers of *Neisseria meningitidis*.

Pharmacokinetics/Dosing
Rifampin is well absorbed orally and is widely distributed in the body. It is lipid soluble and therefore may reach and kill intracellular

Acetylation Polymorphism

Acetylation polymorphism, a well-known example of a genetic defect in drug metabolism, was first studied when isoniazid therapy was introduced for the treatment of TB. Individuals were classified as fast or slow eliminators of isoniazid on the basis of a metabolic defect in their ability to metabolize the drug. This polymorphism is especially important in the study of ethnic and racial drug responses, because the proportions of rapid acetylators (RAs) and slow acetylators (SAs) vary dramatically in different ethnic and/or geographic populations. For example, both white and black populations have approximately equal numbers of SAs and RAs, whereas in Chinese, African American, Japanese, and Inuit descent populations the percentage of SAs is particularly low (20.5%) and that of RAs is high (Zaid et al., 2004; Ford, Delaney, Ling, & Erickson, 2001). See Chapter 6 for further discussion of genetic influences in pharmacokinetics.

Critical Thinking Question

- How would knowing whether your client was an RA or an SA affect your clinical management of his or her isoniazid therapy?

and extracellular susceptible bacteria. The time to peak serum levels is 1.5 to 4 hours, and the elimination half-life is up to 5 hours. It is metabolized in the liver by a number of cytochrome P450 enzymes including 2A6, 2C8/9, and 3A4. It is excreted primarily in the feces. The adult oral dosage of rifampin in combination with other agents (for TB) is 600 mg daily. To treat asymptomatic meningococcal carriers, the dosage is 600 mg PO twice daily for 2 days. For children 1 month and older, the dosage to treat TB (with other antituberculous drugs) is 10 to 20 mg/kg PO daily. For asymptomatic meningococcal carriers, the adult dosage is 600 mg PO or IV every 12 hours for a total of four doses.

Adverse Effects
The most serious risk with rifampin is hepatotoxicity, although this risk appears significantly lower than with isoniazid. Other adverse effects of rifampin include gastric distress, hypersensitivity, and a flu-like syndrome. Clients should be educated about the ability of rifampin to produce a red/orange color to urine, saliva, tears, and sweat.

Drug Interactions
Rifampin is a strong inducer of a number of the cytochrome P450 enzyme systems, including 1A2, 2A6, 2B6, 2C19, and 3A4. This accounts for the numerous interactions that are observed with rifampin. In most cases, rifampin is responsible for increased metabolism (and therefore reduced levels or effect) of other drugs metabolized by these systems. Affected drugs include (but not limited to) estrogen and hormonal contraceptives, warfarin, antidysrhythmics, calcium channel blockers, antiepileptic drugs, levothyroxine, fluoroquinolones, antipsychotics, antidepressants, and a number of drugs used in the management of HIV. If other drug therapy is stabilized while on rifampin therapy, toxicity related to those other drugs may be problematic when rifampin is discontinued. Because the scope of drugs affected is so broad, and the degree of impact on metabolism of drugs so significant, the entire drug regimen should be reviewed and managed carefully for all clients who initiate or discontinue rifampin therapy.

Other First-Line Agents to Treat TB

Rounding out the first-line agents used to treat TB are pyrazinamide, ethambutol, rifabutin, and rifapentine. These agents are typically used reserved for treatment of active TB.

Pyrazinamide is an antimycobacterial agent with an unknown mechanism of action. Pyrazinamide can be bacteriostatic or bactericidal depending on its concentration at the site of action and the susceptibility of the mycobacteria. Ethambutol is a bacteriostatic antituberculous agent; it is believed to diffuse into the mycobacteria bacilli and suppress RNA synthesis. Ethambutol is effective only against actively dividing mycobacteria. Rifabutin is an antimycobacterial that inhibits DNA-dependent RNA polymerase in susceptible *Escherichia coli* and *Bacillus subtilis* microorganisms. Rifapentine is an antitubercular with action similar to rifampin and rifabutin, and resistant strains to rifampin or rifabutin are likely to be resistant to rifapentine.

✸▉ pyrazinamide [peer a **zin** a mide]
(Pyrazinamide, Tebrazid✚)
Indications
Pyrazinamide is indicated in combination with other agents for the treatment of TB.
Pharmacokinetics/Dosing
Pyrazinamide is well absorbed orally and is widely distributed in the body. The time to peak serum levels is 1 to 2 hours; the elimination half-life is 9 to 10 hours. Pyrazinamide is primarily metabolized in the liver and is excreted by the kidneys. When given in combination with other agents, the adult oral dosage of pyrazinamide is 15 to 30 mg/kg daily, up to a maximum dosage of 2 g daily.
Adverse Effects
The adverse effects of pyrazinamide include arthralgia related to hyperuricemia.

ethambutol [e **tham** byoo tole]
(Myambutol, Etibi✚)
Indications
Ethambutol is indicated in combination with other drugs for the treatment of TB.
Pharmacokinetics/Dosing
Ethambutol is absorbed orally and distributed to most body tissues and fluids (with the exception of cerebrospinal fluid). High concentrations are found in the kidneys, lungs, saliva, urine, and erythrocytes. The time to peak serum levels is 2 to 4 hours, and the half-life is between 3 and 4 hours. Ethambutol is metabolized in the liver and excreted by the kidneys. The adult oral dosage in combination with other agents is 15 to 25 mg/kg daily.
Adverse Effects
The most serious adverse effect of ethambutol is optic neuritis, which requires regular ophthalmologic evaluations with its use. Other adverse effects of ethambutol include gastric distress, confusion, disorientation, and headache.

rifabutin [**riff** a byoo tin]
(Mycobutin)
Indications
Rifabutin, chemically related to rifampin, is indicated for the prophylaxis for disseminated *M. avium* complex (MAC) in persons with advanced HIV infection.

Pharmacokinetics/Dosing

This drug is absorbed from the GI tract, reaches peak serum levels in 2 to 4 hours, and has a terminal half-life of 45 hours. It is metabolized in the liver and primarily excreted by the kidneys. The usual adult dosage is 450 to 600 mg PO once daily for treatment of MAC and 300 mg PO once daily for prophylaxis.

Adverse Effects

The adverse effects of rifabutin include nausea, vomiting, and skin rash. Rifabutin use typically results in a red/orange coloring to body secretions; clients should be informed of this to prevent alarm.

Drug Interactions

Rifabutin, like rifampin, may have a number of interactions with other drugs affecting the cytochrome P450 enzyme systems (particularly 1A2 and 3A4). It may decrease levels of benzodiazepines, ß blockers, clofibrate, dapsone, opioids, anticoagulants, corticosteroids, cyclosporine, quinidine, hormonal contraceptives, progestins, sulfonylureas, ketoconazole, fluconazole, barbiturates, theophylline, and antiepileptic drugs, resulting in therapeutic failure.

Nursing Management

Rifabutin is not administered to clients with active TB; they are better treated with the therapies previously described. If rifabutin is administered to a client with active TB as a prophylaxis of MAC, there is the risk of the TB becoming resistant to both rifabutin and rifampin. A CBC with a white blood cell (WBC) differential and platelets are required as a part of the baseline assessment, because this drug may cause blood dyscrasias. Rifabutin accelerates the metabolism of protease inhibitors (amprenavir, indinavir, nelfinavir, ritonavir, saquinavir), nonnucleoside reverse transcriptase inhibitors (NNRTIs), and zidovudine, however, in vitro studies have indicated that rifabutin does not affect the inhibition of HIV by zidovudine. Rifabutin also stimulates the metabolism of estrogen-containing hormonal contraceptives; advise clients to use nonhormonal measures of birth control. Platelet counts and WBC counts are performed at periodic intervals to monitor for neutropenia and, rarely, thrombocytopenia. Monitor the client for the development of MAC. Administer on an empty stomach, it can be given with food if GI distress occurs. Body secretions may be discolored as with rifampin.

The expected outcome of rifabutin therapy is that the client will manage the therapeutic regimen effectively and will not contract MAC.

rifapentine [riff a pen teen]
(Priftin)
Indications

Rifapentine is used to treat pulmonary TB in combination with other agents.

Pharmacokinetics/Dosing

Rifapentine is moderately well absorbed orally and bioavailability improves when dosed with food. It is highly bound to plasma albumin, and is eliminated by hepatic metabolism. The adult dose of rifapentine in the treatment of active TB is dependent on protocol, and is always used in combination with other agents.

Adverse Effects

Among the most serious reactions to rifapentine is hepatotoxicity. Elevated uric acid levels, hypertension, headache, GI upset, and joint pain have also been reported. Like rifampin and rifabutin, rifapentine may produce a red or orange tinge to body fluids, including tears, urine, saliva, and sweat.

Drug Interactions

As a strong inducer of cytochrome P-450 2C8/9 and 3A4, rifapentine is responsible for a number of interactions with other drugs; see the discussion under rifampin.

Nursing Management

See discussion under rifampin.

Combinations

For ease of drug administration, isoniazid has been combined with rifampin (Rifamate) and is available in dual packs (Rimactane/INH). A three-drug combination is available that contains rifampin, isoniazid, and pyrazinamide (Rifater). The marketing of combination antituberculous products may help to improve compliance with drug therapy.

✳ How are the drugs for TB selected?

Drug selection is based on the development of drug-resistant organisms and drug toxicity. The usual regimen for the treatment of latent TB is isoniazid given daily for 6 months; HIV-infected clients receive 12 months of isoniazid preventive therapy (CDC, 2003b) (Table 60-1).

General guidelines for the management of active TB include the following:

- To avoid the development of drug-resistant organisms, all individuals diagnosed with active TB (isolated *M. tuberculosis*) should undergo drug susceptibility tests on their first isolation.

TABLE 60-1 Drug Regimens for the Treatment of LTBI

Drugs	Duration (months)	Interval	Minimum Doses
isoniazid	9	Daily	270
		Twice weekly	76
isoniazid	6	Daily	180
		Twice weekly	52
rifampin	4	Daily	120
rifampin/pyrazinamide	Generally should not be offered for treatment of LTBI*		

Data from Centers for Disease Control and Prevention, 2004. (www.cdc.gov/nchstp/tb/pybs/tbfactsheets/250110.htm)
*Because of the reports of severe liver injury and deaths, CDC now recommends that the combination of rifampin and pyrazinamide should generally *not* be offered for the treatment of LTBI. If the potential benefits significantly outweigh the demonstrated risk of severe liver injury and death associated with this regimen and the client has no contraindications, a TB/LTBI expert should be consulted prior to the use of this regimen. Clinicians should continue the appropriate use of rifampin and pyrazinamide in multidrug regimens for the treatment of active TB disease.

- In most instances drug therapy is started before the results of the in vitro susceptibility test are known. It is recommended that a four-drug regimen be instituted (especially in areas in which primary isoniazid resistance occurs), because this regimen provides adequate therapy that will be at least 95% effective, even in the presence of drug-resistant organisms. The recommended drugs are INH, rifampin, pyrazinamide (PZA), and ethambutol (EMB), or streptomycin (Table 60-2).

TABLE 60-2 DRUG REGIMENS FOR CULTURE-POSITIVE PULMONARY TUBERCULOSIS CAUSED BY DRUG-SUSCEPTIBLE ORGANISMS

	Initial Phase		Continuation Phase			Range of Total Doses (Minimal Duration)	Rating* (Evidence)†	
Regimen	Drugs	Interval and Doses‡ (Minimal Duration)	Regimen	Drugs	Interval and Doses‡§ (Minimal Duration)		HIV⁻	HIV⁺
1	INH RIF PZA EMB	7 days/wk for 56 doses (8 wk) or 5 days/wk for 40 doses (8 wk)¶	1 a	INH/RIF	7 days/wk for 126 doses (18 wk) or 5 days/wk for 90 doses (18 wk)¶	182-130 (26 wk)	A (I)	A (II)
			1 b	INH/RIF	Twice weekly for 36 doses (18 wk)	92-76 (26 wk)	A (I)	A (II)#
			1 c**	INH/RPT	Once weekly for 18 doses (18 wk)	74-58 (26 wk)	B (I)	E (I)
2	INH RIF PZA EMB	7 days/wk for 14 doses (2 wk), then twice weekly for 12 doses (6 wk) or 5 days/wk for 10 doses (2 wk),¶ then twice weekly for 12 doses (6 wk)	2 a	INH/RIF	Twice weekly for 36 doses (18 wk)	62-58 (26 wk)	A (II)	B (II)#
			2 b**	INH/RPT	Once weekly for 18 doses (18 wk)	44-40 (26 wk)	B (I)	E (I)
3	INH RIF PZA EMB	Three times weekly for 24 doses (8 wk)	3 a	INH/RIF	Three times weekly for 54 doses (18 wk)	78 (26 wk)	B (I)	B (II)
4	INH RIF EMB	7 days/wk for 56 doses (8 wk) or 5 days/wk for 40 doses (8 wk)¶	4 a	INH/RIF	7 days/wk for 217 doses (31 wk) or 5 days/wk for 155 doses (31 wk)¶	273-195 (39 wk)	C (I)	C (II)
			4 b	INH/RIF	Twice weekly for 62 doses (31 wk)	118-102 (39 wk)	C (I)	C (II)

From ATS, CDC, & IDSA. (2003). Treatment of Tuberculosis. *Morbidity and Mortality Weekly Report 52,* (RR-11), 1-50.

EMB, ethambutol; INH, isoniazid; PZA, pyrazinamide; RIF, rifampin; RPT; rifapentine.

* Definitions of evidence ratings: A, preferred; B, acceptable alternative; C, offer when A and B cannot be given; E, should never be given.

† Definition of evidence ratings: I, randomized clinical trial; II, data from clinical trials that were not randomized or were conducted in other populations; III, expert opinion.

‡ When DOT is used, drugs may be given 5 days/week and the necessary number of doses adjusted accordingly. Although there are no studies that compare five with seven daily doses, extensive experience indicates this would be an effective practice.

§ Clients with cavitation on initial chest radiograph and positive cultures at completion of 2 months of therapy should receive a 7-month (31 week; either 217 doses [daily] or 62 doses [twice weekly]) continuation phase.

¶ Five-day-a-week administration is always given by DOT. Rating for 5 day/week regimens is A III.

Not recommended for HIV-infected clients with CD4⁺ cell counts less than 100 cells/mcL.

** Options 1 c and 2 b should be used only in HIV-negative clients who have negative sputum smears at the time of completion of 2 months of therapy and who do not have cavitation on initial chest radiograph. For clients started on this regimen and found to have a positive culture from the 2-month specimen, treatment should be extended an extra 3 months.

- The drug regimen can be adjusted when drug susceptibility results are available.
- Monitor the prescribed therapy regimen closely to support client compliance, detect adverse effects, and register progress of the treatment program.

✳ **J.L. returns to the physician's office 48 hours later to have her Mantoux test read. She has an area of induration of 7 mm, which is considered positive given her recent contact with individuals with active TB. Active TB is ruled out for J.L. by history, physical examination, and chest radiograph. However, those recently infected with *M. tuberculosis* are at greatest risk for developing the active disease shortly after infection occurred, so J.L. is to be treated for latent tuberculosis infection (LTBI). After reviewing the available regimens (see Table 60-1) and their adverse effect profiles, isoniazid 300 mg PO daily and pyridoxine 50 mg PO daily are prescribed.**

✳ **What are the nursing implications for the use of anti-TB drugs for J.L.'s LTBI?**

Assessment Before being treated for LTBI, J.L. had active TB ruled out by history, physical examination and a negative chest radiograph for active disease. Assess for hypersensitivity to isoniazid (INH), niacin, ethionamide, and pyrazinamide. Assess whether J.L. is at risk for developing INH-associated peripheral neuropathy; clients with diabetes mellitus, uremia, malnutrition, alcoholism, HIV infection, pregnancy, and seizure disorders are at greater risk. INH should be administered cautiously to clients who have a history of alcoholism and/or hepatic function impairment, because there is increased risk of hepatitis. A history of seizures will also increase the risk of neurotoxicity with a decreased seizure threshold. J.L. opts for the daily dosing of INH because the twice weekly dosing involves DOT. DOT involves providing the anti-TB drugs directly to the client and watching as the drug is swallowed. DOT is the preferred management strategy to promote adherence for clients who are at high risk for noncompliance.

Review J.L.'s current medication regimen for the risk of significant drug interactions, which may be contraindicated or involve closer monitoring of the client. Daily use of alcohol may result in increased isoniazid metabolism and an increased risk of hepatotoxicity. Monitor clients, because a dosage adjustment may be necessary. INH inhibits liver metabolism, which may decrease alfentanil (Alfenta) metabolism and lead to increased serum levels of alfentanil and prolong its duration of action. Concurrent use of INH and carbamazepine (Tegretol) may result in increased carbamazepine serum levels and toxicity. The use of INH and disulfiram (Antabuse) may increase the incidence of CNS adverse effects, such as ataxia, irritability, dizziness, or insomnia. Monitor closely for these symptoms, because a dosage reduction or even the discontinuation of disulfiram may be required. Other hepatotoxic drugs may increase the potential for hepatotoxicity; avoid concurrent use or a po-

tentially serious drug interaction may occur. INH with ketoconazole (Nizoral) may decrease serum levels of ketoconazole. Combining INH with phenytoin (Dilantin) may result in impaired phenytoin metabolism, leading to increased serum levels and toxicity. The dosage of phenytoin may need to be adjusted. Monitor serum phenytoin closely. Rifampin (Rifadin) with isoniazid may increase the potential for hepatotoxicity, especially in clients with liver impairment. Monitor closely for hepatotoxicity, especially during the first 90 days of therapy.

Hepatic function determinations, CBC, weight, blood pressure (BP), vision and neurological assessment, and the status of the underlying TB should also be documented as part of the baseline assessment.

Nursing Diagnosis While J.L. is taking INH, she is at risk for the following nursing diagnoses/collaborative problems: deficient fluid volume related to anorexia, nausea, vomiting, and diarrhea; disturbed sensory perception related to peripheral neuritis (numbness and tingling of the fingers and toes) and optic neuritis (blurred vision or loss of vision); ineffective protection related to leukopenia, thrombocytopenia, and anemia (fever, sore throat, fatigue, unusual bruising, or bleeding); and the potential complications of hepatitis (yellow skin and sclera), neurotoxicity (depression, psychosis, seizures), and hypersensitivity (fever, rash, arthralgia).

Planning The goals for J.L.'s INH therapy for LTBI are that she will:
- Not develop active TB.
- Remain free of adverse effects of INH.
- Effectively manage her therapeutic regimen, including medication compliance, reporting adverse drug effects appropriately, and maintain scheduled visits with the health team for monitoring and treatment.

Implementation

Monitoring Routine laboratory monitoring (AST and ALT) during treatment of LTBI is indicated only if J.L.'s baseline tests suggest a liver disorder or if there were a risk of hepatic disease. Laboratory testing should be performed to evaluate possible adverse effects that occur during the treatment regimen. Observe J.L. for symptoms of jaundice and hepatitis prodromal syndrome (anorexia, nausea, or fatigue). If J.L. were older than 50 years of age, she would be more prone to the development of hepatitis. INH should be discontinued at the first signs of hepatotoxicity.

Although its incidence is rare, optic neuritis (blurred vision, vision loss, and/or eye pain) does occur. J.L. should undergo an ophthalmologic examination at the first indication of symptoms related to vision changes.

Monitor J.L.'s compliance with her medication, and for symptoms of developing active TB (e.g., malaise, anorexia, weight loss, fever, night sweats, cough, presence of sputum).

Intervention Administer oral INH with meals or antacids to minimize GI distress. If aluminum-containing

CHAPTER 60 Other Antimicrobial Drugs and Antiparasitic Drugs **1107**

antacids are used, administer them at least 1 hour after INH. Oral absorption may be decreased if the drug is taken with food or antacids. Pyridoxine may be prescribed concurrently to help prevent peripheral neuritis.

There are slow and fast acetylators of isoniazid. Slow acetylators may require lower dosages and are more apt to develop adverse effects, particularly peripheral neuritis. The highest prevalence of slow acetylators is found in Egyptian, Israeli, Scandinavian, and other Caucasian and black populations; the lowest prevalence of slow acetylators is found in Eskimo, Asian, and Native American populations.

Education Encourage J.L. to comply with the full course of INH therapy. Regular visits to the health care provider are necessary for monitoring progress and for periodic eye examinations. Any symptoms related to changes in vision should be promptly reported to the prescriber. Because alcohol decreases the effects of INH by increasing its metabolism and INH-associated hepatotoxicity, alert J.L. not to drink alcohol while taking INH. Advise J.L. to use an alternative form of contraception if she is using hormonal contraception.

Evaluation The expected outcome of isoniazid therapy for J.L.'s LTBI is that she will not develop the active form of the disease and will be able to manage the therapeutic regimen effectively (e.g., complying with the medication regimen, reporting adverse drug effects appropriately, maintaining scheduled visits with the health team). She will not experience any adverse effects of the drug (e.g., GI disturbances, peripheral neuritis, optic neuritis, hepatotoxicity, blood dyscrasias).

✱ **L.M., a 21-year-old nursing student, is admitted to the hospital with a 3-month history of cough. She smokes, but her cough has recently become more productive. She is also experiencing fatigue, night sweats, and an unintentional weight loss of 10 pounds in the last 2 months. L.M. has been working in a nursing home on weekends and two of the clients for whom she recently cared have been diagnosed with TB. Although her physical exam was essentially negative, her chest radiograph revealed bibasilar infiltrates. A Mantoux test was administered and sputum collected for acid-fast bacteria (AFB) smear and culture and sensitivity. Her other laboratory tests were within the normal limits.**

✱ **L.M.'s sputum smear was positive for AFB and at 48 hours her Mantoux was positive at 12 mm induration. Although a positive culture for M. tuberculosis is necessary to definitely diagnose active TB, the decision is made to initiate treatment. L.M. is placed in respiratory isolation.**

The overall goals of antitubercular therapy for active TB are both to cure the individual client and to prevent transmission of TB to other persons. Combination antitubercular chemotherapy is used to kill the tubercula bacilli rapidly,

prevent the emergence of drug resistance, and eliminate persistent bacilli from the client's tissues to prevent relapse (CDC, 2003b). Currently, four basic regimens are recommended for the treatment of adults with TB caused by organisms that are known or presumed to be drug-susceptible (see Table 60-2).

✱ **What are the nursing management issues for the anti-TB therapy for L.M.?**

Assessment Obtain cultures for *Mycobacterium* and tests for the organism's susceptibility to the antituberculous drugs before and periodically during the course of drug therapy. Sputum specimens can help confirm active TB and help to estimate the degree of infectiousness. If the client has suspected pulmonary TB, at least three sputum specimens should be examined by smear and culture. The smear test can detect mycobacterial organisms, but culture and sensitivity testing takes much longer—from 1 to 3 weeks to detect growth and 8 to 12 weeks to be certain. In the initial assessment, a client may exhibit as L.M. has, nonspecific symptoms, such as fatigue, weakness, anorexia, weight loss, night sweats, or low-grade fever. Radiographs may show nodular lesions, patchy infiltrates (many in the upper lobes), cavity formation, scar tissue, and calcium deposits. Ascertain any drug hypersensitivities that may affect L.M.'s antitubercular chemotherapy.

In addition to the basic assessment related to antitubercular drugs, each of the drugs within the treatment regimen also requires additional assessment to initiate safe drug therapy: INH was discussed in J.L.'s treatment of her latent TB infection, but the others will be listed here.

Rifampin (RIF), pyrazinamide, and INH carry a high risk for hepatotoxicity, assess L.M. for impaired hepatic function and/or active alcoholism (or a history of it). Hepatic function studies (ALT, AST, serum alkaline phosphatase, serum bilirubin levels) should be obtained before initiating drug therapy.

Pyrazinamide (PZA): Use PZA with caution if a client has a history of gout because PZA increases serum uric acid concentrations

Ethambutol (EMB): Assess L.M. for preexisting optic neuritis. The risk for neurotoxicity (e.g., optic and peripheral neuritis) is increased if EMB is administered concurrently with other neurotoxic agents. A baseline ophthalmic examination should be performed before initiating EMB therapy. It also increases uric acid concentrations, so it carries the same cautions as PZA in clients with gout. Weigh L.M. carefully, because the dosage is based on weight.

Review L.M.'s current medication regimen for the risk of significant drug interactions in relation to rifampin. Daily use of alcohol may increase the risk of rifampin-induced hepatotoxicity and increase the rate of rifampin metabolism. Rifampin increases levels of hepatic enzymes and therefore may decrease the effectiveness of some medications which are metabolized by the liver: antidysrhythmics (disopyramide [Norpace], mexiletine [Mexitil], tocainide [Tonocard], quinidine), anticoagulants, antidiabetic agents (oral), azole antifungals, chloramphenicol, corticosteroids, digoxin, estrogen-containing hormonal contraceptives, methadone, nonnucleoside reverse transcriptase inhibitors (NNRTIs), phenytoin (Dilantin), protease inhibitors, theophylline, and verapamil. Other hepatotoxic drugs, such as INH, increase the risk of hepatotoxicity.

Nursing Diagnosis L.M., as a client receiving chemotherapy for TB will have the nursing diagnosis of risk for infection transmission (at least initially). The following should also be considered: ineffective airway clearance related to copious tracheobronchial secretions; risk of infection related to the ineffectiveness of the antituberculous drug; risk for infection transmission; deficient knowledge related to unfamiliarity with the disease process and treatment methods; ineffective therapeutic regimen management; and any collaborative problems that might relate to complications of TB.

INH: See the nursing diagnoses for the previous case on p. 1106.

RIF: The client receiving rifampin should be assessed for the following nursing diagnoses/collaborative problems: impaired comfort related to rash (hypersensitivity) and flu-like syndrome (chills, fever, headache, generalized discomfort); diarrhea; ineffective protection related to fungal overgrowth (sore mouth and tongue) and blood dyscrasias; deficient fluid volume related to nausea and vomiting; impaired urinary elimination related to interstitial nephritis as evidenced by greatly decreased frequency of urination and amount of urine; and the potential complications of hepatitis and red-orange discoloration of the skin, mucous membranes, and sclera.

PZA: The client receiving pyrazinamide should be assessed for the following nursing diagnoses/collaborative problem: impaired skin integrity (rash and itching); impaired comfort related to hyperuricemia (gouty arthritis [pain and swelling of joints, especially the big toe, ankle, and knee]); and the potential complication of hepatotoxicity (anorexia, fatigue, yellow skin, and sclera).

EMB: The client receiving ethambutol should be assessed for the following nursing diagnoses/collaborative problems: impaired comfort (headache); disturbed thought processes (confusion); deficient fluid volume related to anorexia, nausea, and vomiting; disturbed sensory perception related to retrobulbar optic neuritis (red-green color blindness, blurred vision, or vision loss); and the potential complications of hypersensitivity (rash, fever, arthralgia), hyperuricemia and gout (pain and swelling of joints, particularly the big toe, ankle, and knee), and peripheral neuritis (numbness, tingling of the fingers and toes).

Planning The goals for L.M.'s antitubercular chemotherapy are that she will:
- Show improvement in her disease state.
- Remain free of adverse effects of the antitubercular drugs.
- Effectively manage her therapeutic regimen, including medication compliance, reporting adverse drug

effects appropriately, and maintain scheduled visits with the health team for monitoring and treatment.

Implementation

Monitoring Sputum cultures and radiographs are used to monitor L.M.'s status. Monitor the client for symptoms that indicate resolution of the infection: diminished cough and sputum production, decreased fever and night sweats, reduction of cavitation on chest x-ray examination, reduction of anorexia with concomitant weight gain, and decreased AFB in sputum specimens. (See the Community and Home Health Considerations box on p. 1109 for information regarding medication monitoring in the community.)

RIF: Monitor hepatic function studies closely with rifampin, because dosage adjustments may be necessary. Monitor L.M. for anorexia, nausea, fatigue, jaundice, yellow sclera, and dark urine, which may indicate hepatotoxicity.

PZA: Monitor L.M. for hepatotoxicity as above. Monitor serum uric acid levels to help prevent an acute episode of gout in clients at risk and observe for symptoms of acute gouty arthralgia (pain and swelling of joints such as the big toe, knee, and ankle).

EMB: Ethambutol is known to decrease visual acuity and the ability to see red and green. This presents a safety hazard, especially in driving motor vehicles, and L.M. should be tested for these visual disturbances at frequent intervals during drug therapy. Discontinuation of the drug is usually indicated when visual acuity is disturbed. Monitor for elevated serum uric acid and gout symptoms as with PZA.

Intervention Administer antitubercular drugs with consideration for L.M.'s comfort. For example, GI disturbances following administration can be reduced by the concurrent administration of food or antacids.

Some settings have instituted DOT to prevent multidrug-resistant therapy (CDC, 2003b).

RIF, PZA, and EMB are administered concurrently with other antituberculous drugs to minimize bacterial resistance. The treatment period may be 6 months to 2 years. The regimen is altered as appropriate when the results of susceptibility for these medications are available.

Education For maximum therapeutic effectiveness, L.M. must take prescribed medications regularly and without interruption. Instruct L.M. who is responsible for self-medication about the necessity of taking these drugs (three or more concurrently) according to the prescribed regimen and not discontinuing them when feeling better. Alert L.M. to the adverse effects of the specific drugs and the need to report these effects immediately. Instruct her about the necessity for periodic medical evaluations to evaluate the effectiveness of therapy.

Remind L.M. to get sufficient rest. Stress the importance of having a well-balanced diet. Encourage her to eat small, frequent meals if she is anorexic. Have her record her

Antituberculous Medication Management in the Community

Nursing management of an antituberculous therapeutic regimen has the following expected outcomes: completion of an effective course of therapy that consists of at least two drugs to which the organism is susceptible; keeping the course of therapy as short as possible to promote client adherence; and preventing the transmission of outbreaks (Neff, 2003):

1. Monitor the client's response to therapy. A client with pulmonary TB should have sputum tested at 2 months to determine the course of therapy, and monthly thereafter until two consecutive sputum culture results are negative. Follow-up sputum testing is necessary to determine the client's response to therapy and how long therapy should last. Once effective antituberculous therapy begins, the number of organisms in the smear tests will decrease, and the client's symptoms will improve. If specimens remain positive after 3 months of therapy, the disease may be the result of a drug-resistant organism, or the client is not taking medications as prescribed.
2. Ensure client adherence. Instruct the client in the importance of taking the medication for the duration of therapy, even if client is feeling better. Assess for adherence at every follow-up visit. Pill counts are helpful. Urine tests

are available as a dipstick test that can detect INH in the urine 24 to 48 hours after the drugs are taken. Rifampin also turns the urine orange-colored for several hours after a dose. The most effective way to ensure client compliance is "directly observed therapy." DOT requires that someone actually observe the client take every dose of medication for the entire therapeutic regimen. DOT programs increase adherence in both rural and urban settings. One hospital in New York City reported that only 11% of clients under care for TB reported to an outpatient clinic for further treatment when discharged from the hospital. In contrast, a program in which DOT is routinely used for all clients had a completion rate of 98%. Although an expanded use of DOT may require additional resources, intermittent and directly observed regimens are cost-effective (CDC, 2003b). DOT can be conducted with regimens given once daily, two times weekly, or three times weekly.

3. Monitor for adverse drug reactions. Because of the long-term nature of drug therapy for TB, clients may need support in maintaining the therapeutic regimen and in managing the adverse effects of the TB drugs.

---

weekly weights and review them with her on clinical visits. Instruct L.M. in the importance of measures to minimize disease transmission, such as covering the mouth when coughing and sneezing.

If peripheral neuritis appears as an adverse effect of the antituberculous drugs, teach L.M. precautionary strategies to avoid injury from burning agents and sharp objects until the alteration in sensation is remedied. Use of pyridoxine is recommended with INH to reduce this risk.

RIF: Have L.M. take her rifampin with a full glass of water on an empty stomach, 1 hour before or 2 hours after a meal, of with food if GI distress occurs. Alert her that there may be a reddish brown discoloration of urine, feces, saliva, sputum, sweat, and tears but that this effect is not hazardous. However, if she wears soft contact lenses, this effect may permanently discolor the lens.

If L.M. is using an estrogen-containing hormonal contraceptives concurrent with rifampin or INH, she should be cautioned to use an alternate form of contraception.

Advise her to avoid alcoholic beverages while taking rifampin because it increases the risk of hepatotoxicity.

PZA: Teach L.M. measures to prevent gout, such as maintaining a fluid intake of 2500 mL daily, adjusting to an optimum weight, and limiting the intake of alcohol and foods high in purines, such as organ meats (liver, kidneys, hearts, sweetbreads), shellfish, and sardines.

EMB: Alert L.M. to notify her prescriber if no improvement occurs in 2 to 3 weeks. Report promptly signs of optic neuritis (blurred vision, any loss of vision or red-green

perception, or eye pain) or peripheral neuritis (numbness, tingling, or weakness in the hands and feet).

Evaluation The expected outcome of antituberculous therapy is that L.M.'s will have a negative sputum culture and chest radiograph and the signs and symptoms of the disease (e.g., cough, sputum production, fever, night sweats, weight loss) diminish or do not reappear, and she effectively self-manages the therapeutic regimen (e.g., medication compliance, adequate diet and rest, prevention of disease transmission).

Second-Line Agents for Drug-Resistant TB

The second-line drugs used to treat TB are typically reserved for drug-resistant cases. These include aminosalicylic acid (PAS), capreomycin, cycloserine, ethionamide, and the aminoglycoside, streptomycin. Although not officially indicated for the treatment of TB, some of the fluoroquinolones (gatifloxacin, levofloxacin, and moxifloxacin), and the aminoglycosides (amikacin, kanamycin) are occasionally used in drug resistant cases. See Chapter 58 for a discussion of these agents. New agents are under study to treat drug-resistant TB. One promising class of agents includes the diarylquinolones, which may provide a welcome addition in the fight against this disease (Andries et al., 2005).

Aminosalicylic acid is a bacteriostatic agent closely related to para-aminobenzoic acid (PABA); thus it competitively inhibits folic acid formation and results in the suppression of the growth and reproduction of *M. tuberculosis*.

Capreomycin is an antimycobacterial agent with an unknown mechanism of action. Cycloserine is a broad-spectrum antibiotic that can be bacteriostatic or bactericidal depending on drug concentration at the infection site and the susceptibility of the organism. It is an antimycobacterial agent that interferes with synthesis of the bacterial cell wall. The mechanism of action of ethionamide is unknown, but it is believed to inhibit peptide synthesis. Streptomycin is an aminoglycoside antimicrobial (see Chapter 58) and was one of the first effective agents used in the late 1940s to treat TB. It remains an important agent in managing severe TB.

aminosalicylic acid [a mee noe sa **lis** i lic **as** id]
(PAS, Paser granules, Tubasal, Nemasol)
Indications
Aminosalicylic acid is indicated for the treatment of pulmonary and extrapulmonary *M. tuberculosis* in combination with other antituberculous drugs.

Pharmacokinetics/Dosing
Aminosalicylic acid is well absorbed orally and distributed to various body fluids, with high levels accumulating in the pleural fluids, kidney, lungs, and liver tissues. The half-life is between 45 and 60 minutes, although it may extend up to 23 hours in clients with impaired renal function. Peak serum levels are reached within 1 to 2 hours. This drug is metabolized in the liver and excreted by the kidneys. The adult oral dosage given in combination with other antimycobacterials is 3.3 to 4 g every 8 hours. The maximum daily dose is 20 g. The pediatric dosage in combination with other antimycobacterials is 50 to 75 mg/kg PO every 6 hours.

Adverse Effects
The adverse effects of aminosalicylic acid therapy include a hypersensitivity reaction and gastric distress.

Nursing Management
See previous discussion about antitubercular therapy, p. 1107. A history of allergic reaction to other salicylates and sulfonamides may indicate a cross-intolerance for aminosalicylic acid, in which case the drug is contraindicated. Aminosalicylic acid should be used with caution if the client has any of the following preexisting conditions: anemia (this drug competes successfully with vitamin B_{12} and worsens anemias) or severe renal or hepatic function impairment (reduced dosages are required). Aminosalicylic acid in the Paser granule form has no significant drug interactions. Perform a baseline assessment as described in the previous section on antituberculous drug therapy.

Assess the client receiving aminosalicylic acid for the following nursing diagnoses/collaborative problems: deficient fluid volume related to anorexia, nausea, vomiting, and diarrhea; ineffective protection related to leukopenia or thrombocytopenia; activity intolerance related to hemolytic anemia or an infectious mononucleosis-like syndrome (fever, headache, rash, sore throat, fatigue); and the potential complications of hepatitis (yellow sclera and skin) and crystalluria.

Urinalyses should be performed at periodic intervals during drug therapy to monitor for crystals, casts, cells, and decreased specific gravity. The Paser extended-release granules of aminosalicylic acid may be administered by sprinkling them on applesauce or yogurt or by mixing them in a glass to suspend them in an acidic drink such as orange, grapefruit, grape, cranberry, apple or tomato juice, or fruit punch. Encourage the client to have a fluid intake of 3000 mL daily, and the urine should be maintained at a neutral or alkaline pH to minimize crystalluria. Advise the client that the skeleton of the granules may be seen in the stool but that this is not significant. The drug should not be used if the packets are swollen or if the granules have changed from tan to dark brown or purple.

The expected outcome of aminosalicylic acid therapy is that the client will eventually be free of infection (negative sputum or other culture for AFB) without experiencing any adverse effects of the drug (e.g., hypersensitivity, GI distress).

capreomycin [kap ree oh **mye** sin]
(Capastat)
Indications
Capreomycin is indicated in combination therapy for the treatment of pulmonary TB caused by *M. tuberculosis* after primary medications (streptomycin, isoniazid, rifampin, pyrazinamide, and ethambutol) fail or when these medications cannot be used because of resistant bacilli or drug toxicity.

Pharmacokinetics/Dosing
Administered IM, capreomycin has a half-life between 3 and 6 hours and reaches peak serum levels in 1 to 2 hours. It is excreted primarily unchanged by the kidneys. The adult dosage in combination with other antituberculous agents is 1 g IM daily for 2 to 4 months, followed by 1 g two or three times weekly for 18 to 24 months.

Adverse Effects
The adverse effects of capreomycin include nephrotoxicity, hypokalemia, neuromuscular blockade, ototoxicity, and hypersensitivity.

Nursing Management
See the discussion of the general management of antitubercular therapy. Assess the client to determine if the client has the following preexisting conditions: dehydration (increases the risk of toxicity because of increased serum levels of the drug), myasthenia gravis and parkinsonism (neuromuscular deficits may increase), impairment of the eighth cranial nerve (may cause increased auditory and vestibular toxicity), and renal impairment (may increase because of the nephrotoxic effects of this drug). Because of these effects, assess fluid balance, audiograms, and vestibular and renal function determinations before therapy.

Review the client's medication regimen for the risk of potentially life-threatening drug interactions, such as parenteral aminoglycosides (increased risk for developing ototoxicity, nephrotoxicity, and neuromuscular blockade). Hearing loss may progress to deafness, even after the drug is stopped. Avoid methoxyflurane or parenteral polymyxins as the potential for nephrotoxicity and/or neuromuscular blockade is increased. Other nephrotoxic or ototoxic medications, such as amphotericin B parenteral, bacitracin parenteral, bumetanide parenteral (Bumex), cisplatin (Platinol), cyclosporine (Sandimmune), ethacrynic acid (Edecrin), furosemide parenteral (Lasix), paromomycin (Humatin), or vancomycin (Vancocin) for concurrent or even sequential use with may increase the risk of ototoxicity and/or nephrotoxicity. Concurrent use of neuromuscular blocking agents may result in increased neuromuscular blocking effects, resulting in respiratory depression or paralysis. Monitor closely, especially during surgery or in the postoperative period. Avoid this combination if possible. If not, closely monitor and keep anticholinesterase agents or calcium salts on hand to reverse the blockade.

The client receiving capreomycin should be assessed for the following nursing diagnoses/collaborative problems: impaired tissue integrity related to the injection of capreomycin (pain, bleeding, or induration at the injection site); disturbed sensory perception related to auditory ototoxicity (tinnitus or hearing loss) or vestibular ototoxicity (dizziness or unsteadiness); and the potential complications of hypersensitivity (rash, swelling, fever), hypokalemia (dysrhythmia, anorexia, nausea and vomiting, muscle cramps, fatigue), nephrotoxicity (increased or decreased frequency of urination or amount of urine), and neuromuscular blockade (fatigue, weakness, drowsiness, dyspnea).Weekly renal function studies should be performed. Monitor fluid intake and output throughout therapy. Monitor liver function studies and serum potassium levels that are performed at periodic intervals. Review the results of weekly or twice-weekly audiograms and periodic vestibular function determinations. Symptoms of tinnitus, hearing deficits, and/or vertigo should be reported to the prescriber.

To prepare for IM administration, add 2 mL of 0.9% sodium chloride injection or sterile water for injection to the vial. Allow 2 to 3 minutes for dissolution to occur. Reconstituted solutions may darken, but this does not affect their potency. These solutions are stable for 48 hours at room temperature or for 14 days if refrigerated. Administer capreomycin intramuscularly deep into a large muscle mass to increase absorption and minimize pain and the risk of sterile abscesses.

As with other antitubercular medications, the expected outcome of capreomycin is that the client will be free of infection (negative sputum culture for AFB) without experiencing any adverse effects of the drug (e.g., nephrotoxicity, hypokalemia, neuromuscular blockade, ototoxicity). The client will manage the therapeutic regimen effectively.

cycloserine [sye kloe **ser** een]
(Seromycin)
Indications
In combination with other drugs, cycloserine is indicated for the treatment of active pulmonary and extrapulmonary TB after failure of the primary antituberculous medications.

Pharmacokinetics/Dosing
Cycloserine is well absorbed orally and is widely distributed in body tissues and fluids. It reaches peak serum levels between 3 and 4 hours and has a half-life of 10 hours. Approximately 35% of cycloserine is metabolized, with excretion primarily via the kidneys. The adult oral dosage used in combination with other drugs is 250 mg every 12 hours for 2 weeks; the dosage is then increased as necessary up to 250 mg every 6 to 8 hours. The maximum daily dose is 1 g. The pediatric dosage is 10 to 20 mg/kg daily in divided doses.

Adverse Effects
The adverse effects of cycloserine include headache and dose-related CNS toxicity.

Nursing Management
Cycloserine should be used with caution if the client has the following preexisting conditions: severe renal impairment, alcoholism, or seizure disorders (the risk for seizures is greater); or severe anxiety, depression, or psychosis (these conditions may be worsened). Blood urea nitrogen (BUN) and serum creatinine concentrations should be determined before administering cycloserine. The CBC will serve as a baseline, because this drug has been associated with deficiencies of vitamin B_{12} and/or folic acid, resulting in anemia. In clients with a history of chronic alcohol abuse, cycloserine may increase the risk of seizures. Avoid concurrent use or a potentially serious drug interaction may occur. The concurrent use of ethionamide (Trecator-SC) may increase CNS adverse effects such as seizures. Monitor closely, because dosage adjustments may be necessary.

The client receiving cycloserine should be assessed for the following nursing diagnoses/collaborative problems: impaired comfort (headache); disturbed sensory perception related to peripheral neuritis (numbness, tingling in the fingers and toes); and the potential complications of hypersensitivity (rash) and CNS toxicity (anxiety, confusion, dizziness, drowsiness, irritability, depression, nightmares, mood swings, suicidal ideation, seizures).

Renal function studies and CBCs may be required periodically. Serum cycloserine levels may also be required; levels should be 25 to 30 mcg/mL, and levels above 30 mcg/mL are to be avoided. Administer cycloserine after meals if the client experiences GI irritation. The daily administration of pyridoxine will help to prevent drug-related neurotoxicities. Caution the client to avoid alcohol while taking this medication, because it increases the risks of CNS toxicity such as dizziness, mental disturbances, and seizures. Advise the client to report immediately to the prescriber any signs of dizziness, drowsiness, numbness or tingling of the fingers and toes, or thoughts of suicide.

The expected outcome of cycloserine therapy is that the client will manage the therapeutic regimen effectively and eventually be free of infection (negative sputum or other culture for AFB) without experiencing any adverse effects of the drug (e.g., headache, CNS toxicity).

ethionamide [e thye on **am** ide]
(Trecator-SC)
Indications
Ethionamide is an antimycobacterial agent indicated for the treatment of TB after failure of the primary antituberculous agents (streptomycin, isoniazid, rifampin, and ethambutol).

Pharmacokinetics/Dosing
Ethionamide is well absorbed orally and is distributed to most body tissues and fluids, including cerebrospinal fluid. It has a half-life of 2 to 3 hours and may be metabolized in the liver and excreted primarily by the kidneys. The adult oral dosage in combination with other agents is 250 mg every 8 to 12 hours. The pediatric dosage is 4 to 5 mg/kg PO every 8 hours.

Adverse Effects
The adverse effects of ethionamide include gastric distress, orthostatic hypotension, and peripheral neuritis.

Nursing Management
Administer ethionamide cautiously to clients with diabetes mellitus because hypoglycemia related to its administration makes the management of diabetes more difficult. Clients with severe hepatic dysfunction have a higher risk of adverse hepatic reactions. Determine the client's tolerance for ethionamide. The concurrent use of cycloserine will increase the risk for CNS toxicity, especially seizures. Dosage adjustments may be necessary, and the client should be monitored closely for CNS toxicity. A baseline assessment should include cultures, an ophthalmologic examination, a neurologic examination, and hepatic function determinations.

The client receiving ethionamide should be assessed for the following nursing diagnoses/collaborative problems: impaired comfort (rash and metallic taste); deficient fluid volume related to anorexia, nausea, and vomiting; risk for injury related to orthostatic hypotension (dizziness on standing); disturbed thought processes related to CNS toxicity (psychiatric disturbances, mood and mental changes, confusion); disturbed body image related to gynecomastia (in males); disturbed sensory perception related to optic neuritis (blurred vision or loss of vision) or peripheral neuritis (numbness or tingling of the fingers and toes); and the potential complications of hepatitis (yellow sclera and skin), hypoglycemia (tachycardia, shakiness, confusion), mental depression, and goiter/hypothyroidism (weight gain, dry, puffy skin, lethargy, coldness).

Although its incidence is rare, optic neuritis (blurred vision, vision loss, and/or eye pain) does occur. The client should have a thorough ophthalmologic examination at periodic intervals and at the first indication of symptoms related to vision changes. To monitor for hepatotoxic effects, AST and ALT should be performed at least monthly during the course of therapy. Observe the client for jaundice. Administer ethionamide with meals to minimize GI distress. GI upset may be minimized by a divided dosage schedule, but serum concentrations may not be adequate. Pyridoxine may be prescribed concurrently to prevent peripheral neuritis. Bacterial resistance develops rapidly if this drug is administered alone; therefore it is administered in combination with other antimycobacterial drugs. Regular visits to the health care provider are necessary to monitor progress and to receive periodic eye examinations. Any symptoms related to changes in vision should be reported to the prescriber promptly. Advise the client that ethionamide may cause dizziness, drowsiness, or weakness; hazardous activities requiring mental alertness (e.g., driving) should be avoided until the response to the medication has been ascertained. Alert the client to other potential adverse effects, such as mental depression or mood changes.

The expected outcome of ethionamide therapy is that the client will manage the therapeutic regimen effectively and will eventually be free of infection (negative sputum or other culture for AFB) without experiencing any adverse effects of the drug (e.g., gastric distress, orthostatic hypertension, peripheral neuritis).

streptomycin injection [strep toe **mye** sin]
Indications
Streptomycin is indicated as part of combined therapy in the treatment of active TB. It is occasionally used for other infections, including gram-positive endocarditis, mycobacterial infections, brucellosis, tularemia, and plague.

Pharmacokinetics/Dosing
Streptomycin and other aminoglycosides are very water soluble and not absorbed systemically when administered by the oral route. The

adult dosage for streptomycin is 1 g IM daily. As soon as possible, reduce the dosage to 1 g two or three times weekly. The dosage for older adults is 500 to 750 mg daily in combination with other antituberculous agents. The dosage for children is 20 mg/kg daily in combination with other antituberculous agents. The maximum daily dose is 1 g.

Adverse Effects
As with other aminoglycosides, the major toxicities of streptomycin include ototoxicity and nephrotoxicity, especially when given to clients with impaired renal function or with other medications with the same toxicities. Refer to Chapter 58 for a further discussion of aminoglycoside toxicity.

Nursing Management
See Chapter 58 for nursing management of streptomycin.

Amebicidals

⊛ **J.S. is a 27-year-old male who returns with profuse diarrhea after a 2-week backwoods camping trip. A stool sample is sent to the lab for analysis of amebic antigen and confirms the presence of *Entamoeba histolytica*.**

⊛ **What are the key pathogenic and epidemiologic features of amebiasis?**
Amebiasis is an infection of the large intestine produced by a protozoan parasite, *Entamoeba histolytica*. This infestation is found worldwide but is prevalent and severe in tropical areas. It has been detected in poorly sanitized areas, including some rural communities, Native American reservations, and migrant labor farm camps; it is also common in homosexual males. Transmission is usually through the ingestion of cysts (fecal to oral route) from contaminated food or water or from person-to-person contact. Poor personal hygiene can increase the spread of this parasite.

Life Cycle of the Ameba The protozoan has two stages in its life cycle: (1) the trophozoite (vegetative ameba), which is the active, motile form; and (2) the cyst, or inactive, drug-resistant form that appears in intestinal excretion. The *trophozoite stage* is capable of amoeboid motion and sexual activity. Because of its susceptibility to injury, it generally succumbs to an unfavorable environment. The trophozoite protects itself under certain circumstances by entering the *cystic stage*. During this phase the protozoan becomes inactive by surrounding itself with a resistant cell wall within which it can survive for a long time, even in an unsuitable environment.

The complete life cycle of the ameba occurs in humans, the main host. It begins when the human ingests cysts that are present on hands, in food, or in water contaminated by feces. The hydrochloric acid of the stomach does not destroy the swallowed cysts; they pass unharmed into the small intestine. The digestive juices penetrate the cystic walls, and the trophozoites are released. The motile amoebae later pass into the colon, where they live and multiply for a time, feeding on the bacterial flora of the gut. The presence of bacteria is essential for the survival of amoebae.

Before excretion, the trophozoites move toward the terminal end of the bowel and again become encysted. The cysts remain viable and infective after being eliminated in the feces. The cycle may begin again when the cysts that appear in fecal excretion are ingested through the contamination of food or water.

The parasite causing amebiasis replicates in three major locations: (1) the lumen of the bowel, (2) the intestinal mucosa, and (3) extraintestinal sites. Amebiasis is classified according to its primary site of action: intestinal amebiasis, where amebic activity is restricted to the bowel lumen or intestinal mucosa; or extraintestinal amebiasis, where parasitic invasion occurs outside the intestine.

Intestinal Amebiasis Intestinal amebiasis may be manifested as an asymptomatic intestinal infection or as a symptomatic intestinal infection that may be mild, moderate, or severe.

Asymptomatic Intestinal Amebiasis In asymptomatic intestinal amebiasis the action of the parasite is restricted to the lumen of the bowel. The individual is asymptomatic but becomes a carrier of the disease by passing mature cysts of the parasite in formed stools. The cysts can live for several weeks outside the body and can survive dry, freezing, or high-temperature conditions. The infection is transmitted from person to person by flies or contaminated food or water. Ordinary concentrations of chlorine in water purification do not destroy the cysts. Serious GI pathologic problems eventually develop if the carrier fails to follow any drug treatment. Mild symptoms occasionally exist and include vague abdominal pain, nausea, flatulence, fatigue, and nervousness.

Symptomatic Intestinal Amebiasis Symptomatic amebiasis occurs when the trophozoites in the lumen of the bowel penetrate the mucosal lining of the colon. After they multiply and thrive on bacterial flora, a large infestation occurs and produces diarrhea and abdominal pain. The increased loss of fluid may cause prostration. Ulcerative colitis may also result. This state of the disease is called intestinal amebiasis and is usually diagnosed as mild, moderate, or severe according to the intensity of the symptoms and the extent of the disease.

Extraintestinal Amebiasis The term *extraintestinal amebiasis* means the parasites have migrated to other parts of the body, such as the liver or occasionally the spleen, lungs, or brain. When the parasites are in the liver, necrotic foci develop because of the parasites' destructive effect on tissues. The terms *liver abscess* and *hepatic amebiasis* are usually used when there is liver involvement.

⊛ **What agents are available for the treatment of amebiasis?**
Drugs for the treatment of amebiasis are classified according to the site of the previously described amebic action. Luminal amebicides act primarily in the bowel lumen and in general are ineffective against parasites in the bowel wall or tissues. Tissue amebicides are drugs that act primarily in

the bowel wall, liver, and other extraintestinal tissues. Although metronidazole has activity for both luminal and tissue sites, combination therapy is often prescribed. The intestinal amebicides are considered to be iodoquinol, metronidazole, and paromomycin; the extraintestinal amebicides are chloroquine and metronidazole.

Metronidazole (Flagyl) is an antibacterial, antiprotozoal, and anthelmintic agent. It is used for the treatment of extraintestinal and intestinal amebiasis. When used for the treatment of invasive amebiasis, it is recommended that it be administered with a luminal amebicide, such as iodoquinol or paromomycin. See Chapter 58 for a discussion of metronidazole.

Chloroquine (Aralen) is used to treat amebic liver abscess, usually in combination with other drugs. See the discussion of chloroquine earlier in this chapter for further information. Dehydroemetine (Mebadin) is an additional antiinfective agent used to treat amebiasis. However, it is associated with significant adverse effects, including cardiac toxicity, and therefore must be administered only when clients can be monitored in the hospital.

Paromomycin and iodoquinol are presented here. Paromomycin is both an amebicidal and an antibacterial agent. The drug is an aminoglycoside antibiotic with antibacterial properties similar to that of neomycin. Paromomycin acts directly on intestinal amoebae and on bacteria such as *Salmonella* and *Shigella*. Because the drug is poorly absorbed from the GI tract, it exerts no effect on systemic infections such as extraintestinal amebiasis. Iodoquinol is an antiprotozoal with a direct action on intestinal forms of amebiasis, but may produce vision problems in high doses with children.

paromomycin [par oh moe **mye** sin]
(Humatin)
Indications
Paromomycin is indicated for the treatment of acute and chronic intestinal amebiasis and for adjunct therapy in the management of hepatic coma.
Pharmacokinetics/Dosing
Paromomycin is poorly absorbed from the intestinal tract; thus most of the drug is excreted in the feces. The adult and pediatric dosage to treat intestinal amebiasis is 25 to 35 mg/kg daily, administered in 3 divided doses with meals for 5 to 10 days. To manage hepatic coma, the adult dosage is 4 g daily in divided doses at regular intervals for 5 or 6 days.
Adverse Effects
The adverse effects of paromomycin include nausea, diarrhea, and gastric distress. Paromomycin is an aminoglycoside, and the drug interactions possible with this family of medications may also occur with paromomycin but are unlikely given the minimal systemic absorption. (See the discussion of aminoglycoside antibiotics in Chapter 58.)
Nursing Management
For general nursing management of amebiasis, see the case of J.S. below. Chapter 58 discusses aminoglycosides. However, paromomycin is contraindicated for use in intestinal obstruction and in ulcerative bowel lesions because of possible systemic absorption. It is to be used only for luminal amebiasis. Assess the client receiving paromomycin for the risk of the following nursing diagnoses: deficient fluid volume related to nausea, vomiting, and diarrhea; diarrhea; activity intolerance related to light-headedness and dizziness; and disturbed sensory perception (auditory disturbances) related to tinnitus

and hearing loss. Notify the prescriber of any ringing in the ears or dizziness, because this drug is ototoxic. Administer paromomycin after meals to minimize GI distress. Teach the client proper personal hygiene to help prevent reinfection. After the end of therapy, examine fresh, warm stools for the presence of amoebae at weekly intervals for 6 weeks, then monthly for 2 years to indicate that the client is not harboring the parasite. The expected outcome of paromomycin therapy is that the client will manage the therapeutic regimen effectively and be free of amoebas in stools for 2 years.

iodoquinol [eye oh do **kwin** ole]
(diiodohydroxyquin, Yodoxin)
Indications
Iodoquinol is indicated for the treatment of intestinal amebiasis in asymptomatic carriers of *E. histolytica*.
Pharmacokinetics/Dosing
Iodoquinol is poorly absorbed from the intestinal tract; thus it produces its effect against the trophozoites of *E. histolytica* at the site of intestinal infestation. Following administration and local effect, iodoquinol is excreted in the feces. The adult oral dosage is 650 mg three times daily after meals for 20 days. The pediatric dosage is 40 mg/kg PO in three divided doses after meals for 20 days.
Adverse Effects
The adverse effects of iodoquinol include gastric distress, hypersensitivity, fever, and chills. High doses in children with chronic diarrhea have been associated with optic atrophy and permanent loss of vision (Tracy & Webster, 2001c).

✴ **J.S.'s acute amoebic dysentery is treated with a combination of metronidazole, 750 mg PO three times daily × 10 days to eliminate invasive amebiasis, followed by a luminal agent to eliminate intraluminal encysted organisms, iodoquinol 650 mg PO three times daily × 10 days.**

✴ **Metronidazole was discussed in Chapter 58, but what are the nursing management issues in the use of iodoquinol as a antiamebiasis agents for J.S.?**

Assessment Iodoquinol should be used with caution if J.S. has the following preexisting conditions: intolerance to iodoquinol, iodine, or 8-hydroxyquinolines; optic neuropathy; peripheral neuropathy; or thyroid, hepatic, or renal disease.

Perform a baseline assessment for antiinfective administration as described in Chapter 57. Stool specimens should be collected and taken directly to the laboratory for the detection of amebic antigen or for microscopic examinations of stools, collect three specimens at 2-day intervals or longer, one of which needs to be following after a laxative. J.S. should undergo an ophthalmologic examination before initiating iodoquinol therapy because optic neuropathy and optic atrophy are risks of therapy.

Nursing Diagnosis While receiving iodoquinol, J.S. is at risk for the following nursing diagnoses/collaborative problems: impaired comfort (rash, itching of rectal area, or headache); deficient fluid volume related to nausea, vomiting, and diarrhea; hyperthermia; diarrhea; disturbed sensory perception, such as visual disturbances related to optic atrophy, optic neuritis, or subacute optic neuropathy, or sensory disturbances related to numbness and tingling of the fingers and toes from the development of peripheral neuropathy; and the potential complication of thyroid enlargement.

Planning The goals for J.S.'s antiamebiasis drug therapy are that he will:

- Reestablish normal bowel patterns, appetite, weight, and body temperature
- Have three consecutive negative stools at 2- to 3-day intervals, starting 2 to 4 weeks after the end of treatment.
- Remain free of adverse effects of the antiamebiasis drugs.
- Effectively manage his therapeutic regimen, including medication compliance, reporting adverse drug effects appropriately, and maintaining scheduled visits with the health team for monitoring and treatment.

Implementation

Monitoring Document intake and output, and the frequency and character of stools. Fresh, warm stools should be monitored for the presence of amoebae. Diarrhea may occur during the first few days of therapy with iodoquinol. Alert the prescriber if it continues for more than 3 days. Ophthalmologic examinations are required periodically during long-term therapy. The development of neurologic disorders such as optic neuropathy, optic atrophy, optic neuritis, and peripheral neuropathy has been implicated in treatment with prolonged high doses.

Iodoquinol may cause thyroid enlargement and interferes with certain thyroid function tests by increasing protein-bound serum iodine levels for as long as 6 months after discontinuing therapy. This drug contains approximately 64% iodine.

In children, the administration of iodoquinol for chronic diarrhea has been responsible for causing optic atrophy and permanent vision loss. Thus the administration of this drug is not advocated for the treatment or prophylaxis of "traveler's diarrhea" or for use in chronic nonspecific diarrhea.

Intervention Administer iodoquinol after meals to minimize GI irritation. This course of therapy may be repeated if necessary after a 2- to 3-week rest period.

Tablets may be crushed and mixed with applesauce, gelatin dessert, or ice cream for ease of administration to children and to clients who may have difficulty swallowing.

Education Instruct J.S. in proper hygiene to prevent reinfection, including frequent handwashing and handwashing before meals and after using the bathroom. Alert him to report any rash, fever, chills, headache, or vision disturbances to his prescriber. Inform him that any results of thyroid function studies completed within 6 months of discontinuing iodoquinol may be distorted.

Evaluation The expected outcome of iodoquinol therapy is that J.S. will be free of amoebae in stools at the end of the

year following therapy without adverse effects of the drug (e.g., peripheral neuropathy, optic neuritis).

✱ What other protozoan infections are observed in North America?

Several other protozoan diseases are widespread throughout the world and may be encountered in clinical practice in the United States and Canada. These are often more pronounced in clients who are immunocompromised. These include balantidiasis, babesiosis, cryptosporidiosis, giardiasis, leishmaniasis, and toxoplasmosis.

- **Balantidiasis**: The intestinal parasite *Balantidium coli* is responsible for this infection. Manifestations include diarrhea, abdominal cramping and weight loss. It is treated with tetracycline, iodoquinol, or metronidazole.
- **Babesiosis**: In North America, *Babesia microti* is the tick-borne pathogen responsible for this condition. Symptoms of infection include fever, fatigue, shaking chills, sweating, and GI complaints. When present in immunocompromised clients, it is treated with clindamycin and quinine.
- **Cryptosporidiosis**: Infections with *Cryptosporium* produce diarrhea, but good treatments are lacking. Occasionally paromomycin and azithromycin are used in management.
- **Giardiasis**: Giardia lamblia infections often occur in clients who drink infected water supplies and often result in a profuse diarrhea or abdominal cramping. Metronidazole is considered the treatment of choice, but furazolidone, paromomycin or tinidazole are also used.
- **Leishmaniasis**: *Leishmania braziliensis* and other species produce various types of disease including cutaneous manifestations, mucosal and intestinal symptoms. Cutaneous leishmaniasis infections are treated with fluconazole, whereas more deep-seated infections may require amphotericin B.
- **Toxoplasmosis:** Toxoplasma gondii infections may be clinical or subclinical. Significant disease is more common in immunocompromised clients. Symptomatically the individual may experience lymphadenopathy, fever, and occasionally a rash on the palms and soles. The most serious complication of toxoplasmosis is meningoencephalitis. Toxoplasmosis is treated with a combination of sulfadiazine and pyrimethamine.
- **Trichomoniasis:** Trichomoniasis iss a vaginal disease caused by *Trichomonas vaginalis*. Its characteristic presentation consists of a wet, inflamed vagina, a "strawberry" cervix, and a thin, yellow, frothy malodorous discharge. Both sexual partners are usually infected by this organism, which can be identified microscopically in the semen, prostatic fluid, or exudate from the vagina. Infections often recur, which indicates that the protozoa persist in the extravaginal foci, male urethra, or periurethral glands and ducts of both genders. Metronidazole (Flagyl) is the drug of

choice, and treatment must be given simultaneously to both partners involved.

Anthelminthics

✳ **T.P. is a 5-year-old boy brought to the pediatrician's office because of irritability and vague complaints of abdominal discomfort. His mother has observed him scratching his anal area. A cellophane tape swab placed over the perianal area shows evidence of *E. vermicularis* (pinworm) eggs.**

✳ **What are the important helminth infections in humans?**

The disease-producing helminths are classified as metazoa, or multicellular animal parasites. Unlike the protozoa, these parasites are large organisms that have a complex cellular structure and feed on host tissue. They may be present in the GI tract, but several types also penetrate the tissues; some undergo developmental changes, during which they wander extensively in the host. Because most anthelmintic used today are highly effective against specific parasites, the organism must be accurately identified before treatment is started, usually by finding the parasite ova or larvae in the feces, urine, blood sputum, or tissues of the host.

Helminth infestations do not necessarily cause clinical manifestations, but they may be injurious for a number of reasons:

- Worms may cause mechanical injury to the tissues and organs. Roundworms in large numbers may cause obstruction in the intestine; filariae may block lymphatic channels and cause massive edema; and hookworms often cause extensive damage to the wall of the intestine and considerable loss of blood.
- Toxic substances produced by the parasite may be absorbed by the host.
- The tissues of the host may be traumatized by the presence of the parasite and made more susceptible to bacterial infections.
- Heavy infestation with worms will rob the host of food. This is particularly significant in children.

Helminths that are parasitic to humans are classified as (1) *Platyhelminthes* (flatworms), which include two subclasses: cestodes (tapeworms) and trematodes (flukes); and (2) *Nematoda* (roundworms).

Platyhelminthes (Flatworms)

Cestodes Cestodes are tapeworms, of which there are four varieties: (1) *Taenia saginata* (beef tapeworm), (2) *Taenia solium* (pork tapeworm), (3) *Diphyllobothrium latum* (fish tapeworm), and (4) *Hymenolepis nana* (dwarf tapeworm). As indicated by the name of the worm, the parasite enters the intestine by way of improperly cooked beef, pork, or fish or, in the case of the dwarf tapeworm, contaminated food.

Cestodes are segmented flatworms with a head or scolex (which has hooks or suckers used to attach to tissues) and a number of segments, or proglottids, which in some cases may extend for 20 to 30 feet in the bowel. Drugs affecting the scolex allow the organisms to be expelled from the intestine. Each of the proglottids contains both male and female reproductive units. Fertilized eggs are expelled from the worm into the environment. On ingestion, the infected larvae develop into adults in the small intestine of the human. The larvae may travel to extraintestinal sites and enter other tissues such as the liver, muscle, and eye. With the exception of the dwarf tapeworm, tapeworms spend part of their life cycle in a host other than humans—pigs, fish, or cattle. Dwarf tapeworms do not require an intermediate host.

The tapeworm has no digestive tract; it depends on the nutrients intended for the host. The host suffers by eventually developing a nutritional deficiency.

Trematodes Trematodes, or flukes, are flat, nonsegmented parasites with suckers that attach to and feed on host tissue. The life cycle begins with the egg, which is passed into fresh water following fecal excretion from the body of the human host. The egg containing the embryo forms into a ciliated organism (the *miracidium*). In the presence of water the miracidium escapes from the egg and enters the intermediate host—the freshwater snail, which exists extensively in rice paddies and irrigation ditches. After entry, the fluke forms a cyst in the lungs of the snail, and many organisms develop in this cyst. The organisms can penetrate other parts of the snail and grow into worms called *cercariae*. Eventually the cercariae are released from the snail into the water, where they attach themselves to blades of grass to encyst. A human, the final host, then becomes infected by the parasite.

When humans swallow encysted organisms in snails (or even in fish and crabs), they develop into adult flukes in different structures of the body. The flukes are classified according to the type of tissues they invade. Following ingestion, the eggs of *Schistosoma haematobium* appear in the urinary bladder and cause inflammation of the urogenital system. This can result in chronic cystitis and hematuria. Infestations with *S. japonicum* and *S. mansoni* produce intestinal disturbances with resultant ulceration and necrosis of the rectum. *S. japonicum* is more concentrated in the veins of the small intestine. If the liver and spleen become infected, the disease is usually fatal. *S. mansoni* prefers the portal veins that drain the large intestine, particularly the sigmoid colon and rectum. Unlike the other parasites, the cercariae of *S. mansoni* are not ingested but burrow through the skin, especially between the toes of a human host who is standing in contaminated water. They then make their way to the portal system, where they mature into adult flukes.

Schistosomiasis (bilharziasis) is endemic to Africa, Asia, South America, and the Caribbean islands. The disease can be controlled largely by eliminating the intermediate host, the snail. Travelers to these areas must avoid contact with contaminated water for drinking, bathing, or swimming. Unfortunately, immigrants or individuals who have traveled to the endemic areas have introduced the disease in the United States and Canada.

Nematoda (Roundworms)

Nematoda are nonsegmented, cylindrical worms that consist of a mouth and complete digestive tract. The adults reside in the human intestinal tract; there is no intermediate host. Two types of nematode infection exist in the human: the egg form and the larval form.

Egg Infective Form *Ascaris lumbricoides* is a large nematode (approximately 30 cm in length) that is known as the "roundworm of humans."

The adult *Ascaris* usually resides in the upper end of the small intestine of the human, in which it feeds on semidigested foods. When excreted with feces, the fertilized egg can survive in the soil for a long time. When inadvertently ingested by another host, the embryos escape from the eggs and mature into adults in the new host. To prevent the disease, proper sanitary conditions and meticulous personal habits must be observed.

Infection with *Enterobius vermicularis*, or pinworm, is highly prevalent among children and adults in the United States. Adult pinworms reside in the large intestine. The female migrates to the anus and deposits her eggs around the skin of the anal region. This causes intense itching and can be noted especially in children.

Diagnosis is made by finding the eggs deposited in the perianal region; these eggs are detected by applying clear cellulose acetate tape to the perianal region in the morning. The ingestion of excreted eggs can infect an individual. Additionally, eggs that contaminate clothing, bedding, furniture, and other items may be responsible for reinfecting an individual and initiating the infection of others.

Larval Infective Form *Necator americanus* (New World) or *Ancylostoma duodenale* (Old World) hookworms are somewhat similar in action. They reside in the small intestine of humans. When the eggs are excreted in the feces, the larvae hatch in the soil. The larvae can penetrate the skin of humans, particularly through the soles of the feet, and produce dermatitis (ground itch). On entry into the small intestine, they develop into adult worms. During this process they extravasate blood from the intestinal vessels and cause a profound anemia in the victim. The presence of eggs in the feces indicates a positive test for hookworm disease. This type of infection can be avoided by wearing shoes.

Trichinella spiralis is a small pork roundworm that causes trichinosis. In humans the disease begins by ingesting insufficiently cooked pork or bear meat. After the entry of encysted meat into the small intestine, the larvae are released from the cysts. Following maturation, the females develop eggs that later form into larvae. The larvae migrate through the bloodstream and lymphatic system to the skeletal muscles, where they encyst. Encapsulation and eventually calcification of the cysts occur. Diagnosis of trichinosis is made by muscle biopsy, in which microscopic examination reveals the presence of larvae. This disease is prevented by cooking pork and bear meat thoroughly before eating.

✴ **T.P. is started on a course of mebendazole (Vermox) 100 mg once; repeat in 2 weeks.**

✴ **What agents are available to treat helminth infections?**

Anthelmintic drugs are used to rid the body of worms (helminths). Anthelmintics are among the most primitive types of chemotherapy. It has been estimated that one third of the world's population is infested with these parasites.

A number of drugs are available and are chosen based on the specific infection noted. Included among the anthelmintics are benzimidazoles, mebendazole, and chemically related albendazole and thiabendazole. Other anthelmintics include diethylcarbamazine, ivermectin, niclosamide, oxamniquine, praziquantel, and pyrantel.

Benzimidazoles

The benzimidazoles are fairly broad spectrum against a number of GI nematodes. Mebendazole is vermicidal and may also be ovicidal for most helminths. It causes degeneration of a parasite's cytoplasmic microtubules that results in blocking glucose uptake in the helminth and leads to the death of the parasite. Albendazole is similar in action to mebendazole. The mechanism of action of thiabendazole is unknown but has been reported to inhibit specific enzymes (fumarate reductase) in the helminth, and it is vermicidal.

✴▼ **mebendazole** [me **ben** da zole]
(Vermox)
Indications
Mebendazole is indicated for the treatment of single or mixed infestations of *Trichuris* (whipworm), *Enterobius* (pinworm), *Ascaris* (roundworm), *Ancylostoma* (common hookworm), and *Necator* (American hookworm).
Pharmacokinetics/Dosing
The oral absorption of mebendazole is increased if given with fatty foods. It is distributed to the serum, cyst fluid, liver, hepatic cysts, and muscle tissue, and it has a half-life of 2.5 to 5.5 hours. It is metabolized in the liver and excreted primarily in the feces. The adult and pediatric dosage (children 2 years of age and older) is 100 mg PO twice daily for 3 days. This dosage may be repeated in 2 to 3 weeks if necessary.
Adverse Effects
The adverse effects of mebendazole are uncommon and include gastric distress, diarrhea, nausea, and vomiting.

✴ **What are the nursing management issues for anthelmintic therapy with mebendazole for T.P.?**

Assessment Review T.P.'s health history for Crohn's disease or ulcerative colitis because there is increased absorption with mebendazole and therefore greater risk for toxicity. Those with hepatic function impairment may require lower dosages.

To assist in diagnosis (already done in T.P.'s case), collect pinworm specimens for a baseline assessment. To do so, wrap a transparent strip of cellophane tape (sticky side out) around a tongue blade and press it against the perianal area.

Place the sticky side of the tape on a glass slide and send it to the laboratory. The female worm emerges from the rectum during the night to lay eggs in the perianal area. This causes the client to become restless during sleep. The emerging worms can be seen at night with a flashlight. If T.P. were to have other types of helminths, such as roundworm and whipworm, send a baseline warm stool sample to the laboratory.

A CBC is required as a baseline before therapy, because mebendazole may cause leukopenia. Also assess T.P. for insomnia, restlessness, enuresis, and irritability.

Nursing Diagnosis While T.P. is receiving mebendazole, he is at risk for the following nursing diagnoses/collaborative problems: impaired comfort (dizziness); diarrhea; ineffective protection related to leukopenia (sore throat, fever, and fatigue); and the potential complication of hypersensitivity.

Planning The goals for T.P.'s anthelmintic drug therapy are that he will:

- Have three consecutive negative stools at 2- to 3-day intervals, starting 2 to 4 weeks after the end of treatment.
- Remain free of adverse effects of anthelmintic drug.
- With his caregivers, effectively manage his therapeutic regimen, including medication compliance, reporting adverse drug effects appropriately, and maintaining scheduled visits with the health team for monitoring.

Implementation

Monitoring Continue to monitor T.P.'s progress. The therapy should be repeated at 2 and 4 weeks. For helminths other than pinworm, collect the stool specimen in a clean, dry, and properly labeled container, and send it to the laboratory. Do not contaminate the specimen with water, urine, or chemicals, because the parasite may be destroyed. Monitor for fever and sore throat, to assess the need for a repeat CBC for neutropenia.

Intervention For ease of administration, tablets may be crushed and mixed with applesauce or other food. No dietary restrictions, laxatives, or posttreatment enemas are necessary.

Treat all family members for pinworm infestation, because it is readily transmitted from person to person. Clients with heavy infestation may require more prolonged therapy.

Education Stress the importance of handwashing and sanitary disposal of the feces. Instruct the client to take frequent showers rather than baths; to change underclothes, nightclothes, bedclothes, and towels daily; and to disinfect toilet facilities daily. Instruct T.P. and his caregivers to wash the perianal area daily to prevent reinfestation.

For pinworm infestation, instruct T.P.'s caregivers to wash (not shake) all the bed clothing and nightclothes after treatment.

For hookworm or whipworm infestation, instruct the client that iron supplements may be required treatment for up to 6 months afterward if anemia is diagnosed. Avoid walking barefoot to prevent hookworm infestation; the larvae hatch in the soil and penetrate through the skin.

Evaluation The expected outcome of mebendazole therapy is that T.P. will have negative perianal swabs for 7 days. Clients with other helminths will have three negative stool samples after completion of the therapy. Clients and their caregivers will be able to manage the therapeutic regimen effectively by treating all family members at the same time, washing all the night clothing and bed linens to prevent reinfestation, and using appropriate hygiene measures.

albendazole [al **ben** da zole]
(Albenza)
Indications
Albendazole is used to treat a number of intestinal roundworm infections, including *Ascaris lumbricoides* (ascariasis), *Enterobius vermicularis* (pinworm), *Necator americanus* (hookworm), *Trichostrongylus*, and *Trichuris trichiura* (whipworm). It has activity against other nematodes as well.

Pharmacokinetics/Dosing
Albendazole is poorly absorbed orally, but oral absorption may increase when dosed with a fatty meal. It undergoes extensive first-pass metabolism in the liver. The dosage varies based on indication. The typical adult dose is between 400 mg once or twice daily with duration ranging from a single dose to six months depending on pathogen. It is also used in children with daily doses up to 7.5 mg/kg twice daily depending on pathogen.

Adverse Effects
Adverse effects include hypersensitivity reactions, headache, elevated liver function tests, and leukopenia. Abdominal pain, nausea, and vomiting are also reported. Inflammatory reactions associated with CNS infections usually require pretreatment for 1 to 2 days with corticosteroids and antiepileptic drugs before using albendazole.

Nursing Management

Assessment
Albendazole should be used with caution in clients with a hypersensitivity to the benzimidazole class. Use with caution if the client has retinal lesions.

Nursing Diagnosis
The client receiving albendazole should be assessed for the following nursing diagnoses/collaborative problems: altered comfort (headache); deficient fluid volume related to anorexia, nausea, and vomiting; and the potential complications of hypersensitivity, Stevens-Johnson syndrome, agranulocytosis, and hypersensitivity (rash, urticaria).

Planning
The goals for albendazole are as for T.P.'s therapy with mebendazole discussed above.

Implementation
Monitoring
Monitor stool examinations approximately 2 to 3 weeks after therapy. Observe the client for hypersensitivity reactions to detect severe erythema multiforme (Stevens-Johnson syndrome). Monitor WBC count, absolute neutrophil count, and liver function tests. Withhold dose and notify prescriber if WBC falls below normal or if liver enzymes become elevated.

Intervention
Give with meals to increase absorption, particularly fatty meals. Do not exceed the maximum total daily dose of 800 mg. If the client is being treated for neurocysticercosis, steroid and antiepileptic therapy are also prescribed.

Education

Encourage the client to comply with the full course of treatment and to visit the prescriber to monitor progress. Teach proper hygiene, both personal and environmental. Do not breastfeed while taking this drug or become pregnant during and for 1 month after therapy.

Evaluation

The expected outcome of albendazole therapy is that the client will manage the therapeutic regimen effectively and have a negative stool examination for eggs, larvae, or worms without experiencing adverse effects of the drug.

thiabendazole [thye a **ben** da zole]
(Mintezol)

Indications

Thiabendazole is indicated for the treatment of cutaneous and visceral larva migrans (creeping eruption), strongyloidiasis, and trichinosis.

Pharmacokinetics/Dosing

Thiabendazole is rapidly absorbed orally and reaches peak serum levels in 1 to 2 hours. The half-life ranges from 0.9 to 2 hours, with metabolism in the liver and excretion by the kidneys. For cutaneous larva migrans, the dosage of thiabendazole for adults and children weighing 13.6 kg and over is 25 mg/kg PO twice daily for 2 days. If lesions are still present, the dosage may be repeated 2 days after completion of the initial treatment. For other dosing recommendations, see a current package insert or the *USP DI.*

Adverse Effects

The adverse effects of thiabendazole include a dry mouth and eyes, gastric distress, and neuropsychiatric and CNS adverse effects.

Nursing Management

Assessment

Thiabendazole should be used with caution in clients with hepatic or renal dysfunction, a hypersensitivity to thiabendazole, severe dehydration, when vomiting may be dangerous, and children weighing less than 15 Kg. Concurrent administration with theophylline decreases theophylline clearance, which may result in elevated serum levels and toxicity. Monitor theophylline levels.

Nursing Diagnosis

The client receiving thiabendazole should be assessed for the following nursing diagnoses/collaborative problems: deficient fluid volume related to anorexia, nausea, vomiting, and diarrhea; diarrhea; disturbed sensory perception—visual (blurred vision), and tactile (numbness or tingling in the hands and feet); disturbed thought processes related to neuropsychiatric toxicity (irritability, disorientation, depression, hallucinations); and the potential complications of hypersensitivity, Stevens-Johnson syndrome, crystalluria, hepatotoxicity, and CNS toxicity (seizures).

Planning

The goals for thiabendazole are as for T.P.'s therapy with mebendazole discussed above.

Implementation

Monitoring

Sputum examinations will monitor the progress of treatment of strongyloidiasis; for all other organisms, monitor stool examinations approximately 2 to 3 weeks after therapy. Observe the client for hypersensitivity reactions to detect severe erythema multiforme (Stevens-Johnson syndrome). A transient rise in liver function tests has occurred in clients receiving thiabendazole.

Intervention

Thiabendazole should be administered after meals to minimize anorexia, nausea, and vomiting; no dietary restrictions, laxatives, or enemas are required with this drug. For the oral suspension form, shake well and use the calibrated measuring device provided to ensure accurate dosage. Chew or crush the tablet form before swallowing.

Education

Encourage the client to comply with the full course of treatment and to visit the prescriber to monitor progress. Because of the adverse effects of dizziness and drowsiness, caution the client to avoid hazardous activities that require alertness, such as driving. Teach proper hygiene, both personal and environmental. Do not breastfeed while taking this drug.

Evaluation

The expected outcome of thiabendazole therapy is that the client will manage the therapeutic regimen effectively and have a negative sputum examination for strongyloidiasis or a negative stool examination for eggs, larvae, or worms without experiencing adverse effects of the drug.

Other Anthelmintics

Other available anthelmintics work by various mechanisms and include diethylcarbamazepine, ivermectin, niclosamide, oxamniquine, praziquantel, and pyrantel.

Diethylcarbamazine has microfilaricidal and macrofilaricidal effects. The microfilaricidal action increases the loss of microfilariae and inhibits the rate of embryogenesis from nematodes. It has no sterilizing effect on adult worms.

Ivermectin is a semi-synthetic anthelmintic that interferes with chloride ion channels and leads to altered nerve and muscle cell function and ultimately death in affected parasites. It is primarily used for nematode infections such as strongyloidiasis.

Niclosamide is an anthelmintic that affects the mitochondria of the cestode, inhibiting aerobic metabolism and possibly anaerobic metabolism, on which many cestodes depend for survival. Contact with the drug results in destruction of the scolex and proximal segments of the organism, the proglottids. When loosened from the intestinal wall, the scolex is usually digested in the intestine. Consequently, the worm cannot be identified in the feces.

Oxamniquine is schistosomicidal against both immature and mature worms, and it produces its effect by causing worms to shift from the mesenteric veins to the liver, where they are destroyed. Although male schistosomes appear to be more susceptible to this drug than female schistosomes, female schistosomes do stop laying eggs after successful treatment with this agent.

Praziquantel is an anthelmintic that penetrates cell membranes and increases cell permeability in susceptible worms. This results in an increased loss of intracellular calcium, contractions, and muscle paralysis of the worm. The drug also disintegrates the schistosome tegument (covering). Subsequently, phagocytes are attracted to the worm and ultimately kill it.

Pyrantel is an anthelmintic that is a depolarizing neuromuscular blocking agent; it causes contraction and then paralysis of the helminth muscles. The helminths are dislodged and expelled from the body by peristalsis.

diethylcarbamazine [dye eth il **kar** ba ma zeen]
(Hetrazan)

Indications

Diethylcarbamazine is indicated for the treatment of lymphatic filariasis, loiasis, onchocerciasis, and tropical eosinophilia. It is not distributed for use in the United States but can be obtained from the CDC under an Investigational New Drug (IND) protocol.

Pharmacokinetics/Dosing

Diethylcarbamazine is absorbed after oral administration and is distributed to nonfatty tissues. Peak serum levels are reached in 1 to 2 hours, and the half-life is 8 hours. Excretion is via the kidneys. The adult dosage of diethylcarbamazine is 2 to 3 mg/kg PO three times daily. For tropical eosinophilia, the dosage is 6 mg/kg PO daily for 4 to 7 days.

Adverse Effects
The adverse effects of diethylcarbamazine include joint pains, fever, increased weakness, headache, dizziness, nausea and vomiting, facial swelling (especially around the eyes), and pruritus. Less often reported are a rash and painful, tender glands (especially in the neck, armpits, or groin area).

Nursing Management
The treatment of pregnant clients should be deferred until after delivery. Treatment is also contraindicated with ocular onchocerciasis, because long-term therapy may cause inflammation and then degenerative changes in the optic disc and retina. Ophthalmologic examinations should be part of the baseline assessment. Additionally, microfilarial blood concentrations and skin biopsy for intradermal microfilariae should be obtained before therapy if diethylcarbamazine is administered for lymphatic filariasis and loiasis.

Contact the prescriber if allergic reactions (swelling and itching of the skin, fine papular rash, tenderness of lymph nodes, headache, fever, tachycardia, conjunctivitis, uveitis) occur as the result of the substances released when the microfilariae are destroyed. Microfilarial blood concentrations are used to monitor this effect, and antihistamine therapy or corticosteroids are usually prescribed to relieve these symptoms. Ophthalmoscopic examinations are performed on clients treated for onchocerciasis. Report immediately any signs of itching or swelling of eyes. Under the guidance of an ophthalmologist, corticosteroid eye drops may be administered for the treatment of this condition. Blood and skin samples are obtained periodically to monitor the client's progress. If a severe reaction occurs after a single dose, discontinue use.

Stress the importance of remaining under the prescriber's care during the treatment of filariasis. Failure to follow the drug regimen can eventually obstruct lymph flow, thereby producing hydrocele, elephantiasis of the limbs, an enlarged scrotum or breasts, and chyluria (milk-like urine).

ivermectin [eye ver **mek** tin]
(Stromectol)
Indications
Ivermectin is indicated for the treatment of intestinal tract infections caused by *Strongyloides stercoralis* and immature forms of *Onchocerca volvulus*.

Pharmacokinetics/Dosing
Ivermectin is well absorbed orally, and undergoes extensive hepatic metabolism. The typical oral dose for the treatment of strongyloidiasis in adults and children over 15 kg is 200 mcg/kg as a single dose. Treatment of onchocerciasis in adults and children over 15 kg is 150 mcg/kg as a single oral dose, with retreatment every 3 to 12 months until the infection is clear.

Adverse Effects
Hypersensitivity reactions with ivermectin may be related to the drug itself, or secondarily to the death of the microfilariae. Hypersensitivity reactions include dermatologic, ophthalmic and systemic effects and may be mild or severe. Dermatologic effects include pruritus and urticaria. Hypotension, conjunctivitis, blurred vision and punctate opacity have also been reported. Central nervous system effects include dizziness, headache, and insomnia. Abdominal pain, nausea, vomiting, and diarrhea are also reported.

Nursing Management
Ivermectin is contraindicated in clients with a hypersensitivity to the drug. Safety and efficacy in children less than 15 kg are not established. Clients may experience the nursing diagnoses of altered comfort (dizziness, rash); hyperthermia; diarrhea; and the potential complications of hypotension, arthralgia and lymphadenopathy. Monitor for hypotension and drug efficacy evidenced by negative stools. Retreatment is usually necessary. Give tablets with water rather than other fluids. Do not breastfeed while taking this medi-

cine. The expected outcome is that the client will have negative stools for helminths.

praziquantel [pray zi **kwon** tel]
(Biltricide)
Indications
Praziquantel is indicated for the treatment of schistosomiasis, opisthorchiasis (liver flukes), and clonorchiasis (Chinese or Oriental liver fluke) infestations.

Pharmacokinetics/Dosing
Praziquantel is absorbed orally and reaches peak serum levels in 1 to 3 hours. The half-life is 0.8 to 1.5 hours for praziquantel and 4 to 6 hours for its metabolites. It is excreted by the kidneys and is generally well tolerated. For clonorchiasis, the dosage for adults or children 4 years of age and older is 25 mg/kg three times daily for 1 day (total of three doses).

Adverse Effects
The adverse effects of praziquantel include headache, light-headedness, gastric distress, sweating, and fever.

Nursing Management
Assessment
Praziquantel is contraindicated in clients with ocular cysticercosis because the destruction of the parasites in the eye by the medication may cause severe ocular damage. Use with caution in clients with liver disease. Document the client's hypersensitivity to the drug.

Nursing Diagnosis
The client receiving praziquantel should be assessed for the following nursing diagnoses/collaborative problem: impaired comfort (headache, nausea and vomiting); diarrhea; hyperthermia; risk for injury related to light-headedness, weakness, and dizziness; and the potential complication of hypersensitivity (rash).

Planning
The goals for praziquantel therapy are that the client will:
- Have negative specimens without adverse effects of the drug.
- Effectively manage his therapeutic regimen, including medication compliance, reporting adverse drug effects appropriately, and maintaining scheduled visits with the health team for monitoring and continued treatment.

Implementation
Monitoring
Urine examinations for the eggs of *S. haematobium* are necessary at 1, 3, and 12 months after therapy to provide proof of a cure. Examinations of stool specimens for tapeworms, flukes, and other *Schistosoma* are required at 1, 3, and 12 months after treatment to determine the efficacy of the drug.

Intervention
No special preparations such as fasting, dietary restrictions, or laxatives are necessary for the administration of praziquantel. However, the tablets should be taken with meals and swallowed whole with a small amount of fluid to avoid the extremely bitter taste. Chewing the tablets may cause gagging and vomiting.

Education
The client should be encouraged to comply with the medication regimen and to visit the prescriber regularly to monitor progress. Because of the adverse effects of dizziness and drowsiness, caution the client to avoid hazardous activities such as driving until the response to the medication has been ascertained.

Evaluation
To monitor the expected outcomes of praziquantel therapy, stool examinations are completed at specific intervals depending on the parasite. These examinations should be negative for eggs or worm segments:
- Intestinal, liver, and blood flukes: 1 week and 1, 6, and 12 months after treatment
- Lung flukes: 1 month after treatment
- Tapeworms: 1 and 3 months after treatment

For *S. haematobium* and *S. mekongi*, urine examinations are required at 1, 3, and 6 months to determine proof of a cure. A client is not considered cured unless examination results have been negative for several months.

pyrantel [pi **ran** tel]
(Antiminth, Combantrin)
Indications
Pyrantel is indicated for the treatment of ascariasis, enterobiasis, and helminth infestations.
Pharmacokinetics/Dosing
This product is poorly absorbed from the GI tract. Pyrantel reaches peak serum levels in 1 to 3 hours and is primarily excreted in the feces. For ascariasis and enterobiasis, the dosage for adults and children 2 years of age and over is 11 mg/kg PO as a single dose (maximum dose is 1 g). This may be repeated in 2 to 3 weeks if necessary.
Adverse Effects
These effects include gastric distress and CNS adverse effects.
Nursing Management
Use pyrantel with caution in clients who are hypersensitive to it. Perianal swabs and stool examinations confirm the presence of the helminth. The client receiving pyrantel should be assessed for the following nursing diagnoses/collaborative problem: impaired comfort (headache, nausea and vomiting); diarrhea; risk for injury related to CNS effects (drowsiness, light-headedness, and dizziness); and the potential complication of hypersensitivity. For pinworms, monitor the perianal area with cellophane tape swabs starting 1 week after treatment; this should be performed every morning before bathing or defecation. For roundworms, stool examinations are checked 2 weeks after therapy. The administration of pyrantel does not require any special preparation such as fasting, dietary restrictions, laxatives, or enemas. It may be taken with or without food or at any time of day. Shake well and use the calibrated measuring device provided to measure the dosage accurately. Encourage the client to take the full course of therapy and to visit the prescriber on a regular basis to monitor progress. Alert the client to avoid hazardous tasks that require mental alertness (e.g., driving) until the response has been determined. For pinworm infestation, it is important to wash (without shaking) all of the bed linens and nightclothes to prevent reinfestation. All household members should be treated simultaneously. Stress proper hygiene, both personal and environmental, with the client. The expected outcome of pyrantel therapy for pinworms is that the client's perianal examinations using cellophane tape swabs will demonstrate negative results for 7 consecutive days. For roundworms, stool examination results should be negative for ova, larvae, or worms 2 to 3 weeks after the completion of therapy.

Leprostatic Drugs

✱ What are the key features of leprosy?
Leprosy, or **Hansen's disease**, is a chronic infectious disease that is caused by *M. leprae* in humans. Leprosy is considered to be a special public health problem, owing to the permanent disabilities it causes and its social consequences such as discrimination and stigma. It currently affects over 1 million people in Africa, Asia, South America and the Pacific, and the WHO estimates that between 2 and 3 million individuals are permanently disabled as a result of it. Although all the registered cases are on treatment, it is estimated that during the period 2000 to 2005, about 2.5 million people affected by leprosy need to be detected and treated.

Because of the substantial progress in leprosy control through multidrug therapy (MDT), the World Health As-

sembly (WHA) was prompted in 1991 to call for the "elimination of leprosy as a public health problem by the year 2000," defining elimination as attaining a level of prevalence below 1 case per 10,000, but has fallen short of that goal. At the beginning of 2004, the number of leprosy clients under treatment in the world was around 460,000. About 515,000 new cases were detected during 2003. Among them, 43% were multibacillary cases, 12% were children, and 3% were diagnosed with severe disabilities. During the past two years, the global number of new cases detected continued to decrease dramatically (a reduction of about 20% per year) (WHO, 2005a). Although the precise mode of transmission is unknown, the incubation period for leprosy ranges from a few months to decades. Large numbers of leprosy bacilli are generally shed from skin ulcers, nasal secretions, the GI tract and, perhaps, biting insects.

M. leprae is a bacillus that in humans first presents as a skin lesion—a large plaque or macule that is erythematous or hypopigmented in the center. More numerous lesions, peripheral nerve trunk involvement, and the common complications of plantar ulceration of the feet, foot drop, loss of hand function, and corneal abrasions may follow.

✱ What drugs are available to treat *M. leprae* infections?
Most cases can be arrested, if not cured, by appropriate therapy and management. The drugs of choice are dapsone and clofazimine. Thalidomide (Thalomid) was approved in 1998 for the treatment and prevention of cutaneous manifestations of erythema nodosum leprosum (ENL).

Dapsone is an antibacterial (antileprosy) agent that is bacteriostatic and has an action similar to that of the sulfonamides. Dapsone may also be a dihydrofolate reductase inhibitor and is effective against *M. leprae* (the cause of leprosy). Clofazimine has a slow bactericidal effect on *M. leprae*, inhibits mycobacterial growth, and tends to bind preferentially to mycobacterial DNA.

Despite its history of causing thousands of deformed infants (birth defects) in the 1960s and being withdrawn from the market in Germany, Great Britain, Japan, Canada, and many other countries, thalidomide has been studied as an investigational drug for the past 30 years. As a result, thalidomide has exhibited some promising new uses for clinical practice. It is indicated for the treatment of erythema nodosum leprosum, and is also under study for the treatment of immune related conditions, including Crohn's disease, treatment of graft-versus-host reactions with bone marrow transplantation, AIDS-related aphthous stomatitis, discoid lupus erythematosus, erythema multiforme, and RA.

Most clients today are treated with dapsone, rifampin, and clofazimine (in multibacillary [MB] cases) (Table 60-3.) However, ofloxacin and levofloxacin, minocycline, and clarithromycin are also being used in select cases or drug trials. Streptomycin, ethionamide, prothionamide, thiambutosine, and thiacetazone were occasionally administered in the past, but their toxicity, limited effectiveness,

TABLE 60-3 WHO-RECOMMENDED TREATMENT OF LEPROSY FOR ADULTS

Disease	Dapsone	Rifampin	Clofazimine	Interval
Paucibacillary (PB)	100 mg daily	600 mg daily		1 yr
Multibacillary (MB)	100 mg daily	600 mg daily	50 mg daily	2 yr

and/or requirement for intramuscular administration have effectively eliminated them from consideration for therapy of leprosy today.

Multidrug therapy (MDT) has been the standard treatment for leprosy in the United States since introduced at Carville in the early 1970s. At that time, 3 years of dapsone plus rifampin (with the addition of clofazimine if there was any suspicion of dapsone resistance), followed by indefinite dapsone monotherapy was recommended for all MB cases. These protocols required longer treatment than the MDT regimen introduced by the WHO in 1982. Short-term therapy was introduced in the United States under FDA-approved protocols in 1990. No new drugs were introduced, but the treatment periods have been shortened considerably. Selected clients have been treated under these protocols since 1990, and, thus far, the regimens have proven effective and without significant toxicity. Newly diagnosed leprosy clients are now treated according to the protocol shown in Table 60-3.

Treatment for 99% of clients worldwide is with the standard WHO paucibacillary (PB) and MB regimens, which basically differ from the United States regimens by giving rifampin only once monthly instead of daily and by treating clients for a somewhat shorter period of time. Because clients seen in the United States on the average have more active disease than those seen elsewhere, physicians in the United States continue to utilize daily rifampin and a longer duration of therapy.

The standard WHO regimen for PB clients is rifampin (600 mg PO monthly under supervision) plus dapsone (100 mg PO daily); therapy is continued for 6 months and then stopped. The 7th WHO Expert Committee on Leprosy recommended that single lesion PB disease could be treated with ROM therapy, which consists of single doses of rifampin (600 mg), ofloxacin (400 mg), and minocycline (100 mg) based on a multicenter trial (WHO, 2003). In this trial, the single dose of ROM showed slightly less clinical improvement compared to those taking the standard WHO PB regimen during 18 months of follow-up, all other parameters including relapse rate were similar.

Multibacillary cases receive rifampin (600 mg) plus clofazimine (300 mg) both monthly under supervision in conjunction with dapsone (100 mg) plus clofazimine (50 mg) both daily. Until recently, WHO recommended that treatment be continued for 24 months. The 7th Expert Committee noted that the recommendation of 24 months of therapy for MB disease remains valid but indicated that 12 months might be sufficient based on an ongoing trial and several reports in clients who had defaulted from therapy before completion of 24 months. Thus, WHO now recommends only 12 months of treatment for MB clients; although this length of therapy is probably adequate for most cases, concern has been expressed that it is not sufficient for higher bacterial index (BI) cases, although these are a minority of MB cases worldwide.

Early diagnosis and chemotherapy for leprosy and prompt treatment for all reactive episodes will prevent most leprosy complications and indeed, a decrease in disabilities has occurred. The clofazimine component of the MB regimen may have some protective effect in preventing reactions because ENL has become less common. In the affected hands and feet, in which loss of protective sensation has occurred, clients need to be taught to evaluate their hands and feet daily for any evidence of injury and to promptly obtain treatment. Protective measures may be necessary, particularly for the feet, utilizing special shoes to avoid injury and ulceration. Motor loss leading to deformed hands and/or feet will require corrective surgery.

Follow-up visits may be required during treatment at weekly intervals, if a severe leprosy related reaction is present, up to every three months in those without complications. Routine follow-up studies in the laboratory would include compete blood count, urinalysis, serum creatinine, and liver function tests while on treatment. However, drug toxicity is uncommon after the first year of treatment, and serious toxicity may manifest itself clinically before it is detected in the laboratory. Skin scrapings should be done from three or four of the most active sites yearly if possible. Routine follow-up biopsies are not necessary unless new lesions appear.

Follow-up visits should consist of a clinical examination and annual skin smears from previously positive sites for MB cases plus skin biopsies, if indicated. Additionally, clients should be advised to report at once any new skin lesions, reactions, further sensory or motor loss, iritis, or other symptoms possibly related to leprosy.

Clinically, there is a gradual clearance of skin lesions, mostly within the first year. The bacillary index on skin scrapings or biopsy specimens falls slowly; approximately 0.5 to 1 per year. Thus, it might take a decade for a client with very active disease to completely clear the bacilli.

★ ▢ **dapsone [dap** sone]
(DDS, Avlosulfon)
Indications
Dapsone is indicated for the treatment of all types of leprosy and for dermatitis herpetiformis.
Pharmacokinetics/Dosing
Dapsone is absorbed orally, distributed throughout the body, and found in fluids and in all body tissues. The time to peak serum levels is 2 to 6 hours; the half-life is approximately 30 hours. It is

acetylated by *N*-acetyltransferase in the liver; thus slow acetylators are more apt to develop higher serum levels and adverse effects than fast acetylators. Excretion is via the kidneys. The adult dosage for leprosy (given in combination with other antileprosy drugs) is 50 to 100 mg PO daily. As a suppressant for dermatitis herpetiformis, the adult dosage is 50 mg PO daily initially, which is increased as necessary until symptoms are controlled. As an antileprosy agent, the dosage for children is 1.4 mg/kg PO daily.

Adverse Effects

The adverse effects of dapsone include hypersensitivity, hemolytic anemia, and methemoglobinemia.

Nursing Management

Assessment

Administer dapsone cautiously in clients with severe anemia, G6PD deficiencies, and methemoglobin reductase, because hemolytic anemia may occur. Use caution in clients with hepatic or renal function impairment. This drug is also contraindicated with clients who are hypersensitive to dapsone and sulfonamides. A CBC and platelet count, and ALT and AST levels, should be completed before dapsone therapy for a baseline assessment.

Review the client's current medication regimen for the risk of significant drug interactions, such as those that may occur when dapsone is given with didanosine (ddI) as concurrent drug administration may reduce the absorption of dapsone. Dapsone requires an acid media for absorption, whereas didanosine is given with a buffer to neutralize stomach acid to increase absorption. Administer dapsone at least 2 hours before ddI. Hemolytic agents increase the potential for serious adverse blood reactions.

Nursing Diagnosis

The client receiving dapsone therapy should be assessed for the following nursing diagnoses/collaborative problems: impaired comfort (headache); deficient fluid volume related to anorexia, nausea, and vomiting; disturbed thought processes (mood and mental changes); ineffective protection related to leukopenia, thrombocytopenia, and anemia; and the collaborative problems of methemoglobinemia (bluish discoloration of the skin and lips), exfoliative dermatitis, peripheral neuritis (numbness and tingling of the hands and feet), hypersensitivity (rash), hepatic damage, and a "sulfone syndrome"—a hypersensitivity reaction that occurs after 6 to 8 weeks of therapy with fever, malaise, lymphadenopathy, exfoliative dermatitis, and anemia.

Planning

The goals for dapsone therapy are that the client will:
* Have negative skin scrapings without adverse effects of the drug.
* Effectively manage the therapeutic regimen, including medication compliance, reporting adverse drug effects and any new lesions appropriately, and maintaining scheduled visits with the health team for monitoring and continued treatment.

Implementation

Monitoring

Once therapy has started, a CBC should be determined monthly for 1 to 3 months and then semiannually for the remainder of dapsone therapy. The dosage may be reduced or suspended if CBC values are diminished: RBCs, below 2.5 million/mm³; hemoglobin, below 9 g/dL; WBCs, below 3500/mm³. Additionally, the client should be observed for the development of hemolytic anemia; symptoms are pale skin, fever, and unusual tiredness and weakness. During the first few weeks of therapy, monitor temperature. Approximately 25% of clients will develop a leprosy reactional state. If mild, a reduction of dosage and symptomatic treatment may resolve the fever. Severe reactions to therapy with neuritis, ulceration, and other significant symptoms require prompt treatment with corticosteroids if permanent nerve damage is to be avoided.

Hepatic function studies should be performed if the client develops anorexia, nausea, vomiting, or jaundice. Peripheral neuritis (numbness and tingling of the hands and feet) and exfoliative dermatitis (itching and scaling of the skin and loss of hair) are also indications for dosage interruption. Monitor client for cyanotic appearance or brownish color of mucous membranes for methemoglobinemia.

Intervention

Because of bacterial resistance, dapsone is usually given with other antimycobacterial agents. Therapy is continued for according to the type of leprosy, see Table 60-3.

Education

Encourage the client to comply with the dapsone regimen, and stress that the use of the drug is long-term. Dosage should not be omitted, increased or decreased without advice of physician. Taking the medication at the same time each day will assist in compliance. Stress the importance of regular visits to the prescriber to monitor progress. Caution the client to report any new lesions. Do not breastfeed without consulting the prescriber.

Evaluation

The expected outcome of dapsone therapy is that the client will effectively manage the therapeutic regimen. The skin scrapings will be negative without the client experiencing no or only a mild leprosy reactional state.

clofazimine [kloe **fa** zi meen]
(Lamprene)
Indications

Clofazimine is indicated as a secondary drug for the treatment of leprosy, especially for the dapsone-resistant type of leprosy.

Pharmacokinetics/Dosing

Clofazimine has a variable oral absorption and is distributed primarily in fatty tissues and cells. Macrophages take up this drug and further distribute it throughout the body. The half-life is approximately 2 to 3 months with chronic therapy, with time to peak serum levels between 1 and 6 hours. It is excreted primarily in the feces. The adult dosage in dapsone-resistant leprosy, in combination with one or more other agents, is 50 to 100 mg PO daily.

Adverse Effects

The adverse effects of clofazimine include gastric distress, ichthyosis, and discoloration of the skin, feces, sweat, tears, and urine.

Nursing Management

In addition to the following discussion, see the nursing management of dapsone therapy above. Clients with preexisting GI problems are at risk for GI bleeding, bowel obstruction, splenic infarction, and enteritis. There are no known significant drug interactions with this drug.

The client receiving clofazimine should be assessed for the following nursing diagnoses/collaborative problems: impaired comfort (photosensitivity, rash and itching, and change in taste); deficient fluid volume related to anorexia, nausea, and vomiting; disturbed thought processes (mood and mental changes, especially depression and suicidal thoughts related to skin discoloration); disturbed body image related to pink, red, or brownish-black discoloration of the skin and lips; and the potential complications of GI bleeding, clofazimine toxicity, and hepatitis. Administer with milk or meals to reduce GI irritation. Alert the client that a reddish-brown discoloration of skin, cornea, conjunctiva and body fluids may occur, which will resolve months or years after the drug is discontinued.

thalidomide [tha **lid** oh myde]
(Thalomid)
Indications

Thalidomide is approved in the United States for the treatment and prevention of a painful skin problem caused by leprosy (erythema nodosum leprosum). Although not approved for use by the FDA, thalidomide is also sometimes used in the management of AIDS-related aphthous stomatitis, Crohn's disease, discoid lupus erythematosis, graft-versus-host reactions after bone marrow transplantation, erythema multiforme, and rheumatoid arthritis.

Pharmacokinetics/Dosing

Thalidomide reaches peak serum levels in approximately 3 to 6 hours. It has a half-life of 5 to 7 hours and is excreted primarily in urine. The usual dosage of thalidomide is 100 to 300 mg daily initially and is adjusted or tapered by 50 mg every 2 to 4 weeks when the symptoms subside. It is recommended the dose be taken with water at bedtime.

Adverse Effects

The adverse effects of thalidomide include sedation, peripheral neuropathy, hypotension, hypersensitivity, rash, and bradycardia (*Drug Facts and Comparisons*, 2005). The most serious toxicity is its human teratogenic effects (the FDA Pregnancy Category is X). It is recommended that women who take this medication during their childbearing years use two reliable methods of birth control for 1 month before taking thalidomide, during therapy, and for 1 month after the last dose. Men should use a latex condom even if they have had a vasectomy, and they should continue using condoms for at least 30 days after taking their last dose of thalidomide. Advise clients that they cannot donate blood while taking this drug.

Nursing Management

Thalidomide is contraindicated for clients with peripheral neuropathy because that condition is a serious adverse effect of the drug. For this same reason, concurrent administration of other medications associated with peripheral neuropathy is contraindicated. Thalidomide has CNS depressant effects; therefore use caution whenever other CNS depressants are prescribed and when driving and engaging in potentially hazardous activities. Alert both male and female clients in effective methods of birth control, starting 1 month before and 1 month following discontinuation of thalidomide therapy. Other nursing management is similar to that for dapsone therapy.

Summary

Malaria is still prevalent despite the WHO's attempts to eradicate it by controlling the insect vector and the causative parasite. Although it is essentially considered a tropical disease, nurses in the United States and Canada may come into contact with imported cases; both countries have populations that travel extensively, and both countries provide havens for refugees and immigrants from areas in which the disease is endemic. Chloroquine, hydroxychloroquine, mefloquine, primaquine, quinine, and other drugs are commonly used for the prevention and treatment of malaria.

The incidence of TB is increasing because of the increasing numbers of persons with AIDS, persons who are living in the street or are homeless, malnourished individuals, and those taking immunosuppressant drugs. For acute tuberculosis, three or more antituberculous agents are administered concurrently for their additive effect and to minimize the risk of the organism becoming drug-resistant. Isoniazid, rifampin, ethambutol, and pyrazinamide are among the more commonly used antitubercular agents.

Amebiasis, an infection of the large intestine by *E. histolytica*, is prevalent in tropical areas and is again imported by travel; it is also found in poorly sanitized areas of Canada and the United States. Transmission is fecal to oral and occurs through the ingestion of cysts from contaminated food and water. Antiamebiasis agents in current use are metronidazole, paromomycin, chloroquine, and iodoquinol. Other protozoan diseases of concern include giardiasis, toxoplasmosis and trichomoniasis.

Helminths (worms parasitic to man) may be flatworms (platyhelminthes) or roundworms (nematodes). There are two types of flatworms: tapeworms (cestodes) and flukes (trematodes). They cause injury to the host in a variety of ways: by causing damage to and loss of blood from the intestinal wall, by producing toxic substances absorbed by the host, by traumatizing the host's tissues and making the host more susceptible to infection, and by competing with the host for sustenance within the bowel. The anthelmintic agents most commonly used are mebendazole, albendazole, thiabendazole, diethylcarbamazine, ivermectin, praziquantel, and pyrantel.

Leprosy, or Hansen's disease, is caused by *M. leprae* and is treated with dapsone, clofazimine, and thalidomide.

Although these diseases and the therapeutic agents used in their prevention and treatment are not commonly dealt with by most U.S. and Canadian nurses, familiarity with them is necessary to manage them appropriately when they do occur.

✴ Critical Thinking Questions

- Why is it necessary to determine whether an antimalarial is being used prophylactically, for the suppression of symptoms, or for the acute phase of malaria?

- Why are three or more antituberculous drugs administered concurrently?

- What advice would you provide for someone who was traveling to a place where malaria is endemic? Amebiasis? Leprosy?

Bibliography

American Association of Blood Banks. (2002). *Standards for blood banks and transfusion services* (21st ed.). Bethesda, MD: American Association of Blood Banks.

ℓ-LEARNING SUPPLEMENTS

Student CD-ROM
- Final Exam questions
- NCLEX® Examination review questions
- Pharmacology animations
- Printable chapter summary

Evolve Website (http://evolve.elsevier.com/mckenry)
- Case study on antimicrobial and antiparasitic drugs
- Content updates, including information on new drugs

- WebLinks corresponding to this chapter
- Answers to the critical thinking questions in this chapter
- *Elsevier ePharmacology Update* newsletter
- Mosby's Drug Consult Internet Edition
- Supplemental and reference information

Anandan, J.V. (2005). Parasitic infections. In M.A. Koda-Kimble, L.Y. Young, W.A. Kradjan, B.J. Guglielmo, B.K. Alldredge, & R.L. Corelli (Eds.), *Applied therapeutics: The clinical use of drugs.* (8th ed.) Philadelphia: Lippincott, Williams & Wilkins.

Anderson, D.M., Keith, J., & Novak, P.D. (Eds.) (2002). *Mosby's medical, nursing, and allied health dictionary* (6th ed.). St. Louis: Mosby.

Andries, K., Verhasselt, P., Guillemont, J., Gohlmann, H.W., Neefs, J.M., Winkler, H., et al. (2005). A diarylquinolone drug active on the ATP synthase of Mycobacterium tuberculosis. *Science, 307,* 223-227.

Blood Centers of the Pacific. (2002). Infectious risks of blood transfusion. *Blood Developments, 16,* 1-3.

Centers for Disease Control and Prevention, National Center for HIV, STD, and TB Prevention, Division of Tuberculosis Elimination Core Curriculum on Tuberculosis. (2000). Retrieved October 5, 2005, from http://www.cdc.gov/nchtp/tb/pubs/corecurr/Chapter9/Chapter_9_Recommendations.htm.

Centers for Disease Control and Prevention. (2003a). Reported tuberculosis in the United States. Atlanta, GA: Department of Health and Human Services.

Centers for Disease Control and Prevention (2003b) Treatment of tuberculosis - Official Joint Statement of the American Thoracic Society, CDC, and Infectious Diseases Society of America. *MMWR Morbidity and Mortality Weekly Report, 52*(RR11), 1-77.

Centers for Disease Control and Prevention. (2004). Areas where Malaria is No Longer Endemic. Retrieved January 22, 2005, from http://www.cdc.gov/malaria/distribution_epi/areas_eliminated.htm.

Centers for Disease Control and Prevention. (April 2004). Malaria surveillance - United States, 2002. *MMWR Morbidity and Mortality Weekly Report, 53,* SS1.

Centers for Disease Control and Prevention. (2005). Health information for international travel. Retrieved January 22, 2005, from http:.//www.cdc.gov.

Centre for Infectious Disease Prevention and Control. (2003). Tuberculosis in Canada 2000. Ottawa: Health Canada.

Drug facts and comparisons (58th ed.). (2005). St. Louis: Facts and Comparisons.

Ford, M.D., Delaney, K.A., Ling, L.J., & Erickson, T. (2001). Clinical toxicology. Philadelphia: W.B. Saunders Co.

Health Canada, Bureau of HIV/AIDS, STD, & TB. (2000). Retrieved March 7, 2005, from http://www.phac-aspc.gc.ca/publicat/epiu-aepi/tb/epi0100/tbdrug_e.html.

Itokazu, G.S., Bearden, D.T., & Danziger, L.H. (2005). Infectious diarrhea. In M.A. Koda-Kimble, L.Y. Young, W.A. Kradjan, B.J. Guglielmo, B.K. Alldredge, & R.L. Corelli (Eds.), *Applied therapeutics: The clinical use of drugs.* (8th ed.) Philadelphia: Lippincott, Williams & Wilkins.

Kain, K.C., MacPherson, D.W., Kelton, T., Keystone, J.S., Mendelson, J. & MacLean, J.D. (2001). Malaria deaths in visitors to Canada and in Canadian travelers: a case series. Canadian *Medical Association Journal, 164*(5), 654-659.

Kays, M.B. (2005). Tuberculosis. In M.A. Koda-Kimble, L.Y. Young, W.A. Kradjan, B.J. Guglielmo, B.K. Alldredge, & R.L. Corelli

(Eds.), *Applied therapeutics: The clinical use of drugs.* (8th ed.) Philadelphia: Lippincott, Williams & Wilkins.

Lacy, C.F., Armstrong, L.L., Goldman, M.P., & Lance, L.L. (2004). *Lexi-Comp's Drug Information Handbook* (12th ed) Hudson, Ohio: Lexi-Comp.

Leder, K., & Weller, P.F. (2004). Epidemiology, pathogenesis, clinical feature and diagnosis of malaria. Wellesley, MA: UpToDate.

MacLean, J.D., Demers, A.M., Ndao, M., Kokoskin, E., Ward, B.J. & Gyorkos, T.W. (2004). Malaria epidemics and surveillance systems in Canada. *Emerging Infectious Disease, 10*(7), 1195-1201.

Neff, M. (2003). ATS, CDC, and IDSA update recommendations on the treatment of tuberculosis. *American Family Physician, 68*(9), 1854, 1857-8, 1861-2.

Petri, W.A. (2001). Antimicrobial agents (Continued) - Drugs used in the chemotherapy of tuberculosis, mycobacterium avium complex disease, and leprosy. In Hardman, J.G. & Limbird, L.E. (Eds.), *Goodman & Gilman's The pharmacological basis of therapeutics* (10th ed.). New York: McGraw-Hill.

Tracy, J.W., & Webster, L.T. (2001a). Chemotherapy of parasitic infections - Introduction. In Hardman, J.G. & Limbird, L.E. (Eds.), *Goodman & Gilman's The pharmacological basis of therapeutics* (10th ed.). New York: McGraw-Hill.

Tracy, J.W., & Webster, L.T. (2001b). Drugs Used in the chemotherapy of protozoal infections - Malaria. In Hardman, J.G. & Limbird, L.E. (Eds.), *Goodman & Gilman's The pharmacological basis of therapeutics* (10th ed.). New York: McGraw-Hill.

Tracy, J.W., & Webster, L.T. (2001c). Drugs used in the chemotherapy of protozoal infections (Continued) - Amebiasis, giardiasis, trichomoniasis, trypanosomiasis, leishmaniasis, and other protozoal infections. In Hardman, J.G. & Limbird, L.E. (Eds.), *Goodman & Gilman's The pharmacological basis of therapeutics* (10th ed.). New York: McGraw-Hill.

USP DI: Drug information for the health care professional (25th ed.). (2005). Greenwood Village, CO: MICROMEDEX Thomson Healthcare.

Vincent, W.F. (2000). Overview of malaria: Infectious disease update. *Medical News, 11*(8), 53-59.

World Health Organization. (2003). Leprosy Prevalence: Global Leprosy Situation in 2003. Retrieved March 10, 2005, from http://w3.whosea.org/en/Section10/Section20/Section55.htm.

World Health Organization. (2004). Fact Sheet on Tuberculosis. Retrieved March 7, 2005, from http://www.who.int/mediacentre/factsheets/fs104/en/.

World Health Organization. (2005a). Elimination of leprosy as a public health problem. Retrieved March 28, 2005, from http://www.who.int/lep/.

World Health Organization. (2005b). Tuberculosis (TB). DOTS: The internationally recommended TB control strategy. Retrieved October 5, 2005, from http://www.who.int/tb/dots/en/.

Zaid, R.B., Nargis, M., Neelotpol, S., Hannan, J.M., Islam, S., & Akhter, R., et al. (2004). Acetylation phenotype status in a Bangladeshi population and its comparison with that of other Asian population data. *Biopharmaceutics and Drug Disposition 25*(6), 237-241.

OVERVIEW OF THE IMMUNOLOGIC SYSTEM

CHAPTER FOCUS

The immunologic system is composed of cells and organs that defend the body against invasion by foreign biologic and/or chemical substances. The immunocompetent cells in the body have an inherent ability to distinguish foreign protein substances from the body's own cells. This chapter reviews the organs and tissues of the immune system, the immunocompetent cells, and the types of immunity.

LEARNING OBJECTIVES

- Identify the lymphoid organs of the immune system.
- Describe the role of each lymphoid organ in defending the body against foreign biologic and/or chemical substances.
- Identify the immunocompetent cells involved in the immune response.
- Compare and contrast the functions of the three major groups of T cells.
- Describe the action of B cells in responding to foreign antigens.
- Identify the five classes of antibodies and their functions.
- Compare and contrast humoral immunity and cell-mediated immunity.
- Describe the two types of active immunity and two types of passive immunity.

▲ KEY TERMS

antibodies, p. 1129
B lymphocytes (B cells), p. 1126
complement system, p. 1130
cytokines, p. 1126

immunity, p. 1130
immunocompetent cells, p. 1126
polymorphonuclear leukocytes (PMLs), p. 1126
T lymphocytes (T cells), p. 1126

✱ What are the organs of the lymphatic system and their roles?

The lymphoid organs consist of the spleen, tonsils, lymph nodes, and thymus. The lymphoid tissues are mainly lymphocytes and plasma cells that travel freely throughout the human system. The two major classes of lymphocytes are T-cell and B-cell lymphocytes, which are discussed under Immunocompetent Cells. Figure 61-1 identifies the organs and tissues of the immune system.

Spleen

The spleen, the largest lymphatic organ in the body, is located on the left side of the body in the extreme superior, posterior corner of the abdominal cavity. It has the following two main functions: (1) a storage site or reservoir for blood, and (2) a processing station for red blood cells (RBCs) (i.e., RBCs break down in the spleen near the end of their life cycle). The spleen intercepts foreign matter or

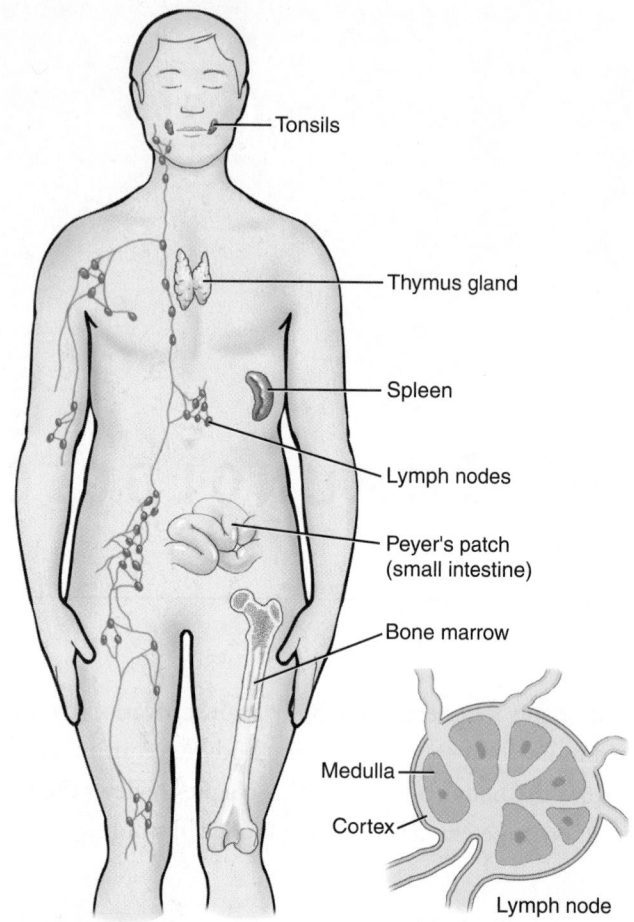

FIGURE 61-1 Location of organs and tissues of the immune system.

antigens that have reached the bloodstream. Macrophages lining the pulp and sinuses of the spleen remove cellular debris and process hemoglobin in the red pulp area of the spleen. The white pulp area of the spleen contains lymphocytes and plasma cells that are involved in the immune process.

Tonsils

The tonsils are an accumulation of lymphoid tissue and are named according to their location: lingual, palatine, and pharyngeal tonsils. They intercept foreign bodies or antigens that enter the body by way of the respiratory tract. Similar lymphoid tissue is located in the submucosal areas of the gastrointestinal (GI) tract (Peyer patches) to intercept antigens (bacteria and viruses) entering from the gut. Other lymphoid tissues are located in the bone marrow and help to intercept antigens in the blood and in the lymph nodes.

Lymph Nodes

The lymph nodes are capsulated organs that are located throughout the body and are involved with lymph circulation. The outer portion of the lymph node is the cortex, and the inner portion is the medulla. The thymus-depend-

ent zone exists in the deep area or middle cortex. This area contains mainly **T lymphocytes (T cells);** T cells are lymphocytes formed or seeded from the thymus gland that when exposed to an antigen divide rapidly and produce large numbers of new T cells sensitized to that antigen.

Lymph nodes are essentially a row of in-line filters that screen the lymph flowing through it. Many lymphocytes and macrophages are located throughout the lymph nodes, especially in the cortical, paracortical, and medullary areas. T lymphocytes are located mainly in the paracortical region, whereas plasma cells are found in the medullary sinuses.

Thymus Gland

The thymus gland is located in the mediastinal area. It processes lymphocytes and, in the early years up to puberty, rapidly produces lymphocytes. The immune system is developed when immature lymphocytes from the bone marrow are processed in the thymus gland and then sent to the spleen, lymphatic system, and other tissues and organs in the body to mature. The lymphocytes are active against some bacteria and viruses, allergens, fungal infections, and foreign tissue.

At birth, the thymus gland is larger than it is in an adult. By the time a person reaches puberty, the thymus has grown to nearly six times its original size. After puberty, this gland undergoes involution; in older adults, it is usually a small mass of reticular fibers with some lymphocytes and connective tissue. Although its importance was largely discounted over the years, today it is one of the most important areas for medical research. Scientists are searching for answers to the many questions about the thymus gland and its relationship to the other tissues and organs in the immune system.

✱ What are the immunocompetent cells and how are they differentiated?

Mononuclear T cells and B cells and the **polymorphonuclear leukocytes (PMLs)** are involved in the immune response. The PMLs are nonspecific cells that interact with lymphocytes to produce an inflammatory response, whereas T cells and B cells are capable of recognizing specific antigens and initiating the immune response. However, only mononuclear T cells and B cells are **immunocompetent cells**—cells with the ability to mobilize and deploy antibodies and other responses to stimulation by an antibody.

In humans, stem cells from the bone marrow are transformed to T cells (T lymphocytes) in the thymus gland and B cells (B lymphocytes) elsewhere in the body. As stated previously, the T lymphocytes then migrate to lymphoid tissue and organs. When in contact with an antigen, T lymphocytes form specialized cells to provide cellular immunity. **B lymphocytes (B cells)** are small, agranulocytic leukocytes that form antibodies to search out, identify, and bind with specific antigens to provide humoral immunity.

Cytokines are biologic factors released from T cells, macrophages, mast cells, and other cells in the body. Included among the cytokines are the interferons, interleukins, and tumor necrosis factors. They each interact with components of the immune system in complex ways. They are critically involved in host defense against infection, tumors or foreign substances, and are also important in many inflammatory conditions. The interferons and interleukins, for example, foster maturation and/or stimulate T cells, B cells, and other components of the immune system. Some were briefly introduced in Chapter 57 in relation to inflammation and fever; Table 61-1 presents some of these.

T Lymphocytes (T Cells)

T cells are generally long-lived. When they are not in their special areas, they circulate continuously through the body by way of the bloodstream and lymphatic system. They are involved with the B lymphocytes (B cells) by cooperating with them (helper T cells) or inhibiting them (suppressor T cells). The B cells do not interact with the thymus. Clones of B cells or T cells are groups of lymphocytes capable of responding to a specific type of antigen; only the specific antigen can activate the specialized clones.

When the T cells first contact an antigen, the lymphocytes that recognize the foreign substance proliferate, which gives rise to larger numbers of cells that have the capacity to recognize and respond to this antigen. Some of the cells trigger B-cell antibody production or cell-mediated immune-type responses, whereas others increase the population of antigen-sensitive memory cells. This is called acquired immunity, an immunity that is not innate but is obtained during life. A second exposure to this antigen will provoke a more powerful response by the specific T cells.

Three major groups of T cells include (1) cytotoxic T cells, (2) helper T cells, and (3) suppressor T cells (Figure 61-2).

Cytotoxic T Cells Cytotoxic T cells can bind tightly to organisms or cells that contain their binding-specific antigen, and they release cytotoxic (probably lysosomal) enzymes directly into the cell. Cytotoxic T cells are capable of killing microorganisms, cancer cells, viruses, heart transplant cells, and other cells that are foreign to the body. Body tissue that contains viruses or foreign cells may also be attacked by the killer cells.

Helper T Cells Helper T cells account for the majority of T cells and help the immune system in many ways (Box 61-1). They increase the activation of B cells, cytotoxic T cells, and suppressor T cells by antigens. Helper T cell clones are activated by very small amounts of antigens, quantities that may not activate B cells, cytotoxic T cells, or suppressor T cells. Once helper T cells are activated, they secrete cytokines; these chemical factors attract macrophages to the site of infection or inflammation and increase the response of the B cells, cytotoxic T cells, and suppressor T cells to the antigen.

Helper T cells may also secrete interleukin-2, a cytokine that is capable of stimulating the action of other T cells, such as cytotoxic T cells and some suppressor T cells. Helper T cells also secrete macrophage migration inhibition factor, another cytokine. This substance slows or stops the migration of macrophages into the affected area and also activates the macrophages that are present to be more effective phagocytotic agents. The activated macrophages can attack and destroy a vastly increased number of invading organisms.

Acquired immunodeficiency syndrome (AIDS) is the final outcome of an infection with the human immunodeficiency virus (HIV). This virus binds to protein on the cell membranes of the helper T lymphocytes (T4 cells), monocytes, macrophages, and colorectal cells. The helper T cells

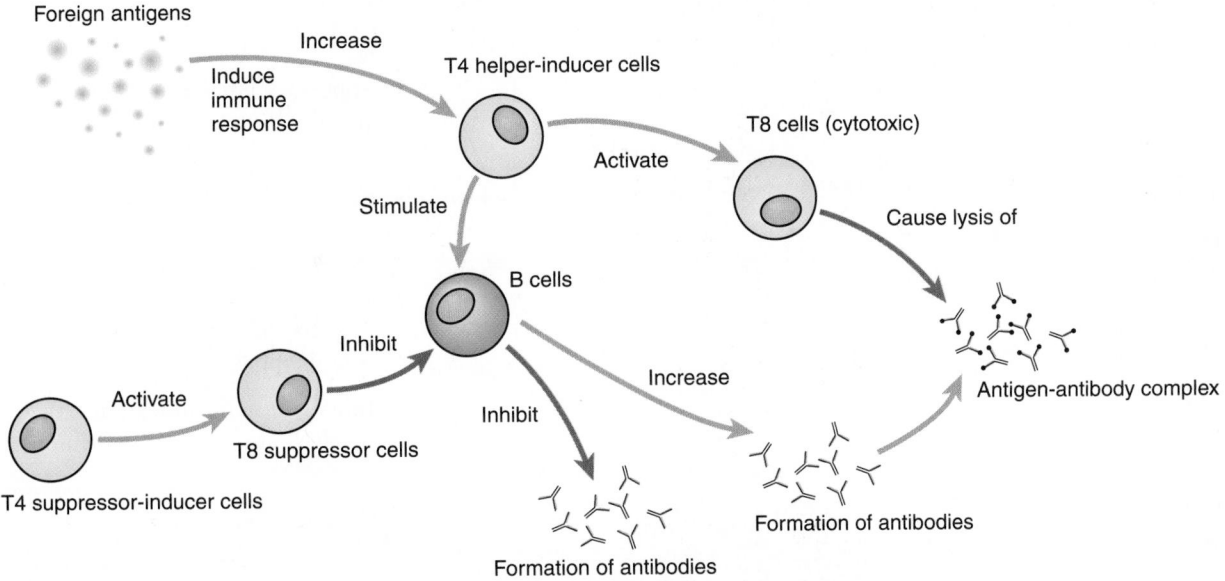

FIGURE 61-2 T4 cell effects in the body. T4 cells are mainly the helper-inducer type of cells and increase when antigens are present. T4 suppressor-inducer cells do not respond to antigens. They act indirectly to suppress antibody formation.

Cytokine	Activates/Stimulates and/or Promotes Maturation					Other Action
	T Cell	B Cell	Natural Killer Cell	Macrophage	Mast Cell	
INF-α Interferon-α			X	X		Active against viruses
INF-γ Interferon-Gamma			X	X		
IL-1 Interleukin-1	X	X				Important in inflammation
IL-2 Interleukin-2	X	X	X			
IL-3 Interleukin-3					X	Involved in maturation of hematopoietic cells
IL-4 Interleukin-4	X	X		X		Stimulates IgE production
IL-5 Interleukin-5		X				Activates eosinophils Stimulates IgE production
IL-6 Interleukin-6	X	X				Important in inflammation
IL-7 Interleukin-7	X					
IL-8 Interleukin-8	X					Triggers chemotaxis for T cells, neutrophils
IL-9 Interleukin-9	X				X	
IL-10 Interleukin-10					X	
IL-11 Interleukin-11		X				Promotes maturation megakaryocytes
IL-12 Interleukin-12	X		X			
IL-13 Interleukin-13		X				Suppresses inflammatory cytokines Involved in IgE production
IL-14 Interleukin-14		X				
IL-15 Interleukin–15	X					
IL-16 Interleukin-16	X					Triggers chemotaxis of CD4 T cells and eosinophils.
TNF-α Tumor Necrosis Factor-Alpha						Important in inflammation Involved in production of acute phase proteins
TNF-β Tumor Necrosis Factor-Beta						Toxic to tumor cells

Modified from Hall, P.D., & Karlix, J.L. (2002). Function and evaluation of the immune system. In J.T. DiPiro, R.L. Talbert, G.C. Yee, G.R. Matzke, B.G. Wells & L.M. Posey (Eds.), *Pharmacotherapy: A pathophysiological approach* (5th ed.). Norwalk, CT: Appleton & Lange.

T4 cells are responsible for a variety of immune functions, some of which include the following:

1. Release of colony-stimulating factors and cytokines to stimulate the production of leukocytes, and activate cells in the immune system
2. Activation of the natural killer cells (cytotoxic NK cells), which are large lymphocytes in the blood that have non–antigen-specific antitumor and antibacterial properties
3. Activation of T8 suppressor cells by T4 helper-inducer cells can, which will stop antibody production, or activation of T8 cytotoxic T cells and stimulation of B cells by T4 suppressor-inducers to increase the production of antibodies

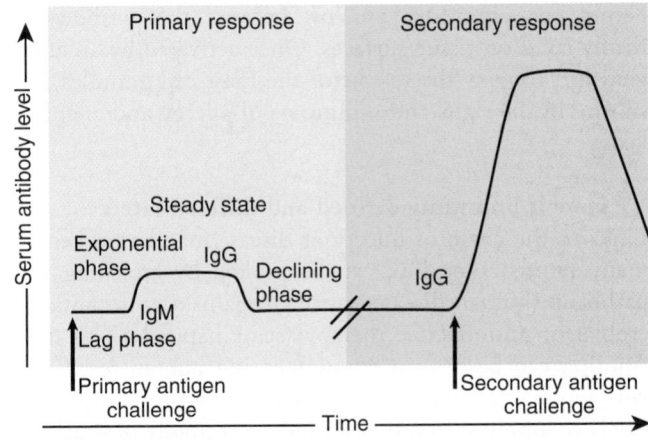

FIGURE 61-3 Primary and secondary immune response.
From Mudge-Grout, C.L. (1993). *Immunologic disorders*. St. Louis: Mosby.

are destroyed by the virus, which leads to the immunodeficiency syndrome known as AIDS. (See Chapter 59 for additional information on this disease and its treatment.)

Suppressor T Cells Less is known about suppressor T cells, but it is known that they can suppress the function of both cytotoxic and helper T cells. This suppression may be useful in preventing excessive immune reactions that can cause severe body damage. These cells are often called regulatory T cells.

B Lymphocytes (B Cells)

B lymphocyte clones lie dormant in lymphoid tissue until a foreign antigen appears. The macrophages in the lymphoid tissue phagocytize the foreign substance, and the adjacent B lymphocytes and perhaps the T cells are activated. B cells specific for the antigen enlarge, and some differentiate to form plasmablasts (a plasma cell precursor) and memory cells. The plasmablasts proliferate and divide, and in 4 days approximately 500 plasma cells are present for each original plasmablast. The plasma cells rapidly produce gamma globulin antibodies that are secreted into the lymph and transported by the blood.

Cells similar to those in the original clone are called memory cells. The first response to an antigen may be slow, weak, and of short duration. The second response is much more rapid and far more potent and prolonged, and antibodies are formed for months rather than only for a few weeks. This is why vaccinations that use several doses given weeks or months apart are so effective (Figure 61-3).

✴ What are the roles of the immunoglobulins?

Antibodies are gamma globulins (a type of protein) called immunoglobulins. They are specific for particular antigens and are produced by lymphoid tissue in response to antigens. At the present time, five classes of antibodies have

been identified: IgG, IgM, IgA, IgD, and IgE. (The "Ig" stands for immunoglobulin, and the other letters designate the classes.)

IgG is the major immunoglobulin in the blood (approximately 75% to 80% of the total antibodies in the normal person) and is capable of entering tissue spaces, coating microorganisms, and activating the complement system, thus accelerating phagocytosis. It is the only immunoglobulin capable of crossing the placenta to provide the fetus with passive immunity until the infant can produce its own immune defense system.

IgM is the first immunoglobulin produced during an immune response. It is located primarily in the bloodstream and develops in response to an invasion of bacteria or viruses. IgM activates complement and can destroy foreign invaders during the initial antigen exposure. Its level decreases in approximately 1 week, whereas IgG levels progressively increase.

IgA is located primarily in external body secretions—saliva, sweat, tears, mucus, bile, and colostrum—and it is found in respiratory tract mucosa and in plasma. It helps to provide a defense against antigens on exposed surfaces and antigens that enter the respiratory and GI tracts. The plasma cells in the intestinal area secrete IgA and secretory components to defend the body against bacteria and viruses.

The function of IgD is unknown. It is found in the plasma and has been located on lymphocyte surfaces together with IgM; therefore it may be associated with binding antigens to the cell surface. Although levels of IgD are increased in chronic infections, IgD does not appear to have a particular affinity for specialized antigens.

IgE binds to histamine-containing mast cells and basophils. It can mediate histamine release in the immune response to parasites (helminths) and in some allergic conditions. It is often called the *reaginic antibody* because of its involvement in immediate hypersensitivity reactions.

Serum concentrations are low because the antibody is firmly fixed on tissue surfaces. Once activated by an antigen, IgE triggers the release of the mast cell granules, resulting in the signs and symptoms of allergy and anaphylaxis.

How is immunity defined and differentiated?

Links in the chain of infectious disease may be broken at many points. One link can be broken by attacking the pathogen (human disease–causing organism) with antimicrobial or antiinfective therapy (see Chapters 57 to 60). Another can be broken by augmenting human resistance with biologic agents such as vaccines and serums, which artificially supply antibodies or catalyze antibody production by the immune system (see Chapter 62). Agents that enhance immunity, called immunomodulators, are also used in the treatment of some cancers and viral diseases (see Chapters 55, 56, 59, and 63). An immunologic reaction that destroys or resists foreign cells or their products (antigens) is termed immunity. The most successful antigens, or immunogens, are protein or polysaccharide macromolecules that are usually bacterial, viral, fungal, or rickettsial in origin.

Antigens may be recognized by T-helper cells that activate specific B cells, by a strong B-cell response to the invasion of certain antigens (e.g., large polymers, *Escherichia coli*, dextrans), or by a macrophage intermediary. Macrophage interactions often enhance the antigen recognition by both T cells and B cells in the body.

The primary types of immunity are humoral immunity and cell-mediated immunity.

Humoral Immunity

Humoral immunity is critical in the immune response and refers to the involvement of immunoglobulins, cytokines, and other protein mediators (especially complement). Humoral response is described as a primary or secondary immune response.

Primary Response A foreign antigen in the body will bind to specific B cells to produce specialized antibody-producing plasma cells. Antibodies specific to the antigen can be found in the blood, usually within 6 days. The initial immunoglobulin is IgM, which increases in quantity for up to 2 weeks; production then declines so that very little IgM is present in a few weeks. After the initial IgM elevation, IgG antibodies start to appear at approximately day 10; these levels peak in several weeks and maintain high levels for a much longer time period (see Figure 61-3).

Secondary Response The secondary response is often called the *memory* response because the immune system responds so much faster to a second exposure to the same antigen. Both T and B memory cells are involved in beginning the immediate production of antibodies in large amounts.

The second part of humoral immunity is activation of the complement system, a series of approximately 20 proteins that circulate in the blood in an inactive form. When an antigen-antibody complex triggers complement, each component in the cascade is activated in precise order. This reaction causes the mast cells to release substances that produce redness, increased heat, and the edema of inflammation. It may also cause bacterial cell death and damage to normal tissue that surrounds the affected area.

Cell-Mediated Immunity

Cell-mediated immunity is the result of contact between T cells and antigens. Receptors on the T-cell surface are capable of recognizing foreign antigens, and antigen destruction may occur through one of the two following processes: (1) directly, by injecting chemical compounds into the target cell membrane (killer activity by cytotoxic T cells, often called natural killer cells); or (2) by secreting cytokines. The cytokines can enhance or suppress the action of other lymphocytes, or they can create a chemotactic gradient in the area that will attract macrophages (and eosinophils, basophils, and neutrophils) to the site (see Table 61-1). Cell-mediated immunity (delayed hypersensitivity) involves only the direct action of T cells without humoral assistance.

Natural and Acquired Immunity

The body has certain inherited and innate abilities to resist encounters with antigens. This ability is known as *natural* resistance or *natural immunity*, which is not to be confused with naturally acquired immunity. Some general defenses inherent to natural resistance come from factors familiar to the focus of nursing, such as adequate rest, nutrition, exercise, and freedom from undue stress. Others are physiologic factors that discourage the proliferation of microbes, including the acidity of gastric secretions, respiratory tract cilia, and bactericidal lysozymes in tears. During his or her lifetime, an individual may also acquire further immune capabilities through both natural and artificial means. Acquired immunity is conferred by either active or passive action (Figure 61-4).

Unbroken skin is extremely effective in barring entry to microorganisms. If invasion does succeed, a barrage of defenses is mounted by the inflammatory response. The immune system identifies the threatening antigens or allergens and creates specific gamma globulins directed against the particular species of antigen. These gamma globulins (also called antibodies or immunoglobulins) are proteins that are chemically complementary and specifically configured to lock into the foreign antigen and inactivate it.

Antibodies also activate cellular defenses to phagocytize invading microorganisms. Custom-made gamma globulins, or antibodies, provide acquired immunity to the specific antigen for varying lengths of time. Those antibodies will gradually disappear from the serum, but the potential for their rapid replication in response to a repeat challenge by that specific antigen continues to exist after the initial exposure. Consequently, the result is known as *naturally acquired* immunity, which is a process of *naturally acquired active* immunity because of the body's active involvement in creating the antibodies. *Naturally acquired passive* immunity is a process of immunity that occurs when antibodies made by the mother's body are passively transferred through the placenta or breast milk (especially colostrum, the breast milk produced shortly after delivery) to the fetus or infant.

Artificial induction of the immune state, *artificially acquired* immunity, is initiated purposefully to protect the susceptible individual. It may also be induced either actively or passively. Artificially acquired *active* immunity is evoked by the deliberate administration of antigens, either live partially modified organisms, killed organisms, or their toxins. The parenteral route is the predominant mode of administration, although the nasal route may be used for influenza or the oral route for polio and typhoid. Periodic reactivation of actively acquired artificial immunity against certain organisms by booster doses (e.g., tetanus) is sometimes necessary. Artificially acquired *passive* immunity is conferred by the parenteral administration of antibody-containing immune serum from immune humans or animals (see Figure 61-4).

In general, artificially acquired active immunity secures protection for a longer duration than any type of passive immunity and is usually the prophylactic treatment of choice for populations at risk. Adverse effects may include local pain at the injection site and headache with mild to moderate fever. Because of the agents used, *active* immunity results in fewer adverse effects than passive immunity. Artificially acquired *passive* immunity is often chosen for susceptible individuals following a known exposure. A combination of active and passive approaches is also occasionally used. A number of products used in artificial passive immunization cause adverse effects because of individual hypersensitivities to animal products (especially horse serum or eggs), to the preservative used in a medication, or to an antibiotic. The products of bacterial metabolism are the agents responsible for other adverse effects.

The presence of mild to moderate upper respiratory tract infection or pregnancy does not always prohibit immunization. However, an immunosuppressed state (as a result of cancer chemotherapy or disease) may prohibit or limit immunization. Current manufacturers' instructions should always be consulted. Table 61-2 compares the capabilities and effects of active and passive immunity.

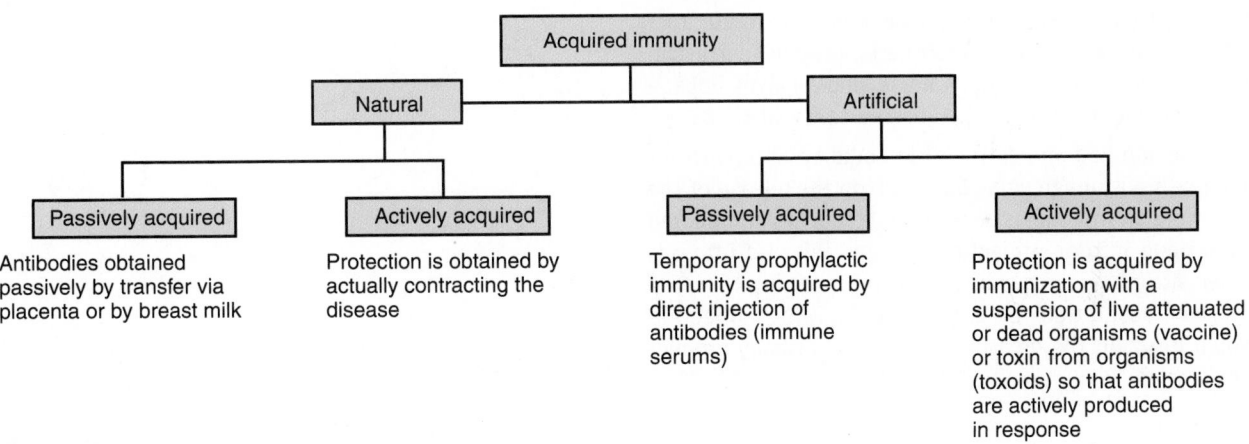

FIGURE 61-4 The process of acquired immunity.

TABLE 61-2 COMPARISON OF ACTIVE AND PASSIVE IMMUNITY

	Active Immunity	Passive Immunity
Source	Individual	Other human or animal
Efficacy	High	Low to moderate
Method	Contracting disease or stimulating host immune system	Administer preformed antibody by injection, maternal transplacental transfer, or in breast milk
Time to develop	5-21 days	Immediate effect
Duration	Long, up to years	Usually shorter in time
Ease of reactivation	Easy with booster dose	Can be dangerous, anaphylaxis may occur, especially if animal sources are used
Purpose	Prophylaxis	Prophylaxis and therapy

Summary

The immunologic system consists of lymphoid organs (the spleen, tonsils, lymph nodes, and thymus), immunocompetent cells known as T lymphocytes (T cells) and B lymphocytes (B cells), and related cytokines. All of these components defend the body against the invasion of foreign biologic and chemical substances. Antibodies are immunoglobulins that are specific for particular antigens. Immunity is the immunologic reaction that destroys or resists foreign cells or their products. It may be natural or artificial and actively or passively acquired. Pharmacologic therapy is usually aimed at strengthening the body's immunologic status for the prevention of disease.

✳ Critical Thinking Questions

- As a bacterium entering a human body, what do you expect to experience when encountering T cells? You have invited a friend, a virus, to meet you by entering via the respiratory system. What will be the virus's experience with the various antibodies?

- What type of immunity do the following have: A child recovering from the measles? A 6-week-old nursing infant? A first-grader with a DTaP (diphtheria, tetanus, pertussis) and polio vaccine booster? A nurse who receives hepatitis B immune globulin after exposure to hepatitis B?

- Suppose you had an additive that could be used with injectable solutions to delay but not stop the release of the drug from an injection site into the blood. If you injected an antigen into one injection site and injected into another site an antigen mixed with the additive to cause delay of absorption for 2 to 3 weeks, which injection would result in the greater response of antibody production? Why?

Bibliography

Anderson, D.M., Keith, J., & Novak, P.D. (Eds.) (2002). *Mosby's medical, nursing, and allied health dictionary* (6th ed.). St. Louis: Mosby.

Guyton, A.C., & Hall, J.E. (2000). *Textbook of medical physiology* (10th ed.). Philadelphia: W.B. Saunders.

Hall, P.D., & Karlix, J.L. (2002). Function and Evaluation of the Immune System. In J.T. DiPiro, R.L. Talbert, G.C. Yee, G.R. Matzke, B.G. Wells & L.M. Posey (Eds.), *Pharmacotherapy: A pathophysiological approach* (5th ed.). Norwalk, CT: Appleton & Lange.

Hardman, J.G., & Limbird, L.E. (Eds.). (2001). *Goodman and Gilman's The pharmacological basis of therapeutics* (10th ed.). New York: McGraw-Hill.

Herlihy, B., & Maebius, N.K. (2003). *The human body in health and illness* (2nd ed.). Philadelphia: W.B. Saunders.

McCance, K.L., & Huether, S.E. (2002). *Pathophysiology: The biological basis for disease in adults and children* (4th ed.). St. Louis: Mosby.

Thibodeau, G.A., & Patton, K.T. (2003). *Anatomy and physiology* (5th ed.). St. Louis: Mosby.

e-LEARNING SUPPLEMENTS

Student CD-ROM
- Final Exam questions
- NCLEX® Examination review questions
- Pharmacology animations
- Printable chapter summary

Evolve Website (http://evolve.elsevier.com/mckenry)
- Content updates, including information on new drugs
- WebLinks corresponding to this chapter
- Answers to the critical thinking questions in this chapter
- *Elsevier ePharmacology Update* newsletter
- Mosby's Drug Consult Internet Edition
- Supplemental and reference information

SERUMS, VACCINES, AND OTHER IMMUNIZING AGENTS

CHAPTER FOCUS

More than 200 years ago, Edward Jenner observed that milkmaids who developed cowpox were rarely victims of smallpox. This finding prompted him to develop the first vaccine. A modern version of this vaccine led to the eradication of smallpox as a naturally acquired disease in 1980—a health success for the world. The development of vaccines against more than 20 infectious diseases has revolutionized the approach to public health. A number of new or improved vaccines have become available in the last two decades. Today advances in molecular biology are enabling scientists to develop new vaccines against diseases that continue to plague the world.

LEARNING OBJECTIVES

- Explain the present status of immunization and anticipated future developments.
- State the appropriate immunization schedule for children 2 years of age and younger.
- Identify immunizations recommended for adults.
- Describe the recommended use of tetanus toxoid and tetanus immune globulin in wound management.
- Describe the nursing management of serums, vaccines, and other immunizing agents as immunotherapy.
- List the adverse effects of immunizations, and correlate them with client education.
- Compare the advantages and disadvantages of live attenuated and inactivated biologic products.

▲ KEY TERMS

active immunity, p. 1133
antibody titer, p. 1139
herd immunity, p. 1134
passive immunity, p. 1134

The body's first defense against invasion by potentially lethal microorganisms is intact skin and mucous membranes. The antiinflammatory process and/or a competent immune system are the body's defense against microbes that break this barrier.

✳ How are the terms active immunity and passive immunity defined?

Active immunity exists when the body produces specific antibodies to combat infections caused by specific antigens or microbes. This immunity may be referred to as *naturally acquired immunity,* because a person who recovers from an infectious disease produces antibodies and memory cells against that specific antigen. The next time the body is in contact with the same antigen, the immune system will be primed to destroy the antigen. Vaccines and toxoids also confer active immunity artificially.

Passive immunity occurs when antibodies are transferred from a human or animal to a susceptible person. Newborn infants usually have passively acquired immunization that is naturally acquired from their mothers. However, this type of immunity protects for only short periods of time (weeks to several months). Intravenous (IV) or intramuscular (IM) administration of immune globulin confers passive immunity artificially.

Occasionally, reference is made to the concept of herd immunity. Herd immunity is a public health concept that reflects the degree to which members of a society who are vulnerable to a particular infectious disease are protected from that disease when a high percentage of the community is immune to the condition. Increasing vaccination rates in the general population serve to reduce risk for clients who are not vaccinated by reducing exposure risk.

What modalities exist to induce immunity?

Vaccines and toxoids are available to provide artificially acquired active immunity. Vaccines contain whole microbes (dead or attenuated) that are not pathogenic but can induce the formation of antibodies. Toxoids contain detoxified microbe by-products that are antigenic and also induce antibody production. Different manufacturing techniques are utilized to optimize the ability to induce an immune response with reduced toxicity. Such techniques include attenuation, inactivation, use of a subunit of the pathogen, conjugation, and use of genetic recombinant interventions. Table 62-1 differentiates advantages, disadvantages, and examples of each.

Sera and antitoxins, which contain exogenous antibodies or immunoglobulins, are used to provide artificially acquired passive immunity.

What adverse effects are associated with immunizations?

Although being protected from debilitating infectious disease is important, immunization is not without some risk. Adverse effects (e.g., slight fever, discomfort at injection

TABLE 62-1 EXAMPLES OF DIFFERENT MODALITIES IN MANUFACTURING VACCINES

	Description	Example	Advantages	Disadvantages
Live attenuated vaccines	Microbe is weakened or "attenuated"	Oral Polio Vaccine (OPV) Measles, Mumps, Rubella (MMR) Vaccine Nasal Influenzae Vaccine	Often long-lasting immunity Resistance to disease similar to that seen with natural disease	Increased risk of inducing disease Cannot be used is immunocompromised clients Some products cannot be used in pregnant women Higher risk for contamination Product is more labile and often requires special storage conditions
Inactivated vaccines or toxoids	Whole organism is killed or toxin from bacteria is inactivated	Inactivated Polio Vaccine (IPV) Tetanus and Diphtheria Toxoids (TD)	Highly purified, low contamination risk Easier to ship and store Little risk for inducing disease	Often shorter acting immunity requiring more frequent reimmunization. May be less effective in preventing disease.
Subunit vaccines	Portion of microbe is used	Acellular Pertussis (aP)	Fewer adverse reactions	May be more costly to produce
Conjugate vaccines	Protein or other key component is linked to outer coating of microbe or toxin	*Haemophilus influenza* type b (Hib)	Improved recognition by immature immune system in infants and young children	Ineffective in immunocompromised clients
Recombinant vaccines	Alter genetic makeup of microbe used in production of vaccine to reduce or eliminate active disease risk	Hepatitis B vaccine (HB)	Improved safety	May be less effective in immunocompromised clients Risk-benefit to be considered in clients with allergy to yeast

site, or minor rash) are usually mild and transient; more serious effects (e.g., encephalitis and seizures) are occasionally reported. Although the adverse effects of immunizations can be observed, serious reactions are rare. The benefit of vaccine administration almost always outweighs the risk unless an absolute contraindication to the vaccine/toxoid is present. This is particularly true for individuals at high risk for vaccine-preventable disease (Box 62-1).

Joint pains and malaise may be seen with some products, especially with certain live and inactivated vaccines. Although rare, an allergy to the egg protein providing the culture medium for the organism involved, to antisera or antitoxins, to the mercury preservative, or to contained antibiotics causes a reaction that is usually controllable by antihistamines. When any unusual or severe reaction occurs, the nurse should contact the prescriber, and an informational form should be sent to the Centers for Disease Control and Prevention (CDC) (available at http://www.vaers.org/) in the United States or the Division of Immunization (http://www.phac-aspc.gc.ca/dird-dimr/pdf/hc4229e.pdf) in Canada. The nurse should also give information to those vaccinated on how to contact the health care provider if they become sick. They should also follow up with their health care provider, hospital, or clinic within 4 weeks of immunization.

Monitoring for adverse effects is part of a surveillance system to detect uncommon, severe, previously unrecognized, and rare reactions to vaccination. Past examples are the Guillain-Barré syndrome (which accompanies a small percentage of influenza vaccinations), encephalitis following a measles vaccine, and peripheral neuropathy after rubella vaccinations. All of these occurrences are very rare.

Although uncommon, a large number of benign, expected reactions could indicate a "hot" lot of vaccine. Data are collected by the CDC for comparison with national data and are published in the *Quarterly Adverse Reaction Report*.

Minor expected reactions can be treated with acetaminophen and rest. Severe fevers (temperatures more than 103°F) can be treated with acetaminophen and tepid sponge baths to reduce body temperature; occasionally a seizure may accompany a high temperature, and parents need to be advised. Serum sickness sometimes occurs after repeated serum injections and consists of a rash, urticaria, arthritis, adenopathy, and fever that start hours or even days after the injection. Treatment consists of analgesics, antihistamines, or corticosteroids.

Rare but serious anaphylactic reactions constitute an emergency situation; they are characterized by urticaria, dyspnea, cyanosis, shock, or unconsciousness that occurs within minutes of injection. Therefore a nurse or someone responsible should observe any recipient of immunotherapy for up to one half hour after therapy. Treatment for anaphylaxis may require the administration of epinephrine. Vasopressors and intermittent positive-pressure breathing (IPPB) oxygen, antihistamines, and corticosteroids may help.

Nurses often find themselves in charge of vaccination programs and clinics. Because nurses are often the first to be consulted by clients, it is important to keep current on immunization recommendations and adverse effect monitoring.

✳ What biologic agents to enhance immunity are commonly used in North America?

A number of products are available for use in North America to prevent infectious diseases. A representative sampling of agents that produce active and passive immunity are briefly presented below. Review package inserts or other prescribing information for schedules and dosing for different populations.

Products Inducing Active Immunity

Products that induce active immunity interact with the host to stimulate the client's immune system to produce antibodies. They may also have various other actions to allow the client to respond to infection more appropriately in the future. The advantage of inducing active immunity is that this approach often leads to long-term protection (months

---

BOX 62-1 RISKS FROM DISEASE VERSUS RISK FROM VACCINES

MEASLES/RUBELLA

DISEASE	VACCINE
Measles	**MMR**
Pneumonia: 6 in 100	Encephalitis or severe allergic reaction: 1 in 1,000,000
Encephalitis: 1 in 1000	
Death: 2 in 1000	
Rubella	
Congenital Rubella Syndrome: 1 in 4 (if woman becomes infected early in pregnancy)	

DIPHTHERIA/TETANUS/PERTUSSIS

DISEASE	VACCINE
Diphtheria	**DTaP**
Death: 1 in 20	Continuous crying, then full recovery: 1 in 1000
Tetanus	
Death: 2 in 10	Seizures or shock, then full recovery: 1 in 14,000
Pertussis	
Pneumonia: 1 in 8	Acute encephalopathy: 0-10.5 in 1,000,000
Encephalitis: 1 in 20	
Death: 1 in 200	Death: None proven

Data from Centers for Disease Control and Prevention, National Immunization Program. *Six common misconceptions about vaccination and how to respond to them.* Available at http://www.cdc.gov/nip/publications/6mishome.htm.

in the case of influenza vaccine, years to a lifetime in the case of inactivated polio vaccine).

Efficacy when administered after exposure is variable and depends on the time course of the disease and the ability of the product to quickly produce an active immune response. Agents that are used postexposure include tetanus toxoid, hepatitis B vaccine, and rabies vaccine, although supportive immunoglobulin therapy to provide passive immunity is often used concurrently.

diphtheria and tetanus toxoids, and acellular pertussis vaccine [dif **theer** ee a, **tet** a nus **toks** oyds, and ay **cel** yoo lar per **tus** sis vak **seen**]
(DTaP, Daptacel, Infanrix, Tripedia, Adacel✦)
Formulation
The DTaP formulations are mixes of toxoids of diphtheria and tetanus and inactivated antigens of pertussis. The inactivated antigens of pertussis (referred to as "acellular") are associated with significantly fewer adverse effects than were older formulations, which included the whole pertussis pathogen in an attenuated state. Variations of this formulation are also available, including diphtheria and tetanus toxoids combined (know as DT, or Td), and combinations of DTaP with inactivated poliovirus vaccine (PEDIARIX) and DTaP with *Haemophilus influenzae* b conjugate vaccine (TriHIBit).

Indications
The DTaP formulation is indicated for active immunization in children and adolescents against diphtheria, pertussis, and tetanus. Diphtheria is an acute contagious disease caused by the bacterium *Corynebacterium diphtheriae*. This infection is characterized by the production of a system toxin and an adherent false membrane lining of the mucous membrane of the throat that may interfere with eating, drinking and breathing; untreated it is often fatal. Pertussis is an acute highly contagious respiratory disease that lasts 6 to 8 weeks characterized by paroxysmal coughing that ends in a loud whooping inspiration. Tetanus is an acute potentially fatal infection of the central nervous system (CNS) characterized by irritability, headache, fever, and painful spasms of the muscles resulting in lockjaw, risus sardonicus, opisthotonus, and laryngeal spasm.

The DT formulation of the vaccine without acellular pertussis is often used as prophylaxis in adults and is administered regularly at 10-year intervals in adulthood and more frequently as part of postwound prophylaxis against tetanus. The other combined formulations are also used as part of pediatric immunization protocols.

Contraindications
DTaP is contraindicated in clients with hypersensitivity to the product or any ingredients, or in clients with active febrile reactions. DTaP is assigned to the Food and Drug Administration (FDA) Pregnancy Category C.

Adverse Effects
Local swelling or redness at the injection site is among the most commonly reported adverse effects. Others include drowsiness, irritability, fever, and gastrointestinal (GI) complaints. The pertussis component may increase the likelihood for an encephalopathic or anaphylactic syndrome (including high fever, hypotension/unresponsive state, or seizures), but this risk is probably reduced with the acellular formulation. Infants with inconsolable crying beyond 3 hours should be evaluated for this syndrome as well.

Haemophilus influenzae type b conjugate vaccine [he **mof** fi lus bee **kon** joo gate vak **seen**]
(ActHIB, HibTITER, Pedvax HIB)
Formulation
These are inactive vaccines using a protein or saccharide conjugate to render improved response with an immature immune system.

Indications
Haemophilus influenzae type b conjugate vaccine is routinely used in children aged 2 months to 5 years to reduce risk of *H. influenzae* infection, a severe destructive inflammation of the larynx, trachea, and bronchi that may be life-threatening. The vaccine is also used in children older than 5 years of age with other chronic illnesses in which *H. influenzae* infection could be problematic.

Contraindications
Haemophilus influenzae type b conjugate vaccine administration is contraindicated in clients with active febrile illness or active infection. It is also avoided for clients who have hypersensitivity to the vaccine or any ingredients (e.g., thimerosal) or are immunosuppressed. Although not typically used in adults, it has a pregnancy risk rating of C.

Adverse Effects
Adverse effects include edema, local irritation at the injection site, and fever or irritability. Refer to package insert for more complete information.

hepatitis A vaccine [hep a **tye** tis aye vak **seen**]
(Havrix, VAQTA)
Formulation
Hepatitis A vaccine is an inactivated virus vaccine.

Indications
For individuals at high risk for hepatitis A, including travelers to regions where hepatitis A is prevalent, workers or others in areas in which exposure risk may be higher (e.g., child day care, institutional workers), and those for whom lifestyle factors may increase risk (intravenous [IV] drug use, sexually active clients with multiple partners). Hepatitis A may be spread through fecally contaminated food or water.

Contraindications
Hepatitis A vaccine is contraindicated in clients who have hypersensitivity to the vaccine or components of the vaccine. It has a pregnancy risk rating of C.

Adverse Effects
Headache and local pain at injection site is commonly observed. Other rare events include pharyngitis and abdominal pain. Refer to package insert for more complete information.

hepatitis B vaccine [hep a **tye** tis bee vak **seen**]
(Engerix-B, Recombivax-HB)
Formulation
Hepatitis B vaccine is an inactivated virus vaccine (via recombinant deoxyribonucleic acid [DNA] technology)

Indications
Hepatitis B vaccine is indicated for immunization against hepatitis B. It is commonly administered in North America to all newborns. Hepatitis B virus is transmitted by transfusion of contaminated blood or blood products, by sexual contact with an infected person, or by the use of contaminated needles and instruments. Severe infection may cause prolonged illness, destruction of liver cells, cirrhosis, increased risk of liver cancer, or death. Immunization is also recommended to those at higher risk, including health care workers, those in the military, those undergoing hemodialysis, clients with multiple sexual partners, residents of institutions in which risk is high (institutions for mentally handicapped, prisons), and intravenous drug users.

Contraindications
Hepatitis B vaccine is contraindicated for clients who have a hypersensitivity to yeast, hepatitis B vaccine, or any ingredient in the formulation. Hepatitis B vaccine has a category C rating for pregnant women.

Adverse Effects
Multiple adverse effects are possible, and include injection site reactions. Hypotension and anaphylaxis are rare. Also refer to package insert for a more complete listing.

influenza-virus vaccine [in floo **en** za **vye** rus vak **seen**]
(Fluvirin, Fluzone, FluMist)
Formulation
Formulations and activity vary each year based on isolation of likely strains expected to impact the next influenza season. Of great concern are case reports of outbreaks of Avian influenza strains (including HSN1), which are associated with high mortality rates (Ungchusak et al., 2005); de Jong et al., 2005). Both of the injectable formulations are not live virus, with Fluzone made from purified split-virus and Fluvirin comprised of purified split-virus antigen. The nasal formulation, FluMist is a trivalent live virus which has a more limited indication.

Indications
The injectable forms of influenza vaccine are recommended for individuals at high risk for influenza-related complications, including those older than 65 years of age, residents of institutional settings, health care workers, individuals with pulmonary conditions or chronic disease, and children and adolescents who receive chronic aspirin therapy (to reduce the risk of developing Reye syndrome). Live nasal influenza vaccine is contraindicated in children under 2 years of age, and the inactivated vaccine does not offer protection to those under 2 years of age (Jefferson et al., 2005). Influenza is a highly contagious myxoviral infection of the respiratory tract characterized by sore throat, cough, fever, muscular pains and weakness; it may be complicated by bacterial pneumonia among high risk clients such as the very young, the older adult, and clients with chronic pulmonary disease. The CDC in the United States (www.cdc.gov) and the Public Health Agency of Canada (http://www.phac-aspc.gc.ca/im/index.html) often update their recommendations from year to year.

The nasal formulation is a live vaccine and must be avoided in both immunocompromised individuals and those who have contact with them for a period of 21 days after administration. Influenza virus vaccine live, intranasal contains live attenuated influenza viruses that replicate in the nasopharynx of the recipient and are shed in respiratory secretions. As such, a number of individuals, including health care workers, should not receive the nasal formulation as it may put immunocompromised contacts at risk for the disease. Its use is also limited to otherwise healthy individuals who are between the age of 18 and 49 years.

Contraindications
The influenza vaccine is contraindicated for clients with a history of hypersensitivity reactions to it, presence of an acute infection or respiratory condition, an acute neurologic condition, or hypersensitivity to ingredients (including egg or egg protein). The live nasal product should be avoided in youth or adolescents taking aspirin containing products, in clients with a history of Guillain-Barré syndrome, and those with asthma or reactive airway disease. Influenza vaccine has a pregnancy risk rating of C, but its use appears safe in pregnancy (Munoz et al., 2005).

Adverse Effects
Adverse effects are numerous, but usually mild. They include local tenderness, fever, malaise, and sometimes mild flu-like symptoms (Skowronski et al., 2003). Such flu-like symptoms may be more common with the attenuated nasal formulation. Refer to package insert for more complete information.

measles, mumps, and rubella vaccines (combined) [**mee** zels, mumpz and roo **bel** a vak seen]
(MMR)
Formulation
The combined measles, mumps, and rubella vaccine is a live virus vaccine.

Indications
MMR combined vaccine is indicated to prevent measles, mumps and rubella in children and nonpregnant adults. Measles is an acute, highly contagious viral disease involving the respiratory tract characterized by a spreading maculopapular cutaneous rash with the complications of pneumonia, obstructive laryngitis, laryngotracheitis, and occasionally, encephalitis. Mumps is an acute viral disease characterized by the swelling of the parotid glands, with the complications of arthritis, pancreatitis, myocarditis, oophoritis, orchitis, and nephritis. Rubella is a contagious viral disease characterized by fever, symptoms of a mild upper respiratory tract infection, lymph node enlargement, arthralgia, and a diffuse, fine red maculopapular rash, but if contracted by a woman in the first trimester of pregnancy, it may cause fetal anomalies, such as heart defects, cataracts, deafness, and mental retardation.

Contraindications
MMR combined vaccine should not be used in pregnant women because the live rubella (German measles) component has a high risk for inducing teratogenic effects. Other contraindications include prior hypersensitivity to the product, hypersensitivity to egg or egg protein, immunocompromised status or clients receiving immunosuppressant therapy, and clients with tuberculosis. Although possessing a Pregnancy Category C rating, most clinicians strongly recommend avoiding this product in pregnancy. Refer to CDC protocols regarding avoiding dosing with other live vaccinations.

Adverse Effects
Moderate fever (e.g., up to 102° F) for up to 12 days is common. Rash, malaise, sore throat, and rarely orchitis have been reported. Refer to package insert for more complete information.

meningococcal polysaccharide vaccine [me **nin** joe kok al pol i **sak** a ride vak **seen**]
(Menomune)
Formulation
The meningococcal polysaccharide vaccine contains inactivated antigen for several groups of *Neisseria meningitidis*, including groups A, C, Y, and W-135.

Indications
The use of this vaccine is primarily limited to preventing and controlling outbreaks of susceptible groups of *N. meningitidis* infection, and is used for at-risk clients older than 2 years of age. It is also used in targeted populations in which rates of infection may be high, or for travelers who may visit an area with higher risk. Although it is not highly contagious, its manifestations are severe, a bacterial meningitis, and/or meningococcemia, both of which are life-threatening.

Contraindications
Meningococcal polysaccharide vaccine is contraindicated in clients with a history of hypersensitivity to the product, in clients younger than 2 years of age, and in those with active febrile illness. It is rated as a C category agent via the FDA pregnancy risk classification.

Adverse Effects
The most frequently reported adverse effect is local irritation at the injection site. Other adverse effects include headache, fever, and malaise. Refer to the package insert for complete information.

pneumococcal conjugate vaccine [noo moe **kok** al **kon** ju gate vak **seen**]
(Prevnar)
pneumococcal polysaccharide vaccine [noo moe **kok** al pol i **sak** a ride vak **seen**]
(Pneumovax 23, Pnu-Immune 23, Pneumo 23✤)
Formulation
Both of these vaccines are inactivated products. The pneumococcal conjugate vaccine contains saccharides to antigens of seven types of pneumococci and is recommended for infants age 2 to 23 months because of improved response for this formulation with immature

immune systems. The polysaccharide version offers protection against 23 of the most commonly observed pathogenic types of pneumococci and is recommended for adults.

Indications

The conjugate formulation is indicated as part of routine childhood immunization protocols. It is also used in children up to 59 months of age with other concurrent chronic disease states who are at higher risk for pneumococcal infection. The conjugate formulation may also be considered for splenectomized adults who do not respond to the polysaccharide vaccine (Musher et al., 2005). The polysaccharide version is used in adults and children older than 2 years of age who are at high risk for pneumococcal disease, including those older than 65 years of age, those with underlying chronic conditions with increased risk (e.g., cochlear implants, asplenic clients). Pneumococcal pneumonia is an acute respiratory infection with fever, productive cough vomiting, malaise, weakness, pleuritic chest pain, and atelectasis with a high risk of pleural effusion and bacteremia. There may be metastatic infection to the meninges, joints, and heart valves. Other pneumococcal infections, including otitis media, appear to be reduced with use of this vaccine (Fireman et al., 2003; Jackson et al., 2003), as are macrolide-resistant strains of streptococcal pneumonia (Stephens et al., 2005).

Contraindications

These vaccines are contraindicated for clients with a history of hypersensitivity to the product or any ingredient in the product, or clients with thrombocytopenia or current febrile illness. Both formulations carry a FDA Pregnancy Category C rating.

Adverse Effects

The most common adverse effects include fever, irritability, restlessness, GI complaints, and local irritation at the injection site. Anaphylaxis to both formulations has been reported. Refer to package inserts for more complete listings.

poliovirus vaccine (inactivated) [**poe** lee oh **vye** rus vak **seen**, in ak ti **vay** ted]
(IPOL)
Formulation

The inactivated polio vaccine is an inactive form of polio administered subcutaneously also known as the Salk vaccine. The active oral polio formulation (OPV) is no longer used in the United States and Canada, because it is a live vaccine product and poses risks for clinical or subclinical disease in immunocompromised clients who either receive the oral product or come in contact with a recently vaccinated individual. OPV use is recommended by the World Health Organization (WHO) in those countries in which wild poliovirus remains, or recently has been endemic for its ease of distribution and economies associated with immunization programs.

Indications

Inactivated polio vaccine (IPV) is indicated as part of routine childhood and adolescent immunizations to prevent poliomyelitis and travelers to countries in which polio is still endemic. Poliomyelitis is an infectious disease caused by poliovirus; asymptomatic, mild, and paralytic forms of the disease occur.

Contraindications

Hypersensitivity to the product or to any ingredients in the vaccine (including neomycin, streptomycin, or polymyxin B) are reasons for avoiding use. Use should be delayed for clients with febrile illness.

Adverse Effects

The IPV is generally well tolerated, with fever, rash, and local irritation at the injection site being the most frequently reported events. Refer to package insert for a more complete discussion of risks and benefits of use.

rabies virus vaccine [**rab** beez **vye** rus vak **seen**]
(Imovax Rabies, RabAvert)
Formulation
Rabies virus vaccine is an inactivated product.

Indications

Rabies virus vaccine is indicated for preexposure prophylaxis in clients with high occupational risk for rabies (e.g., animal handlers) or travelers to rural areas of countries in which rabies is still endemic. Rabies is an acute, usually fatal viral disease of the CNS. Postexposure, it is used as part of a protocol with rabies immune globulin in the prevention of rabies.

Contraindications

Hypersensitivity to any component of the product is a contraindication for use, although as part of life-threatening use postexposure, risk and benefit are carefully assessed. Like other vaccines, rabies virus vaccine is assigned to FDA Pregnancy Category C.

Adverse Effects

The most frequent adverse effects include edema, dizziness, and other CNS effects. Refer to package insert information for complete information on its use and risks.

varicella virus vaccine [var i **sel** a **vye** rus vak **seen**]
(chicken pox vaccine, varicella-zoster vaccine, Varivax)
Formulation

The varicella virus vaccine is a live vaccine that is administered subcutaneously.

Indications

Varicella virus vaccine is used as part of routine childhood immunization protocol to prevent varicella infection. Varicella (chickenpox) is an acute, highly contagious viral disease caused by a herpes virus, varicella zoster virus (VZV) characterized by fever, malaise, and a generalized vesicular rash. Although an attack usually confers life-long immunity, the virus lies dormant in certain sensory nerve roots after the primary infection, and may result in recurring episodes of herpes zoster, especially in older adults and debilitated or immunocompromised individuals.

Morbidity and mortality in both children and adults have declined since the addition of varicella vaccine to childhood vaccination schedules in 1995 (Nguyen, Jumaan, & Seward, 2005). The existing vaccine does not appear to have an impact on future outbreaks of herpes zoster later in life (Jumaan et al., 2005). A different vaccine (similar to the varicella virus vaccine) is under study to prevent herpes zoster in older adults (Oxman et al., 2005).

Contraindications

Varicella virus vaccine is contraindicated in clients who have a history of hypersensitivity to the vaccine or any component (including neomycin). It also should not be used in pregnant women or in clients who are immunocompromised or are receiving immunosuppressant drug therapy. Despite the FDA Pregnancy Category C rating, most clinicians do not recommend its use in pregnancy.

Adverse Effects

The most common adverse effects are local reactions at the injection site and fever. Other effects include a varicella-like rash, chills, malaise, and insomnia. Refer to the package insert for more complete information.

Products Providing Passive Immunity

Providing passive immunity (administering immunoglobulin therapy directed against a targeted pathogen), is a common modality to treat clients with known exposure, or high likelihood of exposure, to life-threatening infectious diseases. The benefit of such therapy is that a near immediate effect can be observed. Unfortunately, this therapy has only a short benefit (typically weeks) and often poses some risk for blood-borne pathogen transmission because they are often blood products. In addition to unfractionated immune globulin (see Chapter 63), more specific immunoglobulin or related therapy with a known reaction to targeted antigens (e.g., hepatitis B, rabies) is also used. Three examples are presented in the following monographs.

hepatitis B immune globulin [hep a **tye** tis **bee** i **myun glob** yoo lin]
(Bay Hep B, H-BIG, Nabi-HB)

Formulation
Hepatitis B immune globulin is derived from plasma of donors with known hepatitis B antibodies. Each particular formulation or brand undergoes different purification techniques before being marketed.

Indications
Hepatitis B immune globulin is used to provide passive immunity to individuals exposed to hepatitis B.

Contraindications
Hypersensitivity to the product or any ingredient in the formulation is considered a contraindication to use. Clients with immunoglobulin A (IgA) deficiency should also avoid the product. Hepatitis B immune globulin is rated FDA Pregnancy Category C.

Adverse Effects
The most common adverse effects include pain on injection, fever, chills, dizziness, urticaria, GI disturbances, and joint and muscle pain. As with other immunoglobulin therapy, hypersensitivity reactions, including angioedema and anaphylaxis, have been reported.

palivizumab [pah li **viz** u mab]
(Synagis)

Formulation
Palivizumab is a monoclonal antibody with activity against respiratory syncytial virus (RSV). It is manufactured utilizing recombinant DNA technology and is not derived directly from blood or a blood product.

Indications
Palivizumab is indicated for the prevention of serious or life-threatening RSV infection in high risk neonates and infants younger than 2 years of age. It is typically administered as a monthly intramuscular (IM) injection during RSV season (e.g., typically October through April in North America, but may be different in local areas). High risk infants typically are those who were born prior to 26 to 29 weeks gestation and displayed respiratory difficulties during their first few weeks or months of life.

Contraindications
Palivizumab is contraindicated in clients with prior history of serious hypersensitivity reactions. It has an FDA Pregnancy Category C rating, but is only used in clients younger than 2 years of age.

Adverse Effects
Adverse effects of palivizumab are infrequent. Rare but serious hypersensitivity reactions have been reported.

rabies immune globulin [**ray** beez i **myun glob** yoo lin]
(BayRab, Imogam)

Formulation
This immune globulin is derived from human plasma in which donors have been immunized to rabies and have high titers of antibody.

Indications
Rabies immune globulin is indicated for postexposure prophylaxis in individuals with a documented risk for rabies exposure.

Contraindications
Hypersensitivity to the product or to any ingredient (e.g., thimerosal) is considered a contraindication to use, although risk and benefit must be evaluated. Rabies Immune Globulin has an FDA Pregnancy Category C rating.

Adverse Effects
Fever and soreness at the injection site are the most common adverse effects to rabies immune globulin.

✳ What psychosocial issues impact on vaccine and toxoid use?

The critical age period for immunization is from birth through grade school entry and during the school years (most states and provinces now require maintenance of immunizations as a criterion for retention in the school system). Groups at particular risk include adolescents, new parents (if they are not immunized or have waning immunity, because they are exposed to childhood illness or vaccines), debilitated persons, and health care providers. Other groups such as migrant workers and recent immigrants to the United States and Canada are predictably at high risk for infectious diseases.

International political and economic upheavals and the refugee influx to the United States and Canada have illustrated the major problems encountered in other countries: diphtheria, measles, hepatitis B, tuberculosis, and malaria carrier status. Immunization programs that are taken for granted in the United States, Canada, and other countries are not as well funded in developing countries.

As a group, adolescents also seem to be at high risk for preventable infections. Of these, certain subgroups may be particularly in need of immunization, such as athletes, those with a history of substance abuse, runaways, foreign travelers, and those isolated from or rejecting allopathic health care. Millions of children in North America are not adequately immunized against measles, polio, rubella (German measles), mumps, diphtheria, pertussis (whooping cough), and tetanus.

Newspapers and television news programs have reported the adverse effects associated with the pertussis vaccine and other vaccines; such reports have served to bias some individuals against vaccination. It is important to stress that, although vaccines are not without some risks, the risks associated with not being vaccinated and actually contracting the disease are even more serious. Table 62-2 illustrates the impact of diseases before immunizations. Diphtheria, tetanus, polio, and other diseases can cause crippling and death, and most of these diseases are very contagious.

Other perceived barriers to immunization are living in medically underserved areas, not having health insurance, having problems accessing immunization clinics, and having insufficient information about the value of immunizations. The incidence rates of traditional vaccine-preventable diseases are at an all-time low, and corresponding vaccination coverage rates are at an all-time high; however, a system to ensure the timely vaccination of newborn infants that also incorporates newly recommended vaccines is incomplete. Schedules for immunizations for these diseases have been developed as guidelines for the practitioner and for parents to ensure adequate protection for their children (Figure 62-1).

With some of these diseases, obtaining a valid history of clinical disease or an antibody titer (the concentration of antibodies in the serum) is useful in determining disease exposure and immunity. Proven exposure to the disease does not always guarantee immunity. Therefore timely immunizations are even more important if the person's potential

Recommended Childhood and Adolescent Immunization Schedule — UNITED STATES • 2005

Vaccine ▼ / Age ▶	Birth	1 month	2 months	4 months	6 months	12 months	15 months	18 months	24 months	4–6 years	11–12 years	13–18 years
Hepatitis B[1]	HepB #1	HepB #2			HepB #3						HepB Series	
Diphtheria, Tetanus, Pertussis[2]			DTaP	DTaP	DTaP		DTaP	DTaP		DTaP	Td	Td
Haemophilus influenzae type b[3]			Hib	Hib	Hib	Hib	Hib					
Inactivated Poliovirus			IPV	IPV	IPV	IPV	IPV	IPV		IPV		
Measles, Mumps, Rubella[4]						MMR #1	MMR #1			MMR #2	MMR #2	
Varicella[5]						Varicella	Varicella	Varicella	Varicella	Varicella	Varicella	
Pneumococcal[6]			PCV	PCV	PCV	PCV	PCV		PCV	PPV	PPV	
Influenza[7]						Influenza (Yearly)	Influenza (Yearly)			Influenza (Yearly)	Influenza (Yearly)	
Hepatitis A[8]									Hepatitis A Series	Hepatitis A Series	Hepatitis A Series	

Vaccines below red line are for selected populations

Legend:
- Range of recommended ages
- Preadolescent assessment
- Only if mother HBsAg(−)
- Catch-up immunization

This schedule indicates the recommended ages for routine administration of currently licensed childhood vaccines, as of December 1, 2004, for children through age 18 years. Any dose not administered at the recommended age should be administered at any subsequent visit when indicated and feasible. ▨ Indicates age groups that warrant special effort to administer those vaccines not previously administered. Additional vaccines may be licensed and recommended during the year. Licensed combination vaccines may be used whenever any components of the combination are indicated and other components of the vaccine are not contraindicated. Providers should consult the manufacturers' package inserts for detailed recommendations. Clinically significant adverse events that follow immunization should be reported to the Vaccine Adverse Event Reporting System (VAERS). Guidance about how to obtain and complete a VAERS form are available at www.vaers.org or by telephone, 800-822-7967.

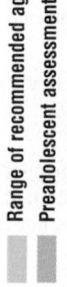

DEPARTMENT OF HEALTH AND HUMAN SERVICES · CENTERS FOR DISEASE CONTROL AND PREVENTION

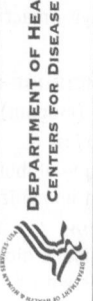

The Childhood and Adolescent Immunization Schedule is approved by:
Advisory Committee on Immunization Practices www.cdc.gov/nip/acip
American Academy of Pediatrics www.aap.org
American Academy of Family Physicians www.aafp.org

FIGURE 62-1 Recommended childhood and adolescent immunization schedule.

From Centers for Disease Control and Prevention, National Immunization Program. Available at http://www.cdc.gov/nip/recs/child-schedule.pdf

Footnotes
Recommended Childhood and Adolescent Immunization Schedule
UNITED STATES • 2005

1. **Hepatitis B (HepB) vaccine.** All infants should receive the first dose of HepB vaccine soon after birth and before hospital discharge; the first dose may also be administered by age 2 months if the mother is hepatitis B surface antigen (HBsAg) negative. Only monovalent HepB may be used for the birth dose. Monovalent or combination vaccine containing HepB may be used to complete the series. Four doses of vaccine may be administered when a birth dose is given. The second dose should be administered at least 4 weeks after the first dose, except for combination vaccines which cannot be administered before age 6 weeks. The third dose should be given at least 16 weeks after the first dose and at least 8 weeks after the second dose. The last dose in the vaccination series (third or fourth dose) should not be administered before age 24 weeks.

   Infants born to HBsAg-positive mothers should receive HepB and 0.5 mL of hepatitis B immune globulin (HBIG) at separate sites within 12 hours of birth. The second dose is recommended at age 1-2 months. The final dose in the immunization series should not be administered before age 24 weeks. These infants should be tested for HBsAg and antibody to HBsAg (anti-HBs) at age 9-15 months.

   Infants born to mothers whose HBsAg status is unknown should receive the first dose of the HepB series within 12 hours of birth. Maternal blood should be drawn as soon as possible to determine the mother's HBsAg status; if the HBsAg test is positive, the infant should receive HBIG as soon as possible (no later than age 1 week). The second dose is recommended at age 1-2 months. The last dose in the immunization series should not be administered before age 24 weeks.

2. **Diphtheria and tetanus toxoids and acellular pertussis (DTaP) vaccine.** The fourth dose of DTaP may be administered as early as age 12 months, provided 6 months have elapsed since the third dose and the child is unlikely to return at age 15-18 months. The final dose in the series should be given at age ≥4 years. **Tetanus and diphtheria toxoids (Td)**is recommended at age 11-12 years if at least 5 years have elapsed since the last dose of tetanus and diphtheria toxoid-containing vaccine. Subsequent routine Td boosters are recommended every 10 years.

3. **Haemophilus influenzae type b (Hib) conjugate vaccine.** Three Hib conjugate vaccines are licensed for infant use. If PRP-OMP (PedvaxHIB or ComVax [Merck]) is administered at ages 2 and 4 months, a dose at age 6 months is not required. DTaP/Hib combination products should not be used for primary immunization in infants at ages 2, 4 or 6 months but can be used as boosters after any Hib vaccine. The final dose in the series should be administered at age ≥12 months.

4. **Measles, mumps, and rubella vaccine (MMR).** The second dose of MMR is recommended routinely at age 4-6 years but may be administered during any visit, provided at least 4 weeks have elapsed since the first dose and both doses are administered beginning at or after age 12 months. Those who have not previously received the second dose should complete the schedule by age 11-12 years.

5. **Varicella vaccine.** Varicella vaccine is recommended at any visit at or after age 12 months for susceptible children (i.e., those who lack a reliable history of chickenpox). Susceptible persons age ≥13 years should receive 2 doses administered at least 4 weeks apart.

6. **Pneumococcal vaccine.** The heptavalent **pneumococcal conjugate vaccine (PCV)** is recommended for all children age 2-23 months and for certain children age 24-59 months. The final dose in the series should be given at age ≥12 months. **Pneumococcal polysaccharide vaccine (PPV)** is recommended in addition to PCV for certain high-risk groups. See *MMWR* 2000;49(RR-9):1-35.

7. **Influenza vaccine.** Influenza vaccine is recommended annually for children age ≥6 months with certain risk factors (including, but not limited to, asthma, cardiac disease, sickle cell disease, human immunodeficiency virus [HIV], and diabetes), health care workers, and other persons (including household members) in close contact with persons in groups at high risk (see *MMWR* 2004;53[RR-6]:1-40). In addition, healthy children age 6-23 months and close contacts of healthy children age 0-23 months are recommended to receive influenza vaccine because children in this age group are at substantially increased risk for influenza-related hospitalizations. For healthy persons age 5-49 years, the intranasally administered, live, attenuated influenza vaccine (LAIV) is an acceptable alternative to the intramuscular trivalent inactivated influenza vaccine (TIV). See *MMWR* 2004;53(RR-6):1-40. Children receiving TIV should be administered a dosage appropriate for their age (0.25 mL if age 6-35 months or 0.5 mL if age ≥3 years). Children age ≤8 years who are receiving influenza vaccine for the first time should receive 2 doses (separated by at least 4 weeks for TIV and at least 6 weeks for LAIV).

8. **Hepatitis A vaccine.** Hepatitis A vaccine is recommended for children and adolescents in selected states and regions and for certain high-risk groups; consult your local public health authority. Children and adolescents in these states, regions, and high-risk groups who have not been immunized against hepatitis A can begin the hepatitis A immunization series during any visit. The 2 doses in the series should be administered at least 6 months apart. See *MMWR* 1999;48(RR-12):1-37.

FIGURE 62-1 Recommended childhood and adolescent immunization schedule.

From Centers for Disease Control and Prevention, National Immunization Program. Available at http://www.cdc.gov/nip/recs/child-schedule.pdf

TABLE 62-2 IMPACT OF SELECTED DISEASES BEFORE IMMUNIZATION

Disease	Comments
Measles	• Before vaccinations, nearly everyone in the United States contracted measles (an estimated 3 to 4 million cases annually). • The average annual number of measles-related deaths was 450 (1953 to 1963). • A low rate of vaccination in preschool children in 1995 resulted in more than 55,000 cases, 11,000 hospitalizations, and 120 deaths. • The risk for measles in African American and Hispanic children was 8 to 10 times greater than in white children, because vaccination rates in African American and Hispanic children were lower.
H. influenzae type b (Hib) meningitis	• Before the release of this vaccine in December 1987, Hib was the most common cause of meningitis in infants and children in the United States. • Approximately 8000 new cases were seen annually (with 600 deaths), and many survivors were left with deafness, seizures, or mental retardation. • Since the release of the vaccine, the incidence of Hib meningitis has decreased 97% to 99% from previous reports.
Pertussis (whooping cough)	• Before this vaccine, 150,000 to 260,000 children had pertussis annually, and there were approximately 9000 deaths. • Pertussis is a serious illness; it can cause weeks of prolonged coughing and vomiting. Infants may contract pneumonia. Pertussis may also cause seizures, brain damage, and mental retardation. • The new acellular pertussis (DTaP) vaccine is safer than the older, whole-cell DTP vaccine; it has been available in the United States since 1991. • Countries have reported epidemics of pertussis that correspond to decreased immunization levels; for example, Japan's immunization dropped from 80% to 20% from 1974 to 1979, and in 1979 a pertussis epidemic resulted in 13,000 new cases and 41 deaths.
Rubella	• This is usually a mild disease in children and adults but is a serious problem in pregnant women during the first trimester. Teratogenic effects may occur in up to 90% of the exposed fetuses; that is, they may contract congenital rubella syndrome (CRS), which causes heart defects, cataracts, deafness, and mental retardation. • A rubella epidemic occurred during 1964 and 1965 (before rubella vaccinations were used regularly in the United States). Nearly 20,000 infants were born with CRS, 2100 died, and 11,250 miscarriages were reported. Of the 20,000 infants with CRS, 11,600 were born deaf, 3580 were blind, and 1800 were mentally retarded.

Data from Centers for Disease Control and Prevention. (2000). What would happen if we stopped vaccinations. Retrieved July 15, 2000, from http://www.cdc.gov/nip/publications/fs/gen/whatifstop.htm.

for developing the disease is imminent or increased, such as with traveling to foreign countries in which some diseases are endemic or indigenous to a geographic area or population. Required and recommended immunizations for foreign travel are constantly changing and are best obtained before travel from the local public health department or the National Center for Infectious Disease, CDC (www.cdc.gov/travel/), or, in Canada, the Travel Medicine Program (http://www.phac-aspc.gc.ca/tmp-pmv/index.html).

The client's tetanus immunization status must be assessed any time a traumatic wound (especially a puncture wound) is encountered. A booster dose of tetanus toxoid may be in order if the client has not been fully immunized within the past 10 years or if the wound is contaminated and an immunization is more than 5 years old. Tetanus and diphtheria toxoid is recommended for adults, because diphtheria protection is enhanced by this combination.

Most new parents today are too young to remember the fear engendered by the very mention of childhood illnesses a few decades ago. For example, measles, the most common

childhood disease, can cause pneumonia, encephalopathy, deafness, blindness, and seizures in 1 out of every 1000 children. If parents are not convinced, outbreaks of communicable diseases (e.g., poliomyelitis) may make the argument for us. Complacency about childhood illnesses and their current and potential threats must be shaken. The initial effects of childhood illnesses can be very serious, and more potential future hazards are currently being discovered (e.g., the possible association of mumps with eventual diabetes and of chickenpox with shingles).

A request for exemption from the immunizations required for school entry on medical grounds can be obtained from the child's physician. A model form for exemption on religious grounds can be obtained from the Christian Science Committee on Publications. However, it is *theoretically* possible that the right to exempt certain children could interfere with "herd immunity" by sustaining a continued pool of susceptible individuals, thereby maintaining a hazard that would be unacceptable to other parents, who might apply legal and other pressures.

TABLE 62-3 GUIDELINES FOR SPACING THE ADMINISTRATION OF LIVE AND KILLED ANTIGENS

Antigen Combination	Recommended Minimum Interval Between Doses
2 or more killed antigens	None. May be administered simultaneously or at any interval between doses.*
Killed and live antigens	None. May be administered simultaneously or at any interval between doses.†
2 or more live antigens	4-week minimum interval if not administered simultaneously.

From Centers for Disease Control and Prevention. (2005). Retrieved March 21, 2005, from http://www.cdc.gov/travel/vaccinations/recommendations.htm#spacing.

*If possible, vaccines associated with local or systemic side effects (e.g., cholera, parenteral typhoid, and plague vaccines) should be administered on separate occasions to avoid accentuated reactions.

†A cholera vaccine with yellow fever vaccine is the exception. If time permits, these antigens should not be administered simultaneously, and at least 3 weeks should elapse between the administration of the yellow fever vaccine and the cholera vaccine. If the vaccines must be administered simultaneously or within 3 weeks of each other, the antibody response may not be optimal.

Community health nurses, school nurses, teachers, local public health departments, the Department of Health and Human Services, and the WHO need to work together to share expertise in educating the public, in case finding and reporting, in screening, and in mass immunization programs.

✲ When are vaccines administered, and what is their optimal sequencing?

Immunization schedules are recommended for children and for adults by the CDC's National Immunization Program (see Figure 62-1).

When multiple doses of a particular immunization are recommended to achieve an adequate antibody response, the recommended time interval between doses should be followed. Although an interval that is longer than recommended is acceptable and does not require starting over, shorter intervals are not acceptable because the overall antibody response will be decreased, and some persons will experience an increased frequency in local or systemic adverse effects. Although live vaccines such as the yellow fever vaccines can be given at any time with an immune globulin, there is some evidence that high doses of immune globulin can inhibit the immune response to a measles vaccine for more than 3 months. There are instances in which an inactivated vaccine interferes with other killed or live antigens. Table 62-3

lists the recommended guidelines for spacing the administration of live and killed antigens and immune globulin.

✲ What special circumstances must be considered with vaccine use?

Issues related to vaccine use during pregnancy, breastfeeding, and use in premature infants may raise questions for health care providers and clients alike. Vaccinations during pregnancy depend on weighing the potential risk of the vaccine against the result of disease exposure. For example, tetanus and diphtheria toxoids are routinely used for susceptible pregnant women; hepatitis B vaccine, influenza, and pneumococcal vaccines are also recommended for pregnant women at risk for the infection or complications of the disease. The use of live measles, mumps, and rubella vaccine is contraindicated in pregnancy because of the potential for low-grade rubella infections, which can be highly teratogenic. There is no contraindication to breastfeeding and vaccinations. Premature infants should be vaccinated on the same chronologic age schedule as full-term infants and with the same recommended vaccine dose.

Contraindications to all vaccines include a history of anaphylaxis to the individual vaccine or a component of it, or the presence of moderate to severe illness with or without a fever. In general, immunocompromised individuals should not receive any live vaccines. Special exceptions for immunocompromised clients and specific recommendations for their household contacts are available (CDC, 2004a). (Table 62-4.)

✲ D.S., a 2-month-old baby boy, is brought to the clinic for a scheduled well-baby visit. D.S.'s parents ask about immunizations for their son. D.S.'s mother tested negative for HBsAg and D.S. received his first immunization with hepatitis B vaccine before he left the hospital after birth. At this visit, he will receive Hep B #2, DTaP, Hib, IPV, and PVC.

✲ What are the nursing management issues involved in the use of vaccines and toxoids for D.S.?

Assessment Assess D.S.'s age, current physical condition and general resistance to disease, history of exposure to infectious diseases (both past and potential), and previous immunizations. Providers are required to provide detailed information on the risks and benefits of immunization. Before immunization, obtain a signed consent form or a note indicating that the parents (or client) has read and understood the information regarding the specific immunization. Share printed information at this time to ensure that the parent/client is aware of the adverse effects and how to manage them. Assess D.S. for general contraindications to immunization:

- Current acute or severe febrile illness
- Immunosuppressive therapy in progress or an immunodeficient state
- Recent immune serum globulin (ISG), plasma, or blood transfusions

TABLE 62-4 CHECKLIST OF CONTRAINDICATIONS FOR VACCINE USE AS RECOMMENDED BY CENTERS FOR DISEASE CONTROL AND PREVENTION

Check For	Reason*
Anaphylactic allergies	Contraindicates some vaccines
Anaphylactic reaction to previous dose of any vaccine	Contraindicates that vaccine
Anthrax (prior infection)	Contraindicates anthrax vaccine
Antimicrobial therapy (current)	Precaution for several vaccines
Eczema or atopic dermatitis in client or household contact	Contraindicates vaccinia vaccine
Guillain-Barré syndrome, history of	Precaution for DTaP and influenza vaccines
Hematopoietic stem cell transplant	Contraindicates varicella vaccine, precaution for several other vaccines
HIV (in recipient)	Contraindication or precaution for several vaccines
Immune globulin (IG) administration, recent	Precaution for MMR and varicella vaccines
Illness (moderate to severe acute illness, fever, otitis, diarrhea, vomiting)	Deferral of vaccination until recovery may be prudent
Immunodeficiency:	
Family history	Precaution for varicella vaccine
In household contact	Contraindicates vaccinia and live flu vaccines
In recipient	Contraindication of precaution for several vaccines
Neurologic disorder	Precaution for DTaP
Pregnancy:	
In mother or household contact of recipient	Contraindicates vaccinia vaccine
In recipient	Contraindication or precaution for several vaccines
Reaction to previous vaccine dose	May be contraindication or precaution for that vaccine
Skin condition (acute, chronic or exfoliative)	Contraindication for vaccinia vaccine
Thrombocytopenic purpura (history)	Precaution for MMR vaccine

Data from Guide to Contraindications to Vaccines. (2003). Retrieved February 10, 2005, from http://www.cdc.gov/nip/recs/contraindications.htm#Check.
*Refer to http://www.cdc.gov/nip/recs/contraindications.htm#allergies for more specific updated information.

- Certain malignancies that leave the client susceptible to infection (e.g., leukemias, lymphomas)
- Simultaneous administration of another single live virus, unless proved safe
- Prior unusual or allergic reaction to the same vaccine or a similar vaccine
- Allergy to constituents in the vaccine, including thimerosal used as a preservative

Minor afebrile infections such as the common cold are not usually contraindications to immunization. Immunizations should not be delayed in a child with other minor illnesses (e.g., otitis media, diarrhea) with or without a low grade fever. A family history of seizures and allergies are not contraindications (Luedtke, Condren, & Haase, 2005). Assess clients (especially children) for immune status at routine intervals. High-risk groups include adolescents, new parents, individuals not vacci-

nated with the live measles vaccine, migrant workers, and recent immigrants. Older adults (especially those in nursing homes) and anyone with chronic health problems are at particular risk for respiratory infections and should be encouraged to obtain an annual influenza virus vaccination.

Individuals are also candidates for immunization if they have been exposed to or are at risk of exposure to one of the childhood diseases or serious communicable diseases or if they have incurred a traumatic wound.

Be aware that a history of hypersensitivity reactions to the biologic agent or to any contained constituents or preservatives is a contraindication to immunotherapy.

Always assess the client's allergy history carefully and test for hypersensitivity before administering animal sera. Keep epinephrine on hand to counter any potentially dangerous event (e.g., anaphylaxis).

Nursing Diagnosis While receiving immunotherapy, D.S. is at risk for the following selected nursing diagnoses/collaborative problems: impaired comfort (malaise, headache, rash, lymphadenopathy, and pain and tenderness at the injection site); ineffective thermoregulation (fever); and the potential complications of allergic reaction and encephalopathy.

Planning During immunotherapy, D.S.'s parents will:
- State the risks and benefits and complete any informed consents.
- Manage minimal discomfort as a result of the administration of a vaccine or toxoid.
- Return for completion of immunization series and boosters.
- State the adverse effects of the immunizing agent that are reportable and to whom to report them.

Implementation

Monitoring Because of the risk of anaphylaxis after any immunization, ask D.S.'s parents to keep the baby in the immediate area for up to half an hour for observation of any developing adverse reactions. Be alert for the early symptoms of such a reaction—hives, shock-like appearance, confusion, and hypotension.

Intervention Complete any informed consent documentation that may be required. Be aware that a crying, wriggling baby or child presents a challenging moving target for injection, and therefore D.S. must be restrained temporarily. This can often be accomplished just as effectively in the warmth and security of another's arms (D.S.'s parent's, if feasible) rather than on a hard table surface. For children old enough to understand, taking out the needle and syringe and explaining that "this may hurt for only a minute" *just* before the actual injection will lessen the fear of pain.

Record immunization dates and lot numbers at the time of administration, and give a copy to D.S.'s parents (or recipient) for permanent safekeeping. Explain that this record may be invaluable later, when these dates may be required on applications to school, summer camp, college, or visas for travel to other countries.

Almost all immunotherapy is parenteral and must be given by the specified route and with the specified diluent to avoid local reactions (especially when the intracutaneous route is used) or possible anaphylaxis. All needles should be changed after the vaccine is withdrawn from a multidose vial, if possible. Aspiration after insertion is, of course, also necessary to prevent the danger of depositing the dose into the bloodstream.

Immune antisera and globulin are administered IM unless otherwise noted. Passive immunization or immunoprophylaxis should always be administered as soon as possible after exposure to the agent.

Be aware that most products lose their potency at temperatures higher than 35.6°F to 46.4°F (2°C to 8°C). Therefore most immunization agents should be stored in a medical refrigerator and replaced immediately after use. They should not be stored near a heat source, on a windowsill, or on a refrigerator door shelf because of unpredictable temperatures.

Education Clarify perceptions and misconceptions concerning immunization. Discuss the relative safety and merits of immunization vs. the risks of the disease process itself (both short-range and long-range), and use statistics where appropriate. The correlation between vaccine use, thimerosal (a preservative historically used and remaining in some vaccinations) and autism is unfounded, despite widespread belief in many communities (Madsen et al., 2003; Smeeth et al., 2004). Tell the client and/or family that a repeat immunization is usually not contraindicated if records are unclear; the risk with the repeat immunization is usually minimal, and in this way future protection is ensured. Unimmunized parents should be identified and immunized.

Noncompletion of an immunization series may occasionally be prevented if vaccinees or their parents know that a prolonged period between phases of immunization makes no difference to eventual antibody levels as long as they have the entire series. Giving a copy of the immunization schedule to the client or family also enhances compliance with the immunization series.

Complete, written, and accurate documentation of immunizations remains problematic. The CDC provides vaccine management software (VAC MAN) used by a number of governmental vaccine programs, which assists in this documentation (http://www.cdc.gov/nip/vacman/about.htm). Many health care practice settings utilize other electronic information systems to assist with documentation of vaccine administration dates, doses, lot numbers, and client response. Unfortunately, whether electronic or not, this data may not always be readily accessible to health care providers, clients, or parents/guardians. It is crucial to teach parents/guardians or those vaccinated to keep careful written records for each vaccination, especially in view of the high mobility of today's population. Simple blank forms are available for this purpose and should be given to parents or the vaccinee with an explanation and advice to keep them updated and in a safe place (e.g., with health record files at home) and to bring them to each child's appointment.

Teach clients or their parents how to recognize and differentiate between anticipated side effects and serious adverse reactions. Acetaminophen may be taken for the aches, local pain and swelling, or mild temperature elevations that may occur within 24 hours. Recipients of immunotherapy should understand whom to contact if complications later occur.

Evaluation The expected outcome of immunotherapy associated with vaccines, toxoids, and immunoglobulins is that the client will receive immunity without experiencing adverse effects of the drug (e.g., rash, chills, GI disturbances, encephalopathy, anaphylactic response). The client (or caregivers) will effectively manage any local injection site tenderness and low-grade fever with acetaminophen and state adverse effects that are reportable to the health care provider.

• • •

Primary sources of information on immunization include the Public Health Service Advisory Committee on Immunization Practices (ACIP), which advises public health agencies; and the Committee on Control of Infectious Diseases (the Red Book Committee), which is drawn from the members of the American Academy of Pediatrics and advises the private health sector. The ACIP can be contacted through the CDC. Because the two groups maintain a slightly different perspective, minor inconsequential variations in recommendations may occasionally be noted. Other sources include local public health departments and printed package inserts included with the vaccine or serum. Biologic preparations and the accompanying inserts are regulated by the Bureau of Biologics of the FDA.

The state of the art of immunotherapy is in rapid flux. The only constant in immunization practice is change itself. To read, attend seminars, and consult with experts is to keep pace.

✳ What recent trends have been observed in vaccine development?

Research is continually evolving to expand the role of vaccines in preventing and/or treating disease. A vaccine against human papilloma virus (HPV) has demonstrated efficacy, and may prevent HPV infection and cervical cancer (Simon, 2005). A conjugate vaccine for meningococcal may reduce the risk for meningitis (Healy & Baker, 2005). Vaccines for malaria and herpes zoster are also on the horizon (Hampton, 2004; Oxman et al., 2005). For decades, attempts to develop a successful vaccine against HIV have been less than fruitful at prevention, and have been examined to evaluate whether they could alter the course of the disease by stimulating the immune system (Smith & Blower, 2004).

Interest in development of vaccines against potential bioterrorist agents has gained significant interest since the events of September 11, 2001. Vaccines against anthrax and small pox are available, but their routine use requires weighing risk and benefit (Karwa, Currie, & Kvetan, 2005). Smallpox vaccine, for example, has been associated with significant cardiovascular and noncardiac risk (CDC, 2004b; Talbot et al., 2004) and hampers willingness of candidates to receive it (Gershon, Gemson, Qureshi, & McCollum, 2004). (See the Pharmacologic Issues in an Age of Terrorism box below).

⣿ Pharmacologic Issues in an Age of Terrorism

Role of Vaccines and Antitoxins in Response to a Bioterrorism Threat

Vaccines and antitoxins may play an important role in responding to bioterrorist treats. Among the available vaccines and antitoxins which may be employed in preparing for bioterrorist threats are smallpox vaccine, botulinum toxoid, yellow fever vaccine, and anthrax vaccine. Vaccines for tularemia and other viral hemorrhagic fevers are under study.

Smallpox Vaccine

Smallpox infection is discussed in the Pharmacologic Issues in an Age of Terrorism box in Chapter 59 on pp. 1063 to 1064. The vaccine for smallpox is part of a national strategy to manage risk of widespread smallpox exposure. Variations of a vaccine for smallpox have been available since Jenner first studied vaccination in 1796. The current smallpox vaccine is a live vaccinia virus and poses potential risks with use.

Efficacy

The smallpox vaccine provides high levels of immunity for 3 to 5 years after an initial dose, with approximately 95% of those vaccinated being fully protected from smallpox. Administered within 3 days of exposure is believed to offer significant benefit and may prevent symptoms of smallpox infection. Dosing 4 to 7 days after exposure may also offer some benefit. Administering once symptoms appear probably offers little benefit.

Dosing

Smallpox vaccine is administered intradermally with a bifurcated (two-prong) needle that is impregnated with vaccine solution. The upper arm is the most common site of administration. Successful dosing produces a draining blister which produces a scab (see figure). The resultant scab typically falls away after 2 to 3 weeks. The inoculation site must be carefully covered because viral shedding may occur. Many cases of contact vaccinia, particularly in the ocular region, have occurred as a result of a poorly covered inoculation site. This may pose a greater risk for immunocompromised household contacts.

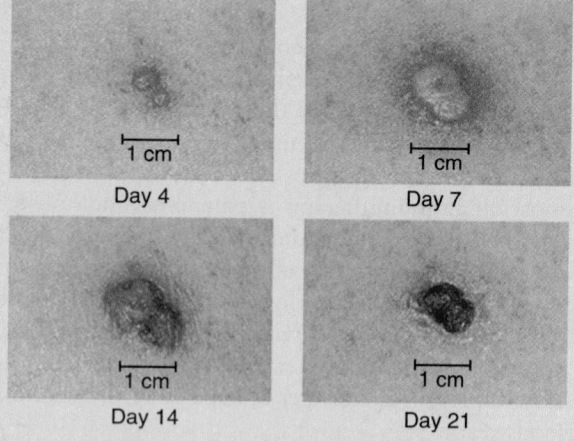

Primary Vaccination Site Reaction

Day 4   Day 7

Day 14   Day 21

From Centers for Disease Control and Prevention: Emergency Preparedness and Response. *Vaccine Overview*. Retrieved April 7, 2005, from http://www.bt.cdc.gov/images/VAXSIT5 A.jpg.

Data from Emergency Preparedness and Response: Centers for Disease Control and Prevention. Retrieved March 6, 2005, from http://www.bt.cdc.gov; http://www.cdc.gov/ncidod/dbmd/diseaseinfo/botulism.PDF; http://www.bt.cdc.gov/agent/anthrax/vaccination/index.asp and http://www.cdc.gov/mmwr/preview/mmwrhtml/rr4915 a1.htm.

Role of Vaccines and Antitoxins in Response to a Bioterrorism Threat—cont'd

Safety

Safety concerns regarding smallpox vaccination have surfaced with its use since the terrorist attack at the World Trade Center in New York on September 11, 2001. Local soreness and aches are common following vaccination. Specific concerns include a low but real risk for cardiovascular events including myocardial infarction, heart failure, cardiomyopathy, and stroke. Other serious risks include hypersensitivity reactions and erythema multiforme. Individuals with immune deficiencies or on immunosuppressive agents may pose a greater risk for adverse effects with this live vaccine. Risk is also greater for those younger than 1 year of age, women who are pregnant or breastfeeding, and those with high risk for cardiovascular events. In general, these individuals are not candidates for smallpox vaccine.

Given safety concerns, it is likely that smallpox vaccine will not be administered to the population at large unless the risk for infection is high. However, in a mass outbreak, or immediate postexposure, vaccine may be administered to most at risk individuals.

Availability

Smallpox vaccine is not available to the general public for regular use. The U.S. government has stockpiled adequate vaccine to allow for full vaccination of the general public in the event of a smallpox emergency. Further information on the U.S. government's response plan for smallpox vaccine can be found at http://www.bt.cdc.gov/agent/smallpox/response-plan/index.asp.

Botulinum Antitoxin (ABE) and Botulinum Toxoid (ABCDE)

Botulinum toxin is one of the most potent neurotoxins known. Risks and effects of botulinum toxin are discussed in the Pharmacologic Issues in an Age of Terrorism box on p. 1035 in Chapter 58.

Efficacy

Seven different neurotoxins have been identified, each with designation A through G. Botulinum antitoxin provides passive immunity against types A, B, and E, and is sometimes used postexposure. Immediate use after exposure improves health outcomes.

Botulinum toxoid is an investigational agent that stimulates active immunity against types A, B, C, D, and E. Its use is limited to laboratory workers who may come in contact with *Clostridium botulinum* cultures. Although data are limited, early treatment is expected to offer improved outcomes.

Safety

Safety data for both products are lacking. Botulinum antitoxin is derived from equine serum and hypersensitivity reactions are possible.

Availability

Both botulinum antitoxin and botulinum toxoid are available from the CDC. Botulinum toxoid is available on a limited basis from the CDC primarily for laboratory workers who are frequently exposed to *C. botulinum* cultures and is not currently recommended for other at risk individuals. Information on availability from the CDC can be found at: http://www.cdc.gov/ncidod/srp/drugs/formulary.html.

Yellow Fever Vaccine

Yellow fever vaccine offers protection against one of the causes of viral hemorrhagic fever (See the Pharmacologic Issues in an Age of Terrorism box on pp. 1063 to 1064 in Chapter 59). It is primarily indicated for individuals who plan to travel to endemic areas (e.g., Central and South America, Sub-Saharan Africa), or responders who may be at risk for exposure in a bioterrorist attack. Its role in postexposure circumstances is not clear.

Efficacy

Yellow fever vaccine provides active immunity against yellow fever.

Dosage

The adult dose is 0.5 mL administered subcutaneously. It is dosed 10 days to 10 years before anticipated exposure, with boosters obtained every 10 years. Yellow fever vaccine is very temperature sensitive and is inactivated at room temperature. Consult package insert data for storage and reconstitution information.

Safety

Yellow fever vaccine should not be used for individuals with impaired immune status, pregnant women, infants younger than 4 months of age, or individuals with hypersensitivity to eggs.

Anthrax Vaccine

The presentation and management of anthrax is discussed in the Pharmacologic Issues in an Age of Terrorism box on p. 1035 in Chapter 58. Anthrax vaccine has been formulated for limited use for individuals who work directly with the organism in the laboratory, those who work with imported animal hides or infected animal products, and military personnel deployed to areas with a high risk for exposure. A newer anthrax vaccine (recombinant protective antigen anthrax vaccine) is being produced and will be added to the U.S. Strategic National Stockpile.

Efficacy

Vaccination is primarily effective when given in advance of exposure, and immunity is short lived. Protection postexposure to anthrax is best achieved with antimicrobial therapy, including ciprofloxacin or doxycycline.

Dosing

A total of six subcutaneous injections are recommended for anthrax vaccine. Three subcutaneous injections are given 2 weeks apart, with the fourth, fifth, and sixth injection administered at 6, 12, and 18 months. Annual boosters are recommended after completing the series.

Safety

Mild local reactions are observed in about one third of those vaccinated. Systemic reactions have rarely been reported.

Refinement of existing vaccines to improve safety and efficacy is also an ongoing trend. The vaccine against rotavirus infection, a sometimes life-threatening gastroenteritis with dehydration, was associated with intussusception and removed from the North American Market nine months after release in 1998. Alternatives to avoid toxicity are under study (Bines, 2005). Continuous evaluation of influenza and related avian strains are made by a number of researchers in developing revised formulations of influenzae vaccine each year (Hien, de Jong, & Farrar, 2004).

The development of vaccines to stimulate the immune system for altering health status or treating noninfectious diseases is also under study. Potential areas of study include contraception, the prevention or treatment of diabetes mellitus, substance abuse, dental caries, and cancer (Plotkin, 2005).

Summary

Immunization is available for a number of diseases whose prevalence has abruptly declined because of the availability of vaccines and sera; such diseases include measles, polio, rubella, mumps, diphtheria, and tetanus. Smallpox has been publicly eradicated because of a WHO campaign of near-universal vaccination, although the threat of bioterrorism has resurrected interest in smallpox vaccination. Vaccines are also available for yellow fever, hepatitis B, influenza, rabies, cholera, typhoid, plague, and other diseases. Although such preparations are available, and more are in the pipeline, nurses must still educate the public to minimize complacency regarding the diseases for which they provide protection and to promote immunization.

(✳) Critical Thinking Questions

- An adolescent mother brings her infant to the clinic for the first well-baby checkup at 6 weeks. What would you include when teaching her about the infant's immunizations?

- As an adult and as a nursing student, what immunizations should you have and why?

Bibliography

Anderson, D.M. (2002). *Mosby's medical, nursing, & allied health dictionary* (6th ed.). St. Louis: Mosby.

Bertino, Jr., J.S., & Hayney, M.S. (2002). Vaccines, toxoids, and other immunobiologics. In J.T. DiPiro, R.L. Talbert, G.C. Yee, G.R.Matzke, B.G. Wells & L.M. Posey. (Eds.), *Pharmacotherapy: A pathophysiologic* approach (3rd ed.). New York: McGraw Hill.

Bines, J.E. (2005). Rotavirus vaccines and intussusception risk. *Current Opinion in Gastroenterology, 21*(1), 20-25.

Centers for Disease Control and Prevention (2004a). Recommended childhood and adolescent immunization schedule, 2005. Retrieved June 20, 2005, from http://www.cdc.gov.

Centers for Disease Control and Prevention. (2004b). Update: adverse events following civilian smallpox vaccination—United States 2003. *Morbidity and Mortality Weekly Report, 53*, 106.

de Jong, M.D., Bach, V.C., Phan, T.Q., Vo, M.H., Tran, T.T., Nguyen, B.H., et al. (2005). Fatal avian influenza A (H5N1) in a child presenting with diarrhea followed by coma. *New England Journal of Medicine, 352*, 686-691.

Drug facts and comparisons (57th ed.). (2004). St. Louis: Facts and Comparisons.

Fireman, B., Black, S.B., Shinefield, H.R., Lee, J., Lewis, E., & Ray, P. (2003). Impact of the pneumococcal conjugate vaccine on otitis media. *The Pediatric Infectious Disease Journal, 22*, 10-16.

Gershon, R.R., Gemson, D.H., Qureshi, K., & McCollum, M.C. (2004). Terrorism Preparedness Training for Occupational Health Professionals. *Journal of Occupational & Environmental Medicine, 46*(12), 1204-1209.

Hampton, T. (2004). Malaria vaccine shows promise. *Journal of the American Medical Association, 292*(22), 2703-2704.

Healy, C.M., & Baker, C.J. (2005). The Future of meningococcal vaccines. *Pediatric Infectious Disease Journal, 24*(2), 175-176.

Hien, T.T., de Jong, M., & Farrar, J. (2004). Avian influenza - A challenge to global health care structures. *New England Journal of Medicine, 351*(23), 2363-2365.

Jackson, L.A., Neuzil, K.M., Yu, O., Benson, P., Barlow, W.E., & Adams, A.L., et al. (2003). Vaccine safety datalink. Effectiveness of pneumococcal polysaccharide vaccine in older adults. *New England Journal of Medicine, 348*, 1747-55.

Jefferson, T., Smith, S., Demicheli, V., Harnden, A., Rivetti, A., Di Pietrontonj, C. (2005). Assessment of the efficacy and effectiveness of influenza vaccines in healthy children: Systematic review. *Lancet, 365*, 773-780.

Jumaan, A.O., Yu, O., Jackson, L.A., Bohlke, K., Galil, K., Seward, J.F. (2005). Incidence of herpes zoster before and after varicella vaccination-associated decreases in the incidence of varicella, 1992-2002. *Journal of Infectious Disease, 191, 2002-2007.*

𝑒-LEARNING SUPPLEMENTS

Student CD-ROM
- Final Exam questions
- NCLEX® Examination review questions
- Pharmacology animations
- Printable chapter summary

Evolve Website (http://evolve.elsevier.com/mckenry)
- Case study on serums, vaccines, and other immunizing agents
- Content updates, including information on new drugs

- WebLinks corresponding to this chapter
- Answers to the critical thinking questions in this chapter
- *Elsevier ePharmacology Update* newsletter
- Mosby's Drug Consult Internet Edition
- Supplemental and reference information

Karwa, M., Currie, B., & Kvetan, V. (2005). Bioterrorism: Preparing for the impossible or the improbable. *Critical Care Medicine,* *33*(1) Supplement, S75-S95.

Krensky, A.M., Strom, T.B., & Bluestone, J.A. (2001). Immunomodulators: Immunosuppressive agents, tolerogens, and immunostimulants. In Hardman, J.G. & Limbird, L.E. (Eds.), *Goodman & Gilman's The pharmacological basis of therapeutics* (10th ed.). New York: McGraw-Hill.

Lacy, C.F., Armstrong, L.L., Goldman, M.P., & Lance, L.L. (2004). *Lexi-Comp's Drug Information Handbook,* (12th ed). Hudson, Ohio: Lexi-Comp.

Luedtke, S., Condren, M., & Haase, M. (2005). Pediatric immunizations. In M.A. Koda-Kimble, L.Y. Young, W.A. Kradjan, B.J. Guglielmo, B.K. Alldredge, & R.L. Corelli (Eds.), *Applied therapeutics: The clinical use of drugs.* (8th ed.) Philadelphia: Lippincott, Williams & Wilkins.

Madsen, K.M., Lauritsen, M.B., Pedersen, C.B., Thorsen, P., Plesner, A.M., & Andersen, P.H., et al. (2003). Thimerosal and the occurrence of autism: Negative ecological evidence from Danish population-based data. *Pediatrics, 112,* 604-606.

McCormack, J.P., & Brown, G. (2005). Traumatic skin and soft tissue infections. In M.A. Koda-Kimble, L.Y. Young, W.A. Kradjan, B.J. Guglielmo, B.K. Alldredge, & R.L. Corelli (Eds.), *Applied therapeutics: The clinical use of drugs.* (8th ed.) Philadelphia: Lippincott, Williams & Wilkins.

Mosby's drug consult (15th ed.). (2005). St. Louis: Mosby.

Munoz, F.M., Greisinger, A.J., Wehmanen, O.A., Mouzoon, M.E., Hoyle, J.C., Smith, F.A., et al. (2005). Safety of influenza vaccination during pregnancy. *American Journal of Obstetrics and Gynecology, 192,* 1098-1106.

Musher, D.M., Ceasar, H., Kojic, E.M., Musher, B.L., Gathe, J.C., Jr., Romero-Steiner, S., White, A.C., Jr. (2005) Administration of protein-conjugate pneumococcal vaccine to patients who have invasive disease after splenectomy despite their having received 23-valent pneumococcal polysaccharide vaccine. *Journal of Infectious Disease, 191,* 1063-1067.

Nguyen, H.Q., Jumaan, A.O., Seward, J.F. (2005). Decline in mortality rate due to varicella after implementation of varicella vaccination in the United States. *New England Journal of Medicine, 352,* 450-458.

Oxman, M.N., Levin, M.J., Johnson, G.R., Schmader, K.E., Straus, S.E., Gelb, L.D., et al. (2005). A vaccine to prevent herpes zoster and postherpetic neuralgia in older adults. *New England Journal of Medicine, 352,* 2271-2284.

Plotkin, S.A. (2005). Six revolutions in vaccinology. *Pediatric Infectious Disease Journal, 24*(1), 1-9.

Simon, P. (2005). Progress towards a vaccine for cervical cancer. *Current Opinion in Obstetrics & Gynecology, 17*(1), 65-70.

Skowronski, D.M., Strauss, B., De Serres, G., MacDonald, D., Marion, S.A., & Naus, M., et al. (2003). Oculo-respiratory syndrome: A new influenza vaccine-associated adverse event? *Clinical Infectious Diseases, 36,* 705-713.

Smeeth, L., Cook, C., Fombonne, E., Heavey, L., Rodrigues, L.C., & Smith, P.G., et al. (2004). MMR vaccination and pervasive developmental disorders: A case-control study. *Lancet, 364,* 963-969.

Smith, R., & Blower, S.M. (2004). Could disease-modifying HIV vaccines cause population-level perversity? *The Lancet Infectious Diseases, 4,* 636–639.

Stephens, D.S., Zughaier, S.M., Whitney, C.G., Baughman, W.S., Barker, L., Gay, K. (2005). Incidence of macrolide resistance in *Streptococcus pneumoniae* after introduction of the pneumococcal conjugate vaccine: Population-based assessment. *Lancet, 365,* 855-863.

Talbot, T.R., Stapleton, J.T., Brady, R.C., Winokur, P.L., Bernstein, D.I., & Germanson, T., et al. (2004). Vaccination success rate and reaction profile with diluted and undiluted smallpox vaccine: A randomized controlled trial. *Journal of the American Medical Association, 292*(10), 1205-1212.

Ungchusak, K., Auewarakul, P. Dowell, S.F., Kitphati, R., Auwanit, W., Puthavathana, P. (2005). Probable person-to-person transmission of avian influenza A (H5N1). *New England Journal of Medicine, 352,* 333-340.

USP DI: Drug information for the health care professional (25th ed.). (2005). Greenwood Village, CO: MICROMEDEX Thomson Healthcare.

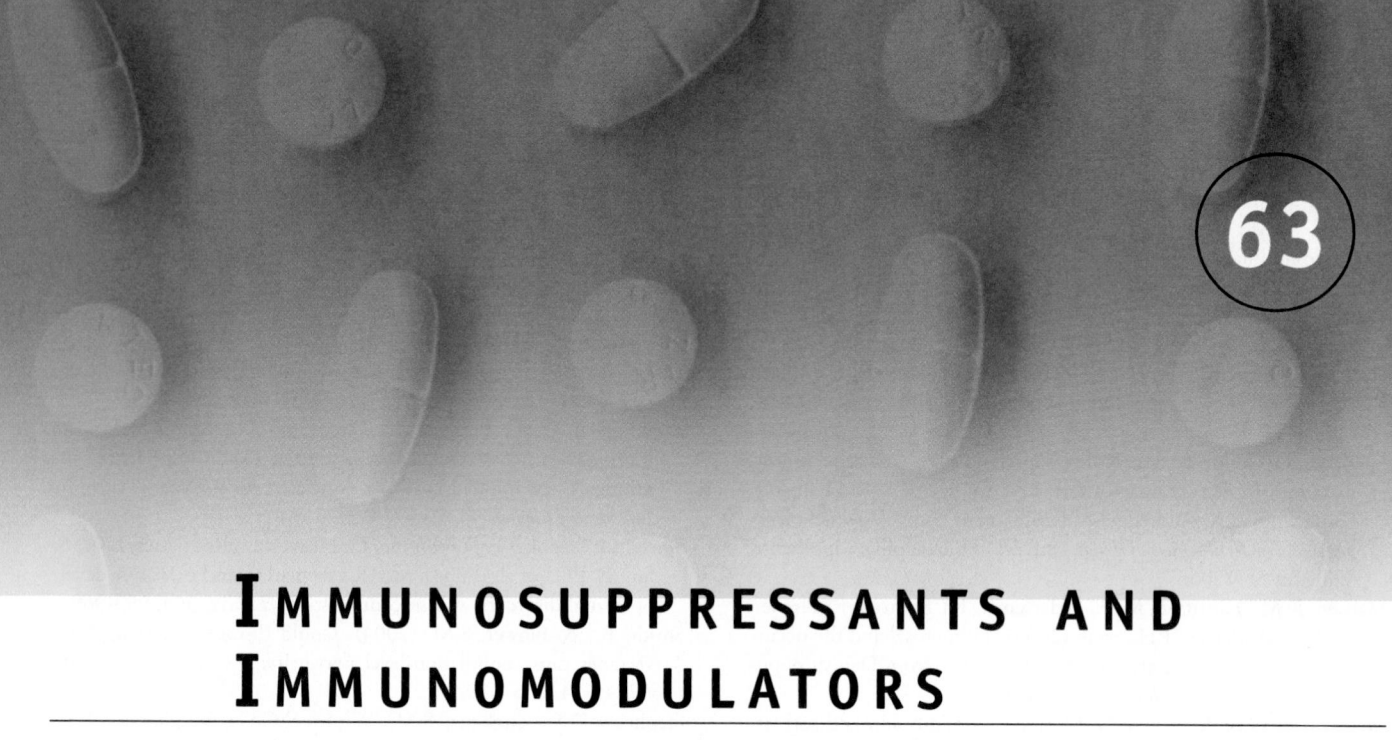

IMMUNOSUPPRESSANTS AND IMMUNOMODULATORS

CHAPTER FOCUS

As client acuity levels increase and treatments become more complex, nurses are increasingly aware of the impact of the immune system on the treatment regimens of clients. **Immunomodulating agents** affect the immune system. Because nurses administer treatments that decrease immunity (immunosuppressants) or enhance immune function (immunoglobulins, interferons), they need to maintain a working understanding of the immune system, how it relates to the clinical presentation of clients, and the agents that affect it.

LEARNING OBJECTIVES

- Identify four factors relating to the immune system that can lead to an immunocompromised state.
- Describe the general nursing management of the immunosuppressed client.
- Compare and contrast the nursing management of clients receiving azathioprine, basiliximab, cyclosporine, daclizumab, muromonab-CD3, mycophenolate mofetil, and tacrolimus.
- Implement the nursing management of clients receiving immunomodulators.

▲ **KEY TERMS**

immunocompromised state, p. 1151
immunomodulating agents, p. 1150
immunosuppressant agents, p. 1151
immunosuppression, p. 1150

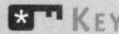 **KEY DRUGS**

cyclosporine, p. 1153
immune globulin, p. 1159

✳ **F.K. is a 43-year-old female with end-stage renal disease who is scheduled for a kidney transplant over the next 6 months. She understands that she will be required to take immunosuppressant drugs to help prevent organ rejection, but is concerned about the effects, which may decrease her ability to fight infection.**

✳ **What is immunosuppression?**

Immunosuppression is a state of reduced T-cell and/or B-cell function and may be related to disease or drugs. Im-

munodeficiency or immunosuppression may occur from a genetic or an acquired disorder of the immune system. Although genetic disorders such as agammaglobulinemia or severe combined immune deficiency syndrome (SCIDS) are usually diagnosed shortly after birth, acquired disorders may occur at any time throughout life. Acquired immunodeficiency may be induced by a variety of drugs, such as chemotherapeutic and immunosuppressant agents or radiation therapy, or through viral infections such as acquired immunodeficiency syndrome (AIDS). Because AIDS often has devastating complications, much research interest has been directed toward the development of immunomodulating or immunostimulating medications.

Although immunosuppression contributes to morbidity in many conditions, it can be helpful in cases in which an overactive immune response is problematic. **Immunosuppressant agents,** drugs that decrease or prevent an immune response, are sometimes used in the treatment of Crohn's disease, rheumatoid arthritis (RA), and psoriasis, but they are most commonly used to prevent or treat organ rejection in a transplant recipient.

The body activates an immune response by releasing macrophages to phagocytize and process foreign substances. Additionally, a number of cytokines are involved in the immune response (see Table 61-1). Among the cytokines involved is interleukin-1 (IL-1), which activates helper T cells containing a surface receptor or CD3. The activated T cell stimulates the production of killer or cytotoxic T lymphocytes and B lymphocytes, in part by producing interleukin-2 (IL-2). T cells are necessary for cellular immunity (attacking the foreign substance directly and with released toxic substances), and B lymphocytes are responsible for humoral immunity or the production of antibodies. Figure 63-1 notes the primary sites of action of the immunosuppressant agents.

An **immunocompromised state** may result from one or more of the following: (1) inhibition of granulocyte formation leading to severe neutropenia; (2) impairment of synthesis and antibody production; (3) loss of mucocutaneous barriers that permit bacteria or microorganisms access to internal organs, which may occur in a variety of therapeutic situations, such as postinsertion of medical devices (central venous catheters, Foley catheters, endotracheal tubes) or after chemotherapy; and (4) impairment of cellular immunity such as macrophages and T-cell lymphocytes (usually seen in clients receiving immunosuppressants such as corticosteroids or cyclosporine, clients with certain types of cancer [Hodgkin's lymphoma], or organ transplant recipients).

In the majority of clients, combinations of these defects are common because several immune functions may be affected at the same time. For example, chronic therapy with antineoplastic medications will affect granulocytes and cellular immunity. Chemotherapy may result in the loss of mucocutaneous barriers or the development of mucositis and ulcers in the mouth and gastrointestinal (GI) tract. These individuals are at greater risk for developing bacterial, fungal, or viral infections. Chapters 56 and 59 discuss concepts related to the management of clients with immunocompromised states. This chapter reviews some of the primary agents that suppress, modify, or stimulate the human immune system.

✳ **What are the nursing management issues for F.K. and other clients receiving immunosuppressant therapy?** The care of F.K., a client with secondary immunodeficiency (immunosuppression caused by the therapeutic regimen), focuses on immunotherapy and on treatment of the underlying condition.

Assessment Assess F.K. for her understanding of the condition and her feelings about the illness. In assisting F.K.

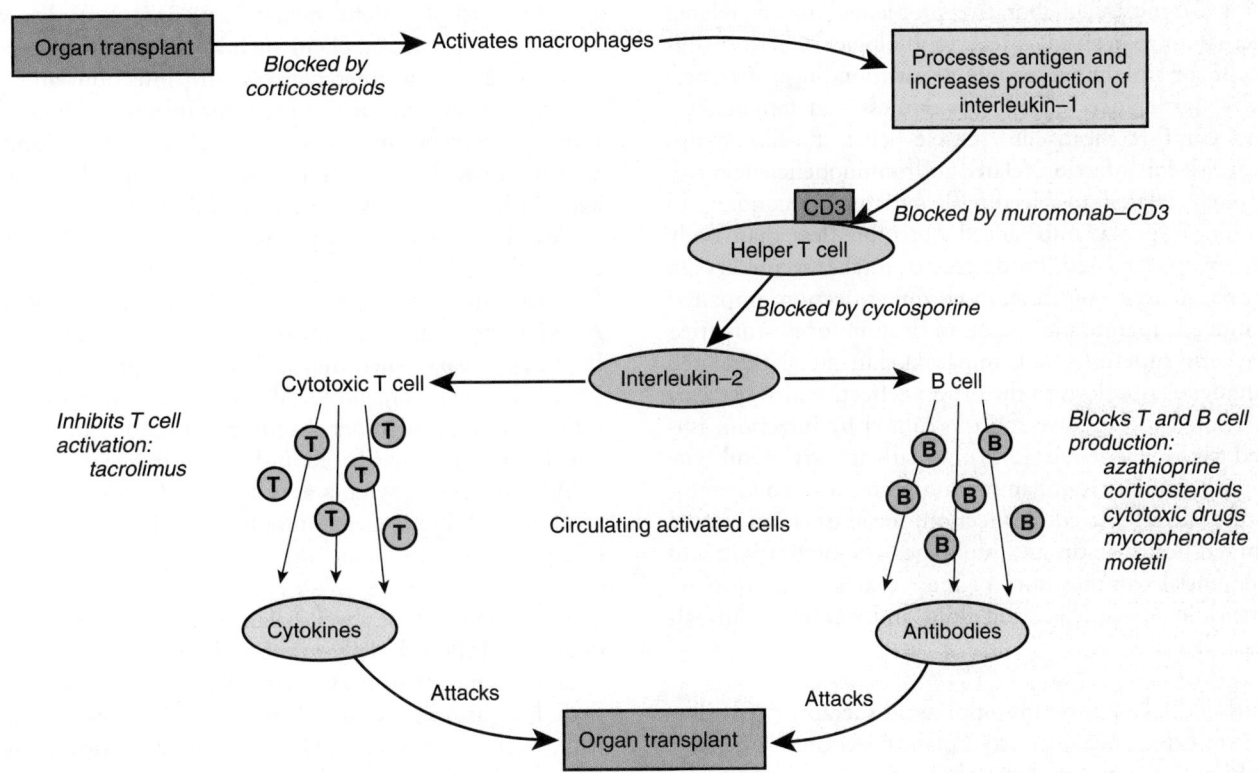

FIGURE 63-1 Sites of action for immunosuppressive agents.

with the effective management of her therapeutic regimen, the availability of a support system is a primary consideration.

Before administering an immunosuppressant drug, determine that F.K. does not have or has not recently had or been exposed to either chickenpox, herpes zoster, tuberculosis, or other infection, because there is the risk for the occurrence of severe generalized disease when an immunosuppressant is administered. Determine also whether F.K. has a current malignancy, history of malignancy, or premalignant skin lesions because there is an increased susceptibility to malignancies with immunosuppression.

Assess nutritional status and F.K.'s likes and dislikes so that nutritional counseling will be effective; these clients usually have had some weight loss or require a modified diet. Determine level of comfort regarding activity tolerance and participation in therapies.

If F.K. is taking other immunosuppressant drugs, the additive effects will be greater, requiring closer monitoring for nontherapeutic effects. There is also increased risk of renal or hepatic toxicity if she is taking other renal or hepatotoxic medications.

A full health examination will provide a baseline for monitoring clinical issues once therapy has begun. Renal (blood urea nitrogen [BUN] and serum creatinine) and hepatic (aspartate aminotransferase [AST] and alanine aminotransferase [ALT]) impairment studies will determine if dosage adjustments are required. A complete blood count (CBC) and platelet count are required for baseline.

Nursing Diagnosis The administration of immunosuppressive agents will increase F.K.'s risk for the following nursing diagnoses/collaborative problems: anxiety related to actual or perceived threat to biologic integrity, self-concept, or unfamiliar people or surroundings; diarrhea; activity intolerance related to weakness and fatigue; impaired comfort (headache, muscle aches, flu-like symptoms); risk for infection related to immunodeficiency; risk for injury related to bleeding/hemorrhage secondary to thrombocytopenia; imbalanced nutrition (less than body requirements) related to decreased intake secondary to anorexia, nausea, vomiting, or chronic infection; impaired oral mucous membrane related to drug-induced stomatitis or mycotic superinfection; impaired skin integrity related to cutaneous reactions to the drug; ineffective airway clearance related to excessive sputum caused by infection; impaired gas exchange related to alveolar-capillary membrane changes secondary to inflammation; imbalanced body temperature (fever) related to infection; social isolation related to altered health status and prolonged hospitalization; and the potential complications of renal toxicity, hepatotoxicity, neurologic sequelae, and fluid and electrolyte imbalances.

Planning During immunosuppressant therapy, F.K. will:
- Not experience organ transplant rejection.
- Experience minimal complications related to her drug therapy.

- Effectively manage her therapeutic regimen, including drug compliance and use of supportive therapies.
- Collaborate with her health care providers including reporting adverse effects appropriately and maintaining visits for monitoring and continued treatment.

Implementation

Monitoring Assess for symptoms of opportunistic infections, such as night sweats, fever, fatigue, involuntary weight loss, persistent diarrhea, headache, persistent cough, white patches on the tongue and oral mucosa (thrush), and the presence of green or yellow sputum. Monitor F.K.'s temperature and the results of any cultures at frequent intervals. Auscultate the lungs for crackles, consolidation, and pleural friction rub. Monitor pulse oximetry and the CBC. White blood cell (WBC) counts indicate the effectiveness of the drug; drug dosage is usually titrated according to leukocyte and platelet counts. Monitor renal and hepatic function tests.

Assess nutritional status daily; note weight, fluid intake and output, caloric intake, hematocrit, hemoglobin, and serum protein and albumin values. Monitor F.K. for dehydration (decreased urine output, increased specific gravity, poor skin turgor, confusion). Assess stool, urine, emesis, and secretions for the presence of occult blood. Assess and document skin for redness and purulent drainage, and mucous membrane integrity for redness, creamy white patches, and a black furry tongue. Monitor skin color and capillary refill. Assess F.K.'s tolerance to activity by assessing blood pressure, respiratory rate, and pulse rate before and immediately after activity. Monitor her for verbal or nonverbal indications of anxiety and social isolation.

Intervention Careful medical asepsis is a priority with an immunosuppressed client such as F.K. Thorough handwashing, avoiding other persons with infection, and promoting her own resources to prevent infection are essential nursing interventions. Provide meticulous mouth, skin, and perianal care. Proper mouth care with a topical antifungal agent will help to prevent oral candidiasis.

Avoid injections when possible; if necessary, cleanse the skin with povidone-iodine and allow to dry for 30 seconds. Clean all cuts and scrapes immediately with antiseptic soap. Avoid unnecessary and invasive procedures (e.g., biopsy, barium enemas); when they are necessary, prophylactic antibiotic coverage is required. Also avoid having irrigating solutions, vases, and other standing collections of water in which organisms may breed in the immediate environment.

Administer antipyretics as ordered and monitor F.K.'s response. In children, acetaminophen should be used instead of aspirin.

Education Advise a well-balanced diet and a fluid intake of at least 1500 mL daily to minimize the risk of tissue dehydration and of urinary tract infection (UTI) associated with low urinary output. Instruct F.K. to avoid trauma (e.g., breaks in the skin) and to seek medical treatment for wounds that do not heal quickly. Encourage meticulous oral hygiene, including the cautious use of toothbrushes, dental floss, and toothpicks, and regular dental care to minimize gingival inflammation and to detect early any altered oral mucous membranes. Promote pulmonary hygiene by encouraging F.K. to perform frequent breathing or incentive spirometry exercises. Encourage ambulation; if she is unable to ambulate, reposition her at frequent intervals. To minimize the risk of GI bleeding, she should avoid ingestion of alcohol, aspirin, and other NSAIDs.

Instruct F.K. to report any signs and symptoms of infection (sore throat, malaise, headache, fever, dysuria, urinary frequency), bleeding gums, bruising, or signs and symptoms of hepatic dysfunction (abdominal pain, jaundice, pruritus, clay-colored stools). Advise her to consult with the prescriber before taking any over-the-counter (OTC) medications (including aspirin) or receiving any vaccinations while taking immunosuppressant medications. Do not give live viral vaccines to F.K., and no one in her household should receive a nasal influenza vaccine. Reinforce the importance of keeping appointments with the health care provider for follow-up care and laboratory examinations.

Teach F.K. and her family to monitor her blood pressure at home. Instruct her to report any significant changes in blood pressure, hematuria, cloudy urine, decreased urinary output, sudden weight gain, edema of the face or ankles, headache, or unusual fatigue.

Caution F.K. that raw oysters or other shellfish may contain microbes that can cause serious illness. Even though such seafood comes from a good restaurant or "clean" water, there is the possibility that it may be contaminated. Although eating this seafood is not risky for most healthy individuals, clients with immunosuppression are at risk for serious disease.

Instruct F.K. to take her drugs at the same time each day and as directed, emphasizing the need for life-long therapy to prevent rejection. Inform her of symptoms of organ rejection and the need to seek medical attention at once if they occur. Reinforce the importance of keeping appointments for laboratory work and follow-up care. Advise her of the risks of taking immunosuppressant drugs during pregnancy, and instruct her about contraception as needed.

Because F.K. will be taking the immunosuppressant to prevent transplant rejection, emphasize the importance of life-long therapy.

Evaluation The expected outcome of F.K.'s immunosuppression therapy is that she will not experience rejection of the transplanted tissue, the presence of infection, or impaired skin integrity. If she experiences adverse effects, they will be minimal and she will notify the prescriber, if fever, sore throat, or fatigue occurs. F.K. will also be able to describe methods of preventing infection, the need to maintain optimal nutrition, and other issues for effective management of her therapeutic regimen.

✪ What agents are used in transplant medicine to suppress the immune system?

The primary immunosuppressant drugs used to prevent transplant organ rejection include azathioprine (Imuran),

basiliximab (Simulect), cyclosporine (Neoral, Sandimmune), daclizumab (Zenapax), muromonab-CD3 (Orthoclone OKT3), mycophenolate mofetil (CellCept), sirolimus (Rapamune), and tacrolimus (FK 506, Prograf). Cyclosporine is considered the prototype drug for this class. Use of corticosteroids and thymoglobulin (an immunoglobulin used in transplant medicine) may also be indicated.

✱▢ cyclosporine [**sye** klow spor een]
(Neoral, Sandimmune)

Cyclosporine inhibits the formation and release of IL-2, the substance necessary to induce the response of cytotoxic T lymphocytes to an antigenic challenge. It does not cause significant myelosuppression or bone marrow suppression.

Indications

Cyclosporine is a potent immunosuppressant used to prevent organ transplant rejection (renal, hepatic, or cardiac allografts). It is usually administered in combination with corticosteroids. It is also used to treat advanced autoimmune diseases unresponsive to alternate therapies, including RA and psoriasis. An ophthalmic preparation (Restasis) is used topically to increase tear production due to specific ocular inflammatory states.

Pharmacokinetics/Dosing

Cyclosporine is available in oral and parenteral dosage forms. Orally, its bioavailability is variable (approximately 30%) and is based on the specific oral dosage formulation and brand used. Bioavailability may improve with increasing dosages and chronic administration. Absorption may decrease after a liver transplant or in clients with liver impairment or GI dysfunction (e.g., diarrhea or vomiting). It has a half-life of approximately 7 hours in children and 19 hours in adults; orally it reaches peak serum levels in 3.5 hours. It is metabolized extensively in the liver by cytochrome P450 3 A4 with some genetic differences in metabolic rates noted (see the Special Considerations for Pharmacogenetics box on p. 1154). It is excreted primary in the bile and feces.

The oral dosage for adults and children varies based on dose form and indication. Children may need higher or more frequent dosing because they seem to metabolize this drug rapidly. Refer to package insert for appropriate dosage guidelines based on indication and drug formulation.

Because of variability in drug absorption and metabolism, and the impact of concurrent drug therapy on cyclosporine pharmacokinetics, drug levels are routinely used to evaluate the effective dose of cyclosporine. When used for organ transplant management, subtherapeutic levels greatly increase the risk for organ rejection, whereas elevated drug levels are associated with nephrotoxicity. The therapeutic range for cyclosporine is dependent on organ transplant and laboratory variation, and is often between 100 and 400 ng/mL. Most often a trough level (lowest expected level of the day) is used and it obtained 12 hours after the prior dose. Refer to information provided by the laboratory in which the specimen was analyzed for more detailed information.

Adverse Effects

The adverse effects of cyclosporine are dose related and include nausea, vomiting, leg cramps, acne or oily skin, hirsutism, and tremors. Adverse effects include nephrotoxicity, gingival hyperplasia (bleeding, swollen gums), and severe hypertension; the latter is usually associated with 25 to 50 mg/kg doses of cyclosporine. Lymphomas and other lymphoproliferative-type disorders have been reported; some regress when immunosuppression is discontinued (*USP DI*, 2005). Gingival hyperplasia, a common problem with the use of this drug, is generally reversible approximately 6 months after discontinuing cyclosporine administered for nontransplant purposes.

Drug Interactions

Cyclosporine drug interactions are significant and require careful monitoring to assure client safety. Two areas of concern are drugs

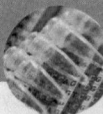

Special Considerations for Pharmacogenetics | IMMUNOSUPPRESSIVE THERAPY

PHARMACODYNAMICS

The very basis for organ rejection is related to genetics. Matches for transplanted organs are based on the degree of genetic similarity of the transplant organ to the recipient, with fewer rejection reactions observed when this match is close (or in the case of donation from an identical twin, a complete match). For most immunosuppressive drugs, therapeutic and toxic responses in organ transplantation are highly dependent on drug levels. As such, pharmacokinetic variables have been better studied.

PHARMACOKINETICS

A genetic explanation for variation in azathioprine levels has been well established since the 1980s. The enzyme responsible its metabolism (thiopurine methyltransferase) is highly influenced by genetics (Anglicheau, Legendre, & Thervet, 2004; von Ahsen, Oellerich, & Armstrong, 2004).Cyclosporine is significantly metabolized by P450 3 A4, an enzyme system that is known to be influenced by genetics. Reports differ on whether there is a strong correlation with pharmacokinetics of cyclosporine and genetically determined P450 3 A4 activity. One analysis correlates differences in kinetics to genetics with differences in metabolism noted with African Americans compared to those of Northern European descent (Min, Ellingrod,

Marsh, & McLeod, 2004). Other analysis has noted no significant correlation between genetic markers for 3 A4 and cyclosporine metabolism (Buchler & Johnston, 2005; Kreutz et al., 2004). Tacrolimus levels are highly correlated with the genetically determined availability of P450 3 A isoenzymes (MacPhee et al., 2002; Goto et al, 2004). Genetic testing will likely play some role in predicting azathioprine and tacrolimus dosing in the future (van Gelder, Hesselink, van Hest, Mathot, & van Schaik, 2004), but the role of genetic testing in assisting clinicians with cyclosporine dosing may be less straightforward (Haufroid et al., 2004).

ADVERSE EFFECTS

Adverse effects of azathioprine are correlated with drug levels, which are highly influenced by genetics (see the previous section). Similar observations can be made for tacrolimus, and to a lesser extent, cyclosporine. Genetic markers specific for predicting adverse effects per se, however, have yet to be identified (Gearry, Roberts, Barclay, & Kennedy, 2004). The risk for hepatic and gastrointestinal toxicity to mycophenolate may be higher is some individuals with variation in the gene HNF4 (McCaughan, 2004), although the clinical importance of this finding has yet to be determined.

---

that affect cyclosporine levels by interfering with cytochrome P450 3 A4 activity or otherwise affect cyclosporine pharmacokinetics, and agents that may increase the risk for toxicity to the kidney.

Drugs that increase cyclosporine levels include allopurinol, metoclopramide, and a host of drugs that interfere with 3 A4 activity, including amiodarone, cimetidine, macrolide antimicrobials, calcium channel blockers, the HMG CoA reductase inhibitors ("statins"), azole antifungals, antidepressants, and drugs used to treat HIV. Grapefruit juice also is noted to decrease intestinal metabolism and therefore increase levels of cyclosporine. Alternately, many antiepileptic drugs, isoniazid, rifampin, and rifabutin increase metabolism and therefore decrease levels of cyclosporine.

Concurrent drugs that may increase the risk for renal toxicity include aminoglycosides, amphotericin B, acyclovir, nonsteroidal antiinflammatory agents (NSAIDs), and tacrolimus. Because other drugs also interact with cyclosporine, careful assessment and referral to the package insert is warranted.

Nursing Management

The nursing management of cyclosporine is the same as the nursing management of an immunosuppressant in the case of F.K. discussed above, with the following additions or exceptions.

Assessment

For the treatment of psoriasis and RA, two baseline serum creatinine determinations should be performed before initiating therapy. Blood pressure, BUN, cholesterol, CBC, serum magnesium, serum potassium, and uric acid should also be documented. Hepatic function studies are performed before initiating therapy. The results of a dental examination should be documented for baseline data.

Nursing Diagnosis

In addition to the nursing diagnoses cited earlier in the chapter, the client taking cyclosporine has the potential for disturbed body im-

age related to acne, gingival hyperplasia, and hirsutism, and the potential complications of hypertension, posttransplant lymphoproliferative disorder (PTLD), nephrotoxicity, hepatotoxicity, and pancreatitis.

Implementation

Monitoring

Baseline assessments, except for hepatic studies and dental examinations, should be performed every 2 weeks during the first 3 months of therapy, and then monthly if the client has stabilized. Serum cyclosporine levels are evaluated periodically during a course of therapy, and dosages are adjusted accordingly. Significant changes in renal and hepatic function may necessitate a reduction in dosage or a discontinuation of cyclosporine. Dental examinations should be performed at 3-month intervals for the early detection and treatment of gingival hyperplasia.

Monitor the client for signs and symptoms of hypersensitivity (dyspnea, wheezing, hypotension), and have resuscitation equipment near when the drug is administered IV.

Intervention

When administering the oral solution, use the calibrated measuring device supplied by the manufacturer. Because cyclosporine solution is prepared with a mixture of alcohol and vegetable oil and has an unpleasant taste, mix the Sandimmune oral solution thoroughly with milk, chocolate milk, or orange juice or the Neoral oral solution with apple juice or orange juice at room temperature, and administer it at once. Use a glass container to prevent the drug from binding to the container, and rinse with additional juice or milk to ensure that the entire dose is taken. Wipe the measuring device dry; do not wash it after use.

The IV infusion is begun 4 to 12 hours before surgery and continued postoperatively until the client can tolerate an oral dosage form. The drug is prepared for IV infusion by diluting each 1 mL in 20 to 100 mL of 0.9% sodium chloride injection or 5% dextrose injection. Glass containers are preferred to prevent the leaching of diethylhexylphthalate (DEHP) from the polyvinyl chloride (PVC) infusion bags into the cyclosporine solution. However, some agencies will use PVC containers and prepare the drug just before it is administered. Significant amounts of the drug are lost when administered through PVC tubing. The solution is stable for 24 hours in 5% dextrose injection. In 0.9% sodium chloride injection at room temperature, cyclosporine is stable for 6 hours in a PVC container and for 12 hours in a glass container. Infuse over 2 to 6 hours using an infusion pump or continuously over 24 hours.

Education
Advise the transplant client about the need to adhere to the drug regimen to prevent rejection. Instruct the client to maintain good dental hygiene and to visit a dentist frequently for teeth cleaning to help prevent gingival hyperplasia. Alert the client not to drink grapefruit juice or eat grapefruit; it inhibits the metabolism of cyclosporine, resulting in toxic blood levels of the drug.

Clients receiving cyclosporine therapy for RA may continue to take corticosteroids, NSAIDs, and salicylates. For clients with psoriasis, any skin lesion that is not typical of that condition should be biopsied for malignancy.

Evaluation
The expected outcome of cyclosporine therapy for clients being treated for psoriasis is that they will experience some improvement within 2 weeks; satisfactory control of symptoms may take 12 to 16 weeks. The client taking cyclosporine as part of the therapeutic regimen for transplantation will not demonstrate signs of organ rejection and will remain free of hepatotoxicity and nephrotoxicity. The client will also manage the therapeutic regimen effectively, including complying with the medication regimen, stating reportable symptoms, and maintaining scheduled visits to the prescriber for monitoring and treatment.

azathioprine [ay za **thye** oh preen]
(Imuran, Alti-Azathioprine✦)
The mechanism of action for azathioprine is unknown, but it appears primarily to suppress T-cell and B-cell production; that is, it suppresses cell-mediated hypersensitivity and antibody production. In combination with steroids, this drug appears to have a steroid-conserving effect; a lower dosage of steroid may be used to treat chronic inflammatory processes when given with azathioprine.

Indications
Azathioprine is indicated as an adjunct medication to prevent rejection in renal organ transplants and for severe, active RA in clients who have not responded to other therapies.

Pharmacokinetics/Dosing
Azathioprine is available in oral and parenteral dosage forms. The oral dosage form is well absorbed from the intestinal tract and has a half-life of 5 hours and an onset of action of 6 to 8 weeks for RA and perhaps 4 to 8 weeks for other inflammatory disease states. It is metabolized in the liver to active metabolites (6-mercaptopurine and 6-thioinosinic acid), with further metabolism by xanthine oxidase. This metabolism appears to be highly influenced by genetics (see the Special Considerations for Pharmacogenetics box on p. 1154). It is primarily excreted via the biliary system. The immunosuppressant dosage for adults and children is 3 to 5 mg/kg PO 1 to 3 days before or at the time of surgery; if administered IV, this dose is given before, during, or immediately after surgery for transplantation. The maintenance dosage is 1 to 3 mg/kg/day. For RA, the adult oral dosage is 1 mg/kg daily and is adjusted every 1 to 2 months as necessary.

Adverse Effects
The adverse effects of azathioprine include anorexia, nausea, vomiting, leukopenia or infection, megaloblastic anemia (usually asymptomatic, but the client may also have fever, chills, cough, low back or side pain, pain on urination, or increased weakness), hepatitis, hypersensitivity, pneumonitis, sores in the mouth and on the lips,

and skin rash. The risk of hepatotoxicity is greater when the dosage of azathioprine exceeds 2.5 mg/kg/day but also varies based on genetically determined ability to metabolize the drug.

Nursing Management
The nursing management of azathioprine is as for the nursing management of an immunosuppressant in the case of F.K. discussed above with the following additions or exceptions.

Assessment
If azathioprine is administered for RA, assess the client's range of motion, status of affected joints (swelling, pain, and strength), and ability to accomplish activities of daily living before and at periodic intervals during therapy. A significant drug interaction occurs with allopurinol; it inhibits xanthine oxidase that may result in increased azathioprine activity and toxicity.

Nursing Diagnosis
In addition to the earlier discussion, the client receiving azathioprine may experience the following nursing diagnoses/collaborative problems: impaired mucous membranes (mouth ulcers); and the potential complications of hepatitis, pancreatitis, and skin rash.

Implementation
Monitoring
CBCs should be performed weekly during the first month, twice a month for the next 2 to 3 months and monthly thereafter. Notify the prescriber if the leukocyte count is less than 3000/mm³ or if platelets are less than 100,000/mm³; therapy will be reinstituted at reduced dosages when these counts reach an acceptable level, usually after 7 to 10 days. A decrease in hemoglobin may indicate bone marrow suppression. Renal and hepatic function studies should be monitored with the same frequency. Increased alkaline phosphatase, bilirubin, AST, ALT, and amylase concentrations may indicate hepatotoxicity. Because of the delayed action of azathioprine, the dosage will be reduced at the first indication of serious bone marrow depression (leukocyte count less than 3000/mm³ or platelet count less than 100,000/mm³).

Intervention
Azathioprine is usually started 1 to 5 days before transplantation and restarted within 24 hours after transplantation. Administer oral doses of azathioprine with or after meals to minimize GI distress. Reconstitute each 100 mg for IV use by adding 10 mL of sterile water for injection to the vial and swirling to dissolve. It may be administered by IV push or further diluted with 0.9% sodium chloride injection or 5% dextrose and 0.9% sodium chloride injection for IV infusion. It may be administered over a time period of 5 minutes to 8 hours. Once reconstituted, azathioprine is stable at room temperature for 24 hours.

Handle this drug with caution because of its potential mutagenicity, teratogenicity, and carcinogenicity. Consult the policies and procedures of the health care agency.

Education
If azathioprine is being administered for RA, the client should be advised to continue physical therapy and other concurrent therapy (salicylates, nonsteroidal antiinflammatory drugs, glucocorticoids) as prescribed. Because azathioprine has teratogenic effects, advise fe-

PREGNANCY SAFETY IMMUNOSUPPRESSANTS AND IMMUNOMODULATORS	
Category	**Drug**
B	basiliximab
C	cyclosporine, daclizumab, muromonab-CD3, mycophenolate mofetil, tacrolimus
D	azathioprine

Data from *Mosby's drug consult* (15th ed.). (2005). St. Louis: Mosby.

male clients who are of childbearing age to practice contraception during the course of therapy and for at least 4 months after its completion (see the Pregnancy Safety box on p. 1155).

Alert the client to report to the prescriber unusual bleeding or bruising; blood in the urine or stools; black, tarry stools; or pinpoint red spots on the skin.

Evaluation

The expected outcome of azathioprine therapy prescribed for RA is that the client will experience decreased pain, stiffness, and swelling of the affected joints in 6 to 8 weeks. If administered to prevent transplant rejection, the client will not experience rejection of the transplanted organ and will manage the therapeutic regimen effectively as described in F.K.'s case.

basiliximab [bas i **licks** i mab]
(Simulect)

Basiliximab is an IL-2 receptor antagonist; it binds to the alpha subunit on the IL-2 receptor to inhibit IL-2 binding. This binding prevents IL-2–mediated lymphocyte activation, thus impairing the response of the immune system to antigens.

Indications

Basiliximab is an immunosuppressant used in combination with other immunosuppressants to prevent kidney transplant rejection. It is primarily used during the perioperative period when the organ is first transplanted.

Pharmacokinetics/Dosing

Basiliximab is administered by IV infusion; it has a half-life of 7.2 ± 3.2 days in adults and 11.5 ± 6.3 days in children. The duration of action is 36 ± 14 days. The usual adult dosage is 20 mg administered by IV infusion 2 hours before the transplantation surgery and repeated 4 days later. The pediatric dosage is 12 mg/m^2 of body surface area by IV infusion administered 2 hours before the transplantation surgery. This dose is repeated 4 days later.

Adverse Effects

The adverse effects of basiliximab include weakness, headache, nausea, vomiting, stomach and/or back pain, pulmonary edema (shortness of breath), edema (swelling of the lower extremities, weight gain), hypertension, infection (fever, chills, candidiasis, pharyngitis, cough, dysuria), neuropathy (numbness or pain in legs), tremors, acne, and insomnia.

Nursing Management

The nursing management of basiliximab is as for other immunosuppressants with the following additions or exceptions.

Assessment

In clinical trials, basiliximab was used concurrently with clients receiving other immunosuppressants; no drug interactions have been reported with its use.

Implementation

Intervention

Vials of basiliximab should be used within 4 hours of preparation, because basiliximab does not contain preservatives. Avoid shaking the vial because doing so may cause foaming. Keep medications and equipment for the emergency management of acute hypersensitivity reactions in the immediate area.

Education

Advise women of childbearing age to use effective contraception before, during, and for 2 months after receiving basiliximab. Although basiliximab is listed as Pregnancy Category B, the manufacturer recommends the use of contraception during its use.

Evaluation

The client will not experience rejection of the transplant kidney and will manage the therapeutic regimen effectively as described in F.K.'s case on p. 1153.

daclizumab [dak lih zoo mab]
(Zenapax)

Daclizumab shares the same mechanism of action as basiliximab.

Indications

Daclizumab is an immunosuppressant agent combined with other immunosuppressants to prevent kidney transplant rejection. Its use is not recommended for clients who have undergone cardiac transplantation because of increased reports of severe infections and mortality associated with its use (Gordon, 2003).

Pharmacokinetics/Dosing

Daclizumab is administered by IV infusion and has a half-life of 11 to 38 days. The therapeutic serum level is between 5 and 10 mcg/mL. The adult dosage is 1 mg/kg body weight administered over 15 minutes every 2 weeks for five doses. The first dose should be administered no earlier than 24 hours before the transplantation.

Adverse Effects

The most serious adverse effects of daclizumab include hypersensitivity (including anaphylaxis) and severe infections (Gordon, 2003). Other adverse effects include headache, nausea, vomiting, gas, constipation, diarrhea, shortness of breath, hypertension or hypotension, peripheral edema, tachycardia, tremor, muscle and/or joint pain, dizziness, weakness, insomnia, and wound infection.

Nursing Management

The nursing management of daclizumab is as for basiliximab.

muromonab-CD3 [myoo roe **moe** nab-CD3]
(Orthoclone, OKT3)

Muromonab-CD3 is a monoclonal antibody that reacts with CD3 receptors on the surface of T lymphocytes. It blocks the activation and functions of the T cells in response to an antigenic challenge. Thus it functions as an immunosuppressant and does not cause myelosuppression.

Indications

Muromonab-CD3 is indicated for the treatment of acute renal organ transplant rejection and is usually given in combination with azathioprine, cyclosporine, and/or corticosteroids. It is also administered to treat steroid-resistant acute rejection in cardiac and hepatic transplants.

Pharmacokinetics/Dosing

Available parenterally, muromonab-CD3 acts to reduce activated T cells within minutes of administration. It reaches steady-state plasma levels in approximately 3 days and has a duration of action of approximately 7 days. In other words, the number of circulating CD3-positive T cells will return to baseline levels within a week of discontinuing muromonab-CD3. The adult IV dosage is 5 mg daily for 10 to 14 days. Children under 12 years of age receive 0.1 mg/kg/day for 10 to 14 days (not to exceed the adult dose).

Adverse Effects

The most common adverse effects of muromonab-CD3 occur with the first course. The first-dose effect consists of light-headedness, elevated temperature, chills, nausea, vomiting, diarrhea, headache, dyspnea, chest pain, and tremors and trembling. These effects may be repeated to a lesser degree after the second dose but are rarely encountered with later doses. Fever and chills that occur later may be caused by infection. Anaphylaxis, hypersensitivity, encephalopathy, seizures, cerebral edema, and aseptic meningitis syndrome are reported less frequently.

Nursing Management

In addition to the nursing management presented earlier for F.K., the following content is in addition to or exceptions from that content.

Assessment

The client's temperature should be taken before drug administration. A temperature above 100° F (37.8° C) should be lowered with antipyretics, and infection should be ruled out before muromonab-CD3 is administered. Uncompensated heart failure or fluid volume excess is a contraindication for this drug because of the risk of life-threatening pulmonary edema if administered. There is an increased risk of hypersensitivity to muromonab-CD3 if the antimouse titer is 1:1000 or more.

Nursing Diagnosis

In addition to the nursing diagnoses/collaborative problems cited in the general nursing management for immunosuppressed clients (see pp. 1151 to 1153), the client receiving muromonab-CD3 has the potential for the following: hyperthermia; risk for injury related to cytokine release syndrome (chest pain, dizziness, fever and chills, tachycardia, dyspnea, tremors); and the potential complication of anaphylaxis, aseptic meningitis syndrome, cerebral edema, pulmonary edema, and encephalopathy (confusion, hallucinations, coma, seizures).

Implementation

Monitoring

Monitor the client's temperature at frequent intervals for several hours after administration, especially with the first two doses. A cytokine release syndrome may occur as evidenced by chest pain, dizziness, fever and chills, tachycardia, dyspnea, and tremors. These symptoms occur in most clients 30 minutes to 48 hours after the first dose and may last several hours; they may occur to a lesser extent with each subsequent dose. Fever and chills occurring later in therapy may be caused by infection. The client should also be assessed for headache, stiff neck, and photosensitivity, because aseptic meningitis syndrome may occur in the first 3 days of therapy. CBCs should be monitored periodically throughout the course of treatment.

Observe the client for fluid volume excess: auscultate the lungs, check for peripheral edema, monitor daily weights, and monitor fluid intake and output ratios. Monitor vital signs and observe for signs of infection.

Notify the oncologist if the client has greater than 25 CD3 antigen or Muromonab-CD3 serum concentrations less than 800 ng/mL.

Intervention

Ensure that cardiopulmonary resuscitation equipment and medications are immediately available during administration of the first dose. Muromonab-CD3 should be administered by IV push over a period of less than 1 minute by a health care provider who is experienced in immunosuppressive therapy.

Methylprednisolone may be administered intravenously before the first dose to minimize cytokine release syndrome. IV hydrocortisone sodium succinate may be given 30 minutes after the first dose (and possibly the second dose) for the same reason. Antihistamines may also be used to minimize this reaction. The client's temperature should be maintained below 100° F (37.8° C) with acetaminophen.

Muromonab-CD3 is prepared for IV administration by drawing the solution through a low protein-binding 0.2- or 0.22-μm filter, then discarding the filter and attaching the appropriate needle for administration. The drug is not administered by IV infusion or with other drug solutions. Do not agitate the solution, because it will foam.

Education

Prepare the client for the possibility of the cytokine release syndrome and the client to report any of the adverse signs and symptoms of that reaction or of aseptic meningitis syndrome (e.g., fever, headache, altered mental status, stiff neck, photophobia).

Evaluation

The evaluation is the same as for F.K.'s case (see p. 1153).

mycophenolate mofetil [mye koe **fen** oe late **moe** fe till] (CellCept)

Mycophenolate is metabolized to MPA, an active metabolite that inhibits the response of T and B lymphocytes to mitogenic and allospecific stimulation. Therefore this drug has a cytostatic effect on lymphocytes. It also suppresses antibody formation by B lymphocytes and may inhibit the influx of leukocytes into inflammatory and graft rejection sites.

Indications

Mycophenolate is used in conjunction with cyclosporine and corticosteroids and is indicated for the prophylaxis of renal transplant and allogenic cardiac rejection.

Pharmacokinetics/Dosing

Available orally, mycophenolate is rapidly metabolized to the active metabolite MPA and other inactive metabolites. The half-life of MPA is 18 hours, with excretion primarily in the kidneys. For renal transplant prophylaxis, an oral dosage of 1 g twice daily is administered as soon as possible after surgery in combination with cyclosporine and corticosteroids. For cardiac transplant rejection prophylaxis, the

dosage is 1.5 g twice daily in combination with cyclosporine and corticosteroids.

Adverse Effects

The major adverse effects of mycophenolate include diarrhea, vomiting, and respiratory infections (leukopenia, sepsis). Peripheral edema, urinary tract infections, anemia, hepatotoxicity, hypertension, and abdominal pain are also reported.

Nursing Management

Refer to the nursing management of the immunosuppressed client F.K.; the following discussion is in addition to or exceptions from that content.

Assessment

It is essential to assess exposure to or the presence of infection. Although mycophenolate mofetil has enhanced immunosuppression for both acute and chronic rejection, the client is at higher risk for infection than with other similar agents. Any current infection may become life threatening with the administration of mycophenolate. This drug is contraindicated for clients who are hypersensitive to the drug and should be used cautiously in clients with serious disease of the GI tract or a history of ulcer disease or GI bleeding. Clients with impaired renal function will experience reduced excretion of the drug with an increased risk of mycophenolate toxicity; dosages may need to be reduced. Baseline assessment should include a negative pregnancy test.

Nursing Diagnosis

Clients receiving mycophenolate may experience the following nursing diagnoses/collaborative problems: impaired comfort (headache, heartburn, nausea, vomiting); disturbed sleep pattern (insomnia); impaired skin integrity (acne, rash); diarrhea; constipation; ineffective protection related to leukopenia or thrombocytopenia; activity intolerance related to anemia; ineffective airway clearance (cough); excess fluid volume (dyspnea, peripheral edema); risk for infection; and the potential complications of GI bleeding, heart failure (HF), and increased risk of malignancy.

Implementation

Monitoring

CBCs should be performed weekly during the first month, twice a month for the next 2 to 3 months, and monthly thereafter. Notify the prescriber if the absolute neutrophil count (ANC) is less than 1300/mm³ (1.3×10^3). Renal and hepatic function studies and electrolytes should be monitored periodically during therapy. Increased alkaline phosphatase, bilirubin, AST, ALT, and amylase concentrations may indicate hepatotoxicity. Increased serum creatinine, hypercalcemia, hypocalcemia, hyponatremia, hyperglycemia, hypoglycemia, and hyperlipidemia may occur.

Intervention

Mycophenolate is given within 72 hours of transplantation. Administer oral doses on an empty stomach, 1 hour before or 2 hours after meals. Capsules should be swallowed whole, not opened, crushed, or chewed.

Education

Female clients who are of childbearing age need to practice two reliable forms of contraception or abstinence both during the course of therapy and for 6 weeks following the end of therapy.

Evaluation

The evaluation is the same as for F.K.'s case (see p. 1153).

sirolimus [sir **oh** li mus] (Rapamune)

Sirolimus inhibits the activation and proliferation of T lymphocytes.

Indications

Sirolimus is used in combination with corticosteroids and cyclosporine to prevent organ rejection in clients undergoing renal transplant.

Pharmacokinetics/Dosing

Bioavailability of sirolimus is moderate, but adequate for oral administration. It is metabolized hepatically by cytochrome P450 3 A4 and is primarily eliminated in the feces. The adult dose for clients over

40 kg is 2 mg daily taken 4 hours after cyclosporine with loading dose of 6 mg on day 1.

Adverse Effects

Among the more serious adverse effects of sirolimus are nephrotoxicity, bone marrow suppression, cardiac dysrhythmias, HF, and respiratory distress. Sirolimus is associated with a number of dose related adverse effects, including hypertension, edema, fever, headache, GI complaints (abdominal pain, nausea, vomiting, constipation, diarrhea, heartburn), and joint/muscle pain.

Drug Interactions

Sirolimus is both metabolized by cytochrome p450 3 A4 and interferes with other drugs metabolized by this isoenzyme. Other drugs may inhibit metabolism of sirolimus (leading to elevated sirolimus levels and toxicity) including cyclosporine, calcium channel blockers, azole antifungals, macrolides, and HIV protease inhibitors. Concurrent rifampin or antiepileptic drugs may result in increased metabolism of sirolimus and subtherapeutic levels. Sirolimus may also interfere with the metabolism of other drugs, including cyclosporine. Consult the package insert for interactions and their management.

Nursing Management

Refer to the nursing management of the immunosuppressed client, F.K.; the following discussion is in addition to or exceptions from that content.

Assessment

Because sirolimus is a known CYP3 A4 metabolite, other drugs such as cyclosporine, diltiazem, or ketoconazole, or grapefruit juice, also metabolized by CYP3 A4 may lead to elevation of sirolimus blood concentrations and toxicity, whereas rifampin increases sirolimus clearance and decreases serum levels of the drug.

Implementation

Monitoring

In addition to monitoring other lab studies to determine drug toxicity, trough sirolimus whole blood concentrations should be monitored with clients weighing less than 40 kg, those with hepatic impairment or those receiving P450 3 A4 inducers or inhibitors.

Evaluation

The evaluation is the same as for F.K.'s case (see p. 1153).

tacrolimus [ta **kroe** li mus]

(FK 506, Prograf)

Tacrolimus inhibits the activation of T lymphocytes. Although its exact mechanism of action is unknown, it is believed to bind to FKBP-12 protein and form complexes that prevent the activation of T lymphocytes.

Indications

Tacrolimus in conjunction with corticosteroids is indicated for the prophylaxis of organ rejection (kidney, liver and, investigationally, other organs). Atopical ointment (Protopic) is also available for short-term treatment of atopic dermatitis (eczema), but long-term potential cancer risks are unknown (U.S. Food and Drug Administration [FDA], 2005).

Pharmacokinetics/Dosing

Tacrolimus is available orally and parenterally. Oral absorption is variable, with peak blood levels reached in 1.5 to 3.5 hours. It is metabolized in the liver (primarily by the cytochrome P450 system) to a number of metabolites, including several active ones. Metabolism is highly influenced by genetics (see the Special Considerations for Pharmacogenetics box on p. 1154). Less than 1% is excreted in the urine. The initial adult dosage by IV infusion is 0.03 to 0.05 mg/kg/day; the client is converted to the oral dosage form as soon as possible, usually in 2 to 3 days of therapy. The initial oral adult dosage is 0.1 to 0.2 mg/kg/day. Dosing is further refined based on indication and trough levels.

Adverse Effects

The adverse effects of tacrolimus include headaches, nausea, diarrhea, hypertension, tremors, and renal dysfunction. Hyperglycemia that requires insulin therapy, hyperkalemia, hypomagnesemia, and hyperuricemia have also been reported (*Drug Facts and Comparisons*,

2005). Tacrolimus and related agents appear to increase cancer risk in animal models, but the risk for humans has not yet been quantified (FDA, 2005).

Drug Interactions

Like sirolimus, tacrolimus affects and is affected by drugs that interfere with cytochrome P450 enzyme systems. Interactions as similar to those observed with sirolimus. Tacrolimus may be more likely to produce renal toxicity if administered concurrently with other nephrotoxic drugs, including amphotericin, aminoglycosides, or NSAIDs. Refer to package labeling for more complete information.

Nursing Management

Refer to the nursing management of the immunosuppressed client F.K.; the following discussion is in addition to or exceptions from that content.

Assessment

The use of tacrolimus is contraindicated for clients with hypersensitivity to the drug or to HCO-60 polyoxyl hydrogenated castor oil (which is contained in the injection solution).

Review the client's current drug regimen for the risk of significant drug interactions, such as those that may occur when tacrolimus is given concurrently with the following drugs. Danazol (Danocrine), erythromycin, fluconazole (Diflucan), itraconazole (Sporanox), and ketoconazole (Nizoral) increase tacrolimus blood levels; monitor tacrolimus blood levels at frequent intervals. Dosage adjustments may be necessary. Rifampin (Rifadin) decreases blood levels of tacrolimus. With concurrent use of cyclosporine (Sandimmune) the risk of nephrotoxicity increases. Allow 24 hours to pass after discontinuing cyclosporine before starting tacrolimus. Monitor renal function studies carefully. With potassium-sparing diuretics, concurrent use increases the risk of hyperkalemia. Monitor serum potassium levels. A baseline assessment should include serum creatinine, serum electrolytes, CBC and platelet counts, and blood glucose. The client's clinical status should be documented.

Implementation

Monitoring

Observe the client for a hypersensitivity response for at least 30 minutes after IV tacrolimus and frequently thereafter. Monitor blood pressure closely during therapy. Monitor CBCs and platelet counts, blood glucose, serum electrolytes, serum creatinine levels, and tacrolimus blood levels. Monitor children closely, because higher dosages are necessary to maintain adequate blood levels.

Intervention

Tacrolimus therapy should be initiated no sooner than 6 hours after transplantation. Concurrent glucocorticoid therapy may occur. IV administration is by continuous infusion over 24 hours. The client should be changed to oral administration of tacrolimus as soon as possible to reduce the risk of adverse effects from IV tacrolimus—usually 8 to 12 hours after the last IV dosing.

Education

Alert the client to avoid grapefruit and grapefruit juice; both increase the serum levels of tacrolimus.

Evaluation

The evaluation is the same as for F.K.'s case (see p. 1153).

✪ What agents serve to support or stimulate the immune response?

A number of modalities have been utilized to stimulate immune response as part of treatment of cancers, viral infections, and other conditions. The oldest and most common means utilized to stimulate immune response is the use of vaccines (see Chapter 62). Other, newer modalities include the use of biologic response modifiers, interferons and interleukins, in the treatment of cancers and viral hepatitis B and C (see Chapters 56 and 59, respectively). Chapter 56 presents a host of other biologic response modifiers also available in the treatment of cancers. The granulocyte or granulocyte-macrophage colony-stimulating factors (G-CSF or filgrastim [Neupogen] and sargramostim [GM-CSF; Leukine]) are used to induce WBC production in a number of conditions, particularly after chemotherapy (see Chapters 30 and 56). Specific immune globulins are used as postexposure treatment for a particular infectious condition, including hepatitis B, rabies, and tetanus (see Chapter 62). Nonspecific immune globulins are used to treat a number of conditions, including congenital agammaglobulinemia and idiopathic thrombocytopenic purpura (ITP).

✳◩ intravenous immune globulin [in tra vee nus i myun glob you lin]
(Carimmune, Gammagard, Gammar-P, Iveegam, Polygam)
✳◩ intramuscular immune globulin [in tra mus kyoo ler i myun glob you lin]
(BayGam✦)
Immune globulin is derived from pooled human plasma and undergoes processing to purify the product. Different formulations provide subtle differences in the percentage of IgG subclasses 1, 2, 3, and 4.

Indications
Primary indications for IV immune globulin are the treatment of primary immunodeficiency states (e.g., congenital agammaglobulinemia), idiopathic thrombocytopenic purpura (ITP), Kawasaki syndrome and B-cell chronic lymphocytic leukemia. Immune globulin is used for a number of non-FDA approved indications with varying efficacy, including management of autoimmune diseases, Guillain-Barré syndrome, and as adjunct therapy for bacterial and viral infections for clients with suppressed immune systems. The IM formulation is most often used for prophylaxis of viral infections, including hepatitis A, hepatitis B, measles, poliomyelitis, rubella, and varicella.

Pharmacokinetics/Dosing
The IV administration of the IV immune globulin formulation provides effects for up to 4 weeks depending on dosage, indication, and client status. The IM formulation provides similar effects. Dosage varies widely based on indication and formulation. Refer to package labeling for dosing.

Adverse Effects
Multiple adverse events have been reported with immune globulin administration, and include cardiovascular, central nervous system, dermatologic, hematologic, renal, respiratory, and muscle/joint effects. Hypersensitivity reactions are the most concerning and may be most problematic for clients with IgA deficiencies. Refer to package labeling for specific types of events and rates.

❋ **What are the nursing implications of the use of immune globulins?**

Assessment Interview the client and family before giving an immunoglobulin. Assess the individual's age, current physical condition and general resistance to disease, history of exposure to infectious diseases (both past and potential), and previous immunizations. Providers are required to provide detailed information on the risks and benefits of passive immunization. Before giving immunoglobulin, a signed consent form or a note indicating that the individual has read and understood the information regarding the specific product may be obtained. Share printed information at this time to ensure that the parent/client is aware of the adverse effects and how to man-

age them. Immune globulin has the following contraindications: anaphylactic reaction to immune globulin and immunoglobulin A (IgA) deficiency and it is used cautiously in clients with thrombocytopenia and other blood clotting disorder. Sensitivity to sucrose and maltose is of concern with immune globulin IV (IGIV). Exercise caution when administering IGIV to clients with preexisting renal insufficiency, diabetes mellitus, age older than 65, volume depletion, paraprotein sepsis, or concomitant nephrotoxic drugs, because there is an increased risk for developing acute renal failure.

Nursing Diagnosis The client receiving immunoglobulin has the potential for the following selected nursing diagnoses/collaborative problems: impaired comfort (nausea, vomiting, malaise, headache, migraine, rash, lymphadenopathy, and pain and tenderness at the injection site); imbalanced body temperature (fever); and the potential complications of allergic reaction, arthralgia, acute renal failure, and encephalopathy.

Planning After receiving immune globulin, the client will:
- Not contract the illness to which he has been exposed.
- Not experience adverse effects of the immunization and state reportable ones (e.g., fever, chills, myalgias, bronchospasm).
- Use supportive measures, such as acetaminophen or diphenhydramine, as recommended by the prescriber to manage minimal adverse effects.

Implementation
Monitoring Because of the risk of anaphylaxis after any immunization, ask clients to remain in the immediate area for up to half an hour for observation of any developing adverse reactions. Be alert for the early symptoms of such a reaction—hives, shock-like appearance, confusion, and hypotension.

Intervention Passive immunization or immunoprophylaxis should always be administered as soon as possible after exposure to the agent.
Keep epinephrine on hand to counter any potentially life-threatening adverse event (e.g., anaphylaxis).

Education If the client has had a vaccination for measles, mumps, rubella, or chickenpox in the previous 14 days, it may have to be repeated and the client should not receive any other vaccinations until at least 3 months after receiving immune globulin. Because this medication only provides protection for a limited time (1 to 3 months), additional doses may be necessary based on the situation.
Teach clients or their parents how to recognize and differentiate between anticipated side effects and serious adverse reactions. Acetaminophen may be taken for aches, local pain and swelling, or mild temperature elevations, which may occur within 24 hours. Recipients of im-

munotherapy should understand whom to contact if complications later occur. As a product of human plasma, this product may potentially transmit disease. An outbreak of hepatitis C in 1993-1994 related to the use of immunoglobulin prompted FDA action to improve viral inactivation steps, with no new cases noted (Park & Chandhok, 2004).

Evaluation The expected outcome of immunotherapy is that the client will receive immunity to the disease of exposure or anticipated exposure without experiencing adverse effects of the drug (e.g., tenderness at injection sites, aches, low-grade fever, anaphylaxis).

Summary

Immunomodulators (both those that suppress and those that enhance immune function) are relatively new products. The immunosuppressant agents are primarily used in transplant medicine, although some have a role in the management of autoimmune conditions. Many various types of agents serve to support or stimulate immune function, including vaccines, toxoids, and immunoglobulins. Nursing management centers on careful medical asepsis, proper diet and oral hygiene, and prevention of infection. As new drugs continue to be introduced, the nurse's role in this important therapy is likely to continue to expand.

✱ Critical Thinking Questions

- Susan Goode, 35 years old, has just received a kidney transplant. Her physician has prescribed cyclosporine, 15 mg/kg PO daily. What is the mechanism of action by which cyclosporine prevents transplant rejection? What nursing care is required to support Susan's cyclosporine regimen?

Bibliography

Anderson, D.M., Keith, J., & Novak, P.D. (Eds.) (2002). *Mosby's medical, nursing, and allied health dictionary* (6th ed.). St. Louis: Mosby.

Anglicheau, D., Legendre, C., & Thervet, E. (2004). Pharmacogenetics in Solid Organ Transplantation: Present Knowledge and Future Perspectives. *Transplantation, 78*(3), 311-315.

Bosker, G. (Ed.). (2004). *Primary and acute care medicine: Practice, protocols, pathways*, (2nd ed.). Atlanta: Thomson American Health Consultants.

Buchler, M., & Johnston, A. (2005). Seeking optimal prescription of cyclosporine ME. *Therapeutic Drug Monitoring, 27*(1), 3-6.

Drug facts and comparisons (58th ed.). (2005). St. Louis: Facts and Comparisons.

Gearry, R.B., Roberts, R.L., Barclay, M.L., & Kennedy, M.A. (2004). Lack of association between the ITPA 94 C>A polymorphism and adverse effects from azathioprine. *Pharmacogenetics, 14*(11), 779-781.

Gordon, R.D. (August 2003). Zenapax Dear Heath Care Provider Letter. Retrieved February 12, 2005, from http://www.fda.gov/medwatch/SAFETY/2003/zenapax.htm.

Goto, M., Masuda, S., Kiuchi, T., Ogura, Y., Oike, F., & Okuda, M., et al. (2004). CYP3 A5*1-carrying graft liver reduces the concentration/oral dose ratio of tacrolimus in recipients of living-donor liver transplantation. *Pharmacogenetics, 14*(7), 471-478.

Hardman, J.G., & Limbird, L.E. (Eds.). (2001). *Goodman & Gilman's The pharmacological basis of therapeutics* (10th ed.). New York: McGraw-Hill.

Haufroid, V., Mourad, M., Van Kerckhove, V., Wawrzyniak, J., De Meyer, M., & Eddour, D.C., et al. (2004). The effect of CYP3 A5 and MDR1 (ABCB1) polymorphisms on cyclosporine and tacrolimus dose requirements and trough blood levels in stable renal transplant patients. *Pharmacogenetics, 14*(3), 147-154.

Johnson, H.J., & Heim-Duthoy, K. (2002). Renal transplantation. In J.T. DiPiro, R.L. Talbert, G.C. Yee, G.R. Matzke, B.G. Wells & L.M. Posey (Eds.), *Pharmacotherapy: A pathophysiological approach* (5th ed.). Norwalk, CT: Appleton & Lange.

Kishiyama, J.L., & Adelman, D.C. (2003). Allergic and immunologic disorders. In L.M. Tierney, Jr., S.J. McPhee & Papadakis, M.A. (Eds.), *Current Medical Diagnosis & Treatment*. New York: Lange Medical Books/McGraw-Hill.

Krensky, A.M., Strom, T.B., & Bluestone, J.A. (2001). Immunomodulators: Immunosuppressive agents, tolerogens, and immunostimulants. In Hardman, J.G. & Limbird, L.E. (Eds.), *Goodman & Gilman's The pharmacological basis of therapeutics* (10th ed.). New York: McGraw-Hill.

Kreutz, R., Zurcher, H., Kain, S., Martus, P., Offermann, G., & Beige, J. (2004). The effect of variable CYP3 A5 expression on cyclosporine dosing, blood pressure and long-term graft survival in renal transplant patients. *Pharmacogenetics, 14*(10), 665-671.

Lacy, C.F., Armstrong, L.L., Goldman, M.P., & Lance, L.L. (2004). *Lexi-Comp's Drug Information Handbook* (12th ed.). Hudson, Ohio: Lexi-Comp.

e-LEARNING SUPPLEMENTS

Student CD-ROM
- Final Exam questions
- NCLEX® Examination review questions
- Pharmacology animations
- Printable chapter summary

Evolve Website (http://evolve.elsevier.com/mckenry)
- Case study on immunosuppressants and immunomodulators
- Content updates, including information on new drugs

- WebLinks corresponding to this chapter
- Answers to the critical thinking questions in this chapter
- *Elsevier ePharmacology Update* newsletter
- Mosby's Drug Consult Internet Edition
- Supplemental and reference information

MacPhee, I.A., Fredericks, S., Tai, T., Syrris, P., Carter, N.D., & Johnston, A., et al. (2002). Tacrolimus pharmacogenetics: Polymorphisms associated with expression of cytochrome p4503 A5 and P-glycoprotein correlate with dose requirement. *Transplantation, 74*(11), 1486–1489.

McCaughan, G. (2004). Molecular approaches to the side effects of immunosuppressive drugs. *Transplantation, 78*(8),1114-1115.

Min, D.I., Ellingrod, V.L., Marsh, S., & McLeod, H.(2004). CYP3 A5 Polymorphism and the Ethnic Differences in Cyclosporine Pharmacokinetics in Healthy Subjects 1. *Therapeutic Drug Monitoring, 26*(5), 524-528.

Mosby's drug consult (15th ed.). (2005). St. Louis: Mosby.

Park, K.W., & Chandhok, D. (2004). Transfusion-associated complications. *International Anesthesiology Clinics, 42*(3), 11-26.

Taber, D.J., & Dupuis, R.E. (2005). Solid organ transplantation. In M.A. Koda-Kimble, L.Y. Young, W.A. Kradjan, B.J. Guglielmo, B.K. Alldredge, & R.L. Corelli (Eds.), *Applied therapeutics: The clinical use of drugs* (8th ed.). Philadelphia: Lippincott Williams & Wilkins.

U.S. Food and Drug Administration. (2005). FDA Public Health Advisory: Elidel (pimecrolimus) cream and Protopic (tacrolimus) ointment. Retrieved July 28, 2005, from http://www.fda.gov/cder/drug/advisory/elidel_protopic.htm.

USP DI: Drug information for the health care professional (25th ed.). (2005). Greenwood Village, CO: MICROMEDEX Thomson Healthcare.

van Gelder, T., Hesselink, D.A., van Hest, R., Mathot, R.A.A., & van Schaik, R. (2004). Pharmacogenetics in Immunosuppressive Therapy: The Best Thing Since TDM? *Therapeutic Drug Monitoring, 26*(4), 343-346.

von Ahsen, N., Oellerich, M., & Armstrong, V.W. (2004). Thiopurine pharmacogenetics: the inosine triphosphate pyrophosphohydrolase (itpase) intronic ivs2+21 a>c mutation affects purine synthesis/salvage pathways by acting on mRNA splicing efficiency. *Transplantation, 78*(2) Supplement 1, 597.

OVERVIEW OF THE INTEGUMENTARY SYSTEM

CHAPTER FOCUS

The skin is the body's largest organ and forms a protective boundary between the internal environment and external world. Drugs are applied to the skin in the case of impaired skin integrity, and the skin is also being increasingly used as a route of drug administration for systemic purposes. The nurse must know the structure and function of the skin to administer drugs for both purposes.

LEARNING OBJECTIVES

- Describe the two layers of the skin.
- Differentiate among the three types of exocrine glands.
- Explain five major functions of the skin.
- Name three appendages of the skin.

▲ KEY TERMS

apocrine glands, p. 1163
dermis, p. 1163
eccrine glands, p. 1163
epidermis, p. 1162

exocrine glands, p. 1163
melanin, p. 1163
sebaceous glands, p. 1163

The skin (or integument) has been described as the largest organ in the body. In most disease states, medications are administered at a site that is distant from the target organ. In dermatology, medications can be applied directly to the target site; some skin conditions, however, may require systemic medications. Because skin functions are vital to survival and are also quite diverse, this chapter reviews the structure and function of the skin. Chapter 65 discusses issues related to hair, nails, and skin glands.

✳ What are the structural components of the skin?

The skin is made up of two layers: the epidermis and the dermis (Figure 64-1). The **epidermis,** or outer skin layer, consists of four strata or layers:

- *Stratum corneum (horny layer).* This layer contains dead outer cells that have been converted to keratin, a water-repellent protein. This layer forms a protective cover for the body; it will desquamate or shed and be replaced by new cells from the bottom layers.
- *Stratum lucidum or clear layer.* This area contains translucent flat cells; keratin is formed here.
- *Stratum granulosum or granular layer.* Granules are located in the cytoplasm of these cells. Cells die in this layer of skin.
- *Stratum germinativum.* This layer is divided into two layers; the top layer is the stratum spinosum, and the innermost layer is the stratum basale. The latter two names were devised to describe the cellular structure

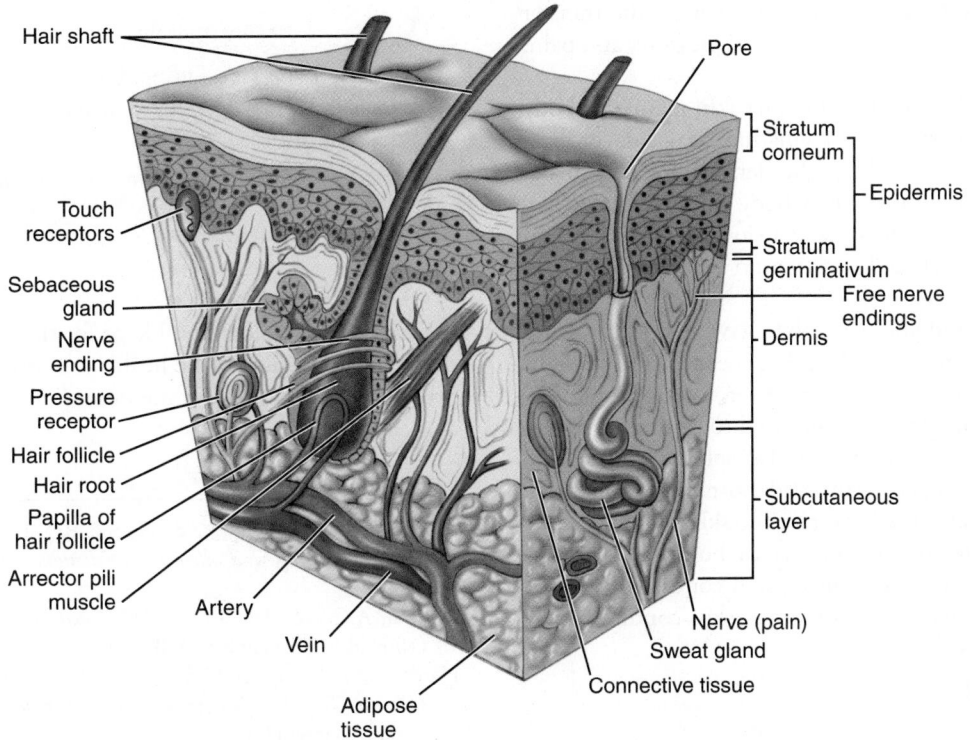

FIGURE 64-1 Structures of the skin.

Modified from Herlihy, B., & Maebius, N.K. (2003). *The human body in health and illness* (2nd ed.). Philadelphia: W.B. Saunders.

of the two layers; the stratum spinosum contains spine-like cells, whereas the stratum basale has column-shaped cells. The cells in the latter area germinate; they undergo cellular mitosis to generate new cells for the skin.

Melanocytes, which are responsible for synthesizing **melanin,** a skin color pigment that occurs naturally in the hair and skin, are also located deep in the stratum germinativum. The more melanin that is present, the deeper the brown skin color. Melanin also is a protective agent; it blocks ultraviolet rays, thus preventing injury to the underlying dermis and tissues.

The epidermis has no direct blood supply of its own; it is nourished only by diffusion. The **dermis** lies between the epidermis and subcutaneous fat. It is thicker than the epidermis, and it contains and provides skin support from its blood vessels, nerves, lymphatic tissue, and elastic and connective tissues. The two main divisions of the dermis are the papillary dermis and the reticular dermis. Sweat glands, sebaceous glands, and hair follicles originate in the reticular dermis, and their structures branch out in the papillary dermis.

Below the dermis layer is the hypodermis or subcutaneous layer, which contributes flexibility to the skin. Subcutaneous fat tissue is an area for thermal insulation, nutrition, and cushioning or padding.

The skin contains three types of **exocrine glands:** sebaceous, eccrine, and apocrine. These exocrine glands are multicellular glands that open on the surface of the skin through ducts in the epithelium.

Sebaceous glands are large, lipid-containing cells that produce sebum, the oil or film layer that covers the epidermis; these glands are especially abundant in the scalp, face, anus, and external ear. Sebum protects and lubricates the skin; it is not only water-repellent but also has some antiseptic effects. The sebaceous fluid travels by way of a short duct (sebaceous duct) to the hair follicles in the upper dermis. Therefore hair, which is located everywhere on the skin except the palms of the hands, soles of the feet, and mucous membrane tissues, is lubricated.

The **eccrine glands,** or sweat glands, are also widely distributed on the skin surface, including the soles and palms. These glands help to regulate body temperature by promoting cooling through evaporation of their secretion; they also help to prevent excessive skin dryness.

The **apocrine glands** are located mainly in the axillae, genital organs, and breast areas. They are odoriferous and are believed to represent scent or sex glands.

Normal skin is weakly acidic, with a pH of 4.5 to 5.5. This acid mantle is a protective mechanism, because microorganisms grow best at a pH 6.0 to 7.5. Infected areas of the skin usually have a higher pH.

✷ What are the functions of the skin?

The skin serves many functions in the body. The following are some of the major functions:

Protector The skin forms a protective covering for the entire body. It protects the internal organs and their environment from external forces. Thus it is a barrier against invasion by microorganisms and chemicals.

Organ of Sensation Nerve endings permit the transfer of stimuli sensations, such as heat, cold, pressure, and pain.

Body Temperature Regulator The skin maintains body temperature homeostasis by regulating heat loss or heat conservation. Blood vessels in the dermis area can dilate, and perspiration increases when body temperature is elevated. If the body temperature is below normal, the skin blood vessels constrict, and perspiration is decreased to conserve body heat.

Skin excretes fluid and electrolytes (sweat glands), stores fat, synthesizes vitamin D (when skin is exposed to sunlight or ultraviolet rays, 7-dehydrocholesterol—a steroid normally present in the skin—is converted to vitamin D_3), and provides a site for drug absorption. Fat-soluble vitamins (A, D, E, and K), estrogens, corticoid hormones, and some chemicals can be absorbed through the skin.

Skin contributes to the concept of body image and a feeling of well-being. A disfiguring skin condition can lead to emotional problems, and a chronic skin condition may also lead to depression.

Summary

The skin, the largest organ of the body, consists of two layers: the epidermis and the dermis. The pharmacologic activity of dermatologic agents occurs at the target site. The skin is also used as a route of administration for systemically acting drugs. Skin injuries, lesions, and disorders result in a

Critical Thinking Questions

- Johnny, 10 years of age, is outside playing ball on a hot summer day. How does his skin serve to regulate his body temperature?
- In what other ways does the skin function to protect the body?

variety of dermatologic problems for the client, and various nursing care issues for the health care provider. Major skin problems are discussed in the next chapter.

Bibliography

Anderson, D.M., Keith, J., & Novak, P.D. (Eds.) (2002). *Mosby's medical, nursing, and allied health dictionary* (6th ed.). St. Louis: Mosby.

Guyton, A.C., & Hall, J.E. (2000). *Textbook of medical physiology* (10th ed.). Philadelphia: W.B. Saunders.

Hardman, J.G., & Limbird, L.E. (Eds.). (2001). *Goodman and Gilman's The pharmacological basis of therapeutics* (10th ed.). New York: McGraw-Hill.

Herlihy, B., & Maebius, N.K. (2003). *The human body in health and illness* (2nd ed.). Philadelphia: W.B. Saunders.

McCance, K.L., & Huether, S.E. (2002). *Pathophysiology: The biological basis for disease in adults and children* (4th ed.). St. Louis: Mosby.

Thibodeau, G.A., & Patton, K.T. (2003). *Anatomy and physiology* (5th ed.). St. Louis: Mosby.

e-LEARNING SUPPLEMENTS

Student CD-ROM
- Final Exam questions
- NCLEX® Examination review questions
- Pharmacology animations
- Printable chapter summary

Evolve Website (http://evolve.elsevier.com/mckenry)
- Content updates, including information on new drugs
- WebLinks corresponding to this chapter

- Answers to the critical thinking questions in this chapter
- *Elsevier ePharmacology Update* newsletter
- Mosby's Drug Consult Internet Edition
- Supplemental and reference information

DERMATOLOGIC DRUGS

CHAPTER FOCUS

The integumentary system is the largest organ system in the body. As such, the skin performs a number of vital functions, such as protecting internal structures from mechanical and chemical damage, preventing entry of infectious agents, providing protection against ultraviolet radiation from the sun, preventing dehydration, regulating temperature, producing vitamin D, and detecting stimuli. Additionally, the skin often contributes to our definition of who we are through color, aging processes, scarring, and other conditions. Clients with skin disorders may experience a disturbed body image along with their physical conditions. The nurse needs to be not only skilled at various procedures used to treat skin disorders but also sensitive to the client as a whole.

LEARNING OBJECTIVES

- State the principles of skin absorption.
- Describe different types of lesions and some conditions associated with each.
- Identify common drug-induced dermatologic conditions.
- Identify life-threatening, drug-induced skin eruptions.
- Identify the general goals of dermatologic therapy.
- Describe general dermatologic preparations, including baths, soaps, solutions, lotions, and cleansers, and clinical indications for their use.
- Implement the nursing management of clients receiving therapy with topical antiinfectives, antiinflammatory corticosteroids, topical anesthetics, and acne and burn products.
- Describe ectoparasitic diseases and the use of topical ectoparasiticidal drugs in their treatment.

▲ KEY TERMS

ectoparasites, p. 1192
keratolytics, p. 1190
sun protection factor (SPF), p. 1177

☒⚑ KEY DRUGS

isotretinoin, p. 1185
permethrin, p. 1192
silver sulfadiazine, p. 1188

✳ P.G. is a 32-year-old female who presents to her primary care provider with a skin eruption on her lower arms. She complains of intense itching, which has been present for the past 2 days. The nurse observes erythematous, vesicular lesions in a linear pattern on the inner aspect of both forearms and both her hands.

✳ **How do dermatologic conditions present?**
Reactions or disorders of the skin are manifested by symptoms such as itching, pain, or tingling, and by signs such as swelling, redness, papules, pustules, blisters, and hives. Common dermatologic disorders in the United States and Canada include acne vulgaris (cystic acne and acne scars), atopic dermatitis, eczema, folliculitis, fungus infections,

herpes simplex, lichen simplex chronicus, psoriasis, seborrheic dermatitis, verruca (warts), and vitiligo. The nurse is often the first health team member to observe and assess these conditions. The nurse should also be familiar with the dermal effects of vesicants used in chemical warfare or as a weapon in a terrorist attack (see the Pharmacologic Issues in an Age of Terrorism box below.)

A skin reaction that makes the client uncomfortable or has an unsightly appearance may be due to a drug sensitivity, allergy, infection, emotional conflict, genetic disease (e.g., atopic eczema, psoriasis), hormonal imbalance, or degenerative disease. Sometimes the cause is unknown; in such cases treatment may be empiric in the hope that the right remedy is found.

Dermatologic diagnosis includes physical assessment, personal and family medical history, drug history (includ-ing over-the-counter [OTC] medications), and laboratory tests, biopsy, and cytodiagnosis.

When the nature of the lesion has been established, its characteristics should be defined according to size, shape, surface, and color (Box 65-1).

The next step is to discover the distribution of the condition; sometimes the diagnosis can be made from the distribution alone. However, a disease should not be ruled out as a possible diagnosis based on lack of the usual pattern of distribution. For example, psoriasis is commonly found on the extensors, but occasionally it is seen as a solitary lesion in the external ear. A basal cell carcinoma is most common on the face, but occasionally it occurs on the trunk. On the other hand, rosacea attacks only those areas of the face that flush.

Box 65-2 is a summary of common drug-induced dermatologic conditions. Some may even be life-threatening.

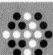 **Pharmacologic Issues in an Age of Terrorism**

Vesicants

Vesicants are agents capable of inducing blisters and include mustards, and lewisite. Chlorine and phosgene are primarily considered pulmonary toxins (see the Pharmacologic Issues in an Age of Terrorism box on p. 711 in Chapter 37) but may also induce blisters.

Mustards

Sulfur and nitrogen mustards were used extensively in World War I, and more recently were reportedly used by Iraq against Iran. Mustards are oily liquids, have a low volatility, and are heavier than water. Mustard becomes a solid at 58° F.

Presentation

Mustards have many damaging effects to tissue. Skin, eye, and pulmonary toxicity are all common with mustard exposure, and systemic effects on bone marrow, the GI tract, CNS, and lymphatic tissue can occur. Doses as low as 10 micrograms can form blisters, and as little as 5 mL of undiluted liquid mustard can be lethal. Typical effects on each body system are noted below:

- Skin: blistering, tissue sloughing
- Eyes: range from conjunctivitis to edema, corneal ulcers, and blindness
- Pulmonary: upper airway pain, hoarseness, bronchospasm, hemorrhagic edema
- GI: nausea, vomiting, abdominal pain, diarrhea within the first 24 hours, necrosis and bleeding noted over time.
- CNS: lethargy and euphoria are noted with lower exposures. Higher exposures can produce seizures, coma or death.

Management

The principles of management include limiting or preventing further exposure, maintaining airway patency, administering analgesics for pain, and preventing infection. Fluid replacement is often required because fluid loss through damaged skin is extensive. Treatment of skin lesions is similar to the management of thermal burns. Hydrating eye drops may improve eye symptoms in mild cases. Pulmonary manifestations may require bronchodilators and oxygen, and in more severe cases, intubation and respiratory support. Atropine, antiemetics, and fluid/electrolyte replacement are often required for GI symptoms.

Lewisite

Lewisite is an arsenic compound that can produce blisters on exposure to tissue and systemically may contribute to arsenic poisoning. There have been no confirmed battlefield uses of Lewisite.

Presentation

Lewisite produces immediate local and systemic toxicity. Lewisite produces an immediate stinging pain on contact. In addition to dermal and mucous membrane toxicity, systemically absorbed lewisite results in increased capillary permeability, hypotension, and shock. Lewisite is likely to produce immediate blepharospasm, but the extent of ocular exposure and toxicity unknown.

Management

Management is similar to mustard exposure. Immediate decontamination is more critical with lewisite because its toxic effects are noted more quickly than with mustards. Topical application of 2,3-dimercaptopropanol (also known as British Anti-Lewisite or BAL) inactivates lewisite immediately.

Data from Evison, D., Hinsley, D., & Rice, P. (2002). Chemical weapons. *British Medical Journal, 324*(72333), 332–335; Emergency Preparedness and Response: Centers for Disease Control and Prevention. Retrieved February 22, 2005, from http://www.bt.cdc.gov; and Stokes, E., Gilbert-Palmer, D., Skorga, P., Young, C., & Persell, D. (2004). Chemical agents of terrorism: Preparing nurse practitioners. *Nurse Practitioner, 29*(5), 30-39.

BOX 65-1 TYPES OF LESIONS AND CONDITIONS ASSOCIATED WITH THEM

Macule—flat; nonpalpable; circumscribed; less than 1 cm in diameter; brown, red, purple, white, or tan in color
Examples: Freckles; flat moles; rubella; rubeola; drug eruptions

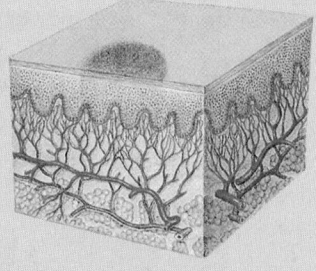

Vesicle—elevated; circumscribed; superficial; filled with serous fluid; less than 1 cm in diameter
Examples: Blister varicella

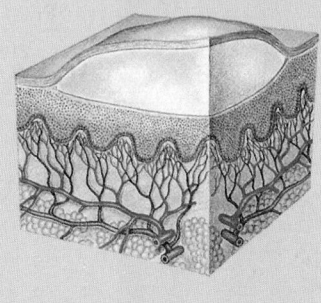

Papule—elevated; palpable; firm; circumscribed; less than 1 cm in diameter; brown, red, pink, tan, or bluish red in color
Examples: Warts; drug-related eruptions; pigmented nevi; eczema

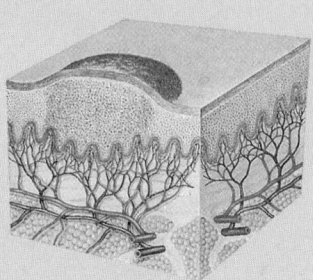

Bulla—vesicle greater than 1 cm in diameter
Examples: Blister; pemphigus vulgaris

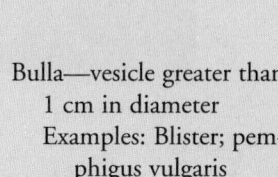

Plaque—elevated; flat topped; firm; rough; superficial papule greater than 1 cm in diameter, may be coalesced papules
Example: Psoriasis; seborrheic and actinic keratoses; eczema

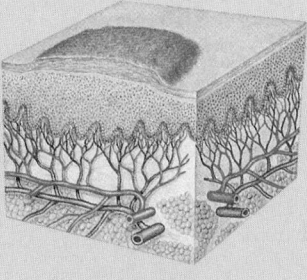
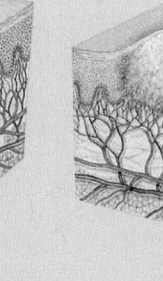

Pustule—elevated; superficial; similar to vesicle but filled with purulent fluid
Examples: Impetigo; acne; variola; herpes zoster

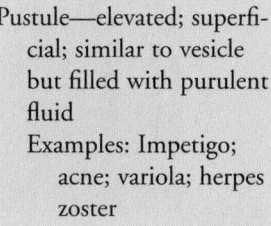

Wheal—elevated, irregular-shaped area of cutaneous edema; solid, transient, changing variable diameter; pale pink in color
Examples: Urticaria; insect bites

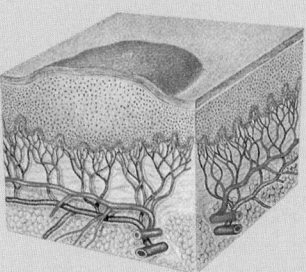

Cyst—elevated; circumscribed; palpable; encapsulated; filled with liquid or semi-solid material
Example: Sebaceous cyst

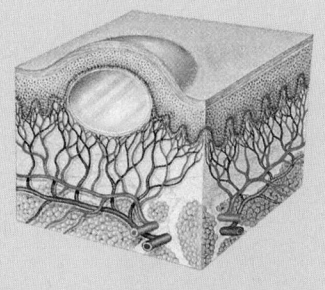

Nodule—elevated; firm; circumscribed; palpable; deeper in dermis than papule; 1 to 2 cm in diameter
Examples: Erythema nodosum; lipomas

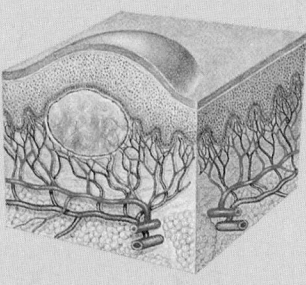

Scale—heaped-up keratinized cells; flaky exfoliation; irregular; thick or thin; dry or oily; varied size; silver, white, or tan in color
Examples: Psoriasis; exfoliative dermatitis

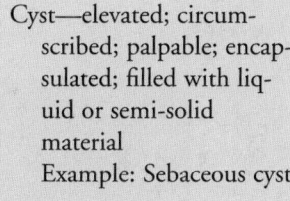

Tumor—elevated; solid; may or may not be clearly demarcated; greater than 2 cm in diameter; may or may not vary from skin color
Example: Neoplasms

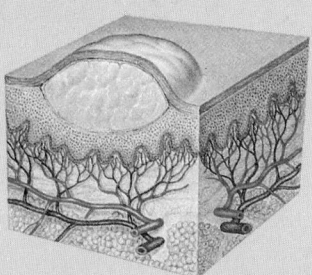

Lichenification—rough, thickened epidermis; accentuated skin markings because of rubbing or irritation; often involves flexor aspect of extremity
Example: Chronic dermatitis

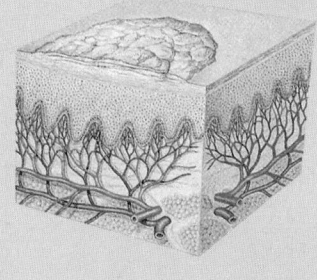
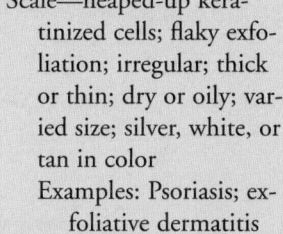
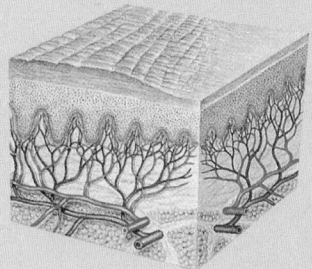

From Seidel, H.M., Ball, J.W., Dains, J.E., & Benedict, G.W. (2003). *Mosby's guide to physical examination* (5th ed.). St. Louis: Mosby.

Box 65-2 Common Drug-Induced Dermatologic Conditions

Acneform Reaction

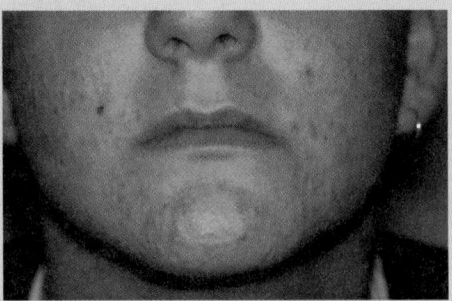

From Lemmi, F., & Lemmi C. (2000). *Physical assessment findings CD-ROM*. Philadelphia: W.B. Saunders.

Alopecia

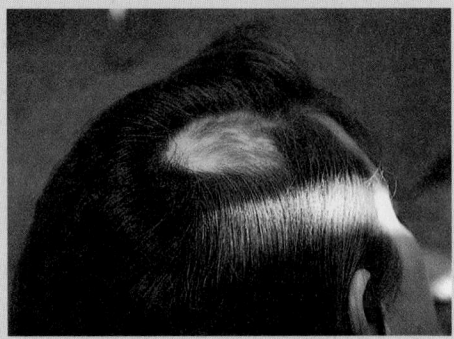

From Goldstein, B.G., & Goldstein, A.O. (1997). *Practical dermatology*. (2nd ed.). St. Louis: Mosby.

Lichenoid Reactions

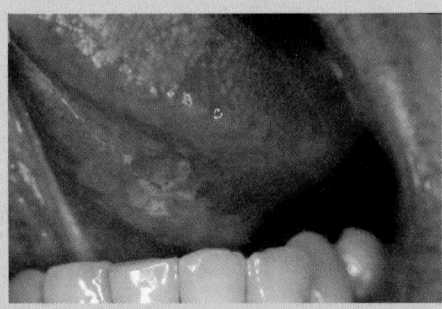

From Lemmi, F., & Lemmi C. (2000). *Physical assessment findings CD-ROM*. Philadelphia: W.B. Saunders.

Contact Dermatitis

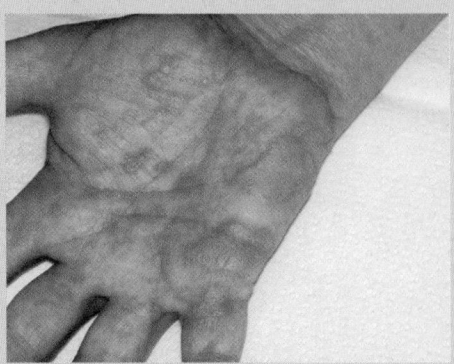

From Lemmi, F., & Lemmi C. (2000). *Physical assessment findings CD-ROM*. Philadelphia: W.B. Saunders.

Purpura

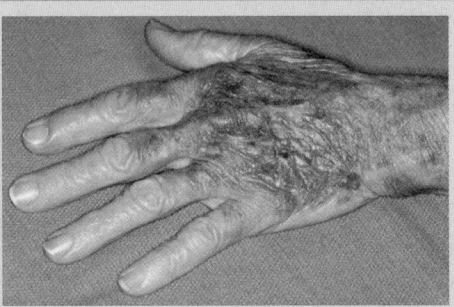

From Lemmi, F., & Lemmi C. (2000). *Physical assessment findings CD-ROM*. Philadelphia: W.B. Saunders.

Morbilliform Reactions

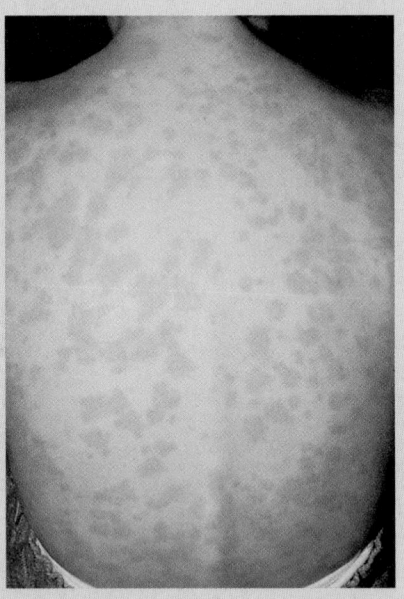

From Zitelli, B.J., & Davis, H.W. (2002). *Atlas of pediatric physical diagnosis*. (4th ed.). St. Louis: Mosby.

Urticaria

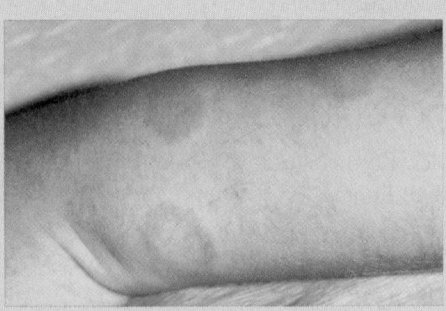

From Lemmi, F., & Lemmi C. (2000). *Physical assessment findings CD-ROM*. Philadelphia: W.B. Saunders.

BOX 65-2 COMMON DRUG-INDUCED DERMATOLOGIC CONDITIONS—CONT'D

FIXED DRUG ERUPTIONS

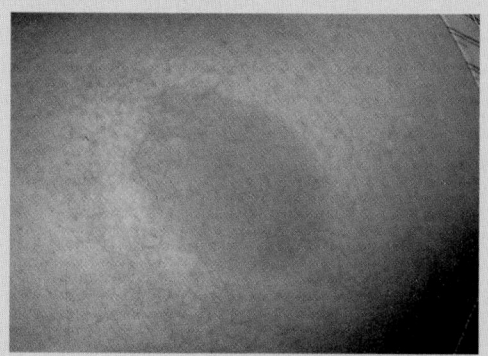

From Zitelli, B.J., & Davis, H.W. (2002). *Atlas of pediatric physical diagnosis.* (4th ed.). St. Louis: Mosby.

PHOTOSENSITIZERS

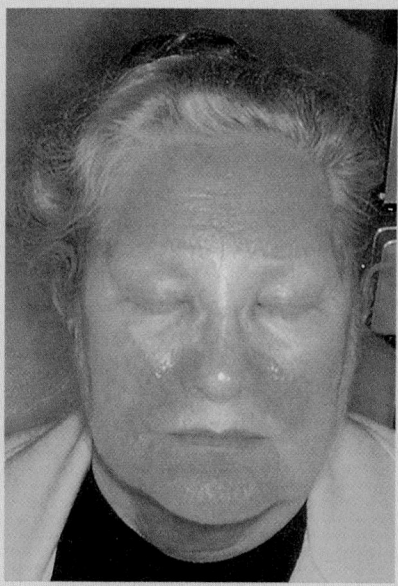

From Goldstein, B.G., & Goldstein, A.O. (1997). *Practical dermatology.* (2nd ed.). St. Louis: Mosby. (Courtesy Marshall Guill, MD.)

See Table 65-1 for the drugs most commonly involved in life-threatening, drug-induced skin eruptions.

The nurse always needs to be cognizant of a client's drug history and current therapy to correlate such lesions and sequelae with the appropriate cause; simply discontinuing a particular drug can often resolve a complicated dermatologic problem or sequelae of unknown origin.

✸ **What skin disorders observed in clinical practice respond to drug therapy?**

Many common skin disorders are treated with various topical or systemic therapies. See Table 65-2 for some dermatologic conditions for which drugs may be indicated.

✸ **P.G. is interviewed by her health care provider and indicates that she has not been walking in the woods. However, her puppy had broken his leash near the woods. When she had found him, she picked him up and carried him home. The provider explains that poison ivy contains an oil that readily coats the fur of animals, which explains why people often get the dermatitis from their outdoor pets. P.G. is diagnosed with poison ivy contact dermatitis.**

✸ **What nursing management issues are involved in the treatment of P.G.'s dermatologic conditions?**

Assessment Both a thorough history and an objective examination of the dermatologic condition are essential for the initial assessment and ongoing evaluation of care. Elicit information regarding the onset of the problem,

changes in the condition since onset, specific cause if known (or if not, recent exposures to new or different activities that might provide a clue about cause), client-determined or prescriber-prescribed factors that may have alleviated the condition, and the P.G.'s psychologic response to the problem. Accomplish direct inspection and observation with a good light source. Palpation may be necessary, particularly when assessing dark skin, in which erythema may not be noticeable but warmth and edema can be determined. Observations should be systematic and thorough, and the left side should be compared with the right. Descriptions need to be specific, using the metric system for measurement, and recorded. It may be helpful to take a photograph of the affected area as a baseline observation. Recorded changes will determine P.G.'s progress toward the desired outcome of resolution of the dermatologic problem.

Nursing Diagnosis While P.G. is using dermatologic agents, she is at risk for the following nursing diagnoses: impaired skin integrity; impaired comfort (pain, burning, or itching of the affected areas); risk for infection related to open skin areas; self-care deficits related to the location of the affected areas; deficient knowledge related to new or altered dermatologic therapy; and disturbed body image related to perceived and actual disfigurement of the affected areas.

Planning While on dermatologic therapy, P.G. will:
• Experience relief from the symptoms of her disorder (e.g., itching, pain, erythema, and vesicles).

TABLE 65-1 LIFE-THREATENING DRUG INDUCED SKIN ERUPTIONS

Skin Eruption	Description	Drugs Involved
Exfoliative dermatitis 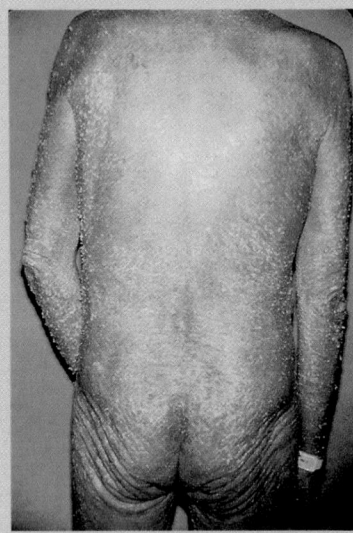 From Goldstein, B.G., & Goldstein, A.O. (1997). *Practical dermatology.* (2nd ed.). St. Louis: Mosby. (Courtesy Department of Dermatology, University of North Carolina at Chapel Hill.)	Entire surface of skin is red and scaly and eventually sloughs off. Hair and nails may also be affected. Eruption may take weeks or months to resolve after causative agent is stopped. If not resolved, it may be fatal.	barbiturates, carbamazepine, demeclocycline, furosemide, gold, griseofulvin, penicillin, phenothiazines, phenytoin, sulfonamides, tetracyclines
Stevens-Johnson syndrome (erythema multiforme) 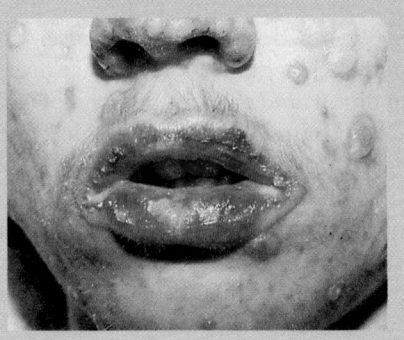 From Zitelli, B.J., & Davis, H.W. (2002). *Atlas of pediatric physical diagnosis.* (4th ed.). St. Louis: Mosby.	Severe form that involves widespread eruptions or lesions, usually on the face, neck, arms, legs, hands, and feet. May also involve mucosa, and may produce fever and malaise. Syndrome may last for months and is life threatening.	May result from the use of many drugs, especially carbamazepine, penicillin, phenytoin, sulfonamides, tetracyclines
Lupus erythematosus 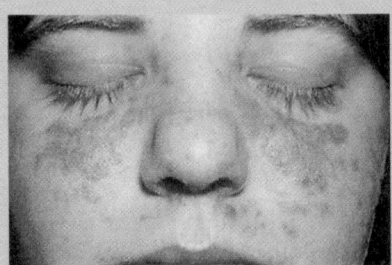 From Goldstein, B.G., & Goldstein, A.O. (1997). *Practical dermatology.* (2nd ed.). St. Louis: Mosby. (Courtesy Department of Dermatology, University of North Carolina at Chapel Hill.)	Erythematous rash that may be flat or elevated (butterfly) on cheek (malar), and across nose. Joint swelling and pain, rash, oral ulcers, serositis, renal, hematologic, pulmonary, and other systems may be affected. Condition is reversible when drug is stopped.	hydantoins, hydralazine, isoniazid, procainamide, quinidine, trimethadione

TABLE 65-2 DERMATOLOGIC CONDITIONS THAT MAY RESPOND TO DRUG THERAPY

NONINFECTIOUS DERMATOLOGIC CONDITIONS

Eczema and dermatitis are noninfectious inflammatory dermatoses. Contact dermatitis has clinical features that include a skin rash with eczema (red, thick, crusty, fissured, suppurating area) in various stages. The causes may be from contact with a primary irritant (acids, oils, soaps) in the environment, home, or work place or from a delayed allergic reaction (as seen with poison ivy contact).

Eczema

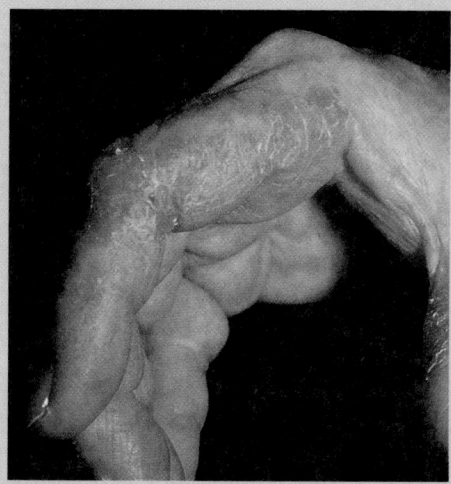

From Goldstein, B.G., & Goldstein, A.O. (1997). *Practical dermatology*. (2nd ed.). St. Louis: Mosby.

Contact Dermatitis

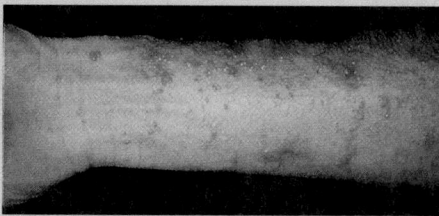

From Goldstein, B.G., & Goldstein, A.O. (1997). *Practical dermatology*. (2nd ed.). St. Louis: Mosby.

Atopic Dermatitis

Atopic dermatitis appears as general eczema dermatitis, usually on the flexor body surfaces; it has genetic associations with hay fever or asthma.

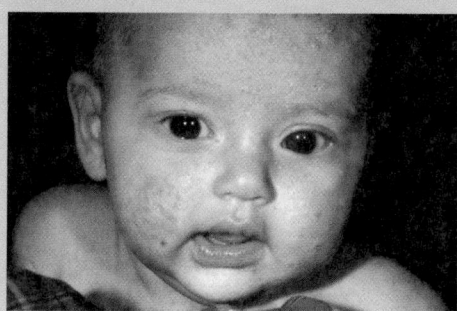

From Lemmi, F., & Lemmi C. (2000). *Physical assessment findings CD-ROM*. Philadelphia: W.B. Saunders.

Seborrheic Dermatitis

Seborrheic dermatitis often appears on the scalp, eyebrows, ears, or sternum as a brown to red scaly rash.

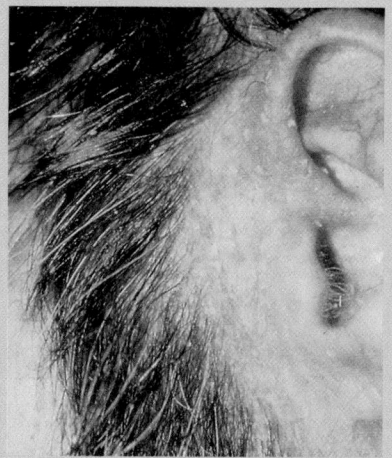

From Goldstein, B.G., & Goldstein, A.O. (1997). *Practical dermatology*. (2nd ed.). St. Louis: Mosby. (Courtesy Department of Dermatology, University of North Carolina at Chapel Hill.)

Stasis Dermatitis

Stasis dermatitis often preceding a venous stasis ulcer is found on the lower legs secondary to venous stasis and poor vascularity; it is brown and eczematous in appearance.

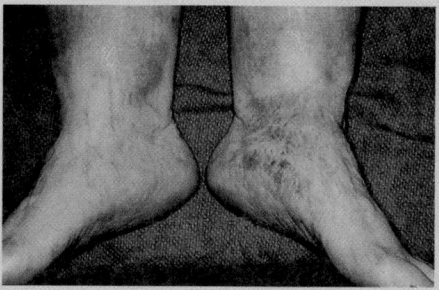

From Goldstein, B.G., & Goldstein, A.O. (1997). *Practical dermatology*. (2nd ed.). St. Louis: Mosby. (Courtesy Department of Dermatology, University of North Carolina at Chapel Hill.)

Continued

TABLE 65-2 DERMATOLOGIC CONDITIONS THAT MAY RESPOND TO DRUG THERAPY—CONT'D

NONINFECTIOUS DERMATOLOGIC CONDITIONS—CONT'D

Papulosquamous eruptions are noninfectious inflammatory dermatoses that include urticaria (hives), psoriasis, pityriasis rosea, lichen planus, and exfoliative dermatitis. Acute urticaria appears as an insidious, itchy erythematous wheal resulting from an allergen. Chronic urticaria appears as a large hive without the sensation of itch or pruritus, and it is often accompanied by angioneurotic edema.

Psoriasis

Psoriasis often appears as erythematous plaques and orange-red-brown lesions covered with silvery scales. Psoriasis is often found on the scalp and extensor surfaces of the limbs and neck. The nails often become thick and irregular.

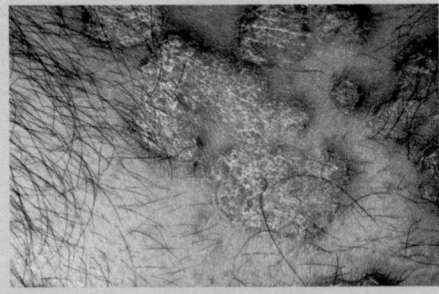

From Lemmi, F., & Lemmi C. (2000). *Physical assessment findings CD-ROM*. Philadelphia: W.B. Saunders.

Pityriasis Rosea

Pityriasis rosea is a self-limited, oval salmon-colored patch that follows the axis of the skin cleavage lines. The major patches appear on the trunk, and smaller scales appear on the peripheral areas.

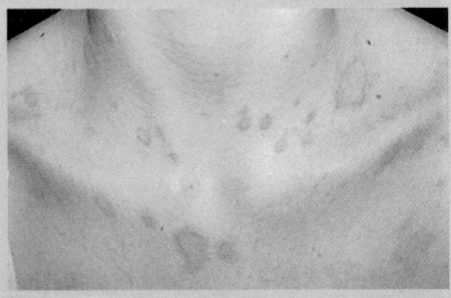

From Goldstein, B.G., & Goldstein, A.O. (1997). *Practical dermatology*. (2nd ed.). St. Louis: Mosby. (Courtesy Department of Dermatology, University of North Carolina at Chapel Hill.)

INFECTIOUS INFLAMMATORY DERMATOSES (VIRAL)

Infectious inflammatory dermatoses include viral diseases (verruca [wart], herpes simplex, varicella zoster/chickenpox, bacterial diseases (impetigo, folliculitis, furuncle [boil]), and fungal diseases. Herpes simplex and infectious inflammatory dermatoses appear as vesicles with an inflamed base and have an incubation period of up to 2 weeks in the primary infection. Late antibody development occurs. The herpes virus type 1 affects the skin and the oral cavity, whereas herpes virus type 2 affects the skin of neonates and genital mucosa. A recurrent infection is a reactivation of the older infection or new infection; antibodies appear early.

Herpes Simplex

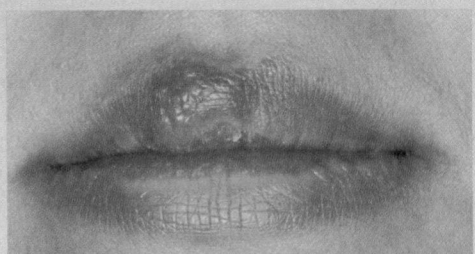

From Lemmi, F., & Lemmi C. (2000). *Physical assessment findings CD-ROM*. Philadelphia: W.B. Saunders.

Herpes Zoster

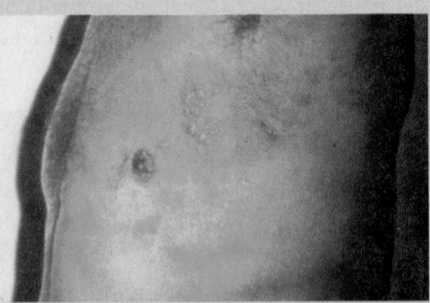

From Lemmi, F., & Lemmi C. (2000). *Physical assessment findings CD-ROM*. Philadelphia: W.B. Saunders.

TABLE 65-2 DERMATOLOGIC CONDITIONS THAT MAY RESPOND TO DRUG THERAPY—CONT'D

INFECTIOUS INFLAMMATORY DERMATOSES (FUNGAL)

Fungal diseases, which include tinea or dermatophytosis, appear in the following various clinical classifications: tinea capitis (caused by either a *Trichophyton* or *Microsporum* fungal infection in children or adults); tinea corporis (or *Microsporum* in children; *Trichophyton* in adults); tinea cruris *(Epidermophyton* or *Trichophyton)*; and tinea pedis; onychomycosis *(Trichophyton)*; and tinea versicolor *(Malassezia furfur)*. Tinea or dermatophytosis often appears as a scaly, erythematous circular lesion. Tinea versicolor appears as a brown discoloration. Hair breakage is seen in tinea capitis or tinea barbae. The client with onychomycosis has thick, discolored nails.

Tinea Pedis

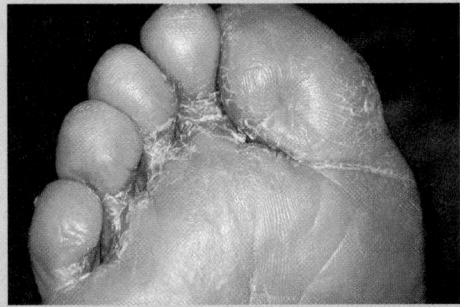

From Lemmi, F., & Lemmi C. (2000). *Physical assessment findings CD-ROM*. Philadelphia: W.B. Saunders.

Onychomycosis

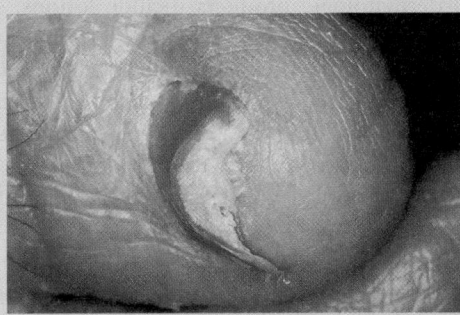

From Lemmi, F., & Lemmi C. (2000). *Physical assessment findings CD-ROM*. Philadelphia: W.B. Saunders.

Tinea Versicolor

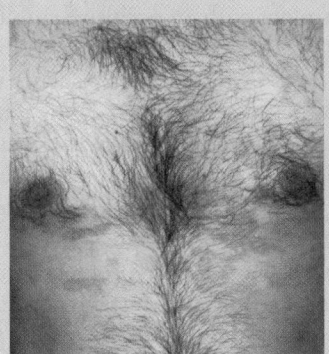

From Lemmi, F. & Lemmi C. (2000). *Physical assessment findings CD-ROM*. Philadelphia: W.B. Saunders.

Tinea Capitis

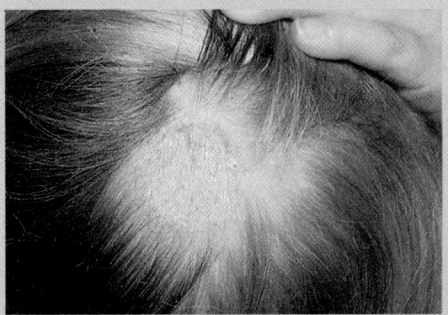

From Goldstein, B.G., & Goldstein, A.O. (1997). *Practical dermatology.* (2nd ed.). St. Louis: Mosby. (Courtesy Department of Dermatology, Medical College of Georgia.)

Tinea Corporis

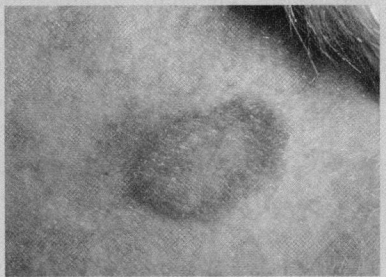

From Goldstein, B.G., & Goldstein, A.O. (1997). *Practical dermatology.* (2nd ed.). St. Louis: Mosby.

Tinea Cruris

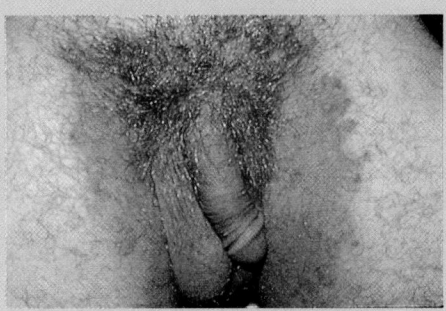

From Goldstein, B.G., & Goldstein, A.O. (1997). *Practical dermatology.* (2nd ed.). St. Louis: Mosby. (Courtesy Department of Dermatology, University of North Carolina at Chapel Hill.)

- Effectively manage her regimen, including avoidance of the cause of the skin disorder (if possible), medication compliance, and proper hygiene of the affected area.

Implementation

Monitoring Observation and, if required, palpation, are essential in evaluating P.G.'s progress toward resolving the dermatologic condition. Monitor and document the description of the dermatologic condition, including its area, body part involvement, depth, surface appearance, color, drainage, sensation, healing, and any systemic effects such as fever. Also document the effectiveness of the prescribed therapy.

Intervention Follow the manufacturer's instructions in detail for application of the various preparations used for dermatologic conditions. Additionally, some conditions may be severe enough to require supportive therapy that is more systemic in nature. See also Box 65-3 regarding skin absorption principles of dermatologic drug therapy.

Education Because the etiology of P.G.'s condition is known, counsel her on avoiding exposure to the causative agent to prevent future episodes (unless the condition is genetic). Because the cause of P.G.'s contact dermatitis is known, exposure to poison ivy is treated with cleansing of the exposed skin with isopropyl (rubbing) alcohol, washing with water, and only then showering with soap and water. Soap is not used before this point because it will pick up urushiol (the noxious ingredient in the sap) and spread it around (U.S. Food and Drug Administration [FDA], 1996). Advise her to maintain good hygiene of the unaf-

fected areas of the body and to cleanse the affected area only in the prescribed fashion. Instruct her not to touch the affected areas and to dress to avoid or minimize contact with the involved area. Apply only prescribed preparations to the area and follow through with therapy, even when the improvement may not be immediate. Avoid exposing the involved areas to direct sunlight unless advised as part of therapy. Instruct P.G. to report any adverse effects to the prescriber.

Evaluation The expected outcome for therapy with dermatologic agents is that P.G.'s lesions will decrease in size and eventually disappear without adverse effects of her drug therapy. P.G. will state the importance of avoidance of poison ivy and appropriate measures to take if she does have contact.

•   •   •

As previously stated, so many dermatologic products are available that it would be difficult to discuss all of them in this chapter. For the sake of simplicity, this chapter discusses three selected groups of dermatologic products: general products, prophylactic agents, and therapeutic agents.

General Dermatologic Preparations

General dermatologic products include lotions, solutions, baths, soaps, wet dressings, and soaks. Prophylactic agents include sunscreens, protectives, and antiseptics and disinfectants. Therapeutic agents include antiinfectives, antiinflammatory corticosteroids, keratolytic agents, acne products, stimulants and irritants, topical anesthetics, products for second- and third-degree burns, antiaging products, and ectoparasiticidal topical drugs.

✴ **How do dermatologic formulations affect response?** Many dermatologic preparations are available to treat the numerous and common skin disorders. Certain ointments, creams, powders, or specific vehicles often provide a desired effect without the addition of an active ingredient. For example, an ointment with an occlusive emollient effect (e.g., petrolatum base is desired for clients with the dry, scaly skin found in psoriasis or dry eczema. Clients with a moist or dry skin condition may receive a cooling emollient preparation that is also moisturizing, such as a cream formulation.

Clients with an acute inflammation that is weeping or oozing often need a drying and soothing lotion, such as a saline solution, aluminum acetate solution, or calamine lotion. A lichenified, oozing skin problem (eczema) may need a protective and drying agent, such as coal tar paste, Lassar's paste, or zinc compound paste. If the skin problem is sore, wet, and located on an elbow or knee, a dusting powder such as talcum or starch may be appropriate to reduce friction and help to dry the area.

Specific formulations can be classified in a number of ways. This section refers to single and combination formu-

---

BOX 65-3 PRINCIPLES OF SKIN ABSORPTION

- Keratin in the outer skin layer provides a waterproof barrier. To enhance drug absorption, the epidermis (keratin skin layer) needs to be hydrated. Therefore some medications are placed under an occlusive dressing (e.g., plastic wrap) or administered in an occlusive type of ointment (petroleum jelly), because both trap and prevent the loss of water (sweat) from the skin, thus increasing epidermis hydration.
- Fat- or lipid-soluble drugs are better absorbed through the skin than water-soluble drugs. In specific body areas, the skin is very thin (e.g., eyelids, scrotum area, or the skin of a child) or very thick. The palms of the hands and soles of the feet are nearly impenetrable by topical agents.
- Products with alcohol content may be administered for drying effects.
- Corticosteroid products thin the skin, and many are contraindicated for the face, groin, and axillae. Fluorinated corticosteroids should not be used for these areas. Hydrocortisone is generally recommended if a corticosteroid is necessary.

lations used as bath preparations, cleansers, soaps, solutions and lotions, emollients (including ointments, emulsions, and creams), skin protectants, wet dressings and soaks, and rubs and liniments.

Baths Baths may be used to cleanse the skin, medicate, or reduce temperature. The usual method of cleansing the skin by using soap and water may not be tolerated in skin diseases. In some cases even water is not tolerated; in such cases inert oils must be substituted. Persons with dry skin should bathe less frequently than those with oily skin. Frequent bathing tends to stimulate oil production, causing oily skin to remain oily. It is possible to keep the skin clean without a daily bath. Overbathing can cause the skin to become dry and itchy. Explain to clients that bathing dries the skin through the evaporation of water.

However, bathing also hydrates the skin, when moisturizer is applied immediately after bathing before the water has a chance to evaporate (within 3 minutes), thus retaining the hydration and keeping the skin soft and flexible. Pat the skin dry before moisturizer application. Daily bathing is possible if the 3-minute moisturizing rule is followed. Use of unscented moisturizers, such as an ointment like petrolatum or a cream, is ideal, whereas lotions are less effective emollients (Tofte & Hanifin, 2001).

To render baths soothing in irritative conditions, oatmeal, starch, or gelatin may be added—usually 1 to 2 ounces per gallon of water. Oils such as Alpha-Keri and Aveeno Oilated Oatmeal (in a proportion of 1 ounce to a tub of water) decrease the drying effect of water and help to relieve the itching of sensitive, xerotic skin. A lubricating topical medication or bland emollient should be applied immediately after the bath while skin is still moist; this increases absorption and hydration.

Soaps Ordinary soap (the sodium salt of palmitic, oleic, or stearic acids alone or in a mixture) is made by saponifying fats or oils with alkalies. The oil used for castile soap is supposed to be olive oil; some soaps are made with coconut oil. The consistency of the soap depends on the major acid and alkali used.

Although all soaps are relatively alkaline, an excess of free alkali or acid is a potential source of skin irritation. Medicated soaps contain antiseptics, but soaps per se are antiseptic only to the degree that they mechanically clean the skin. Many people believe that soap and water are bad for the complexion; this belief is erroneous, because clean skin helps to promote healthy skin. The soap used in maintaining clean skin should be mild and contain a minimum of irritating materials. Perfumed or medicated soaps may be harmful if the skin is extra sensitive to soap products or if the soap is not adequately rinsed off the skin, stimulates excess production of natural skin oils, or dries the skin excessively. Soaps are irritating to mucous membranes; they are used in enemas mainly because of this action.

Solutions and Lotions Soothing preparations may be liquids that carry an insoluble powder or suspension, or

they may be mild acid or alkaline solutions, such as acetic acid or aluminum acetate used as wet dressings and soaks. Bismuth salts and starch are also commonly used for their soothing effect. Aluminum acetate solution (Burow's Solution, Modified Burow's Solution) is a mild antiseptic for acute inflammation and poison ivy, insect bites or athlete's feet. It is diluted with 10 to 40 parts of water before application. Acetic acid 1% to 2.5% is bacteriostatic for certain gram-negative bacteria (e.g., *Pseudomonas aeruginosa*), otitis externa, *P. intertrigo*. Vinegar is 5% acetic acid; make a 1% solution by adding one half cup of vinegar (white or brown) to 1 pint of water (Habif, 2004).

Calamine lotion contains calamine, zinc oxide, bentonite magma, and glycerin in a calcium hydroxide solution. It is a soothing lotion used for the dermatitis caused by conditions such as poison ivy, insect bites, and prickly heat.

Cleansers Cleansers are usually free of soap or are modified soap products recommended for clients with sensitive, dry, or irritated skin or for those who have had a previous reaction to a soap product. These cleansers are less irritating, may contain an emollient substance, and may also have been adjusted to a slightly acidic or neutral pH. Included in this category are Aveeno Cleansing Bar, Lowila Cake, and others.

Emollients Emollients are fatty or oily substances that soften or soothe irritated skin and mucous membranes. An emollient is often used as a vehicle for other medicinal substances. Emollients can be further divided into four distinct types: ointments, water in oil emulsions, oil in water emulsions, and creams.

Ointments are typically petrolatum or mineral oil based, are greasy and provide a high degree of occlusion or protection. The classic ointment is petroleum jelly (Vaseline), and a number of topical agents are prepared in an ointment base. Lanolin, derived from wool fatty acids and cholesterol, is sometimes used as an ointment base, but its use may increase risk for hypersensitivity reactions. Ointments are particularly good for keeping moisture near the skin and are often used for dry, brittle lesions. The occlusive nature of ointments increases drug penetration into skin for drugs that are delivered in an ointment base. Many clients, however, do not find ointments cosmetically appealing, as they stain clothing and bed linen.

Water in oil emulsions are preparations in which very small beads of a water based product are evenly dispersed in an oil base. They tend to be greasy, but are more appealing to clients than pure petrolatum based ointments.

Oil in water emulsions are similar, with very small beads of oil dispersed in a water base; they are less slippery and also less occlusive than ointments or water in oil products.

Creams are the least occlusive of the four types of emollients listed here. They are a very common vehicle, are appealing to clients in that they are not overly greasy, can be rubbed into the skin and tend to disappear. They are less occlusive, and are good choices as a drug delivery vehicle when the treated area has some degree of moisture.

Skin Protectants Skin protectants are used to coat minor skin irritations or to protect the person's skin from chemical irritants. There are several products currently available for use in hospitals and extended care facilities to prevent skin breakdown from irritants such as urine or stool. These products are available in the form of wipes, barrier films, swabs, and sprays. Small prep pads that resemble alcohol wipes can be rubbed on the skin for their protective function before affixing tape or ostomy bags, thus reducing the chance of skin breakdown. Another protectant less commonly used in hospitals today is tincture of benzoin (Aerozoin, Benzoin, Benzoin Compound).

Wet Dressings and Soaks Wet dressings and soaks include some of the preparations discussed under Solutions and Lotions. These liquids are either a wet or an astringent type of dressing used to treat inflammatory skin conditions such as insect bites and poison ivy. Aluminum acetate solution, Domeboro Powder, and others are available for this use. The temperature of the compress solution should be cool when an antiinflammatory effect is desired and tepid when the purpose is to debride an infected, crusted lesion. Avoid covering the compress; covering a wet compress with a towel or plastic inhibits evaporation, promotes maceration, and increases skin temperature, which facilitates bacterial growth (Habif, 2004).

Rubs and Liniments Rubs and liniments are indicated for pain relief for intact skin. Pain caused by muscle aches, neuralgia, arthritis, and sprains are the types of pain that usually respond to these products. The ingredients in the preparations may include a counterirritant (e.g., camphor, oil of cloves, methyl salicylate), an antiseptic (chloroxylenol, eugenol, thymol), a local anesthetic (benzocaine), or analgesics (salicylate-containing substances). Examples from this category include Aspercreme, Ben-Gay, and Icy Hot. See Chapter 14 for information on capsaicin topical.

Prophylactic Agents

❋ **What agents are available to prevent skin trauma or irritation?**

Agents used prophylactically to prevent skin injury include the protectives, which form a barrier to the skin and sunscreens, which block the damaging effects of sunlight. Most of these agents are OTC products (see Chapter 11 for a discussion of OTC status).

Protectives

Protectives are soothing, cooling preparations that form a film on the skin. To be useful, they must not macerate the skin, must prevent drying of the tissues, and must keep out light, air, and dust. Nonabsorbable powders are usually listed as protectives, but they are not particularly useful because they stick to wet surfaces and need to be scraped off, and they do not stick to dry surfaces at all. Nonabsorbable powders include zinc stearate, zinc oxide, certain bismuth preparations, talcum powder, and aluminum silicate. Collodion is a 5% solution of pyroxylin in a mixture of ether and alcohol. When collodion is applied to the skin, the ether and alcohol evaporate, leaving a transparent film that adheres to the skin to protect it. Flexible collodion is a mixture of collodion with 2% camphor and 3% castor oil. The addition of the latter makes the resulting film elastic and more tenacious. Styptic collodion contains 20% tannic acid and therefore is both astringent and protective. Although no substances known at present can stimulate healing at a more rapid rate than is normal under optimal conditions, preparations that act as bland protectives may help by preventing crusting and trauma. In some instances they may reduce offensive odors.

Sunscreen Preparations

❋ **T.Y. is a 26-year-old mother of twin 4-year-old girls who seeks advice about sunscreens and their use for her family.**

Sunscreens are agents that reduce the damaging effects of ultraviolet light to skin when applied topically before exposure. Whether from sunbathing, or as a normal consequence of an outdoor occupation, extended exposure to the sun may lead to sunburn and/or premature aging of the skin (photoaging). Certain chemicals (e.g., tetracyclines, sulfonamides, thiazides, phenothiazines), plants, cosmetics, and soaps may cause photosensitivity or phototoxicity when an ultraviolet wavelength substance (UVA-absorbing compound) is present on the skin in sufficient amounts and is also exposed to a particular sunlight wavelength. The substance absorbs the offending wavelength, and energy is transferred; as a result, it becomes destructive to surrounding tissues. The exposed skin rapidly becomes red, painful, prickling, or burning, with a peak skin reaction reached within 24 to 48 hours of exposure. This reaction does not involve the immune system.

A photoallergy reaction is different from a phototoxic reaction; it is less common and requires prior exposure to the photosensitizing agent. The immune system is involved; a delayed hypersensitivity reaction occurs when the photosensitizers react with UVA. The reaction occurs several days after exposure and presents as severe pruritus and a rash that can spread to skin areas that were not exposed to sunlight.

Cutaneous malignant melanoma has been associated with excessive sun exposure, especially during childhood, whereas large cumulative ultraviolet ray (UVR) doses over a lifetime appear to increase the incidence of nonmelanoma skin cancers (Box 65-4). Excessive exposure to ultraviolet rays (UVRs) may result in skin damage that progresses from minor irritation to a precancerous skin condition and, perhaps, to skin cancer later in life. Significant sun exposure occurs during the early years of life when children spend hours playing outside. A study showed that regular use of a sunscreen with a sun protection factor (SPF) (see later definition) of 15 during the first

18 years of life reduces the lifetime incidence of basal and squamous cell carcinoma by 78% (Habif, 2004). All children should be protected with high-number SPF sunscreens. One-piece bathing suits that cover the trunk, upper arms, and legs are ideal for children.

Sunscreen preparations are applied either to absorb or to reflect the sun's harmful rays. Absorbing agents are chemicals such as aminobenzoic acid (para-aminobenzoic acid [PABA]), benzophenones, cinnamates, and anthranilates; reflectors are physical agents such as titanium dioxide and zinc oxide. The latter agents are opaque (i.e., look like thick paste) and must be applied heavily; thus they are not cosmetically acceptable to most persons.

The spectrum for ultraviolet radiation includes UVA, UVB, and UVC. UVA, or long-wave radiation, has a wavelength of 320 to 400 nm and is the closest to visible light. UVB has also been determined to be responsible for inducing skin cancer, although the carcinogenic properties of UVB appear to be augmented by UVA. Approximately 90% of UVB radiation is blocked by the earth's ozone layer, with the balance absorbed by the epidermal skin layer. UVB has a wavelength between 290 and 320 nm, which causes erythema and is also associated with the synthesis of vitamin D_3. The UVC radiation from the sun does not appear to reach the earth's surface; therefore this type of radiation is usually emitted by artificial ultraviolet sources. UVC can cause some erythema but will not stimulate tanning. Not all agents block the full spectrum of ultraviolet rays. Aminobenzoic acid (PABA) has fallen out of favor and is less frequently used, partly because it is only effective in absorbing UVB rays and it is also more likely to be sensitizing and produce contact dermatitis.

The **sun protection factor (SPF)** is a ratio between the exposures to ultraviolet wavelengths required to cause erythema with and without a sunscreen. This is expressed as the minimal erythema dose (MED), which has been defined as the quantity of erythema-effective energy (expressed in Joules per square meter) required to produce the first perceptible redness reaction with clearly defined borders. Therefore if a person experiences 1 MED with 25 units of UV radiation (in an unprotected state) but requires 250 units of radiation to produce 1 MED after applying a sunscreen, then this sunscreen is given an SPF rating of 10. In general, the higher the SPF, the longer it takes to develop a tan. If a person normally burns within 30 minutes with 1 MED, then applying a sunscreen with an SPF of 6 allows that person to stay in the sun six times longer, or for nearly 3 hours, before reaching 1 MED. The following are current SPF values according to individual requirements:

SUN PROTECTION REQUIRED	SPF RECOMMENDED
Minimal	2 to 11
Moderate	12 to 29
High	30 or above (30+)

The best way to choose a sunscreen agent is according to skin type, the length of time spent in the sun, the usual intensity of the sun's rays in the particular geographic area,

BOX 65-4 SKIN CANCER

INCIDENCE

Skin cancers are composed essentially of nonmelanoma (basal and squamous cell carcinomas) and malignant melanoma. Nonmelanoma skin cancer is the most prevalent cancer in the United States. The American Cancer Society data indicates that more than 1 million cases of nonmelanoma skin cancer are found in this country each year. Melanoma is the most common cause of death from skin cancer.

BASAL CELL CARCINOMA

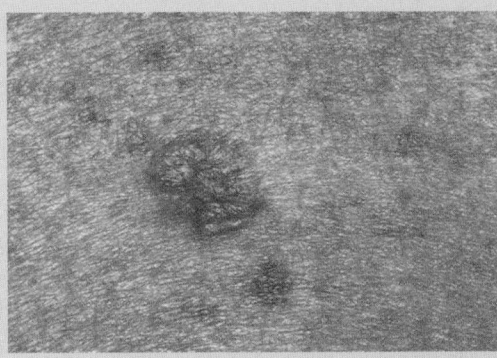

From Lemmi, F., & Lemmi C. (2000). *Physical assessment findings CD-ROM*. Philadelphia: W.B. Saunders.

MELANOMA

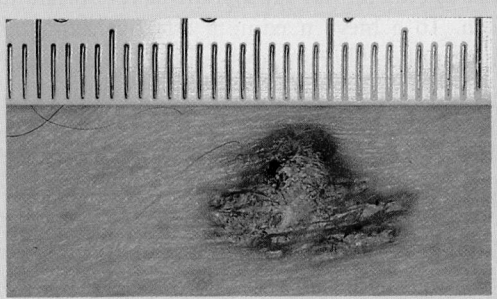

From Lemmi, F., & Lemmi C. (2000). *Physical assessment findings CD-ROM*. Philadelphia: W.B. Saunders.

PREVENTATIVE MEASURES

Sun protection is necessary because the 10- to 20-year period between ultraviolet (UV) light exposure (especially UVB) and the appearance of the skin cancer.

The primary source of protection is to avoid sunburns, especially in childhood and adolescence. If possible, avoid outdoor activities when the sun is strongest (10 AM to 2 PM), wear protective clothing (hat and long sleeves) and, if exposed to sun, use a sunscreen that blocks exposure to UV light (SPF 15 or 30). Reapply every 1 to 2 hours and after swimming.

UV radiation can also affect the eyes, increasing risk for cataracts and other eye disorders, and it can also suppress the immune system. It is recommended that sunglasses that block 99% to 100% of UV radiation be worn.

and the preferred type of preparation or formulation. For example, if an individual's skin turns red after being in the sun for 10 minutes, then an SPF of 15 may permit him or her to stay in the sun 15 × 10, or 150 minutes. A SPF of 30 is recommended for use in the tropics.

A sunscreen that contains ingredients that absorb at least 85% of the radiation in the UV range of 290 to 400 nm is known as a sunscreen with active ingredients. According to the Food and Drug Administration (FDA), the previous category of opaque sunblock is no longer an acceptable term for label use. The term sunblock implies an agent that blocks all sun rays (e.g., titanium dioxide), which most sunscreens do not do. As such, the term sunblock cannot appear on the label of a sunscreen product.

A topical sunscreen can be either chemical (absorbs and blocks UV radiation) or physical (opaque; reflects and scatters UV radiation but does not absorb it). Most products are a combination of these. The primary difference between a preventive agent and a suntanning agent might be the concentration of the active ingredient.

The effectiveness of a sunscreening agent depends on its ability to remain effective during vigorous exercise, sweating, and swimming. Historically, products may have been labeled as water resistant (maintaining their SPF after 40 minutes in the water) or very water-resistant (maintaining their SPF after 80 minutes of water activity or sweating). Because testing of these products was done in ideal instead of realistic conditions, this type of labeling has been questioned (Ives, 2005).

Advise clients on the appropriate selection and use of a sunscreen. To achieve maximum effectiveness, sunscreens should be applied liberally to all exposed body areas (except eyelids) and reapplied as frequently as recommended. Teach clients to do the following:

- Use a sunscreen SPF of at least 12 to 30 daily. Apply the sunscreen to exposed areas 15 to 30 minutes before sun exposure (Diffey, 2001).
- Reapply sunscreen to exposed areas 15 to 30 minutes after beginning exposure to the sun (Diffey, 2001).
- Reapply every 2 hours or after activity that could result in removal of sunscreen, such as excessive sweating, swimming, or towel drying (Diffey, 2001).
- Avoid peak sunlight hours between 10 AM and 3 PM, when the sun's rays are most direct and damaging.
- Wear sunscreen and limit exposure on overcast or cloudy days. Very little UV radiation is blocked by cloud cover, although the infrared radiation that contributes to the sensation of heat is usually reduced. This heat reduction might give a false sense of security against sunburn.
- Be aware of reflective surfaces; the sun's rays can be reflected on skin from water, concrete, snow, and sand.
- Wear a broad-brimmed hat, dark, loose clothing with a tight weave, a long-sleeved shirt, and long pants.
- Keep infants out of the sun, and always use sunscreens on children over 6 months of age.

- Consider taking oral antioxidant supplements daily: 25,000 international units of vitamin A and 1 to 2 g daily of L-ascorbic acid (vitamin C) (Habif, 2004).

See Table 65-3 for examples of sunscreen preparations, including their SPFs.

Therapeutic Agents

✱ What types of topical agents are available for therapeutic use?

A number of topical agents exist for treating many dermatological conditions, including topical antibacterials, antivirals, antifungals, corticosteroids, keratolytics (agents that soften scales), products for the treatment of acne, agents for treating burns, topical anesthetics, analgesics, and agents to treat ectoparasites like lice and scabies. Many are available over-the-counter (OTC), and clients will often self-treat a condition prior to seeking advice from a health care professional.

Antibacterials

✱ T.P. is a camp counselor who is asked to prepare a first aid kit for a day camp in her town. She seeks advice of the community nurse regarding which topical antibiotic cream should be part of the kit.

✱ What antibacterials are available for topical use?

The most common causative organisms of skin infections (xerodermas) are *Streptococcus pyogenes* and *Staphylococcus aureus*. Folliculitis, impetigo, furuncles, carbuncles, and cellulitis often result from these organisms. These common skin disorders are infections for which topical prophylaxis antibacterials may be applied but for which efficacy is questionable. Cellulitis, in particular, requires systemic antibacterial therapy (see Chapter 58).

Bacitracin and a combination of bacitracin-neomycin-polymyxin B are among the more common OTC agents used topically to help prevent wound infection with minor scrapes and cuts. Their use is limited to superficial wounds and is not a substitute for systemic antimicrobials for existing infections. A third agent, mupirocin (Bactroban) re-

TABLE 65-3 SELECTED SUNSCREEN PREPARATIONS	
Name	**Sun Protection Factor (SPF)**
Banana Boat Sunblock	15, 30, 50
Coppertone Moisturizing Sunblock	30 or 45
Hawaiian Tropic Baby Faces Sunblock	50+ or 60+
Panama Jack	8, 15, 30, 45, 50, 75

quires a prescription and is used to treat impetigo caused by *S. aureus*. A topical form of gentamicin is also available. Other antibacterials used to treat acne (including topical clindamycin and topical erythromycin) and burns (silver sulfadiazine) are discussed later in this chapter.

bacitracin [bass i **tray** sin]
(Baciguent)
Bacitracin is a topically applied antibacterial that inhibits bacterial cell wall synthesis. It is primarily effective against gram-positive cocci.

Indications
Bacitracin use is primarily limited to topical use in treating local lesions that may become or are infected. The ointment form (Baciguent) is most commonly used, although it has also been used in solution to moisten wet dressings or as a dusting powder.

Adverse Effects
Topically applied bacitracin is very well tolerated. It is odorless and nonstaining, and its use seldom results in sensitizing; however, allergic contact dermatitis is common.

neomycin [nee oh **mye** sin]
(Myciguent)
Neomycin is an aminoglycoside antimicrobial with a gram negative spectrum of activity. Its use is primarily limited to topical therapy, and it is considered highly sensitizing, which limits its use. An ointment (Mycitracin), which combines neomycin, bacitracin, and polymyxin B, may be more efficacious in mixed infections than when these agents are used singly.

Indications
Neomycin has been used in the treatment of superficial infections of the skin and mucous membranes.

Adverse Effects
Applied topically, neomycin occasionally irritates the skin; allergic contact dermatitis is often reported, especially when neomycin is used on stasis ulcers. In conditions in which the absorption of neomycin may occur (including burns and trophic ulceration), there is the potential for nephrotoxicity, ototoxicity, and neomycin hypersensitivity reactions. This risk is seen more often in clients with compromised renal function or extensive burns, and in clients using systemic aminoglycosides. Sensitization may occur, and prolonged use may produce a superinfection with an overgrowth of nonsusceptible organisms such as fungi.

mupirocin [**myoo** peer oh sin]
(Bactroban)
Mupirocin inhibits bacterial protein and ribonucleic acid (RNA) synthesis and is used topically for limited infections.

Indications
Mupirocin is indicated for the treatment of impetigo caused by *S. aureus* and other β-hemolytic streptococci. It is also used intranasally to eradicate nasal colonization of methicillin-resistant *S. aureus* (MRSA) or other susceptible pathogens.

Adverse Effects
Topical mupirocin is well tolerated, with local irritation being the most frequently reported adverse effect.

✳ **For her first aid kit, T.P. is advised to stock cleansing wipes to clean any superficial wounds, and plain bacitracin ointment in single use packaging to prevent cross-contamination.**

Antivirals

✳ **B.L. is a 28-year-old office worker with a new onset herpes simplex lesion (cold sore) on his upper lip. He questions a friend who is a nurse regarding how he should treat it.**

✳ **What dermal antiviral therapies are available?**
Dermal antiviral therapy is fairly limited in scope. Two prescription agents, acyclovir (Zovirax) and penciclovir (Denavir) and an OTC agent, docosanol (Abreva), are available to treat herpes simplex labialis (cold sores). In each case, treatment must begin at the first sign of prodromal symptoms (tingling and burning) and must be applied frequently throughout the day.

acyclovir [ay **sye** kloe ver]
(Zovirax Ointment 5%, Avirax✱)
Acyclovir inhibits the viral enzymes necessary for deoxyribonucleic acid (DNA) synthesis.

Indications
Topical acyclovir is used to treat initial episodes of herpes genitalis and for herpes simplex in immunocompromised clients. In many instances systemic acyclovir is much more effective and may be the preferred formulation (see Chapter 59).

Dosing
The dosage is adequate covering of the lesions with ointment every 3 hours six times daily for 7 days.

Adverse Effects
The more common adverse effects of acyclovir include local pain, pruritus, or stinging.

docosanol [doe **koe** san ole]
(Abreva)
Docosanol is a topical antiviral that prevents viral cell entry and viral replication and is available over the counter.

Indications
Docosanol is used to treat cold sores of the face and lips.

Dosage
Docosanol is applied five times daily to the affected area.

Adverse Effects
Docosanol is well tolerated with few adverse events reported.

penciclovir [pen **sye** kloe veer]
(Denavir)
Penciclovir is like acyclovir in action and indication.

Indication
Penciclovir is used topically to treat herpes simplex labialis (cold sores). As with other antiviral therapy, treatment should be initiated as soon as symptoms appear.

Pharmacokinetics/Dosing
Penciclovir is the active metabolite of famciclovir, and is only available for topical use. It is typically dosed every 2 hours while awake for up to 4 days. To be effective, it must be started within a few hours of onset of symptoms.

Adverse Effects
Topical penciclovir is well tolerated. The most frequently observed adverse effect is mild erythema.

✳ **What are the nursing implications for dermal antivirals?**

The dose per application will vary depending on the lesion area; a one half–inch ribbon of ointment covers approximately 4 inches of surface area. Store the ointment at 15° C to 25° C (59° F to 78° F).

Instruct the client to use a finger cot or rubber glove when applying the ointment to prevent autoinoculation to other sites. It is applied as soon as symptoms of herpes infection begin. Avoid contact with eyes. Advise an annual or more frequent Papanicolaou (Pap) smear, because women with herpes genitalis are more likely to be sexually active, and that is correlated with an increased risk for human papillomavirus and cervical cancer. Recommend that the client wear loose clothing and keep the affected areas clean and dry to prevent further irritation. Advise the client to avoid sexual activity if either partner has active lesions. The disease can still be sexually transmitted even if the partner is asymptomatic; depending on the location of the lesion, the use of a condom may help to prevent the transmission of herpes.

Antifungals

✳ **S.T. is a 19-year-old college freshman who reports to the college health service with itchy and burning feet and toes. His nurse practitioner assesses the affected areas and diagnoses tinea pedis (athlete's foot) infection.**

✳ **What are key features of dermal fungal and yeast infections?**

A few fungi produce keratinolytic enzymes to provide for their existence on the skin. Three infectious fungi can cause local fungal infections without producing systemic effects: *Microsporum*, *Trichophyton*, and *Epidermophyton*. The possibility of a mixed infection with these fungi must never be overlooked.

Fungi exist in a moist, warm environment, preferably in dark areas such as skin areas covered by shoes and socks (tinea pedis or athlete's foot). Immunologic mechanisms may have an important role in fungal control. The triad of suspicion for fungal infections is an immunologic deficit, a specific fungal involvement, and the skin condition.

The stratum corneum is a layer of dead, desquamated cells that are shed normally or are dissolved in sebum. The fungi invade this layer and cause inflammation and induce sensitivity when they penetrate the epidermis and dermis. Because the stratum corneum is shed daily, the ability to spread or transmit the fungi is by contact.

✳ **S.T. asks his nurse practitioner about what treatments are effective.**

✳ **What drugs are available to treat fungal and dermatophytic infections of the skin?**

A number of topical treatments are available for fungal or dermatophyte infections, with many available over the counter. The most commonly used OTC topical agents include terbinafine (Lamisil, Lamisil AT), and butenafine (Lotrimin Ultra, Mentax). Both agents have gained popularity because each is often effective with a 7- or 14-day course of therapy. Other OTC topical antifungals include clotrimazole (Lotrimin, Lotrimin AF), ketoconazole (Nizoral), miconazole (Lotrimin AF Spray, Micatin, Monistat Derm), selenium sulfide (Selsun, others) and tolnaftate (Tinactin). Prescription topical agents include ciclopirox (Loprox), econazole (Spectazole), naftifine (Naftin, nystatin (Mycostatin), oxiconazole (Oxistat, sertaconazole (Ertaczo), sulconazole (Exelderm). Ciclopirox topical nail lacquer (Penlac) has been used for the topical management of onychomycosis, whereas oral terbinafine has been used for the same indication (see Chapter 59). Older agents, like undecylenic acid products (Desenex and others) and gentian violet, have been largely replaced by newer more effective agents.

The most commonly reported adverse effects with the use of topical antifungals include local irritation, pruritus, a burning sensation, and scaling. Erythema, blistering, stinging, peeling, urticaria, pruritus, and general irritation may occur with products such as clotrimazole. Three representative agents will be presented.

butenafine [byp **ten** a feen]
(Lotrimin Ultra; OTC, Mentax)
Butenafine is a topical antifungal that inhibits the synthesis of ergosterol in dermatophytes. It also affects cell membranes in fungi at high concentrations.
Indications
Butenafine is used to treat various tinea infections, including tinea corporis (ringworm), tinea cruris (jock itch), tinea pedis (athlete's foot) and tinea versicolor.
Dosing
Butenafine is applied once daily for 4 weeks or twice daily for 1 week in the treatment of tinea pedis. Other tinea conditions respond to once-daily application for 2 weeks.
Adverse Effects
Dermal administration of butenafine is well tolerated with burning, stinging, and itching being occasionally reported with use.

clotrimazole [kloe **trim** a zole]
(Cruex, Lotrimin AF, Mycelex, Clotrimaderm✲)
Clotrimazole exerts is antifungal effects by increasing the permeability of fungal cell walls. In addition to dermal preparations, oral and vaginal formulations are available.
Indications
Clotrimazole is used to treat superficial fungal infections.
Dosing
Clotrimazole is available as a 1% cream or solution and is dosed twice daily for up to 4 weeks.
Adverse Effects
Infrequent reports of local irritation or burning have been reported.

terbinafine [**ter** bin a feen]
(Lamisil AT)
Terbinafine is similar to butenafine. An oral formulation is also available (see Chapter 59).
Indications
Indications for terbinafine are identical to butenafine.
Dosing
Dermal application of terbinafine twice daily for 1 to 4 weeks is the typical regimen for tinea pedis. Once- or twice-daily application for 1 to 4 weeks is recommended for tinea corporis and tinea cruris infections.

Adverse Effects
Dermal reactions are occasionally noted with topical application of terbinafine.

✳ **S.T. begins a 1-week twice-daily course of terbinafine (Lamisil AT) with recommendation to return to Health Services if improvement is not noted in 7 days.**

✳ **What are the nursing implications of using dermal antifungal agents for S.T.?**

Assessment Carefully note skin characteristics, symptoms, and predisposing factors such as trauma, suppressed immunity, general health, hygiene practices, or exposure to an infecting agent. Laboratory tests (e.g., cultures of exudate or tissue) may be obtained before the topical agent is applied.

Nursing Diagnosis While S.T. is using a topical antifungal agent, he is at risk for the following nursing diagnoses: impaired skin integrity; impaired comfort (pain, burning, or itching of the affected areas); risk for infection related to open skin areas; and deficient knowledge related to new or altered dermatologic therapy.

Planning While on topical antifungal therapy, S.T. will:
- Experience relief from the symptoms of his disorder (e.g., itching, pain, erythema, and vesicles).
- Effectively manage the therapeutic regimen, using measures to support the drug (e.g., appropriate hygiene, cotton socks, keeping the area dry).

Implementation
Monitoring The use of these agents may lead to skin sensitization and result in symptoms of hypersensitization, such as increasing redness and swelling, weeping, and itching and burning not present at the beginning of therapy. The client needs to be reevaluated if no improvement is seen within 4 weeks depending on the treatment regimen used.

Intervention Topical substances for antifungal purposes should be applied liberally to a clean, dry, affected skin area. An occlusive dressing should not be applied unless directed by the prescriber. Avoid contact of these substances with the eyes. Store them below 30° C (85° F), but do not freeze them.

Education Encourage S.T. to comply with his full course of therapy. In general, fungal infections require prolonged therapy. Encourage S.T. to practice adequate hygiene to discourage growth. Principles of hygiene include the following: (1) keep the affected areas dry and aerated, and avoid clothing that is warm or that causes an occlusive environment of moisture; (2) keep body areas dry with powders (with or without antifungal ingredients) to prevent maceration; (3) before applying the antifungal medication, wash the area with mild soap and water and then dry it; (4) avoid friction or trauma of the area by not wearing tight-fitting clothing; clothing should be laundered daily. For infants with anogenital lesions, avoid tight diapers, disposable diapers, and plastic pants. Advise clients with foot infections to wear cotton socks and well-ventilated shoes or sandals.

Evaluation The expected outcome of topical antifungal therapy is that S.T. will experience a resolution of the fungal infection (e.g., absence of itching and burning of feet and toes). He will effectively manage his therapeutic regimen with by using appropriate hygiene, wearing cotton socks, and keeping the area dry to prevent recurrence.

Corticosteroids

✳ **K.L. is a 14-year-old high school freshman who presents with intense pruritus and papules/plaques on the inner aspects of his arms and ankles. He has a longstanding history of atopic dermatitis since early childhood. He has historically used hydrocortisone cream, but this has not been effective for his current symptoms. He visits his health care provider accompanied by his father for a "stronger" treatment.**

✳ **What is the role of topical corticosteroids?**
Topical corticosteroids are generally indicated for the relief of inflammatory and pruritic dermatoses, including those of atopic dermatitis (Ellsworth & Smith, 2005). They also offer the benefit of fewer systemic adverse effects, and they allow direct contact with the localized lesion.

The effectiveness of topical corticosteroids is a result of their antiinflammatory, antipruritic, and vasoconstrictor actions. Topical corticosteroids may also stabilize lysosomes in the epidermis, and fluorinated steroids are antiproliferative.

Fluorinated topical corticosteroids (fluocinonide, betamethasone, and others) are used to treat dermatologic disorders such as psoriasis because of their antiinflammatory, antipruritic, and vasoconstrictive actions, and their ability to decrease cell proliferation. They are very potent agents and are less likely to cause sodium retention.

A correlation exists between the potency and the therapeutic efficacy of corticosteroids. The vehicle in which the corticosteroid is placed (aerosol, cream, gel, lotion, ointment, solution, or tape) may alter the vasoconstrictor property and therapeutic efficacy. Corticosteroid skin penetration is enhanced by the following vehicles (in decreasing order of effectiveness): ointments, gels, creams, and lotions.

Ointment bases and propylene glycol both enhance the penetration of the corticosteroid and its vasoconstrictor effects. As a result of their occlusive nature, ointments hydrate the stratum corneum, permitting granular steroid penetration. Lotions are well suited for hairy areas or for lesions that are oozing and wet. Creams and ointments are well suited for dry, scaling, thickened, and pruritic areas. Sprays, lotions, and gels are suited for the scalp or for hairy areas. Sprays are aesthetically suitable for acute weeping lesions; they are cooling and have antipruritic effects. All of these vehicles influence absorption and have a therapeutic effect.

The rate of percutaneous penetration after application also influences therapeutic efficacy. The percutaneous penetration of a steroid increases with its vehicle base solubility. Also affecting the rate of drug penetration are the rate of drug dissolution in the vehicle and the rate of passive diffusion through the skin. The thickness and nature of cell layers in different areas of the body will have a considerable effect on these rates. The skin is selectively permeable by regional variations in absorptive capacity. Most topical corticosteroids are in suspension vehicles (ointments, creams, lotions), so the addition of a solvent (propylene glycol) to the product enhances drug dissolution, which may improve absorption. Sebum, enzymes, and perspiration partially convert topical suspensions to solutions; thus they need the inclusion of a solvent, surfactant, or emulsifier in the vehicle to increase the rate of dissolution and distribution. Inflamed skin absorbs topical steroids to a greater degree than thick or lichenified skin.

The adverse effects of topical corticosteroids include acneiform eruptions, allergic contact dermatitis, burning sensations, dryness, itching, hypopigmentation, purpura, hirsutism (usually facial), folliculitis, a round and swollen face, alopecia (usually of the scalp), immunosuppression, and overgrowth of bacteria, fungi, and viruses.

Most topical corticosteroids require a prescription. The adult dosage is one or two applications daily as directed. The frequency of application depends on the site, response of the cutaneous eruption to medication, and application technique. Table 65-4 presents a comparison of a number of available dermal corticosteroids and their relative poten-

TABLE 65-4 REPRESENTATIVE SAMPLING OF AVAILABLE TOPICAL CORTICOSTEROIDS AND THEIR RELATIVE POTENCY

Relative Potency	Generic	Brand	Formulations
Very High	betamethasone dipropionate[a,b,d]	Diprolene	Ointment, gel, lotion
	clobetasol	Clobex, Olux, Temovate	Foam, cream, ointment, gel
	halobetasol	Ultravate	Cream, ointment
High	amcinonide[b]	Cyclocort	Cream, lotion, ointment
	desoximetasone[b]	Topicort	Cream, gel, ointment
	diflorasone[b]	Maxiflor, Psorcon E	Cream, ointment
	fluocinonide[b]	Lidex	Cream, gel, lotion, ointment
	halcinonide[b]	Halog, Halog-E	Cream, ointment, solution
	mometasone[c]	Elocon	Cream, lotion, ointment
Moderately High	betamethasone valerate[c,d,e]	Valisone	Cream, lotion, ointment, foam
	fluticasone[d]	Cutivate	Cream, ointment, oil
	triamcinolone[c,d,e]	Aristocort A, Kenalog	Cream, ointment
Medium	clocortolone	Cloderm	Cream
	fluocinolone[d,e]	Synalar	Cream, ointment, solution
	flurandrenolide[d]	Cordran	Cream, ointment, lotion, tape
	hydrocortisone[f], hydrocortisone valerate	Hydrocort, Westcort	Cream, ointment, lotion
Moderately Low	desonide[e]	DesOwen	Cream, lotion, ointment
	hydrocortisone butyrate	Locoid, Locoid Lipocream	Cream, ointment, solution
	prednicarbate	Dermatop	Cream
Low	alclometasone	Aclovate	Cream, ointment

Data from ePocrates Rx Version 6.6. Retrieved September 7, 2004, from http://www.epocrates.com.
[a] Some formulations categorized as High potency.
[b] Some formulations categorized as Moderately High potency.
[c] Some formulations categorized as Medium potency.
[d] Some formulations categorized as Moderately Low potency.
[e] Some formulations categorized as Low potency.
[f] Some formulations categorized as Very Low potency.

cies. Appropriate strength preparations should be used to control the condition. For maintenance, most dermatologic conditions requiring topical corticosteroids can be managed with medium- or low-strength corticosteroid preparations.

✴ **Because K.L.'s lesions are dry and plaque-like, he may be a candidate for an ointment-based formulation of a corticosteroid. A more potent agent is also indicated. His prescriber orders fluocinolone (Synalar) ointment to be applied twice daily.**

✴ **What nursing management issues are involved in the use of dermal corticosteroids for K.L.?**

Assessment Assess the skin for conditions that would be worsened by the application of topical corticosteroids (e.g., acne vulgaris, ulcers, scabies, warts, molluscum contagiosum, fungal infections, balanitis). The age of the skin affects absorption of the potent fluorinated corticosteroids; the very young and the very old have skin that is more permeable and so more susceptible to adverse effects.

Nursing Diagnosis While K.L. is using a topical antifungal agent, he is at risk for the following nursing diagnoses: impaired skin integrity; impaired comfort (pain, burning, or itching of the affected areas); risk for infection related to open skin areas; and deficient knowledge related to new or altered dermatologic therapy.

Planning While on topical corticosteroid therapy, K.L. will:

- Experience relief from the symptoms of his disorder (e.g., itching, pain, erythema, and crusting).
- Effectively manage the therapeutic regimen, using measures to support the drug (e.g., appropriate hygiene, dosing compliance, reporting to the prescriber appropriately).

Implementation

Monitoring Occluded areas and certain, thin-skinned areas of the body, such as the face and flexures, are more prone to the development of adverse effects (epidermal and dermal atrophy, telangiectasis, localized fine hair growth, bruising, hypopigmentation, striae). Check with the prescriber if no improvement in the appearance of the lesions is noticeable after 1 week.

Intervention Topical corticosteroids should be applied twice daily. Increasing the application from twice daily to four times daily does not produce superior responses and is more expensive. Rub ointment in thoroughly and when possible, apply while the skin is moist (e.g., after bathing). Hydration of the skin increases absorption and the therapeutic effect of the corticosteroid (Ellsworth & Smith, 2005). To help prevent adverse effects if prolonged treatment is required, treatment may be interrupted periodically, small amounts of the drug can be applied, or one area of the body can be treated at a time. Most adverse effects are temporary

and are resolved when the topical steroid is discontinued.

For some conditions, gradual withdrawal of therapy may be indicated after high-dose or prolonged therapy to help prevent a rebound flare-up, as may be seen with psoriasis.

Use occlusive dressings only if ordered by the prescriber. Occlusive dressings may cause folliculitis from a bacterial or candidal infection, hyperthermia from heat retention, or systemic effects related to increased drug absorption. Do not use an occlusive dressing if the client has a fever. If the site becomes infected, discontinue the use of topical corticosteroids, and initiate the appropriate treatment.

Education To enhance client compliance, explain to the client the reasons for the occlusive dressing procedure. This technique intensifies percutaneous penetration of the topical steroid and concentrates the medication in the area in which it is most needed.

Evaluation The expected outcome of topical corticosteroid therapy is that K.L. will experience resolution of his skin lesions with diminished plaques, itching, redness, and size without adverse drug effects (e.g., increased discomfort, infection). He will maintain appropriate hygiene, appropriate application of the drug, and scheduled visits with his provider for monitoring and treatment.

✴ **What noncorticosteroid alternatives exist for the treatment of atopic dermatitis?**

Intense pruritus associated with atopic dermatitis is often treated with oral antihistamines. It is occasionally treated with topical antihistamines or other agents that affect dermal serotonin, histamine, or norepinephrine action. A topical formulation of the antidepressant drug, doxepin (Zonalon), is available as a 5% cream and applied four times daily for pruritus. A number of OTC dermal products containing antihistamines, including diphenhydramine, are also available.

The topical immunosuppressants pimecrolimus (Elidel) and tacrolimus (Protopic) are available to treat atopic dermatitis in clients who do not respond adequately to conventional therapies. Pimecrolimus inhibits T cell activation by interfering with dermal cytokines including interleukin 2, interferon-gamma, interleukin 4, and interleukin 10. Tacrolimus, also used systemically as an immunosuppressant for organ transplant recipients, is discussed more fully in Chapter 63. Cancer risk in laboratory animals has been noted with these agents, but the extent of human risk is not known (FDA, 2005a, b).

pimecrolimus [pim e **kroe** li mus]
(Elidel)

Indications
Pimecrolimus is used in the short to intermediate term treatment of atopic dermatitis. It is typically reserved for clients not responsive to other modalities. It has been used in children as young as 2 years of age.

Dosing
It is applied topically to affected areas twice daily up to 6 weeks. It should not be used with occlusive dressings.

Adverse Effects

Headache, fever, burning at application site, and upper respiratory tract infections have been associated with the topical use of pimecrolimus. Exacerbation of warts, herpes simplex dermatitis, or dermal infections, otitis, ocular infections, and other viral infections have been reported with the use of this topical immunosuppressant. It should not be used for clients with underlying immunosuppressive states, with Netherton's syndrome, or current infection. Cancer risk may also be increased with its use (FDA, 2005a, b).

Nursing Management

Instruct the client to minimize exposure of the treated area to natural or artificial sunlight. Stop application of pimecrolimus once signs of the dermatitis have disappeared. Caution the client to wash his hands after applying the drug unless the hands are the affected areas. Advise him to report any significant irritation that is the result of the application of the cream.

Acne Products

✴ **H.P. is a 15-year-old male who has asked his mother to bring him to see the prescriber "to get something for his 'zits.'"** He has no other health problems. After school he plays on the varsity basketball team and works in a fast food restaurant. H.P. has tried OTC benzoyl peroxide cream 5% "once in a while" when he feels his acne is particularly bad, but has not used it consistently. At present, he has two pustules and three closed comedones on his forehead, three excoriated lesions on his cheeks, and two healing areas on his chin.

✴ **What treatments are available to manage acne?**
Acne vulgaris is a skin disease that involves increased sebum production and abnormal keratinization and leads to the formation of a keratin plug at the base of the pilosebaceous follicle; it affects up to 90% of adolescents (Seaton, 2005). The reduction and removal of sebum and bacteria, specifically *Propionibacterium acnes*, is the goal of acne vulgaris therapy.

Treatment of acne therapy may include (1) removing keratin plugs, (2) decreasing the amount of *P. acnes*, (3) lowering the amounts of free fatty acid, (4) decreasing sebum production, and (5) effectively improving the appearance of the client for psychosocial benefits.

Topical and systemic antibacterials used to treat acne have an unknown mechanism of action. Acne is not an infection nor is it contagious, but *P. acnes* appears to convert comedones to inflamed pustules or papules. Antibacterials may decrease the colonization of *P. acnes*, thus decreasing the formation of sebaceous fatty acid byproducts and preventing the formation of new acne lesions. The antibacterials used include clindamycin, erythromycin, tetracycline, and doxycycline (see Chapter 58). Topical erythromycin and clindamycin are most commonly prescribed for mild to moderate acne, whereas oral antibacterials (tetracyclines) are generally reserved for severe acne and for clients who are intolerant of or did not respond to topical agents. Metronidazole is also used topically for treating acne rosacea. Treatment failures have been associated with antibacterial resistance (Seaton, 2005).

Oral use of isotretinoin (Accutane, Amnesteem, Sotret) is used for severe nodular acne vulgaris not response to other interventions. Because of its high potential to produce teratogenic effects, it is contraindicated in women who are pregnant, and generally avoided in other women of childbearing age unless other modalities are not effective, effective birth control or abstinence is assured, and informed consent is obtained.

✴ **H.P. is assessed to have mild acne with papules and pustules; he is started on topical clindamycin.**
Of the many treatment modalities in acne therapy, the more commonly used agents are discussed here.

Topical Antibacterial Acne Treatments

clindamycin [klin da **mye** cin]
(Cleocin T topical solution, Dalacin✷)
Topical clindamycin may be as effective as low-dose, oral tetracycline therapy for inflammatory acne. It is believed to lower the free fatty acid concentration on the skin and to suppress the growth of *P. acnes*. It has an antibacterial effect.

Indications
Topical clindamycin is used in the treatment of moderate to severe acne vulgaris.

Pharmacokinetics/Dosing
Systemic absorption of topically administered clindamycin is relatively low (about 10%). By hydrolysis, skin phosphatases convert inactive clindamycin phosphate to active clindamycin base, which is excreted by the kidneys. It is dosed topically to affected areas twice daily.

Adverse Effects
Adverse effects of topical clindamycin include dry, scaly and/or peeling skin, a stinging or burning sensation, and a hypersensitive skin reaction.

erythromycin topical solution [er ith roe **mye** sin]
(A/T/S, EryDerm)
Indications
Erythromycin topical solution is indicated for the treatment of acne vulgaris.

Pharmacokinetics/Dosing
Systemic absorption of topically applied erythromycin is low. It is applied twice daily.

Adverse Effects
Adverse effects include skin reactions such as erythema, desquamation, tenderness, dryness, pruritus, burning, oiliness, and acne.

metronidazole [meh troe **nid** a zole]
(MetroCream, MetroGel, MetroLotion, Apo-Metronidazole✷, Nida-Gel✷)
Metronidazole is an antibacterial/antiprotozoan agent with activity against anaerobic pathogens (see Chapter 58).

Indications
Topical metronidazole is used to treat inflammatory acne rosacea. It is not used to treat acne vulgaris.

Pharmacokinetics/Dosing
Systemic absorption of topically applied metronidazole is low. Topical metronidazole is applied to affected lesions once or twice daily depending on concentration.

Adverse Effects
The most common effects with topical administration include local irritation, burning, and dryness. Systemic effects, including headache, altered taste and nausea have also been reported.

Other Topical Acne Treatments

azelaic acid [a zeh **lay** ik **as** id]

(Azelex, Finacea, Finevin)
Azelaic acid is derived from yeast and possesses antiinflammatory and keratolytic properties. It also has some antibacterial action (DermNetNZ, 2004).

Indications
Azelaic acid is a prescription product indicated for the treatment of mild to moderate acne vulgaris and acne rosacea.

Dosing
Azelaic acid is administered to affected areas twice daily.

Adverse Effects
Topical burning and irritation are the most frequently reported adverse events.

adapalene [a **dap** a leen]

(Differin)
Adapalene is a retinoid similar to tretinoin. It alters the inflammation and cell differentiation.

Indications
Adapalene is used to treat acne vulgaris.

Pharmacokinetics/Dosing
Systemic absorption is minimal and therefore relatively safe to use for women of childbearing age. It is applied to lesions once daily.

Adverse Effects
Like tretinoin, adapalene is associated with relatively high rates of erythema, scaling, dryness, pruritus, and burning.

benzoyl peroxide [**ben** zoe ill **per oks** eyde]

(Benzac, Brevoxyl, Desquam-X 5, Desquam-X 10)
Benzoyl peroxide slowly and continuously liberates active oxygen to produce an antibacterial, keratolytic, and drying effect in the treatment of acne vulgaris. The release of oxygen into the pilosebaceous and comedone area creates unfavorable growth conditions for *P. acnes* and reduces the release of fatty acids from the sebum. Additionally, the drying vehicle aids in shrinking the papules or pustules but does not have an effect on comedones or cysts.

Indications
Benzoyl peroxide is used to treat acne vulgaris. It is available in OTC formulations and also prescription formulations alone, or in combination with hydrocortisone, clindamycin, or erythromycin.

Pharmacokinetics/Dosing
Benzoyl peroxide is absorbed and metabolized in the skin to benzoic acid. Approximately 5% of the benzoic acid is absorbed and excreted by the kidneys. Acne improvement is usually noted after 4 to 6 weeks of therapy. In adults and children 12 years of age and older, benzoyl peroxide lotion (5% or 10%) is applied one to four times daily. Benzoyl peroxide 5% applied twice daily is as effective as topical and oral antimicrobials in treating mild to moderate acne (Ozolins et al., 2004).

Adverse Effects
Adverse effects are uncommon and include dry or peeling skin, red skin, a sensation of warmth of the skin, severe redness, pruritus, blisters, and burning or swelling of the skin caused by an allergic reaction. No significant drug interactions are reported.

tazarotene [taz **ar** oh teen]

(Avage, Tazorac)
Tazarotene is a synthetic retinoid similar to adapalene and tretinoin.

Indications
Tazarotene is used to treat facial acne vulgaris and stable plaque psoriasis. It has also been used cosmetically to reduce facial wrinkles.

Pharmacokinetics/Dosing
After topical administration, systemic absorption is low, but is enough to render this agent contraindicated in pregnancy (FDA Pregnancy Category X). It is dosed in adults once daily, with frequency and strength of formulation adjusted based on indication and response to therapy.

Adverse Effects
The gravest concern with this agent is the potential to produce teratogenicity in women of childbearing age, and as such, must be avoided in pregnancy. Like tretinoin, tazarotene is associated with relatively high rates of erythema, scaling, dryness, pruritus, and burning.

tretinoin topical [**tret** i noyn]

(retinoic acid, vitamin A acid, Retin-A, Renova)
Tretinoin is a retinoid that stimulates the turnover of epidermal cells. This results in skin peeling. The primary effect of tretinoin is to reduce the hyperkeratinization that results in comedone formation, a lesion in acne.

Indications
Tretinoin is used to treat acne vulgaris in which comedones, pustules, and papules are predominant. Tretinoin emollient cream (Renova) is used to treat facial wrinkles caused by aging or sun exposure. This product contains 0.05% tretinoin and is the first prescription drug with this indication (*Drug Facts and Comparisons*, 2005).

Pharmacokinetics/Dosing
Systemic absorption of topically applied tretinoin is minimal but does carry an FDA Pregnancy Category C rating. It is dosed once daily or every other day, with strength of preparation and frequency of application adjusted based on response and tolerability.

Adverse Effects
The most common and significant reactions of topical tretinoin include red and edematous blisters; crusted, stinging, or peeling skin; and temporary alterations in skin pigmentation. Concomitant topical use with drying or peeling agents such as benzoyl peroxide, resorcinol, salicylic acid, and sulfur may result in excessive keratolytic and peeling effects. This FDA Pregnancy Category C topically applied agent is not routinely recommended for women of childbearing age, but may be considered if the benefit outweighs the risk.

Systemically Administered Acne Treatments

★⬛ isotretinoin [eye soe **tret** i noyn]

(Accutane, Roche✦)
Isotretinoin is an oral retinoid indicated for the treatment of severe, recalcitrant, cystic acne. This product inhibits sebaceous gland activity, thereby decreasing the formation and secretion of sebum. It also has antikeratinizing and antiinflammatory effects. Its FDA Pregnancy Category X rating limits its use.

Indications
Isotretinoin is reserved to treat severe acne and has induced prolonged remissions in severe cystic acne.

Pharmacokinetics/Dosing
Isotretinoin is absorbed orally and distributes well into tissue including placental tissue in pregnant women. It is highly plasma protein bound, and is eliminated by hepatic metabolism via cytochrome P450 2D6, 3A4, and other cytochrome P450 isoenzymes. It is usually dosed in adults at 0.25 to 1 mg/kg twice daily for up to 20 weeks. Lower doses have been used.

Adverse Effects
Women who are pregnant or are planning to become pregnant should not use this drug. Many spontaneous abortions have been reported in pregnant women, and premature birth, birth defects, and neonatal death. Abstinence or effective birth control and informed consent are required if used in women of childbearing age. Other adverse effects include tachycardia, flushing, edema, dizziness, seizures, depression, psychosis, agitation, rash, elevated triglycerides, hyperglycemia, bone marrow suppression, osteopenias, and bronchospasm. Refer to prescribing literature for a full listing of adverse effects possible with this agent.

Drug Interactions

Isotretinoin may increase metabolism of carbamazepine. Low dose progesterone only hormonal contraceptives may not be adequate birth control with concurrent isotretinoin. Refer to package labeling for full discussion of interactions with isotretinoin.

✳ **What are the nursing implications with the use of therapies for acne?**

Clindamycin Topical Therapy

Cross-resistance exists with lincomycin. Contraindications demonstrated by hypersensitivity to any form of clindamycin or lincomycin may apply to the topical preparation. During the client interviews, inquire about any previous sensitivity not only to clindamycin but also to other antimicrobials or allergens, and obtain a history of regional enteritis. In particular, clients with a history of drug allergies or asthma should be questioned, because some absorption may occur through the skin. Some clients develop antibiotic-associated pseudomembranous colitis (AAPC) caused by *Clostridium difficile* during or following topical clindamycin therapy. The client should report any diarrhea to the prescriber. Mild cases may resolve by discontinuing the clindamycin; more severe cases may require fluid and electrolyte replacement. For adults and children, the dosage is an application of a thin film twice daily to the affected area. Shake the topical suspension well before applying.

Erythromycin Topical Solution Therapy

Hypersensitivity to erythromycin or the other components of the solution (alcohol, propylene glycol, or acetone) is a contraindication to its use. A cumulative irritant effect may occur with the concomitant use of peeling, desquamating, or abrasive agents. Noticeable improvement may be seen in 3 to 4 weeks, but the maximum effects may take 8 to 12 weeks. Erythromycin topical solution is applied to the affected areas morning and evening. Wait at least 1 hour before applying any other topical preparation to the skin. Caution the client that erythromycin solution should not be used near the eyes, nose, mouth, and other mucous membranes.

Tretinoin Topical Therapy

Irritation and desquamation are most likely during the first 1 to 3 weeks of treatment. For acne, therapeutic results can be seen after 2 to 3 weeks of therapy, with an optimal response after 3 months. If used for the effects of photoaging, the improvement continues for 2 months after therapy, with a partial and gradual regression.

Apply this drug each night by covering the area lightly at bedtime. Some clients require less frequent applications or the use of a lower-percentage strength, whereas others may respond to the higher percentage forms. Tretinoin should be applied after a thorough cleansing of the area. Allow a minimum of 30 minutes for the skin to dry before applying tretinoin, because an increased drying effect and redness may occur if it is applied to wet skin. After application, wait 1 hour before applying any other preparation to the same area.

Clients with sunburned skin, skin that is sensitive to ultraviolet light, or skin exposed to weather extremes must exercise caution and avoid tretinoin until the skin has recovered. The client must avoid medicated or abrasive cleansers, astringents, soaps, and cosmetics that have a drying effect and a high alcohol concentration. The client will be excessively sensitive to the sun and should wear a sunscreen of at least 15 SPF during therapy.

✳ **B.C. is a 32-year-old female bank executive who visits the dermatologist because she has had moderate acne for over 10 years. Over this time, she has tried several medications without success, or she experienced intolerable adverse effects and the medications had to be discontinued. Now B.C. feels that her acne is affecting her social life and may be keeping her from a promotion. Her blood chemistries, blood counts, and a lipid panel were normal. The dermatologist and B.C. discuss various therapies, and the decision is to begin isotretinoin therapy.**

✳ **What nursing management of B.C.'s isotretinoin therapy is essential?**

Assessment Because isotretinoin has been demonstrated to cause fetal abnormalities, a negative pregnancy test and an appropriate history and physical examination should be used to determine that the client is not pregnant. Because B.C. is of childbearing age, assess her capability to comply with mandatory contraceptive measures; these should be accomplished for at least 1 month before therapy, during therapy, and for 1 month after the end of therapy (see the Pregnancy Safety box below).

PREGNANCY SAFETY DERMATOLOGIC DRUGS	
Category	**Drug**
B	adalizumab, alefacept, topical clindamycin, erythromycin, etanercept, malathion topical, meclocycline topical, permethrin, silver sulfadiazine
C	benzoyl peroxide, corticosteroids (topical), crotamiton, efalizumab, lindane, mafenide, tretinoin
D	tetracycline
X	acitretin, isotretinoin, tazarotene

Data from *Mosby's drug consult* (15th ed.). (2005). St. Louis: Mosby.

Review B.C.'s medication regimen. Isotretinoin should not be used concurrently with acitretin, oral tretinoin, or vitamin A, because additive toxic effects may result. The use of tetracyclines with isotretinoin increases the risk for the development of pseudotumor cerebri—a condition characterized by increased intracranial pressure, headache, blurring of the optic disc margins, vomiting, and papilledema without neurologic findings (except palsy of the sixth cranial nerve).

B.C. should have baseline measurements of complete blood count (CBC), blood lipid levels, blood glucose levels, and hepatic function studies. These should also be monitored throughout therapy.

Nursing Diagnosis While receiving isotretinoin, B.C. is at risk for the following nursing diagnoses/collaborative problems: impaired comfort (headache; heartburn; inflammation of the eye; pain, tenderness, and stiffness of the muscles, bones, or joints; dryness of the mouth, skin, and eyes; difficulty wearing contact lenses); fatigue; impaired skin integrity (scaling, redness, inflammation of the skin); and the potential complications of mental depression, nosebleeds, cataracts, optic neuritis, corneal opacities, pseudotumor cerebri, hepatitis, and inflammatory bowel disease.

Planning While on isotretinoin therapy, B.C. will:
* Experience relief from the symptoms of acne.
* Effectively manage her therapeutic regimen, including birth control measures, dietary changes, compliance with medications, maintaining appointments with the dermatologist for monitoring).

Implementation

Monitoring Monitor laboratory reports, nursing diagnoses, and potential complications as mentioned previously.

Education Provide B.C. with both oral and written instructions regarding the hazards of use during pregnancy, and evaluate her understanding and acceptance of the written warnings. Alert her not to donate blood during or for 30 days after isotretinoin therapy, because there is a risk to the fetus of a pregnant woman who may receive the blood. Because isotretinoin may increase concentrations of plasma triglycerides, clients at particular cardiovascular risk should be cautioned; this includes clients with a history of high alcohol intake, obesity, or a history or family history of hypertriglyceridemia or diabetes mellitus.

To minimize additive toxic effects, alert B.C. to avoid concurrent use of vitamin A unless prescribed by a physician. Avoid ingestion of alcohol because of possible hypertriglyceridemia and consequent cardiovascular risks. Caution her about a decrease in night vision; she should alert the prescriber if this occurs. B.C. may also be intolerant of contact lenses because of dryness of the eyes. Contact lens use may need to be discontinued during therapy if an ocular lubricant is not successful in relieving dryness. Sips of water or sugar-free gum or candies may be recommended to relieve mouth dryness.

Advise B.C. to contact the prescriber if there is no improvement in 1 to 2 months; full improvement may take 5 to 6 months. Skin irritation may occur during the first several weeks of therapy. Stress the need for protection from exposure to wind and sun, with the use of protective clothing and a sunscreen of at least 15 SPF at all times.

Advise B.C. that dental problems may occur from mouth dryness; regular dental appointments are necessary to minimize dental complications.

Evaluation The expected outcome of B.C.'s isotretinoin therapy is that her acne should improve after 1 to 2 months; 5 to 6 months of therapy may be required. She will effectively manage her therapeutic regimen by not becoming pregnant, by not donating blood during or for 30 days after therapy, by avoiding alcohol, and by maintaining scheduled visits to her dermatologist.

Burn Products

Burn injuries range from mild and superficial to very severe, with extensive skin loss associated with systemic and metabolic complications. In America each year, approximately 2 million people are burned, 80,000 are hospitalized, and 6500 die (Sheridan, 2002). The chief cause of death is shock; this fact is of considerable significance in any effective plan of treatment.

Burns cause skin lesions accompanied by pain. The burn may be caused by heat (thermal burn), chemical cauterizing agents (chemical burns), or electricity (electrical burns). Sources may be friction, lightning, or electromagnetic energy (ultraviolet light, x-rays, lasers, or atomic explosion). The types of burns that result from various sources are relatively specific and diagnostic.

A consideration of what takes place in the damaged tissues clarifies many points of treatment. Capillary permeability is initially increased in the local injured area, which results in plasma loss and weeping of the surface tissues. If the burn is at all extensive, considerable amounts of plasma fluid may be lost in a relatively short time.

This plasma loss depletes blood volume and causes a decreased cardiac output and diminished blood flow. Unless the situation is brought under control quickly, irreparable damage may result from rapidly developing tissue anoxia. The lack of sufficient oxygen and accumulation of waste products from inadequate oxidation results in a loss of tone in the small blood vessels. Increased capillary permeability then extends to tissues beyond those suffering the initial injury. A generalized edema often develops; once established, the vicious cycle tends to be self-perpetuating. One of the aims of burn treatment is to stop the loss of plasma and to replenish lost fluid as quickly as possible.

Partial- or full-thickness burns must be thought of as open wounds with the accompanying danger of infection. The infection must be prevented or treated. The treatment, however, must not cause any further destruction of tissue or of the small islands of remaining epithelium from which growth and regeneration can take place.

Burns are classified by degree, which is determined by the depth of skin involved within a geographic designation. First-degree burns involve only the epidermis, causing erythema with characteristic dry, painful reddening and edema without blistering or vesiculation (e.g., overexposure to sun or a flash burn). Second-degree burns involve the epidermis and extend into the dermis; they may be superficial or involve a deep dermal necrosis. Epithelial regeneration may extend from deep skin appendages, such as hair follicles and sebaceous glands that penetrate the dermis. This burn is characterized by a moist, blistered, very painful surface (e.g., flash or scald burns from nonviscous liquids). Third-degree burns involve destruction of the entire dermis and epidermis and are characterized by white, lustrous, or opaque skin; dry, leathery skin; or coagulated, charred skin without sensation as a result of the destruction of nerve endings (e.g., flame burns or hot, viscous liquids). Fourth-degree burns extend into subcutaneous fat, muscle, or bone; they appear black and dry in appearance and cause scarring.

The severity of electrical burns depends on the amount of voltage received, the condition of the skin (e.g., cuts, abrasions, and moisture, which lower resistance), and the contraction of flexor muscles, which inhibits release from the power source. Electrical burns result in the necrosis of more tissue than thermal burns and are of three types:

- *Type I.* The electrical current causes effects on blood vessels such as occlusion, thrombosis, or tissue destruction.
- *Type II.* Electrical burns from high-tension currents (e.g., an electrical arc) produce a crater in the skin.
- *Type III.* These burns are similar to flame burns because the arc flame ignites the victim's clothes.

Chemical burns occur after contact with an acid or alkali; the initial treatment is water irrigation of the affected area followed by neutralization. Chemical burns may occur in the mouth and appear as a white slough because of necrosis of the epithelium and underlying connective tissues.

✷ What strategies are used to manage burns?

Regardless of the cause (chemical, electric, thermal), an important first-aid treatment for minor and major burns is to cool the wound immediately to remove irritants, decrease inflammation, and constrict blood vessels; this reduces the permeability of the blood vessels and checks the formation of edema. Cool tap water can be used to flush the wound thoroughly and to cool hot clothing. The more quickly the wound is cooled, the less tissue damage there is likely to be, and the more rapid the recovery. Greasy ointments, lard, butter, or dressings should not be applied, because they inhibit the loss of heat from the burn and increase both discomfort and tissue damage. The burn may be left exposed to the air, or cold, wet compresses may be applied until the victim can be transported for medical attention.

Burn victims treated in an emergency department or burn unit are stabilized with IV fluids, given analgesics for pain, and sedated if necessary. These individuals are immunized with tetanus toxoid and/or tetanus immunoglobulin depending on their immunization status. Catheterization may be necessary to measure urinary output. Following stabilization, the burn wound is gently cleaned with sterile saline, and a sterile, nonadherent gauze dressing is applied. In some settings, synthetic dressings (DuoDERM, OpSite) may be used. Topical antiinfective therapy may also be indicated. Silver sulfadiazine is usually preferred because of its broad-spectrum activity; this product is easy and painless to apply and remove from the burn (Ives, 2005).

✷ ▪ silver sulfadiazine [sul fa **dye** a zeen]
(Silvadene, Demazin❖, Flamazine❖)

Silver sulfadiazine is an antiinfective agent with broad antimicrobial activity against many gram-negative and gram-positive bacteria (similar to mafenide). It acts only on the cell membrane and cell wall to produce its bactericidal effect. It softens eschar, facilitating its removal and preparation of the wound for grafting.

Indications
Silver sulfadiazine is used in second- and third-degree burns for the prevention and treatment of sepsis.

Dosing
Silver sulfadiazine is available as a 1% cream to be applied topically.

Adverse Effects
Pain, burning, and itching occur infrequently after application of the silver sulfadiazine cream. Silver sulfadiazine may cause a hypersensitivity reaction, in which case the drug should be discontinued. Hemolysis may occur in persons with glucose-6-phosphate dehydrogenase (G6PD) deficiency. When silver sulfadiazine is applied to extensive areas of the body, significant amounts of the drug may be absorbed, reaching therapeutic serum levels and producing adverse effects characteristic of the sulfonamides. Renal function in these clients should be monitored and the urine examined for sulfa crystals.

mafenide [**ma** fe nide]
(Sulfamylon)

Mafenide (sulfonamide), a broad-spectrum, antibacterial (bacteriostatic) topical agent, penetrates eschar even in the presence of pus and serum. It is a carbonic anhydrase inhibitor that can alter acid-base balance, resulting in metabolic acidosis. In contrast to silver sulfadiazine, it is usually painful on application.

Indications
Mafenide is used in combination with other drug and nondrug modalities to treat second- and third-degree burns and to prevent associated infection.

Pharmacokinetics/Dosing
On application, mafenide rapidly diffuses through partial (second-degree) and full-thickness (third-degree) burns and has proved to be an effective means for preventing and slowing bacterial invasion in burn wounds. It is rapidly metabolized to a metabolite and eliminated by way of the kidneys.

Adverse Effects
Mafenide is relatively nontoxic, but burning or pain on application and allergic reactions have been reported.

nitrofurazone [nye troe **fyoor** a zohn]
(Furacin)

Nitrofurazone is a broad antibacterial topical agent and is active against many bacteria that cause local infections, including *S. aureus*, *Streptococcus*, *Escherichia coli*, and others.

Indications
Nitrofurazone is indicated as adjunct therapy to clients with second- and third-degree burns when bacterial resistance to other agents is a problem; it is also used during skin grafting when bacterial contamination may result in graft rejection or a donor site infection.

Dosing
The 0.2% cream, ointment, or solution may be applied directly on the area or to a gauze dressing for application. Efficacy is reduced in the presence of heavy microbial contamination, plasma, or blood. Resistance seldom develops.

Adverse Effects
Rash, itching, local edema (dermatitis), and allergic reactions have been reported. Hypersensitivity occurs early in the treatment of a few individuals. Bacterial and fungal superinfections may occur. Furacin is not absorbed significantly through mucosal or burned tissues, and systemic toxicity is rare. However, its polyethylene glycol base may be absorbed and may challenge the client with renal dysfunction.

✳ What are the nursing management issues in regard to burn treatments?

Assessment Ascertain the client's sensitivity to the agent to be used for burn care; for mafenide, allergy to sulfites may be an issue and there is a potential cross-sensitivity between silver sulfadiazine and other sulfonamides. Because sulfonamide therapy is known to increase the possibility of kernicterus, silver sulfadiazine cream 1% should not be used on pregnant women approaching or at term, on premature infants, or on newborn infants during the first 2 months of life. The use of silver sulfadiazine cream 1% in some cases of glucose-6-phosphate dehydrogenase-deficient individuals may be hazardous, as hemolysis may occur. Pregnant women should avoid using nitrofurazone unless the potential benefits outweigh the possible risks to the fetus. Judgment should be used in treating with nitrofurazone if a client has a renal disorder; these preparations include polyethylene glycol and may produce adverse effects. Older adults are at a higher risk for allergic responses to nitrofurazone. For all burn preparations, renal and hepatic impairment may cause drug accumulation, because systemic absorption of these agents may be significant at the wound site.

Vital signs, blood chemistries, and blood counts are included in the baseline assessment. A detailed documentation of the burn(s) is also included.

Nursing Diagnosis While on burn therapy, the client is at risk for infection and impaired skin integrity related to allergic contact dermatitis (erythema, pruritus, and burning) and the potential complications of transient leukopenia (silver sulfadiazine), blood dyscrasias, allergic reactions, gastrointestinal (GI) reactions, hepatitis, CNS reactions, and toxic nephrosis.

Planning While on burn therapy, the client will:
- Not evidence infection.
- Experience wound granulation and healing by primary intention or split-thickness skin grafting within an acceptable time frame.
- Collaborate with health care providers with dressing changes, application of medication, and pain management.

Implementation

Monitoring Evaluate the affected areas daily. If areas do not seem to be responding to treatment by nitrofurazone, consider the possibility of overgrowth by nonsusceptible organisms such as fungi and *Pseudomonas* or an allergic response. Watch for dermatitis or other manifestations of hypersensitivity to this product.

Because mafenide and its metabolite are strong carbonic anhydrase inhibitors, acidosis (metabolic) may occur and is usually compensated by hyperventilation. Observe the client carefully for any signs of respiratory alkalosis. If rapid or labored respirations occur, the ointment should be removed from the wound.

Intervention Apply the preparation to cleansed, debrided burn wounds once or twice daily; whirlpools and showers are helpful. Apply with a sterile gloved hand to a thickness of approximately 1.5 mm. Avoid cross-contamination of multi-use containers. Burn wounds should be continuously covered with the preparation; reapply it to burned areas from which it has been removed by client activity. Daily bathing and debriding are important, and a dressing may or may not be used. Therapy is usually continued until satisfactory healing has occurred or until the wound is ready for grafting.

Because silver sulfadiazine inhibits bacterial growth, delayed eschar separation may occur, which necessitates an escharotomy to prevent contractures.

Mafenide may cause some discomfort when first applied; a burning or pain sensation may occur that lasts from a few minutes to as long as an hour. It is not necessary to discontinue mafenide therapy if infection occurs. Mafenide therapy can be interrupted for 2 to 3 days without impairing bacterial control of the wound while continuing fluid therapy and acid-base restoration. Mafenide is a highly stable drug. It remains active for several years and does not need to be refrigerated except in tropical countries.

As a solution, nitrofurazone may be sprayed directly on the wound. If the solution is cloudy, it may be warmed to restore clarity. Meticulous sterile technique is essential during dressing changes and when opening and withdrawing nitrofurazone-saturated dressings from their sterile packets. Nitrofurazone darkens on exposure to light, but such discoloration does not affect drug potency. Severe skin reactions to nitrofurazone may require application of topical steroids or short-term administration of systemic corticosteroids.

Education Instruct client in role during dressing changes and application of topical burn preparations, adverse effects of preparations, and pain management.

Evaluation The expected outcome of burn preparation therapy is that the client's wound will show granulation and healing by primary intention or split-thickness skin grafting within an acceptable time frame without evidence of infection.

Keratolytics

Keratolytics (keratin dissolvers) are drugs that soften scales and loosen the outer horny layer of the skin. Salicylic acid and resorcinol are the drugs of choice. Their action makes the penetration of other medical substances possible by cleaning the involved lesions. Salicylic acid is particularly important for its keratolytic effect in the local treatment of scalp conditions, warts, corns, fungous infections, acne, and chronic types of dermatitis. It is used up to 20% in ointments, plasters, or collodion for this purpose. Examples of salicylic acid products include Panscol Ointment, Wart-Off, and Dr. Scholl's Corn/Callus Remover.

✿ **M.N. is a 32-year-old man who visits his primary care provider with a skin disorder he has been treating for the last 6 months without success. He has several thick, well-defined erythematous plaques on his elbows that are covered with silvery scales. M.N. has applied skin lotion and kept them covered but now that summer is coming, he would like to be able to wear short sleeved shirts. His prescriber diagnoses his lesions as psoriasis. M.N. is prescribed desoximetasone (Topicort 0.25%) for twice a day application to the affected areas.**

✿ **What agents are available to treat psoriasis?**
Treatments for psoriasis have evolved over the past decade and include topical therapies, phototherapy, and systemic agents.

Topical therapies are aimed at improving symptoms. Dermal corticosteroids are among the more frequently used topical modalities. Other topical therapies include anthralin and retinoids (e.g., tazarotene). Moisturizers, baths, and keratolytics (e.g., salicylic acid) round out the topical treatments used to manage mild to moderate psoriasis.

Moderate to severe psoriasis often requires systemic therapy for adequate response. Oral and parenteral agents may both improve symptoms and modify disease progression. Systemic agents include oral retinoids (e.g., acitretin), immunosuppressants like cyclosporine (Chapter 63), methotrexate (Chapter 56), and biologic response modifiers (alefacept, etanercept, adalimumab, efalizumab, infliximab; see Chapters 40 and 63). The biologic response modifiers vary in indication, and are used for other autoimmune diseases such as Crohn's disease and rheumatoid arthritis. Not all biologic response modifiers have official indications for psoriasis, but may be used in severe cases. A brief review of selected agents will be presented here.

Retinoids

The systemic retinoids are vitamin A–related compounds that affect cell turnover rates. Their use is associated with a significant number of adverse effects and is contraindicated in pregnancy because of their high risk to injure the developing fetus. The systemic retinoid most often used to treat psoriasis is acitretin.

acitretin [ah sea **tray** tin]
(Soriatane)
Acitretin is an oral synthetic retinoid used to alter the rate of cell growth and shedding. As with other systemically administered retinoids, the risk for teratogenicity with its use is high.

Indications
The use of acitretin limited to the treatment of severe psoriasis.

Pharmacokinetics/Dosing
Acitretin is reasonably orally well absorbed when dosed with food. It is highly bound to plasma albumin, and is eliminated by metabolism. The oral adult dose is typically 25 to 50 mg daily with adjustments made based on response and toleration of adverse effects.

Adverse Effects
Acitretin is teratogenic and possesses an FDA Pregnancy Category X rating. Women who take acitretin must not be pregnant, nor become pregnant for 3 years after completion of therapy. Other adverse effects include hair loss, skin peeling, altered tactile sensation, hyperlipidemias, hyperglycemia, hypoglycemia, dry mouth, bone marrow changes, altered hepatic function tests, hematuria, and rhinitis. Many of these effects can limit use of acitretin. Review package labeling for a more complete listing of adverse effects.

Biologic Response Modifiers

✿ **M.N. is returning to the clinic after 6 months because despite corticosteroid therapy, his lesions have increased. In addition to his previous lesions, there are now several scattered, circumscribed, erythematous, scaly plaques on the flexural surfaces of both arms and legs. The dermatologist discusses the option of efalizumab (Raptiva) and the anticipated results, cost, route of administration and adverse effects. They decide to proceed with an efalizumab drug regimen. M.N. is initiated with a single 0.7 mg/kg subcutaneous conditioning dose followed by weekly subcutaneous doses of 1 mg/kg.**

A number of biologic response modifiers are used to help regulate immune function for clients with autoimmune diseases. Topical pimecrolimus and tacrolimus are presented above in the treatment of mild to moderate atopic dermatitis. Parenterally administered immunomodulators are presented here. In psoriasis, these are primarily monoclonal antibodies or related proteins, which bind to T-lymphocytes or mediators of inflammation such as TNF. Because of the nature of different autoimmune diseases, some agents may be effective in one condition but data supporting its use in another may be lacking. Adalimumab is included in the discussion here because its mode of action is similar to other agents, but it is rarely used in the management of psoriasis. Infliximab, used primarily in the treatment of Crohn's disease and rheumatoid arthritis, is discussed in Chapter 40. Among the risks in using most of these agents is the risk for serious infection secondary to immunosuppression. These agents may also increase the risk for certain cancers.

alefacept [ah **le** fa sept]
(Amevive)
Alefacept is a monoclonal antibody that binds to CD2 lymphocytes and results in suppressed immune response and improved symptoms of psoriasis. It also suppresses CD4 and CD7 T-lymphocyte counts and function.

Indications

Alefacept is used to treat moderately severe psoriasis in adults.

Pharmacokinetics/Dosing

Alefacept is administered intramuscularly (IM) or intravenously (IV) and the elimination half-life is approximately 10 to 14 days. The typical adult dose is 7.5 mg IV or 15 mg IM once weekly for 12 weeks. A repeat 12-week course of therapy may be considered after a 3-month drug-free period if T-lymphocyte counts are within normal limits.

Adverse Effects

The most serious effects of alefacept relate to immunosuppression and risk for infection. Other adverse effects include injection site pain, and potentially higher risk for malignancies, 1% with treatment compared to 0.2% with placebo (Lacy, Armstrong, Goldman, & Lance, 2004).

etanercept [eh **tan** er sept]

(Enbrel)

Etanercept is a protein that binds to tumor necrosis factor (TNF) and blocks its action. This renders etanercept effective in the treatment of conditions in which TNF plays a role, including rheumatoid arthritis, psoriatic arthritis, and Crohn's disease.

Indications

Etanercept is used to treat moderate to severe rheumatoid arthritis, juvenile arthritis, and psoriatic arthritis. Its use in Crohn's disease is considered investigational.

Pharmacokinetics/Dosing

Administered subcutaneously, etanercept has an onset of action of 14 to 21 days and an elimination half-life of about 5 days. Adult dose is 50 mg once weekly or 25 mg twice weekly by subcutaneous injection. In children with juvenile rheumatoid arthritis, it is dosed subcutaneously at 0.8 mg/kg once weekly or 0.4 mg/kg twice weekly not to exceed the adult doses listed above. Doses above 25 mg should be administered as two single injections.

Adverse Effects

Etanercept is associated with a relatively high risk for infection and is the major concern with its use. Other adverse effects include headache, injection site pain or inflammation, and respiratory distress. Consult package labeling for a more complete listing of effects.

adalimumab [a da **lim** yoo mab]

(Humira)

Adalimumab is a monoclonal antibody with affinity for TNF. Its use is primarily limited to treating rheumatoid arthritis, but it has occasionally been used in other autoimmune conditions.

Indications

Adalimumab is indicated for the treatment of moderate to severe active rheumatoid arthritis.

Pharmacokinetics/Dosing

Adalimumab is administered subcutaneously and has an elimination half-life of approximately 14 days. For clients with rheumatoid arthritis, it is dosed at 40 mg subcutaneously every other week.

Adverse Effects

Adalimumab, like other biologic response modifiers, increases risk for infections. The most frequently observed infections associated with its use are upper respiratory and sinus infections. Other adverse effects include headache, rash, and hyperlipidemia. See package insert for a more thorough discussion of adverse effects.

efalizumab [e fa li **zoo** mab]

(Raptiva)

Efalizumab is a monoclonal antibody that binds to the CD11 a site of T-lymphocytes and interferes with T-lymphocyte–induced inflammation associated with psoriasis.

Indications

Efalizumab is used to treat chronic plaque psoriasis that is considered moderate to severe.

Pharmacokinetics/Dosing

Administered via subcutaneous injection, efalizumab is associated with therapeutic benefit within 3 months of initiation of therapy. The adult dose of psoriasis is 0.7 mg/kg by subcutaneous injection on week one, then 1 mg/kg weekly thereafter.

Adverse Effects

A reaction associated with fever, chills, headache, muscle pain and nausea is noted in about one third of clients who receive full dosing initially; such reactions are less common when the first dose is reduced to 0.7 mg/kg. Immune-mediated hemolytic anemia has also been reported and may be observed 4 to 6 months after starting therapy (Genentech, 2005). Other adverse effects include headache and nausea. Unlike other biologic modifiers, efalizumab is associated with elevated lymphocyte and leukocyte counts. It, however, may also predispose to infection risk and package labeling recommends the same cautious monitoring for infection as other biologic modifiers.

✳ What are the issues of nursing management with biologic response modifiers for M.N.?

Assessment Assess M.N.'s allergy history for hypersensitivity to efalizumab or any of its components. No formal drug interaction studies have been performed with efalizumab. Document a baseline status of M.N.'s lesions. Obtain complete cell count, particularly white blood cell (WBC), and platelets.

Nursing Diagnosis While on biologic response modifier therapy, M.N. has the potential for the following nursing diagnoses: increased risk of infection, altered comfort (nausea, headache, chills, myalgias); excess fluid volume (peripheral edema); and potential complication of first dose reaction (headache, fever, nausea, vomiting, myalgias), acne, arthralgia, and thrombocytopenia.

Planning As a consequence of efalizumab therapy, M.N. will:

- Experience a decrease in plaque induration, scaling and erythema without adverse drug effects.
- Effectively manage his therapeutic regimen (e.g., self-administer efalizumab, appropriately report adverse symptoms to the prescriber).

Implementation

Monitoring Monitor M.N. for signs and symptoms of infection (e.g., cellulitis, pneumonia, abscess, sepsis, bronchitis, gastroenteritis, aseptic meningitis, Legionnaires' disease, vertebral osteomyelitis). Obtain monthly platelet counts to determine if thrombocytopenia develops. WBCs increase with therapy and take about 8 weeks to normalize following the discontinuation of efalizumab therapy. Psoriasis lesions should begin to diminish by week 4.

Intervention Administer M.N. a reduced initial dose to prevent "first dose reaction" that may include headache, fever, nausea, and vomiting. Reconstitute efalizumab immediately before use. Use a prefilled syringe with sterile water for injection and inject its contents slowly into the vial.

Swirl the syringe, but don't shake it, to obtain a pale yellow solution without particulate matter. Following administration, discard any unused reconstituted efalizumab solution. Replace the needle on the syringe before administration. Inject subcutaneously; rotating sites for each weekly injection. Do not administer acellular, live and live-attenuated vaccines during the time M.N. is taking efalizumab.

Education Discuss the expected results, with M.N., and cost, route of administration, and adverse drug effects. In clinical studies, 52% to 61% of participants experienced over a 50% improvement in plaque induration, scaling, and erythema (*Mosby's Drug Consult*, 2005). Efalizumab costs over $1200 for a 28-day supply. The route of administration is subcutaneous so teach M.N. the subcutaneous injection technique so that he may self-administer his medications. Efalizumab is an immunosuppressive agent and has the potential to increase the risk of malignancy and infection, and reactivate latent, chronic infections. Advise M.N. to report any symptoms of infection, such as fever, abscess, or sore throat), symptoms of thrombocytopenia (bleeding from gums, bruising, and petechiae), or worsening of psoriasis. Alert M.N. that the prescriber may monitor platelet counts during therapy. Advise him not to get any live virus vaccines without consulting his prescriber while taking the efalizumab.

If M.N. were female, she should notify her physician immediately if she should become pregnant while taking or within 6 weeks of taking efalizumab. Consult the prescriber before breastfeeding.

Evaluation During efalizumab therapy, M.N. will experience a decrease in the size of psoriasis lesions, plaque induration, scaling, and erythema without adverse drug effects (e.g., fever, headache, muscle pain, nausea, infection). He will successfully demonstrate a subcutaneous injection of efalizumab and appropriately report any signs or symptoms of infection to his prescriber.

Topical Antipruritics

Antipruritic agents are given to allay itching of the skin and mucous membranes. The need for these preparations is declining as the constitutional treatment skin disorders are increasingly understood. Dilute solutions containing phenol have been widely used. Dressings wet with potassium permanganate 1:4000, aluminum subacetate 1:16, boric acid, or physiologic saline solution may cool and soothe and thus prevent itching. Lotions such as calamine or calamine with phenol (phenolated calamine), and cornstarch or oatmeal baths, may also be used to relieve itching.

Local anesthetics such as dibucaine and benzocaine may decrease pruritus, but their use is not recommended because of their high sensitizing and irritating effects. The application of hydrocortisone in a lotion or ointment in a strength of 0.5% to 1% has proved to be one of the best methods of relieving pruritus and decreasing inflammation. An additional advantage is its low sensitizing index.

Topical Ectoparasiticidal Drugs

❋ **L.G., an 8-year-old, comes home with a handout from school indicating that there have been two cases of head lice in her class. The information sheet alerts L.G.'s mother of symptoms for which to check L.G. and how to manage the infestation if L.G. has head lice.**

❋ **What are the key considerations with ectoparasite infestation?**

Ectoparasites are insects that live on the outer surface of the body, and ectoparasiticides are drugs used against those animal parasites. For human use, these drugs are more commonly referred to as *pediculicides* and *scabicides (miticides)*; these names reflect the parasite treated with each group.

Pediculosis is a parasitic infestation of lice on the skin of a human. Lice are transmitted from one person to another by close contact with infested persons, clothing, combs, and towels. There are three different varieties of infestations: (1) pediculosis pubis, caused by *Phthirus pubis* (pubic or crab louse); (2) pediculosis corporis, caused by *Pediculus humanus corporis* (body louse), and (3) pediculosis capitis, caused by *P. humanus* capitis (head louse) (Figure 65-1). Except in individuals with heavy infestation, a characteristic finding of *P. corporis* is that the parasite is absent from the body but inhabits seams of clothing that come in contact with the axillae or that are in the belt line or collar.

Common findings in a person who is infested include pruritus, nits (eggs of louse) on hair shafts, lice on skin or clothes and, with pubic lice, occasional sky-blue macules on the inner thighs or lower abdomen. The drug of choice is the pediculicide lindane (gamma benzene hexachloride).

Scabies is a parasitic infestation caused by the itch mite *Sarcoptes scabiei*. It is transmitted from one person to another by close contact, such as sleeping next to an infested individual. It bores into the horny layers of the skin in cracks and folds, causing irritation and pruritus. Itching occurs almost exclusively at night. The adult infestation is usually generalized over the body, especially in the webbed spaces between the fingers, wrists, elbows, and buttocks.

❋ **What drugs are used topically to treat these infestations?**

The drug of choice is permethrin cream because it is considered to be more effective than crotamiton and safer than lindane. Dimeticone is a newer agent that may be an effective alternative, but it is not available in the United States at press time (Burgess, Brown, & Lee, 2005).

❋▭ **permethrin** [per **meth** rin]
(Nix, Elimite)
Permethrin acts on the nerve cell membranes of lice, ticks, mites, and fleas. It disrupts sodium channel repolarization, thus paralyzing the parasites. Although it has a high cure rate after only a single application, head lice in children who reside where pediculicides are readily available are less susceptible to permethrin.

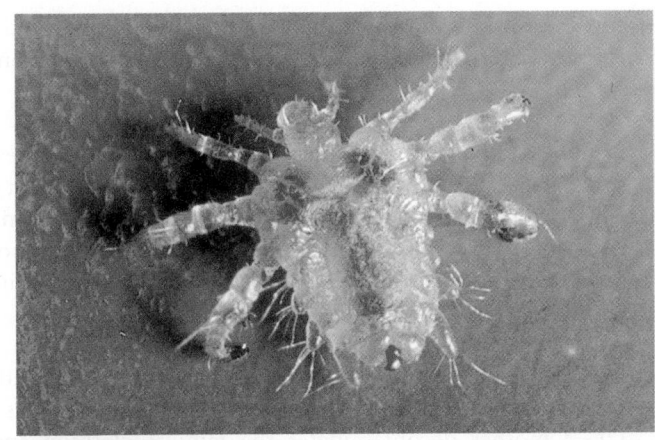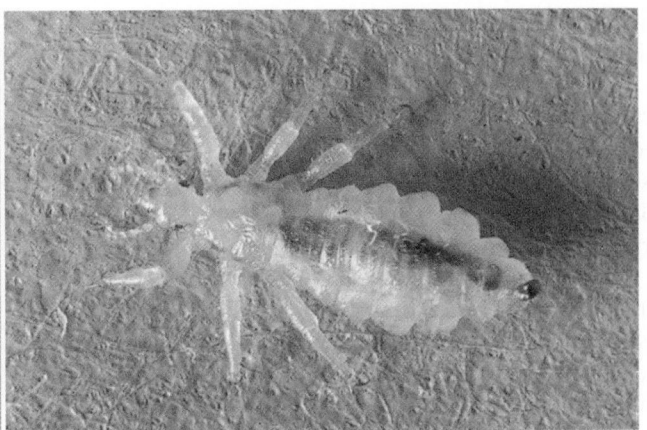

FIGURE 65-1 **A,** Pubic louse (*Phthirus pubis*). **B,** Body louse (*Pediculus humanus*). Notice that the first pair of legs on the pubic louse are thinner than the second and third pairs, and the abdomen is shorter. On the body louse, all legs are approximately the same length, and the abdomen is longer.

From Habif, T.B., Campbell, J.L., Quitadamo, M.J., & Zug, K.A. (2001). *Skin disease: Diagnosis and treatment.* St. Louis: Mosby.

Indications
Permethrin is used to treat scabies in adults and children older than the age of 2 months. Its efficacy in the treatment of lice is variable.

Dosing
Permethrin is applied to affected areas and left on for 8 to 14 hours before removal by washing.

Adverse Effects
The most common adverse effects of permethrin include pruritus, mild burning on application, transient erythema, edema, and rash.

lindane [**lin** dane]
(gamma benzene hexachloride [Kwell])
Lindane is both a scabicide and a pediculicide because it is effective in the treatment of both lice and mite infestations. Its use, however, is limited to second line therapy because of the potential for toxicity (U.S. Food and Drug Administration, 2003).

Indications
Lindane is used to treat both scabies and lice infestations in adults and children older than the age of 1 month when other therapies are not effective or tolerated.

Dosing
Lindane is available in a 1% cream, lotion, and shampoo. To treat pediculosis pubis and infestations of *P. humanus capitis,* the cream or lotion is applied in a sufficient quantity to cover the skin and hair of the infected and surrounding areas; it is left on for 12 hours and then washed out thoroughly. It seldom needs to be applied more than once. The shampoo is worked into the hair and left on for 4 minutes. The hair is then rinsed and dried, and the nits (eggs) are combed from the hair shafts. Retreatment is usually not necessary.

Lindane cream or lotion is used for the treatment of scabies. If crusted lesions are present, a warm bath preceding the application of lindane is recommended. Lindane is applied over the entire body from the neck down. It is left on for 8 hours and then washed off. One application is usually sufficient. It is common to have pruritus after application, but this does not indicate a need for reapplication unless live mites can be demonstrated.

Adverse Effects
Lindane penetrates human skin and has a potential for producing central nervous system (CNS) toxicity (e.g., seizures, increased irritability, dizziness), especially in children, adults under 110 pounds, and older adults (U.S. Food and Drug Administration, 2003). Lindane occasionally will cause an eczematous skin rash. Pruritus or rash associated with lindane is occasionally observed. Although clients may confuse pruritus with ineffective management of lice or mite infes-

tation, they should *not* reapply lindane because this greatly increases risk for toxicity.

crotamiton [kroe **tam** i ton]
(Eurax)
Indications
Crotamiton is indicated for the treatment of scabies in adults.

Dosing
Crotamiton is rubbed into the skin from the chin down, particularly in the folds and creases of the body and moist areas, such as the axillae and groin. It is reapplied in 24 hours and is washed from the body surface 48 hours after the second application. Two applications of crotamiton usually eradicate most infestations. In resistant cases it may be reapplied in 1 week.

Adverse Effects
The most common reactions associated with the use of crotamiton are allergic dermatitis, rash, and pruritus.

malathion [mal i **thye** on]
(Ovide)
Malathion is an organophosphate cholinesterase inhibitor available for the treatment of head lice and ova. This product is usually effective in lice-infested individuals within 24 hours and is well tolerated.

Indications
Malathion is used to treat pediculosis in adults and children older than the age of 2 years.

Dosing
Malathion lotion is rubbed into the scalp and left to air dry. Because the drug is flammable, the client must be warned to avoid open flames, smoking, or using a hairdryer. The hair is shampooed 8 to 12 hours after application, and the dead lice are combed out.

Adverse Effects
Although rare, bronchospasm has been reported. Other adverse effects include skin irritation, conjunctivitis and contact dermatitis.

✱ **L.G.'s mother asks her if she feels "itchy" around her head and ears. When she says "yes," her mother checks L.G.'s head and finds nits. She calls L.G.'s pediatrician who calls a prescription into the pharmacy for lindane (Kwell) shampoo.**

✳ What are the nursing management issues for topical ectoparasiticidal therapy for L.G.?

Assessment The first step in the treatment of both pediculosis and scabies is identification of the source of infestation. For scabies, pay particular attention to intertriginous areas (finger webs and other body creases and folds), wrists, elbows, and belt line. Burrows made by scabies may or may not be visible as linear, curved, or S-shaped burrows, 2 to 15 mm. They are pink-white and slightly elevated. A vesicle or the mite may look like a black dot at the end of the burrow. The main feature of head louse infestation is scalp itching, although secondary bacterial infection is not uncommon. The diagnosis is made by finding empty egg cases ("nits") stuck to the base of hair follicles; the highest concentration is usually in the occipital and parietal regions. In heavy infestations, developing eggs, nymphs and adult lice may be seen. Body lice and pubic lice "crabs" are considered sexually transmitted diseases.

Nursing Diagnosis After receiving lindane, L.G. is at risk for altered comfort (itching) and the potential complication of CNS toxicity.

Planning After receiving the lindane shampoo, L.G. will be free of ectoparasites without adverse drug effects.

Implementation
Monitoring Reexamine in 7 days, reapply lindane if necessary.

Intervention
Pediculosis Capitis (Head Lice) Lindane shampoo is the most convenient dosage form but the lotion and cream are also effective. Apply a quantity sufficient to cover only the affected and adjacent hairy areas. The cream should be rubbed into scalp and hair and left in place for 12 hours followed by thorough washing. Retreatment is usually not necessary.

Pediculosis Pubis (Crab Lice) Apply a sufficient quantity only to cover thinly the hair and skin of the pubic area, and if infested, the thighs, trunk, and axillary regions. The material should be rubbed into the skin and hair, and left in place for 12 hours followed by a thorough washing. Sexual contacts should be treated simultaneously. Retreatment is usually not necessary.

Sarcoptes scabiei (Scabies) Apply the cream to dry skin in a thin layer and rub in thoroughly. If crusted lesions are present, a warm bath preceding the medication is helpful. If a warm bath is used, allow the skin to dry and cool before applying the cream. Usually 1 oz is sufficient for an adult. A total body application should be made from the neck down. Scabies rarely affects the head of children or adults but may occur in infants. The cream should be left on 8 to 12 hours and should then be removed by thorough washing. Many clients exhibit persistent pruritus after treatment;

this is rarely a sign of treatment failure and is not an indication for retreatment, unless living mites can be demonstrated.

Education Decontamination of the clothing and personal articles used by the infested person is also necessary. This can be performed by washing clothing and bedding with hot, soapy water or by dry cleaning items that cannot be washed. Usually all persons involved (e.g., the entire family) are treated to prevent reinfestation.

Evaluation L.G. will be free of ectoparasites without adverse CNS drug effects (e.g., dizziness, irritability, seizures). L.G.'s mother decontaminates the family's clothing and bedding appropriately.

Miscellaneous Therapeutic Agents

✳ **S.F. is a 63-year-old female with a longstanding history of type 2 diabetes mellitus. She has lost some sensation in her lower extremities over the past year, and visits the wound clinic over the past 3 months with an ongoing 4-cm ulcer on her right toe not responsive to oral antimicrobial therapy, topical dressings, elevation, and avoidance of weightbearing. Her health care provider initiates becaplermin (Regranex) topically daily to ulcer.**

✳ What is the role of becaplermin in the treatment of diabetic neuropathic ulcer?

Becaplermin is a recombinant form of human platelet-derived growth factor used to promote the formation of new granulation tissue. Applied to wound tissue of diabetic neuropathic ulcers, it stimulates fibroblasts to proliferate and differentiate and improves wound healing. The use of becaplermin is associated with moderate improvement in wound healing over 20 weeks, but its use is often limited to those ulcers not responsive to conventional care (Boulton, Kirsner, & Vileikyte, 2004). A 15-gram tube of 0.01% gel costs approximately $465 (Drugstore.com, 2005).

becaplermin [be **kap** ler min]
(Regranex)
Indications
Becaplermin is used as an adjunct to debridement in treatment of lower limb or foot ulcers in clients with diabetes mellitus. Treatment continues until healed, although is not considered successful unless the ulcer has reduced in size by at least 30% by week 10 or completely healed by week 20.
Dosing
Becaplermin is applied sparingly to the ulcer daily with the use of a cotton swab. The amount applied is dependent on ulcer size. Specific dosing is based on ulcer length × width × 0.6 for 7.5- or 15-gram tubes and ulcer length × width × 1.3 for 2-gram tube. The difference in multiplying factor is a function of the size of ribbon of gel delivered by different size tubes.
Adverse Effects
Erythema, local pain, and infection have infrequently been reported with becaplermin use.

TABLE 65-5 MISCELLANEOUS TOPICAL AGENTS

Generic (Trade Name)	Indication(s)	Comment(s)
eflornithine (Vaniqa)	Unwanted facial hair in women	Applied twice daily to affected area. Improvement noted after 4 to 8 weeks, but hair growth returns after discontinuation.
imiquimod (Aldara)	external genital and vaginal warts	Concurrent use with a condom or diaphragm is not recommended. Avoid sexual contact when cream is on skin. Wash treatment area with a mild soap and water 6 to 10 hours after application. Local skin reaction may occur (e.g., redness, flaking, erosion, pruritus, and edema).
masoprocol (Actinex)	actinic keratoses	Do not apply near the eyes or the mucous membranes of the nose or mouth. Apply morning and evening for 28 days. Transient burning, flaking, pruritus, and dryness have been reported.
minoxidil (Rogaine)	androgenetic alopecia	Advise the client that hair growth usually takes up to 4 months to appear. If treatment is stopped, new growth will probably shed in a couple of months. Do not use on an irritated or sunburned scalp. Do not use with other topical medications on the scalp.
podofilox (Condylox)	external genital and perianal warts	Do not use to treat mucous membrane warts. Adverse effects include burning, pain, inflammation, and pruritus.

Data from *Drug facts and comparisons* (58th ed.). (2005). St. Louis: Facts and Comparisons.

Nursing Implications

Consult wound care provider who will adjust the dosage weekly or biweekly. Follow the package directions carefully. The gel may be measured on waxed paper provided by the manufacturer. Do not allow the tip of the tube to contact the ulcer or skin surface. Report the appearance of a rash or a worsening of the ulcer.

✳ What other topical agents are available for use?

Numerous other topical products are available alone or in combination. An example of an older product is coal tar or its derivatives, which are antipruritic and antieczematous and therefore are used to treat psoriasis and other skin conditions. Examples of products with coal tar as an ingredient include Medotar, Tegrin Lotion for Psoriasis and Polytar. See Table 65-5 for other miscellaneous topical agents.

Summary

Many dermatologic agents are available and are used to treat numerous skin disorders. Three major groups of preparations were discussed: general products, prophylactic agents, and therapeutic agents. General dermatologic preparations include bath substances, cleansers, soaps, solutions and emollients, skin protectants, wet dressings and soaks, and rubs and liniments. Many are soothing and are used to promote the comfort of clients who have a dermatologic condition. Prophylactic agents form a film on the skin to keep out sun, light, air, or dust. Therapeutic agents may be antiinfectives (antibiotics, antivirals, and antifungals), corticosteroids, keratolytics, acne products, burn products, preparations for psoriasis, antipruritics, ectopara-

siticidal drugs, and a growth factor for diabetic lower extremity ulcers. The nurse must apply these preparations correctly and safely and instruct the client (or caregiver) to do likewise if they are to be self-administered. Evaluating the effectiveness of dermatologic agents is based on improvement without adverse effects.

✳ Critical Thinking Questions

- Ronald Jones, 48 years old, comes to the clinic with a superficial skin infection as the result of an abrasion he received on the job as a construction worker. The health care provider orders the wound to be cleansed and dressed with bacitracin ointment (500 units/gram, which the client is to continue three times daily) and also orders culture and sensitivity testing. As the nurse, what action will you take and in what sequence?

- What teaching would you provide to a mother who has discovered a pediculosis infestation in one of her children?

Bibliography

American Cancer Society. Skin cancer. Retrieved March 23, 2005, from http://www.cancer.org/docroot/PE dischargeontent/ped_7 _1 _What_You_Need_To_Know_About_Skin_Cancer.asp?sitearea=PEDAs.

Anandan, J.V. (2005). Parasitic infections. In M.A. Koda-Kimble, L.Y. Young, W.A. Kradjan, B.J. Guglielmo, B.K. Alldredge, & R.L. Corelli (Eds.), *Applied therapeutics: The clinical use of drugs.* (8th ed.). Philadelphia: Lippincott Williams & Wilkins.

Anderson, D.M., Keith, J., & Novak, P.D. (Eds.) (2002). *Mosby's medical, nursing, and allied health dictionary* (6th ed.). St. Louis: Mosby.

Boulton, A.J.M., Kirsner, R.S., & Vileikyte, L. (2004). Neuropathic diabetic foot ulcers. *New England Journal of Medicine, 351*(1), 48-55.

Burgess, I.F., Brown, C.M., & Lee, P.N. (2005). Treatment of head louse infestation with 4% dimeticone lotion: Randomised controlled equivalence trial. *British Medical Journal, 330*, 1423-1426.

DermNetNZ, New Zealand Dermatological Society. (2004). Azelaic acid. Retrieved September 10, 2004, from http://dermnetnz.org/treatments/azelaic-acid.html.

Diffey, B.L. (2001). When should sunscreen be reapplied? *Journal of the American Academy of Dermatology, 45*, 882-885.

Drug facts and comparisons (58th ed.). (2005). St. Louis: Facts and Comparisons.

Drugstore.com. (2005). Regranex. Retrieved September 30, 2005, from http://www.drugstore.com/pharmacy/prices/drugprice.asp?ndc=00045081015&trx=1Z5006.

Ellsworth, A. (2005). Psoriasis. In M.A. Koda-Kimble, L.Y. Young, W.A. Kradjan, B.J. Guglielmo, B.K. Alldredge, & R.L. Corelli (Eds.), *Applied therapeutics: The clinical use of drugs.* (8th ed.). Philadelphia: Lippincott Williams & Wilkins.

Ellsworth, A., & Smith, R.E. (2005). Dermatology and drug induced skin disorders. In M.A. Koda-Kimble, L.Y. Young, W.A. Kradjan, B.J. Guglielmo, B.K. Alldredge, & R.L. Corelli (Eds.), *Applied therapeutics: The clinical use of drugs.* (8th ed.). Philadelphia: Lippincott Williams & Wilkins.

Genentech. (July 2005). Dear Healthcare Provider letter. Important drug warning regarding RAPTIVA (efalizumab).

Habif, T.B. (2004). *Clinical dermatology.* (4th ed.). St. Louis: Mosby.

Hanifin, J.M., & Chan, S. (1999). Biochemical and immunologic mechanisms in atopic dermatitis: New targets for emerging therapies. *Journal of the American Academy of Dermatology, 41*(1), 72-77.

Ives, T.J. (2005). Photosensitivity and burns. In M.A. Koda-Kimble, L.Y. Young, W.A. Kradjan, B.J. Guglielmo, B.K. Alldredge, & R.L. Corelli (Eds.), *Applied therapeutics: The clinical use of drugs.* (8th ed.). Philadelphia: Lippincott Williams & Wilkins.

Lacy, C.F., Armstrong, L.L., Goldman, M.P., & Lance, L.L. (2004). Lexi-Comp's Drug Information Handbook, (12th ed.). Hudson, Ohio: Lexi-Comp.

Mosby's drug consult (15th ed.). (2005). St. Louis: Mosby.

Ozolins, M., Eady, E.A., Avery, A.J., Cunliffe, W.J., Po, A.L., O'Neill, C, et al. (2004). Comparison of five antimicrobial regimens for treatment of mild to moderate inflammatory facial acne vulgaris in the community: Randomised controlled trial. *Lancet, 364*, 2188-2195.

Pollack, R.J., Kiszewski, A., Armstrong, P., Hahn, C., Wolfe, N., & Rahman, H.A., et al. (1999). Differential permethrin susceptibility of head lice sampled in the United States and Borneo. *Archives of Pediatric & Adolescent Medicine, 153*(9), 969-973.

Seaton, T.L. (2005). Acne. In M.A. Koda-Kimble, L.Y. Young, W.A. Kradjan, B.J. Guglielmo, B.K. Alldredge, & R.L. Corelli (Eds.), *Applied therapeutics: The clinical use of drugs.* (8th ed.). Philadelphia: Lippincott Williams & Wilkins.

Sheridan, R.L. (2002). Burns. *Critical Care Medicine, 30*(11), S500-S514.

Strange, C.J. (1998). Thwarting skin cancer with sun sense. *FDA Consumer, 29*(6). Retrieved July 23, 1998, from, http://www.fda.gov/fdac/features/695 skincanc.html.

Tofte, S., & Hanifin, J. (2001). Current management and therapy of atopic dermatitis. *Journal of American Academy of Dermatologists, 44*(1), S13.

U.S. Food and Drug Administration. (March 2003). FDA Public Health Advisory: Safety of topical lindane products for the treatment of scabies and lice. Retrieved February 13, 2005, from http://www.fda.gov/cder/drug/infopage/lindane/lindanePHA.htm.

U.S. Food and Drug Administration. (1996). Outsmarting poison ivy and its cousins. *FDA Consumer.* Retrieved August 22, 2005, from http://www.fda.gov/fdac/features/796_ivy.html).

U.S. Food and Drug Administration. (March 2005a). FDA Talk Paper: FDA issues public health advisory informing health care providers of safety concerns associated with the use of two eczema drugs, Elidel and Protopic. Retrieved July 28, 2005, from http://www.fda.gov/bbs/topics/ANSWERS/2005/ANS01343.html.

U.S. Food and Drug Administration. (March 2005b). FDA Public Health Advisory: Elidel (pimecrolimus) cream and Protopic (tacrolimus) ointment. Retrieved July 28, 2005, from http://www.fda.gov/cder/drug/advisory/elidel_protopic.htm.

USP DI: Drug information for the health care professional (25th ed.). (2005). Greenwood Village, CO: MICROMEDEX Thomson Healthcare.

Wyatt, E.L., Sutter, S.H., & Drake, L.A. (2001). Dermatological pharmacology. In Hardman, J.G. & Limbird, L.L. (Eds.). *Goodman & Gilman's The pharmacological basis of therapeutics* (10th ed.). New York: McGraw-Hill.

e-LEARNING SUPPLEMENTS

Student CD-ROM
- Final Exam questions
- NCLEX® Examination review questions
- Pharmacology animations
- Printable chapter summary

Evolve Website (http://evolve.elsevier.com/mckenry)
- Case study on dermatologic drugs
- Content updates, including information on new drugs

- WebLinks corresponding to this chapter
- Answers to the critical thinking questions in this chapter
- *Elsevier ePharmacology Update* newsletter
- Mosby's Drug Consult Internet Edition
- Supplemental and reference information

66

DEBRIDING AGENTS

CHAPTER FOCUS

Nurses have the major responsibility of assessing the client's risk for pressure ulcers and planning the care needed to prevent them. Cleansing, debridement, and dressing of the wounds are necessary when pressure ulcers do occur. Knowledge of the various debriding agents allows the nurse to apply the most appropriate agent for the client's pressure ulcer according to the location, size, presence of eschar, or state of granulation.

LEARNING OBJECTIVES

- Use preventive and treatment measures to reduce the occurrence of pressure ulcers.
- Describe a classification system for grades of pressure ulcers.
- State the purpose of proteolytic enzyme preparations in the treatment of pressure ulcers.
- Implement the nursing management of clients receiving topical enzymatic agents.
- Describe the mechanism of action of nonenzymatic agent therapy for pressure ulcers.
- Implement the nursing management of clients receiving nonenzymatic agent therapy for pressure ulcers.

▲ KEY TERMS

debridement, p. 1197
eschar, p. 1203
granulation tissue, p. 1203
pressure ulcer, p. 1197
proteolytic enzymes, p. 1202

This chapter covers debriding agents, which are agents used to remove dirt, foreign objects, damaged tissue, and cellular debris from a wound or burn to prevent infection and promote healing. Preliminary assessment determines the process for appropriate cleansing of the wound. Wound cleansing itself is the process of using fluid to remove inflammatory contaminants from the wound surface. If such materials cannot be removed gently with fluids then more specific mechanical or biologic techniques are required. These techniques are termed "debridement." Debridement allows for a more thorough assessment of the wound including the wound bed (necrotic and granulation tissue,

fibrin slough, epithelium, exudate, odor), surrounding skin (color, moisture, suppleness), wound edges (undermining and condition of margins), and size (width, depth). After debridement, the wound assessment provides the foundation for a plan of care. Its thorough documentation is the only means of determining the effectiveness of the interventions.

✳ What are the key issues involved in the development, assessment, and management of pressure ulcers?

The **pressure ulcer** (formerly bed sore or decubitus ulcer) is a break in the skin and underlying subcutaneous and muscle tissue. It is caused by abnormal, sustained pressure or friction exerted over the bony prominences of the body by the object on which the body part rests. Exposure to moisture weakens the outer layers of skin and nutritional depletion contributes to the risk of pressure ulcers. These factors result in vascular insufficiency and ischemic necrosis, and it most commonly affects debilitated, comatose, immobilized, or paralyzed clients.

According to results of the Fifth National Prevalence and Incidence Study, the prevalence of pressure ulcers in acute care facilities ranged from 14% to 17% annually from 1999 to 2004 (Whittington & Briones, 2004). Agostini, Baker, and Bogardus (2004) reported that prevalence rates in skilled care facilities have declined by about 25% in the mid 1990s from the 13.2% prevalence rate (range 7% to 23%) in the early 1990s. In addition to increasing length of stay, hospital costs, and nursing care time, pressure ulcers can lead to cellulitis, osteomyelitis, sepsis, and possibly death.

Many causes contribute to this condition and must be treated. Among the local and systemic causes are the following: obesity or malnutrition; debilitation; a pressure and shearing force (friction drag between body tissues and underlying surfaces) on the lower body if the head of the bed is raised more than 30 degrees (Krasner, Rodeheaver, Sibbald, & Price, 2001); a loss of sensation of pressure or pain; muscle atrophy and motor paralysis; a reduction in the amount of adipose tissue between the skin and underlying bone; emaciation and dehydration; poor nutrition because of inadequate intake of vitamins, minerals, and trace elements (such as copper and zinc); friction; local anatomic defects; trauma; incontinence; edema; infections; heat and moisture (maceration); hypertension; septicemia; and local circulatory interference.

The bacterial flora of pressure ulcers (present in stages II, III and IV) are both gram-negative and gram-positive organisms and include *Staphylococcus aureus*, *Streptococcus* groups A and D, *Escherichia coli*, *Clostridium tetani*, and *Bacteroides*, *Proteus*, *Pseudomonas*, *Klebsiella*, and *Citrobacter* organisms. Parenteral antimicrobials may be needed in infected pressure sores that are difficult to treat because adequate levels in granulating wounds are not reached. These antibiotics are used as adjunct therapies prior to, during, and after surgical management.

Vacuum assisted closure (VAC) devices are also used to treat wounds or to prepare them for surgery. A VAC device uses a reticulated foam dressing cut to conform to an individual wound. The foam is covered by an occlusive drape under which a vacuum tube is placed. The tube is connected to a pump, which provides 50 to 125 mm of negative pressure to the occluded wound environment. The device has been shown to enhance local blood flow, diminish edema, limit bacterial proliferation, and accelerate granulation tissue formation in wounds. It has been used successfully in a wide variety of wounds either to facilitate complete wound closure or to prepare the wound for a reconstructive procedure (Lionelli & Lawrence, 2003).

Maggots have had a historical and resurgent role in debridement for wound healing. Maggots are fly larvae that have been raised in sterile conditions can be applied to a wound for debridement of necrotic tissue. It is not clear why the maggots spare the normal tissue, but they are able to do so and effectively work in deep and irregular wounds that are otherwise difficult to address with surgical debridement. In addition to the stimulation of host healing through debridement and resultant cytokine release, the maggots are known to secrete calcium salts and other antimicrobial agents (Mostow, 2003).

Although less frequently observed, surgical management is considered for those selected clients whose length of healing would be extraordinarily long in months and years and whose health status is appropriate for more rapid healing options. Surgical decisions include the underlying disease, the ability of the client to withstand surgery, and the condition or prognosis of the pressure ulcer (especially those in which all soft tissue is destroyed and bone is exposed).

✳ **J.D., an 84-year-old poorly nourished man is admitted to the hospital for a general workup. He was found on the floor in his home in a confused state by his neighbor. During his admission assessment, a Grade 2, 5 × 7 cm, sacral pressure ulcer with purulent discharge was noted.**

✳ **What are the nursing management issues for J.D.?**

Assessment To assess a client's risk for developing pressure sores, or to attempt to treat impaired skin integrity, it is necessary to determine the probable causes. Most health care agencies have assessment guides by which to assess risk (Figure 66-1). Use of this type of assessment tool with J.D. addresses common risk factors such as mobility, activity, mental status, medications that affect blood circulation or cognition, incontinence, nutritional status, and other current illnesses. He is assessed and given a score of 13 of a possible 24 using the Skin Integrity High Risk Form (see Figure 66-1); the higher the score, the higher the risk. These assessment guides are usually completed on admission to the agency and will be used to continue to monitor J.D. for the risk of impaired skin integrity during his stay with the health care agency. As J.D. has an ulceration, accurate assessment determines the intervention. See the clinical guideline algorithm for the treatment of pressure ulcers developed by the Agency for Healthcare Research and Quality (formerly the Agency for Health Care Policy and Research) (Figure 66-2).

Nursing Diagnosis The pertinent nursing diagnosis is either risk for impaired skin integrity (given a client's assessment score) or actual impairment of skin integrity if the client, such as J.D., demonstrates skin changes such as erythema that does not resolve in 30 minutes, blisters, or tissue erosion. Risk for infection and impaired comfort (pain) may also occur.

SKIN INTEGRITY HIGH RISK FORM

	PARAMETERS	0	1	2	3	4	5	SCORE
1.	General state of health	Good	Fair	Poor	Moribund			
2.	Predisposing diseases	Absent	Slight	Moderate	Severe			
3.	Mental status	Alert	Lethargic	Semicoma	Comatose			
4.	Nutrition	Good	Fair	Poor	None			
5.	Fluid intake	Good	Fair	Poor	None			
6.	Activity	Ambulates	Needs help			Chairfast	Bedfast	
7.	Mobility	Full	Limited			Very limited	Immobile	
8.	Incontinence	None	Occasional			Frequent	Total	
							TOTAL	

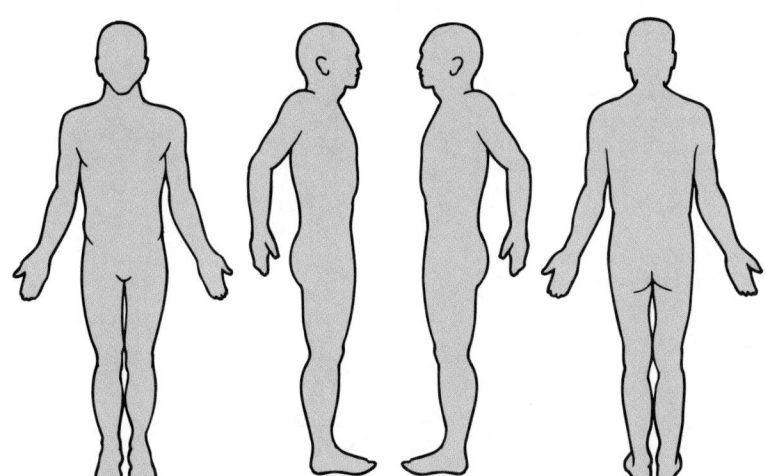

Draw and Number Impairments

		#1
Stage:		
Size:		
Shape:		
Drainage:		
		#2
Stage:		
Size:		
Shape:		
Drainage:		
		#3
Stage:		
Size:		
Shape:		
Drainage:		

Date/Signature: _____

PARAMETERS:
1. GENERAL STATE OF HEALTH:
   0—Good: injury limited to one area, no major health problems
   1—Fair: minor surgery or controlled health problems
   2—Poor: major surgery or serious health problems
   3—Moribund: prognosis fatal, death within 3 months
2. PREDISPOSING DISEASE:
   0—Absent: no vascular disease, anemia, diabetes, neuropathies
   1—Slight: controlled diabetes, anemia, mild vascular diseases, mild skin disorder
   2—Moderate: brittle diabetes, advanced vascular disease, unhealed ulcers, absent peripheral pulses
   3—Severe: uncontrolled diabetes/anemia, severe vascular disease manifested by decreased sensation, edema of ankles and feet, thin atrophic skin, brown pigmentation with stasis dermatitis
3. MENTAL STATUS:
   0—Alert: oriented, communicates appropriately
   1—Lethargic: listless, sluggish, slow to respond
   2—Semicoma or confused: responds to painful stimuli, unable to cooperate with pressure relief
   3—Comatose: no verbal response, no response to pain
4. NUTRITION:
   0—Good: weight within normal limits
   1—Fair: under or overweight, enternal or parenteral nutrition meeting RDA
   2—Poor: losing weight slowly or obese, seldom eats 1/2 served portion, enteral feeding tolerated poorly, i.e., high gastric residual, diarrhea
   3—None: losing weight rapidly, emaciated, unable to eat, refuses to eat, no nutritional support

5. FLUID INTAKE:
   0—Good: 1500 mL, skin warm resilient, normal turgor
   1—Fair: 1000-1500 mL, dry skin and flaccid, concentrated urine output
   2—Poor: ↓1000 mL, skin dry, cracked and flaky, mouth dry, lips parched, decreased urine output in the absence of renal disease
   3—None: no fluid intake
6. ACTIVITY:
   0—Ambulates: walks without help
   1—Needs help: requires assistance, uses crutch, walker
   2—Chairfast: cannot ambulate, confined to chair
   3—Bedfast: remains in bed constantly
7. MOBILITY:
   0—Full: voluntarily changes position
   1—Limited: cannot voluntarily move all extremities, cast on arm or leg, pain with movement
   2—Very limited: move only with assistance, severe pain with movement, body cast, paraplegia, hemiparesis
   3—Immobile: never voluntarily changes position, contractures prevent movement, quadriplegia
8. INCONTINENCE:
   0—None: control of bowel and bladder
   1—Occasional: stress incontinence, occasional diarrhea with the continent patient
   2—Frequent: usually of urine and/or bowels
   3—Total: no control of bowel or bladder

FIGURE 66-1 Assessment guide. A score of 12 or greater is an indication that the client is at risk for impaired skin integrity. The nursing diagnosis should be included in the client's care plan.

Planning During pressure ulcer treatment, J.D. will:
- Evidence intact skin/or decrease in size of pressure sore without infection or complications of therapy.
- Effectively manage the therapeutic regimen (by self or caregiver) including, adequate hydration and nutrition, changing position, and wound care.

Implementation

Monitoring Monitor the bony prominences of the ankles, coccyx, elbows, heels, hips, knees, shoulders, ears (cartilaginous areas), and other areas having thin layers of subcutaneous tissue. Continue to assess J.D. for the presence or worsening of the risk factors previously discussed. Assess the wound on a daily basis for a gradual reduction in size; meas-

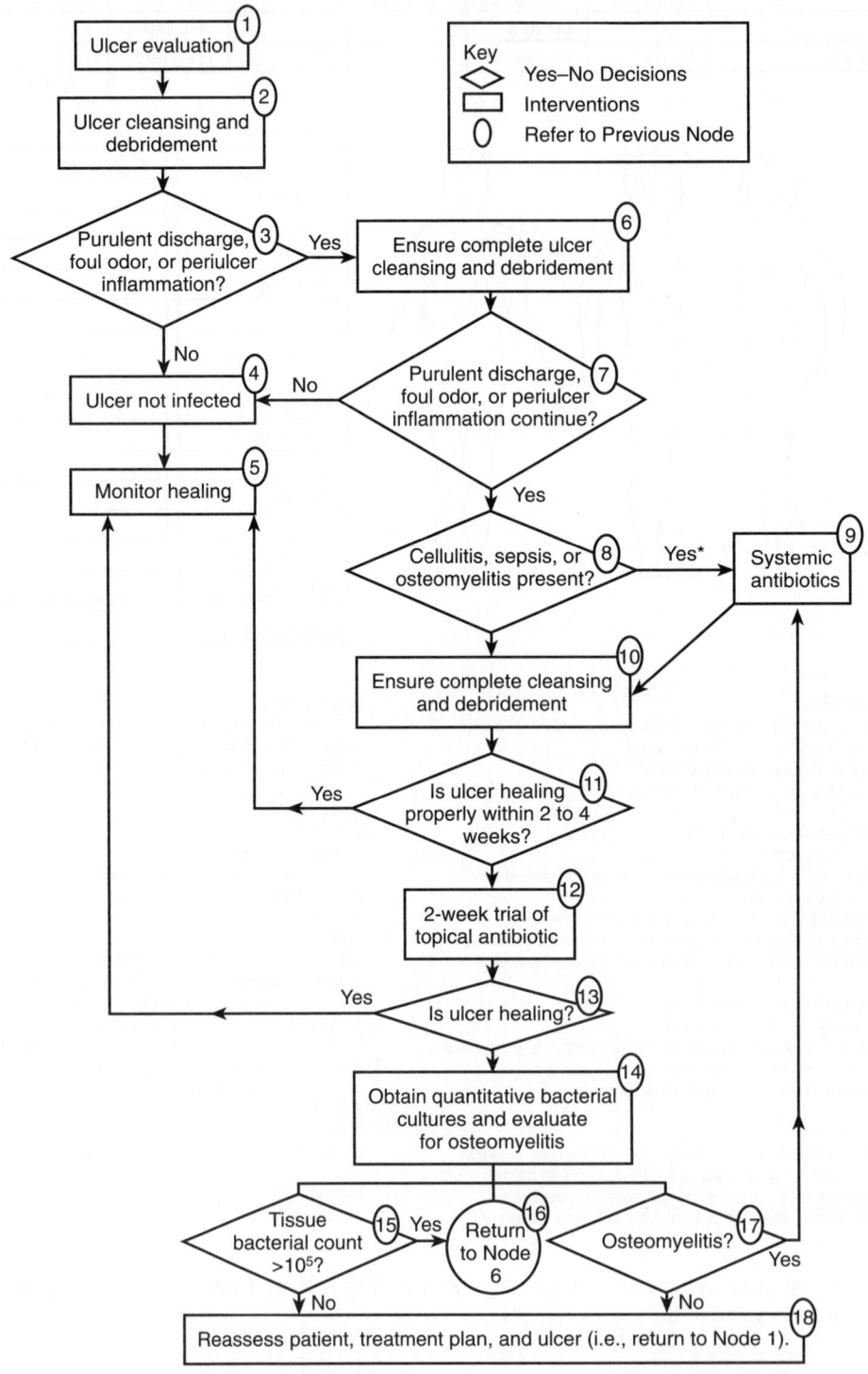

FIGURE 66-2 Clinical guideline algorithm for the treatment of pressure ulcers. *Suspicion of sepsis requires urgent medical evaluation and treatment. The treatment of sepsis is not discussed in this guideline.

From Agency for Health Care Policy and Research (1994). *Pressure ulcer treatment: Quick reference guideline.* No. 15. AHCPR Pub. No. 95-0653. Rockville, MD: Agency for Health Care Policy and Research, Public Health Service, U.S. Department of Health and Human Services.

ure and record the size at its greatest length, width, and depth. Determine the stage of the wound and describe its appearance regarding necrotic debris, eschar, granulation tissue, drainage, color, and odor. Assess for pockets, tracts, and undermining. Observe the wound margins for induration or tenderness. Photographs provide excellent documentation by which to monitor the efficacy of nursing interventions.

Intervention The prevention and treatment of pressure ulcers are focused on treating the underlying causes, providing a well-balanced nutritional state, and minimizing or eliminating the pressure or friction that is causing the tissue damage. The following are some preventive and treatment measures that can be used to reduce the occurrence of impaired skin integrity:

- Change J.D.'s position frequently (every 1 to 2 hours day and night) for pressure relief.
- Maintain a clean, dry, and wrinkle-free bed. Bedclothes should be smooth rather than coarse and should be changed frequently.
- Provide active and passive exercise to increase muscle and skin tone and to improve vascularity, or use a whirlpool for hydrotherapy.
- Position the client with pillows and pads; do not exceed a 30-degree elevation of the head.
- Use hydrofloat devices, silica gel pads, polystyrene, and convoluted foam pads and heel protectors to reduce pressure. Place them on a mattress in direct contact with the client's skin. The mattress should be free of surface bulges and indentations and should have a uniform, flat surface to prevent friction or wrinkles.
- Use an alternating pressure mattress pad covered with one layer of sheet to promote circulation and to reduce the occurrence of tissue ischemia.
- Provide meticulous skin hygiene, with frequent inspections for abnormal alterations. Wash the skin gently with warm water and, if needed, mild nondetergent soap; rinse the skin and blot it dry with a soft towel. An emollient lubricating lotion may be used after washing to keep the skin soft.
- J.D. is not incontinent, but if he were the nurse would need to keep his skin dry and clear of urine and fecal contamination, because maceration from moisture promotes tissue breakdown and predisposes to infection. Perspiration in the continent client is also a cause of maceration. Trimmed nails prevent self-inflicted injury caused by scratching of the skin.
- Maintain nutritional support for a positive nitrogen balance, tissue turgor, and adequate fluid intake with 3800 to 4600 cal/24 hours and a diet high in protein, vitamins, minerals, and trace elements. J.D.'s hemoglobin level should be at least 12 g/100 mL, and serum protein levels should be above 6 g/100 mL.
- Necrotic pressure ulcers often require meticulous wound care and debridement by surgical or drug methods.

- J.D. should be offered analgesics before pressure ulcer care depending on the extent of the wound and his preferences.
- Treatment regimens are based on the extent of skin involvement.

Education Teach preventive measures to J.D., family members, or other caregivers of chair-bound or bedridden clients or other clients at risk for developing pressure ulcers. Inform J.D. that the preparations used are to promote healing, and describe the procedure involved in cleansing and dressing the wound (see the Community and Home Health Considerations below).

Evaluation The expected outcome of pressure ulcer care is that J.D.'s wound will diminish in size and form a healthy, clean surface. Other areas of skin will remain warm, without erythema, and intact.

✱ **How should therapy for pressure ulcers be approached?**
A treatment plan for pressure ulcers should consider four basic principles: (1) providing assessment and interventions

---

✱✱✱ **Community and Home Health Considerations**

Wound Care at Home

Instruction should be provided for the caregiver if decubitus care is to be performed in the home. This should include all of the supportive care to the client, such as positioning, nutrition, and hydration discussed in the interventions. Pressure sore dressings should be changed as ordered by the prescriber or when soiled.

Dressing supplies, the debriding agent, gloves, and a bag for disposal or the soiled dressings should be gathered together before the dressing change is begun. Consider the client's anticipated need for analgesia for the dressing change and/or debridement. A waiting period after analgesic administration should ensure that the client has less discomfort. The client should be positioned for comfort and for good access to the pressure sore. The pressure sore should be assessed each time the dressing is changed; the size and character of the wound is recorded to monitor progress. Any increase in drainage or foul smell should be reported to the nurse.

Expose the pressure sore, and drape the client for modesty as much as possible. Glove hands and remove the soiled dressing, pulling the adhesive tape in the direction of the pressure sore. Mineral oil may be used to loosen the adhesive tape. Discard the old dressings and gloves in the bag. Glove hands to clean the wound from the center out, using one stroke each time until crusting and old drainage are removed. Apply a pharmacologic agent as ordered using swabs, a tongue blade, or gloved fingers. Apply outer dressings. Remove gloves, and secure dressing with tape. Discard soiled gloves in the bag.

to improve the client's general health, which may help to reduce factors contributing to the problem, such as incontinence, anemia, or edema; (2) reducing pressure sites through positioning or the use of padding, special beds, and other items, thus increasing blood flow to the site; (3) maintaining a clean wound site; and (4) using an appropriate agent for treatment or stimulation of granulation tissue.

The treatment of pressure ulcers depends on the stage of the ulcer and condition of the wound bed. In many instances, cleansing and debridement prevents bacterial colonization from progressing to an infection. A 2-week trial with topical antibiotics should be considered if a clean ulcer has exudate or does not heal after 2 to 4 weeks of treatment. The topical agent should be effective against gram-positive, gram-negative, and anaerobic bacteria, such as triple antibiotic or silver sulfadiazine.

If the ulcerated area does not respond, a tissue biopsy may be needed. For ulcers with exudates, a bacterial culture is often recommended to evaluate for osteomyelitis. Clients with osteomyelitis may present with bone pain, drainage, and/or systemic manifestations of infection including fever, chills, leukocytosis, and bacteremia. Osteomyelitis, as a complication, of pressure ulcers, may result in amputation. Systemic antimicrobials are necessary for sepsis, osteomyelitis, bacteremia, and advancing cellulitis.

Saline solutions are considered safe and effective in cleaning most pressure ulcers. Unless prescribed by the practitioner, avoid the use of povidone-iodine, iodophor, Dakin's solution, acetic acid, and hydrogen peroxide, as they may be cytotoxic (i.e., toxic to fibroblasts) and interfere with the granulation process.

Pressure ulcers are classified into four grades or stages (Figure 66-3):

- Stage I: A red area that overlies a bony or tendinous (tendons) site that remains even when the pressure is relieved
- Stage II: A partial-thickness skin loss that involves the epidermis and/or dermis
- Stage III: A skin ulcer that extends into exposed subcutaneous tissue; it may include necrotic tissue, sinus tract formation, exudate, and/or infection
- Stage IV: A deep skin ulcer that exposes muscle and bone; the body enzymes usually separate the eschar. The sloughing of tissue results in an ulcer and may include necrotic tissue, sinus tract formation, exudate, and/or infection

In addition to the nursing management previously reviewed, numerous treatment protocols have been applied. The treatment approach can vary considerably depending on the evaluation of the wound, the physician, the nurse, and local practice. Table 66-1 is a recommended treatment protocol based on the staging system previously noted.

⬤ What is the role of debriding agents?

Debridement is used to remove necrotic and sloughing tissue in a pressure ulcer. This tissue delays healing and provides a media for bacterial infestation. Although commonly used for debridement, wet-to-dry saline dressings can be irritating, painful, and disruptive to healthy tissue. Proteolytic enzymes are used for chemical debridement; they digest or liquefy necrotic tissue. The drawback with these preparations is that 2 or 3 days are usually needed to remove an eschar. However, their use is appropriate for uninfected necrotic sites and for clients unable to tolerate surgical intervention. If these preparations are used for in-

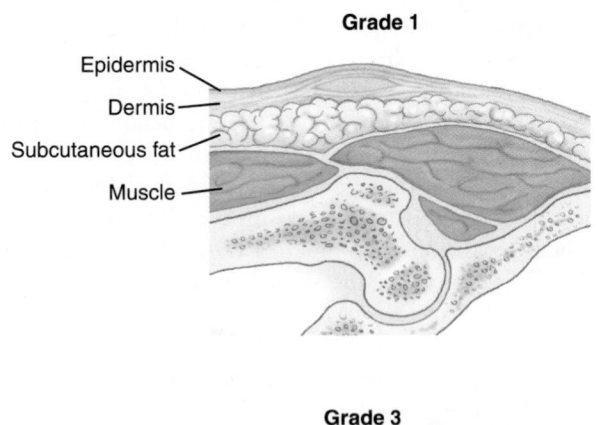

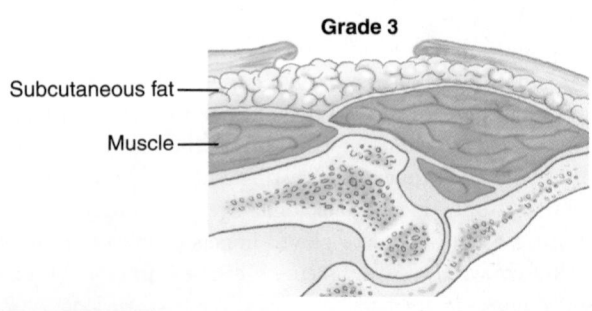

FIGURE 66-3 The four grades of pressure ulcers.

TABLE 66-1 PRESSURE ULCERS—RECOMMENDED TREATMENT PROTOCOL	
Staging	**Typical Treatment Modalities**
Stage I or II	Silicone spray, transparent or hydrocolloidal
Stage III	Wet-to-dry dressings until wound is clean, enzymatic debridement, hydrocolloidal dressing
Stage IV	As for Stage III and surgical debridement/intervention

Modified from Brem, H., & Lyder, C. (2004). Protocol for the successful treatment of pressure ulcers, *American Journal of Surgery*, 188(1A Supplement), 9-17; Duthie, E.H., Jr., & Katz P.R. (1998). *Practice of Geriatrics*. Philadelphia: W.B. Saunders.

fected necrosis tissue, a systemic antibiotic may also be necessary.

The enzyme preparation should be discontinued when granulation tissue is evident or if bleeding occurs during gentle cleansing. Surgical debridement may be required for very serious ulcerations or if complications (e.g., osteomyelitis) are present.

Most enzymes contain the suffix "ase" in their name plus the name of the substrate on which they act. For example, collagenase acts on and degrades collagen, and hyaluronidase acts on hyaluronic acid (a ground substance of connective tissue). Enzymes are also grouped according to the reactions they catalyze. For example, proteolytic enzymes hasten the hydrolysis of proteins. Because enzymes are proteins, they may be antigenic and cause immunologic-type toxic reactions.

The enzymes discussed in this chapter are used topically for medical or *chemical debridement*—the removal, by enzymatic digestion, of necrotic and injured tissue, clotted blood, purulent exudates, or fibrinous accumulations in wounds. This action cleans the wounds and facilitates healing. Other modalities used in wound management include the use of topical antibacterial therapies, including topical metronidazole (see Chapter 65).

✻ **A regimen is established for the initial treatment of J.D.'s wound; daily sterile normal saline cleansing to cleanse the ulcer base with a daily application of papain-urea debriding ointment with evaluation of this therapy on day 4.**

✻ **What are the nursing management issues involved in the use of debriding agents for J.D.?**
The following are aspects of care for clients being treated with topically applied enzymatic drugs (not the nonenzymatic agents). These are in addition to the aspects of J.D.'s care previously discussed. Before the topical aseptic application of enzymes, the wound should be thoroughly cleansed (flushing away necrotic debris and fibrinous exudates) with a solution that does not inactivate the enzyme (e.g., physiologic saline or sterile distilled water). Healing wounds

should be cleansed gently; high-pressure irrigation or aggressive scrubbing with gauze pads should be avoided, because they can cause tissue trauma and delayed healing. Solutions containing heavy metals, detergents, and antiseptics should be avoided to prevent inactivation of the enzymes. As much necrotic tissue, as can be readily removed, a wound care specialist should remove it with forceps and scissors. All previously applied ointment should be removed before new ointment is applied to the wound bed.

Although J.D.'s wound eschar was minimal, dense, dry, and thick eschar, or crust, should be crosshatched by the physician with a No. 10 or No. 11 blade for adequate contact of the enzyme with the substrate of necrotic debris. Ointment should be applied directly to the wound with a sterile tongue depressor or spatula and then covered with sterile petrolatum gauze or sterile gauze (or other nonadhering dressing); ointment can also be applied with a sterile gauze pad that is then placed over the wound. A bandage and/or tape should be used to hold the dressing in place.

Ointment or jelly preparations should be confined to the wound. The surrounding healthy tissue (or skin) should be protected from the enzyme (e.g., zinc oxide paste can be used). The treated lesion should be kept moist and protected from drying. The enzyme must be in direct contact with the wound for a sufficient length of time—usually about 4 days. To avoid delayed healing, the enzyme should be discontinued when the wound is cleaned and débrided and when granulation tissue (healthy pink, soft new tissue) is evident. If required, secondary skin closure or grafting may follow debridement.

Topical enzymes used for debriding theoretically may increase the risk of bacteremia in the debilitated client; this may necessitate monitoring J.D. for systemic bacterial infections (*Mosby's Drug Consult*, 2005). He should be observed for allergic or sensitivity reactions (e.g., dermatitis and febrile reactions).

Proteolytic Enzymes

collagenase [**kole** a jen aze]
(Santyl)
Collagenase is an enzymatic debriding agent capable of degrading both native and denatured collagen. Other proteolytic enzymes act only on denatured collagen. Thus it is claimed that collagenase produces more effective debridement by acting on collagen at the wound edges, in which necrotic slough is anchored.
Indications
Collagenase product is used to debride necrotic lesions and severe burns.
Dosing
This ointment should be applied only within the area of the lesion and should not be applied more frequently than twice daily.
Adverse Effects
A transient erythema has been reported as a cutaneous reaction on the wound surface or the area adjacent to the lesion. Applying a protectant (e.g., zinc oxide paste) may prevent this reaction around the lesion.
Nursing Management
The use of collagenase is based on the general care and that of proteolytic enzymes already discussed.

Assessment

By client history, determine that the client is not sensitive to collagenase before initiating therapy. In the use of concurrent medication, Burow's solution and other acidic solutions can inactivate collagenase by irrigating the lesion with acidic solutions such as Burow's solution (pH 3.6 to 4.4). The optimal pH range for collagenase is 6 to 8; an alteration outside this range decreases the activity of the enzyme. Nitrofurazone (Furacin) also inactivates the activity of collagenase.

Implementation

Intervention

Cleanse the wound area of debris by gentle irrigation with sterile normal saline. Pat the ulcer dry with a sterile gauze pad. If infection is present, apply a topical antibacterial agent (e.g., neomycin, bacitracin-polymyxin B solution or powder) directly to the ulcer surface before the collagenase. Collagenase should be applied once daily. If the wound is deep, collagenase should be applied directly with a wooden tongue depressor or spatula. The application should be repeated if the dressing area becomes soiled (e.g., because of incontinence). Adherent dressings or moisture barriers help prevent the introduction of stool and urine.

The average time for complete debridement of dermal ulcers and decubiti with collagenase is approximately 11 days. This time permits debridement of necrotic tissue and the establishment of granulation tissue. Careful observation of the wound bed is indicated. The enzyme should be stopped when granulation tissue is evident. The ointment does not need to be refrigerated; it is stored at room temperature.

fibrinolysin and desoxyribonuclease [fye bri noe **lye** sin/des ock see rye bo **nu** klee aze]

(Elase)

The proteolytic enzymes fibrinolysin and desoxyribonuclease have individual effects; fibrinolysin digests fibrin or blood clots, and desoxyribonuclease digests deoxyribonucleic acid (nucleic acids). Because purulent exudates are composed mainly of fibrin and nucleic acids, this product produces its effects on denatured proteins (devitalized tissue); the protein elements of living cells remain unaffected.

An ointment that contains the two enzymes in combination with chloramphenicol is also available. The added antibiotic bacteriostatic properties inhibit the synthesis of bacterial protein in infected lesions. Systemic antibiotics are also indicated when clinical infection has been verified by positive culture results.

Indications

Fibrinolysin and desoxyribonuclease is used to debride inflamed and/or infected lesions, including surgical wounds, ulcerative lesions, second- and third-degree burns, and wounds resulting from circumcision or episiotomy. The combination product with antibiotic is preferred for infected lesions.

Dosing

The ointment is typically dosed one to three times daily to affected area or as part of routine wound management protocols.

Adverse Effects

Local erythema and irritation are the most commonly reported adverse effects.

Nursing Management

The use of fibrinolysin and desoxyribonuclease is based on the general care and that of proteolytic enzymes already discussed.

Assessment

Obtain the client's sensitivity history, because allergic reactions have been observed in clients who are sensitive to bovine source materials or mercury compounds (thimerosal, a mercury derivative, is used as a preservative in the ointment base of Elase). When using the ointment formulation containing chloramphenicol, monitor the wound for superinfection. This preparation may be used in Canada but is not available in the United States.

Proteolytic Enzyme Combination Products

Trypsin and papain (proteolytic enzymes), balsam of Peru (a mild antibacterial agent that aids in improving circulation in the wound area by stimulating the capillary bed), castor oil (provides protective covering and improves epithelialization), urea (emollient and keratolytic), and chlorophyll derivatives (aid in controlling wound odor and healing) have been formulated into various combinations and marketed. For example, Granulex contains trypsin, balsam of Peru, and castor oil, whereas Panafil contains papain, urea, and chlorophyll derivatives.

Such products may be ordered for administration once or twice daily. The wound area should be cleansed by flushing it with physiologic saline before each application. Be aware that hydrogen peroxide solution can inactivate papain and is not generally used in ulcer care because of destructive effects on granulation tissue.

Nonenzymatic Agents

flexible hydroactive dressings and granules

(DuoDERM)

Flexible hydroactive dressings and granules are available as a sheet dressing. Many variations of this type of dressing are available on the market. DuoDERM is one such product.

Indications

Controlling the absorption of wound fluid exudate is a function of the rate at which the dressing interacts with the exudate. Flexible hydroactive dressings are indicated for necrotic wounds only after the thick eschar at the wound margin is removed. They provide local management of venous stasis ulcers, ulcers secondary to arterial insufficiency, diabetes mellitus, trauma, pressure ulcers, and superficial wounds. The granule form is for the local management of exudating dermal ulcers in association with the dressings.

Dosing

Varies with product. Frequency of dressing change is dependent on condition of wound and recommendations by the dressing manufacturer.

Adverse Effects

Irritation to the dressing material is possible with many dressings. Maceration may occur if the wound is not dry and/or not allowed adequate ventilation.

Nursing Management

The use of flexible dressings is based on the general care and that of proteolytic enzymes already discussed.

Assessment

The use of flexible hydroactive dressings should be avoided with the following dermal conditions: tissue of muscle, tendon, or bone; ulcers with infection (tuberculosis, syphilis, or deep fungal infections); and active vasculitis (periarteritis nodosa, systemic lupus erythematosus, and cryoglobulinemia).

Implementation

Intervention

During the initial phase of treatment, the wound increases in size and depth because of the cleaning away of necrotic debris. The liquefied material left in the wound, which is seen when the dressing is removed, has a purulent appearance and should be washed away before proceeding with further wound evaluation.

Clean the wound site before applying this product, and follow the specific instructions outlined in the package labeling. Dressings are designed to remain in place from 1 to 7 days. During periods of infection, the dressings should be discontinued and antimicrobial treatment started until the infection is completely treated.

Summary

Pressure ulcers add greatly to the length and cost of a hospital stay. They are best prevented; when they do occur they are treated with nonpharmacologic measures (e.g., debridement, positioning) and with proteolytic enzyme or nonenzymatic preparations depending on the cause and extent of the wound.

⊛ Critical Thinking Questions

- How do the indications for the use of proteolytic enzyme preparations differ from the uses for flexible hydroactive dressings and granules?
- How might a nurse determine that it is time to discontinue the use of proteolytic enzyme preparations?

Bibliography

Agostini, J.V., Baker, D.I., & Bogardus, S.T. (2004). Chapter 27. Prevention of Pressure Ulcers in Older Patients. Retrieved April 2, 2005, from, http://www.ahrq.gov/clinic/ptsafety/chap27.htm.

Alvarez, O.M., Fernandez-Obregon, A., Rogers, R.S., Bergmamo, L. Masso, J., & Black, M. (2002a). A prospective, randomized, comparative study of collagenase and papain-urea for pressure under debridement, *Wounds, 14*(8), 293-301.

Alvarez, O.M., Fernandez-Obregon, A., Rogers, R.S., Bergmamo, L. Masso, J., & Black, M. (2002b). Chemical debridement of pressure ulcers: A prospective, randomized, comparative trial of collagenase and papain/urea formulations. *Wounds, 12*(2), 15-25.

Anderson, D.M., Keith, J., & Novak, P.D. (Eds.) (2002). Mosby's medical, nursing, and allied health dictionary (6th ed.). St. Louis: Mosby.

Drug facts and comparisons (58th ed.). (2005). St. Louis: Facts and Comparisons.

Krasner, D.L., Rodeheaver, G.T., Sibbald, R.G., & Price, P.E. (Eds.). (2001). *Chronic wound care: A clinical source book for healthcare professionals (3rd ed.).* Wayne PA: HNP Communications.

Lawrence, W.T., Bevin, A.G., & Sheldon, G.F. (2002). Acute wound care, ACS Surgery: Principles and Practice. Elmwood Park, NJ: WebMD.

Lionelli, G.T., & Lawrence, W.T. (2003). Wound dressings. *Surgical Clinics of North America 83*(3), 617-638.

Mosby's drug consult (15th ed.). (2005). St. Louis: Mosby.

Mostow, E.N. (2003). Wound healing: a multidisciplinary approach for dermatologists, *Dermatology Clinics, 21*(2), 371-387.

National Institute for Clinical Excellence, National Health Service. (2001). Guidance on the use of debriding agents and specialist wound care clinics for difficult to heal surgical wounds, Technical Appraisal Guidance, No. 24. London: National Institute for Clinical Excellence.

USP DI: Drug information for the health care professional (25th ed.). (2005). Greenwood Village, CO: MICROMEDEX Thomson Healthcare.

Whittington, K.T., & Briones, R. (2004). National Prevalence and Incidence Study: 6-year sequential acute care data. *Advances in Skin & Wound Care, 17*(9), 490-494.

e-LEARNING SUPPLEMENTS

Student CD-ROM
- Final Exam questions
- NCLEX® Examination review questions
- Pharmacology animations
- Printable chapter summary

Evolve Website (http://evolve.elsevier.com/mckenry)
- Interactive concept map on the client with a pressure ulcer
- Content updates, including information on new drugs

- WebLinks corresponding to this chapter
- Answers to the critical thinking questions in this chapter
- *Elsevier ePharmacology Update* newsletter
- Mosby's Drug Consult Internet Edition
- Supplemental and reference information

67

VITAMINS AND MINERALS

CHAPTER FOCUS

Over-the-counter (OTC) vitamin and mineral preparations are very popular in the United States and Canada. However, these dietary supplements possess the capacity for producing toxic reactions if used inappropriately. Consumers often do not perceive vitamins and minerals as being drugs. It is imperative that nurses incorporate the assessment and instruction of vitamin therapy into their practice to be supportive of appropriate nutrient management for their clients.

LEARNING OBJECTIVES

- Review the recommended daily allowances of vitamins and minerals.
- Describe factors that might contribute to the inadequate intake of vitamins and minerals.
- Explain the difference between fat-soluble and water-soluble vitamins.
- Cite the results of a deficiency or excess of each vitamin.
- Implement the nursing management essential for clients receiving vitamin therapy.
- Compare the contents of over-the-counter vitamin and mineral preparations with recommended daily allowances.

▲ KEY TERMS

avitaminosis, p. 1208
fat-soluble vitamins, p. 1215
hypervitaminosis, p. 1215
vitamins, p. 1208
water-soluble vitamins, p. 1215

■▬ KEY DRUGS

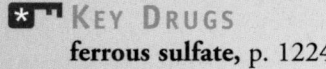

ferrous sulfate, p. 1224

✱ **What are the consequences of nutritional deficiencies?** The nutritional needs of the individual are best met by adequate oral ingestion of fluids and regular, balanced meals. Dietary recommendations are revised every 5 years by the U.S. Department of Health and Human Services and the U.S. Department of Agriculture (http://www.healthierus.gov/dietaryguidelines/). Box 67-1 presents key points. There is a growing body of research that demonstrates that the prevalence of vitamin deficiency in usual Western diets is higher than generally believed. Subtle deficiencies in several vitamins (at levels below those that cause classic vitamin deficiency syndromes such as scurvy or pellagra) put the individual at risk for chronic degenerative diseases such as atherosclerosis, cancer, and osteoporosis. Progression of other diseases may also be linked to vitamin and nutritional status. Concurrent multivitamin use in underdeveloped countries is associated with slowed progression from human immunodeficiency virus (HIV) to advanced acquired immune deficiency syndrome (AIDS) (Fawzi et al., 2004).

Breast milk or formula meets the normal nutritional needs of the infant, and strained and chopped table foods are added to the diet as tolerated by the growing child. Throughout life, challenges to nutrition status can occur, requiring replacement or supplementation of nutrients, vitamins, minerals, electrolytes, and fluids. Debilitation from nutritional deprivation may impair wound healing; reduce

ADEQUATE NUTRIENTS WITHIN CALORIE NEEDS

- Consume a variety of nutrient-dense foods and beverages within and among the basic food groups while choosing foods that limit the intake of saturated and trans fats, cholesterol, added sugars, salt, and alcohol.
- Meet recommended intakes within energy needs by adopting a balanced eating pattern, such as the U.S. Department of Agriculture (USDA) Food Guide or the Dietary Approaches to Stop Hypertension (DASH) Eating Plan.

WEIGHT MANAGEMENT

- To maintain body weight in a healthy range, balance calories from foods and beverages with calories expended.
- To prevent gradual weight gain over time, make small decreases in food and beverage calories and increase physical activity.

PHYSICAL ACTIVITY

- Engage in regular physical activity and reduce sedentary activities to promote health, psychological well-being, and a healthy body weight.
  - To reduce the risk of chronic disease in adulthood: Engage in at least 30 minutes of moderate-intensity physical activity, above usual activity, at work or home on most days of the week.
  - For most people, greater health benefits can be obtained by engaging in physical activity of more vigorous intensity or longer duration.
  - To help manage body weight and prevent gradual, unhealthy body weight gain in adulthood: Engage in approximately 60 minutes of moderate- to vigorous-intensity activity on most days of the week although not exceeding caloric intake requirements.
  - To sustain weight loss in adulthood: Participate in at least 60 to 90 minutes of daily moderate-intensity physical activity although not exceeding caloric intake requirements. Some people may need to consult with a health care provider before participating in this level of activity.
- Achieve physical fitness by including cardiovascular conditioning, stretching exercises for flexibility, and resistance exercises or calisthenics for muscle strength and endurance.

FOOD GROUPS TO ENCOURAGE

- Consume a sufficient amount of fruits and vegetables while staying within energy needs. Two cups of fruit and 2 and one half cups of vegetables per day are recommended for a reference 2000-calorie intake, with higher or lower amounts depending on the calorie level.
- Choose a variety of fruits and vegetables each day. In particular, select from all five vegetable subgroups (dark green, orange, legumes, starchy vegetables, and other vegetables) several times a week.
- Consume 3 or more ounce-equivalents of whole-grain products per day, with the rest of the recommended grains coming from enriched or whole-grain products. In general, at least half the grains should come from whole grains.
- Consume 3 cups per day of fat-free or low-fat milk or equivalent milk products.

FATS

- Consume less than 10% of calories from saturated fatty acids and less than 300 mg daily of cholesterol, and keep trans fatty acid consumption as low as possible.
- Keep total fat intake between 20% to 35% of calories, with most fats coming from sources of polyunsaturated and monounsaturated fatty acids, such as fish, nuts, and vegetable oils.
- When selecting and preparing meat, poultry, dry beans, and milk or milk products, make choices that are lean, low-fat, or fat-free.
- Limit intake of fats and oils high in saturated and/or trans fatty acids, and choose products low in such fats and oils.

CARBOHYDRATES

- Choose fiber-rich fruits, vegetables, and whole grains often.
- Choose and prepare foods and beverages with little added sugars or caloric sweeteners, such as amounts suggested by the USDA Food Guide and the DASH Eating Plan.
- Reduce the incidence of dental caries by practicing good oral hygiene and consuming sugar- and starch-containing foods and beverages less frequently.

SODIUM AND POTASSIUM

- Consume less than 2300 mg (approximately 1 teaspoon of salt) of sodium per day.
- Choose and prepare foods with little salt. At the same time, consume potassium-rich foods, such as fruits and vegetables.

ALCOHOLIC BEVERAGES

- Those who choose to drink alcoholic beverages should do so sensibly and in moderation—defined as the consumption of up to one drink per day for women and up to two drinks per day for men.
- Alcoholic beverages should not be consumed by some individuals, including those who cannot restrict their alcohol intake, women of childbearing age who may become pregnant, pregnant and lactating women, children and adolescents, individuals taking medications that can interact with alcohol, and those with specific medical conditions.
- Alcoholic beverages should be avoided by individuals engaging in activities that require attention, skill, or coordination, such as driving or operating machinery.

FOOD SAFETY

- To avoid microbial foodborne illness:
  - Clean hands, food contact surfaces, and fruits and vegetables. Meat and poultry should not be washed or rinsed.
  - Separate raw, cooked, and ready-to-eat foods while shopping, preparing, or storing foods.
  - Cook foods to a safe temperature to kill microorganisms.
  - Chill (refrigerate) perishable food promptly and defrost foods properly.
  - Avoid raw (unpasteurized) milk or any products made from unpasteurized milk, raw or partially cooked eggs or foods containing raw eggs, raw or undercooked meat and poultry, unpasteurized juices, and raw sprouts.

NOTE: The Dietary Guidelines for Americans 2005 contains additional recommendations for specific populations. The full document is available at www.healthierus.gov/dietaryguidelines.

United States Department of Health and Human Services, Department of Agriculture. (2005). Dietary guidelines for Americans 2005. Retrieved August 20, 2005, from http://www.healthierus.gov/dietaryguidelines.

collagen, hormone, and enzyme synthesis; and decrease essential protein production, reducing circulating albumin, fibrinogen, and hemoglobin. Malnutrition or mild-to-moderate starvation produces serious cellular biochemical changes, including diminished liver glycogen stores that start the first day of deprivation. Protein stores are more diminished via gluconeogenesis because amino acids are converted into glucose as an energy source. Tissue proteins are depleted and short-lived in the intestinal mucous membranes, liver, pancreas, and kidney tubular epithelia. Muscle proteins are converted to provide energy, and adipose tissues are metabolized to produce free fatty acids for energy substrates. The byproducts of fatty acid oxidation (ketones) are used as energy for the brain if starvation is prolonged.

Unusual or abnormal circumstances that necessitate the administration of various nutritional modalities (e.g., vitamin replacement and enteral or parenteral feedings) are discussed in the following sections.

⚹ **T.L. is a 34-year-old single woman who reports to clinic for her regular checkup. On obtaining a history, the nurse asks T.L. about her nutritional habits and whether she takes vitamins and minerals. T.L. indicates that she "doesn't eat properly with fruits and vegetables." She frequently eats fast foods because she lives alone and does not like to cook for herself, and then she "diets" by cutting back on calories and skipping meals.**

⚹ **What are vitamins and their role in health?**

Vitamins are organic compounds that help to maintain normal metabolic functions, growth, and tissue repair. Mechanisms of action, specific indications for use, and pharmacokinetics are not well understood for all vitamins, nor have dosages been established for all vitamins. However, vitamin supplement therapy may be essential during periods of nutritional challenge, typically during rapid growth, pregnancy, lactation, or convalescence. Other challenges to nutrition occur with inadequate nutrient ingestion, malabsorption syndromes, and increased nutrient requirements caused by specific disease states, such as celiac sprue and ulcerative colitis. An increase in cellular proliferation in the latter conditions may result in the depletion of key nutrients, such as folic acid.

Insufficient dietary intake of vitamins and other essential nutrients may be occasionally traced to impoverished diets resulting from cultural, religious, or personal beliefs; fad diets; alcoholism; poverty; ignorance; or a lack of available food. Mild forms of **avitaminosis** (vitamin deficiency) are more common in the United States and Canada (often as a result of alcoholism) than are the pronounced deficiency states of beriberi, pellagra, rickets, or scurvy. The potential for iatrogenic starvation exists because of ignorance or oversight on the part of health care personnel who routinely fail to assess their clients' nutrition status or do not know how to correct it when neces-

TABLE 67-1 VITAMIN REVIEWS*

Vitamin	Sources	Adverse Effects†
FAT-SOLUBLE VITAMINS		
A	Fish-liver oil, liver, butter, darkly colored fruit, green leafy vegetables, milk	*Acute*: confusion, irritation, diarrhea, dizziness, visual alterations, skin peeling, severe vomiting *Chronic*: Bone pain, dry/cracked skin or lips; fever, increased urination, anorexia, hair loss, seizures, vomiting, liver toxicity *Teratogenic effects*
D	Fish-liver oil, fortified milk products and fortified cereals, fatty fish, exposure to sunlight	*Early with hypercalcemia:* constipation (mostly in children), diarrhea, headache, increased thirst and urination, metallic taste, nausea, vomiting

Data from USDA. Retrieved April 7, 2005, from http://www.nal.usda.gov.

AI, Adequate intakes; *DRI*, dietary reference intakes; *FNB*, Food and Nutrition Board; *GI*, gastrointestinal; *ND*, not determinable; *RDA*, recommended dietary allowance.

*Bold type** indicates RDAs; *italics* indicates AIs.

†Adverse effects include acute and chronic early and late overdose symptoms, when available.

sary. Many medical procedures, such as nothing by mouth (NPO) orders to prepare the person for various gastrointestinal (GI) x-rays and procedures, may also potentiate client malnutrition.

A commonly prescribed intravenous (IV) solution of dextrose 5% in water delivers only 170 calories/L, and it is delivered purely in the form of a carbohydrate. Multiple cleansing enemas or prolonged GI suction robs the body of essential electrolytes. Only a perfunctory medical assessment may be made of the effects of intraoperative blood losses or of wound drainage on nutrition needs, and surgery is always accompanied by increased nitrogen excretion. Common nursing problems that result when the client does not, cannot, or will not eat are often not given adequate medical attention to enable satisfactory nursing care.

Vitamin preparations and other more aggressive and supportive nutrition therapies are needed for the hospitalized client more often than is recognized, because only a few vitamins are synthesized in the body—bacteria in the gut form vitamin K, vitamin D is produced when skin is exposed to sunlight, and small and insufficient amounts of vitamin B are made in the gut. Most vitamins must either be ingested in food or taken as dietary supplements. There are two schools of thought concerning the consumption of vitamin supplements. In the past it was generally believed that the average American diet contains adequate vitamins and that additional supplements are unnecessary. Achievement of the recommended daily allowances (RDAs) was considered appropriate. However, the RDAs are established by the National Academy of Sciences and National Research Council as the amount necessary to prevent gross deficiency syndromes. It is now becoming apparent that some vitamins aid in preventing chronic disease. There is also concern regarding surveys that indicate specific segments of our society—older adults, smokers, nursing home residents, and teenagers—reportedly do not consume the RDA levels of all vitamins and minerals. The most effective approach to correct such deficiencies is through diet, perhaps with the help of a dietitian.

A strong rationale for a daily multivitamin for all adults is developing. Homocystinemia, a major risk factor for cardiovascular disease, can be lowered by one RDA of folic acid daily (Woo et al., 2002). Vitamin D deficiency is common in older adults; supplements of vitamin D with calcium have been shown to reduce fracture sites and increase bone density (Bischoff-Ferrari et al., 2004). Vitamin B_{12} deficiency in older adults may account for some cases of neurologic disease, such as peripheral neuritis and dementia (Andrès, 2004). Antioxidant supplements may reduce coronary events, improve immune function, and prevent dementia and macular degeneration. Multivitamins are inexpensive, convenient, and safe. Table 67-1 reviews vitamins and recommended their RDAs.

Deficiency Effects	Age of Individuals	Daily Dietary Reference Intakes (DRIs/RDAs/AIs)	Daily Tolerable Upper Intake Levels (ULs)
Night blindness, xerophthalmia, keratomalacia, skin lesions	Infants and children		
	Birth to 6 months	*400 mcg*	600 mcg
	7-12 mo	*500 mcg*	600 mcg
	1-3 yr	**300 mcg**	600 mcg
	4-8 yr	**400 mcg**	900 mcg
	9-13 yr	**600 mcg**	1700 mcg
	Adolescent and adult males	**900 mcg**	2800-3000 mcg
	Adolescent and adult females	**700 mcg**	2800-3000 mcg
	Pregnant females	**750-770 mcg**	2800-3000 mcg
	Breastfeeding females	**1200-1300 mcg**	2800-3000 mcg
Bone-muscle pain, pain, weakness, and softening of the bones that may result in fractures	Infants and children		
	Birth to 3 yr	*5 mcg*	25 mcg
	4-6 yr	*5 mcg*	25 mcg
	7-10 yr	*5 mcg*	50 mcg
	Adolescents and adults	*5 mcg*	50 mcg
	Adults 50-70 yr	*10 mcg*	50 mcg
	Adults greater than 70 yr	*15 mcg*	50 mcg
	Pregnant and breastfeeding females	*5 mcg*	50 mcg

Continued

TABLE 67-1 VITAMIN REVIEWS*—cont'd

Vitamin	Sources	Adverse Effects[†]
FAT-SOLUBLE VITAMINS—cont'd		
E	Nuts, green leafy vegetables, wheat and rice germ	*Acute*: Visual disturbances, headache, nausea, stomach pain, weakness, blurred vision *Chronic*: Increased bleeding tendencies in vitamin K-deficient clients, altered thyroid metabolism, impaired sexual function
K	Liver, green leafy vegetables	Hypersensitivity (flushing, dyspnea, chest pain), taste alterations
WATER-SOLUBLE VITAMINS		
Cyanocobalamin (B_{12})	Fortified cereals, meat, fish, poultry	No toxicity
Niacin (B_3)	Meats, eggs, milk, dairy products	Flushing, pruritus, feelings of warmth *High doses:* Dizziness, dysrhythmias, dry skin, hyperglycemia, myalgia, nausea, vomiting, diarrhea
Pyridoxine (B_6)	Liver, meats, whole grain breads and cereals, soybeans, eggs, vegetables	Acute: Low toxicity *Chronic high doses:* neurotoxicity—ataxia, numb feet, clumsiness

Data from USDA. Retrieved April 7, 2005, from http://www.nal.usda.gov.

AI, Adequate intakes; *DRI,* dietary reference intakes; *FNB,* Food and Nutrition Board; *GI,* gastrointestinal; *ND,* not determinable; *RDA,* recommended dietary allowance.

***Bold type** indicates RDAs; *italics* indicates AIs.

[†]Adverse effects include acute and chronic early and late overdose symptoms, when available.

Deficiency Effects	Age of Individuals	Daily Dietary Reference Intakes (DRIs/RDAs/AIs)	Daily Tolerable Upper Intake Levels (ULs)
Hyporeflexia, ataxia, myopathy, anemia; may increase cancer risk	Infants and children	(mg of alpha-TE)	(mg of alpha-TE)
	Birth to 6 mo	*4 mg*	ND
	7-12 mo	*5 mg*	ND
	1-3 yr	**6 mg**	200 mg
	4-8 yr	**7 mg**	300 mg
	9 to 13 yr	**11 mg**	600 mg
	Adolescent and adult males	**15 mg**	800-1000 mg
	Adolescent and adult females	**15 mg**	800-1000 mg
	Pregnant females	**15 mg**	800-1000 mg
	Breastfeeding females	**19 mg**	800-1000 mg
Increased bleeding (e.g., ecchymoses, hematuria, GI bleeding)	Infants and children		
	Birth to 6 mo	*2 mcg*	ND
	7-12 mo	*2.5 mcg*	ND
	1-3 yr	*30 mcg*	ND
	4-8 yr	*55 mcg*	ND
	9-13 yr	*60 mcg*	ND
	14-18 yr	*75 mcg*	ND
	Adult males	*120 mcg*	ND
	Adult females	*90 mcg*	ND
	Pregnant females	*75-90 mcg*	ND
	Breastfeeding females	*75-90 mcg*	ND
Irreversible nervous system damage (paresthesia, ataxia), memory loss, confusion, dementia, abnormal hematopoiesis	Infants and children		
	Birth to 6 mo	*0.4 mcg*	ND
	7-12 mo	*0.5 mcg*	ND
	1-3 yr	**0.9 mcg**	ND
	4-8 yr	**1.2 mcg**	ND
	9-13 yr	**1.8 mcg**	ND
	Adolescent and adult males	**2.4 mcg**	ND
	Adolescent and adult females	**2.4 mcg**	ND
	Pregnant females	**2.6 mcg**	ND
	Breastfeeding females	**2.8 mcg**	ND
Skin eruptions, stomatitis, diarrhea, enteritis, headache, dizziness, insomnia, memory impairment, dementia	Infants and children		
	Birth to 6 mo	*2 mg*	ND
	7-12 mo	*4 mg*	ND
	1-3 yr	**6 mg**	10 mg
	4-8 yr	**8 mg**	15 mg
	9-13 yr	**12 mg**	20 mg
	Adolescent and adult males	**16 mg**	30-35 mg
	Adolescent and adult females	**14 mg**	30-35 mg
	Pregnant females	**18 mg**	30-35 mg
	Breastfeeding females	**17 mg**	30-35 mg
Seborrhea-like skin lesions, stomatitis, seizures, peripheral neuritis	Infants and children		
	Birth to 6 mo	*0.1 mg*	ND
	7-12 mo	*0.3 mg*	ND
	1-3 yr	**0.5 mg**	30 mg
	4-8 yr	**0.6 mg**	40 mg
	9-13 yr	**1 mg**	60 mg
	Adolescent and adult males	**1.3-1.7 mg**	80-100 mg
	Adolescent and adult females	**1.2-1.5 mg**	80-100 mg
	Pregnant females	**1.9 mg**	80-100 mg
	Breastfeeding females	**2 mg**	80-100 mg

Continued

Table 67-1 Vitamin Reviews*—cont'd

Vitamin	Sources	Adverse Effects[†]
Water-Soluble Vitamins—cont'd		
Riboflavin (B$_2$)	Milk, cheese, eggs, green leafy vegetables, whole grain and enriched cereals and breads, organ meats	Low toxicity
Thiamine (B$_1$)	Whole grain and enriched cereals, beef, pork, peas, beans, nuts	Low oral toxicity
Folic acid, folate	Enriched cereal grains, dark leafy vegetables, enriched and whole grain breads and bread products, fortified ready-to-eat cereals	Allergic reaction, red skin, fever, skin rash, pruritus
C (ascorbic acid)	Citrus fruits, tomatoes, potatoes, strawberries, cabbage	Kidney stones, dizziness *High doses:* diarrhea, red skin, headache, nausea, vomiting

Data from USDA. Retrieved April 7, 2005, from http://www.nal.usda.gov.
AI, Adequate intakes; *DRI,* dietary reference intakes; *FNB,* Food and Nutrition Board; *GI,* gastrointestinal; *ND,* not determinable; *RDA,* recommended dietary allowance.
*__Bold type__ indicates RDAs; *italics* indicates AIs.
[†]Adverse effects include acute and chronic early and late overdose symptoms, when available.

Deficiency Effects	Age of Individuals	Daily Dietary Reference Intakes (DRIs/RDAs/AIs)	Daily Tolerable Upper Intake Levels (ULs)
Sore throat; stomatitis; red, painful, or swollen tongue; facial dermatitis; anemia	Infants and children		
	Birth to 6 mo	*0-3 mg*	ND
	7-12 mo	*0.4 mg*	ND
	1-3 yr	**0.5 mg**	ND
	4-8 yr	**0.6 mg**	ND
	9-13 yr	**0.9 mg**	ND
	Adolescent and adult males	**1.3 mg**	ND
	Adolescent and adult females	**1-1.1 mg**	ND
	Pregnant females	**1.4 mg**	ND
	Breastfeeding females	**1.6 mg**	ND
Peripheral neuritis, loss of muscle strength, depression, memory loss, anorexia, poor memory, dyspnea	Infants and children		
	Birth to 6 mo	*0.2 mg*	ND
	7-12 mo	*0.3 mg*	ND
	1-3 yr	**0.5 mg**	ND
	4-8 yr	**0.6 mg**	ND
	9-13 yr	**0.9 mg**	ND
	Male adolescents and adults	**1.2 mg**	ND
	Females 14-18 yr	**1 mg**	ND
	Adult females	**1.1 mg**	ND
	Pregnant females	**1.4 mg**	ND
	Breastfeeding females	**1.4 mg**	ND
Megaloblastic anemia	Infants and children		
	Birth to 6 mo	*65 mcg*	ND
	7-12 mo	*80 mcg*	ND
	1-3 yr	**150 mcg**	300 mcg
	4-8 yr	**200 mcg**	400 mcg
	9-13 yr	**300 mcg**	600 mcg
	Adolescent and adult males	**400 mcg**	800-1000 mcg
	Adolescent and adult females	**400 mcg**	800-1000 mcg
	Pregnant females	**600 mcg**	800-1000 mcg
	Breastfeeding females	**500 mcg**	800-1000 mcg
Scurvy (loosening of teeth, gingivitis), anemia; infants: irritability, pain if touched	Infants and children		
	Birth to 6 mo	*40 mg*	ND
	7-12 mo	*50 mg*	ND
	1-3 yr	**15 mg**	400 mg
	4-8 yr	**25 mg**	650 mg
	9-13 yr	**45 mg**	1200 mg
	Males 14-18 yr	**75 mg**	1800 mg
	Adult males	**90 mg**	2000 mg
	Females 14-18 yr	**65 mg**	1800 mg
	Adult females	**75 mg**	2000 mg
	Pregnant females	**80-85 mg**	1800-2000 mg
	Breastfeeding females	**115-120 mg**	1800-2000 mg

Many multivitamin capsules and tablets vary in their contents. "Optional vitamins" (E, B$_6$, folic acid, pantothenic acid, and B$_{12}$) may or may not be included as ingredients in over-the-counter (OTC) multivitamin preparations. The most popular OTC multivitamin preparations contain all of the vitamins needed by humans. Most OTC vitamin preparations are designed to meet the daily needs of the body completely without regard for the amounts of various vitamins contained in the daily diet.

✱ **T.L. asks the nurse about what vitamins she should be taking for good health.**

✱ **What are the nursing management issues for vitamin therapy for T.L.?**
Good nutrition is essential for good health. The nurse's participation in health promotion includes providing information regarding all aspects of nutrition. With the many misconceptions regarding the role of vitamins and minerals in health and the prevention of illness prevalent today, the nurse has an important role in providing accurate dietary counseling regarding vitamins and minerals.

Assessment A dietary history for the client provides the nurse with insights into T.L.'s eating patterns (e.g., in the last 24 hours). Additionally, obtain information related to food source and preparation, living arrangements, financial status, coping patterns, knowledge of nutrition, and physiologic alterations that the client is experiencing as background for client teaching. This will also provide T.L. with more specifics regarding her dietary planning. Assess concurrent medications; mineral oil interferes with the absorption of fat-soluble vitamins. Obtain T.L.'s height and weight. Assess for signs of the specific vitamin or mineral deficiency throughout therapy. (Refer to the specific vitamin for relevant nursing management.) Consider that vitamin and mineral requirements may change with age and health status (e.g., in pregnancy). (See the Pregnancy Safety box below for the Food and Drug Administration's [FDA] categories for vitamins.) For clients with suspected deficiencies, baseline diagnostic studies can be obtained for the specific vitamin or mineral deficiency (e.g., serum folic acid and hemoglobin determinations). Assess pregnancy status with women of childbearing age.

Nursing Diagnosis The general nursing diagnosis for clients with vitamin and mineral deficiencies is imbalanced nutrition: less than body requirements. Depending on the type and severity of the deficiency and the nature of the signs and symptoms, other nursing diagnoses or collaborative problems are also relevant.

Planning While on multivitamin and mineral therapy, T.L. will:
- Experience good health with an absence of signs and symptoms of vitamin and/or mineral deficiency.
- Effectively manage her lifestyle to include a nutritionally adequate diet.

Implementation
Monitoring A food diary will assist in monitoring T.L.'s effective management of the therapeutic regimen. Note any signs and symptoms of nutritional deficiency. Record weight at every visit; and record height for children.

Intervention Assist T.L. to select a multivitamin/mineral supplement that is cost effective. For pediatric clients, use the calibrated measuring device provided by the manufacturer for accurate dosing. Chewable tablets should be chewed or crushed thoroughly before swallowing. Use caution in administering fat-soluble vitamins to children, because they are more sensitive to high doses.

Education Discuss with T.L. the function of vitamins and minerals in the body, signs of vitamin deficiency, and unproven uses. Diet is the treatment of choice for vitamin deficiencies; vitamins are not a substitute for a balanced diet.
Instruct T.L. about the recommended dietary guidelines (see Table 67-1) and, in particular, about specific foods that supply the vitamin in which she is deficient. Encourage a diet with at least five fruits and vegetables a day. Fruits and vegetables not only provide known vitamins, but they also contain fiber and other poorly defined nutrients. They may also be filling and limit her intake of meat and animal fats. Advise T.L. to take a daily multivitamin that meets the RDA for all adults. Megadoses are not recommended, and there is the risk of toxicity with chronic overdoses; the RDA should not be exceeded. There is a great deal of ongoing research about the prophylactic role for vitamins.

Evaluation The expected outcome of vitamin and mineral therapy is that T.L. will not demonstrate any signs or symptoms of vitamin or mineral deficiency or hypervitaminosis.

PREGNANCY SAFETY VITAMINS	
Category	**Drug**
A	cyanocobalamin, ferrous fumarate, ferrous gluconate, ferrous sulfate, folic acid, pyridoxine, riboflavin, thiamine, vitamin A (less than 6000 international units), vitamin E,
B	iron sucrose injection
C	ascorbic acid, calcifediol, calcipotriene, calcitriol, cyanocobalamin (parenteral), ergocalciferol, iron dextran, niacin, pyridoxine (if over RDA), riboflavin (if over RDA),

Data from *Mosby's drug consult* (15th ed.). (2005). St. Louis: Mosby.

✱ **T.L. indicates that she has considered taking a number of vitamin supplements, including one formu-**

lation she obtains from her health-food store with high doses of both fat- and water-soluble vitamins.

✳ What are the fat- and water-soluble vitamins?

Vitamins are important components of enzyme systems that catalyze the reactions for protein, fat, and carbohydrate metabolism. They are classified as being fat-soluble or water-soluble. The **fat-soluble vitamins** are A, D, E, and K. They are stored in the liver and fatty tissue in large amounts. A deficiency in these vitamins occurs only after a long deprivation from an adequate supply or as a result of disorders that prevent their absorption. **Water-soluble vitamins** include the B-complex group and vitamin C. These vitamins are not stored in the body in large amounts, and short periods of inadequate intake can lead to a deficiency.

Hypervitaminosis is also of concern today, especially with the large consumption of vitamins in the United States and Canada. **Hypervitaminosis** is defined as an abnormal condition that results from the consumption of high or excessive amounts of one or more vitamins, usually over an extended period. The effects produced are discussed under each vitamin monograph in the later sections, but is most problematic with the fat-soluble vitamins because they accumulate with time.

Fat-Soluble Vitamins

The fat-soluble vitamins A, D, E, and K produce variable effects, but can accumulate with chronic administration. Vitamins A and D possess antioxidant properties, although health benefits related to their antioxidant activity have been questioned. Vitamin A, often thought of as the important vitamin to maintain vision is related to the retinoids, which are used in dermal conditions and may increase risk for fetal harm if used in very high doses for pregnant women. Vitamin D helps regulate calcium and phosphate balance and is used in treating osteoporosis, osteomalacia, parathyroid dysfunction, and other related conditions. The role of vitamin E is less clear, with cardiovascular benefits being claimed in the 1990s and disputed more recently. Chapter 30 discusses Vitamin K, which is a key factor in the synthesis of clotting factors II, VII, IX and X.

vitamin A
[Aquasol A]

Vitamin A, the fat-soluble, growth-promoting vitamin, is essential for growth in the younger age groups, for normal function of the retina, and for health maintenance at all ages. Vitamin A (retinol) is derived from animals, whereas the provitamin A carotenoids are found in plants. Beta-carotene, the most active carotenoid from plants, is hydrolyzed in the body to form two molecules of vitamin A. Animal fats, such as those found in butter, milk, eggs, and fish liver, are sources of carotenoids that were originally derived from plants and stored in animal tissues.

Vitamin A is essential for promoting normal growth and the development of bones and teeth and for maintaining the health of epithelial tissues of the body. Its function in relation to normal vision and the prevention of night blindness has been studied carefully. Vitamin A actually is part of one of the major retinal pigments, rhodopsin, and thus is required for normal "rod vision" in the retina of human beings and many animals.

Beta-carotene, as an antioxidant, has been studied in clients with coronary artery disease. Unfortunately, analysis of multiple trials including 138,000 clients identifies no benefit of beta-carotene therapy in improving cardiac status (Vivekananthan et al., 2003).

Indications

Vitamin A is used to treat or relieve symptoms associated with a deficiency of vitamin A, such as night blindness (nyctalopia), hyperkeratosis, delayed growth, xerophthalmia, keratomalacia, weakness, and increased susceptibility of the mucous membranes to infection. Retinoids, which are analogs of vitamin A, (e.g., tretinoin) are used to treat acne and psoriasis, and are considered teratogenic (see Chapter 65).

Pharmacokinetics/Dosing

Vitamin A and carotene are readily absorbed from the normal GI tract. Efficient absorption depends on fat absorption and therefore on the presence of adequate bile salts in the intestine. Certain conditions, such as obstructive jaundice, some infectious diseases, and the presence of mineral oil in the intestine, may result in vitamin A deficiency even if a normal amount is ingested.

Vitamin A is stored to a greater extent in the liver than elsewhere. The liver also functions in changing carotene to vitamin A; this function is inhibited by liver diseases and diabetes. The amount of vitamin A stored depends on dietary intake. When intake is high or excessive, the stores formed in the liver may be sufficient enough to last several years. Vitamin A is metabolized by the liver and excreted by the feces and kidneys. Table 67-1 provides the RDA, adverse effects, and deficiency effects for vitamin A.

The dosage for vitamin A depends on the age, gender, purpose (prophylaxis or treatment), and condition of the individual. Refer to a current reference for dosing information.

Adverse Effects

Large doses of vitamin A may cause neurologic and skin damage in adults, and excessive doses are known to produce highly toxic effects in rats and in young children. High blood levels of retinol or beta-carotene may be associated with increased fracture risk (Michaëlsson, Lithell, Vessby, & Melhus, 2003). Although vitamin requirements increase during pregnancy and during breastfeeding, high doses of vitamin A are generally avoided because of the potential for vitamin A analogs to be injurious to the developing fetus.

Nursing Management
Assessment

Vitamin A is contraindicated for clients with hypervitaminosis A or sensitivity to any of the in gradients in the preparation, and is administered cautiously to clients with renal function impairment, because serum vitamin A levels are increased. Assess the client's concurrent drug therapy because women on oral contraceptives have shown a significant increase in plasma vitamin A levels when the drugs are taken concurrently. Obtain a complete diet and drug history to identify risk for vitamin A deficiency. Obtain a baseline of the client's vision, including night blindness, and the appearance of the eyes, skin, and mucous membranes. In addition to dry skin and corneal changes, infants may show failure to thrive and apathy. Serum vitamin A levels less than 20 mcg/dL in adults and 10 mcg/dL in children indicate a vitamin A deficiency.

Nursing Diagnosis

The client undergoing vitamin A deficiency therapy is at risk for the following nursing diagnoses related to the effectiveness/ineffectiveness of therapy: disturbed sensory perception (night blindness), fatigue, impaired skin integrity, and impaired oral mucous membrane. Nursing diagnoses associated with vitamin A toxicity are impaired comfort (headache, bone or joint pain, general feeling of discomfort, irritability); impaired oral mucous membrane (dry mouth, drying or cracking of lips); imbalanced body temperature (fever); deficient fluid volume (anorexia, nausea, vomiting); disturbed body image related to hair loss or yellow-orange patches on the palms of the hands, soles of the feet, or skin around the nose and mouth; hyperthermia; and fatigue; and the potential complication of hepatosplenomegaly. With infants there is the potential complication of bulging fontanel.

Planning

The client receiving vitamin A therapy will:

• Maintain a well-balanced dietary intake, including adequate vitamin A intake.
• Not evidence signs and symptoms of vitamin A deficiency or hypervitaminosis A.

Implementation

Monitoring

Monitor the client's diet and serum levels of vitamin A. Monitor for signs and symptoms of vitamin A deficiency, hypercarotenemia (orange coloration of the skin and eyes), and hypervitaminosis A (see the Nursing Diagnosis section for this vitamin). Plasma levels of vitamin A may not be indicative of vitamin A status because of significant hepatic storage; however, a vitamin A deficiency does correlate with low serum levels.

Intervention

Administer oral vitamin A with or after meals. Parenteral administration is indicated when oral administration is not feasible as in anorexia, nausea, vomiting, or it is not available as in "malabsorption syndrome." Do not administer IV unless contained in a total parenteral nutrition (TPN) solution. Exposure to light causes vitamin A to degrade, and therefore TPN solutions containing vitamin A should be protected from the light.

Education

Provide the client with nutritional counseling. The best sources of dietary vitamin A are fish liver oil, liver, kidney, egg yolk, butter, milk, cream, cheese, and fortified margarine, and its precursor carotene, which is found in dark green leafy vegetables and yellow and orange fruits and vegetables. Water-miscible products are available for clients with fat malabsorption. Avoid the use of mineral oil while on vitamin A therapy. Consult with physician before breastfeeding while taking high doses of vitamin A.

Evaluation

The expected outcome of vitamin A therapy is that the client will achieve adequate serum concentrations of vitamin A, consume adequate dietary vitamin A, and maintain normal vision and intact skin without vitamin A toxicity.

vitamin D (ergocalciferol) [er goe kal **sif** e role]

(Calciferol, Drisdol, Ostoforte✣)
Related forms: calcitriol (Rocaltrol, Calcijex) dihydrotachyserol (DHT, Hytakerol), paricalcitol (Zemplar)

The term *vitamin D* is applied to two substances that affect the proper use of calcium and phosphorus in the body. Both substances have the ability to prevent or cure rickets. Although an essential vitamin, vitamin D is found in only a few foods in the average diet of North Americans (see Table 67-1). The plant vitamin D is referred to as vitamin D₂, or ergocalciferol; the natural form of vitamin D is produced in the skin by ultraviolet irradiation of 7-dehydrocholesterol and is referred to as vitamin D₃, or cholecalciferol. Although ergocalciferol contains a chemical double bond and an extra methyl group, the difference between these two substances is not physiologically significant.

Both cholecalciferol and ergocalciferol are metabolized in the liver to calcifediol. Calcifediol is transported to the kidney and converted to calcitriol, which is believed to be the most active analogue. Calcitriol appears to bind to a receptor in the intestinal mucosa; it is incorporated into the cell nucleus, which results in the formation of a calcium-binding protein that increases calcium absorption from the intestine. Parathyroid hormone and calcitriol act to control the transfer of calcium ions from bones into the extracellular fluid; therefore they maintain calcium homeostasis in the extracellular fluid (Marcus, 2001).

In addition to ergocalciferol, other available vitamin D analogues include calcitriol (Rocaltrol), dihydrotachysterol (DHT, Hytakerol), and paricalcitol (Zemplar). They are primarily used in end-stage renal disease (ESRD) because they do not require conversion for their action. They also have shorter half-lives, which makes any toxic adverse effects easier to manage. Calcifediol (Calderol) appears to have some vitamin D activity in addition to its conversion to the active metabolite calcitriol. See Chapter 35 for a discussion of the use of these agents in renal failure, and Chapter 47 for review of drug therapy with parathyroid dysfunction.

Vitamin D is necessary for the absorption and use of calcium and phosphorus in the body and for the normal calcification of bone. Rickets in children and osteomalacia in adults may result in the absence of vitamin D—even if the intake of calcium and phosphate is adequate. Vitamin D is used to treat and prevent nutritional rickets, osteomalacia, hypoparathyroidism, and osteoporosis. Use of single high dose orally administered vitamin D (100,000 units once every three months) is associated with reduced fracture risk in older adults (Trivedi, Doll, & Khaw, 2003). Vitamin D use may also reduce falls risk and associated fractures secondary to falls (Bischoff-Ferrari et al., 2004), although other trials note no benefit in fracture reduction (Bischoff-Ferrari et al., 2005; Grant et al., 2005; Porthouse et al., 2005). Variation in response to vitamin D is sometimes observed, and may partially be explained by genetics. (See the Special Considerations for Pharmacogenetics box below.)

The incidence of rickets is low in the United States and Canada but can occur in young children who are restricted to vegetarian diets without milk supplementation or in infants who are breastfed by moth-

---

Special Considerations for Pharmacogenetics | VITAMINS AND MINERALS

PHARMACODYNAMICS

Responses to calcium and analogs of vitamin D in the prevention and treatment of osteoporosis appear to be correlated with genetic variation in the vitamin D receptor (Morrison et al., 2005). Genetically related differences in the vitamin D receptor are also correlated with breast cancer risk (Sillanpaa et al., 2004) and may be a factor in the risk for colon cancer (Makishima et al., 2002), although the clinical importance of these findings is unclear.

PHARMACOKINETICS

Although not well studied, it is likely that genetic variation in nutrient absorption and metabolism occurs (Anderson & Milner, 2004). Future study may assist in the identification of nutritional recommendations which are specific for client need based on individual specific genetic information (Hasselmann & Reimund, 2004).

ADVERSE EFFECTS

Excessive body iron stores are correlated with genetic markers for P450 2 A6 in a subset of Southeast Asian populations (Ujjin et al., 2002). Clinical importance of this observation, however, is unclear. Chronic elevated body iron may be a risk factor for iron toxicity, including GI hemorrhage and hepatic failure, but it is premature to suggest a direct link between genetics and the potential for iron toxicity.

ers who did not take prenatal vitamins or drink milk. Vitamin D deficiency results in an inadequate intake and perhaps an excessive loss of calcium from the body. The prevalence of vitamin D deficiency is high in older adults as a result of a combination of decreased dietary intake, diminished absorption, and limited exposure to sunlight. Long-term use of some anticonvulsants (phenytoin, phenobarbital, perhaps carbamazepine) increase vitamin D metabolism and increase the risk for osteomalacia (see Chapter 17). Adequate vitamin D and calcium is associated with reduced colorectal cancer (Grau et al., 2003).

Indications
Ergocalciferol is indicated for the treatment of rickets and vitamin D deficiency. It is also used for treating hypoparathyroidism, and as part of management of osteoporosis and osteomalacia. Active vitamin D analogs, including calcitriol and paricalcitol are indicated for the management of secondary hyperparathyroidism secondary to renal failure.

Pharmacokinetics/Dosing
Vitamin D is absorbed from the small intestine (ergocalciferol requires the presence of bile salts for absorption). It is protein bound and is stored mainly in fat and in the liver. The serum half-life for calcifediol is approximately 16 days; for calcitriol, from 3 to 6 hours; and for ergocalciferol, within 19 to 48 hours. Ergocalciferol can be stored in fat sites for longer periods. For calcitriol, the onset of hypercalcemic effects is within 3 to 6 hours; for dihydrotachysterol, within hours (although the maximum effect is seen in 7 to 14 days); for ergocalciferol, within 12 to 24 hours (although the therapeutic response may not be seen until 10 to 14 days later). The duration of effect after oral administration is calcifediol, 15 to 20 days; calcitriol, 3 to 5 days; dihydrotachysterol, up to 9 weeks; and ergocalciferol, up to 6 months. Excretion is via the bile and kidneys.

The usual adult dose of ergocalciferol is 10 to 15 mcg (400 to 600 units) per day. Higher doses are often used to prevent osteomalacia (e.g., secondary to concurrent drugs with increase vitamin D metabolism such as phenytoin, and phenobarbital). Because of its long duration of action, very high doses (e.g., 10,000 to 60,000 units) weekly or monthly are sometimes used to treat hypoparathyroid states, resistant rickets, or other related conditions. The usual adolescent and adult dosage for calcifediol is 50 to 100 mcg daily; for calcitriol, 0.25 mg daily, and for dihydrotachysterol, 125 mcg to 2 mg daily. Dosages are adjusted periodically as necessary, with monitoring of calcium and phosphate levels when high doses are used. Pediatric dosages vary. Refer to a current reference for recommendations.

Adverse Effects
The most serious adverse effects of high doses of vitamin D are hypercalcemic states. Hypercalcemia can present with nausea, vomiting, flank pain, constipation, flank pain, and other symptoms, and if markedly elevated, can lead to coma and death. Such presentation is very rare with usual doses of vitamin D, but may be seen with very high dosing of these agents. See Table 67-1 for adverse effects, deficiency effects, and the RDA of vitamin D.

Nursing Management
Assessment
The administration of vitamin D is contraindicated in clients with hypercalcemia, hypervitaminosis D, malabsorption syndrome, or abnormal sensitivity to the toxic effects of vitamin D. Use assessment findings to rule out these conditions before initiating vitamin D therapy. Also use caution when administering vitamin D to clients with arteriosclerosis, hyperphosphatemia, hypersensitivity to vitamin D, and renal or cardiac impairment. Hyperphosphatemia must be controlled before the start of vitamin D therapy.

Review the client's current medication regimen for the risk of significant drug interactions, such as those that may occur when vitamin D products are given concurrently with antacids containing magnesium, as it may result in hypermagnesemia, especially in clients with chronic renal failure. Avoid concurrent administration of magnesium containing products and calcium if possible. If concurrent use is required, monitor closely for diminished reflexes, muscle weakness, drowsiness, confusion, lethargy, bradycardia, and hypotension. Calcium preparations in high doses or thiazide diuretics increase the risk for hy-

percalcemia. Monitor closely for drowsiness, lethargy, weakness, muscle flaccidity, hypertension, anorexia, nausea, constipation, polyuria, and flank pain. The range between therapeutic and toxic doses is narrow so other vitamin D products increase the risk for toxicity.

A baseline assessment of the client's skeletal status by x-ray examination and the appearance of bone malformations should be obtained. Serum calcium levels under 7.5 mg/dL, serum inorganic phosphorus levels under 3 mg/dL, serum citrate levels under 2.5 mg/dL, and elevated serum alkaline phosphatase levels indicate a vitamin D deficiency. Obtain a complete diet, drug and sunlight exposure history to identify risk for vitamin D deficiency.

Nursing Diagnosis
Clients receiving vitamin D therapy may experience the following nursing diagnoses because of their underlying vitamin D deficiency: impaired comfort related to ineffective drug therapy (pain in the legs and lower back); risk for injury related to motor deficits resulting from skeletal deformities and weakness; and impaired physical mobility related to poorly developed muscles. Nursing diagnoses related to the drug toxicity itself are constipation; fatigue; deficient fluid volume related to anorexia, nausea, or vomiting; and impaired comfort (headache, metallic taste); and the potential complications of anemia, nephrocalcinosis, dwarfism (infants and children) and mental retardation.

Planning
The client receiving vitamin D therapy will:
- Maintain a well-balanced dietary intake, including adequate vitamin D intake.
- Not evidence signs and symptoms of vitamin D deficiency or hypervitaminosis D.

Implementation
Monitoring
Because vitamin D has a narrow therapeutic range, monitor serum calcium levels weekly during early therapy along with periodic evaluations of renal function; this will help to establish the dosage. Serum calcium values should be in the 8 to 9 mg/dL range, and the product of calcium and phosphorus (Ca $\times$ P [mg/dL]) should not be greater than 60. Other examinations may be required according to the client's response to therapy.

Children should have their growth monitored during therapy because growth may be inhibited by prolonged administration of vitamin D. X-ray studies are recommended every 3 to 6 months until the client is stable. Additionally, assess for signs of toxicity as described in the Nursing Diagnosis section for this vitamin.

Intervention
If calcitriol is given for hypothyroidism, give the dose in the morning. Capsules should be protected against light, heat, and moisture.

Education
Stress the importance of regular visits to the health care provider to monitor progress. Review with the client any instructions for a special diet or for a calcium supplement if prescribed. Foods high in vitamin D include fish and fish liver oils, egg yolks, and vitamin D–fortified milk. Judicious exposure to sunlight is helpful. Vitamin D content is not altered with cooking.

The daily intake of vitamin D in older adults should be at least 800 international units, with at least 1.2 g of elemental calcium in the diet or as a supplement. If prescribed a supplement, caution the client not to use any OTC products that contain calcium, phosphorus, or vitamin D unless approved by the prescriber. Clients taking calcifediol or calcitriol should avoid the use of antacids containing magnesium.

Evaluation
The expected outcome of vitamin D therapy is that the client will consume adequate dietary vitamin D and remain pain free without vitamin D toxicity. The child or infant will maintain adequate growth.

vitamin E
(d-Alpha-tocopherol, dl-Alpha-tocopherol)
(Aqua Gem E, Aquasol E, Key-E)
Vitamin E is a fat-soluble vitamin that is present in margarine made from plant oils such as cottonseed oil; it is also present in green,

leafy vegetables and whole grains. Although a number of compounds have been found to exhibit vitamin E activity, the most active of these is α-tocopherol; it is the substance used to calculate the food content of vitamin E.

Studies have variably reported the beneficial effects of large doses of vitamin E on the progression of coronary artery disease. The hypothesis is that the oxidation of lipoproteins reduces atherogenesis. Individuals without cardiovascular disease who consume a high intake of vitamin E have a lower risk of developing coronary artery heart disease. However, analysis of seven trials with about 82,000 clients failed to reveal a mortality benefit from the use of vitamin E for clients with existing cardiovascular disease (Vivekananthan et al., 2003). Existing cardiovascular disease does not appear to be positively impacted by vitamin E, but many people take supplemental vitamin E because some evidence suggests it prevents cardiovascular disease and cancer. Megadoses of this vitamin, however, may actually increase the risk of all-cause mortality, according to a meta-analysis (Miller et al., 2005). Overall, there was a significant dose-response relationship between vitamin E dosages greater than 150 international units/day and an increased risk of all-cause mortality. However, the effect of lower-dosage vitamin E supplementation on all-cause mortality was not clear. Other studies correlate vitamin E use with an increased risk of accelerating cancer progression (Bairati et al., 2005) and heart failure (Lonn et al., 2005).

Vitamin E is an essential nutrient, but its exact function is unknown. It has been reported to have antioxidant properties when used in conjunction with dietary selenium, to prevent the effects of peroxidase on unsaturated bonds in the cell membranes, and to protect red blood cells (RBCs) from hemolysis. It is also known to be a cofactor for several enzyme systems in the body.

Indications
Vitamin E is used as a dietary supplement, and is used to prevent and treat hemolytic anemia secondary to vitamin E deficiencies. Vitamin E has also been used in the treatment of tardive dyskinesia secondary to long term typical antipsychotic use with variable effect. Its role in preventing coronary artery disease is unclear.

Pharmacokinetics/Dosing
The absorption of vitamin E from the GI tract requires the presence of bile salts, dietary fats, and normal pancreatic functioning. Vitamin E binds to beta lipoproteins in the blood and is stored in all body tissues, especially in fat deposits (which contain up to a 4-year requirement of this vitamin). It is metabolized in the liver and excreted in the bile and kidneys.

The usual adult dosage for vitamin E deficiency is 100 to 400 units daily. Pediatric dosages vary. Refer to a current reference for recommendations. The oxidation of vitamin E increases when given concurrently with large doses of iron supplements; this increases the daily requirement for vitamin E. If given concurrently, monitor closely to determine an appropriate intervention.

Adverse Effects
Blurred vision and contact dermatitis are among the potential adverse effects observed with acute vitamin E ingestion. Vitamin K deficiency may be induced which may lead to bleeding tendencies. See Table 67-1 for adverse effects and deficiency effects for vitamin E.

Nursing Management
Assessment
Before the initiation of vitamin E therapy, ascertain whether the client has hypoprothrombinemia as a result of vitamin K deficiency; vitamin E in doses over 400 units will aggravate this condition. Advise clients who are taking anticoagulants against taking high doses of vitamin E. There may be an impaired hematological response to iron in children with iron-deficiency anemia (*Mosby's Drug Consult*, 2005).

A baseline assessment should include the presence or absence of edema, skin condition, and extent of muscle weakness. A serum α-tocopherol level below 0.5 mg/dL in adults and below 0.2 mg/dL in infants confirms a vitamin E deficiency. Obtain a complete diet and drug history to determine risk for vitamin E deficiency.

Nursing Diagnosis
The client with a vitamin E deficiency may experience the following selected nursing diagnoses: excess fluid volume; impaired skin integrity; and impaired physical mobility. Nursing diagnoses associated with vitamin E toxicity are disturbed sensory perception (visual) related to blurred vision; diarrhea; fatigue; impaired comfort (headache, nausea or stomach cramps, dizziness); and risk for injury related to increased bleeding tendencies.

Planning
The client receiving vitamin E therapy will:
- Maintain a well-balanced dietary intake, including adequate vitamin E intake.
- Not evidence signs and symptoms of vitamin E deficiency or hypervitaminosis E.

Implementation
Monitoring
Monitor the client's dietary intake, regression of symptoms, and serum α-tocopherol levels.
Intervention
Water-miscible forms are more readily absorbed from the GI tract. Assess the client taking large doses of vitamin E for prolonged periods for signs of toxicity (see the Nursing Diagnosis section for this vitamin).
Education
Although a vitamin E deficiency is uncommon, dietary instruction for clients may be necessary. Foods high in vitamin E are vegetable oils, wheat germ, whole-grain cereals, egg yolks, and liver. Alert clients that dosages greater than 150 international units/day for individuals without vitamin E deficiency have been linked to an increased risk of all-cause mortality.
Evaluation
The expected outcome of vitamin E therapy is that the client will maintain a diet adequate in vitamin E and will experience normal muscle strength, intact skin, and α-tocopherol levels within normal limits without symptoms of vitamin E toxicity (e.g., disturbed vision, diarrhea, fatigue, increased bleeding tendencies).

vitamin K
Vitamin K is a fat-soluble vitamin. Because of its importance in blood coagulation, it is covered in detail in Chapter 30, but see Table 67-1 for a review of this vitamin.

Water-Soluble Vitamins

The water-soluble vitamins are ascorbic acid (vitamin C) and B vitamins. The B vitamins are often found together in food and are referred to as vitamin B complex. However, they are chemically dissimilar and have different metabolic functions. This B grouping is largely based on their having been discovered in sequential order. A sensible and increasingly popular trend promotes discarding names such as vitamin B_1 and B_2 and referring to these vitamins as thiamine and riboflavin, respectively. The vitamin B complex includes thiamine, riboflavin, nicotinic acid, pyridoxine, folic acid, pantothenic acid, biotin, choline, inositol, and vitamin B_{12} (cyanocobalamin).

This discussion will be limited to the B vitamins that are associated with deficiency states and for which information on therapeutic application is available: thiamine (vitamin B_1), riboflavin (vitamin B_2), niacin (nicotinic acid), pyridoxine (vitamin B_6), vitamin B_{12} (cyanocobalamin), and folic acid.

thiamine [**thye** a min]
(vitamin B_1, Biamine)
Thiamine in combination with adenosine triphosphate (ATP) results in thiamine pyrophosphate coenzyme, a substance necessary for carbohydrate metabolism.

Indications

Thiamine is used to prevent and treat thiamine deficiencies that can result in beriberi or Wernicke's encephalopathy. It is routinely used for clients with nutritional deficiencies (e.g., recent history of alcohol abuse) prior to administration of carbohydrates (e.g., IV dextrose solutions).

Pharmacokinetics/Dosing

Thiamine is well absorbed from the GI tract, except in malabsorption syndrome or in the presence of alcohol, which inhibits absorption. It is metabolized in the liver and excreted by the kidneys. The usual adult dosage is determined by the age, gender, and degree of vitamin deficiency and ranges from 5 to 30 mg daily. Refer to a current reference for recommended pediatric dosages.

Adverse Effects

Adverse effects with thiamine use are usually rare. Skin rash, pruritus, or respiratory difficulties (wheezing) may occur after a large IV dose is administered (anaphylactic reaction) but are rare.

Nursing Management

Assessment

Thiamine rarely causes toxicity in clients who have normal renal function. Because a deficiency of a single B vitamin is uncommon, assess the client for multiple deficiencies. Serious sensitivity reactions can occur; assess drug history carefully.

A baseline assessment of the client should include neurologic and mental status, pulse rate, blood pressure, and 24-hour urinary thiamine levels. Deficiency levels vary by age; less than 27 mcg/dL indicates a deficiency in adults. Obtain a complete diet and drug history and determine alcohol drinking patterns to identify poor dietary habits. Total absence of dietary thiamine results in a deficiency state in about 3 weeks.

Nursing Diagnosis

The client with a thiamine deficiency may exhibit the following nursing diagnoses: disturbed thought processes (confusion, psychosis); decreased cardiac output (tachycardia, palpitations); and disturbed sensory perception (neuropathy, ataxia, nystagmus). The only potential complication with the administration of thiamine is an anaphylactic reaction (rare), usually after a large IV dose.

Planning

The client receiving thiamine therapy will:
- Maintain a well-balanced dietary intake, including adequate thiamine intake.
- Not evidence signs and symptoms of thiamine deficiency or sensitivity reaction.

Implementation

Monitoring

Continue to monitor the client with the indicators in the baseline assessment.

Intervention

In most instances thiamine is administered as an oral preparation; if this is not acceptable or possible, parenteral forms are available. An intradermal test dose is recommended prior to administration in clients suspected of being sensitive to the drug.

Education

Instruction for the client should include sources that are high in thiamine, such as whole grain or enriched cereals and meats, particularly yeast, pork, nuts, fish, organ/muscle meat, poultry, rice bran, dried beans, and fresh vegetables. Nutritional loss during cooking is variable and may be as high as 50%.

Evaluation

The expected outcome of thiamine therapy is that the client will maintain a diet adequate in thiamine, normal neurologic and cardiovascular status, and normal levels of urinary thiamine without experiencing anaphylaxis.

riboflavin [**rye** boo flay vin]

(vitamin B₂)

Riboflavin is converted in the body into two coenzymes: flavin mononucleotide (FMN) and flavin adenine dinucleotide (FAD). Both of these substances are necessary for normal tissue respiration. Riboflavin is also necessary to activate pyridoxine and to convert tryptophan to niacin, and it may be associated with the maintenance of erythrocyte integrity.

Indications

Riboflavin is used to prevent and treat riboflavin deficiency; usually this deficiency does not occur in healthy persons, but it may be detected as a result of malnutrition or intestinal malabsorption.

Pharmacokinetics/Dosing

Riboflavin is well absorbed in the GI tract and has a half-life of approximately 1 to 1.5 hours. It is metabolized in the liver and excreted by the kidneys. The usual adult dosage to treat riboflavin deficiency ranges from 5 to 10 mg. Refer to a current reference for additional dosing information.

Adverse Effects

Adverse effects are rare with riboflavin. No significant drug interactions have been reported.

Nursing Management

Assessment

A baseline assessment of the client with riboflavin deficiency should include examining the skin and mucous membranes, checking the appearance of the eyes and the client's vision status, and monitoring levels of RBCs, hemoglobin, and hematocrit. Riboflavin deficiency may be detected by measuring erythrocyte or urinary riboflavin concentrations. Obtain a complete diet and drug history and determine alcohol drinking patterns to identify poor dietary habits.

Nursing Diagnosis

The client with a riboflavin deficiency and ineffective riboflavin therapy may experience the following nursing diagnoses: impaired oral mucous membrane (cracking of the lips and corners of the mouth, glossitis); impaired skin integrity (seborrheic dermatitis in nasolabial folds, scrotum, labia; generalized dermatitis); and disturbed sensory perception (light sensitivity, burning of the eyes).

Planning

The client receiving riboflavin therapy will:
- Maintain a well-balanced dietary intake, including adequate riboflavin intake.
- Not evidence signs and symptoms of riboflavin deficiency.

Implementation

Monitoring

Water-soluble vitamins rarely cause toxicity in clients with normal kidney function. Monitor indicators within the baseline assessment.

Intervention

Give with food to enhance absorption.

Education

Alert the client that large doses of riboflavin may cause the urine to become yellow in color. The best food sources of riboflavin are milk and dairy products, meats, eggs, fish, poultry, enriched grains/cereals, and green, leafy vegetables (see Table 67-1). There is little loss of riboflavin with cooking.

Evaluation

The expected outcome of riboflavin therapy is that the client will maintain an adequate dietary intake of riboflavin and will have intact skin and mucous membranes, normal vision, and urinary riboflavin concentration values within the normal range.

niacin [**nye** a sin]
(nicotinic acid)
niacin extended-release
(Nicobid, Slo-Niacin)
niacinamide tablets/injection

Niacin is converted to niacinamide in the body and is part of two coenzymes: nicotinamide adenine dinucleotide (NAD) and nicotinamide adenine dinucleotide phosphate (NADP), which are necessary for glycogenolysis, tissue respiration, and lipid, protein, and purine metabolism. As an antihyperlipidemic agent, niacin lowers serum cholesterol and triglyceride levels by reducing the synthesis of very-low-density lipoproteins (VLDLs). VLDL is the precursor to low-density lipoprotein, the main carrier of cholesterol in the blood. Chapter 31 presents its use as an antihyperlipidemic more fully.

Indications

Niacin and niacinamide are used to prevent and treat vitamin B₃ deficiency conditions. A niacin deficiency may result in pellagra. Only niacin is indicated as a treatment adjunct for hyperlipidemia, but its acceptability may be limited by its vasodilating effects. Niacinamide does not cause direct peripheral vasodilation.

Pharmacokinetics/Dosing

With the exception of the malabsorption syndromes, both niacin and niacinamide are readily absorbed orally and have a half-life of 45 minutes. The onset of action to reduce triglyceride serum levels is several hours, whereas reducing cholesterol levels takes several days. Niacin is metabolized by the liver and excreted in the kidneys. For antihyperlipidemia, the usual adult dosage for niacin is 1 g PO daily, increased every 2 to 4 weeks as necessary up to a total of 4 to 6 grams daily. Refer to a current reference for additional information, because the dosages of niacin and niacinamide vary according to age and gender of the client.

Adverse Effects

Flushing is the most troublesome adverse effect of niacin in the higher doses observed for treatment of hyperlipidemias. Strategies to reduce or eliminate flushing include initiation of low doses, using formulations with inositol, and using concurrent aspirin therapy. The risk for hepatotoxicity has also been noted with slow release formulations of niacin. See Table 67-1 for additional information. Chapter 31 presents a more complete discussion of high dose niacin, adverse effects, and interactions.

Nursing Management

Assessment

Before large doses are administered, determine whether the client has arterial bleeding, diabetes mellitus (niacin only), peptic ulcer, or hepatic disease; all of these conditions will be aggravated by niacin and niacinamide. A baseline assessment should include activity tolerance, skin status, bowel status, and neurologic and mental status. Obtain a complete diet and drug history and determine alcohol drinking patterns to identify poor dietary habits.

Nursing Diagnosis

The client with a niacin deficiency and ineffective niacin therapy may experience the following nursing diagnoses: activity intolerance (fatigue, muscle weakness); impaired comfort (headache, indigestion); impaired skin integrity (dermatitis); impaired mucous membranes (red and sore mouth, tongue, and lips); diarrhea; and disturbed thought processes (confusion, disorientation, hallucinations). Clients undergoing niacin and niacinamide therapy may experience impaired comfort (flushing, headache [niacin only]); risk for injury (dizziness); impaired skin integrity (pruritus); and the potential complication of hepatitis (with the long-term use of extended-release niacin).

Planning

The client receiving niacin and niacinamide therapy will:
- Maintain a well-balanced dietary intake, including adequate niacin intake.
- Not evidence signs and symptoms of niacin deficiency.

Implementation

Monitoring

Monitor the client's progress by indicators within the baseline assessment. Assess blood glucose and hepatic function periodically if clients are receiving large doses of niacin or niacinamide for prolonged periods. Monitor clients with diabetes; hyperglycemia may occur, which increases insulin requirements.

Intervention

Administer with milk or food to help prevent GI distress. Oral administration of niacin is preferred. Parenteral niacin is used only when the oral route is not acceptable or possible. If administered IV, do not exceed a rate of 2 mg/min.

Education

Alert the client to expect a feeling of warmth and a flushing of the skin of the face and neck shortly after taking the tablets for the first 2 weeks of therapy. This sensation may be reduced by starting with a low dosage and gradually increasing it to the therapeutic level. Niacinamide is preferred because it lacks this blushing effect. Alcohol and niacin cause increased flushing. Avoid direct exposure to direct sunlight, while you have skin manifestations. Stress the importance of regular visits to the health care provider to monitor the effectiveness of the medication and the client's progress. Because one of the adverse effects is dizziness, caution the client to avoid hazardous tasks that require mental alertness until the response to the medication has been determined. Do not breastfeed while taking niacin.

The best food sources of niacin are meats, eggs, whole grain and enriched cereal/bread/flour, milk, and other dairy products (see Table 67-1).

Evaluation

The expected outcome of niacin and niacinamide therapy is that the client will maintain an adequate dietary intake of niacin and will not show any signs of niacin deficiency or toxicity.

pyridoxine [peer i **dox** een]
(vitamin B₆)
pyridoxine extended-release
(Rodex)

Pyridoxine is taken up by erythrocytes and converted into pyridoxal phosphate, a coenzyme necessary for many metabolic functions that affect proteins, carbohydrates, and lipid use in the body. Pyridoxine is also involved with converting tryptophan to niacin or serotonin.

Indications

Pyridoxine is indicated to treat or prevent pyridoxine deficiency. A deficiency state can lead to sideroblastic anemia, neurologic disturbances, seborrheic dermatitis, cheilosis, and xanthurenic aciduria. Vitamin B₆, folic acid, and vitamin B₁₂ are required for the metabolism of homocysteine; an increased level of homocysteine may be a major risk factor for vascular disease.

Pharmacokinetics/Dosing

Oral pyridoxine is well absorbed from the jejunum and is converted in the erythrocytes to pyridoxal phosphate, which is totally protein bound in the plasma. It has a half-life of 15 to 20 days and is metabolized by the liver and excreted in the kidneys. The usual dosage of pyridoxine varies according to age, gender, and degree of vitamin deficiency. Refer to a current reference for dosing recommendations.

Adverse Effects

The adverse effects of pyridoxine are very rare. Adverse effects are seen only when dosages of 200 mg daily are given for more than a month, leading to a dependency-type syndrome. Megadoses can cause problems (see Table 67-1).

Nursing Management

Assessment

Determine during the initial assessment whether the client has Parkinson's disease, which is treated with levodopa. A significant drug interaction occurs when pyridoxine is given with levodopa—the antiparkinsonian effects of levodopa may be reduced or reversed. This effect is not reported with the carbidopa-levodopa combination. Larobec is a vitamin B complex with vitamin C (without pyridoxine) for use prophylactically or therapeutically with clients undergoing treatment with levodopa. Obtain a complete diet and drug history and determine alcohol drinking patterns to identify poor dietary habits.

A baseline assessment of the client with a pyridoxine deficiency should include an inspection of the skin and mucous membranes and neurologic status. A pyridoxine deficiency is indicated by decreased serum transaminase and RBC levels and reduced urinary excretion of pyridoxic acid.

Nursing Diagnosis

The client with a pyridoxine deficiency and ineffective pyridoxine therapy may experience the following nursing diagnoses: impaired skin integrity (dermatitis); fatigue; activity intolerance related to anemia (weakness); risk for injury related to unsteady gait; and disturbed sleep pattern (drowsiness).

Planning

The client receiving pyridoxine therapy will:
- Maintain a well-balanced dietary intake, including adequate pyridoxine intake.
- Not evidence signs and symptoms of pyridoxine deficiency.

Implementation

Monitoring

Observe for improvement of deficiency symptoms. Evaluate the client for nutritional adequacy.

Intervention

IV pyridoxine may be administered undiluted at a rate of 50 mg/min and may be added to most IV solutions. If administered IM, inject into a large muscle.

Education

Large doses of pyridoxine for a period of several months may result in sensory neuropathy, which affects gait and causes numbness of the hands and feet.

The best food sources of pyridoxine are yeast, wheat germ, glandular and muscle meats (especially liver), eggs, bananas, potatoes, sweet potatoes, lima beans, and whole grain cereals.

Evaluation

The expected outcome of pyridoxine therapy is that the client will maintain an adequate dietary intake of pyridoxine, intact skin and mucous membranes, and a normal neurologic and mental status.

cyanocobalamin [sye an oh koe **bal** a min]
(vitamin B₁₂)
hydroxocobalamin [hye drox oh koe **bal** a min]
(Alphamin)

Cyanocobalamin is a coenzyme for a variety of metabolic functions, including protein synthesis and fat and carbohydrate metabolism. It is also needed for growth, cell replication, hematopoiesis, and nucleoprotein and myelin synthesis. A deficiency of vitamin B₁₂ (along with folic acid and pyridoxine [vitamin B₆] deficiencies) is a cause of abnormal homocysteine metabolism.

Indications

Cyanocobalamin is used to treat pernicious anemia (caused by a lack of intrinsic factor) and to prevent and treat vitamin B₁₂ deficiency caused by malabsorption or strict vegetarianism. Vitamin B₁₂ deficiency can lead to macrocytic megaloblastic anemia and irreversible neurologic damage.

Pharmacokinetics/Dosing

Intrinsic factor must be present in the intestinal tract in order for vitamin B₁₂ to be absorbed orally. It is highly protein bound, has a half-life of 6 days, and reaches peak serum levels in 8 to 12 hours. It is metabolized (and stored) by the liver and excreted in the bile and urine. The usual dosage of vitamin B₁₂ varies according to age, gender, and degree of vitamin deficiency. See Box 67-2 for information on the nasal spray form of vitamin B₁₂. Refer to a current reference for dosing recommendations.

Adverse Effects

Anaphylactic reactions are possible but are rare after a parenteral injection (see Table 67-1). No significant drug interactions are reported.

Nursing Management

Assessment

Cyanocobalamin is contraindicated for Leber hereditary optic neuropathy (a rare type of blindness resulting from an autosomal recessive trait); cyanocobalamin levels are already elevated in this condition, and optic nerve atrophy can occur rapidly after the administration of more cyanocobalamin. Ascertain the client's sensitivity to cyanocobalamin before initiating therapy; sensitization to the drug can take as long as 8 years to develop.

Plasma levels of vitamin B₁₂ should be determined before initiating therapy and on approximately the sixth day of therapy. A diagnosis of vitamin B₁₂ deficiency should be confirmed by the laboratory (serum B₁₂ levels under 150 pg/mL); otherwise the initiation of B₁₂ therapy may mask pernicious anemia or a folic acid deficiency.

A baseline assessment should include activity tolerance, neurologic status, RBC count, hemoglobin, hematocrit, and serum cobalamin levels. Obtain a complete diet and drug history and determine alcohol drinking patterns to identify poor dietary habits.

Nursing Diagnosis

The client with a cyanocobalamin deficiency and ineffective cyanocobalamin therapy may experience the following nursing diagnoses: activity intolerance related to anemia; and disturbed sensory perception (peripheral neuritis, hyperactive reflexes). Clients undergoing cyanocobalamin therapy may also experience diarrhea, impaired comfort (pruritus), and the potential complication of anaphylaxis.

Planning

The client receiving cyanocobalamin therapy will:
- Maintain a well-balanced dietary intake, including adequate cyanocobalamin intake.
- Not evidence signs and symptoms of cyanocobalamin deficiency.

Implementation

Monitoring

During the first 48 hours of therapy, monitor serum potassium levels closely for the possibility of severe hypokalemia. Hypersensitivity, which is rare, is demonstrated by a skin rash and, after parenteral administration, wheezing. Serum B₁₂ levels should be obtained on the fifth and seventh days of therapy. Reticulocyte concentration increases in 3 to 4 days, peaks in 5 to 8 days, and then gradually declines as erythrocyte count and hemoglobin rise to normal levels in 4 to 6 weeks.

Intervention

Administer oral forms of cyanocobalamin with meals to enhance absorption. Parenteral cyanocobalamin is administered intramuscularly (IM) or subcutaneously, not IV. Small amounts are sometimes included in TPN. An intradermal test dose is recommended before cyanocobalamin injection is administered to clients suspected of being sensitive to this drug. The parenteral product contains benzyl alcohol, which has been reported to be associated with a fatal "Gasping Syndrome" in premature infants.

Education

Stress compliance with the medication regimen if the client is undergoing life-long therapy following a gastrectomy or ileal resection or for pernicious anemia. For these conditions the drug is administered IM because of the absence of intrinsic factor.

The best food sources of vitamin B₁₂ are fortified breakfast cereals, organ meats, clams, oysters, crab, salmon, sardines, muscle meat, egg yolk, milk, fermented cheeses and other dairy products. There is little loss of the vitamin with ordinary cooking, but severe heating may cause its destruction.

Evaluation

The expected outcome of cyanocobalamin therapy is that the client will maintain an adequate dietary intake of B₁₂, a normal neurologic status, serum B₁₂ levels above 150 pg/mL, and RBC, hemoglobin, and hematocrit values that are within normal limits.

BOX 67-2 VITAMIN B₁₂ NASAL SPRAY

Nascobal, a vitamin B₁₂ nasal spray, was approved as a maintenance drug for persons in remission after undergoing IM therapy for conditions such as pernicious anemia. The dose is usually 500 mcg intranasally once weekly. A warning on the product states that the resumption of IM vitamin B₁₂ is necessary if the client is not properly maintained on the nasal spray. Adverse effects include infection, headache, glossitis, nausea, and rhinitis.

Data from *Drug facts and comparisons* (58th ed.) (2005). St. Louis: Facts and Comparisons.

folic acid

(vitamin B₉, Folvite, Apo-Folic)

Folic acid is converted to tetrahydrofolic acid in the body, which is necessary for normal erythropoiesis, the metabolism of amino acids, and nucleoprotein synthesis. A folic acid deficiency may result in megaloblastic and macrocytic anemias and glossitis. A deficiency of maternal folic acid is associated with neural tube defects. Although most women of childbearing age may be familiar with the importance of folic acid supplementation prior to becoming pregnant, only about one third of those women actually receive adequate folate supplementation (Cleves et al., 2004). The fortification of flour (as is done in the United States and Canada) may do more to improve folate intake than client education (Botto et al., 2005).

Folic acid and vitamins B₆ and B₁₂ supplements lower plasma homocysteine levels by 25% to 50% in clients with normal levels of homocysteine and in clients with hyperhomocysteinemia (Schnyder, Roffi, & Flammer, 2001). Although this reduction in homocysteine levels is hoped to reduce cardiovascular risks, folic acid has not demonstrated any significant benefit for clients with coronary artery disease or stroke (Liem et al., 2003, Lange et al., 2004). A Japanese trial of folic acid and vitamin B₁₂ significantly reduced hip fractures (Sato, Honda, Iwamoto, Kanoko, & Satoh, 2005), but additional data are warranted before routine recommendation of folate and vitamin B₁₂ supplementation can be advocated.

Indications

Folic acid is used to treat and prevent folic acid deficiency. Folic acid should not be administered until pernicious anemia has been ruled out as a potential diagnosis. If administered to clients with undiagnosed pernicious anemia, folic acid will correct the hematologic changes and mask pernicious anemia while the underlying neurologic damage progresses.

Pharmacokinetics/Dosing

Folic acid is absorbed mostly from the upper duodenum; it is highly protein bound, metabolized (and stored) in the liver, and excreted by the kidneys. In the presence of vitamin C, folic acid (ascorbic acid) is converted in the liver and serum to its active form, tetrahydrofolic acid, by dihydrofolate reductase. The usual dosage of folic acid varies according to age, gender, and degree of vitamin deficiency. The U.S. Preventive Services Task Force of the U.S. Department of Health and Human Services (2004) recommends a folic acid supplement of 400 mcg daily for all women in the childbearing years.

Adverse Effects

These effects are rare. An allergic reaction (elevated temperature and rash) or yellow discoloration of urine may occur.

Nursing Management

Assessment

Determine whether the client has pernicious anemia, because folic acid will reverse hematologic abnormalities while the neurologic aspects of the disease continue to progress. No significant drug interactions are reported. Ascertain if the client has a sensitivity to the vitamin before initiating therapy. A baseline assessment should include the client's activity tolerance, RBC count, hemoglobin, and hematocrit. Obtain a complete diet and drug history and determine alcohol drinking patterns to identify poor dietary habits. Drugs reported to cause folate deficiency include alcohol, barbiturates, methotrexate, hormonal contraceptives, phenytoin, primidone, and trimethoprim.

Nursing Diagnosis

Clients with folic acid deficiency will probably experience activity intolerance and ineffective protection secondary to anemia. Those receiving folic acid may experience the potential complication of anaphylaxis.

Planning

The client receiving folic acid therapy will:
- Maintain a well-balanced dietary intake, including adequate folic acid intake.
- Not evidence signs and symptoms of folic acid deficiency.

Implementation

Monitoring

Monitor the client's progress using the indicators in the baseline assessment.

Intervention

Folic acid is available as oral tablets, IM, subcutaneous, or may be given undiluted IV over 1 minute. It may be added to most IV solutions. The injection preparation contains benzyl alcohol as a preservative and should not be administered to newborns and immature infants.

Education

Alert the client that large doses of folic acid may turn the urine yellow. The best food sources of folic acid are yeast, liver, whole grains, bran, fresh leafy vegetables, fruits, nuts, dried beans, and lentils. Consult with physician before breastfeeding while taking folic acid.

Evaluation

The expected outcome of folic acid therapy is that the client will maintain an adequate dietary intake of folic acid, a tolerance for desired activities, and an RBC count, hemoglobin, and hematocrit within normal limits. If the client is pregnant, the infant will be born without a neural tube defect.

ascorbic acid

(vitamin C)

Ascorbic acid is necessary for collagen formation in fibrous tissue (including bone) and in development of teeth, blood vessels, and blood cells. It also plays a role in carbohydrate metabolism. It is believed to stimulate the fibroblasts of connective tissue and thus promote tissue repair and wound healing. It may also help to maintain the integrity of the intercellular substance in the walls of blood vessels; the capillary fragility associated with scurvy is explained on this basis. Preliminary data suggests a benefit of reducing rates of preterm labor may be linked with adequate ascorbic acid intake (Siega-Riz et al., 2003). Vitamin C may also help prevent gout by lowering uric acid levels (Huang et al., 2005). Ascorbic acid may be necessary for the metabolism of phenylalanine, tyrosine, folic acid, norepinephrine, histamine, and iron. The effectiveness of ascorbic acid in preventing or relieving cold symptoms or in treating cancer, infertility, aging, or peptic ulcer is primarily unproven. Studies performed over the years have not substantiated these claims (USP DI, 2005).

Indications

Ascorbic acid is used to prevent and treat vitamin C deficiency (scurvy) and, in larger doses, for urine acidification.

Pharmacokinetics/Dosing

Ascorbic acid is well absorbed from the GI tract and is stored in the plasma and cells, with the highest concentration found in glandular sites. It is metabolized in the liver and excreted by the kidneys (see Table 67-1). The adult dosage as a nutritional supplement is 50 to 100 mg daily. The dosage to treat a vitamin C deficiency varies according to the age of the client and the severity of the vitamin deficiency. Doses as high as 1000 to 4000 mg four times daily have been used for urinary acidification, but such high doses may increase the potential for crystal formation in the urine and urinary obstruction.

Adverse Effects

Standard doses of ascorbic acid are well tolerated by most clients. Clients with glucose-6-phosphate dehydrogenase (G6PD) deficiency may be predisposed to hemolytic anemia with the use of ascorbic acid. High doses of ascorbic acid may cause diarrhea, cramps, headache, nausea, vomiting, and red skin. Very high doses may precipitate hyperoxaluria and calcium oxalate kidney stones.

Nursing Management

Assessment

Determine that the client does not have cystinuria, oxalosis, or a history of gout or urate renal stones, because there is a risk for urinary stone formation when large doses of vitamin C are given to clients with these conditions. Large doses may also precipitate a crisis in sickle cell anemia.

If the purpose of administering vitamin C is to acidify the urine, urinary pH needs to be monitored to determine the effectiveness of the drug.

A baseline assessment of the client should include an inspection of the skin and mucous membranes, comfort levels, mental status, and serum levels of ascorbic acid. Check the bowel status and temperature in children. Serum ascorbic acid levels less than 0.2 mg/dL confirm a deficiency. Obtain a complete diet and drug history and determine alcohol drinking patterns to identify poor dietary habits.

Nursing Diagnosis

The client with a vitamin C deficiency and ineffective ascorbic acid therapy may experience the following nursing diagnoses: impaired comfort (limb and joint pain); impaired oral mucous membrane (swollen or bleeding gums); ineffective protection related to capillary fragility (petechiae, ecchymoses); and disturbed thought processes (irritability, depression, hysteria). Clients receiving ascorbic acid therapy may experience diarrhea; impaired comfort (headache, flushing of the skin, nausea, vomiting, stomach cramps); and the potential complication of oxalate kidney stones.

Planning

The client receiving ascorbic acid therapy will:
- Maintain a well-balanced dietary intake, including adequate ascorbic acid intake.
- Not evidence signs and symptoms of ascorbic acid deficiency.

Implementation

Monitoring

Monitor the client using the indicators in the baseline assessment.

Intervention

Ascorbic acid can be added to IV solutions and given as a continuous infusion. Bolus therapy that is administered too rapidly may cause dizziness and syncope. Ensure that the oral effervescent tablet form is dissolved in water just before administering. For IM and subcutaneous injections, open ampules with caution; prolonged storage may cause the release of carbon dioxide resulting in increased pressure within ampule. The injection solution may gradually darken on exposure to light; a slight discoloration does not affect its efficacy.

Education

Clients taking more than 600 mg of ascorbic acid daily may experience a small increase in urination; with more than 1 g daily, diarrhea; and with more than 2 to 3 g daily of prolonged therapy, withdrawal scurvy. Take large doses in divided amounts because the body does not store what it cannot use at a particular time and the rest is excreted in the urine. Vitamin C increases the absorption of iron when taken with iron rich foods. Consult with physician before breastfeeding while taking this vitamin.

The best food sources of vitamin C are citrus fruits, tomatoes, strawberries, cantaloupe, potatoes, and green vegetables (green peppers, broccoli, cabbage). Cooking destroys the vitamin C content of food by 30% to 50%, especially if copper pots are used. A gradual loss occurs in fresh foods in storage, but not with freezing unless over prolonged periods. Chopping fresh vegetables also causes some loss.

Evaluation

The expected outcome of ascorbic acid therapy is that the client will maintain an adequate intake of dietary vitamin C; healthy skin, mucous membranes, and mental state; and serum levels of ascorbic acid that are within the normal limits.

Multivitamin Preparations

Numerous multivitamin preparations are available in the United States and Canada. Supplemental preparations should provide 100% of the United States RDA to meet the needs of the vast majority of clients. Daily use of a multivitamin preparation is associated with reduced infection risk in adults (El-Kadiki & Sutton, 2005), and this benefit appears particularly true for clients with diabetes (Barringer et al., 2003). Extra-potency or high-potency vitamins are rarely necessary for routine supplementation. Additionally, the nurse should be aware that many preparations contain chemicals not yet known to be associated with any deficiency states.

✱ **T.L. does not currently take a vitamin or mineral supplement. The nurse advises her to compare prices and ingredients of the vitamins she is considering in the health food stores with other retailers. She advises a daily vitamin and mineral supplement that contains the daily recommended allowances of vitamins and calcium supplementation to a total of 1000 mg of elemental calcium daily.**

Minerals used for therapeutic supplementation include calcium, iron, phosphate, and magnesium. Chapter 40 presents calcium, magnesium and aluminum that are used therapeutically as antacids for treating dyspepsia. See Chapters 35 and 47 for their use for clients with renal failure and parathyroid dysfunction, respectively. The discussion in this chapter is limited to iron which is prescribed for iron-deficiency anemia. Other minerals are reviewed in other sections of this text.

✱ **L.S., a 21-year-old female, presents to her health care provider with weakness, loss of energy, and pale appearance. On history, her nurse notes she is a vegetarian and also reports a heavy monthly menstrual flow. A complete blood count is taken with a work up for anemia. Her labs are as follows: hemoglobin: 8 g/dL (normal, 14 to 18); hematocrit: 27% (normal, 40% to 44%); serum ferritin: 9 ng/mL (normal, 15 to 200); serum B$_{12}$: 450 pg/mL (normal 200 to 1000); and folate: 12.2 ng/dL (normal 3.6 to 20 ng/dL).**

✱ **What are the common types of anemias?**

Chapter 29 briefly presents anemias, or reduced red blood cell counts. Anemias typically result in reduced oxygen carrying capacity of blood, and contribute to weakness or lethargy. Anemias can also contribute to reduced respiratory and cardiovascular reserve for clients with asthma, chronic obstructive pulmonary disease (COPD), coronary artery disease, heart failure, and a number of other conditions. Anemias can be related to increased destruction or loss and/or decreased production of erythrocytes. Table 67-2 presents common etiologies and related lab findings. Loss of RBCs may be secondary to blood loss of trauma, surgery, or menses, or because of destruction of erythrocytes via hemolysis. Hemolytic anemias may result from genetic predisposition (e.g., G6PD deficiency) or antibody/antigen interactions (e.g., hemolytic anemia of the newborn related to RH factor, drug induced hemolytic anemia). Decreased production of red blood cells may be because of direct bone marrow suppression (e.g., cancer chemotherapy, other drugs), chronic illness (e.g., anemia of chronic disease), or to deficiency of a substance required for erythrocyte production (e.g., erythropoietin, iron, folic acid, cyanocobalamin).

TABLE 67-2 TYPES OF ANEMIAS AND RELATED LAB FINDINGS

↑ RBC Destruction/Loss		↓ RBC Production	
Etiology	**Typical Lab Findings**	**Etiology**	**Typical Lab Findings**
Acute or chronic blood loss G6PD deficiency Hemolytic anemia of the newborn Drug-induced hemolytic anemia	↓ Hct ↓ Hgb Normal iron/ferritin Normal B_{12} Normal folate Normal MCV Normal MCH **If Hemolytic:** ↓ Bilirubin-indirect (hemolysis) + Coombs Test (autoimmune hemolysis)	Iron deficiency	**Microcytic (Small RBC)** **Hypochromic (Pale RBC)** ↓ MCV ↓ MCH ↓ Hct ↓ Hgb ↓ Iron/ferritin Normal B_{12} Normal folate
		Erythropoietin deficiency Renal failure	**Normocytic (Normal size RBC)** **Normochromic (Normal color RBC)** Normal MCV Normal MCH ↓ Hct ↓ Hgb Normal/↓ Iron/ferritin Normal B_{12} Normal folate
		Vitamin B_{12} deficiency Folate deficiency	**Macrocytic (Small RBC)** **Normochromic (Normal color RBC)** ↑ MCV Normal MCH ↓ Hct Normal/↓ Hgb Normal iron/ferritin ↓ B_{12} (B_{12} deficiency) ↓ Folate (folate deficiency)

Hct, Hematocrit; *Hgb,* hemoglobin; *MCH,* mean corpuscular hemoglobin; *MCV,* mean corpuscular volume.

The deficiency anemias may present differently based on which factor is lacking (see Table 67-2). Management revolves around identifying the deficient factor, and supplementing the factor or factors. Chapter 35 discusses erythropoietin, which is administered for clients with reduced erythrocyte production secondary to renal failure, cancer chemotherapy, and other selected states. Folic acid and cyanocobalamin are discussed above. Iron supplements are discussed below.

Based on history and lab results, L.S. is diagnosed with iron deficiency anemia.

What are the treatments for iron deficiency anemia? Iron deficiency is the most common nutritional deficiency in the United States and Canada that results in anemia. Young children and women, especially pregnant women, are most commonly affected.

Iron is an essential mineral for the proper functioning of many biologic systems in the body. It functions as an oxygen carrier in hemoglobin and myoglobin and is also involved in tissue respiration and in many enzyme reactions in the body. It is also stored in various body sites such as the liver, spleen, and bone marrow.

Iron is supplied through diet (lean red meats) and iron supplements. Ingested iron is converted to the ferrous state by gastric juices; it is then more readily absorbed in the body. The absorption of iron is increased if it is taken with ascorbic acid (vitamin C), orange juice, veal, and other animal tissues. Coffee, tea, milk, eggs, whole grain breads, and cereals decrease iron absorption. For clients who are not able to tolerate oral iron, or who need large doses of iron (e.g., clients undergoing renal dialysis), parenteral forms of iron (ferric gluconate, iron dextran) are sometimes used.

Oral Iron Salts

ferrous sulfate [**fer** us **sul** fate]
(Feratab, Fer-In-Sol, Fer-Iron, Slow-FE)
ferrous gluconate [**fer** us **gloo** koe nate]
(Fergon)
ferrous fumarate [**fer** us **fyoo** ma rate]
(Femiron, Feostat, Ferro-Sequels)

polysaccharide-iron complex [pol i **sak** a ride **eye** ern **kom** pleks]
(Niferex, Hytinic)
Indications
Iron is indicated for the treatment of iron-deficiency anemia.
Pharmacokinetics/Dosing
In iron deficiency, 10% to 30% of iron is absorbed; in normal individuals, approximately 5% to 15% is usually absorbed. Ferrous iron is better absorbed than the ferric dosage form. Iron binds to transferrin and is transported to bone marrow to aid in RBC production. Iron is not eliminated physiologically by the body. Excess iron intake can result in accumulation and iron toxicity. Small amounts are lost daily in the shedding of skin, nails, and hair; in breast milk; in urine; and in menstrual blood. The daily iron loss in healthy adults is approximately 1 mg daily for males and postmenopausal females and 1.5 to 2 mg daily in healthy premenopausal females. Dose used

in the treatment of iron deficiency anemia is dependent on salt form used and degree of anemia. Dosage range is often 60 mg of elemental iron once to three times daily. Table 67-3 compares different iron formulations.
Adverse Effects
The most common adverse effects of iron therapy include nausea, vomiting, constipation (diarrhea is less commonly reported), and abdominal cramps. For the treatment of iron toxicity, see the Management of Drug Overdose box below.

Parenteral Iron Formulations

Parenteral formulations of iron are used on occasion for clients who are significantly deficient in iron stores and, either require large doses or, cannot tolerate oral formulations.

TABLE 67-3 ORAL IRON SALTS

Formulation/ Salt Form	Tablet Strength (mg)	Iron Content (mg)	Typical Adult Dose for Salt Form
ferrous sulfate	325	65	325 mg (65 mg elemental) one to four times daily
ferrous gluconate	220, 300	27, 35	220-600 mg (27-70 mg elemental) one to four times daily
ferrous fumarate	63, 100, 150, 200, 325	20, 33, 50, 66,106	63-325 mg (10-106 mg elemental) one to two times daily
polysaccharide-iron complex	50, 150	50, 150	50-150 mg (50-150 mg elemental) one to two times daily

---

Management of Drug Overdose

Iron Salts

The body is unable to effectively eliminated large amounts of ingested iron. Acute iron overdose is primarily seen in children (e.g., toxic ingestion of iron supplements or vitamins with iron by toddlers) although chronic iron overload is more often observed in adults who receive high doses of iron supplements long term (Daram & Hayashi, 2005). Intentional overdose, however, can also be observed. Significant iron overdose can lead to multiple complications including GI bleeding (Abraham, Yardley, & Wu, 1999) and liver failure (Smith, Simpson, Garden, & Wigmore, 2005).

Signs and Symptoms

Diarrhea (often with blood), fever, severe abdominal cramps/pain and vomiting are early indications of over overdose. Late signs/symptoms include pale, cold skin, cardiac dysrhythmias, hypertension, metabolic acidosis, seizures, increased weakness, sedation, and blue tint to lips, fingernails, and palms. Cardiovascular collapse is also possible.

Treatment

Treatment of iron overdose includes the following principles:
- Obtaining immediate medical attention.
- Utilizing gastric lavage (often with sodium bicarbonate) in the case of acute ingestion.
- Maintaining fluid and electrolyte status.
- Administering the parenteral antidote deferoxamine (Desferal). Deferoxamine binds to ferric ions which are renally removed. Reduced doses are required for clients with renal insufficiency.
- Monitoring laboratory tests, including serum iron, complete blood counts (with hemoglobin and hematocrit), electrolytes, blood gasses, blood glucose, and total iron binding capacity. Monitoring of liver function tests, including bilirubin, alanine aminotransferase (ALT), aspartate aminotransferase (AST), and international normalized ratio (INR) is also warranted. If liver failure is suspected, monitoring of mental status is also prudent.
- Occasionally, implementing exchange transfusions are also sometimes utilized in management.

ferric gluconate [**fer** ik **gloo** koe nate]
(Ferrlecit)
Indications
Ferric gluconate is used to replace total body iron stores in clients undergoing hemodialysis with concurrent erythropoietin. It is contraindicated for clients who have demonstrated hypersensitivity to it or related products.

Pharmacokinetics/Dosing
Ferric gluconate is administered by IV injection and about 50% of administered iron is bound to plasma protein or tissue storage sites within one hour. Prior to initiating IV iron gluconate therapy in adults, a one-time test dose of 25 mg should be given IV. Typical doses are 125 mg of elemental iron (10 mL ferric gluconate) administered IV with each hemodialysis treatment (typically three times weekly) for a total of 8 doses.

Adverse Effects
Hypersensitivity and anaphylaxis are the most important adverse effects with ferric gluconate. Flushing, transient hypotension, chest pain, headache, and pain on injection have been noted. Refer to package insert for the most complete information regarding adverse effects.

iron dextran complex [**eye** ern **deks** tran **kom** plex]
(DexFerrum, InFeD, DexIron✤, Infurer✤)
Indications
Iron dextran complex is indicated for treatment of iron deficiency anemia in clients who cannot tolerate oral iron therapy. It is contraindicated in clients who have demonstrated a hypersensitivity reaction to injectable forms of iron. Because of its higher risk for hypersensitivity than ferric gluconate and iron sucrose, its use is should be restricted to selected clients in whom there is a particular need to treat with this compound (Fishbane, 2003).

Pharmacokinetics/Dosing
Iron dextran is usually administered IM by Z-track injection or IV. On IM administration, the majority of iron is quickly absorbed within a few hours. IV administration may pose a higher risk for immediate hypersensitivity reactions and is usually diluted in 250 to 1000 mL normal saline and infused over 1 to 6 hours. Direct IV push is not recommended. Dosing is based on degree of iron loss and the package insert identifies a formula for calculating dose based on blood loss, hematocrit and lean body weight. Test doses of 0.5 mL (25 mg) IM or IV are often utilized prior to initiating full therapeutic doses. Full adult doses are typically in the range of 50 to 100 mg of iron (1 to 2 mg) up to once daily depending on response and indication.

Adverse Effects
The most serious adverse effects are hypersensitivity reactions including anaphylaxis. Other adverse effects include flushing, dizziness, pain, nausea, vomiting, and staining at the IM site. Refer to package labeling for complete information.

iron sucrose [**eye** ern **sue** krose]
(Venofer)
Indications
Iron sucrose is indicated for hemodialysis associated iron deficiency anemia.

Pharmacokinetics/Dosing
Iron sucrose is administered in doses of 100 mg IV with each hemodialysis treatment for a total of 10 doses (1000 mg) over approximately 3 to 4 weeks. Additional dosing beyond the initial 1000 mg dose over 4 weeks is determined by client response.

Adverse Effects
As with other parenteral iron formulations, iron sucrose has the potential for serious hypersensitivity reactions, including anaphylaxis. Other adverse events are similar to the above noted parenteral iron formulations.

✴ What are the nursing management issues involved with iron therapy for L.S.?

Assessment Complete a thorough dietary history, and assess L.S.'s nutritional status to ascertain the possible causes of anemia and the need for client education. See Table 67-3 for typical adult doses of oral iron salts.

Iron should be administered for iron-deficiency anemias specifically rather than for all anemias in general. Some anemic conditions, such as thalassemia, may actually result in excess deposits of iron in the body. Determine that L.S. does not have a disorder of iron metabolism such as hemochromatosis, which causes an excess deposition of iron in the tissues, skin pigmentation, cirrhosis of the liver, and decreased carbohydrate tolerance; or hemosiderosis, an increase in tissue iron stores without associated tissue damage. Porphyria cutanea tarda may be caused by an excess accumulation of iron in the liver. All of these conditions contraindicate the use of iron. Clients receiving repeated blood transfusions are also at risk for iron overload as a result of the addition of high erythrocytic iron content.

Some older adults may need larger doses of iron than the usual daily adult dose for iron deficiency anemia, because the reduction of gastric secretions and achlorhydria that accompanies aging also inhibits the ability to absorb iron.

A baseline assessment of L.S. should include activity tolerance; a hemoglobin, hematocrit, and reticulocyte count; and plasma iron and ferritin values. Obtain a complete diet and drug history to identify poor dietary habits.

Review L.S.'s current medication regimen for the risk of significant drug interactions, such as those that may occur when iron salts are given concurrently with acetohydroxamic acid (Lithostat) as iron may be chelated by acetohydroxamic acid, resulting in reduced absorption of both drugs. If iron therapy is necessary for a client receiving acetohydroxamic acid, it is suggested that iron be administered parenterally. Decreased iron absorption may result if given with antacids, calcium supplements, milk or dairy products, coffee, fiber or selected food products. Schedule iron supplements at least 1 hour before and 2 hours after the administration of these substances. Concurrent administration of iron with etidronate (Didronel) may result in decreased absorption of oral etidronate. Teach clients to avoid the consumption of iron products within 2 hours of etidronate. Iron may reduce the absorption of fluoroquinolones; take these antimicrobials at least 2 hours before or 2 hours after iron supplements. Oral iron may decrease the absorption of fluoroquinolones and tetracycline, which may result in reduced antimicrobial effectiveness and also impair hematologic effectiveness of the iron supplement; administer iron supplements 2 hours after fluoroquinolones and tetracyclines. Concurrent administration of vitamin E with iron may reduce the client's hematologic response to iron therapy. If larger iron doses are administered, vitamin E requirements may also need to be increased. Close monitoring is suggested when concurrent therapy is administered.

Nursing Diagnosis While L.S. is receiving iron therapy, she is at risk for the following nursing diagnoses/collaborative problems: activity intolerance related to ineffectiveness of the therapy (anemia); constipation; diarrhea; impaired comfort (heartburn); disturbed body image related to stained teeth from liquid forms of iron; altered comfort (nausea and vomiting); and the potential complications of allergic reaction (backache, chills, dizziness, fever, headache, nausea, tingling of the hands or feet) or toxicity (fever, nausea, stomach pain, vomiting, and diarrhea, sometimes with blood). If L.S. were receiving parenteral iron, impaired tissue integrity (pain, redness at the injection or infusion site), would also be an issue.

Planning The client receiving iron therapy will:
- Maintain a well-balanced dietary intake, including adequate iron intake.
- Not evidence signs and symptoms of iron deficiency anemia.

Implementation

Monitoring Monitor the hemoglobin, hematocrit, reticulocyte count, and plasma iron values every 3 weeks during the first 2 months of oral iron therapy or for a few days after the initiation of parenteral therapy. It usually takes 1 to 2 months of oral therapy for the hemoglobin concentration of a client with iron deficiency anemia to reach normal levels. L.S.'s diagnosis should be reconsidered if a 1 g/100 mL increase in hemoglobin does not occur during the first 2 weeks of therapy. With iron sucrose injection, withhold the drug and notify physician when serum ferritin level equals or exceeds established guidelines or hypotension, edema, headache, dizziness, nausea, vomiting or abdominal, joint or bone pain occur.

Monitor L.S.'s bowel pattern, because more than 10% of clients report constipation with iron administration.

Intervention The ferrous rather than ferric preparation of iron provides for the most efficient absorption of iron. Iron is best administered on an empty stomach. When taken with food, its absorption may be decreased by as much as one half to one third. Administer liquid iron preparations with a full glass of water to prevent staining of the teeth. A drinking straw or a dropper may be used to place the dose far back on the tongue to prevent contact with the teeth. Oral preparations of iron should be discontinued before parenteral iron therapy begins. Some clients may require laxatives if iron supplement–induced constipation occurs.

Anaphylaxis has been known to occur up to 24 hours after parenteral administration. Epinephrine should be available during the injection of iron dextran, particularly in clients with asthma and known allergies. A test dose of 25 mg should be administered IM or IV to all clients at least 1 hour before their first therapeutic parenteral dose of iron dextran. Closely monitor clients receiving IV iron sucrose injection for the first 30 minutes of administration.

Do not mix the IV administration of iron dextran with other medications or add it to parenteral nutrition solutions. It should be administered undiluted and at a rate of no more than 1 mL/min. Flush the IV line with normal saline for injection. Maintain the client in a recumbent position for 30 minutes in case orthostatic hypotension should occur.

It is recommended that iron dextran be administered into the muscle mass of the upper outer quadrant of the buttock using the Z-track technique and a 2- to 3-inch, 19- or 20-gauge needle. The preparation should never be injected into the upper arm or any other exposed area because of the possibility that it will stain the skin dark brown. To minimize staining of the flesh, use a separate needle to withdraw the drug from the vial.

Education Alert L.S. that iron preparations cause black stools, which are medically insignificant. However, she should notify the prescriber if she experiences other symptoms of internal blood loss, such as bloody streaks in the stool, abdominal tenderness, cramping, or pain. If a client experiences dental discoloration from iron therapy, recommend a baking soda toothpaste or one that contains 3% hydrogen peroxide. Advise L.S. to increase dietary fiber and fluid intake if constipation becomes a problem. Instruct L.S. to maintain a diet rich in sources of iron, such as liver, green leafy vegetables, potatoes, dried peas and beans, dried fruit, and enriched flour, breads, and cereals. For prophylaxis, 300 mg daily of elemental iron is recommended.

Evaluation The expected outcome of iron therapy is that L.S. will maintain an adequate dietary intake of iron, tolerate activities as desired, and maintain hemoglobin, hematocrit, reticulocyte count, and plasma iron values within normal limits.

Summary

Nutritional requirements are best met by the oral ingestion of adequate fluids and regular, balanced meals. When clients experience altered nutrition: less than body requirements, the nurse may participate in various nutritional modalities, such as vitamin replacement and enteral or parenteral feedings. Vitamins are essential to help maintain normal metabolic functions, growth, and tissue repair.

Most vitamin deficiencies are not singular but are multiple and result from impoverished diets because of alcoholism, poverty, fads, or ignorance. Replacement therapy is available for the water-soluble vitamins (vitamin C and the B-complex groups) and the fat-soluble ones (vitamins A, D, E, and K). Because water-soluble vitamins are not stored in the body, deficiencies can appear after short periods of inadequate intake. Fat-soluble vitamins, on the other hand, are stored in the liver and fatty tissue in large amounts; deficiencies occur only after a long period of deprivation. However, toxic levels are easier to reach with supplements of fat-soluble vitamins. Iron deficiency is a very common nutritional deficiency in the United States and Canada, especially in young children and women. Supplement therapy is practical but, as in prophylaxis of nutritional deficiencies, the best remedy is dietary intake.

✳ Critical Thinking Questions

- How would you plan to incorporate the U.S. RDA requirements for vitamins and minerals into a day's diet for a vegetarian? For a Latino client? For an edentulous client? For an older adult on a limited income with only biweekly access to transportation?

- Take 10 minutes and write down your diet for the last 24 hours. Using your nutrition books, analyze the diet's vitamin and mineral content. Did you meet the U.S. RDA requirements for vitamins and minerals? How would you modify your diet to do so? What are the barriers to these modifications?

Bibliography

Abraham, S., Yardley, J.H., & Wu, T.T. (1999). Mucosal injury to the upper gastrointestinal tract due to iron medication is an under-recognized entity. *Laboratory Investigation, 79*(1), 71A.

Anderson, P., & Milner, J. (2004). Highlights of ILSI Functional Foods Meeting: Reports From the Special Conference on Functional Foods for Health Promotion: Making sense of the science. *Nutrition Today, 39*(3), 122-127.

Anderson, D.M., Keith, J., & Novak, P.D. (Eds.) (2002). *Mosby's medical, nursing, and allied health dictionary* (6th ed.). St. Louis: Mosby.

Andrès, E. (2004). Vitamin B12 (cobalamin) deficiency in elderly patients. *Canadian Medical Association Journal, 171*(3), 251-259.

Bairati, I., Meyer, F., Gelinas, M., Fortin, A., Nabid, A., Brochert, F., et al. (2005). A randomized trial of antioxidant vitamins to prevent second primary cancers in head and neck cancer patients. *Journal of the National Cancer Institute, 97,* 481-488.

Barringer, T.A., Kirk, J.K., Santaniello, A.C., Foley, K.L., & Michielutte, R. (2003). Effect of a multivitamin and mineral supplement on infection and quality of life: A randomized, double-blind, placebo-controlled trial. *Annals of Internal Medicine, 138*(5), 365-371.

Bischoff-Ferrari, H.A., Dawson-Hughes, B., Willett, W.C., Staehelin, H.B., Bazemore, M.G., & Zee, R.Y., et al. (2004). Effect of Vitamin D on falls: A meta-analysis. *Journal of the American Medical Association, 291*(16), 1999-2006.

Biscoff-Ferrari, H.A., Willett, W.C., Wong, J.B., Giovannucci, E., Dietrich, T., Dawson-Hughes, B. (2005). Fracture preventions with vitamin D supplementation: A meta-analysis of randomized controlled trials. *Journal of the American Medical Association, 293,* 2257-2264.

Botto, L.D., Lisi, A., Robert-Gnanisa, E., Erickson, J.D., Vollset, S.E., Mastroiacovo, P., et al. (2005). International retrospective cohort study of neural tube defects in relation to folic acid recommendations: Are the recommendations working? *British Medical Journal, 330,* 571-573.

Cleves, M.A., Hobbs, C.A., Collins, H.B., Andrews, N., Smith, L.N., & Robbins, J.M. (2004). Folic acid use by women receiving routine gynecologic care. *Obstetrics & Gynecology, 103*(4), 746-753.

Daram, S.R., & Hayashi, P.H. (2005). Acute liver failure due to iron overdose in an adult. *Southern Medical Journal, 98*(2), 241-244.

El-Kadiki, A., & Sutton, A.J. (2005). Role of multivitamins and mineral supplements in preventing infections in elderly people: Systematic review and meta-analysis of randomised controlled trials. *British Medical Journal, 330,* 871-874.

Fawzi, W.W., Msamanga, G.I., Spiegelman, D., Wei, R., Kapiga, S., & Villamor, E., et al. (2004). A randomized trial of multivitamin supplements and HIV disease progression and mortality. *New England Journal of Medicine, 351*(1), 23-32.

Fishbane, S. (2003). Safety in iron management, *American Journal of Kidney Disease, 41*(5 Supplement), 18-26.

Grant, A.M., Avenell, A., Campbell, M.K., McDonald, A.M., MacLennan, G.S., McPherson, G.C,. et al. (2005). Oral vitamin D₃ and calcium for secondary prevention of low-trauma fractures in elderly people (Randomised Evaluation of Calcium Or vitamin D, RECORD): A randomised placebo-controlled trial. *Lancet, 365,* 1621-1628.

Grau, M.V., Baron, J.A., Sandler, R.S., Haile, R.W., Beach, M.L., & Church, T.R., et al. (2003). Vitamin D, calcium supplementation, and colorectal adenomas: results of a randomized trial. *Journal of the National Cancer Institute, 95*(23), 1765-1771.

Hasselmann, M., & Reimund, J.M. (2004). Lipids in the nutritional support of the critically ill patients. *Current Opinion in Critical Care, 10*(6), 449-455.

Huang, H.Y., Appel, L.J., Choi, M.J., Gelber, A.C., Charleston, J., Norkus, E.P., et al. (2005). The effects of vitamin C supplementation on serum concentrations of uric acid: Results of a randomized controlled trial. *Arthritis and Rheumatology, 52,* 1843-1847.

Kritharides, L., & Stocker, R. (2002). The use of antioxidant supplements in coronary heart disease. *Atherosclerosis, 164*(2), 211-219.

Lange, H., Suryapranata, H., De Luca, G., Borner, C., Dille, J., & Kallmayer, K., et al. (2004). Folate therapy and in-stent restenosis after coronary stenting. *New England Journal of Medicine, 350*(26), 2673-2681.

Liem, A., Reynierse-Buitenwerf, G.H., Zwinderman, A.H., Jukema, J.W., & van Veldhuisen, D.J., (2003). Secondary prevention with

---

𝓔-LEARNING SUPPLEMENTS

Student CD-ROM
- Final Exam questions
- NCLEX® Examination review questions
- Pharmacology animations
- Printable chapter summary

Evolve Website (http://evolve.elsevier.com/mckenry)
- Content updates, including information on new drugs
- WebLinks corresponding to this chapter
- Answers to the critical thinking questions in this chapter
- *Elsevier ePharmacology Update* newsletter
- Mosby's Drug Consult Internet Edition
- Supplemental and reference information

folic acid: Effects on clinical outcomes. *Journal of the American College of Cardiology, 41*(12), 2105-2113.

Lonn, E., Bosch, J., Yusuf, S., Sheridan, P., Pogue, J., Arnold, J.M., et al. (2005). Effects of long-term vitamin E supplementation on cardiovascular events and cancer: A randomized controlled trial. *Journal of the American Medical Association, 293,* 1338-1347.

Makishima, M., Lu, T.T., Xie, W., Whitfield, G.K., Domoto, H., & Evans, R.M., et al. (2002). Vitamin D receptor as an intestinal bile acid sensor. Science. RNA Silencing and Noncoding RNA. *Science, 296*(5571), 1313-1316.

Marcus, R. (2001). Agents affecting calcification and bone turnover: calcium, phosphate, parathyroid hormone, vitamin D, calcitonin and other compounds. In J.F. Hardman & L.E. Limbird (Eds.), *Goodman & Gilman's The pharmacological basis of therapeutics* (10th ed.). New York: McGraw-Hill.

Michaelsson, K., Lithell, H., Vessby, B., & Melhus, H. (2003). Serum Retinol Levels and the Risk of Fracture. *New England Journal of Medicine, 348*(4), 287-294.

Miller, E.R., Pastor-Barriuso, R., Dalal, D., Riemersma, R.A., Appel, L.J., & Guallar, E. (2005). Meta-Analysis: High dosage vitamin E supplementation may increase all cause mortality, *Annals of Internal Medicine 142*(1):37-46.

Morrison, N.A., George, P.M., Vaughan, T., Tilyard, M.W., Frampton, C.M., & Gilchrist, N.L. (2005). Vitamin D receptor genotypes influence the success of calcitriol therapy for recurrent vertebral fracture in osteoporosis. *Pharmacogenetics & Genomics, 15*(2), 127-135.

Mosby's drug consult (15th ed.). (2005). St. Louis: Mosby.

National Kidney Foundation-Kidney Disease Outcomes Quality Initiative (NKF-K/DOQI) Clinical Practice Guidelines for Anemia of Chronic Kidney Disease. (2001). *American Journal of Kidney Disease, 37*(1 Suppl 1), S182-S238.

Porthouse, J., Cockayne, S., King, C., Saxon, L., Steele, E., Aspray, T., et al. (2005). Randomised controlled trial of calcium and supplementation with cholecalciferol (vitamin D3) for prevention of fractures in primary care. *British Medical Journal, 330,* 1003-1005.

Sato, Y, Honda, Y., Iwamoto, J., Kanoko, Y., & Satoh, K. (2005). Effect of folate and mecobalamin on hip fractures in patients with stroke: A randomized controlled trial. *Journal of the American Medical Association, 293,* 1082-1088.

Schnyder, G., Roffi, M., Pin, R., Flammer, Y., Lange, H., Eberli, F.R., et al. (2001). Decreased rate of coronary restenosis after lowering of plasma homocysteine levels. *New England Journal of Medicine, 345*(22), 1593-1600.

Siega-Riz, A.M., Promislow, J.H., Savitz, D.A., Thorp, J.M. Jr., & McDonald, T. (2003). Vitamin C intake and the risk of preterm delivery. *American Journal of Obstetrics & Gynecology, 189*(2), 519-525.

Sillanpaa, P., Hirvonen, A., Kataja, V., Eskelinen, M., Kosma, V.M., & Uusitupa, M., et al. (2004). Vitamin D receptor gene polymorphism as an important modifier of positive family history related breast cancer risk. *Pharmacogenetics, 14*(4), 239-245.

Smith, I., Simpson, K.J., Garden, O.J., & Wigmore, S.J. (2005). Non-paracetamol drug-induced fulminant hepatic failure among adults in Scotland. *European Journal of Gastroenterology & Hepatology, 17*(2), 161-167.

Toole, J.F., Malinow, M.R., Chambless, L.E., Spence, J.D., Pettigrew, L.C., & Howard, V.J., et al. (2004). Lowering homocysteine in patients with ischemic stroke to prevent recurrent stroke, myocardial infarction, and death: the Vitamin Intervention for Stroke Prevention (VISP) randomized controlled trial *Journal of the American Medical Association, 291*(5), 565-575.

Trivedi, D.P., Doll, R., & Khaw, K.T. (2003). Effect of four monthly oral vitamin D3 (cholecalciferol) supplementation on fractures and mortality in men and women living in the community: randomised double blind controlled trial. *British Medical Journal, 326*(7387), 469.

Tucker, K.L., Olson, B., Bakun, P., Dallal, G.E., Selhub, J., & Rosenberg, I.H. (2004). Breakfast cereal fortified with folic acid, vitamin B6, and vitamin B12 increases vitamin concentrations and reduces homocysteine concentrations: a randomized trial, *American Journal of Clinical Nutrition, 79*(5), 805-811.

Ujjin, P., Satarug, S., Vanavanitkun, Y., Daigo, S., Ariyoshi, N., & Yamazaki, H., et al. (2002). Variation in coumarin 7-hydroxylase activity associated with genetic polymorphism of cytochrome P450 2 A6 and the body status of iron stores in adult Thai males and females. *Pharmacogenetics, 12*(3), 241-249.

United States Department of Health and Human Services, Agency for Healthcare Research and Quality. (2004). *Guide to clinical preventive services.* (3rd ed.). Retrieved July 28, 2005, from, http://www.ahrq.gov/clinic/gcpspu.htm.

United States Department of Health and Human Services, Department of Agriculture. (2005). Dietary guidelines for Americans 2005. Retrieved August 20, 2005, from http://www.healthierus.gov/dietaryguidelines.

USP DI: Drug information for the health care professional (25th ed.). (2005). Greenwood Village, CO: MICROMEDEX Thomson Healthcare.

Vivekananthan, D.P., Penn, M.S., Sapp, S.K., Hsu, A., & Topol, E.J. (2003). Use of antioxidant vitamins for the prevention of cardiovascular disease: Meta-analysis of randomised trials. *Lancet, 361,* 2017-2023.

Woo, K.S., Chook, P., Chan, L.L., Cheung, A.S., Fung, W.H., & Qiao, M., et al. (2002). Long-term improvement in homocysteine levels and arterial endothelial function after 1-year folic acid supplementation. *American Journal of Medicine, 112*(7), 535-539.

68

FLUIDS AND ELECTROLYTES

CHAPTER FOCUS

The concept of fluid and electrolyte balance cuts across the nursing care of all clients. It is essential that nurses have an understanding of the physiology involved. With this knowledge, nurses can accurately identify clients at risk for specific imbalances so that derangements can be detected early and corrective measures taken.

LEARNING OBJECTIVES

- Identify the various therapeutic reasons for the infusion of intravenous (IV) solutions.
- Describe the role of water in human physiology.
- Explain the process of water transport in the body.
- Describe the four categories of parenteral solutions, and give examples of particular solutions in each category.
- Identify abnormal states of fluid balance.
- Describe the symptoms of hypertonic dehydration by clinical grading.
- State the normal requirements, dietary sources, specific functions, and problems associated with an excess or deficiency of sodium, potassium, calcium, and magnesium.
- Implement the nursing management of clients receiving IV therapy.

▲ KEY TERMS

dehydration, p. 1231
extracellular fluid, p. 1231
intracellular fluid, p. 1231
milliequivalent (mEq), p. 1241
osmosis, p. 1232
overhydration, p. 1231

❋ **What is the role of intravenous fluid management in client care?**

The intravenous (IV) administration of parenteral fluids has become more prevalent during the past 75 years. Historically, some of the early solutions tended to be unsafe because of pyrogens. Once this issue was resolved, advances in the technology of IV therapy resulted in products that have significantly improved client safety (Box 68-1).

There has also been a vast increase in outpatient and home administration of IV medications, total parenteral nutrition (TPN), and fluids. Over the past 50 years, newer and more sophisticated delivery systems have been developed, and different methods of application are constantly

being conceived. IV solutions are infused for various therapeutic reasons, including the following:

- Replacing fluids and electrolytes
- Correcting acid-base imbalances
- Administering medications, blood products, and diagnostic aids
- Administering essential nutrients
- Maintaining ready access to the venous system if any of the first four measures is anticipated
- Measuring changes in venous pressure

Blood and its components are transfused intravenously to (1) replace blood volume or plasma fractions; (2) restore the blood's capabilities for carrying oxygen, clotting, or oncotic

---

BOX 68-1 INTRAVENOUS THERAPY: 1930S TO TODAY

EARLY 1930S

- IV injections are reserved only for seriously ill clients.
- Only a physician can perform venipuncture.

1940S

- Massachusetts General Hospital becomes one of the first hospitals to assign a nurse to IV therapy.
- The job description includes administering IV solutions and blood transfusions, cleaning the infusion sets for reuse, and cleaning and sharpening needles for reuse.
- The primary responsibility is of a technical nature: administering and maintaining the infusions and keeping the equipment clean and functional.

1950S

- Improvements and innovations in equipment (e.g., pumps and monitors), needles (e.g., Intracaths), and tubing; the development of plastic and disposable equipment; and an increased variety of commercially prepared IV fluids increase the safety of IV therapy.

1960S

- A variety of IV solutions are developed.
- In addition to IV fluids, the IV route is used to administer many medications and hyperalimentation fluids.

1970S

- The Centers for Disease Control and Prevention (CDC) develop standards for infection control related to IV therapy.

- Hickman-Broviac and Groshong tunneled catheters are developed for long-term access.
- IV nurse specialists, IV departments or teams in the hospital, standards for client care, and professional organizations to promote IV therapy as a specialty area in nursing are developed.

1980S

- The National Intravenous Therapy Association (NITA) publishes recommended practices for therapy.
- Implantable ports are developed for long-term access.

1990S

- The role of the nurse is to incorporate IV skills in all settings, including community.
- The role for IV therapy is extended to LPNs/LVNs.

2000S

- Home infusion is increasingly more common as lengths of hospital stay decline.
- Subtle refinements continue to be made in IV-related procedures and techniques using evidence gained from nursing research about site care, frequency of dressing and tubing changes, flushes, and prevention of complications.
- Use of pumps for IV infusion is widely recommended to prevent speed-related complications.

Data modified from Phillip, L.D. (1997). *Manual of IV therapeutics* (2nd ed.). Philadelphia: F.A. Davis.

---

pressure; or (3) cleanse the plasma of harmful constituents by exchanges (see Chapter 30). IV total parenteral nutrition solutions (formerly referred to as hyperalimentation) are infused to complement or supplement the dietary intake of clients in deprived nutritional states (see Chapter 69).

✹ What are the types of fluids and their locations in the body?

Depending on the amount of adipose tissue present, water accounts for 45% to 75% of the total body weight in humans. Infants and young children have more water per unit of body weight than adults, and female adults have less water content than male adults. The greatest amount of body water (up to 45% of body weight) is to be found in the intracellular fluid; the remainder of body water is located in the extracellular fluid. **Intracellular fluid** is the fluid inside the cells, in which the chemical reactions of all metabolisms essential to life occur. **Extracellular fluid** is the fluid surrounding the cells—plasma, interstitial fluid, and lymph—and extracellular portions of dense connective tissue, cartilage, and bone. The volume of fluid in the two body fluid compartments varies with age and differs in the genders.

Metabolic exchanges between the cells and tissues and the external environment occur in this fluid.

✹ How is hydration status maintained?

The importance of body water is highlighted by two facts: (1) it is the medium in which all metabolic reactions occur, and (2) the precise regulation of volume and composition of body fluid is essential to health. In healthy individuals, body water remains remarkably constant and is maintained by a balance between intake and excretion—the water gained each day is equal to the water lost. If the water gained exceeds the water lost, excess fluid volume (**overhydration**) and edema occur. If the water lost exceeds the water gained, deficient fluid volume (**dehydration**) occurs. If 20% to 25% of body water is lost, death usually occurs.

Water is an excellent solvent that permits many substances to be dispersed through it and permits the ionization of electrolytes. These electrolytes are important in maintaining physiologic processes and the volume and distribution of body fluid. These electrolytes include the cations sodium (Na^+), potassium (K^+) and magnesium (Mg^{++}), and the anions chloride (Cl^-) and bicarbonate (HCO_3^-) for phosphate

(PO_4^{--}). Calcium is also an important cation for many cellular functions and is found in lower concentrations throughout the body. Although each of these electrolytes is found through the body, the primary intracellular ions are potassium, magnesium, and phosphate, whereas sodium, chloride and bicarbonate are found in higher concentrations in the plasma and extracellular fluid (Table 68-1). Water is also an excellent lubricant between membranes, and it functions well as a heat insulator and heat exchanger. The daily intake of water in some form is essential to maintain water balance. Human beings can go several weeks without food but can survive only a few days without water. The average volume of water consumed daily is 120 to 150 mL/kg body weight in neonates and infants, 120 to 130 mL/kg in children, and 30 mL/kg in adults.

Thirst, the subjective desire to ingest water, helps to maintain water balance. Although thirst is complex and not well understood, it is induced by a decrease in saliva and dryness of the mouth and throat. The dehydration of thirst receptors may lead to their stimulation. The sensation of thirst is often reduced for older adults and thus puts them at greater risk for further dehydration.

Water intake occurs primarily by (1) drinking fluids, (2) ingesting food containing moisture (most foods contain a high percentage of water), and (3) absorbing water formed by the oxidation of hydrogen in the food during metabolic processes. This third process produces approximately 0.5 L of water per day.

Water is lost from the body in five principal ways, through: (1) the kidneys (urine), (2) the skin (insensible perspiration and sweat), (3) expired air (as water vapor), (4) feces, and (5) tears and saliva. Urine excretion accounts for 50% to 60% of the total daily water loss. Urine output, of course, varies with the amount of water ingested.

Water loss by the kidney varies with the solute (molecular ions or particles) load and the antidiuretic hormone (ADH or vasopressin) level. If an increase in solute load occurs, such as with diabetes mellitus or following the ingestion of excessive amounts of food (especially those that gen-erate solutes, such as sodium from salty foods), the kidney excretes sufficient urine to transport the solutes into the bladder. The reabsorption of water in the distal convoluted tubules is controlled by vasopressin (ADH). An increase in ADH levels leads to an increase in water reabsorption, which produces more concentrated urine. ADH is secreted by the posterior pituitary gland; this secretion is regulated by osmoreceptors located in the supraoptic nucleus. ADH acts on specific vasopressin receptors on the medullary tubular cell to stimulate the production of cyclic adenosine monophosphate (cAMP). cAMP activates an enzyme that alters the structure of protein in the cell membrane to increase the permeability of the tubular cell to water. This increases water resorption and urine osmolality.

How is water transported in the body?

Water travels from less concentrated areas to areas with higher concentrations of solutes or dissolved substances by **osmosis.** The solutes may be electrolytes (e.g., potassium chloride or sodium chloride), which yield potassium cations and chloride anions when dissolved in water or nonelectrolytes such as dextrose, urea, or creatinine. Each fluid compartment in the body—intracellular and extracellular compartments—has its own electrolyte composition (see Table 68-1). Disturbances in electrolyte composition can be reflected in clinical symptoms in the client.

Osmolality refers to the total solute concentration usually expressed per liter of serum. The number of solutes in solution determines the osmotic pressure. For example, if the extracellular fluid contains a large number of dissolved particles and the intracellular fluid has a small number of dissolved particles, then the osmotic pressure from the intracellular fluid forces water to pass from the less concentrated intracellular area to the more concentrated extracellular area. This process occurs until both concentrations are equal.

Deciding on the appropriate IV therapy for a client requires knowledge of the client's fluid status and electrolyte values. Accurate assessment of fluid status (e.g., dehydration, overhydration) will help the clinician determine the amount and type of fluid replacement that best meets the needs of the client. Evaluation of plasma sodium levels, the principal electrolyte in the extracellular fluid, is essential in initial evaluation. Potassium levels, serum osmolality, current disease state or illness, other laboratory values and the initial signs and symptoms are also important in assessment.

What solutions are available for parenteral administration?

Parenteral solutions must contain similar numbers of dissolved or dispersed particles so as not to produce excessive fluids across cell membranes. Sterile water for injection, for example, must not be administered in large volumes intravenously, because it contains no solutes and will contribute to RBC swelling and hemolysis. Solutions with very high amounts of dissolved or disperse components (e.g., dextrose 50% or parenteral nutrition solutions) are typically given

Electrolytes	Extracellular (mEq/L)		Intracellular (mEq/L)
	Plasma	Interstitial	
sodium (Na$^+$)	142	146	15
potassium (K$^+$)	4	5	150
calcium (Ca^{++})	5	3	2
magnesium (Mg^{++})	2	1	27
chloride (Cl$^-$)	103	114	1
bicarbonate (HCO$_3^-$)	27	30	10

TABLE 68-1 NORMAL DISTRIBUTION OF ELECTROLYTES IN THE BODY

Additionally, phosphates, sulfates, and other substances are located in the extracellular and intracellular fluids.

via central or large-bore peripheral lines to allow for rapid dissolution and reduced tissue irritation.

In general, parenteral solutions may be divided into four broad categories: *blood products* (e.g., blood, plasma, platelets); *colloids* like albumin; *combinations of carbohydrates, proteins, fats, nutrients and electrolytes* for nutritional supplementation, and *crystalloids* like saline and dextrose. Chapter 30 discusses blood products that are used primarily to replace cellular or chemical components (erythrocytes, platelets, clotting factors in fresh frozen plasma) in maintaining oxygen-carrying capacity or coagulation. Colloids are large molecular weight substances like albumin, dextran, or hetastarch that remain in the intravascular compartment drawing fluid into the vasculature by oncotic pressure, and maintain blood pressure. Albumin, although appearing to offer a theoretical advantage by preferentially increasing intravascular volume, is no more clinically effective than crystalloids in fluid resuscitation of critically ill clients (Finfer et al., 2004). Furthermore, albumin and blood products are in limited supply, and despite careful processing to reduce contamination, can pose some risk for transmission of blood-borne disease. Dextran and hetastarch are also associated with other potential adverse effects including inhibition of platelet function and potential for hypersensitivity. As such, the use of blood products and colloids are usually limited to serious or life-threatening conditions such as posttrauma or bleeding, or circumstances refractory to crystalloid therapy. Chapter 69 discusses nutritional solutions that are primarily used to provide IV support for clients who have limited or no enteral access.

Crystalloids are the most commonly administered solutions in acute care and are subdivided into four categories: (1) hydrating solutions, (2) isotonic solutions, (3) maintenance solutions, and (4) hypertonic solutions (Table 68-2).

Hydrating solutions include those that are preferentially drawn into the intracellular space with lower amounts remaining in the vascular or interstitial space (Table 68-3). Hydrating solutions include various concentrations of dextrose solutions and 0.45% sodium chloride. Hydrating solutions are used to hydrate or to prevent dehydration. They are often used to assess kidney status before specific electrolytes are ordered as replacement and maintenance therapy, and also to help increase diuresis in dehydrated clients. They are less effective for volume replacement when clients have low intravascular volumes (e.g., trauma, severe dehydration accompanied by hypotension) because little of the solution remains in the intravascular space.

Dextrose is a source of calories (1 L of 5% dextrose = approximately 170 calories) that is rapidly metabolized in the body. Dextrose 5% solution is considered isotonic. A 50% dextrose solution is available for the emergency management of hypoglycemia (e.g., excessive insulin or oral hypoglycemic dosage) (see Chapter 49). Dextrose 50% IV is also used in combination with insulin in the acute management of hyperkalemia, because this combination enhances the transfer of potassium into the cell. Dextrose is metabo-

TABLE 68-2 TYPES OF CRYSTALLOID SOLUTIONS FOR INTRAVENOUS ADMINISTRATION*

	Na⁺	K⁺	Mg⁺⁺	Ca⁺⁺	Cl⁻	Osmolarity
HYDRATING SOLUTIONS (MAY BE HYPOTONIC, ISOTONIC, OR HYPERTONIC)						
dextrose 2.5%, 5%, 10%						126, 252, 505
dextrose 2.5% in 0.45% NaCl injection†	56				56	280
dextrose 5% in 0.45% NaCl injection‡	77				77	405
ISOTONIC SOLUTIONS						
normal saline or sodium chloride injection (0.9% NaCl)	154				154	310
Ringer's injection	147	4		4	155	310
lactated Ringer's injection	130	4		3	109	275
MAINTENANCE SOLUTIONS (GENERALLY ISOTONIC)						
Plasmalyte 56	40	13	3		40	111
Plasmalyte 148 (or Normosol-R, Isolyte S)	140	5		3	98	295
HYPERTONIC SOLUTIONS						
sodium chloride, 3% injection	513				513	1025
sodium chloride, 5% injection	855				855	1710

*Normal plasma contains Na⁺ (135-147 mEq/L), K⁺ (3.5-5 mEq/L), Mg⁺⁺ (1.8-3.0 mg/dL), Ca⁺⁺ (8.8-10.3 mg/dL), Cl⁻ (95-105 mEq/L), HCO3⁻ (27 mEq/L); normal osmolarity is 280-300 mOsm/L. Normal values from Ferri, F.F. (2004). Practical guide to the medical patient (6th ed.). St. Louis: Mosby.
†Dextrose 2.5% = 25 g dextrose/L or 85 calories.
‡Dextrose 5% = 50 g dextrose/L or 170 calories.

TABLE 68-3 DISTRIBUTION OF VARIOUS INTRAVENOUS FLUIDS AFTER INTRAVENOUS ADMINISTRATION

Solution	Hypotonic	Isotonic	Hypertonic	Distribution After IV Administration Intravascular	Interstitial	Intracellular
CRYSTALLOIDS						
Dextrose 5% (D5W)		X[a]		0 to +	+	++ to +++
Dextrose 5%/0.45% Sodium Chloride (D5/.45)			X[a]	0 to +	++	+ to ++
Sodium Chloride 0.45% (Half Normal Saline [½ NS])	X			0 to +	++	+
Sodium Chloride 0.9% (Normal Saline [NS])		X		+ to ++	+++	0
Lactated Ringer's (LR)		X		+ to ++	+++	0
Sodium Chloride 3%			X[b]	0 to +	+++[c]	+[c]
COLLOIDS						
Albumin 5%		X		++++	0	0
Albumin 25%			X[b]	++++[c]	0	0
Dextran		X[d]	X[d]	++++	0	0
Hetastarch		X[d]	X[d]	++++	0	0

0, None; +, minimal; ++, moderate; +++, significant; ++++, extensive.

[a] Reflects isotonicity of this solution in the bottle. Once in the body, dextrose pulls water into the interstitial and intracellular spaces, is metabolized and may result in hypotonic or "free" water in the interstitial and intracellular spaces.

[b] Considerably hypertonic and may require administration via a central or large bore peripheral line.

[c] Typically draws additional fluid into this space.

[d] Degree of isotonicity depends on concentration and other ingredients in formulation.

lized internally, which leaves water that decreases the osmotic pressure of the plasma, easily transfers to body cells, and provides water immediately to dehydrated tissues.

Isotonic solutions are usually prescribed to replace extracellular fluid losses that occur from blood loss, severe vomiting episodes, or any situation in which the chloride loss is equal to or greater than the sodium loss. Isotonic or normal saline is also the preferred agent to be used before and after a blood transfusion as this avoids dextrose related hemolysis of red blood cells (RBCs).

Isotonic sodium chloride is also used to treat metabolic alkalosis, especially when it occurs in the presence of fluid loss. The increased administration of chloride ions helps to decrease the number of bicarbonate ions in the client. Other solutions that are considered isotonic include Ringer's injection and lactated Ringer's injection. A major difference between Ringer's injection and lactated Ringer's injection is the 28 mEq of lactate (a precursor of bicarbonate) in the lactated injection. Therefore lactated Ringer's is preferred for clients with metabolic acidosis perhaps caused by burns or infections. Ringer's injection has more chloride ions and is more useful in treating dehydration from reduced water intake, vomiting, or diarrhea or for clients with hypochloremia.

Maintenance solutions or multiple electrolyte solutions have been formulated to replace daily electrolyte and extracellular needs and water. Such solutions may also be indicated to replace electrolytes and water loss from severe vomiting or diarrhea. With these preparations, the extracellular replacement is usually achieved within 2 days (usually 1 to 3 L daily is administered) with close monitoring of electrolytes. If maintenance solutions are continued after the client's deficits have been corrected, the excess sodium may lead to circulatory overload, pulmonary edema, and heart failure. Examples of maintenance solutions include Plasma-lyte and Normosol. Many settings avoid these "fixed" dose combinations of fluids/electrolytes because adjustment of electrolytes is more difficult when client needs change. Instead, most acute care facilities use saline or saline and dextrose combinations with additions of potassium and/or other electrolytes tailored to client need.

Hypertonic solutions are sometimes used to treat hypotonic expansion (water intoxication) when increased body fluid volume is caused by water only. This can happen under several different circumstances: (1) hospitalized clients who receive large amounts of dextrose 5% in water or electrolyte-free solutions to replace fluid and electrolytes that

TABLE 68-4 DIFFERENCES AMONG THE THREE TYPES OF DEHYDRATION

	Hypotonic	Isotonic	Hypertonic
Cause	Loss of salt (NaCl)	Blood loss	Water loss or lack of sufficient fluid intake
Effect on ICF and ECF compartments	Volume ICF↑ Volume ECF↓	Decrease in ECF volume	Decrease in ICF and ECF volume
Significant signs:			
Rate of water elimination	Increased	Decreased	Decreased
Thirst			Early warning because of cell dehydration
Pulse rate	Increased, weak, thready	Regular	Regular in early stages
Behavioral signs	May see vomiting, abdominal cramps		Confusion, irritability, agitation
Late stages	Skin turgor poor Weak pulse, lethargy, confusion, death due to circulatory failure	Shock, weak Weak, thready pulse	Skin turgor poor Dry, furrowed tongue; death
Clinical laboratory results			
Hematocrit	Increased	Increased	Increased
Hemoglobin	Increased	Increased	Increased
Sodium levels	Decreased		Increased

ECF, Extracellular fluid; *ICF*, intracellular fluid.

have been lost from vomiting, diarrhea, diuresis, or gastric suction, or (2) more commonly in older adults during the postoperative period, when water is retained in response to stress (endocrine response to stress).

Overhydration should be considered when behavioral changes such as lethargy, confusion and, perhaps, disorientation occur postoperatively in an older adult. Central nervous system (CNS) signs and symptoms such as increased tiredness, muscle twitching, headaches, nausea, vomiting, and even seizures have been noted. Weight gain is always present, and the blood pressure may be normal or elevated.

In milder cases of overhydration, the treatment usually includes withholding all fluids until excess fluids are excreted. In severe cases of hyponatremia, small quantities of hypertonic sodium chloride are sometimes administered to (1) increase the osmotic pressure, (2) increase the water flow from body cells to the extracellular compartment, and (3) to enhance the excretion of fluids by the kidneys.

The typical hypertonic saline is a 3% or 5% solution that must be administered slowly via central or large-bore peripheral lines with close supervision to prevent pulmonary edema. Close monitoring of laboratory tests for electrolytes is also required.

✺ How are hydration status and fluid-electrolyte balance assessed and maintained?

A dynamic relationship exists in the body between water and sodium. Abnormal states of hydration can be classified as (1) dehydration (deficient fluid volume), (2) overhydration (excess fluid volume or hypervolemia), (3) loss of water in excess of sodium (hypernatremia), and (4) loss of sodium in excess of water (hyponatremia). Overhydration was reviewed in the preceding section under the description of hypertonic solutions. The other three abnormal states may be viewed as various types of dehydration.

Table 68-4 illustrates the differences between the three types of dehydration. Note that the causes of the three dehydration states are different, as are the effects on fluid compartments in the body and some of the initial signs and laboratory values, especially sodium concentration. This is important information because it aids the provider not only in diagnosing the initial condition but also in choosing the appropriate IV therapy.

Hypertonic dehydration caused by heat exhaustion and resulting from water depletion can occur on land or sea. Many boaters lost at sea or refugees fleeing their countries overseas for another country run out of water for days before being rescued or reaching land. Such persons require intensive care for their dehydration, and some may die from this deprivation (Table 68-5).

The nurse should be aware that older adults with decreased renal function are more vulnerable to dehydration and electrolyte imbalance. The additional physiologic changes experienced by older adults because of the aging process may also make them more susceptible to the adverse effects of fluid and electrolyte administration, such as overhydration or decreased renal excretion of exogenous potas-

TABLE 68-5 SYMPTOMS OF HYPERTONIC DEHYDRATION	
Clinical Grading	**Symptoms**
Mild or early	Increased thirst. Usually a 2% loss in body weight.
Moderate to severe	Very dry mouth, difficulty swallowing, scant urine output (highly concentrated urine), increased pulse rate and body temperature, poor skin turgor, an approximate 6% body weight loss.
Extreme or very severe	All previous symptoms plus impaired mental and physical capabilities, very high rectal temperature, respiratory difficulties (hyperventilation that may lead to tetany), cyanosis, severe oliguria or anuria, circulatory failure, loss of more than 7% in body weight. Coma and death usually occur when approximately 15% of body weight is lost.

sium or magnesium, with resultant toxic accumulation in the body.

✱ What are the major electrolytes?

The major electrolytes in the body are sodium, potassium, calcium, and magnesium. This section reviews the normal requirements, sources, and specific functions of these electrolytes, and the problems associated with their excess or deficiency.

Sodium

Sodium is the major electrolyte in the extracellular fluid. Sodium is necessary for the control of body water; for the electrophysiology of nerve, muscle, and gland cells; and for the regulation of pH and isotonicity. The normal range is from 136 to 145 mEq/L of plasma. Sodium content in the body is regulated by sodium consumption (dietary) and sodium excretion by the kidneys. In the average person with normal renal function, sodium excretion closely matches sodium intake. This helps to keep sodium content in the body at a constant level, even if sodium intake is somewhat varied. Major dietary sources of sodium are table salt (sodium chloride) and many processed foods (including tomato juice, canned soups and vegetables, cured or processed meats, many cheeses, pickles, olives, and savory snacks like potato chips and popcorn). Healthy 19- to 50-year-old adults require 1.5 grams of sodium and 2.3 grams of chloride each day—or 3.8 grams of salt—to replace the amount lost daily on average through perspiration. This is easily exceeded with the typical North American diet. Elevated blood pressure, which may lead to stroke, coronary

heart disease, and kidney disease, is associated with elevated sodium intake. On average, blood pressure rises progressively as salt intake increases. A tolerable upper intake level (UL)—a maximum amount that people should not exceed—is set at 5.8 grams of salt (2.3 grams of sodium) per day. Older individuals, African Americans, and people with chronic diseases including hypertension, diabetes, and kidney disease are especially sensitive to the blood pressure-raising effects of salt and should consume less than the UL. More than 95% of American men and 90% of Canadian men ages 31 to 50, and 75% of American women and 50% of Canadian women in this age range regularly consume salt in excess of the UL (National Academies News, 2004).

Hyponatremia Hyponatremia may be detected when serum levels fall below 135 mEq/L. This condition may be induced by excessive sweating when only the water is replaced, by the infusion of large quantities of nonelectrolyte parenteral fluids, by syndrome of inappropriate antidiuretic hormone (SIADH), and by adrenal insufficiency or gastrointestinal (GI) suctioning with replacement fluids limited to water by mouth.

Symptoms include lethargy, hypotension, stomach cramps, vomiting, diarrhea and, possibly, seizures. Deficiency states are usually treated with Ringer's solution or normal saline injection.

Hypernatremia Hypernatremia is seen when serum sodium levels are higher than normal (usually greater than 150 mEq/L). This excess may be induced by the excessive use of saline infusions, inadequate water consumption (as described previously), diabetes insipidus, or excess fluid loss without a corresponding loss of sodium.

The signs and symptoms of hypernatremia include edema; hypertonicity; red, flushed skin; dry and sticky mucous membranes; increased thirst; elevated temperature; and a decrease in or absence of urination. Treatment includes reducing salt intake and using dextrose in water IV to promote diuresis and increase the excretion of both salt and water from the blood.

Potassium

Potassium is the major electrolyte in the intracellular fluids. The amount of potassium in the intracellular fluid is approximately 150 mEq/L, whereas the amount in the plasma is between 3.5 and 5 mEq/L. Even though this plasma amount appears to be low, it is of great importance—serum potassium must be maintained between 3.5 and 5 mEq/L for survival. The diet of most individuals contains from 35 to 100 mEq of potassium daily, with any excess potassium normally excreted by the kidney in the urine. Potassium plays an important part role in (1) skeletal, smooth and cardiac muscle contraction, (2) conduction of nerve impulses, (3) enzyme action, and (4) cell membrane function.

Hypokalemia Hypokalemia, or a potassium deficit, may be caused by the chronic administration of IV solutions containing little or no potassium; diuretic therapy with potassium-depleting medications; reduced dietary intake (e.g., in persons on "starvation diets"); poor absorption because of steatorrhea, regional enteritis, or short bowel syndrome; loss of GI secretions (which are very rich in potassium) due to vomiting, diarrhea, GI suction, or fistula drainage; extensive burn conditions; or the presence of excessive amounts of adrenocorticotropic hormone (ACTH).

Unlike sodium, which is reabsorbed when the serum sodium level is low, potassium ions continue to be excreted in the urine even when the serum potassium level is low. As potassium loss continues, the individual's condition deteriorates unless potassium intake is increased and normal levels are reestablished.

With hypokalemia, impaired skeletal muscle function may cause profound weakness or paralysis, including paralysis of the respiratory muscles. Impaired smooth muscle function may result in ileus. The cardiac effects of hypokalemia include an increased sensitivity to digoxin with potential toxicity and electrocardiogram (ECG) changes. Early potassium deficiency may be detected by the use of the ECG, because the T wave tends to flatten when serum potassium levels are below 3.5 mEq/L and tends to elongate vertically (become "tall and tented") when the serum potassium level is 5.8 mEq/L or higher. Atrioventricular block and cardiac arrest may occur. The renal manifestations of hypokalemia include polyuria, polydipsia, and impaired ability to concentrate urine or excrete an acid load.

Hypokalemia also causes the movement of Na^+ and H^+ from the extracellular fluid and the excretion of H^+, which may elevate plasma pH and result in metabolic alkalosis. In response to a low serum potassium level, potassium moves out of the cell in exchange for H^+, causing an extracellular alkalosis and an intracellular acidosis. In response to the drop in intracellular pH, renal tubular cells excrete H^+, leading to paradoxical aciduria and exacerbating the extracellular alkalosis (Marx, Hockberger, & Walls, 2002).

Other effects include increased risk of electrolyte abnormalities, elevated serum enzymes, and other systemic effects.

Treat hypokalemia by replacing potassium orally or parenterally. Be aware, however, that one hazard of parenteral correction is potassium poisoning, or hyperkalemia which can cause fatal cardiac dysrhythmias (see the Medication Safety Alert box above).

Parenteral or IV Supplementation The dosage of potassium supplements depends on the individual requirement and requires close supervision. IV potassium must always be diluted and administered slowly, see Safety Box, this page. *Undiluted or rapid administration of potassium is fatal.* In general, potassium is given only to clients with a documented adequate urine flow. In dehydrated clients, it is best to administer a potassium-free fluid first to hydrate the client and determine urinary output.

It is recommended that for adults parenteral fluids not contain more than 40 mEq/L of potassium, and the rate of administration should not be more than 20 mEq/hour.

⁂ Medication Safety Alert

Intravenous Potassium Administration

Every dose of IV potassium must be diluted in a larger volume of suitable IV solution and given as an infusion at a controlled rate. Potassium is readily soluble in commonly used IV solutions. Forty mEq/liter or less is the preferred dilution, although agency policy may allow a maximal concentration of 60 mEq/L when there is a specific need for greater replacement therapy and the IV catheter gauge is suitably large. When large doses are required, continuous cardiac monitoring is recommended, particularly at rates greater than 10 mEq/hr in adults or comparable rates in children. Even in critical care settings, rates greater than 20 mEq/hr in adults are avoided. Intravenous solutions containing potassium should be administered using an infusion pump to reduce the risk of medication overdosage, cardiac arrest, or extravasation leading to necrosis as a result of IV infiltration. In all clients, assess the line for patency when beginning a potassium infusion and at least hourly thereafter.

Direct injection of any concentrated solution of potassium can be instantly fatal. Gently agitate the prepared IV solutions to prevent concentration of potassium in any part of the container. Never add potassium to an IV container in the hanging position; remove from the hanger to disperse potassium throughout the solution.

Have the client report burning at the IV site promptly. Monitor IV flow and the site; monitor client's serum potassium, ECGs, adequate hydration, adequacy of urinary output and health status (bradycardia, confusion, weakness, nausea and vomiting, and respiratory distress indicate hyperkalemia). Progression of symptoms may cause death.

Data from Gahart, B.L., & Nazareno, A.R. (2005). *Intravenous Medications.* (21st ed.) St. Louis: Mosby.

However, for adults with life-threatening hypokalemia-induced dysrhythmias or those with a serum potassium level less than 2 mEq/L, a more concentrated potassium solution (60 mEq/L can be infused at a rate not exceeding 40 mEq/hour) accompanied by continuous cardiac monitoring in a critical care setting (Lau, 2005). Potassium infusions must always be administered via a controller or pump to prevent rapid infusion. The potassium concentration should be monitored every 4 hours, more frequently in clients with severe potassium depletion or when a rapid infusion is given. Many facilities have internal policies that require cardiac monitoring when rates of administration exceed 10 mEq/hour. Whenever possible, the oral preparations or the consumption of foods high in potassium should replace the IV potassium solutions (see Chapter 33).

Parenteral potassium salts are available as acetate, chloride, and phosphate salts. In general, potassium chloride is the preferred preparation, because the chloride helps to correct the hypochloremia often seen with hypokalemia. In general, the alkalinizing potassium salts (acetate, bicarbonate, citrate, or gluconate) may be necessary to treat the hypokalemia associated with metabolic acidosis (a rare situation).

Oral Supplementation The potassium salts available for oral administration include acetate, bicarbonate, chloride, citrate, and gluconate, either alone or in combination. Liquid preparations are generally preferred for oral therapy, and most contain 10, 20, or 40 mEq of potassium/15 mL. These preparations must be diluted with fruit juice or water before ingestion and taken after meals with a full glass of water to minimize GI irritation. For powder preparations, follow the manufacturer's instructions closely. Liquids, effervescent forms, powders, and extended-release dosage forms (wax matrix, microencapsulated) are the currently available preparations. GI ulceration has been reported with the extended-release products, although much less often than with the other products; therefore these preparations should be reserved for clients who cannot or will not take the liquid or effervescent potassium.

Extended-release potassium should be discontinued immediately and the prescriber contacted if the client complains of stomach pain, swelling, or severe vomiting, or if GI bleeding is noted. Potassium supplements are contraindicated with severe renal impairment, untreated chronic adrenocortical insufficiency (Addison's disease), hyperkalemia, and severe burn conditions or acute dehydration. They should also be avoided or used with extreme caution in clients who are taking potassium-sparing diuretics or angiotensin-converting enzyme (ACE) inhibitors. Solid dosage forms of potassium should not be administered to clients with esophageal compression caused by an enlarged left atrium or other anatomic variation that results in increased compression in this area. In such cases, the ingestion of potassium-rich foods may also be helpful (see Table 33-2).

K-Dur 20 and Micro-K (both controlled release), and Klor-Con (potassium chloride powder) are among the more commonly prescribed oral potassium supplements. The dosage of potassium supplements depends on individual requirements. The daily allowance for adults varies based on condition and concurrent drugs but is often considered 40 to 50 mEq; for infants, approximately 1 to 3 mEq/kg body weight daily.

Hyperkalemia Hyperkalemia, or potassium excess, can be caused by acute or chronic renal failure; the release of large amounts of intracellular potassium in burns, crush injuries, or severe infections; overtreatment with potassium salts; or metabolic acidosis, including diabetic ketoacidosis, which causes a shift of potassium from the cells into the extracellular fluids.

Hyperkalemia interferes with neuromuscular function and may result in abdominal distention, diarrhea, weakness, and paralysis. The cardiac effects caused by hyperkalemia result from impaired conduction. The ECG shows a widening and slurring of the QRS complexes, peaked T waves, depressed ST segments and, possibly, a disappearance of P waves. Ventricular fibrillation and cardiac arrest may occur.

The treatment of hyperkalemia depends on the serum level of potassium and on the ECG patterns. Mild hyperkalemia usually involves serum levels below 6.5 mEq/L, with ECG changes limited to peaking of the T waves. Moderate hyperkalemia involves potassium serum levels between 6.5 and 8 mEq/L, and severe hyperkalemia involves serum levels above 8 mEq/L with an ECG pattern of absent P waves, widened QRS complexes, or ventricular dysrhythmias. Management and treatment of hyperkalemia involves careful monitoring, and the use of a number of agents, including dextrose, insulin, calcium salts, and sodium polystyrene sulfonate. See the Management of Drug Overdose box on p. 1239 for more details. A brief discussion of sodium polystyrene sulfonate is presented below.

sodium polystyrene sulfonate [**sow** de um pol ee **stye** reen **sul** fon ate]
(Kayexalate, Kionex, SPS)

Sodium polystyrene sulfonate is an orally or rectally administered cation exchange resin which exchanges sodium ions for potassium ions in the gut. After binding potassium, it is expelled in the feces.

Indications
Sodium polystyrene sulfonate is used as an adjunct to the acute management of cardiovascular complications of hyperkalemia, but does not replace acute measures to preserve cardiac function.

Pharmacokinetics/Dosing
Sodium polystyrene sulfonate is not absorbed after oral or rectal administration. Observable declines in serum potassium levels may be observed in as soon as 2 hours, but are more commonly observed within the first 24 hours of dosing. Laxatives such as sorbitol are routinely used concurrently but may increase the risk for colon necrosis (see Adverse Effects below). The adult dose of sodium polystyrene sulfonate is 15 grams one to four times daily in water or 25% sorbitol. The pediatric dose is 1 gm/kg/dose one to four times daily, with doses not to exceed the adult dose. Chilling the solution improves client palatability. Although less effective, it can also be given as a rectal retention enema in doses of 30 to 50 grams every 1 to 2 hours until hypokalemia is corrected, then every 6 hours. Each dose is followed by normal saline irrigation to prevent localized necrosis. Treatment with sodium polystyrene sulfonate is usually discontinued when serum potassium levels return to the normal range.

Adverse Effects
The most serious adverse effect of sodium polystyrene sulfonate is colonic necrosis. This appears more probable with the concurrent use of sorbitol in critically ill clients or those with renal insufficiency (Rogers & Li, 2001), although other clients may also be at risk. Other adverse effects include anorexia, nausea, vomiting, constipation, hypokalemia, and hypocalcemia. Fecal impaction has also been reported.

Calcium

Calcium (Ca^{++}) is essential for the growth and ossification of bones, neuromuscular transmission, cell membrane permeability, maintenance of excitability in nerve fibers, hormone secretion and action, muscle contraction, maintenance of cardiac and vascular tone, many enzyme activities, and the normal coagulation of blood. Chapter 47 discusses more fully the regulation of calcium levels by the parathyroid.

Almost all of the 1000 to 1200 grams of calcium in the normal adult is found in the skeletal tissue; only about 1% of the total body calcium is in solution in body fluids. Approximately half the calcium in plasma is bound to complex organic anions (e.g., bicarbonate and phosphate) or plasma proteins (albumin). Nearly all unbound serum calcium is ionized. The normal serum concentration of calcium is 4.5 to 5.5 mEq/L or 9 to 11 mg/100 mL.

The recommended dietary allowance of calcium for adults is 0.8 to 1.2 g daily. Pregnant or lactating women need 1.2 g; children 1 to 3 years of age, 0.4 to 0.8 g; and children 4 to 10 years of age, 0.8 g. Although many individuals have sufficient calcium from dietary sources, calcium supplementation to prevent bone loss seems reasonable for women. There is modest epidemiologic evidence for an inverse relationship between dietary calcium intake and colorectal adenoma and cancer risk (Gatof & Ahnen, 2003).

The absorption of calcium depends on how well it is kept in solution in the digestive tract; an acid medium favors calcium solubility and absorption in the upper intestinal tract. Absorption is decreased by the presence of alkalis and large amounts of fatty acids. Adequate intake of vitamin D appears to promote calcium absorption. Calcium is excreted in the urine and feces and in perspiration. Estrogen deficiency promotes calcium loss.

The maintenance of normal concentrations of serum calcium depends on the interactions of three agents: parathyroid hormone, vitamin D, and calcitonin. Parathyroid hormone and vitamin D mobilize the removal of calcium from bone—the principal source of calcium for extracellular fluids. Parathyroid hormone also promotes renal tubular reabsorption of calcium and a slight increase in intestinal absorption of calcium. Calcitonin synthesized in the thyroid gland moderates, or decreases, the rate of removal of calcium from the bone.

Hypocalcemia Hypocalcemia, or a decrease in serum calcium, results from: (1) hypoparathyroidism, (2) chronic renal insufficiency, (3) hypoalbuminemia, (4) malabsorption syndrome, and (5) a deficiency of vitamin D. Hypoparathyroidism may follow a thyroidectomy, because several parathyroid glands are often removed with this surgery. If the function of the remaining gland(s) is impaired, the result is depressed parathyroid activity.

Clients who are bedridden tend to develop a negative calcium balance—the ion is lost from the bones and excreted. This effect is likely to be serious when the client needs to be immobilized for long periods.

Hypocalcemia increases the excitability of the nerves and neuromuscular junction; this leads to muscle cramps, muscle twitching, and tetany. Numbness and tingling of the fingers, toes, and lips occurs. Hypertonicity of muscle may cause tonic contractions of the hands and feet (carpopedal spasm), whereas increased neural excitability may cause

---

Management of Drug Overdose

Potassium

Clients with underlying renal dysfunction, those receiving potassium sparing diuretics, angiotensin converting enzyme (ACE) inhibitors or angiotensin 2 receptor blockers (ARBs), and those who are receiving supplemental potassium are at the highest risk for developing hyperkalemia. Immediate recognition and management is critical.

Signs and Symptoms

Neuromuscular
- Muscle cramps
- Weakness
- Paralysis
- Paresthesias
- Focal neurologic deficits

Cardiovascular
- Peaked T waves leading to progressive ECG changes (e.g., loss of P waves and widening and slurring of QRS complex)
- Dysrhythmias (e.g., second- and third-degree heart block, wide complex tachycardia, ventricular fibrillation, asystole)

Treatment

Treatment of all cases of hyperkalemia includes:
- Obtaining immediate medical attention.
- Remove or treat the cause, including discontinuing potassium supplements or drugs contributing to elevated potassium levels (e.g., ACE inhibitors).
- Treat underlying metabolic acidosis if present.
- Monitor cardiac function with ECG, especially if hyperkalemia is moderate or severe.

For moderate to severe hyperkalemia:
- Treatment with dextrose 50% and IV insulin may be used to shift potassium into the cells.
- Addition of parenteral sodium bicarbonate may be used to correct acidosis and also help shift potassium into cells
- Calcium gluconate may be administered to counteract the effects of elevated potassium on neuromuscular membranes, although this is only a temporary measure.

To reduce serum potassium levels, one or more of the following interventions may be considered:
- Dialysis, including hemodialysis, can serve to correct elevated potassium levels, particularly in clients with underlying renal insufficiency.
- Administer sodium polystyrene sulfonate (Kayexalate) resin orally or rectally.
- Occasionally, the use of loop diuretics with fluid administration may serve to reduce serum potassium levels.

TABLE 68-6 CALCIUM CONTENT OF VARIOUS CALCIUM SALTS

	Percentage of Salt or Elemental Calcium	Amount of Elemental Calcium per Tablet	Number of Tablets Needed to Provide 1000 mg of Calcium
calcium carbonate	40	260 mg/650 mg	4
calcium gluconate	9	45 mg/500 mg	22
calcium lactate	13	42 mg/325 mg	24
calcium phosphate tribasic	39	608 mg/1600 mg	2

Data from Medline Plus. (2005). Calcium supplements (systemic). Retrieved August 22, 2005, from http://www.nlm.nih.gov/medlineplus/druginfo/uspdi/202108.html.

seizures, abnormal behavior, and personality changes. Prolonged hypocalcemia in children has resulted in mental retardation. The ECG shows a prolonged QT interval and an inverted T wave. In prolonged hypocalcemia, defects can occur in the nails, skin, and teeth; cataracts may appear; and calcification of the basal ganglia may occur.

Regardless of the underlying cause, severe hypocalcemia is treated initially with the IV administration of rapidly available calcium ions. An oral calcium salt is administered for latent tetany, mild symptoms of hypocalcemia, and maintenance therapy. Vitamin D may also be prescribed. An overdose of calcium may cause hypercalcemia, which results in anorexia, nausea, vomiting, weakness, depression, polyuria, and polydipsia.

Calcium must be administered cautiously to clients undergoing digoxin therapy, because calcium potentiates the effect of digoxin and may precipitate dysrhythmias. ECG monitoring of the client is recommended when parenteral calcium is administered.

Calcium salts are used as a nutritional supplement, particularly during pregnancy and lactation. They are specific in the treatment of hypocalcemic tetany. They have also been used for their antispasmodic effects in cases of abdominal pain, tenesmus, and colic resulting from disease of the gallbladder or painful contractions of the ureters. The basic salts of calcium are also used as antacids. Approximately 1 to 1.5 g calcium daily has been recommended to prevent postmenopausal bone loss or osteoporosis (Sayegh & Stubblefield, 2002).

The most widely used calcium salt is calcium carbonate, which requires an acid medium to form soluble calcium salts because it is nearly insoluble in water. The absorption or dissolution of calcium phosphate and calcium sulfate is also pH dependent, whereas calcium lactate, calcium citrate, and calcium gluconate are considered pH independent. Impaired stomach acid production is common in older adults and postmenopausal women; the high stomach pH or achlorhydric state results in a decreased solubility of pH-dependent calcium salts.

Because the different calcium salts contain different amounts of calcium, many professionals choose the calcium salt with the highest percentage of calcium per gram; in this

TABLE 68-7 FOODS WITH HIGH CALCIUM CONTENT

Food	Calcium Content
Yogurt, low fat (1 cup)	275-400 mg
Skim milk (1 cup)	300 mg
Cheese, Swiss (1 ounce)	272 mg
Cheese, cottage (1 cup)	215 mg
Cheese, cheddar (1 ounce)	200 mg
Broccoli, raw (1 cup)	100 mg
Ice cream (½ cup)	100 mg
Ice milk (¾ cup)	132 mg

way, a smaller quantity of drug may be administered. For example, if the recommended daily dose of calcium is 1000 mg daily, it would be necessary to administer nearly 10 g of calcium gluconate to reach this amount, whereas only 2.5 g of calcium carbonate per day would be required. This would require the consumption of smaller quantities of tablets to obtain the same amount of calcium, assuming of course that the calcium is soluble under the conditions present in the client (Table 68-6).

To improve the solubility of calcium carbonate tablets, especially in achlorhydric conditions, it is recommended the tablets be taken with meals, when acid secretion is highest. Avoid taking the tablets on an empty stomach or at night, because acid secretions are minimal at these times. Calcium phosphates and tricalcium phosphate have little usefulness in possible achlorhydric states and, perhaps, even in individuals with normal production of stomach acid. Both products have a very poor dissolution rate or pattern, thus reducing the possibility of calcium absorption. Soluble calcium salts (lactate or citrate) might be the appropriate form to use in clients with known achlorhydric states, even though it is necessary to use more tablets to provide sufficient quantities of calcium. Selected food consumption is another source for calcium (Table 68-7).

Hypercalcemia Neoplasms with or without bone metastases may cause hypercalcemia, or elevated serum calcium levels (Deftos, 2002). Carcinoma of the ovary, kidney, or lung can synthesize and secrete a parathyroid-like hormone, causing hypercalcemia. Other common causes are hyperparathyroidism, thiazide diuretic therapy, multiple myeloma, sarcoidosis, and vitamin D intoxication.

The clinical manifestations of hypercalcemia are highly variable and involve many organ systems, because calcium may be deposited in various body tissues. Symptoms may include the following:

- GI: anorexia, nausea, vomiting, constipation, and abdominal pain.
- Neurologic: weakness, apathy, depression, amnesia, confusion, stupor, and coma may occur.
- Renal: polyuria and nephrocalcinosis may occur, seriously impairing renal function; this may lead to edema, uremia, and hypertension, which may be irreversible.
- Cardiovascular: increased cardiac contractility, ventricular extrasystoles, and heart block. ECG changes include a short QT segment and characteristic signs of heart block.

Treatment is variable and aimed at controlling the underlying disease. For dehydrated clients, restore extracellular fluid volume with normal saline infusions; this also increases calcium excretion. Furosemide may be prescribed to enhance diuresis, but thiazide diuretics should be avoided because they block or lower calcium excretion. Chelating (binding) agents, such as disodium edetate, have been used to treat acute hypercalcemia in selected individuals. It increases the renal excretion of calcium by forming soluble complexes with the calcium that is not reabsorbed by the renal tubules. Chapter 47 discusses calcitonin and the bisphosphonates (including etidronate and pamidronate), which are important in the treatment of hypercalcemia.

Magnesium

Magnesium (Mg^{++}) is an important ion for the function of many enzyme systems. Magnesium salts are widely used therapeutically, including their use as antacids/laxatives and topical soaks, and their use in the treatment of ventricular dysrhythmias, preeclampsia, seizures, and magnesium deficiencies.

Hypomagnesemia Hypomagnesemia, a deficit of magnesium, may be encountered in chronic alcoholism, severe malabsorption, starvation, diarrhea, prolonged GI suction, vigorous diuresis, acute pancreatitis, and primary aldosteronism. Drug-induced hypomagnesemia may also be noted with a number of agents, including loop diuretics, cisplatin, aminoglycosides, digoxin, and amphotericin B therapy (Moe, 2005). Magnesium, the second most abundant intracellular cation, plays an important role in regulating the function of the sodium-potassium adenosine triphosphatase (ATPase) pump, neuromuscular transmission, cardiovascular function, and mitochondrial and other cellular functions in the body.

A magnesium deficiency may result in additional electrolyte problems (hypokalemia, hypocalcemia), cardiac dysrhythmias, and neurotoxicity. It may also cause an increase in neuromuscular irritability and contractility, coarse tremors, muscle spasm, delirium, athetoid movements, nystagmus, and tetany. It also causes tachycardia, hypertension, and vasomotor changes and increases the risk of digoxin toxicity in clients who are taking cardiac glycosides.

Hypomagnesemia may be treated with IV fluids containing magnesium (10 to 40 mEq daily for a severe deficit) followed by 10 mEq daily for maintenance. The use of IV fluids containing from 3 to 5 mEq magnesium/L may avert a magnesium deficiency that arises from the prolonged administration of IV solutions that do not contain magnesium.

Hypermagnesemia Hypermagnesemia occurs primarily in clients with chronic renal insufficiency. Administration of magnesium containing laxatives or antacids for clients with renal failure contributes to elevated magnesium levels. The adverse effects of hypermagnesemia include lethargy, nausea, confusion, hypoventilation, hypotension, dysrhythmias, muscle weakness and decreased deep tendon reflexes and other depression of cardiac, CNS, and respiratory functions. Decreased muscle cell excitability is caused by blockade of the myoneural junction (inhibition of acetylcholine release). Cardiac depression effects result in an increase in conduction time, with the ECG showing a lengthened PR segment and a prolonged QRS complex. If the Mg^{++} concentration continues to increase, third-degree atrioventricular block and cardiac arrest may occur.

An excess of Mg^{++} may require dialysis. Because calcium acts as an antagonist to Mg^{++}, calcium salts may be given parenterally. Normal serum concentration is 1.5 to 2.5 mEq/L, with one third bound to protein and two thirds free. A toxic blood level involves a magnesium level greater than 4 mEq/L. Magnesium has physiologic effects on the nervous system that are similar to those of calcium. See Chapter 17 for the drug monograph of magnesium as an anticonvulsant.

✱ How are electrolytes monitored?

Laboratory tests are used to monitor the client's electrolyte levels and to help determine replacement therapies when necessary for electrolyte deficiency. Table 68-1 lists the normal plasma values. Health care professionals should be aware of the difference between milligrams (mg), which reflects weight, and milliequivalents (mEq), which measures the number of chemically active ions in solution. A **milliequivalent (mEq)** is the number of grams of solute or electrolyte that is dissolved in 1 mL of a normal solution. It is a more precise measure of the relative potency of an electrolyte solution and is the method the prescriber uses to order electrolytes.

✱ What other salts are administered intravenously?

In addition to the previously discussed salt preparations, ammonium chloride injection and sodium lactate injection are also available for use.

Ammonium chloride injection is indicated to treat hypochloremia and metabolic alkalosis (not associated with severe liver disease) to prevent tetany or renal damage. Most cases respond to sodium chloride solution, but ammonium chloride is available for the rare, nonresponsive situation. Ammonium chloride has been used as a urinary acidifier to promote the excretion of alkaline substances. This product is available in 20-mL vials (100 mEq). The dose selected depends on the client—usually 1 to 2 vials, which is added to normal saline and infused slowly.

Sodium lactate injection available as a one sixth molar solution contains 167 mEq/L each of sodium and lactate ions. It is used to treat metabolic acidosis when no evidence of an elevated level of lactic acid exists. Sodium lactate is converted to sodium bicarbonate in the liver. Sodium bicarbonate is preferred for clients with lactic acidosis or impaired liver function.

✳ **C.S., a 21-year-old college student, presents to University Health Services with complaints of anorexia, nausea, vomiting, diarrhea, and generalized weakness for the past 3 days. She denies other medical problems and states she has not used any drugs. Her mucous membranes are dry, but her skin turgor is normal. Her sitting BP is 104/70 mm Hg with a pulse of 80. Her standing BP is 84/58 mm Hg, and she states she feels dizzy when she stands. Her serum electrolytes are within the normal limits. It is decided that C.S.'s signs and symptoms are consistent with volume depletion. Because she is neither hyponatremic nor hypernatremic, normal saline is administered IV to replenish the extracellular volume and improve tissue perfusion while the etiology of her symptoms is determined.**

✳ **What are the nursing management issues involved with intravenous therapies for C.S.?**
IV fluid and dextrose or electrolyte replacement by infusion continues to be the most common application of intravascular therapy. Although the dosage and choice of solution is tailored to C.S.'s needs by the prescriber according to the disorder and body surface area, monitoring the therapy is the nurse's responsibility. With the increasing prevalence of clients receiving some type of intravascular therapy in hospitals, and in home settings, the role of the nurse in IV therapy has also grown and developed. See the Community and Home Health Considerations box above for additional information on IV therapy in the home.

Consider intravascular therapy as a closed-system sterile procedure. Because it is invasive, and its effects are relatively irreversible, intravascular therapy is important to take care to perform and maintain it precisely.

Assessment Assessment begins with an understanding of the purpose of C.S.'s IV therapy and the potential risks to her. Clients who are debilitated, have a renal or cardiovascular problem, are prone to infection, or have very sclerotic veins are particularly at risk for complications related to IV therapy.

Factors to be considered for site selection include the following: suitable location, purpose of infusion, expected du-

✤ Community and Home Health Considerations

Home IV Therapy Clients

The provision of IV therapy to clients in their homes is growing in practice. It allows the client to remain in a home setting, be more comfortable, and to perform many daily activities. There may also be cost benefits for clients and health care agencies.

Clients should be carefully selected to receive home IV therapy. Instruction should begin in the hospital and be completed before the client is discharged. If the nurse is to provide the IV therapy on a home visit, all of the nursing processes applicable to institutional care will be adapted for the home setting. If the IV therapy is to be self-administered or administered by a caregiver in the home, it should be determined that the client/caregiver is willing and capable of administering the therapy safely. This capability includes the economics and transportation to obtain supplies; fine movement coordination to manipulate the equipment; understanding of asepsis, rationale for therapy, the interventions, potential complications and whom to contact in case of emergency. The home environment must also have some basic features (running water, electricity, refrigerator space for drug and supplies storage [if needed], a clean area in which aseptic catheter and simple wound care can be performed and access to a telephone to contact the home infusion team). Instruct the client in any activity limitations; how to check the venipuncture site for any complications; what to do if redness, swelling, or pain occurs, if the dressing becomes soiled, if blood appears in the tubing, or if the alarm on the electronic infusion device goes off. If the client is using a heparin lock, teach the client how and when to flush it. Have the client document a daily check of the venipuncture site. Have the client/caregiver return demonstrations. Develop a number of "what if . . ." scenarios to test the client's understanding and decision-making skills before an urgent situation occurs. Encourage the client/caregiver to contact the health care provider for assistance if required.

ration of therapy, condition of veins, restrictions imposed by the client's current health status and past health history, and the dominant extremity. C.S. is left-handed, so the IV site is placed on the right. Unless contraindicated, it is most appropriate to use veins in the nondominant upper extremity. When more than one puncture is anticipated, it is better to make the first venipuncture distally and work proximally. Avoid venipuncture in the affected arm of clients who have undergone axillary dissection (as in radical mastectomy) or have impaired mobility of the upper extremity (as in unilateral paralysis secondary to a cerebrovascular accident). In both instances circulation may not be adequate and affects the flow of the infusion, causing increased edema.

Nursing Diagnosis With an IV infusion C.S. is at risk for the following nursing diagnoses: impaired tissue integrity related to infiltration, thrombosis, thrombophlebitis, and necrosis; pain at the administration site; and the potential complications of pulmonary edema, pyrogenic reaction, speed shock, and sepsis. Because of their smaller body size, infants and children are especially at risk for overhydration.

Planning During fluid and electrolyte therapy, C.S. will experience serum electrolyte determinations returning to or remaining within the normal limits; she will not experience any adverse effects of IV therapy.

Implementation

Monitoring Continued reassessments of laboratory data reports are essential for clients who are receiving electrolyte replacement therapy. Serum electrolytes should not exceed the following accepted ranges during IV therapy:

Sodium	135 to 145 mEq/L
Chloride	95 to 108 mEq/L
Potassium	3.5 to 5 mEq/L
Calcium	4.5 to 5.8 mEq/L
Magnesium	1.5 to 2.5 mEq/L

Watch carefully for fluctuations in potassium, calcium, and magnesium during IV electrolyte therapy, because even a small deviation in these electrolytes creates a much greater risk than in those electrolytes with a wider range of normal values. Understand that milliequivalents (mEq) are not related to milligrams; and that "mEq" does not reflect a measure of weight, but the number of chemically active ions in solution (a more precise measure of the relative potency of an electrolyte solution than weight-by-volume measurements). Remember that an ongoing assessment of C.S's response is essential to preventing complications from IV therapy. Monitor the entire IV system—from the fluid container to her infusion site at frequent intervals. Flow rates may change 20% to 40% during an infusion; check the flow rate every hour if not using an infusion pump. Occasionally the nurse may be responsible for calculating hourly the need for changes in IV flow rates based on individual fluid output. The nurse may also need to titrate infusion fluid intake according to the amount of urine, gastric, or other outputs over specified periods.

Ongoing assessment of C.S. while receiving IV therapy should include observations for the complications described in the following sections. The assessment for some clients may include whether IV fluids should be used at all (Box 68-2). The client should be assessed for the following:

- **Infiltration.** Infiltration occurs when the needle is dislodged from the vein; this permits the solution to enter the surrounding tissues and causes pain and edema. Check the infusion site at frequent intervals for signs of infiltration (painful, blanched, cool swelling at infusion site without blood return). There may also be a significant decrease in flow rate, or it may stop altogether if the infiltration is extensive.

  To detect infiltration in a questionable IV site, locate the vein in which the parenteral solution is infus-

---

BOX 68-2 SHOULD INTRAVENOUS FLUIDS BE GIVEN TO THE DYING?

Over the past 20 years, the question of administering intravenous fluids to dying clients has been examined. IV fluids are sometimes provided to terminally ill client in the belief that electrolyte imbalance and dehydration are painful, agonizing events. It is also feared that the lack of medical intervention may be interpreted as abandonment, provoking familial condemnation and raising the specter of malpractice.

From a legal standpoint, however, IV fluids may be withheld or withdrawn in the same manner as other medical treatments with the proviso that the client requests such limitations. A study by Andrews and Levine (1989) reports that dehydration is not painful and may even be beneficial to the dying client. Although the administration of IV fluids may produce a temporary sense of well-being, it often aggravates the client's symptoms. Hydration increases urinary output, often necessitating the insertion of an indwelling catheter and exposing the client to infection. Pulmonary and pharyngeal secretions increase and precipitate a cough, dyspnea, and pulmonary edema. Increased GI secretions exacerbate nausea and vomiting. IV fluids may also produce peripheral edema and increase the risk for skin breakdown. All of these symptoms increase the client's discomfort, and the IV fluids may prolong the dying process.

Fluid deprivation reduces these symptoms. The fluid and electrolyte imbalance produced by dehydration may be a natural anesthetic, thereby reducing discomfort associated with the dying process. Most experts believe that dehydration in the last hours of life does not cause distress. It may stimulate endorphin release and add to the client's sense of well-being (Ferris, 2004). It has become more widely accepted to withhold IV fluids in late palliative care (Hurwitz, Duncan, & Wolfe, 2004).

Once a client decides to undergo terminal dehydration, the nurse's role is to provide scrupulous oral hygiene to reduce inflammation and minimize discomfort and to provide the client and family with emotional support.

CRITICAL THINKING QUESTIONS

- As a nurse, what feelings do you have about participating in the care of a dying client for whom IV hydration is being withheld?
- How would you respond when asked about the rationale for this approach to the care of a dying client?

---

ing. Place two fingers on the vein, approximately 3 to 4 inches above the injection, depending on the length of the needle or catheter that is in place. Observe the drip chamber while applying digital pressure. If the flow of solution in the drip chamber stops, the needle is in the vein. If there is no alteration of flow in the drip chamber, the needle is probably in the tissue, because flow continues into the tissues even if the vein is occluded. If infiltration is confirmed, stop the infusion.

- **Thrombosis.** An intravascular blood clot occurs when platelets agglutinate and fibrin strands and RBCs and white blood cells (WBCs) adhere to the platelet mass. A thrombus may form any time a blood vessel is injured, including injury by venipuncture. A thrombus may form in or around the needle or catheter, plugging the lumen; if this occurs, the infusion stops.
- **Thrombophlebitis.** Formation of a blood clot and inflammation of the vein may result from several factors: chemical as a result of the pH of the solution or the toxicity of the drug being administered; mechanical as a result of injury of the vein by movement of the cannula; and septic as a result of contamination. Thrombophlebitis is manifested by pain, heat, swelling, and redness along the course of the vein, and loss of motion of the affected part.
- **Pain at administration site.** Pain occurs when (1) the needle touches the venous wall, (2) too much tension is put on the needle or tubing, and (3) irritating drugs are administered too rapidly.
- **Necrosis.** Death and sloughing of tissue can occur when irritating drugs or solutions, such as epinephrine or norepinephrine, infiltrate into the tissues.
- **Pulmonary edema.** Pulmonary edema occurs when the circulatory system is overloaded with fluids. Careful monitoring of flow rate and urinary output is necessary. Central venous pressure monitoring, particularly in clients with cardiac disease, can help to prevent this hazardous complication. The client will exhibit dyspnea on exertion, orthopnea, and coughing. Tachycardia, tachypnea, dependent crackles, neck vein distention, and diastolic (S3) gallop may be heard. Coughing produces frothy, sometimes bloody sputum. Dysrhythmias may occur. The client becomes cold, clammy, sweaty, and cyanotic; blood pressure falls, and the pulse becomes thready.
- **Pyrogenic reactions.** Pyrogenic reactions occur when pyrogens, or fever-producing substances, are introduced into the circulatory system. Bacterial pyrogens are filterable, thermostable products of bacterial origin and activity that may accumulate and tend to cause a severe rigor when injected into the body. Pyrogenic reactions are characterized by fever and chills, malaise, headache, backache, nausea, vomiting and, if severe, vascular collapse with hypotension.
- **Air emboli.** Although they rarely occur, air emboli have a 40% to 50% mortality rate. Cannulation of the central veins is far more likely to be associated with air embolism than is cannulation of the peripheral veins. The occurrence of the following symptoms in a client receiving an infusion may indicate the presence of an air embolism: dyspnea, cyanosis, hypotension, weak/rapid pulse, loud and continuous churning sound over the precordium (not always present), and loss of consciousness.

Intervention Maintain a steady, even flow at the rate ordered; do not speed up rates to make up for lost time (watch the literature, however, for a resolution of the question about slowed rates being more compatible with basal metabolic rates during the before-dawn hours). Use every aid to facilitate therapy, such as calculating drops to be infused per minute and then time-taping the container. The use of an electronic infusion device (EID) is the standard for practice in many institutions, with either a controller that regulates IV flow rates by gravity or a controller that uses positive pressure to maintain flow. Accidental, uncontrolled free flow of medication when an IV administration set is removed from an EID has been reported. Ensure that you are familiar with the EIDs on your unit. Avoid using restraints and checking blood pressures on the arm receiving the infusion; the cuff interferes with fluid flow, forces blood back into the needle, and may cause clot formation.

Changes in solutions may require changes in equipment. Be aware of the options available in selecting a filter for the specific IV infusion. Several different IV filter products are designed for different filtration needs. Filters are available in a range of sizes and in add-on or in-line form:

- A 5-μm filter removes *particulate* material and is designed to filter gross particulate matter. The smallest particle visible to the unaided eye is approximately 30 μm in diameter.
- A 0.5-μm filter is considered a *bacteria-retention* filter, which is designed to prevent the passage of most particulate matter and certain fungi and bacteria. A yeast cell is approximately 3 μm in diameter.
- The 0.22-μm filter is called a *sterilizing* filter, because it is designed to prevent the passage of virtually all particulate matter and most bacteria for at least 24 hours. Bacteria range in size from 0.2 to 2 μm in diameter. Travenol Laboratories and other manufacturers provide these filters for use with the add-on or in-line systems. Select a 0.22-μm filter for parenteral nutrition solutions.

Tightly secure all connections in the administration setup to prevent air from being drawn in. Do not allow containers to empty completely, because air in the tubing could be driven into the vein when another full container is attached. Keep containers approximately 3 feet above the site during all client activities. If not using an infusion device, a higher position will cause the solution to infuse too rapidly; if too low, blood may find its way into the needle or tubing and clot there. Avoid using areas of flexion (e.g., the wrist or antecubital fossa); if such a site must be used, consider the use of an armboard.

Take the necessary precautions to prevent thrombophlebitis by doing the following: using sterile aseptic technique with proper cleansing of skin before inserting the needle; checking solutions for precipitation, debris, sediment, or color changes before and during IV therapy; ascertaining that no IV bottle or tubing is left in place for more than 24 hours, because some organisms proliferate at room temperature in IV fluids; and changing and dating the IV setup and site dressings every 24 hours to reduce the possibility of sepsis. Additionally, especially with the administration of irritating drugs, use veins with ample blood volume, use a cannula smaller than the vein to provide for greater hemodilution, administer irritating drugs slowly, rotate venipuncture sites every 48 to 72 hours, and avoid injecting IV infusions into leg veins or small veins.

Discontinue the infusion and restart it at another site if infiltration, thrombus, thrombophlebitis, or necrosis occur. If the IV has infiltrated, elevate the arm and apply heat to promote absorption of the infiltrated solution. Infiltration is especially serious when infusions of vasopressors (e.g., norepinephrine, dopamine) or vesicants (e.g., many antineoplastic agents) are involved; this is usually known as extravasation. If extravasation occurs, stop the infusion *immediately* and inject the known antidote immediately and subcutaneously in small amounts at many sites in the edematous area. Dress the wound, elevate the extremity, and apply heat or cold (depending on the infiltrated agent) for the client's comfort. See Chapter 56 for specific antineoplastic agents and their antidotes.

If a thrombus has occurred, restart the infusion at a new site with a new needle or catheter. It is unwise and unsafe to attempt to unplug the needle by forcing a bolus of solution in a syringe through the needle into the vein. Theoretically, the thrombus may become an embolus and lodge in a vital organ, causing more serious complications (e.g., pulmonary embolus). Although most hospital policies discourage irrigating, this practice is widespread; however, no confirmed pulmonary embolism has been reported with this technique. Elevate the affected extremity and apply heat to enhance resorption of the thrombus. Occasionally, very low doses of fibrinolytic (e.g., alteplase-TPA) are used to clear a thrombosed line. Such use typically requires following institutional protocol carefully.

When thrombophlebitis occurs, stop the infusion, withdraw the needle, and immediately report and record the condition. Treatment usually consists of applying moist heat to the affected area and resting the body part; anticoagulant therapy may also be ordered.

If pain occurs at the venipuncture site in the absence of other symptoms, adjust the needle and relieve the tension by readjusting the needle support or relaxing the pull on the tubing, and administer irritating drugs at a slow rate. These actions may alleviate the pain and discomfort.

Pulmonary edema is considered to be a medical emergency; the prescriber needs to be notified as soon as the client's fluid volume excess is noted. Slow the IV infusion to a "keep open" (KVO, keep vein open) rate to provide access for emergency medications. Oxygen can be started to improve gas exchange. Monitor vital signs every 15 to 30 minutes, and intake and output and arterial blood gas results. The following may be ordered: bronchodilators to decrease bronchospasm; diuretics to mobilize extravascular fluid; digoxin or pressor agents to increase cardiac contractility; nitroprusside to decrease peripheral vascular resistance, preload, and afterload; and morphine to reduce anxiety and dyspnea. Provide support for the client, who will be fearful because of decreased respiratory capacity.

If a pyogenic reaction is suspected, stop the infusion *at once*. Do not discard the solution, but instead send it to the pharmacist. Pyrogenic reactions are treated symptomatically but must be reported and recorded. Note the stock/lot number, because an entire batch of solutions may be contaminated.

When difficulties are encountered, consult agency infusion specialists, such as members of the IV therapy team, when available.

Education Inform C.S. and/or family members to notify the nurse if pain or swelling occurs at the infusion site or if any symptoms of the previously mentioned complications occur. Instruct C.S. to ambulate with the involved arm held lightly at the waist and with the unaffected arm guiding the IV pole. Advise her to avoid actions that elevate the arm with the venipuncture, such as using that arm to comb the hair or to shave.

Evaluation The expected outcome of IV therapy is that C.S. will receive fluid and electrolyte therapy as ordered, with serum electrolyte determinations returning to or remaining within normal limits; she will not experience any adverse effects of IV therapy (e.g., infiltration, thrombosis, thrombophlebitis, pulmonary edema, pyogenic reaction).

Summary

The administration of IV fluids and electrolytes has become commonplace in the experience of hospitalized clients. IV fluids are administered for a variety of reasons: to replace fluids and electrolytes, to correct acid-base imbalance, to administer medications, to maintain access to the venous system, to measure changes in venous pressure, to measure renal function, and to administer essential nutrients. With the increased prevalence of intravascular therapy, the role of nursing management in IV therapy has also grown and developed.

⊛ **Critical Thinking Questions**

- How do water, potassium, sodium, calcium, and magnesium contribute to survival?
- How would you minimize the risk of the various complications of IV therapy?

Bibliography

Anderson, D.M., Keith, J., & Novak, P.D. (Eds.) (2002). *Mosby's medical, nursing, and allied health dictionary* (6th ed.). St. Louis: Mosby.

Andrews, M.R., & Levine, A.M. (1989). Dehydration in the terminal patient: Perception of hospice nurses. *American Journal of Hospice Care, 6*(1), 31-34.

Deftos, L.J. (2002). Hypercalcemia in malignant and inflammatory diseases, *Endocrine & Metabolism Clinics of North America, 31*(1), 141-158.

Drug facts and comparisons (58th ed.). (2005). St. Louis: Facts and Comparisons.

Ferris, F.D. (2004). Last hours of living. *Clinics in Geriatric Medicine, 20*(4), 641-667.

Finfer, S., Bellomo, R., Boyce, N., French, J., Myburgh, J., & Norton, R., et al. (2004). A comparison of albumin and saline for fluid resuscitation in the intensive care unit. *New England Journal of Medicine, 350*, 2247-2256.

Gatof, D., & Ahnen, D. (2003). Primary prevention of colorectal cancer: Diet and drugs. *Acta Oncology, 42*(8), 809-815.

Hurwitz, C.A., Duncan, J., & Wolfe, J. (2004). Caring for the child with cancer at the close of life: "There Are People Who Make It, and I'm Hoping I'm One of Them." *Journal of the American Medical Association, 292*(17), 2141-2149.

Lacy, C.F., Armstrong, L.L., Goldman, M.P., & Lance, L.L. (2004). *Lexi-Comp's Drug Information Handbook* (12th ed.). Hudson, Ohio: Lexi-Comp.

Lau, A.H. (2005). Fluids and electrolytes. In M.A. Koda-Kimble, L.Y. Young, W.A. Kradjan, B.J. Guglielmo, B.K. Alldredge, & R.L. Corelli(Eds.), *Applied therapeutics: The clinical use of drugs* (8th ed.). Philadelphia: Lippincott Williams & Wilkins.

Marx, J., Hockberger, R., & Walls, R. (Eds.). (2002). *Rosen's Emergency medicine: Concepts and clinical practice* (5th ed.). St. Louis: Mosby.

Moe, S.M. (2005). Disorders of calcium, phosphorus and magnesium. *American Journal of Kidney Diseases, 45*(1), 213-218.

Mosby's drug consult (15th ed.). (2005). St. Louis: Mosby.

National Academies News. (2004). Report sets dietary levels for water, salt and potassium to maintain health and reduce chronic disease risk. Retrieved August 20, 2005, from http://www4.nationalacademies.org/news.nsf/isbn/0309091691 OpenDocument.

Rogers, F.B., & Li, S., (2001). Acute colonic necrosis associated with sodium polystyrene sulfonate (Kayexalate) enemas in a critically ill patient: Case report and review of the literature. *Journal of Trauma-Injury Infection & Critical Care, 51*(2), 395-397.

Sayegh, R.A., & Stubblefield, P.G. (2002). Bone metabolism and the perimenopause: Overview, risk factors, screening, and osteoporosis preventive measures, *Obstetrics & Gynecology Clinics, 29*(3), 495-510.

USP DI: Drug information for the health care professional (25th ed.). (2005). Greenwood Village, CO: MICROMEDEX Thomson Healthcare.

e-LEARNING SUPPLEMENTS

Student CD-ROM
- Final Exam questions
- NCLEX® Examination review questions
- Pharmacology animations
- Printable chapter summary

Evolve Website (http://evolve.elsevier.com/mckenry)
- Content updates, including information on new drugs
- WebLinks corresponding to this chapter
- Answers to the critical thinking questions in this chapter
- *Elsevier ePharmacology Update* newsletter
- Mosby's Drug Consult Internet Edition
- Supplemental and reference information

ENTERAL AND PARENTERAL NUTRITION

CHAPTER FOCUS

Enteral and parenteral feedings are commonly used to provide nutritional support to clients who, for some reason, cannot consume adequate nutrients through the normal processes of ingestion. The nursing focus for the nursing diagnosis "Imbalanced Nutrition" is on assisting the client or family to improve nutritional intake; this diagnosis should not be used to describe clients who are prescribed nothing by mouth (NPO) or cannot ingest food (Carpenito-Moyet, 2004). Because enteral and parenteral nutrition is used most commonly for clients who are NPO or cannot ingest food, this chapter considers the potential complications of electrolyte imbalances and negative nitrogen balance.

LEARNING OBJECTIVES

- Describe the techniques commonly used to deliver enteral feedings.
- Distinguish among elemental, polymeric, modular, and altered amino acid formulations for enteral feedings.
- Identify major drug-food interactions to be aware of when administering enteral nutrient formulations.
- Implement the nursing management of clients receiving enteral formulations.
- Describe parenteral protein-sparing nutrition and peripheral vein and central parenteral nutrition and the indications for their use.
- Describe the components of total parenteral nutrition solutions and the function of each element in the attainment of body requirements.
- Cite the possible complications of parenteral nutrition therapy.
- Implement the nursing management of clients receiving parenteral nutritional therapy.

▲ KEY TERMS

What is the role of nutritional supplementation in health care?

To achieve and maintain good health requires a regular intake of sufficient amounts of protein (amino acids), carbohydrates, fats, vitamins, and minerals. Under normal conditions adequate nutrition can be achieved by the ingestion of a balanced diet, but there are situations in which the nutritional needs of the body are not met. Such conditions include malnutrition, severe inflammatory bowel disease and other gastrointestinal (GI) diseases, coma, postsurgical complications, major burns, and others. Nutritional support is necessary for clients with these problems.

Over the past 50 years many advances have been recorded in the fields of both enteral and parenteral nutrition. Clinical nutrition is now a recognized and active entity for improving health care in all settings, including the home, long-term care facilities, and hospitals. Today nutritional programs or specific products have been developed for clients with specific disease states or illnesses. In this chapter, enteral and parenteral nutrition are reviewed along with selected disease states and criteria for the use of specific nutritional products.

How is nutritional supplementation via enteral means achieved?

Malnutrition among hospitalized persons and nursing home residents is associated with complications such as muscle atrophy, slow wound healing, impaired immunocompetence, infection, and death. Other complications include peripheral edema caused by reduced plasma proteins and its resultant decreased oncotic pressure, dry and flaky skin, and hair loss.

Malnutrition is also reflected in reduced total lymphocyte count, serum albumin, and transferrin levels (or iron-binding capacity). An increase in the concentration of 24-hour urine urea nitrogen reflects the protein catabolism that occurs with malnutrition.

Stress in relation to hospitalization may alter a client's usual eating habits. Unfamiliar foods and the general malaise resulting from illness also may cause clients to lose their appetites. An inadequate oral intake may result from oropharyngeal surgery, trauma, neoplasm, paralysis, or esophageal fistula. Fasting before surgery or for a diagnostic workup may also be nutritionally depleting. Energy needs may be doubled when sepsis, trauma, major surgery, inflammation, infection, or severe burns occur. Enteral or tube feedings may effectively supply essential nutrition if the GI tract is functional.

Enteral nutrition is the provision of liquid formula diets into the GI tract. Nasogastric or nasoenteric tubes are ideal for clients who require short-term (less than 2 weeks) enteral nutrition. The stomach is the preferred route of delivery but the nasoenteric tube may be advanced into the jejunum in clients with gastroparesis or with a high risk of aspiration (Rombeau, 2004). Permanent access through tube enterostomies is the preferred route of delivery for long-term (more than 2 weeks) (Figure 69-1). Tube enterostomies are inserted either endoscopically, laparoscopi-

cally, or operatively into the stomach and jejunum. Enteral nutrition has many advantages compared to parenteral nutrition; it has fewer serious complications. Enteral nutrition can supply gut-preferred fuels (e.g., glutamine, glutamate, short-chain fatty acids) not available in parenteral formulations. It maintains the structural and functional integrity of the GI tract. Cholelithiasis is prevented by stimulating gallbladder motility, and enteral nutrition is probably less expensive than parenteral nutrition (Klein & Rubin, 2002). Tube feedings may also be used to supplement inadequate oral intake and parenteral nutrition as it is being tapered.

Enteral feedings may be administered by bolus doses, typically 250 to 400 mL of formula every 4 to 6 hours; by intermittent feedings using a 20- to 30-minute drip; or by continuous gravity or enteral pumps. The continuous method over 16 to 24 hours has had more success because it helps to prevent complications such as dumping syndrome and avoids the need for frequent tube irrigations. Dumping syndrome is the result of a sudden influx of feeding and the creation of a high osmotic gradient within the small intestine; this causes a sudden shift of fluid from the

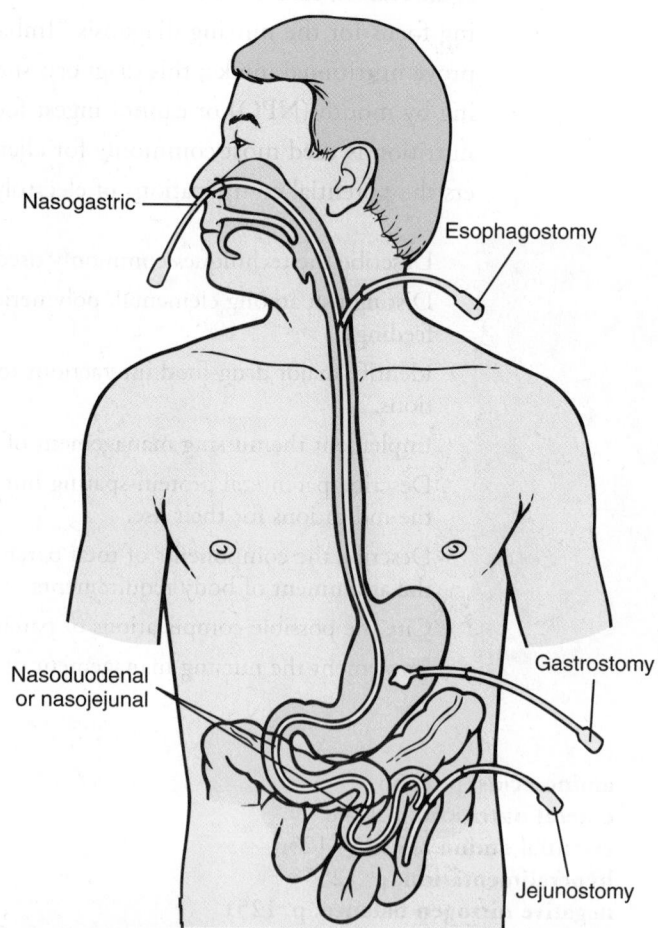

FIGURE 69-1 Tube feeding routes. The name of each tube denotes its terminus.

From Lewis, S.M., Heitkemper, M.M., & Dirksen, S.R. (2004). *Medical-surgical nursing: Assessment and management of clinical problems* (6th ed.). St. Louis: Mosby.

vascular compartment to the intestinal lumen. Plasma volume decreases, causing vasomotor responses such as increased pulse rate, hypotension, weakness, pallor, sweating, and dizziness. Rapid distention of the intestine produces a feeling of fullness, cramping, nausea, vomiting, and diarrhea.

Enteral feedings can be administered by the following routes: nasogastric, nasoduodenal, esophagostomy, gastrostomy, and jejunostomy. The last three are more invasive and require surgically created stomas; therefore they are less preferred routes for short-term enteral feeding. Nasogastric, esophagostomy, and gastrostomy feedings allow for more natural digestion in the stomach. Aspiration is a risk with nasogastric tubes because incomplete closure of the esophageal sphincter may result in gastric reflux.

Administering feedings directly into the small intestine reduces the risk of aspiration, but GI distress and diarrhea may develop because of the sudden influx of the enteral nutrition preparation. Skin excoriation and infection are potential risks with gastrostomies and jejunostomies, because the surgical opening penetrates the peritoneum. These complications are avoided in the cervical esophagostomy, which is a surgically created, skin-lined canal that is tunneled from the lower neck border and extends to below the cervical esophagus.

The selection of a tube feeding formula depends on the client's nutritional needs, concomitant disease states, lactose intolerance, and GI competence, and on convenience, feasibility, and cost. Nutritional assessment may be based on anthropometric parameters, biochemical data, and physical findings, and on medical, diet, drug, and socioeconomic histories. Ideal body weight (IBW) can be obtained from tables or by estimation as shown below:

- *Men:* 106 pounds (48 kg) for the first 5 feet (150 cm) plus 6 pounds (2.7 kg) per inch (2.5 cm) over 5 feet (plus or minus 10%)
- *Women:* 100 pounds (45 kg) for the first 5 feet plus 5 pounds (2.2 kg) per inch over 5 feet (plus or minus 10%)

IBW can be used instead of actual weight for determining nutritional requirements, because adipose tissue requires less energy for maintenance; if actual weight is used in the calculations, a client who is obese would receive excessive calories.

What types of enteral formulations are available?

Numerous different enteral formulations are available, and they can be broadly divided into modular, monomeric, oligomeric, polymeric, and disease specific formulations (Klein & Rubin, 2002):

- *Modular formulations* are single-nutrient formulas (i.e., protein, carbohydrate, or fat). Such a formula can be added to a monomeric or polymeric formulation to provide a more individualized and specialized nutrient formulation.
- *Monomeric formulations,* also known as "elemental" diets contain nitrogen in the form of free amino acids, carbohydrates as glucose polymers, and mini-

mal amounts of fat as long-chain triglycerides, usually accounting for 3% or less of total calories. Used for a variety of GI diseases, but in the absence of pancreatic insufficiency, nutrient absorption has no advantage over oligomeric or polymeric formulations.
- *Oligomeric formulations* are chemically defined formulations that require minimum digestion and produce minimal fiber in the colon. The two oligomeric subgroups include true elemental formulations that contain free amino acids and peptide-based formulations that contain dipeptides and tripeptides and/or crystalline amino acids. These formulations are indicated for clients with partial bowel obstruction, inflammatory bowel disease, radiation enteritis, bowel fistulas, and short bowel syndrome.
- *Polymeric formulations* are the most commonly prescribed complete formula, enteral preparations. Such formulations contain complex nutrients: protein (e.g., casein and soy protein), carbohydrates (e.g., corn syrup solid, maltodextrins), and fat (vegetable oil or milk fat) and are preferred for clients who have a fully functional GI tract and few or no specialized nutrient requirements. They should not be used in clients with a malabsorption problem. These formulations are preferred because the hyperosmolarity of the oligomeric preparations causes more GI problems than the polymeric formulations.
- *Specialized formulations* are indicated for clients with specific disease states such as genetic errors of metabolism (e.g., phenylketonuria, homocystinuria, maple syrup urine disease) or acquired disorders of nitrogen accumulation (e.g., cirrhosis or chronic renal failure), and for clients who are catabolic because of injuries or infection (Table 69-1).

Enteral formulas with high amounts of omega-3 fatty acids, arginine, glutamine and nucleotides are often referred to as "immunonutrients." These compounds are added to formulations to enhance immune response. Treatment with such formulas in an attempt to improve immunity is often referred to as immunonutrition (Jeebjeebhoy, 2005). Immunonutrition is correlated with reduced rates on infection and shorter lengths of hospital stay (Montejo et al., 2003), but formulations with high concentrations of arginine have been associated with increased mortality rates in critically ill clients, presumably related to elevated nitric oxide levels secondary to metabolism of arginine (Heyland & Samis, 2003). As such, the role of immunonutrition is still being determined.

Drug-Food Interactions

A number of drug–enteral nutrient interactions have been identified, and these interactions can be clinically significant. However, this possibility is often overlooked when enteral nutrient formulations are being administered. Table 69-2 lists the major drug interactions with enteral or tube feedings.

TABLE 69-1 EXAMPLES OF COMMERCIAL ENTERAL FORMULATIONS

Formulations	Comments
OLIGOMERIC	
Elemental	
Vivonex TEN	Contains free amino acids, linoleic acid, vitamins, minerals
Peptide-Based	
Peptamen Liquid	Composed of hydrolyzed whey proteins, amino acids, carbohydrates, fat, vitamins, and minerals
POLYMERIC	
Nutrient Source	
Blenderized	Prepared by dietary department
Compleat Modified	Has beef, amino acids, soy protein isolate, soy fiber, maltodextrin, pureed fruits and vegetables, canola oil, mono- and diglycerides, vitamins, and minerals
Milk-Based	
Nutrament Liquid	Composed of calcium and sodium caseinates, skim milk, soy protein isolates, sugars, canola oil, high oleic sunflower oil, corn oil, soy lecithin, vitamins, and minerals
Lactose-Free	
Ensure-Plus	Higher caloric formulation of protein, carbohydrates, fat, vitamins, and minerals that is lactose-free
MODULAR COMPONENTS	
Carbohydrate	
Polycose	Glucose polymers derived from cornstarch; high source of calories from carbohydrate
Protein	
Amin-Aid	Contains essential amino acids, carbohydrates, and fat; has high caloric formula indicated for acute or chronic renal failure
Fats	
MCT Oil	Medium chain triglycerides (MCT) that need less bile acid for digestion; does not provide any essential fatty acids
SPECIALIZED FORMULATIONS	
Renal Failure	
Amin-Aid	See above
Hepatic Failure	
Hepatic-Aid II	Contains amino acids (about 50% protein as branched-chain amino acids or BCAA), carbohydrates, and fat. Hepatic encephalopathy reportedly improved by increased serum levels of BCAA; used for chronic liver disease
Pulmonary Disease	
Pulmocare	Composed of calcium and sodium caseinate, amino acids, carbohydrates, fats, vitamins, minerals; has high caloric content; fat in this preparation is primarily from canola oil and corn oil (60%) plus 40% from MCT; persons with respiratory disease that received high fat, low carbohydrate diets demonstrated improvement in respiratory monitoring parameters

Data from *Drug facts and comparisons* (58th ed.). (2005). St. Louis: Facts and Comparisons.

✱ V.L., a 72-year-old woman, was admitted to the hospital 3 days ago after her daughter had found her semiconscious at home alone. Her admission assessment revealed left-sided paralysis. She is confused and disoriented and has dry mucous membranes and poor skin turgor. V.L. is diagnosed with a cerebrovascular accident and dehydration with little change from admission.

✱ What are the nursing management issues involved in enteral nutrition for V.L.?

Assessment A baseline assessment of V.L. should include body weight, weight loss history, and any clinical manifestations of impaired nutrition, less than required. The nutritional history should include (along with the cause if possible) inadequate nutrient intake, excessive nutrient losses or a

TABLE 69-2 DRUG INTERACTIONS WITH ENTERAL AND TUBE FEEDINGS*

Drug	Comments
Fluoroquinolone antimicrobials (ciprofloxacin, levofloxacin, moxifloxacin, gatifloxacin)	Interact with select metals such as calcium, magnesium, and iron via a chelation effect. The bioavailability of the fluoroquinolones will be significantly reduced when given simultaneously with most enteral feedings.
phenytoin (Dilantin)	The bioavailability of the liquid preparation is often reduced by the drug's ability to bind with the protein component of the enteral feeding, leading to less drug availability and inadequate therapeutic levels.
warfarin (Coumadin)	Warfarin resistance is reported when warfarin is administered with an enteral preparation. Interaction may be due to vitamin K in the feeding or due to warfarin binding to the protein ingredients in the formulation.

*When necessary, enteral feeding may be stopped for 1 hour before and 2 hours after the dose; alternatively, a higher dose of the affected drug may be considered. Closely monitor clients receiving the above and any other drugs in combination with enteral formulations. Laboratory tests such as serum drug levels or INR, when appropriate, may be ordered (Society of Hospital Pharmacists of Hong Kong, 2004).

failure to absorb nutrients, increased metabolic requirements, or medications that might have a catabolic effect, such as corticosteroids or antineoplastic agents. Baseline laboratory determinations, such as serum albumin, serum electrolytes, serum transferrin, serum prealbumin, urine creatinine clearance, and total lymphocyte count are indicators of protein nourishment. Hemoglobin, hematocrit, mean corpuscular volume (MCV), mean corpuscular hemoglobin (MCH), mean corpuscular hemoglobin concentration (MCHC), and the various blood levels of specific vitamins and minerals are indicators of vitamin and mineral nourishment. In general, enteral feedings are contraindicated for clients who are capable of oral intake or who have adynamic ileus, intestinal obstruction, intractable vomiting, or esophageal fistulas.

✱ V.L.'s daughter indicates that V.L. is 5'2" and her weight when taken on the bed scale is 93.5 lbs (42.5 kg). She has been receiving a maintenance IV of 5% dextrose/0.45% sodium chloride with KCL 20 mEq at 100 mL/hr. V.L.'s blood chemistries are within normal limits. Because V.L. has mild malnutrition and is not likely to take adequate nutrition in the next few days, it is decided to initiate continuous tube feedings with a full strength formula with a goal of 1440 mL daily (1-kcal/mL) or 60 mL/hr. The feeding is to start at 50 mL/hr for 8 hrs, then increased to 60 mL/hr if tolerated.

Nursing Diagnosis See the Nursing Care Plan on p. 1252 for nursing diagnoses related to a client with enteral tube feedings. Additionally, the potential complications of **negative nitrogen balance** (a condition in which more nitrogen is excreted than is taken in, indicating the wasting of tissue) and electrolyte imbalances exist.

Planning While V.L. is receiving enteral therapy, she will:
- Maintain blood chemistries within normal limits and a normal fluid balance without aspiration or other adverse effects.

- Achieve a body mass index (BMI) within normal limits for her height.

Implementation

Monitoring Ensure that there is an abdominal radiograph, or CO_2 monitoring device result to confirm tube location before feeding (Burns, Carpenter, & Truwit, 2001). Nasally or orally placed feeding tubes are generally anchored to the nose or face with tape. Check tube length and security of tape every 4 hours. Assess her for respiratory distress, frothy sputum, abnormal lung sounds, or new pulmonary infiltrates on x-ray examination. The addition of dye, particularly Food Drug and Cosmetic Blue No. 1, to enteral feedings is commonly employed for the detection of aspiration in the critical care setting. However, evidence suggests that this dye is potentially toxic under some clinical conditions (Lucarelli, Shire, Julian, & Crouser, 2004; Maloney and Metheny, 2002). Alternative approaches should be considered and glucose measurement in tracheal aspirates appears the most promising. This technique utilizes glucose oxidase reagent strips to detect increases in glucose concentrations in tracheal secretions attendant to aspiration of enteral nutritional formula. Clinical trials comparing enteral food dye administration and glucose testing of tracheal secretions demonstrate the latter to have better sensitivity (Lucarelli et al., 2004). Monitor the temperature, volume, and flow rate of the feeding.

Monitor V.L.'s nutritional status using the indicators mentioned in the baseline assessment. Weigh her 3 times a week.

Assess periodically for residual gastric volume and tube placement, particularly before each feeding or before administering a dose of a medication into the feeding tube. Although this procedure is frequently performed with tube fed clients, there is no standard definition regarding what constitutes a significant residual volume (RV). It is widely assumed that monitoring RV indicates GI tolerance of enteral nutrition and may prevent aspiration if kept below a certain

NURSING CARE PLAN SELECTED POTENTIAL NURSING DIAGNOSES FOR THE CLIENT WITH ENTERAL TUBE FEEDINGS

Nursing Diagnosis	Outcome Criteria	Interventions
Diarrhea	The client will have soft, formed stools fewer than three times daily.	• Record the frequency and consistency of stools. • If not contraindicated, decrease the hypertonicity of the feedings by diluting. • Check the client's medication regimen for diarrhea-causing drugs. • Assess the hygiene used in the administration of the feedings. • Perform a digital examination to ensure that the client does not have a fecal impaction. • Administer antidiarrheals as prescribed.
Risk for aspiration	The client will not experience aspiration.	• Assess the client for respiratory distress, frothy sputum, abnormal lung sounds, and new infiltrates on x-ray examination. Glucose testing of tracheal secretions assists assessment. • Elevate the head of bed at least 30 degrees during and for 1 hour after feeding. • Verify placement of the nasogastric or nasojejunal feeding tube with air auscultation. • Aspirate for residual contents every 4 to 8 hours or halfway between intermittent feedings. Hold the feeding and notify the prescriber if residuals are greater than the amount of 2 hours of continuous feeding or 50% of the volume of the previous intermittent feeding.
Deficient fluid volume	Fluid balance will be maintained. Hematocrit, BUN, and urine specific gravity will be within normal limits.	• Assess the client for poor skin turgor, dry mucous membranes, and thirst. • Monitor fluid intake and output. • Monitor laboratory values for increases in BUN, hematocrit, and urine specific gravity. • Provide increased amounts of water through feeding tube.

volume. However, evidence for this has not been substantiated by prospective, randomized studies. It may be that the tip of the feeding tube has settled into the fundus of the stomach and turning V.L. onto her right side for 15 to 20 minutes may allow the contents to flow out the pylorus, before reassessing the RV. Monitor continuous feedings every 4 to 8 hours; simply stop the feeding and measure the residual by aspirating the stomach contents with a syringe. In 2002, the North American Summit on Aspiration in the Critically Ill Patient evaluated the evidence and made the following consensus recommendations regarding RV.

• Total enteral nutrition (TEN) should be held for overt regurgitation or aspiration of gastric contents.
• TEN should be held for RV greater than 500mL and GI tolerance reassessed.
• RV of 200 to 500 mL should prompt careful bedside evaluation and steps should be taken to minimize aspiration risk.
• RV of less than 400 to 500 mL does not ensure tolerance of TEN or prevention of aspiration.

• RV less than 500 mL should be returned to the client.
• Clinical assessment should be always be used in combination with RV (McClave, 2002). Assess for abdominal distention, fullness, bloating, or discomfort.

For intermittent administration, measure the residual volume halfway between feedings.

Monitor bowel sounds to ensure that the client has good bowel function, although many experts feel that TEN can safely be initiated even when bowel sounds are not present (Charney, 2001). Bowel elimination patterns and fluid intake and output ratios should be carefully documented.

Many types of enteral formulas are lactose-free (nonmilk proteins are the base) for clients who lack sufficient lactase in intestinal microvilli for lactose absorption. Blacks, Asians, Native Americans, and Jews are particularly prone to lactase deficiency. Lactose ingestion causes varying degrees of diarrhea, abdominal cramps, bloating, and flatulence. Isotonic formulas administered at a continuous rate may be useful in preventing dumping syndrome. Commercially prepared enteral formulas have been developed and are designed for many specific disease states.

Intervention Although the GI tract is the optimal route for nutrient administration, in many ill clients the normal ingestion of food is difficult, if not nearly impossible, to achieve. Enteral nutrient preparations were designed for such clients. These formulations may be administered by the nasoenteral route through thin, flexible tubing that is generally well tolerated by clients. These feeding tubes are made from silicone or polyurethane compounds and have small lumen sizes (5 to 10 French). However, aspirating for residual GI contents and irrigating may be difficult with these small-lumen tubes. Change the administration tubing daily. See Box 69-1 for guidelines for enteral feedings.

Small-diameter feeding tubes also get clogged more easily. To prevent the buildup of formula residue, flush the tube with 20 mL of water at the completion of each intermittent feeding, when the tube is disconnected after the delivery of crushed medications, if feeding is stopped for any reason, and every 4 hours, with 20 mL of cranberry juice followed by 10 mL of water. The acidity of the juice breaks up the formula residue, and the water prevents sugar from crystallizing. Elevate the head of the bed 30 degrees when feeding into the stomach.

Surgical placement of a gastrostomy (G) tube or a jejunostomy (J) tube can be instituted if tube feedings must be administered for long periods of time. This helps to reduce the need for frequent flushing and replacement of the nasoenteral tube, and it is more comfortable for the client. A more common procedure in use today is the placement of a G tube percutaneously using endoscopic guidance; this is known as percutaneous endoscopic gastrostomy (PEG).

The enteral preparation may be given continuously or by cyclic administration. Cyclic feedings are similar to a person's normal feeding cycle and are the preferred method in some settings. Additional water may be added to the enteral formulations if the client cannot or does not drink additional water while receiving the formulations. In general, enteral formulations that have 1 kcal/mL usually contain approximately 80% water, whereas the formulations with more concentrated kcal/mL contain less than 70% water.

Although it is often recommended that continuous TEN begin at a lower amount than is prescribed and increase the amount gradually, there are no clinical studies to support this approach (Parrish & McCray, 2003). Based on current research, the University of Virginia Health System has developed the following guidelines (Parrish, Krenitsky, & McCray, 2003):

- *Continuous/nocturnal feeding.* Initiation: full strength (all products except 2 cal/mL) at 50 mL/hour and increase by 25 mL every 8 hours to goal rate. A 2 cal/mL is started at 25 mL/hour. The final goal rate depends on the client's caloric requirements and GI comfort.
- *Bolus/intermittent feeding.* Initiation: 125 mL, full strength (regardless of product) every 3 hours for 2

feedings; increase by 125 mL every 2 feedings to final goal volume per feeding during waking hours.

Nursing efforts should be maintained to encourage intake; milk-based formulas, for example, contain 1 kcal/mL, and the client must take 1000 to 2000 mL of formula to achieve their caloric needs and to obtain the Recommended Dietary Allowance (RDA) or Reference Nutrient Intake (RNI) for vitamins and minerals. Elevate the head of the bed at least 30 to 45 degrees during and for 1 hour after the feeding to reduce the risk for aspiration (Ibanez et al., 2000). Warm the feeding to room temperature before administering.

If the client develops diarrhea, it is often related to medications or other treatments, infectious causes, the underlying disease state, or altered anatomy, rather than the TEN. Many clients are switched to liquid forms of medications with TEN; these preparations may contain sorbitol and the client may be taking a number of them. There may also be an association between antibiotics, *C. difficile,* and diarrhea in clients receiving TEN (Parrish & McCray, 2003).

Record the name, volume, and strength of the formula and duration and rate (mL/hr) of feeding. Monitor intake and output totals daily. Every 8 hours, chart the volume of formula administered separately from water or other oral intake.

Education The self-administration of tube feedings is now possible with the advent of smaller tubes and infusion instrumentation that incorporates improved human engineering features. If V.L. is to go home on TEN, the necessary preparation of the caregivers (or client) should begin as soon as possible after admission. Individualized instruction with return demonstrations of learning take approximately 3 to 6 hours, perhaps more if insertion and removal of the tube is learned. Coughing, choking, difficulty speaking, or cyanosis signify incorrect tube placement. The concept of correct tube placement cannot be overemphasized. Written and verbal instructions related to possible secondary effects are also necessary (Table 69-3). Resuming daily activities at home is more inconvenient for the tube-fed ostomy client who must loosen clothing or undress for each feeding.

Clients receiving tube feedings are deprived of the usual personal and social gratifications of the eating act. They may feel "different" and alienated from others. To some, it may be symbolic of a rapidly deteriorating state of health and a last resort for survival. They especially need to understand the procedure, its rationale, and what to expect from it. Once given the opportunity to discuss its meaning, many can go on to participate actively in their feedings and express greater satisfaction.

Evaluation The expected outcome of enteral nutrition therapy is that the client will experience adequate nutrition as evidenced by blood urea nitrogen (BUN), serum protein, hemoglobin, and hematocrit levels that are within normal limits. The client will maintain or progress to a weight-for-height ratio normal for age and will not experience diarrhea, aspiration, or deficient fluid volume.

BOX 69-1 GUIDELINES FOR ENTERAL FEEDINGS

FEEDING SYSTEM DESIGN

Evaluate the design of the feeding system, including the container of the formula and the delivery set, on an ongoing basis. Closed systems, and those that minimize the risk of providers touching parts that come in contact with the formula, are recommended, as are systems with fewer connections. Evidence is mounting that closed enteral systems are also highly effective in reducing costs because they reduce nursing time and formula waste. Systems with medication ports are also recommended.

PROVIDER GUIDELINES FOR ENTERAL FEEDING PREPARATION

Wash hands with an antimicrobial soap or an alcohol-based hand rub for at least 10 seconds before preparing, assembling, and handling any part of a feeding system. Wear nonsterile disposable gloves, and change them when they become soiled. Wear a mask if you have a cold or other upper respiratory infection.

PREPARING ENTERAL FORMULAS

- With open systems, use prepackaged, ready-to-use, sterile feeding formulas—avoid those formulas that require dilution, reconstitution, or additions. Required mixing or formula preparation should take place in the dietary department using aseptic technique. Discard dented or damaged cans and those that are past their expiration dates. Cover, label, and refrigerate opened or prepared formula at a temperature lower than 4° C, and use it within 24 hours.
- For dilution and irrigation, the use of tap water as opposed to sterile water remains controversial; use tap water when its safety can be reasonably assumed; otherwise, use sterile water (which should always be considered when the client is critically ill or immunocompromised).
- Maintain irrigation sets with medical asepsis, and replace them every 24 hours.
- Assemble feeding systems on a surface disinfected with 70% isopropyl alcohol; using the same strength solution, disinfect the opening and the rim of the can of formula before opening.
- Label each feeding container with the expiration date, and discard the container after that date.

ADMINISTERING ENTERAL FEEDINGS

- Handle the feeding system and the ports as little as possible. Parts of the feeding system that come in contact with the formula should never touch the hands, clothes, or skin. Disinfect ports with 70% isopropyl alcohol before and after manipulation (before irrigation or drug administration, for example).
- With open systems, handle formula as little as possible, and avoid adding new formula to that remaining in the container from previous administration. Keep formula at room temperature, and use it within 12 hours.
- With closed systems, formula stored at room temperature can be used for at least 24 hours—there is evidence that some formulas can be used for up to 48 hours. Always check the manufacturer's guidelines.

DRUG ADMINISTRATION

- Enteral administration of drugs should be avoided whenever possible; use the oral route if possible. If it's unavoidable, use liquid medications when available (diluted with a minimum of 30 mL of water to decrease osmolality). Don't enterally administer enteric-coated tablets, buccal or sublingual medications, syrups, or sustained-release medications. Check with the pharmacist or appropriate references to establish which solid dosing forms can be crushed or opened and administered via an enteral tube. Crush tablets to a fine powder with a mortar and pestle or commercially available medication crushing device and mix it with at least 30 mL of water before administration. Whenever possible, administer medication through a medication port. (If one isn't available, then, wearing nonsterile gloves, draw the diluted solution into a syringe and administer into an administration port that has been thoroughly washed with alcohol.) Iron and potassium preparations are incompatible when mixed with enteral formula, and liquid medications that are acidic or with a pH of 5 or less should be avoided because of possible precipitation. Other known drug–nutrient interactions in enteral feeding occur with phenytoin (Dilantin), warfarin (Coumadin), ciprofloxacin (Cipro), carbidopa–levodopa (Sinemet), and carbidopa-levodopa-entacapone (Stalevo).
- Systems with medication ports are recommended. Before and after administering drugs through the feeding tube, disinfect the port with 70% isopropyl alcohol and flush the tube with 30 mL of water.

CLIENT MONITORING

To assess gastric emptying, check gastric residual volumes every 4 to 6 hours in clients receiving continuous feeding or before intermittent feedings. Additionally, check the tube placement using gastric pH before administering an intermittent feeding. A flush with 30 mL of water before and after fluid is aspirated from a feeding tube can reduce precipitation of acid from the formula, which clogs the tube, and is recommended every four to six hours during continuous feeding.

From Padula C.A., Kenny A., Planchon C., & Lamoureux C. (2004). Enteral feedings: What the evidence says: Avoid contamination of feedings and its sequelae with this research-based protocol. *American Journal of Nursing, 104*(7), 62-69.

TABLE 69-3 MOST COMMON SECONDARY EFFECTS OF TUBE FEEDINGS

Condition	Cause	Preventive Action
Aspiration	Impaired gag reflex	Position head of bed at 30-60 degrees for feedings and for 1 hour after.
	Uncuffed tracheostomy tube	Stop; suction trachea; inflate cuff before feedings.
	Decreased gastric motility	Check for residual of feedings and tube placement.
	Misplaced tube	Check taping and placement of tube. Advance tube through pyloric sphincter. Conduct glucose testing of tracheal secretions.
Obstructed tube	Plugged tube end-ports	Flush tubing before and after feedings or instillation of medications. Shake or mix formula well.
Hyperglycemia, dumping syndrome: nausea, vomiting, diaphoresis, cramping	Osmotic intolerance to hyperosmolar load of feeding, rapid rate, or high concentration	Change volume or rate of delivery, and dilute feeding temporarily.
	Ice-cold feeding	Allow feedings to warm slightly.

✳ What parenteral options exist for nutritional supplementation?

Enteral nutrition is always considered first-line therapy for clients who have a functioning gut. Parenteral nutrition is the treatment of choice for selected clients who are unable to tolerate and maintain adequate enteral intake. Historically called hyperalimentation, **total parenteral nutrition (TPN)** is the IV approach to complete nutrition. TPN is the administration of a nutritionally adequate hypertonic solution that consists of glucose, protein hydrolysates, minerals, and vitamins. Fat is also provided in a three-in-one solution or "piggy-backed." TPN can supply all of the calories, dextrose, amino acids, fats, trace elements, and other essential nutrients needed for growth, weight gain, wound healing, convalescence, immunocompetence, and other health-sustaining functions. It provides these components in the same ratio as a regular diet, and it promotes anabolism by supplying all necessary nutrients in excess of those needed for energy expenditure. TPN may be infused through a central vein, a peripheral vein or, rarely, both simultaneously.

Although the related nomenclature has not yet been standardized, partial parenteral nutrition has come to denote parenteral nutrition therapy with IV solutions that are lacking some essential elements, notably fats. Although insulin and heparin (and several other medications) have been added to parenteral nutrition preparations for specific clients, the addition of medications to TPN solutions should generally be avoided because of the potential incompatibilities of the medication with the nutrients in the solution. The following are the major parenteral systems for nutritional support:

- Peripheral vein parenteral nutrition
- Central-line venous total parenteral nutrition

Peripheral Vein Parenteral Nutrition

Peripheral vein parenteral nutrition (PPN) is prescribed for clients who need modest nutritional support. Peripheral vein total parenteral nutrition (PTPN) is prescribed for clients for whom insertion of a central venous line for total parenteral nutrition may not be possible. The client with PPN may be nutritionally healthy or have slight to moderate nutritional deficits without being in a hypermetabolic state. The client's current health status indicates that a nutritional deficit will probably occur if nutritional therapy is not instituted.

PPN is considered a temporary measure to provide an appropriate nitrogen balance in clients who have mild deficits or have orders for nothing by mouth (NPO) and have no or only a slightly elevated metabolic rate. It may be prescribed to precede a procedure that imposes restrictions on oral feedings; for GI illnesses that prevent oral food ingestion; for anorexia caused by radiation or chemotherapy in cancer treatment programs; or following surgery if the client's nutritional deficits are minimal but oral food consumption will not be instituted for 5 or more days. It is not indicated for nutritionally depleted clients in a hypermetabolic state. If used for such clients, it should be a temporary measure until central vein total parenteral nutrition can be initiated.

PPN solution is composed of 3% to 5% isotonic amino acids mixed with a carbohydrate solution (usually dextrose 5% to 10%), vitamins, minerals, and electrolytes for administration through a peripheral vein, providing less than 1kcal/mL, so several liters may be needed daily to meet energy and protein needs. The major advancement in this therapy is the use of a lipid as a nonprotein source of calories. When administered peripherally, dextrose must be limited to a 10% solution to avoid sclerosing of the veins. For the same reason, most institutions also limit the concentration of electrolytes to be infused.

Peripherally administered lipid preparations or IV fat emulsions (Liposyn, Intralipid, and others) are a source of additional calories for the client.

Central Total Parenteral Nutrition (TPN)

In central TPN, a catheter is placed in a central vein, most commonly the subclavian vein, to administer solutions that contain hypertonic glucose and amino acids. Because of its blood flow, the central vein can accept the high-osmolar concentrated solutions. Central TPN is usually composed of the three major nutrients—dextrose, crystalline amino acids, and lipid emulsions—plus vitamins, minerals, trace elements, electrolytes, and water. The solutions may vary according to the client's requirements and, in general, according to the supplier of the basic amino acid solution. Special preparations of amino acids are also available for the client with a specific disease state.

Central TPN is used primarily for clients with nonfunctioning GI tracts, those that should not use the oral route for more than 7 days, or for clients who either have a limited peripheral access or whose needs cannot be met by peripheral formulations (Holcombe & Gervasio, 2005). For example, clients with conditions of short bowel syndrome, acute pancreatitis, enteric or enterocutaneous fistulas, active inflammatory process, GI tract obstruction, major trauma, or burns—with whom enteral feedings are not possible—may need central TPN for survival.

✱ What solutions are used in parenteral nutrition?
The basic total parenteral solution contains amino acids, carbohydrates (dextrose), lipids, and micronutrients (e.g., trace elements, vitamins).

Amino Acids

Amino acids are necessary to promote the production of proteins (anabolism), to reduce protein breakdown (catabolism), and to help promote wound healing. Protein is composed of essential and nonessential amino acids. The body cannot synthesize **essential amino acids,** but **nonessential amino acids** can be synthesized from a nitrogen source (amino acids, ammonium salts, urea). A negative nitrogen balance is a situation in which more nitrogen is excreted than taken in, which leads to a wasting of body tissue.

All natural amino acids are needed for growth and development and must be present concurrently in the proper amounts for protein synthesis to occur. Adults can synthesize all but eight of these amino acids; these eight are considered essential in adults. To the extent that the oral intake

of amino acids is limited, protein synthesis depends on an exogenous source. The **semiessential amino acids** (histidine, arginine) are not synthesized in adequate amounts during growth periods; thus 10 amino acids are considered essential in infants.

At a minimum, a healthy adult usually requires approximately 0.9 g protein/kg, whereas an infant or child needs between 1.4 and 2.2 g protein/kg. This requirement can increase substantially in undernourished or traumatized clients; for example, it can increase up to sixfold in a traumatized or seriously ill client, because the daily need is approximately 3 g/kg body weight. A nonprotein source of calories must be provided with the amino acids to offset their use as an energy source.

Amino acid solutions contain crystalline amino acid (Aminosyn and many others); solutions are also available with electrolytes. Amino acid crystalline solutions contain synthetic amino acids but not peptides. This is the preferred form of amino acid, because most clients are able to tolerate this formulation. Dextrose usually is administered with these solutions because of the protein-sparing action of carbohydrates. If the protein is administered without adequate calories in the form of carbohydrates, the protein will be used for the body's caloric needs rather than for the repair and regeneration of tissue.

Protein-sparing nutrition is usually reserved for clients who have minimal protein deficiencies and sufficient fat stores. A 3% to 5% isotonic amino acid is mixed with carbohydrate-free fluids, vitamins, minerals, and electrolytes that are administered by peripheral vein. The solution will provide approximately 400 to 600 calories/day. The client will meet many energy requirements by using the free fatty acids and ketones derived from their endogenous adipose tissue, thereby preserving their protein compartment in the body. This type is usually used for short-term periods for clients who are not nutritionally compromised and are not in a hypermetabolic state.

Specially formulated amino acid preparations are available for clients with special disease conditions, such as renal failure, high metabolic stress, encephalopathy, and liver failure. For example, formulas such as HepatAmine are used for hepatic failure, and NephrAmine and others are used for renal failure.

Carbohydrates

Carbohydrates and lipids are used as the primary source of calories for the client. One gram of D-glucose provides 3.4 calories, whereas fat supplies 9 cal/g and protein supplies 4 cal/g. Concentrations of dextrose solutions above 10% are hyperosmolar and are too irritating to be given continuously peripherally; thus they should be administered through central venous catheters. Centrally, the concentration of infused dextrose solutions is usually between 25% and 35%.

Hyperglycemia usually occurs when dextrose is administered without lipids as the primary source of calories. Because dextrose requires insulin for utilization, a combination of caloric sources, dextrose, and lipids will help to decrease the potential for hyperglycemia and the extra need for insulin in some clients. Dextrose alone also increases the rate of metabolism and production of carbon dioxide, which may increase the client's respiratory demands. Administering a combination caloric preparation of dextrose and lipids will reduce the increase in respiratory demands.

Although not as prevalent in usage, other sources of available calories include alcohol in dextrose solution and invert sugar and electrolytes solution (*Drug Facts and Comparisons,* 2005). The dextrose used in formulations is derived from corn sugar; invert sugar derived from cane or beet sugar is an alternative for the very small portion of the population who may be sensitive to corn derivatives. Alcohol is another substrate that provides 7 kcal/g, and it does not require insulin for peripheral utilization. However, providing enough calories would necessitate a quantity of alcohol that would produce a potential for intoxication and hepatotoxicity.

Because dextrose is inexpensive and readily available, it is almost always the preferred product for administration.

Lipid Emulsions

Fat constitutes 40% to 50% of the total calories supplied in the average North American diet. The American Heart Association recommends the following: fat should constitute 30% or less of total calories in the diet; carbohydrates, 55% or more; and protein, approximately 15%. Similar recommendations are made by the United States Departments of Health/Human Services and Agriculture (see http://www.healthierus.gov/dietaryguidelines/).

Fat emulsions are derived from either soybean or safflower oil, which provides a mixture of neutral triglycerides and unsaturated fatty acids. The two functions of IV fat emulsions in parenteral nutrition are to supply essential fatty acids and to be a source of energy or calories (9 cal/g).

Linoleic, linolenic, and arachidonic acids are essential in humans. Linoleic acid cannot be synthesized in the body, and it is the precursor to both linolenic and arachidonic acid. If linoleic acid is either unavailable or deficient, the enzyme system will act on oleic acid to synthesize

icosatrienoic acid, which is incapable of functioning like arachidonic acid. Essential fatty acid deficiency (EFAD) is noted with clinical signs of hair loss, scaly dermatitis, slowed growth, reduced wound healing, decreased platelets, and fatty liver. This necessitates the IV administration of a fat emulsion to correct the biochemical alteration.

The fat emulsions currently available are either safflower oil (Liposyn) or soybean oil (Intralipid) or a combination of both (Liposyn II). Fat emulsion particles are thought to be metabolized from the bloodstream in a manner similar to that of chylomicrons, which appear in the blood postprandially. Fat emulsions may minimize hyperglycemia, hyperinsulinemia, and hyperosmolar syndrome, which often occur in clients who are given dextrose as the only source of parenteral caloric nutrition. Additionally, they may augment immune and inflammatory responses in a number of conditions (Hasselmann & Reimund, 2004). Fat emulsions pose some dangers for clients with severe liver disease, pulmonary disease, anemia, or blood coagulation disorders and for acutely ill clients with elevated serum concentrations of C-reactive protein. Fat emboli and the accumulation of intravascular fat may occur in the lungs of premature, preterm, or low-birth-weight infants (the infusion rate is not to exceed 1 g/kg in 4 hours).

Trace Elements and Electrolytes

Although some of the commercial parenteral nutrition solutions contain trace elements, or minerals, clients who are placed on long-term administration should be evaluated for deficiencies in trace elements. Trace element solutions are available individually (zinc, copper, manganese, chromium, and selenium) and in combination formulations (M.T.E. formulations and others). Several trace metal formulations are also available in combination with electrolytes (Tracelyte and others).

Table 69-4 notes examples of the signs and symptoms of trace element deficiency, normal serum levels, and primary excretion sites. It is also critical to monitor serum electrolyte levels, especially the cations of sodium, potassium, calcium, and magnesium and the anions of chloride, phosphate, bicarbonate, and acetate. In general, serum levels of trace elements are not routinely monitored.

TABLE 69-4 TRACE ELEMENTS

Elements	Dose*	Deficiency Symptoms
copper	0.5-1.5 mg	Decrease in red and white blood cells; hair and skeletal abnormalities; defective tissue growth
chromium	10-15 mcg	Neuropathy, confusion, impaired glucose tolerance, ataxia
manganese	150-800 mcg	Defective growth, nausea, vomiting, weight loss, skin rash, CNS alterations (ataxia, seizures)
selenium	40-80 mcg	Muscle aches, pain or tenderness, cardiomyopathy, kwashiorkor
zinc	2.5-4 mg	Nausea, vomiting, diarrhea, weakness, anorexia, growth retardation, anemia, hypogeusia, rash, depression, eye lesions, defective wound healing, and hepatosplenomegaly

*Recommended daily adult dose.

If iron replacement is necessary, oral replacement is the preferred route of administration. If iron cannot be administered orally, it can be given by IM Z-track injection or by IV injection or infusion. Do not mix iron with other drugs or add it to parenteral nutrition solutions. For additional information on iron [Iron Dextran], refer to a current package insert.

Vitamins

The client receiving parenteral feedings will also need additional vitamins. A combination of multivitamin infusion (MVI) and, perhaps, additional vitamins is usually given on alternate days to meet the client's needs for fat-soluble vitamins A and D and the water-soluble vitamins B and C. Such preparations, if prescribed, can be added to the parenteral nutrition solution. Vitamin K is usually administered weekly by IM or subcutaneous injection. The specific dosage and frequency for vitamin regimens depend primarily on the individual client's needs and on the usual protocols of the prescriber.

✲ What are the nursing management issues in the use of parenteral nutrition?

Assessment A baseline assessment of the client should include body weight, weight loss history, and any clinical manifestations of undernutrition. Parenteral nutrition is used for hospitalized and home care clients who are below their ideal body weight or have a weight change of 10% or more in less than 6 months or children whose weight or height is less than the 5th percentile. TPN is also routinely used in neonatal intensive care units to meet the nutritional needs of preterm neonates.

The nutritional history should include, with cause if possible, inadequate nutrient intake, excessive nutrient losses or failure to absorb nutrients, increased metabolic requirements, or medications that might have a catabolic effect, such as corticosteroids or antineoplastic agents. A dietitian usually assesses the client's nutritional needs. Basal energy needs are calculated from client's weight, height, and age. Additional energy needs are based on an assessment of activity and metabolic needs. Protein needs are determined by client weight and metabolic state (e.g., burn, sepsis, renal disease). Fluid requirements are 30 to 35 mL/kg (average sized adults), or 25 mL/kg (65 years of age or older) (Al-Turf & the Total Parenteral Nutrition Subcommittee, 2003). Fluid requirements vary with neonates, infants, and children depending on age and status.

Baseline laboratory determinations, such as serum albumin, serum electrolytes, serum transferrin, serum prealbumin, urine creatinine clearance, and the total lymphocyte count are indicators of protein nourishment. Hemoglobin, hematocrit, MCV, MCH, MCHC, and the various blood levels of specific vitamins and minerals are indicators of vitamin and mineral nourishment.

If the TPN is to be administered in the home setting, evaluate whether the client/caregiver is able to perform home parenteral nutrition support procedures and is knowledgeable about therapeutic expectations, risks, and benefits of home TPN. Evaluate if the home environment is suitable for home TPN (e.g., electricity, phone availability). Assess and evaluate insurance coverage.

Nursing Diagnosis The client receiving parenteral nutrition therapy may experience the following nursing diagnoses/collaborative problems: risk for infection; deficient fluid volume; excess fluid volume; and the potential complications of negative nitrogen balance related to the underlying condition, hyperglycemia/hypoglycemia, depressed levels of the electrolytes potassium/phosphate/calcium/magnesium, trace element deficiencies, and essential fatty acid deficiency (EFAD) caused by prolonged fat-free total parenteral nutrition therapy. See Box 69-2 for a list of potential complications of parenteral nutrition.

Planning While receiving parenteral therapy, the client will:

- Maintain blood chemistries within normal limits and a normal fluid balance without infection or other adverse effects.
- Achieve a BMI within normal limits for height and age.

Implementation

Monitoring Close, ongoing reassessment of clients' responses to this complex therapy is essential. In particular, monitor the development of circulatory fluid overload or electrolyte imbalance through assessments of vital signs and fluid balance ratios. Elevated body temperature may be an indication of sepsis. Maintain a uniform infusion rate at all times as prescribed. Infusion instrumentation does not eliminate the need for alert nursing care, because this equipment has the same potential for malfunction as all other equipment. In addition, fat emulsions or TPN containing fat emulsions can occasionally separate, with a thin layer of oil rising to the top of the infusion container. Such a condition necessitates immediate halting of the infusion to prevent a fat emboli.

The monitoring of the unstable client in acute condition with early nutrition support is intensive; usually electrolytes, BUN, and serum creatinine are determined 3 to 7 times per week; calcium, magnesium, phosphate, 1 to 3 times per week; liver function tests (LFTs), total protein (TP), albumin, once weekly or every other week; and triglycerides, weekly or as appropriate for IV fat emulsion use. For the stable hospitalized client with prolonged parenteral nutrition support, the monitoring may include electrolytes, BUN, and serum creatinine are determined 1 to 3 times per week; calcium, magnesium, phosphate, once weekly or every other week; LFTs, TP, serum albumin, every 2 to 4 weeks; and complete blood count (CBC)/differential, platelets and red blood cell (RBC) indices, every 2 to 4 weeks. Blood glucose levels are determined every 6 to 8 hours for hypo/hyperglycemia until the client's glucose is stable and then at least every day. Assess the infu-

BOX 69-2 COMPLICATIONS OF PARENTERAL NUTRITION

COMPLICATIONS ARISING FROM INFECTION AND SEPSIS

- Catheter seeding from bloodborne or distant infection
- Contamination of catheter entrance site during insertion or long-term catheter placement
- Solution contamination

COMPLICATIONS THAT ARE METABOLIC IN ORIGIN

- Azotemia
- Cholelithiasis
- Dehydration from osmotic diuresis
- Electrolyte imbalance
- Hyperammonemia
- Hyperosmolar, hyperglycemic, nonketotic coma (HHNC)
- Hyperphosphatemia and hypophosphatemia
- Hypocalcemia
- Hypomagnesemia
- Rebound hypoglycemia or sudden cessation of parenteral nutrition
- Trace element deficiencies

COMPLICATIONS ARISING FROM SUBCLAVIAN CATHETERIZATION

- Air embolism
- Arteriovenous fistula
- Brachial plexus injury
- Cardiac perforation, tamponade
- Catheter embolism
- Catheter misplacement
- Central vein thrombophlebitis
- Endocarditis
- Hemothorax
- Hydromediastinum
- Hydrothorax
- Pneumothorax
- Subclavian artery injury
- Subclavian hematoma
- Subcutaneous emphysema
- Tension pneumothorax
- Thoracic duct injury

sion site for local infection at every dressing change. Suspect thrombosis if the client complains of pain or swelling in the extremity or surrounding area on the side where the catheter is located. Leakage at catheter insertion site may also occur. A venogram is needed to confirm a thrombosis. Weigh the client on a daily basis at the same time of day (preferably the first thing in the morning after voiding), wearing the same type of clothing, and on the same scale.

Monitor clients with diabetes mellitus carefully; insulin may be required to control hyperglycemia. Clients with cardiac insufficiency need to be watched closely for excess fluid volume. Observe the infusion site regularly for inflamma-

tion and infection, and monitor the peripheral infusion lines for phlebitis.

It is critical to record daily the following data and to notify the prescriber of abnormal values: blood glucose in excess of 200 mg/100 mL; weight loss; change in pulse and blood pressure; sweating; elevated temperature; swelling and edema over the puncture site or on the head, neck, or face; abnormal serum electrolytes; distended veins in the neck, arms, and hands; seizures, coma; or other radical changes in the client's condition.

Intervention Starting and weaning the TPN should be done gradually. The starting rate should be no more than 50 mL/hour for 4 to 6 hours. The rate can be increased 25% every 4 to 6 hours. Weaning is accomplished by decreasing the rate by 25% every 4 to 6 hours (Al-Turf & the Total Parenteral Nutrition Subcommittee, 2003).

Standard TPN solution is recommended for general use because it can fulfill most clients' nutritional requirements and be cost effective. Its final concentration is typically 4.25% amino acids and 25% dextrose and its calorie: nitrogen ratio is 125:1 (1 Kcal/mL solution). Peripheral infusions are limited to amino acids 2.5% and dextrose 10%.

A centrally placed catheter is essential for TPN to be infused into the client. These catheters are usually divided into the nontunneled catheters, tunneled catheters, and the implanted ports.

Nontunneled Catheters These are usually placed in the subclavian or jugular veins for short term therapy of less than 8 weeks. A peripherally inserted central catheter (PICC) line may be inserted via the cephalic or basilica vein; these are often the access sites of choice for home TPN. Insertion of these catheters must be done with sterile technique but can be done at the client's bedside. Once the catheter is inserted, a stat portable chest radiograph should be taken to assure correct placement of the catheter and the absence of insertion complications. The tip of the catheter must be in the superior or inferior vena cava to infuse TPN through the catheter. There is a decreased risk of infection with single-lumen catheters although multiple-lumen catheters can be used. If multiple-lumen catheters are used, care must be taken to administer TPN in a lumen in which no other solutions could have contaminated that lumen.

Tunneled Catheters These catheters are more commonly known as Hickman, Groshong, Broviac, and so on, which are brand names for these catheters. They are used with longer term TPN therapy and intermittent infusions of drugs and other adjunctive therapies. These catheters are made of silicone. They are placed most commonly in the chest area. The catheter is tunneled under the skin and enters a large vein and then is threaded into the superior vena cava.

Implanted Ports These catheters are referred to as Infus-a-port, Port-a-cath, and so on, which are brand names. They are used for more intermittent therapies but can be used for TPN infusion both in the hospital and in the home setting. The septum of these catheters is sutured under the skin in the subcutaneous tissue. The silicone catheter that attaches to the septum is then threaded into a major vein.

Consult the pharmacist regarding drug compatibility for simultaneous administration of two or more drugs through a single lumen of the catheter.

When parenteral nutrition infusion is being cycled, a heparin flush is needed to maintain patency of central venous catheter when solution is not infusing. The dosage volume and frequency of heparin is determined by type, size, and number of lumens of the central venous catheter. Resistance to flushing may be corrected with the use of a fibrinolytic instilled into the catheter. See Chapter 30 on the use of fibrinolytics.

Because these balanced nutritional solutions provide an excellent medium for the growth of microorganisms, strict asepsis must be used when preparing solutions (usually done by pharmacists, and ideally in a designated "clean room" under a laminar flow hood) and when handling solutions or the insertion site.

Fat emulsions may be administered either peripherally or centrally. If fat emulsions are co-infused from separate containers that flow into the same vein as the dextrose and amino acid solutions, a Y-connector is used and is positioned just in front of the infusion site. The lipid infusion line should be at least 6 inches higher than the dextrose–amino acid line, because the lipid emulsion has a lower specific gravity. If not administered in this order, the lipid emulsion may flow backward into the amino acid-dextrose line.

The intake of parenteral nutrition may begin at a rate less than 1 L/12 hr for the first 2 days. If tolerated, the rate may be increased gradually during the first 5 days to the final goal rate. Do not shake lipid emulsion infusions that have separated in solution to mix them; instead discard them according to agency policy. Additionally, the fats in lipid emulsions have been found to leach out the plasticizer di(2-ethylhexyl) phthalate (DEHP) in polyvinyl chloride tubing. Because the toxic potential for DEHP is not known, it is wise to use the administration sets provided by the manufacturer for fat emulsions in parenteral nutrition therapy.

Change dressings if they become wet or dislodged; they are designed to be air-occlusive. Specific protocols changing various types of dressings can be found in selected references. Report any elevation of the client's temperature to the physician. Cultures (fungal, bacterial) should be taken of the insertion site, tubing, parenteral solutions, and the client's blood.

Air embolism is a potential hazard with central venous lines because of the low pressure in the venous system. Keep tubing connections taped to prevent their separation. When necessary, change tubing quickly while the client is in a supine position and is executing a Valsalva's maneuver (forced exhalation against a closed glottis). Central line in-

sertions should be accomplished with the client in Trendelenburg position.

Education Parenteral nutrition is often administered in a home setting, usually in one single container per day. Whenever possible, all the necessary nutrients are combined and administered on a cycling basis, depending on the client. Cyclic therapy is the infusion of the feeding over less than 24 hours; this frees the client from constant therapy. Such preparations are often administered during the evening and night hours. TPN is usually infused over 12 to 14 hours depending on how well the infusion of TPN is tolerated; this should begin in the hospital so that tolerance can be properly evaluated before discharge. TPN should have a taper up and a taper down of half rate of the infusion to decrease any glucose intolerance problems. Blood glucose monitoring should be done while initiating cycling approximately 3 to 4 hours into the infusion, when the infusion is complete, and 1 hour after completion of the infusion. If the client experiences blood glucose problems, the taper up or down or the length of cycling may need to be adjusted.

Parenteral nutrition can now be continued at home for indefinite periods of time for those who need ongoing nutritional support and who meet the criteria. The client/caregivers should be familiar with the infusion pump used to administer the TPN, heparin flush, dressing change to the catheter exit site, and sign and symptoms of problems/complications. Client and family education is essential regarding the purposes and techniques of the following: preventing infection, caring for the solution, regulating flow rate, recording daily weights, recording intake and output, monitoring blood for glycemia, and keeping close contact with community health nurses and other personnel. The client and family/caregiver must understand infusion pump monitoring before assuming full responsibility for this technology. Every attempt should be made to resume the usual activities of daily living and to integrate this therapy into the client's lifestyle. See the Community and Home Health Considerations box on p. 1261 for the nursing care of a client who is receiving TPN in the home.

Evaluation The expected outcome of parenteral nutrition therapy is that the client's nutritional status will be improved. If therapy is successful, weight increases of 2 to 3 pounds a week can be expected until the client's weight is within the normal limits for height and age. The client should also demonstrate improved strength and activity tolerance and healthy gums and oral mucous membranes. If administered in a home setting, the client or caregiver will effectively manage, with guidance, the therapeutic regimen associated with parenteral nutrition therapy. Laboratory values should be within the normal limits for BUN and serum albumin, protein, hematocrit, hemoglobin, vitamin B_{12}, folic acid, cholesterol, lymphocytes, and transferrin.

Community and Home Health Considerations

Total Parenteral Nutrition in the Home Setting

The client and family/caregiver should have the opportunity to practice the procedures in the hospital under nursing supervision. Review the procedures for storage of the solution, which should be picked up or delivered every day for the client. Instruct the client to keep the containers refrigerated but to allow them to come to room temperature before administering the solution. Advise the client to check the expiration date, the label of contents, and the appearance of the solution.

The dressing is to be changed at least every 2 days. Instruct the family/caregiver to use aseptic technique when changing the dressing. The site should be inspected for swelling, redness, or drainage; these should be reported to the health care provider if found. Demonstrate to the family how to irrigate the catheter. Instruct the client in how to set the pump to the appropriate settings, how the infusion pump works, how to care for the pump, and what to do if the alarm sounds. Also demonstrate how to change the solution bag, tubing, and filter.

Explain that the client should be weighed daily and the client's intake and output monitored. Ask the client and family to observe for edema, and show them how to check urine glucose levels. Review the potential complications of TPN, such as chills, fever, dyspnea, chest pain, and coughing as an adverse effect of lipid infusion; dyspnea, chest pain, and coughing with air embolism; nervousness, faintness, and tachycardia with hypoglycemia; and nausea, vomiting, polyuria, polydipsia, and positive urine glucose or acetone with hyperglycemia. Instruct the client to discontinue the infusion and to contact the prescriber if any of these occur. Recommend that the client keep the telephone number of the prescriber, nursing service, and community emergency services within easy reach.

Summary

Nutrition in the form of enteral or parenteral solutions plays a vital role in the treatment of clients. Enteral nutrition bypasses the upper GI tract and introduces liquid enteral formula or pureed foods directly into the stomach or small intestine by way of a feeding tube. Enteral feeding is indicated for clients who have a functional GI tract but cannot take sufficient food by mouth. The complications of enteral nutrition may be mechanical or metabolic.

Parenteral nutrition refers to the IV administration of a solution containing dextrose, proteins, electrolytes, vitamins, and trace elements in amounts that exceed the client's energy needs. It is used for instances in which enteral feeding is contraindicated or ineffective. In both enteral and parenteral nutrition, the nurse has an important role to ensure that clients are nourished adequately and safely.

Critical Thinking Questions

- Jean Sims, 76 years old, has been admitted to the hospital with several health problems, including asthma, emphysema, and esophageal motility problems. She has been losing weight rapidly because of difficulty swallowing and is working so hard to breathe that she is not getting enough to eat. Rather than insert a nasogastric tube, the physician has inserted a gastrostomy tube percutaneously. What are the advantages for this client of the PEG compared to a nasogastric tube?

- Would TPN have any advantages for Mrs. Sims? Why or why not?

Bibliography

Al-Turf, Dillion, K., & the Total Parenteral Nutrition Subcommittee. (2003). *Total Parenteral Nutrition: Policies, Procedures, and Prescribing Information. Virtual Hospital.* Retrieved August 24, 2005, from http://www.vh.org/adult/provider/surgery/totalpareteralnutrition/index.html.

Anderson, D.M., Keith, J., & Novak, P.D. (Eds.) (2002). *Mosby's medical, nursing, and allied health dictionary* (6th ed.). St. Louis: Mosby.

Burns, S., Carpenter, R., & Truwit, J. (2001). Report on the development of a procedure to prevent placement of feeding tubes into lungs using end-tidal CO_2 measurements. *Critical Care Medicine, 29*, 936-939.

Carpenito-Moyet, L.J. (2004). *Nursing diagnosis: Application to clinical practice* (10th ed.). Philadelphia: J.B. Lippincott.

Charney, L.J. (2001). Enteral nutrition: Indications, options, and formulations. In: M.M. Gottschlich (Ed.). *The Science and Practice of Nutrition Support.* Dubuque, IA: Kendall/Hunt Publishing.

 e-LEARNING SUPPLEMENTS

Student CD-ROM
- Final Exam questions
- NCLEX® Examination review questions
- Pharmacology animations
- Printable chapter summary

Evolve Website (http://evolve.elsevier.com/mckenry)
- Content updates, including information on new drugs
- WebLinks corresponding to this chapter
- Answers to the critical thinking questions in this chapter
- *Elsevier ePharmacology Update* newsletter
- Mosby's Drug Consult Internet Edition
- Supplemental and reference information

Drug facts and comparisons (58th ed.). (2005). St. Louis: Facts and Comparisons.

Hasselmann, M., & Reimund, J.M. (2004). Lipids in the nutritional support of the critically ill patients. *Current Opinion in Critical Care, 10*(6), 449-455.

Heyland, D.K., & Samis, A. (2003). Does immunonutrition in patients with sepsis do more harm than good? *Intensive Care Med, 29*, 669-671.

Holcombe, B.J., & Gervasio, J.M. (2005). Adult parenteral nutrition. In M.A. Koda-Kimble, L.Y. Young, W.A. Kradjan, B.J. Guglielmo, B.K. Alldredge, & R.L. Corelli (Eds.), *Applied therapeutics: The clinical use of drugs.* (8th ed.). Philadelphia: Lippincott, Williams & Wilkins.

Ibanez, J., Penafiel, A., Marse, P., Jorda, R., Raurich, J.M., & Mata, F. (2000). Incidence of gastroesophageal reflux and aspiration in mechanically ventilated patients using small-bore nasogastric tubes. *Journal of Parenteral & Enteral Nutrition 24*:103-6.

Jeejeebhoy, K.N. (2005). Enteral feeding. Current Opinion in Gastroenterology, 21(2), 187-191.

Klein, S., & Rubin, D.C. (2002). Enteral and parenteral nutrition. In: Feldman, M. (Ed.), *Sleisenger & Fordtran's Gastrointestinal and Liver Disease* (7th ed.). St. Louis: Elsevier.

Lucarelli, M.R., Shire, M.B., Julian, M.W., & Crouser, E.D. (2004). Toxicity of Food Drug and Cosmetic Blue No. 1 Dye in critically ill patients. *Chest, 125*(2), 793-795.

Maloney, J., & Metheny, N. (2002). Controversy in using blue dye in enteral tube feeding as a method of detecting pulmonary aspiration. *Critical Care Nurse, 22* (5), 84-85.

McClave, S.A. (2002). Clinical use of gastric residual volumes as a monitor for patients on enteral feeding. *Journal of Parenteral & Enteral Nutrition, 26*, S43-S50.

McClave, S.A., DeMeo, M.T., DeLegge, M.H., DiSario, J.A., Heyland, D.K., Maloney, J.P., et al. (2002). North American Summit on Aspiration in the Critically ill Patient: Consensus statement. *Journal of Parenteral & Enteral Nutrition, 26*, S80-S85.

Montejo, J.C., Zarazaga, A., Lopez-Martinez, J., Urrutia, G., Roque, M., & Blesa, A.L., et al. (2003). Immunonutrition in the intensive care unit. A systematic review and consensus statement. *Clinical Nutrition*, 22(3), 221-233.

Opilla, M. (2003). Aspiration risk and enteral feeding: A clinical approach. *Practical Gastroenterology, XX*, 89,90,92-94,96.

Parrish, C.R. & McCray, S. (2003). Enteral feeding: Dispelling myths, *Practical Gastroenterology XX*:33, 37, 39, 43-44, 46, 48, 50.

Parrish, C.R., Krenitsky, J., & McCray, S. (2003). *University of Virginia Health System Nutritional Support Traineeship Syllabus.* University of Virginia Medical Center Nutrition Services Department, Charlottesville, VA.

Rollins, C.J., Huckleberry, Y., & Cawley, P. (2005). Adult enteral nutrition. In M.A. Koda-Kimble, L.Y. Young, W.A. Kradjan, B.J. Guglielmo, B.K. Alldredge, & R.L. Corelli (Eds.), *Applied therapeutics: The clinical use of drugs.* (8th ed.). Philadelphia: Lippincott, Williams & Wilkins.

Rombeau, J.L. (2004). Enteral nutrition. In: L. Goldman & D. Ausiello (Eds.), *Cecil's textbook of medicine.* (22nd ed.). Philadelphia: W. B. Saunders.

Society of Hospital Pharmacists of Hong Kong. (2004). Drug–enteral tube feeding interaction. Retrieved August 24, 2005, from http://www.shphk.org.uk.

Taylor, S.J., Fettes, S.B., Jewkes, C., & Nelson, R.J. (1999). Prospective, randomized, controlled trial to determine the effect of early enhanced enteral nutrition on clinical outcome in mechanically ventilated patients suffering head injury, *Critical Care Medicine, 27*, 2525-2431.

USP DI: Drug information for the health care professional (25th ed.). (2005). Greenwood Village, CO: MICROMEDEX Thomson Healthcare.

70

ANTISEPTICS, DISINFECTANTS, AND STERILANTS

CHAPTER FOCUS

Most infectious diseases are transmitted in one of four ways: airborne transmission (inhalation of contaminated, evaporated droplets); vector-borne transmission of an organism by an intermediate carrier, such as a mosquito; contact transmission (direct or indirect contact with the source); and enteric transmission (oral-fecal transmission through direct or indirect contact with feces or objects heavily contaminated with feces). To inhibit the transmission of infection, nurses both practice and teach good aseptic and sterile technique. Nurses work to break the cycle of contact and enteric transmission by using antiseptics, disinfectants, and sterilant agents to decontaminate surfaces and equipment to prevent the spread of infection.

LEARNING OBJECTIVES

- Compare nosocomial infections and community- or home-acquired infections.
- Differentiate between medical asepsis and surgical asepsis.
- Describe the characteristics of an ideal antiseptic/disinfectant.
- Explain the mechanisms of action of antiseptics and disinfectants.
- List the indications for use of common antiseptics and disinfectants.
- Describe the uses and limitations of silver nitrate and silver sulfadiazine.
- Describe the effectiveness of iodine compounds and iodophors.
- Explain the mechanism of action of oxidizing agents.
- List the current uses of sterilants.
- Implement nursing management for the safe and effective use of antiseptics, disinfectants, and sterilants.

▲ KEY TERMS

antiseptics, p. 1264
bactericidal, p. 1264
bacteriostatic, p. 1264
disinfectants, p. 1264

medical asepsis, p. 1264
nosocomial infections, p. 1264
sterilization, p. 1264
surgical asepsis, p. 1264

How are infections in the clinical setting characterized?

Infections and infectious diseases, although differing in type and character, occur in people in all settings—hospitals, institutions, the community at large, and the home.

Community-acquired infections in usually healthy individuals are often benign and are relatively responsive to treatment. *Streptococcus pneumoniae* or *Mycoplasma pneumoniae* infections are common in this population. Nosocomial infections are acquired in the hospital and most commonly result from gram-negative infections including *Pseudomonas, Proteus, Serratia, Providencia,* and others. Virulent, drug-resistant, Gram positive microorganisms such as methicillin-resistant staphylococcus aureus (MRSA) and vancomycin resistant enterococci (VRE) are now also commonly observed nosocomial pathogens.

Urinary tract infections and postoperative wound infections account for the majority (approximately 70% or more) of the nosocomial infections detected in a hospital setting. High-risk areas, such as critical care units, burn units, and dialysis units, usually have the highest incidence of infection outbreaks and antibiotic resistance, but these pathogens are now found in all settings. Nurses must be aware of this problem and of the methods used to reduce the incidence of nosocomial infections in their practice.

What are the principles of medical and surgical asepsis?

Medical asepsis (the absence of pathogenic organisms) and surgical asepsis (the absence of all microorganisms) are used in health care to reduce the number and spread of organisms. These approaches presume the presence of pathogens (organisms capable of inducing disease or infection in human beings) or potential pathogens in the immediate environment and seek to limit their transmission.

Methods in surgical asepsis destroy *all* microorganisms, including spores; in medical asepsis, only *pathogens* are destroyed or inhibited. The focus in surgical asepsis is to keep all organisms out of a designated area (e.g., fresh wound), whereas in medical asepsis the goal is to remove or destroy the pathogens in the area and to contain the remaining nonpathogens by conscious efforts. Surgical asepsis uses "sterile technique" (the use of sterile equipment or sterile fields), and medical asepsis uses "clean technique" (e.g., hygienic measures, cleaning agents, antiseptics, disinfectants, and barrier fields). The technique used in a given situation depends largely on the susceptibility of the host, the organism's virulence, and other factors in the infectious cycle.

An object is sterile if it is free of all forms and types of life. Sterilization is a process that destroys all forms of life on an instrument or utensil, in a liquid, or within a substance. Living tissue (of clients, nurses, or surgeons) cannot be sterilized by any known means without damaging that tissue; therefore sterilization is applied only to objects. It is also important to grasp the concept put forth by the Council on Pharmacy and Chemistry that the terms *sterile, sterilizer,* and *sterilization* can be used only in the absolute sense—there is no acceptable concept of relative sterility.

However, just because a piece of equipment is labeled "sterilizer" does not mean that it is totally and permanently effective for sterilizing. Nor does the term *sterilized* testify to an object's current condition of purity.

Several acceptable and practicable sterilization methods now exist. Steam under pressure (autoclaving) is preferred as the most effective method. Ethylene oxide is a gas sterilant used for heat-labile materials, for sharp-edged instruments that could be dulled by steam, for electrical and anesthesia equipment, and for bedding. Hot air ovens are used to sterilize glassware. Chemical sterilants are also used when necessary.

What chemical agents are used to support medical and surgical asepsis?

Antiseptics and disinfectants are chemical agents used to kill many pathogens within a given population of microorganisms. In general, their mechanisms of action are not very effective against spores of bacteria and fungi, many viruses, and some very resistant bacterial strains. As a group, the effects of disinfectants and antiseptics differ from sterilization largely in the type of organisms destroyed and the degree to which they are destroyed. Disinfectants and antiseptics kill only pathogens, but sterilizing kills all types of organisms.

Although some of the literature use the terms *disinfectant* and *antiseptic* interchangeably, such use is erroneous and confusing. Disinfectants differ from antiseptics in the matter on which they are used and in their ability to destroy organisms. Disinfectants are used only on nonliving objects; they are toxic to living tissue. Antiseptics are typically applied only to living tissue; they must be less potent or made more dilute to prevent cell damage. Such lessening of potency, although crucial to viable tissue, decreases their effectiveness accordingly. Some definitions of antiseptics emphasize their inhibiting rather than their destructive effects. The narrow range of tolerance by tissues to antiinfective topical preparations tends to limit the variety and number of acceptable antiseptic agents available. Antiseptics may differ markedly from disinfectants in chemical composition or may simply be a dilute version of a disinfectant for use on intact tissue. Thus some chemical substances may be used either as an antiseptic or as a disinfectant, depending on concentration.

Antiseptics and disinfectants are further categorized as bacteriostatic or bactericidal in character. Antiseptics are most often bacteriostatic; they slow the growth and replication of bacteria but do not kill off the entire bacteria population. Disinfectants are bactericidal (bactericides); they actually kill bacteria, but perhaps not all types (depending on the disinfectant, its specificity, and so on) and often not fungi, viruses, or spores. Other disinfectants—fungicides, virucides, and sporicides—act specifically on these organisms. *Germicides* is an all-encompassing term for agents that work against many types of "germs"—bacteria, fungi, viruses, and spores.

Organisms vary in their sensitivity to disinfectants and antiseptics (Box 70-1). However, factors such as the dormant and impervious spore forms of some bacteria; the waxy en-

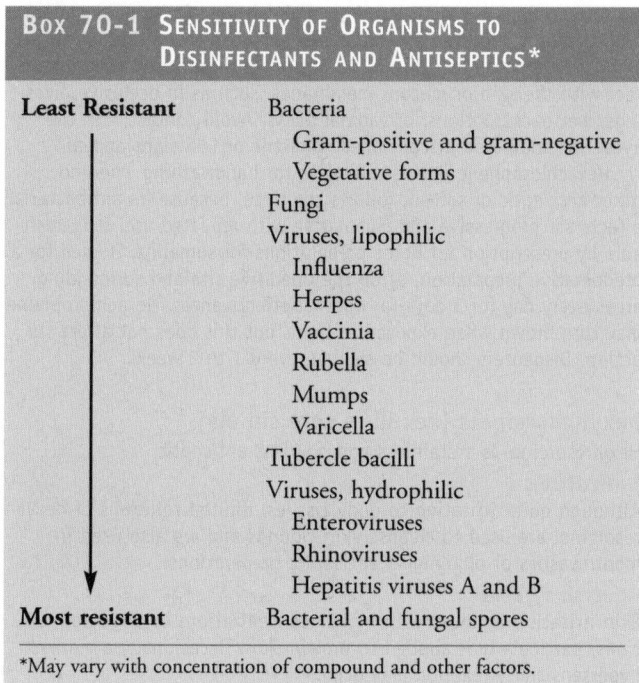

velopes of the tubercle bacilli; and certain properties of some types of gram-positive bacteria (staphylococci and enterococci), some gram-negative bacteria (*Salmonella* and *Pseudomonas* species), and hepatitis viruses make them highly refractory to many forms of disinfectants or antiseptics.

The ideal all-around antiseptic/disinfectant does not yet exist. Such an ideal agent would need to do the following:

- Be destructive to all forms of microorganisms without being toxic to human cells
- Have a low incidence of hypersensitivity
- Be active in the presence of organic matter and soaps
- Be stable, noncorrosive, nonstaining, and inexpensive

The current criteria for an effective disinfectant include the ability to destroy within 10 minutes all vegetative bacteria (not spores) and fungi, tubercle bacilli, animal parasites, and viruses (not hepatitis viruses). Many variables affect the relative efficiency of a product, including the ingredients' ability to dissolve, mix, and work in the presence of organic matter such as blood or other exudate and its ability to penetrate into recesses. Other properties include chemical composition, concentration, pH, ionization, surface tension, temperature, and length of time required for action. In actual clinical use, there may be extreme variability in the effectiveness of any given product; this variability depends on the specific application and situation. Although several standard tests for the efficacy of these products are available, the results are subject to the same variables and may also be difficult to administer.

Currently, there are few established guidelines for specific approved use of any particular disinfectant—an agent is considered a disinfectant whether it is used on corridor floors or on surgical instruments. This method of classifying permits widespread practices such as the common use of iodophor solutions as disinfectants when they have earned approval by the Food and Drug Administration (FDA) as antiseptics. Antiseptics are not required to be as potent as disinfectants.

The relative usefulness of various antiseptics can be compared based on their therapeutic index. This index is the relationship between the specific antiseptic concentration proved to be effective against microorganisms without irritating tissues or interfering with healing. Other decisive factors are the potential for causing hypersensitivity reactions or systemic absorption. *Thorough handwashing still predominates as the most effective measure for controlling the spread of infection.*

To place the concepts of sterilization, disinfection, and antisepsis in perspective, it should be made clear that these processes differ in the degree to which they destroy organisms. Anything that is sterile can also be considered both disinfected and antiseptic. (The converse is, of course, not true.) All of these processes correctly begin with handwashing, even when gloves are to be worn. It has been repeatedly demonstrated that clean, washed hands are crucial deterrents to the growth, reproduction, and transmission of microorganisms in any environment.

Antiseptics and disinfectants may act in three ways:

- They may bring about a change in the structure of the protein of the microbial cell (denaturation), which often proceeds to coagulation of protein with increased concentration of the chemical agent.
- They may lower the surface tension of the aqueous medium of the parasitic cell, which increases the permeability of the plasma membrane. This results in the lysis or destruction of cellular constituents. (The surface-active agents are thought to act this way.)
- They may alter a metabolic process in the microbial cells that interferes with the cell's ability to survive and multiply.

✴ What antiseptics and disinfectants are available for use in clinical practice?

A number of agents are available for use as antiseptics and disinfectants. A number of agents that were historically used (e.g., mercury compounds, hexachlorophene) are less common in clinical practice because of toxicity concerns. Other agents, such as triclosan, are found in many consumer soaps and touted for their antibacterial properties. Consumer products containing triclosan do not offer significant protection against common respiratory, gastrointestinal (GI) or dermal infections observed in typical households (Larsen, Lin, Gomez-Pichardo, & Della-Latta, 2004). Despite evidence lack of protection against infection by these products, consumer demand remains high. Classes of available antiseptics and disinfectants include phenols, dyes, halogens, oxidizing agents, biguanides, surface acting agents, alcohols, and acids. Sterilants that are used to sterilize equipment are discussed at the end of the chapter.

Phenols and Phenol Derivatives

Phenol was used for more than 100 years as an antiseptic and disinfectant, but today it may be used in some facilities as a disinfectant. All phenols are deadly poisons if taken internally or applied topically to abraded skin. Phenol itself is no longer used because of its toxicity on absorption, its carcinogenic effect, and its corrosive effect on equipment. Its derivatives are used, and these compounds disrupt cell walls and membranes, precipitate proteins, and inactivate enzymes; this makes them bactericidal, fungicidal, and capable of inactivating lipophilic viruses.

Phenols

Phenol and phenolic compounds are intended for disinfectant use only. These disinfectants should not come in contact with the skin in concentrations stronger than 2%, and they should never come in contact with broken skin. If accidental skin contact is made or if a burning sensation is noted, the area should be washed with copious amounts of water. Phenolic disinfectants used to clean bassinets and mattresses in poorly ventilated nurseries have produced epidemics of neonatal hyperbilirubinemia, and fatalities have been documented in infants. Phenol in concentrations above 5% has been implicated in the promotion of tumor growth, and therefore studies are underway to determine the carcinogenic, mutagenic, and teratogenic safety of this agent. A derivative of phenol, triclosan, is not nearly as toxic, and is discussed here as well.

Phenol Derivatives

hexachlorophene [**heks** a klo roe feen]
(pHisoHex, Septisol)
Hexachlorophene is a bacteriostatic agent that at one time was incorporated into detergent creams, soaps, lotions, shampoos, and other topical products to reduce the incidence of pathogenic bacteria on the skin. A single skin washing with hexachlorophene is no more effective than soap in reducing the number of bacteria; however, this product has a cumulative antibacterial property and steadily decreases bacterial flora with repeated use. Cleansing with alcohol and repeated washing with soap removes its antibacterial residue.

Indications
Because of its toxicity, especially in infants, it is currently available only by prescription for surgical scrub purposes and as a bacteriostatic skin cleanser against staphylococci and other gram-positive bacteria. It is used as a surgical scrub and bacteriostatic skin cleansing agent, although other antiseptics such as chlorhexidine are more effective and are safer to use.

Pharmacokinetics
Some systemic absorption of hexachlorophene is possible, particularly when applied to broken skin, mucous membranes or neonatal/infant skin.

Adverse Effects
Hexachlorophene is a toxic agent that can be absorbed through the skin, causing gastric symptoms and central nervous system (CNS) toxicity. Daily topical use on newborns or application several times daily to the skin or vagina in adults has resulted in confusion, diplopia, lethargy, seizures, respiratory arrest, and death. Hexachlorophene is usually not used routinely or recommended for use in bathing infants or pregnant or hypersensitive persons. It also should not be used on mucous membranes or burned or denuded skin or for any prolonged skin contact without rinsing. Dermatitis and photosensitivity have also been reported.

Nursing Management
There is a potential for poisoning; a resultant CNS toxicity may occur if there is accidental excessive exposure to hexachlorophene. Observe clients with prolonged exposure for signs of CNS toxicity: a change in

sensorium, double vision, lethargy, and seizures. These products are highly toxic if ingested and are easily absorbed (even through intact skin) if not thoroughly rinsed. Do not leave these substances in contact with the skin or mucous membranes, such as in occlusive dressings, wet packs, lotions, or vaginal packs. Avoid contact with the eyes. Use should be discontinued if gastric or CNS signs appear.

Hexachlorophene is most effective for handwashing when no other antiseptic or solvent follows the rinse, because its antibacterial effects are progressive and cumulative with repeated use. It is available by prescription for home preparations for surgeries. If used for a preoperative preparation, scrub the operative site and surrounding areas every day for 3 days for optimal effectiveness. Hexachlorophene may turn brown when exposed to light, but this does not affect its action. Dispensers should be cleaned every 1 to 2 weeks.

hexylresorcinols [hex ill re **sore** sin ole]
Hexylresorcinol is a stainless and odorless antiseptic.

Indications
Although quite irritating to body tissues, diluted solutions of hexylresorcinol are used to cleanse skin wounds and are also used in mouthwashes or pharyngeal antiseptic preparations.

Adverse Effects
Skin irritation is noted with higher concentrations or large applications, particularly if applied to broken skin. Occasionally a marked hypersensitivity reaction may occur.

Nursing Management
Monitor for signs of inflammation or irritation. Advise that this product be discontinued if such signs are evident, because they may indicate hypersensitivity rather than simple dermal irritation.

triclosan [tri **kloe** san]
Triclosan is an antiseptic found in a number of consumer products including soaps, dishwashing liquids, detergents, toothpastes, lotions, creams, cosmetics, and plastics. It acts by entering the bacterial cell and preventing fatty acid production. It displays activity bacteriostatic against gram-positive and gram-negative pathogens, although it is not effective against *Pseudomonas aeruginosa* (Russel, 2004). The role of this consumer product is considered controversial, with some data demonstrating no significant long-term difference in hand flora compared to plain soap (Larson et al., 2003) and no difference in risk for developing common infections when widely used in household consumer products (Larson et al, 2004). The widespread inclusion of triclosan in many consumer products may have negative environmental influence as well (Aiello & Larson, 2003; Sabaliunas et al., 2003).

Indications
The FDA has allowed the inclusion of triclosan in toothpaste for gingivitis and plaque control since 1997 (FDA, 1997), but its inclusion was undergoing re-evaluation in 2004 (FDA, 2004).

Adverse Effects
Contact dermatitis has been reported with use (Dastychova, Necas, Pencikova, & Cerny, 2004).

Dyes

Rosaniline dyes are a group of basic dyes used only occasionally today as antibacterial and antifungal agents. Most of these dyes (gentian violet, methyl violet, and others) have been removed from the market or have been replaced by other topical products.

Mercury Compounds

The FDA has banned all first-aid antiseptic mercury products, including thimerosal (Merthiolate) and merbromin (Mercurochrome), because they lack evidence of safety and effectiveness.

Silver Compounds

Many inorganic silver compounds have antiseptic qualities when applied locally. Silver salts that are highly ionizable and soluble produce astringent or caustic actions. Free silver ions precipitate bacterial cellular proteins, which results in bactericidal effects. The effectiveness of these agents is directly proportional to their concentration and duration of contact time. An immediate bactericidal effect occurs when silver solutions are applied to tissue. The silver proteinate that is formed slowly liberates small amounts of ionic silver, which provides continued bacteriostatic action. An unexplained and strongly bactericidal quality resides in distilled water when it is in contact with metallic silver. Silver sulfadiazine (Silvadene) is bactericidal for many gram-positive and gram-negative organisms and yeast, and it also inhibits bacteria that are resistant to other agents (see Chapter 65). It is used to prevent and treat infections in partial- and full-thickness burns.

silver nitrate [**sil** ver **nye** trate]

Silver nitrate reacts with soluble chloride, iodides, and bromides to form insoluble salts that inactivate the action of silver nitrate. Therefore its action can be halted if necessary by irrigating the area with sodium chloride solutions. This chemical characteristic explains why solutions of silver salts penetrate tissues slowly; chlorides apparently precipitate the silver ions and inactivate them.

Indications

Silver nitrate is used to cauterize wounds and ulcers, and remove granulation tissue and warts. It also is used in the management of burns. The American Academy of Pediatrics has endorsed a recommendation to eliminate eye irrigation after instillation of silver nitrate (*Drug Facts and Comparisons*, 2005). In many hospitals, topical erythromycin or tetracycline ophthalmic ointments have replaced silver nitrate because they are effective against chlamydial and gonococcus eye infections. However, silver nitrate is the only one of these agents in preventing ophthalmia caused by penicillinase-producing *Neisseria gonorrhoeae* (Knodel, 2002).

Pharmacokinetics/Dosing

With silver nitrate 1% solution, two drops are instilled and allowed to remain in the eyes for no more than 30 seconds.

Adverse Effects

With silver nitrate 1% solution, eye redness or irritation is the primary adverse effect; with other silver nitrate preparations, it is skin irritation. The long-term use of silver salts can permanently discolor the skin because of the deposit of reduced silver (argyria). Prolonged use of mild silver protein can result in permanent skin discoloration and conjunctival argyria.

Nursing Management

Question the client about hypersensitivity to silver, blood dyscrasias, porphyria, or a glucose-6-phosphate dehydrogenase (G6PD) deficiency; these conditions may preclude treatment with silver compounds. The effects in children and in pregnant or breastfeeding women are not known.

The client receiving silver compound therapy may be at risk for impaired comfort (an itching or burning feeling on treated areas). Evaluate the affected mucous membranes daily, and note any changes. Perform an ongoing evaluation of clients treated with these compounds to limit the adverse effects related to hypersensitivities.

Store silver nitrate solutions at temperatures between 15° C and 30° C (59° F and 86° F), and protect them from light. Use only the appropriate concentrations for antiseptic purposes to avoid irritation and burns to tissue. Sodium chloride can be used to flood the area should this occur accidentally.

Take care with silver solutions to keep spills and stains to a minimum. Gloves are advised when working with silver solutions. Most tissue stains gradually disappear. Stains may be removed from linens, clothing, and shoes by applying household chlorine bleach.

Alert the client that rarely the skin may stain a brownish black. Instruct in the proper application technique. Instruct the client to store silver nitrate solutions out of reach of children and never to take them internally. The expected outcome of silver compound therapy is that the client's mucous membrane will be moist, pink, and intact without drainage or other signs of inflammation or infection.

Halogens

Chlorine Compounds

Although chlorine can be bactericidal (it is ineffective against acid-fast bacteria), sporicidal, viricidal, and amebicidal, the elemental form of chlorine itself has limited usefulness as a disinfectant because the gas is difficult to handle. The antibacterial action of chlorine is said to be caused by the formation of hypochlorous acids, which results when chlorine reacts with water. Therefore chlorine-containing products that can release hypochlorous acid are in use today.

sodium hypochlorite solution

Common household bleaches are usually 5% solutions of sodium hypochlorite. Therapeutic solutions are unstable and must be freshly prepared before use.

Indications

Sodium hypochlorite solution, 1% is used to sterilize equipment; the 0.5% solution is sometimes used as an antiseptic for wound irrigation (see Nursing Management of Chlorine Compounds below).

Adverse Effects

This solution is of limited usefulness for wound irrigations, except for debridement purposes, because they are irritating to the skin and delay the clotting process.

oxychlorosene
(Clorpactin WCS-90)

Oxychlorosene is a combination product that contains hypochlorous acid, which when released is effective (bactericidal) against both gram-negative and gram-positive organisms, fungi, yeast, viruses, molds, and spores.

Indications

Oxychlorosene is indicated for the treatment of localized infections, especially if caused by resistant organisms, and for cleansing and irrigating necrotic debris, wounds, sinus tracts, and empyemas. Dilutions of this product are also used in urology and ophthalmology.

Adverse Effects

Local irritation or discomfort is the most common adverse effect of oxychlorosene.

Nursing Management of Chlorine Compounds Dakin's solution, a diluted 0.5% sodium hypochlorite solution adjusted to a neutral pH with sodium bicarbonate, was once widely used to treat suppurating wounds, but its solvent action delays clotting.

Store chlorine products in marked containers and out of the reach of children. If a chlorine agent is swallowed, a poison control center should be contacted and emergency treatment sought. Store these products away from light and in airtight containers if possible. Avoid spills on skin or delicate tissues because it will cause irritation. Avoid spills on clothing or contact with hair because of its bleaching properties. Rinse thoroughly with clear water if a spill occurs.

See the Evidence-Based Practice box below for information on the use of hypochlorite solutions for preventing the spread of acquired immune deficiency syndrome (AIDS) among intravenous (IV) drug users.

Iodine and Iodophors

Iodine is slightly soluble in water but is soluble in alcohol and in aqueous solutions of sodium and potassium iodide. Iodine is volatile, and solutions should not be exposed to air except during use. In its elemental or free form, iodine is very rapidly bactericidal, viricidal, fungicidal, and lethal to protozoa; it is less effective against spores. It is one of the most efficient chemical disinfectants and antiseptics currently in use.

Some iodine compounds are believed to be superior to other antiseptics, because all types of bacteria may be destroyed with a single concentration of iodine and because it is effective over a wide pH range. Organic matter interferes with the potency of iodine only when it is first applied; effectiveness later increases because of diffusion as the iodine complexes dissociate. This initial delayed effect in the presence of organic material may also be offset by the increased strengths of solution concentrations now on the market.

Iodine solution is used for the treatment of minor wounds, abrasions, and infected wounds; iodine tincture is preferred for intact skin procedures, such as skin preparation before invasive procedures, Hickman catheter and parenteral nutrition dressing changes, and IV needle insertions. Aqueous solutions are thought to be as effective as tincture of iodine for similar therapeutic purposes; because they are less irritating, they are used for abraded skin areas. The various iodine compounds marketed for antisepsis and disinfection include Iodine Topical and Iodine

 Evidence-Based Practice

Effectiveness of Bleach Distribution to Prevent HIV Transmission

IV drug users risk human immunodeficiency virus (HIV) infection from sexual contact and from sharing injection equipment—needles, syringes, or other items—with infected individuals. Although protective changes in behavior have been reported among other high-risk populations in the late 1990s, most IV drug users continue to place themselves at risk. The growing importance of drug use as a mode of HIV transmission has led to increased attention to AIDS prevention among IV drug users. However, the Centers for Disease Control and Prevention (CDC) (2005) reports a resurgence of risky behavior and high rates of new infection among young men who have sex with men.

Siegel, Weinstein, and Fineberg (1991) were among the earlier researchers to examine the effectiveness of bleach distribution, which is a program to prevent HIV transmission via shared needles. Bleach programs employ outreach workers to distribute small bottles of bleach, which IV drug users use to disinfect their injection equipment. An important argument for the implementation of bleach programs has been that they are more politically feasible than needle exchange programs. They examined whether and to what extent the initial HIV prevalence among IV drug users influences program effectiveness. Because of the difficulty of conducting longitudinal surveys of transient populations of IV drug users prevents studies of existing programs, they used a Markov model to provide a practical means for studying the conditions that determine the success of bleach programs.

This model incorporates survey data on risk behaviors and published information describing HIV incubation and mortality. It predicts life expectancy for cohorts of IV drug users with and without a bleach program to estimate program effectiveness.

They found that bleach programs can produce the greatest life-year savings in areas of low HIV prevalence. In the lowest-prevalence scenario (0.02 initial prevalence), initiation of the program resulted in a projected savings of 2.3 life years per HIV-negative drug user, compared with 1.7 and 1.3 years under medium- (0.25) and high- (0.60) prevalence scenarios, respectively. The investigators concluded that bleach programs are beneficial to all groups of IV drug users and that these results highlight the advantages of introducing bleach programs early—when prevalence is still comparatively low in a drug-user population.

In 2000, Romanelli, Smith, and Pomeroy reviewed controlled studies cited in MEDLINE between 1966 and 1999 to review the efficacy, safety, and proper methods for the use of bleach for needle disinfection. They concluded that, used properly, undiluted bleach reduces the risk of HIV transmission from needle sharing among IV drug users. Those who receive more education about safe needle use and/or those involved in needle exchange programs are less likely to share needles, and if they do, to consistently use bleach with used needles (Ouellet, Huo, & Bailey, 2004).

Critical Thinking Questions

- Because HIV prevalence among drug users can increase rapidly, what do you think the opportunities are for early intervention with bleach programs?
- In your own community, what types of programs are available for IV drug users to prevent the spread of HIV? If a bleach program is not available, how would you go about instituting one?

Tincture (the most commonly used iodine antiseptic). Although they both contain 2% iodine and 2.4% sodium iodide, the solution is in water, whereas the tincture has 47% alcohol.

Iodine is toxic if taken internally. It is locally corrosive to GI tissues but is inactivated by GI contents. Iodine tincture may be transiently quite painful when applied to open skin areas, but the aqueous solution form stings only slightly. These agents may be absorbed through the skin and may affect thyroid function with chronic use. Neonates have developed hypothyroidism following the topical application of povidone-iodine. Marked hypersensitivity reactions occasionally occur, even with topical application; they are manifested by severe systemic reactions of fever and generalized skin eruptions.

iodophor: povidone-iodine
(Betadine, Operand)
Indications
Povidone-iodine is considered an iodophor that is widely used as an antiseptic. This is the only purpose for which it has FDA approval, although in practice iodophors continue to be used to disinfect certain equipment.
Pharmacokinetics/Formulations
Iodophors are a group of iodine compounds combined with povidone (carrier), which increases the water solubility of iodine and provides a slow release of iodine. It has the same germicidal action of iodine without irritating the skin and mucous membranes. Povidone-iodines are available in many formulations, such as solution, 2% scrub, spray, foam, vaginal gel and suppositories, ointment, mouthwash, or perineal wash.
Adverse Effects
Rash, pruritus, and local edema are the most common adverse effects of povidone-iodine. Ingested orally, it is highly toxic and sodium thiosulfate is used as an antidote.
Nursing Management
Iodine compounds and iodophors are exceptionally valuable because of their efficiency, low toxicity, and low cost. Before applying iodine compounds and iodophors, ask the client about any past allergic reactions to iodine, shellfish, or iodine-containing diagnostic agents. If there is any doubt, substitute another product. Do not use povidone-iodine as a vaginal douche during pregnancy.

The client is at risk for impaired skin integrity related to hypersensitivity or local irritation, and impaired comfort with iodine tincture related to pain and stinging on application of the agent. Observe the area for irritation not present at the initiation of therapy. Monitor the lesions on a periodic basis for healing. Do not bandage or tape areas treated with tincture of iodine. A cover dressing may be applied if necessary after treatment with povidone-iodine. Wash the skin if irritation develops.

Artificially elevated blood glucose determinations have been noted when povidone-iodine swabs are used for skin preparation. Soap and water cleansing of the fingertips before skin puncture for blood glucose monitoring by some reagent strips is recommended.

Iodophors will stain only starched linen or clothing. Tinctures and solutions of iodine may stain more freely.

Advise the client to purchase iodine preparations in very small quantities and to discard them routinely after a short time, because evaporation of the solvent or vehicle will leave a concentrated iodine preparation that may burn tissues on application. The expected outcome of using iodine compounds and iodophors is that the client will demonstrate signs of wound healing within an appropriate time frame. If the agent is used as an antiseptic to prepare for a procedure, there will be no evidence of sepsis following the procedure.

Oxidizing Agents

Hydrogen peroxide is the most commonly used oxidizing antiseptic. Similar agents include carbamide peroxide (Debrox) used for ear wax removal, and benzoyl peroxide used in the treatment of acne.

hydrogen peroxide
Hydrogen peroxide is a weak antiseptic; when in contact with a tissue enzyme (catalase), it is converted to effervescent oxygen to produce an antibacterial action and cleansing effect on the wound. The presence of blood and pus decreases the efficacy of hydrogen peroxide. The antiseptic action of hydrogen peroxide is fairly fast acting and short-lived; it acts as an antibacterial agent only as long as the bubbling action continues.

The oxygen that is released is particularly suited for destroying aerobic microorganisms in wounds, but as an antibacterial it is weak and slow. However, its effervescent action provides a mechanical effect to aid in removing foreign tissue debris. Several products containing hydrogen peroxide are marketed.
Indications
Hydrogen peroxide topical solution is available in a 3% solution in water and is used to irrigate suppurating wounds and some extensive traumatic wounds, and disinfect soft contact lens. It should be used in areas in which the oxygen can escape and therefore should not be instilled into closed body spaces or abscesses. It is not recommended for use in pressure ulcers, because it and many other antiseptic agents are considered to be cytotoxic to normal tissues. The official hydrogen peroxide solution has been further diluted with water into a one-half or one-fourth strength for most applications. The mouth rinse or mouthwash (Peroxyl) is a 1.5% solution.
Adverse Effects
If a small amount of diluted hydrogen peroxide solution is swallowed, it rapidly decomposes in the stomach into relatively harmless molecular oxygen and water. Repeated use as a mouthwash may cause hypertrophied papillae of the tongue ("hairy tongue"), a reversible condition. The concentrated solutions used for hair bleaching may cause skin irritation and contact dermatitis.
Nursing Management
To delay deterioration of the contents, store solutions in tightly capped, amber containers to protect them from light and air. Solutions in containers should be discarded frequently, and fresh solutions should be used. The rapidity and vigor with which bubbling occurs may be used as a general guide to the freshness of the solution. The bubbling action makes hydrogen peroxide useful for removing mucus secretions from equipment (e.g., inner cannulae of tracheostomy tubes).

Do not leave paper cups containing hydrogen peroxide where clients can reach them. Because the solution looks like water, clients have mistakenly drunk it despite the unusual taste. Although very small amounts are not harmful, large amounts in the stomach can be harmful because of the resultant effervescence in the stomach, a closed cavity. As with all medications, these compounds should be kept secured and out of children's reach.

Biguanides

The most commonly used biguanide is chlorhexidine.

chlorhexidine [klor **hex** i deen]
(Hibiclens)
Chlorhexidine is a biguanide with antiseptic action against both gram-positive and gram-negative bacteria, such as *Pseudomonas*

aeruginosa. Chlorhexidine acts by disrupting the plasma membrane of the bacterial cell (particularly gram-positive organisms).

A bactericidal skin cleansing solution containing chlorhexidine (Hibiclens) is useful as a surgical scrub, as a handwashing agent for personnel, and as a skin wound cleanser. Chlorhexidine oral rinse (Peridex, PerioGard) is also used as an antibacterial dental product to treat gingivitis between dental visits.

Indications
Chlorhexidine is used as a skin cleaner prior to surgery, as a cleaner for superficial wounds, and as an oral rinse for dental conditions.

Dosing
As a hand wash, Hibiclens solution is applied, water added, and friction applied for 15 seconds. Skin wounds should be washed gently with Hibiclens and rinsed. For surgical scrubs, a brush or sponge is used to scrub the hands and forearms with approximately 5 mL Hibiclens for 3 minutes without water. After the hands and forearms are rinsed, the washing is repeated for 3 more minutes.

Adverse Effects
Chlorhexidine is a relatively safe antiseptic. There have been reports of deafness occurring when these products came into contact with the middle ear through a perforated eardrum. Rare secondary effects include dermatitis, photosensitivity, and irritation of mucosal tissue. The physiochemical properties of these agents suggest that absorption through the skin is minimal.

Nursing Management
Use judgment when diluting these agents, because their effectiveness may be greatly reduced in proportion to the dilution. Certain solutions less than 4% may actually support bacterial growth. Chlorhexidine-treated areas should not be wiped with alcohol; this will neutralize the intended residual action. Do not use chlorhexidine on delicate tissues such as eyes and mucous membranes; these areas should be rinsed promptly if contact occurs. Advise clients not to swallow chlorhexidine compounds (especially when used for mouth care).

Surface-Active Agents

As wetting agents, emulsifiers, or detergents, surface-acting agents are considered superior to soap because they can be used in hard water, are stable in acid or alkaline solutions, decrease surface tension more effectively, and are less irritating to the skin. Benzalkonium chloride is the most commonly used of the surface-acting agents.

benzalkonium chloride [benz al **koe** nee um]
(Zephiran Chloride)
Benzalkonium chloride is a cationic (has a positive electric charge on the active portion of the agent) quaternary ammonium compound used in solution as a topical antiseptic or as a disinfectant. In general, it is believed that benzalkonium chloride is not very reliable in either role. As an antiseptic it has a limited antibacterial spectrum, because it lacks fast action and has a potential for inducing toxicity. As a disinfectant, it must be changed regularly to maintain concentration and effectiveness. It is also inactivated by anionic substances such as soap and organic materials.

The mechanism of action is not known for certain, but it may be due to the inactivation of bacterial enzymes. Benzalkonium chloride is slow acting in comparison to iodine. The therapeutic effects are thought to be in direct relation to the concentration of the solution used. Depending on the purpose and tissues or equipment to be treated, recommended dilutions range from 1:750 (tincture or aqueous solutions) on intact skin, minor wounds, and abrasions to 1:5000 or 1:10,000 (aqueous solution) for mucous membranes and broken or diseased skin. A variety of gram-positive and gram-

negative organisms and many fungi and viruses (not hepatitis) are said to be susceptible to this agent. Tap water that contains metallic ions, organic matter, or resin-unionized water may reduce its effectiveness.

Indications
Benzalkonium chloride is used as an antiseptic for topical use. Because of its limited spectrum of activity and duration of action, the use of this agent has waned.

Adverse Effects
Chemical burns may occur if benzalkonium chloride is allowed to stay in contact with tissues, as in wet packs or occlusive dressings. Delicate tissues may be injured if specified dilution recommendations are not used. Ingestion only rarely causes toxicity. Hypersensitivity reactions can occur. The tincture and the spray formulations are flammable.

Nursing Management
If benzalkonium chloride has been used, continue to monitor the area or utensil critically for contamination. In view of the highly questionable efficacy of surface-active agents, especially benzalkonium chloride, question an order or a suggestion to use them as antiseptics or disinfectants. Suggest the substitution of an iodophor, alcohol, or other compound. Use only the concentration recommended for each specified area. Do not use them with occlusive dressings.

Do not apply these compounds to areas previously treated with soaps or anionic agents. Do not apply them to delicate tissues. Flood the area with water if these agents are accidentally introduced. Do not reuse solutions after soaking cotton balls, dressings, or instruments.

Avoid using benzalkonium chloride to disinfect thermometers. If it must be used, use not less than the recommended 1:750 concentration. Do not use the tincture of spray formulation near an open flame.

Alcohols

ethanol [**eth** a nole]
(ethyl alcohol)
isopropanol [eye soe **proe** pa nole]
(isopropyl alcohol)
Ethyl alcohol and isopropyl alcohol are the two more frequently used antiseptics. Ethyl alcohol is slightly less effective as an antiseptic than isopropyl alcohol. Its efficacy may depend on the concentration used and the amount of mechanical friction applied. The most effective solutions of ethyl alcohol are concentrations of 50% to 70%; stronger solutions are less effective. At concentrations of 70%, almost 90% of the bacteria on the skin are killed within 2 minutes if the wet surface is allowed to dry naturally. Inadequate disinfection may occasionally result, even if friction is conscientiously applied to surfaces.

Isopropyl alcohol is used in aqueous solutions of 70% concentration or undiluted as 99% concentration (isopropyl rubbing alcohol). It may be combined with other disinfectants such as iodine and formaldehyde to improve efficiency.

A 70% alcohol solution is antiseptic. The 70% aqueous solution is more effective than absolute alcohol in reducing the surface tension of bacterial cells, which precipitates protoplasm at the periphery of the cell and thus tends to inhibit penetration of the agent. Alcohol also inhibits the growth of bacteria, and thus it is often used as a preservative of biologic specimens and in some prepackaged injectables and medications. Alcohols are potent viricidal agents and may precipitate cellular proteins.

Indications
Alcohol is used topically as a bactericidal agent; to prepare skin for minor invasive procedures (using commercially packaged skin wipes); and for disinfection of heat-labile instruments, polyethylene tubing, catheters, implants, prostheses, smooth/hard-surfaced objects,

hinged instruments, and inhalation and anesthesia equipment. Because of their rapid evaporation rate, dilute solutions of alcohols are still used occasionally as sponge baths to reduce fever, although systemic absorption may be especially harmful to neonates and children. Alcohols are also used as preservatives in solutions, as diluents, to dissolve other drugs, and in combination with many other drugs for over-the-counter (OTC) purchase (often without rationale). Ethyl alcohol is also ingested purposefully as an intoxicating beverage.

Adverse Effects
Depending on the dose, essentially all alcohols are poisonous drugs when taken internally. Isopropyl alcohol is inherently highly poisonous. Ethyl alcohol is pure alcohol made from vegetables, fruits, canes, and grains, and it is used in alcoholic beverages. The degree to which fractional distillation is carried out determines the resultant concentration.

Alcohols can cause intoxication when continuously inhaled or absorbed through the skin. Ethyl alcohol is irritating if left in contact with the skin for prolonged periods. If ethyl alcohol is applied to open skin, a film develops and can harbor microorganisms. Isopropyl alcohol causes subcutaneous vasodilation, which can cause needle sites and incisions to bleed somewhat more freely.

Nursing Management
Do not use alcohols to disinfect wounds, because they cause tissue irritation with painful burning and stinging and because they precipitate protein in which bacteria may grow. The use of alcohol to reduce body temperature is more for the management of hyperthermia in heat stroke or malignant hyperthermia than fever secondary to infection. Use alcohols as a rub with caution for children, because the inhalation of fumes may be intoxicating, and absorption through the skin is possible. There is a risk for poisoning in children and debilitated clients, because they are at risk for accidental exposure to or ingestion of these agents. If alcohol is applied externally to reduce fever in an adult, the client's temperature should be monitored regularly; such use in children should be avoided. Applying an emollient alleviates the dry feeling of the skin after an alcohol rub.

The antiseptic action of alcohols can be enhanced by mechanically cleansing the skin with water and a detergent before applying them, by gently rubbing the skin with a sterile gauze during application, and by allowing the area to dry for 2 minutes without fanning. Be prepared to apply more pressure and possibly a small pressure dressing after giving an injection or discontinuing an IV infusion if alcohol has been applied to the site, because evaporation of the alcohol may cause localized surface vasodilation. If the client is also receiving anticoagulant therapy, the bleeding may be extensive.

If alcohol is used in a home setting to disinfect thermometers, cleanse them with detergent and tepid water before placing them to soak in an alcohol solution; any adherent organic matter will inhibit the action of the solution. Alcohol solutions themselves may harbor organisms and may rust instruments; therefore they are often not the best solution for disinfecting or for sterile storage of equipment.

Alert personnel, clients, and parents that all alcohols are inherently or potentially poisonous and that intoxication or dangerous poisoning can occur as a result of their absorption, inhalation, or ingestion. Keep alcohols secured and out of the reach of children.

Although not recommended, topical alcohol has been used for fever reduction with the expected outcome of normalizing the client's temperature. If it is used as an antiseptic to prepare the skin for a procedure, there will be no evidence of sepsis following the procedure.

Acids

Various acids have been used as antiseptics or as cauterizing agents; of these, vinegar is the most commonly used, especially in community health nursing, because of its practicality, availability, and low cost. Other acids used as anti-

septics include benzoic acid (0.1%), which prevents bacterial and fungous growth; lactic acid, which is used primarily as a component of spermatocides in the United States; and boric acid, which is so mild that it is used in eye and ear preparations. Of these other acids, most have lost credibility as effective antiseptics; for example, boric acid has been implicated in cases of serious systemic intoxication by absorption.

acetic acid (vinegar)
Acetic acid provides an acid medium that inhibits the growth of organisms dependent on a neutral or alkaline medium. In a 5% concentration, acetic acid is germicidal to many organisms and is bacteriostatic at lower concentrations. A mild vinegar solution is often recommended as a vaginal douche for antisepsis in the prevention or suppression of vaginal infections. Acetic acid may also be used as a mild antiseptic-deodorant for many other applications, such as bladder irrigation (0.25% concentration) and diaper soaks.

Nursing Management
A mildly effective, soothing vaginal douche can be prepared by adding 1 to 2 tablespoons of white household vinegar (5%) to 1 quart of warm water. Stronger concentrations are no more effective and may irritate mucosal tissues. The residual pungent odor of acetic acid may be a deterrent to its use.

The use of aseptic technique is essential when irrigating solutions are used for urethral catheters. The solution should not be used unless it is clear and the container is undamaged and has an intact seal. To minimize bacterial growth, the solution is to be used promptly after opening the container. Unused portions of the solutions should be discarded. Antiseptics instilled in urinary collection bags should be of concentrations that are not injurious to bladder mucosa in case the bag is inadvertently raised so that contents reflux into the bladder.

⚙ **How are sterilants differentiated from antiseptics and disinfectants?**
Sterilants are highly effective at killing microorganisms and spores and are used to sterilize surgical or other equipment. They differ from antiseptics in that they should not be directly applied to living tissue. They are more effective against a broad range of pathogens compared to disinfectants. The aldehydes, formaldehyde and glutaraldehyde, are the two most commonly used chemical sterilants. Other means to sterilize equipment include gas and temperature or steam procedures, which are beyond the scope of this text.

Aldehydes

formaldehyde solution
Formaldehyde solution is a 37% concentration of formalin (by weight). It is a clear, colorless disinfectant liquid that liberates a pungent, irritating gas on exposure to air. In a concentration of 1% to 10%, it kills microorganisms and spores within 1 to 6 hours. It is effective against bacteria, fungi, and viruses and acts by combining with them to precipitate protein. It has been widely used as a disinfectant for instruments.

glutaraldehyde [gloo tuh **ral** dah hyde] (Cidex)
Glutaraldehyde (Cidex), 2% alkaline solution, is a liquid disinfectant used as a germicidal agent to disinfect and sterilize some rigid opti-

cal instruments and prosthetic equipment. It kills some microorganisms in 10 minutes and kills spores in 10 hours. However, the solution is unstable, and contact with skin should be avoided.

Summary

Medical asepsis and surgical asepsis are used in health care settings to reduce the number and spread of organisms. Although thorough handwashing is still the best method for accomplishing this reduction, antiseptics, disinfectants, and sterilants need to be used. Antiseptics are chemicals typically applied to living tissue to decrease the microbial population; disinfectants are used only on nonliving objects because they are caustic to living tissue. Antiseptics and disinfectants may be bacteriostatic, bactericidal, or both depending on the concentrations used. Sterilants free objects of all forms and types of life. Although these substances are used for therapeutic purposes, they still are caustic and therefore require careful handling to prevent irritation and injury.

✳ Critical Thinking Questions

- Given the criteria for the ideal antiseptic/disinfectant, which of the agents in this chapter would be closest to the ideal? Why?

- Mrs. Taylor, 24 years old, was prescribed pHisoHex for her preoperative facial scrubs for the rhinoplasty she was having as a day-stay case. When she comes to the clinic for a postoperative follow-up visit, she asks about using the leftover pHisoHex for her baby's diaper rash. How do you respond?

Bibliography

Abate, B.J., & Barriere, S.L. (2002). Antimicrobial regimen selection. In J.T. DiPiro, R.L. Talbert, G.C. Yee, G.R. Matzke, B.G. Wells & L.M. Posey (Eds.), *Pharmacotherapy: A pathophysiological approach* (5th ed.). Norwalk, CT: Appleton & Lange.

Aiello, A.E., & Larson E. (2003). Antibacterial cleaning and hygiene products as an emerging risk factor for antibiotic resistance in the community. *The Lancet Infectious Diseases, 3*(8), 501-506.

Anderson, D.M., Keith, J., & Novak, P.D. (Eds.) (2002). *Mosby's medical, nursing, and allied health dictionary* (6th ed.). St. Louis: Mosby.

Centers for Disease Control and Prevention. (2005). HIV prevalence, unrecognized infection, and HIV testing among men who have sex with men: Five U.S. cities, June 2004—April 2005. *Morbidity and Mortality Weekly Report, 52,* 597-601.

Dastychova, E., Necas, M., Pencikova, K., & Cerny, P. (2004). [Contact sensitization to pharmaceutic aids in dermatologic cosmetic and external use preparations]. [Czech] *Ceska a Slovenska Farmacie, 53*(3), 151-156.

Drug facts and comparisons (58th ed.). (2005). St. Louis: Facts and Comparisons.

FDA Talk Paper T97-31. (July 14, 1997). FDA approves first toothpaste for gum disease. Retrieved September 19, 2004, from http://www.fda.gov/bbs/topics/ANSWERS/ANS00807.html.

Guglielmo, B.J. (2005). Principles of infectious diseases. In M.A. Koda-Kimble, L.Y. Young, W.A. Kradjan, B.J. Guglielmo, B.K. Alldredge, & R.L. Corelli (Eds.), *Applied therapeutics: The clinical use of drugs* (8th ed.). Philadelphia: Lippincott Williams & Wilkins.

Knodel, L.C. (2002). Sexually transmitted diseases. In J.T. DiPiro, R.L. Talbert, G.C. Yee, G.R. Matzke, B.G. Wells & L.M. Posey (Eds.), *Pharmacotherapy: A pathophysiological approach* (5th ed.). Norwalk, CT: Appleton & Lange.

Larson, E., Aiello, A., Lee, L.V., Della-Latta, P., Gomez-Duarte, C. & Lin, S. (2003) Short- and long-term effects of handwashing with antimicrobial or plain soap in the community. *Journal of Community Health, 28*(2), 139-150.

Larson, E.L., Lin, S.X., Gomez-Pichardo, C., & Della-Latta, P. (2004). Effect of antibacterial home cleaning and handwashing products on infectious disease symptoms: a randomized, double-blind trial. *Annals of Internal Medicine, 140*(5), 321-329.

Ouellet, L., Huo, D., Bailey, S.L. (2004). HIV risk practices among needle exchange users and nonusers in Chicago. *JAIDS Journal of Acquired Immune Deficiency Syndromes, 37*(1), 1187-1196.

Romanelli, F., Smith, K.M., & Pomeroy, C. (2000). Reducing the transmission of HIV-1: needle bleaching as a means of disinfection. *Journal of the American Pharmaceutical Association, 40*(6), 812-817.

Russell, A.D. (2004). Whither triclosan? *Journal of Antimicrobial Chemotherapy, 53*(5), 693-695.

Sabaliunas, D., Webb, S.F., Hauk, A., Jacob, M., & Eckhoff, W.S. (2003). Environmental fate of triclosan in the River Aire basin, UK. *Water Research, 37*(13), 3145-3154.

Siegel, J.E., Weinstein, M.C., & Fineberg, H.V. (1991). Bleach programs for preventing AIDS among IV users: Modeling the impact of HIV prevalence. *American Journal of Public Health, 81*(10), 1273-1279.

U.S. Food and Drug Administration. (2004). Over-the-counter drug products: Safety and efficacy review; additional antigingivitis/antiplaque ingredient (July 6, 2004). Retrieved September 19, 2004, from http://www.fda.gov/OHRMS/DOCKETS/98fr/04-15136.htm.

USP DI: Drug information for the health care professional (25th ed.). (2005). Greenwood Village, CO: MICROMEDEX Thomson Healthcare.

ℓ-LEARNING SUPPLEMENTS

Student CD-ROM
- Final Exam questions
- NCLEX® Examination review questions
- Pharmacology animations
- Printable chapter summary

Evolve Website (http://evolve.elsevier.com/mckenry)
- Content updates, including information on new drugs
- WebLinks corresponding to this chapter

- Content updates, including information on new drugs
- WebLinks corresponding to this chapter
- Answers to the critical thinking questions in this chapter
- *Elsevier ePharmacology Update* newsletter
- Mosby's Drug Consult Internet Edition
- Supplemental and reference information

DIAGNOSTIC AGENTS

71

CHAPTER FOCUS

Diagnostic and laboratory tests are a key source of information for the nurse in the assessment and ongoing monitoring of clients. The nurse is also responsible for preparing the client for diagnostic studies and for coordinating their completion. Many of these examinations require diagnostic agents with which the nurse must be knowledgeable to provide appropriate instruction and care for clients undergoing diagnostic testing.

LEARNING OBJECTIVES

- Describe the mechanism of action of a radiopaque contrast medium.
- State the method of absorption, metabolism, and excretion of barium sulfate and iodinated contrast media.
- Describe the nursing assessments necessary to detect adverse effects of iodinated contrast medium and the appropriate nursing interventions to manage the initial symptoms.
- Explain the pharmacokinetics of diagnostic agents used as radioactive tracers and imaging agents.
- State the indications, secondary effects, and nursing management of common nonradioactive agents used for evaluating organ function and challenging glandular response.
- Identify the common tests used to screen selected health conditions.

▲ KEY TERMS

computed tomography (CT), p. 1279
diagnostic agents, p. 1273
nuclear magnetic resonance imaging (MRI), p. 1279

radionuclides, p. 1277
radiopharmaceutical agents, p. 1277
scintigraph, p. 1275
ultrasonography, p. 1279

✴ What is the role of diagnostic agents in clinical medicine?

Diagnostic agents are chemical substances used to diagnose or monitor a client's condition or disease. With diagnostic agents, certain secondary chemical characteristics are used to confirm a diagnosis or prognosis or to guide therapy. One type of diagnostic agent may interact with a bodily fluid specimen as a reagent to produce a color as an indicator, whereas another may induce an inflammatory response or enhance the functioning of a particular gland.

Other agents may act by contrasting and enhancing visibility on an x-ray film of the lumens or cavities of internal body structures. Some permit critical assessment of organ function because of a special affinity and uptake by certain organs. As with any drug, diagnostic agents may have adverse effects. Thus it is necessary that the nurse know the agent used, its mechanism of action, and its indications for use. Secondary effects are equally important, because many agents have a somewhat narrow range of safety. In some instances, nurses are responsible for correctly collecting and testing specimens and interpreting the results. Specialized training and professional education are necessary to administer some types of agents; others are packaged in simple kit form for over-the-counter (OTC) sale. Because the field of diagnostics and its products is burgeoning, always consult manufacturers' instructions to ensure the most current information is obtained.

✱ **P.S. is a 52-year-old female with unstable angina who is undergoing cardiac catheterization to evaluate her coronary artery disease (CAD). As part of the cardiac catheterization procedure, the interventional cardiologists are planning to use radiocontrast dye to better visualize her coronary arteries.**

✱ **What radiopaque agents are used to visualize organ and vessel structures?**
Ordinary radiograph examinations are useful only for studies of dense materials such as bone. However, when injected or instilled, radiopaque agents make the body cavity, compartment, or blood vessels more radiographically dense or opaque than neighboring anatomic structures. They are used when the structural integrity of a soft-tissue organ system is under study. Radiopaque contrast media may also permit visualization of the functional dynamics of organs as part of associated diagnostic tests.

Many of these agents contain molecular iodine in the radiopaque contrast medium to provide the opacity necessary for outlining internal organ cavities, lumens, or ducts that would otherwise be invisible by radiograph or fluoroscopy. Because many iodinated radiopaque agents can produce hypersensitivity reactions and contribute to renal failure, except for angiography, they have largely been replaced by other tests such as ultrasonography, computed tomography (CT) scans, and magnetic resonance imaging (MRI). Newer, lower osmolar, low ionic agents are also more frequently used to prevent renal toxicity when a contrast agent is required (see Chapter 35).

Barium contrast media consist of barium sulfate powder and a vehicle such as hydrosol gum, that are mixed with a prescribed volume of water to provide a suspension for oral or rectal administration. Iodinated radiopaque agents consist of substituted, triiodinated, benzoic acid derivatives or water-soluble, triiodinated, benzoic acid salts. Check the manufacturers' instructions for ingredients.

Consult with the prescriber when a client reports a history of idiosyncratic response; a hypersensitivity to iodine, shellfish, or contrast media; or a history of multiple radiographic or radionuclide studies. The most common radiopaque contrast agents are barium sulfate suspensions and iodinated contrast materials.

Barium Salts

barium sulfate
Indications
Barium-containing preparations are typically used to opacify the gastrointestinal (GI) tract. In general, these preparations are used when peptic ulcers, inflammatory bowel disease, or cancer are suspected. One of the most common uses of barium contrast media is in "double-contrast" studies for GI tract evaluation. "Double contrast" is a method of making an radiograph image by using two contrast agents—usually a gaseous medium and a water-soluble radiopaque agent.

Pharmacokinetics
Barium sulfate preparations are typically administered enterally and not absorbed.

Adverse Effects
Because they are not absorbed internally, barium sulfate preparations are only potentially hazardous when administered to persons with bowel perforations or fistulas. Barium sulfate may cause constipation if allowed to remain in the colon. Hospitalization and close observation during the procedures are recommended for clients who have a high potential for reactions or complications.

Iodinated Contrast Agents

These agents vary in their ionic states and degree of osmolality. These factors may affect their tolerability (specifically their ability to induce renal toxicity). Refer to package inserts for more complete information on each product.

diatrizoate/iopidamide [dye a tri **zoe**-ate/eye-oh **di** pa mide]
(Sinografin)
iohexol [eye oh **hex** ole]
(Omnipaque-140, Omnipaque-180, Omnipaque-210, Omnipaque-240, Omnipaque-300, Omnipaque-350)
iopamidol [eye oh **pa** mi dole]
(Isovue-128, Isovue-200, Isovue-250, Isovue-300, Isovue-370, Isovue-M 200, Isovue-M 300)
iothalamate [eye oh **thal** a mate]
(Angio-Conray, Conray 325, Conray 400)
ioversol [eye oh **ver** sole]
(Optiray 160, Optiray 240, Optiray 300, Optiray 320, Optiray 350)
ioxaglate [eye **oks** a glate]
(Hexabrix, Hexabrix-200, Hexibrix-320)
ioxilan [eye **oks** ee lan]
(Oxilan)
metrizamide [me **tri** za mide]
(Amipaque)
Indications
The most common clinical use of iodinated contrast media is angiography. Iodinated contrast media are often used during CT of the head and body to visualize vascular structures and to detect tumors.

Pharmacokinetics
Radiopaque agents may be administered by the oral, vaginal, rectal, IV, or intraarterial routes, or they may be instilled into other body cavities. Orally administered iodinated agents for visualization of the gallbladder are absorbed across gastrointestinal (GI) mucosa and enter the systemic circulation through the portal venous system. Orally or rectally administered iodinated media for delineation of the GI tract are absorbed only minimally but are absorbed enough that the renal tract may also be visualized. They are metabolized by the liver and gallbladder and excreted by the kidneys.

Adverse Effects
Radiopaque agents are not without risk. The effects are diverse, mild to moderate in severity, and usually occur within 1 to 3 minutes. Delayed reactions may occur up to 1 hour after injection. Anaphylaxis and hypersensitivity reactions are also reported.

Serious reactions are rare with excretory urography. Although oral preparations to visualize the gallbladder are still available, these drugs have been replaced by ultrasonography and nuclear cholescintigraphy. A **scintigraph** is a photographic recording that shows the distribution and intensity of radioactivity in various tissues and organs following administration of a radiopharmaceutical. Certain radiopaque agents are more likely to cause secondary effects than others; consult the manufacturers' information.

A client with a history of allergy is at twice the risk of reaction to contrast media although, paradoxically, these are not true hypersensitivity reactions. Clients with a previous anaphylactoid reaction to contrast media may have an increased risk of tenfold or more (*Drug Facts and Comparisons*, 2005).

The most commonly reported adverse effects are nausea or flushing, with feelings of warmth over the abdomen and chest. Severely dehydrated clients, older adults, infants, and the seriously ill tolerate these hemodynamic and hyperosmolar changes less well than others.

Rare adverse effects include cerebral hematomas, hemodynamic alterations, sinus bradycardia, transient electrocardiogram (ECG) changes, ventricular fibrillation, and petechiae.

Renal system involvement may be manifested by nephrosis of the proximal tubular cells in excretory urography; this condition may proceed to renal failure. Acute tubular necrosis (ATN) is among the more common adverse effects observed with contrast dyes. Factors associated with higher risk for developing ATN include preexisting renal disease, heart failure, diabetes with nephropathy, dehydration, and frequent use or high dose of contrast media. The risk for ATN may be lower when using agents with lower osmolality or nonionic agents and may therefore be preferred for clients with these risks (Brophy, 2005).

Altered respiratory status may include rhinitis, cough, dyspnea, bronchospasm, asthma, laryngeal or pulmonary edema, and subclinical pulmonary emboli.

The senses may be impaired (e.g., distorted taste sensations; irritated, itching, tearing eyes; conjunctivitis). Hypersensitivity reactions and anaphylaxis may occur.

Table 71-1 lists the iodine content of and indications for selected agents.

✱ What are the nursing implications for the use of radiopaque agents with P.S.?

Assessment Radiographic examinations are not without hazard to clients or to personnel. The risk-benefit ratio must be established on an individual basis for P.S. Reactions may arise from either the physical or the chemical properties of the compounds used. Almost any organ system may be affected (see Adverse Effects on p. 1274). Conduct a careful history with P.S. related to kidney, thyroid, or liver disease. Obtain her allergy history, and pay particular attention to any previous reactions she may have had to contrast media or iodine-containing foods (e.g., shellfish or iodized table salt). For clients with a history of iodine hypersensitivity and those with a generally positive allergy history, pretreatment with prednisone, diphenhydramine (Benadryl), and an H_2 blocker has minimized the incidence of a severe reaction (e.g., bronchospasm, shock) to less than one percent (Carroza & Baim, 2004). Do not mix these pretreatment medications for concurrent administration with the contrast media; they are physically incompatible.

Assess if at 52 years of age if P.S. has experienced menopause. It is recommended that radiography, fluoroscopy, or CT not be performed on female clients if they are pregnant or if it has been 10 days since their last menstrual period.

Withhold medications during the preparation period for examinations using radiopaque agents. Although not a concern for P.S., consult with the prescriber for instructions with other clients for essential medications, such as antivirals or medications for epilepsy.

Perform a baseline assessment of P.S.'s vital signs, mental status, and level of consciousness before the testing procedure.

Nursing Diagnosis While P.S. is receiving radiopaque agents for diagnostic testing, she is at risk for the following nursing diagnoses/collaborative problems: impaired comfort (flushing of the skin, nausea); impaired tissue integrity related to irritation or extravasation at the injection site; and the potential complications of hypersensitivity to the agent, nephrotoxicity, and adverse cardiovascular and central nervous system (CNS) effects of the agent. If she were receiving barium for a GI diagnosis, she would be at risk for barium-related concerns, such as constipation.

Planning As the result of being administered a radiopaque preparation, P.S. will:
- Undergo successful diagnostic testing without experiencing adverse effects.

Implementation

Monitoring Monitor levels of consciousness and vital signs during and after the procedure according to protocol. Monitor for flushing of the skin, nausea, symptoms of anaphylaxis, extravasation, and other untoward effects of the agents.

Intervention Prepare P.S. appropriately for her examination using protocols from the cardiac interventionist.

Tests involving barium are performed in radiology. Barium sulfate compounds are noniodinated, and most are prepared from powders for suspensions to be taken orally or instilled rectally. The volume of orally administered reconstituted agents is approximately 8 ounces; the enema volume may range from 500 to 1500 mL. Older adults should be hydrated before and after barium tests to help prevent posttest constipation.

Ask for lead shielding devices and client-supporting devices before participating in radiographic examinations. Nurses who are often involved in such examinations should monitor their cumulative exposure by wearing a dosimeter badge that is checked monthly or quarterly. It is worn outside any shields, and reports are obtained.

A bedpan, an emesis basin, tissues, and a warm blanket are transported with P.S. to the testing area (the room temperature and the equipment in testing facilities are often noted to be cold). Have drugs, equipment, and medical assistance readily available in case of an emergency such as anaphylaxis or cardiac arrest.

TABLE 71-1 SELECTED DIAGNOSTIC AGENTS, INDICATIONS, AND IODINE CONTENT

Agent	Indications	Iodine Content
CONTRAST MEDIA		
diatrizoate meglumine 30% (Reno-Dip)	Computed tomography Pyelography Venography	141 mg/mL
diatrizoate meglumine 60% (Reno-60)	Computed tomography Cerebral angiography Venography	282 mg/mL
diatrizoate meglumine 66% and diatrizoate sodium 10% (Gastrografin)	Radiography of GI tract Computed tomography	367 mg/mL
diatrizoate sodium injection (Hypaque Sodium)	Angiography Aortography Cholangiography Computed tomography	300 mg/mL (50% solution)
iodipamide meglumine (Cholografin)	Cholangiography Cholecystography	257 mg/mL

iodixanol (Visipaque 270; Visipaque 320)*	Angiocardiography
	Visceral arteriography
	Cerebral arteriography
	  (Visipaque 320 only)
	Peripheral venography
	  (Visipaque 270 only)
		270 mg/mL
		320 mg/mL

iohexol (Omnipaque 140, Omnipaque 240, Omnipaque 300, Omnipaque 350)*	Myelography Computed tomography Angiocardiography	140 mg/mL 240 mg/mL 300 mg/mL 350 mg/mL
iopamidol (Isovue-200, Isovue-250, Isovue-300, Isovue-370)*	Myelography Computed tomography	200 mg/mL 250 mg/mL 300 mg/mL 350 mg/mL
iopanoic acid (Telepaque)	Oral cholecystography	333 mg/500 mg tablet
iopromide (Ultravist 150, Ultravist 240, Ultravist 300, Ultravist 370)	Peripheral angiography Cerebral arteriography Coronary arteriography	150 mg/mL 240 mg/mL 300 mg/mL 370 mg/mL
ioversol (Optiray 160, Optiray 240, Optiray 300, Optiray 320)*	Angiography Venography Urography Computed tomography	160 mg/mL 240 mg/mL 300 mg/mL 320 mg/mL
OTHER AGENTS		
amiodarone (Cordarone)	Antidysrhythmic	9 mg/300 mg dose
iodoquinol (Yodoxin)	Antiprotozoal	134 mg/210 mg/tablet
echothiophate iodide ophthalmic (Phospholine Iodide)	Antiglaucoma Cyclostimulant Diagnostic aid	5-41 mcg/drop
idoxuridine ophthalmic (Herplex, Stoxil)	Antiviral	18 mcg/drop

Data from *Mosby's drug consult* (15th ed.). (2005). St. Louis: Mosby; *Drug facts and comparisons* (58th ed.). (2005). St. Louis: Facts and Comparisons; and *USP DI: Drug information for the health care professional* (25th ed.). (2005). Greenwood Village, CO: MICROMEDEX Thomson Healthcare.

* Nonionic iodine contrast media; more hydrophilic than ionic agents; associated with a lower incidence of adverse effects and anaphylactoid reactions.

After a barium enema, obtain an order for a laxative to prevent constipation, or similarly instruct the client.

Education Apprise P.S. and other clients and all those working in an environment of ionizing radiation that there may be current and long-term effects of radiation, that are cumulative. There is no established safe dosage, single or cumulative; therefore keep exposure to a minimum. The risks and benefits of each procedure should be weighed carefully by the clinician and the informed client.

Instruct clients, as appropriate, to prepare for the specific examination. This may require the client to take the agent with water the night before the procedure, to receive an enema, or not to ingest anything but water until the test is completed. For barium, explain as appropriate that the procedure may include the administration of approximately 8 ounces of a fairly thick oral suspension or a retention enema and that position changes may be necessary during the procedure. Advise the client to take a laxative to help prevent constipation following a procedure that uses barium.

Evaluation The expected outcome of the use of a radiopaque agent is that P.S. will complete the diagnostic procedure successfully without experiencing any adverse reactions to the agent (e.g., ECG changes, ATN, anaphylaxis).

⚙ What agents are used to evaluate organ function?

Some diagnostic agents can be used to track and visualize the functional processes of organ systems. Inferences can be made about organ function by measuring the degree to which or the rate at which the agent is distributed, taken up, sequestered, secreted, or excreted from the target organ system or by measuring the volume or flow rates. Some diagnostic agents are **radionuclides** (a species of radioactive atom characterized by a higher atomic number than bodily tissues) whose gamma-ray emissions can be tracked or whose residues can be sampled. Other nonradioactive agents are dyes, polysaccharides, or other substances whose dissemination may be traced by color changes or chemical analysis.

Radioactive Agents

A radionuclide is an unstable form of a chemical element. **Radiopharmaceutical agents** are those in which one of the nonradioactive atoms has been replaced by a radioactive atom. They are either of natural origin or are produced by particle accelerators or generators. The process of neutron activation used in nuclear medicine to produce radionuclides describes the capture of a slow neutron into a stable nucleus with the subsequent emission of a gamma ray. Transmutation is a similar operation but uses a fast neutron. After the injection or ingestion of the resultant nuclide, its distribution can be followed by a gamma-ray detector combined with a rectilinear scanner, scintillation camera, or other radiation-display device. Substances such as glucose, ^{14}C, air, blood, lymph, spinal fluids, urine, or biopsy specimens may be collected and the residual radioactivity analyzed or counted as it is excreted. These data are used to make inferences about organ disorders and the body's ability to absorb, metabolize, or excrete substances.

Ionizing Radiation Through the use of radiation, much can be learned that could not otherwise be discovered or diagnosed. As with any other diagnostic technique, a risk-benefit ratio must be determined. Ionizing radiation has the ability to knock electrons out of atoms to create electrically charged ions. This radiation may be defined as electromagnetic radiation (x-rays and gamma rays) or particulate radiation (electrons, occasionally β particles, protons, neutrons, or atomic nuclei with kinetic energy).

Impact by emitted radiation energy may disrupt bonds between atoms in crucial biologic molecules such as deoxyribonucleic acid (DNA). Disruption can lead to cell death, mutations, or defective mitosis. Energy that is absorbed by tissues can lead to acute effects (as in radiotherapy or radiation accidents) or chronic effects (as from multiple low-radiation doses). Effects such as cataracts may appear only after long periods or in subsequent generations.

The amount of radiation absorbed by the tissues during radiologic tests is determined by the dose administered, the half-life of the radionuclide, the energy, the mode of decay, and the length of time the agent dwells in the body. There is no known safe dosage of ionizing radiation, despite limits set by the Nuclear Regulatory Commission and the National Council on Radiation, Protection and Measurements.

Estimations of the amount of radiation emitted, the effect, and the dose absorbed may be denoted by the following terms:

- *Roentgen:* the amount of gamma or x-ray radiation that creates 1 electrostatic unit of ions in 1 mL of air at 0°C
- *Rem:* the predicted effect on the human body of a 1-roentgen dose
- *Rad:* a unit of measurement of absorbed ionizing radiation energy; one rad equals 100 ergs of radiation energy per gram of matter

Although arbitrary, the annual limits of radiation for the general population and for any single gestational period are set at 0.5 rem (for x-rays, 1 rem is equal to 1 rad) and for closely monitored occupational workers at approximately 3 rem/year. Most nurses, physicians, and other health care personnel are not routinely monitored for radiation exposure unless assigned to an area with a high potential for exposure. Their risk for cumulative exposure is nonetheless higher than that of the general population. Very little is known about the full effects of radiation. Certain increased risks are associated: infertility, birth defects, potential for certain malignant neoplasms, and manifestations of aging. Exposure to low-level ionizing radiation (e.g., from radiographic examinations) and agents containing radionuclides add to the individual's total radiation history. The effects may be insidious, perhaps manifesting themselves in crucial enzyme defects many years after exposure. There is some evidence of the body's ability to repair chromosomal damage, but the scope of this ability is unknown.

The term *excessive radiation exposure* describes any unnecessary exposure above natural background levels. Although natural background radiation adds to the cumulative risk, medical and dental therapies account for the largest proportion of artificially generated exposure.

Indications for Radionuclides Most radionuclides in use today in radiology are for imaging organs, evaluating organ function, or detecting or treating cancer. The role of nuclear imaging is gradually diminishing because of increased reliance on CT, ultrasound, and MRI.

Radionuclides are used as tracers to evaluate the physiologic and biochemical functioning of organ systems. With imaging methods, extremely sensitive radioactivity sensing devices make it possible to detect, count, visualize, and analyze minute amounts of radionuclides. Uniquely useful applications of nuclear imagery include the following:

- *Assessing thyroid enlargement or disease:* Agents currently used include ^{131}I and ^{123}I. These iodine isotopes emit a type of radiation that can be mapped externally. A 24-hour uptake study is usually used to determine the extent and areas of thyroid activity. A scan is then performed to evaluate any thyroid mass or enlargement. "Cold" tumors have a 20% to 25% probability of representing a thyroid cancer. Tumors that localize the radionuclide well are usually benign.
- *Screening clients with diagnosed malignancies for metastases:* Many clients treated for breast cancer, colon cancer, malignant melanoma, lymphoma, prostate cancer, lung cancer, and other cancers are often successfully evaluated by periodic scintigrams of the liver, spleen, and skeletal system. The risk-benefit ratio is very high, and information about new or recurrent disease can help the oncologist and the client make crucial decisions about goals, management, prognosis, and so forth.
- *Evaluating heart disease:* This is a primary application of nuclear imagery. Computers are used to analyze data from the images to detect the extent of myocardial damage and wall motion abnormalities and to estimate the ejection fraction of the ventricles. Underlying CAD can also be estimated with radionuclides before catheterization or other invasive procedures.
- *Tracking physiologic substances and assessing the status of an organ:* Radiopharmaceuticals are sometimes used to evaluate or follow biliary excretion or renal function. In addition to diagnostic uses, some radiopharmaceuticals may be administered therapeutically to deliver radiation to internal body tissues (e.g., ^{131}I to destroy thyroid tissue in hyperthyroidism). Radioactive tracer substances may also be incorporated into a nonradioactive drug to track the pharmacokinetics of the second drug for research purposes.

Pharmacokinetic/Dosing Issues for Radionuclides
Each type of radionuclide emits α or β particles or γ rays or a combination of these. This spontaneous emission of charged particles is termed *radioactive decay* and eventually results in disintegration of the nucleus. The time it takes for the original radioactivity to decay to one half its original value is known as the physical or radioactive *half-life* of the particular radionuclide. As with drugs, the rate at which a tracer substance is excreted from the body also influences its effects, both valuable and undesirable.

The manufacturers' current directions should be reviewed. Dosages are not detailed here because they vary with the needs of the client. The major considerations in radionuclide dosing are the amount of radioactivity that is administered to produce effective readings and secondary radionuclide effects. Although the radioactive material is in the body, it irradiates even after the study has been completed; in contrast, x-rays irradiate from an external source and do so only while the body is exposed during the examination. The radionuclide dosage unit for imaging or nonimaging doses of radionuclide is a *microcurie* (one millionth of a curie). A *curie* is a specified measure of radioactivity associated with a specific amount of a radioactive substance (e.g., a radionuclide). Recommended dosages are spelled out in the manufacturers' literature. The client's absorbed dose of each radionuclide has been predicted for each procedure, with the following three factors being considered: (1) the biologic parameters that describe the uptake, distribution, retention, and release of the radiopharmaceutical in the body; (2) the energy released by the radionuclide and whether it is penetrating or nonpenetrating; and (3) the fraction of emitted energy that is absorbed by the target.

The ultimate radiation dose to both the target organ and the entire body is somewhat less in radionuclide nonimaging procedures than in imaging procedures. It is considerably more in radiation therapy, which is not discussed here.

Protecting the Client and Staff Against Unnecessary Radiation Exposure Shielding is a practical method to prevent or reduce the excess radiation exposure of staff or clients during certain diagnostic examinations. Shielding reduces the intensity of radiation to acceptable limits in body areas not intended for exposure during the radiologic examination. α and β radiation require very little shielding. An α particle can be blocked by the thickness of a sheet of paper, and a β particle can be blocked by an inch of wood; however, several feet of concrete or several inches of lead are necessary to stop γ ray or x-ray radiation. *Half-value layer* is the term describing the thickness of any material required to reduce the intensity of an x-ray or gamma-ray beam to half its original value. Because of its characteristic density, lead is the material typically used for radiation shielding equipment and for coverings such as aprons and gloves.

Imaging Technologies

A number of imaging technologies are commonly utilized in diagnostics. Computer tomography uses radiation, whereas ultrasound and magnetic resonance imaging do not.

Computed tomography (CT) scans body parts in a series of contiguous slices with pencil-thin x-ray beams; after these beams pass through the body, they produce data from detectors positioned diametrically across from the beam source. Huge amounts of data are integrated and displayed by the computer as a video image. CT presents a series of two-dimensional images that represent a reconstructed "slice" in the axial plane. By viewing a series of these images, the anatomy can be perceived in a three-dimensional sense. CT therefore often conveys more information than other modalities about lesion density, location, and size.

CT has largely replaced older techniques such as pneumoencephalography and angiography in the diagnosis of intracranial disease, although angiography is still used for this application. CT may eliminate the need for other x-ray examinations, but it is not considered a first-line or screening technique. Radionuclide scans continue to be used for initial diagnostic screening and for specific tests in which their results are more fruitful. Radiation exposure from CT varies depending on the equipment used and the frequency of testing, but it is said to be equal to or sometimes considerably higher than ordinary x-ray techniques or radionuclides. Although CT is considered to be a noninvasive procedure, IV contrast material is often injected to enhance structures for differential diagnosis. This is referred to as CT with infusion.

Ultrasonography is a nonradioactive diagnostic modality with cardiovascular, abdominal, obstetric, and other applications. It is used with anatomic and physiologic information obtained by other nuclear medicine techniques. Ultrasound examinations yield data about organ contours and tissue consistency or, in the case of Doppler scanning, blood flow patterns. Results can be distorted by the presence of bone or gases in the body. The secondary effects of high-frequency sound waves on cellular structures and functions are not fully known, but such tests are considered to be noninvasive and innocuous by many in the field.

Nuclear magnetic resonance imaging (MRI) is a diagnostic modality that uses radio waves and a magnet, rather than radiation, drugs, biopsy specimens, or body fluids. Like CT, MRI provides sectioned imagery but gives more than the gross anatomic information gained by CT scanning. MRI supplies extremely detailed images of internal heart and brain structures, and it is capable of imaging areas of the spine, abdomen, and extremities. It can differentiate between lesions and normal tissue. Persons ineligible for diagnosis with MRI include those with metal prostheses or pacemakers, because the strong magnetic field surrounding the client may move some metallic devices, or the metallic object may result in a distorted test image.

✳ What are the nursing management issues involved in these technologies?

The basic principles of radiation exposure safety are relative to the source of radiation, the *time* spent in the radioactive field, the *distance* from the source, and *shielding*. The amount of radiation absorbed is directly proportional to the time spent in a radioactive field and inversely related to the distance from the source of radioactive emission. Thus quality nursing care requires careful planning so that limitations on time spent in the radioactive field do not reduce the quality of client care.

Wear rubber or plastic gloves when handling bedpans, urine specimens, or continuous drainage bags of clients within a day or two after nuclear medicine procedures. Wherever radionuclides are used, one person (designated the radiation safety officer) has the responsibility for safety in case of spills or accidents with radioactive materials. Consult this officer if there is a break in safety procedures or if, for example, linen has been contaminated by vomitus or excreta within 24 hours of administration of a radiopharmaceutical. Although it may be determined that unusual precautions are not needed, it is wise to seek consultation as needed.

Follow the instructions of the radiopharmaceutical manufacturers about radionuclide storage (some require refrigeration), security, dosage, and technique. Errors in technique must not be tolerated, especially regarding handling radiopharmaceuticals, disposing of contaminated equipment, and properly shielding all who are present for radiologic and imaging procedures. Monitoring badges are worn by those who regularly participate in these procedures. Protection should be ensured for those who are unfamiliar with these procedures. Women of childbearing age who had their last menstrual period more than 10 days ago or who are pregnant should not assist. (*Radiation therapy* requires other precautions.)

The client's anxiety may be heightened by the uncertainty of unknown diagnosis, a fear of radiation, and cold or unfamiliar surroundings. Give clients written instructions explaining the procedure and how to prepare for it. At the time of the exam, introduce them to the personnel and orient them to the surroundings and large equipment before the scheduled examination, with an opportunity for questions and explanations.

Teach clients that there might be some discomfort at the site of injection, taste alterations, or a feeling of warmth or discomfort in various parts of the body if the administered agent contains an iodine preparation. If a counter or rectilinear scanner is used, advise clients that it may typically emit irregular clicks as it collects data; it does not emit radiation. Clients may be required to maintain a single position on a hard surface for extended periods, or they may be restrained for a brief period; supply foam wedge supports and coverings as necessary. Explain that personnel may wear strange-looking apparel to shield them from excess radiation and that clients will also be protected according to established protocols.

Give clients written instructions, especially about the specific time they should return for the examination after the nuclide dose. Explain that the test must be performed at a very specific time after the medication is administered (at the point of a specific half-life).

Follow the policies of the health care agency regarding the length, frequency, and duration of exposure to clients in the posttest period. Additionally, provide instructions for caring for the client at home.

✷ What alternatives are available to evaluate organ function?

Nonradioactive Agents for Evaluating Organ Function via Volumes and Flows

These relatively biologically inert and nonradioactive substances are commonly used to measure flow rates, fluid volumes, diffusion, concentration ability, and organ function. These compounds are mostly dyes, polysaccharides, or other substances that can be assayed chemically or detected by characteristic colors after administration. Many of the dye tests determine the rate of plasma clearance of the dye by the organ under study. The ability to measure certain parameters against known normal values at defined points in the procedure makes these compounds useful as diagnostic aids. They are used variously to evaluate processes such as cardiac output, liver or kidney function, blood flow, circulation time, and intestinal absorption. Urine testing prod-

ucts are commonly used by nurses in primary care settings (e.g., the Multistix 10 SG, a dipstick that tests for the presence of glucose, protein, blood, ketones, bilirubin, urobilinogen, nitrites, and leukocytes, as well as the pH and specific gravity).

Some nonradioactive compounds are administered primarily by the intravenous (IV) or intramuscular (IM) routes. They are rapidly absorbed by the organ system under examination and are usually excreted by that system. These drugs are relatively pharmacologically inert and are used to measure specific physiologic functions without themselves significantly altering those functions (Table 71-2).

Nonradioactive Agents for Challenging Glandular/Organ Response

Certain compounds are used diagnostically to challenge a particular system (often glandular) to produce measurable responses. Secretory responses indicate whether or not there is functional integrity within the secreting gland or system.

TABLE 71-2 SELECTED NONRADIOACTIVE AGENTS FOR EVALUATION OF ORGAN FUNCTION

Agent	Indication(s)	Secondary Effects	Nursing Management
aminohippurate sodium	Measures effective renal plasma flow (ERPF) and the functional capacity of the renal tubular secretory mechanism.	Vasomotor disturbances, flushing, nausea, vomiting, cramping, and tingling	Give IV at a constant rate. Use caution with clients with low cardiac reserve; because a rapid increase in plasma volume can precipitate heart failure. Clients may have a sensation of warmth or the desire to defecate or urinate during or shortly following initiation of infusion. Have atropine at hand to relieve severe cholinergic reactions.
D-xylose (Xylo-Pfan)	Evaluates intestinal absorption; aids in providing an index of degree of impairment and extent of therapy in malabsorption syndromes.	Infrequent: nausea, intestinal bloating, vomiting, cramps, and diarrhea	A number of medical conditions give false-positives with this test; check the literature.
indocyanine green (IC Green)	Measures cardiac output, hepatic function and liver blood flow, used for ophthalmic angiography	Anaphylactic or urticarial reactions have been reported in clients with or without history of allergy to iodides.	Use caution with clients who have a history of iodide allergy. If such reactions occur, treatment with the appropriate agents, e.g., epinephrine, antihistamines, and corticosteroids should be administered. Radioactive iodine uptake studies should not be performed for at least a week following the use of indocyanine green. IV injection.

Data from *Mosby's drug consult* (15th ed.). (2005). St. Louis: Mosby.

Many of these testing agents are protein substances that mimic the action of naturally occurring bodily chemicals, such as secretagogues for exocrine gland response and stimulants for endocrine secretion. Because most of these agents are administered intramuscularly or intravenously, they move rapidly to the site of action. The degradation of these agents is equally rapid.

Nonradioactive agents are used to evaluate or enhance capabilities such as thyroid secretion, gallbladder contraction, insulin response, and gastric acid secretory function. These testing agents act on the targeted gland or site as releasing factors. Thus the secondary effects may be as widespread and disruptive to bodily chemical balance as a large dose of the secretion or hormone itself (Table 71-3).

Epinephrine, antihistamines, corticoids, and a tourniquet should be readily available for all tests in case of severe reactions. Analgesics, nasogastric suction equipment, vasodilators (for histamine agents), IV glucose solutions (for tolbutamide), and atropine (for edrophonium) should also be kept available. Follow the manufacturers' instructions very closely, because nearly all of these compounds are administered parenterally and in very small doses.

✳ What agents are available to screen or alter immune reactions?

Extracts of common allergens (ragweed, grasses, trees, molds, animal dander, and foods) are used by allergists to screen for specific allergies. Administered in minute doses by regular injection, such agents may serve to alter the degree of reactivity to the specific allergen administered. Purified derivatives or concentrates of microbial antigens are used to diagnose exposure to conditions (e.g., intradermal tuberculin) or to test for immune function (e.g., intradermal extracts of *Candida* or *Trichophyton*).

Antigens applied topically or intradermally cause antigen-antibody reactions that may be manifested by a local

TABLE 71-3 SELECTED NONRADIOACTIVE AGENTS FOR EVALUATION OF BODY RESPONSE

Agent	Indication	Secondary Effects	Nursing Management
dipyridamole (Persantine)	Diagnostic aid for coronary artery disease	Coronary artery vasodilator, antiplatelet	Dosed at 0.14 mg/kg/minute for four minutes up to a maximum dose of 60 mg during cardiac stress testing. Monitor for bronchospasm and unstable angina. Bronchospasm may be reversed with aminophylline.
edrophonium (Tensilon)	Myasthenia gravis, cholinergic stimulant	Severe cholinergic reaction, bradycardia or cardiac standstill, dysrhythmias	Have 1 mg IV atropine available to relieve the adverse muscarinic effects of edrophonium. Monitor vital signs carefully. Have facilities available for CPR, cardiac monitoring, and respiratory assistance. A placebo may be administered first as if it were the test dose to evaluate baseline muscular capabilities. A number of drugs may be withheld for at least 8 hours; check with the prescriber.
protirelin (Thypinone)	Thyroid function	Blood pressure alterations, breast enlargement, nausea, increased urination, dizziness, dry mouth, headache	Have client urinate and assume a supine position. Drug is administered as a bolus over 15-30 seconds. Measure blood pressure at frequent intervals for the first 15 minutes. Increases in blood pressure (less than 30 mm Hg) are more common than decreases. Use caution in clients for whom rapid changes in blood pressure would be dangerous.
sincalide (Kinevac)	Gallbladder and pancreatic function	Hypersensitivity, nausea, cramps, dizziness, flushing	Administered IV. Adverse effects usually occur immediately after the injection and last for a few minutes.
tolbutamide (Orinase Diagnostic)	Pancreatic islet cell function	Severe hypoglycemia	Instruct the client to adhere to a 150-300 g/day carbohydrate diet for 3 days before the test and to fast overnight. Avoid smoking during fasting and during the test. Tolbutamide is not administered to clients who have known sensitivities to the drug or other sulfonylurea drugs. For 3 days before the examination, withhold salicylates and other drugs known to potentiate the hypoglycemic action of tolbutamide (see Chapter 49). If severe hypoglycemia occurs during the test, administer 12.5-25 g of glucose in a 25%-50% IV.

inflammatory response at the test site. The test site is assessed after a prescribed time interval. A positive response is indicated by the presence of erythema and induration (a firm lump under the skin). In the case of microbial antigen challenge, this positive response may merely indicate a previous exposure to the microbe or its products; it does not necessarily indicate the presence of an active disease process. False negative results may also occur, and further investigation may be necessary. The size of the erythematous area or induration may be measured to estimate the degree of the client's sensitivity or immune response. These responses may be short lived or of lifelong duration. (See also Chapter 62.)

Clients who are immunosuppressed because of cancer chemotherapy or radiation treatments, malnutrition, debilitation, or congenital or acquired immunodeficiency syndrome (AIDS) may demonstrate no response (anergy) when tested with a prescribed battery of antigen challenges. These clients are extremely vulnerable to infection and may need metabolic support and precautions to avoid infection. Test results may not be reliable in those who have viral infections, are febrile or uremic, or have recently received live viral vaccinations.

Indications Some diagnostic agents measure a client's physiologic response or hypersensitivity to the agent as a specific chemical challenge. These agents are typically used in simple baseline screening procedures as part of an initial diagnostic workup. Some are used in skin tests by patch, prick, scratch, or intradermal injection to assess hypersensitivity (allergy), anergy (congenital or acquired inability to develop a cell-mediated reaction), cellular immunity, or antibody response (Table 71-4). Others are used as reagents in specimens of blood, urine, and bodily discharges to detect the levels of certain components to facilitate diagnosis or to monitor known conditions (Table 71-5).

Adverse Effects Local reactions to skin tests do not usually cause discomfort. Occasionally a highly positive reaction will result in vesiculation and necrosis of the overlying skin, and corticosteroids may be ordered. Transient tachycardia, malaise, or low-grade fever may occur separately from a local reaction. Occasionally a client may report systemic allergic reactions of urticaria, sneezing, or dyspnea. An overwhelming antigen-antibody response (anaphylactic response) is rare but can occur; such a reaction calls for emergency measures such as the administration of epinephrine and respiratory and circulatory support. These secondary effects are more likely to occur if hyposensitization therapy is begun, because this includes a well-controlled program of increasing dosages of the allergen in question.

Dosage For certain standardized tests such as that for coccidioidomycosis, the dosage is fixed (0.1 mL of a 1:100 dilution). Dosages for allergy testing are also very small (0.02 to 0.05 mL) and typically are extensively diluted but may be individualized. The manufacturers' instructions for all these diagnostic agents should be followed carefully.

✷ What are the nursing management issues for these agents?

Assessment Depending on the diagnostic agent used and the procedure in which it is administered, determine a clinical baseline for the physiological factors being tested and systems that might be affected by an adverse effect.

Nursing Diagnosis While clients are receiving nonradioactive or screening agents, they may experience the following nursing diagnoses/collaborative problems: impaired comfort (flushing of the skin, nausea, rash); impaired tissue integrity related to irritation or extravasation at the injection site; and the potential complications of hypersensitivity to the agent, nephrotoxicity, and adverse cardiovascular effects of the agent.

Planning After being administered a nonradioactive or screening agent, the client will have an accurate diagnosis made without experiencing adverse effects.

Implementation
  Monitoring Be prepared for major allergic manifestations such as angioedema, urticaria, serum sickness, or anaphylactic shock, which can occur. Have the client wait for 30 minutes to observe for development of an allergic reaction.

TABLE 71-4 BIOLOGIC AGENTS USED FOR DIAGNOSTIC TESTS

Biologic Product*	Indication/Adult Dosage
Tuberculin (purified protein derivative [PPD])	Indication: tuberculosis. Adult dosage: 5 U.S. units (Tu), intradermal following specific instructions as noted by manufacturer or *USP DI*.
Allergenic extracts	Several hundred individual purified fluid allergens are available for diagnosis and hyposensitization of allergies: pollens, poison ivy, foods, dusts, yeast, and other allergens. Treatment: periodic subcutaneous injection of gradually increasing potent dilutions of a specific allergen.

*See the nursing management for each of these agents.

TABLE 71-5 COMMON TESTS FOR SCREENING SELECTED CONDITIONS

Identifies/Detects	Test(s)	Available Forms
Ketones in blood or urine	Acetone tests: Acetest, Chemstrip K, Ketostix	Tablets, strips
Protein in urine	Albumin tests: Albustix, Chemstrip Micral	Strips
Nitrates, nitrite, uropathogens, bacteria	Microstix-3, Uricult, Isocult for Bacteriuria, UTI Urinary Tract Infection Urine Test Strips	Culture paddles, strips
Bilirubin in urine	Ictotest	Tablets
Urea nitrogen in blood	Azostix	Strips
Candida albicans, vaginal	Isocult for *Candida*, CandidaSure	Culture paddles, reagent slides
Chlamydia trachomatis for urogenital, rectal, conjunctival or nasopharyngeal specimens	Chlamydiazyme, Amplicor, Sure Cell Chlamydia	Reagent kits
Cholesterol in blood	Advanced Care Cholesterol Test—for home use	Cassette
Color allergy screening for serum	CAST	Reagent sticks
Cryptococcus neoformans in cerebrospinal fluids and serum	Crypto-LA	Slide tests
Drugs of abuse in urine	Dr. Brown's Home Drug Testing System	Kits
Gastrointestinal: duodenal fluid or stomach acid	Entero-Test, Gastro-Test,	String capsules
H. pylori test of gastric urease in breath samples	PYtest	Capsules
Glucose in blood	Chemstrip bG, Diascan, Glucostix, Glucometer Encore, and others	Strips
Glucose in urine	Clinitest, Chemstrip bG, Chemstrip UG, Clinistix, Diastix	Tablets, strips
N. gonorrhoeae in urogenital, rectal and oropharyngeal specimens	Biocult-GC, Gonozyme Diagnostic, and others	Kits
Hemoglobin, glycated for blood	A1cNow	Kits
Human immunodeficiency virus (HIV) tests	HIV-1 LA Recombigen HIV-1 Latex Agglutination Test, HIVAB HIV-1 EIA, and others	Kits
Mononucleosis in serum or plasma	Mono-Diff, Mono-Latex, and others	Reagent kits
Occult blood screening	ColoCARE, Colo-Screen, and others	Reagent kits, slide tests
Ovulation tests to measure luteinizing hormone for prediction of ovulation	Answer Ovulation, Clearplan Easy, Ovu-Quick Self-Test, Color Ovulation Test, and others	Kits
Human chorionic gonadotropin pregnancy tests	Advance, Answer Plus, Answer Quick & Simple, Fact Plus, and others	Kits, sticks
Rheumatoid factor in blood	Rheumatex, Rheumaton	Slide tests
Hemoglobin S sickle cell test	Sickledex	Kit
Staphylococcus aureus in exudate	Isocult for *Staphylococcus aureus*	Culture paddles
Streptococci tests	Sure Cell Streptococci, Bactigen B Streptococcus-CS, and others	Kits, slide tests
Virus tests, miscellaneous	Human T-Lymphotropic Virus Type, Sure Cell Herpes, Rubazyme for Rubella, and others	Reagent kits, slide tests

Data from *Drug facts and comparisons* (58th ed.). (2005). St. Louis: Facts and Comparisons.

Intervention Administer screening agents with care because of their propensity to trigger allergic reactions. Question the client regarding any previous reactions to skin testing. If the client responds positively, contact the prescriber to clarify orders. Often a dilute test dose of less than one tenth the usual concentration may be administered.

For skin testing for allergies, inspect the liquid extract of the antigen for clarity; do not use it if particles are seen. As appropriate, administer these diagnostic test agents using one of the methods described in the following paragraphs.

A sterile needle or other instrument may be used to prick or scratch the skin after a drop of the extract is placed on the skin. Depending on the approach used, the results may be read directly or after removing the testing patch.

Intradermal injections are commonly administered on the ventral surface of the forearm. Use a tuberculin syringe with a 25- to 27-gauge needle. Inject intradermally with the needle nearly parallel to the skin surface, making certain that the needle does not penetrate deeper into subcutaneous tissue. This intradermal insertion will increase the precision with which the results may be interpreted; it will also prevent febrile reactions to tuberculin tests.

Stop inserting the needle as soon as the tip of the needle, with its bevel up, has entered the skin but is still visible. Inject the antigen with steady pressure. A correctly administered intradermal injection will immediately raise a small, colorless bleb or lump.

Have medications available for emergency administration, such as antihistamines (e.g., diphenhydramine and epinephrine, 0.2 mL for subcutaneous use). Equipment for full circulatory and respiratory support should also be available.

After the injection there is a prescribed wait—often 20 minutes or several days (depending on the antigen)—before the local reaction is assessed for erythema and induration. A positive reaction to some antigens is determined by the presence of induration alone; erythema is not always a criterion. *Erythema* (redness) is categorized as follows:

Trace	Faint discoloration
+ (one plus)	Pink
+ +	Red
+ + +	Purplish red
+ + + +	Vesiculation or necrosis

Measure the single largest induration (area of hardness) or the largest coalesced induration. Induration can be measured with precision by using the following technique:

- Place your index, middle, and ring fingers together, and stroke the test site to determine the presence of induration.
- To delimit the indurated area, use a ballpoint pen to draw a line toward the indurated area in four direc-

tions. The edges of the induration can easily be perceived as the ballpoint tip touches them; stop each marking when the edge is perceived.
- Measure the diameter of the remaining unmarked indurated area in millimeters, or use the following criteria for indurations:

Trace	Barely palpable
+	Palpable, but not visible
+ +	Easily palpable and visible; indurated area buckles when squeezed gently
+ + +	Easily palpable and visible; does not buckle when squeezed gently
+ + + +	Vesiculation or necrosis

Criteria used to categorize Mantoux tuberculin test results according to the induration diameter are as follows: less than 5 mm is a negative result; 5 to 9 mm is a questionable result (retesting by another method may be necessary), and more than 9 mm is a positive result.

Indurations resulting from multiple-puncture tuberculin testing devices are interpreted as positive if they have a diameter of more than 2 mm. Results from multiple-puncture tuberculin tests are considered less reliable than the results of Mantoux tests.

Education Instruct the client about the nature of the test and the possible benefits and adverse effects (e.g., localized vesiculation or necrosis, anaphylaxis). Advise the client of the time frame for returning to the site to have the results of a skin test determined.

Evaluation The client will be accurately diagnosed without experiencing adverse effects from the testing procedure.

Summary

Diagnostic agents are chemical substances used to diagnose or monitor a condition or disease. As with other drugs, they may also produce adverse effects. Radiopaque agents are used for visualizing organ or vascular structure. Examinations used for evaluating organ function involve radioactive agents, computed tomography, ultrasonography, and nuclear magnetic resonance imaging. Nonradioactive agents may be used for evaluating organ function via volumes and flows and for challenging a glandular response. Other agents are available for screening and monitoring immune status and disorders. It is essential that the nurse know the agent used, its mechanism of action and indications, and how to prevent or minimize any adverse effects.

✴ Critical Thinking Questions

- Bobby Brown, 24 years old, a newly hired teacher, is required by the school board to have a medical history and physical examination, including diagnostic skin testing with tuberculin (the PPD test), before his employment is finalized. Why would the PPD be included? What would constitute a positive response for a PPD? What would a positive response indicate? Suppose Mr. Brown tells the nurse who is about to administer his PPD that he has had a positive response to the test in the past. What action should the nurse take?

- Sally Grey, 54 years old, has been advised by her health care provider to get a mammogram every year. She confesses to you that she is concerned about excessive radiation exposure. How will you respond?

Bibliography

Anderson, D.M., Keith, J., & Novak, P.D. (Eds.). (2002). *Mosby's medical, nursing, and allied health dictionary* (6th ed.). St. Louis: Mosby.

Brophy, D.F. (2005). Acute renal failure. In M.A. Koda-Kimble, L.Y. Young, W.A. Kradjan, B.J. Guglielmo, B.K. Alldredge, & R.L. Corelli (Eds.), *Applied therapeutics: The clinical use of drugs* (8th ed.). Philadelphia: Lippincott Williams & Wilkins.

Carroza, J.P., & Baim, D.S. (2004). Complications of diagnostic cardiac catheterization. Wellesley, MA: *UpToDate.*

Drug facts and comparisons (58th ed.). (2005). St. Louis: Facts and Comparisons.

Kee, J.L. (2005). *Laboratory and diagnostic tests with nursing implications* (7th ed.). Upper Saddle River, NJ: Pearson Education, Inc.

Mosby's drug consult (15th ed.). (2005). St. Louis: Mosby.

USP DI: Drug information for the health care professional (25th ed.). (2005). Greenwood Village, CO: MICROMEDEX Thomson Healthcare.

e-LEARNING SUPPLEMENTS

72

POISONS AND ANTIDOTES

CHAPTER FOCUS

As with most critical illnesses, an assessment followed by the appropriate interventions will influence the ultimate outcome for the client with poisoning. The role of the nurse is important not only in the assessment and treatment of such clients but also in the teaching of safety promotion and accident prevention to keep poisonings from occurring. In an age of terrorism preparedness, recognition and management of widely disseminated toxin exposure is also an important nursing role.

LEARNING OBJECTIVES

- Identify the major causes of poisoning in children of various ages.
- List at least five objective and/or subjective nursing assessments of a client presenting with a suspected poisoning.
- Describe the four grades of drug overdose–induced coma.
- Identify the major drugs causing organ or tissue damage resulting from chemical poisoning.
- Implement the nursing management for a client with suspected poisoning.
- Implement the nursing management for the pharmacologic treatment of methanol, cyanide, iron, and insecticide overdose.

▲ KEY TERMS

acute poisoning, p. 1287
chronic poisoning, p. 1287
gastric lavage, p. 1294

poison, p. 1287
toxicology, p. 1287
toxidromes, p. 1290

✳ What is the nature of poisonings in North America?
On an average day, more than 6000 poison exposures related to drugs, plants or chemicals are reported to poison control centers in the United States. Between 2000 and 2500 exposures per day are related to pharmaceuticals. Nonpharmaceuticals account for between 3000 and 5000 exposures per day, with higher rates noted during summer. In Canada, 100,000 children and youth less than 15 years of age fall victim to poisoning each year (Sanfacon, 2001). Ninety percent of exposures take place in the home (Watson et al., 2004).

Of the nearly 2.4 million poisoning exposures reported in the United States in 2003, 1106 resulted in death. Although children less than 6 years of age account for 52% of exposures reported, they only account for 3.1% of fatalities. Those aged 20 to 49 years of age account for 58% of fatalities. The majority of fatal exposures in children are unintentional whereas most fatal cases in adults are intentional and are the result of a suicide attempt or substance abuse. Among children less than 6 years of age, cosmetics and personal care products are the most frequent poison exposure. Cleaning substances, analgesics, topical agents, and foreign bodies are also frequently observed in reports to poison control centers for this age group. Ingestions of cough and cold preparations, plants, and pesticides are also observed frequently. Careful storage inaccessible to children and use of child-resistant packaging can prevent many of these exposures (Watson et al., 2004).

Almost two thirds of exposures for those less than 5 years of age are observed with toddlers 1 to 2 years of age. Toddlers are at the greatest risk of accidental ingestions because they tend to put many things in their mouths as part of how they interact with their environment. Miniature button or disc batteries commonly used in video games, personal data assistants, cameras, hearing aids, watches and other devices are among the foreign body ingestants observed in toddlers. They contain very caustic substances such as potassium hydroxide. In most cases they pass uneventfully through the gastrointestinal (GI) tract intact over 2 to 3 days while is child is monitored with sequential x-rays to assess passage. In children aged between two and four household chemicals like liquid polish, bleach, and lavatory disinfectants are also the likely cause of poisoning.

For adults, analgesics and drugs with sedative properties are the most frequent agents involved in poisoning. Ingestion of cleaning supplies and insect/animal bites are also often reported. Food poisonings, chemicals/pesticides, and personal care products are also among the more common implicated agents. Drugs of abuse, although not as frequently reported to poison control centers as other substances, are associated with higher risk for death (Watson et al., 2004). Chapter 9 reviews drug overdoses resulting from substance abuse. Complementary and alternative therapies are also pose risks for toxicity from either their active ingredients or from contaminants used in processing such as lead and arsenic (refer to Chapter 12).

Terrorism threats involving chemical, biological, or nuclear agents must also be considered. Issues related to terrorism are discussed throughout this text. Chapter 21 discusses the parasympathomimetic nerve gases. Most of these agents bind to acetylcholinesterase, the enzyme responsible for the breakdown of acetylcholine. Treatment involves the immediate use of antimuscarinic therapy (e.g., atropine) and/or agents that break the bond between the agent and acetylcholinesterase (e.g., 2-PAM). Chapter 38 discusses pulmonary toxins, including chlorine and phosgene. Chapter 47 discusses the use of potassium iodide in response to radioactive iodine exposure. Chapters 58 and 59 present a review of the acute management of bacterial threats such as anthrax and plague, and viral threats, such as smallpox and Ebola. Chapter 62 presents the role of vaccines in preparing or responding to a terrorist threat. Chapter 65 presents vesicants such as nitrogen mustard and Lewisite, which can cause damage to dermal tissue and mucous membranes. Principles of poison management, and management of other potential threats, including cyanide, are discussed later in this chapter. Finally, the Pharmacologic Issues in an Age of Terrorism box on p. 1288 reviews the role of the nurse in disaster preparedness, and principles. The nurse must be well versed in these issues in advance of an imminent threat to best respond in an emergency situation.

⊛ **R.J., a 19-year-old college freshman, is brought to the hospital by his roommate who found him in the dorm, covered with vomitus, smelling of alcohol, and unresponsive to repeated attempts to awaken him. He believes R.J. had been partying with some of his buddies and got involved in a drinking contest.**

⊛ **How are poisons or toxic exposures detected?**
Toxicology is the study of poisons and their action and effects, methods of detection, and diagnosis and treatment. To paraphrase Paracelsus, the sixteenth-century pharmacologist considered the father of toxicology: "Every substance is a poison. There is none which is not. The only thing that differentiates a poison from a remedy is the dose." A **poison** is defined as any substance that can injure or kill a living organism. All drugs are potential poisons when used improperly or in excess doses. Poisoning may be acute or chronic. In **acute poisoning** the effects are usually observed within a few hours, although may be delayed for many hours. **Chronic poisoning** is usually related to cumulative exposures over time. Chronic poisoning can produce acute effects as the threshold level of toxicity is exceeded.

Nurses may be confronted with a suspected poisoning in many ways. A mother may call, upset that her small child has taken one of her contraceptive pills; a nursing home resident may accidentally drink the glass of peroxide mixture intended as a mouthwash; or an adolescent who cannot be aroused may be brought into the emergency department.

Clues that typically point to poisoning include sudden, violent symptoms of severe nausea, vomiting, diarrhea, collapse, or seizures. If possible, it is important to find out what poison has been taken and how much. Additional information that might prove helpful to the health care provider in making a diagnosis includes answers to questions or reports of observed phenomena, with the nurse noting the following:

- Any reports of poison contact by the victim
- Age of victim (note "at-risk" age-group, 1 to 5 years of age)
- Report of a history of previous poisonings or the ingestion of foreign substances
- Diverse symptoms or signs indicating multiple organ system involvement that defy diagnosis
- A history of suicidal intent or thought
- Symptoms that appear suddenly in an otherwise healthy individual or in a number of persons who become ill at approximately the same time, as might occur in food poisoning
- Anything unusual about the individual, his or her clothing, or the surroundings; evidence of burns around the lips and mouth; discolored gums; needle (hypodermic) pricks, pustules, or scars on the exposed and accessible surfaces of the body or dilated or constricted pupils, as may be seen in individuals with a history of IV drug abuse; any skin rash or discoloration
- The odor of the breath, the rate of respiration, any difficulty in respiration, and cyanosis
- The quality and rate of the pulse

Pharmacologic Issues in an Age of Terrorism

Disaster Preparedness

The Centers for Disease Control and Prevention (CDC) support web-based information for consumers and health care providers regarding emergency preparedness and response. This website (available at http://www.bt.cdc.gov/) provides a wealth of information on biologic, chemical, radiation, and other disaster issues related to terrorist and natural events. The CDC website links to other sites including the ReadyAmerica website (http://www.ready.gov/overview.html) that provides consumer information related to preparing for and recognizing chemical, biologic, radiation, and other threats.

The nurse plays an important role in both disaster preparedness, and implementation of disaster protocols should they be activated. Clients will often require reassurance and direction from the nurse in a disaster situation. The nurse is a key player in assuring a coordinated response in disaster management. The nurse should review what his/her role would be in the event of different disasters, and be familiar with the plan before it is implemented. The school nurse, for example, may have a very different role in a disaster plan than a critical care nurse, or a home care based nurse. Each should be aware of the likely response that will be required, and be familiar with appropriate management of potential disaster issues in which they may participate. All health care organizations have a disaster plan, and may institute mock drills to test the plan and its implementation.

In a disaster, the nurse may be called to:
• Assess clients and the environment
• Reassure and direct clients to resources and care
• Prevent or limit exposure to clients and caregivers
• Triage care and resources
• Provide physical and psychological support
• Implement treatments
• Monitor interventions
• Provide follow up care
• Evaluate the effectiveness of interventions

The nation's disaster preparedness response is guided through designated federal agencies. Health care professions training programs are sponsored by the CDC, the Department of Health and Human Services (DHHS), Department of Defense and many other federal agencies. To prepare for participation, individual nurses can contact the American Red Cross (http://www.redcross.org), their state nurses association, or the National Nurses Response Team (NNRT), a part of the National Disaster Medical System (NDMS) (http://www.oep-ndms.dhhs.gov/federal.html). The NDMS website also provides links to the numerous agencies involved in guiding and assisting communities and health care professionals throughout the response process. Also specific to health care provider participation is the Medical Reserve Corps (http://www.citizencorps.gov/medical.html) created to assist health care professionals to augment local health care capacity during an emergency. This project is being managed under the auspices of the Federal Emergency Management Agency (FEMA) and the Department of Health and Human Ser-

vices. The American Nurses Association (ANA) strongly recommends that if you want to respond to a disaster, do so as part of a team. This helps to ensure that you have the proper specialized training, are credentialed, and that the appropriate protective equipment and coordination are in place to make the best use of your skill and expertise.

The nurse should be familiar with symptoms of various chemical, biologic, and radiation exposures, and the management strategies in responding to each exposure. Log on to any of the websites cited above for current information and in-depth educational programs. The table below provides a review of some of the more likely threats and their pharmacologic management:

THREAT	CHAPTER	PAGE NUMBER
Nerve Agents		
Tabun	21	432-433
Sarin		
Soman		
VX		
Novichok		
Pulmonary Toxins		
Chlorine	37	711
Phosgene		
Perfluoroisobutylene		
Radiation Exposure and the Thyroid		
Radioactive Iodine	47	845
Bacterial Agents and Related Toxins		
Anthrax	58	1035-1036
Plague		
Tularemia		
Botulinum toxin		
Viral Agents		
Smallpox	59	1063-1064
Hemorrhagic Fever Viruses		
The Role of Vaccines in Terrorism Response		
Smallpox vaccine	62	1146-1147
Botulinum antitoxin and toxoid		
Yellow fever vaccine		
Anthrax vaccine		
Vesicants		
Mustards	65	1166
Lewisite		
Antidotes		
Cyanide	72	1301-1302

BOX 72-1 TOXIDROMES*

anticholinergics (atropine, scopolamine): dry skin, dry mucous membranes, tachycardia, beet-red skin color, agitation, mydriasis (dilated pupils), urinary retention, hyperthermia, and mental status changes including delirium, hallucinations, and/or coma. (A simple mnemonic, "hot as a hare, blind as a bat, dry as a bone, red as a beet, mad as a hatter, bloated as a bladder," describes many of the features of the anticholinergic toxidrome.)

barbiturates, sedative-hypnotics: ataxia, drowsiness, slurred speech (without an alcohol breath odor), respiratory depression, hypotension

cholinergics (such as organophosphates), mushrooms (*Amanita* or *Galerina*): salivation, lacrimation, involuntary urination and defecation, diarrhea, miosis, mental status changes, pulmonary congestion, bronchospasm, and seizures. Severe cases present with respiratory muscle depression or paralysis. (Also see the Pharmacologic Issues in an Age of Terrorism box on pp. 432 and 433.) DUMBELS is a mnemonic used to recall many of the muscarinic effects: defecation, urination, miosis, bronchorrhea, bronchospasm, bradycardia, emesis, lacrimation, and salivation.

opioids: pinpoint pupils, respiratory depression, hypotension, bradycardia, hypothermia, hyporeflexia, mental status depression, sedation, coma and needle marks may be present.

salicylates: fever, vomiting, GI bleeding, dehydration, hypoglycemia, hypokalemia, tinnitus, seizures, central hyperventilation, concretions (solid drug mass), mixed respiratory alkalosis and metabolic acidosis, coma

sympathomimetics (cocaine, amphetamine, OTC decongestants [phenylpropanolamine, ephedrine, pseudoephedrine], theophylline, caffeine β₂-adrenergic receptor agonists [ephedra, ma huang]): hypertension, diaphoresis, tachycardia, tachypnea, hyperthermia, mydriasis; restlessness, agitation, excessive speech, tremors, and insomnia also occur. Severe cases are associated with dysrhythmias and seizures. This toxidrome may be difficult to distinguish from the anticholinergic syndrome. However, sweating and normal to hyperactive bowel sounds are associated with sympathomimetic overdose, and dry skin and diminished bowel sounds with the anticholinergic toxidrome (Ford, 2001).

tricyclic antidepressants: anticholinergic signs and symptoms [see above], vomiting, hypotension (often profound), tachycardia and dysrhythmias (prolonged QRS duration on ECG report), seizures, mental status changes including confusion and coma

Modified from Graber, M.A., & Lanternier, M.L. (2001). *University of Iowa: the family practice handbook* (4th ed.). St. Louis: Mosby.
*The drugs or drug types in bold are followed by clusters of signs of poisonings.

- The appearance and odor of vomitus, if any, and accompanying diarrhea or abdominal pain
- Any abnormalities of stool and urine; change in color or the presence of blood
- For signs of involvement of the nervous system, the presence of excitement, muscular twitching, delirium, speech difficulty, stupor, coma, constriction or dilation of the pupils, and elevated or subnormal temperature

Coma caused by a drug overdose is characterized by the following categories:

- *Grade I.* The individual is asleep but is easily aroused and reacts to painful stimuli. Deep tendon reflexes are present, pupils are normal and reactive, ocular movements are present, and vital signs are stable.
- *Grade II.* Pain response is absent, deep tendon reflexes are depressed, pupils are slightly dilated but reactive, and vital signs are stable.
- *Grade III.* Deep tendon and pupillary reflexes are absent, and vital signs are stable.
- *Grade IV.* Respiration and circulation are depressed.

All specimens of vomitus, urine, or stool for examination and possible submission to the proper authority for analysis are placed in a labeled covered container, refrigerated, and securely stored. This is of particular importance not only in making or confirming a diagnosis but also in the event that the case has medicolegal significance.

Any of the signs listed earlier should be noted carefully for reporting to the poison control center or physician in charge. However, a complete reliance on the signs and symptoms for a clear-cut diagnosis and poison identification is fraught with danger, because these incidents may occur concurrently with an episode of acute disease, especially in children (e.g., aspirin intoxication), and the symptoms may be similar or otherwise confusing. Additionally, more than one substance may be responsible for the signs of poisoning observed.

The term "nontoxic" is a misnomer in that all substances could potentially produce toxic response based on dose. Poison control should always be contacted immediately if there is uncertainty regarding risk or if there is *any* question about the potential for injury. Never wait for symptoms to appear before calling poison control.

Obtaining an accurate estimate of the nature, amount and duration of exposure is critical. Poison control center professionals are very careful in obtaining victim histories, asking probing questions such as bottle size and spill size with comparisons made to common objects familiar to the caller. For example, terms like "mouthful" are imprecise with variation in interpretation of what is full, and differences in mouth capacity with age. The assessment may be improved by assessing how much was in the container before and after the exposure event. Such an approach improves communication and assessment without wasting valuable time.

In assisting with the poisoning diagnosis and in the identification of a toxic substance, nurses (especially emergency department nurses and nurse practitioners) should familiarize themselves with certain clusters of signs associated with common drug poisonings or overdoses. Box 72-1 lists these clusters, called **toxidromes**. Table 72-1 lists

TABLE 72-1 SINGLE SIGNS THAT SUGGEST THE PRESENCE OF CERTAIN TOXINS

Sign	Possible Inferences	Sign	Possible Inferences
Abdominal pain/ discomfort	Acetaminophen Black widow spider bite Heavy metals Mushrooms Withdrawal from opioid	Paralysis	Botulism Heavy metals Plants (e.g., poison hemlock) Triorthocresyl phosphate (plasticizer)
Ataxia	Alcohol Antiepileptic drugs (e.g., carbamazepine, phenytoin) Barbiturates Bromides Carbon monoxide Hallucinogens Heavy metals Organic solvents Sedative/hypnotics	Pupillary changes Dilated	Amphetamines Antihistamines Atropine Barbiturates (when combined with coma) Cocaine Ephedrine LSD (occasionally) Methanol Withdrawal from opioids (occasionally)
Breath Odors Acetone	Acetone Alcohol (methyl or isopropyl) Phenol Salicylates	Constricted, pinpoint pupils	Mushrooms (muscarinic) Opioids Organophosphate insecticides
Alcohol	Ethyl alcohol	Nystagmus on lateral gaze	Barbiturates Benzodiazepines Phencyclidine (PCP) Phenytoin
Bitter almonds	Cyanide		
Garlic	Arsenic Dimethyl sulfoxide (DMSO) Phosphorus Organophosphate insecticides Thallium	Respiratory alterations Increased	Amphetamines Aspirin Carbon monoxide Methanol Petroleum distillates
Coma and drowsiness	Alcohol (ethyl) Antiepileptic drugs Antidepressants Antihistamines Barbiturates Carbon monoxide Opioids Salicylates Sedative/hypnotics	Paralysis Slowed or depressed	Botulism Alcohol (late sign) Barbiturates Benzodiazepines Opioids Organophosphate insecticides Sedative/Hypnotics
		Wheezing/pulmonary edema	Mushrooms (muscarinic) Opioids Organophosphate insecticides Petroleum distillates
Oliguria/anuria	Carbon tetrachloride Ethylene glycol (antifreeze) Heavy metals Hemolysis caused by naphthalene, plants, and so on Methanol Mushrooms Oxylates Petroleum distillates Solvents	Salivation	Alkaline cleaners Corrosive substances Mercury Nicotine Organophosphate insecticides Thallium

other common single signs and their associated causative toxins.

What is the role of the poison control center?

There are approximately 80 poison control centers in the United States and Canada. The national 800 telephone number in the United States is 800-222-1222, and, like 911, your call will be routed to your regional poison center. Regional poison control centers in Canada each have different telephone numbers. Poison centers are staffed with highly trained health care professionals who have extensive knowledge of clinical toxicology. The doctors, pharmacists, and nurses who staff these centers have immediate access to a wealth of information and assist in the medical management of people exposed to any toxic or potentially toxic substance.

How are poisons classified?

The classification of poisons is as broad as the classification of drugs, because any drug is a potential poison when used in excess. Poisons may be classified in various ways. They may be grouped according to chemical classifications as organic and inorganic poisons; as alkaloids, glycosides, and resins; or as acids, alkalis, heavy metals, oxidizing agents, halogenated hydrocarbons, and so on. Poisons may also be classified according to the organ or tissue of the body in which the most damaging effects are produced. Some poisons injure all cells they contact; these are sometimes called protoplasmic poisons or cytotoxins. Others have a greater effect on the kidney (nephrotoxins), the liver (hepatotoxins), or the blood-forming organs.

Poisons that mainly affect the nervous system are called neurotoxins. They must be studied separately, because different symptoms characterize each one. Symptoms of toxicity are mentioned with each of these drugs in previous chapters. Although the symptoms of this group of poisons are specific to some extent, certain symptoms are encountered repeatedly and are associated with many poisons. Drowsiness, dizziness, headache, delirium, coma, and seizures always indicate central nervous system (CNS) involvement. On the other hand, dry mouth, dilated pupils, and difficulty swallowing are associated with an overdose of atropine or one of the atropine-like drugs. Ringing in the ears, excessive perspiration, and gastric upset may be associated with an overdose of salicylate.

Often the precise mechanism of action of a poison is not known. For example, death may be caused by respiratory failure, but exactly what happens to cause depression of the respiratory center may not be known. The human body depends on a constant supply of oxygen if various physiologic functions are to proceed satisfactorily. Anything that interferes with the use of oxygen by the cells, or with the transportation of oxygen, will produce damaging effects faster in some cells than in others. Carbon monoxide (CO) from automobile engines and unvented gas heaters is one of the most widely distributed toxic agents. It poisons by producing hypoxia and finally asphyxia. CO has a great affinity for

TABLE 72-1 SINGLE SIGNS THAT SUGGEST THE PRESENCE OF CERTAIN TOXINS—cont'd

Sign	Possible Inferences	Sign	Possible Inferences
Seizures or muscle twitching	Alcohol Amphetamines Antihistamines Camphor Chlorinated hydrocarbon insecticides (DDT) Cyanide Lead Organophosphate insecticides Plants (azalea, iris, water hemlock) Salicylates Strychnine Tricyclic antidepressants Withdrawal from drugs: barbiturates, benzodiazepines	Flushing	Alcohol Antihistamines Atropine Boric acid Carbon monoxide Nitrites Sympathomimetics Tricyclic antidepressants Yellow phosphorus
		Cyanosis	Aniline dyes Carbon monoxide Cyanide Nitrites Strychnine
Skin color changes Jaundice	Aniline dyes/coal tar colors Arsenic Carbon tetrachloride Castor bean Fava bean Mushroom Naphthalene (moth repellent/insecticide)	Violent emesis (with or without hematemesis)	Aminophylline Bacterial food poisoning Boric acid Corrosives Fluoride Heavy metals Phenol Salicylates

hemoglobin and forms carboxyhemoglobin; this interferes with the production of oxyhemoglobin and the free transport of oxygen, and oxygen deficiency soon develops in the cells. Anoxia may produce serious brain damage unless exposure to the CO is terminated before 40% of hemoglobin has been changed to carboxyhemoglobin. Death occurs when 60% of the hemoglobin has been changed to carboxyhemoglobin.

The cyanides act somewhat similarly in that they bring about cellular anoxia, but they do so differently. They inactivate certain tissue enzymes so that cells are unable to use oxygen. Death from cyanide may occur very rapidly. Curare and the curariform drugs in toxic amounts bring about paralysis of the diaphragm, and again the victim dies from lack of oxygen.

Certain drugs have a direct effect on muscle tissue of the body, such as that of the myocardium or the smooth muscle of the blood vessels; therefore death results from the failure of circulation or cardiac arrest. The nitrites, potassium salts, and digoxin may exert such toxic effects.

Strong acids and alkalis denature and destroy cellular proteins. Examples of corrosive acids are hydrochloric, nitric, and sulfuric acids. Sodium, potassium, and ammonium hydroxides are examples of strong and caustic alkalis. Locally, these substances cause destruction of tissue, and death may result from hemorrhage, perforation, or shock. Corrosive poisons may also cause death by altering the pH of the blood or other body fluids, or they may produce marked degenerative changes in vital organs such as the liver or kidney.

✲ What steps are involved in the management of poisonings?

Poison management involves assessment, support of vital functions, and may involve attempts to remove, eliminate, or counteract the poison. Prevention of further complications related to the existing event, and preventing future events is also important in management.

Assessment Because the emphasis is on *prompt* treatment, health care may be best served by the quick action of informed bystanders at the scene who administer first aid while help is sought from the poison control center and while transportation to a hospital or other health care setting is arranged. Box 72-2 provides first aid instructions for possible poisoning.

The caller to the poison control center should have the following information, if available:
- Physical appearance of the substance
- Odor, color, texture, and distinguishing characteristics of the substance
- Trade name or chemical name, if known
- Purpose of the substance or how the substance was meant to be used
- Label statements relating to "poison" content or flammability
- Container or pill to verify identification

After the events of the suspected poisoning have been assessed, prompt medical interventions must be instituted.

Nursing management is therefore guided by the four major goals:
- Vital functions (respirations, circulation, and others) will be maintained, supported, or restored.
- The toxic substance will be removed or eliminated from the system as soon as possible.
- The action of certain specific poisons may be counteracted, reversed, or antagonized by specific antidotes.
- Recurrences will be reduced or prevented.

Support of Vital Functions Basic to the treatment of poisoning is intensive supportive therapy, good nursing care, and minimal dangerous invasive interventions. Nursing care of the poisoned client should focus on the restoration, support, and maintenance of vital functions such as ventilation, circulation, and acid-base and fluid-electrolyte balance. Emotional support for the client and others involved in this crisis is crucial.

A general assessment and history is performed quickly and competently to determine the extent of any impairments of body systems or particular susceptibilities. Expert nursing care is essential for observing the following for information that indicates impending complications:
- Level of consciousness.
- Vital signs. Temperature may be elevated with certain CNS stimulants and salicylates and depressed with others. Transient cardiac dysrhythmias may occur; anticipate obtaining an electrocardiogram (ECG). Pulmonary congestion, airway obstruction, or apnea is common; aspiration of vomitus can occur.

Implemented plans may include the following:
- Turning, deep breathing, coughing, and suctioning
- Auscultation to demonstrate a need for chest radiograph examination, suctioning, tracheostomy, endotracheal intubation, blood gas determinations, supplemental oxygen, and a respirator/ventilator

It is also essential that the victim be positioned to prevent aspiration of vomitus and that mouth care be provided promptly after emesis. Moderate amounts of plain water by mouth (if a gag or swallow reflex is present) may be all that is needed to dilute or effectively inactivate many ingested poisons. Close attention to developing problems and responsive interventions can often prevent the need for more aggressive medical therapies that tax the already tenuous condition of the poisoned individual.

Removal or Elimination of Poison Carefully evaluate the client who has been affected by a toxic substance to determine which of the foregoing steps take priority and by which route the poison should be removed or eliminated, if necessary. The route is largely determined by the manner of the poisoning. The removal of ingested substances can be attempted in several ways: (1) by directly removing it from the stomach, if the poisoning is discovered early; (2) by increasing the rate of transit of the poison through the colon, even though little or no absorption occurs there and thus may not be effective; or (3) by attempting to remove or fil-

BOX 72-2 FIRST AID FOR POSSIBLE POISONING

Remember: any nonfood substance may be poisonous.

1. Keep all potential poisons—household products and medicines—out of children's reach.
2. Use "safety caps" (child-resistant containers) to avoid accidents.

Keep the phone number of your poison center and your physician handy.

If you think an accidental ingestion has occurred, do the following:

1. Keep calm. Do not wait for symptoms. Call the poison center immediately.
2. Have the following information available:
   a. The name, age, and gender of the poisoning victim.
   b. The exact name of the product or substance involved in the poisoning. Bring the container to the telephone with you, if possible.
   c. An estimate of the amount of substance that may have been involved.
   d. When the poisoning occurred.
   e. The physical condition of the victim, including any preexisting medical problems
   f. How the poisoning occurred.
   g. Any additional information you feel the staff member needs to know.
   h. Any treatment implemented prior to calling poison control center.
3. Find out if the substance is toxic; the poison control center can tell you if a risk exists and what you should do.

4. Take appropriate action.
   a. If a poison is on the skin:
   Immediately remove affected clothing.
   Flood involved body parts with water and rinse thoroughly.
   b. If a poison is in the eye:
   Immediately flush the eye with water for up to 20 minutes.
   c. If a poison is inhaled:
   Immediately get the victim to fresh air. Give mouth-to-mouth resuscitation if necessary.
   d. Never induce emesis unless specifically directed to do so by the poison control center or qualified practitioner.

Never induce vomiting in the following situations:

1. The victim is in a *coma* (obtunded, reduced level of consciousness).
2. The victim is *convulsing* (having a seizure).
3. The victim has swallowed a caustic or corrosive substance (e.g., lye).

For reemphasis:

1. Call poison control immediately for any event where toxicity is suspected or possible. Do not wait for symptoms to appear.
2. Always call the poison control center before undertaking treatment.
3. Never induce vomiting unless you are instructed to do so.
4. Do not rely on the label's antidote information, because it may be out of date. Instead call poison control.
5. If you need to go to an ED, take the tablets, capsules, container, and/or label with you.

---

ter it from the bloodstream if the substance has probably already been assimilated into the system or was injected. Contact poisons may be flushed from the skin, eyes, and other external areas with copious volumes of plain, flowing water from a pitcher or other container. Inhaled toxins are treated by placing the individual in fresh air and by administering artificial respiration or oxygen and other supportive measures as necessary.

Various methods exist for the removal or elimination of poisons from the GI tract or systemic circulation: emesis, gastric lavage, cathartics, diuretics, dialysis or, occasionally, blood exchange transfusions or hemoperfusion through charcoal or exchange resins.

Emesis Vomiting may be a natural response of the client to many poisoning events. Although emesis may be an effective method of removing some ingested toxins, many toxins are rapidly absorbed and emesis occurs too late to be effective. Complications associated with emesis are also problematic—particularly for agents that suppress CNS function (multiple

CNS depressants), produce local irritation (e.g., acids, bases, and other caustic agents), or agents which are more likely to be aspirated (e.g., gasoline, petroleum-based products). The risk for aspiration and further tissue damage often outweighs the benefit of inducing emesis in the client, and must be avoided if harm is likely (Box 72-3). Emesis is no longer recommended as a treatment in most poison exposures because of its limited effectiveness and potential for complications.

✷ What interventions are used for removal or elimination in poison management?

Of the nearly 2.4 million calls to U.S. poison control centers in 2003, nearly 75% were managed in the home or from a nonhealth care facility. Of those exposures requiring treatment, dilution and/or irrigation is by far the most common intervention utilized. Dilution or irrigation often reduces the injury and can usually be implemented immediately in the setting in which the intervention occurs. Plain water is the recommended universal diluent. With health care assistance (e.g., emergency medical services, in a health

care setting), activated charcoal is also frequently administered in decontamination procedures (Committee on Injury, Violence, and Poison Prevention, AAP, 2003). Gastric
lavage, use of ipecac syrup, alkalinization of the urine, and
hemodialysis are also utilized in management, but are usually reserved for severe poisonings not responsive to other
modalities in which these interventions demonstrate benefit (Watson et al., 2004).

activated charcoal [**ak** ti vat id **char** kole]
(Actidose-Aqua)
activated charcoal with sorbitol [**ak** ti vat id **char** kole
with **sor** bi tole]
(Actidose with Sorbitol)
Activated charcoal adsorbs many substances and therefore is used as
an adjunct in the treatment of oral poisonings with heavy metals, mercuric chloride, strychnine, phenol, atropine, phenolphthalein, oxalic
acid, poisonous mushrooms, aspirin, and most drugs. It is not effective
for poisoning with ethanol, methanol, caustic alkalis, ferrous sulfate,
boric acid, gas, kerosene, lithium, and mineral acids. The charcoal mixture need not be removed from the stomach afterward because no serious adverse effects exist. Activated charcoal can also serve as a stool
marker to indicate when further GI absorption of the ingested poison
has ended. Tablets or capsules of charcoal should not be used to treat
poisoning, because they are less effective than the powder.

Indications
Activated charcoal is used in the emergency treatment of oral poisonings for a number of drugs and chemicals. The addition of sorbitol results in increased hyperosmotic colonic elimination, but may
contribute to fluid and electrolyte imbalance.

Contraindications
Activated charcoal should not be used in cases of intestinal obstruction or GI perforation. It is not effective for management of acid or
alkali, cyanide, organic solvent, iron, ethanol, methanol, or lithium
poisonings.

Pharmacokinetics/Dosing
Activated charcoal remains in the GI tract and is not systemically
absorbed. For acute poisonings, approximately 10 g of activated
charcoal are administered for each 1 g of ingested toxin. Repeat
doses may be needed. Alternately, a single 1 g/kg body weight is
given orally. Sorbitol dose should not exceed 1.5 g/kg. Aqueous suspensions of activated charcoal are available in 15-, 25-, and 50-g
dosage units. Formulations of activated charcoal suspended in sorbitol are available in 25- and 50-g dosage units as well. Capsule and
granular formulations are available, but are generally not recommended for acute poison management because reduced surface area
on ingestion reduces their efficacy to bind toxins.

Adverse Effects
Vomiting and diarrhea are among the more common adverse effects,
and may be more pronounced with formulations containing sorbitol.
This is an important consideration for toxic ingestions in which
vomiting may be contraindicated (e.g., multiple agent ingestion in
which petroleum distillates or caustic agents are involved). Altered
fluid and electrolyte balance can also be problematic and is more
likely with sorbitol use. Black-colored stools are typically observed
after administration of activated charcoal.

Drug Interactions
Ipecac delays the administration of activated charcoal, which is the
preferred treatment in most poisonings. Cathartics/laxatives are
used in many cases if increased elimination is recommended. Most
commonly, sorbitol is used in combination with activated charcoal
as noted above. Chapter 40 discusses other cathartic/laxatives.

Gastric lavage involves washing out the stomach with sterile water or a saline solution. (Refer to a basic nursing text
for the procedure.) Until recently, gastric lavage was a time-
honored element of the management of poisoned clients,
but its routine use is no longer recommended by the American Academy of Clinical Toxicology or the European Association of Poison Centres and Clinical Toxicologists (Vale &
Kulig, 2004). Gastric lavage is less effective than activated
charcoal in reducing the absorption of simulated toxins but
is roughly equivalent in efficacy to ipecac (Burns &
Schwartzstein, 2005). Gastric lavage is generally reserved
for large, potentially life-threatening ingestions and for substances not absorbed by charcoal. The procedure itself can
sometimes contribute to complications during management. It is important to maintain the client's airway during
lavage. Gastric lavage is most effective when initiated within
one hour of ingestion, and is almost always conducted with
concurrent activated charcoal administration. Lavage may
be contraindicated in the presence of cardiac dysrhythmias.

An Ewald orogastric tube, No. 16 to 30 French, may be
used for lavage in children; tube sizes for an adult lavage range
from No. 34 to 42 French. The newer, clear-plastic Lavacuator tube also may be used. A standard nasogastric tube is too
narrow for the extraction of particulate matter such as intact
tablets (Figure 72-1). Stomach contents should be aspirated
first and saved for toxicologic analysis if necessary.

Several liters of half-strength saline solution may be used
in increments of 50 to 100 mL for children and 150 to 200
mL for adults during repeated lavage until the return flow is
clear. (Remember that dead space in the tube itself accounts
for 20 to 25 mL of the fluid instilled.) Neither emesis nor
lavage is guaranteed to empty the stomach completely.

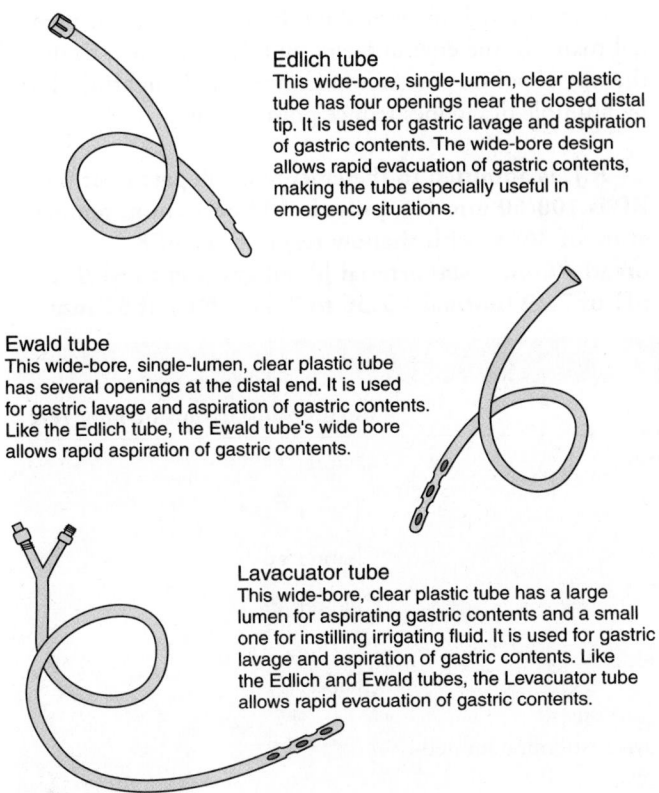

Edlich tube
This wide-bore, single-lumen, clear plastic tube has four openings near the closed distal tip. It is used for gastric lavage and aspiration of gastric contents. The wide-bore design allows rapid evacuation of gastric contents, making the tube especially useful in emergency situations.

Ewald tube
This wide-bore, single-lumen, clear plastic tube has several openings at the distal end. It is used for gastric lavage and aspiration of gastric contents. Like the Edlich tube, the Ewald tube's wide bore allows rapid aspiration of gastric contents.

Lavacuator tube
This wide-bore, clear plastic tube has a large lumen for aspirating gastric contents and a small one for instilling irrigating fluid. It is used for gastric lavage and aspiration of gastric contents. Like the Edlich and Ewald tubes, the Levacuator tube allows rapid evacuation of gastric contents.

FIGURE 72-1 Various tubes used for lavage.

Historically, emesis was frequently induced with the use of syrup of ipecac. Ipecac syrup is rarely utilized today because it is of questionable efficacy and often significantly complicates management. The American Academcy of Pediatrics advises against the routine use of ipecac in the home (Burns & Schwartzstein, 2005). Ipecac syrup acts both centrally and locally by stimulating the vomiting center and by irritating the gastric mucosa.

ipecac syrup [**ip** e kak]
(PMS Ipecac Syrup�)

Indications
Ipecac syrup is for emergency use to cause vomiting in poisoning when specifically recommended by a poison control center. Do not use if strychnine, corrosives such as alkalis (lye) and strong acids, or petroleum distillates such as kerosene, gasoline, fuel oil, coal oil, paint thinner, or cleaning fluid have been ingested. It may be considered in an alert, conscious client who has ingested a substantial amount of a toxic substance within 60 minutes of presentation (Position Paper: Ipecac Syrup, 2004). (See also Box 72-3.)

Pharmacokinetics/Dosing
The usual dosage for adults is 15 to 30 mL, which is followed immediately by 240 mL of water. Four to 8 ounces of water is given with the following dosages: children 6 months to 1 year of age, 5 to 10 mL (under special circumstances only); and children 1 to 12 years of age, 15 mL. Vomiting usually occurs in 15 to 30 minutes. The dose may be repeated once after 20 minutes if the first dose is not effective.

Adverse Effects
In addition to the expected nausea and vomiting, ipecac syrup is cardiotoxic if absorbed. It may cause conduction disturbances, atrial fibrillation, or myocarditis.

Whole bowel irrigation (WBI) with a polyethylene glycol electrolyte solution (PEG-ELS) is another method of GI decontamination. PEG-ELS is administered orally or infused by a nasogastric tube at a rate of 1.5 to 2 L/hour for adults and at a rate of 25 mL/kg/hr for children. WBI is continued until the rectal effluent is clear, which may take many hours (Alsop, 2005).

Changing the pH of the urine by alkalinization (sodium bicarbonate) may enhance the excretion of certain drugs, such as salicylates and, possibly, tricyclic antidepressants. Forced acid diuresis is probably more potentially hazardous but is often recommended for poisoning with amphetamines and fenfluramine (Pondimin).

Poisons are occasionally cleared directly from the bloodstream by peritoneal dialysis or hemodialysis, hemoperfusion, or transfusion to augment the other measures previously discussed. Peritoneal dialysis is less effective than hemodialysis or hemoperfusion. The degree to which these methods may be useful depends in part on the properties of the substance (e.g., whether it freely circulates or whether it is bound to plasma proteins or to tissues). Various lists of substances amenable to dialysis exist; some substances for which hemodialysis has *not* proved useful include diazepam (Valium), cyclosporine, digoxin (Lanoxin), phenytoin (Dilantin), and propranolol (Inderal) (*USP DI*, 2005).

✱ What antidotes are available for managing poisonings?
The number of antidotes for specific toxins is minimal; no widely accepted "universal antidote" exists. Nevertheless, some general statements can be made about antidotes. For orally ingested poisonings, antidotes are more effective after the stomach is empty. The correct dosage to reverse toxicity depends on the specific drug involved, its half-life, and the severity of toxicity shown.

Antidotes work by any of the following mechanisms: (1) antagonizing or stimulating receptor sites that have been rendered hyperfunctional or dysfunctional by the poison, (2) interfering with enzyme inhibition, (3) administering the product of metabolism that has been interfered with, (4) inhibiting the biotransformation of a substance to a poisonous metabolite, (5) giving an agent that inactivates the toxic product, (6) chelation (forming highly stable complexes, tying up the substance—usually a heavy metal such as iron), and (7) producing immunotherapy—the use of antidrug antibodies to bind and inactivate drugs (e.g., severe digoxin poisoning reversed with digoxin-specific antibodies). Many of these antidotes have been discussed throughout this text. Table 72-2 lists common poisonings or toxic exposures and available antidotes.

✱ How are poisonings prevented?
The focus of nursing on primary care and its corollary, prevention, applies readily to poisonings. The nursing profession has always emphasized prevention, and now other disciplines are beginning to take part. Combined efforts with drug information centers and other health care professionals and creative approaches have already had an impact on

the frequency of certain categories of drug poisoning, notably aspirin poisoning.

Various creative graphic symbols appear on the labels of poisonous substances to alert the adult and/or nonreading child to the potential hazard contained therein. "Mr. Yuk," an ugly, green-faced, scowling image, is one of these. "Childproof" caps appear to delay if not completely prevent children's indiscriminate use of medicines. Others who do not have a need for these caps can request medication in the familiar easy-to-open caps.

There is much to learn about both apparent and potential toxins in the environment, and there is much to do in the way of poison prevention. Concerted, thoughtful efforts by multiple disciplines reduce poison events.

✱ **R.J. is admitted to the emergency department. His BP is 100/60 mm Hg, pulse is 100 beats/min, temperature of 36° C with shallow respirations of 8 breaths/min. A stat arterial blood gas result reveals a pH of 7.29 (normal – 7.36 to 7.44), P_{CO_2} of 52 mm**

TABLE 72-2 COMMON POISONINGS AND THEIR ANTIDOTES

Poisoning/Toxin	Antidote	Further Discussion in This Text
acetaminophen	acetylcysteine (Mucomyst)	Chapter 14
anticholinergic, neuromuscular blockers	physostigmine sulfate	Chapter 21
benzodiazepine	flumazenil (Romazicon)	Chapter 16
β blockers/propranolol	glucagon	Chapter 49
cholinergics • nerve agent poisoning – Soman • organophosphates/insecticides • mushrooms with muscarine • anticholinesterase overdose	atropine pralidoxime [2-PAM] (Protopam) [pretreatment with pyridostigmine limited to military applications]	Chapter 21
cyanide	amyl nitrate methylene blue sodium thiosulfate	Chapter 72
digoxin	digoxin immune FAB (Digibind, DigiFab)	Chapter 25
heavy metal	arsenic, gold, mercury, lead: • dimercaprol (BAL in Oil) arsenic, lead, mercury: • D-penicillamine (Cuprimine) • succimer (Chemet) iron: • deferoxamine (Desferal) • edetate calcium disodium (Versenate) copper: • trientine (Syprine)	Chapter 72
heparin	protamine sulfate	Chapter 30
insulin, oral hypoglycemics	dextrose glucagon	Chapter 49
isoniazid	pyridoxine (Vitamin B_6)	Chapter 67
methotrexate	leucovorin	Chapter 56
opioids	naloxone (Narcan) nalmefene (Revex)	Chapters 9, 14
toxic alcohols: • methanol • ethylene glycol	ethanol fomepizole (Antizol)	Chapter 72
warfarin	fresh frozen plasma (FFP) phytonadione (Vitamin K)	Chapter 30

Modified from Lacy, C.F., Armstrong, L.L., Goldman, M.P., & Lance L.L (2004). *Lexi-Comp's Drug Information Handbook*, (12th ed.). Hudson, Ohio: Lexi-Comp.

Hg (normal – 35 to 45), and HCO₃⁻ of 19 mEq/L (normal – 21 to 27). His blood ethanol is 475 mg/dL (see Tables 9-7 and 9-9 for the relationship of blood alcohol to clinical status). R.J. receives endotracheal intubation for respiratory support.

✱ **What are the nursing management issues involved in poisoning care for R.J.?**

Assessment As discussed previously, perform an assessment quickly to determine what substance is involved so that immediate action can be taken to prevent or minimize its effects. Even with R.J.'s case, it is not certain that alcohol is the only substance involved. Depending on the causative agent, symptoms may include nausea and vomiting, abdominal cramping, seizures, a change in the level of consciousness, and decreased rates of pulse and respiration. Assess cardiopulmonary and respiratory function. Poisoning should be suspected in any unconscious individual with no history of diabetes, seizure disorders, or trauma. Death in ethanol-intoxicated client, such as R.J., most often results from respiratory depression and is often accompanied by aspiration of vomitus. Assess breath sounds for crackles at the bases of the lungs and review any radiographic studies of the chest that are done.

To assist in determining the ingested agent, check R.J.'s lips and mouth for excessive salivation, burns, or difficulty swallowing. Assess his breath for its odor. Some petroleum and cleaning products have distinct smells that can be identified. With R.J., the odor of alcohol is strong. His pupils are checked for dilation or constriction, which may also help to indicate what substances are involved.

If R.J. were conscious, it would be important to question him about what substance was taken and in what quantity. As R. J. is unconscious, use clues in the environment to facilitate identification the substance. Empty containers, open bottles or medication containers, or syringes should be gathered and taken to the hospital with the victim. Containers often list the ingredients of the substance to assist the health care provider in choosing the treatment or antidote. R.J.'s roommate did indicate that there were empty vodka bottles in the room, but as he had not been present at the party and he had no idea how much alcohol R.J. had ingested or whether other substances had been involved.

Toxicologic studies that include drug screens can determine poison levels in the mouth, vomitus, urine, feces, or blood or on R.J.'s hands and clothing and confirm the diagnosis. For inhalation poisoning or aspiration, chest radiograph studies might show pulmonary infiltrates or edema. R.J.'s breath, vomitus and clothing smelled of alcohol, so a drug screen of his blood was obtained and it determined ethanol was the sole responsible substance. See Table 72-3 for the relationship between alcohol consumption, alcohol blood levels, and clinical manifestations. See also Chapter 9 for a discussion of alcohol as a substance of abuse.

Nursing Diagnosis While receiving care for poisoning, R.J. is at risk for the following nursing diagnoses/collaborative problems: disturbed thought processes (confusion); risk for aspiration; ineffective breathing patterns; impaired gas exchange; and the potential complications of hypoglycemia, dehydration, seizures, coma, and death.

Planning Following treatment for poisoning, R.J. will:
- Return to normal functioning without any continuing adverse effects of the ethanol, or any adverse effects of the detoxification therapies.
- Collaborate with health care providers to prevent future poisoning events and monitoring and treatment for this event.

TABLE 72-3 RELATIONSHIP BETWEEN ALCOHOL CONSUMPTION, BLOOD ALCOHOL LEVELS, AND CLINICAL MANIFESTATIONS

Alcohol Consumption (Drinks)*		Approximate Blood Alcohol Concentrations, mg/dL (mmol/L)†	Probable Clinical Manifestations
55-kg person	90-kg person		
1-3	2-5	50-100 (10.9-21.7)	Impaired sensation, incoordination
3-5	5-8	100-150 (21.7-32.6)	Behavioral changes, ataxia, cognitive and memory difficulties
5-7	8-11	150-200 (32.6-43.4)	Marked incoordination, worsening ataxia, cognitive impairment
7-9	11-14	200-300 (43.4-65.1)	Nausea, vomiting, diplopia, lethargy, aspiration risks (impairment of protective reflexes)
More than 10	More than 15	300-400 (65.1-86.8)	Decreased respiratory drive, hypoventilation, amnesia, hypothermia, cardiac dysrhythmias
Extreme		Greater than 400 (greater than 86.8)	Coma, respiratory arrest, death

Data from Marco, C.A., & Kelen, G.D. (1990). Acute intoxication. *Emergency Medicine Clinics of North America, 8*(4), 731-748.
*One drink equals 1 oz (one shot) of 80-proof liquor, 12 oz of beer, or 4-5 oz of wine.
†1 oz of 80-proof liquor in a 70-kg person raises BAC by 25 mg/dL (5.4 mmol/L).

Implementation

Monitoring Carefully monitor R.J.'s vital signs and level of consciousness. Observe him for nausea, vomiting, diarrhea, and abdominal cramping. Assess his vomitus, stool, and urine for abnormalities such as the presence of blood. In intentional suicide, malicious administration or therapeutic error, these body substances need to be retained for analysis for both medical and legal reasons.

Intervention With poisoning, immediate action is required to prevent the absorption of the substance. If the individual is unconscious, as with R.J., transport him as soon as possible to a hospital. If the individual is conscious, a physician and/or the poison control center should be contacted immediately. The telephone number of the nearest poison control center is usually listed in the front of the telephone directory with other emergency numbers for the community (800-222-1222 in the United States; Canadian Poison Control Centers are listed separately by province).

If the poison has been inhaled (e.g., a toxic gas or CO), remove the individual from the source to the fresh air, and administer oxygen if available. If indicated, start cardiopulmonary resuscitation. Call 911; the victim will need to be transported to the hospital.

If the substance is a contact poison absorbed through the skin and mucous membranes, the individual should be rinsed off immediately with copious amounts of water. The clothing should then be removed, and the skin is rinsed again. A shower is the best method for removing the agent from the skin.

If the poison is ingested, the objective is to prevent absorption of the substance by following the instructions of the Poison Control Center. If lavage is attempted with an unconscious client within the institutional setting, a cuffed endotracheal tube should be in place to prevent aspiration. Vomiting or lavage should not be attempted for the ingestion of caustic substances or hydrocarbons (found in petroleum products). Care for the ingestion of these substances is to give nothing by mouth and to seek urgent medical assistance.

If the substance has a known antidote, that antidote will likely be administered.

Other nursing interventions relate to the supportive care of the acutely ill client. Monitor vital signs and report any changes immediately. For R.J., administer oxygen and suction as necessary. Maintain IV fluids as ordered. Keep him warm and turn him at frequent intervals to promote drainage from the respiratory tract.

If the poisoning was intentional, such as a suicide attempt, safety precautions should be instituted to protect the client from further self-destructive behavior. Additionally, a psychiatric referral should be considered.

Education To prevent accidental poisoning, families should be assisted to evaluate environmental hazards in the home and place the nearest poison control center telephone number by the phone. Toddlers are at the greatest risk.

Cleaning agents, especially furniture polish and products containing caustic agents, should be stored in high cabinets with childproof locks. In homes in which children live or visit, all medications should be stored in locked cabinets or boxes. Remind parents that pocketbooks containing medications should be kept out of the reach of youngsters. Substances such as insecticides or alcohol should be inaccessible to children. All medications should be clearly labeled with the type, dosage, and storage requirements. Additionally, the client's ability to safely self-medicate should be assessed before there is an expectation for self-medication.

Caution clients not to store toxic substances in food containers or improperly labeled containers or in a place that is accessible to children. Medications should not be stored beyond the date of expiration. Poisonous plants should not be kept in households in which there are small children.

When interacting with clients, nurses should be alert to the presence of anger, depression, withdrawal, and faulty judgment, which may precede intentional or unintentional poisoning.

Evaluation The expected outcome of poisoning treatment is that R.J. will experience a regression of his symptoms, which indicates the successful elimination and inactivation of the poison.

✳ For what types of poisonings should the nurse be prepared?

Ethanol and acetaminophen are among the most common agents associated with significant consequences in overdose for adults. Chapter 9 reviews ethanol, and Chapters 11 and 14 review acetaminophen. Management of overdose of many other agents is presented throughout the text (see Table 72-2). CO, iron, toxic alcohols (isopropyl, methyl), cyanide, and organophosphate insecticides/nerve gas are reviewed here.

✳ B.D., 86 years old, has been despondent over the recent death of his wife and has been diagnosed with a steadily progressing cancer of his prostate. He also is concerned that he will be a burden to his children who have moved out of state. Just before Christmas, he puts his house in order, leaves a note, connects a hose from his car exhaust to the interior of his car, and goes to sit in his car with the engine running in a closed garage.

✳ How does carbon monoxide (CO) poisoning present?

Carbon monoxide is an odorless gas produced by the incomplete combustion of carbon or carbonaceous materials. Sources of this gas include improperly maintained heating systems, improperly ventilated charcoal cookers, wood stoves, heaters, or fireplaces, and industrial furnaces, such as those in steel mills. Automobile exhaust contains 3% to 7% CO. CO causes more deaths in the United States and Canada than any other poison. The inhalation of automobile exhaust is a common method of suicide, and accidental home and industrial exposure to CO is much more common than generally appreciated.

CO poisoning is the result of pulmonary absorption of the gas and it readily combines with hemoglobin to form carboxyhemoglobin. The oxygen in hemoglobin is replaced, thus lowering the available oxygen carried by the blood to the body tissues. With the addition of each CO molecule, the oxygen molecules remaining on the hemoglobin become so tightly bound that they are not readily released to the oxygen-starved tissues. CO is measured in the blood as the percent carboxyhemoglobin (%HbCO). Additionally, CO gas that is dissolved in blood but not bound to hemoglobin diffuses into the body tissues and poisons the cytochrome enzymes necessary for the use of oxygen by cells.

In general, the symptoms of CO poisoning are related to %HbCO. Clinically, only mild (if any) symptoms occur at 10% HbCO; cigarette smokers may have a CO level of this percentage. The initial signs of poisoning usually occur at 10% to 30% HbCO and include a throbbing headache, nausea, vomiting, dizziness, weakness, and visual disturbances. These early symptoms of intoxication are nonspecific and may be attributed to a number of other causes unless a history of CO is available or laboratory tests demonstrate an elevated %HbCO. At 40% to 50% HbCO, syncope, tachycardia, tightness in the chest, and tachypnea occur. HbCO has a cherry pink color rather than the red color of oxyhemoglobin; therefore the client may have a cherry pink coloration to the skin. A level of HbCO in excess of 50% causes life-threatening seizures, coma, dangerously compromised cardiopulmonary function, and possible death. Fatalities in victims of suicide or fire often have a %HbCO of 60% to 80%.

Treatment for CO poisoning is based on a client's symptoms and %HbCO. Hyperbaric oxygen is the antidote of choice, because oxygen under pressure is capable of replacing CO from hemoglobin and from the iron containing respiratory cytochrome enzymes in the tissues.

Ninety-five percent of absorbed CO is excreted by the lungs; once removed from the source of exposure, the half-life of CO in normal ambient air is 4 hours. If 100% oxygen is administered, the half-life ($t^1/_2$) decreases to 40 minutes. Hyperbaric oxygen at 3 atmospheres of pressure decreases the $t^1/_2$ of CO to only 23 minutes. In severe poisoning, cardiopulmonary support is maintained throughout therapy. Additional drug therapy to control dysrhythmias, cerebral edema, and seizures may be indicated.

B.D. is found by a neighbor who hears his car engine running in the closed garage and calls 911. The neighbor pulls B.D. from his car and drags him out into the fresh air. The emergency medical services workers arrive and place B.D. on high-dose oxygen using a face mask attached to an oxygen reserve bag. He is transported to the hospital.

Nursing Management The nursing management for B.D.'s CO poisoning is as discussed with the previous care for poisoning, except that B.D. will receive a psychiatric evaluation as part of his evaluation and therapy.

A.W., a 19-month-old boy, begins to vomit while his mother is breastfeeding his 1-month-old sister. He was left alone in his room for about 10 minutes to take a nap and is discovered with some red tablets. His mother calls the poison control center and indicates that A.W. has probably taken about 10 tablets of her prenatal iron supplement. Emergency medical services transport A.W. and his mother to the emergency department (ED); she has brought the prescription container with the remaining medication. Although A.W. has no symptoms other than vomiting, his serum iron concentration was 450 mcg/mL (normal – 60-160 mcg/dL) 2 hours after ingestion.

What are the issues involved in iron overdose?
Iron supplements are a leading cause of pediatric poisoning in the United States. From 1986 to 1996, more than 110,000 accidental ingestions of iron preparations have been reported, with 33 deaths (Morris, 2000). And despite safety campaigns, there were 3371 exposures to iron overdose and 2 deaths in 2003 (Watson et al., 2004). Iron overdoses have also been noted to result in profound mental retardation; therefore such products should be dispensed in child-resistant containers and stored in an area that is not readily accessible to small children.

Iron deficiency is a primary cause of anemia in both infants and adults. Thus iron is often added to infant formulas and foods and is available in more than 100 commercial products for adults, including multiple and prenatal vitamins. Available products use a number of forms of iron and various salts and chelates. The toxic effects of iron are caused by its elemental form; therefore the relative toxicity of iron salts is related to the percentage of elemental iron in the substance. For example, ferrous fumarate (33% iron) is more toxic on a weight basis than ferrous gluconate (12% iron).

On ingestion, large amounts of iron cause local corrosive actions on the gastric and duodenal mucosa and upper GI tract. Initial symptoms of iron poisoning include nausea, vomiting, upper abdominal pain, and bloody diarrhea. The corrosive action destroys the normal mucosal barrier to iron absorption, allowing the rapid absorption of large amounts of iron into the general circulation. These overdose concentrations of iron exceed the binding capacity of transferrin, the iron-carrying protein of the blood. The excess free iron readily diffuses into various tissues and binds to the sulfhydryl (SH) radicals of numerous enzymes and structural proteins. This binding of iron to compounds necessary for normal cellular function poisons the tissue cells.

Symptoms of systemic intoxication—cyanosis, pulmonary edema, and possible cardiovascular collapse—start to occur within 6 to 24 hours after ingestion. Coagulation defects, hepatic necrosis, and renal failure may develop within a few days. As with adults, the initial symptoms of pediatric iron poisoning are characterized by repeated vomiting, abdominal pain, and diarrhea. A latent phase often occurs—the initial symptoms abate and the child appears well for a 6- to 12-hour period; this is followed by rapid illness and the development of shock. The determination of serum iron value will indicate the severity of the intoxication and prevent the possible dangerous misinterpretation of this latency period.

Additionally, serum iron values indicate the necessity of initiating antidotal therapy. Serum iron concentrations of 350 mcg/dL or less are rarely associated with clinical illness. Concentrations between 350 and 500 mcg/dL call for observation of the client for the development of clinical signs of intoxication. Deferoxamine (an iron chelating agent) therapy is recommended for concentrations above 500 mcg/dL. Deferoxamine is a specific chelator that binds free serum iron and the iron associated with hepatic and splenic stores. It does not bind with zinc, copper, or other trace metals. The deferoxamine-iron complex is nontoxic and is freely excreted by the kidneys.

The treatment for iron poisoning includes general supportive measures, and a specific antidote to bind the ingested iron. Emesis may be induced (if not contraindicated) to expel unabsorbed iron tablets in the stomach; a sodium bicarbonate lavage is also indicated, because bicarbonate converts ferrous iron to ferrous carbonate, which is poorly absorbed. After lavage, 200 to 300 mL of the bicarbonate solution should be left in the stomach.

✴ **A.W. alternately cries and sleeps throughout his stay in the ED. After gastric lavage and whole bowel irrigation with polyethylene glycol electrolyte solution administered through a nasogastric tube for 3 hours until his bowel effluent was clear, A.W. begins to vomit again. A second serum iron concentration obtained 6 hours after ingestion has increased to 525 mcg/mL. A.W. is admitted to the pediatric intensive care unit (ICU) and an infusion of deferoxamine 10 mg/kg/hr is started. A.W. becomes more alert and his vomiting stops and his IV deferoxamine is discontinued after 8 hours. A serum iron level the next morning is 160 mcg/mL and A.W. is discharged home that afternoon.**

Nursing Management In addition to the following discussion, which is specific to iron poisoning, see the general nursing management of poisoning as described in the case of R.J., pp. 1297 and 1298.

Institute emesis if indicated or gastric lavage as soon as possible. Initiate supportive measures, including maintaining a clear airway and providing interventions related to the presence of shock and to acidosis. Deferoxamine is sometimes administered IM using a long needle and the Z-track method; 0.2 to 0.3 mL of air may be added to the medication in the syringe to prevent pain and induration at the site of injections. However, carefully controlled, slow IV infusion rates are preferred and are more effective. Alert A.W.'s mother that he will have a reddish brown coloration of urine and stools. Review poisoning prevention with her before A.W.'s discharge from the hospital.

✴ **P.D. is a 18-month-old boy who has ingested approximately 30 mL of windshield washer fluid (methanol) from his garage. He is brought immediately to the ED by ambulance for assessment.**

✴ **How does methanol toxicity present?**
Ingestion of toxic alcohols (e.g., methanol, isopropyl alcohol and ethylene glycol) can result in short- and long-term complications. Symptoms of methanol poisoning include muscle weakness and cramps, rapid and shallow respirations, blurred vision, cyanosis, headache, dizziness, nausea, vomiting, hypotension, and may occur up to 12 to 24 hours after ingestion. Higher levels can result in seizures, respiratory arrest, and coma. Metabolites of methanol include formaldehyde and formic acid which are toxic to the optic nerve and can lead to blindness. Fatalities have been noted in children with doses as low as 30 mL of pure methanol in a child or 60 to 240 mL in an adult.

Methanol may be found in a number of products, including antifreeze, windshield washer fluid, cleaners, paint thinners, and varnishes. The actual methanol content varies dramatically in different products, so it is most helpful for poison control to obtain the label for the original product in assessing risk. Methanol content in windshield washer fluid varies from 5% to over 50%, with some products containing no methanol at all.

Toxicity of other alcohols differs from methanol. Ethylene glycol ingestion, for example, results in nephrotoxicity as its primary major organ toxicity, although also produces metabolic acidosis. Isopropyl alcohol toxicity is often less severe than methanol, but may present with similar symptoms.

✴ **What agents are available to treat methanol poisoning?**
The management of methanol overdose typically requires critical care support and involves blocking the metabolism of methanol by alcohol dehydrogenase. This is achieved with the administration of ethanol orally or by gastric tube in doses of up to 1 g/kg of absolute ethanol. An IV ethanol dose of 0.6 grams/kg diluted to a 15% solution may also be administered over 30 minutes. Metabolic acidosis is treated with IV sodium bicarbonate. Hemodialysis is used if methanol plasma levels exceed 20 mmol/L.

As an alternative to ethanol, fomepizole is sometimes used. Its expense and lack of cost effectiveness data, however, render fomepizole a second line agent by many critical care specialists (Zimmerman, 2003). Fomepizole is a competitive inhibitor of alcohol dehydrogenase which is used manage ethylene glycol or methanol overdoses and prevents accumulation of their toxic metabolites. Left untreated, ethylene glycol is metabolized to glycoaldehyde, glycolate, glyoxylate, and oxalate, the latter two being nephrotoxic. Formic acid, the metabolite of methanol, is toxic to the optic nerve. Each of these metabolites also contributes to metabolic acidosis.

fomepizole [foe **me** pi zole]
(Antizol)
Indications
Fomepizole is used alone or in combination with hemodialysis for the treatment of methanol and ethylene glycol poisoning. Although

not officially indicated for their use, case reports suggest it may be safe and effective for use in infants and children (Detaille et al., 2004).

Pharmacokinetics/Dosing
Administered IV, it is rapidly distributed throughout the body and is metabolized extensively in the liver. The adult dose is 15 mg/kg IV, followed by 10 mg/kg every 12 hours for four doses. Additional doses of 15 mg/kg may be continued beyond the initial five doses based on response.

Adverse Effects
Headache and nausea are the most frequently reported effects, with bradycardia, dizziness, agitation, altered taste, and hypersensitivity have also been reported.

✱ **P.D. is assessed with frequent plasma methanol levels and observation of vital signs. Identification of the ingested product revealed a very low concentration of methanol and no other toxic alcohols. P.D. is observed for 24 hours and discharged to home uneventfully.**

•   •   •

✱ **L.F. is the new safety officer for a metal processing plant. He is evaluating emergency preparedness in the event of a cyanide exposure at the facility. L.F. contacts the regional poison control center to identify the latest recommendations and resources in prevention and management of cyanide poisoning.**

✱ **How is cyanide poisoning manifested?**
At high concentrations, cyanide is a very rapid and lethal poison. Significant cyanide exposures are rare, but may be more likely in occupational settings where high amounts of cyanide are present. The disaster at the Union Carbide plant in Bhopal, India in December 1984 resulted in over 3000 deaths because of cyanide gas exposure. Concerns for the use of cyanide as a weapon of mass destruction is also a concern (see the Pharmacologic Issues in an Age of Terrorism box on p. 1288).

Cyanide can exist in various forms, including hydrogen cyanide gas or crystal forms of sodium or potassium cyanide. Cyanide is also a metabolic byproduct of nitroprusside therapy (see Chapter 27). It may or may not have a "bitter almond" smell that is not always easily detected. Forms of cyanide are used in a number of manufacturing procedures, including paper, plastics, textiles, and metal electroplating. Cyanide gas is sometimes used to exterminate pests in ships and buildings. Small amounts of cyanide are present in natural substances and are released in cigarette smoke, but these small amounts typically do not pose an immediate risk to health. More concentrated forms, however can pose a significant risk, with exposures through inhalation, skin or mucous membrane, and/or via ingestion.

Cyanide has a high affinity for trivalent form of iron (ferric) and inhibits cellular respiration by binding to trivalent iron in cytochrome oxidase in cellular mitochondria. Lactic acidosis and cytotoxic hypoxia are consequences of cyanide exposure.

Symptoms of low exposures to cyanide may occur within minutes of exposure and include tachypnea, restlessness, dizziness, weakness, headache, nausea, vomiting, and tachycardia. Higher exposures, including exposure to high concentrations of cyanide gas, also has a rapid presentation which may include seizures, hypotension, bradycardia, loss of consciousness, pulmonary toxicity, and respiratory failure with an imminent risk for death within minutes. Cardiac and brain injury may be noted with significant or long-term exposures because of cellular hypoxia.

✱ **How is cyanide poisoning treated?**
Because inhaled and dermal exposures to cyanide can be rapidly lethal, caregivers or responders must protect themselves from cyanide exposure before attending to the needs of the victim. This typically includes protective clothing for the caregiver, moving the client to an uncontaminated area, and removing contaminated clothing from the client. Treatment for cyanide poisoning must be implemented immediately and involves interrupting the ability of cyanide to bind to trivalent iron and converting cyanide to the minimally toxic thiocyanate.

Concurrent administration of amyl nitrite, sodium nitrite, and sodium thiosulfate is often utilized in the management of cyanide toxicity, and is typically initiated at the site of exposure if possible because cyanide toxicity is rapidly fatal. Amyl nitrite inhalation and IV sodium nitrite oxidize hemoglobin to methemoglobin, which competes with cytochrome oxidase for cyanide. This results in the release of cyanide from cytochrome oxidase in mitochondria and allows for more normal cellular respiration. Sodium thiosulfate helps convert cyanide to the less toxic thiocyanate that is eliminated in the urine. Methylene blue is sometimes used in the management of cyanide poisoning as well, but has complicated concentration dependent effects on cyanide binding and methemoglobin levels.

Cyanide antidote kits often include nitrite salts and sodium thiosulfate. Administration of oxygen is also helpful. Work sites where cyanide is present typically carry such kits in the event of a cyanide exposure to allow trained responders or emergency medical personnel to administer these agents immediately in the field.

amyl nitrite [am il **nye** trite]
Indications
Amyl nitrite is used as an adjunct in the management of cyanide poisoning. It is also used as a coronary vasodilator in angina pectoris. See Chapter 54 for a discussion of its illicit use as an enhancer of sexual experience.

Pharmacokinetics/Dosing
It is absorbed systemically after nasal inhalation. The usual dose for cyanide poisoning is inhalation of the contents of a 0.3 mL crushed ampule for 15 to 30 seconds. Repeat the one-ampule dose every minute until sodium nitrite infusion is initiated.

Adverse Effects
Adverse effects of amyl nitrite are similar to nitroglycerin and include hypotension, headache, and dizziness.

Drug Interactions
Significant hypotension is noted when combined with phosphodiesterase type 5 inhibitors (e.g., sildenafil [Viagra]).

methylene blue [meth **i** leen bloo]
(Urolene Blue)
Indications
Methylene blue is used as an antidote for cyanide poisoning and methemoglobinemia. It has also been historically used as a dye in diagnostics.
Pharmacokinetics/Dosing
Although it possesses extensive absorption on oral administration, it is dosed intravenously for cyanide poisoning to result in a more rapid onset of effect. The typical IV dose is 1 to 2 mg/kg over several minutes.
Adverse Effects
Hypotension, chest pain, confusion, headache, nausea, vomiting, and diaphoresis have all been reported with methylene blue use.

sodium nitrite [**sow** dee um **nye** trite]
Indications
Sodium nitrite is indicated for treatment of cyanide poisoning in combination with sodium thiosulfate.
Pharmacokinetics/Dosing
IV sodium nitrite has an immediate effect, but the full effects may not be observed for up to one hour. The adult dose is typically 300 mg administered at 75 to 150 mg/min. The pediatric dose is 6 mg/kg not to exceed the adult dose.
Adverse Effects
Adverse effects of sodium nitrite are similar to amyl nitrite and other nitrates. Cyanosis and CNS depression may also be noted.

sodium thiosulfate [**sow** dee um thye oh **sul** fate]
Indications
Sodium thiosulfate is used in the treatment of cyanide and arsenic poisoning. It is also used with cisplatin to prevent renal toxicity. A topical formulation is sometimes used for the treatment of tinea versicolor.
Pharmacokinetics/Dosing
IV sodium thiosulfate is rapidly eliminated in the urine. The typical adult dose for cyanide poisoning is 12.5 grams (2.5 to 5 mL/min of 250 mg/mL solution). A dose of 412.5 mg/kg is recommended for children.
Adverse Effects
Hypotension, CNS depression, dermatitis, tinnitus, and muscle weakness are possible.

✳ **L.F. works with public health officials and poison control to identify and minimize risks for exposure at the plant. He also assures an adequate supply of cyanide antidote kits, and makes sure that there are trained responders well acquainted with the use of the kits working on each shift. He has also contacted the emergency medical services in his region to review his disaster preparedness plan.**

•   •   •

✳ **D.O. is a 47-year-old sheep farmer in England. In preparing to dip his sheep in organophosphates for the control of scab, blow-fly, ticks, and lice, he loses his footing and falls into the dipping pool. He showers immediately in copious amounts of water and reports to the local hospital for care.**

✳ **How do cholinergic agents produce toxicity?**

Chapter 21 discusses both organophosphates and nerve gas exposures threatened by terrorists, which involve cholinergic excess. Organophosphate compounds are highly effective insecticides. Their chemical structure is unstable, which results in their disintegration into nontoxic radicals within days of their application. Therefore they do not persist or accumulate in the environment or animal tissues as do the chlorinated insecticides such as DDT. This accounts for their addition to numerous commercial products—from flea collars, bug bombs, and flypapers to most home and commercial insect sprays. Their popularity accounts for their high potential for accidental poisoning.

Organophosphates and nerve gases are powerful inhibitors of the enzyme acetylcholinesterase (AChE), which breaks down the neurotransmitter acetylcholine (ACh) (see Chapter 21). In general, organophosphates are rapidly absorbed in the body by all routes. Individual organophosphates display a wide variation in their ability to penetrate the skin and in oral absorption, and thus in their toxicity. For example, malathion does not penetrate the skin well and its oral toxicity is low; this makes it a popular insecticide for use in home products.

The signs and symptoms of organophosphate insecticide poisoning are related to inhibition of AChE, which results in an accumulation of ACh in the parasympathetic nervous system. As a result, all organs affected by ACh are overstimulated. The expected results of organophosphate poisoning are as follows: bradycardia, hypotension, dyspnea, wheezing, miosis, blurred vision, seizures, muscular fasciculations, and profuse sweating. A common mnemonic for symptoms of organophosphate intoxication is SLUDGE: **s**alivation, **l**acrimation, **u**rination, **d**efecation, **G**I distress, and **e**mesis. The usual mode of death is respiratory arrest caused by bronchospasm, decreased pulmonary muscle strength, and finally depression of the CNS control of respiration. The sequence in which specific systems develop is related to the route of exposure. Respiratory tract effects appear first after inhalation, whereas GI effects appear initially after ingestion. Skin absorption results in immediate profuse sweating and muscle weakness.

Therapy for organophosphate poisoning involves the support of cardiopulmonary function, the clearance of respiratory tract secretions to maintain a clear airway, and the use of appropriate antidotes, atropine and pralidoxime (2-PAM, Protopam). Atropine competitively antagonizes the action of ACh at muscarinic receptors on the organs innervated by postganglionic parasympathetic nerves and cholinergic sympathetic nerves (Chapter 21).

Although atropine is effective in blocking the muscarinic symptoms of bradycardia, bronchoconstriction, and excess secretions, muscular fasciculations are refractory to this antidote. These involuntary contractions, twitching and respiratory paralysis are best treated with 2-PAM, a cholinesterase reactivator that removes organophosphates bound to AChE. This frees AChE to break down the accumulated ACh, thereby resuming normal activity at the neuromuscular junction. 2-PAM also directly detoxifies certain organophosphates. The adverse effects of 2-PAM include dizziness, nausea, headache, and tachycardia.

✳ D.O. is asymptomatic, but is admitted to the hospital for observation.

Nursing Management Monitor D.O. for SLUDGE symptoms. Closely monitor both respiratory status and the production of secretions, because doses of atropine may be predicated on this information. Plan to monitor D.O.'s status closely for 72 hours. If he develops copious secretions, this may initially necessitate suctioning; anticipate supplemental oxygen therapy. If D.O.'s organophosphates had been ingested, gastric lavage would be considered. As it is, D.O. is placed in a chemical detoxification shower for 15 minutes to cleanse the skin if any insecticide contaminant is present. Anticipate the need to administer atropine and/or pralidoxime (Protopam) if poisoning is severe.

Summary

Poisoning, either accidental or intentional, is a commonplace reason for admission to a hospital emergency department. Children make up the majority of the accidental poisoning population, whereas intentional poisoning is more likely to be the result of a suicide attempt or an overdose of an abused substance. No matter how poisonings are classified, the care provided focuses on prompt treatment, identification of the substance (if possible), the support of vital functions, the removal or elimination of the poison, and the prevention of future occurrences.

✳ Critical Thinking Questions

- In what poisoning situations would the following be the most appropriate therapy: Emesis? Gastric lavage? Refraining from induced vomiting?

- Two-year-old Samantha Rogers has been brought to the ED by her mother, who found Samantha in the bathroom with a container of toilet bowl cleaner (alkali base) in her hands. She is crying and her lips are swollen and excoriated. Mrs. Rogers believes that Samantha has ingested some of the liquid. What sequence of actions should the nurse take?

Bibliography

Alsop, J.A. (2005). Managing acute drug toxicity. In M.A. Koda-Kimble, L.Y. Young, W.A. Kradjan, B.J. Guglielmo, B.K. Alldredge, & R.L. Corelli (Eds.), *Applied therapeutics: The clinical use of drugs* (8th ed.). Philadelphia: Lippincott Williams & Wilkins.

Anderson, D.M., Keith, J., & Novak, P.D. (Eds.) (2002). *Mosby's medical, nursing, and allied health dictionary* (6th ed.). St. Louis: Mosby.

Bosker, G. (Ed.). (2004). *Primary and acute care medicine: Practice, protocols, pathways*, (2nd ed.). Atlanta: Thomson American Health Consultants.

Burns, M.J., & Schwartzstein, R.M. (2005). Decontamination of poisoned adults-1. Wellesley, MA: UpToDate.

Chyka, P.A. (2002). Clinical toxicology. In J.T. DiPiro, R.L. Talbert, G.C. Yee, G.R. Matzke, B.G. Wells & L.M. Posey (Eds.), *Pharmacotherapy: A pathophysiological approach* (5th ed.). New York: McGraw-Hill.

Committee on Injury, Violence, and Poison Prevention. American Academy of Pediatrics. (2003). Policy statement: Poison treatment in the home. *Pediatrics, 112*(5), 1182-1185.

Detaille, T., Wallemacq, P., de Clety, S.C., Vanbinst, R., Dembour, G., & Hantson, P. (2004). Fomepizole alone for severe infant ethylene glycol poisoning. *Pediatric Critical Care Medicine, 5*(5), 490-491.

Drug facts and comparisons (58th ed.). (2005). St. Louis: Facts and Comparisons.

ePocrates Rx, version 6.6 as updated September 15, 2004. Available at http://www.epocrates.com.

Ford, M.D. (2001). *Clinical Toxicology.* Philadelphia: W.B. Saunders.

Hardman, J.G., & Limbird, L.E. (Eds.). (2001). *Goodman & Gilman's The pharmacological basis of therapeutics* (10th ed.). New York: McGraw-Hill.

Lacy, C.F., Armstrong, L.L., Goldman, M.P., & Lance, L.L. (2004). *Lexi-Comp's Drug Information Handbook* (12th ed.). Hudson, Ohio: Lexi-Comp.

Marco, C.A., & Kelen, G.D. (1990). Acute intoxication. *Emergency Medicine Clinics of North America, 8*(4), 731-48.

Morris, C.C. (2000). Pediatric iron poisoning in the United States. *Southern Medical Journal, 93*(4), 351-358.

Mosby's drug consult (15th ed.). (2005). St. Louis: Mosby.

Olson, K.R. (2003). Poisoning. In L.M. Tierney, Jr., S.J. McPhee & Papadakis, M.A. (Eds.), *Current Medical Diagnosis & Treatment.* New York: Lange Medical Books/McGraw-Hill.

Position Paper: Ipecac syrup. (2004). *Journal of Toxicology and Clinical Toxicologists, 42*(2), 133-143.

Sanfacon, G. (2001). *PROTOX: A powerful tool for poison control centre and surveillance users.* Retrieved March 9, 2004, from http://www.pmra-arla.gc.ca/english/pdf/pmac/pmac_27032001_h-e.pdf.

𝑒-LEARNING SUPPLEMENTS

Student CD-ROM
- Final Exam questions
- NCLEX® Examination review questions
- Pharmacology animations
- Printable chapter summary

Evolve Website (http://evolve.elsevier.com/mckenry)
- Content updates, including information on new drugs
- WebLinks corresponding to this chapter
- Answers to the critical thinking questions in this chapter
- *Elsevier ePharmacology Update* newsletter
- Mosby's Drug Consult Internet Edition
- Supplemental and reference information

USP DI: Drug information for the health care professional (25th ed.). (2005). Greenwood Village, CO: MICROMEDEX Thomson Healthcare.

Vale, J.A., & Kulig, K. (2004). Position paper: Gastric lavage. *Journal of Toxicology and Clinical Toxicologists, 42*(7), 933-943.

Watson, W.A., Litovitz, T.L., Klein-Schwartz, W., Rodgers, G.C., Youniss, J., & Reid, N., et al. (2004). 2003 annual report of the American Association of Poison Control Centers toxic exposure surveillance system. *American Journal of Emergency Medicine, 22*(5), 335-376.

Zimmerman, J.L. (2003). Poisonings and overdoses in the intensive care unit: General and specific management issues. *Critical Care Medicine, 31*(12), 2794-2801.

Disorders Index

Comprehensive Index

---

b indicates boxed material, *f,* indicates illustrations, and *t* indicates table.